Pharmacotherapeutics for Advanced Practice

A PRACTICAL APPROACH

FOURTH EDITION

Pharmacotherapeutics for Advanced Practice

A PRACTICAL APPROACH

FOURTH EDITION

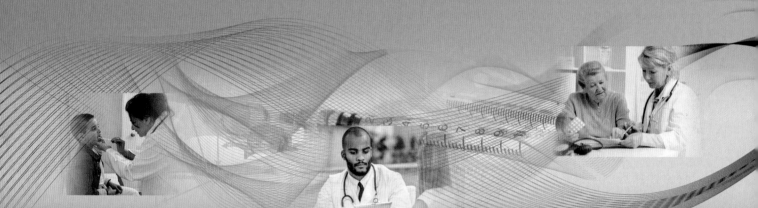

EDITORS

Virginia P. Arcangelo, PhD, NP
Family Nurse Practitioner, Retired
Berlin, New Jersey

Andrew M. Peterson, PharmD, PhD, FCPP
John Wyeth Dean
Professor of Clinical Pharmacy and
Professor of Health Policy
University of the Sciences in Philadelphia
Philadelphia, Pennsylvania

Veronica F. Wilbur, PhD, APRN-FNP, CNE, FAANP
Assistant Professor of Graduate Nursing
West Chester University
West Chester, Pennsylvania

Jennifer A. Reinhold, BA, PharmD, BCPS, BCPP
Associate Professor of Clinical Pharmacy
Philadelphia College of Pharmacy
University of the Sciences in Philadelphia
Philadelphia, Pennsylvania

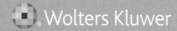

Wolters Kluwer

Philadelphia · Baltimore · New York · London
Buenos Aires · Hong Kong · Sydney · Tokyo

Executive Editor: Shannon W. Magee
Product Development Editor: Maria M. McAvey
Developmental Editor: Tom Conville
Senior Marketing Manager: Mark Wiragh
Production Project Manager: Marian Bellus
Design Coordinator: Elaine Kasmer
Manufacturing Coordinator: Kathleen Brown
Prepress Vendor: SPi Global

4th edition

Library of Congress Cataloging-in-Publication Data
  Names: Arcangelo, Virginia P, editor. | Peterson, Andrew M., editor. | Wilbur, Veronica, editor. | Reinhold, Jennifer A., editor.
  Title: Pharmacotherapeutics for advanced practice : a practical approach / editors, Virginia P. Arcangelo, Andrew M. Peterson, Veronica F. Wilbur, Jennifer A. Reinhold.
  Description: Fourth edition. | Philadelphia : Wolters Kluwer, [2017]
  Identifiers: LCCN 2016002801 | ISBN 9781496319968
  Subjects: | MESH: Drug Therapy—methods | Pharmaceutical Preparations—administration & dosage
  Classification: LCC RM262 | NLM WB 330 | DDC 615.5/8—dc23 LC record available at http://lccn.loc.gov/2016002801

We dedicate this book to all our students.
This book never would have come to fruition without
the impact of the students who have touched our lives.
It is our hope that this book and its evolution into
the fourth edition has influenced more than just our students
but that it has helped to promote excellence in patient
care through all of its users.

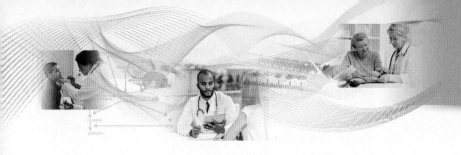

CONTRIBUTORS

Virginia P. Arcangelo, PhD, NP
Family Nurse Practitioner, Retired
Berlin, New Jersey

Laura Aykroyd, PharmD
Clinical Pharmacy Specialist–Neurocritical Care
Department of Pharmacy
IU Health Methodist Hospital
Indianapolis, Indiana

Kelly Barranger, MSN, RN, CRNP
Certified Registered Nurse Practitioner
Department of Nursing
Veterans Affairs
Philadelphia, Pennsylvania

John Barron, PharmD
Staff Vice President and Clinical Research Advisor
HealthCore, Inc.
Wilmington, Delaware

Laura L. Bio, PharmD, BCPS
Assistant Professor
Department of Pharmacy Practice
Philadelphia College of Pharmacy
Philadelphia, Pennsylvania
Clinical Pharmacist
Department of Pharmacy
Children's Regional Hospital at Cooper University Hospital
Camden, New Jersey

Lauren M. Czosnowski, PharmD, BCPS
Assistant Professor
Department of Pharmacy Practice
Butler University
Clinical Specialist
Pharmacy Department
IU Health Methodist Hospital
Indianapolis, Indiana

Quinn A. Czosnowski, PharmD
Clinical Pharmacy Specialist
Pharmacy Department
IU Health Methodist Hospital
Indianapolis, Indiana

David Dinh, PharmD, BCPS
Clinical Pharmacy Specialist, Emergency Medicine
Department of Pharmacy
Yale New Haven Hospital
New Haven, Connecticut

Amy M. Egras, PharmD, BCPS, BC-ADM
Associate Professor
Department of Pharmacy Practice
Jefferson School of Pharmacy
Clinical Pharmacist
Jefferson Family Medicine Associates
Thomas Jefferson University
Philadelphia, Pennsylvania

Kelleen N. Flaherty, MS
Adjunct Assistant Professor
Department of Biomedical Writing
University of the Sciences in Philadelphia
Philadelphia, Pennsylvania

Maria C. Foy, PharmD, BCPS, CPE
Clinical Specialist, Palliative Care
Pharmacy Department
Abington Memorial Hospital
Abington, Pennsylvania

Steven P. Gelone, PharmD
Chief Development Officer
Nabriva Therapeutics
King of Prussia, Pennsylvania

Andrew J. Grimone, PharmD, BCPS-AQ ID
Assistant Professor
Department of Nursing
Clarion University of Pennsylvania
Clarion, Pennsylvania
Clinical Pharmacy Manager
Department of Pharmacy
Saint Vincent Hospital
Allegheny Health Network
Erie, Pennsylvania

Anisha B. Grover, PharmD, BCACP
Assistant Professor of Clinical Pharmacy
Department of Pharmacy Practice and Pharmacy Administration
Philadelphia College of Pharmacy
University of the Sciences
Philadelphia, Pennsylvania

Diane E. Hadley, PharmD, BCACP
Assistant Professor of Clinical Pharmacy
Department of Pharmacy Practice and Pharmacy Administration
University of the Sciences
Philadelphia, Pennsylvania

Emily R. Hajjar, PharmD, BCPS, BCACP, CGP
Associate Professor
Department of Pharmacy Practice
Jefferson School of Pharmacy
Philadelphia, Pennsylvania

Amalia M. Issa, PhD, MPH, FCPP
Professor of Health Policy
Department of Health Policy and Public Health
Director
Program in Personalized Medicine and Targeted
Therapeutics
University of the Sciences
Philadelphia, Pennsylvania

Tep Kang, PharmD, BCPS
Adjunct Instructor
Department of Nursing
University of Delaware
Newark, Delaware
Wilmington University
New Castle, Delaware
Critical Care Pharmacist
Department of Pharmacy
Christiana Care Health Services
Newark, Delaware

Alice Lim, PharmD, BCACP
Assistant Professor of Clinical Pharmacy
Department of Pharmacy Practice and Pharmacy
Administration
Philadelphia College of Pharmacy
Philadelphia, Pennsylvania

Laura A. Mandos, BS, PharmD, BCPP
Professor of Clinical Pharmacy
Department of Pharmacy Practice and Pharmacy
Administration
Philadelphia College of Pharmacy
University of the Sciences
Philadelphia, Pennsylvania

Lauren K. McCluggage, PharmD
Associate Professor
Lipscomb University College of Pharmacy
Clinical Pharmacist
Department of Pharmacy
St. Thomas West Hospital
Nashville, Tennessee

Karleen Melody, PharmD, BCACP
Assistant Professor of Clinical Pharmacy
Department of Pharmacy Practice and Pharmacy
Administration
Philadelphia College of Pharmacy
University of the Sciences
Philadelphia, Pennsylvania

Isabelle Mercier, PhD
Associate Professor
Pharmaceutical Sciences
University of the Sciences
Philadelphia, Pennsylvania

Carol Gullo Mest, PhD, RN, ANP-BC
Professor of Nursing
Director of Graduate Program
DeSales University
Center Valley, Pennsylvania

Samir K. Mistry, PharmD
Senior Director
Specialty Product Strategy
CVS Health
Minneapolis, Minnesota

Lorraine Nowakowski-Grier, MSN, APRN, BC, CDE
Adjunct Faculty
Department of Nursing
College of Health Professions
Wilmington University
New Castle, Delaware
Nurse Practitioner, Diabetes Educator
Department of Nursing Education
and Development
Christiana Care Health Services
Newark, Delaware

Judith A. O'Donnell, MD
Associate Professor of Medicine
Division of Infectious Diseases
Perelman School of Medicine at the University of
Pennsylvania
Chief, Division of Infectious Diseases
Hospital Epidemiologist and Director, Infection Prevention
& Control
Penn Presbyterian Medical Center
Philadelphia, Pennsylvania

Staci Pacetti, PharmD
Assistant Professor
Department of Nursing
Rutgers University School of Nursing
Camden, New Jersey

Andrew M. Peterson, PharmD, PhD, FCPP
John Wyeth Dean
Professor of Clinical Pharmacy and Professor
of Health Policy
University of the Sciences in Philadelphia
Philadelphia, Pennsylvania

Louis R. Petrone, MD
Clinical Assistant Professor
Family and Community Medicine
Sidney Kimmel Medical College
Attending Physician
Family and Community Medicine
Thomas Jefferson University Hospital
Philadelphia, Pennsylvania

Melody D. Randle, DNP, FNP-C, MSN, CCNS, CNE
Chair
Nurse Practitioner Program
College of Health Professions
Wilmington University
New Castle, Delaware

Troy L. Randle, DO, FACC, FACOI
Assistant Program Director of Cardiology
Department of Cardiology
School of Osteopathic Medicine
Rowan University
Cardiologist
Lourdes Cardiology
Cherry Hill, New Jersey

Jennifer A. Reinhold, BA, PharmD, BCPS, BCPP
Associate Professor of Clinical Pharmacy
Philadelphia College of Pharmacy
University of the Sciences in Philadelphia
Philadelphia, Pennsylvania

Christopher C. Roe, MSN, ACNP-BC
Nurse Practitioner Manager
Center for Heart and Vascular Health
Christiana Care Health Systems
Newark, Delaware

Cynthia A. Sanoski, PharmD, BCPS, FCCP
Department Chair and Associate Professor
Department of Pharmacy Practice
Jefferson School of Pharmacy
Thomas Jefferson University
Philadelphia, Pennsylvania

Briana L. Santaniello, MBA, PharmD
PGY1 Managed Care Pharmacy Resident
University of Massachusetts Medical School's Clinical
Pharmacy Services
Shrewsbury, Massachusetts

Jason J. Schafer, PharmD, MPH
Associate Professor
Department of Pharmacy Practice
Jefferson School of Pharmacy
Thomas Jefferson University
Philadelphia, Pennsylvania

Shelly Schneider, APN
Nurse Practitioner
Woodbury Dermatology
Woodbury, New Jersey

Jean M. Scholtz, BS, PharmD, BCPS, FASHP
Associate Professor, Vice Chair
Department of Pharmacy Practice
Philadelphia College of Pharmacy
Philadelphia, Pennsylvania

Anita Siu, PharmD
Clinical Associate Professor
Department of Pharmacy Practice and Pharmacy Administration
Rutgers, The State University of New Jersey
Piscataway, New Jersey
Neonatal/Pediatric Pharmacotherapy Specialist
Department of Pharmacy
Jersey Shore University Medical Center
Neptune, New Jersey

Sarah A. Spinler, PharmD
Professor of Clinical Pharmacy
Department of Pharmacy Practice and Pharmacy Administration
Philadelphia College of Pharmacy
University of the Sciences
Philadelphia, Pennsylvania

Joshua J. Spooner, PharmD, MS
Associate Professor of Pharmacy
College of Pharmacy
Western New England University
Springfield, Massachusetts

Linda M. Spooner, PharmD, BCPS, FASHP
Professor of Pharmacy Practice
Department of Pharmacy Practice
MCPHS University School of Pharmacy–Worcester/Manchester
Clinical Pharmacy Specialist in Infectious Diseases
Saint Vincent Hospital
Worcester, Massachusetts

Richard G. Stefanacci, DO, MGH, MBA, AGSF, CMD
Faculty
School of Population Health
Thomas Jefferson University
Philadelphia, Pennsylvania
Chief Medical Officer
The Access Group
Berkeley Heights, New Jersey
Senior Physician
Mercy LIFE
Trinity Health System
Philadelphia, Pennsylvania

James C. Thigpen Jr, PharmD, BCPS
Associate Professor
Department of Pharmacy Practice
Bill Gatton College of Pharmacy
East Tennessee State University
Johnson City, Tennessee

Tyan F. Thomas, PharmD
Associate Professor of Clinical Pharmacy
Department of Pharmacy Practice and Pharmacy
Administration
Philadelphia College of Pharmacy at the University of the
Sciences
Clinical Pharmacy Specialist
Department of Pharmacy
Philadelphia VA Medical Center
Philadelphia, Pennsylvania

Karen J. Tietze, PharmD
Professor of Clinical Pharmacy
Philadelphia College of Pharmacy
University of the Sciences in Philadelphia
Philadelphia, Pennsylvania

Elena M. Umland, PharmD
Associate Dean, Academic Affairs
Professor, Pharmacy Practice
Jefferson School of Pharmacy
Thomas Jefferson University
Philadelphia, Pennsylvania

Sarah F. Uroza, PharmD
Assistant Professor
Department of Pharmacy Practice
Lipscomb University
Clinical Pharmacist
Faith Family Medical Clinic
Nashville, Tennessee

Craig B. Whitman, PharmD, BCPS
Clinical Associate Professor of Pharmacy Practice
Temple University School of Pharmacy
Clinical Specialist, Critical Care
Temple University Hospital
Philadelphia, Pennsylvania

Veronica F. Wilbur, PhD, APRN-FNP, CNE, FAANP
Assistant Professor of Graduate Nursing
West Chester University
West Chester, Pennsylvania

Vincent J. Willey, PharmD
Staff Vice President, Industry Sponsored Research
HealthCore, Inc.
Wilmington, Delaware

Eric T. Wittbrodt, PharmD, MPH
Director, Health Economics and Outcomes Research
at AstraZeneca

Angela A. Allerman, PharmD, BCPS

Kelly Barranger, MSN, RN, CRNP

John Barron, BS Pharmacy, PharmD

Laura L. Bio, PharmD, BCPS

Tim A. Briscoe, PharmD, CDE

Debra Carroll, MSN, CRNP

Quinn A. Czosnowski, PharmD, BCPS

Lauren M. Czosnowski, PharmD, BCPS

Elyse L. Dishler, MD

Amy M. Egras, PharmD, BCPS

Heather E. Fean, MSN, APN-C

Kelleen N. Flaherty, MS

Maria C. Foy, PharmD, CPE

Stephanie A. Gaber, PharmD, CDE

Jomy M. George, PharmD, BCPS

Ellen Boxer Goldfarb, CRNP

Andrew J. Grimone, PharmD, RPh, BCPS

Emily R. Hajjar, PharmD, BCPS, CGP

Andrea M. Heise, MSN, APN-C

Lauren K. McCluggage, PharmD, BCPS

Carol Gullo Mest, PhD, RN, ANP-BC

Samir K. Mistry, PharmD

Angela Cafiero Moroney, PharmD

Betty E. Naimoli, MSN, CRNP

Jessica O'Hara, PharmD

Dharmi Patel, PharmD

Jeegisha R. Patel, PharmD

Louis R. Petrone, MD

Jennifer A. Reinhold, BA, PharmD, BCPS

Alicia M. Reese, PharmD, MS, BCPS

Cynthia A. Sanoski, BS, PharmD, BCPS, FCCP

Matthew Sarnes, PharmD

Jason J. Schafer, PharmD, BCPS, AAHIVE

Susan M. Schrand, MSN, CRNP

Henry M. Schwartz, BSc Pharm, PharmD, CDE

Anita Siu, PharmD

Joshua J. Spooner, PharmD, MS

Linda M. Spooner, PharmD, BCPS

Liza Takiya, PharmD, BCPS

Jim Thigpen, PharmD, BCPS

Tyan F. Thomas, PharmD, BCPS

Craig B. Whitman, PharmD, BCPS

Veronica F. Wilbur, PhD, FNP-BC

Eric T. Wittbrodt, PharmD

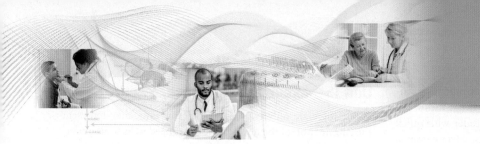

Pharmacotherapeutics for Advanced Practice originated from our combined experience in teaching nurse practitioners and in practice in primary care. As a nurse practitioner and educator herself, Virginia saw a need for practical exposure to the general principles of prescribing and monitoring drug therapy, particularly in the Family Practice arena. As a PharmD, Andrew saw a need to be able to teach new prescribers how to think about prescribing systematically, regardless of the disease state. For this edition, we have expanded the editorial staff to include Veronica F. Wilbur and Jennifer Reinhold. Veronica, a Family Nurse Practitioner and PhD in Nursing, has extensive experience in education of Advanced Practice Nurses and primary care practice. Jennifer, a PharmD, has expertise in pharmacotherapy and prescribing in primary care. Both of these colleagues were contributors in previous editions and understand the focus, intent, and direction of this text.

This edition still provides basic pharmacology, while also providing a process and framework through which learners can begin to think pharmacotherapeutically. The text still allows learners to identify a disease, review the drugs used to treat the disease, select treatment based on goals of therapy and special patient considerations, and adjust therapy if it fails to meet goals.

This text meets the needs of both students and practitioners in a practical approach that is user friendly. It teaches the practitioner how to prescribe and manage drug therapy in primary care. The book has evolved over the years, based on input from students, academicians, and practitioners. Long-standing contributors were asked to update their chapters, and new contributors were selected based on their academic or practice expertise to provide a combination of evidence-based medicine and practical experience. The text considers disease- and patient-specific information. With each chapter, there are tables and evidence-based algorithms that are practical and easy to read and that complement the text.

Additionally, the text guides the practitioner to a choice of second- and third-line therapy when the first line of therapy fails. Since new drugs are being marketed continually, drug classes are discussed with a focus on how the broader, class-specific properties can be applied to new drugs. Each chapter ends with a simple case study or series of questions designed to prompt the learner to think systematically and the teacher to ask critical questions. Also, the disorder chapter's case study asks the same questions; reinforcing a clinical decision-making process and promoting critical thinking skills. There are no answers to the questions in the text since the authors believe that the purpose of the case studies is to promote discussion and that there may be more than one correct answer to each question, especially as new drugs are developed. However, one potential answer to each question in the case is available online for use by faculty. Additionally, there is an additional case with several sample multiple-choice questions for each chapter online. We realize that there may be several answers to these questions and the authors have just provided one option. To assist faculty in the classroom, there are power point slides available online for each chapter. To assist the student, the acronyms contained in each chapter are defined in a separate file online as well.

ORGANIZATION OF THE BOOK

Unit 1—Principles of Therapeutics

As with previous editions, the Principles Unit of the book reviews basic elements of therapeutics necessary for safe and effective prescribing. The first chapter introduces the prescribing process, including how to avoid medication errors. The next two chapters provide the foundation of therapeutics, including information on the pharmacokinetics and pharmacodynamics of drugs and drug–drug/drug–food interactions. The following three chapters review how these foundations change in pediatric, pregnant, and geriatric patients. Similarly, the basics of the principles of pain management and infectious disease therapy are reviewed in the next two chapters so that the reader can learn how these concepts are applied to the disorders discussed in the following units. Updated Complementary and Alternative Medicine (CAM) and Pharmacogenomics chapters are included in this unit, recognizing the growing use of these modalities in all aspects of patient care.

Units 2 through 12—Disorders

This section of the book, consisting of 41 chapters, reviews commonly seen disorders in the primary care setting. Although not all-inclusive, the array of disorders allows the reader to gain an understanding of how to approach the pharmacotherapeutic treatment of any disorder. The chapters are designed to give a brief overview of the disease process, including the causes and pathophysiology, with an emphasis placed on how drug therapy can alter the pathologic state. **Diagnostic Criteria** and **Goals of Therapy** are discussed and underlie the basic principles of treating patients with drugs. Osteoarthritis and rheumatoid arthritis have been split and each has a chapter devoted to it. A new chapter on Parkinson Disease has been added since this is frequently treated in primary care. Each chapter has been updated with the newest therapies available at the time of writing.

The drug sections review the agents' uses, mechanism of action, contraindications and drug interactions, adverse effects, and monitoring parameters. This discussion is organized primarily by drug class, with notation to specific drugs within the text and the tables. The tables provide the reader with quick access to generic and trade names and dosages, adverse events, contraindications, and special considerations. Used together, the text and tables provide the reader with sufficient information to begin to choose drug therapy.

The section on **Selecting the Most Appropriate Agent** aids the reader in deciding which drug to choose for a given patient. This section contains information on first-line, second-line, and third-line therapies, with rationales for why drugs are classified in these categories. Accompanying this section is an algorithm outlining the thought process by which clinicians select an initial drug therapy. Again, the text organization and the illustrative algorithms provide readers with a means of thinking through the process of selecting drugs for patients. In the third edition, we have kept the **Recommended Order of Treatment tables** and updated them, along with the algorithms and drug tables, to reflect current knowledge. Each chapter has been updated to reflect the most current guidelines available at the time of writing. However, medicine and pharmacotherapy are constantly changing, and it remains the clinician's responsibility to identify the most current information.

Included in each chapter is a section on **Monitoring Patient Response**. This encompasses clinical and laboratory parameters, times when these items should be monitored, and actions to take in case the parameters do not meet the specified goals of therapy. In addition, special patient populations are discussed when appropriate. These discussions include pediatric and geriatric patients but may also include ethnic- or sex-related considerations. Last, this section includes a discussion of patient education material relevant to the disease and drugs chosen. In each chapter, there is a patient education section that includes information on CAM related to that disorder as well as sections on external information for patients and practitioners.

Each of the case studies has been reviewed and updated as appropriate. However, the pedagogical style of reasoning remains the same. As previously stated, answers to these case studies are not supplied since the purpose is to promote discussion and evoke a thought process. Also, as time changes, so do therapies. The cases are short, compelling the learner to ask questions about the patient and allowing flexibility for multiple correct answers to be developed by the instructor as they work through the clinical decision-making process.

Units 13 and 14—Pharmacotherapy in Health Promotion and Women's Health

These units discuss several areas of interest for promoting health or maintaining a healthy lifestyle using medications, including smoking cessation, immunizations, and weight management; the chapter on travel medicine has been eliminated since there are specialty clinics that provide this service, and it is not done frequently in primary care. The four chapters in Women's Health assist the learner to recognize the special nature of care that this population deserves.

Unit 15—Integrative Approach to Patient Care

While there are only two chapters in this unit, they represent the culmination of the text. Practitioners need to have an understanding of the economics of pharmacotherapeutics in order to effectively prescribe medications and treat patients. This chapter is updated with information on the Affordable Care Act and its impact on therapeutic decision making while still being anchored in the basics of pharmacoeconomics, formulary decision making, co-pays, prior authorizations, and Medicare as well as managed care as it applies to prescribing medications.

The last chapter, Integrative Approaches to Pharmacotherapy, is an attempt to examine real-life, complex cases. Each case addresses the nine questions posed in the individual chapter case studies, but now provides the reader with examples of how to approach the case studies and examines issues to consider when presented with more than one diagnosis. These cases are more complex, requiring the reader to think through multiple diseases and therapies instead of a single disorder in isolation. Within this chapter, we do offer potential answers to the cases. These may not be the only answers but indicate some of the thought processes that go into the decision-making process in the pharmacologic management of a problem.

Chapter Organization

This edition continues the consistent format approach throughout each disorder chapter. Each chapter begins with the background and pathophysiology of the disorder, followed by a discussion of the relevant classes of drugs. These broad categories are then integrated in the section on **Selecting the Most Appropriate Agent**.

Drug Overview Tables are also organized consistently, giving the reader much information on each drug, including the usual dose, contraindications and side effects, and any special considerations a prescriber should be aware of during therapy. **Algorithms** provide the reader with a visual cue on how to approach treating a patient.

Recommended Order of Treatment tables provide the reader with basic drug therapy selection, from first-line to third-line therapies for each disorder. These, coupled with the algorithms and the drug tables, are the core of the text.

A **Case Study** is provided for each disorder discussed. These short cases are designed to stimulate discussion among students and with instructors. The nine questions at the end of each case are tailored to each disorder but remain similar across all cases to reinforce the process of thinking pharmacotherapeutically.

Pharmacotherapeutics for Advanced Practice continues to provide primary care students with a reasoned approach to learning pharmacotherapeutics and to serve as a reference for the seasoned practitioner. Prescribing is becoming more and more complex, and the information in this book has helped us in our own practices. As experienced educators and practitioners, we are dedicated to providing you with a textbook that will meet your needs.

Virginia P. Arcangelo
Andrew M. Peterson
Veronica F. Wilbur
Jennifer A. Reinhold

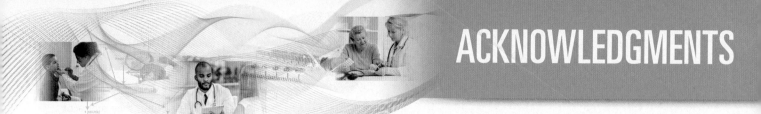

ACKNOWLEDGMENTS

We would like to thank Shannon Magee, Maria McAvey, and Marian Bellus, from Wolters Kluwer/Lippincott Williams & Wilkins and Tom Conville, Development Editor, for all their invaluable assistance. We are also forever indebted to the contributors who spent countless hours on this project. Without them, this would never have become a reality.

In addition, we would like to thank our families who supported us throughout the project and understand the importance of this book to us.

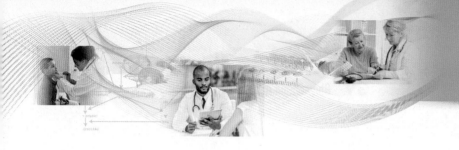

CONTENTS

UNIT 1

Principles of Therapeutics

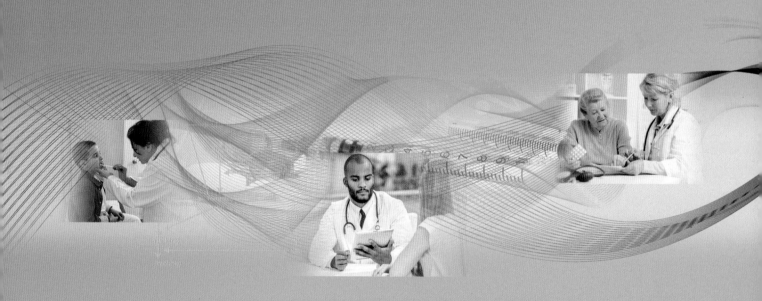

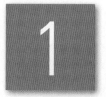

1 Issues for the Practitioner in Drug Therapy

Virginia P. Arcangelo ■ Veronica F. Wilbur

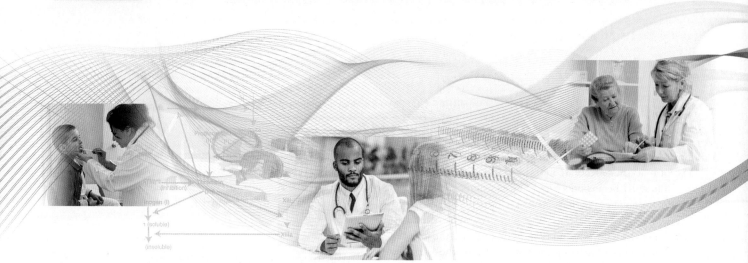

Drug therapy is often the mainstay of treatment of acute and chronic diseases. An important role of health care practitioners is to develop a treatment plan with the patient; an integral part of the treatment plan of disease and health promotion is drug therapy. According to the Health in the United States (2014), from 2009 to 2012, of those persons aged 55 to 64, 55.6% used one to four prescription drugs and 20.3% used five or more during the last 30 days. Additionally, according to the National Ambulatory Medical Survey (2010), there were 2.6 billion drugs (75.1%) prescribed during office visits, 329.2 million drugs (72.5%) prescribed during visits to a hospital outpatient department, and 286.2 million drugs (80.3%) prescribed during visits to a hospital emergency department. The overall growth in spending on prescription drugs has slowed to 2.9% by 2011, but the overall spending equals $263 billion and accounts for a large share of national health care expenditures (CDC, FastStats, 2014). Therefore, it is imperative that prescribers have the best knowledge about principles of prescribing.

In developing a treatment plan that includes drug therapy, the prescribing practitioner considers many issues in achieving the goal of safe, appropriate, and effective therapy. Among them are drug safety and product safeguards, the practitioner's role and responsibilities, the step-by-step process of prescribing therapy and writing the prescription, and follow-up measures. Particularly important are promoting adherence to the therapeutic regimen and keeping up-to-date with the latest developments in drug therapy.

DRUG SAFETY AND MARKET SAFEGUARDS

In the United States, drug safety is ensured in many ways, but primarily by the U.S. Food and Drug Administration (FDA),

which is the federal agency charged with conducting and monitoring clinical trials, approving new drugs for market and manufacture, and ensuring safe drugs for public consumption. Although the federal government provides guidelines for a pure and safe drug product, guidelines for prescribers of drug therapy are dictated both by state and federal governments and by licensing bodies in each state.

Clinical Trials

Various legislated mechanisms are in place to ensure pure and safe drug products. One of these mechanisms is the clinical trial process by which new drug development is carefully monitored by the FDA. Every new drug must successfully pass through several stages of development (see **Figure 1.1**). The first stage is preclinical trials, which involve testing in animals and monitoring efficacy, toxic effects, and untoward reactions. Application to the FDA for investigational use of a drug is made only after this portion of research is completed.

Clinical trials, which begin only after the FDA grants approval for investigation, consist of four phases and may last up to 9 years before a drug is approved for general use. During clinical trials, performed on informed volunteers, data are gathered about the proposed drug's purity, bioavailability, potency, efficacy, safety, and toxicity.

Phase I of clinical trials is the initial evaluation of the drug. It involves supervised studies on 20 to 100 healthy people and focuses on absorption, distribution, metabolism (sometimes interchangeable with biotransformation), and elimination of the drug. In phase I, the most effective administration routes and dosage ranges are determined. During phase II, up to several hundred patients with the disease for which the drug is

3

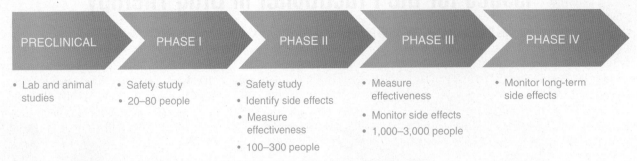

PRECLINICAL	PHASE I	PHASE II	PHASE III	PHASE IV
• Lab and animal studies	• Safety study • 20–80 people	• Safety study • Identify side effects • Measure effectiveness • 100–300 people	• Measure effectiveness • Monitor side effects • 1,000–3,000 people	• Monitor long-term side effects

FIGURE 1.1 Phases of drug development.

intended are subjects. The testing focus is the same as in phase I, except that drug effects are monitored on people with disease.

Phase III begins once the FDA determines that the drug causes no apparent serious adverse effects and that the dosage range is appropriate. Double-blind research methods (in which neither the study and control subjects nor the investigators know who is receiving the test drug and who is not) are used for data collection in this phase, and the proposed drug is compared with placebo. Usually several thousand subjects are involved in this phase, which lasts several years and during which most risks of the proposed drug are discovered. At the completion of phase III, the FDA evaluates data presented and accepts or rejects the application for the new drug. Approval of the application means that the drug can be marketed—but only by the company seeking the approval.

Once on the market, the drug enters phase IV or postmarketing surveillance. Objectives at this stage are (1) to compare the drug with others on the market, (2) to monitor for long-term effectiveness and impact on quality of life, and (3) to analyze cost-effectiveness (Center Watch, 2015). During postmarketing surveillance, drugs can be taken off the market or restricted due to additional findings about the drug and side effects.

Prevention of Harm and Misuse

The passage of the FDA's Controlled Substances Act of 1970 established the schedule of ranking of drugs that have the potential for abuse or misuse. Drugs on the schedule are considered controlled substances. These drugs have the potential to induce dependency and addiction, either psychologically or physiologically. **Box 1.1** defines the five categories of scheduled drugs, with Schedule 1 drugs having the greatest potential for abuse and Schedule 5 drugs the least.

Schedule drugs can be prescribed only by a practitioner who is registered and approved by the U.S. Drug Enforcement

---

BOX 1.1   Scheduled Drugs

Schedule 1 drugs have a high potential for abuse. There is no routine therapeutic use for these drugs, and they are not available for regular use. They may be obtained for "investigational use only" by applying to the U.S. Drug Enforcement Agency. Examples include heroin and LSD.

Schedule 2 drugs have a valid medical use but a high potential for abuse, both psychological and physiologic. In an emergency, a Schedule 2 drug may be prescribed by telephone if a written prescription cannot be provided at the time. However, a written prescription must be provided within 72 hours with the words *authorization for emergency dispensing* written on the prescription. These prescriptions cannot be refilled. A new prescription must be written each time. Examples include certain amphetamines and barbiturates.

Schedule 3 drugs have a potential for abuse, but the potential is lower than for drugs on Schedule 2.

These drugs contain a combination of controlled and noncontrolled substances. Use of these drugs can cause a moderate to low physiologic dependence and a higher psychological dependence. A verbal order can be given to the pharmacy, and the prescription can be refilled up to five times within 6 months. Examples include certain narcotics (codeine) and nonbarbiturate sedatives.

Schedule 4 drugs have a low potential for abuse. They can cause psychological dependency but limited physiologic dependency. Examples include nonnarcotic analgesics and antianxiety agents, such as lorazepam (Ativan).

Schedule 5 drugs have the least potential for abuse. They contain a moderate amount of opioids and are used mainly as antitussives and antidiarrheals. Examples include antitussives and antidiarrheals with small amounts of narcotics.

Agency (DEA), and in some states, practitioners must possess a controlled substance (CS) license as well. The DEA issues approved applicants a number, which must be written on the prescription for a controlled substance for the prescription to be valid. The prescriber's DEA number must also appear on a prescription that is being filled in another state.

Currently, in the United States, overdose emergencies and abuse of schedule drugs have become epidemic with over 259 million prescriptions written for painkillers (CDC Vital Statistics, 2014). To assist health care providers with safe prescribing practices, many states have enacted prescription drug monitoring programs (PDMPs). These programs are established and run by individual states through electronic databases that collect information on designated substances dispensed in the state. The DEA does not have involvement in any state PDMP program. According to the National Association of State Controlled Substance Authorities (NASCSA), in 2014, only one state did not have a PDMP. The program allows prescribers of controlled substance to look up patients for previous prescriptions of controlled substances including type of medication, amount, and name of the prescriber. The information obtained from this program helps to reveal those patients who prescriber shop and are receiving too many controlled substances. It also helps to start a conversation with the patients, exploring their health care needs.

National Provider Identifier

The Administrative Simplification provisions of the Health Insurance Portability and Accountability Act of 1996 (HIPAA) mandated the adoption of standard unique identifiers for health care providers and health plans. This identification system improves the efficiency and effectiveness of electronically transmitting health information. The Centers for Medicare & Medicaid Services (CMS) has developed the National Plan and Provider Enumeration System (NPPES) to assign each provider a unique National Provider Identifier (NPI). Covered health care providers and all health plans and health care clearinghouses must use NPIs in the administrative and financial transactions adopted under HIPAA. The NPI is a 10-position, intelligence-free numeric identifier (10-digit number). The NPI does not carry other information about the health care provider, such as the health care provider's specialty or in which state he or she practices. The NPI must be used in lieu of legacy provider identifiers in HIPAA standard transactions. Covered providers must also share their NPI with other providers, health plans, clearinghouses, and any entity that may need it for billing purposes.

The purpose of the NPI is to identify all health care providers by a unique number in standard transactions such as health care claims. NPIs may also be used to identify health care providers on prescriptions, in internal files to link proprietary provider identification numbers and other information, in coordination of benefits between health plans, in patient medical record systems, in program integrity files, and in other ways. HIPAA requires that covered entities (i.e., health plans, health care clearinghouses, and those health care providers who transmit health information in electronic form in connection with a transaction for which the Secretary of Health and Human Services has adopted a standard) use NPIs in standard transactions. The NPI is the only health care provider identifier that can be used in standard transactions by covered entities.

A health care provider may apply for an NPI through a web-based application process at https://nppes.cms.hhs.gov or by filling out and mailing a paper application to the NPI Enumerator. A copy of the application (CMS-10114), which includes the NPI Enumerator's mailing address, is available upon request through the NPI Enumerator at 1-800-465-3203, TTY 1-800-692-2326.

When applying for an NPI, providers are asked to include their Medicare identifiers as well as those issued by other health plans. A Medicaid identification number must include the associated state name. The legacy identifier information is critical for health plans to aid in the transition to the NPI. When the NPI application information has been submitted and the NPI assigned, NPPES sends the health care provider a notification that includes their NPI. This notification is proof of NPI enumeration and helps to verify a health care provider's NPI.

Prescription versus Nonprescription Drugs

Many drugs may now be obtained that were previously available only with a prescription, and at the prescription dosage. Although these drugs are commonly and legally obtained over the counter (OTC) without a prescription, approval for the drug must still be obtained from the FDA for specific uses in specific doses.

These drugs carry user warnings on the labels. Many have the potential for interacting adversely with prescribed drugs or complicating existing disease. The self-prescribed use of OTC drugs may delay diagnosis and treatment of potentially serious problems. On the other hand, the use of OTC drugs can be beneficial for treatment of self-limiting disorders that are not serious.

Generic Drugs versus Brand Name Drugs

Substituting a generic drug for a brand name drug is a common practice. In many states, it is required. When the patent on a brand name drug expires, other drug manufacturers can then produce the same drug formula under its generic name (the generic name and formula of a drug are always the same; only the brand names change). This practice not only benefits the manufacturer but also decreases the cost to the consumer.

To ensure safety, the FDA must grant approval for these drugs, and rigorous testing is again required to ensure that all generic drugs meet specifications for quality, purity, strength, and potency. Generic drugs must demonstrate therapeutic equivalence to the brand name equivalent. They must be manufactured under the same strict standards and meet the same batch requirements for identity, strength, purity, and quality as the brand name drug. To obtain FDA approval, the generic drug is administered in a single dose to at least 18 healthy human subjects. Next, peak serum concentration and the area under the plasma concentration curve (AUC) are measured. The values obtained for the generic drug must be within 80% to 125% of those obtained for the brand name drug. Most generic drugs have a mean AUC within 3% of the brand name drug. There has been no reported therapeutic difference of a serious nature between brand name products and FDA-approved generic products. For more information, see **Table 1.1**, which presents FDA equivalency ratings for brand name and generic drugs.

Complementary and Alternative Medicine

In the United States, the use of herbal preparations as treatments for disease and disease prevention has increased tremendously. According to the National Center for Complementary and Integrative Health, in 2012 approximately 33% of adults and 11% of children use some form of complementary approach to health care. The findings mirror similar surveys from 2007. The most popular products for adults (7.8%) and children (1.1%) are fish oils/Omega-3 fatty acids. These are followed by glucosamine and/or chondroitin (2.6%), probiotics/prebiotics (1.6%) and melatonin (1.3%) for adults, and for children melatonin (0.7%) (Clarke et al., 2015).

Historically, herbs were the first healing system used. Herbal medicines are derived from plants and thought by many to be harmless because they are products of nature. Some prescription drugs in current use, however, such as digitalis, are also "natural," which is not synonymous with "harmless." Before 1962, herbal preparations were considered to be drugs, but now they are sold as foods or supplements and therefore do not require FDA approval as drugs. Hence, there are no legislated standards on purity or quantity of active ingredients in herbal preparations. The value of herbal therapy is usually measured by anecdotal reports and not verified by research. Like synthetic products, herbal preparations may interact with other drugs and may produce undesirable side effects as well.

The Dietary Supplement Health and Education Act (1994) requires labeling about the effect of herbal products on the body and requires the statement that the herbal product has not been reviewed by the FDA and is not intended to be used as a drug. Complementary and alternative medicine (CAM) is discussed in Chapter 9.

Foreign Medications

In today's global society, practitioners will experience encounters with patients from many countries. These individuals may request refills of drugs for treating their chronic conditions. These drugs may have unrecognizable names, different dosages/dosage forms, or different active ingredients. Additionally, patients may get their drugs from online pharmacies in other countries because they are less expensive. Today, there is a proliferation of these online pharmacies, and only 3% comply with U.S. pharmacy laws (FDA, 2013). According to the World Health Organization, 80% of drugs are counterfeited in some countries (FDA, 2014). The Food and Drug Administration (FDA) has many resources for the practitioner to guide patients toward sound decision making about prescription drug acquisition.

TABLE 1.1

FDA Therapeutic Equivalence Ratings

Rating Scale	Definition
A	*Therapeutically Equivalent*
AA	Products in conventional dosage forms not presenting bioequivalence problems
AB	Products meeting necessary bioequivalence requirements
AN	Solutions and powders for aerosolization
AO	Injectable oil solutions
AP	Injectable aqueous solutions and, in certain instances, intravenous nonaqueous solutions
AT	Topical products
B	*Not Therapeutically Equivalent*
BB	Drug products requiring further FDA investigation and review to determine therapeutic equivalence
BC	Extended-release dosage forms (capsules, injectables, and tablets)
BD	Active ingredients and dosage forms with documented bioequivalence problems
BE	Delayed-release oral dosage forms
BN	Products in aerosol–nebulizer drug delivery systems
BP	Active ingredients and dosage forms with potential bioequivalence problems
BR	Suppositories or enemas that deliver drugs for systemic absorption
BS	Products having drug standard deficiencies
BT	Topical products with bioequivalence issues
BX	Drug products for which the data are insufficient to determine therapeutic equivalence
AB	Potential equivalence problems have been resolved with adequate in vivo or in vitro evidence supporting bioequivalence

U.S. Department of Health and Human Services, Food and Drug Administration, Center for Drug Evaluation and Research, Office of Pharmaceutical Science, Office of Generic Drugs. (2010). *Approved drug products with therapeutic equivalence evaluation* (30th ed.).

Disposal of Medications

Many medications can be potentially harmful if taken by someone other than the person for whom they are prescribed. Understand that improperly disposed drugs can leak into the environment, and the best disposal method is through community drug take-back programs. Almost all medicines can be safely disposed of if they are mixed with an undesirable substance, such as cat litter or coffee grounds, and placed in a closed container. Any personal information should be removed from the container by using a black marker or duct tape. Many communities have a drug take-back program for disposal, or drugs can be disposed of when the community collects hazardous material. Drugs should not be flushed down the toilet or drain unless the dispensing directions say this is permitted. Drugs permitted to be flushed can be found on the Web site http://www.fda.gov/Drugs/ResourcesForYou/Consumers/BuyingUsingMedicineSafely/EnsuringSafeUseofMedicine/SafeDisposalofMedicines/ucm186187.htm.

PRACTITIONER'S ROLE AND RESPONSIBILITIES IN PRESCRIBING

Before prescribing therapy, the practitioner has a responsibility to gather data by taking a thorough history and performing a physical examination. Once the data are gathered and evaluated, one or more diagnoses are formulated and a treatment plan established. As noted, the most frequently used treatment modality is drug therapy, usually with a prescription or OTC drug.

If a drug is deemed necessary for therapy, it is essential for the practitioner to understand the responsibility involved in prescribing that drug or drugs and to consider seriously which class of medication is most appropriate for the patient. The decision is reached based on a thorough knowledge of diagnosis and treatment.

Drug Selection

To determine which therapy is best for the patient, the practitioner conducts a risk–benefit analysis, evaluating the therapeutic value versus the risk associated with each drug to be prescribed. The practitioner then selects from a vast number of pharmacologic agents used for treating the specific medical problem. Factors to consider when selecting the drug or drugs are the subtle or significant differences in action, side effects, interactions, convenience, storage needs, route of administration, efficacy, and cost. Another factor in the decision may involve the patient pressuring the practitioner to prescribe a medication (because that is the expectation of many patients at the beginning of a health care encounter). Clearly, many responsibilities are inherent in prescribing a medication, and serious consequences may result if these responsibilities are not taken seriously and the prescription is prepared incorrectly.

BOX 1.2 Questions to Address When Prescribing a Medication

- Is there a need for the drug in treating the presenting problem?
- Is this the best drug for the presenting problem?
- Are there any contraindications to this drug with this patient?
- Is the dosage correct? Or is it too high or too low?
- Does the patient have allergies or sensitivities to the drug?
- What drug treatment modalities does the patient currently use, and will the potential new drug interact with the patient's other drugs or treatments?
- Is there a problem with storage of the drug?
- Does the dosage regimen (schedule) interfere with the patient's lifestyle? For example, if a child is in school, a drug with a once- or twice-daily dosing schedule is more realistic than one with a four-times-daily schedule.
- Is the route of administration the most appropriate one?
- Is the proposed duration of treatment too short or too long?
- Can the patient take the prescribed drug?
- Has the patient been informed of possible side effects and what to do if they occur?
- Is there a genetic component to consider?
- What is the cost of the drug?
- What, if any, prescription plan does the patient have?

Initial questions to ask when selecting drug therapy include "Is there a need for this drug in treating the presenting problem or disease?" and "Is this the best drug for the presenting problem or disease?" Additional questions are listed in **Box 1.2.**

Concerns Related to Ethics and Practice

Certain ethical and practical issues must be considered as well. One overriding issue may be the lack of a clinical indication for using a medication. As mentioned, many patients visit a practitioner with the sole purpose of obtaining a prescription. In seeking medical attention, the ill patient expects the health care provider to promote relief from symptoms. In today's world, an abundance of information available in books, magazines, television, Web sites, and other media suggests that the health care provider can do this by prescribing a special medication. This expectation—that a magic pill or potion—the prescription—is the ticket that will relieve reflux, kill germs, end pain, and restore health—puts pressure on the practitioner to prescribe for the sake of prescribing. A common example of this involves the patient with a cold who seeks an antibiotic, such as penicillin. In such a situation, the practitioner has a responsibility to prescribe only medications that are necessary for the well-being of the patient and that will be effective in treating the problem. In the example of the patient with an uncomplicated head cold, an antibiotic would not be effective, and the responsible practitioner must be prepared to make an ethical and judicious decision not to prescribe an antibiotic and explain it to the patient.

Patient Education

An integral part of the practitioner's role and responsibility is educating the patient about drug therapy and the intended therapeutic effect, potential side effects, and strategies for dealing with possible adverse drug reactions. This may be explained verbally, with written instructions given, when appropriate. Instructions that are printed and handed to the patient must be readable, in a language that the patient can understand, and at the appropriate health literacy. If side effects are discussed in advance, the patient will know what to expect and will contact the prescriber with symptoms. There may be less likelihood that the patient will discontinue the drug before discussing it with the prescriber.

Medications can also have a placebo effect. Patients must believe that the drug will work for them to be committed to taking it as recommended. If that belief is not instilled in patients, the drug may not be perceived as effective and may not be taken as directed.

The practitioner may want to advise the patient to use only one pharmacy when filling prescriptions. The choice of only one pharmacy has several advantages, which include maintaining a record of all medications that the patient currently receives and serving as a double-check for drug–drug interactions.

Prescriptive Authority

Prescribing practices of each practitioner are regulated by the state in which he or she practices. Each state determines practice parameters by statutes (laws enacted by the legislature), rules, and regulations (administrative policies determined by regulatory agencies). Each practitioner is responsible for knowing the laws and regulations in the state of practice.

Prescriptive authority is regulated by the State Board of Nursing, Board of Medicine, or Board of Pharmacy, depending on the state. States allow full practice authority, collaborative practice, supervised practice, or delegated practice. Full practice authority has no requirements for mandatory physician collaboration or supervision. Collaborative practice requires a formal agreement with a collaborating physician, ensuring a referral–consultant relationship. Supervised practice is overseen or directed by a supervisory physician. Delegated practice means that prescription writing is a delegated medical act. Regulations can be found at the Division of Professional Regulation for prescribers in each state.

Related to prescriptive authority issues is the issue of drug samples. Most drug companies engage in the promotional practice of distributing sample drugs to practitioners for use by patients. The Prescription Drug Marketing Act (PDMA), which was enacted in 1988 to protect the American consumer from ineffective drugs, also affects the receipt and dispensing of sample drugs. Prescription drugs can be distributed only to licensed practitioners (one licensed by the state to prescribe drugs) and health care entity pharmacies at the request of a licensed practitioner. PDMA protects the public in several ways. It forbids foreign countries to reimport prescription drugs; bans the sale, trade, and purchase of drug samples; prohibits resale of prescription drugs purchased by hospitals, health care entities, and charitable organizations; requests practitioners to ask for drug samples in writing; and regulates wholesale distributors of prescription drugs by requiring licensing in states where facilities are located. There are penalties for violation of the act. This act affects the distribution and use of pharmaceutical samples.

Because these samples are freely available, it might be assumed that they can be distributed by all practitioners, but this is not the case. The practitioner must be aware of the rules that govern requesting, receiving, and distributing these agents because the rules vary from state to state.

Specific procedures are required with drug samples. The pharmaceutical representative's Sample Request Form must be signed. It includes the name, strength, and quantity of the sample. The sample must be then recorded on the Record of Receipt of Drug Sample sheet. The samples must be stored away from other drug inventory and where unauthorized access is not allowed or in a locked cabinet or closet in a public area. Samples are to be inspected monthly for expiration dates, proper labeling and storage, presence of intact packaging and labeling, and appropriateness for the practice. If a sample has expired, it must be disposed of in a manner that prevents accessibility to the general public. It cannot be disposed into the trash.

When distributing samples, each must be labeled with the patient's name, clear directions for use, and cautions. All samples are to be dispensed free of charge along with pertinent information. The medication is then documented in the patient's chart with dose, quantity, and directions.

ADVERSE DRUG EVENTS

Prescription and nonprescription drugs are an increasing part of life in the United States. Between the years of 2009 and 2012, there were 48.7% of individuals who took at least one prescription drug in the last 30 days (CDC, FastStats, 2015). Adverse drug events (ADE) have consequently become an increasing problem resulting in adverse events both in the inpatient and outpatient settings. Due to the magnitude of the problem, the Home of the Office of Disease and Health Promotion have created a National Action Plan for Adverse Drug Event Prevention 2014 (http://health.gov/hcq/ade.asp). Therefore, the prudent prescriber must always be aware of any medications presenting for health care. Chapter 3 reviews the impact of ADE in depth.

Lack of Drug Knowledge

There can be a lack of knowledge about indications and contra-indications for drugs. This includes underuse, overuse, and mis-use of drugs. An example of underuse is failure to prescribe an inhaled corticosteroid for an asthmatic patient who uses his alb-uterol daily. An example of overuse is prescribing an antibiotic for a cold or prescribing an antihypertensive drug for someone whose blood pressure is elevated because he is taking pseudoephedrine (Sudafed). An example of misuse is prescribing penicillin to some-one for a strep throat who has identified a clear allergy to the drug.

Dosing errors occur when a larger dose is prescribed than needed or the conversion from oral to intravenous is too high. This is especially problematic with pediatrics for antibiotics (Aseeri, 2013). For example, prescribing a dose of Augmentin that is greater than the suggested amount or starting a patient on 30 mg paroxetine instead of 20 mg may increase anxiety.

Lack of knowledge about drug–drug interactions can also cause errors. For example, many drugs interfere with warfarin and cause increased bleeding if taken together. The prescriber must be aware of the potential for drug–drug interactions (see Chapter 3 for more information).

Lack of Patient Information

A common error in prescribing is failure to obtain an adequate history from the patient. Often an adequate drug history is not obtained and the provider does not specifically inquire about herbal preparations or OTC medications. Also, information on allergies to medications is not always obtained. In addition to allergies, it is imperative to ascertain the reaction to the medi-cation. Nausea is not considered an allergic reaction. An allergy history should be taken and documented at each visit before a new medication is prescribed. Additionally, asking multiple times about allergies or reactions to drugs during a visit is a safety cross-check to responsible prescribing.

Poor Communication

Poor communication between health care providers, pharma-cists, and patients can be a result of poor handwriting, incor-rect abbreviations, misplaced decimals, and misunderstanding of verbal prescriptions. These potential errors can be mitigated through the use of electronic health record (EHR); however, new errors can occur if the practitioner does not click on the correct medication. Additionally, there are areas in the United States where providers still handwrite prescriptions. Poor communica-tion also results when the prescriber fails to discuss potential side effects or ask about side effects at subsequent visits.

SPECIAL POPULATION CONSIDERATIONS

Doses for children are usually based on weight in kilograms. The prescriber has a responsibility to calculate the dose and write the correct dose, rather than relying on the pharmacist to calculate the dose. See Chapter 4 for more information about pediatric drug dosing.

Elderly patients may have some difficulty hearing or reading small print. Additionally, they may be taking multiple prescrip-tion medications and OTC medications. The prescriber needs to be specific about when the patient should take each medication and if one drug cannot be taken with others. When the practi-tioner prescribes for the elderly, he or she must consider renal function because some medications can cause toxicity, even in small doses, with decreased renal function. Chapter 6 reviews the considerations necessary for good prescribing in the elderly.

PHARMACOGENOMICS

Recently, pharmacogenomics has gained importance in pre-scribing medication. The way a person responds to a drug is influenced by many different genes. Without knowing all of the genes involved in drug response, it has not been possible to develop genetic tests that could predict a person's response to a particular drug. Knowing that people's genes show small variations in the DNA base makes genetic testing for predict-ing drug response possible. Genetic factors can account for 20% to 95% variability of the patient's reaction to a drug. Pharmacogenomics examines the inherited variations in genes that dictate drug response and explores the ways these variations can be used to predict the response a patient will have to a drug. Pharmacogenetic testing may enable providers to understand why patients react differently to various drugs and to make better decisions about therapy. This understand-ing may allow for highly individualized therapeutic regimens. This concept is discussed in detail in Chapter 10.

STEPS OF THE PRESCRIBING PROCESS

At each visit, a medication history is obtained with the name of the drug, dosage, and frequency of administration. Information on any allergies should also be obtained. It is also helpful if the patient brings his or her actual drugs to the visit.

Multiple steps (**Figure 1.2**) are involved in prescribing drugs and evaluating their effectiveness. Again, the first step is determining an accurate diagnosis based on the patient's his-tory, physical examination, and pertinent test findings.

Next, in selecting the best agent, the practitioner thor-oughly evaluates the patient's condition, taking into consid-eration the effect that various medications may have on the patient and the disorder, the expected outcomes of therapy, and other variables (**Box 1.3**). When prescribing any drug therapy, the practitioner must have a solid knowledge and background in the pathophysiology of disease, pharmacotherapeutics, pharmacokinetics, pharmacodynamics, and any interactions (see Chapters 2 and 3).

The practitioner needs to be knowledgeable about the best class of drugs for the diagnosed disorder or presenting problem,

FIGURE 1.2   Process for prescribing.

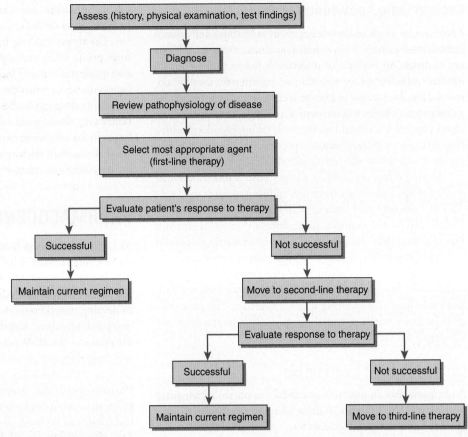

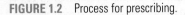

BOX
1.3
Variables to Consider in Prescribing a Medication

Age
Sex
Race
Weight
Culture
Allergies
Pharmacogenomics
Other diseases or conditions
Other therapies
　　Prescription medications
　　Over-the-counter medicines
　　Alternative therapies
Previous therapies
　　Effectiveness
　　Adverse effects
　　Adherence
Socioeconomic issues
　　Insurance status
　　Income level
　　Daily schedule
　　Living environment
　　Support systems
Health beliefs

the recommended dosage, potential side effects, possible interactions with other drugs, and special prescribing considerations, such as required laboratory tests, contraindications, and patient instructions. To select the correct medication, the practitioner must thoroughly understand the pathophysiology of the condition being treated and the natural history of the disease. This information allows the practitioner to decide at which point in the disease process intervention with drug therapy is indicated because in many diseases or disorders, nonpharmacologic therapies are tried before drug therapy is initiated.

Next, the practitioner sets goals for therapy. Goals need to be realistic and outcomes measurable. All interventions, nonpharmacologic and pharmacologic, are initiated to meet these goals, and evaluation of the therapy's efficacy is based on these goals.

Selecting Most Appropriate Agent

For most disease entities, there is a recommended first-line therapy—that is, research shows certain agents to be more effective than others. Once initiated, the first-line therapy is evaluated and either continued or changed. If the desired goals are not achieved, or if an adverse reaction occurs, second-line therapy is initiated. The second-line therapy is then evaluated. If this therapy is not tolerated or efficacious, a third-line therapy is initiated, and so on. The practitioner continually evaluates the patient's response to therapy and maintains current therapy or changes it as indicated by the patient's response. For more information, see the case study outlining the prescribing process. Case studies such as this one are used throughout the text.

Consideration of Special Populations

Another step in prescribing drugs is considering specific concerns related to special populations, such as children, pregnant or breast-feeding women, and the elderly. Cultural beliefs are also considered to ensure that the drug regimen honors individual and family customs and preferences. Pharmacogenomics are gaining in popularity when considering which drug to prescribe.

Identifying Outcomes

Expected outcomes can include improvement in clinical symptoms or pathologic signs or changes in biochemistry as determined by laboratory tests. To assess whether expected outcomes have been achieved, the practitioner reviews data collected on subsequent visits, evaluates the effectiveness of drug therapy, and investigates any adverse reactions.

The frequency of follow-up visits is determined by the disease and the patient's response to treatment. While outcomes are being assessed, the practitioner educates the patient about the outcomes of therapy as well. Topics for discussion include drug benefits, side effects, dosage adjustments, and monitoring parameters.

The patient as well as the practitioner must be informed about any undesirable outcomes of therapy with a prescription drug. Reactions that may be expected and must be discussed include side effects, drug or food interactions, and toxicity. Unexpected reactions include allergic reactions or intolerance to a drug. If a patient experiences a serious adverse drug reaction, the practitioner files a report with the FDA's MedWatch program on a special form obtainable from MedWatch (5600 Fishers Lane, Rockville, MD 20852-9787 or it can be reported online at https://www.accessdata.fda.gov/scripts/medwatch/; see Chapter 3 for a sample of the MedWatch form). Similarly, adverse reactions to vaccines are reported through the Vaccine Adverse Event Reporting System (VAERS) online at http://vaers.hhs.gov/esub/index#Online or by mail by completing a VAERS form requested by calling 1-800-822-7967 and mailing it to VAERS, P.O. Box 1100, Rockville, MD 20849-1100. Adverse events are discussed in Chapter 4.

WRITING THE PRESCRIPTION

The practice of handwriting prescriptions is slowly becoming an exercise of the past; however, there are still instances where a practitioner needs to know the steps. The prescription is a form of communication between the practitioner and the pharmacist. It is also the basis for written directions to patients, and it is a legal document. Each prescription should be clearly written to avoid errors of misinterpretation in filling the prescription. Although potentially serious errors occur infrequently, they are avoidable and should not occur at all.

An early step in the prescribing process involves ensuring that common but potentially serious errors are not made. The first is failure to identify a patient's allergies, particularly to a medication. In identifying a drug allergy, the practitioner should also investigate the kind of reaction experienced with the medication to differentiate between a true, life-threatening drug allergy and less serious drug sensitivity. Some cross-sensitivities must also be considered. Another error is failure to instruct the patient to stop a previously prescribed medication that treats the same condition. In some instances, an additional medication may be prescribed to increase the effect for the same problem, but the patient must be made aware of this. Otherwise, the original medication must be canceled. Failure to recognize the effect of a prescribed drug on other diseases or drugs can lead to potentially serious effects. There are now programs that can do multiple checks for interactions. One of these is Epocrates for mobile devices and desktops.

Date, Name, Address, and Date of Birth

There are standard components of any prescription. One is the date and another is the full name, address, and date of birth of the patient. The name should be the patient's given name (the one on the medical record) and not a nickname. If a different name is used each time, the patient could have multiple records in pharmacy record-keeping systems. The address should be the current home address of the patient and not a work address or a post office box.

Prescriber's Name, Address, and Phone Number

The next components are the name, address, and phone number of the prescriber and the collaborating physician if required by state law or regulations. This enables the pharmacist to contact the prescriber if there is a question about the prescription.

Name of Drug

Of course, the name of the drug is the most essential part of the prescription. Ideally, the generic name (with the trade or brand name in parentheses) is used. The name must be legible to avoid errors in filling the prescription correctly. For instance, some drugs have names that are commonly confused or misread, such as Norvasc and Navane, Prilosec and Prozac, carboplatin and cisplatin, and Levoxine and Lanoxin. Severe problems may result if the wrong drug is supplied erroneously. Adding the diagnosis to the prescription, although optional, can help the pharmacist avoid misinterpreting the prescribed drug.

Dose, Dosage Regimen, and Route of Administration

The drug dose is essential because many drugs are available in various strengths. The dose is written in numerals. If the dose is a fraction of 1, it is written in decimal form with a leading zero to the left of the decimal point (e.g., 0.75). However, a whole number should not be followed by a decimal point and a trailing zero (10.0 could be misinterpreted as 100). The numeric dose is followed by the correct metric specification such as milligram (mg), gram (g), milliliter (mL), or microgram (mcg). Many practitioners spell out *microgram* to avoid confusion with *milligram*. Some drugs are manufactured in units that should be specified, and the term *unit* should be written out (insulin 10 units, not 10 U). Usually, the strength of drugs that are combination products or that are manufactured only in one strength do not need to be included. The route of the drug is specified as well. (Routes of administration are discussed in Chapter 2.)

The prescription also specifies how frequently the drug is to be taken. A drug prescribed to be taken as needed is termed a *prn* drug. For example, dosage frequency can be written as "prn every 4 hours" (or another appropriate interval) for the problem for which the drug is prescribed (e.g., "as needed for nausea"). It is good practice to write out the number (10–ten), especially with controlled substances. Any special instructions, such as "after meals," "at bedtime," or "with food," also should be specified. If the dose is once a day it is safer practice to write out daily than to write OD because this can be confused with every other day.

The prescription also includes the number of pills, vials, suppositories, or containers or amount in milliliters or ounces to be dispensed. Prescription reimbursement or health care insurance programs often allow for 30- or 90-day supplies to be dispensed at a time, working with the pharmacist is imperative for optimal prescribing practices. They are the best connection regarding the rules of various prescription plans. The prescription indicates whether the prescription may be refilled and the number of refills permitted.

When prescribing a new drug for a patient, the practitioner may want to consider prescribing just a few doses or a 7-day supply initially. Alternatively, samples may be provided, if allowed by law or regulations. This allows the prescriber to determine if the patient can tolerate the drug and if it is effective. When deciding on the number of refills, the practitioner may decide when the patient should return for a follow-up visit and allow just the number of refills that will take the patient until the next visit to ensure that the patient returns. Some drug prescriptions cannot be refilled. For all Schedule 2 drugs, for example, a new prescription must be written each time.

Allowable Substitutions

There are many generic equivalents for brand name drugs. Indication of whether a substitution is allowed is a part of the prescription. As discussed earlier, a generic drug substitute must have the same chemical composition and dosage as the brand name drug originally prescribed. In many states, a generic drug will automatically be substituted for a brand name drug. If there is a medical reason to require a brand name drug (that has a generic equivalent), "Brand Medically Necessary" must be written on the prescription.

Prescriber's Signature and License Number

The signature of the prescriber is required. It should be legible and should be the person's legal signature. The license number of the prescriber or the collaborating physician is required on the prescription in some, but not all, states depending on the rules and regulations that govern the prescriber. In some instances, the DEA number of the prescriber is also required, especially when prescribing between states or prescribing a controlled substance. **Figure 1.3** illustrates a blank prescription and a completed prescription. Each state has specific requirements for components on a printed prescription. The practitioner must be in compliance with state regulations and may prescribe only in the state in which he or she holds a license. Although the prescription may be filled in another state (if allowed by state regulations), a DEA number is usually required. An NPI number must be on each prescription along with a serial number of the prescription form. If the practitioner is a federal employee, he or she may prescribe in any federal facility.

Any drug prescribed should be clearly documented in the medical record with date of order, dosage, amount prescribed, and number of refills. It is helpful to have a specific area in the record to record all drugs taken by the patient—prescription, OTC, and CAM—for ease of audit, reference, and communication among health care professionals.

Sally Jones, FNP
111 High Street
Hometown, NH 00440
555-432-1111
Serial #00001
NPIH 1234567890

Patient's Name ____________ Date ______
Patient's Address ____________
____
Date of Birth ______
Drug ______ Dosage ______
Number ______
Directions ______
Number of refills ______
Generic substitution yes_____ no_____
Signature ______
License Number ______
DEA Number (if required) ______

Sally Jones, FNP
111 High Street
Hometown, NH 00440
555-432-1111
Serial #00001
NPIH 1234567890

Patient's Name John Smith Date 6/29/00
Patient's Address 13 Comstock Street
Newtown, NH 33300
Date of Birth 1/2/33
Enalapril (Vasotec) 5 mg
#30
Take one daily
Number of refills 5
Substitution yes X no
Signature *Sally Jones, FNP*
License Number RN0000033
DEA Number (if required) 012345-E

FIGURE 1.3 Example of a blank prescription form **(left)** and a completed form **(right)**.

Electronic Prescriptions

Electronic prescribing has become increasingly popular. Health care technology reduces medication errors with the use of drug-checking software, which checks the medication dose, potential interactions with other medications the patient may be taking, and the patient's known allergies. This drug-checking software may be part of the EHR or of a freestanding e-prescribing system. Integrated EHRs can calculate dosing based on a patient's weight and carry out other contextual medication checking against a patient's laboratory results, age, and disease states. In addition, computer systems provide pick lists of each clinician's favorite medications with a precalculated dose, frequency, and route, reducing the opportunity for clinicians to order inappropriate amounts of medications with the wrong frequency and route.

E-Prescribing improves the legibility of prescriptions and the rate of completed prescriptions. Patients no longer need to carry paper copies of a prescription to a pharmacy and are more likely to have formulary-compliant medications prescribed for them and to find their prescriptions waiting for them when they arrive at the pharmacy. This leads to greater patient convenience, shorter wait times, and increased compliance with formulary requirements. Electronic prescribing has been said to show a 12% to 20% decrease in ADEs (Figge, 2009).

With electronically generated prescriptions, there are no handwriting misinterpretations and no manual data entry. Correct dosages are built into the software. They assist with formulary requirements based on the patient's insurance and maintain allergy profiles and ADEs. They also serve to decrease drug–drug interactions.

ADHERENCE ISSUES

A prescribed drug must be used correctly to produce optimal benefits. Patient nonadherence to a prescribed regimen leads to less-than-optimal outcomes, such as progression of the disease state and an increased incidence of hospitalizations. Studies demonstrate that the more complex the treatment regimen, the less likely the patient is to follow it. Benner (2009) studied 5,759 patients taking antihypertensive and lipid-lowering drugs. In patients with 0, 1, and 2 prior medications, 41%, 35%, and 30% of patients were adherent, respectively, to antihypertensive and lipid-lowering therapy. Of patients with 10 or more prior medications, 20% were adherent.

Karter (2009) studied 27,329 subjects prescribed new medications. Pharmacy utilization data were used. It was found that 22% of patients had the prescription filled zero or one times. The proportion of newly prescribed patients who never became ongoing users was eight times greater than the proportion who maintained ongoing use, but with inadequate adherence. Four percent of those who had the prescription filled at least two times discontinued therapy during the 24-month follow-up. Nonadherence was significantly associated with high out-of-pocket costs and clinical response to therapy.

Several variables are associated with improved adherence to a drug regimen. These include variables associated with the patient's perception of the encounter and of the benefit of the treatment. If a patient is nonadherent to the prescribed regimen, it is important to document that in the chart. The risks of nonadherence are discussed, and that discussion is documented. It is essential to ask why the patient is not following the prescribed treatment, and actions to rectify the problem should be taken. All of this is documented. One issue may be that the patient is unable to swallow the pill. The medicine may be available in liquid form, or the pill may be split or crushed. The practitioner needs to review and understand the factors that affect adherence to a regimen (**Box 1.4**).

UPDATING DRUG INFORMATION

Many sources of drug information can be accessed by practitioners who must keep current on changes in drug therapy and continually update their fund of knowledge. Resources include reference books, pharmacists (who are expertly informed about drugs, interactions, dosages, etc.), easy-to-carry drug handbooks and pocket guides for quick reference, and online databases and programs for mobile devices and desktop computers (**Tables 1.2 and 1.3**).

BOX 1.4   Factors Influencing the Patient's Adherence to a Medication Regimen

- Approachability of the health care provider
- Perception of respect with which he or she is treated by the practitioner
- Belief that the therapy is beneficial
- Belief that the benefits of therapy outweigh the risks or side effects
- Degree to which the patient participates in developing the treatment regimen
- Cost of the regimen
- Simplicity of the regimen

- Understanding of the treatment regimen
- Degree to which the patient feels that expectations are being met
- Degree to which the patient perceives his or her concerns are important and being addressed
- Degree to which the practitioner motivates the patient to adhere to the regimen
- Degree to which the regimen is compatible with the patient's lifestyle

TABLE 1.2

Common Drug Reference Books

Reference	Features
American Hospital Formulary Service. Bethesda, MD: American Society of Health System Pharmacists.	Drug entries are indexed by generic and brand names and organized by pharmacologic–therapeutic class.
Drug Facts and Comparisons. Philadelphia, PA: Wolters Kluwer Health.	Drugs are indexed by generic and brand names and organized by major classes of drugs. Updates are issued monthly (in print and CD-ROM).
Physician's Desk Reference (PDR). Montvale, NJ: Medical Economics.	Drugs are indexed by manufacturer, brand name, generic name, and product category. Volume contains product identification section. Information replicates the official package insert from the drug manufacturer.

TABLE 1.3

Online Drug Reference Data

Reference	Address	Features
Agency for Healthcare Research and Quality (AHRQ)	www.ahrq.gov	Guidelines for clinical practice from the Agency for Healthcare Research and Quality (AHRQ), National Guidelines Clearinghouse, U.S. Preventive Services Task Force
Center Watch Clinical Trials	www.centerwatch.com	Lists clinical research trials and drug therapy newly approved by the U.S. FDA and the FDA New Drug Listing Service
Coreynahman	www.coreynahman.com	Pharmaceutical news and information. Gives a choice of many sites for information
Epocrates	www.epocrates.com	Software for PDA with drug information, interactions, etc.
Healthtouch Drug Information	www.healthtouch.com	Information for patient and provider
Mediconsult	www.mediconsult.com	Professional- and consumer-focused. Detailed medical and drug information
Medscape	www.medscape.com	Drug search database. Links to online journals
RxList—The Internet Drug Index	www.rxlist.com	Cross-index of U.S. prescription products

CASE STUDY*

A.J. is a 16-year-old who has just started soccer practice at school. She complains of increased shortness of breath with exercise, and describes having a hard time catching her breath when she runs, which she does five to six times a week. She does not wake up at night with a cough or shortness of breath, and has no problems at any other time except in the spring when the trees start to blossom. The soccer coach advised A.J.'s mother to seek health care because A.J. had a very difficult time breathing at practice that afternoon. A.J. also has a history of eczema and seasonal allergies for which she takes an over-the counter antihistamine when symptoms get severe.

Social History: Nonsmoker. Lives in an urban area with mother, father, and brother. Does not use street drugs.
Family History: Father has a history of asthma.
Physical Examination:

Nose: Mucosa pale and boggy bilaterally
Lungs: Respirations 26 and shallow; diffuse expiratory wheezing; peak flow 340
Diagnosis: Mild persistent asthma

QUESTIONS

1. List specific goals of therapy for A.J.
2. What drug therapy would you prescribe and why?
3. What are the parameters for monitoring success of the therapy?
4. Discuss specific patient education based on the prescribed therapy.
5. List one or two adverse reactions for the selected agent that would cause you to change therapy.
6. What would be the choice for second-line therapy?

* Answers can be found online.

Bibliography

Starred references are cited in the text.

Adler, K. G. (2009). E-prescribing: Why the fuss. *Family Practice Management, 16*(1), 22–27.

Aseeri, M. A. (2013). The impact of pediatric antibiotic standard dosing table on dosing errors. *Journal of Pediatric Pharmacologic Therapeutics, 18*(3), 220–226. doi: 10.5863/1551-6776-18.3.220.

Belle, D. G., & Singh, H. (2008). Genetic factors in drug metabolism. *American Family Physician, 77*(11), 1553–1168.

*Benner, J. S. (2009). Association between prescription burden and medication adherence in patients initiating antihypertensive and lipid-lowering therapy. *American Journal of Health System Pharmacies, 66*(16), 1471–1477.

*Centers for Disease Control and Prevention. (2015). Therapeutic drug use. Retrieved from www.cdc.gov/nchs/fastats/drug-use-therapeutic.htm on August 23, 2015.

*Centers for Disease Control and Prevention. (2014). Vital signs: Variation among states in prescribing of opioid pain relievers and benzodiazepines—United States, 2012. *Morbidity and Mortality Weekly Report, 63*(26), 563–568.

*Center Watch. (2015). Overview of clinical trials: What is clinical research? Retrieved from http://www.centerwatch.com/clinical-trials/overview.aspx

*Clarke, T. C., Black Lindsey, L. I., Stussman, B. J., et al. (2015). Trends in the use of complementary health approaches among adults: United States, 2001–2012. *National Health Statistics Report, 79*, February 10. 1–16. Retrieved from http://www.cdc.gov/nchs/data/nhsr/nhsr079.pdf on August 23, 2015.

Court, M. H. (2007). A pharmacogenomics primer. *Journal of Clinical Pharmacology, 47*(9), 1087–1103.

Cusack, C. M. (2008). Electronic health records and electronic prescribing: Promise and pitfalls. *Obstetric and Gynecology Clinics of North America, 35*(1), 63–79.

DiPiro, J. T., Talbert, R. L., Yee, G.C., et al. (Eds.). (2014). *Pharmacotherapy: A pathophysiologic approach* (9th ed.). New York, NY: McGraw-Hill Medical.

Doherty, K., Segal, A., & McKinney, P. (2004). The 10 most common prescribing errors: Tips on avoiding the pitfalls. *Consultant, 44*(2), 173–182.

*FDA. (2014). Counterfeit drugs: Fighting illegal supply chains. Retrieved from http://www.fda.gov/NewsEvents/Testimony/ucm387449.htm

*FDA. (2013). BeSafeRx: Know your online pharmacy. Retrieved from http://www.fda.gov/Drugs/ResourcesForYou/Consumers/BuyingUsingMedicineSafely/BuyingMedicinesOvertheInternet/BeSafeRxKnowYourOnlinePharmacy/ucm294170.htm

*Figge, H. (2009). Electronic prescribing in the ambulatory care setting. *American Journal of Health System Pharmacy, 66*(1), 16–18.

Hampton, L. M., Ngyuen, D. B., Edwards, J. R., et al. (2013). Cough and cold medications adverse events after market withdrawal and labeling revision. *Pediatrics, 132*(6), 1047–1054. doi: 10.1542/peds.2013-2236.

*Home of Office Disease Prevention & Health Promotion. (2014). National action plan for adverse drug event prevention. [online retrieved on August 23, 2015] http://health.gov/hcq/ade.asp#overview

*Karter, A. J. (2009). New prescription medication gaps: A comprehensive measure of adherence to new prescriptions. *Health Service Research, 44*(5 Pt. 1), 1640–1661.

Keohane, C. A., & Bates, D. W. (2008). Medication safety. *Obstetrics and Gynecology Clinics, 35*(1), 37–52.

Mahoney, D. F. (2010). More than a prescriber: Gerontological nurse practitioners' perspectives on prescribing and pharmaceutical marketing. *Geriatric Nursing, 31*(1), 17–27.

*National Association of State Controlled Substances. (2014). Authorities. Retrieved from http://www.nascsa.org/rxMonitoring.htm

O'Connor, N. R. (2010). FDA boxed warnings: How to prescribe drugs safely. *American Family Physician, 81*(3), 298–303.

Pollock, M., Bazaldua, O., & Dobbie, A. (2007). Appropriate prescribing of medications: An eight-step approach. *American Family Physician, 75*(2), 231–236.

Sadee, W. (2008). Drug therapy and personalized health care: Pharmacogenomics in perspective. *Pharmacology Research, 25*(12), 2713–2719.

Weber, W. W. (2008). Pharmacogenomics: From description to prediction. *Clinics in Laboratory Medicine, 28*(4), 499–511.

Wessell, A. M., Litvin, C., Jenkins, R. G., et al. (2010). Medication prescribing and monitoring errors in primary care: A report from the practice partner research network. *Quality Safety in Health Care, 19*, e21. doi: 10.1136/qshc.2009.034678.

2 Pharmacokinetic Basis of Therapeutics and Pharmacodynamic Principles

Andrew M. Peterson

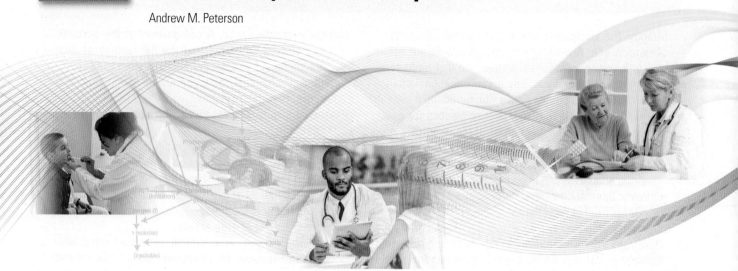

The art and science of clinical practice is based on understanding the relationship between the person and the disease and determining the most appropriate means for alleviating symptoms, curing disease, or preventing severe morbidity or even mortality. Very often, medications are prescribed to accomplish one or more of these goals.

Underpinning this treatment process is the intricate relationship between the body and the medication. Often, practitioners seek to understand the effect a drug has on the body (whether therapeutic or harmful) but neglect to consider the effect that the body has on the drug—even though one cannot be understood without the other. How the body acts on a drug and how the drug acts on the body are the subjects of this chapter.

Pharmacokinetics refers to the movement of the drug through the body—in essence, how the body affects the drug. This involves how the drug is administered, absorbed, distributed, and eventually eliminated from the body. *Pharmacodynamics* refers to how the drug affects the body—that is, how the drug initiates its therapeutic or toxic effect, both at the cellular level and systemically. **Box 2.1** lists terms and definitions used throughout this chapter.

The purpose of pharmacokinetic processes is to get the drug to the site of action where it can produce its pharmacodynamic effect. There is a minimum amount of drug needed at the site of action to produce the desired effect. Although the amount of drug concentrated at the site of action is difficult to measure, the amount of drug in the blood can be measured. The relationship between the concentration of drug in the blood and the concentration at the site of action (i.e., the drug receptor) is different for each drug and each person. Therefore, measuring blood concentrations is only a surrogate marker, an indication of concentration at the receptor.

Figure 2.1 shows the relationship between pharmacokinetics and pharmacodynamics.

PHARMACOKINETICS

Pharmacokinetics relates to how the drug is absorbed, distributed, and eliminated from the body. In reality, it is the study of the fate of medications administered to a person. It is sometimes described as *what the body does to the drug*. In theory, pharmacokinetics not only deals with medications, it deals with the disposition of all substances administered externally to any living organism. Pharmacokinetics can help the clinician determine the onset and duration of a drug's action as well as determine blood levels that would produce therapeutic and toxic effects. As such, one can determine the blood levels necessary to produce a desired effect. This target drug concentration is key to monitoring the effects of many medications. Assuming that the magnitude of the drug concentration at the site of action influences the drug effect, whether desired or undesired, it can be inferred that a range of drug levels produces a range of effects (**Figure 2.2**). Below a specific level, or threshold, the drug exerts little to no therapeutic effect. Above this threshold, the concentration of drug in the blood is sufficient to produce a therapeutic effect at the site of action. However, as the drug concentration increases in the blood, so does the concentration at the site of action. Above a specific level, an increased therapeutic effect may no longer occur. Instead, an unacceptable toxicity may occur because the drug concentration is too high. Between these two levels—the minimally effective level and the toxic level—is the *therapeutic window*. The therapeutic window is the range of blood drug concentration that yields a sufficient therapeutic response without excessively toxic reactions.

BOX 2.1 Definitions of Terms Related to Pharmacokinetics and Pharmacodynamics

Affinity: The attraction between a drug and a receptor.

Allosteric site: A binding site for substrates not active in initiating a response; a substrate that binds to an allosteric site may induce a conformational change in the structure of the active site, rendering it more or less susceptible to response from a substrate.

Bioavailability (F): The fraction or percentage of a drug that reaches the systemic circulation.

Biotransformation: Metabolism or degradation of a drug from an active form to an inactive form.

Chirality: Special configuration or shape of a drug; most drugs exist in two shapes.

Clearance: Removal of a drug from the plasma or organs.

Downregulation: Decreased availability of drug receptors.

Enantiomer (also called isomer): A mirror-image spatial arrangement, or shape, of a drug that suits it for binding with a drug receptor.

Enterohepatic recirculation: The process by which a drug excreted in the bile flows into the gastrointestinal tract, where it is reabsorbed and returned to the general circulation.

First-pass effect: The phenomenon by which a drug first passes through the liver where it may be degraded before distribution to the tissues.

Half-life (t½): The time required for half of a total drug amount to be eliminated from the body.

Hepatic extraction ratio: A comparison of the percentage of drug extracted and the percentage of drug remaining active after metabolism in the liver.

Ligand: Any chemical, endogenous or exogenous, that interacts with a receptor.

Pharmacodynamics: Processes through which drugs affect the body.

Pharmacokinetics: Processes through which the body affects drugs.

Prodrug: A drug that is transformed from an inactive parent drug into an active metabolite; in effect, a precursor to the active drug.

Receptor: The site of drug action.

Second messenger: A chemical produced intracellularly in response to a receptor signal; this second messenger initiates a change in the intracellular response.

Therapeutic window: The range of drug concentration in the blood between a minimally effective level and a toxic level.

Threshold: The level below which a drug exerts little to no therapeutic effect and above which a drug produces a therapeutic effect at the site of action.

Upregulation: Increased availability of receptors.

Volume of distribution (V_d): The extent of distribution of a drug in the body.

This range should not be considered absolute because it varies from individual to individual and therefore serves only as a guide to the practitioner.

Absorption

The first aspect of pharmacokinetics to consider is how drugs are administered, how they are absorbed into the body, and how they eventually reach the bloodstream. Merely introducing the drug into the body does not ensure that the compound will reach all tissues uniformly or even that the drug will reach the target site. Commonly recognized methods of absorption include enteral absorption (after the drug is administered by the oral or rectal route) and parenteral absorption (associated with drugs administered intramuscularly [IM], subcutaneously, or topically). The various administration routes and other factors affect a drug's ability to enter the bloodstream.

The extent to which the drug reaches the systemic circulation is referred to as *bioavailability*, or F, which is defined as the fraction or percentage of the drug that reaches the systemic circulation. Drugs administered intravenously are 100% bioavailable. Drugs administered by other routes (e.g., oral, IM) may be 100% bioavailable, but more often, they are less than

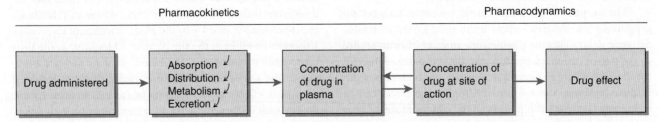

FIGURE 2.1 Relationship between pharmacokinetics and pharmacodynamics. Note the two-way relationship between the concentration of drug in the plasma and the concentration of drug at the site of action, depicting the interrelationship between pharmacokinetics and pharmacodynamics.

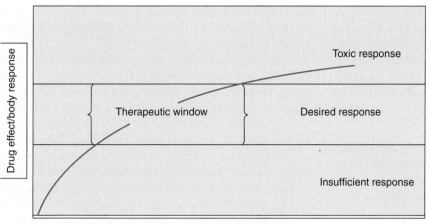

FIGURE 2.2 Therapeutic window: concentration versus response. The concentration of the drug in the body produces specific effects. A low concentration is considered subtherapeutic, producing an insufficient response. As the concentration increases, the desired effect is produced at a given drug level. A drug concentration that exceeds the upper limit of the desired response may produce a toxic reaction. The concentration range within which a desired response occurs is the therapeutic window.

100% bioavailable. Therefore, bioavailability depends on the route of administration and, equally important, the drug's ability to pass through membranes or barriers in the body. **Box 2.2** discusses the specific case of oral bioavailability.

Factors Affecting Absorption

A variety of factors affect absorption, such as the presence or absence of food in the stomach, blood flow to the area for absorption, and the dosage form of the drug. The following sections discuss some of the major factors affecting absorption.

Movement through Membranes and Drug Solubility

Throughout the body, biologic membranes act as barriers, blocking or permitting the passage of various substances. These membranes protect certain areas of the body from harmful chemicals and allow other areas to be accessed as needed.

Biologic membranes composed of cells serve as barriers primarily because of the structure and function of the cells that make up the membrane. Cell membranes are composed of lipids and proteins, creating a phospholipid bilayer. This bilayer acts as a barrier that is almost impermeable to water, other hydrophilic (water-loving) substances, and ionized

BOX 2.2   Oral Bioavailability and the First-Pass Effect

Drugs given orally may be subject to the first-pass effect, by which drugs are metabolized by the liver before passing into circulation. After absorption from the alimentary canal, drugs go directly to the liver through the portal vein. In the liver, hepatic enzymes act on the drug, reducing the amount of active drug reaching the bloodstream and decreasing the amount available to the body. The fraction (or percentage) of medication reaching systemic circulation after the first pass through the liver is referred to as the drug's bioavailability (F).

The first-pass effect is not the only factor contributing to the oral bioavailability of a drug. Poorly soluble drugs and drugs adversely affected by gastric pH or other presystemic factors can also have a low bioavailability.

Drugs not usually subject to the liver's first-pass effect are known as drugs with a low hepatic extraction ratio because the liver does not extract a large percentage of the drug before releasing it into the circulation. Usually, drugs with a low extraction ratio have high oral bioavailability. In contrast, drugs with a high extraction ratio have low oral

bioavailability. For example, lidocaine has a hepatic extraction ratio of 0.7; that is, the liver metabolizes 70% of the drug before the drug reaches the circulation and, as such, only 30% remains available systemically. This is one reason lidocaine is administered parenterally. In other words, the first-pass effect for lidocaine is of such magnitude that an alternative route of administration is required. Giving large oral doses of a drug to compensate for the high extraction ratio is often an alternative to parenteral administration. For example, because of the high extraction ratio of propranolol, a 1-mg dose administered intravenously is approximately equivalent to a 40-mg dose administered orally.

Examples of drugs with a high hepatic extraction ratio (70% or more) are imipramine (Tofranil), lidocaine (Xylocaine), and meperidine (Demerol); drugs with intermediate rankings are codeine, nortriptyline (Aventyl), and quinidine (Quinaglute); and some drugs with a low extraction ratio (30% or less) are barbiturates, diazepam (Valium), theophylline (Theo-Dur), tolbutamide (Orinase), and warfarin (Coumadin).

substances. However, the bilayer does allow most lipid-soluble (hydrophobic) compounds to pass through readily. Interspersed throughout this bilayer are protein molecules and small openings, or pores. The proteins may act as carrier molecules, bringing molecules through the barrier. The pores allow hydrophilic molecules to pass through if they are small enough. Therefore, drugs and other compounds that pass through membrane barriers can do so by passive or active means.

Passive Diffusion Drugs can pass through membrane barriers by diffusion. In passive diffusion, molecules move from one side of a barrier to another without expending energy. In passing, the molecules move down a concentration gradient—that is, they move from an area of higher concentration to an area of lower concentration. The rate of diffusion depends on the differences in concentrations, the relative strength of the barrier, the distance that the molecules must travel, and the size of the molecules. This relationship is known as Fick's law of diffusion. In essence, Fick's law states that the greater the distance to travel and the larger the molecule, the slower the diffusion.

Another major barrier to the absorption of a drug is its solubility. To facilitate drug absorption, the solubility of the administered drug must match the cellular constituents of the absorption site. Lipid-soluble drugs can penetrate fatty cells; water-soluble drugs cannot. For example, a water-soluble drug such as penicillin cannot easily pass through the barrier between the blood and brain, whereas a highly lipid-soluble drug such as diazepam (Valium) can. The relative strength of the barrier is important because the barrier must be permeable to the diffusing substance. Drugs diffuse more readily through the lipid bilayer if they are in their neutral, nonionized form. Most drugs are weak acids or weak bases, which have the potential for becoming positively or negatively charged. This potential is created through the pH of certain body fluids. In the plasma and in most other fluids, most drugs remain nonionized. However, in the gastric acid of the stomach, weak bases become ionized and are more difficult to absorb. As this weak base progresses through the alkaline environment of the small intestines, it becomes nonionized and therefore more easily absorbed. Similarly, weak acids remain nonionized in the stomach and become ionized in the small intestines. The result is reduced absorption by the intestines.

Active Transport In active transport, membrane proteins act as carrier molecules to transport substances across cell membranes. The role of active transport in moving drugs across cell membranes is limited. To be carried through by a protein, the drug must share molecular similarities with an endogenous substance the transport system routinely carries. Cells can accomplish this through the process of endocytosis. In this process, the cell forms a vesicle surrounding the molecule, and it is subsequently invaginated in the cell. Once inside the cell, the vesicle releases the molecule into the cytoplasm of the cell.

Pharmaceutical Preparation

Drugs are formulated and administered in such a way as to produce either local or systemic effects. Local effects (e.g., antiseptic, anti-inflammatory, and local anesthetic effects) are confined to one area of the body. Systemic effects occur when the drug is absorbed and delivered to body tissues by way of the circulatory system.

Depending on how a drug is formulated (e.g., tablet or liquid), the means of drug delivery can target a site of action. Some drug formulations (dosage forms) deliver the drug into the gastrointestinal (GI) tract quickly (immediate release), whereas others release the drug slowly. This strategy for extending the activity of drugs in the body dampens the high and low swings of drug concentrations, thereby yielding a more constant blood level. Many medications are available in these controlled- or sustained-release dosage forms. The aim of sustained-release dosage forms is to administer them as infrequently as possible, improving compliance and minimize hour-to-hour or day-to-day blood level fluctuations. The various release systems available are subject to physiologic and pathophysiologic changes in patient conditions.

Blood Flow

Blood flow ensures that the concentration across a gradient is continually in favor of passive diffusion—that is, as blood flows through an area, it continually removes the drug from the area, thereby maintaining a positive concentration gradient. Many hydrophobic–lipophilic drugs can readily pass through membranes and be absorbed. However, if the blood flow to that area is limited, the extent of absorption is limited. Because of the minimal vascularization in the subcutaneous layer compared with the greater vascularity of the musculature, drugs injected subcutaneously may undergo less absorption compared with drugs delivered by IM injection.

Gastrointestinal Motility

High-fat meals and solid foods affect GI transit time by delaying gastric emptying, which in turn delays initial drug delivery to intestinal absorption surfaces. The administration of agents that delay or slow intestinal motility (e.g., anticholinergic agents) prolongs the contact time. This increased intestinal contact time secondary to prolonged intestinal transit time may increase total drug absorption. Conversely, laxatives or diarrhea can shorten an agent's contact time with the small intestine, which may decrease drug absorption.

Enteral Absorption

Enteral absorption, with the oral route of administration being the most common and probably the most preferred, occurs anywhere throughout the GI tract by passive or active transport of the drug through the cells of the GI tract.

Following Fick's law, low molecular weight, nonionized drugs diffuse passively down a concentration gradient from the higher concentration (in the GI tract) to the lower concentration (in the blood). Active transport across the GI tract occurs more frequently with larger, usually ionized, molecules. These active mechanisms include binding of the drug to carrier molecules in the cell membrane. The molecules carry the drug across the lipid bilayer of the cells. However, most drugs are absorbed passively.

Oral Administration

The oral route of administration refers to any medication that is taken by mouth (per os or PO). The ability to swallow is implicit in oral administration; however, many practitioners consider local action, in which absorption does not occur, also to be "oral" (e.g., troches for fungal infections of the mouth). Common dosage forms administered by mouth include tablets, capsules, caplets, solutions, suspensions, troches, lozenges, and powders.

Absorption after oral administration usually occurs in the lower GI tract (small or large intestine), is slow, and depends on the patient's gastric-emptying time, the presence or absence of food, and the gastric or intestinal pH. Variations in one or more of these factors can affect the stability of the drug, the contact time with the intestinal walls, or the blood flow to the GI tract. Most of the absorption occurs in the small intestine, where the large surface area enhances and controls drug entry into the body.

Drugs administered orally must be relatively lipid soluble to cross the GI mucosa into the bloodstream. The diffusion rate, a function of the lipid solubility of a drug across the GI mucosa, is a major factor in determining the rate of absorption of a drug. The acid pH of the stomach and the nearly neutral pH of the intestines can degrade some medications before they are absorbed. In addition, bacteria in various parts of the intestines secrete enzymes that also can break down drugs before absorption.

Although the GI tract is generally resistant to a variety of noxious agents, considerable irritation and discomfort can arise from certain medications in some people. Nausea, vomiting, diarrhea, and less often mucosal damage are common side effects of medications, and the practitioner should monitor all patients for these effects.

Sublingual Administration

Sublingual (SL, *under the tongue*) drug administration relies on absorption through the oral mucosa into the veins that drain those vascular beds. These veins carry the drug to the superior vena cava and eventually the heart. Drugs administered this way are not subject to the first-pass effect (see **Box 2.2**). This method of administration is limited by the amount of drug that can be placed sublingually and the drug's ability to pass through the oral mucosa into the venous system. Buccal administration, in which the drug is absorbed through the mucous membranes of the mouth, is similar to SL administration.

Rectal Administration

Drugs administered rectally (PR, per rectum) include suppositories and enemas. Primarily used in the treatment of local conditions (e.g., hemorrhoids) and inflammatory bowel disease, this method is less effective than other enteral routes because of the erratic absorption of most agents. Bowel irritation, early evacuation, and minimal surface area contribute to erratic absorption and poor tolerability of this route. Advantages, however, include the ability to administer a medication to an unconscious or nauseated patient.

Parenteral Absorption

All routes of administration not involving the GI tract are considered parenteral. Parenteral routes include inhalation, all forms of injection, and topical and transdermal administration.

Inhalation

Drugs that are gaseous or sprayable in small particles may be delivered by inhalation. The lungs provide a large surface area for absorption and quick entry into the bloodstream. Inhaled medications bypass the first-pass effect and therefore may have a high bioavailability. Examples of inhalants are anesthetic gases and beta-adrenergic agonists (e.g., albuterol) used in treating asthma. Conversely, agents such as inhaled corticosteroids are intended for local action in the lung tissue. Regardless of the intent of inhaled medications, the disadvantages include irritation to the alveolar space and the need for good coordination during self-administration, such as with metered-dose inhalers.

Intravenous Administration

The intravenous (IV) route provides rapid access to the circulatory system with a known quantity of drug. Bypassing the first-pass effect and any GI metabolism or degradation, drug absorption by this route is considered the gold standard with regard to bioavailability. IV bolus injections allow for large amounts of medication to be administered quickly for a high peak drug level and a rapid effect. However, adverse effects from these high levels of medications also occur with this form of administration. Repeated bolus doses of medications, at designated intervals, can produce large fluctuations in peak and trough (lowest concentration before next dose) levels. Although over time these peaks and troughs produce average desired concentrations, significant peak and trough fluctuations may not be desirable in some patients. Continuous administration by an infusion can minimize or eliminate these fluctuations and produce a consistent, steady-state concentration.

Like IV administration, intra-arterial administration produces a rapid effect. However, because the drug is directly instilled in an organ, this route is considered more dangerous than the IV route. Therefore, intra-arterial administration is usually reserved for a time when injection into a specific tissue is indicated (e.g., anticancer treatment for a specific tumor).

Subcutaneous Administration

Subcutaneous (SC or SQ) administration produces a slower, more prolonged release of medication into the bloodstream. Injected directly beneath the skin, a drug must diffuse through layers of fat and muscle to encounter sufficient blood vessels for entry into the systemic circulation. This route is limited by the quantity of the liquid suitable for administration (usually 2 to 3 mL). Caution must also be taken because dermal irritation, or even necrosis, may occur. More recent technological advances allow the practitioner to implant drug-releasing mechanisms under the skin, providing a reservoir of drug for long-term absorption. Levonorgestrel (Norplant), a hormonal contraceptive, is administered in this manner.

Intramuscular Administration

Injecting medications into the highly vascularized skeletal muscle is a way of administering drugs quickly and avoiding the relatively large changes in plasma levels seen with IV administration. Local pain and muscle soreness are drawbacks to this method, as is the wide variability in the rate of absorption resulting from injections given in different muscles and in different patients. Blood flow to the area is the major factor in determining the rate of absorption. This is considered a safe way to administer irritating drugs, although not all IM injections are truly IM: in grossly obese patients, presumed IM injections may actually be intralipomatous, which decreases the rate of absorption because of the lower vascularity of fatty tissue.

Topical Administration

Topical drug administration involves applying drugs, in various vehicles (e.g., liquids, powders), to the site of action, primarily the skin. Topical ointments, creams, drops, and gels typically produce a local effect. Ointments are occlusive, preventing water absorption or evaporation, and therefore have a hydrating effect and typically produce greater local effects than their cream counterparts. Creams are water soluble and therefore can be washed from the skin more readily than ointments. In hairy areas, creams are preferred over ointments because creams are hydrophilic and hence easier to apply and wash off. Gels, the most water-soluble topical dosage form, allow medication to be spread more easily over a larger area.

Transdermal Administration

Transdermal (*across the skin*) administration refers to the systemic delivery of medication through the skin. Several transdermal drug delivery systems are available for a wide range of medications, including estrogens (Estraderm) and fentanyl (Duragesic). In general, this method continuously delivers medication to achieve a constant blood level. The consistent delivery of drug throughout the dosing interval minimizes the peak-to-trough fluctuations seen with other forms of drug administration, thereby minimizing the toxicity associated with high blood levels while maintaining therapeutic concentrations.

Distribution

A discussion of the routes of administration offers the opportunity to consider the factors affecting drug absorption and bioavailability; once the medication is in the body, however, it must distribute to the site of action to be effective.

Distribution of an absorbed drug in the body depends on several factors: blood flow to an area, lipid or water solubility, and protein binding. For an absorbed drug to distribute from the blood to a specific site of action, there must be adequate blood flow to that area. In patients with compromised blood flow (e.g., from shock), relying on the blood to deliver a drug to a site of action, such as the kidney, may be risky.

In addition, drug distribution may be affected by obesity, both immediately after absorption and after achieving an equilibrium or steady state in the body. Lipid-soluble drugs readily distribute into the fatty tissues, where they may be stored and even concentrated. Water-soluble drugs, however, tend to remain in the highly vascularized spaces of the skeletal muscle. Ideal body weight is usually considered the standard for determining drug dosage, which is often adjusted for obese or cachectic patients.

Protein Binding

After absorption into the blood (and lymph), a drug may circulate throughout the body unbound (*free drug*) or bound to carrier proteins such as albumin. The extent of drug binding to carrier proteins depends on the affinity of the drug for the carrier protein and the concentrations of both the drug and the protein. Acidic drugs commonly bind to albumin and basic drugs commonly bind to alpha$_1$-acid glycoprotein or lipoproteins.

Plasma protein binding is typically a reversible phenomenon, with binding and unbinding occurring within milliseconds. Therefore, the bound and unbound forms of the drug can be assumed to be at equilibrium at all times. As such, the degree of binding to plasma proteins can be expressed as a percentage of bound drug to total concentration (bound plus unbound). It is only the unbound or free drug that can exert a pharmacologic effect. If the drug becomes bound, it becomes inactive because it cannot leave the bloodstream or bind to an enzyme or receptor and exert its therapeutic action (**Figure 2.3**).

Once the free drug is eliminated from the body through metabolism or excretion, the bound drug can be released from the protein to become active. In essence, the bound drug may serve as a storage site or reservoir of the drug. The percentage of the free drug usually is constant for a single drug but varies among drugs. Patient-specific factors, such as nutritional status, renal function, and levels of circulating protein or albumin, can change the percentage of the free drug.

Volume of Distribution

The amount of drug in the human body can never be directly measured. Observations are made of the concentration of drug in plasma or sometimes in blood. Over time, the concentration of drug in the plasma depends on the rate and extent of drug distribution to the tissues and on how rapidly the drug is eliminated. For most drugs, distribution occurs more rapidly than elimination. The resultant plasma concentration after

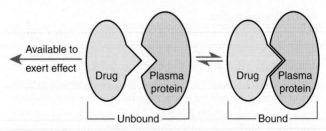

FIGURE 2.3 Relationship between bound and unbound drugs and plasma proteins.

distribution depends on the dose and the extent of distribution into the tissues. This extent of distribution can be determined by relating the concentration obtained with a known amount of administered drug.

For example, if 100 mg of an IV drug is administered to a person and remains only in the plasma, and if that person's total plasma volume measures 5 L, the resulting measured concentration of drug would be 20 mg/L [concentration = dose/volume: 100 mg/5 L]. However, in reality, few drugs distribute solely in the plasma, and many bind to plasma proteins. Drugs commonly bind not only to plasma proteins but also to tissue-binding sites on fat and muscle. In addition, drugs translocate into other "compartments" or spaces throughout the body. The volume into which a drug distributes in the body at equilibrium is called the (apparent) volume of distribution (V_d). This volume does not refer to a real volume; rather, it is a mathematically calculated volume (**Box 2.3**). The V_d is a direct measure of the extent of distribution of a drug in the body and represents the apparent volume that a drug must distribute to contain the amount of drug homogenously.

Drugs that are highly water soluble or highly bound to plasma proteins remain in the blood compartment and do not distribute or bind to fatty tissue. These drugs have a low V_d, usually less than the volume of total body water (approximately 50 L, or 0.7 L/kg). Drugs with a low V_d usually circulate at high levels in the blood. In contrast, drugs that are not highly protein bound and are highly lipophilic have a high V_d (greater than 150 L, which is greater than the volume of total body water). These drugs distribute widely throughout the body and may even cross the blood–brain barrier.

Elimination

All drugs must eventually be eliminated from the body to terminate their effect. Drugs can be eliminated through metabolism (or biotransformation) of the drug from an active form to an inactive form. Drugs can also be eliminated by excretion from the body. Therefore, elimination is a combination of the metabolism and excretion of drugs from the body. Important concepts in understanding drug elimination are half-life, steady state, and clearance. Knowledge of these phenomena in any given patient helps practitioners understand how long a drug will last in the body and how much should be given to maintain therapeutic levels and therefore helps in determining the appropriate dose and dosing intervals.

Metabolism

Metabolism is a function of the body designed to change substances into water soluble, more readily excreted forms. The liver primarily performs the body's metabolic functions because of its high concentration of metabolic enzymes. This is why the first-pass effect is significant to the bioavailability of a drug administered orally.

Other organs, such as the kidneys and intestines, as well as circulating enzyme systems, also contribute to the metabolism of drugs. Metabolic processes are used to detoxify drugs and other foreign substances as well as endogenous substances. Drugs may be metabolized from active components into inactive or less active ones. Some drugs, however, may be biologically transformed from an inactive parent drug into an active metabolite. This type of drug is called a prodrug because it is a precursor to the active drug (**Table 2.1**). Not all drugs are metabolized to the same extent or by the same means. In fact, some drugs, such as the aminoglycosides (e.g., gentamicin [Garamycin]), are not metabolized at all.

Enzyme actions are the primary means for metabolizing drugs, and these actions are broadly classified as phase 1 and phase 2 enzymatic processes. Phase 1 enzymatic processes involve oxidation or reduction, by which a drug is changed to form a more polar or water-soluble compound. Phase 2 processes involve adding a conjugate (e.g., a glucuronide) to the parent drug or the phase 1–metabolized drug to further increase water solubility and enhance excretion.

The oxidative process of phase 1 metabolism is catalyzed by the flavin-containing monooxygenases (FMO), the epoxide hydrolases (EH), and the cytochrome P-450 system (CYP). The FMOs and CYP are composed of superfamilies of more than 100 enzymes each. Three families (about 15 total enzymes) of the CYP enzymes are important contributors to drug metabolism. The common feature of these enzymes is their lipid solubility. Most lipophilic drugs are substrates for

---

BOX 2.3 Calculating the Apparent Volume of Distribution (V_d)

$$V_d = \frac{\text{Amount in body}}{\text{Plasma drug concentration}}$$

V_d is usually measured in liters (L); *amount in body* is usually measured in milligrams (mg); and *plasma drug concentration* is usually measured in milligrams per liter (mg/L).

The apparent volume of distribution is a theoretical parameter calculated by determining the amount of drug in the body (usually the dose administered) divided by the concentration of drug in the plasma taken at an appropriate time interval after administration.

TABLE 2.1 Selected Prodrugs and Metabolites

Parent Drug (Prodrug)	Active Metabolite
allopurinol	oxypurinol
codeine	morphine
enalapril	enalaprilat
prednisone	prednisolone
valacyclovir	acyclovir

TABLE 2.2
Key Cytochrome P-450 Families and Isoforms in Drug Metabolism

Family	Isoform	Example of Drugs Metabolized
CYP1	CYP1A2	theophylline
CYP2	CYP2C	omeprazole
	CYP2D6	dextromethorphan
	CYP2E1	acetaminophen
CYP3	CYP3A4	atorvastatin

one or more of the CYP enzymes (**Table 2.2**). FMOs are not considered major contributors to drug metabolism at this time.

Some drugs can induce or stimulate the production of one or more isoforms of the enzymes by a process called enzyme induction, which increases the amount of enzyme available to metabolize drugs. The result of enzyme induction is an increased metabolism of other drugs, thereby decreasing the amount of drug circulating throughout the body.

Conversely, some drugs inhibit the production of CYP enzymes and thereby decrease the metabolism of drugs and increase circulating levels. This is known as enzyme inhibition. Both enzyme induction and inhibition are the basis of metabolically mediated drug–drug interactions. See Chapter 3 for further discussion of induction and inhibition and their role in drug–drug interactions.

Although the liver is regarded as the primary site of drug metabolism, other tissues also possess the enzymes necessary for metabolism. The kidneys, for example, have several enzymes needed for drug metabolism and can serve as the site of drug inactivation. The GI tract is also known to possess several of the CYP isoforms, contributing to the extrahepatic metabolism of drugs.

The nature, function, and amount of any drug-metabolizing enzyme can be different, resulting in differing drug disposition among patients. Disease-induced changes can affect drug metabolism as well. For example, alterations in liver function induced by long-standing cirrhotic changes can reduce the production of necessary enzymes, resulting in increased concentrations of drugs typically metabolized in the liver. Also, decreased blood flow to the liver, as occurring in congestive heart failure, can decrease the delivery of drug to metabolic sites in the liver. Cigarette smoking on the other hand, can increase the levels of enzymes responsible for drug metabolism, resulting in increased metabolic rates and the need for higher doses of drugs (e.g., theophylline) in smokers than in nonsmokers.

Drug Excretion

Metabolism eliminates a drug from the body by changing the drug molecule into something else, but drugs also can be eliminated from the body by excretion. Excretory organs include the kidneys, lower GI tract, lungs, and skin. Other structures, such as the sweat, salivary, and mammary glands, are active in excretion as well. Drugs may also be removed forcibly by dialysis.

The primary route of excretion is the kidney. After the drug is metabolized, the resultant metabolite may be filtered by the glomerulus. As the drug continues through the proximal tubule, loop of Henle, and distal tubule, several things may occur: the drug may exert action (as in the case of diuretics), be reabsorbed into the bloodstream, or remain in the nephron, eventually reaching the collecting ducts, from which it ultimately leaves the body in the patient's urine. This filtration works well for hydrophilic, ionized compounds and is a common route of elimination. Conversely, active secretion of drugs occurs in the proximal tubule. Two different systems exist, one for organic acids (e.g., uric acid) and one for organic bases (e.g., histamine). Once ionized by the acidic pH of the urine, organic bases are not reabsorbed back into the bloodstream. If the pH rises, then more of the organic base becomes nonionized and thus more readily reabsorbed. Similarly, changes in urine pH can alter the reabsorption of organic acids, increasing or decreasing the circulating levels as the pH changes. Drugs such as penicillin are excreted by the organic acid system.

Drugs are excreted by the liver into the gallbladder, resulting in biliary elimination. Biliary elimination can sometimes result in drug reabsorption. For example, if a drug is excreted in the bile, it goes into the GI tract, where it may be reabsorbed and returned to the general circulation. This is called *enterohepatic recirculation* (**Figure 2.4**). The result of significant enterohepatic recirculation is a measurable increase in the plasma concentration of a drug and a delay in its elimination from the body.

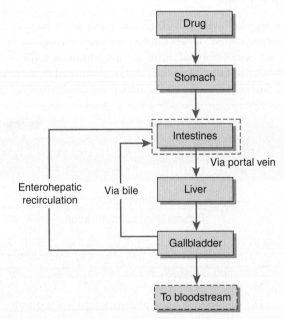

FIGURE 2.4 Enterohepatic recirculation. When a drug is absorbed from the intestine, travels to the liver and gallbladder, and into the bile unchanged, it has the potential for being reintroduced into the intestine and therefore reabsorbed. This is known as enterohepatic recirculation.

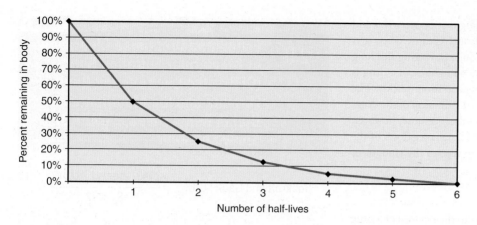

FIGURE 2.5 Drug elimination based on half-life ($t_{\frac{1}{2}}$).

Half-Life

The time required for a drug to be eliminated from the body varies according to the drug and the individual. However, useful generalizations can be made that help practitioners estimate how long a drug will remain in the body. The first generalization has to do with the elimination half-life ($t_{\frac{1}{2}}$), which is the time required for half of the total drug amount to be eliminated from the body. Assuming 100% of a drug exists in the body at time X, then one half-life later, 50% of the original amount would remain in the body. An additional half-life later, 25% would remain and so on. For example, theophylline has a $t_{\frac{1}{2}}$ of approximately 8 hours. If the theophylline concentration in a patient's body is 15 mg/L, then it would take 8 hours to decline to 7.5 mg/L, another 8 hours (16 hours total) to fall to 3.75 mg/L, and another 8 hours (24 hours total) to fall to 1.875 mg/L. The actual rate of elimination of a drug remains constant, but as can be seen in **Figure 2.5**, the actual amount of drug eliminated is proportional to the concentration of the drug—that is, the more drug there is, the faster it is eliminated. This phenomenon, known as first-order kinetics, applies to most drugs. Rate processes can also be independent of concentration, and fixed amounts of drugs, rather than a fractional proportion, are eliminated at a constant rate. This phenomenon is called zero-order kinetics. Alcohol undergoes zero-order elimination.

After five half-lives, according to first-order kinetics, approximately 97% (96.875%) of the drug is eliminated from the body. Even after three half-lives, nearly 90% (87.5%) of the drug is eliminated. In most cases, after three to five half-lives,

the amount of drug remaining is too low to exert any pharmacologic effect, and the drug is considered essentially eliminated. Understanding this concept is useful for practitioners in many situations. For example, if a drug reaches a toxic level, the practitioner knows that it will take three to five half-lives for the drug to be essentially eliminated from the body. The practitioner also can estimate when the drug level will approach a minimally effective concentration and can then calculate when to administer another dose of medication to reach a therapeutic drug level.

Steady State

In reality, patients take medications on a consistent basis, usually somewhere between one and four times daily. By doing so, they are absorbing and eliminating the drug throughout the day. Because the rate of elimination is proportional to the concentration, at some point, equilibrium is reached. **Figure 2.6** demonstrates how doses of a drug with a half-life of 8 hours produce this equilibrium. Note that after approximately three to five half-lives, the curve levels off. This demonstrates equilibrium between the amount of drug entering the body and the amount leaving the body. This point, which is called *steady state*, reflects a constant mean concentration of drug in the body. At steady state, even though the blood levels of a drug fluctuate above and below this mean concentration and the drug level tends to have peaks and troughs during dosing intervals, the fluctuations remain within a constant range.

For some drugs, the time required to achieve steady state may be very long. For example, digoxin (Lanoxin) has a

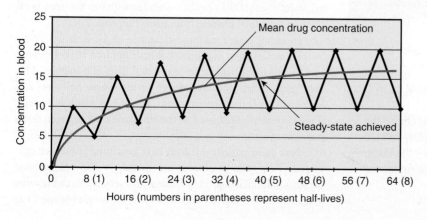

FIGURE 2.6 Steady state achieved with regular dosing (half-life = 8 hours).

half-life of 39 hours (1.6 days), meaning that between 4.8 and 8 days are needed to achieve steady state. Clearly, when it is imperative to gain a therapeutic level quickly, waiting this long is unacceptable. Therefore, an initial loading dose of a drug is needed to reach the desired blood concentration quickly. The loading dose is based on the volume of distribution of the drug, independent of the half-life. The maintenance dose, however, is based on the half-life of the drug. Maintenance doses of the drug are given at scheduled intervals to replace the amount of drug eliminated.

Clearance

The concept of clearance, which refers to the removal of a drug from the plasma or organ, is the final element in the process of elimination. Drugs with high clearances are removed rapidly; those with low clearances are removed slowly. Drugs can be cleared by biliary, hepatic, and renal means. The following discussion highlights renal clearance.

Clearance is related to the volume of distribution and the half-life (**Box 2.4**). Clearance of a drug from the body depends directly on the apparent volume of distribution and is inversely related to the elimination half-life: the greater the volume of distribution and the shorter the half-life, the faster the clearance.

Because most drugs are "cleared" through the kidney, estimating the renal elimination rate or clearance can help the practitioner to understand how fast a drug is being eliminated in an individual patient. The kidney's ability to clear drugs is estimated through a surrogate substrate: creatinine. Creatinine, which is produced through the continual breakdown of muscle tissue and eliminated largely by glomerular filtration, is not significantly secreted or reabsorbed. Therefore, in estimating the creatinine clearance, the practitioner can also estimate the glomerular filtration rate (GFR). The level of creatinine is usually measured through a blood test (serum creatinine), with normal values ranging from 0.8 to 1.2 mg/dL. By combining this information with a patient's

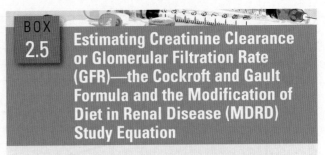

BOX 2.5 Estimating Creatinine Clearance or Glomerular Filtration Rate (GFR)—the Cockroft and Gault Formula and the Modification of Diet in Renal Disease (MDRD) Study Equation

$$\text{Cockroft and Gault} : \text{CrCl}_{est} = \frac{\left[140 - \text{age(y)}\right] \times IBW}{S_{cr} \times 72}$$

$$\text{MDRD} : \text{GFR} = 175 \times \left(\text{Standarized } S_{cr}\right)^{-1.154} \times \left(\text{age}\right)^{-0.203} \times \left(0.742 \text{ if female}\right) \times \left(1.212 \text{ if African American}\right)$$

Note: GFR is expressed in mL/min per 1.73 m², S_{cr} is serum creatinine expressed in mg/dL, and age is expressed in years.

Multiply CrCl_{est} by 0.85 for women.
CrCl_{est} = estimated creatinine clearance
S_{cr} = serum creatinine (mg/dL)
IBW = ideal body weight in kilograms (kg; 2.2 lb = 1 kg)

ideal body weight and age, the practitioner can use the formula of Cockroft and Gault to evaluate creatinine clearance and evaluate the kidney's ability to function and eliminate drugs (**Box 2.5**). For example, for a 40-year-old man of average height weighing 70 kg (154 lb) and having a serum creatinine level of 1 mg/dL, the estimated creatinine clearance is 97 mL/min. (This is only an estimate of this patient's creatinine clearance. The best method of determining the actual value is by a 24-hour urine specimen collection and measurement of excreted creatinine.)

Alternatively, the Modification of Diet in Renal Disease (MDRD) equation can also be employed to estimate the GFR of a patient. This equation, also shown in **Box 2.5**, should be used in adults only. This equation estimates the GFR adjusting for body surface area. There are several studies that show that the MDRD equation is useful in patients with chronic kidney disease, but in patients with a true GFR greater than 90 mL/min, the MDRD equation underestimates the true GFR (National Kidney Disease Education Program, 2012).

In either case, creatinine clearance or GFR values below 50 mL/min suggest significant impairment of renal function and thus possible impairment of renal drug elimination. This may result in administered drugs having longer half-lives and higher steady-state concentrations, which may result in toxicity if the dose is not decreased or the length of time between doses is not increased.

Not every patient needs to have creatinine clearance estimated. Two rules of thumb are useful for the practitioner: patients older than age 65 or those with a serum creatinine value greater than 1.5 mg/dL may be at risk for accumulating drug

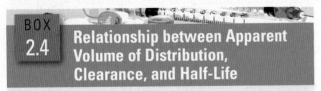

BOX 2.4 Relationship between Apparent Volume of Distribution, Clearance, and Half-Life

$$\text{Clearance} = \frac{0.693 \times V_d}{t_{1/2}}$$

Clearance is usually expressed as L/hour; V_d is in L; $t_{1/2}$ is usually in hours.

Clearance of a drug is directly dependent on the apparent volume of distribution and inversely related to the elimination half-life. The larger the V_d, the faster the clearance. Also, the smaller the $t_{1/2}$, the faster the clearance.

(and therefore toxicity) because of decreased renal function. In patients with either of these characteristics, a baseline and routine evaluation of renal function (e.g., serum creatinine determination) should be performed.

PHARMACODYNAMICS

Pharmacodynamics refers to the set of processes by which drugs produce specific biochemical or physiologic changes in the body. Most often, pharmacodynamic effects occur because a drug interacts with a receptor. Receptors may be cell membrane proteins, extracellular enzymes, cytoplasmic enzymes, or intracellular proteins. A receptor is the component of the cell (or an enzyme) to which an endogenous substance binds, or attaches, initiating a chain of biochemical events. This chain of biochemical events culminates in a change in the physiologic function of the cell or activity of the enzyme. Like endogenous substances, drugs can initiate the biochemical chain of events. For example, a drug stimulating a receptor on the surface of an artery may ultimately cause vasoconstriction or vasodilation; or the drug's binding to a receptor may produce a change in cell wall permeability, thus allowing other substances to enter or leave a cell, such as occurs in nerve cells; or the drug attached to a receptor may initiate an increase or decrease in

the production of an enzyme, thereby changing the amount of enzymatic activity for a given process.

Any chemical, endogenous or exogenous, that interacts with a receptor is called a *ligand*. Regardless of the ligand, or the actual interaction type, a substance can only alter or modify a cell or process, not impart a new function.

Drug Receptors

The capacity of a drug to bind to a receptor depends on the size and shape of the drug and the receptor. The drug acts as a "key" that fits into only a certain receptor or receptor type (**Figure 2.7**). Once the drug fits into the receptor, it may act to "unlock" the activity of the receptor, thus initiating the biochemical chain of events, much like an ignition key initiates the chain of events that starts a car.

Drug receptors are commonly classified by the effect they produce. Some drugs interact with several receptors, causing multiple effects, whereas others interact with only a specific receptor, eliciting a single response. Epinephrine, for example, interacts with the alpha and beta receptors of the sympathetic nervous system. As a result, epinephrine produces vasoconstriction (alpha receptor action) and an increase in heart rate (beta receptor action). Various molecules or enzymes can serve as drug receptors, such as ion channels (calcium channels),

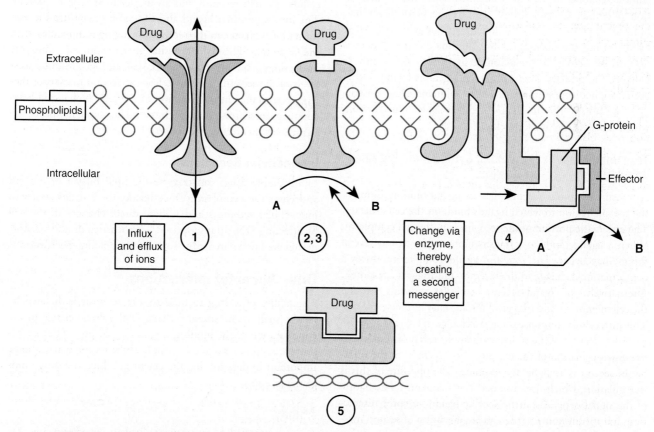

FIGURE 2.7 Drug and drug–receptor interaction and signal transduction. The five primary receptors and their mechanisms of signal transduction include (1) gated ion channels; (2 and 3) transmembranous receptors—cytoplasmic enzyme and tyrosine kinase activated; (4) G protein–coupled receptors; and (5) intracellular receptors.

enzymes (angiotensin-converting enzyme [ACE]), and even receptors that generate intracellular second messengers (substances that interact with other intracellular components).

There are four known types of receptors: gated ion channels, transmembranous receptors, G protein–coupled receptors, and intracellular receptors (see **Figure 2.7**). Understanding these receptors and the signals they generate is central to understanding the actions of many drugs.

Gated Ion Channels

The function of gated ion channel receptors is to open or close channels to allow certain ions to pass through the cell membrane. Binding of ligands to these receptors produces a conformational change that widens or narrows the channel, thereby regulating the access of soluble ions (**Figure 2.7**). The nicotinic acetylcholine receptor is a good example of a gated ion channel receptor. Its function is to translate the signal from acetylcholine into an electrical signal at the neuromuscular endplate. As such, when acetylcholine binds to this receptor, the channel opens, allowing sodium or potassium to enter the cell and cause cellular depolarization.

Other types of gated ion channel receptors are associated with the neurotransmitters. Gamma-aminobutyric acid ($GABA_A$), the primary inhibitory neurotransmitter, opens a chloride channel in the cell, which minimizes the depolarization potential. Certain drugs, such as the benzodiazepines, bind to an allosteric site and enhance the activity of $GABA_A$ by increasing the opening of the chloride channel. There is no intrinsic activity at the allosteric site, and it serves only to enhance the primary action of the endogenous ligand. Other excitatory neurotransmitters, such as L-glutamate and L-aspartate, operate by this mechanism, called signal transduction, which transfers the signal quickly.

Transmembranous Receptors: Cytoplasmic Enzyme or Tyrosine Kinase Activated

A transmembranous receptor has its ligand-binding domain, the specific region to which ligands bind, on the cell's surface. The enzymatic portion of the receptor is in the cell cytoplasm. When a ligand binds to a transmembranous receptor, several things may occur. The receptor–ligand complex produces a conformational change in the receptor and triggers a response. Alternatively, the ligand–receptor complex can pass through the cell membrane and trigger an intracellular response directly. This intracellular response often is a change in enzymatic activity. A key feature of the transmembranous receptor response is the downregulation of the receptors or a decrease in the number of receptors available for response. The opposite of this is upregulation, which does not occur as frequently. The nature of the signal depends on the specific ligand–receptor interaction, but it commonly results in the generation of second messengers. A second messenger is an intracellular chemical that interacts with other intracellular components. Ions such as calcium and potassium, along with cyclic adenosine monophosphate, are common second messengers. Hormones and other endogenous substances, such as growth factors and insulin, often operate with this signaling mechanism.

The receptor tyrosine kinase signaling pathway can bind with a polypeptide hormone or growth factor at the receptor's extracellular domain. This results in enzymatically active tyrosine kinase domains that phosphorylate each other, allowing a single receptor to activate multiple biochemical processes. For example, insulin works by stimulating the uptake of glucose as well as amino acids, resulting in changes in glycogen content within the cell. Alternatively, inhibition of tyrosine kinase processes through blockage of the external receptor can result in a decrease in stimulation of growth factors within the cell. This is particularly important in cancer treatments, when inhibiting the growth of the cell is key to treatment success.

A drawback of this system is the potential for downregulation of the receptors. Activation of these receptors leads to an endocytosis of the receptor and subsequent receptor degradation. When this activity exceeds the production of new receptors, there is a reduction in the number of receptors available for stimulation, thus a decrease in the cell's activity.

G Protein–Coupled Receptors

G protein–coupled receptors are another family of receptors that generate intracellular second messengers. These receptors also exist as transmembranous receptors composed of an extracellular protein receptor and an intracellular type G protein. The interaction of a ligand and the receptor produces a conformational change in the receptor, bringing it in contact with the G protein. This contact results in activation of an enzyme or opening of an ion channel in the cell and, in turn, increased levels of the second messenger. It is the second messenger that triggers a change in the function of the cell. Alpha- and beta-adrenergic receptors, along with several hormone receptors, use G proteins to affect cell function.

Intracellular Receptors

Lipid-soluble drugs can traverse the lipid bilayer of the cell and enter the cytoplasm. Once inside, these drugs attach to intracellular receptors and initiate direct changes in the cell by affecting DNA transcription. Glucocorticoids and sex hormones are known to act by way of this signaling mechanism.

Drug–Receptor Interactions

The ability of a drug to bind to any receptor is dictated by factors such as the size and shape of the drug relative to the configuration of the binding site on the receptor. The electrostatic attraction between the drug and the receptor may also be important in determining the extent to which the drug binds to the receptor.

Affinity

A drug attracted to a receptor displays an *affinity* for that receptor. This affinity, the degree to which a drug is attracted to a receptor, is related to the concentration of drug required to occupy a receptor site. Drugs displaying a high affinity for a given receptor require only a small concentration in the circulation to elicit a response, whereas those with a low affinity require higher circulating concentrations. There exists equilibrium between the blood concentration of a drug, the concentration of drug at the site of action (i.e., near the receptor), and the amount of drug bound to a receptor. The magnitude of a drug's effect can be explained by the receptor occupancy theory—that is, a response from a cell (or group of cells) depends on the fraction of receptors occupied by a drug or endogenous substance. Therefore, one can infer a relationship between the minimally and maximally effective concentrations needed at the site of action and the minimum and maximum blood concentrations.

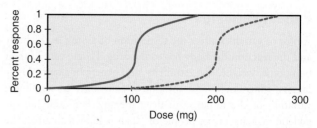

FIGURE 2.8 Two drugs with differing receptor affinities produce similar effects at different dosage ranges. The drug with the greater affinity (*solid line*) requires less drug to produce the same effect as a drug with less affinity (*dotted line*). This demonstrates the relationship between receptor affinity and drug potency.

Chirality

The shape of a drug can influence its interaction with a receptor. Most drugs display chirality—that is, they exist in two forms with mirror-image spatial arrangements called enantiomers, or isomers. Each enantiomer is distinguished from the other through its ability to rotate polarized light in pure solution to the right or left. This results in a dextrorotary, or D-enantiomer, and a levorotary, or L-companion.

A pair of enantiomers is like a left and a right hand. As such, enantiomeric pairs may not fit into a receptor equally well, just as a right hand does not fit well into a left-hand glove. This is called stereoselectivity; one enantiomer may fit better into a receptor than the other and, hence, be more active. For example, the drug dextromethorphan (Robitussin DM) is the D-isomer of a compound. This D-isomer is a common cough suppressant found in most over-the-counter medications. Its L-isomer counterpart, levorphanol (Levo-Dromoran), is an extremely potent narcotic analgesic. Although the L-isomer also possesses cough suppressant activity, the D-isomer is essentially devoid of analgesic activity at commonly used doses. This similarity coincident with dissimilarity illustrates the importance of isomers in pharmacodynamics.

Agonists and Antagonists

Not all drugs with an affinity for a receptor elicit a response. Drugs that display a degree of affinity for a receptor and stimulate a response are considered agonists. Others that display an affinity and do not elicit a response are called antagonists. Antagonists do not have intrinsic activity; they can only block the activity of the endogenous agonist. An antagonist may be viewed as a key that fits into the lock but, because of its different configuration, cannot be turned. Because an antagonist can occupy, or fit into, a receptor, it competes with agonists for that receptor, thereby blocking the effect of the agonist. Antagonists with a high affinity for a receptor may be able to "bump" an agonist off the receptor and reverse the agonist activity. Antagonists usually are used to block the activity of an endogenous substance, but they also can be used to block the activity of exogenously administered drugs. For example, when naloxone (Narcan) is given to a patient taking opioid drugs, the analgesic (and adverse) effects of the opioid are reversed within 1 to 2 minutes. In most cases, naloxone has a higher affinity for the opioid receptor than the opioid itself. This rough explanation of drug–receptor interactions serves only as a basis for understanding the complexity of this interplay.

Dose–Response Relationships

For many drugs, the relationship between the dose and the response is obvious: lower doses produce smaller responses, whereas higher doses increase the response. This correlation is based on the amount of drug occupying specific receptors. As the amount of drug exceeds the number of available receptors, the response reaches a plateau, so that further increases in dose do not increase response. However, dose–response relationships such as these clearly depend on the affinity of a drug for a receptor: a drug with a high affinity for a receptor needs a significantly lower concentration to achieve the same effect compared with a drug with a lower affinity.

This difference in affinity accounts for the varying "potency" of drugs. For example, drugs such as hydromorphone (Dilaudid) and morphine produce the same effect: analgesia. However, hydromorphone is more potent than morphine and therefore requires a smaller concentration to elicit a similar level of analgesia. **Figure 2.8** demonstrates a typical dose–response relationship.

FACTORS AFFECTING PHARMACOKINETICS AND PHARMACODYNAMICS

The goal of pharmacotherapeutics is to achieve a desired beneficial effect with minimal adverse effects. Once a medication has been selected for a patient, the practitioner must determine the dose that most closely achieves this goal. A rational approach to this objective combines the principles of pharmacokinetics with pharmacodynamics to clarify the dose–response relationship. Knowing the relationship between drug concentration and response allows the practitioner to take into account the various pathologic and physiologic features of a particular patient that make his or her response different from the average person's response to a drug.

Patient Variables

A host of variables affect the disposition of a drug in the body and the reaction the body has to the drug. People vary in their body type, weight, diet, ethnicity, and genetic makeup. These factors, individually and combined, contribute to significant variation in the response to drug therapy. For example, the genetic makeup of the people of Japan is known to affect the expression of certain hepatic enzymes involved in the metabolism of drugs. This suggests that, at least pharmacokinetically, some people of Japanese heritage respond differently to certain drugs. The same logic applies to people who are overweight and underweight, people of varying ages, people with various pathophysiologic problems, and even people with different diets and nutritional habits.

Pathophysiology

Structural or functional damage to an organ or tissue responsible for drug metabolism or excretion presents an obvious problem in pharmacology. Diseases that initiate changes in tissue function or blood flow to specific organs can dramatically affect the elimination of various drugs. Certain diseases may also impair the absorption and distribution of the drug, complicating the problem of individualized response. The role of disease in affecting the patient's response is crucial because the response to the medication may be affected by the same pathologic process that the drug is being used to treat. For instance, renal excretion of antibiotics, such as aminoglycosides, is altered radically in many types of bacterial infection, but these drugs are typically administered to treat the same infections that alter their own excretion. Consequently, great care must be taken to adjust the dosage accordingly when administering medications to patients with conditions in which drug elimination may be altered.

Genetics

Genetic differences are a major factor in determining the way that people metabolize specific compounds. Genetic variations may result in abnormal or absent drug-metabolizing enzymes. The anomaly can be harmful or even fatal if the drug cannot be metabolized and therefore exerts a toxic effect from accumulation or prolonged pharmacologic activity. Some people, for example, lack the enzyme that breaks down acetylcholine. In these people, a drug such as succinylcholine (Anectine, an acetylcholine-like drug) is not degraded and therefore accumulates. The result is respiratory paralysis because the undegraded, accumulated succinylcholine has an increased half-life, causing it to remain active longer.

Age

The influence of age on pharmacokinetics and pharmacodynamics is well known. Developmental differences in the neonate, toddler, and young child, for instance, influence how drugs are handled by the GI tract, liver, and kidneys. Of equal importance is how these children respond to drugs in light of the presence or absence of receptors at different stages of development. For example, drug-metabolizing enzymes are deficient in the fetus and premature infant. The fetus can metabolize drugs early in its development, but its expression of drug-metabolizing enzymes differs from that of the adult and is usually less efficient.

Children can metabolize many drugs more rapidly than adults, and as children approach puberty, the rate of drug metabolism approaches that of adults. Similarly, older adults undergo physiologic changes that affect the absorption, distribution, and elimination of many agents. The pharmacodynamic changes imparted by age as well as accompanying diseases pose a greater challenge for the practitioner in understanding the impact a single agent has on a patient's health and well-being. Chapter 4 discusses pediatric considerations, and Chapter 6 discusses geriatric considerations in more depth.

Sex

The role of sex as a distinct patient variable is recognized by some but poorly understood by most. Most of the published clinical drug studies use male subjects as the primary study population, and clinicians then extrapolate the data to women. However, women in general have a higher percentage of body fat, which could ultimately alter the pharmacokinetic disposition of certain drugs. Similarly, the pharmacodynamic response of women may be different because of the presence or absence of hormones such as estrogen and testosterone.

Ethnicity

Ethnicity is a significant factor in both the pharmacokinetic and pharmacodynamic responses of patients. The genetic makeup of various ethnic populations governs the levels of hepatic enzymes expressed in these groups. Equally important are the habits and traditions of certain groups, such as diet or the use of home remedies.

Pharmacodynamically, ethnically based differences exist in the responses to agents. An example is the minimal response of African American patients to monotherapy with some drugs, such as ACE inhibitors. African Americans produce a low level of renin, a key component in the renin–angiotensin–aldosterone system by which the ACE inhibitors work. This low level of renin makes this system unaffected by the ACE inhibitor, thereby negating its effect.

Diet and Nutrition

Diet affects the metabolism of and response to many drugs. Animal and human studies indicate that total caloric intake and the percentage of calories obtained from different sources (carbohydrates, proteins, and fats) influence drug pharmacokinetics. Specific dietary constituents, such as cruciferous vegetables and charcoal-broiled beef, can also alter drug metabolism. Fortunately, most food–drug interactions are not serious and

CASE STUDY*

M.T., a 75-year-old, white 60-kg IBW woman with a serum creatinine of 1.8 mg/dL, has atrial fibrillation. A decision has been made to use digoxin for heart failure. The target concentration of digoxin for the treatment of atrial fibrillation is 0.5 ng/mL to less than 1 ng/mL, but her current level is high at 2 ng/mL.

1. What is her estimated creatinine clearance using the Cockcroft/Gault method? GFR using the MDRD Method?
2. Assuming a 4-day half-life, how long will it take for MT to achieve a 1 ng/mL level? A 0.5 ng/mL level?

* Answers can be found online.

do not alter the clinical effects of the drug. However, a few well-known food and drug combinations should be avoided because of their potentially serious interactions. For instance, certain tyramine-containing foods, such as fermented cheese and wine, should not be ingested with drugs that inhibit the monoamine oxidase enzyme (MAO) inhibitors. Tyramine-rich foods stimulate the body to release catecholamines (norepinephrine, epinephrine). MAO-inhibiting drugs work by suppressing the destruction of catecholamines, thereby allowing higher levels of norepinephrine and epinephrine to accumulate. Consequently, when MAO inhibitors are taken with tyramine-containing foods, excessive catecholamine levels may develop and lead to a dangerous increase in blood pressure (hypertensive crisis). Practitioners should be aware of this and should be on the alert for other such interactions as new drugs arrive on the market.

Bibliography

Starred references are cited in the text.

Goodman, L. S., Gilman, A., Hardman, J. G., et al. (Eds.). (2011). *Goodman and Gilman's the pharmacological basis of therapeutics* (12th ed.). New York, NY: McGraw-Hill.

Katzung, B. G., & Trevor, A. (Eds.). (2014). *Basic and clinical pharmacology* (13th ed.). New York, NY: McGraw-Hill.

*National Kidney Disease Education Program. (2012). Retrieved from http://nkdep.nih.gov/lab-evaluation/gfr-calculators/adults-conventional-unit.asp on February, 13, 2015

Spruill, W., Wade, W., DiPiro, J. T., et al. (2014). *Concepts in clinical pharmacokinetics* (6th ed.). Bethesda, MD: American Society of Health-System Pharmacists.

Wiedersberg, S., & Guy, R. H. (2014). Transdermal drug delivery: 30+ years of war and still fighting! *Journal of Controlled Release, 190*(28), 150–156.

Zanger, U. M., & Schwab, M. (2013). Cytochrome P450 enzymes in drug metabolism: Regulation of gene expression, enzyme activities, and impact of genetic variation. *Pharmacology and Therapeutics, 138*, 103–141.

3 Impact of Drug Interactions and Adverse Events on Therapeutics

Tep Kang ■ Andrew M. Peterson

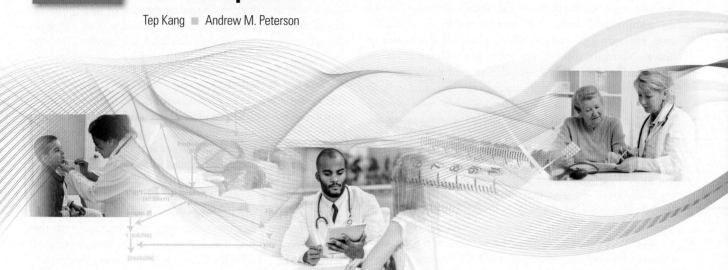

As the quantity and types of pharmacologic agents continue to expand, the likelihood of drug interactions and adverse reactions increases. Currently, more than 8,000 drugs are available to treat various conditions. Each agent is designed to alter the homeostasis of the human body to some degree, and individual responses to these agents can be unpredictable.

In a prospective study, Benard-Laribiere et al. (2014) found that 3.6% (97/2,692) of hospital admissions were due to serious adverse drug reactions (ADRs). Thirty percent of which were preventable and 16.5% of which were potentially preventable. Drug interactions caused 29.9% of ADR-related hospital admissions. According to the Institute for Safe Medicine Practices (ISMP) QuarterWatch (2014), psychiatric adverse drug events, notably suicidal behaviors, represent the major adverse effects reported in children under age 18. In a meta-analysis of observational studies, Martins et al. (2014) reported a 21.3% incidence of adverse drug events among adult inpatients. These data were captured during prospective monitoring whereby the events are detected during the hospital stay and can include interviews of the patient and/or care team and reviews of clinical and laboratory records.

ADRs present an alarming problem that warrants significant attention from health care practitioners. Not only do ADRs affect morbidity and mortality, they also dramatically increase health care costs. In the United States, the impact of ADRs may cost up to $30.1 billion per year. Most of the cost is attributed to increased hospitalization, increased length of stay, and increased cost of performing additional tests (Sultana et al., 2013).

Similarly, drug interactions are potentially preventable ADRs posing a significant problem to the health care community. It has been reported that approximately 10% to 20% of hospital admissions are drug related and about 1% of these are secondary to drug interactions. Others have reported that drug interactions are responsible for up to 3% of hospital admissions (Bjerrum et al., 2008). In addition, the prevalence of a first dispensing of drug–drug interactions in people older than age 70 has been reported to have increased from 10.5% in 1992 to 19.2% in 2005 (Becker et al., 2008). Therefore, a thorough understanding of how drug–drug interactions occur and how they relate to ADRs should help decrease the rate of occurrence and the associated morbidity/mortality. This chapter discusses the mechanisms of drug interactions and their potential consequences. For the purpose of this chapter, these interactions are broken down into four major categories: drug–drug interactions, drug–food interactions, drug–herb interactions, and drug–disease interactions. Each of the interaction categories can affect the drug's pharmacokinetic or pharmacodynamic profile. The definition, identification, and management of ADRs are discussed at the end of the chapter.

DRUG–DRUG INTERACTIONS

When a person takes two or more medications concomitantly, the potential exists for one or more drugs to change the effect of other drugs. The drug whose effect is altered by another drug is termed the *object* or *target* drug. Although minor interactions between drugs probably occur frequently, these interactions may not be significant enough to alter the effect of either drug. However, it is important for the practitioner to understand the mechanisms behind these interactions to predict more accurately when clinically significant (and potentially fatal) drug interactions may occur.

Pharmacokinetic Interactions

Absorption

Because most medications in the ambulatory care setting are administered orally, this route is the focus of discussion. For a drug to exert its effect, it must reach its site of action. Normally, this requires access to the bloodstream. As discussed in Chapter 2, drugs administered orally must be absorbed into the portal vein, through the intestinal wall, to reach the systemic circulation. The oral tablet must dissolve in the gastrointestinal (GI) tract before it can penetrate the intestinal wall.

Acidity (pH)

For some drugs, this process depends on the acidity in the GI tract. Therefore, if a drug that alters the gastric pH is administered concomitantly with a drug that depends on a normal gastric pH for dissolution, the absorption of the object drug will be affected. An example of this type of interaction is the concurrent administration of a histamine-2 (H_2) receptor antagonist (e.g., ranitidine) and ketoconazole, an imidazole antifungal agent. Ketoconazole is the object drug that requires an acidic pH for absorption. When ranitidine is administered along with ketoconazole, the increase in gastric pH hinders the dissolution of ketoconazole and, therefore, decreases its absorption. Similarly, this change in pH can increase the absorption of other drugs that require a more alkaline environment for absorption.

Adsorption

Another mechanism of absorptive drug–drug interactions is adsorption. Adsorption occurs when one agent binds the other to its surface to form a complex. The most common agents associated with this type of interaction are divalent and trivalent cations (Mg^{2+}, Ca^{2+}, Al^{3+}, found in antacids and some vitamin preparations) and anionic-binding resins (colestipol, cholestyramine). This type of interaction occurs when certain medications such as tetracyclines or fluoroquinolones are given with antacids. The metal ions in the antacid chelate (form a complex with) the antibiotic, preventing absorption of both components (ion and antibiotic). Adsorbents can interact with a variety of drugs; therefore, appropriate intervals between doses of the interacting medications are warranted. In general, with agents known to interact in this manner, the object drug should be administered at least 2 hours before or 4 to 6 hours after the interacting agent.

Gastrointestinal Motility and Rate of Absorption

Drugs that affect the motility of the GI tract produce a less common absorption-altering mechanism. These agents tend to affect the rate of absorption and not the amount of drug absorbed. Any agent—for example, metoclopramide—that stimulates peristalsis and increases gastric-emptying time can affect the rate of absorption of other medications. In most cases, an increase in the rate of absorption occurs because the target drug reaches the duodenum faster, allowing absorption to occur sooner. However, in some cases such as with metoclopramide and digoxin, a decrease in digoxin concentrations

may occur (American Society of Health-System Pharmacists, 2008).

Conversely, anticholinergic agents and opiates decrease gastric motility, thereby decreasing the rate of absorption of object drugs. Because this type of interaction does not usually affect the amount of drug absorbed, it is usually clinically insignificant.

GI Flora and Absorption

The bacteria present in the GI tract are also responsible for a portion of the metabolism of some agents. An example of this is digoxin; concomitant administration with antibiotics (such as erythromycin or tetracycline) may alter the normal bacterial flora and reduce digoxin metabolism, thereby increasing bioavailability and serum concentrations in some patients (Susla, 2005). To the contrary, GI bacteria produce enzymes that deconjugate inactive unabsorbable ethinyl estradiol metabolites of oral contraceptives that have been excreted into the GI tract via the bile. Deconjugation allows reabsorption of active ethinyl estradiol back into the bloodstream. By disrupting the GI flora, anti-infectives may decrease or eliminate reabsorption of active ethinyl estradiol, thereby decreasing plasma concentrations and the effectiveness of oral contraceptives (Weaver & Glasier, 1999). However, in a case-crossover study of 1,330 failure cases, Toh et al. (2011) did not find an association between concomitant antibiotic use and the risk of breakthrough pregnancy among combined oral contraceptive users.

Table 3.1 summarizes some of the major drug interactions that occur in the absorptive process.

Distribution

After drugs are absorbed into the bloodstream, most of them, to some degree, are bound to plasma protein such as albumin or α_1-acid glycoprotein. As described in Chapter 2, only an unbound drug is free to interact with its target receptor site and is therefore active. The percentage of drug that binds to plasma proteins depends on the affinity of that drug for the protein-binding site. If two drugs with high affinity for circulating proteins are administered together, they may compete for a single binding site on the protein. In fact, one drug may displace the other from the binding site with the result being an increase in the unbound (free) fraction of the displaced drug. This increase in free drug may trigger an exaggerated pharmacodynamic response or toxic reaction. However, because the excess unbound drug is now subject to elimination processes, the increases in both free drug fraction and the effects produced are usually transient.

Clinically significant drug displacement interactions normally occur only when drugs are more than 90% protein bound and have a narrow therapeutic index. For example, warfarin is 99% protein bound, and therefore, only 1% of the drug in the bloodstream is free to induce a pharmacodynamic response (inhibition of clotting factors). If a second drug is administered that displaces even 1% of the warfarin bound to albumin, the amount of free warfarin is doubled, to 2% free.

TABLE 3.1

Drugs Affecting Absorption

	Mechanism of Action	Object Drug	Results
Absorption Inhibitors			
activated charcoal	Binding agent	digoxin	Decreased absorption
aluminum hydroxide	Unknown	allopurinol	Decreased absorption
antacids (Mg^{2+}, Ca^{2+}, Al^{3+})	Chelating agent	quinolones, tetracyclines, levodopa, levothyroxine	Decreased absorption
aluminum and Mg hydroxide	Binding agent	digoxin	Decreased absorption
bismuth (Pepto-Bismol)	Binding agent	tetracycline, doxycycline	Decreased absorption
antibiotics (i.e., erythromycin, tetracycline)	Altered GI flora	digoxin	Increased absorption
	Altered GI flora	oral contraceptives	Decreased reabsorption, decreased enterohepatic recycling
anticholinergics	Decreases gastric emptying	acetaminophen, atenolol, levodopa	Decreased absorption
cholestyramine	Binding agent	acetaminophen, diclofenac, digoxin, glipizide, furosemide, iron, levothyroxine, lorazepam, methotrexate, metronidazole, piroxicam	Decreased absorption
colestipol	Binding agent	carbamazepine, diclofenac, furosemide, tetracycline, thiazides	Decreased absorption
desipramine	Decreases GI motility	phenylbutazone	Decreased absorption
didanosine	Binding agent	ciprofloxacin	Decreased absorption
	Increases gastric pH	imidazole, antifungals	Decreased absorption
ferrous sulfate	Chelating agent	quinolones, tetracyclines, levodopa, levothyroxine	Decreased absorption
histamine-2 receptor antagonists/proton pump inhibitors	Increases gastric pH	imidazole, antifungals, enoxacin	Decreased absorption
phenytoin	Unknown	furosemide	Decreased absorption
sucralfate	Binding agent	quinolones, tetracyclines, phenytoin, levothyroxine	Decreased absorption
sulfasalazine	Unknown	digoxin	Decreased absorption
Absorption Enhancers			
cisapride	Increases gastric emptying	disopyramide	Increased absorption
histamine-2 receptor antagonists	Increases gastric pH	pravastatin, glipizide, dihydropyridine, calcium antagonists	Increased absorption
metoclopramide	Increases gastric motility	cyclosporine	Increased absorption
	Increases GI motility	acetaminophen, cefprozil, ethanol	Increased absorption

GI, gastrointestinal.

This can result in a significant increase in its pharmacodynamic action, leading to excessive bleeding. **Table 3.2** lists examples of several displacement interactions.

Metabolism

Lipophilicity (fat solubility) enables drug molecules to be absorbed and reach their site of action. However, lipophilic drugs are difficult for the body to excrete. Therefore, they must be transformed by the body to more hydrophilic (water-soluble) molecules. This is accomplished primarily through phase I, or oxidation, reactions. The main sites of metabolism in the body are the liver (hepatocytes) and small intestine (enterocytes). Other tissues, such as the kidneys, lungs, and brain, play a minor role in the metabolism of drug molecules (Michalets, 1998). These sites of metabolism contain enzymes called cytochrome P-450 isoenzymes. This group of isoenzymes has been identified as the major catalyst of phase I metabolic reactions in humans.

The nomenclature of the cytochrome P-450 system classifies the isoenzymes (designated CYP) according to family (greater than 36% homology in amino acid sequence), subfamily (77% homology), and individual gene (Brosen, 1990; Guengerich, 1994; Nebert et al., 1987). For example, the isoenzyme CYP3A4 belongs to family 3, subfamily A, and gene 4. As one moves down the classification system from family to gene, the structures of the isoenzymes become more similar.

TABLE 3.2

Distribution Drug Interactions

Displacing Agent	Object Drug
aspirin	meclofenamate, tolmetin
salicylates	methotrexate
TMP-SMZ	
sulfaphenazole	phenytoin
tolbutamide	
valproic acid	
halofenate	sulfonylureas
quinidine	digoxin
aspirin	warfarin
chloral hydrate	
diazoxide	
etodolac	
fenoprofen	
lovastatin	
nalidixic acid	
phenylbutazone	
phenytoin	
sulfinpyrazone	

TMP-SMZ, trimethoprim–sulfamethoxazole.

This enzyme system has evolved to form new isoenzymes that metabolize foreign substrates (i.e., drugs) that are presented to the body. These enzymes are structured to recognize and bind to molecular entities on substrates. Many different substrates may have molecular structures that differ only slightly; therefore, an isoenzyme can bind to any one of these substrates. Although several different substrates may compete for the same enzyme receptor, the substrate with the highest affinity binds most often. The converse of this is also true. Two isoenzymes can bind to the same substrate (**Figure 3.1**), but the substrate binds more often to the isoenzyme to which it has the most affinity. However, not every drug molecule ("substrate") can be metabolized by every enzyme with which it binds; therefore, it is not a true substrate. These concepts form the backbone for the drug interactions that are expanded on later.

Six isoenzymes have been determined to be responsible for most metabolism-related drug interactions. They are the isoforms CYP1A2, CYP2C9, CYP2C19, CYP2D6, CYP2E1, and CYP3A4. The CYP3A4 isoform is responsible for 40% to

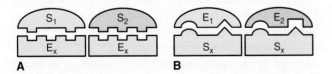

FIGURE 3.1 Substrate binding. **A.** Different substrates. Although Enzyme X (E_x) can bind to both Substrate 1 (S_1) and Substrate 2 (S_2), S_2 has greater affinity for E_x than S_1. Therefore E_x will bind to S_2 most often. **B.** Different enzymes. Although Substrate X (S_x) can bind to both Enzyme 1 (E_1) and Enzyme 2 (E_2), E_1 has a greater affinity for S_x than E_2. Therefore, S_x will bind to E_1 most often.

45% of drug metabolism, the CYP2D6 for the next 20% to 30%, CYP2C9 about 10%, and CYP2E1 and CYP1A2 each responsible for about 5% (Ingelman-Sundberg, 2004). The remaining 5% to 20% is accounted for by several lesser important isoforms. Because there are so few enzymes that transform a multitude of substrates, it is easy to see how there would be a great potential for interactions.

There are some genetic variations with respect to the distribution of the enzymes. For example, about 10% of Europeans lack the CYP2D6 enzyme and are therefore considered poor metabolizers of drugs using this pathway for biotransformation. These individuals are at greater risk for ADRs related to drugs metabolized by CYP2D6. In addition, prodrugs requiring this enzyme for activation (e.g., codeine, tamoxifen) may be less effective or have no effect. In contrast, about 5% of this population are considered ultrametabolizers, have too rapid metabolism, and may show little to no response related to drugs metabolized by the CYP2D6 pathway (Ingelman-Sundberg, 2004). Similarly, there is variability within the CYP2C19 isoform, with about 14% of Chinese, 2% of Whites, and 4% of Blacks being poor metabolizers (Scott et al., 2011). The effectiveness of certain prodrugs (e.g., clopidogrel) that require metabolic activation by this enzyme system may be reduced (Holmes et al., 2010).

There has been increasing interest in genetic testing to identify strategies to reduce the risk of ADRs and to optimize therapy for individuals. Pharmacogenomic information has been incorporated into about 10% of labels for drugs approved by the U.S. Food and Drug Administration (FDA) in an effort to identify responders and nonresponders, avoid toxicity, and adjust doses of medications to optimize efficacy and ensure safety (FDA Table of Pharmacogenomic Biomarkers in Drug Labeling accessed July 16, 2015). In addition, regulatory authorities have recently recommended genetic testing to aid the clinician in determining if an agent is safe and effective in certain individuals (e.g., abacavir) (Highlights of Prescribing Information: Ziagen (abacavir sulfate) Tablets and Oral Solution accessed July 16, 2015). While commercial assays are available for genetic testing, turnaround time for the results varies, testing can be expensive, data on the validation of techniques used and reliability and reproducibility are limited, and, to date, there is limited evidence-based data on which to develop specific recommendations on the role of genetic testing in routine care (Holmes et al., 2010).

There are two types of metabolic drug interactions: drugs that inhibit the action of an enzyme and those that induce the activity of the enzyme.

Inhibition

Inhibition of drug metabolism occurs through competitive and noncompetitive inhibition. When two drugs, administered concurrently, are metabolized by the same isoenzyme, they are defined as competitive inhibitors of each other. In essence, they compete for the same binding site on an enzyme to be metabolized.

Noncompetitive inhibition also occurs when both drugs compete for the same binding site, but one drug is metabolized by that isoenzyme and the other drug is not. The best known example of a noncompetitive inhibitor is quinidine. Quinidine is metabolized by the CYP3A4 isoenzyme but can also bind to the CYP2D6 enzyme. Therefore, although quinidine does not compete for metabolism by the CYP2D6 isoenzyme, it does compete for the CYP2D6 isoenzyme binding site.

In both competitive and noncompetitive inhibition, the drug with the greatest affinity for the isoenzyme receptor is usually the inhibiting drug because it binds in the receptor site, preventing the other drug from being bound and metabolized (**Figure 3.2**). The significance of the drug interaction depends on several characteristics of the inhibiting drug.

Affinity The first characteristic, affinity, has already been mentioned. Many drugs may inhibit the same isoenzyme but not to the same extent. The greater the affinity of an inhibiting drug for an enzyme, the more it blocks binding of other drug molecules.

Half-Life Along with affinity, the half-life ($t_{1/2}$) of the inhibiting drug determines the duration of the interaction. The longer the half-life of the inhibiting drug, the longer the drug interaction lasts. For example, after a regimen of ketoconazole ($t_{1/2}$ = 8 hours) is discontinued, its ability to inhibit the CYP3A4 enzyme lasts until it is eliminated, in three to five half-lives or approximately 1 day. However, the inhibiting effect of amiodarone, with a $t_{1/2}$ of approximately 53 days, lasts for weeks to months after its discontinuation.

Concentration The third major factor contributing to a drug's ability to inhibit hepatic enzymes is the concentration of the inhibiting drug. A threshold concentration must be reached or exceeded to inhibit an enzyme. This is similar to the threshold concentration discussed in Chapter 2 regarding minimally effective concentrations and therapeutic responses. This minimally effective threshold concentration, or concentration-dependent inhibition, is exhibited by a variety of drugs. The dose yielding

this concentration-dependent inhibition varies based on volume of distribution, drug and receptor affinity, and characteristics of the individual patient. An example of a dose- or concentration-dependent inhibitor is cimetidine. In most patients, a dose of 400 mg/d results in only weak enzyme inhibition. However, at higher doses, it interacts significantly with both the CYP2D6 and CYP1A2 isoenzymes (Shinn, 1992).

Some enzyme inhibitors may affect one enzyme at a smaller concentration and more than one isoenzyme at higher concentrations. These enzyme inhibitors demonstrate that some isoenzymes have differing thresholds. For example, fluconazole at a dose of 200 mg/d significantly inhibits only the 2C9 isoenzyme, but as the dose increases above 400 mg/d, it also inhibits the 3A4 isoenzyme (Hansten & Horn, 2015; Kivisto et al., 1994).

Toxic Potential Another consideration with regard to inhibition interactions is the toxic potential of the object drug. For example, nonsedating antihistamines (i.e., terfenadine and astemizole) are metabolized by the CYP3A4 isoenzyme to a nontoxic metabolite. The parent compound of both drugs is cardiotoxic. If a potent CYP3A4 inhibitor (e.g., erythromycin) is administered concurrently with these agents, the parent compound accumulates in the body and causes a potentially fatal arrhythmia, such as torsades de pointes (Mathews et al., 1991; Woosley, 1996). Because of their serious toxic potential, both terfenadine and astemizole have been removed from the market.

Efficacy An additional consideration related to inhibition interactions is the effectiveness of the object drug. This is particularly important for prodrugs that require cytochrome P-450 metabolism to the active metabolite in order for the drug to be effective. An example of this is clopidogrel, an antiplatelet agent, which requires CYP2C19 enzymes to be metabolized to the active form. When administered with omeprazole, a CYP2C19 inhibitor, a reduction in plasma concentrations of the active metabolite of clopidogrel as well as reduced platelet function occur (clopidogrel [Plavix] prescribing information). In addition, tamoxifen, an agent used for breast cancer, is converted to its active metabolite by CYP2D6. Women may have a higher risk of breast cancer recurrence if they take tamoxifen in combination with CYP2D6 inhibitors such as the serotonin reuptake inhibitors paroxetine, fluoxetine, or sertraline (The Medical Letter, 2009).

Not all inhibition reactions result in harmful effects, however. Some interactions may be inconsequential or even beneficial. For example, ketoconazole (a potent inhibitor of the CYP3A4 isoenzyme) can be given with cyclosporine. The consequent interaction enables practitioners to give less cyclosporine to achieve the same immunosuppressive response (Hansten & Horn, 2015).

The cytochrome P-450 system is complex, but an understanding of the basic concepts of inhibitory interactions leads to the ability to anticipate which agents are likely to interact. The affinity, half-life, and drug concentration determine the potency of the inhibiting drug. A potent enzyme inhibitor inhibits most drugs metabolized by that enzyme. A clinically significant drug interaction also depends on the toxic potential of the drug being inhibited. **Table 3.3** lists several enzyme inhibitors.

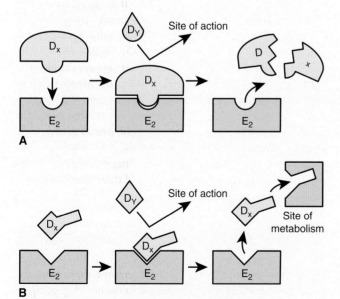

FIGURE 3.2 Inhibition. **A.** Competitive inhibition. Drug X (D_X) and Drug Y (D_Y) are both metabolized by Enzyme 2 (E_2). **B.** Noncompetitive inhibition. Although D_X and D_Y compete for the binding site on E_2, only D_Y is metabolized by E_2. Therefore, D_X noncompetitively inhibits D_Y.

TABLE 3.3

Drugs Affecting Metabolism through Cytochrome P-450 Isoenzymes

Inhibitors	Inducers	Substrates	Inhibitors	Inducers	Substrates
Isoenzyme 1A2			*Isoenzyme 3A4*		
cimetidine	carbamazepine	theophylline	amiodarone	carbamazepine	alprazolam
ciprofloxacin	phenobarbital		azole antifungals	dexamethasone	atorvastatin
clarithromycin	phenytoin	tricyclic antidepressants	clarithromycin	ethosuximide	calcium channel blockers
enoxacin	rifampin	benzodiazepines	erythromycin	phenobarbital	carbamazepine
erythromycin	ritonavir	warfarin	fluoxetine	phenytoin	clindamycin
norfloxacin	smoking		fluvoxamine	rifabutin	clomipramine
oral contraceptives	polycyclic		imidazole	rifampin	clonazepam
SSRIs	aromatic		nefazodone		cyclosporine
zileuton	hydrocarbons		norfloxacin		dapsone
			protease inhibitors		dexamethasone
			quinine		dextromethorphan
Isoenzyme 2C (primarily 2C9, 2C19)					
amiodarone	carbamazepine	amitriptyline	telithromycin		disopyramide
cimetidine	phenobarbital	clomipramine	verapamil		erythromycin
fluconazole	phenytoin	diazepam	zafirlukast		oral contraceptives (estrogens)
fluoxetine	rifampin	imipramine			
fluvastatin		losartan			ethosuximide
fluvoxamine		omeprazole			fexofenadine
isoniazid		phenytoin			imipramine
metronidazole		tricyclic antidepressants			ketoconazole
omeprazole		warfarin			lidocaine
sertraline					lovastatin
zafirlukast					miconazole
					midazolam
Isoenzyme 2D6					nefazodone
amiodarone	carbamazepine				ondansetron
					oxycodone
cimetidine	phenobarbital				pravastatin
clomipramine	phenytoin				prednisone
codeine	rifampin				protease inhibitors
desipramine					quinidine
haloperidol					quinine
perphenazine					rifampin
propafenone					sertraline
quinidine					tacrolimus
SSRIs					tamoxifen
thioridazine					temazepam
venlafaxine					triazolam
					verapamil
					warfarin
Isoenzyme 2E1					zileuton
disulfiram	ethanol	acetaminophen			
ritonavir	isoniazid	chloral hydrate			
		ethanol			
		isoniazid			
		ondansetron			
		tamoxifen			

SSRIs, selective serotonin reuptake inhibitors.

Induction

Drug–drug interactions can also result from the action of one drug (inducer) stimulating the metabolism of an object drug (substrate). This enhanced metabolism is thought to be produced by an increase in hepatic blood flow or an increase in the formation of hepatic enzymes. This process, known as *enzyme induction*, increases the amount of enzymes available to metabolize drug molecules, thereby decreasing the concentration and pharmacodynamic effect of the object drug.

Some of the more common enzyme inducers are rifampin, phenobarbital, phenytoin, and carbamazepine. Enzyme induction, like enzyme inhibition, is substrate dependent. Therefore, any drug that is a potent inducer of a cytochrome P-450 system increases the metabolism of most drugs metabolized by that enzyme. Also, in a manner similar to that of enzyme inhibitors, inducers may affect more than one cytochrome P-450 isoform; for example, phenobarbital is a potent inducer of the CYP3A4, CYP1A2, and CYP2C isoforms.

Some enzyme inducers, such as carbamazepine, also increase their own metabolism. Over time, carbamazepine stimulates its own metabolism, thereby decreasing its half-life and frequently resulting in an increased dose requirement to maintain the same therapeutic drug level. This process is termed *autoinduction*.

The onset and duration/cessation of enzyme induction depend on both the half-life of the inducer and the half-life of the isoenzyme that is being stimulated. For example, rifampin ($t_{1/2}$ = 3 to 4 hours) results in enzyme induction within 24 hours, whereas the enzyme induction capacity of phenobarbital ($t_{1/2}$ = 53 to 140 hours) is not evident for approximately 7 days. The level of induction remains constant while the drugs are being administered. However, on discontinuation of the respective inducers, the inducing action of rifampin ends more rapidly because of its shorter half-life. This occurs because rifampin is removed from the body at a faster rate than phenobarbital and therefore is not available to inhibit hepatic enzymes for as long.

The initiation and duration of enzyme induction also depend on the half-life of the induced isoenzyme. It takes anywhere from 1 to 6 days for a cytochrome P-450 enzyme to be degraded or produced. Therefore, even if a drug achieves a high enough concentration to produce induction of liver enzymes, the increase in metabolism of an object drug may not be evident until more liver enzymes have formed. The effect of rifampin on warfarin metabolism is a good example of this. Although induction begins within 24 hours of rifampin administration, its effect on warfarin metabolism is not evident for approximately 4 days. On discontinuation of rifampin, the remaining drug is metabolized to negligible levels before the effect on warfarin metabolism dissipates. This occurs because the half-life of the liver enzymes is greater than the half-life of rifampin, and therefore, the enzymes remain to metabolize warfarin after rifampin is eliminated from the body.

These concepts are important to remember when monitoring laboratory values that demonstrate the effectiveness of the object medication. For example, the international normalized ratio (INR), which is a surrogate marker of warfarin levels, fluctuates significantly within a couple of days of the initiation or discontinuation of rifampin. However, no change in the INR is evident for approximately 1 week after administration of phenobarbital. This is also true when measuring levels of certain antibiotics and other agents that may be affected by inducers. **Table 3.3** lists several enzyme inducers and the drugs they affect.

Excretion

Although most drugs are metabolized by the liver, the primary modes of elimination from the body are biliary and renal excretion. Drugs are removed from the bloodstream by the kidneys by filtration or by urinary secretion. However, reabsorption from the urine into the bloodstream may also occur.

Changes in these processes become important when they affect drugs that are unchanged or still active. Excretion of drug molecules can be affected in a number of ways; these include, but are not limited to, acidification or alkalinization of the urine and alteration of secretory or active transport pathways. For example, amphetamine is excreted predominantly via the urine. Thirty percent of the drug can be recovered from the urine after 24 hours of administration. Acidic urine increases while alkaline urine slows down the renal excretion of amphetamine (Jones & Karlsson, 2005). Although they are not discussed here for various reasons, there are a select number of other mechanisms of renal drug interactions.

The ionization state of drug molecules plays a key role in the excretion process. The urine pH determines the ionization state of the excreted molecule. Because lipophilic membranes are less permeable to ionized molecules (hydrophilic), ionized molecules become "trapped" in the urine and are subsequently excreted. Drugs that are nonionized in the urine may be reabsorbed and then recirculated, effectively decreasing their elimination and increasing their half-lives.

Acidic drugs remain in their nonionized state in an acidic urine and become ionized in an alkaline urine. The opposite is true for basic drug molecules, which remain nonionized in an alkaline urine and are ionized in an acidic urine. When a drug is administered that alters the urine pH, it may promote an increased reabsorption or excretion of another drug. For example, the administration of bicarbonate can potentially increase the urine pH. This leads to the increased excretion of acidic drugs (e.g., aspirin) and the increased reabsorption of basic drugs (e.g., pseudoephedrine).

Although most drugs cross the membrane of the renal tubule by simple diffusion, some drugs are also secreted into the urine through active transport pathways. These pathways, however, have a limited capacity and can accommodate only a set amount of drug molecules. Therefore, if two different drugs using the same pathway are coadministered, the transport pathway may become saturated. This causes a "traffic jam" and the excretion of one or both of the drugs is inhibited.

These interactions can be beneficial or detrimental, depending on the agents that are administered. For example, when probenecid and penicillin are given together, they compete for secretion through an organic acid pathway in the renal tubule. The probenecid blocks the secretion of the penicillin, thereby increasing the therapeutic concentration of penicillin in the bloodstream. This is a prime example of drug interactions benefiting the patient. In contrast, digoxin and verapamil also share an active transport pathway. When they are administered concomitantly, their interaction leads to an increase in digoxin levels resulting in potential cardiotoxicity (e.g., arrhythmia). **Table 3.4** lists some other clinically important excretion interactions.

The other common pathway of excretion, the biliary tract, allows for the elimination of drugs and their metabolites into the feces. This route of excretion is involved in interactions with drugs that undergo enterohepatic recirculation. Drugs subject to this process are excreted into the GI tract through the biliary ducts and have the potential to be reabsorbed through the intestinal wall into the bloodstream. Some of these drugs depend on enterohepatic recirculation to achieve therapeutic concentrations. An example of a drug class that undergoes enterohepatic recirculation is the oral contraceptive. As previously described, antibiotics can adversely affect reabsorption

of the estrogen components of oral contraceptives, potentially rendering them ineffective. In addition, drugs that undergo enterohepatic recirculation may also be affected by binding agents. An example of this is warfarin in combination with the bile acid sequestrants colestipol and cholestyramine. Warfarin undergoes enterohepatic recirculation. Once warfarin has been excreted in the bile, the bile acid sequestrant binds with warfarin, preventing its reabsorption and increasing its clearance, decreasing its efficacy. This has been shown to occur even when warfarin is administered intravenously (Jahnchen et al., 1978). Therefore, it is not only important to administer warfarin 2 hours before or 6 hours after cholestyramine, but consistency in the administration time of these agents is important as well (Mancano, 2005).

Pharmacokinetic interactions make up a large part of the interactions that practitioners must contend with every day. These interactions are the most studied because they have an objective measurable outcome (e.g., drug concentrations, enzyme concentrations). However, a drug's pharmacodynamic profile must also be considered when it is administered with other agents.

P-Glycoprotein Interactions

Inhibition or induction of P-glycoprotein (P-gp), an energy-dependent efflux transporter, can result in interactions involving absorption or excretion (biliary or renal). P-gp pumps drug molecules out of cells and is found in the epithelial cells of the intestine (enterocytes), liver, and kidney. As a drug passes through the enterocyte in the intestine to be absorbed into the systemic circulation, P-gp can pick up the molecule and carry it back to the intestinal lumen, preventing absorption. P-gp in the liver and kidney act to increase the excretion of drugs by transporting the molecules into the bile and urine, respectively (Hansten & Horn, 2015).

If P-gp is inhibited, more drugs will be absorbed through the enterocytes. This will result in an increase in plasma concentrations of the object drug. An example of this interaction is when quinidine is administered with digoxin. Quinidine inhibits intestinal P-gp, which results in increased absorption of digoxin. In addition, quinidine inhibition of renal P-gp results in reduced elimination of digoxin by the kidney. The end result is increased concentrations of serum digoxin (Horn & Hansten, 2004).

If P-gp is induced, less drug will be absorbed through the enterocytes. An example of an induction interaction of P-gp is when rifampin is given with digoxin. Rifampin induces intestinal P-gp, resulting in reduced absorption and reduced serum digoxin concentrations (Hansten & Horn, 2015).

Table 3.5 provides examples of common substrates, inhibitors, and inducers of P-gp (Hansten & Horn, 2015; Kim, 2002).

Pharmacodynamic Interactions

The responses or effects produced by a drug's actions are referred to as the drug's *pharmacodynamic profile*. Although drugs are administered to elicit a specific response or change

TABLE 3.4

Drugs Affecting Excretion

Renal Elimination	Mechanism	Object Drug	Results
acetazolamide	Increases urine pH	salicylates	Increased elimination
losartan	Unknown	lithium	Decreased elimination
salicylates	Unknown	acetazolamide	Decreased elimination
cetazolamide	Increases urine pH	quinidine	Decreased elimination
triamterene	Unknown	amantadine	Decreased elimination
amiodarone	Unknown	digoxin	Decreased elimination
	Unknown	procainamide	Decreased renal and hepatic elimination
antacids	Increase urine pH	dextroamphetamine, quinidine, pseudoephedrine	Decreased elimination
diuretics	Inhibit sodium reabsorption with subsequent renal tubular reabsorption of lithium	lithium	Decreased elimination
salicylates	Inhibit renal tubular secretion of methotrexate	methotrexate	Decreased elimination

TABLE 3.5

Examples of Substrates, Inhibitors, and Inducers of P-Glycoprotein*

Substrates	Inhibitors	Inducers
aldosterone	amiodarone	indinavir
cimetidine	atorvastatin	morphine
colchicine	clarithromycin	nelfinavir
cyclosporine	cyclosporine	phenothiazine
digoxin	diltiazem	rifampin
diltiazem	erythromycin	ritonavir
erythromycin	felodipine	saquinavir
fexofenadine	indinavir	St. John's wort
indinavir	itraconazole	
itraconazole	ketoconazole	
morphine	methadone	
nelfinavir	nelfinavir	
quinidine	nicardipine	
ranitidine	quinidine	
saquinavir	ritonavir	
tetracycline	sirolimus	
verapamil	tacrolimus	
	verapamil	

*Data from Horn, J. R., & Hansten P. D. (2004). Drug interactions with digoxin: The role of P-glycoprotein. *Pharmacy Times* (October). Retrieved from http://www.hanstenandhorn.com/hh-article10-04.pdf and Kim, R. B. (2002). Drugs as P-glycoprotein substrates, inhibitors, and inducers. *Drug Metabolism Reviews, 34*, 47–54.

in dynamics, an agent usually causes several changes in the body. When one or more drugs are coadministered, the entire pharmacodynamic profile of each drug must be considered because of the potential for each to interact. Drugs that have a similar characteristic in their pharmacodynamic profile may produce an exaggerated response. For example, when a benzodiazepine (e.g., alprazolam) is administered with a muscle relaxant (e.g., cyclobenzaprine), the sedative effects of both drugs combine to produce excessive drowsiness. A less obvious pharmacodynamic interaction occurs with the coadministration of angiotensin-converting enzyme (ACE) inhibitors (e.g., enalapril) and potassium-sparing diuretics (e.g., triamterene). These agents individually can both produce an increase in the potassium (K^+) level. Unless the prescriber is aware of the pharmacodynamic profile of both drugs, the potential for an excessive increase in the potassium level may go unnoticed and arrhythmia may ensue.

In contrast, drugs may also produce opposing pharmacodynamic effects. This type of interaction may cause the expected drug response to be diminished or even abolished. Unfortunately, these interactions are often overlooked. Instead of the lack of response being interpreted as a pharmacodynamic drug interaction, it is suspected to be due to an ineffective dose or drug. This often leads to an increase in the amount of drug administered and consequent unwanted side effects or interactions. This type of interaction is illustrated by the concomitant administration of an antihypertensive agent (e.g., a diuretic)

and a nonsteroidal anti-inflammatory drug (NSAID). Thiazide diuretics produce their hypotensive effects by blocking sodium reabsorption in the distal tubule of the kidney, which leads to increased sodium and water excretion. If NSAIDs are administered concomitantly, the sodium and water retention effects of the NSAIDs may reduce or nullify the hypotensive action of the diuretic.

DRUG–FOOD INTERACTIONS

The interaction between food and drugs can affect both pharmacokinetic and pharmacodynamic parameters. The mechanism of these pharmacokinetic interactions is mediated by alteration of drug bioavailability, distribution, metabolism, or excretion, as seen with drug–drug interactions. The potential for pharmacodynamic drug–food interactions warrants concern about proper diet for patients on certain drugs. Although practicing clinicians often overlook drug–food interactions, these interactions can significantly affect efficacy of drug therapy. Awareness of significant drug–food interactions can reduce the incidence of these effects and optimize drug therapy.

Effect of Food on Drug Pharmacokinetics

Absorption

Food can affect the absorption of drugs in two ways: first, by altering the extent of drug absorption and second, by changing the rate of drug absorption. Usually, changes in the rate of drug absorption have less significance if only the rate of absorption is delayed without affecting bioavailability. The underlying mechanisms that mediate these interactions are highly variable and depend on both the content of food and the properties of the drug involved.

Food can either increase or decrease the amount (extent) of drug absorption, potentially altering the bioavailability of a drug. One mechanism, similar to drug–drug interactions, is adsorption. For example, tetracycline and fluoroquinolone antibiotics (e.g., ciprofloxacin, ofloxacin) can chelate with calcium cations found in milk or milk products, thus significantly limiting the drug's bioavailability.

A second type of drug–food interaction occurs when food serves as a physical barrier and prevents the absorption of orally administered drugs. The absorptive capacity of the small intestine is related to the accessibility of a drug to the GI mucosal surfaces, the site where absorption occurs. When food is coadministered with a drug, access to the mucosa is reduced, resulting in delayed or decreased drug absorption. For example, the bioavailability of azithromycin is reduced by 43% when the drug is taken with food (Zithromax (Pfizer Pharmaceuticals) Package Insert, 2013). Similar types of interactions can be seen when erythromycin, isoniazid, penicillins, and zidovudine are given orally. To avoid such interactions, these drugs can be administered 2 hours apart from mealtime. **Box 3.1** identifies some commonly prescribed drugs that should be taken on

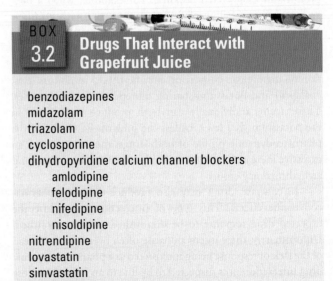

Drugs to Be Taken on an Empty Stomach

azithromycin
captopril
erythromycin
fluoroquinolones (e.g., ciprofloxacin, ofloxacin)
griseofulvin
isoniazid
oral penicillins
sucralfate
tetracycline
theophylline, timed release (e.g., Theo-Dur Sprinkle, Theo-24, Uniphyl)
zidovudine

an empty stomach. Note, however, if patients cannot tolerate these medications on an empty stomach (because of GI side effects like diarrhea), coadministration with food may be advisable.

In contrast, food can also decrease the absorption of some drugs. For example, phenytoin is known to bind to protein source, heavy metals such as calcium carbonate, and enteral feeding formulas (Sacks, 2004). Doses of phenytoin may have to be increased up to 1,000 mg/d compared to 300 mg/d when it is given without food. To avoid the drug–food interaction, phenytoin doses can be given 1 hour before or 2 hours after eating.

Metabolism

Food can also affect drug metabolism. Grapefruit juice, for example, can affect the metabolism of many drugs. Grapefruit juice specifically inhibits the 3A4 subset of intestinal cytochrome P-450 enzymes and thus increases the serum concentration of drugs dependent on these enzymes for metabolism (Ameer & Weintraub, 1997; Huang et al., 2004).

The extrahepatic cytochrome enzymes are found in highest concentrations in the proximal two thirds of the small intestine. These enzymes are located at the distal portion of the villi that line the small intestine and are responsible for the extrahepatic metabolism of more than 20 drugs (Ameer & Weintraub, 1997; Huang et al., 2004). The component in grapefruit juice that is responsible for this interaction remains undetermined; however, the flavonoid naringin, found in high concentrations in grapefruit juice, is suspected. Increases in the bioavailability of verapamil and dihydropyridine calcium channel blockers such as felodipine, nisoldipine, nitrendipine, nifedipine, and amlodipine have been documented with the coadministration of grapefruit juice (Bailey et al., 1991, 1992, 1993; Rashid et al., 1993). The bioavailability of carbamazepine and midazolam is markedly increased when taken with grapefruit juice (Sacks, 2004). However, unlike verapamil and dihydropyridine calcium channel blockers, diltiazem does

not demonstrate an increase in bioavailability with grapefruit juice.

The amount of grapefruit juice required to increase plasma concentrations can vary between agents. A single glass of grapefruit juice can increase the area under the curve and maximum concentration (C_{max}) of felodipine by several fold (Bailey et al., 1998) while the warnings in the product labeling for some HMG CoA reductase inhibitors metabolized by CYP3A4 say to avoid quantities greater than 1 quart per day (Zocor Package Insert, 2015). The extent of the increase in felodipine plasma concentrations is maximal between simultaneous and 4 hours before administration of grapefruit juice. However, higher C_{max} concentrations were evident even when grapefruit juice is consumed 24 hours before felodipine. Therefore, separating doses may reduce but does not eliminate the potential for the interaction (Bailey et al., 1998). Because grapefruit juice appears to inhibit mostly intestinal CYP3A4 and not hepatic CYP3A4 enzymes, the metabolism of drugs administered intravenously is unlikely to be altered. Further, the data suggest that only those agents given at doses higher than usual or if the patients' livers are severely damaged result in the intestinal CYP3A4 as the primary metabolic pathway (Huang et al., 2004). **Box 3.2** identifies some drugs that may interact with grapefruit juice.

In contrast to the ability of grapefruit juice to inhibit drug metabolism, other components of food may induce drug metabolism and therefore decrease drug efficacy. For example, in the treatment of Parkinson disease, dopamine in the brain needs to be replenished. However, exogenous dopamine does not cross the blood–brain barrier, but its precursor, levodopa, does. Unfortunately, much of the levodopa is lost to metabolism when given orally and only approximately 1% of the administered amount enters the brain to be converted to dopamine (Trovato et al., 1991). Concomitant administration with

Drugs That Interact with Grapefruit Juice

benzodiazepines
midazolam
triazolam
cyclosporine
dihydropyridine calcium channel blockers
    amlodipine
    felodipine
    nifedipine
    nisoldipine
nitrendipine
lovastatin
simvastatin
theophylline
verapamil
17 β-estradiol

CHAPTER 3 | IMPACT OF DRUG INTERACTIONS AND ADVERSE EVENTS ON THERAPEUTICS 43

food containing pyridoxine (or vitamin B$_6$) can potentially further enhance the peripheral metabolism of levodopa, thus decreasing drug efficacy (Trovato et al., 1991). Patients taking levodopa should therefore be educated about moderate intake of pyridoxine-rich foods, such as avocados, beans, bacon, beef, liver, peas, pork, sweet potatoes, and tuna. Similarly, charcoal-broiled meats can induce the activity of the CYP1A2 isoenzymes, thus increasing the metabolism of drugs such as theophylline.

Excretion

Ingestion of certain fruit juices can alter the urinary pH and affect the elimination and reabsorption of drugs such as quinidine and amphetamine. Orange, tomato, and grapefruit juices are metabolized to an alkaline residue, which can increase the urinary pH. For drugs that are weak bases, making the urine more alkaline by raising the pH increases the proportion of nonionized drug and enhances the reabsorption of the drug systemically. (Recall that the ionization of drugs helps promote water solubility and ultimately enhances drug elimination into the urine.)

Effect of Food on Pharmacodynamics

Food affects the pharmacodynamics of drugs either by opposing or potentiating a drug's pharmacologic action. For example, warfarin exerts its anticoagulant effects by inhibiting synthesis of vitamin K–dependent clotting factors. Vitamin K is required for activation by several protein factors of the clotting cascade, namely, factors II, VII, IX, and X. When foods rich in vitamin K are ingested, they can significantly oppose the anticoagulatory efficacy of warfarin. Leafy green vegetables, such as collard greens, kale, lettuce, spinach, mustard greens, and broccoli, are generally recognized to contain large quantities of vitamin K. Health care providers should educate patients who are taking warfarin about this interaction. More importantly, however, practitioners should stress maintaining a balanced diet without abruptly changing the intake of foods rich in vitamin K.

Another significant drug–food interaction occurs between monoamine oxidase (MAO) inhibitors and foods containing tyramine, an amino acid that is contained in many types of food. Tyramine can precipitate a hypertensive reaction in patients taking MAO inhibitors, such as phenelzine, tranylcypromine, or isocarboxazid. MAOs are enzymes located in the GI tract that inactivate tyramine in food. When patients are taking MAO inhibitors, the breakdown of tyramine is prevented and therefore allows for more tyramine to be absorbed systemically. Because of the indirect sympathomimetic property of tyramine, this amino acid provokes the release of norepinephrine from sympathetic nerve endings and epinephrine from the adrenal glands, resulting in an excessive pressor effect. Clinically, patients may complain of diaphoresis, mydriasis, occipital or temporal headache, nuchal rigidity, palpitations, and elevated blood pressure. Examples of foods that contain tyramine are listed in **Box 3.3**.

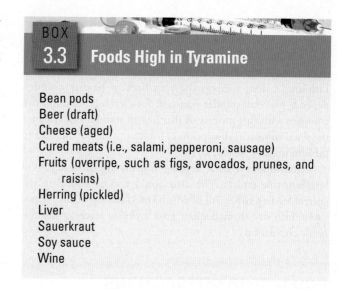

BOX 3.3 Foods High in Tyramine

Bean pods
Beer (draft)
Cheese (aged)
Cured meats (i.e., salami, pepperoni, sausage)
Fruits (overripe, such as figs, avocados, prunes, and raisins)
Herring (pickled)
Liver
Sauerkraut
Soy sauce
Wine

Effect of Drugs on Food and Nutrients

Many of the aforementioned examples indicate that food can precipitate an interaction with a drug, but in some cases, a reciprocal relationship also holds true. First, some drugs can cause a depletion of nutrients or minerals found in food through various mechanisms. For example, drugs such as cholestyramine and colestipol, which were designed to bind bile acid in the GI tract, could also potentially bind to fat-soluble vitamins (i.e., vitamins A, D, E, and K) and folic acid when taken with food, resulting in the decreased absorption of these vitamins. Orlistat, an over-the-counter and prescription medication used for weight loss, reduces fat absorption. In addition to reducing fat absorption, it can also decrease the absorption of fat-soluble vitamins and beta-carotene. Similarly, the chronic use of mineral oil as a laxative reduces the absorption of fat-soluble vitamins. Careful monitoring of the INR in patients taking warfarin and drugs that affect vitamin K absorption is warranted to avoid changes in bleeding times.

Second, drug-induced malabsorption can occur in patients with pre-existing poor nutritional status. For example, long-term use of isoniazid can cause pyridoxine (vitamin B$_6$) deficiency. Pyridoxine supplementation is recommended for patients who are malnourished or predisposed to neuropathy (e.g., patients with diabetes or alcoholism) when treated with isoniazid. Metformin is associated with vitamin B$_{12}$ deficiency in about 7% of patients, which may lead to anemia. In general, the clinical significance of these interactions may depend on the baseline nutritional status of the patient. Patients with poor nutrition or inadequate dietary intake (e.g., elderly or alcoholic patients) are potentially at greater risk for drug-induced vitamin and mineral depletion.

Third, drugs can change nutrient excretion as well. Both thiazide and loop diuretics can enhance the excretion of potassium, possibly leading to hypokalemia. Digoxin, in the presence of diuretic-induced hypokalemia, can lead to digoxin-induced arrhythmias. Spironolactone, an aldosterone antagonist and potassium-sparing diuretic, can increase potassium levels, especially in the presence of an ACE inhibitor or angiotensin receptor blocker. Loop diuretics can increase urinary excretion of calcium, whereas thiazide diuretics can decrease it. In addition, ascorbic acid and potassium depletion can occur with high doses of long-term aspirin therapy (Trovato et al., 1991). Lithium, a drug used in the treatment of bipolar disorder, depends on renal tubular transport for clearance. Sodium can compete with this process. A diet low in sodium can enhance the renal tubular reabsorption of lithium, which could lead to lithium toxicity (Chan, 2013).

Continuous enteral feeding impairs the dissolution of levothyroxine tablets. The drug could also be bound to the enteral feeding tubes. All of which could lead to further hypothyroidism due to inadequate levothyroxine reaching the systemic circulation.

DRUG–HERB INTERACTIONS

In today's society, the search for a "natural way" to treat and prevent diseases has become commonplace. This potentially stems from the misconception that "natural" means "safer." Among U.S. adults aged 18 years and older, 33.2% of the population has used some form of herbal products in 2012 (Clarke et al., 2015). For the most part, these herbal supplements are not regulated by the FDA. In many cases, little research has been conducted to assess the efficacy and safety of these agents or the potential for pharmacokinetic or pharmacodynamic interactions. Some clinical trials have been conducted to evaluate the safety and efficacy of certain herbal medications; however, much of available data are based on animal studies, case reports, and the potential for interactions derived from what is known about the chemical characteristics and pharmacokinetic parameters of the herbs.

Pharmacokinetic Interactions

Absorption

As discussed earlier in the chapter, certain agents can interact with other medications in the GI tract to prevent absorption. Likewise, some herbs can prevent absorption of medications and reduce the effectiveness of those medications. For example, acacia, marketed as a fiber supplement, has been shown to impair the absorption of amoxicillin. This may be secondary to the fiber content of acacia. Doses of acacia and amoxicillin should be separated by 4 hours. Dandelion has a high mineral content and has been shown to reduce the effectiveness of quinolones in animals (Ulbricht et al., 2008). **Table 3.6** summarizes some of the potential herb–drug interactions that can occur in the absorptive process.

Distribution

Meadowsweet and black willow contain salicylates that have the potential to displace highly protein-bound drugs. To avoid toxicity, coadministration of these products with highly protein-bound drugs with a narrow therapeutic index, such as warfarin and carbamazepine, should be avoided.

Metabolism

Certain herbs can be inducers or inhibitors of the cytochrome P-450 enzyme system. St. John's wort, an herbal medication often used to treat depression, has consistently been shown to induce CYP3A4, CYP2E1, and CYP2C19. In addition, St. John's wort induces intestinal P-gp and has been shown to lower plasma concentrations of common P-gp substrates such as digoxin and fexofenadine. Induction of these enzymes is secondary to hyperforin, an ingredient in St. John's wort. St. John's wort has been shown to clinically interact with a number of drugs, including

TABLE 3.6

Herb–Drug Interactions Affecting Absorption

Herbal Medication	Mechanism of Action	Object D	Results
Acacia	Fiber content may slow or reduce absorption of medications	Amoxicillin	Decreased absorption (separate doses by at least 4 h)
Carob	Decreased bowel transit time	Oral medications	Decreased absorption (separate doses by several hours)
Citrus pectin	Fiber content may slow or reduce absorption of medications	Oral medications	Take 1 h before or 2 h after intake of other oral medications
Dandelion	High mineral content (chelation)	Ciprofloxacin and potentially other medications affected by chelation	Decreased absorption; dandelion and quinolone coadministration should be avoided
Flaxseed	Fiber content may decrease absorption of oral agents	Oral agents/vitamins/minerals	Decreased absorption; oral agents should be taken 1 h before or 2 h after flaxseed
Psyllium	Fiber content may decrease absorption of oral agents	Carbamazepine, digoxin, lithium	Decreased absorption

Data from Ulbricht, C., Chao, W., Costa, D., et al. (2008). Clinical evidence of herb–drug interactions: A systematic review by the Natural Standard Research Collaboration. *Current Drug Metabolism, 9*, 1063–1120.

immunosuppressants, hypoglycemics, anti-inflammatory agents, antimicrobial agents, antimigraine medications, oral contraceptives, cardiovascular agents, and antiretroviral and anticancer drugs as well as drugs affecting the central nervous, GI, and respiratory systems (Izzo & Ernst, 2009).

In contrast, kava, used as an anxiolytic, and garlic, used to treat dyslipidemia, have both been shown in pharmacokinetic studies to inhibit the cytochrome P-450 enzyme system, specifically CYP2E1 (Izzo & Ernst, 2009). **Table 3.7** shows some common herb–drug interactions affecting metabolism.

Pharmacodynamic Interactions

Herbs may contain ingredients that potentiate the pharmacodynamic effects of certain medications, which may lead to adverse effects. The causative mechanism of these effects may not be well understood in many cases.

Several herbal medications have been shown to inhibit platelet activity and/or have an effect on increasing the INR. Case reports of increased bleeding in patients taking herbal medications with nonsteroidal anti-inflammatory agents, antiplatelet agents, and anticoagulants have been reported (Ulbricht et al., 2008). **Box 3.4** shows herbal medications that may increase the potential for bleeding when given concomitantly with medications that inhibit platelets or alter coagulation.

Some herbal medications have been shown to potentiate the central nervous system (CNS) depressant effects of some medications. Kava, lavender, and valerian may potentiate the effects of CNS depressants, such as barbiturates, benzodiazepines, and narcotics. In addition, kava may interfere with the effects of dopamine or dopamine antagonists and it is potentially hepatotoxic (Kuhn, 2002; Ulbricht et al., 2008).

Aloe has been associated with hypoglycemia in patients taking glibenclamide (glyburide). Bitter orange contains MAO inhibitor substrates such as tyramine and octopamine, and concomitant use with an MAO inhibitor may increase the potential for hypertensive effects (Ulbricht et al., 2008).

While many patients may believe herbal medications are safe because they are "natural" and are available over the counter, the potential for herb–drug interactions still exists. Clinicians must be aware of the potential for these interactions and encourage patients to disclose all medications they are taking, including herbal remedies.

TABLE 3.7

Drug–Herb Metabolism Interactions

Herbal Medication	Mechanism of Action	Object Drug	Results
Garlic	Inhibitor of CYP2E1	Chlorzoxazone	Increased chlorzoxazone levels and potentially other 2E1 substrates
Ginkgo	Inducer of CYP2C19	Antiseizure medications, omeprazole	Decreased levels of valproic acid, phenytoin, and omeprazole possible
Goldenseal (berberine)	Inhibitor of CYP3A4	Cyclosporine	Increase in cyclosporine levels
Kava	Inhibitor of CYP2E1	Chlorzoxazone	Increased chlorzoxazone levels and potentially other 2E1 substrates
Licorice	Inhibitor or inducer of CYP3A4	CYP3A4 substrates	Potential increase or decrease in CYP3A4 substrate levels
Red yeast rice	CYP3A4 inhibitors can increase plasma concentrations of Monacolin K	Monacolin K	Increased plasma concentrations of Monacolin K can result in muscle toxicity
Scotch broom	Haloperidol (CYP2D6 inhibitor) has been shown to increase levels of sparteine	Sparteine	Increased levels of sparteine, which may be potentially cardiotoxic
St. John's wort	Inhibitor of CYP3A4	Alprazolam, amitriptyline, atorvastatin, erythromycin, imatinib, indinavir, irinotecan, ivabradine, methadone, midazolam, nevirapine, nifedipine, oral contraceptives, quazepam, simvastatin, tacrolimus, verapamil, warfarin	May result in decreased efficacy and/or effectiveness of the object drugs listed
	Inducer of CYP2C19	Omeprazole	Decreased levels of omeprazole possible
	Inducer of CYP2E1	Chlorzoxazone	Decreased chlorzoxazone levels and potentially other 2E1 substrates

Data from Ulbricht, C., Chao, W., Costa, D., et al. (2008). Clinical evidence of herb–drug interactions: A systematic review by the Natural Standard Research Collaboration. *Current Drug Metabolism, 9,* 1063–1120 and Izzo, A. A., & Ernst, E. (2009). Interactions between herbal medicines and prescribed drugs: An updated systematic review. *Drugs, 69,* 1777–1798.

BOX 3.4 Herbal Supplements That Potentially Increase Bleeding When Taken with Antiplatelets/Anticoagulants*

Borage seed oil
Clove
Danshen
Devil's claw
Dong quai
Feverfew
Garlic
Ginger
Ginkgo
Ginseng
Goji
Omega-3 fatty acids
Papaya
Peony
Policosanol
Pycnogenol
Saw palmetto
Turmeric

*Data from Ulbricht, C., Chao, W., Costa, D., et al. (2008a). Clinical evidence of herb–drug interactions: A systematic review by the Natural Standard Research Collaboration. *Current Drug Metabolism, 9,* 1063–1120.

DRUG–DISEASE INTERACTIONS

Certain drug–disease interactions can change drug pharmacokinetic and pharmacodynamic parameters, leading to less-than-optimal drug therapeutic outcomes and greater risk of toxicity. In addition, certain drugs can exacerbate a patient's coexisting disease.

Effect of Disease on Pharmacokinetics of Drugs

Absorption

As already discussed, the absorption of drugs may be affected by the presence of other drugs and food in the GI tract. However, drug absorption also depends on the physiologic processes that maintain normal GI function. These processes can include enzyme secretion, acidity, gastric emptying, bile production, and transit time. Thus, any disease that alters the normal physiologic function of the GI system potentially alters drug absorption.

Vitamin B_{12} deficiency is common in patients undergoing stomach surgery. Stomach acid and intrinsic factor play a critical role in the absorption of vitamin B_{12}. Without acid, vitamin B_{12} is not able to be cleaved and released from proteins in food. Vitamin B_{12} and intrinsic factor form a complex and are absorbed in the duodenum. Without intrinsic factor, vitamin B_{12} absorption is impaired (Goldenberg, 2008).

As an example, the gastric-emptying rate can be reduced in patients with duodenal or pyloric ulcers and hypothyroidism. In addition, long-term diabetes can result in diabetic gastroparesis, which delays gastric emptying. This results in later or fluctuating maximal serum concentrations and has been documented with oral hypoglycemic agents. This may become particularly important when a rapid acting drug is required. However, drugs with longer half-lives may be less likely to be affected (Jing et al., 2009). Another example includes bowel edema and intestinal hypoperfusion from advancing heart failure, which can delay the absorption of diuretics prescribed to control edema (Hunt et al., 2009). Finally, diarrhea, a manifestation of many diseases, can pose a problem for oral absorption of drugs as well as food and nutrients.

Distribution

The distribution of drugs can be affected by certain disease states. Of significance are conditions that change plasma albumin levels and therefore can increase or decrease the concentration of drugs usually bound to albumin. Examples of conditions that may decrease plasma albumin levels include burns, bone fractures, acute infections, inflammatory disease, liver disease, malnutrition, and renal disease. Examples of conditions that may increase plasma albumin levels include benign tumors, gynecologic disorders, myalgia, and surgical procedures.

Metabolism

The metabolism of drugs can often be altered by diseases that affect the functions of the liver, such as cirrhosis. Failure of the liver (the primary organ responsible for drug metabolism) not only impairs drug metabolism but can cause a reduction in albumin synthesis. Therefore, the clinical impact of liver failure includes a strong potential for interactions with drugs. Heart failure is another disease that can cause direct reduction in the ability of the liver to metabolize drugs. In patients with heart failure, however, decreased metabolic capacity of the liver is also caused by a decrease in blood flow to the liver owing to changes in cardiac output.

In some cases, normal liver function is needed to activate a drug rather than to inactivate it. Certain drugs like enalapril are called *prodrugs*, meaning the drug needs to be converted by the liver to its active form (enalaprilat) to achieve maximal therapeutic effect. Therefore, use of a prodrug in patients with liver dysfunction can potentially reduce the efficacy of the drug.

Excretion

Renal function can influence serum drug concentrations because most drugs are eliminated by the kidneys either as unchanged drug or as metabolites. Chronic renal diseases that compromise the function of the kidney to clear drugs can result in drug accumulation. Glomerulonephritis, interstitial nephritis, long-term and uncontrolled diabetes, and hypertension are primary causes of declining renal function. In clinical practice, once the patient's estimated creatinine clearance has declined to less than 50 mL/min, dose adjustments usually are required for drugs that are primarily renally cleared. For example, drugs such as H_2 receptor antagonists and fluoroquinolone antibiotics commonly require dose adjustments for patients with renal insufficiency. In particular, the drug regimen of elderly patients or those with an elevated serum creatinine level above 1.5 mg/dL should be evaluated to detect any ADRs from possible drug accumulation secondary to declining renal clearance.

Effects of Drugs on Coexisting Disease

Drugs used to treat one medical condition can sometimes exacerbate the status of another comorbid disease. Practitioners, therefore, should be aware of potential drug–disease interactions. This is of particular importance in elderly individuals who have multiple concomitant diseases and often take multiple medications. Detected rates of drug–disease interactions range from 6% to 30% in older adults (Lindblad et al., 2006). A complete discussion of this topic is beyond the scope of this chapter. However, a consensus statement has been published from a multidisciplinary panel of health care providers whose members specialize in geriatric medicine. The statement identifies several drug–disease interactions that are common in older individuals and are considered to have a deleterious impact on coexisting disease in older individuals. **Table 3.8** lists these common and clinically significant drug–disease interactions in the elderly (American Geriatrics Society, 2012).

PATIENT FACTORS INFLUENCING DRUG INTERACTIONS

The outcomes of drug interactions are highly variable from one person to another. Many patient factors can influence the propensity for an interaction to occur, such as genetics, diseases, environment, smoking, diet/nutrition, and alcohol. An understanding of these factors can help to identify potential sources of drug interactions.

Heredity

As discussed previously, the cytochrome P-450 system can display genetic polymorphism. That is, the variable metabolism of drugs by cytochrome P-450 enzymes from one person to another in the population can be partly explained by genetic differences. For example, approximately 8% of Americans lack the gene to form the isoenzyme CYP2D6 and therefore are at greater risk for toxicity from psychotropic drugs and, potentially, other drugs that are metabolized by these isoenzymes. The metabolism of isoniazid also demonstrates variation among different people; some acetylate isoniazid very rapidly, whereas others acetylate it slowly.

Warfarin is a widely used oral anticoagulant. Its dose depends on age and CYP2C9 genotype. It works by depleting the supply of vitamin K. The formation of vitamin K depends on a protein known as vitamin K epoxide reductase complex

TABLE 3.8

Drug–Disease Interactions Common in the Elderly*

Disease/Condition	Drug/Drug Class
Benign prostatic hyperplasia	Anticholinergics
	Tricyclic antidepressants
Chronic renal failure	Nonaspirin NSAIDs
Heart failure (systolic dysfunction)	First-generation calcium channel blockers
Constipation	Anticholinergics
	Opioid analgesics
	Tricyclic antidepressants
Dementia	Anticholinergics
	Barbiturates
	Benzodiazepines
	Tricyclic antidepressants
Diabetes	Corticosteroids
Falls	Antipsychotics (thioridazine/haloperidol)
	Benzodiazepines
	Sedative hypnotics
	Tricyclic antidepressants
Heart block	Digoxin
	Tricyclic antidepressants
Narrow-angle glaucoma	Anticholinergics
Parkinson disease	Metoclopramide
Peptic ulcer disease	Aspirin
	Nonaspirin NSAIDs
Postural hypotension	Thioridazine
	Tricyclic antidepressants
Seizures	Bupropion
Syncope	Alpha-blockers (e.g., doxazosin, terazosin, methyldopa)

*Data from Lindblad, C. I., Hanlon, J. T., Gross, C. R., et al. (2006). Clinically important drug–disease interactions and their prevalence in older adults. *Clinical Therapeutics, 28*, 1133–1143.

subunit 1 gene (VKORC1). Mutations of this particular gene have been associated with a decrease in formation of clotting factors and warfarin resistance (Sconce et al., 2005).

Disease

Another important factor that influences drug interactions is the patient's existing disease state. Any disease affecting liver or kidney function can potentially predispose the patient to drug interactions and ADRs because these organs are primary sites of drug metabolism and elimination, respectively. Significant deterioration in drug metabolism or elimination can lead to increased serum drug concentrations and therefore increase the likelihood for drugs to interact. Consequently, elderly patients and those with a history of liver disease or renal insufficiency should be evaluated for dose adjustments of drugs significantly cleared by the liver and kidneys. For example, enoxaparin is a drug used to treat various clotting disorders. It is renally cleared from the body. Poor kidney function could lead to its accumulation. If the dose is not lowered in these patients, they could be exposed to too much enoxaparin resulting in excessive bleeding (Nutescu et al., 2009).

Environment

Environmental factors, such as DDT and other pesticides, can increase the activity of liver enzymes, potentially causing an increase in drug metabolism. Although the general significance of the effect of environmental exposure on the clinical outcome of drug therapy has not been well studied, people working in occupations with prolonged exposure to toxins and chemicals should be more closely observed.

Smoking

Studies show that smoking can increase the liver's metabolism of certain drugs, including diazepam, propoxyphene, chlorpromazine, and amitriptyline. For example, the polycyclic aromatic hydrocarbons in cigarettes can induce CYP1A2 metabolism, resulting in decreased theophylline serum concentrations (Schein, 1995).

Diet and Nutrition

The nutritional status and dietary intake of the patient can influence the importance of a drug–nutrient interaction. Drugs can deplete valuable vitamins and minerals from food; however, these interactions are often difficult to recognize and may go undetected. Patients with poor baseline nutrition (e.g., alcoholics) may experience more pronounced effects mainly because of underlying nutritional deficiency. Practitioners should be aware of potential drug–nutrient interactions by identifying patients who have poor dietary intake and who concurrently take medications that can deplete vitamins and minerals.

Alcohol Intake

Alcohol can complicate drug therapy on many different levels. Alcohol has a variable effect on drug metabolism depending on acute or chronic intake. Acute alcohol ingestion can inhibit drug metabolism, thus increasing serum drug concentrations; it also can enhance the pharmacodynamic effect of drugs with properties of CNS depression. Patients concurrently taking narcotics, antihistamines, antidepressants, antipsychotics, and muscle relaxants with alcohol are at greatest risk for CNS depression and should be warned of this interaction (Trovato et al., 1991). In addition, acute ingestion of alcohol can increase the potential for hypoglycemia in diabetic patients taking insulin or insulin secretagogues (e.g., sulfonylureas). Metronidazole is an antibiotic used to treat intra-abdominal infections. When taken with alcohol, it inhibits the enzyme, aldehyde dehydrogenase, which is responsible for metabolizing alcohol. This results in an accumulation of the intermediate metabolite, acetaldehyde, causing a disulfiram-like reaction such as facial flushing, headache, nausea and vomiting, weakness, dizziness, blurred vision, confusion, and hypotension.

In contrast, chronic alcohol intake tends to increase the synthesis of drug-metabolizing enzymes, leading to induction. Enzyme induction causes decreases in serum drug levels. Enzyme induction secondary to chronic alcohol use increases conversion of acetaminophen to hepatotoxic metabolites. Chronic use of alcohol in combination with high doses of acetaminophen (often from several sources) above that recommended in the labeling may result in liver damage (Jang & Harris, 2007). In addition, chronic use of alcohol in combination with NSAIDs or aspirin increases the risk of GI bleeding. Long-term abuse of alcohol leads to liver cirrhosis, which ultimately impairs drug metabolism by destruction of functional hepatocytes.

ADVERSE DRUG REACTIONS

An ADR can be defined as an undesirable clinical manifestation that is consequent to and caused by the administration of a particular drug. ADRs are basically drug-induced toxic reactions. The World Health Organization defines an ADR as "a response to a medicine which is noxious and unintended, and which occurs at doses normally used in man" (Nebeker et al., 2004).

There are two general types to consider. The first type of ADR is an exaggeration of the principal pharmacologic action of the drug. The ADR is simply a more pronounced drug response than normal. These reactions usually are dose dependent and predictable. These are often referred to as type A reactions.

In the second type, type B reactions, the ADR is unrelated to the principal pharmacologic action of the drug itself. These reactions are precipitated by the secondary pharmacologic actions of the drug, may be unpredictable, and may or may not be dose dependent. In either type, the ADR can result from overdosage of drug or administration of therapeutic doses to a patient hyperreactive to the drug or as an indirect consequence of the primary action.

ADRs are sometimes referred to as side effects. A side effect is also recognized as an undesirable pharmacologic effect that accompanies the primary drug action and usually occurs within the therapeutic dosing range. ADRs or side effects can have varying levels of intensity. For example, the dry mouth and blurred vision that occur from drugs with anticholinergic properties are considered routine side effects of that class of medication. In contrast, drug-induced liver damage would be an uncommon and severe ADR or side effect not routinely associated with that class of medication. Patients experiencing ADRs or side effects from drugs do not necessarily require discontinuation of therapy; however, proper drug selection emphasizing agents with minimal side effect profiles may help improve patient acceptance of and compliance with the drug.

TABLE 3.9

Potential Causes of Medication Errors

Potential Causes of Medication Errors	Example
Dosage conversion	When converting from oral to IV medications and vice versa, it is often not a 1 to 1 conversion. Levothyroxine 100 mcg oral dose is equal to ~50 mcg IV dose.
Foreign drugs	Dilacor is the brand name drug for diltiazem in the United States. In Serbia, it is the brand name drug for digoxin.
Illegible handwriting	Isordil was mistakenly filled with Plendil.
Look-alike and soundalike	Phenylephrine vial mistaken for metoclopramide vial.
Unacceptable abbreviations	Insulin 5.0 units was mistaken for 50 units.

Medication Errors

Medication errors are also a potential cause of ADRs. These errors could range from switching from one dosage form to another to using foreign drugs. **Table 3.9** lists some potential causes of ADRs. Some drugs may look-alike and soundalike. The Institute for Safe Medication Practices (2015) provides a list of drugs with confused drug names. For example, **Figure 3.3** shows two look-alike vials of drugs were mixed-up and a patient inadvertently received phenylephrine instead of metoclopramide. Phenylephrine is a potent blood vessel vasoconstrictor often used to manage hypotension. Metoclopramide is a drug often used to treat nausea and vomiting. The event can lead to pulmonary edema and cardiac arrest.

Tracking Drug Interactions and Adverse Drug Reactions

The initial source of documented ADRs comes primarily from the experience gained while using a drug during clinical trials. Usually, the number of people taking the drug in clinical trials, on the order of hundreds to several thousands, is too few to detect all the possible adverse reactions from the drug. However, after a drug is approved by the FDA, it becomes readily available for public use in hundreds of thousands to millions of people. The potential for drug interactions and ADRs then becomes much greater than during clinical trials. Therefore, practitioners should have a basic understanding of drug interactions and ADRs and report these events to the FDA when they occur.

MedWatch is a medical product reporting program conducted by the FDA (**Figure 3.4**). The purpose of the MedWatch program is to enhance the effectiveness of surveillance of drugs and medical products after they are marketed and as they are used in clinical practice. The benefit to health care providers for reporting drug interactions and ADRs is to ensure that drug safety information is rapidly communicated to health care professionals, thus improving patient care. Health care providers should also be aware of programs in their own institutions that collect and report ADRs or drug interactions.

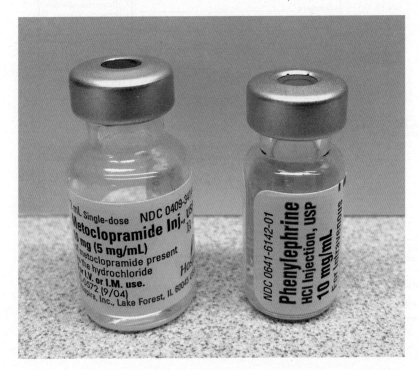

FIGURE 3.3 Look-alike drugs: Phenylephrine vial was mistaken for a metoclopramide vial.

MEDWATCH
THE FDA MEDICAL PRODUCTS REPORTING PROGRAM

For VOLUNTARY reporting
by health professional of adverse
events and product problems

Page ___ of ___

Form Approved OMB No. 0910-0291 Expires: 12/31/94
See OMB statement on reverse
FDA Use Only **(DAVIS)**
Triage unit
sequence #

A. Patient information

1. Patient identifier In confidence

2. Age at time of event:
or ___
Date of birth

3. Sex ☐ female ☐ male

4. Weight ___ lbs or ___ kgs

B. Adverse event or product problem

1. ☐ Adverse event and/or ☐ Product problem (e.g., defects/malfunctions)

2. Outcomes attributed to adverse event (check all that apply)
☐ death ___ (mo day yr)
☐ life-threatening
☐ hospitalization - initial or prolonged
☐ disability
☐ congenital anomaly
☐ required intervention to prevent permanent impairment/damage
☐ other: ___

3. Date of event (mo day yr)

4. Date of this report (mo day yr)

5. Describe event or problem

6. Relevant tests/laboratory data, including dates

7. Other relevant history, including preexisting medical conditions (e.g., allergies, race, pregnancy, smoking and alcohol use, hepatic/renal dysfunction, etc.)

PLEASE TYPE OR USE BLACK INK

C. Suspect medications(s)

1. Name (give labeled strength & mfr/labeler, if known)
#1
#2

2. Dose, frequency & route used
#1
#2

3. Therapy dates (if unknown. give duration) from (to or best estimate)
#1
#2

4. Diagnosis for use (indication)
#1
#2

5. Event abated after use stopped or dose reduced
#1 ☐ yes ☐ no ☐ doesn't apply
#2 ☐ yes ☐ no ☐ doesn't apply

6. Lot # (if known)
#1
#2

7. Exp. date (if known)
#1
#2

8. Event reappeared after reintroduction
#1 ☐ yes ☐ no ☐ doesn't apply
#2 ☐ yes ☐ no ☐ doesn't apply

9. NDC # (for product problems only)

10. Concomitant medical products and therapy dates (exclude treatment of event)

D. Suspect medical device

1. Brand name

2. Type of device

3. Manufacturer name & address

4. Operator of device
☐ health professional
☐ lay user/patient
☐ other: ___

5. Expiration date (mo day yr)

6.
model # ___
catalog # ___
serial # ___
lot # ___
other #

7. If implanted, give date (mo day yr)

8. If explanted, give date (mo day yr)

9. Device available for evaluation? (Do not send to FDA)
☐ yes ☐ no ☐ returned to manufacturer on ___ (mo day yr)

10. Concomitant medical products and therapy dates (exclude treatment of event)

E. Reporter (see confidentiality section on back)

1. Name, address & phone #

2. Health professional? ☐ yes ☐ no

3. Occupation

4. Also reported to
☐ manufacturer
☐ user facility
☐ distributor

5. If you do NOT want your identity disclosed to the manufacturer, place an "X" in this box. ☐

Mail to: MEDWATCH
5600 Fishers Lane
Rockville, MD 20852-9787

or **FAX to :**
1-800-FDA-0178

FDA Form 3500 (6/93)   Submission of a report does not constitute an admission that medical personnel or the product caused or contributed to the event.

FIGURE 3.4 MedWatch form for reporting an adverse event or product problem to the U.S. FDA.

CASE STUDY*

A.C. is a 60-year-old Caucasian woman with newly diagnosed peptic ulcer disease, generalized anxiety disorder, and iron deficiency anemia. She also has a long history of asthma and depression. She is a strong believer of herbal medicine. She takes St. John's wort for her depression, iron pills for her anemia, and alprazolam (Xanax) as needed for her anxiety. During her asthma exacerbation, she is instructed to take prednisone for at least 5 days. She also takes esomeprazole (Nexium) for her peptic ulcer disease. Three months later, she experienced severe fatigue, shortness of breath, dizziness, and swelling/soreness in the tongue. Her asthma is well controlled with the occasional use of albuterol (Proventil) inhaler. During her physical exam, her physician suspected that she had bacterial vaginosis and gave her a prescription for a 1-week course of metronidazole (Flagyl). She drinks at least two to three cans of beer per day.

DIAGNOSIS: DRUG–DRUG INTERACTIONS

1. St. John's wort is known to inhibit which of her medication that is known to be metabolized by cytochrome P-450 (CYP3A4) and could potentially cause her to experience significant fatigue?
2. Which of her medication could interfere with the absorption of her iron pills?
3. Which of her medication could potentially cause her to develop vitamin B_{12} deficiency?
4. How does metronidazole interfere with alcohol?
5. If she was given a prescription for ketoconazole, which of her medication could interfere with its absorption?

* Answers can be found online.

Bibliography

Starred references are cited in the text.

*Ameer, B., & Weintraub, R. A. (1997). Drug interactions with grapefruit juice. *Clinical Pharmacokinetics, 33*(2), 103–121.

*American Geriatrics Society (AGS). (2012). Updated beers criteria for potentially inappropriate medication use in older adults. *Journal of the American Geriatrics Society, 60*(4), 616–631.

*American Society of Health-System Pharmacists. (2008). *AHFS drug information 2008.* (1961, 3062). Bethesda, MD: Author.

*Bailey, D. C., Arnold, J. M. O., Strong, H. A., et al. (1993). Effect of grapefruit juice and naringin on nisoldipine pharmacokinetics. *Clinical Pharmacology and Therapeutics, 54*, 589–594.

*Bailey, D. G., Malcolm, J., Arnold, O., et al. (1998). Grapefruit juice–drug interactions. *British Journal of Clinical Pharmacology, 46*, 101–110.

*Bailey, D. G., Munoz, C., Arnold, J. M. O., et al. (1992). Grapefruit juice and naringin interaction with nitrendipine [Abstract]. *Clinical Pharmacology and Therapeutics, 51*, 156.

*Bailey, D. G., Spence, J. D., Munoz, C., et al. (1991). Interaction of citrus juices with felodipine and nifedipine. *Lancet, 337*, 268–269.

*Becker, M. L., Visser, L. E., van Gelder, T., et al. (2008). Increasing exposure to drug–drug interactions between 1992 and 2005 in people aged ≥55 years. *Drugs and Aging, 25*, 145–152.

Benard-Laribiere, A., Miremont-Salame, G., & Perault-Pochat, M. (2014). Incidence of hospital admissions due to adverse drug reactions in France: The EMIR study. *Fundamental and Clinical Pharmacology, 29*, 106–111.

*Bjerrum, L., Lopez-Valcarcel, B. G., & Petersen, G. (2008). Risk factors for potential drug interactions in general practice. *European Journal of General Practice, 14*, 23–29.

*Braun, L. D. (1997). Therapeutic drug monitoring. In L. Shargel, A. H. Mutnick, P. F. Souney, et al. (Eds.). *Comprehensive pharmacy review* (3rd ed., pp. 586–597). Baltimore, MD: Lippincott Williams & Wilkins.

*Brosen, K. (1990). Recent developments in hepatic drug oxidation: Implications for clinical pharmacokinetics. *Clinical Pharmacokinetics, 18*, 220–239.

Chan, L. (2013). Drug–nutrient interactions. *Journal of Parenteral and Enteral Nutrition, 37*, 450–459.

Clarke, T., et al. (2015). National Health Statistics Report. Trends in the use of complementary health approaches among adults: United States, 2002–2012. *National Health Statistics, 79*, 1–15.

*Clopidogrel (Plavix®) prescribing information. Retrieved from http://products.sanofi-aventis.us/PLAVIX/PLAVIX.html on July 29, 2010.

Cupp, M., & Tracy, T. (1997). Role of the cytochrome P450 3A subfamily in drug interactions. *US Pharmacist, 22*, HS9–HS21.

Deppermann, K. M., & Lode, H. (1993). Fluoroquinolones: Interaction profile during enteral absorption. *Drugs, 45*(Suppl. 3), 65–72.

Drew, R. H., & Gallis, H. A. (1992). Azithromycin—Spectrum of activity, pharmacokinetics, and clinical applications. *Pharmacotherapy, 12*, 161–173.

FDA Drug Safety Communication: Reduced effectiveness of Plavix (clopidogrel) in patients who are poor metabolizers of the drug. Retrieved from http://www.fda.gov/Drugs/DrugSafety/PostmarketDrugSafetyInformationforPatientsandProviders/ucm203888.htm on July 16, 2015.

*FDA Table of Pharmacogenomic Biomarkers in Drug Labeling. Retrieved from http://www.fda.gov/Drugs/ScienceResearch/ResearchAreas/Pharmacogenetics/ucm083378.htm on July 16, 2015.

Fraser, A. G. (1997). Pharmacokinetic interactions between alcohol and other drugs. *Clinical Pharmacokinetics, 33*(2), 79–90.

*Goldenberg, L. (2008). Nutritional deficiencies following bariatric surgery. *Gastroenterology and Endoscopy*, 31–37.

*Guengerich, F. (1994). Catalytic selectivity of human cytochrome P450 enzymes: Relevance to drug metabolism and toxicity. *Toxicology Letters, 70*, 133–138.

Hansten, P. D. (1998). Understanding drug–drug interactions. *Science and Medicine*, (Jan/Feb), 16–20.

*Hansten, P. D., & Horn, J. R. (2015). *Drug interactions: Top 100 drug interactions: A guide to patient management.* Freeland, WA: H&H Publications.

Harder, S., & Thurmann, P. (1996). Clinically important drug interactions with anticoagulants: An update. *Clinical Pharmacokinetics, 30*, 416–444.

Herb Fact Sheet. (2006). National Toxicology Program. Retrieved from http://ntp.niehs.nih.gov/ntp/Factsheets/HerbalFacts06.pdf on July 24, 2010.

*Highlights of Prescribing Information: Ziagen (abacavir sulfate) Tablets and Oral Solution. Retrieved from http://www.accessdata.fda.gov/drugsatfda_docs/label/2008/020977s019,020978s022lbl.pdf on July 27, 2010.

*Holmes, D. R., Dehmer, G. J., Kaul, S., et al. (2010). ACCF/AHA clopidogrel clinical alert: Approaches to the FDA "Boxed Warning": A report of the American College of Cardiology Foundation Task Force on Clinical Expert Consensus Documents and the American Heart Association. *Journal of the American College of Cardiology, 56*, 321–341.

52 UNIT 1 | PRINCIPLES OF THERAPEUTICS

*Horn, J. R., & Hansen, P. D. (2004). Drug interactions with digoxin: The role of P-glycoprotein. *Pharmacy Times (October)*. Retrieved from http://www.hanstenandhorn.com/hh-article10-04.pdf

*Huang, S. M., Hall, S. D., Watkins P., et al. (2004). Drug interactions with herbal products and grapefruit juice: A conference report. *Clinical Pharmacology and Therapeutics, 75*, 1–12.

*Hunt, S. A., Abraham, W. T., Chin, M. H., et al. (2009). 2009 Focused update incorporated into the ACC/AHA 2005 guidelines for the diagnosis and management of heart failure in adults. *Circulation, 119*, e391–e479.

*Ingelman-Sundberg, M. (2004). Pharmacogenetics of cytochromes P450 and its applications in drug therapy; the past, present and future. *Trends in Pharmacological Sciences, 25*(4), 193–200.

Institute for Safe Medication Practices (ISMP). 2015. *ISMP's list of confused drug names*. Retrieved from https://www.ismp.org/tools/confuseddrugnames.pdf

ISMP Quarter Watch. (2014). Adverse drug events in children under age 18. Retrieved from www.ismp.org/quarterwatch

*Izzo, A. A., & Ernst, E. (2009). Interactions between herbal medicines and prescribed drugs: An updated systematic review. *Drugs, 69*, 1777–1798.

*Jahnchen, E., Meinertz, T., Gilfrich, H.-J., et al. (1978). Enhanced elimination of warfarin during treatment with cholestyramine. *British Journal of Clinical Pharmacology, 5*, 437–440.

*Jang, G. R., & Harris, R. Z. (2007). Drug interactions involving ethanol and alcoholic beverages. *Expert Opinion on Drug Metabolism and Toxicology, 3*, 719–731.

*Jing, M., Rayner, C. K., Jones, K. L., et al. (2009). Diabetic gastroparesis diagnosis and management. *Drugs, 69*, 971–986.

Johnson, K. A., Strum, D. P., & Watkins, W. D. (1995). Pharmacology and the critical care patient. In P. L. Munson, R. A. Mueller, & G. R. Breese (Eds.), *Principles of pharmacology: Basic concepts and clinical application* (pp. 1673–1688). New York, NY: Chapman & Hall.

*Jones, A.W., Karlsson, L. (2005). Relation between blood- and urine amphetamine concentrations in impaired drivers as influenced by urinary pH and creatinine. *Human and Experimental Toxicology, 24*, 615–622.

*Kim, R. B. (2002). Drugs as P-glycoprotein substrates, inhibitors, and inducers. *Drug Metabolism Reviews, 34*, 47–54.

Kirk, J. K. (1995). Significant drug–nutrient interactions. *American Family Physicians, 51*(5), 1175–1182.

*Kivisto, K., Neuvonen, P., & Koltz, U. (1994). Inhibition of terfenadine metabolism: Pharmacokinetic and pharmacodynamic consequences. *Clinical Pharmacokinetics, 27*, 1–5.

*Kuhn, M. A. (2002). Herbal remedies: Drug–herb interactions. *Critical Care Nurse, 22*, 22–32.

Lazarou, J., Pomeranz, B., & Corey, P. (1998). Incidence of adverse drug reactions in hospitalized patients: A meta-analysis of prospective studies. *Journal of the American Medical Association, 279*, 1200–1205.

*Lindblad, C. I., Hanlon, J. T., Gross, C. R., et al. (2006). Clinically important drug–disease interactions and their prevalence in older adults. *Clinical Therapeutics, 28*, 1133–1143.

*Lovastatin (Mevacor®) prescribing information. Retrieved from http://www.merck.com/product/usa/pi_circulars/m/mevacor/mevacor_pi.pdf on July 30, 2010.

*Mancano, M. A. (2005). Clinically significant drug interactions with warfarin. *Pharmacy Times*. Retrieved from https://secure.pharmacytimes.com/lessons/200301-01.asp on July 27, 2010.

*Mathews, D., McNutt, B., Okerholam, R., et al. (1991). Torsades de pointes occurring in association with terfenadine use. *Journal of the American Medical Association, 266*, 2375–2376.

Martins A. C., Giordani, F., & Rozenfeld, S. (2014). Adverse events among adult patient inpatients: A meta-analysis of observational studies. *Journal of Clinical Pharmacy and Therapeutics, 39*, 609–620.

May, R. J. (1993). Adverse drug reactions and interactions. In J. T. DiPiro, R. L. Talbert, P. E. Hayes, et al. (Eds.), *Pharmacotherapy: A pathophysiologic approach* (2nd ed., pp. 71–83). East Norwalk, CT: Appleton & Lange.

*Michalets, E. (1998). Update: Clinically significant cytochrome P-450 drug interactions. *Annals of Pharmacotherapy, 18*, 84–112.

*Nebeker, J. R., et al. (2004). Clarifying adverse drug events: A clinician's guide to terminology, documentation, and reporting. *Annals of Internal Medicine, 140*, 795–801.

*Nebert, D., Adesnich, M., Coon, M., et al. (1987). The P450 gene superfamily: Recommended nomenclature. *DNA, 6*, 1–11.

*Nutescu, E., Spinler, S., Wittkowsky, A., et al. (2009). Low-molecular weight heparins in renal impairment and obesity: Available evidence and clinical practice recommendations across medical and surgical settings. *Annals of Pharmacotherapy, 43*, 1064–1083.

Olivier, P., Bertrand, L., Tubery, M., et al. (2009). Hospitalizations because of adverse drug reactions in elderly patients admitted through the emergency department: A prospective survey. *Drugs and Aging, 26*, 475–482.

Pharmacist's Letter. (2008). Alcohol-related drug interactions. *24*, 1–11.

Plaa, G. L., & Smith, R. P. (1995). General principles of toxicology. In P. L. Munson, R. A. Mueller, & G. R. Breese (Eds.), *Principles of pharmacology: Basic concepts and clinical application* (pp. 1537–1543). New York, NY: Chapman & Hall.

*Rashid, J., McKinstry, C., Renwick, A. G., et al. (1993). Quercetin, an in vitro inhibitor of CYP3A, does not contribute to the interaction between nifedipine and grapefruit juice. *British Journal of Clinical Pharmacology, 36*, 460–463.

*Sacks, G. (2004). Drug–nutrient considerations in patients receiving parenteral and enteral nutrition. *Practical Gastroenterology*, 39–48.

*Schein, J. R. (1995). Cigarette smoking and clinically significant drug interactions. *Annals of Pharmacotherapy, 29*, 1139–1147.

*Sconce, E. A., Khan, T. I., Wynne, H. A., et al. (2005). The impact of CYP2C9 and VKORC1 genetic polymorphism and patient characteristics upon warfarin dose requirements: Proposal for a new dosing regimen. *Blood, 106*(7), 2329–2333.

*Scott, S. A., Sangkuhl, K., Gardner, E., et al. (2011). Clinical pharmacogenetics implementation consortium guidelines for cytochrome P450-2C19 genotype and clopidogrel therapy. *Clinical Pharmacology and Therapeutics, 90*(2), 328–332.

Shargel, L., & Yu, A. B. C. (1993). *Applied biopharmaceutics and pharmacokinetics* (3rd ed.). East Norwalk, CT: Appleton & Lange.

*Shinn, A. F. (1992). Clinical relevance of cimetidine drug interactions. *Drug Safety, 7*, 245–267.

Simvastatin (Zocor®) prescribing information. Retrieved from http://www.merck.com/product/usa/pi_circulars/z/zocor/zocor_pi.pdf on July 29, 2010.

Spinler, S., Cheng, J., Kindwall, K., et al. (1995). Possible inhibition of hepatic metabolism of quinidine by erythromycin. *Clinical Pharmacology and Therapeutics, 57*, 89–94.

*Sultana, J., Cutroneo, P., & Trifiro, G. (2013). Clinical and economic burden of adverse drug reactions. *Journal of Pharmacology and Pharmacotherapeutics, 4*(Suppl.), S73–S77.

*Susla, G. M. (2005). Miscellaneous antibiotics. In S. C. Piscitelli, K. A. Rodvold (Eds.), *Drug interactions in infectious diseases* (2nd ed., pp. 358–359). Totowa, NJ: Humana Press, Inc.

Tegretol (carbamazepine USP) Label. Retrieved from http://www.accessdata.fda.gov/drugsatfda_docs/label/2009/016608s101,018281s048lbl.pdf on July 27, 2010.

*The Medical Letter. (2009). In brief: Tamoxifen and SSRI interactions. *The Medical Letter on Drugs and Therapeutics, 51*, 45.

*Toh, S., Mitchell, A., Anderka, M., et al. (2011). Antibiotics and oral contraceptive failure—A case-crossover study. *Contraception, 83*(5), 418–425.

*Trovato, A., Nuhlicek, D. N., & Midtling, J. E. (1991). Drug–nutrient interactions. *American Family Practitioner, 44*, 1651–1658.

*Ulbricht, C., Chao, W., Costa, D., et al. (2008). Clinical evidence of herb–drug interactions: A systematic review by the Natural Standard Research Collaboration. *Current Drug Metabolism, 9*, 1063–1120.

*Weaver, K., & Glasier, A. (1999). Interaction between broad-spectrum antibiotics and the combined oral contraceptive pill: A literature review. *Contraception, 59*, 71–78.

*Woosley, R. (1996). Cardiac actions of antihistamines. *Annual Review of Pharmacology and Toxicology, 36*, 233–252.

*Zithromax (Pfizer Pharmaceuticals). Package insert. (2013).

*Zocor (Merck & Co.). Package insert. (2015).

4 Principles of Pharmacotherapy in Pediatrics

Anita Siu ■ James C. Thigpen Jr

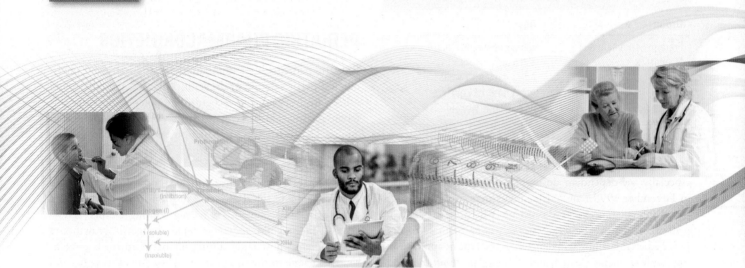

When treating pediatric patients, many health care practitioners use the terms *infant*, *child*, or even *kid* interchangeably. However, there are currently accepted terms that define the different age categories of pediatric patients (**Table 4.1**). These terms should be used for accuracy when describing young patients and especially when determining drug dosages. Safe and effective drug therapy in pediatric patients is based on a firm understanding of three concepts:

- Ongoing maturation and development in pediatric patients and their effect on a drug's absorption, distribution, metabolism, and excretion. Interpatient variabilities may be attributed to physiologic changes throughout childhood.
- Short- and long-term effects that the prescribed drug will have on a pediatric patient's growth and development
- Effects of underlying congenital, chronic, or current diseases on the prescribed drug, and vice versa

The popular concept that the pediatric patient is merely a "little or small adult," and therefore, pediatric pharmacokinetics, drug dosing, and even adverse effects can be extrapolated from the results of adult clinical drug trials is a serious misconception. Although many drugs do exhibit similarities between the adult and pediatric populations, the assumption of resemblance should not be applied to all drugs. Several tragic drug misadventures in the 1960s and 1970s illustrate this. Extrapolated data from adult responses to chloramphenicol (Chloromycetin) led to its use in neonates in the 1960s. When given chloramphenicol, these neonates developed gray baby syndrome, hypotension, and hypoxemia, leading eventually to shock and death (Haile, 1977). This occurred because neonates, unlike adults, lack the enzyme needed to metabolize chloramphenicol. Another tragedy in the 1970s involved the topical antimicrobial cleanser hexachlorophene.

Used routinely and safely in adults, hexachlorophene caused vacuolar encephalopathy of the brain stem in premature neonates after they were repeatedly bathed in a 3% solution (Anonymous, 1972).

Several barriers exist for pharmaceutical manufacturers in conducting pediatric clinical trials, such as fears of unforeseen adverse events affecting growth or development or difficulties in obtaining informed consent or blood samples. In turn, the lack of clinical trials in pediatric patients prevents the U.S. Food and Drug Administration (FDA) from approving drugs for use in the pediatric population. As such, the prescribing information commonly states "Pediatric Use: Safety and effectiveness in pediatric patients has not been established."

Without FDA approval or adequate documented information, many practitioners are uncertain how to use drugs in pediatrics. This leaves prescribers little choice but to use drugs in pediatric patients in an off-label capacity, based on adult data, uncontrolled pediatric studies, or personal experience. In 1997, the FDA took the initiative to increase the quantity and quality of clinical drug trials in the pediatric population by proposing alternate ways to obtain FDA approval. The FDA would waive the need for well-controlled clinical drug trials if drug manufacturers provided other satisfactory data for drugs already approved for the same use in adults. These data could include the results of controlled or uncontrolled pediatric studies, pharmacodynamic studies, safety reports, and premarketing or postmarketing studies. Alternatively, the drug manufacturer could provide evidence demonstrating that the disease course and drug effects are sufficiently similar in adult and pediatric patients in order to support extrapolation of data from adult clinical trials. In addition, pediatric pharmacokinetic studies are necessary to provide

TABLE 4.1

Age Groups of Pediatric Population

Group	Age
Preterm or premature	<36 wk gestational age
Neonate	<30 d old
Infant	Age 1 mo until 1 y old
Child	Age 1 until 12 y old
Adolescent	Age 12 until 18 y old

data for an appropriate pediatric dosage recommendation, especially age-dependent dosing. An FDA regulation issued in December 1998 required manufacturers to provide additional information about the use of their drug products in pediatric patients. The nature of the studies required to support pediatric labeling will depend on the type of application, the condition being treated, and existing data about the product's safety and efficacy in pediatric patients. Manufacturers will be required to study the drug in all relevant pediatric age groups (U.S. FDA, 1998a). Over the years, the FDA has encouraged more well-controlled trials on drug efficacy and safety in pediatrics. The FDA Modernization Act of 1997 and the Best Pharmaceuticals for Children Act of 2002 offered support for the pharmaceutical industries to conduct and submit pediatric clinical trials. Companies that conduct appropriate clinical trials are eligible to receive a 6-month patent extension on their product. The Pediatric Research Equity Act of 2003 mandated that drugs used in pediatrics require literature or clinical trials supporting their use, even

if the original patent did not have a pediatric indication. As a result, pediatric pharmacotherapy will evolve with additional clinical trials.

PEDIATRIC PHARMACOKINETICS

Pediatric patients differ from adults, anatomically and physiologically. For safe use of drugs in pediatrics, prescribers and other caregivers need to recognize the potential for very different pharmacokinetics in pediatric patients as opposed to adults. The differences are based on developing body tissues and organs, which affect a drug's absorption, distribution, metabolism, and excretion.

Changes in a pediatric patient's body proportions and composition and the relative size of the liver and kidneys can alter the pharmacokinetics of a drug. During the first several years of life, a child undergoes rapid changes in growth and development, most rapid during infancy. Growth is a quantitative change in the size of the body or any of its parts, and development is a qualitative change in skills or functions. Maturation, a genetically controlled development independent of the environment, is a slower process, lasting until late childhood. **Table 4.2** summarizes pharmacokinetic differences in pediatric patients.

By the end of the first year of life, an infant's weight triples, whereas body surface area (BSA) and length double. Accompanying these changes in growth and development are changes in body composition, intracellular and extracellular body water, fat, and protein. Approximately 75% to 80% of a full-term neonate's body weight is total body water (Friis-Hansen, 1957). By age 3 months, total body water constitutes

TABLE 4.2

Age-Related Pharmacokinetic Differences in Children Compared with Adults

	Premature Neonate	Neonate	Infant	Child	Adolescent
Absorption					
Gastric acidity	↓	↓	↓	=	=
Gastric emptying time	↓	↓	=	=	=
GI motility	↓	↓	↓	=	=
Pancreatic enzyme activity	↓↓	↓	↓	=	=
GI surface area	↑	↑	↑	↑	=
Skin permeability	↑↑	↑	=	=	=
Distribution					
Blood–brain barrier	↓	↓	=	=	=
Plasma proteins	↓↓	↓	=	=	=
Metabolism					
Liver	↓	↓	↓	=/↑	=
Elimination					
Renal blood flow	↓	↓	↓	=	=
Glomerular filtration	↓	↓	↓	=	=
Tubular function	↓	↓	↓	=	=

approximately 65% of the patient's body weight. Extracellular water progressively declines and intracellular water increases faster than total body water, exceeding extracellular water (Friis-Hansen, 1957). The decreasing percentage of body weight from total body water is replaced by an increase in body fat during the first 5 months of life. In fact, the percentage of body weight from fat doubles in these 5 months. The protein percentage increases during the second year of life as fat is lost, primarily because of ambulation. The liver and kidney reach their maximum size relative to body weight by age 2, producing a "peak" in the child's metabolism and elimination. After age 2, the child's liver and kidney size/body weight ratios steadily decrease until adult liver and kidney ratios are reached by adolescence.

Oral Absorption

The extent of a drug's absorption in a pediatric patient depends on a variety of factors: gastric pH, gastric and intestinal transit time, gastrointestinal surface area, enzymes, and microorganism flora or any combination thereof.

Gastric pH

Basal and stimulated secretion of gastric acid controls the pH of the stomach. The stomach pH is alkaline at birth (greater than 4) because of residual amniotic fluid and the immaturity of parietal cells. As gastric acid is produced, the pH falls. By the end of the first day of life, the basal and stimulated rates are equal, although lower than the rates in adults. An increased stomach pH (alkaline) adversely affects the absorption of weakly acidic drugs and improves the absorption of weakly basic drugs. This phenomenon results from increased ionization of the weakly acidic drug, producing more ionized (polar) drug, which moves poorly across the nonpolar gastric membrane, and vice versa for weakly basic drug. For example, the bioavailability of phenobarbital (a weak acid) is decreased in neonates, infants, and young children because their alkaline gastric pH produces more ionized phenobarbital, which crosses the gastric membrane poorly.

For weakly basic drugs, the alkaline stomach pH increases the nonionized form of the drug, which then easily moves across the gastric membrane. By the second year of life, the child's gastric acid output on a per kilogram body weight basis is similar to that observed in the adult (Deren, 1971). As a result, gastric pH affects the degree of drug ionization, thus changing the amount of drug absorbed.

Gastric Emptying Time and Surface Area

The gastric emptying time is delayed in both preterm and full-term neonates during the first 24 hours of life. No studies have been conducted beyond the immediate neonatal period. The combination of delayed gastric emptying time and gastroesophageal reflux can result in the regurgitation of orally administered drugs, producing irregular drug absorption. In general, gastric emptying is more prolonged in neonates and infants than in children.

The characteristics of a drug's movement through the intestines can drastically affect the rate and extent of drug absorption because most drugs are absorbed in the duodenum. Both neonates and infants have irregular peristalsis, which can lead to enhanced absorption. In addition, the type of feeding an infant receives can affect intestinal transit time. For instance, the intestinal transit time in breast-fed infants is greater than in formula-fed infants (Cavell, 1981).

The relative size of the absorptive surface area in the duodenum can significantly influence the rate and extent of drug absorption. In the young, the greater relative size of the duodenum compared with adults enhances drug absorption.

Gastrointestinal Enzymes and Microorganisms

The absorption of drugs that are fat soluble or carried in fat vehicles depends on lipase. Premature neonates have low lipase concentrations and no alpha amylase. The reduced activity of bile acids, lipase, alpha amylase, and protease continues until approximately age 4 months. Vitamin E absorption is decreased in neonates because of the diminished bile acid pool and biliary function; therefore, supplementation of this vitamin may be necessary.

The development of the intestinal microorganism flora depends more on diet than on age (Yaffe & Juchau, 1974), which may account for the more rapid development of flora in breast-fed infants than in formula-fed infants. The reduction of digoxin (Lanoxin) to inactive metabolites by anaerobic intestinal bacteria can be used as a marker for the development or changes in intestinal flora (Lindenbaum et al., 1981). Digoxin metabolites are not detected in children until 16 months, and an adult-like reduction of digoxin does not occur until age 9 (Linday et al., 1987).

Rectal Absorption

The rectal route of administration is seldom used; it usually is reserved for patients who cannot tolerate oral drugs or who lack intravenous access. In rectal administration, the drug is absorbed by the hemorrhoidal veins, which are not part of the portal circulation, therefore avoiding first-pass hepatic elimination. Unfortunately, most drugs administered by this route are erratically and incompletely absorbed. Feces in the rectum, frequent bowel movements in neonates and infants, and lack of anal sphincter muscle contribute to the poor absorption profile of drugs administered rectally.

Although rectal administration may not be appropriate for routine dosing of drugs, the rectal administration of diazepam (Valium), valproic acid (Depakote), or midazolam (Versed) has been used to control seizures when intravenous access could not be quickly established in infants or children with status epilepticus (Brigo et al., 2015; Graves & Kriel, 1987).

Intramuscular and Subcutaneous Absorption

Both the characteristics of the patient and the properties of the drug influence the absorption of intramuscularly or subcutaneously administered drugs. Patient characteristics include blood flow to the muscle, muscle mass, tone, and activity. Important properties of the drug are its solubility, the pH of extracellular fluid, its ease in crossing capillary membranes, and the amount of drug administered at the injection site.

In pediatric patients, all the patient characteristics are highly variable. Neonates have decreased muscle mass, and their limited muscle activity decreases blood flow to and from the muscle. Collectively, these factors produce erratic and poor intramuscular drug absorption. On the contrary, infants possess a greater density of skeletal muscle capillaries than older children, allowing for more efficient drug absorption. Some drugs, such as erythromycin, can cause pain at the injection site and should not be administered intramuscularly. However, many drugs, such as the penicillins, reach concentrations in the serum with intramuscular administration that are comparable with those achieved after intravenous administration, with minimal adverse effects.

Percutaneous Absorption

Adverse effects resulting from the inadvertent systemic absorption of percutaneously administered hexachlorophene emulsion, salicylic acid ointment, and hydrocortisone creams in neonates have limited the use of this route of drug administration. The absorption of compounds is inversely related to the thickness of the stratum corneum and directly related to hydration of the skin (Morselli et al., 1980). Relative to body mass, the BSA is greatest in the infant and young child compared with older children and adults. The decreased thickness of the skin with increased skin surface hydration relative to body weight produces much greater percutaneous drug absorption in neonates than in adults. The percutaneous administration of drugs in neonates does pose some risks of toxic effects. Neonatal skin is structurally immature, resulting in less subcutaneous fat and a thinner stratum corneum and epidermis (Rutter, 1987). Since a greater skin surface area/body weight ratio is observed during the neonatal period, percutaneous drug absorption is also superior. Both the advantages and subsequent disadvantages of enhanced percutaneous absorption disappear after infancy, however.

Mucosal Absorption

Mucosal administration of medications, whether via the nasal or buccal route, has become a viable method for use in children. Some medications, such as nasal corticosteroids, are intended for a local effect and have almost no systemic absorption or effects. However, some medications, such as midazolam (Versed) and ketamine (Ketalar), have been administered by nasal aerosolization with good absorption and systemic effect (Hosseini Jahromi et al., 2012; Klein et al., 2011). Administration by these routes avoids the trauma of placing an intravenous line and the associated costs. Also, in urgent situations where there may be considerable difficulty placing an intravenous line (i.e., status epilepticus), nasal administration can be utilized with great effectiveness (Thakker & Shanbag, 2013).

Pulmonary Absorption

Aerosolized drug delivery to the lungs continues to be a favorite technique in many respiratory disorders, such as asthma. Factors affecting drug deposition in the lungs include particle size, lipid solubility, protein binding, drug metabolism in the lungs, and mucociliary transport (American Academy of Pediatrics, 1997). Aerosol particle size and lipid solubility are factors in determining whether the drug is deposited in the upper or lower airways; smaller particle size and lipid-soluble drugs are more likely to be absorbed and deposited in the lower airways (Bond, 1993).

Besides drug considerations, pediatric characteristics also affect aerosol drug delivery. Infants and children have lower tidal volumes and increased respiratory rates (especially while crying), reducing drug delivery and absorption in the lungs. Studies have shown that less than 2% of aerosolized drugs are deposited in young infants and toddlers (Fok et al., 1996; Salmon et al., 1990). Therefore, adult dosing may be necessary to counteract these effects.

Distribution

Six factors affect drug distribution in the pediatric population: vascular perfusion, body composition, tissue-binding characteristics, physicochemical properties of the drug, plasma protein binding, and route of administration (Stewart & Hampton, 1987). During the neonatal period, most of these factors are significantly different from those in the adult population, while children and adolescents are very similar to or the same as adults.

Vascular Perfusion

Changes in vascular perfusion are common in neonates. For example, in neonatal respiratory distress syndrome and postasphyxia, a right-to-left vascular shunt may occur and divert blood from the lungs to the tissues and organs, potentially changing the Vd of some drugs.

Body Composition

Neonates have increased total body water (75% to 80%) with decreased fat compared with adults, resulting in a higher water-to-lipid ratio. After the neonatal period, fat increases and total body water decreases steadily until puberty, especially in girls. For instance, neonates and infants have increased total body and extracellular water, creating a larger volume of distribution and affecting the pharmacokinetics of some drugs, such as aminoglycoside. The larger volume, in turn, requires administering a larger milligram-per-kilogram dose of aminoglycosides to neonates and infants than to adults.

Tissue-Binding Characteristics

The mass of tissue available for binding can affect drug distribution. Drugs extensively bound to tissues exhibit increased "free" blood levels when the mass of tissue is reduced by disease or degeneration or immaturity, as in pediatrics.

Physicochemical Properties

The physicochemical properties of a drug include lipid solubility (ionized vs. nonionized) and molecular configuration. These properties affect the ability of a drug to move across membranes into target cells or tissues. Drugs that display favorable properties for absorption may pose a greater risk for toxicity in neonates, who have enhanced percutaneous drug absorption.

Plasma Protein Binding

Preterm neonates have lower circulating amounts of alpha$_1$ acid glycoprotein, which binds alkaline drugs, than full-term neonates, who have lower alpha$_1$ acid glycoprotein levels than adults. Neonates also have a reduced amount of circulating albumin compared with adults. Albumin is responsible for binding acidic drugs, fatty acids, and bilirubin. While the affinity of drugs for either of these plasma proteins is harder to determine, theoretically a neonate's affinity for protein binding is reduced, resulting in the likelihood of displacing drugs or bilirubin bound to albumin and leading to increased serum concentrations. All these factors produce a larger volume of distribution and increased free drug concentrations (e.g., phenytoin [Dilantin]) in neonates than in adults.

Route of Administration

The route by which a drug is administered has a primary influence on the drug's distribution. If the drug is administered orally, the liver becomes the primary distribution site. However, if a drug is administered intravenously, the heart and lungs act as the primary distribution sites. This is important because when a drug passes through the liver before reaching its site of activity, it is subject to the first-pass effect of extensive hepatic metabolism, which typically reduces the amount of circulating active drug and thus limits its effects. Therefore, to achieve an equal effect, the dosage of a drug administered by the oral route usually needs to be higher than the dosage of a drug administered intravenously.

Metabolism

Clearance of many drugs is mainly reliant on hepatic metabolism. The two phases of drug metabolism in the liver are the oxidation, reduction, and hydrolysis reactions (phase I) and conjugation reactions (phase II). Age-related changes in metabolism affect how drugs are broken down or transformed in pediatric patients and how certain metabolic enzymes are activated (**Table 4.3** summarizes developmental patterns in phase I oxidation reactions). Phase I and II reactions are delayed in neonates, infants, and young children, with consequential drug toxicities.

The P-450 cytochrome (CYP) is the most important component of phase I drug metabolism. Cytochromes in the CYP1, CYP2, and CYP3 families have been identified as important in human drug metabolism. Additional information suggests there is substantial genetic variability in the quantity and quality of CYP in the human body (Kearns, 1995). For example, codeine is metabolized to morphine via the CYP2D6 and can result in high levels of morphine in ultrarapid metabolizers to the enzyme. Deaths in children who are ultrarapid metabolizers have been reported after receiving codeine postoperatively from tonsillectomy and/or adenoidectomy. These reports led to the FDA to create a boxed warning avoiding the use of codeine in children undergoing these procedures.

The metabolism of caffeine and theophylline, the prototypic substrate for CYP1A2, is reduced at birth; the drug concentration increases linearly over the first year of life and exceeds adult levels in older infants and children. To maintain therapeutic serum theophylline concentrations, smaller doses are prescribed and administered less frequently in neonates than in older infants and children.

In pediatrics, phase II reactions are less well studied than phase I reactions. In adults, acetaminophen (Tylenol) (a substrate for glucuronosyltransferase 1A6 and 1A9) is metabolized by a phase II glucuronidation reaction. In neonates and infants, however, this metabolic pathway is deficient. As a result, acetaminophen metabolism is shifted to sulfate conjugation, which results in a half-life for acetaminophen that is similar to its half-life in adults.

TABLE 4.3

Summary of Age-Related Changes in Metabolism

P-450 Cytochromes	Reduced Activity versus Adults	Increased Activity versus Adults	Age at Which Adult Activity Is Reached
CYP1A2	Until age 4 mo	1–2 y old	End of puberty
CYP2C19			
CYP2C9	First week of life	3–4 y old	End of puberty
CYP2D6	Until age 3–5	3–5 y old	
CYP2E1	Unknown	Unknown	Unknown
CYP3A4	First month of life	1–4 y old	End of puberty

Based on data from Leader, J. S., & Kearns, G. L. (1997). Pharmacogenetics in pediatrics: Implications for practice. *Pediatric Clinics of North American, 44*, 55–77.

Elimination

Almost all drugs and their metabolites are excreted through the kidneys. The kidney eliminates drugs by glomerular filtration (passive diffusion) or tubular secretion (energy-dependent channels or pumps). The glomerular filtration rate (GFR) increases quickly during the first 2 weeks of postnatal life and does not approach adult rates until age 2 (Rubin et al., 1949); tubular secretion and reabsorption rates do not reach adult values until age 5 to 7 months. The proximal tubules are characterized by an inability to concentrate urine or reabsorb various filtered compounds and a reduced ability to secrete organic acids. This immaturity of the renal system in neonates and infants results from restricted blood flow and a resultant decrease in cardiac output to the kidneys, combined with incomplete glomerular and tubular development. As a result, plasma clearance of many drugs via the kidneys is altered. For example, during infancy, the response to thiazide diuretics, which require a GFR greater than 30 mL/minute to be effective, is diminished. Often, a larger dosage of a thiazide diuretic or substitution by a loop diuretic is required to produce adequate diuresis. Because the elimination of aminoglycosides is directly related to the GFR, aminoglycosides have a longer half-life in neonates and infants, thus requiring a longer dosing interval than in adults. In addition, decreased tubular secretion in neonates and infants can lengthen the elimination half-life of other antibiotics, such as the penicillins and sulfonamides. Selecting the appropriate dosing regimen based on age, weight, and kidney maturation and identifying concomitant agents renally eliminated are important factors to prevent toxicity. In general, renal excretion of many drugs is directly proportional to age.

DRUG SELECTION

Various factors are considered when prescribing a drug for a pediatric patient. Among them are the benefits of the drug in relation to the risks of administration, the long-term effects, the dosage form, and the route and frequency of administration (**Figure 4.1**).

Risks and Benefits

The classic medication when discussing risks and benefits in the pediatric population is ciprofloxacin (Cipro), a fluoroquinolone. Ciprofloxacin was brought to market in 1987 and carried a risk of severe degenerative arthropathy. This effect was seen in juvenile study animals during drug development. The potential for this problem led to these drugs being contraindicated in all pediatric populations. Numerous studies over the past 20 years disputing this risk has led to over 500,000 prescriptions for the drug being written annually for children younger than age 18. The American Academy of Pediatrics developed a policy statement that provides an outline for the use of fluoroquinolones in children (American Academy of

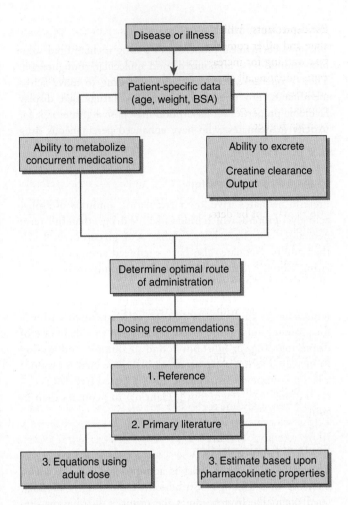

FIGURE 4.1 Approach to prescribing drug therapy for the pediatric patient.

Pediatrics, 2011). The use of the drug class in children is driven more by resistance patterns in pathogens covered by the class than the potential risk of arthropathy to the patient.

Cardiovascular safety and adverse psychiatric effects are a concern with the use of psychostimulants in the treatment of attention deficit hyperactivity disorder (ADHD). A very small number of case reports of sudden cardiac death have been reported in children prescribed psychostimulants for ADHD. The risk has been found to be greater in patients with underlying cardiac structural abnormalities. However, the risk is similar to that of strenuous exercise in this population, and the use in the general population does not necessitate additional testing beyond normal screening. There is also a small risk of psychosis and mania-type reactions in children. As a result, the FDA requires the pharmaceutical industry to provide medication guides to patients and prescribers explaining the risks of ADHD drug treatments and information on their potential side effects.

Another widely used drug class with specific safety concerns in the pediatric population is antidepressants. There is a very slight increase in suicide risk in patients started on antidepressants, which likely reflects the current depressed state and other comorbidities. The FDA has included a black box warning for increased suicidality for children and adolescents initiating all classes of antidepressants. Although this is a statistically significant increased risk compared to the normal population, the risk of suicide in untreated depressed patients is much higher.

Long-Term Effects

Drugs administered to pediatric patients may take a longer time to produce adverse effects than in adults. Certain adverse effects may not be detected until decades after treatment. For example, secondary cancers, growth retardation, hypogonadism, and sterility have all been reported as late adverse effects associated with certain antineoplastic therapies. Inhaled and intranasal corticosteroids may decrease growth velocity, which is a means of comparing growth rates among children of the same age. Studies with inhaled steroids showed approximately a 1-cm/year reduction in growth velocity. The FDA suggests that the reduction is related to dose and how long the child takes the drug (U.S. FDA, 1998b). Lone and Pederson (2000) evaluated the long-term effect on growth of inhaled or intranasal budesonide in pediatric asthma patients. At the end of this 10-year study, the researchers concluded that normal adult height was achieved in patients receiving these corticosteroids. More recently, the Children Asthma Management Program (CAMP) Research Group showed a reduction of 1.2 cm in adult height in the inhaled budesonide versus placebo group (Kelly et al., 2012).

Potential long-term effects of medications used in children create a concern. The 5-year survival rates of most pediatric malignancies are approaching 80%. This has led to a focus on the late effects of therapy and the quality of life in this growing population of childhood cancer survivors (Shankar et al., 2008). Nearly two thirds of all childhood cancer survivors will experience some physical or psychological outcome that develops or persists beyond 5 years from the initial diagnosis (Shankar et al., 2008). Other medications used in pediatrics may also carry risks for long-term effects. Unfortunately, these effects may not be seen for years after the medication is stopped, and there are likely other factors that could cause or at least contribute to the effect. Studies that evaluate the long-term effect of a medication are very difficult to perform and often yield conflicting results.

Dosage Formulation

Commercially available dosage formulations often limit the drugs that can be prescribed to children and are not always child friendly. Many drugs are available only as an oral tablet, capsule, or intravenous dilution in adult dosage strengths. Prescribing a drug as a tablet or capsule for a pediatric patient has several drawbacks. He or she may have difficulty swallowing a whole or intact tablet or capsule, and attempting to break a tablet into smaller pieces or emptying part of a capsule to

provide an appropriate dose leads to questionable accuracy of the administered dose. It is important to provide a dosage form that can be administered easily, accurately, and safely to a pediatric patient. A method to improve administration is via extemporaneous formulations, especially if a product is not commercially available as an elixir, solution, suspension, or syrup. However, these oral liquid formulations also have drawbacks such as an unfavorable taste. Other alternatives to oral liquid formulations include tablet dispersion, powdered papers, and repacked capsules. Combination products are available to reduce pill burden and improve medication adherence. However, these agents contain fixed dosage forms in tablets or capsules, making it difficult for a child less than age 5 to swallow.

Ideally, a practitioner who is prescribing a dosage formulation not commercially available for a pediatric patient ought to work with a pharmacist who is willing and able to compound accurate pediatric drug dosages and formulas. Practitioners can familiarize themselves with additional drugs that can be extemporaneously compounded for use in pediatrics by a pharmacist in such publications as *Pediatric Drug Formulations* (Nahata & Hipple, 2010); *Teddy Bear Book: Pediatric Injectable Drugs* (Phelps, 2013); *Pediatric Dosage Handbook* (Taketomo et al., 2014); *Extemporaneous Formulations for Pediatric, Geriatric, and Special Needs Patients* (Jew et al., 2010); or *Trissel's Stability of Compounding Formulations* (Trissel, 2012). A Medline search should be conducted for drugs not contained in these publications.

Dosage

In adult drug therapy, one standard dose of a drug can be used for almost all adults, but the opposite is true in pediatric drug therapy: a pediatric drug dose changes for different illnesses or as the patient grows or develops and requires age-dependent adjustments.

When writing or assessing a pediatric medication order, the following process is recommended to ensure safe and effective pharmaceutical care:

1. Determine the patient type (i.e., neonate, pediatric, adolescent).
2. Assess the appropriateness of the drug therapy selected in this patient type, patient population, and/or disease state.
3. Establish the appropriate dose, route, formulation, and frequency based on the recommended references mentioned below.
4. If all resources have been exhausted or further information is needed regarding the pediatric dosage, contact a pharmacist. It is important to ensure that the dose is appropriate or reasonable based on his or her knowledge of pediatric pharmacokinetics and available resources.

Many drugs currently in use in pediatrics have established dosing recommendations based on body weight, BSA, concurrent drug therapy, and stage of development or physiologic function (age). Body weight–based dosing is the most common method for pediatric dosing. A total daily dose, milligrams per kilogram per day (mg/kg/day), is divided by the dosing interval to calculate each individual dose. Analgesics, antipyretics, and emergency drugs are often administered on a dose-by-dose method; as such, the recommended pediatric dose is reported as milligrams per kilogram per dose (mg/kg/dose). The starting or maximum doses for pediatric intravenous infusions are usually reported as micrograms per kilogram per minute (mcg/kg/minute) or micrograms per kilogram per hour (mcg/kg/hour). Drug dosages based on a patient's BSA are usually reserved for antineoplastic agents or critically ill patients. BSA correlates closely with many factors that influence drug elimination, including cardiac output, respiratory metabolism, blood volume, extracellular water volume, GFR, and renal blood flow. Dosages of several drugs, including docusate (Colace) and montelukast (Singulair), are based on age.

General pediatric drug references such as the *Pediatric Dosage Handbook* (Taketomo et al., 2014) and Micromedex (MICROMEDEX Solutions, 2015) provide comprehensive drug monographs, including dosage formulations, adverse events, pharmacology, and pharmacokinetics. *The Harriet Lane Handbook* (Engorn & Flerlage, 2014) provides drug monographs based on the Johns Hopkins Hospital formulary and special drug topics. A specialty pediatric reference such as the *Red Book* (Pickering et al., 2012) covers only antimicrobial agents and vaccines; *Neofax* (Neofax, 2015) provides information about drug dosing in neonates.

Obesity

Obesity, defined in children as a body mass index (BMI) at or above the 95th percentile for age, is considered a public health crisis in the United States (Ogden et al., 2010). Since 1980, the percentage of school-age children and adolescents that are considered obese has tripled and is approximately 17% (Ogden et al., 2010). Children with a BMI at or above the 85th percentile are considered "at risk for overweight," and nearly 32% of U.S. children ages 2 to 19 fall into this category (Ogden et al., 2010). While it is known that there is an overall lack of information on dosing most medications in children, there is far less information on proper medication dosing in the overweight child. Obesity can affect the pharmacokinetics, dosing, half-life, and metabolism of a medication. Medications originally intended for adult use are now being utilized to treat hypertension, hyperlipidemia, and type 2 diabetes as these diseases are on the rise secondary to the increase in obesity (Kennedy et al., 2013). There is a greater risk of dosing errors in overweight children, specifically for underdosing and overdosing of antimicrobials (Pediatric Pharmacy Advocacy Group, 2010). The Pediatric Pharmacy Advocacy Group recommends that weight-based dosing be utilized for all children less than age 18 and weighing less than 88 lb (40 kg). For children who weigh over 40 kg, weight-based dosing should be used, unless the patient's dose or dose/day exceeds the recommended adult dose for the specific indication (Johnson et al., 2010).

Routes of Administration

Oral

When prescribing or administering oral drugs for pediatric patients, the caregiver needs to consider not only the drug's flavor and ease of delivery but the frequency of administration, dosage form, and "inactive" ingredients, such as alcohol and sugar. A liquid dosage form is preferred for most pediatric patients.

To ensure the accuracy of each dose administered, the drug should be measured and then administered with an oral syringe or a calibrated drug cup, with the base of the meniscus viewed at eye level. If the drug is available only in tablet form, and the tablet can be broken, the tablet may be crushed and mixed in compatible syrup. However, mixing a crushed or whole tablet with food should be done cautiously because many foods interfere with drug absorption.

If the patient is an infant, the head should be raised to prevent aspiration of the drug. Applying gentle downward pressure on the chin with a thumb helps open the patient's mouth. If a syringe is used, the tip of the syringe should be placed in the pocket between the patient's cheek and gum and the drug administered slowly and steadily to reduce the risk of aspiration.

For bottle-fed infants, the drug can be placed in a nipple and the infant allowed to suck the contents. However, a drug should never be mixed with the contents of a baby's bottle because the correct dose will not be received if the infant does not consume the full contents of the bottle. In addition, a drug–nutrient interaction may occur if a drug is mixed with formula. A classic example of a drug–nutrient interaction is the significant reduction of oral phenytoin absorption after concurrent administration with an enteral feeding formula (Sacks & Brown, 1994).

Rectal

Toddlers being toilet trained, especially children experiencing stress or difficulty, often resist the rectal administration of drugs. Older children may perceive the procedure as an invasion of privacy and may react with embarrassment or anger and hostility. The best approach to reducing anxiety and increasing cooperation is to spend time explaining the procedure and to reassure the child that giving drugs by this route will not hurt. It may be necessary, after placing a suppository, to hold the child's buttocks together for a few minutes to prevent expulsion of the drug.

Parenteral

Establishing venous access, venipuncture for blood samples, and intramuscular injections are a great source of distress and pain for children. Several local anesthetic agents have been developed to help manage the pain and anxiety brought on by these procedures. The ideal product would have needle-free or topical administration, a rapid onset of anesthetic, and no dermal or systemic adverse effects, and

TABLE 4.4
Topical Anesthetics

Method	Product(s)	Medication(s)	Onset of Topical Anesthesia	Adverse Reactions
Injection of local anesthetics	Lidocaine Lidocaine buffered with sodium bicarbonate	Lidocaine	<1 min	Pain associated with initial needle stick for injection of medication
Lidocaine needle-free injection	J-Tip	Lidocaine	<1 min	"Popping noise" with administration (may frighten some children)
Passive diffusion with topical creams or gels	EMLA, generic	Lidocaine 2.5%, prilocaine 2.5%	30 min (minimum), 60 min for more complete effect	Skin blanching, rare methemoglobinemia in infants
	LMX4	Liposomal lidocaine 4%	30 min	Erythema, blanching
Needle-free strategies to accelerate onset	Synera	Lidocaine/tetracaine	10 min	Local reactions (erythema, 71%; blanching; and edema)
Lidocaine iontophoresis	Numby Stuff	Lidocaine	10–15 min	Intolerable tingling, itching, burning sensation, and discomfort, potential for burn
Lidocaine HCl monohydrate powder intradermal injection system	Zingo	Lidocaine HCl monohydrate	1–3 min	Local reactions (erythema, 62%; petechiae, 52.8%) and edema
Vapocoolant sprays	Pain Ease	Liquid refrigerant (ethyl chloride)	Immediate (may require two providers as effect lasts <1 min)	Some skin pigmentation changes (temporary)

the product would have no impact on the success rate of the procedure. No commercially available product has all these qualities. The three general delivery methods used to bypass the stratum corneum layer include direct injection of local anesthetics, passive diffusion from topically applied gels or creams, and several needle-free methods that hasten the rate of drug passage through the skin and speed the time to onset of action. **Table 4.4** lists the methods of drug delivery, the available agents, and the advantages and disadvantages of each (Zempsky, 2008).

Pulmonary
Nebulizers, metered-dose inhalers (MDIs), and dry powder inhalers (DPIs) can be used to deliver bronchodilators, aminoglycosides, and corticosteroids in the treatment of asthma or cystic fibrosis. Nebulized drugs require connecting an air or oxygen tube to the nebulizer machine and are often used in infants and young children. MDIs require coordination between actuation and inhalation; this is difficult in any age group, so a tube spacer is recommended for children less than age 5 (National Heart, Lung, and Blood Institute, 2007). Spacer devices have expanded the use of MDIs even to the neonatal population. A DPI such as budesonide powder (Pulmicort Turbuhaler) involves coordination with the patient's inspiratory flow; therefore, the delivery mechanism

is not recommended in children less than age 4. **Table 4.5** summarizes the recommended population for aerosol delivery devices (National Heart, Lung, and Blood Institute, 2007).

Topical
The topical delivery of medications is common in the pediatric population with diseases such as eczema and acne as well as other skin disorders that appear during childhood. Caution

TABLE 4.5
Recommended Age Groups of Aerosol Delivery Devices

Device	Age
Metered-dose inhaler (MDI)	• ≥5 y old • <5 y old (+ spacer or valved holding chamber)
Breath-actuated MDI	• ≥5 y old
Dry powder inhaler	• ≥4 y old
Spacer or valved holding chamber (VHC)	• ≥4 y old • <4 y old (VHC + face mask)
Nebulizer	• Any age

is warranted in this population due to several factors that may lead to a higher rate of drug absorption. When compared to adults, infants and children have a higher ratio of skin surface to body weight. This increases the risk of accumulating significant serum drug levels (Metry & Herbert, 2000). It is especially true in the newborn and infant because the barrier function of their skin is immature. Parents must be cautioned to follow the directions for administration of all topical medications to prevent toxic drug levels. A fatal case of diphenhydramine toxicity was reported in the literature, largely due to excessive application following a bath in a child with eczema (Turner, 2009).

Medication Adherence

The term "medication adherence" is used to describe the extent to which patients take medication as prescribed by their health care providers (Osterberg & Blaschke, 2005). Adherence (or nonadherence) to prescribed therapy is multifactorial and includes simply forgetting, busy lifestyle, complexity of the regimen, taste, education, and motivation, among others. Practitioners must consider these factors when prescribing therapy and must strive to find the balance that will help the patient and family achieve necessary adherence to the prescribed therapy. It is practical to select medications that can be administered once or twice daily because adherence falls dramatically when medications are to be administered more than twice per day (Richter et al., 2003). Establishing a good relationship with honest communication between the prescriber and the patient/family is an important factor in medication adherence and positive outcomes. Practitioners should always look for poor adherence as a cause of less-than-optimal outcomes. Better adherence can often be achieved by additional education, simplifying the regimen, and customizing the regimen to the patient's/family's lifestyle (Osterberg & Blaschke, 2005).

CONCLUSION

In summary, pediatric pharmacotherapy poses a unique challenge. The lack of medications approved by the FDA, insufficient literature resources, pharmacokinetic parameters compared to adults, individual drug dosing calculations, lack of dosage forms, and inappropriate drug delivery systems are a few examples (Levine et al., 2001). Ensuring effective and safe delivery of drugs in pediatrics involves understanding the physiologic changes that occur throughout childhood. Since the start of the Institute for Safe Medication Practices in 1994, pediatric medication safety movements have progressed over time. In 2004, the Institute of Healthcare Improvement (IHI) introduced the 100K Lives Campaign to protect patients from medical harm. Two years later, the IHI launched the 5 Million Lives Campaign with a pediatric initiative to reduce adverse drug events and decrease harm from high-alert medications (i.e., anticoagulants, sedatives, opioids, insulin) (IHI, 2006). The Joint Commission Sentinel Event Alert stated that harm caused by medication errors is three times greater in pediatric patients than adults (The Joint Commission, 2008). As a result, the Joint Commission Issue 39 recommends initiatives to prevent medication errors and suggests risk reduction strategies. **Box 4.1** gives some recommendations to assist health care professionals in reducing medication errors (American Academy of Pediatrics, 2003; The Joint Commission, 2008). In the future, pediatric pharmacotherapy will evolve with additional legislation and safety movements.

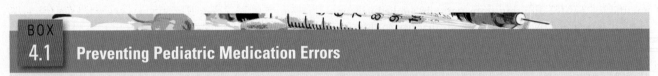

BOX 4.1 Preventing Pediatric Medication Errors

AMERICAN ACADEMY OF PEDIATRICS

- Maintain an up-to-date patient allergy profile.
- Confirm the validity of a patient's weight for medications that are dosed by body weight (or body surface area [BSA] for medications dosed by BSA).
- State specific dosage strengths or formulation.
- Do not use abbreviations for drug names or patient instructions.
- Avoid using abbreviations for dosage units.
- Use a zero before a decimal point.
- Avoid a zero after a decimal point.

THE JOINT COMMISSION

- Standardize concentrations of high-alert medications (i.e., heparin, insulin, or narcotics).
- Utilize oral syringes to administer liquid formulations.
- Create drug order pathways for protocols.
- Collaborate and educate all health care members involved with the patients' care.
- Use technology such as automated dispensing cabinets, smart infusion pumps, bar coding.

CASE STUDY*

M.T. is an 18-month-old, 20-kg male who presents to the emergency department in status epilepticus, which has continued for approximately 20 minutes. He was brought to the emergency department from a small community via a family vehicle. He has not received any care at this point. The nursing staffs has attempted several intravenous line insertions but were unable to gain access. M.T. continues to convulse without interruption.

1. Which of the following would be the most appropriate route of administration for an anticonvulsant to consider for M.T.?
   a. Intramuscular
   b. Percutaneous
   c. Subcutaneous
   d. Rectal
2. Midazolam is a benzodiazepine that can be used effectively for status epilepticus. Which of the following routes of administration has been used effectively for the delivery of midazolam when intravenous access is unobtainable?
   a. Percutaneous
   b. Mucosal
   c. Oral
   d. Subcutaneous

3. Which of the following is true regarding the percutaneous absorption of medications?
   a. The absorption of compounds is inversely related to the thickness of the skin.
   b. The absorption of compounds is inversely related to the hydration of the skin.
   c. Body surface area (BSA) is decreased, relative to body mass, in the infant and young child when compared with older children and adults.
   d. The percutaneous administration of medications is reliable and safe in the infant and young child.
4. What are the advantages of utilizing the mucosal route of administration?
   a. Some medications have very good absorption and systemic effect when administered by nasal spray.
   b. Nasal (mucosal) administration avoids the trauma of intravenous line placement.
   c. Nasal administration of medication is typically less expensive than intravenous administration.
   d. All of the above are advantages of the mucosal route of administration.

* Answers can be found online.

Bibliography

Starred references are cited in the text.

*American Academy of Pediatrics. (1997). Alternative routes of drug administration—Advantages and disadvantages (subject review). *Pediatrics, 100,* 143–152.

*American Academy of Pediatrics. (2003). Prevention of medication errors in the pediatric inpatient setting. *Pediatrics, 112,* 431–436.

*American Academy of Pediatrics. (2011). The use of systemic and topical fluoroquinolones. *Pediatrics, 128,* e1034–e1045.

*Anonymous. (1972). American Academy of Pediatrics committee on fetus and newborn: Hexachlorophene and skin care of newborn infants. *Pediatrics, 49,* 625–626.

*Bond, J. A. (1993). Metabolism and elimination of inhaled drugs and airborne chemicals from the lungs. *Pharmacology and Toxicology, 72,* 23–47.

*Brigo, F., Nardone, R., Tezzon, F., et al. (2015). Nonintravenous midazolam versus intravenous or rectal diazepam for the treatment of early status epilepticus: A systemic review with meta-analysis. *Epilepsy and Behavior, 25,* pii: S1525-5050(15)00090-6.

*Cavell, B. (1981). Gastric emptying in infants fed human milk or infant formula. *Acta Paediatrica Scandinavica, 70,* 639–641.

*Deren, J. S. (1971). Development of structure and function of the fetal and newborn stomach. *American Journal of Clinical Nutrition, 24,* 144–159.

*Engorn, B., & Flerlage, J. (2014). *The Harriet Lane handbook* (20th ed.). San Francisco, CA: Elsevier.

*Fok, T. F., Monkman, S., Dolovich, M., et al. (1996). Efficacy of aerosol medication delivery from a metered-dose inhaler versus jet nebulizer in infants with bronchopulmonary dysphasia. *Pediatric Pulmonology, 21,* 301–309.

*Friis-Hansen, B. (1957). Changes in body water compartment during growth. *Acta Paediatrica, 46*(Suppl. 110), 1–68.

*Graves, N. M., & Kriel, R. L. (1987). Rectal administration of antiepileptic drugs in children. *Pediatric Neurology, 3,* 321–326.

*Haile, C. A. (1977). Chloramphenicol toxicity. *Southern Medical Journal, 70,* 479–480.

*Hosseini Jahromi S. A., Hosseini Valami S. M., Adeli, N., et al. (2012). Comparison of the effects of intranasal midazolam versus different doses of intranasal ketamine on reducing preoperative pediatric anxiety: A prospective randomized clinical trial. *Journal of Anesthesia, 26,* 878–882.

*Institute of Healthcare Improvement. (2006). Protecting 5 million lives from harm. Retrieved from http://www.ihi.org/IHI/Programs/Campaign/Campaign.htm?TabId=1 on August 16, 2010.

*Jew, R. K., Soo-Hoo, W., & Erush, S. C. (2010). *Extemporaneous formulations for pediatric, geriatric, and special needs patients* (2nd ed.). Bethesda, MD: American Society of Hospital Pharmacists.

*Johnson, P. N., Miller, J. L., & Boucher, E. A. (2010). Medication dosing in overweight and obese children. Retrieved from www.ppag.org/obesedose/ on Accessed August 16, 2010.

*Kearns, G. L. (1995). Pharmacogenetics and development: Are infants and children at increased risk for adverse outcomes? *Current Opinion in Pediatrics, 7,* 220–233.

*Kelly, H.W., Sternberg, A.L, Lescher, R., et al. (2012). Effect of inhaled glucocorticoids in childhood on adult height. *New England Journal of Medicine, 367,* 904–912.

*Kennedy, M. J., Jellerson, K. D., Smow, M. Z., et al. (2013). Challenges in the pharmacological management of obesity and secondary dyslipidemia in children and adolescents. *Pediatric Drugs, 15,* 335–342.

*Klein, E. J., Brown, J. C., Kobayashi, A., et al. (2011). A randomized clinical trial comparing oral, aerosolized intranasal, and aerosolized buccal midazolam. *Annals of Emergency Medicine, 58*, 323–329.

*Levine, S. R., Cohen, M. R., Blanchard, N. R., et al. (2001). Guidelines for preventing medication errors in pediatrics. *Journal of Pediatric Pharmacologic Therapies, 6*, 426–442.

*Linday, L., Dobkin, J. F., Wang, T. C., et al. (1987). Digoxin inactivation by the gut flora in infancy and childhood. *Pediatrics, 79*, 544–548.

*Lindenbaum, J., Rund, D. G., Butler, V. P., et al. (1981). Inactivation of digoxin by gut flora; reversal by antibiotic therapy. *New England Journal of Medicine, 305*, 789–794.

*Lone, A., & Pederson, S. (2000). Effect of long-term treatment with inhaled budesonide on adult height in children with asthma. *New England Journal of Medicine, 343*, 1064–1069.

*Metry, D. W., & Herbert, A. A. (2000). Topical therapies and medications in the pediatric patient. *Pediatric Clinics of North America, 47*, 867–876.

*MICROMEDEX® Solutions (electronic version). Truven Health Analytics, Greenwood Village, Colorado. Retrieved from http://www.micromedex-solutions.com/home/dispatch on May 12, 2015.

*Morselli, P. L., Franco-Morselli, R., & Bossi, L. (1980). Clinical pharmacokinetics in newborns and infants: Age-related differences and therapeutic implications. *Clinical Pharmacokinetics, 5*, 485–527.

*Nahata, M. C., & Hipple, T. F. (2010). *Pediatric drug formulations* (6th ed.). Cincinnati, OH: Harvey Whitney.

*National Heart, Lung, and Blood Institute. (2007). Expert panel report 3: Guidelines for the diagnosis and the management of asthma. Retrieved from http://www.nhlbi.nih.gov/guidelines/asthma/ on May 12, 2015.

*Neofax® (electronic version). Truven Health Analytics, Greenwood Village, Colorado. Retrieved from http://neofax.micromedexsolutions.com/neofax/neofax.php on May 12, 2015.

*Ogden, C. L., Carroll, M. D., Curtin, L. R., et al. (2010). Prevalence of high body mass index in U.S. children and adolescents, 2007–2008. *Journal of the American Medical Association, 303*, 242–249.

*Osterberg, L., & Blaschke, T. (2005). Adherence to medication. *New England Journal of Medicine, 353*, 487–497.

*Pediatric Pharmacy Advocacy Group. (2010). Medication dosing in overweight and obese children. Retrieved from http://www.ppag.org/obesedose/ on May 12, 2015.

*Phelps, S. J. (2013). *Teddy bear book: Pediatric injectable drugs* (10th ed.). Bethesda, MD: American Society of Hospital Pharmacists.

*Pickering, L. K., Baker, C. J., Kimberlin, D. W., et al. (2012). *Red Book: 2012 Report of the Committee on Infectious Diseases* (29th ed.). Elk Grove Village, IL: American Academy of Pediatrics.

*Richter, A., Anton, S. F., & Pierce, C. (2003). A systematic review of the associations between dose regimens and medication compliance. *Clinical Therapeutics, 25*, 2307–2335.

*Rubin, M. I., Bruck, E., & Rapoport, M. J. (1949). Maturation of renal function in childhood: Clearance studies. *Journal of Clinical Investigation, 28*, 1144–1162.

*Rutter, N. (1987). Percutaneous drug absorption in the newborn: Hazards and uses. *Clinical Perinatology, 14*, 911–930.

*Sacks, G. S., & Brown, R. O. (1994). Drug-nutrient interactions in patients receiving nutritional support. *Drug Therapy, 24*, 35–42.

*Salmon, B., Wilson, N. M., & Silverman, M. (1990). How much aerosol reaches the lungs of wheezy infants and toddlers? *Archives of Disease in Childhood, 65*, 401–404.

*Shankar, S. M., Marina N., Hudson, M. M., et al. (2008). Monitoring for cardiovascular disease in survivors of childhood cancer: Report from the cardiovascular disease task force of the children's oncology group. *Pediatrics, 121*, 387–396.

*Stewart, C. F., & Hampton, E. M. (1987). Effect of maturation on drug disposition in pediatric patients. *Clinical Pharmacy, 6*, 548–564.

*Taketomo, C. K., Hodding, J. H., & Kraus, D. M. (2014). *Pediatric dosage handbook* (21st ed.). Hudson, OH: Lexi-Comp.

*Thakker, A., & Shanbag P. (2013). A randomized controlled trial of intranasal-midazolam versus intravenous-diazepam for acute childhood seizures. *Journal of Neurology, 260*, 470–474.

*The Joint Commission. (2008). Preventing pediatric medication errors. Retrieved from http://www.jointcommission.org/sentinelevents/sentinel-leventalert/sea_39.htm on August 16, 2010.

*Trissel, L. (2012). *Trissel's stability of compounded formulations* (5th ed.). Washington, DC: American Pharmacist Association.

*Turner, J.W. (2009). Death of a child from topical diphenhydramine. *American Journal of Forensic Medical Pathology, 30*, 380–381.

*U.S. Food and Drug Administration. (1998a). Rules and regulations. *Federal Register, 63*(231), 66631–66672.

*U.S. Food and Drug Administration. (1998b). *FDA talk paper.* Rockville, MD: Author.

U.S. Food and Drug Administration. (2013). FDA drug safety communication: Safety review update of codeine use in children; new Boxed Warning and Contraindication on use after tonsillectomy and/or adenoidectomy. Retrieved from http://www.fda.gov/Drugs/DrugSafety/ucm339112.htm on May 12, 2015.

*Yaffe, S. J., & Juchau, M. R. (1974). Perinatal pharmacology. *Annual Review of Pharmacology, 14*, 219–238.

*Zempsky, W. T. (2008). Pharmacologic approaches for reducing venous access pain in children. *Pediatrics, 122*, S140–S153.

5 Principles of Pharmacotherapy in Pregnancy and Lactation

Andrew M. Peterson ■ Lauren M. Czosnowski

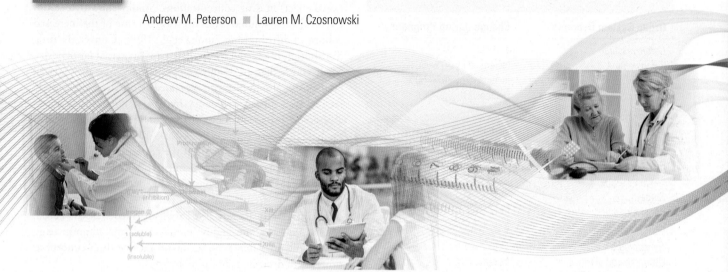

Although very little is known about the effects of medications on the fetus, many women ingest drugs during their pregnancy. The World Health Organization states "there can be no doubt that at present some drugs are more widely used in pregnancy than is justified by the knowledge available" (Collaborative Group on Drug Use in Pregnancy, 1991). Although considerable attention has been given recently to complementary and alternative medicine use during pregnancy, the use of these ubiquitous substances continues and poses significant challenges to today's health care practitioner (Briggs et al., 2014).

ISSUES IN MEDICATION USE DURING PREGNANCY

Studies have determined that about 90% of women will use one medication during pregnancy, and about 70% will use one or more prescription medications (CDC, 2014). As the number of medications being prescribed during pregnancy increases, the practitioner needs a solid understanding of the physiologic changes that occur during pregnancy and the effects that these changes have on medication use. The practitioner must also balance the need to treat the mother against the potential risk to the fetus. Because there are few studies available discussing the pharmacokinetic changes that occur during pregnancy, appropriate dosing of medications may be difficult. Understanding these changes will assist the practitioner in making recommendations during drug therapy. The maternal and fetal response to medications ingested during pregnancy may be influenced by two factors:

- Changes in the absorption, distribution, and elimination of the drug in the mother, which are altered by physiologic changes.

- The placental–fetal unit, which affects the amount of drug that crosses the placental membrane, the amount of drug metabolized by the placenta, and the distribution and elimination of the drug by the fetus.

Pregnancy-Induced Maternal Physiologic Changes

Women undergo many physiologic changes during pregnancy (**Table 5.1**). These changes affect the way a medication exerts its effects on both the mother and fetus.

Absorption

Drug absorption into the maternal bloodstream can occur by different processes, including the gastrointestinal (GI) tract, skin, or lungs, or the drug may be directly placed into the bloodstream via intravenous administration.

Gastrointestinal Absorption

Pregnancy-induced maternal physiologic changes may affect GI function, and therefore, the absorption of some drugs may be altered. Of the many factors that can affect GI absorption of drugs, one is the decrease in GI tract motility, especially during labor. It is believed that an increase in plasma progesterone levels causes this decrease in motility, which may delay the absorption of orally administered drugs.

In addition, pregnant women experience a reduction in gastric acid secretions (up to 40% less than in nonpregnant women) as well as an increase in gastric mucus secretion (Fredericksen, 2001; Loebstein et al., 1997). Together, this may lead to an increase in gastric pH and a decrease in the absorption of medications that need an acidic pH for appropriate absorption.

TABLE 5.1	
Physiologic Changes in Pregnancy	
Organ System Dynamic	**Change during Pregnancy**
Cardiovascular	
Blood volume	Increased by 30%–50%
Cardiac output	Increased by 30%–50%
Systemic vascular resistance	Decreased
Gastrointestinal	
pH of intestinal secretions	Increased
Gastric emptying time	Increased
Gastric acid secretions	Decreased
Intestinal motility	Decreased
Kidney	
Renal blood flow rate	Increased
Glomerular filtration rate	Increased
Gynecologic	
Uterine blood flow	Increased

Adapted with permission from Kraemer, K., et al. (1997). Placental transfer of drugs. *Neonatal Network, 16*(2), 65–67. Copyright 1997 Springer Publishing Company, Inc., with permission.

Another reason for decreased GI absorption may be the nausea and vomiting that is common during the first trimester of pregnancy and that is thought to be associated with increased progesterone levels. Therefore, pregnant women may be well advised to take their medications at times when nausea is minimal.

Lung Absorption

Physiologic changes in pregnancy favor the absorption of medications administered through the inhalation route. Both cardiac and tidal volumes are increased by approximately 50% in pregnancy; this results in hyperventilation and increased pulmonary blood flow (Loebstein et al., 1997). These alterations aid in the transfer of medications through the alveoli into the maternal bloodstream (Loebstein et al., 1997).

Transdermal Absorption

An increase in the absorption of medications through the skin is evident during pregnancy. The increase in peripheral vasodilation and increase in blood flow to the skin (Kraemer et al., 1997) enhance this increase in absorption. Because of an increase in total body water, there is increased water content in the skin, therefore favoring an increased rate and extent of absorption to water-soluble medications like lidocaine, which is used as a topical anesthetic during pregnancy (Yankowitz & Niebyl, 2001).

Distribution

Maternal blood volume increases significantly during pregnancy. The 30% to 50% increase in blood volume (Guyton & Hall, 1996; Loebstein et al., 1997) is characteristically distributed to various organ systems serving the needs of the growing fetus. The full increase in total body water during pregnancy is 8 L, with 60% distributed to the placenta, fetus, and amniotic fluid and 40% going to maternal tissues (Loebstein et al., 1997). It is these increases that cause the volume of distribution of medications to increase, resulting in a decrease (dilutional effect) in drug concentrations. Studies show that serum levels of water-soluble drugs decrease because of the increased volume of distribution (Simone et al., 1994). Conversely, drug distribution is affected by an increase in maternal fat deposits. Medications that are highly lipophilic distribute to maternal fat deposits, also resulting in decreased serum drug levels. Body fat increases during pregnancy by 3 to 4 kg and may act as a reservoir for medications that favor a fat-soluble environment (Yankowitz & Niebyl, 2001). Another factor that may affect medication distribution is the concentration of albumin in the maternal blood. The concentration of plasma albumin decreases during pregnancy. This decrease is believed to be caused by a reduction in the rate of albumin in synthesis or an increase in its rate of catabolism (Fredericksen, 2001). Medications that are highly bound to plasma albumin (e.g., anticonvulsants) may have an increased free drug concentration due to decreased albumin binding.

Elimination

Hormonal changes that normally occur during pregnancy can affect the elimination of various medications. The normal increase in progesterone levels can stimulate hepatic microsomal enzyme systems, thereby increasing the elimination of some hepatically eliminated medications (e.g., phenytoin [Dilantin]). Progesterone may also decrease the elimination of some medications (e.g., theophylline [Theo-Dur]) by inhibiting specific microsomal enzyme systems. Therefore, depending on the elimination pathway of a specific medication, the elimination rate may not be predictable. The extent of these physiologic changes is difficult to quantify, and it is unknown whether changes in dosages are required.

As plasma volumes increase, so does renal blood flow (Fredericksen, 2001; Guyton & Hall, 1996; Loebstein et al., 1997). With the increase in renal blood flow by 50% (Loebstein et al., 1997) and increased glomerular filtration rate, drugs excreted primarily by the kidney show increased elimination. Again, the magnitude of these increases in elimination is not known, and therefore, dosage adjustment may not be required.

Factors in Placental–Fetal Physiology

Until the 1960s, it was widely believed that the uterus provided a secure and protected environment for the developing fetus. Very little thought was given to the potential harm posed to the fetus from maternal drug use. After the thalidomide tragedy in the 1960s, the government required testing of drugs before human use. It is now known that by the fifth week of fetal development, virtually every drug has the ability to cross the placenta (Kraemer et al., 1997).

The treatment of medical conditions is complicated during pregnancy by various factors that must be considered before initiating drug therapy. A key factor is whether the drug will cross the placenta and potentially cause fetal harm.

Placental Transfer of Medications

The following factors affect a drug's ability to cross the placenta:

- Lipid-soluble drugs can cross the placenta more freely than water-soluble drugs because the outer layers of most cell membranes are made up of lipids. Many antibiotics and opiate compounds are highly soluble in lipids and can therefore easily cross the placental membrane.
- The ionization status of the drug affects placental transfer. Drugs with high lipid solubility tend to remain in a nonionized state; therefore, placental transfer is increased. Heparin, for example, is a highly ionized drug, and therefore, it does not readily cross the placental membrane.
- The molecular weight of the drug can determine the ease of placental transfer. The lower the molecular weight or the smaller the drug molecule, the more readily the drug crosses the placenta (**Table 5.2**).
- Only drugs that are not bound to a protein (e.g., albumin) can cross the placenta. Albumin is the most abundant protein in the human body. During pregnancy, the concentration of albumin decreases, and therefore, fewer proteins are present, allowing for more unbound or "free" drug to cross the placental membrane.

Placental and Fetal Metabolism

Evidence exists to support the theory that the human placenta and fetus are capable of metabolizing medications. Research findings suggest that liver enzyme systems are present in fetal livers as early as 7 to 8 weeks' gestation (Juchau & Choa, 1983). Although these enzyme systems are present, they are immature, and any drug elimination that occurs is a result of drug diffusing back into maternal blood.

Fetal Physiology

Not all drugs that cross the placental barrier cause fetal harm. Therefore, the practitioner needs to ask whether a specific drug will cross the placenta and cause fetal harm. Fetal factors to be

TABLE 5.2
Effect of Molecular Weight on Placental Transfer of Drugs

Molecular Weight	Drug Example	Rate of Placental Transfer
<500 g/mol	acetaminophen, caffeine, cocaine, labetalol, morphine, penicillins, theophylline	Readily crosses the placenta
600–1,000 g/mol	digoxin	Crosses the placenta at a slower rate
>1,000 g/mol	heparin, insulins	Transfer across the placenta severely impeded

considered in answering the question include the gestational age at the time of exposure to the drug, which is important because some drugs can exert their effects on the fetus throughout gestation. On the other hand, some drugs exert their effects on the fetus at different stages of gestation. For example, angiotensin-converting enzyme inhibitors, such as captopril (Capoten), quinapril (Accupril), and enalapril (Vasotec), vary in their fetal risk during pregnancy, being a lesser risk in the second trimester and higher risk in the third trimester. In other words, they become less safe as the pregnancy advances.

Within the first 14 days after conception, the embryo is protected from exogenous toxicity (Kraemer et al., 1997; Rayburn, 1997). The cells at this time are totipotential, meaning that if one cell is damaged or killed, another cell can perform the dead cell's function, and the embryo remains unharmed (Dicke, 1989). After this point, the developing fetus is susceptible to the effects of drugs. The first 3 months of gestation are the most crucial in terms of abnormalities and malformations (Briggs et al., 2014). Some medications that may be relatively safe during the middle trimester of pregnancy may not be safe in the last trimester or during delivery. For example, aspirin use late in pregnancy is associated with increased bleeding at the time of delivery. Moreover, the effect that aspirin has on prostaglandins may delay labor.

Fetal total body water and fat deposition are associated with gestational age, and they affect the absorption and distribution of drugs. As the fetus matures, total body water decreases and fat deposition increases, and the fetus is more likely to be affected by medications that are highly lipophilic (e.g., opiates) than by medications that are water soluble (e.g., ampicillin [Principen]).

Fetal circulatory patterns can alter the amount of drug distributed to the fetus. In early gestation, a disproportionately large percentage of the fetal cardiac output is presented to the brain, and consequently, the concentration of drug in the fetal circulation is increased (Kraemer et al., 1997).

Teratogenicity of Medications

The word *teratogenicity* is derived from the Greek root *teras*, meaning "monster." Teratogenicity is the ability of an exogenous agent to cause the dysgenesis of fetal organs as evidenced either structurally or functionally (Koren et al., 1998; Kraemer et al., 1997).

The risk of fetal abnormality depends on many factors, including not only the gestational age of the fetus at the time of exposure but the agent or medications the fetus is exposed to and the length of exposure.

The health care provider must therefore balance the risk of exposing the fetus to the drug with the benefit of treatment to the mother. If it is determined that the drug is necessary, the drug with the safest profile should be used at the lowest effective dose. The practitioner always keeps in mind that the mother is not the only recipient of the drug—the fetus is as well. It is estimated that approximately 2% or 3% of all malformations and abnormalities in the developing fetus result from drug ingestion (Oakley, 1986). In addition, it is important to

TABLE 5.3

FDA Pregnancy Risk Categories

Category	Risk Summary	Example
A	Controlled studies in women fail to demonstrate a risk to the fetus in the first trimester (and there is no evidence of a risk in later trimesters), and the possibility of fetal harm appears remote.	folic acid, thyroid hormone
B	Either animal reproduction studies have not demonstrated a fetal risk but there are no controlled studies in pregnant women or animal reproduction studies have shown an adverse effect (other than decrease in fertility) that was not confirmed in controlled studies in women in the first trimester (and there is no evidence of a risk in later trimesters).	erythromycin, penicillin
C	Either studies in animals have revealed adverse effects on the fetus and there are no controlled studies in women or studies in women and animals are not available. Drugs should be given only if the potential benefit justifies the potential risk.	labetalol, nifedipine, angiotensin-converting enzyme (ACE) inhibitors
D	There is positive evidence of human fetal risk, but benefits from the use in pregnancy may be acceptable despite the risk.	glyburide, diazepam, aspirin, ACE inhibitors
X	Studies in animals or human beings have demonstrated fetal abnormalities, or there is evidence of fetal risk based on human experience, or both, and the risk of the use of the drug in pregnant women clearly outweighs any possible benefit. The drug is contraindicated in women who are or may become pregnant.	oral contraceptives, lovastatin, isotretinoin

remember that any illnesses or chronic medical conditions that go untreated during pregnancy could potentially cause harm to the mother and fetus, even though treating the illness or condition may be potentially harmful to the fetus. Therefore, weighing the benefit of drug therapy to the mother with the risk of drug therapy to the fetus needs to be as balanced as possible.

To help prevent drug-induced abnormalities in the fetus, starting in 1979, the U.S. Food and Drug Administration (FDA) categorized drugs according to fetal risks. The categories were based on the presence or absence of controlled studies in women to determine the level of fetal risk (**Table 5.3**). Health care providers have used these categories to determine the appropriate drug therapy that will effectively treat the mother but carries the least potential for fetal harm, but the pregnancy categories had inherent flaws. Because the drug categories were based on animal data and controlled trials in pregnant women, which are scarce, these drug categories often oversimplified a complex medical decision and did not inform the provider or patient about the risk–benefit profile of the drug. The new FDA rule, entitled the Pregnancy and Lactation Labeling Rule (PLLR), was passed in December 2014 and took effect in June 2015. The new rule includes three separate sections that are required in package labeling: pregnancy, lactation, and females and males of reproductive age. The third section was not required previously.

The updated requirements for these new sections in the package labeling are summarized in **Table 5.4**. All new drugs will have to include the current labeling requirements and will not be assigned a pregnancy category. Pregnancy risk categories should be removed from existing drugs by 2018. It will still be important to understand the pregnancy categories until

the new changes are completely adopted and may take some extra effort from practitioners to interpret the data for clinical decision making. All drugs approved after June 2001 will be required to submit new labeling information within a minimum of 3 years, and manufacturers are also required to update labeling when new information is available under the new rule. It is important to note that OTC products were not affected by this new legislation. Drugs approved before 2001 must remove pregnancy categories, but are not required to conform to the new labeling requirements. The manufacturers of these drugs are encouraged to voluntarily use the new labeling sections.

TABLE 5.4

Pregnancy and Lactation Labeling Rule

Labeling Section	Requirements
8.1 Pregnancy (Includes Labor and Delivery)	Includes risk summary, clinical considerations, and data (to support the risk summary) Must include information for a pregnancy exposure registry if one is available
8.2 Lactation	Also includes risk summary, clinical consideration, and data, including the amount of drug appearing in breast milk and potential effects on the infant
8.3 Females and Males of Reproductive Potential	Includes information about need for pregnancy testing, contraception recommendations, and infertility information when applicable

DRUG THERAPY IN THE BREAST-FEEDING MOTHER

With the number of women who choose to breast-feed their infants increasing yearly, the number of questions presented to health care practitioners concerning the safety of medication use while breast-feeding is also increasing. Recommendations to discontinue or interrupt breast-feeding while taking a medication are far too common. Health care practitioners are reluctant to recommend medication use while the mother is breast-feeding because of the potential adverse effects on the infant. Most research on lactation has been conducted in small groups or on animal models. The American Academy of Pediatrics has previously published lists of medications that are safe for use while breast-feeding (**Boxes 5.1** and **5.2**), although recently they have placed less emphasis on these lists, last updated in 2001, and published that the benefits of breast-feeding usually outweigh the risks of many drugs (Sachs, 2013).

Human Breast Milk as a Drug Delivery System

Human breast milk is complex, nutrient-enriched fluid. Containing approximately 80% water, breast milk also has immunologic properties and proteins, fats, carbohydrates, minerals, and vitamins needed for normal development. The availability of the drug to be distributed into breast milk depends on many factors. For a drug to be distributed into

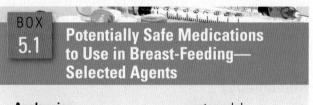

BOX 5.1 Potentially Safe Medications to Use in Breast-Feeding— Selected Agents

Analgesics
  acetaminophen
Narcotic analgesics
  codeine
  morphine
  fentanyl
  methadone
Anticoagulants
  warfarin
Anticonvulsants
  carbamazepine
  ethosuximide
  phenytoin
Antihistamines
  brompheniramine
  diphenhydramine
  triprolidine
Antihypertensives
  diltiazem
  enalapril

metoprolol
hydralazine
hydrochlorothiazide
Anti-infectives
  cephalosporins
  penicillins
  macrolides
  tetracyclines
  trimethoprim/sulfa-
    methoxazole
  nitrofurantoin
Nonsteroidal anti-inflammatory drugs
  ibuprofen
  indomethacin
  naproxen
Sedatives–hypnotics
  zolpidem
Vitamins

BOX 5.2 Medications Contraindicated or Cautioned in Breast-Feeding

Anticonvulsants
  phenobarbital
  primidone
Antidepressant
  lithium (use with caution)
Chemotherapeutic agents
  cyclosporine
  cyclophosphamide
  methotrexate
  doxorubicin
Radioactive isotopes
Recreational drugs
  alcohol (in large amounts)
  amphetamines
  cocaine
  heroin, methadone
  lysergic acid diethylamide (LSD)
  marijuana

breast milk, it must first be absorbed into the maternal circulation. The concentration or level of the drug in the mother's plasma influences the amount and degree of drug distributed into breast milk. Once drug is available for distribution into breast milk, several other factors need to be considered. These factors are similar to those determining whether a drug will cross the placental membrane and include (Dillon et al., 1997):

- Blood flow to the breast—the greater the blood flow to the breast, the greater the drug level in breast milk.
- Plasma pH (7.45) and milk pH (7.08)—the medication will stay in the maternal plasma if the medication favors a higher pH.
- Mammary tissue composition—high adipose or fat content of the breast tissue causes lipophilic medications to be distributed into the breast tissue and then into breast milk.
- Breast milk composition—breast milk contains proteins, fat, water, and vitamins. Any medication that has a high affinity for any component will have an increased distribution into breast milk.
- Physicochemical properties (i.e., lipophilicity, molecular weight, ionization of medication in plasma and breast milk) of the drug—drug characteristics that favor transfer of medication into breast milk are low molecular weight, low ionization in plasma, low protein binding, and high lipophilicity.
- Extent of drug protein binding in plasma and breast milk—medications that are highly protein bound in the plasma are less likely to be distributed into the breast milk.
- The rate of breast milk production—the more breast milk produced, the more diluted the medication will be in the breast milk.

CASE STUDY*

K.F. is a 23-year-old female with a history of acne and bipolar disorder. She currently takes lithium to treat her bipolar disorder and isotretinoin (Accutane) for her acne. She also occasionally takes famotidine for reflux.

1. Should K.F. become pregnant, which of the following would be considered safe for her to continue taking?
   a. Accutane
   b. Lithium
   c. Famotidine

2. One year later, K.F. is seen again in your clinic. Her acne and bipolar medications have been discontinued, and she now presents 4 months pregnant with a complaint of pain and rising fever since the last 5 days. Lab tests show gram-negative bacilli and Widal test comes out positive. Which one of the following drugs will most likely be administered?
   a. Ampicillin
   b. Ciprofloxacin
   c. Levofloxacin
   d. Tetracycline

* Answers can be found online.

When considering these factors, it can easily be appreciated that different medications distribute into breast milk at different rates and to different extents. That is one factor that makes prescribing medications to the breast-feeding woman problematic at best. Health care providers need to ask themselves many questions before selecting a drug therapy.

First, is there a need to treat the maternal condition? Many prescriptions are written for conditions that do not need to be treated. Second, what medication can be prescribed that is least likely to be secreted into the breast milk, and for which there is the greatest information about its use in breast-feeding mothers? Third, would it be possible to treat the condition with a different route of therapy that is not systemic?

Answers to these questions are often difficult or elusive. Referring to the FDA guidelines for medication use in pregnancy and lactation is helpful. A database called LactMed is available to all practitioners that has comprehensive and up-to-date information regarding the known concentrations of drug reaching the infant through breast milk, possible adverse reaction, and potential alternatives. This is an excellent resource that is powered by the National Library of Medicine. Consulting the known pharmacokinetic parameters of medications can also be helpful in prescribing medications. Selected drugs should have short half-lives, and the use of sustained-release products should be discouraged. Dosing schedules also help in minimizing the amount of drug reaching the infant. Scheduling the mother to take the medication immediately after breast-feeding minimizes the dose to the infant by circumventing peak breast milk levels (Dillon et al., 1997).

Patients with chronic conditions, such as hypertension, epilepsy, or diabetes, need to consult their health care practitioners about continuing treatment and minimizing risk to the infant. If a medication is for short-term use, the clinician can also consider if the medication could be postponed until the mother is finished breast-feeding and limiting the medication to the shortest possible duration. Without other options, patients with short-term illnesses can temporarily interrupt breast-feeding for the duration of treatment and resume breast-feeding a

few days after therapy is completed if the risk of the drug to the infant is thought to outweigh the benefits. By this time, no residual drug should be concentrated in the breast milk. During the interruption, however, the mother must pump the breast and discard the milk. Doing so relieves engorgement and promotes continued milk production and flow.

Balancing Benefits and Risks

Although the health benefits of breast-feeding are established, there remain a few medications that are unsafe to use during breast-feeding. As with medication use during pregnancy, the risk–benefit ratio needs to be assessed. Choice of the best medication to treat the maternal condition needs to be balanced against the risk of adverse effects to the infant.

Bibliography

*Starred references are cited in the text.

Anderson, G. D. (2006). Using pharmacokinetics to predict the effects of pregnancy and maternal-fetal transfer of drugs during lactation. *Expert Opinion on Drug Metabolism and Toxicology, 2*(6), 947–960.

*Briggs, C. G., Freeman, R. K., & Yaffe, S. J. (2014). *Drugs in pregnancy and lactation* (10th ed.). Philadelphia, PA: Lippincott Williams & Wilkins.

*Centers for Disease Control and Prevention. (2014). Treating for Two: Data and Statistics. Updated: February 19, 2014. Retrieved from http://www.cdc.gov/pregnancy/meds/treatingfortwo/data.html on July 15, 2015.

*Collaborative Group on Drug Use in Pregnancy. (1991). An international survey on drug utilization during pregnancy. *International Journal of Risk and Safety in Medicine, 2*(6), 345–349.

Cordero, J. F., & Oakley, G. P. (1983). Drug exposure during pregnancy: Some epidemiological considerations. *Clinical Obstetrics and Gynecology, 26,* 418–428.

Dawes, M., & Chowienczyk, P. J. (2001). Drugs in pregnancy. Pharmacokinetics in pregnancy. *Best Practice and Research. Clinical Obstetrics and Gynaecology, 15*(6), 819–826.

Department of Health and Human Services. Food and Drug Administration. 21 CFR Part 201. Content and Format of Labeling Human Prescription Drug and Biological Products; Requirements for Pregnancy and Lactation Labeling. Published December 04, 2014. Retrieved from http://www.fda.gov/OHRMS/DOCKETS/98fr/06-545.pdf on July 20, 2015.

*Dicke, J. M. (1989). Teratology: Principles and practice. *Medical Clinics of North America, 73,* 567–582.

*Dillon, A. E., et al. (1997). Drug therapy in the nursing mother. *Obstetrics and Gynecology Clinics of North America, 24*, 676–697.

*Fredericksen, M. C. (2001). Physiologic changes in pregnancy and their effect on drug disposition. *Seminars in Perinatology, 25*(3), 120–123.

Gonsalves, L., & Scheuremeyer, I. (2009). Treating depression in pregnancy: Practical suggestions. *Cleveland Clinical Journal of Medicine, 73*(12), 1098–1104.

*Guyton, A. C., & Hall, J. C. (1996). *Human physiology and mechanisms of disease* (6th ed.). Philadelphia, PA: Saunders.

*Juchau, M. R., & Choa, S. T. (1983). Drug metabolism by the human fetus. In M. Gibaldi, & L. Prescott (Eds.), *Handbook of clinical pharmacokinetics* (pp. 58–78). New York, NY: Adis.

*Koren, G., et al. (1998). Drugs in pregnancy. *New England Journal of Medicine, 338*, 1128–1137.

*Kraemer, K., et al. (1997). Placental transfer of drugs. *Neonatal Network, 16*(2), 65–67.

*Loebstein, R., et al. (1997). Pharmacokinetic changes during pregnancy and their clinical relevance. *Clinical Pharmacokinetics, 33*, 328–343.

McElhatton, P. R. (2003). General principles of drug use in pregnancy. *The Pharmaceutical Journal, 270*, 232–234.

Mosley, J. F., II, Smith, L. L., & Dezan, M. D. (2015). An overview of upcoming changes in pregnancy and lactation labeling information. *Pharmacy Practice, 13*(2), 605.

*Oakley, G. P. (1986). Frequency of human congenital malformations. *Clinics in Perinatology, 13*, 545–554.

*Rayburn, W. F. (1997). Chronic medical disorders during pregnancy. *Journal of Reproductive Medicine, 42*, 1–24.

*Sachs, H., & Committee on Drugs. (2013). The transfer of drugs and therapeutics into human breast milk: An update on selected topics. *Pediatrics, 132*, e796–e809.

Scott, J. R., DiSaia, P. J., Hammond, C. B., et al. (Eds.). (1999). *Danforth's obstetrics and gynecology* (8th ed.). Philadelphia, PA: Lippincott Williams & Wilkins.

*Simone, G., Derewlany, L., & Koren, G. (1994). Drug transfer across the placenta. *Clinics in Perinatology, 21*, 463–482.

Tettenborn, B. (2006). Management of epilepsy in women of childbearing age: Practical recommendations. *CNS Drugs, 20*(5), 373–387.

Wyska, E., & Jusko W. J. (2001). Approaches top pharmacokinetic/pharmacodynamic modeling during pregnancy. *Seminars in Perinatology, 25*, 124–132.

*Yankowitz, J., & Niebyl, J. R. (2001). *Drug therapy in pregnancy* (3rd ed.). Philadelphia, PA: Lippincott Williams & Wilkins.

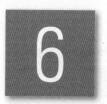

6

Pharmacotherapy Principles in Older Adults

Richard G. Stefanacci

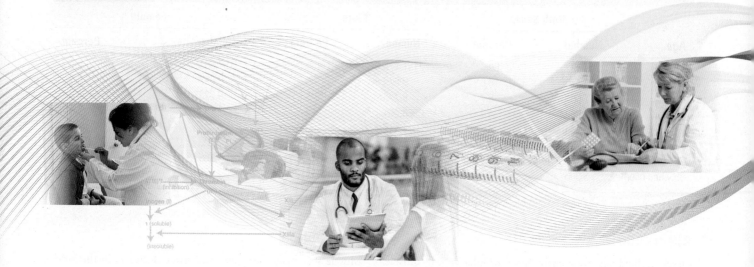

Older adults are the most pharmacotherapeutically challenging population because of the requirement to take into consideration their unique physiology and other factors in the face of the need to treat multiple chronic comorbid conditions. This warrants an understanding of aging and its effects on the body. Some of the other factors impacting this population include changes such as cognitive and social issues affecting proper adherence resulting in suboptimal outcomes. In addition, part of this challenge is the fact that many pharmaceuticals have not been testing in this population. As a result, practitioners need to rely on their knowledge of basic principles of pharmacotherapy in the older and monitor on an individual patient basis.

This expertise of managing pharmacotherapy in the older adults is crucial given that the older population is the fastest growing of any age group. By the year 2050, the "oldest old," those aged 85 and older, will approach 19 million and 4.3% of the U.S. population (Vincent & Velhoff, 2010). The latest numbers available from the Centers for Disease Control and Prevention (CDC) reveal that 14.1% of the U.S. population is over the age of 65. Specifically, that population breaks down as shown in **Table 6.1**.

A report from National Center for Health Statistics, Division of Vital Statistics at the Centers for Disease Control and Prevention, finds an increase in overall life expectancy from 78.7 years in 2011 to 78.8 years in 2012. This is the longest life expectancy ever recorded, which they attribute to a reduction in many major causes of death, such as cancer, heart disease, and stroke. While decreasing in frequency, these remain significant health issues for older adults, which is a concern given the rise in obesity. Specifically, the CDC

has identified certain overall health issues for older adults as described in **Box 6.1**.

The consequences of longevity are evidenced by the rising number of older adults living with multiple chronic diseases, contributing to disability, frailty, and decline in function and presenting significant challenges for medical management (Norris et al., 2008). This has led to an increased use of health care utilization, which the CDC reports as described in **Box 6.2**.

Treating multiple problems with prescription as well as over-the-counter (OTC) medications can result in adverse drug reactions (ADRs) and interactions related to changes produced by aging. Problems of polypharmacy (the use of an inappropriate amount of medications to treat a host of medical conditions), improper dosing for an older adult, and a lack of understanding by adults about medications can lead to significant but preventable adverse effects, such as falls, fractures, and delirium. This chapter discusses basic physiologic changes of aging, proper prescribing principles, and social concepts pertaining to safe medication use for the older adult.

BODY CHANGES AND AGING

Every body system is affected by the aging process, although homeostasis is often maintained despite less-than-optimal functioning of organ systems. Certain systems are more vitally affected by aging and play significant roles in the pharmacokinetic and pharmacodynamic changes in drug effects. **Box 6.3** summarizes the impact of aging on the pharmacokinetics of drugs.

TABLE 6.1							
Population by Age and Sex: 2012							
	Both Sexes		**Male**		**Female**		
Age	Number	Percent	Number	Percent	Number	Percent	
All ages	308,827	100.0	151,175	100.0	157,653	100.0	
55–59 y	20,470	6.6	9,879	6.5	10,592	6.7	
60–64 y	17,501	5.7	8,278	5.5	9,223	5.8	
65–69 y	13,599	4.4	6,461	4.3	7,139	4.5	
70–74 y	9,784	3.2	4,519	3.0	5,265	3.3	
75–79 y	7,331	2.4	3,122	2.1	4,209	2.7	
80–84 y	5,786	1.9	2,421	1.6	3,365	2.1	
85 y and over	5,006	1.6	1,809	1.2	3,196	2.0	

Numbers in thousands. Civilian noninstitutionalized population.

Absorption

Older individuals frequently have oropharyngeal muscle dysmotility and altered swallowing of food. Reductions in esophageal peristalsis and lower esophageal sphincter (LES) pressures are also more common in the aged. Delayed motility and gastric emptying have been reported in some cases as well as the propulsive motility of the colon is also decreased, which may impact absorption. Decreased gastric secretions (acid, pepsin) and impairment of the mucous–bicarbonate barrier are frequently described in the older and may impact absorption. The prolonged transit time in the GI tract still allows for adequate drug absorption.

Distribution

Muscle that makes up lean body tissue decreases in the older adult, shifting to increased fat stores, and body water content decreases by 10% to 15% by age 80. Aging results in some reduction in serum albumin (by approximately 20%), leading to an increase in free drug concentration of drugs such as warfarin (Coumadin) and phenytoin (Dilantin).

There are two important plasma-binding proteins in drug metabolism: albumin and α-acid glycoprotein. Albumin has an affinity for acid compounds or drugs such as warfarin, whereas α_1-acid glycoprotein binds more readily with lipophilic and alkaline drugs such as propranolol (Inderal). The effects of chronic disease, nutritional deficits, immobility, and age-related liver changes contribute to the changes in serum proteins. The significance of decreased serum proteins is realized when highly protein-bound drugs compete for decreased protein-binding sites. The result can be greater levels of free or unbound circulating drug and, therefore, potential toxicity.

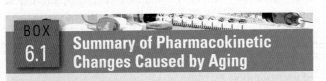

BOX 6.1   Summary of Pharmacokinetic Changes Caused by Aging

Absorptive Changes
  Decreased blood flow
  Increased gastric pH
  Delayed gastric emptying
Distribution Changes
  Decreased albumin
  Decreased lean body mass
  Increased total body fat
  Decreased total body water
Metabolic Changes
  Decreased liver blood flow
  Decreased liver mass
  Decreased enzymatic activity
Excretion Changes
  Decreased glomerular filtration
  Decreased secretion

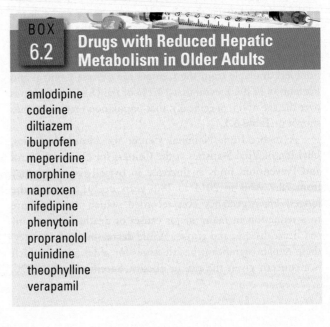

BOX 6.2   Drugs with Reduced Hepatic Metabolism in Older Adults

amlodipine
codeine
diltiazem
ibuprofen
meperidine
morphine
naproxen
nifedipine
phenytoin
propranolol
quinidine
theophylline
verapamil

BOX 6.3 Guidelines for Safe Prescribing for Older Adults

INITIATION OF THERAPY

- Review the risks and benefits of adding a medication. Explore nonpharmacologic options first.
- If possible, choose one medication that treats two coexisting problems.
- Always start with the lowest dose possible and titrate up slowly. "Start low; go slow."
- Choose a drug with the fewest daily required doses (i.e., daily vs. twice daily).
- Remember to consider the cost of the brand name drug and consider generic equivalents if cost issues will deter compliance.

ONGOING PHARMACOTHERAPY ASSESSMENT

- Schedule routine follow-up examinations for the patient who has multiple chronic illnesses and who takes multiple medications.
- Reduce dosages or discontinue medications if possible to avoid polypharmacy.
- Advise adults to bring all medications (prescription or OTC) to each office visit for review.
- Document accurately all current medications and dosages.

- Review medications added by other practitioners and specialists. Inform these professionals of changes made by the primary health care provider.
- Schedule blood tests regularly to monitor levels of such medications as diuretics, ACE inhibitors, antiseizure medications, anticoagulants, antiarrhythmics, and digitalis.

PATIENT SUPPORT

- Give a written list and instructions to the patient after each office visit of the medications to be taken.
- Provide the written medication instructions and changes in large print in terms easily understood by older adults.
- Explain and document both the generic and brand name of the prescribed drug to avoid confusing the patient as well as the important reason for each medication.
- Review medications and changes in the regimen with family/caregivers especially for those caring for loved ones with cognitive impairments.
- Recommend or provide medication planners or weekly/daily dosage containers to improve compliance and promote safe medication administration.

Body mass changes may lead to changes in total body content of drugs in older adults. A water-soluble drug (low volume of distribution [V_d]) is taken up more readily by lean tissue or muscle and attains higher serum concentrations in adults with less body water or lean tissue. Conversely, a lipid-soluble drug is retained in body fat, resulting in a higher V_d for some drugs. Coupled with a decrease or no change in total body clearance, this increase in V_d can lead to increased half-lives and drug accumulation in older adults. For example, diazepam (Valium) has a half-life ($t_{1/2}$) of approximately 20 hours in a young adult, but the $t_{1/2}$ can exceed 70 hours in the older adult. In addition, some drugs, such as tricyclic antidepressants (TCAs) and long-acting benzodiazepines, pass more readily through the blood–brain barrier, causing more pronounced central nervous system (CNS) effects. Older adults who are treated for depression and anxiety may experience fatigue and confusion from drug therapy because antidepressant and antianxiety agents more readily cross their blood–brain barrier.

Elimination

The liver is the major organ of drug metabolism in the body. With aging comes a decrease in blood flow and liver size. However, in the absence of disease, function is maintained.

Decreased size and hepatic blood flow may slow the clearance of certain drugs, and reduced dosages may be required. This is particularly important for drugs with high hepatic extraction ratios. Phase I metabolism, particularly oxidation, is affected by aging. The result is decreased oxidation of drugs, which in turn results in a decreased total body clearance (**Box 6.3**). The phase II metabolism of drugs by conjugation, which promotes drug elimination by breaking the drug into water-soluble components, is not affected by age.

After the liver, the kidneys are the most important organs for drug metabolism and excretion. After age 40, renal blood flow declines and the glomerular filtration rate (GFR) drops approximately 1% a year and accelerates with advancing age. Function is usually maintained despite decreased filtration unless illness or disease overstresses the kidney (Kelleher & Lindeman, 2003). In older adults, drugs excreted primarily by the kidney are given in smaller doses, or the time between doses is extended.

A serum creatinine level alone cannot be used to estimate renal function in the aging person because reductions in lean body mass result in decreased rates of keratinase formation. This, coupled with the decreased GFR, makes the serum keratinase appear normal. It cannot be assumed that the GFR is normal from a normal serum creatinine value. The most

TABLE 6.2

Examples of Dose Adjustments Based on Estimated Creatinine Clearance

Drug	Usual Oral Dose (Nonrenally Impaired)	Dose Based on Estimated CrCl*		
		CrCl >50 mL/min	CrCl 10–50 mL/min	CrCL <10 mL/min
amantadine	100 mg q12h	Usual dose	Increase interval to q24–72h	Increase interval to q7 days
amoxicillin	250–500 mg q8h	Usual dose	Increase interval to q12h	Increase interval to q24h
cefaclor	250 mg tid	Usual dose	Decrease dose to 50%–100% of usual	Decrease dose to 50% of usual
ciprofloxacin	250–750 mg q12h	Usual dose	Reduce dose to 50% of usual	Reduce dose to 33% of usual or extend to q24h
codeine	30–60 mg q4–6h	Usual dose	Reduce dose to 75% of usual	Reduce dose to 50% of usual
digoxin†	0.125–0.5 mg q24h	Usual dose	Reduce dose to 25%–75% of usual OR increase interval to q48h	Reduce dose to 10%–25% of usual
enalapril	5–10 mg q12h	Usual dose	Reduce dose to 75% of usual 300 mg daily (for CrCl 15–30 mL/min)	Reduce dose to 50% of usual
gabapentin†	400 mg tid (for CrCl >60)	300 mg bid (for CrCl 30–60 mL/min)		300 mg every other day (for CrCl 15 mL/min)
nadolol	80–120 mg/d	Usual dose	Reduce dose to 50% of usual	Reduce dose to 25% of usual
procainamide‡	350–400 mg q3–4h	Usual dose	Increase interval to 6–12h	Increase interval to q8–24h
ranitidine	150 mg q12h or 300 mg qhs	Usual dose	Decrease dose to 50% of usual OR increase interval to q24h	Decrease dose to 25% of usual OR increase interval to q48h

*Dose adjustments based on actual creatinine clearance or creatinine clearance estimated by the Cockroft and Gault formula (see Chapter 2).
†These drugs are best monitored using actual drug levels, and dose adjustments should be made based on these results.
‡Based on manufacturer's information.

accurate means of measuring renal function is a 24-hour urine test for creatinine clearance; however, this is not standard procedure before ordering a medication. When there is a need to determine a drug choice in the setting of a potential reduction in creatinine clearance, the Cockcroft and Gault or the MDR formula (see Chapter 2) provides an estimate based on age, weight, and serum creatinine level with an adjustment for sex. **Table 6.2** lists drugs eliminated by the kidney and recommended dosage adjustments based on estimated creatinine clearance.

PHARMACODYNAMIC CHANGES IN THE OLDER ADULT

Many of the changes that occur due to aging affect major organ systems and therefore affect the pharmacokinetic disposition of the drug. However, the clinician also must consider the impact drugs have on the aging body, the pharmacodynamic effect. Although few data are available regarding age-related pharmacodynamic changes in older adults, it is known that the older adult may be more sensitive to drug–receptor interactions, because of either increased sensitivity of the receptor to the drug or decreased capacity to respond to drug-induced innervation of receptors. In addition, the number or affinity of receptors may be reduced. Nevertheless, it is commonly accepted that the CNS effects of drugs appear to be exaggerated in the older patient. Particularly egregious are the agents with anticholinergic effects, such as the TCAs, antihistamines, and antispasmodics. The anticholinergic

effect induced by these agents can lead to excessive dry mouth, blurred vision, constipation, and even an exacerbation of benign prostatic hyperplasia in men. Caution should be used if these agents are prescribed at all.

Similarly, the sedative effects of agents may be intensified in older adults. The benzodiazepines and potent analgesic agents are examples of drugs for which older adults are particularly susceptible to this adverse effect. Overprescribing, or typical prescribing without considering the potential for exaggerated effect, can lead to oversedation and a greater risk of falls and fractures.

The cardiovascular system also can be affected by changes due to aging. Orthostatic hypotension is more common in the older adult because of a loss of the baroreceptor reflex and changes in cerebral blood flow. Moreover, drugs that lower blood pressure or decrease cardiac output put the older patient at risk for a syncopal episode.

POLYPHARMACY

Polypharmacy is a significant factor in the morbidity and mortality of older adults. Increasing age puts the person at risk for multiple chronic illnesses, many of which require drug therapy For example, the most common chronic disease in the United States, osteoarthritis, affects 40 million people, the majority being older adults. The costs in terms of morbidity are staggering. Chronic stiffness and pain from arthritis have an impact on function, prompting the routine use of nonsteroidal anti-inflammatory drugs (NSAIDs) and aspirin products. Long-term use of NSAIDs lowers the prostaglandin level in the GI tract, which may result in esophagitis, peptic ulcerations, GI hemorrhage, and GI perforation. In an older adult, treatment with histamine-2 blockers or proton pump inhibitors to relieve the side effects of aspirin or other NSAIDs may cause additional side effects, such as confusion and mental status changes, in turn requiring more treatment. This demonstrates how easily adverse events occur and snowball in an older patient. ADRs account for 30% of hospital admissions for persons older than age 65; approximately 106,000 deaths are attributed to medication problems. Sadly, 15% to 65% of these events are preventable (Shiyanbola & Farris, 2010) by avoiding potentially inappropriate medications, effective communication, and patient education.

Several factors contribute to polypharmacy. Among them are the varied symptoms and complaints associated with multiple chronic illnesses. In addition, adults often believe that a "pill will fix what ails them," and the health care provider feels pressured to "prescribe something" to satisfy the adults' expectations of a prescription for medication. When a particular medication regimen is unsuccessful, the health care provider typically prescribes another drug, this is referred to as the prescribing cascade. Dr. Jerry Gurwitz, a noted geriatrician, has attributed the caveat that "Any symptom in an elderly patient should be considered a drug side effect until proved otherwise," although his wife, Leslie Fine, a pharmacist, is actually believed to have first described this approach (Smith, 2013).

Polypharmacy is also the effect from many older adults stockpiling their discontinued medications in case they may be needed again—primarily because of the cost of prescription drugs. Many providers who visit older adults in their homes have seen evidence of stockpiled medications. Some older adults keep a drawer or cabinet full of old prescription drug bottles. Some contain the same medication, differing only in brand name. Some adults may place a current medication (prescription or OTC) in a labeled prescription bottle that was used for another drug. In addition, the stockpile may reveal prescription bottles for other family members. Adults may be sharing medications or may have received medications from others who believed that the drug that helped them would help the patient.

Other sources of polypharmacy are "polyproviders." Many older adults see multiple specialists for various chronic diseases. Medications prescribed without the provider carefully reviewing the patient's other medications can lead to drug overuse and complications. Without a primary care provider overseeing the care of the older adult seeing multiple specialists, ADRs are sure to occur.

The health care provider sometimes creates a polypharmacy situation because multiple drugs are used to treat several chronic illnesses. The provider who is not astute in the principles of safe geriatric prescribing practices may create avoidable side effects and complications. In addition, the patient, who may be a great consumer of OTC medications or home remedies, often self-prescribes without knowing the consequences of mixing these treatments with current prescription drugs.

Drug Interactions in the Older Adult

Because of normal, age-related physiologic changes, the older adult is at greater risk for complications from medications. Complications related to drug–disease, drug–drug, and drug–food interaction are all commonly encountered. (For more information on drug–drug interactions, see Chapter 3.)

Adverse Drug Reactions

ADRs often result in significant negative health outcomes, such as falls and fractures, costing billions of dollars in hospital and nursing home care (Shiyanbola & Farris, 2010). Although age itself creates a risk for ADRs, polypharmacy and the multiplicity of drugs taken by older adults present the greater risk. The older adult with multiple chronic illnesses and medications must be identified as a potential candidate for ADRs (Fick et al., 2003). Older women in particular are at great risk for ADRs because they often receive more prescription drugs and have a more significant loss of muscle mass than older men.

There is a paucity of information on safety and efficacy of drugs for the older patient. Most research and clinical trials are performed with younger subjects. It often is difficult or impossible to predict the consequences of a medication for its intended use on an older adult because few data may be available. In an effort to better understand the effects of drugs on older adults, the U.S. Food and Drug Administration published guidelines in 1997 recommending older adults be included in clinical trials of drugs specifically being developed to treat prevalent diseases affecting older adults (Murray & Callahan, 2003).

Contributing Lifestyle Factors

Preventing adverse events or failed treatments begins with being unaware of potential drug interactions resulting from older adults commonly taking OTC medications and prescription drugs without alerting their health care providers. Additional combinations of foods or nutritional supplements can slow absorption, prolonging the time for medications to reach peak levels (see Chapter 3). Fatty foods, in particular, can increase intestinal drug absorption because of the longer time required to digest a fatty meal. This, in turn, potentially leads to increased drug levels or toxicity.

Alcohol and Other Drugs

The ingestion of alcohol and other drugs can alter the metabolism of many medications in older adults. The combination of comorbid conditions, physiological changes with age, and concomitant medications is often potentiated with alcohol usage. CNS effects such as lethargy and confusion occur, as does hypotension, when alcohol is combined with nitrates and some cardiovascular drugs. Alcohol can be found in many OTC products such as cough and cold syrups and mouthwashes.

Alcohol abuse may be overlooked as a potential problem in the older adult, but abuse among community-dwelling (noninstitutionalized) people age 65 and older has a prevalence of 14% for men and 1.5% for women. High numbers of older alcoholics are treated in emergency departments and medical offices or are hospitalized for medical or psychiatric admissions. Depression, which is more prevalent in the older, often coexists with alcohol abuse. Moderate-to-heavy drinkers older than 65 are 16 times more likely to die of suicide. Practitioners need to be more aware of the potential for alcohol abuse in older adults. Although alcohol use and abuse decline with age, approximately 40% of older adults use alcohol, with between 2% and 4% meeting the criteria for alcohol abuse/dependency. The use of alcohol is anticipated to increase as baby boomers age. The baby boomer cohort has a history of greater alcohol, tobacco, and nonmedical substance usage than previous generations. Life stressors such as retirement, loss of loved ones, dependency, and chronic illness are contributors to potential alcohol abuse. Also, as more and more states follow Washington and Colorado's lead in legalizing the recreational use of marijuana, it should be expected that older adults will also be among the users. So the inclusion of this potential drug–drug interaction needs to be taken into account as well.

Caffeine and Nicotine Use

Caffeine and nicotine are among some of the most commonly used products that have the potential to interact with certain drugs, thereby altering efficacy and therapeutic drug levels. Besides its presence in coffee, tea, and some sodas, caffeine is found in many OTC drug products. The interaction of caffeine and certain medications may alter drug absorption, cause CNS effects, or decrease drug effectiveness. **Table 6.3** summarizes selected caffeine–medication interactions.

TABLE 6.3

Medication–Caffeine Interactions

Type of Interaction	Example of Interaction Effect
Caffeine-induced increase in gastric acid secretion	Decreased absorption of iron
Caffeine-induced gastrointestinal irritation	Decreased effectiveness of cimetidine; increased gastrointestinal irritation from corticosteroids, alcohol, and analgesics
Altered caffeine metabolism	Prolonged effect of caffeine when combined with ciprofloxacin, estrogen, or cimetidine
Caffeine-induced cardiac arrhythmic effect	Decreased effectiveness of antiarrhythmic medications
Caffeine-induced hypokalemia	Exacerbated hypokalemic effect of diuretics
Caffeine-induced stimulation of CNS	Increased stimulation effects from amantadine, decongestants, fluoxetine, and theophylline
Caffeine-induced increase in excretion of lithium	Decreased effectiveness of lithium

TABLE 6.4

Medication–Nicotine Interactions

Type of Interaction	Example of Interaction Effect
Nicotine-induced alteration in metabolism	Decreased efficacy of analgesics, lorazepam, theophylline, aminophylline, β-blockers, and calcium channel blockers
Nicotine-induced vasoconstriction	Increased peripheral ischemic effect of β-blockers
Nicotine-induced CNS stimulation	Decreased drowsiness from benzodiazepines and phenothiazines
Nicotine-induced stimulation of antidiuretic hormone secretion	Fluid retention and decreased effectiveness of diuretics
Nicotine-induced increase in platelet activity	Decreased anticoagulant effectiveness (heparin, warfarin); increased risk of thrombosis with estrogen use
Nicotine-induced increase in gastric acid	Decreased or negated effects of H_2 antagonists (cimetidine, famotidine, nizatidine, ranitidine)

Many older adults have lifelong smoking addictions and are unsuccessful in stopping. Adults and providers alike are frequently unaware of the effects of nicotine and medications. Nicotine alters the metabolism of many drugs, causes CNS effects, and interferes with platelet activity. **Table 6.4** reviews nicotine–medication effects and interactions.

ADHERENCE ISSUES

One reason older adults, similar to all patients, do not achieve the optimum outcome from their treatments is their failure to adhere to the medication regimen. In many cases, prescription drugs are not taken as prescribed: up to 40% of older adults take their medications improperly. More than 40% of ambulatory adults age 65 and older take at least 5 medications per week, with 12% taking at least 10 per week. Studies have shown that as the complexity of the medication regime increases, improper drug usage rises proportionately. In some cases, they may not take enough of the medication, either because they think that they will save money by making the prescription last longer or because they believe that the medicine is not needed at the prescribed dose. In other situations, a medication may not be taken if it interferes with the patient's lifestyle, for example, not taking a diuretic for fear of incontinence on certain days.

Cost Factors

Cost is actually becoming less of an issue for some of the more commonly used medications while it is still an issue especially for older adults requiring innovative biologics. For the more commonly used medications today, many are available in a generic formulation such as those needed for hypertension, diabetes, and hypercholesterolemia. The addition of the Medicare Part D prescription drug benefit provides older adults drug coverage. When this Medicare benefit was first introduced in 2006, there was a coverage gap or as it is more commonly referred to as "the doughnut hole." During this gap period in the Medicare Part D benefit, beneficiaries were responsible for 100% of the cost of their medication. As a result, this sudden increase in cost from 25% during the initial benefit period to 100%, many older adults abandoned their medication at the pharmacy counter (Tseng et al., 2009). Follow on legislation has moved to close the coverage gap, so by 2020, it will no longer exist and older adults will continue to only be responsible for a maximum of 25% through their benefit until they reach the catastrophic period where they are only responsible for 5% of the cost of their medication (Stefanacci & Spivack, 2010). The savings on prescription drugs is even greater for older adults with low income who qualify for extra help. These individuals only pay a little over $2 per prescription for generic medications and $6 for branded products. This exact co-payment is adjusted annually.

Side Effects

Other reasons for nonadherence to drug treatments include the unpleasant or inconvenient side effects accompanying some medications. Dry mouth, change in taste sensations, fatigue, or frequent urination are reported as reasons for stopping a medication. The form of the medication and ease of administration are reasons as well. Large tablets and capsules may be difficult to swallow. Swallowing problems may be compounded by insufficient fluid being taken with medications. Taking several oral medications at one dosing time with too little fluid may result in the medications "getting stuck," leading to chronic esophageal irritation. Presbyesophagus (the slowing of esophageal motility with advancing age) makes it difficult and frustrating to swallow multiple medications, and it can also lead to choking or aspiration.

Many times, perceived side effects are not truly related to the medications resulting in an inappropriate discontinuation of a needed therapy. Critical in the management of side effects are education and communication. Education requires that health care providers inform patients of the expected side effects of their medications. Communication is required to assure that patients openly describe their concerns regarding any and all real and perceived side effects. It is only through effective education and communication that side effects are appropriately managed.

Physical and Mental Changes

Functional deficits, especially those affecting the senses, can also challenge adherence to the medication regimen. Poor vision leads to difficulty reading labels and consequently taking the wrong pills or too many of the same pills. Arthritic hands and safety caps can make opening prescription bottles difficult and frustrating for an older adult.

The prevalence of dementia, which manifests in symptoms of cognitive impairment and poor short-term memory and recall, slowly progresses with age, affecting a substantial percentage of those residing in the community. The condition may be unrecognized by the family because the patient may remain seemingly independent and functional despite mental deficits. The family may be fooled into believing the loved one is fine until the condition affects the person's ability to manage basic, daily routines. Unfortunately, the affected older adult is often responsible for taking his or her own medications. Poor memory results in not taking medication properly, forgetting doses, or taking too many doses of the same drug. Approximately 30% of hospital admissions in the older adult are attributed to toxicity from medications or ADRs. Of prescription medications, almost one third are for those age 65 and older. While technology including personal mechanical medication management systems is providing a wide range of solutions to assist in overcoming these challenges, having engaged caregivers is often required to overcome these issues in assuring adherence to therapy.

Self-Medication Issues

The use of OTC drugs and home remedies is another significant issue. Noninstitutionalized older adults consume between 40% and 50% of all OTC medications sold. Of more concern is the fact that 70% of those OTC medications were consumed without the patient consulting the health care provider. Approximately 20% of ADRs in the older are due to OTC medications. On average, the older take two OTC medications with 3.8 to 6.7 prescription drugs. Many OTC medications are taken without the medical provider's awareness in order to treat symptoms they do not want to report. Family members and friends often borrow medications believed to treat a particular ailment, again without consultation with their medical provider.

The use of herbal preparations contributes to ADRs, especially when taken with prescription medications. Of those over age 65 taking herbal preparations, 49% do not divulge this information to their medical providers, compounding the risk of drug interactions and toxicity.

Many OTC medications are products that were once available only by prescription. Now, despite their decreased strength, these medications that once required medical supervision and monitoring present a potential hazard for side effects.

The most common OTC medications used by the older adult include analgesics, vitamins and minerals, antacids, and laxatives. Cough and cold products and sleeping aids such as Tylenol PM are frequently used by older adults. Combining these products may result in confusion, change in mental status, fluid and electrolyte imbalances, dysrhythmias, and nervousness. Cold medications may worsen hypertension without the patient's knowledge or worsen glucose control in a patient with diabetes.

The older adult must be educated to use OTC drugs safely and to do so only after consulting with the health care provider.

If an alternative to drug use is feasible, such as initiating sleep hygiene practices versus taking a sleeping pill, the patient should be encouraged to try these measures first because of their limited negative side effects.

LIFE EXPECTANCY AND GOALS OF CARE

Appreciating an older adult's life expectancy and goals of care is critical for determination of when discontinuation of treatments would be appropriate. To aid in the determination of prognosis, there is a calculator available to health care providers through www.ePrognosis.org.

The information on ePrognosis is intended as a rough guide to inform health care providers about possible mortality outcomes. This information can assist in making a determination when a medication such as a statin may no longer be appropriate because of a limited life expectancy. This situation is unique to older adults, for in the care of younger adults, discontinuation because of limited effectiveness secondary to a shortened life expectancy is typically not an issue. Understanding this dynamic such that recommendations can be made for discontinuation is essential to prevent unnecessary adverse events from occurring as well as a waste of health care resources.

SPECIAL CONSIDERATIONS IN LONG-TERM CARE

Advanced age and years of multiple illnesses and mental decline result in frailty and disability. Transitioning to a long-term care (LTC) facility occurs when an older adult requires assistance with daily functions, such as bathing and dressing, shows cognitive impairment, or has a significant nursing need such as wound care. The national percentage of older adults in nursing homes is about 5%, rising to 20% for age 85 and older. With a wide array of physical, psychiatric, neurologic, and behavioral problems, the LTC resident is the most complex of all older adults. Consequently, the complexity of prescribing medications for the nursing home resident can be challenging. As a result, there is a federal requirement that all residents of skilled nursing facilities receive a drug regimen review by a consultant pharmacist on a monthly basis. All of these practices described for older adult residents of skilled nursing facilities apply to those living in the community as well. This is especially true given that LTC needs are increasing being served in the community. Programs such as the Program of All-Inclusive Care for the Elderly (PACE) service nursing home eligible older adults in the community. Additionally, states are using home and community waivers to provide LTC services outside of the nursing home. This has forced clinicians to be able to apply LTC practices outside of the nursing home to serve this increasingly community-based frail older adults.

Falls and Medication

One of the most serious problems in LTC facilities are traumatic falls. Approximately half of nursing home residents fall annually, sustaining fractures and soft tissue and other injuries. Among the multiple causes of falls are medications, in particular psychotropic agents (e.g., sedatives, hypnotics, antidepressants, and neuroleptics). These medications are useful for treating the depression, anxiety, and behavioral problems that are not unusual in the LTC resident. However, their use presents an ongoing treatment challenge. Medication-related falls are often caused by orthostatic hypotension, sedation, extrapyramidal side effects, myopathy, and pupil constriction. **Table 6.5** lists drug classes leading to instability (Hile & Studenski, 2007).

Antipsychotics

Significant reduction of antipsychotic use in nursing home residents suffering from dementia is a high priority of legislators, regulators, and LTC providers (Smith, 2013). Currently, the Food and Drug Administration (FDA) has approved the use of certain antipsychotic drugs only for schizophrenia, bipolar disorder, and major depressive disorder (in the latter case, when used as adjunctive treatment). Yet, almost 40% of people with dementia living in nursing homes receive antipsychotic medications for management of a wide variety of behavioral/neuropsychiatric symptoms, many of which fall outside the indications approved by the FDA.

Since the launch of the National Partnership to Improve Dementia Care in early 2012, the Centers for Medicare and Medicaid Services (CMS) set an ongoing goal of reducing the use of antipsychotics in LTC facilities by 15%. The overall goal of the partnership is to improve the quality of life for the 1.5 million nursing home residents in the United

TABLE 6.5	
Medications That Contribute to Instability	
Mechanism	**Classes of Medications**
Orthostatic hypotension	Antihypertensives, antianginals, Parkinsonian drugs, TCAs, and antipsychotics
Sedation, decreased attention	Benzodiazepines, sedating antihistamines, narcotic analgesics, TCAs, SSRIs, antipsychotics, anticonvulsants, and ethanol
Extrapyramidal side effects	Antipsychotics, metoclopramide, phenothiazines for nausea such as prochlorperazine, and SSRIs
Myopathy	Corticosteroids; colchicine; high-dose statins, especially in combination with fibrates; ethanol; and interferon
Miosis (pupil constriction)	Glaucoma medications, especially pilocarpine

States by improving the quality of care. Disruptive behavior by LTC residents is problematic beyond the resident themselves. Disruptive behavior is troubling to family, caregivers, providers, and the LTC community as a whole—disruptive behavior is truly disruptive. All too often in the past, this behavior has been addressed with antipsychotic medications but studies show that there will be 1 premature death for every 53 frail elderly patients with dementia who are treated with antipsychotics. To improve the management of disruptive behavior and reduce antipsychotic medication in LTC, several regulations and guidance have been developed. This included a bill entitled Improving Dementia Care Treatment for Older Adults Act of 2012 (Act), which was enacted to establish requirements relating to antipsychotic administration to residents of skilled nursing facilities under Medicare and Medicaid and for the implementation of prescriber education programs.

These risks were previously noted when the Food and Drug Administration (FDA) issued black box warnings in 2005 (for "atypical" antipsychotics) and 2008 (for "conventional" antipsychotics), stating that elderly patients with dementia-related psychosis who are administered antipsychotics face a 1.6 to 1.7 times greater risk of death than patients treated with placebo. However, antipsychotic prescription rates in LTC facilities for patients with dementia and no diagnosis of psychosis remained high despite these significant warnings. A study in 1999 showed that within a 1-week period, 39% of elderly nursing home residents with dementia and aggressive behavioral symptoms received antipsychotics.[1] By 2006, some facilities had more than 50% of nursing home residents with dementia using antipsychotics, which was an increase of approximately 33%. Despite the FDA black box warning, the State Operations Manual tag F329, and consultant pharmacist medication regimen review (MRR) requirements, inappropriate use of antipsychotics continues to be an issue.

According to the CMS Online Survey, Certification and Reporting (OSCAR) data from 2012, the national average utilization rate of antipsychotics was more than 25% among all long-stay residents (**Table 6.6**) (CMS, 2012).

In May 2012, CMS set a goal to reduce the use of antipsychotic drugs in LTC facilities by 15% by the end of that year. A 15% reduction in that rate would have meant a national prevalence of 20.3%. This does not mean that each facility across the country should have a prevalence of 20.3% but that the national average should not be higher. This initial target was to ensure that rapid progress was made and that systems and infrastructure were put in place to continue to work toward lower rates of antipsychotic medication use. It does not mean that a rate of 20.3% is acceptable, since tag F329 requires the lowest dose possible to improve the targeted symptoms. Thus, it is believed by CMS, the Department of Health and Human Services (HHS) Office of Inspector General (OIG), and others that a much lower percentage is achievable and more appropriate. In addition, although the goal was a reduction in the use nationally, facilities with use

TABLE 6.6

National Average Utilization Rate of Antipsychotics among All Long-Stay Residents, Reported February 1, 2012 (CMS, 2012)

Category	Value
Antipsychotic medications	25.2%
Antianxiety medications	22.0%
Antidepressant medications	48.5%
Hypnotic medications	7.6%
All psychoactive medications	65.6%
Total residents	1,388,058
Total facilities	15,712

higher than the national or state norm will be more closely scrutinized during routine surveys.

This goal of reducing psychotropic drug use was followed by reporting requirements tied to the Nursing Home Five-Star Quality Rating System. Specifically, new quality measures related to antipsychotic medications for both the short- and long-stay residents will be posted on the Nursing Home Compare (NHC) Web site. For short-stay residents, the measure covers those who are given an antipsychotic medication after admission to the nursing home; the focus therefore is on new starts. A separate prevalence measure assesses the percentage of long-stay residents who are receiving an antipsychotic medication without regard to when it was initially ordered. The Pharmacy Quality Alliance (PQA) has endorsed a similar measure—Antipsychotic Use in Persons with Dementia—which measures the percentage of older individuals with dementia (age ≥65 years) who are taking an antipsychotic medication and who show no evidence of a psychotic disorder or related condition.

The Interdisciplinary Team (IDT) approach to caring for patients includes many professionals performing a variety of specialized functions designed to meet the physical, emotional, and psychological needs of the patient. The collaborative efforts of the members are focused on delivering patient-centered coordinated care. A number of experts have said that IDT collaboration improves safety and quality of care. This approach can be used to optimize individual resident management assuring appropriate use of antipsychotic medications, which should result in the CMS goal of a 15% reduction.

The goals for this team are as follows:

1. Prevent initiation of inappropriate use of psychotropic medications in residents.
2. Taper and discontinue inappropriate psychotropic medications, to ensure that use of the medications is appropriate and that monitoring and documentation are properly conducted.
3. Improve disruptive behaviors while limiting/diminishing the use of psychotropic medications, by educating and

encouraging prescribers and nursing facility staff to adopt a more structured and broader approach to management of behavioral symptoms.

The team approach to management of older adults with disruptive behaviors should emphasize certain key principles:

- Individuals who exhibit disruptive symptoms should be thoroughly assessed by a qualified health professional.
- The assessment should seek to identify possible underlying causes that may contribute to disruptive symptoms, so that treatment can target the underlying cause.
- Disruptive symptoms should be objectively and quantitatively monitored by caregivers or facility staff and documented on an ongoing basis.
- If the behaviors do not present an immediate and serious threat to the patient or others, the initial approach to management should focus on environmental modifications, behavioral interventions, psychotherapy, or other nonpharmacologic interventions.
- When medications are indicated, an appropriate agent should be selected only after consideration of the underlying diagnosis or condition, effectiveness of the medication, and risk of side effects.

While developed for antipsychotic medications, these practices should be applied to all classes of medications when managing pharmacotherapy in older adults.

Anxiolytics

Anxiety is a problem frequently confronted in the nursing home setting. It may be precipitated by physical causes such as pain, infection, or chronic illness. Other stressors that contribute to anxiety include fatigue or change, such as a change in a daily routine or change of caregiver. An overly stimulating environment or expectations of staff members hurrying the older resident through daily routines may evoke anxiety. Initially, nonpharmacologic measures should be used to assess and ameliorate anxiety; prescribing a medication to relieve anxiety should be a last choice.

Several nonpharmacologic antianxiety treatments may be beneficial. They include establishing daily routines in a structured environment, consistently providing the same caregiver for bathing and hygiene assistance, avoiding overstimulation from activities, limiting social visits, and scheduling quiet time with rest or naps.

When anxiolytic drugs are prescribed, the benzodiazepines are often chosen for adults age 65 and older. Unfortunately, side effects are prevalent, among which are the discomforts of discontinuing the therapy. Benzodiazepines can impact cognitive function and psychomotor performance in older adults. The patient may experience increased agitation, anxiety, and insomnia. More serious symptoms include tremors, tachycardia, diaphoresis, nausea, vomiting, and alterations in perception, anterograde amnesia, and seizures. The benzodiazepines have a propensity for

dependence by accumulating in the older body. For this reason, they should be prescribed for short courses of up to 2 weeks at most.

The older patient receiving benzodiazepine therapy often experiences significant daytime sedation, dizziness, and subsequent falls. Studies indicate the "oldest old," those older than age 85, have a 15-fold increased risk of falls with benzodiazepine use. When a benzodiazepine with a long half-life is prescribed, the fall rate is 10-fold greater than when a benzodiazepine with a short to moderate half-life is prescribed. Benzodiazepines with a long half-life include diazepam and flurazepam (Dalmane); benzodiazepines with a shorter half-life include lorazepam (Ativan), alprazolam (Xanax), and oxazepam (Serax). When a benzodiazepine is prescribed, it should have a short half-life, be for short-term use, and be given in the lowest dose possible.

The selective serotonin reuptake inhibitors (SSRIs), which treat depression, general anxiety, and panic and obsessive–compulsive disorders, are now considered the better choice for treating anxiety in the frail older adult due to their favorable side effect profile (Sheikh & Cassidy, 2003). There is often comorbid depression with anxiety, so an SSRI may treat both conditions, such as sertraline (Zoloft) for panic and depression.

An alternative anxiolytic is buspirone (BuSpar). It is nonsedating and has minimal drug interactions and a slow onset of action, 2 to 3 weeks. For that reason, it is not indicated for acute anxiety but works well as an add-on drug. Caution must be used with buspirone in adults with Parkinson disease because EPSs can occur. For anxiety with underlying depression and insomnia, trazodone (Desyrel) is an alternative. Because of its sedating properties, it promotes sleep and treats underlying depression that may exacerbate anxiety.

Antidepressants

The prevalence of depression increases with age, as evidenced by 25% of those with chronic illness and a 15% to 25% rate of depression among nursing home residents (Bergman et al., 2009). Older adults with late life depression exhibit more psychotic symptoms, delusions, insomnia, and somatic complaints. In such settings, older adults with depression should be treated because antidepressant treatment usually improves nutrition and function and decreases symptoms of pain and insomnia. Better choices for antidepressants include SSRIs (e.g., paroxetine, fluoxetine [Prozac], sertraline [Zoloft], citalopram [Celexa], and escitalopram [Lexapro]). SSRIs have the advantage of daily dosing and fewer side effects than TCAs, which were used frequently before the advent of SSRIs. Although the TCAs are still used, they are associated with many side effects that can lead to cognitive impairment and falls. Cardiovascular effects include hypotension, arrhythmias, and sudden death. Other troublesome side effects include sedation, dry mouth, urinary retention, and dizziness from anticholinergic properties.

Significant drug interactions and toxicity may occur with SSRI use because these drugs inhibit oxidative metabolism. Drugs that may be affected by SSRIs include warfarin, phenytoin, and class 1C antiarrhythmics. Studies indicate that older adults taking SSRIs have a greater risk of falls than older adults not taking antidepressants (Leipzig et al., 1999) and suggest higher doses of combined CNS medications, such as SSRIs, benzodiazepines, and antipsychotics, can lead to cognitive decline in older adults (Wright et al., 2009). Common side effects of SSRIs in the older include headache, nausea, dry mouth, dizziness, constipation, dyspepsia, diarrhea, asthenia, insomnia, decreased appetite, tachycardia, and abnormal taste. Hyponatremia has been increasingly noted to occur in older adults on SSRIs. On withdrawal of the SSRI, sodium levels return to normal within days to weeks (Kirby & Ames, 2001). The prescriber needs to be aware of early signs of hyponatremia: lethargy, fatigue, muscle cramps, anorexia, and nausea.

Other Disorders and Drug Therapies

Studies have shown that, in general, older adults are more vulnerable to severe or persistent pain and that the inability to tolerate severe pain increases with age. Further, older adults are far more likely to experience pain associated with surgical procedures, such as knee and hip replacements, arthritis, cancer, and end-of-life symptoms. Compounding the problem of pain in the elderly is the well-documented fact that pain in the institutionalized older adult population, particularly among minorities and those with dementia, is far more likely to be undertreated. According to the IOM report, "a study of more than 13,000 people with cancer aged 65 and older discharged from the hospital to nursing homes found that, among the 4,000 who were in daily pain, those aged 85 and older were more than 1.5 times as likely to receive no analgesia than those aged 65-74; only 13 percent of those aged 85 and older received opioid medications, compared with 38 percent of those aged 65-74".

While many drug precautions have been in effect since the passage of the Comprehensive Drug Abuse Prevention and Control Act of 1970, they have now taken the form of forced restrictions. Some of these new restrictions are resulting in issues in managing pain for SNF residents. For example, in 2011, the U.S. Food and Drug Administration (FDA) asked drug manufacturers to limit the strength of acetaminophen in combination prescription drugs to 325 mg per tablet by January, 2014, in an attempt to reduce incidences of potentially fatal liver damage. Even though acetaminophen has been commercially available since 1953, it was not until 2009 that the FDA required manufacturers of OTC Tylenol and its generic equivalents to post a warning label for liver damage, due in large part to deaths attributable to acetaminophen use and heavy alcohol consumption. According to the FDA, more than half of manufacturers have voluntarily complied with this request. However, some prescription combination drug products containing more than 325 mg of acetaminophen per dosage unit remain available, prompting the FDA to eventually withdraw approval of any prescription combination drug products containing more than 325 mg of acetaminophen that remain on the market. The result of all of this focus is a limitation on access of higher dose acetaminophen preparations, and as a result, appropriate adjustments for patients receiving these treatments may need to occur. To avoid hepatotoxicity, caution should be taken not to exceed 4,000 mg in 24 hours, especially with known liver disease, alcoholism, or malnutrition.

The chronic pain of degenerative joint disease unrelieved by acetaminophen can be treated with an NSAID. Long-term treatment with NSAIDs can result in GI bleeding, anemia, and renal insufficiency. Caution should be taken when on highly bound drugs, such as warfarin, digoxin, and anticonvulsants, because increased bioavailability occurs due to NSAIDs being highly protein bound. The cyclooxygenase 2 (COX-2) inhibitor celecoxib (Celebrex) is a nontraditional anti-inflammatory drug developed to prevent GI bleeding by not affecting platelet aggregation and bleeding. Although the risk of bleeding with COX-2 inhibitors may be lower than traditional NSAIDs, such as naproxen or ibuprofen, it can still occur. Cardiovascular safety issues led to the withdrawal of rofecoxib and valdecoxib from the market in the United States.

Neuropathic pain from postherpetic neuralgia or diabetic neuropathy can be treated with mixed serotonin and norepinephrine uptake inhibitors, such as duloxetine (Cymbalta) and venlafaxine (Effexor), with a better side effect profile than older TCAs. The anticonvulsant agents gabapentin (Neurontin) and carbamazepine (Tegretol) are also effective in treating neuropathic pain. Pregabalin (Lyrica) is indicated for diabetic peripheral neuropathy; however, it can cause somnolence and dizziness.

Topical analgesics can be effective in pain management in the LTC setting. The 5% lidocaine patch may help with neuralgia pain, although it is often used off label for localized back pain or arthritis. A newer topical NSAID diclofenac (Flector) is indicated for chronic pain management with less systemic absorption than oral NSAIDs (American Geriatrics Society [AGS] Panel on Pharmacological Management of Persistent Pain in Older Persons, 2009).

Other commonly encountered drug-related problems in LTC are urinary incontinence and recurrent urinary tract infections (UTIs), evidenced by confusion and mental status changes. Respiratory infections such as bronchitis and pneumonia quickly spread through a facility because of the compromised immune state of frail residents. Thus, antibiotic use is called on more frequently than for the community-residing adult. The frail older patient with pneumonia may not have typical signs of illness. For example, the patient may not have a cough or fever. Moreover, the frail older patient becomes ill more quickly and decompensates rapidly if untreated. Dehydration, sepsis, or even death may result.

Constipation is another concern, and sometimes an obsession, of older adults. In many instances, they think they need medications to promote bowel movements. However, alternate methods of treating this problem may be judicious, including increasing physical activity and consumption of fluids, fiber, and fruit. One or two tablespoons of a mixture of prune juice, unprocessed bran, and applesauce taken daily is an alternative to stool softeners and laxatives. When assessing constipation, a review of current medications may yield clues to drug use that contributes to the constipation. For example, anticholinergics, such as oxybutynin (Ditropan) used for urinary incontinence; antidepressants, such as the TCAs; and calcium channel blockers may all cause constipation in the frail older patient.

In summary, the older resident in LTC is usually the frailest and at greatest risk for complications related to improper drug administration. The health care provider should attempt to keep medications at a minimum with the lowest dosage possible. A monthly or bimonthly review of all medications should be done to review medical necessity. A pharmacist from within the facility or from the company supplying the facility with medications should routinely review charts and write recommendations to decrease or stop medications. The suggestions should be evaluated by the health care provider and acted on if appropriate to reduce polypharmacy, side effects, and costs for the resident.

GUIDELINES FOR SAFE PRESCRIBING

Guidelines for safe prescribing apply not only to residents of LTC facilities but all older adults. The goal of prescribing for adults in LTC should be to prevent adverse events, falls, and injuries that will further degrade the patient's function, both physical and mental. The provider must prescribe cautiously and keep the patient's safety in mind while promoting his or her comfort and dignity. Providers in LTC need to familiarize themselves with the Beers Criteria, a consensus-based document listing potentially inappropriate medications for use in older adults and guidelines for safe-prescribing practices. This extensive list of medication guidelines was created by a consensus panel of nationally recognized experts in geriatrics and updated in 2015 (AGS, 2015).

In addition to the Beers Criteria, an additional opportunity to improve outcomes comes from the Choosing Wisely initiative. In response to the challenge of improving health care, national organizations representing medical specialists have asked their members to "choose wisely" through the identification of tests or procedures commonly used in their field, whose necessity should be questioned and discussed. The resulting list of "Things Providers and Patients Should Question" is meant to discuss about the need—or lack thereof—for many frequently ordered tests or treatments.

The AMDA–The Society for Post-Acute and LTC Medicine developed 5 things to question, while the AGS developed 10. Taking these 15, one can identify five common themes that clinicians should focus their attention. These five center on the following critical areas for management of pharmacotherapy in older adults:

1. Dementia and behavioral and psychological symptoms of dementia (BPSD)
2. Screening and medication management
3. Antibiotic use
4. Diabetes management
5. Nutritional management

These five areas come from extensive work done by both AMDA and AGS and are refined here with a special focus toward the care of older adults. The result is five Choosing Wise initiatives that when followed will serve clinicians caring for older adults well. Choosing wisely starts and often ends with a "wise" clinician; one that understands these five initiatives is a step in that direction.

Dementia and Behavioral and Psychological Symptoms of Dementia

A starting point is the management of dementia and BPSD for perhaps nothing is more critical given the increasing prevalence of dementia. Several of the AMDA and AGS Choosing Wise directives are focused in this area. These include appropriate management of dementia through not prescribing cholinesterase inhibitors for dementia without periodic assessment for perceived cognitive benefits and adverse gastrointestinal effects. In randomized controlled trials, some patients with mild-to-moderate and moderate-to-severe Alzheimer disease (AD) achieve modest benefits in delaying cognitive and functional decline and decreasing neuropsychiatric symptoms. The impact of cholinesterase inhibitors on institutionalization, quality of life, and caregiver burden is less well established. Clinicians, caregivers, and patients should discuss cognitive, functional, and behavioral goals of treatment prior to beginning a trial of cholinesterase inhibitors. Advance care planning, patient and caregiver education about dementia, diet and exercise, and nonpharmacologic approaches to behavioral issues are integral to the care of patients with dementia and should be included in the treatment plan in addition to any consideration of a trial of cholinesterase inhibitors. If goals of treatment are not attained after a reasonable trial (e.g., 12 weeks), then consider discontinuing the medication. Benefits beyond a year have not been investigated and the risks and benefits of long-term therapy have not been well established resulting in a need for ongoing assessment.

Regarding other treatments for agitation and delirium, two items were raised regarding the use of chemical and physical restraints. Both the AGS and AMDA called out the use of antipsychotic medications because of their adverse effects and consideration as chemical restraints, specifically not to use antipsychotic medications for BPSD in individuals with dementia as first choice or without an assessment for an underlying cause of the behavior. People with dementia often exhibit aggression, resistance to care, and other challenging or disruptive behaviors. In such instances, antipsychotic medicines are often prescribed, but they often provide limited benefit and can cause serious harm, including stroke and premature death. Use of these drugs should be limited to cases where nonpharmacologic measures have failed and patients pose an imminent threat to themselves or others. Identifying and addressing causes of behavior change can make drug treatment unnecessary.

Careful differentiation of cause of the symptoms (physical or neurological vs. psychiatric, psychological) may help better define appropriate treatment options. The therapeutic goal of the use of antipsychotic medications is to treat patients who present an imminent threat of harm to self or others or are in extreme distress—not to treat nonspecific agitation or other forms of lesser distress. Treatment of BPSD in association with the likelihood of imminent harm to self or others includes assessing for and identifying and treating underlying causes (including pain, constipation, and environmental factors such as noise, being too cold or warm, etc.), ensuring safety, reducing distress, and supporting the patient's functioning. If treatment of other potential causes of the BPSD is unsuccessful, antipsychotic medications can be considered, taking into account their significant risks compared to potential benefits. When an antipsychotic is used for BPSD, it is advisable to obtain informed consent.

Also regarding chemical restraints in older adults, using benzodiazepines or other sedative–hypnotics as first choice for insomnia, agitation, or delirium is discouraged. Large-scale studies consistently show that the risk of falls and hip fractures leading to hospitalization and death can more than double in older adults taking benzodiazepines and other sedative–hypnotics. Older patients, their caregivers, and their providers should recognize these potential harms when considering treatment strategies for insomnia, agitation, or delirium. Use of benzodiazepines should be reserved for alcohol withdrawal symptoms/delirium tremens or severe generalized anxiety disorder unresponsive to other therapies.

And lastly, avoiding physical restraints to manage behavioral symptoms of hospitalized older adults with delirium was called out. Persons with delirium may display behaviors that risk injury or interference with treatment. There is little evidence to support the effectiveness of physical restraints in these situations. Physical restraints can lead to serious injury or death and may worsen agitation and delirium. Effective alternatives include strategies to prevent and treat delirium, identification and management of conditions causing patient discomfort, environmental modifications to promote orientation and effective sleep–wake cycles, frequent family contact, and supportive interaction with staff. Educational initiatives and innovative models of practice have been shown to be effective in implementing a restraint-free approach to patients with delirium. This approach includes continuous observation; trying reorientation once, and if not effective, not continuing; observing behavior to obtain clues about patients' needs; discontinuing and/or hiding unnecessary medical monitoring devices or IVs; and avoiding short-term memory questions to limit patient agitation. Pharmacological interventions are occasionally utilized after evaluation by a medical provider at the bedside, if a patient presents harm to him or herself or others. Physical restraints should only be used as a very last resort and should be discontinued at the earliest possible time (**Box 6.4**).

> ### BOX 6.4 Guidelines for Safe Prescribing
>
> 1. Assure that dementia and BPSD are properly managed through use of physical and chemical restraints such as antipsychotics and benzodiazepines as well as cholinesterase inhibitors.
> 2. Assist in the reduction of inappropriate screening and medications that are not beneficial because of limited effectiveness and dangerous adverse effects.
> 3. Do not request a urine analysis or order for an antibiotic unless there is clear indication of a bacterial infection.
> 4. Assure appropriate diabetes management through a reasonable HgbA1c target and use of regularly scheduled antidiabetic medications thus avoiding SSI.
> 5. Assist in the promotion of oral feeding such that percutaneous feeding tube and appetite stimulants are only used in rare situations.

Screening and Medication Management

Consider the true benefits for each and every individual resident before recommending a screening test or medication. All too often, treatments are ordered based on an overestimate of the benefits and under valuation of the risks. This includes such actions as not recommending screening for breast or colorectal cancer or prostate cancer (with the PSA test) without considering life expectancy and the risks of testing, overdiagnosis, and overtreatment. Cancer screening is associated with short-term risks, including complications from testing, overdiagnosis, and treatment of tumors that would not have led to symptoms. For prostate cancer, 1,055 men would need to be screened and 37 would need to be treated to avoid one death in 11 years. For breast and colorectal cancer, 1,000 patients would need to be screened to prevent one death in 10 years. For patients with a life expectancy under 10 years, screening for these three cancers exposes them to immediate harms with little chance of benefit.

In addition, a resident's life expectancy should be taken into account such that there is not routine use of lipid-lowering medications in individuals with a limited life expectancy. There is no evidence that hypercholesterolemia, or low HDL-C, is an important risk factor for all-cause mortality, coronary heart disease mortality, or hospitalization for myocardial infarction or unstable angina in persons older than 70 years. In fact, studies show that elderly patients with the lowest cholesterol have the highest mortality after adjusting other risk factors. In addition, a less favorable risk–benefit ratio may be seen for patients older than 85, where benefits may be more diminished and risks from statin drugs more increased (cognitive impairment, falls, neuropathy, and muscle damage).

Drug regimen reviews are done monthly by consultant pharmacist within the nursing home and these assessments are critical in assuring appropriate medication use. Older patients disproportionately use more prescription and nonprescription drugs than other populations, increasing the risk for side effects and inappropriate prescribing. Polypharmacy may lead to diminished adherence, ADRs, and increased risk of cognitive impairment, falls, and functional decline. Medication review identifies high-risk medications, drug interactions, and those continued beyond their indication. Additionally, medication review elucidates unnecessary medications and underuse of medications and may reduce medication burden (**Box 6.4**).

Antibiotic Use

The CDC and others are increasingly sensitive to the overuse of antibiotics. This overuse has led to dangerous drug-resistant organisms. As a result, both the AGS and AMDA made recommendations to not use antimicrobials to treat bacteriuria in older adults unless specific urinary tract symptoms are present. Cohort studies have found no adverse outcomes for older men or women associated with asymptomatic bacteriuria. Antimicrobial treatment studies for asymptomatic bacteriuria in older adults demonstrate no benefits and show increased adverse antimicrobial effects. Consensus criteria have been developed to characterize the specific clinical symptoms that, when associated with bacteriuria, define UTI.

The inappropriate treatment of positive urine cultures starts with an inappropriate urine analysis; as such, it is recommended not to obtain a urine culture unless there are clear signs and symptoms that localize to the urinary tract. Chronic asymptomatic bacteriuria is frequent in the LTC setting, with prevalence as high as 50%. A positive urine culture in the absence of localized UTI symptoms (i.e., dysuria, frequency, urgency) is of limited value in identifying whether a patient's symptoms are caused by a UTI. Colonization (a positive bacterial culture without signs or symptoms of a localized UTI) is a common problem in LTC facilities that contributes to the overuse of antibiotic therapy, leading to an increased risk of diarrhea, resistant organisms, and infection due to *Clostridium difficile*. An additional concern is that the finding of asymptomatic bacteriuria may lead to an erroneous assumption that a UTI is the cause of an acute change of status, hence failing to detect or delaying the more timely detection of the patient's more serious underlying problem. A patient with advanced dementia may be unable to report urinary symptoms. In this situation, it is reasonable to obtain a urine culture if there are signs of systemic infection such as fever (increase in temperature of equal to or greater than 2°F [1.1°C] from baseline), leukocytosis, or a left shift or chills in the absence of additional symptoms (e.g., new cough) to suggest an alternative source of infection. Remember it often starts with clinicians believing a patient's change in condition and requesting a urine analysis despite their not being any signs of a urinary infection. Thoughtful recommendations in this area can go a long way in assuring appropriate antibiotic use (**Box 6.4**).

Diabetes Management

Diabetes management was another area where both the AGS and AMDA found common ground. The inappropriate treatment of residents with diabetes can result in falls from hypoglycemia as well as painful frequent fingersticks and injections from the overuse of sliding scale insulin (SSI). As a result, it is recommended to avoid using medications to achieve hemoglobin A1c less than 7.5% in most adults age 65 and older; moderate control is generally better. There is no evidence that using medications to achieve tight glycemic control in older adults with type 2 diabetes is beneficial. Among nonolder adults, except for long-term reductions in myocardial infarction and mortality with metformin, using medications to achieve glycated hemoglobin levels less than 7% is associated with harms, including higher mortality rates. Tight control has been consistently shown to produce higher rates of hypoglycemia in older adults. Given the long time frame to achieve theorized microvascular benefits of tight control, glycemic targets should reflect patient goals, health status, and life expectancy. Reasonable glycemic targets would be 7% to 7.5% in healthy older adults with long life expectancy, 7.5% to 8% in those with moderate comorbidity and a life expectancy less than 10 years, and 8% to 9% in those with multiple morbidities and shorter life expectancy.

SSI was called out to avoid using for long-term diabetes management for individuals residing in the nursing home. SSI is a reactive way of treating hyperglycemia after it has occurred rather than preventing it. Good evidence exists that neither SSI is effective in meeting the body's insulin needs nor is it efficient in the LTC setting. Use of SSI leads to greater patient discomfort and increased nursing time because patients' blood glucose levels are usually monitored more frequently than may be necessary and more insulin injections may be given. With SSI regimens, patients may be at risk from prolonged periods of hyperglycemia. In addition, the risk of hypoglycemia is a significant concern because insulin may be administered without regard to meal intake. Basal insulin, or basal plus rapid-acting insulin with one or more meals (often called basal/bolus insulin therapy), most closely mimics normal physiologic insulin production and controls blood glucose more effectively. Clinicians can raise awareness of inappropriate SSI with recommendations for changes to scheduled dosing or oral or insulin treatments (**Box 6.4**).

Nutritional Support

Lastly, appropriate nutritional support is often critical at the end of life. This involves avoiding inappropriate nutritional interventions. One such intervention is percutaneous feeding tubes. As such, it is recommended not to use percutaneous feeding tubes in individuals with advanced dementia. Instead, offer oral-assisted feedings. Strong evidence exists that artificial nutrition does not prolong life or improve quality of life in patients with advanced dementia. Substantial functional decline and recurrent or progressive medical illnesses may indicate that a patient who is not eating is unlikely to obtain any significant or long-term benefit from artificial nutrition.

Feeding tubes are often placed after hospitalization, frequently with concerns for aspirations and for those who are not eating. Contrary to what many people think, tube feeding does not ensure the patient's comfort or reduce suffering; it may cause fluid overload, diarrhea, abdominal pain, local complications, and less human interaction and may increase the risk of aspiration. Assistance with oral feeding is an evidence-based approach to provide nutrition for patients with advanced dementia and feeding problems.

Careful hand-feeding for patients with severe dementia is at least as good as tube feeding for the outcomes of death, aspiration pneumonia, functional status, and patient comfort. Food is the preferred nutrient. Tube feeding is associated with agitation, increased use of physical and chemical restraints, and worsening pressure ulcers.

Also called out regarding nutritional support was avoiding the use of prescription appetite stimulants or high-calorie supplements for treatment of anorexia or cachexia in older adults; instead, optimize social supports, provide feeding assistance, and clarify patient goals and expectations. Unintentional weight loss is a common problem for medically ill or frail elderly. Although high-calorie supplements increase weight in older people, there is no evidence that they affect other important clinical outcomes, such as quality of life, mood, functional status, or survival. Use of megestrol acetate results in minimal improvements in appetite and weight gain, no improvement in quality of life or survival, and increased risk of thrombotic events, fluid retention, and death. In patients who take megestrol acetate, one in 12 will have an increase in weight and one in 23 will die. The 2012 AGS Beers Criteria lists megestrol acetate and cyproheptadine as medications to avoid in older adults (AGS, 2012). Systematic reviews of cannabinoids, dietary polyunsaturated fatty acids (DHA and EPA), thalidomide, and anabolic steroids have not identified adequate evidence for the efficacy and safety of these agents for weight gain. Mirtazapine is likely to cause weight gain or increased appetite when used to treat depression, but there is little evidence to support its use to promote appetite and weight gain in the absence of depression. In the end, clinicians can assist by increasing family involvement in feeding and promoting this oral feeding activity to prevent the potential inappropriate use of a pharmacotherapy (**Box 6.4**).

Executing on These Five

These five areas of dementia and BPSD management, screening and medication management, antibiotic use, diabetes management, and nutritional management are critical to improving outcomes for nursing home residents. A common thread through these "Choosing Wisely" initiatives is that prudent use of services such that on an individual resident's care is based on the benefits that clearly exceed the risks. This requires thoughtful assessments to assure that interventions are not encouraged that are truly not of benefit for that particular patient. In the end, all clinicians can play a key role in assuring each resident receives appropriate care. And it's this care that will assist in improving the quality of life and death for older adults.

Exploring Alternatives to Medication

The health care provider must evaluate new problems and determine if a medication is necessary as part of the treatment plan. If there are alternatives to medications, such as diet, exercise, and weight loss for borderline hypertension or antiembolism stockings instead of a diuretic for pedal edema, these options should be explored. Only after nonpharmacologic treatments fail should a medication be initiated. In knowing the patient's overall situation—physically, mentally, and socially—the provider has a baseline from which to consider the risks and benefits of medication therapy. **Table 6.7** lists 20 medications that should not be prescribed to any older patients. All of the drugs in this table are also present in the 2002 Beers Criteria (Fick et al., 2003) except for phenylbutazone, which is no longer marketed.

When deciding on a medication for an older adult, assisting with that decision, or evaluating a selection, a drug that treats two coexisting conditions should be considered. For example, a calcium channel blocker might be selected for the patient with angina and hypertension. An older man with hyperplasia of the prostate and hypertension may benefit from an α-adrenergic blocking agent such as terazosin (Hytrin). Treating two conditions with one medication reduces cost, cuts down on dosing schedules, and improves adherence and patient satisfaction.

Simplifying the Regimen

Simplifying the medication plan is a key to therapeutic adherence and safety. Drugs are started at the lowest dose possible and the dosage increased as needed. Lower doses are often effective and reduce the risk of toxicity. Dosing schedules must be easy to follow and remember. If two drugs are equally suitable to treat the same condition, it is desirable to prescribe the one that requires the least frequent dosing.

Another important concern is cost of the drug, especially if the drug is for long-term use. Many older adults are on fixed incomes and find the cost of prescription drugs unaffordable. If the most suitable medication for the condition is expensive, this is explained to the patient before purchase to prevent "sticker shock" or the embarrassment of not having enough money to pay for the prescription. Understanding the impact of a patient's out of pocket on adherence is important, as Dr. C. Everett Koop, former U.S. Surgeon General, has been quoted—"A medication only works if the patient takes it."

Educating Adults and Caregivers

Potential side effects need to be discussed in a nonthreatening way to prevent needless fear or anticipation when starting a new medication. Many older adults forgo starting a medication for fear of potential side effects that may occur. The media are powerful in alarming adults about potentially undesirable or dangerous adverse effects, proven or not. Many older adults stop taking essential medications after reading or hearing something in the media pertaining to that particular drug.

TABLE 6.7

Twenty Drugs to Avoid in Older Adults

Prescription Drug	Use	Reason for Avoiding
amitriptyline	To treat depression	Other antidepressant medications cause fewer side effects.
carisoprodol	To relieve severe pain caused by sprains and back pain	Minimally effective while causing toxicity. Potential for toxic reaction is greater than potential benefit.
chlordiazepoxide	To tranquilize or to relieve anxiety	Shorter-acting benzodiazepines are safer alternatives.
chlorpropamide	To treat diabetes	Other oral hypoglycemic medications have shorter half-lives and do not cause inappropriate antidiuretic hormone secretion.
cyclandelate	To improve blood circulation	Effectiveness is in doubt. This drug is no longer available in the United States.
cyclobenzaprine	To relieve severe pain caused by sprains and back pain	Minimally effective while causing toxicity. Potential for toxic reaction is greater than potential benefit.
diazepam	To tranquilize or to relieve anxiety	Shorter-acting benzodiazepines are safer alternatives.
dipyridamole	To reduce blood clot formation	Effectiveness at low dosage is in doubt. Toxic reaction is high at higher dosages. Safer alternatives exist.
flurazepam	To induce sleep	Shorter-acting benzodiazepines are safer alternatives.
indomethacin	To relieve the pain and inflammation of rheumatoid arthritis	Other NSAIDs cause fewer toxic reactions.
isoxsuprine	To improve blood circulation	Effectiveness is in doubt.
meprobamate	To tranquilize	Shorter-acting benzodiazepines are safer alternatives.
methocarbamol	To relieve severe pain caused by sprains and back pain	Minimally effective while causing toxicity. Potential for toxic reaction is greater than potential benefit.
orphenadrine	To relieve severe pain caused by sprains and back pain	Minimally effective while causing toxicity. Potential for toxic reaction is greater than potential benefit.
pentazocine	To relieve moderate-to-severe pain	Other narcotic medications are safer and more effective.
pentobarbital	To induce sleep and reduce anxiety	Safer sedative–hypnotics are available.
phenylbutazone	To relieve the pain and inflammation of rheumatoid arthritis	Other NSAIDs cause fewer toxic reactions.
propoxyphene	To relieve mild-to-moderate pain	This drug is no longer available in the United States.
secobarbital	To induce sleep and reduce anxiety	Safer sedative–hypnotics are available.
trimethobenzamide	To relieve nausea and vomiting	Least effective of the available antiemetics

Reviewing Medications

The provider working with a geriatric population should have the patient bring in all of his or her medications to each office visit or review a current medication card if the patient carries one. The current medications taken by the patient are recorded at each office visit as part of the progress note. This review alerts the provider to improper dosing and drug administration, misunderstanding of medications, and changes made by specialists and other professionals. The specialist is not always aware of all the medications or OTC drugs the patient takes and may prescribe a drug that places the patient at risk for interactions. As part of the review, the health care provider should ask about topical creams, vitamins, eye drops, and OTC products that may interact with prescription drugs. Adults do not always view these products as medications.

The provider should review all drugs periodically to determine if the dosage can be reduced or the drug discontinued. The goal should always be to use as little medication as possible to treat the multiple illnesses that challenge the older adult.

At the end of each office visit, the provider needs to give the medication list to the patient. Doses and times to take the medications and any special instructions need to be clearly stated and communicated in writing as appropriate. New medications should be listed by brand and generic name so there is no confusion. Clear writing with large lettering should be used, particularly if the patient has common vision impairments, such as cataracts, glaucoma, or macular degeneration.

The caps of the medication bottles that the patient brings to the office can be labeled with the reason for the drug (e.g., "blood pressure," "water pill," or "diabetes"). This helps to ensure that the patient has a basic understanding of the importance of each drug. If the caregiver of an older patient is available, the provider should explain any new medication changes or special instructions, especially for the patient with cognitive impairment or other changes in mental status.

THERAPEUTIC MONITORING

When memory problems are an issue, a medication planner helps. Labeled with the days of the week and four dosing times per day, the planner is a useful device for preparing medications for a week. A patient who fails to take the medications despite visual cues and careful labeling may be sending a signal that the family or other responsible caregivers need to investigate additional interventions, home care services, or future placement in assisted living or LTC facilities.

It is important routinely to schedule and monitor the results of laboratory tests when the patient is taking medications that may result in fluctuating drug blood levels. For example, older adults taking such drugs as warfarin, theophylline (Theo-Dur), digoxin, and quinidine (Quinaglute) need careful monitoring, as do adults taking anticonvulsant medications, such as phenytoin, carbamazepine (Tegretol), and valproic acid (Depakote), for seizure disorders.

Adults taking diuretics or angiotensin-converting enzyme (ACE) inhibitors require periodic evaluation with a renal profile to detect electrolyte imbalances, as well as renal insufficiency (as evidenced by rising blood urea nitrogen [BUN] and creatinine levels). Adults starting ACE inhibitor therapy should have a baseline BUN/creatinine level documented with a follow-up test in 2 weeks to alert for renal artery stenosis (evidenced by a rise in the BUN/creatinine levels). Because of the potential for elevations in serum potassium concentration with ACE inhibitor therapy, the older adult needs routine renal profiles to detect such changes, especially when drug therapy also includes diuretics and digoxin (Lanoxin). (**Box 6.3** presents guidelines for prescribing drugs safely for older adults.)

SUMMARY

Three quotes help summarize best practices in pharmacotherapy principles in older adults. It begins with determination of the right treatment in the face of new symptoms or issues.

This may not always mean beginning a new medication but rather may mean instead reducing a dose of a current medication, discontinuing a therapy, or starting a nonpharmacologic treatment. The quote from Leslie Fine, RPh, should be remembered and practiced that "Any symptom in an elderly patient should be considered a drug side effect until proved otherwise." This is important to prevent polypharmacy issues in older adults. Also, when determining if a new medication should be started, careful assessment of the benefits versus the costs should be undertaken such that only those treatments that offer benefits over costs should be started. When assessing costs, this includes not only financial but potential side effects, while benefits need to take into account benefits given the life expectancy and other concerns in the older adult.

The second quote deals with starting a new medication. It begins with a standard geriatric quote but with a new addition. The quote is that medications in older adults should "start low and go slow" but, to be complete, should include "but get there." This translates to initiating medications at a low starting dose, titrating slowly but getting to the therapeutic dose. This is not only to prevent adverse events from too quick a titration at too high a dose but also to caution against therapies that are not being used at a therapeutic level.

The final quote comes from C. Evert Koop describing the importance of adherence—"A medication only works if the patient takes it." For after a careful determination and initiation of the "right" medication, at the right dose for the right duration has been made; assurance of adherence is the final step in producing optimum outcomes. Of course, there is no final step; pharmacotherapy management, especially in older adults, requires educated clinicians' ongoing evaluation and support to assure optimum outcomes.

CASE STUDY*

R.S. is an 85-year-old female who has congestive heart failure. Over the past 3 months, she has had four hospitalizations. Like many older adults, R.S. is experiencing difficulty swallowing and psychologic changes affecting her medication absorption.

1. Which of the following would be an appropriate starting point for identifying causes for R.S.'s frequency of hospitalizations?
   a. Simply ask if she is taking her medications as directed.
   b. Assume that her frequent hospitalizations are secondary to expected changes, which are normal parts of aging.
   c. Examine all of R.S.'s medication vials to complete an assessment including pill count for adherence.
   d. Assume that her frequent hospitalizations are the result of undertreating her conditions.

2. In determining the most appropriate course of treatment for R.S., assessing her life expectancy should never be taken into account. Rather, the same course of treatment should be pursued without regard for life expectancy.
   a. True
   b. False

3. Which of the following best describes a concern that R.S. is taking OTCs, which may impact her cardiac function?
   a. Assume that if R.S. has not discussed her taking OTCs with her health care providers that this is most likely not an issue.
   b. Assume because older adults typically do not take OTCs that this is not an issue with R.S.
   c. Because older adults take a significant number of OTCs without knowledge of their physicians, that R.S.'s use is best assessed through a home visit and the asking of open-ended questions.

* Answers can be found online.

Bibliography

Starred references are cited in the text.

AMDA action for improving dementia care in nursing homes. American Medical Directors Association Web site. http://www.amda.com/advocacy/dementiacare.cfm. Accessed January 6, 2014.

American Geriatrics Society 2015 Beers Criteria Update Expert Panel. (November 2015). American Geriatrics Society 2015 updated Beers Criteria for potentially inappropriate medication use in older adults. *Journal of the American Geriatrics Society, 63*(11), 2227–2246.

American Geriatrics Society (AGS) Panel on Pharmacological Management of Persistent Pain in Older Persons. (2009). Retrieved from http://www.americangeriatrics.org/files/documents/2009_Guideline.pdf on February 27, 2016.

American Geriatric Society & American Association for Geriatric Psychiatry. (2003). Consensus statement on improving the quality of mental health care in U.S. nursing homes: Management of depression and behavioral symptoms associated with dementia. *Journal of the American Geriatric Society, 51*(9), 1287–1298.

Arias, E. (2004). United States Life Tables, 2002. *National Vital Statistics Reports, 53*(6). Hyattsville, MD: National Center for Health Statistics.

*Bergman, S., Ronald, K., Gonzales, M., et al (2009). Pharmacotherapy update 2009. Part 1: Cardiology, neurology, and psychiatry. *Annals of Long-Term Care, 17*(12), 30–34.

Brooks, B. R., Crumpacker, D., Fellus, J., et al. (2013). PRISM: A novel research tool to assess the prevalence of pseudobulbar affect symptoms across neurological conditions. *PLoS One, 8*(8), e72232.

Burdick, K., & Goldberg, J. (2002). Cognitive advantages of new anticonvulsants in treating a geriatric population. *Clinical Geriatrics, 10*(10), 25–36.

Caracci, G. (2003). The use of opioid analgesics in the older. *Clinical Geriatrics, 11*(11), 18–21.

Christian, R., Saavedra, L., Gaynes, B. N., et al. Future research needs for first- and second-generation antipsychotics for children and young adults. Future Research Needs Paper No. 13. (Prepared by the RTI-UNC Evidence-based Practice Center under Contract No. 290 2007 10056 I.) Rockville, MD: Agency for Healthcare Research and Quality; February 2012. http://www.effectivehealthcare.ahrq.gov/ehc/products/419/967/FRN13_Antipsychotics_FinalReport_20120427.pdf. Accessed February 10, 2014.

CMS MDS 3.0 for Nursing Homes and Swing Bed Providers. Retrieved from https://www.cms.gov/Medicare/Quality-Initiatives-Patient-Assessment-Instruments/NursingHomeQualityInits/NHQIMDS30.html on February 27, 2016.

CMS National Partnership to Improve Dementia Care in Nursing Homes. Retrieved from https://www.cms.gov/Medicare/Provider-Enrollment-and-Certification/SurveyCertificationGenInfo/National-Partnership-to-Improve-Dementia-Care-in-Nursing-Homes.html on February 27, 2016.

Cooke, C., & Proveaux, W. (2003). A retrospective review of the effect of COX-2 inhibitors on blood pressure change. *American Journal of Therapeutics, 10*(5), 311–317.

Drug Effectiveness Review Project. Drug class review: atypical antipsychotics drugs. Final update3 report. July 2010. https://www.ncbi.nlm.nih.gov/books/NBK50583/pdf/TOC.pdf. Accessed January 17, 2014.

Espinoza, R., & Eslami, M. (2004). Update on treatment for Alzheimer's disease—Part II: Management of noncognitive, psychiatric, and behavioral complications. *Clinical Geriatrics, 12*(1), 45–53.

FDA requests boxed warnings on older class of antipsychotic drugs [news release]. FDA website.http://www.fda.gov/NewsEvents/Newsroom/PressAnnouncements/2008/ucm116912.htm. Accessed February 10, 2014.

*Fick, D., Cooper, J., Wade, W., et al. (2003). Updating the Beers criteria for potentially inappropriate medication use in older adults. *Archives of Internal Medicine, 163*, 2716–2724.

Freedom of Information Act (FOIA) Service Center: contacts by region. CMS website. http://www.cms.gov/center/freedom-of-information-act/regional-contacts.html. Accessed February 4, 2014.

Guralnik, J., & Havlik, R. (2000). Demographics. In M. Beers & R. Berkow (Eds.), *The Merck manual of geriatrics* (3rd ed., pp. 9–21). Whitehouse Station, NJ: Merck Research Laboratories.

Hayes, B., Klein-Schwartz, W., & Barrueto, F. (2007). Polypharmacy and the older adult. *Clinics in Geriatric Medicine, 23*(2), 2007.

Horgas AL. Assessing pain in older adults with dementia. Try this:® Best practices in nursing care to older adults with dementia. ConsultGeriRN website. http://consultgerirn.org/uploads/File/trythis/try_this_d2.pdf. Accessed January 6, 2014.

Hospital Elder Life Program (HELP) website. http://www.hospitalelderlifeprogram.org/public/public-main.php. Accessed January 6, 2014.

Herr K, Bjoro K, Decker S. Tools for assessment of pain in nonverbal older adults with dementia: a state-of-the-science review. *J Pain Symptom Manage, 2006;31*(2):170–192.

*Hile, E., & Studenski, S. (2007). Instability and falls. In E. Duthie, P. Katz, & M. Malone (Eds.), *Practice of geriatrics* (4th ed.). Philadelphia, PA: Saunders.

Horowitz, M. (2000). Aging and the gastrointestinal tract. In M. Beers, & R. Berkow (Eds.), *The Merck manual of geriatrics* (3rd ed., pp. 1000–1052). Whitehouse Station, NJ: Merck Research Laboratories.

Improving Dementia Care Treatment for Older Adults Act of 2012, S 3604, 112th Cong, 2nd Sess. (2012). Website. http://www.gpo.gov/fdsys/pkg/BILLS-112s3604is/pdf/BILLS-112s3604is.pdf. Accessed January 6, 2014.

Jeste, D., Schneider, L., De Deyn, P., et al. (2003). Atypical antipsychotics for the management of adults with dementia and psychotic symptoms. *Clinical Geriatrics and Annals of Long-Term Care, *(Suppl.).

Juurlink, D., Mamdani, M., Kopp, A., et al. (2003). Drug–drug interactions among older adults hospitalized for drug toxicity. *Journal of the American Medical Association, 289*(13), 1652–1658.

*Kelleher, C., & Lindeman, R. (2003). Renal diseases and disorders. In E. Flaherty, T. Fulmer, & M. Mezey (Eds.), *Geriatric nursing review syllabus* (pp. 357–365). New York, NY: American Geriatric Society.

*Kirby, D., & Ames, D. (2001). Hyponatremia and selective serotonin reuptake inhibitors in older adults. *International Journal of Geriatric Psychiatry, 16*(5), 484–493.

Leading Age website. http://www.leadingage.org/. Accessed January 17, 2014.

Leipzig, R., Cumming, R., & Tinetti, M. (1999). Drugs and falls in older people: A systematic review and meta-analysis: Psychotropic drugs. *Journal of the American Geriatrics Society, 47*(1), 30–39.

MDS 3.0 history. CMS website. http://www.cms.gov/Medicare/Quality-Initiatives-Patient-Assessment-Instruments/NursingHomeQualityInits/NHQIMDS30.html. Accessed February 10, 2014.

Moore, A., Karno, M., Grella, C., et al. (2009). Alcohol, tobacco, and nonmedical drug use in older U.S. adults: Data from the 2001/02 national epidemiologic survey of alcohol and related conditions. *Journal of the American Geriatrics Society, 57*(12), 2275–2281.

Murray, M., & Callahan, C. (2003). Improving medication use for older adults: An integrated research agenda. *Annals of Internal Medicine, 139*(5), 425–428.

New data show antipsychotic drug use is down in nursing homes nationwide [news release]. CMS website. http://www.cms.gov/Newsroom/MediaReleaseDatabase/Press-Releases/2013-Press-Releases-Items/2013-08-27.html. Accessed January 2, 2014.

Norris, S., High, K., Gill, T., et al. (2008). Health care for older Americans with multiple chronic conditions: A research agenda. *Journal of American Geriatric Society, 56*(1), 149–159.

Overprescribing antipsychotics. *JAMA.* 2012, *308*(18), 1849.

Pain Assessment in Advanced Dementia Scale (PAINAD). Iowa Geriatric Education Center website. http://www.healthcare.uiowa.edu/igec/tools/pain/PAINAD.pdf. Accessed January 6, 2014.

Quality measures. CMS website. http://www.cms.gov/Medicare/Quality-Initiatives-Patient-Assessment-Instruments/NursingHomeQualityInits/NHQIQualityMeasures.html. Accessed January 13, 2014.

Sheikh, J., & Cassidy, E. (2003). Anxiety disorders. In E. Flaherty, T. Fulmer, & M. Mezey (Eds), *Geriatric nursing review syllabus* (pp. 220–223). New York, NY: American Geriatric Society.

Shiyanbola, O., & Farris, K, (2010). Concerns and beliefs about medicines and inappropriate medications: An internet-based survey on risk factors for self-reported adverse drug events among older adults. *American Journal of Geriatric Pharmacotherapy, 8*(3), 245–257.

*Smith, M. (2013). *Pharmacy and the US healthcare system* (4th ed.). London, UK: Pharmaceutical Press.

*Stefanacci, R., & Spivack, B. (2010). Impact of healthcare reform on today's Medicare beneficiaries—And on those who care for them. *Clinical Geriatrics, 18*(6), 42–48.

*Tseng, C., Dudley, R., Brook, R., et al. (2009). Older adults' knowledge of drug benefit caps and communication with providers about exceeding caps. *Journal of the American Geriatric Society, 57*(5), 848–854.

*Vincent, G., & Velhoff, V. (2010). *The next four decades. The older population in the United States: 2010 to 2050.* Washington, DC: U.S. Census Bureau.

Warden, V., Hurley, A. C., & Volicer, L. 2003. Development and psychometric evaluation of the Pain Assessment in Advanced Dementia (PAINAD) scale. *Journal of the American Medical Directors Associations, 4*(1), 9–15.

*Wright, R., Roumani, Y., Boudreau, R., et al. (2009). Effect of central nervous system medication use on decline in cognition in community-dwelling older adults: Findings from the health, aging and body composition study. *Journal of the American Geriatric Society, 57*(2), 243–250.

Zarowitz, B. J., & O'Shea, T.. (2013). Clinical, behavioral, and treatment differences in nursing facility residents with dementia, with and without pseudobulbar affect symptomatology. *Consultant Pharmacyst, 28*(11), 713–722.

7 Principles of Pharmacology in Pain Management

Maria C. Foy

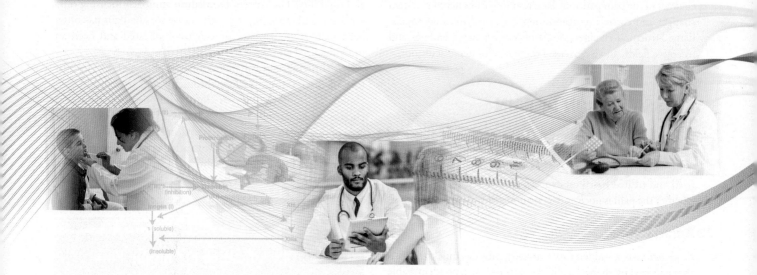

One of the most widely encountered clinical situations is a patient in pain. Treatment of pain is one of the most difficult aspects of patient care. Pain is defined by the International Association for the Study of Pain as "an unpleasant sensory and emotional experience associated with actual or potential tissue damage, or described in terms of such damage" (Merskey & Bogduk, 1994). Pain is subjective, and its intensity varies from patient to patient, day to day. The clinician has a large array of medications available to assist patients in relieving their pain. Principles of managing various types of pain will be described in this chapter and will introduce the practicing nurse to the many types and classes of drugs available for the therapeutic management of pain.

Analgesics represent one of the most frequently prescribed and administered classes of medications used in the treatment of pain. Managing pain in the acutely or chronically ill patient requires both a sound comprehension of the clinical pharmacology of analgesics and a clear understanding of how pain is perceived. Clinicians caring for chronically ill patients not only find themselves assisting the patient in dealing with the physical component of pain but often are confronted by the patient's psychological, spiritual, and social perceptions of pain and pain medications.

Age is a major consideration in assessing pain. For example, elderly patients are less likely to complain about pain and request fewer analgesics to alleviate pain, secondary to incorrect beliefs and biases. A corollary exists in pediatric patients, whose inability to adequately express suffering leads some clinicians to believe that children cannot feel pain. Clinicians, however, now realize that pediatric patients experience as much pain as adults. Because of the identified communication barrier, clinicians need to evaluate a child in pain by utilizing special pain assessment tools developed for children. Similar assessment tools are utilized for adults who may not be able to verbally communicate their pain.

TYPES OF PAIN

Pain can be categorized as nociceptive, neuropathic, or inflammatory based on the presumed underlying cause. Nociceptive pain occurs as a result of nerve receptor stimulation following a mechanical, thermal, or chemical insult. Nociceptive pain is purposeful, where the pain tells you to stop doing whatever is causing the pain. Nociceptive pain can be further classified as somatic or visceral. Somatic pain associated with muscle, skin, or bone injury is often well localized. When pain affects the visceral organs, such as pain seen in pancreatitis, it is referred to as visceral pain. Inflammatory pain is a subtype of nociceptive pain, which results from the release of proinflammatory cytokines at the site of tissue injury. Inflammatory pain may be present in acute pain from bruises or infection and chronically in pain from rheumatoid arthritis or osteoarthritis.

Neuropathic pain is caused by abnormal signal processes in the central nervous system (CNS). Neuropathic pain can be peripheral or central in origin and is no longer protective in nature. Peripheral neuropathies include pain from diabetes and postherpetic neuralgia. Examples of central neuropathic pain syndromes include pain from multiple sclerosis, spinal cord injuries, migraine, and poststroke syndrome. Descriptors of neuropathic pain, such as electric-like, burning, tingling, stabbing, or shooting, can differentiate nerve pain from nociceptive pain and help determine appropriate treatment.

More than one type of pain may occur simultaneously. Failed back surgery syndrome, cancer pain, and chronic regional pain syndrome (CRPS) may have characteristics of a mixed nociceptive/neuropathic pain picture.

New evidence is now leading toward considering pain as a disease of the brain, especially when pain persists long after anticipated healing of the initial injury (Henry et al., 2011).

Noxious stimulants are no longer present and no pathology exists that would explain the pain. This type of pain is often referred to as maldynia, Greek for "bad pain," which results from changes in the pain pathway. Pain resulting from nervous system changes and cortical reorganization is referred to as neuroplasticity. Structural changes consist of increase nerve endings and receptive fields, and a decreased threshold for nerve activation.

CLASSIFICATION OF PAIN

Pain can be classified into two categories, acute and chronic, which help identify the derivation of the pain and provide a framework for treatment. Pain can subsequently be categorized and treated based on expected chronicity of the pain and whether the pain is nociceptive, neuropathic, or mixed in origin.

Acute Pain

Acute pain has a sudden onset, usually subsides quickly, and is characterized by sharp, localized sensations with an identifiable cause. Acute pain is a natural physiologic response to injury, useful in warning individuals of disease or harmful situations. This process is often seen as a signal that the body is invoking critical immunologic and physiologic responses to cellular or tissue damage. Concomitant physiologic responses include excessive sympathetic nervous system activity, such as tachycardia, diaphoresis, and increased blood pressure and respiratory rate. Acute pain is somewhat instructive and purposeful by signaling danger. Pain is usually brief and resolves within a few months of onset. Surgical intervention and trauma are common sources of acute pain.

When acute pain responses become unremitting, constant, or undertreated, the biologic responses outlive their usefulness and can lead to chronic pain. Patients with chronic pain become tolerant to the physiologic response seen in acute pain. In addition, these patients often do not appear to be suffering from pain. The body becomes tolerant to the autonomic indicators where heart rate, blood pressure, and respiratory rate normalize as pain persists. Undesired consequences, such as anxiety and depression, are often associated with constant, long-term pain. The goal of acute pain management is to avoid progression to a chronic pain state. Early pain control will often prevent the development of chronic pain.

Chronic Pain

Chronic pain is defined by the Institute of Clinical Systems Improvement as "pain without biological value that has persisted beyond the normal time and despite the usual customary efforts to diagnose and treat the original condition and injury" (Hooten et al., 2013). Chronic pain may have a verifiable source, as in patients with arthritis, diabetic peripheral neuropathy, and postherpetic neuralgia. In some patients, however, no evidence of structural or nerve damage exists to explain the reason for pain. In these patients, the pain is most likely from peripheral and central sensitization of the pain pathways, explained later in this chapter.

Evidence is now showing that chronic pain is primarily a biopsychosocial disease, with cognitive factors such as pain catastrophizing and anxiety having a strong correlation to pain and disability. The current biomedical approach focusing only on tissue and tissue injury as the cause for the pain has often been ineffective. Patients are often complicated and need an individualized approach to therapy.

Identifying and differentiating pain through careful history of the location, quality, chronicity, and presence of psychological comorbidities is important because treatment choices are dictated by the cause and type of pain. The primary goal of therapy in chronic pain is to decrease the pain to a tolerable level using a combination of various types of therapies to help improve function and quality of life. Examples of types of chronic pain are shown in **Box 7.1**.

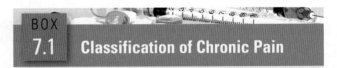

BOX 7.1   Classification of Chronic Pain

NOCICEPTIVE PAIN

Postoperative pain
Mechanical low back pain
Arthropathies (e.g., rheumatoid arthritis, osteoarthritis, gout)
Ischemic disorders
Myalgia (e.g., myofascial pain syndromes)
Nonarticular inflammatory disorders (e.g., polymyalgia rheumatica)
Skin and mucosal ulcerations
Superficial pain (sunburn, thermal burns, skin cuts)
Visceral pain (appendicitis, pancreatitis)

NEUROPATHIC PAIN

Alcoholic neuropathy
Cancer-related pain and some cancer treatments
Vitamin B_{12} deficiency
Chronic regional pain syndrome
Human immunodeficiency virus (HIV)–related pain and some HIV treatments
Multiple sclerosis-related pain
Diabetic peripheral neuropathy
Phantom limb pain
Postherpetic neuralgia
Poststroke pain
Trigeminal neuralgia

MIXED OR UNDETERMINED PATHOPHYSIOLOGY

Low back pain with radiculopathy
Carpal tunnel syndrome
Chronic recurrent headaches
Painful vasculitis

Cancer-Related Pain

Cancer-related pain is pain associated with malignancy and can result from the disease itself or damage to secondary tissue. Disease-induced pain includes pain secondary to direct tumor involvement of bone, nerves, viscera, or soft tissue. In addition, muscle spasm, muscle imbalance, or other body structure/function changes secondary to the tumor are considered disease induced. Pain may be associated with treatment of the disease and may be seen with biopsies, surgeries, and/or chemotherapy and radiation treatments. Pain may be present in sites where cancer has metastasized (i.e., bone pain). Cancer and treatment interventions may activate peripheral nociceptors, causing somatic and visceral nociceptive pain. Neuropathic pain involving the sympathetic nervous system may also be seen.

Chronic Noncancer Pain

Chronic noncancer pain (CNCP) is persistent pain seen in patients not affected by cancer. Some examples of CNCP are rheumatoid arthritis, osteoarthritis, fibromyalgia, and peripheral neuropathies. Alternately, chronic pain may be thought of as the disease itself when no cause of pain is identified. CNCP may be nociceptive, neuropathic, or mixed in origin (see **Box 7.1**). Nociceptive mechanisms usually respond well to traditional approaches to pain management, including common analgesic medications and nonpharmacologic strategies. Neuropathic pain will respond to most traditional approaches including opioid therapy. However, higher doses of opioids are required to control this type of pain. Therefore, adjunctive treatment choices including anticonvulsants, antidepressants, or dual-mechanism medications may be considered to replace or add to traditional treatment modalities.

Breakthrough Pain

Breakthrough pain (BTP) is defined as a transitory pain often seen in conjunction with chronic pain, where moderate to severe pain occurs in patients with otherwise well-controlled pain. True BTP is characterized as brief, lasting minutes to hours, and can interfere with functioning and quality of life. True BTP has historically been associated with cancer pain. BTP can also be seen in many other chronic pain conditions, such as neuropathic pain and chronic lower back pain.

Other types of BTP include pain caused by certain activities (incident pain) or when the duration of analgesia is less than the dosing interval (end-of-dose failure). Giving an analgesic prior to the incident known to cause pain will often allow the activity to be performed with minimal discomfort. Shortening the dosing interval is recommended in patients with end-of-dose failure.

PAIN PATHOPHYSIOLOGY

Several theories exist as to how information resultant from tissue damage is perceived by the brain as pain. Noxious stimuli from the point of the initial injury move through specialized nerve fibers within the spinal cord where the signal reaches the brain and is interpreted by the brain as pain. This transmission of the pain signal through the CNS is termed nociception. Free nerve endings of small myelinated A-delta fibers and larger unmyelinated C fibers are called nociceptors and are responsible for delivering pain signals to the brain. In the past, the "Gate Control Theory" proposed that "closing of the gate" to pain signals was accomplished primarily through stopping the transmission of the pain signal to the brain. However, recent studies theorize that changes in the brain and CNS have a much larger role in the perception of pain (Woo et al., 2015). Anxiety, fear, depression, and previous pain experiences may influence an individuals' perception of pain, especially when pain becomes chronic.

Description of nociception can be divided into four main categories: transduction, transmission, perception, and modulation (**Figure 7.1**).

Transduction

Transduction refers to a process of nociceptor activation due to mechanical, thermal, or chemical injury. Nerve endings are activated through the release of various excitatory chemical neurotransmitters, such as prostaglandins (PGs), substance P, histamine, bradykinin, and serotonin.

Transmission

Transduction results in an action potential transmitted via the myelinated A-delta and unmyelinated C fibers, by way of the dorsal root ganglia, synapsing in the dorsal horn of the spinal cord. Second-order neurons are then activated and convey pain signals to the higher centers of the CNS. Neurotransmitters in the dorsal horn directly or indirectly depolarize the second-order neurons, facilitating transmission of information to the brain leading to the perception of pain. Inhibitory substances are also released in the dorsal horn (see section on modulation) and may decrease the number of signals reaching the brain, thereby lessening transmission.

Perception

Nociceptive information travels through different areas of the CNS to the brain where the pain is perceived. Perception is the end result of the pain transmission to the brain; at this point, we become consciously aware of the pain. Pain perception is not just a manifestation of physical injury but is affected by psychosocial factors and previous experiences of pain. In a chronic pain state, the perception of pain is no longer influenced by the initial noxious stimuli. The presence of psychological comorbidities in many patients with chronic pain may result in fear of the pain and pain catastrophizing, thereby increasing pain perception.

Modulation

Pain modulation occurs at various levels of the CNS. Endogenous opioids work through binding of opioid receptors in both the periphery and CNS. The main central inhibitory neurotransmitters involved in modulation of pain include serotonin and

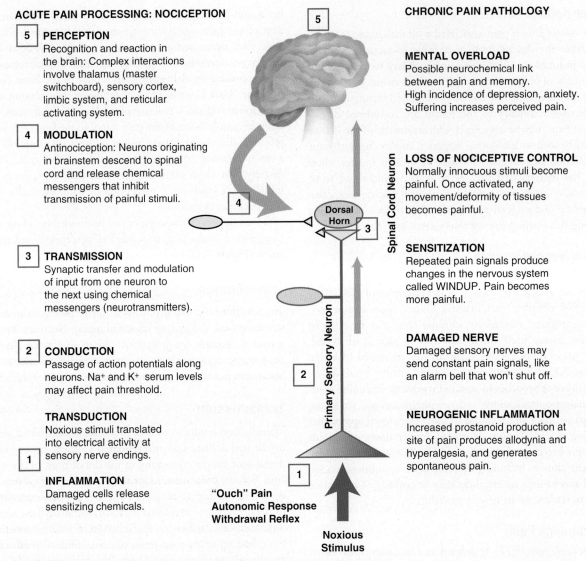

ACUTE PAIN PROCESSING: NOCICEPTION

5 PERCEPTION
Recognition and reaction in the brain: Complex interactions involve thalamus (master switchboard), sensory cortex, limbic system, and reticular activating system.

4 MODULATION
Antinociception: Neurons originating in brainstem descend to spinal cord and release chemical messengers that inhibit transmission of painful stimuli.

3 TRANSMISSION
Synaptic transfer and modulation of input from one neuron to the next using chemical messengers (neurotransmitters).

2 CONDUCTION
Passage of action potentials along neurons. Na+ and K+ serum levels may affect pain threshold.

TRANSDUCTION
Noxious stimuli translated into electrical activity at sensory nerve endings.

1 INFLAMMATION
Damaged cells release sensitizing chemicals.

Dorsal Horn

Spinal Cord Neuron

Primary Sensory Neuron

"Ouch" Pain
Autonomic Response
Withdrawal Reflex

Noxious Stimulus

CHRONIC PAIN PATHOLOGY

MENTAL OVERLOAD
Possible neurochemical link between pain and memory. High incidence of depression, anxiety. Suffering increases perceived pain.

LOSS OF NOCICEPTIVE CONTROL
Normally innocuous stimuli become painful. Once activated, any movement/deformity of tissues becomes painful.

SENSITIZATION
Repeated pain signals produce changes in the nervous system called WINDUP. Pain becomes more painful.

DAMAGED NERVE
Damaged sensory nerves may send constant pain signals, like an alarm bell that won't shut off.

NEUROGENIC INFLAMMATION
Increased prostanoid production at site of pain produces allodynia and hyperalgesia, and generates spontaneous pain.

FIGURE 7.1 Acute and chronic pain pathophysiology. (Reprinted with permission from Whitten, C. E., Donovan, M., & Cristobal, K. (2005). Treating chronic pain: New knowledge, more choices. *The Permanente Journal, 9*(4), 9–18. Retrieved from http://www.thepermanentejournal.org. Copyright 2005 The Permanente Journal.)

norepinephrine. These neurotransmitters fight pain by increasing their concentration in the spinal cord and brainstem.

Peripheral and Central Sensitization

Often, pain persists despite healing, and no reason for the pain can be found. Pain pathways become "broken," and pain is seen without an obvious cause. Modifications occurring in the pain conduction pathways of the peripheral nervous system and CNS where hypersensitivity to pain stimulus and neuronal structural changes result in chronic pain syndromes are referred to as *peripheral* and *central sensitization*.

Peripheral Sensitization

When pain receptors in the periphery are continually stimulated (i.e., untreated acute pain), the threshold for stimulation becomes lowered and increased nerve firing occurs. Increased frequency of nerve impulses results in more pain signals reaching the dorsal horn of the spinal cord. These processes contribute to the development of central sensitization.

Central Sensitization

Central sensitization is defined as "an amplification of neural signaling within the CNS that elicits pain hypersensitivity" (Woolf, 2011). When nociceptive information repeatedly stimulates nerve fibers, increased dorsal horn neuronal activity is seen. With actual or potential nerve damage as in many cases of uncontrolled pain, the increase in firing causes increased excitability and responsiveness, termed central sensitization. The end result is a decrease of central pain inhibition, increased spontaneous neuronal activity in the dorsal horn, formation of neuromas causing an increase in receptive fields, and a decreased threshold for neuronal firing. Sensitization of the NMDA (N-methyl-D-aspartic acid) receptor in the area of the dorsal horn also contributes to central sensitization. Allodynia (pain response to something painless), hyperalgesia (increased response to pain), persistent pain, or referred pain may result.

Central sensitization can occur in many chronic pain states, especially when associated with nerve injury or dysfunction. Alternately, inadequate treatment of acute pain, concomitant psychological comorbidities, and poor coping skills may lead to the development of chronic pain through the sensitization of the CNS. Pain associated with central sensitization often responds poorly to traditional pain therapies. The addition of coanalgesics, reviewed later in this chapter, should be used for the treatment of chronic pain associated with central sensitization.

Chemical Mediators

Coupled with the neuronal component of pain is the release of chemical mediators initiating or continuing the stimulation of pain-conducting fibers. Peripheral chemical mediators include the neurotransmitters norepinephrine, serotonin, and histamine and polypeptides such as bradykinin, PGs, and substance P. Their role in the pain pathway is activating and sensitizing nociceptors and increasing neuronal excitability. Blocking the production of these mediators, particularly inhibiting the production of PGs with anti-inflammatory medications or similar compounds, minimizes nociceptor activation and neuronal firing, thereby lessening the transmission of pain through the CNS. Because of their role in initiating the pain pathway, these chemicals are targets for many of the medications currently available to treat pain.

Both excitatory and inhibitory neurotransmitters can be found in the dorsal horn of the spinal cord. Excitatory amino acids, glutamate and aspartate, along with substance P facilitate activation of second-order neurons in the dorsal horn primarily through activation of the NMDA receptors.

Pain-Modulating Receptors

Historically, pain modulation was thought to be primarily due to descending inhibitory information from the brain. Pain experts now theorize that both descending inhibitory pain pathways and inhibitory neurotransmitters decrease the perception of pain. Inhibitory substances, such as endogenous opioids, norepinephrine, and serotonin are released in various areas of the CNS and attenuate the transmission of pain by modulating the pain signals in the dorsal horn (Pasero & McCaffrey, 2011). Endogenous opioid substances, primarily β-endorphins, stimulate inhibitory neuronal receptors known as the opioid receptors. Stimulation of these receptors, particularly the *mu* opioid receptor, inhibits the transmission of pain signals to and from the higher brain centers. These receptors are stimulated by morphine-like drugs (opioids) and account

for a great deal of the pain relief associated with this class of analgesics.

In contrast, neuropathic pain syndromes do not respond as well to conventional analgesic therapy. Neuropathic pain is often the result of peripheral and central sensitization. Sensitization of the NMDA receptors by various mechanisms is primarily responsible for this type of pain. Use of coanalgesic agents, such as antidepressants, anticonvulsants, and antiarrhythmic agents are recommended for neuropathic pain treatment. Details on the use of coanalgesics are found later in this chapter.

GENERAL PRINCIPLES OF PAIN MANAGEMENT

Treatment of pain in today's society rests on two major principles: appropriate assessment of the severity and intensity of the pain and selection of the most appropriate agent to relieve pain with minimal side effects. Pain relief often requires a multimodal approach, using multiple agents that target different receptors and neurotransmitters in the CNS. Additional mind body approaches such as cognitive–behavioral therapy, massage, acupuncture, and mindful meditation are often recommended to be used in addition to pharmacologic therapy in patients suffering from chronic nonmalignant pain.

Pain Assessment

The individual assessment of pain is extremely important for determining proper treatments as well as monitoring effectiveness over time. According to the National Institutes of Health (NIH), self-reporting by patients is "the most reliable indicator of the existence and intensity of pain" (Herr & Garand, 2001). Along with self-reporting, involving the caregiver's assessment of pain, especially in the very young or noncommunicating older patient, may be helpful. The self-report should include a description of the pain, location, intensity/severity, aggravating and relieving factors, and effect of pain on quality of life. Assessment tools are recommended to be brief and easy to use in order to reliably document pain intensity and pain relief. These tools will also evaluate other factors effecting pain, such as the presence of psychological comorbidities. One routine clinical approach to pain assessment and management is summarized by the mnemonic PQRSTU (**Box 7.2**). Assessment tools should be used initially to obtain a baseline level of pain and impaired function. Follow-up assessments should be performed to measure the progress toward acceptable pain relief based on the individual functional goals of the patient.

Because pain is subjective and is not easily quantifiable, several tools are available to determine the quantity and quality of a patients' pain. The various pain scales can be classified as single or multidimensional and self-report or observational. Common single-dimension tools include the visual analog

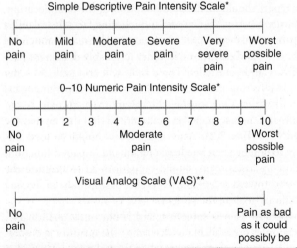

BOX 7.2 P-Q-R-S-T-U Mnemonic for Assessing Pain

P—Presenting, precipitating, palliating. When and how did the pain start? What makes the pain better? What have you used for pain in the past that wasn't effective?

Q—Quality of the pain. What does the pain feel like? (descriptors such as sharp, stabbing, burning)

R—Region, radiation. Where is the pain? Does the pain stay in one location or does the pain radiate?

S—Severity. On a scale of 0 to 10, 0 being no pain, 10 being the worst pain imaginable, what is your pain now? In the last 24 hours? After a pain medication?

T—Temporal pattern. Is the pain constant, intermittent, associated with movement?

U—How does the pain affect *you*? Quality-of-life indicator.

scale (VAS), numerical rating scale (NRS), and verbal description scale (**Figure 7.2**). The single-dimension scales evaluate the intensity of pain. However, single-dimensional scales alone do not take into account function, which may be a more reliable indicator of pain control, especially chronic pain. Multidimensional scales consider location, pattern, and affective responses in addition to a severity score alone. Examples of multidimensional scales include the Brief Pain Inventory and the Initial Pain Assessment Tool (Pasero & McCaffrey, 2011).

The information assessed, particularly from the NRS and VAS, is helpful in determining appropriate treatment and drug selection. The Institute for Clinical Systems Improvement (ICSI) and the NIH have published guidelines on the appropriate evaluation and treatment of acute and chronic pain. Pain

is recommended to be assessed with a 0-to-10 scale to assess a patient's current level of pain. Zero defines a pain-free state, and a 10 describes the most severe pain imaginable by the patient. Pain rated at 1 to 3 is classified as mild; 4 to 7, moderate; and 8 to 10, severe. Other validated scales are available for use in special populations, such as in children and adults unable to self-report.

Subsequent assessments should evaluate the effectiveness of the treatment plan. First, determine if the cause of increased pain is related to the progression of disease, disease treatments, or a new cause of pain, as in cancer that has metastasized. Unrelieved pain may also be due to the development of opioid tolerance where the same amount of pain requires increasing doses of opioids in order to provide relief. The assessment of the patient's pain and the efficacy of the treatment plan should be ongoing, and the pain reports should be documented. Continued use of the same pain scale is crucial to the continued assessment of treatment progress and communication between health care providers.

Pain Management

Treatment options for pain control include nonpharmacologic and pharmacologic therapies. **Box 7.3** lists treatments that complement medication management of pain. Often, a multimodal, multidisciplinary approach using a combination of both pharmacologic and nonpharmacologic treatments is necessary to reduce pain to an acceptable level and provide an improvement in function, especially when opioid therapies are used. Maximizing the patient's quality of life and function, while minimizing adverse effects of treatments, is the goal of the pain management treatment plan. Individualization of drug regimens according to the type and severity of pain is essential principles when using medications to manage both acute and chronic pain states.

For mild to moderate pain, acetaminophen, aspirin, or a nonsteroidal anti-inflammatory drug (NSAID) is usually considered initial therapy. Acetaminophen is used for mild pain across all age groups, mainly due to its favorable side effect profile. NSAIDs are very effective in pain associated with inflammation. However, patients may be at risk for gastrointestinal (GI), cardiac, or renal toxicities. Discussion of risk versus benefits of NSAID therapies will be discussed later in this chapter.

Simple Descriptive Pain Intensity Scale*

No pain | Mild pain | Moderate pain | Severe pain | Very severe pain | Worst possible pain

0–10 Numeric Pain Intensity Scale*

0 1 2 3 4 5 6 7 8 9 10
No pain ... Moderate pain ... Worst possible pain

Visual Analog Scale (VAS)**

No pain ——————— Pain as bad as it could possibly be

*If used as a graphic rating scale, a 10-cm baseline is recommended.
**A 10-cm baseline is recommended for VAS scales.

FIGURE 7.2 Visual analog scales used for ranking pain.

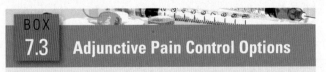

BOX 7.3 Adjunctive Pain Control Options

Physical methods (stretching, exercise, gait training, immobilization, hot or cold applications)
Patient education (Therapeutic Neuroscience Education)
Coping skills training
Cognitive–behavioral therapy
Massage
Transcutaneous electrical nerve stimulation
Acupuncture
Mindful meditation

For pain assessed as moderate to severe, combination opioids, such as oxycodone, hydrocodone, or codeine in combination with acetaminophen or ibuprofen, can be used. More potent opioids, such as morphine, hydromorphone, or fentanyl, are used for the treatment of severe pain. Moderate to severe pain can also be treated with low-dose opioids when a patient has contraindications to NSAIDs or acetaminophen. Opioids may be combined with other coanalgesic medications based on severity, description, and type of pain. The combination of an opioid with a coanalgesic medication may provide more pain control than either of the drug classes alone.

When developing a treatment plan, members of the health care team should take into account the preferences and needs of patients whose education or cultural traditions may impede effective treatment. Certain cultures have strong beliefs about pain and its management. Members of these cultures may hesitate to report unrelieved pain or may have alternative methods of treating pain. Clinicians should be aware of the unique needs and circumstances of patients from different age groups or various ethnic and cultural backgrounds. In addition, many biases to opioids continue to exist in some patients and prescribers. Patient and provider education may be effective in addressing cultural concerns and alleviating biases associated with pain treatments.

Pharmacologic treatment is the most common modality in pain control. However, nonpharmacologic options and therapies have been shown to be effective, especially in patients with chronic pain. Nonpharmacologic approaches include the use of therapies such as heat, cold, exercise, and physical therapy. Complementary therapies such as acupuncture, meditation, and massage may also be effective.

More data is emerging on how CNCP needs to be seen as a biopsychosocial and not a purely biological condition especially when pain has no obvious cause. Behavioral therapies, including systematic coping approaches and relaxation strategies, have been shown to be essential in these patients in order to improve function and quality of life. Transcutaneous electrical nerve stimulation therapy can be used to help control certain types of nerve-related pain. Treatment of difficult pain conditions that cannot be managed by noninvasive and/or pharmacologic treatments may require a consultation with a pain specialist or a pain psychologist to evaluate other options or interventions.

Drug Therapy by Type of Pain

Assessment of pain intensity is important when determining initial analgesic therapies. Mild to moderate pain can be treated with lower-potency medications such as acetaminophen and NSAIDs. These agents can also be part of a multimodal therapy plan in combination with opioids for severe pain. Historically, aspirin had been used as a pain modality for short-term pain treatment. However, increased adverse effects limit its chronic use. Aspirin is mostly used today to prevent cardiac events and is not routinely used as first-line pain management therapy.

Combination opioids, ketorolac, and tramadol are commonly used to treat moderate pain. The combination opioids contain the addition of a "nonopioid," such as acetaminophen or ibuprofen, creating a treatment ceiling dose (maximum dose). Low doses of strong opioids may also be utilized for moderate pain in patients who have contraindications for NSAIDs or tramadol.

Opioids are the most common therapy recommended for severe pain. Morphine is the gold standard and the most studied opioid. When used in equivalent doses, most pure opioids (*mu* receptor agonists) are equally effective in controlling pain, but individual variation may exist among patients. Morphine, oxycodone, hydromorphone, oxymorphone, and fentanyl are pure *mu* opioid agonists indicated for the treatment of severe pain. Morphine is considered the opioid of first choice unless a contraindication exists or the patient has failed prior morphine therapy. Meperidine is another opioid that has historically been utilized for the treatment of severe pain. Use of this agent is no longer recommended due to neurotoxicity associated with accumulation of the active metabolite in patients with renal insufficiency or with chronic use.

In most persistent pain cases, pain medications should be administered around the clock (ATC), with as-needed medications used to treat BTP. This recommendation is based on the finding that regularly scheduled medications maintain a constant level of drug in the body and help prevent a recurrence of pain. BTP medications are indicated when intermittent pain occurs despite ATC therapy.

An essential principle in using medications to manage chronic pain is to individualize medication regimens according to the type and severity of pain. For mild to moderate pain, acetaminophen or an NSAID is usually considered initial therapy. Management of moderate to severe pain may utilize a combination opioid, tramadol, or low doses of opioids. Severe pain is treated with higher-potency opioids, such as morphine, hydromorphone, or oxycodone. Various classes of coanalgesics, such as anticonvulsants and antidepressants, can also be utilized in combination with the opioids (**Table 7.1**).

Acute Pain

Acute pain is often a response to tissue injury or trauma and is usually nociceptive in nature. Treatment includes nonopioids such as NSAIDs and acetaminophen for mild to moderate pain and opioid medications for moderate to severe pain. As acute pain increases and persists, it becomes more difficult to manage. Therefore, it is important to treat acute pain promptly and effectively. Also, untreated acute pain is often the catalyst in the development of chronic pain conditions in which pain persists despite healing of the original injury.

Acetaminophen is the drug of choice for treating minor, noninflammatory pain, especially in patients at risk for GI damage. NSAIDs are also effective as monotherapy in the treatment of mild to moderate pain. Both acetaminophen and NSAIDs are available in combination with opioids for moderate pain. Pure or dual-mechanism opioids are used when pain is severe. The opioids, as a class, generally exhibit equal analgesic effects when given at equipotent doses (adjusted for route of administration and duration of action).

TABLE 7.1

Recommended Order of Pain Treatment Based on Initial Pain Assessment

Pain Rating	Classification	NSAID/APAP	Opioids	Coanalgesics
1–3	Mild	✓	Sometimes	✓
4–7	Moderate	✓	Usually	✓
8–10	Severe	✓	Usually	✓

Supplement each level with nonpharmacologic therapy: *psychological*, cognitive–behavioral therapy, biofeedback, relaxation, imagery, psychotherapy; *physical rehabilitation/alternative therapy*, stretching, exercise, reconditioning, thermotherapy, massage, acupuncture.

PAIN ASSESSMENT TOOLS

SINGLE DIMENSIONAL
Numerical Rating Scale (NRS)
Visual Analog Scale (VAS)
Thermometer Pain Scale
Faces Pain Scale
Painad Scale
FLACC Scale

MULTIDIMENSIONAL
McGill Pain Questionnaire
Brief Pain Inventory
Behavioral Pain Scales
Pain/Comfort Journals
Multidimensional Pain Inventory
Pain Disability Index

Various strategies are currently implemented in the control of pain. Postoperative pain is often treated with multimodal therapies including opioid medications and various coanalgesics for treatment of severe pain. The use of preemptive analgesia, defined as the administration of various analgesics prior to procedures, is often a part of a multimodal treatment plan using two or more medications with different mechanisms to provide benefits to pain control while minimizing adverse effects. Central regional local anesthetic blocks have also been shown to provide additional analgesia when added to opioid therapy. Choice of medications, doses, and use of local interventional techniques should be individualized to the patient (**Box 7.4**).

BOX 7.4 Interventional Techniques for Chronic Pain

Injections
- Nerve blocks
- Epidural steroid injection
- Facet joint injections
- Nerve root blocks
- Sacroiliac joint injection

Spinal fusion
Percutaneous disc decompression
Radiofrequency rhizotomy
Neuromodulatory therapy
- Intrathecal pump implants
- Spinal cord stimulants

Vertebroplasty
Kyphoplasty

Chronic Pain

Noncancer Pain

NSAIDs and salicylates are effective for chronic inflammatory conditions, such as arthritis and musculoskeletal conditions. Efficacy of NSAID treatment varies greatly among patients. Those who do not respond to an NSAID in one class may respond to an NSAID from the same or a different class. Opioids may be considered as an alternative or an addition to NSAID therapy if pain is moderate to severe in appropriately assessed CNCP. Administration of a lower-potency opioid in conjunction with a coanalgesic may be instituted if treatment failure of NSAIDs or acetaminophen occurs.

Historically, opioids were thought to be ineffective in neuropathic pain. It is now known that opioids may be effective against these types of pain but often require higher than usual doses. Utilizing coanalgesics as monotherapy or in combination with opioids may be effective in chronic pain treatment and may decrease opioid requirements.

Care should be taken when administering opioids to the elderly or in patients with renal failure, liver failure, and respiratory diseases because of the increased chance of respiratory depression and oversedation. Lower doses should be initiated in these patients and titrated slowly based on response.

More evidence is emerging that the use of opioids for chronic pain in patients with psychological comorbidities or risk for addiction and/or abuse may not provide long-term benefits and increase in functionality (Franklin, 2014). Historically, opioids were thought to have no ceiling effect. Studies have shown that prolonged use of high-dose opioids in patients at risk may actually facilitate pain and may become pronociceptive. Opioid monotherapy in these patients may not provide functional improvements and a better quality of life.

Physical dependence and fear of addiction should not be the overriding considerations when choosing a pain modality for patients. Appropriate assessment tools may provide guidance on which patients may benefit from opioid therapy. A multidisciplinary approach using medications, physical therapy, massage, acupuncture, meditation, and cognitive–behavioral therapy may be needed in patients where medications alone have not provided benefit in function. Research is currently being conducted on long-term opioid use and optimal treatment approaches for CNCP conditions.

Cancer Pain

The National Comprehensive Cancer Network (NCCN) has released guidelines for the management of cancer pain. In the past, the World Health Organization (WHO) utilized three-step analgesic ladder where therapy is started with mild analgesics, moving to stronger therapies when the current therapy fails (Reidenberg, 1996). We now know that cancer pain is much more complex and needs to be individualized for the patient based on type of pain, degree of pain, and comorbidities that may affect pain and suffering. The NCCN provides an algorithm for a treatment approach with recommendations for therapy. Opioids are the mainstay of cancer pain management. The addition of nonopioids and coanalgesics is advocated as part of a multimodal approach to treatment. The goal of therapy is to safely use medications in order to improve function and quality of life.

Morphine, oxycodone, hydromorphone, and fentanyl are the common used opioids in the management of severe pain. Methadone is a long-acting opioid with a dual mechanism,

working by activating opioid receptors and as an NMDA receptor antagonist. Both actions help to inhibit pain. Methadone can be difficult to dose and has many drug–drug interactions and adverse reactions. Therefore, for safety reasons, methadone should be reserved for treatment failure to other opioids. Referral to a pain professional trained in the safe dosing of methadone is recommended.

MEDICATIONS USED IN PAIN MANAGEMENT

The current pharmacotherapeutic options for pain management include nonopioid and opioid agents. Coanalgesic therapies, such as antidepressants, anticonvulsants, local anesthetics, and topical treatments, are often added especially in neuropathic and/or mixed persistent pain conditions. Selection of the appropriate agent rests on an assessment of the patient's type and source of pain as well as the intensity level of the pain.

Nonopioid Analgesics

The nonopioid analgesics are utilized for mild to moderate pain (**Table 7.2**). Pain is reduced, and beneficial anti-inflammatory action may also be seen with some agents in this class. Onset of analgesia occurs within 1 hour of oral administration, and drug effects last anywhere from 4 to 12 hours. The agents

TABLE 7.2

Pharmacokinetic and Pharmacodynamic Properties of Nonopioid Analgesics

Generic Name	Trade Name	Dosage Forms	Half-Life (h)	Onset (h)	Duration (h)	Route	Usual Starting Dosage	Max Dosage (24 h)
acetaminophen	Tylenol, others	Tablet Suspension Suppository Intravenous	2–7	0.5–0.75 5–10 min	4–6 4–6	PO PR IV	650 mg every 4–6 h 1 g every 6 h	4,000 mg
ibuprofen	Motrin, Advil Caldolor	Tablets Suspension Injection	1.8–2.4	0.5–1	6–8	PO IV	200–400 mg every 4–6 h 400–800 mg every 6 h	3,200 mg
naproxen	Naprosyn	Tablets Suspension	12–15	1	8–12	PO	500 mg × 1, then 250 mg every 8 h	1,250 mg
naproxen sodium	Aleve	Tablets	19	0.5	8–12	PO	550 mg × 1, then 275 mg every 12 h	1,375 mg
diclofenac	Voltaren	Tablets Gel	2 1–2	0.5	8–12	PO Topical	25 mg every 12 h	200 mg
diclofenac epolamine	Flector	Topical patch	12	1	12	Topical	1 patch every 12 h	2 patches
ketorolac	Toradol	Tablets Injection	5.5–7	0.5	5–6 4–6	PO IV, IM	10 mg every 6 h 15–30 mg IV every 6 h	120 mg 40 mg
tramadol	Ultram	Tablet	6–7	1	5–7	PO	50–100 mg every 6 h	400 mg
diflunisal	Dolobid	Tablet	8–12	1	8–12	PO	1 g × 1, then 500 mg every 8–12 h	1,500 mg

can be classified by their mechanism of action, chemical class, and anti-inflammatory activity. When choosing a nonopioid, the lowest effective dose should be used to minimize possible adverse reactions.

Acetaminophen

Acetaminophen is one of the most commonly prescribed analgesic–antipyretic medications.

The mechanism of analgesic activity is unknown, but it is postulated that pain may be mediated through PG inhibition in the CNS as a COX-3 inhibitor. Lack of peripheral PG inhibition makes acetaminophen a weak anti-inflammatory agent and therefore not considered useful in treating inflammatory disorders such as rheumatoid arthritis. Acetaminophen does not adversely affect platelet aggregation or the gastric mucosa and is generally well tolerated.

Acetaminophen is almost completely absorbed from the GI tract and has a quick onset of action with a time-to-peak effect of 1 to 3 hours. Extensive liver metabolism to inactive substances makes acetaminophen a relatively nontoxic agent. However, a small portion (4%) of the drug is converted to a toxic metabolite, normally inactivated by glutathione pathways. Once glutathione stores are depleted, as seen in cases of chronic ingestion or acute overdosage, the toxic metabolite can cause potentially fatal liver necrosis.

Generally, the maximum daily dose of acetaminophen should not exceed 4,000 mg. Lower maximum doses are recommended when two or more drinks per day are ingested or if liver disease is present. In older adults, some experts are recommending reducing the maximum dose to 3,000 mg/d to reduce risk of overdose and to minimize adverse effects (Byrd, 2013).

Nonsteroidal Anti-Inflammatory Drugs

NSAIDs as a class have anti-inflammatory, analgesic, and antipyretic activity. Cyclooxygenase, consisting of the isoforms COX-1 and COX-2, is the enzyme involved in the formation of PGs. Aspirin causes irreversible inactivation of COX-1 and COX-2, where nonaspirin NSAIDs cause reversible inactivation. The COX-1 isoform produces PGs that regulate blood flow to the kidneys and GI tract and decrease platelet aggregation. The COX-2 isoenzyme is usually expressed as a result of tissue injury and is the source of inflammatory pain. First-generation NSAIDs inhibit both isoenzymes, thereby reducing inflammation but also decreasing the gastroprotective effects of COX-1. Pain is decreased but gastroprotection is lost from damage to the GI mucosa, increasing the risk of GI bleeding. COX-2 inhibitors were developed in hopes of relieving pain while reducing the chance for GI toxicities. Unfortunately, a subsequent increase in cardiovascular events was seen. All NSAIDs have some degree of COX-2 inhibition. Those that have a greater proportion of COX-2 versus COX-1 inhibition will have a higher risk of thrombus, heart attack, and stroke.

Some NSAIDs, including aspirin, ketoprofen, and indomethacin, inhibit both COX-1 and COX-2 enzymes but are more selective for inhibiting COX-1. Diflunisal and diclofenac may be more selective for COX-2 inhibition and therefore less likely to cause GI toxicity. Celecoxib is the only available COX-2 inhibitor on the market in the United States (Zarchi et al., 2011).

The analgesic effect of NSAIDs is achieved within 1 hour of administration, with maximal effects within 2 or 3 hours. Anti-inflammatory effect has a longer onset, with maximal effects seen in 7 to 10 days. Decreased pain due to reduced tissue swelling is an indirect response to NSAIDs. Lower doses of nonsteroidal therapies should be used in elderly patients to adjust for the decline in renal function.

Long-term use of NSAIDs at high doses (anti-inflammatory doses) can increase the risk serious adverse effects. Indomethacin (Indocin) is associated with more CNS and ocular adverse effects than other NSAIDs. In patients at risk for a GI bleed or who are taking concomitant aspirin and NSAID therapy, acid suppression therapy preferably with a proton pump inhibitor (PPI) is recommended. Misoprostol, a synthetic PG, is also effective for the prevention of bleeding, but GI adverse reactions (nausea, abdominal cramps, and diarrhea) limit its use.

A black box warning on cardiovascular toxicities has been added to all NSAID products. Unlike NSAIDs, acetaminophen and salicylates have minimal GI toxicity and no effect on platelet aggregation at usual doses. See Chapters 36 and 37 for more discussion of NSAIDs and acetaminophen.

Opioids

Opioids bind to opioid receptors in the CNS (*mu (μ), kappa (κ),* or *delta (δ)*), with analgesic effect primarily associated with *mu* receptor binding. Full agonists include codeine, morphine, hydrocodone, oxycodone, hydromorphone, oxymorphone, fentanyl, and meperidine. Meperidine is associated with significant adverse effects and is no longer recommended as first-line therapy. Meperidine's active metabolite, normeperidine, can accumulate and induce seizures with high doses or in patients with decreased renal function.

Activation of the *mu* opioid receptor produces effective analgesia as well as undesired effects, including respiratory depression, sedation, confusion, nausea/vomiting, pruritus, miosis, constipation, and urinary retention. With the exception of constipation and possibly pruritus, tolerance to adverse effects develops over time. Morphine and other *mu* opioid receptor agonists provide pain relief over a broad dosage range. Multiple *mu* receptor subtypes exist, which may explain why opioids do not have the same outcomes for everyone. Opioid effects may also differ due to individual differences in hepatic metabolism and genetic factors. For example, an adequate concentration of CYP2D6 is needed to convert codeine to morphine, the active agent. Dependent on if a person is a poor or rapid metabolizer based on CYP2D6 concentrations, codeine may be either ineffective or toxic in 5% to 7% of the Caucasian population (Eckhardt et al., 1998). At equianalgesic doses and appropriate dosing intervals, there is no appreciable difference in potency among opioid agents (**Table 7.3**) (McPherson, 2010). The described potency is a reflection of the dose needed to achieve a desired

TABLE 7.3

Pharmacokinetic and Pharmacodynamic Properties of Opioid Analgesics

Generic Name	Trade Name(s)	Route	Onset (min)	Half-Life (h)	Duration (h)	Usual Starting Dose
hydrocodone	Vicodin, Lortab, Lorcet, generic	PO	10–20	3.3–4.5	4–8	1 tablet (5 mg hydrocodone) every 4 h
oxycodone	Percocet, Percodan, generic	PO	15	2–3	4–5	1 tablet (5 mg oxycodone) every 4 h
Moderate to severe						
Morphine-immediate release	Various, generic	PO	30–60	2–3	4–6	10–15 mg every 3–4 h
Sustained release	MS Contin, Kadian, Avinza	PO	15–60	15	8–12 (formulation dependent)	15 mg every 12 h *
Injection	Various, generic	IV, SC	5–10	2–3	2–4	5–10 mg every 3–4 h
Hydromorphone	Dilaudid,	PO	15–30	1–3	3–13	2 mg every 4 h
	Exalgo		6	11		Individualize dose
		IV, SC	5–10	1–3	4–5	0.5 mg every 4 h
Oxycodone-immediate release	Oxy IR, Roxicodone	PO	15–60	2–3	3–4	5 mg every 3–4 h
Sustained release	Oxycontin	PO	50–60	5	8–12	Individualize dose
Fentanyl	Duragesic	Transdermal patch	16–24	1.5–6	48–72	Individualize dose
		IV	0–5	2–4	30–60 min	
	Actiq, Fentora	Transmucosal	5–15	17	Related to blood level	†
Oxymorphone	Opana	PO	30	7–9	4–6	5 mg every 4–6 h
	Opana ER	PO	3	10	12	5 mg every 12 h
Hydrocodone	Vicodin	PO	30–60	7.9	4–6	1 tablet ever 4–6 h
Dual mechanism	Zohydro ER			8	24	Individualize
	Hysingla ER			8	24	Individualize
methadone	Dolophine, others	PO	30–60	8–59	2–10 (acute) >12 (chronic)	2.5–5 mg every 8–12 h
		IV	10–20	8–59	>8 (chronic)	1–2 mg every 8 h
tapentadol	Nucynta	PO	30–45	4	4–6	50 mg every 4–6 h

Opioid Pearls

1. Use lower initial opioid doses in elderly and in patients with respiratory comorbidities.
2. **Hydrocodone** for pain is available in combination with acetaminophen or ibuprofen. A long-acting formulation for chronic pain has recently been approved.
3. **Oxycodone** is available in combination with acetaminophen, aspirin, and ibuprofen.
4. **Morphine** is the opioid of choice unless contraindications exist. Morphine is relatively contraindicated in renal failure.
5. **Hydromorphone** is approximately five times the potency of morphine.
6. **Fentanyl** patch is contraindicated for acute pain and/or opioid naive.
   - Fentanyl patch may not be appropriate for patients with fever, diaphoresis, cachexia, morbid obesity, and ascites, all of which affects absorption and clinical effectiveness.
   - Patch may be appropriate for patients who cannot take long-acting oral opioids.
   - Onset of action is 12–16 hours after application. Utilize breakthrough pain (BTP) medications for pain control until onset of analgesia. Full effect takes 72 hours.
   - Application of external heat sources will increase the release of fentanyl from the transdermal system.
   - Titration of the patch should not occur before 3 days after the initial dose or no more frequent than every 7 days thereafter.
7. **Methadone** has a duration of analgesia much shorter than half-life, making the drug difficult to dose.
   - Conservative dose conversions with careful titration are recommended. Use a higher conversion ratio in patients currently on high-dose opioids.
   - *Steady state is not reached for at least 5–7 days. Use BTP medications early in the titration, as analgesic effects are shorter than the half-life of the drug. Observe for accumulation-related side effects during titration (>2 days treatment).
   - Consult a pain management specialist for dosing.

*Not initial therapy for opioid-naive patients.
†Cancer-related BTP only.

TABLE 7.4

Basic Opioid Conversion Table

Opioid	Oral	Parenteral
Morphine	30 mg	10 mg
Oxycodone	20 mg	—
Hydrocodone	30 mg	—
Hydromorphone	7.5 mg	1.5 mg
Oxymorphone	10 mg	1 mg
Codeine	200 mg	120 mg
Fentanyl	—	0.1 mg
Methadone	Refer to a pain management specialist for methadone dosing	2:1 oral to IV

level of analgesia. In general, the more potent the agent, the fewer milligrams needed (**Table 7.4**).

Opioids are primarily metabolized by the liver to active and inactive metabolites. The metabolites of morphine and hydromorphone are eliminated by the kidneys. In renal failure, morphine's active metabolites may accumulate and cause neurotoxicity, such as myoclonus, confusion, and coma. Death may result if this accumulation is not identified.

Hydromorphone has historically been thought to be safe in renal disease. Data is emerging that hydromorphone metabolites may also accumulate causing neurotoxicity. The metabolites of morphine and hydromorphone differ in that hydromorphone's metabolites are eliminated by dialysis, but morphine metabolites are not dialyzable.

Metabolites of oxycodone are inactive, making this a good option in patients with renal failure. Sustained-release formulations, however, are advised to be used with caution in end-stage renal and liver disease. Fentanyl and methadone do not have active metabolites and are considered the drugs of choice in the treatment of chronic pain in patients with renal failure. Fentanyl is the drug of choice in patients with liver failure.

The onset of the analgesic effects of oral opioids is 30 to 60 minutes, and the peak effect is seen within 1 to 2 hours. Fentanyl has a quicker onset and shorter duration and is considered an ultrashort-acting opioid. Moderate-acting opioids, with duration of actions between 4 and 6 hours, include morphine, codeine, hydromorphone, oxycodone, and oxymorphone. Methadone, a dual-mechanism, long-acting opioid, has a variable duration of action and half-life of approximately 24 to 36 hours. Steady state may take 5 to 7 days to be reached; therefore, upward titration should not occur for at least 5 days after therapy initiation.

Morphine and Congeners

Morphine is a low-cost, readily available agent with well-characterized pharmacokinetic and pharmacodynamic properties. It is the opioid to which all others are compared, due to extensive clinical experience and literature available supporting use. Morphine is absorbed erratically from the GI tract and undergoes significant first-pass hepatic metabolism when given by the oral route. Morphine is distributed throughout the body, and sufficient amounts cross the blood–brain barrier to account for most of its pharmacologic effects. Morphine has a plasma half-life of approximately 3 hours, which is due mainly to its nearly complete metabolism in the liver. Morphine crosses the placental barrier and is excreted in maternal milk.

Morphine may be administered by multiple routes. Oral, injectable, rectal, intrathecal, and intraspinal formulations are available. Dosage forms include immediate-release and sustained-release tablets and capsules. Liquid formulations are also available. With chronic dosing, the potency of the intravenous dose is three times that of the equivalent oral dose.

Morphine effectively relieves severe pain, particularly nociceptive pain, regardless of its cause or anatomic source. Analgesia is due to the drug's binding to *mu* receptors in the CNS. Opioids can cause respiratory depression due to both the drug's actions on the brain's medullary respiratory control center and the drug's ability to suppress the medulla's response to blood carbon dioxide levels. Respiratory depression is seen mainly in opioid-naive patients or with upward dose titration in both acute and chronic pain. Tolerance develops relatively quickly to respiratory depressive effects. A person in whom tolerance has developed may experience only moderate respiratory effects when receiving doses that could cause serious or fatal respiratory depression in a nontolerant person.

Opioids also increase smooth muscle tone in various parts of the GI tract. *Mu* receptors are located throughout the GI tract where receptor binding results in reduced peristalsis and increased tone of the rectal sphincter. The overall resultant effect is constipation. Prophylactic bowel regimens consisting of a stimulant laxative and stool softener is recommended with initiation of opioid therapy.

Hydromorphone is considered more potent and more soluble than morphine; however, it has a similar pharmacologic profile. Hydromorphone is available as an oral immediate-release tablet, a suppository, and an injectable formulation. Recently, a long-acting formulation of hydromorphone was released to the U.S. market.

Oxycodone is slightly more potent than morphine. This agent may be used as monotherapy or in combination with nonopioid analgesics, such as ibuprofen or acetaminophen, for the reduction of moderate pain. Oxycodone is available as an immediate-release tablet, an oral liquid formulation, and a sustained-release tablet. No injectable form of oxycodone is currently available.

Hydrocodone is available in combination with nonopioid analgesics. Hydrocodone is equipotent to morphine on a milligram-to-milligram basis. Hydrocodone is available in combination with acetaminophen or ibuprofen and is used for moderate to severe pain. A long-acting formulation indicated for severe pain has been released in 2013. The DEA has reclassified hydrocodone from Schedule III to Schedule II in 2014.

Oxymorphone, the metabolite of oxycodone, is used to treat moderate to severe pain. Historically, oxymorphone was available as an injectable (Numorphan), but it is now only available as immediate-release and sustained-release tablets. Oxymorphone is approximately twice as strong as oxycodone, with 10 mg of oxymorphone equivalent to 20 mg of oxycodone. Adverse effects and mechanisms of action are similar to other opioids.

Codeine is usually administered orally either alone or in combination with nonopioid analgesics, such as acetaminophen, for moderate pain. Use has fallen out of favor due to increased adverse effects when compared to other opioids. Other more potent and better tolerated pain management modalities are available. At equianalgesic doses, codeine induces greater histamine release than other opioids. This increases the risk of hypotension, cutaneous vasodilation, urticaria, and bronchoconstriction. Currently, codeine is primarily used as an antitussive agent.

Fentanyl and Congeners

Fentanyl is an alternative to morphine and its congeners, with low to no cross-allergenicity in patients with true hypersensitivity to morphine-like drugs. Fentanyl is available for acute pain as injectable and buccal formulations. A long-acting transdermal patch is available for stable chronic pain and is only to be used in opioid-tolerant patients with a chronic pain process. Patients are required to have taken oral morphine 60 mg, oxycodone 30 mg, or hydromorphone 8 mg/d for the previous 7 days or longer to be considered opioid tolerant (Janssen Pharmaceuticals, 2006). Transdermal fentanyl has an onset of effect of 12 to 16 hours after patch placement. Peak systemic concentrations occur between 24 and 72 hours after initial patch application. Duration of effect is approximately 72 hours. However, some patients may require patch changes after 48 hours. Use of the buccal transmucosal formulation is limited to severe BTP associated with cancer. A recent study demonstrated that transmucosal fentanyl formulations (TMF) have better efficacy in cancer BTP when compared to oral short-acting morphine (Maroo et al., 2014). Onset of action is 15 minutes versus 45 to 60 minutes with oral formulations. Practitioners are required to become certified prior to being able to prescribe transmucosal fentanyl as part of a Risk Evaluation Mitigation Strategy (REMS) requirement for safe use.

Other agents, such as sufentanil (Sufenta) and alfentanil (Alfenta), also fall in this class but are used primarily for perioperative and postoperative pain relief and are available only in an injectable formulation.

Meperidine is a synthetic analgesic that binds strongly to both *mu* and *kappa* receptors. Potency is less than that of morphine. Most of the pharmacologic effects of this drug are similar to those of morphine sulfate; however, adverse effects limit its use. Prolonged use of meperidine may cause CNS excitation characterized by tremors and seizures due to the accumulation of its active metabolite, normeperidine. The half-life of normeperidine ranges between 15 and 20 hours and is almost completely renally eliminated. The possibility of accumulation of this metabolite leading to detrimental CNS effects has limited the use of meperidine in the treatment of pain. Meperidine is still used for treatment of rigors and in procedural sedation.

Dual-Mechanism Analgesics

Tramadol is a centrally acting weak *mu* receptor agonist. Pain is also modulated by norepinephrine reuptake inhibition and serotonin release. Tramadol is used to treat moderate to severe pain and is available alone or in combination with acetaminophen. Tramadol may be useful for pain management in patients where a strong opioid is not an option and an NSAID may introduce undue risk (e.g., GI bleeding). In addition, tramadol may have a place in neuropathic pain management due to the additional norepinephrine reuptake inhibition. Maximum dose of tramadol is 400 mg/d. Dosing should be initiated slowly and titrated to an effective dose. Tramadol may have less abuse potential when compared to other opioids but has recently been changed to a Schedule IV medication. Tramadol is rapidly absorbed. Peak serum levels are obtained within 2 hours and have a 4- to 6-hour duration of effect. Tramadol is metabolized in the liver by the cytochrome P450 enzyme system to an active metabolite (O-dimethyl tramadol). Drug–drug interactions are common. Decreased maximum doses are recommended in the elderly and in patients with renal impairment. Increased seizure risk is seen with high doses or in patients with a history of seizure disorders.

Methadone hydrochloride is an effective analgesic alternative when other opioid therapies have failed. Due to different chemical structure, methadone can also be used as an analgesic alternative in patients with a true allergy to morphine-like compounds (anaphylaxis, hives). Methadone is effective both orally and parenterally and has an oral bioavailability exceeding 90%. It is more than 90% bound to plasma tissue proteins and is extensively metabolized by the CYP-450 enzyme system. Patients may be at risk of qTc prolongation and torsades de pointes due to the significant amount of drug–drug interactions seen with methadone. Methadone is most often associated with the treatment of opioid substance abuse but is being used more frequently in the treatment of chronic severe pain. Methadone works as both a *mu* receptor agonist and an NMDA receptor antagonist, making it effective for the treatment of severe neuropathic pain and mixed pain syndromes. The lack of active metabolites makes methadone a viable choice in patients with renal failure. The drug has a long half-life of approximately 24 hours (range between 10 and 60 hours), with an analgesic effect of approximately 4 to 8 hours. Early in methadone titration, pain control may be inadequate until steady state is reached. Aggressive BTP therapies may be required during the first 3 to 5 days of therapy. Tendency to dose methadone aggressively early in titration can lead to serious adverse effects, including fatal respiratory depression. Patients should be monitored carefully for signs of drug accumulation and toxicity. The long biologic half-life also accounts for the mild, but prolonged, withdrawal syndrome if use stops abruptly. Recently, due to a rise in methadone-associated deaths, the *Journal of Pain* released guidelines on methadone safety (Chou et al., 2014). These guidelines provide direction on the appropriate use of methadone for chronic pain and addiction based on the available evidence. Information on dosing, titration, and ECG monitoring are areas covered in the guidelines.

Tapentadol is a newer combination opioid that works on opioid receptors and as a specific norepinephrine reuptake inhibitor. This medication has been shown to be effective in various pain conditions, such as osteoarthritis and postoperative pain. Tapentadol has recently been approved for the treatment of chronic diabetic peripheral neuropathy. Tapentadol has less affinity for the *mu* receptor than morphine, but the analgesic effect is augmented due to norepinephrine reuptake inhibition. Tapentadol may have fewer GI adverse effects (nausea, vomiting, constipation) when compared with other opioids due to less effect on the *mu* receptor.

Opioid Antagonist—Naloxone

Naloxone is a pure opioid antagonist that competitively binds to opioid receptors without producing an analgesic response. Naloxone is inactivated when given orally and therefore is given mainly by injection. Naloxone is indicated for treating opioid-induced respiratory depression.

The duration of naloxone's drug action is approximately 45 minutes. In most cases, this duration is shorter than the offending opioid, and the overdose effect from the opioid may return, requiring readministration of naloxone. Care must be taken to avoid precipitation of withdrawal in opioid-tolerant patients when administering naloxone. Rare adverse effects of naloxone include tachycardia, ventricular fibrillation, and cardiac arrest due to the release of neurotransmitters when naloxone is administered. Opioid withdrawal syndrome may occur in opioid-tolerant patients when excessive or rapid reversal is used.

Safety of Opioids

Side effects common to all opioids include sedation, confusion, respiratory depression, itching, nausea/vomiting, and constipation. Opioid-induced bowel dysfunction develops due to reduced movement through the lower GI tract due to reduction of bowel tone and motility, increased anal sphincter tone, and increased absorption of fluids. Although considered the most dangerous side effect, severe respiratory depression is seen not only in overdose situations but also in patients who are opioid naive. Patients who are at risk for respiratory depression also include elderly patients, patients who have respiratory comorbidities such as obstructive sleep apnea, and patients with kidney/liver failure. Chronic pain patients on opioids usually develop tolerance to the respiratory depression effects. However, if substantial opioid doses are used in addition to chronic therapy, as in the case of a post-op opioid-tolerant patient, risk of respiratory depression is increased. In patients with closed head injury or recent brain surgery, opioids should be used with caution because hemodynamic effects (e.g., hypotension, orthostasis) may be exaggerated.

Bowel Regimen for the Prevention of Constipation

Tolerance usually develops within a few days to most of the adverse reactions associated with opioids except for constipation. Constipation prevention is needed in patients receiving opioids. The general approach for patients requiring opioids is to institute a prophylactic bowel regimen consisting of a mild stimulant +/– a stool softener. Dose of the stimulant can be titrated based on patient response. Initial dosing would consist of senna 2 tablets daily or twice per day. Docusate sodium 100 mg twice per day is often used when stool softening is needed. Polyethylene glycol (PEG) powder packets used daily is another effective alternative. If there is no bowel movement produced in 48 hours, consider using an additional agent (e.g., bisacodyl suppository, lactulose, additional PEG) to stimulate peristalsis. If interventions continue to be ineffective, assess for impaction. If no impaction is present, utilizing an additional method (e.g., enema) is recommended. Once the patient has a bowel movement, titrate the dosage of senna to an effective dose. (Up to 8 tablets per day or the liquid equivalent has been used in the hospice and palliative care population.) Docusate sodium should not be titrated aggressively because sodium salt may affect sodium levels.

Use of bulk-forming laxatives in patients receiving opioids is not recommended. Due to slower peristalsis in patients receiving opioids and potential inadequate fluid intake, the medication may lodge in the colon, causing bowel obstruction.

New novel agents are now available to treat refractory constipation due to opioids by specifically targeting the *mu* receptors in the gut. These medications were developed by altering the structure of naltrexone and naloxone, making them unable to cross the blood–brain barrier preventing reversal of analgesia. Methylnaltrexone is available as an injectable formulation, with effect seen within minutes to a few hours. Naloxegol is an oral agent with time to effect of approximately 12 hours.

Opioid Tolerance, Dependence, Pseudoaddiction, and Addiction

Opioid tolerance develops when chronic use of opioids causes the need for upward dose titration to maintain analgesia. Opioid dependence is defined as an emergence of withdrawal symptoms when the drug is abruptly discontinued or when the dose is rapidly decreased. Tolerance and physical dependence of opioids can develop quickly. Apparent dependence and/or tolerance in a patient with chronic pain should not impede titration of therapy to an effective dose.

Patients taking opioids as briefly as 2 or 3 days may become dependent and can experience withdrawal symptoms upon discontinuation. Withdrawal symptoms range from mild tremors to sweating and fever, and mimic flu-like symptoms. Severe withdrawal in opioid-dependent patients may consist of increased respiratory rate, perspiration, lacrimation, mydriasis, hot and cold flashes, and anorexia.

Patients with pain may demonstrate signs of addictive behavior, which may be a result of undertreated pain or worsening pain due to disease progression, rather than drug abuse or addiction. Pseudoaddiction, defined as drug-seeking behaviors due to inadequate pain management, can be differentiated from true addiction because "pseudoaddictive" behaviors will resolve once adequate pain management is achieved.

Addiction is defined as "a primary, chronic, neurobiological disease with genetic, psychosocial and environmental factors influencing its development and manifestations" (Savage et al., 2003). It is characterized by behaviors that include one or more of the following: impaired control over drug use, compulsive use, continued use despite harm, and cravings. In 2013, an estimated 24.6 million people aged 12 or older (9.4% of the population) live with substance dependence or abuse (National Survey on Drug Use and Health, 2014). Opioid abuse has been reported in chronic pain patients with psychological comorbidities who use opioids to treat pain resulting from depression or anxiety. The concept of substance abuse with respect to opioids is an important consideration in patients presenting with uncontrolled pain but is beyond the scope of this chapter.

Coanalgesics

Several medications have been evaluated for use either alone or in conjunction with other analgesics to treat many persistent pain conditions. The most benefit is seen in chronic pain, neuropathic pain, and postoperative pain syndromes.

Antidepressants

Antidepressants, including tricyclic antidepressants (TCAs) and selective norepinephrine reuptake inhibitors (SNRIs), exhibit analgesic effects by primarily blocking the reuptake of norepinephrine, thereby increasing pain-modulating pathway activity. TCAs also block peripheral sodium channels, which may also help reduce pain. TCAs and SNRIs have been useful in neuropathic pain resulting from cancer or cancer therapies and chronic noncancer, neuropathic pain syndromes (i.e., diabetic or postherpetic neuropathy, chronic low back pain, and fibromyalgia). Several TCAs have beneficial effects in neuropathic pain, including amitriptyline, desipramine, and nortriptyline. Common adverse reactions include dry mouth, weight gain, dizziness, urinary retention, confusion, and sedation. Dosing of TCAs is initiated at 10 to 25 mg nightly and titrated weekly to an effective dose of 75 to 100 mg each evening. Therapy with TCAs should be initiated with caution in the elderly due to an increased incidence of confusion and sedation due to anticholinergic activity and may lead to falls. TCAs should not be used as a first-line agent in the elderly population and should be reserved for patients with treatment failures to other agents.

Amitriptyline is the most studied TCA. The second-generation agent nortriptyline may be better tolerated than amitriptyline because there is less cholinergic and sedative effects. The SNRIs duloxetine and venlafaxine are newer agents used to treat neuropathic pain conditions. Duloxetine dosing is initiated at 20 to 30 mg/d to a target dose of 60 mg/d. Dosing can be titrated to 120 mg/d if indicated. Venlafaxine dose is initiated at 75 mg/d and titrated to a maximum dose of 225 mg/d either once daily or divided twice daily based on dosage form (SR vs. IR) These medications are better tolerated than the TCAs because no cholinergic side effects are seen. GI disturbances, sedation, insomnia, sweating, and confusion may be seen with SNRI use. Venlafaxine has also been associated with increases in blood pressure.

Anticonvulsants

Another group of agents commonly prescribed for neuropathic pain conditions are the anticonvulsants. The most common agents used are gabapentin, pregabalin, and carbamazepine. Gabapentin is the first-line anticonvulsant agent recommended for pain treatment. Pregabalin is structurally similar to gabapentin and has the same mechanism of action. The mechanism of action is not totally understood, but is postulated to be due to the effects of binding to the α-2-delta subunit of voltage-dependent calcium channels, resulting in a reduction of the influx of calcium into the dorsal horn. This results in a decreased release of glutamate, causing less activation of second-order neurons responsible for transmission of the pain signal to the brain. Gabapentin and pregabalin are generally well tolerated. Most common side effects include nausea, sedation, dizziness, weight gain, and ataxia. Peripheral edema has been associated with pregabalin use. Gabapentin has been shown to be effective for many neuropathic pain conditions, including diabetic neuropathy, trigeminal neuralgia, restless leg syndrome, phantom limb pain, and pain after a stroke. Generally, doses are started at 100 to 300 mg daily and titrated up to 1,800 to 3,600 mg daily in three to four divided daily doses. A sustained-release formulation is also available with a lower maximum dose of 1,800 mg/d. The sustained-release and immediate-release products are not interchangeable.

Pregabalin is better absorbed than gabapentin, and efficacy is seen in approximately 1 week, compared to 4 to 6 weeks with gabapentin. The dose should be started low and titrated. Initial doses are 50 mg two to three times daily, titrated to an effective dose. The maximum dose of pregabalin is 600 mg/d. Side effects are similar to gabapentin. Dosing of gabapentin and pregabalin should be reduced in patients with renal impairment.

Carbamazepine and oxcarbazepine are primarily used for trigeminal neuralgia pain and are considered drugs of choice for this indication. Other anticonvulsants including topiramate, lamotrigine, and divalproex may be tried for neuropathic pain treatment if other modalities have failed.

Sodium Channel Blockers (Local Anesthetics)

This class of medications exerts its analgesic effects by blocking sodium channels, thereby slowing pain transmission and lowering the firing threshold of the second-order neurons. Several routes of administration exist and are chosen based on the indication for use. Topical applications help control localized neuropathic pain with minimal absorption. Lidocaine patches and EMLA cream (mixture of lidocaine and prilocaine) are available for topical use. Lidocaine patches are indicated for postherpetic neuralgia, but efficacy is reported in painful conditions such as diabetic peripheral neuropathy and osteoarthritis. Patches may be cut and up to three patches may be used. Application is usually 12 hours on and 12 hours off daily. Systemic absorption is minimal. Safety and tolerability of 24-hour administration were demonstrated in a study in the Annuls of Pharmacotherapy in 2002, which compared safety of 24-hour administration to the recommended 12-hour application. Pharmacokinetic data on

24-hour administration reported in the study showed systemic absorption markedly below the level needed for toxicity and was well tolerated.

Local injections of anesthetics can be utilized as regional anesthesia, injected into tissue or the epidural space. Epidural analgesia is commonly utilized in managing obstetric or postoperative pain. Rarely, lidocaine has been administered intravenously to control refractory pain conditions in subanesthetic dosages. Intravenous infusions must be administered in a monitored setting because of the potential for severe ADRs with possible exceptions in the end-of-life population. Evidence has shown that the use of lidocaine as a palliative measure for refractory pain may be efficacious when other methods have failed.

N-Methyl-D-Aspartate Receptor Antagonists

More evidence is emerging in the use of the NMDA antagonists, specifically ketamine, for both acute and chronic pain. Ketamine, an anesthetic agent, is used as a bolus dose or an intravenous infusion for treatment for a variety of pain conditions, such as postoperative pain, chronic refractory pain, and acute pain in the emergency department. Doses for analgesia are lower than doses used for anesthesia. Cancer and noncancer pain refractory to other treatments may benefit from the addition of ketamine to opioid therapy. Better pain control and an opioid-sparing effect have been demonstrated in studies using this combination. Ketamine reduces firing of the NMDA receptor, thereby decreasing sensitivity to pain impulses. Ketamine, by the oral and topical routes, also shows promise for the treatment of pain. Adverse effects are dose related and increased in patients that have a history of psychiatric comorbidities. The most common side effects with ketamine are vivid dreams and sedation. Delirium, dysphoria, hallucinations, hypotension, hypertension, and increased intracranial pressure have also been associated with its use. Other NMDA antagonists, such as dextromethorphan, memantine, amantadine, and magnesium, have not shown promise for pain reduction in studies related to use as analgesics.

Skeletal Muscle Relaxants

In the past, skeletal muscle relaxants have been one of the most extensively prescribed agents for treatment of musculoskeletal disorders, such as low back pain, muscle sprains, or athletic injury. Currently, muscle relaxants are recommended for the short-term treatment of acute musculoskeletal conditions. Long-term use is not recommended. Two categories of skeletal muscle relaxants exist: antispasmodic agents used for musculoskeletal conditions and antispastic agents for central spasticity in conditions such as multiple sclerosis and cerebral palsy.

Antispasmodic Skeletal Muscle Relaxants

Skeletal muscle relaxants are often used in the treatment of acute low back pain. The most benefit is usually seen within the first few days of treatment. Adverse effects such as drowsiness and dizziness are commonly seen, and some agents in this class have potential for abuse. If a muscle relaxant is indicated, choice should be based on adverse effect profile, drug interaction potential, and identified risk of abuse.

Cyclobenzaprine has been the most studied skeletal muscle relaxant. The manufacturer's recommended dose of cyclobenzaprine is 10 mg. However, a 5-mg dose has been shown to be effective with less toxicity. Its anticholinergic properties must be taken into account if used in the elderly. Tizanidine (Zanaflex) is a centrally acting, α_2-adrenergic agonist, reducing spasticity by increasing presynaptic inhibition of motor neuron excitation. Tizanidine is very sedating and a useful adjunct in patients with sleep disturbances as a result of musculoskeletal pain. Benzodiazepines, such as diazepam, may be effective for acute pain associated with muscle spasms. The predominance of adverse reactions, especially sedation and risk of abuse limit benzodiazepine use for this indication.

Antispastic Agents

Limited evidence exists for using antispastic agents to treat musculoskeletal conditions. Baclofen is the most utilized agent in this class. Baclofen is indicated for managing signs and symptoms of spasticity resulting from multiple sclerosis and for spinal cord injuries or disease. Some anecdotal evidence exists for the use of baclofen in persistent neuropathic states and is used off label for hiccups. It is available as an oral tablet and an injectable formulation for intrathecal administration. Common side effects of the oral form include drowsiness, hypotension, weakness, nausea/vomiting, and headache. Intrathecal administration results in hypotension, somnolence, dizziness, constipation, and headache. Respiratory depression and difficulty with concentration or coordination are also seen with intrathecal administration. Due to possible precipitation of withdrawal with abrupt discontinuation, tapering baclofen is recommended when discontinuing the drug especially with the intrathecal formulation or prolonged oral use. Seizures and delirium may occur and can progress to rhabdomyolysis, disseminated intravascular coagulation (DIC), and hepatic/renal failure with abrupt discontinuation.

CONCLUSION

Pain is difficult to manage and often needs a multidisciplinary approach to therapy. Treatment needs to be individualized for each patient, especially when a chronic pain condition exists. A proper assessment must be performed in order to differentiate the type and chronicity of pain. Once the type of pain is determined, patient-specific factors should be evaluated in order to choose the appropriate analgesic for pain treatment. Combination of therapies is often needed to provide a pain management goal of an acceptable level of pain and improvement in function. By utilizing the information provided in this chapter, the nursing practitioner will obtain the knowledge and the tools to effectively assess, treat, and monitor pain. The subsequent development of the individualized treatment plan will then provide improvement in the quality of life of the patient suffering in pain.

CASE STUDY*

J.T. is a 65-year-old male admitted to the hospital with history of chronic cancer pain using Morphine SR 60 mg PO q8h. On admission, morphine 2 mg IV q4h was ordered. The patient reports his pain only went from a 9 to an 8 after the morphine dose and is asking for more pain medication. The staff begins to question the motivation of the patient and if addiction is present. The resident decides to start a PCA for his pain. In a few hours, the patient is comfortable, resting in bed.

1. J.T.'s behavior is best described as:
   a. Tolerance
   b. Addiction
   c. Pseudoaddiction
   d. Dependence

2. During his hospital stay, J.T. went into acute renal failure. He is increasingly lethargic and is experiencing confusion and some hallucinations. The physician believes the morphine metabolites may be responsible and would like to convert to an alternative regimen. What would be your recommendation?
   a. Change opioid to fentanyl patch 50 mcg q72h.
   b. Decrease morphine SR dose to 60 mg PO q8h.
   c. Switch to hydromorphone 8 mg orally q4h as needed.
   d. Add haloperidol 1 mg PO q6h.

3. Tolerance will not develop to which adverse opioid effect?
   a. Respiratory depression
   b. Sedation
   c. Constipation
   d. Nausea

* Answers can be found online.

Bibliography

Starred references are cited in the text.

*Byrd, L. (2013). Managing chronic pain in older adults: A long-term care perspective. Retrieved from http://www.annalsoflongtermcare.com/article/managing-chronic-pain-older-adult-long-term-care on April 20, 2015.

*Chou, R., Cruciani, R., Fiellin, D., et al. (2014). Methadone safety: A clinical practice guideline from the American Pain Society and College on problems of drug dependence, in Collaboration with the Heart Rhythm Society. *The Journal of Pain, 15*(4), 321–337.

*Eckhardt, K., Li, S., Ammon, S., et al. (1998). Same incidence of adverse drug events after codeine administration irrespective of the genetically determined differences in morphine formation. *Pain, 76*(1–2), 27–33.

*Franklin, G. (2014). Opioids for chronic noncancer pain: A position paper of the American Academy of Neurology. *Neurology, 83*, 1277–1284.

*Henry, D.E., Chiodo, A.E., & Yang, W. (2011). Central nervous system reorganization in a variety of chronic pain states: A review. *American Academy of Physical Medicine and Rehabilitation, 3*(12), 1116–1125.

*Herr, K., & Garand, L. (2001) Assessment and measurement of pain in older adults. *Clinics in Geriatric Medicine, 17*, 457–478.

*Hooten, W. M., et al. (2013). Assessment and management of chronic pain. Retrieved from www.icsi.org/_asset/bw798b/ChronicPain.pdf on April 15, 2015.

*Janssen Pharmaceuticals. (2006). Product Information DURAGESIC® (Fentanyl Transdermal Patch).

Kim, H., & Nelson, L. S. (2015). Reducing the harm of opioid overdose with the safe use of naloxone: A pharmacologic review. *Expert Opinion Drug Safety, 14*(7), 1137–1146.

Manchikanti, L., Falco, F., Singh, V., et al. (2013). An update of comprehensive evidence-based guidelines for interventional techniques in chronic spinal pain. *Pain Physician, 16*, S1–S48.

*Maroo, S., Patel, K., Bhatnagar, S., et al. (2014). Safety and efficacy of oral transmucosal fentanyl citrate compared to morphine sulphate immediate release tablet in management of breakthrough cancer pain. *Indian Journal of Palliative Care, 20*, 182–187.

*McPherson, M. (2010). *Demystifying opioid conversion calculations: A guide for effective dosing.* Bethesda, MD: American Society of Health-System Pharmacists.

*Merskey, H., & Bogduk, N. (2012). Part III: Pain terms: A current list with definitions and notes on usage. *Classification of chronic pain* (2nd ed., pp. 209–214). Seattle, WA: IASP Task Force on Taxonomy.

*Pasero, C., & McCaffery, M. (2011). *Pain assessment and pharmacologic management.* St. Louis, MO: Elsevier/Mosby.

*Reidenberg, M. M., et al. (1996). Assessment of patients' pain. *N Engl J Med, 334*, 59.

*Savage, S., Joranson, D., Covington, E., et al. (2003) Definitions related to the medical use of opioids: Evolution towards universal agreement. *Journal of Pain and Symptom Management, 26*(1), 655–667.

*The NSDUH Report: Substance Use and Mental Health Estimates from the 2013 National Survey on Drug Use and Health: Overview of Findings. (2014). Retrieved from http://www.samhsa.gov/data/sites/default/files/NSDUHresultsPDFWHTML2013/Web/NSDUHresults2013.pdf on April 20, 2015.

Ventafridda, V., & Stjernsward, J. (1996). Pain control and the World Health Organization analgesic ladder. *The Journal of the American Medical Association, 275*, 835–836.

Wilcock, A., & Twycross, R. (2011). Therapeutic reviews: Ketamine. *Journal of Pain and Symptom Management, 41*(3), 640–648.

*Woo, C. W., Roy, M., Buhle, J. T., et al. (2015). Distinct brain systems mediate the effects of nociceptive input and self-regulation on pain. Retrieved from http://wagerlab.colorado.edu/files/papers/Woo_PLOS.pdf on April 15, 2015.

*Woolf, C. (2011). Central sensitization: Implications for the diagnosis and treatment of pain. *Pain, 152*(Suppl. 3), S2–S15.

*Zarchi, A., et al. (2011). Selective COX-2 inhibitors: A review of their structure—activity relationships. *Iranian Journal of Pharmaceutical Research, 10*, 655–683.

8 Principles of Antimicrobial Therapy

Steven P. Gelone ■ Staci Pacetti ■ Judith A. O'Donnell

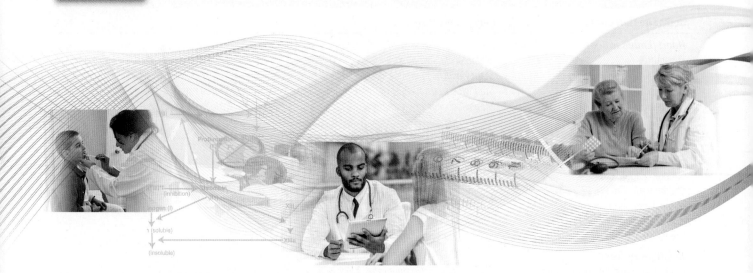

The selection of an appropriate antimicrobial agent to treat an infection is guided by a number of factors. Typically, empiric antimicrobial therapy is based on the epidemiology of the suspected infection, with therapy directed toward the most likely organisms. Laboratory studies, including Gram stain as well as culture and sensitivity testing, help to identify the pathogen and its susceptibility to a variety of antimicrobials. Although there may be several options, efficacy, toxicity, pharmacokinetic profile, and cost ultimately determine the agent of choice. The optimal dose and duration of the antimicrobial therapy are then determined by patient factors such as age, weight, and concurrent disease states as well as the site and severity of infection.

FACTORS IN SELECTING AN ANTIMICROBIAL REGIMEN

Before initiating antibiotic therapy, a systematic approach to identify the source and site of infection must be undertaken. A complete medical history and physical examination should be conducted to identify signs and symptoms consistent with the presence of infection. Identifying underlying medical or social conditions such as diabetes, immunosuppression (cancer, human immunodeficiency virus [HIV] infection), past medications, or intravenous (IV) drug use may help in identifying a predisposition toward infection or the most likely pathogen causing disease. In addition, determining where the infection was acquired (in the community vs. a nursing home or hospital setting) may also help limit the list of most likely pathogens. Health care–acquired pathogens may necessitate broad-spectrum empiric therapy to cover multidrug-resistant (MDR) pathogens.

Identifying the causative pathogen is the ultimate goal because it allows for optimal antibiotic selection and patient outcome. Specimens from the most likely body sites should be properly collected and sent to the microbiology laboratory. Depending on the body site involved, specimens will be stained (e.g., Gram stain) to determine morphology and cell wall structure (gram positive vs. gram negative and cocci vs. bacilli) and analyzed to detect white blood cells (which indicate inflammation and infection). The gold standard of diagnosis in infectious diseases is to be able to grow the causative organism in culture and perform antibiotic susceptibility testing to determine which agents are most likely to be effective in eradicating the pathogen. Susceptibility results often take 48 to 72 hours after cultures are obtained. Newer methods of testing can help identify specific pathogens (such as methicillin-resistant *Staphylococcus aureus* [MRSA] and *Candida*) more quickly.

Often, antibiotic therapy is initiated before culture and sensitivity testing is complete. Empiric antibiotic therapy is based on the premise of providing coverage for the most likely pathogens (**Table 8.1**). In general, the most likely organism is based on the suspected site of the infection. **Table 8.2** outlines key pathogens and spectra of activity for the most commonly prescribed antibiotics.

In most patients treated initially with a parenteral antibiotic who are clinically improving, therapy should be switched to the oral route. This does not apply to certain infections, such as osteomyelitis and endocarditis, in which parenteral antibiotics are continued to ensure adequate concentrations at the infection site. This oral conversion should be based on the following criteria:

- The patient is responding to therapy, as evidenced by a return to normal or a trend toward normal values in the patient's temperature and white blood cell count.

TABLE 8.1

Infection and Most Likely Infecting Organism

Body Site (Infection)	Most Likely Organism
Heart (Endocarditis)	
Subacute	*Streptococcus viridans*
Acute	*Staphylococcus aureus*
Injection drug user	*Staphylococcus aureus*, gram-negative aerobic bacilli, *Enterococcus* spp.
Prosthetic valve	*Staphylococcus epidermidis*
Intra-abdominal tissues	*Escherichia coli*, *Enterococcus* spp., anaerobes (especially *Bacteroides fragilis*), other gram-negative aerobic bacilli
Brain (Meningitis)	
Children <age 2 mo	*E. coli*, group B streptococci, *Listeria monocytogenes*
Children age 2 mo to 12 y	*Streptococcus pneumoniae*, *Neisseria meningitidis*, *Haemophilus influenzae*
Adults (community acquired)	*S. pneumoniae*, *N. meningitidis*
Adults (hospital acquired)	*S. pneumoniae*, *N. meningitidis*, gram-negative aerobic bacilli
HIV coinfected	*Cryptococcus neoformans*, *S. pneumoniae*
Respiratory Tract	
Upper tract, community acquired	*S. pneumoniae*, *H. influenzae*, *Moraxella catarrhalis*, group A streptococci
Lower tract, community acquired	*S. pneumoniae*, *H. influenzae*, *M. catarrhalis*, *Klebsiella pneumoniae* *Mycoplasma pneumoniae*, *C. pneumoniae*, viruses
Aspiration pneumonia	Mouth flora (anaerobic and aerobic)
Lower tract, hospital acquired	*S. aureus (including MRSA)*, *P. aeruginosa*, other gram-negative aerobic bacilli
HIV coinfected	*Pneumocystis jiroveci*, *S. pneumoniae*
Skin and Soft Tissue	
Diabetic ulcer	*Staphylococcus* spp., *Streptococcus* spp., gram-negative aerobic bacilli, anaerobes
Urinary Tract	
Community acquired	*E. coli*, other gram-negative aerobic bacilli, *Enterococcus* spp., *Staphylococcus saprophyticus*
Hospital acquired	*E. coli*, other gram-negative aerobic bacilli, *Enterococcus* spp.

- The patient can take oral medications and absorb them adequately.
- An oral equivalent to the parenteral regimen exists. Not all parenteral agents are available orally. In choosing the oral equivalent, the goal is to select an agent (or agents) that provides a similar spectrum of antimicrobial activity and possesses good oral bioavailability. This may necessitate the use of oral agents that are from a different class from the parenteral agent.

The patient's response to therapy should be monitored regularly. This includes monitoring both efficacy and toxicity. If the patient responds to the prescribed antibiotic regimen, the presenting signs and symptoms of the infection should resolve. Parameters to be considered for response regardless of the site of infection include vital signs, white blood cell count, and, if the culture proved positive for bacteria, subsequent negative cultures. Other signs and symptoms are specific to the body site involved. Monitoring for adverse events is specific to the agents prescribed. (Review the drug overview sections for common adverse events.) All patients should be taught how to recognize the most common adverse events, and they should be advised to notify their health care provider if an adverse reaction occurs. The following sections highlight antimicrobials

used in practice and include pharmacokinetics, pharmacodynamics, mechanism of action, spectrum of activity, common clinical uses, adverse events, drug interactions, and antimicrobial resistance.

PENICILLINS

First isolated in 1928, the penicillins were used successfully to treat streptococcal and staphylococcal infections. Since then, many synthetic penicillins have been developed to address the emerging problem of resistance. Despite resistance, the penicillins remain an important class of antimicrobials. They are classified based on their spectra of activity.

Pharmacokinetics and Pharmacodynamics

Most of the penicillins are unstable in the acid environment of the stomach and must be administered parenterally. Those that are acid stable are given orally. They are widely distributed in the body and penetrate the cerebrospinal fluid (CSF) in the presence of inflammation. Most penicillins are excreted by the kidneys, and renal impairment necessitates dosage adjustment. The half-life of the penicillins in adults with normal renal

TABLE 8.2

Sensitivity of Organisms to Specific Agents

Agent	Staphylococci and Streptococci	Enterococcus	Methicillin-Sensitive S. aureus	Methicillin-Resistant S. aureus (MRSA)	Gram-Negative Aerobes	Pseudomonas	Gram-Negative Anaerobes (Bacteroides fragilis)	Chlamydia pneumoniae, Legionella pneumophila
Penicillins								
amoxicillin	+++	++	+	−	+/++	−	−	−
ampicillin	+++	++	+	−	+/++	−	−	−
dicloxacillin	+++	−	++	−	−	−	−	−
nafcillin	+++	−	++	−	−	−	−	−
penicillin G	+++	++	+	−	+	−	−	−
penicillin V	+++	++	+	−	+	−	−	−
piperacillin	+++	++	++	−	++	++	++	−
ticarcillin	+++	+	++	−	++	++	−	−
Beta-Lactam/Beta-Lactamase Inhibitors								
amoxicillin–clavulanic acid	+++	++	++	−	++	−	++	−
ampicillin–sulbactam	+++	++	++	−	++	−	++	−
ceftazidime–avibactam	+++	++	++	−	+++	+++	++	−
ceftolozane–tazobactam	+++	++	++	−	+++	+++	++	−
piperacillin–tazobactam	+++	++	++	−	+++	+++	+++	−
ticarcillin–clavulanic acid	+++	+	++	−	+++	+++	+++	−
First-Generation Cephalosporins								
cefadroxil	+++	−	++	−	++	−	−	−
cefazolin	+++	−	+	−	++	−	−	−
cephalexin	+++	−	++	−	++	−	−	−
Second-Generation Cephalosporins								
cefotetan	++	−	++	−	++/+++	−	++	−
cefoxitin	++	−	++	−	++	−	++/+++	−
cefuroxime	+++	−	++	−	++	−	−	−
Third-Generation Cephalosporins								
cefotaxime	+++	−	++	−	+++	+	+/++	−
ceftazidime	++	−	+	−	+++	++	−	−
ceftriaxone	+++	−	++	−	+++	+	+	−
Fourth-Generation Cephalosporins								
cefepime	+++	−	++	−	+++	++/+++	−	−
ceftaroline	+++	−	++	−	+++	−	−	−

(Continued)

TABLE 8.2
Sensitivity of Organisms to Specific Agents (Continued)

Agent	Staphylococci and Streptococci	Enterococcus	Methicillin-Sensitive S. aureus	Methicillin-Resistant S. aureus (MRSA)	Gram-Negative Aerobes	Pseudomonas	Gram-Negative Anaerobes (Bacteroides fragilis)	Chlamydia pneumoniae, Legionella pneumophila
Monobactams								
aztreonam	-	-	-	-	++/+++	++/+++	-	-
Carbapenems								
doripenem	++	++	++	-	+++	+++	+++	-
ertapenem	++	++	+++	-	+++	-	+++	-
imipenem	+++	++	+++	-	+++	++/+++	+++	-
meropenem	+++	+	+++	-	+++	++/+++	+++	-
Fluoroquinolones								
ciprofloxacin	+/++	+	++	-	+++	+++	-	+++
gemifloxacin	++/+++	++	++	+/++	+++	+	+	+++
levofloxacin	++/+++	+	++	-	++/+++	++	+/++	+++
moxifloxacin	++/+++	++	++	+/++	+++	+	+	+++
norfloxacin†	++	+	++	-	+++	++	-	-
Macrolides								
azithromycin	++/+++	-	++	-	++	-	-	+++
clarithromycin	++/+++	-	++	-	++	-	-	+++
erythromycin	++/+++	-	++	-	+/++	-	-	+++
telithromycin	++/+++	-	++	-	+++	-	-	+++
Aminoglycosides								
amikacin*	++	-	++	-	+++	++	-	-
gentamicin*	++	++	+/+++	-	+++	++	-	-
tobramycin*	++	-	++	-	+++	++	-	-
Tetracyclines								
doxycycline	++/+++	+	++	+/++	+/++	-	++	+++
minocycline	+++	++	+/+++	+++/+++	++/++	-	++/++	+++
tetracycline	++/+++	+	++	+/++	+	-	+	+++
Glycylcyclines								
tigecycline	+++	++	+++	+++	+	-	++	+
Sulfonamides								
trimethoprim–sulfamethoxazole	+	-	+	++	+/+++	-	-	-

Drug								
Glycopeptides								
dalbavancin	+++	+++	+++	+++	–	–	–	–
oritavancin	+++	+++	+++	+++	–	–	–	–
telavancin	+++	+++	+++	+++	–	–	–	–
vancomycin	+++	+++	++	+++	–	–	–	–
Oxazolidinones								
linezolid	+++	+++	+++	+++	–	–	–	+
tedizolid	+++	+++	+++	+++	–	–	–	–
Lipopeptides								
daptomycin	+++	+++	+++	+++	–	–	–	–
Streptogramins								
quinupristin–dalfopristin	++	++	+++	+++	+	–	–	+
Antianaerobic Agents								
clindamycin	+/++	–	+++	+/++	–	–	+++	–
metronidazole	–	–	–	–	–	–	+++	–
Miscellaneous Agents								
chloramphenicol	+/++	++	–	–	++	–	+++	+
nitrofurantoin†	+++	+++	++	–	+++	–	–	–
rifampin	++/+++	–	+++	++	–	+	–	++

*Provides synergistic activity against gram-positive organisms when combined with a cell wall–active agent.

†Applicable only to organisms isolated in urine.

– = No activity or no information available.

+ = Poor to moderate activity; use only when known to be susceptible.

++ = Good activity; resistance in some strains and geographical location may limit use.

+++ = Excellent activity; generally reliable coverage for empiric therapy.

The PAE is defined as "persistent suppression of bacterial growth after a brief exposure (1 or 2 hours) of bacteria to an antibiotic even in the absence of host defense mechanisms". This delayed growth of bacteria results in an increased efficacy of the drugs and allows for less frequent dosing of medications, potentially lowering toxicity and improving compliance. The duration of the PAE is affected by the class of antibiotic, the relevant exposure time, and the specific bacterial species. Bacteriostatic agents, such as macrolides, clindamycin, streptogramins, tetracyclines, and linezolid, have long PAEs, whereas drugs with relatively slow bactericidal action (e.g., penicillins) have little to no PAE.

function is 30 to 90 minutes. The penicillins are removed by hemodialysis, with the exception of nafcillin and oxacillin. The penicillins exhibit time-dependent bactericidal activity and a postantibiotic effect (PAE) against most gram-positive organisms. See **Box 8.1** for information on PAE. Also, see **Table 8.3** for dosing information.

Mechanism of Action and Spectrum of Activity

The mechanism of action of the penicillins is the inhibition of bacterial cell growth by interference with cell wall synthesis. Penicillins bind to and inactivate the penicillin-binding proteins (PBPs).

Clinical Uses

Although the use of penicillin itself is limited due to widespread resistance, the penicillin class is effective in many infections, including those of the upper and lower respiratory tract, urinary tract, and central nervous system (CNS) as well as sexually transmitted diseases. They are the agents of choice for treating gram-positive infections such as endocarditis caused by susceptible organisms. Both the carboxypenicillins and ureidopenicillins are useful in treating infections caused by *Pseudomonas aeruginosa*.

Adverse Events

There is a low incidence of adverse reactions with penicillin administration. Hypersensitivity reactions characterized by maculopapular rash and urticaria are most common. Gastrointestinal (GI) side effects are most common with oral administration. In the presence of severe renal dysfunction, high-dose penicillins have been associated with seizures and encephalopathy. Thrombophlebitis has occurred with IV administration. The Jarisch-Herxheimer reaction,

TABLE 8.3
Penicillin Dosages

Drug	Adult Dosages	Pediatric Dosages
Natural		
penicillin G	2–4 million units IV q4–6h	100,000–400,000 units/kg/d IV divided q4–6h
penicillin G benzathine	1.2–2.4 million units IM at specified intervals	300,000–2.4 million units IM at specified intervals
penicillin G procaine	0.6–4.8 million units IM in divided doses q12–24h at specified intervals	25,000–50,000 units/kg/d IM divided 1–2 times/d
penicillin VK	250–500 mg PO q6h	25–50 mg/kg/d PO divided q6–8h
Aminopenicillins		
ampicillin	1–2 g IV q4–6h	100–400 mg/kg/d IV divided 4–6h
amoxicillin–ampicillin	250–500 mg PO q8h	400–100 mg/kg/d PO divided q6–12h
	875–1,000 mg PO q12h	
Carboxypenicillins		
ticarcillin sodium	3 g IV q4–6h	200–300 mg/kg/d IV divided q4–6h
Penicillinase Resistant		
cloxacillin	250–500 mg PO q6h	50–100 mg/kg/d PO divided q6h
dicloxacillin	250–500 mg PO q6h	12.5–100 mg/kg/d PO divided q6h
nafcillin	500 mg–1 g IV q4–6h	50–200 mg/kg/d IV divided q4–6h
oxacillin	500–2 g IV q4–6h	100–200 mg/kg/d IV divided q4–6h
Ureidopenicillins		
piperacillin	3–4 g IV q4–6h	200–300 mg/kg/d IV divided q4–6h

Note: Dosage adjustment of all above drugs required in patients with impaired renal function, with the exception of penicillinase-resistant penicillins.

characterized by fever, chills, sweating, and flushing, may occur when penicillin is used in treating spirochetes, in particular syphilis. Release of toxic particles from the organism precipitates the reaction. In rare cases, leukopenia, thrombocytopenia, and hemolytic anemia can occur with penicillins.

Drug Interactions

Drug interactions involving penicillins are rare. Probenecid has been shown to increase the half-life of the penicillins by inhibiting renal tubular secretion. Both the carboxypenicillins and ureidopenicillins have been shown to inactivate the aminoglycosides, and these agents should not be mixed in the same IV solution. Also, the parenteral carboxypenicillins have a high sodium content. Caution should be used in patients with fluid or sodium restrictions.

BETA-LACTAM/BETA-LACTAMASE INHIBITOR COMBINATIONS

Resistance to penicillin develops when the drug is inactivated by the enzymes known as penicillinases or beta-lactamases produced by bacteria. After several attempts over the years to prevent penicillin degradation by this enzyme, clavulanic acid became the first beta-lactamase inhibitor introduced and combined with a beta-lactam. Other beta-lactamase inhibitors, avibactam, sulbactam, and tazobactam, are also available in combination with ampicillin, ceftazidime, ceftolozane, and piperacillin. The role of the beta-lactamase inhibitor is to prevent the breakdown of the beta-lactam by organisms that produce the enzyme, thereby enhancing antibacterial activity. These combinations are suitable alternatives for infections caused by beta-lactamase–producing organisms such as *S. aureus*, *Haemophilus influenzae*, and *Bacteroides fragilis*.

Pharmacokinetics and Pharmacodynamics

The beta-lactam/beta-lactamase inhibitors diffuse into most body tissues, with the exception of the brain and CSF. The half-life of both components in each combination is approximately 1 hour. Because these drugs are eliminated by glomerular filtration, renal dysfunction necessitates dosage changes (**Table 8.4**). The compounds are removed by hemodialysis and peritoneal dialysis.

Mechanism of Action and Spectrum of Activity

The beta-lactam components of the combinations are cell wall–active agents. They interfere with bacterial cell wall synthesis by binding to and inactivating PBPs. The beta-lactamase inhibitors irreversibly bind to most beta-lactamase enzymes, protecting the beta-lactam from degradation and improving their antibacterial activity. The beta-lactamase inhibitors alone lack significant antibacterial activity. The spectrum of activity is similar to the penicillin derivative, with broader coverage against beta-lactamase–producing organisms.

Clinical Uses

Based on their broad spectrum of activity, the beta-lactam/beta-lactamase inhibitors are frequently used in treating polymicrobial infections. They are used extensively to treat intra-abdominal and gynecologic infections, and skin and soft tissue infections, including human and animal bites, as well as foot infections in diabetic patients. Respiratory tract infections, including aspiration pneumonia, sinusitis, and lung abscesses, have been successfully treated with these combinations.

Adverse Events

The addition of the beta-lactamase inhibitor to the penicillins has not resulted in any new or major adverse events. The major effects associated with the beta-lactam/beta-lactamase inhibitor combinations are hypersensitivity reactions and GI side effects

TABLE 8.4

Beta-Lactam/Beta-Lactamase Inhibitor Dosages

Drug	Adult Dosages	Pediatric Dosages
amoxicillin–clavulanic acid	250–500 mg PO q8h 500–875 mg PO q12h 2 g PO q12h*	20–40 mg/kg/d PO divided q8–12h 80–90 mg/kg/d PO divided q12h†
ampicillin–sulbactam	1.5–3 g IV q6h	100–400 mg/kg/d IV divided q6h
piperacillin–tazobactam	4.5 g IV q6–8h or 3.375 g IV q6h	240–300 mg/kg/d IV divided q8h
ticarcillin–clavulanic acid	3.1 g IV q4–6h	200–300 mg/kg/d IV divided q4–6h
ceftazidime–avibactam	2.5 g IV q8h	—
ceftolozane–tazobactam	750 mg IV q8h	—

Note: Dosage adjustment required for all above drugs administered to patients with renal impairment.
* amoxicillin–clavulanic acid (Augmentin XR) extended-release formulation.
† amoxicillin/clavulanic acid (Augmentin ES-600) formulation.

such as nausea and diarrhea associated with oral administration. Elevated aminotransferase levels have been documented for all agents.

Drug Interactions

The combinations are physically incompatible with parenteral aminoglycosides. Each of the penicillins in the combinations has been associated with the inactivation of aminoglycosides in vitro. The clinical significance of this interaction is unknown.

CEPHALOSPORINS

The cephalosporins, a beta-lactam group, are structurally similar to the penicillins. Substitutions on the parent compound, 7-aminocephalosporanic acid, produce compounds with different pharmacokinetic properties and spectra of activity. The cephalosporins are divided into "generations" based on their antimicrobial spectrum of activity. The progression from first to fourth generation in general reflects an increase in gram-negative coverage and a loss of gram-positive activity.

Pharmacokinetics and Pharmacodynamics

The cephalosporins are well absorbed from the GI tract. In some cases, food enhances absorption. They penetrate well into tissues and body fluids and achieve high concentrations in the urinary tract. Noncephamycin second-generation agents and all third- and fourth-generation agents penetrate the CSF and play a role in treating bacterial meningitis. Most of the oral and parenteral cephalosporins are excreted by the kidney, with the exception of ceftriaxone (Rocephin) and cefoperazone (not available in the United States), which are eliminated by the liver. The cephalosporins exhibit a time-dependent bactericidal effect and a prolonged PAE against staphylococci. **Table 8.5** provides dosing information.

Mechanism of Action and Spectrum of Activity

Like other beta-lactams, the cephalosporins interfere with bacterial cell wall synthesis by binding to and inactivating the PBPs.

Clinical Uses

The cephalosporins are used in treating many infections. In general, the first-generation cephalosporins are used in treating gram-positive skin infections, pneumococcal respiratory

TABLE 8.5
Cephalosporin Dosages

Drug	Adult Dosages	Pediatric Dosages
First Generation		
cefazolin	500 mg–1 g IV q8h	50–100 mg/kg/d IV divided q8h
cephalexin	250–1,000 mg PO q6h	25–100 mg/kg/d PO divided q6h
cefadroxil	500 mg–1 g PO q12h	30 mg/kg/d PO divided q12h
Second Generation		
cefotetan	1–2 g IV q12h	40–80 mg/kg/d IV divided q12h
cefoxitin	1–2 g IV q6–8h	80–160 mg/kg/d IV divided q4–8h
cefuroxime	750–1.5 g IV q8h	75–150 mg/kg/d IV divided q8h
cefuroxime axetil	250–500 mg PO q12h	20–30 mg/kg/d PO divided q12h
loracarbef	200–400 mg PO q12–24h	15–30 mg/kg/d PO divided q12h
cefaclor	250–500 mg PO q8h	20–40 mg/kg/d PO divided q8–12h
Third Generation		
cefotaxime	1–2 g IV q8h	100–300 mg/kg/d IV divided q6–8h
ceftazidime	1–2 g IV q8h	90–150 mg/kg/d IV divided q8h
ceftizoxime	1–2 g IV q8h	150–200 mg/kg/d IV divided q6–8h
ceftriaxone*	1–2 g IV q12–24h	50–100 mg/kg/d IV divided q12–24h
ceftibuten	400 mg PO q24h	9 mg/kg/d PO divided q24h
cefpodoxime proxetil	100–400 mg PO q12h	10 mg/kg/d PO divided q12h
cefprozil	250–500 mg PO q12h	15–30 mg/kg/d PO divided q12h
cefdinir	300 mg PO q12h OR 600 mg PO q24h	7–14 mg/kg/d PO divided q12–24h
Fourth Generation		
Cefepime	1–2 g IV q8–12h	50 mg/kg/d IV divided q8h
Ceftaroline	600 mg IV q8h	—

Note: Dosage adjustment necessary for all agents in patients with renal impairment except ceftriaxone.
*Dosage adjustment necessary in patients with liver dysfunction.

infections, urinary tract infections, and for surgical prophylaxis. The second-generation cephalosporins are used in treating community-acquired pneumonia, other respiratory tract infections, and skin infections. Mixed aerobic and anaerobic infections may be treated with the second-generation cephamycins (cefotetan and cefoxitin). In addition, treating community-acquired bacterial meningitis typically includes a third-generation cephalosporin such as ceftriaxone or cefotaxime (Claforan). Nosocomial infections are commonly treated with ceftazidime (Fortaz) or cefepime (Maxipime), whose broad spectrum of activity includes gram-negative organisms, especially *P. aeruginosa*. Ceftaroline fosamil (Teflaro), a new IV cephalosporin, has activity similar to ceftriaxone but is the only cephalosporin that covers MRSA.

Adverse Events

The cephalosporins are a safe class of antimicrobials with a favorable toxicity profile. With a few exceptions, the adverse events are similar across the generations. Hypersensitivity reactions, not unlike those with the penicillins, are characterized by maculopapular rash and urticaria. The cross-reactivity between penicillins and cephalosporins is 3% to 10%. Patients who experience allergic reactions to penicillins (other than a type 1 allergy) can often tolerate a cephalosporin. The most common side effects with oral administration are nausea, vomiting, and diarrhea. GI effects are usually transient. Less common reactions include a positive Coombs test and rarely hemolytic reactions.

Drug Interactions

Drug interactions involving cephalosporins are rare. Probenecid has been shown to increase the half-life of some cephalosporins by inhibiting the renal tubular secretion.

MONOBACTAMS

The monobactams are a unique class of beta-lactams with a four-membered ring but lacking a fifth or sixth member, like other beta-lactams. Because aztreonam (Azactam) is the only agent of its class commercially available, most of the information relates specifically to that agent. With primary activity against gram-negative organisms, including *Pseudomonas*, aztreonam is considered a safer alternative to the aminoglycosides, with a similar spectrum of activity.

Pharmacokinetics and Pharmacodynamics

Aztreonam distributes well into most tissues, with a volume of distribution of 0.16 L/kg. Penetration into the CSF is increased in the presence of inflamed meninges. Aztreonam is not extensively bound to proteins. The approximate half-life is 2 hours, and dosages are typically calculated according to the severity of disease (**Table 8.6**). Aztreonam is excreted primarily unchanged by glomerular filtration, so dosage adjustments are necessary in patients with renal insufficiency. Aztreonam is cleared by hemodialysis and peritoneal dialysis.

TABLE 8.6		
Aztreonam Dosages		
Severity of Infection	**Adult Dosages**	**Pediatric Dosages**
Mild	500 mg IV q8–12h	90–120 mg/kg/d IV divided q6–8h
Moderate	1–2 g IV q8–12h	
Severe	2 g IV q6–8h	

Note: Dosage adjustment required in patients with impaired renal function.

Mechanism of Action and Spectrum of Activity

Aztreonam, like other beta-lactams, interferes with bacterial cell wall synthesis by binding to and inactivating PBPs. The principal activity of aztreonam is against most aerobic gram-negative organisms, including *P. aeruginosa*, *Serratia marcescens*, and *Citrobacter* species. It has virtually no activity against gram-positive organisms. Its gram-negative coverage is similar to that of the aminoglycosides and the third-generation cephalosporin ceftazidime. Aztreonam is not active against anaerobic organisms.

Clinical Uses

Aztreonam is commonly used in treating complicated and uncomplicated urinary tract and respiratory tract infections such as pneumonia and bronchitis when aerobic gram-negative coverage is necessary. To broaden coverage, it is usually used in combination with an agent exhibiting gram-positive activity. It is a reasonable substitute for the aminoglycosides in treating gram-negative infections in patients at high risk for toxicity.

Adverse Events

Aztreonam has a relatively safe toxicity profile. Most of the adverse events associated with aztreonam are local reactions and GI symptoms. Elevated aminotransferase levels have also been documented. Despite its beta-lactam structure, patients allergic to penicillins and cephalosporins usually do not manifest an allergic reaction to aztreonam. A cross-allergy specifically with ceftazidime has been reported and linked to an identical side chain on both compounds.

Drug Interactions

No clinically significant drug interactions have been documented with aztreonam.

CARBAPENEMS

The carbapenems, ertapenem (Invanz), doripenem (Doribax), imipenem (Primaxin), and meropenem (Merrem), are bicyclical beta-lactams with a common carbapenem nucleus (**Table 8.7**). Imipenem is extensively metabolized by renal dehydropeptidases, yielding only limited activity in the urine. Cilastatin,

TABLE 8.7

Carbapenem Dosages

Drug	Adult Dosages	Pediatric Dosages
ertapenem	1 g IV/IM daily	30 mg/kg/d IV divided q12h
doripenem	500 mg IV q8h	Not recommended
imipenem	250–1,000 mg IV q6h	25–100 mg/kg/d IV divided q6h
meropenem	500 mg–1,000 mg IV q8h	30–120 mg/kg/d IV divided q8h

Note: Dosage adjustment required for all above drugs administered to patients with renal impairment.

a competitive inhibitor of the dehydropeptidases, was introduced to overcome imipenem degradation and is commercially available in combination with imipenem in a one-to-one ratio. Subsequently, ertapenem, meropenem, and doripenem were developed; they maintain stability against dehydropeptidase metabolism without the addition of a cilastatin-like agent. The carbapenems are the most broad-spectrum agents commercially available.

Pharmacokinetics and Pharmacodynamics

Carbapenems are not absorbed after oral administration. They exhibit linear pharmacokinetics; thus, peak serum levels increase proportionately as the dose is increased. They are widely distributed into most tissues, with an approximate volume of distribution of 0.25 L/kg. With the exception of ertapenem, they are minimally bound to plasma proteins. Penetration into the CSF varies and depends on the degree of meningeal inflammation. The half-life of the carbapenems is approximately 1 hour. They are primarily eliminated by urinary excretion of unchanged drug. Imipenem, meropenem, and doripenem are removed by hemodialysis and hemofiltration.

The carbapenems, like other beta-lactams, exhibit time-dependent bactericidal effects. Unlike other beta-lactams, they exhibit a PAE against gram-negative aerobes lasting at least 1 to 2 hours.

Mechanism of Action and Spectrum of Activity

Similar to the penicillins and cephalosporins, the carbapenems bind to the PBPs on the cell wall and interfere with bacterial cell wall synthesis. They frequently have stability against beta-lactamases and bind to several PBPs.

Imipenem, meropenem, and doripenem possess the broadest spectrum of activity of any of the beta-lactam compounds. They have excellent activity against aerobic gram-positive organisms, including staphylococci and streptococci and gram-negative organisms such as Enterobacteriaceae, *P. aeruginosa*, and *Acinetobacter* species. They are also active against most gram-negative anaerobic organisms, including *B. fragilis*. Ertapenem has a similar spectrum of activity as the

other carbapenems, with the noted exceptions of *P. aeruginosa* and *Acinetobacter* species, for which ertapenem has no clinically significant activity.

Clinical Uses

Their broad spectrum of activity and stability to many beta-lactamases make the carbapenems useful as single agents in treating polymicrobial infections. They have been used extensively in treating skin and soft tissue, bone and joint, intra-abdominal, and lower respiratory tract infections. In addition, meropenem is used in treating CNS infections because it has a lower risk than imipenem of causing seizures.

Adverse Events

Neurotoxicity, a well-known effect of the carbapenems, is characterized by seizure activity. Imipenem has been reported to lower the seizure threshold more frequently than meropenem and doripenem. Risk factors for seizures include impaired renal function, improper dosing, age, previous CNS disorder, and concomitant agents that lower the seizure threshold. Meropenem and more recently doripenem are the carbapenems of choice in patients with a seizure disorder or underlying risk factors. Such GI side effects as nausea, vomiting, and diarrhea have also been reported. Decreasing the infusion rate may lessen their severity.

Drug Interactions

Concomitant administration of probenecid and meropenem or doripenem results in decreased clearance of these agents and a substantial increase in half-life; therefore, the concurrent administration of meropenem or doripenem with probenecid is not recommended. A similar interaction with imipenem occurs, but to a lesser degree.

FLUOROQUINOLONES

Since 1990, the fluoroquinolones (FQs) have become a dominant class of antimicrobial agents. No other class of antimicrobial agents has grown so rapidly or been developed with such interest by pharmaceutical research companies. Although multiple medications in this class have been approved by the U.S. Food and Drug Administration (FDA), several FQs have been removed from the U.S. market due to the identification of postmarketing adverse events. This emphasizes the importance of postmarketing research and adverse event reporting. **Table 8.8** lists the available FQs. Ciprofloxacin, levofloxacin, and moxifloxacin are most commonly prescribed.

Pharmacokinetics and Pharmacodynamics

The FQs are bactericidal antibiotics. They display a concentration-dependent killing effect. All FQs have excellent bioavailability, making it easy to transition from an IV to an oral formulation. They have a volume of distribution ranging from 1.5 to 6.1 L/kg

TABLE 8.8

Fluoroquinolone Dosages

Drug	Adult Dosage
ciprofloxacin	250–750 mg PO q12h; 200–400 mg IV q12h; 400 mg IV q8h (severe infections)
gemifloxacin	320 mg PO daily
levofloxacin	250–750 mg PO/IV daily
moxifloxacin	400 mg PO/IV daily
norfloxacin	400 mg PO q12h
ofloxacin	200–400 mg PO q12h

Note: With the exception of ciprofloxacin for the treatment of urinary tract infections and anthrax, these drugs are not recommended for use in children younger than age 18. Dosage adjustment required for all above drugs (except moxifloxacin) administered to patients with renal impairment.

and distribute well into most tissues and fluids except the CNS. The half-life for the FQs ranges from 4 to 12 hours, with levofloxacin, gemifloxacin, and moxifloxacin having the longest half-lives. These three agents are dosed once daily. All FQs undergo renal elimination with the exception of moxifloxacin. The FQs are removed by hemodialysis and peritoneal dialysis, with percentages varying between products. All FQs also exhibit a PAE, which also appears to be a concentration-dependent parameter. The newer compounds have been reported to have PAEs of 1 to 6 hours, depending on the pathogen and drug.

Mechanism of Action and Spectrum of Activity

The quinolone antibiotics are strong inhibitors of deoxyribonucleic acid (DNA) gyrase and topoisomerase IV. These enzymes are critical to the process of supercoiling DNA. Without such enzymatic activity, bacterial DNA cannot replicate.

All FQs possess activity against aerobic gram-negative organisms. Ciprofloxacin and levofloxacin have activity against *P. aeruginosa*, representing the only oral antibiotics available to treat this pathogen. However, widespread use of the FQs since the late 1990s have led to increased resistance against gram-negative pathogens and limited use in some parts of the United States. Newer FQs, such as levofloxacin, moxifloxacin, and gemifloxacin, have activity against gram-positive organisms including *Streptococcus* species. These agents are sometimes referred to as the "antipneumococcal" or "respiratory" FQs given their activity against *S. pneumoniae* and usefulness in treating community-acquired pneumonia. Moxifloxacin has some activity against anaerobic bacteria.

Clinical Uses

The FQs have been shown to be effective in treating many infections, including urinary tract infections (for which they are one of the agents of choice), pneumonia, sexually transmitted diseases, skin and soft tissue infections, GI infections (in combination with an agent for anaerobic coverage), traveler's diarrhea, and osteomyelitis. For hospital-acquired infections such as nosocomial pneumonia, ciprofloxacin (Cipro) or levofloxacin (Levaquin) are the preferred agents, as part of a drug combination, because they have the best activity against *P. aeruginosa*. Ciprofloxacin is also recommended for meningococcal prophylaxis as a single 500-mg oral dose.

Adverse Events

The FQs have a relatively safe side effect profile. The most common side effects include nausea, diarrhea, dizziness, and confusion. Rare but serious side effects include QTc prolongation, tendon rupture, tendonitis, and peripheral neuropathy.

Drug Interactions

The FQs have several significant drug–drug interactions. Ciprofloxacin is a potent inhibitor of the cytochrome P-450 (CYP) 1A2 isoenzyme and may increase the effect of other medications, including theophylline, warfarin (Coumadin), tizanidine, propranolol, and others. Antacids, sucralfate, and magnesium, calcium, or iron salts will decrease the absorption of the FQs if given concomitantly. These agents should be separated when administered orally. Due to the risk of QTc prolongation and torsades de pointes, medications that prolong the QTc interval should be used cautiously with the FQs. Prolonged administration of FQs in combination with corticosteroids increases the risk of tendonitis and tendon rupture. Hyperglycemic and hypoglycemic events have been reported with FQs when administered with insulin or other antidiabetic agents.

MACROLIDES AND KETOLIDES

Erythromycin (E-Mycin), the prototypical macrolide, has been used in treating many infections over the years. However, its use has been diminished by its GI side effects. This toxicity has even been used as a means of treating patients with diabetic gastroparesis. Newer agents (clarithromycin and azithromycin) have been developed with improved GI tolerance and longer half-lives. Telithromycin (Ketek) is the only agent in the class known as ketolides. Although separate from macrolides, telithromycin has a similar mechanism of action and antibacterial coverage.

Pharmacokinetics and Pharmacodynamics

The macrolides are usually administered orally and are absorbed from the GI tract if not inactivated by gastric acid. They have good tissue penetration, achieve high intracellular concentrations, and exhibit minimal protein binding. The macrolides are metabolized via the liver and excreted in the urine. Half-lives vary throughout the class, from 2 hours for erythromycin, 4 to 5 hours for clarithromycin (Biaxin), and 50 to 60 hours for azithromycin (Zithromax). The long half-life and high intracellular concentrations of azithromycin permit once-daily dosing and short courses. Dosage adjustment in patients with renal failure is necessary with clarithromycin (Biaxin) and erythromycin (**Table 8.9**).

TABLE 8.9

Macrolide/Ketolide Antibiotic Dosages

Drug	Adult Dosage	Pediatric Dosages
azithromycin	250–500 mg IV/PO daily	5–12 mg/kg IV/PO daily
	2,000 mg (ER) PO single dose	30 mg/kg PO single dose
clarithromycin*	250–500 mg PO q12h or 1,000 mg (ER) PO daily	15 mg/kg/d PO divided q12h
erythromycin base*	250 mg–1 g PO q6h	30–50 mg/kg/d PO divided q6–8h
ethyl succinate	400–800 mg PO q6–12h	30–50 mg/kg/d PO divided q6–8h
estolate, stearate		30–50 mg/kg/d PO divided q6–12h
injection	500–1,000 mg IV q6–8h	15–50 mg/kg/d IV divided q6h
telithromycin*	800 mg PO daily	Not recommended

*Dosage adjustment necessary in patients with renal impairment.
ER, extended-release product.

Telithromycin is well absorbed following oral administration and is moderately protein bound. The half-life of telithromycin is approximately 10 hours. Telithromycin is metabolized in the liver and eliminated in the urine and feces. A dosage adjustment is recommended for patients with renal failure. The macrolides and ketolides are minimally cleared via hemodialysis and peritoneal dialysis.

Mechanism of Action and Spectrum of Activity

The mechanism of action of the macrolides is inhibition of bacterial protein synthesis by binding to the 50S ribosomal subunit. The spectrum of activity of the macrolides includes gram-positive and gram-negative aerobes and atypical organisms, including chlamydia, mycoplasma, legionella, rickettsia, mycobacteria, and spirochetes. Telithromycin is classified as a ketolide and also works by binding to the 50S ribosomal subunit; however, it has a higher binding affinity compared to the macrolides. The spectrum of activity is similar to the macrolides, with coverage against most organisms isolated in respiratory tract infections, including some strains of erythromycin-resistant *S. pneumoniae*.

Clinical Uses

The macrolides are used in several settings. Their broad spectrum of activity makes them useful in treating respiratory tract, skin, and soft tissue infections, sexually transmitted diseases, HIV-related *Mycobacterium avium–Mycobacterium intracellulare* complex infection, and other infections caused by atypical organisms such as chlamydia, rickettsiae, and legionella. Telithromycin is approved for the treatment of community-acquired pneumonia; however, its use is limited due to the risk of hepatotoxicity.

Adverse Events

The macrolides are in general considered safe agents. Particularly with erythromycin, GI effects such as abdominal pain, nausea, and vomiting are most common. The newer macrolides cause fewer GI effects. Hepatotoxicity related to the macrolides is rare but serious; it also is less frequent with the newer agents. Extremely high doses of IV erythromycin and oral clarithromycin have been associated with ototoxicity. Phlebitis may occur with IV erythromycin administration. Telithromycin has been linked to cases of acute hepatic failure and severe liver injury. Common adverse effects of telithromycin include nausea, vomiting, diarrhea, dizziness, and blurred vision.

Drug Interactions

Among the macrolides, erythromycin and clarithromycin are potent inhibitors of the CYP3A4 isoenzyme. When administered concomitantly, they have been shown to prolong the half-life of an extensive list of agents, including cyclosporine, tacrolimus, carbamazepine, theophylline, warfarin, and most statins. Azithromycin does not undergo significant cytochrome P-450 metabolism, so the possibility of similar interactions is low. Telithromycin is also a strong inhibitor of CYP3A4 and has similar interactions and precautions to erythromycin and clarithromycin. Macrolides and ketolides have the potential to increase the QTc interval, so caution should be used in patients receiving concomitant medications that can also prolong the QTc interval.

AMINOGLYCOSIDES

Despite the advent of many new antibiotics over the past several decades, the aminoglycosides remain an important therapeutic drug class. Their major drawback has been their potential for drug-related toxicities (nephrotoxicity and ototoxicity). Because of these, their use or the length of therapy has been restricted. The introduction of a modified dosing regimen that uses once-daily (or extended-interval) dosing of these agents for several infections has provided a way of maximizing their therapeutic effects while minimizing the risk of toxicity.

Pharmacokinetics and Pharmacodynamics

The aminoglycosides are poorly absorbed from the GI tract, and parenteral administration is necessary to treat systemic infections. They are weakly bound to serum proteins (10%) and freely distribute into the extracellular fluid. The approximate volume of distribution is 0.25 L/kg, which may be significantly affected in intensive care patients and in disease states such as malnutrition, obesity, and ascites. The aminoglycosides are excreted unchanged via glomerular filtration. The half-life of aminoglycosides in an adult with normal renal function is approximately 1 to 3 hours. Dosage adjustments are necessary in patients with renal impairment because substantial increases in the half-life are seen. Aminoglycosides can be removed by hemodialysis, peritoneal dialysis, and continuous hemofiltration/dialysis.

Because of a narrow range between efficacy and toxicity, renal function and serum levels are used to monitor therapy with aminoglycosides. **Table 8.10** gives dosage guidelines.

Pharmacodynamically, the bactericidal effect of the aminoglycosides depends on drug concentration. The number of organisms decreases more rapidly when a higher peak concentration is achieved. In addition, the aminoglycosides exhibit a PAE for both gram-positive and gram-negative organisms.

Mechanism of Action and Spectrum of Activity

The aminoglycosides are actively taken up by bacteria and subsequently bind to the smaller 30S subunit of the bacterial ribosome, thus inhibiting bacterial protein synthesis.

The principal activity of the aminoglycosides is against aerobic gram-negative bacilli such as *Escherichia coli*, *Klebsiella* species, *Proteus mirabilis*, *Enterobacter* species, *Acinetobacter* species, and *P. aeruginosa*. They are also generally active against gram-positive cocci, particularly *Staphylococcus*, *Enterococcus*, and *Streptococcus* species, but they must be used in combination (for synergy) with a cell wall–active agent such as ampicillin,

nafcillin, or vancomycin. Streptomycin is also active against *Francisella tularensis* and *Mycobacterium tuberculosis*.

Clinical Uses

The aminoglycosides are primarily used in treating gram-negative infections. They have long been used in the empiric treatment of neutropenic fever and nosocomial infections because of their broad coverage of *P. aeruginosa* and Enterobacteriaceae. They are also frequently used with cell wall–active agents such as penicillins, cephalosporins, and vancomycin to achieve synergy in treating gram-positive infections, including staphylococcal and enterococcal infections. They are routinely used in combination with other agents in treating pneumonia, bacteremia, and intra-abdominal and skin and soft tissue infections. Monotherapy usually is not recommended, with the noted exception of patients with urinary tract infections. The aminoglycosides have been used in treating tuberculosis, with streptomycin having the greatest activity against *M. tuberculosis*. Streptomycin is also the treatment of choice for tularemia, a potential agent of bioterrorism.

Adverse Events

In general, the aminoglycosides have been associated with a variety of adverse events (GI and CNS), most of which are mild and transient. They rarely produce hypersensitivity reactions and are well tolerated at the sites of administration. Nephrotoxicity and ototoxicity are also associated with aminoglycoside use.

Nephrotoxicity results from accumulation of the drug in the proximal tubule cells of the kidney, causing nonoliguric renal failure. This renal failure is usually mild and reversible and rarely progresses to the need for dialysis. Factors that increase the risk of toxicity to the kidney include increased age, renal disease, increased trough levels, dehydration, and concomitant administration of nephrotoxic agents such as amphotericin B,

TABLE 8.10		
Aminoglycoside Dosages		
Aminoglycoside	**Adult Dosages**	**Pediatric Dosages**
Multiple Daily Dosing		
gentamicin, tobramycin	1–1.7 mg/kg IV q8h	6–7.5 mg/kg/d IV divided q8h
netilmicin*	1.7–2 mg/kg IV q8h	
amikacin, kanamycin*	5 mg/kg IV q8h or 7.5 mg/kg IV q12h	15–22.5 mg/kg/d IV divided q8h
streptomycin	0.5–2 g IV q24h	20–40 mg/kg/d IV divided q6–12h
Once-Daily Dosing†		
gentamicin, tobramycin	5–7 mg/kg IV q24h	5–7.5 mg/kg IV q24h
netilmicin*	4–6 mg/kg IV q24h	
amikacin	15–20 mg/kg IV q24h	20 mg/kg IV q24h

Note: Dosage adjustment required for all above drugs administered to patients with renal impairment.
*Not routinely available for use in the United States.
†Once-daily dosing of aminoglycosides is not recommended for enterococcal infections, during pregnancy, in instances of gram-positive synergy, or for endocarditis, meningitis, or ascites.

TABLE 8.11

Aminoglycoside Concentration Monitoring

Aminoglycoside	Target Peak	Target Trough
Multiple Daily Dosing*		
gentamicin, tobramycin	4–10 µg/mL	<2 µg/mL
netilmicin	4–10 µg/mL	<2 µg/mL
amikacin, kanamycin	20–30 µg/mL	<8 µg/mL
streptomycin	20–30 µg/mL	<8 µg/mL
Once-Daily Dosing†		
gentamicin, tobramycin	>15 µg/mL	<1 µg/mL
netilmicin	>15 µg/mL	<1 µg/mL
amikacin	>50 µg/mL	<5 µg/mL

*Serum concentrations based upon steady state for multiple daily dosing. Peak concentrations should be obtained 30–60 min after infusion and trough concentrations 30 min before next infusion.
†Random concentrations routinely measured for once-daily dosing in lieu of peak and trough serum concentrations and dosage adjustments based upon dosing nomograms.

cyclosporine, and vancomycin. Blood urea nitrogen and serum creatinine values are monitored in addition to serum levels to ensure safe and effective therapy. **Table 8.11** provides optimal serum concentrations for aminoglycosides.

Two forms of ototoxicity—auditory and vestibular—may occur alone or simultaneously. Auditory toxicity presents as hearing loss and tinnitus; vestibular toxicity is manifested by nausea, vomiting, and vertigo. Ototoxicity may be irreversible and has been associated with high serum trough levels. The risk of ototoxicity increases when the aminoglycosides are administered in combination with high-dose loop diuretics, high-dose macrolide antibiotics, or vancomycin. Long courses of aminoglycosides warrant baseline and periodic auditory monitoring.

Drug Interactions

The aminoglycosides have the potential to cause or prolong neuromuscular blockade, although this is uncommon. It is recommended that parenteral aminoglycosides be administered over a 30-minute interval. The risk of neuromuscular blockade increases in patients receiving concurrent neuromuscular blockers, general anesthetics, or calcium channel blockers and in those with myasthenia gravis. Administration of calcium gluconate usually reverses the neuromuscular blockade.

TETRACYCLINES

The tetracyclines possess activity against gram-positive, gram-negative, and atypical organisms, including rickettsiae, chlamydia, mycobacteria, and spirochetes. They are separated into short-, intermediate-, and long-acting agents. Doxycycline and minocycline are considered long-acting and the most active of the class. The tetracyclines became the first class of antimicrobials to be labeled "broad spectrum," and they remain a frequently used class of antimicrobials.

Pharmacokinetics and Pharmacodynamics

Absorption from the GI tract along with protein binding varies among agents. The long-acting agents have the highest absorption and are bound to protein to the greatest extent. With the exception of the long-acting agents, absorption is improved with administration on an empty stomach. The tetracyclines have excellent tissue distribution. The primary route of elimination is through the kidney by glomerular filtration, with the exception of doxycycline. In general, the short-acting agents have a half-life of 8 hours, and the long-acting agents, 16 to 18 hours. The tetracyclines are removed to a small degree by hemodialysis. **Table 8.12** provides dosing information.

Mechanism of Action and Spectrum of Activity

The tetracyclines inhibit bacterial protein synthesis by binding to the 30S subunit of the ribosome. The tetracyclines are active against gram-positive and gram-negative bacteria and atypical organisms, including spirochetes, rickettsiae, chlamydia, mycoplasma, and legionella. They typically are bacteriostatic agents.

Clinical Uses

Because of their broad spectrum of activity, the tetracyclines are used extensively in many settings. They are typically used as alternatives when beta-lactams are not an option. They are frequently used in treating rickettsial, chlamydial, and gram-negative infections, in addition to acne vulgaris and pelvic inflammatory disease (PID). Doxycycline is the drug of choice for the treatment of early Lyme disease and used in treating community-acquired pneumonia. Doxycycline and minocycline are used as sclerosing agents for pleurodesis. Additionally, minocycline and doxycycline have gained popularity as a treatment for community-acquired MRSA infections. Though a tetracycline, demeclocycline (Declomycin) is primarily used to treat the syndrome of inappropriate antidiuretic hormone and not as an antibiotic.

TABLE 8.12

Tetracycline Dosages*

Drug	Adult Dosages
demeclocycline	150 mg PO q6h
	300 mg PO q12h
doxycycline	100 mg IV/PO q12h
minocycline	100–200 mg PO q12h
tetracycline	250–500 mg PO q6h

Note: Dosage adjustment for all above drugs necessary in patients with renal impairment, with the exception of doxycycline.
*The tetracyclines are not recommended for use in children less than age 8 or during pregnancy and breast-feeding.

Adverse Events

The most frequent side effects associated with the tetracyclines are anorexia, nausea, vomiting, and epigastric distress. These are typically lessened if the agents are administered with food. Thrombophlebitis is associated with IV administration, and it is recommended that doxycycline be administered in a large volume and infused slowly. Hepatotoxicity is a rare but potentially fatal toxicity. The risk of hepatotoxicity increases if the patient is concurrently receiving other hepatotoxic agents. Gray-brown discoloration of the teeth can be a permanent effect of the tetracyclines. It results from stable tetracycline/calcium complexes in bone and teeth and is related to dose and duration of therapy. Therefore, children younger than age 8 should not receive tetracyclines. Patients receiving tetracyclines are more sensitive to the effects of the sun because of accumulation of the drug in the skin. Minocycline has been associated with dose-related vertigo.

Drug Interactions

There are multiple drug interactions involving the tetracyclines. The absorption of the tetracyclines is affected by several agents. Tetracyclines form chelating complexes with divalent and trivalent cations, decreasing tetracycline absorption. It is recommended that the administration of tetracyclines and antacids, iron, cholestyramine, and sucralfate be separated by at least 1 hour. Likewise, food decreases the absorption of most tetracyclines, with the exception of doxycycline. Milk and dairy products also impair their absorption. Phenytoin and carbamazepine, CYP enzyme inducers, decrease the half-life of doxycycline. Concomitant administration of the tetracyclines and oral contraceptives results in decreased levels of the oral contraceptive, so an additional form of contraception is recommended. The tetracyclines also potentiate the effect of warfarin by impairing vitamin K production by intestinal flora.

GLYCYLCYCLINES

Tigecycline (Tygacil) belongs to a new class of agents known as the *glycylcyclines*. It is structurally related to the tetracycline class. Tigecycline is derived from the addition of a glycyl ring to minocycline, which significantly enhances its antimicrobial spectrum.

Pharmacokinetics and Pharmacodynamics

Tigecycline is available only in a parenteral formulation. Following IV administration, tigecycline has a half-life of 27 to 42 hours. It is moderately protein bound with a volume of distribution of 7 to 9 L/kg. Given its large volume of distribution, it does not result in prolonged serum concentrations. The dose in adults is a single 100-mg IV dose followed by 50 mg IV every 12 hours. Tigecycline is not extensively metabolized in the liver and does not require adjustments for renal

insufficiency; however, the dose should be adjusted for patients with severe underlying liver disease. Tigecycline is not removed by hemodialysis.

Similar to the tetracyclines, tigecycline is bacteriostatic and has a PAE lasting 2 to 4 hours.

Mechanism of Action and Spectrum of Activity

Tigecycline inhibits bacterial protein synthesis by binding to the 30S subunit of the ribosome. It has a fivefold higher binding affinity to these ribosomes compared to the tetracyclines. Tigecycline is active against many gram-positive, gram-negative, and anaerobic organisms, with the exception of *Pseudomonas* and *Proteus* species. Tigecycline has activity against MRSA and vancomycin-resistant enterococci (VRE).

Clinical Uses

Tigecycline is approved by the FDA for treating complicated skin and skin structure infections, intra-abdominal infections, and community-acquired pneumonia; however, given the spectrum of activity, it is also used for gram-negative organisms resistant to alternative agents.

Adverse Events

Tigecycline is generally well tolerated, with nausea and vomiting being the most common adverse effects. Tigecycline has also been reported to cause asymptomatic hyperbilirubinemia. Given the similarity in chemical structure to minocycline, there is the potential for adverse effects seen with the tetracycline class.

Drug Interactions

Concomitant administration of tigecycline and oral contraceptives results in decreased levels of the oral contraceptive, so an additional form of contraception is recommended.

SULFONAMIDES

In 1932, the dye prontosil rubrum was found to be effective in treating streptococcal infections. Subsequent studies found that one of its by-products was sulfanilamide. Manipulation of this by-product created the class of antimicrobials known as the sulfonamides.

Pharmacokinetics and Pharmacodynamics

Oral sulfonamides are readily absorbed from the GI tract. They are distributed through all body tissues and enter the CSF, pleural fluid, and synovial fluid. They are eliminated from the body by glomerular filtration and hepatic metabolism. The half-lives of the sulfonamides vary from hours to days; sulfadoxine (Fansidar) (no longer available in the United States), at 5 to 10 days, has the longest half-life. **Table 8.13** gives dosing information.

TABLE 8.13

Sulfonamide Dosages

Drug	Adult Dosages	Pediatric Dosages
sulfadiazine	4–8 g PO in divided doses q6–12h	100–150 mg/kg/d PO divided q6h
sulfisoxazole	4–8 g PO in divided doses q4–6h	120–150 mg/kg/d PO divided q4–6h
trimethoprim	100 mg PO q12h or 200 mg PO q24h	4–6 mg/kg/d PO divided q12h
trimethoprim–sulfamethoxazole*	160/800 mg PO q12h	6–20 mg/kg/d PO/IV divided q6–12h
	10–20 mg/kg/d IV in divided doses	

Note: Dosage adjustment necessary in patients with renal impairment.
*Dosing recommendations are based on the trimethoprim component.

Mechanism of Action and Spectrum of Activity

The sulfonamides work by inhibiting the incorporation of para-aminobenzoic acid, the basic building block used by bacteria to synthesize dihydrofolic acid, the first step leading to folic acid synthesis, required for bacterial cell growth. Sulfamethoxazole (SMX) competitively inhibits the bacterial enzyme dihydropteroate synthetase.

Trimethoprim (TMP), combined with SMX, inhibits the enzyme dihydrofolate reductase, synergistically inhibiting folic acid formation at another step in the pathway. Because bacterial dihydrofolate reductase is inhibited much more than the mammalian enzyme and because humans obtain exogenous dietary folate, inhibition of folate synthesis by SMX-TMP in humans is not a major problem.

The sulfonamides are active against a wide range of gram-positive and gram-negative organisms, with the exception of *Pseudomonas* species and group A streptococci. In combination with other folate antagonists, they also demonstrate activity against *P. jiroveci* and *Toxoplasma gondii*.

Clinical Uses

The sulfonamides are frequently used in treating many infections. Sulfasalazine (Azulfidine), a sulfonamide derivative lacking significant antimicrobial activity, is poorly absorbed and is used in the management of ulcerative colitis. Because of their limited spectrum of activity and increasing resistance, the sulfonamides are typically used in combination with other agents to increase efficacy or expand coverage. Trimethoprim–sulfamethoxazole (Bactrim) is the combination of choice in treating urinary tract infections, *P. jiroveci* pneumonia (PCP), toxoplasmosis, and some resistant gram-negative infections. Mafenide (Sulfamylon) and silver sulfadiazine (Silvadene) are topical agents frequently used in treating burns.

Adverse Events

Several side effects are reported for sulfonamides. The most common are rash, fever, and GI side effects. The rash occurs within 1 to 2 weeks of initiating therapy. Severe dermatologic reactions, such as Stevens-Johnson syndrome and vasculitis, are uncommon and associated more with longer-acting preparations. Hemolytic anemia can occur in patients with glucose-6-phosphate dehydrogenase deficiency.

Drug Interactions

The sulfonamides potentiate the effects of warfarin, phenytoin, hypoglycemic agents, and methotrexate as a result of drug displacement or decreased liver metabolism.

GLYCOPEPTIDES

Vancomycin, a glycopeptide antibiotic, was first introduced in 1958. Shortly after its introduction, vancomycin became known as "Mississippi Mud" because of the color and impurities in the manufacturing process. The clinical use of vancomycin was initially limited due to its potential for drug-related toxicities, alternative available agents, and concern for the development of resistance. However, since the early 1980s, vancomycin has been an important agent in treating infections. More recent additions to this class include dalbavancin, oritavancin, and telavancin. All of these agents have a narrow spectrum of activity directed toward gram-positive organisms. The newest agents, dalbavancin and oritavancin, have prolonged half-lives that allow for much less frequent dosing.

Pharmacokinetics and Pharmacodynamics

Vancomycin is poorly absorbed from the GI tract. Because of its poor bioavailability, oral administration of vancomycin provides concentrations in the stool sufficient to treat *Clostridium difficile* colitis. The volume of distribution for vancomycin and telavancin, respectively, is 0.6 to 0.9 L/kg and 0.1 L/kg. Vancomycin is minimally bound to proteins; however, telavancin is highly bound to proteins (greater than 90%). They have relatively good penetration into most body fluids and tissues. Unpredictable levels are attained in the CSF and bone. Telavancin is dosed 10 mg/kg IV once daily. Vancomycin is dosed 15 to 20 mg/kg IV with the interval based on kidney function. **Table 8.14** provides an example of a vancomycin-dosing nomogram, and **Table 8.15** provides the dosing of dalbavancin and oritavancin. Monitoring renal function is important in determining proper dosing because dosage adjustments are necessary in patients with renal insufficiency. Both vancomycin and telavancin are renally excreted, primarily as unchanged drug. The vancomycin half-life in adults with normal renal function is 5 to 11 hours. The half-life of telavancin is approximately 8 hours. Neither telavancin nor vancomycin is cleared to a significant extent by hemodialysis or peritoneal dialysis.

Serum drug monitoring is used for vancomycin in patients with unpredictable kidney function or severe infections or those receiving therapy for more than 3 to 5 days. In general, the target trough concentration ranges from 15 to 20 mg/mL for pneumonia, osteomyelitis, meningitis, and endocarditis and from 10 to 15 mg/mL for other infections. Peak concentrations

TABLE 8.14

Vancomycin Dosages

Estimated Creatinine Clearance (mL/min)	Dosing Interval		
	40–55 kg, 500 mg*	55–75 kg, 750 mg*	75–100 kg, 1,000 mg*
>80	q8h	q12h	q12h
54–80	q12h	q18h	q18h
40–53	q18h	q24h	q24h
27–39	q24h	q36h	q36h
21–26	q36h	q48h	q48h
16–20	q48h		

Note: These recommendations represent one of several nomograms used in the empiric dosing of vancomycin. Some prescribers use pharmacokinetic calculations and monitor serum trough levels to evaluate the efficacy and toxicity of a particular regimen. Therapeutic trough levels are typically maintained between 10 and 20 µg/mL.
*Patient's body weight and IV dose of vancomycin.

are generally not recommended. Serum monitoring is not required for dalbavancin, oritavancin, or telavancin. All of these agents exhibit bactericidal activity and a PAE of 1 to 4 hours.

Mechanism of Action and Spectrum of Activity

Glycopeptides are cell wall–active agent. They work by inhibiting the binding of the D-alanyl-D-alanine portion of the cell wall precursor or by interfering with the polymerization and cross-linking of peptidoglycan. The newer agents have more rapid bactericidal activity than vancomycin.

The principal activity of the glycopeptides is limited to gram-positive aerobic and anaerobic bacteria such as methicillin-sensitive and methicillin-resistant staphylococci, streptococci, enterococci, and *Clostridium* species.

Clinical Uses

Vancomycin is used to treat many infections. It is frequently used to treat serious gram-positive infections in patients allergic to or unable to tolerate beta-lactam antibiotics, and it is the drug of choice for MRSA and other resistant gram-positive infections. Neutropenic fever, endocarditis, and meningitis are commonly treated with vancomycin. Oral vancomycin is used in treating severe cases or *C. difficile* colitis or those that have failed to respond to metronidazole. The newer agents are currently indicated only for the treatment of skin and skin structure infections.

TABLE 8.15

Glycopeptide Dosages

Drug	Adult Dosages	Pediatric Dosages
dalbavancin	1,000 mg IV followed by 500 mg IV 1 wk later	—
oritavancin	1,200 mg IV as a single injection	

Adverse Events

The most common side effects associated with vancomycin administration are fever and chills, phlebitis, and "red man" syndrome, a histamine-mediated phenomenon associated with the rate of vancomycin infusion. The typical syndrome consists of pruritus; flushing of the head, neck, and face; and hypotension. It usually resolves when the drug is discontinued. This reaction can also occur with telavancin. Vancomycin and telavancin should be infused over at least 1 hour.

Nephrotoxicity as a result of vancomycin alone is uncommon. Typically, a combination of variables and risk factors precipitates renal insufficiency. Risk factors include age, pre-existing renal disease, and the use of other nephrotoxic agents such as aminoglycosides, amphotericin B, acyclovir, and cyclosporine. In clinical trials evaluating telavancin and vancomycin, an increase in serum creatinine was more common with telavancin. Vancomycin has been classified as an ototoxic agent. Although rare, ototoxicity has occurred in patients receiving high-dose therapy or concurrent ototoxic agents (e.g., aminoglycosides). Hematologic effects from vancomycin such as thrombocytopenia and neutropenia are rare. The most common reported adverse effects of telavancin are taste disturbances, nausea, vomiting, and foamy urine. Due to the risk to the fetus, telavancin is contraindicated during pregnancy.

Drug Interactions

Since the glycopeptides do not undergo significant hepatic metabolism, drug–drug interactions with these two agents are unlikely.

OXAZOLIDINONES

The oxazolidinones are a totally synthetic antibiotic class first investigated in the late 1980s as antidepressant agents. Serendipitously, these agents were discovered to have excellent antibacterial activity. The main reason for their clinical development has been the emergence and spread of resistance in gram-positive pathogens. Linezolid (Zyvox) and tedizolid (Sivextro) are the only agents available in this class.

Pharmacokinetics and Pharmacodynamics

Linezolid and tedizolid are well absorbed from the GI tract. Peak levels are achieved within 1 to 2 hours, and levels increase linearly as the dose is increased. The absolute bioavailability of these agents is greater than 90%. The oral formulation may be administered without regard to meals. Oxazolidinones are predominantly eliminated by nonrenal mechanisms, and their metabolism does not involve the CYP enzyme system. Linezolid is removed by hemodialysis and should be dosed following hemodialysis sessions, while tedizolid is not significantly affected. **Table 8.16** provides dosing information.

Oxazolidinones are considered bacteriostatic agents. A PAE of 3 to 6 hours has been reported, but this has little clinical significance.

Mechanism of Action and Spectrum of Activity

Oxazolidinones bind to the 50S ribosome at a unique binding site and disrupt bacterial protein synthesis. Antagonism has been described with chloramphenicol and clindamycin.

The principal activity of the oxazolidinones is against gram-positive aerobic organisms, including staphylococci, streptococci, and enterococci. In particular, activity against resistant pathogens, including MRSA, penicillin-resistant streptococci, and VRE, is excellent.

Clinical Uses

Linezolid has FDA approval for the treatment of community and nosocomial pneumonia, skin and skin structure infections, and vancomycin-resistant *Enterococcus faecium*, while tedizolid is only approved for the treatment of skin and skin structure infections.

Adverse Events

In general, oxazolidinones are well tolerated when used for short-course therapy. The most common adverse events include diarrhea, nausea, taste perversion, and vomiting. As mentioned earlier, this class of agents was initially investigated for its antidepressant activity. Thrombocytopenia has been reported on average in 3% to 4% of patients in studies of linezolid. Additionally, anemia, leukopenia, and pancytopenia have been reported. A complete blood count should be monitored in patients, especially if receiving linezolid for longer than 2 weeks.

Drug Interactions

Linezolid and tedizolid possess weak monoamine oxidase inhibitory activity. There is a potential for drug interactions with sympathomimetic agents, such as pseudoephedrine, SSRI antidepressants like citalopram, some herbal products, and foods rich in tyramine.

LIPOPEPTIDES

Daptomycin is an antibacterial agent belonging to the class known as the lipopeptides. This class of agents has been studied for its antibacterial activity for several decades; however, daptomycin is the only agent available. Daptomycin is a natural product developed for the treatment of MDR gram-positive pathogens.

Pharmacokinetics and Pharmacodynamics

Daptomycin pharmacokinetics are nearly linear and time independent at doses up to 6 mg/kg administered once daily for 7 days. Its half-life is approximately 8 hours. The apparent volume of distribution in healthy adults is approximately 0.1 L/kg. Daptomycin reversibly binds human plasma proteins, primarily to serum albumin, with a mean serum protein binding of 90%. Because renal excretion is the primary route of elimination, dosage adjustments are necessary in patients with severe renal insufficiency (creatinine clearance less than 30 mL/min). The dose for patients with normal renal function is 4 to 6 mg/kg IV administered daily. There is very limited information to support the use of daptomycin in pediatric patients. Daptomycin exhibits rapid, concentration-dependent bactericidal activity against gram-positive organisms.

Mechanism of Action and Spectrum of Activity

The mechanism of action of daptomycin is distinct from that of any other antibiotic. It binds to bacterial membranes and causes a rapid depolarization of membrane potential. The loss of membrane potential leads to bacterial cell death.

Daptomycin covers most gram-positive pathogens such as *S. aureus* (including methicillin-resistant strains), streptococcus, and enterococcus. It is active against MRSA and VRE.

Clinical Uses

Daptomycin is indicated for the treatment of complicated skin and skin structure infections and *S. aureus* bloodstream infections (bacteremia), including those with right-sided infective endocarditis, caused by methicillin-susceptible and

TABLE 8.16		
Oxazolidinone Dosages		
Drug	**Adult Dosages**	**Pediatric Dosages**
linezolid	400–600 mg PO/IV q12h	20 mg/kg/d PO/IV divided q12h OR 30 mg/kg/d PO/IV divided q8h
tedizolid	200 mg PO/IV daily	—

methicillin-resistant isolates. Daptomycin is a useful alternative to other agents (linezolid, quinupristin/dalfopristin) for treating infections caused by resistant gram-positive pathogens because there are few options at present for treating these infections. For complicated skin and skin structure infections, combination therapy may be clinically indicated if the documented or presumed pathogens include gram-negative or anaerobic organisms. Daptomycin is not indicated for the treatment of pneumonia.

Adverse Events

Daptomycin may cause GI reactions such as constipation, nausea, diarrhea, and vomiting. Injection site reactions and headache may occur. Skeletal muscle toxicity manifested as muscle pain has been reported with daptomycin. This is accompanied by an increase in creatinine phosphokinase (CPK) levels.

Drug Interactions

CPK monitoring should be done at least weekly for patients concomitantly receiving a statin and/or those with renal insufficiency. Otherwise, daptomycin does not have any significant drug–drug interactions.

STREPTOGRAMINS

The streptogramin antibiotics are naturally occurring products that have been used clinically in Europe for more than 40 years. The semisynthetic derivative, quinupristin/dalfopristin (Synercid), is the only streptogramin antibiotic available in the United States. It is a combination of two antibiotics.

Pharmacokinetics and Pharmacodynamics

Quinupristin/dalfopristin is not absorbed from the GI tract. After IV administration, both quinupristin and dalfopristin have a serum half-life of approximately 1 hour. Each drug is moderately protein bound; the volume of distribution is 0.45 and 0.24 L/kg for quinupristin and dalfopristin, respectively. Metabolism of both agents is through the liver. The drug is primarily excreted in the feces.

Quinupristin/dalfopristin is a bactericidal agent against most organisms, with the noted exception of vancomycin-resistant E. faecium. Quinupristin/dalfopristin possesses a PAE ranging from 8 to 18 hours. The dosage for adults and children is 7.5 mg/kg every 8 to 12 hours. It is not significantly removed by hemodialysis or peritoneal dialysis.

Mechanism of Action and Spectrum of Activity

The streptogramins inhibit protein synthesis by binding to the 50S ribosome. The interaction of quinupristin and dalfopristin is synergistic. Either compound alone is bacteriostatic, whereas the combination results in a bactericidal effect.

The principal activity of quinupristin/dalfopristin is against gram-positive aerobic organisms, including staphylococci, streptococci, and enterococci. In particular, its activity against resistant pathogens, including methicillin-resistant staphylococci, penicillin-resistant streptococci, and vancomycin-resistant E. faecium, is excellent. Quinupristin/dalfopristin is not active against Enterococcus faecalis.

Clinical Uses

Quinupristin/dalfopristin is approved by the FDA for treating skin and skin structure infections and vancomycin-resistant E. faecium infections. The use of this agent is limited due to adverse effects and the need for administration through a central venous line. It can be used to treat gram-positive infections caused by methicillin-resistant staphylococci, penicillin-resistant S. pneumoniae, and vancomycin-resistant E. faecium when alternative agents are contraindicated.

Adverse Events

The most common adverse reactions are infusion related. Infusion site reactions, including pain, inflammation, edema, and thrombophlebitis, have been reported in as many as 75% of patients receiving quinupristin/dalfopristin through a peripheral IV catheter. Arthralgias and myalgias have also been reported. They may be severe and result in discontinuation of therapy. They usually occur after several days of therapy. After discontinuation of therapy, these reactions are uniformly reversible. The most common laboratory abnormality is an increased level of conjugated bilirubin.

Drug Interactions

The CYP3A4 isoenzyme (responsible for the metabolism of many drugs) is significantly inhibited by quinupristin/dalfopristin. Close clinical or serum level monitoring of known substrates of the CYP3A4 enzyme is recommended.

ANTIANAEROBIC AGENTS: CLINDAMYCIN

Clindamycin (Cleocin) has been used extensively in treating gram-positive and anaerobic bacterial infections. It was first used orally to treat streptococcal and staphylococcal infections, but it soon became the drug of choice for anaerobic infections. The combination of clindamycin and gentamicin (Garamycin) is still frequently used in treating mixed aerobic and anaerobic infections.

Pharmacokinetics and Pharmacodynamics

Both the hydrochloride and palmitate hydrochloride salts of clindamycin are well absorbed and converted to active forms in the blood. Clindamycin reaches most tissues and bone, but its distribution into CSF is limited. It is 93% bound to proteins. The half-life is approximately 3 hours. Clindamycin is metabolized by the liver, necessitating dosage adjustment in patients with liver impairment (**Table 8.17**). Hemodialysis and peritoneal dialysis do not remove clindamycin to a significant extent.

TABLE 8.17

Clindamycin Dosages

Drug	Adult Dosages	Pediatric Dosages
clindamycin	150–450 mg PO q6–8h	10–30 mg/kg/d PO divided q6–8h
	600 mg IV q8h	25–40 mg/kg/d IV divided q6–8h

Note: Dosage adjustment recommended for patients with liver dysfunction.

Mechanism of Action and Spectrum of Activity

Clindamycin binds to the 50S subunit of the bacterial ribosome and inhibits protein synthesis. It acts at the same site as chloramphenicol and the macrolides.

Clinical Uses

Clindamycin is typically included in regimens for its anaerobic coverage in mixed infections and may also be used in treating gram-positive infections, toxoplasmosis, and PCP or in combination with other agents to treat PID. In addition, it is frequently used to inhibit toxin production as part of the treatment for staphylococcal or streptococcal toxic shock.

Adverse Events

The major side effect associated with clindamycin is diarrhea and associated *C. difficile* colitis. This adverse event is unrelated to dose and may range from acute, self-limiting symptoms to life-threatening toxic megacolon. Pain at the site of IV administration may occur.

Drug Interactions

In rare cases, clindamycin use in combination with skeletal muscle relaxants has been reported to potentiate neuromuscular blockade.

ANTIANAEROBIC AGENTS: METRONIDAZOLE

Metronidazole (Flagyl) was first recognized for its antiprotozoal activity in treating *Trichomonas vaginalis* infections. Subsequently, its utility as an antianaerobic agent was used in treating *B. fragilis* infections. Metronidazole has become a treatment of choice for anaerobic infections, *C. difficile* colitis, and is part of a number of regimens to eradicate *Helicobacter pylori*–associated duodenal ulcers.

Pharmacokinetics and Pharmacodynamics

Metronidazole is completely absorbed from the GI tract after oral administration. It penetrates well into most tissues, with an apparent volume of distribution of 0.3 to 0.9 L/kg.

Its binding to plasma protein is minimal. The liver metabolizes metronidazole, and dosage adjustments are necessary in patients with hepatic impairment (**Table 8.18**). The half-life is approximately 6 to 9 hours. Metronidazole is removed by hemodialysis and peritoneal dialysis.

Mechanism of Action and Spectrum of Activity

Metronidazole is reduced to a toxic product that interacts with DNA, causing strand breakage and resulting in protein synthesis inhibition. Metronidazole has excellent activity against gram-positive and gram-negative anaerobes, *H. pylori*, and protozoa such as *T. vaginalis*.

Clinical Uses

Metronidazole is typically included in regimens for its anaerobic coverage in mixed infections. In addition, metronidazole is the treatment of choice for bacterial vaginosis, trichomoniasis, and *C. difficile* diarrhea.

Adverse Events

Metronidazole is usually safe and well tolerated. GI side effects such as nausea, vomiting, abdominal pain, and a metallic taste are most common. More serious but rare effects include seizures, peripheral neuropathy, and pancreatitis. Seizures have been associated with high doses, whereas peripheral neuropathy has been documented in patients receiving prolonged courses of metronidazole.

Drug Interactions

Metronidazole enhances the anticoagulant effect of warfarin, resulting in a prolonged half-life of warfarin. A disulfiram-like reaction characterized by flushing, palpitations, nausea, and vomiting may occur when alcohol is consumed during metronidazole therapy. Metronidazole is an inhibitor of the CYP3A4 isoenzyme. It has the potential to interact with multiple medications. Additionally, phenobarbital, phenytoin, and rifampin increase the metabolism of metronidazole, which may result in treatment failure. A careful review of a patient's medication list for drug interactions should be done before initiating metronidazole.

TABLE 8.18

Metronidazole Dosages

Drug	Adult Dosages	Pediatric Dosages
metronidazole	250–500 mg PO q6–8h 500 mg IV q6–12h	15–35 mg/kg/d PO/ IV divided q6h

Note: Dosage adjustment recommended for patients with severe liver or kidney dysfunction.

MISCELLANEOUS ANTIMICROBIAL AGENTS: CHLORAMPHENICOL

Chloramphenicol has a wide spectrum of activity against gram-positive, gram-negative, and anaerobic organisms. However, its use has been limited by its toxicity profile, which includes "gray baby" syndrome, optic neuritis, and fatal aplastic anemia. Nonetheless, in selected situations, chloramphenicol remains an important agent.

Pharmacokinetics and Pharmacodynamics

Chloramphenicol is available as an IV succinate ester. The dose is based on age and indication (**Table 8.19**). The ester formulation is hydrolyzed in the body to the active drug. Chloramphenicol penetrates well into most tissues and bodily fluids, including the CSF. Chloramphenicol readily crosses the placenta in pregnant females. It is conjugated in the liver and excreted by the kidney in an inactive, nontoxic form. The serum half-life is 3 to 4 hours. Chloramphenicol is 25% to 50% bound to protein.

Serum levels are frequently monitored in high-risk patients. The therapeutic range of chloramphenicol is 5 to 20 mg/dL. Dose-related myelosuppression typically occurs at serum levels exceeding 25 mg/dL.

Mechanism of Action and Spectrum of Activity

Chloramphenicol reversibly binds to the larger 50S subunit of the ribosome, thereby inhibiting bacterial protein synthesis. It is variably bactericidal.

Chloramphenicol is active against gram-positive and gram-negative aerobes and anaerobes as well as atypical organisms, including mycoplasma, chlamydia, and rickettsiae. Its gram-negative activity includes *E. coli*, *Proteus* species, and *Salmonella* species, but not *P. aeruginosa*.

Clinical Uses

Newer agents have reduced the need to use chloramphenicol in treating infection. However, it can be used as an alternative in treating bacterial meningitis when a patient has a life-threatening penicillin allergy. It is also useful in treating

TABLE 8.19
Chloramphenicol Dosages

Patient Group	Dosage
Older children and adults	50–100 mg/kg/d IV divided q6h (max 4,000 mg daily)
Older children and adults with meningitis	75–100 mg/kg/d IV divided q6h

Note: Chloramphenicol should be used with caution in patients with renal impairment, and serum concentrations should be monitored to guide dosing and prevent toxicity.

rickettsial diseases such as Rocky Mountain spotted fever and typhus fever in patients allergic to tetracyclines or in pregnant women. Chloramphenicol may be used in treating VRE infections as well.

Adverse Events

The major adverse events associated with chloramphenicol are "gray baby" syndrome, blood dyscrasias, and optic neuritis. "Gray baby" syndrome typically occurs in neonates and is manifested by vomiting, lethargy, respiratory collapse, and death. It results from drug accumulation because neonates cannot conjugate chloramphenicol. Two forms of hematologic toxicity may occur with chloramphenicol administration. Dose-related bone marrow suppression has occurred in patients receiving doses exceeding 4 g/d and at serum levels exceeding 25 mg/dL. It may present as a combination of anemia, leukopenia, and thrombocytopenia. Aplastic anemia is an idiosyncratic effect independent of dose and may occur weeks after therapy with chloramphenicol. It is associated with a greater than 50% mortality rate and often necessitates bone marrow transplantation. Optic neuritis is a major neurologic complication and is associated with long courses of chloramphenicol. The toxicity involves red-green color changes and loss of vision. It may be reversible or permanent. GI side effects have been associated with high doses of chloramphenicol.

Drug Interactions

Chloramphenicol is metabolized by the liver and is an inhibitor of the CYP2C19 and CYP3A4 enzymes. It prolongs the half-life of warfarin, phenytoin, and cyclosporine.

MISCELLANEOUS ANTIMICROBIAL AGENTS: RIFAMPIN

Rifampin is a macrocyclic antibiotic used in a variety of settings, and it is a first-line agent in treating tuberculosis. It is typically combined with other antibiotics such as vancomycin in treating MRSA infections.

Pharmacokinetics and Pharmacodynamics

Rifampin is completely absorbed after oral administration. It distributes into most tissues and fluids, including the CSF. The half-life of rifampin is approximately 3 hours. It is metabolized by the liver and is not removed by hemodialysis or peritoneal dialysis. **Table 8.20** provides dosing information.

Mechanism of Action and Spectrum of Activity

Rifampin suppresses initiation of chain formation for RNA synthesis in susceptible bacteria by inhibiting DNA-dependent RNA polymerase. The β-subunit of the enzyme appears to be the site of action.

Rifampin is extremely active against gram-positive cocci. It has moderate activity against aerobic gram-negative bacilli.

TABLE 8.20

Rifampin Dosages

Drug	Adult Dosages	Pediatric Dosages
rifampin	600 mg PO once daily 10–20 mg/kg IV daily	10–20 mg/kg IV generally once daily

Note: Dosage adjustment recommended for patients with liver dysfunction.

Neisseria meningitidis, Neisseria gonorrhoeae, and *H. influenzae* are the most sensitive gram-negative organisms. Rifampin maintains activity against *M. tuberculosis.*

Clinical Uses

Rifampin is commonly used in combination with a cell wall–active agent to treat serious, gram-positive infections that fail to respond to other courses of therapy. This combination is used for synergistic activity and prevents rapid resistance development. It is the drug of choice for postexposure meningitis prophylaxis against *N. meningitidis* and *H. influenzae* type B. Rifampin is a first-line agent in the treatment of *M. tuberculosis* infection, and it is used to treat nontuberculous mycobacterial infections as well.

Adverse Events

The most common side effects associated with rifampin are GI distress (nausea, vomiting, and diarrhea), headache, and fever. Rifampin changes bodily fluids such as sweat, saliva, and tears to a red-orange color. Hepatotoxicity is rare, but the risk increases when it is administered in combination with isoniazid. Liver function tests should be monitored while patients receive rifampin. Anemia or thrombocytopenia also has been reported.

Drug Interactions

Rifampin is a potent inducer of hepatic CYP drug metabolism and precipitates many drug interactions. Rifampin increases the clearance of agents such as antiarrhythmics, azole antifungals, clarithromycin, estrogens, most statins, warfarin, and many HIV medications. A careful review of a patient's medication list for drug interactions should be done before initiating rifampin.

MISCELLANEOUS ANTIMICROBIAL AGENTS: NITROFURANTOIN

Nitrofurantoin is an antimicrobial agent used only for treating and preventing urinary tract infections. Nitrofurantoin has been used in the United States since 1953 and still remains very effective. It is a synthetic nitrofuran-compound derivative, a class that also includes furazolidone, available in Europe.

Pharmacokinetics and Pharmacodynamics

Following oral administration, nitrofurantoin is rapidly absorbed. The bioavailability of nitrofurantoin is approximately 40% to 50%. Absorption can be enhanced with food. Nitrofurantoin serum concentrations are low, with a serum half-life of less than 30 minutes. For this reason, nitrofurantoin should not be used for complicated urinary tract infections or in patients for which a concern of bacteremia exists. Nitrofurantoin undergoes renal elimination. Inadequate urinary concentrations are achieved in patients with renal insufficiency; thus, the drug is ineffective. It is contraindicated in patients with a creatinine clearance of less than 60 mL/min. **Table 8.21** provides dosing information.

Mechanism of Action and Spectrum of Activity

The exact mechanism of nitrofurantoin is poorly understood. The drug does inhibit several bacterial enzymes, which results in impaired bacterial cell wall synthesis.

Nitrofurantoin has adequate antimicrobial coverage against common organisms that cause urinary tract infections such as *E. coli, Citrobacter* species, *Staphylococcus saprophyticus, E. faecalis,* and *E. faecium.* Nitrofurantoin frequently covers strains of VRE. Resistance has increased against some types of bacteria such as *Enterobacter* and *Klebsiella* species.

Clinical Uses

Nitrofurantoin is only used for the treatment and prophylaxis of uncomplicated urinary tract infections. As mentioned earlier, it should not be used for complicated urinary tract infections such as pyelonephritis.

Adverse Events

The most common side effects of nitrofurantoin include nausea and vomiting. Allergic reactions are rare. Pulmonary reactions (pulmonary infiltrates, pneumonitis, pulmonary fibrosis) and hepatic effects (hepatitis, hepatic necrosis) have been reported in rare cases, usually associated with long-term use. Additionally, peripheral neuropathy has been associated with long-term use in patients with renal failure.

TABLE 8.21

Nitrofurantoin Dosages

Drug	Adult Dosages	Pediatric Dosages
nitrofurantoin	50 mg PO q6h (macrocrystal) 100 mg PO q12h (macrocrystal/monohydrate)	5–7 mg/kg/d PO divided q6h

Note: Nitrofurantoin is contraindicated in patients with a creatinine clearance of <60 mL/min.

Drug Interactions

Nitrofurantoin is not associated with significant drug interactions.

ANTIMICROBIAL RESISTANCE

There are multiple mechanisms by which bacteria form or acquire antibiotic resistance. Some types of resistance occur naturally, while others are acquired from another strain of bacteria. Additionally, resistance can sometimes be induced during antibiotic treatment. **Table 8.22** summarizes the most common resistance mechanisms:

1. The first and most common type of resistance is bacterial enzyme production. For example, bacteria frequently produce enzymes that disrupt beta-lactam antibiotics, altering the structure so they cannot bind to the PBPs. There are hundreds of different types of these enzymes known as *beta-lactamases*. Some enzymes have activity only against penicillins (penicillinases), whereas others, such as extended-spectrum beta-lactamases, can render almost all beta-lactam antibiotics ineffective. Separate from beta-lactamases, bacteria also produce enzymes that can alter the chemical structure or inactivate the drug. This can occur with aminoglycosides, chloramphenicol, macrolides, streptogramins, and tetracyclines.
2. Resistance can occur as the bacteria alter their own cell membranes, not permitting antibiotics to enter the bacteria. An example of this is loss of porins on the gram-negative bacterial cell outer membrane. Specifically with beta-lactam antibiotics, loss of these porins alters the ability of the antimicrobial agent to enter the cell.
3. A third, common mechanism of resistance is the activation of efflux pumps that expel antibiotics out of the intracellular space back across the cell membrane. This prevents antibiotics from acting at their intracellular target site. This is a common mechanism of resistance with classes such as tetracyclines and macrolides.
4. A fourth type of resistance is alteration of the antibiotic's target site of action. This occurs with macrolides, among other classes, when mutations alter the ribosomal binding site. The antibiotic does not bind at all or as well to the ribosome anymore. Similarly, VRE is a result of altered cell well precursors. Plasmid-mediated resistance results in a modified peptidoglycan precursor that binds vancomycin, preventing it from binding to its intended target site.
5. A fifth type of resistance is alteration of target enzymes. For example, the FQs work by inhibiting the enzymes DNA gyrase and topoisomerase IV. Mutations to a variety of different chromosomes on these enzymes can reduce the efficacy of the FQs.
6. Last, overproduction of target enzymes can result in resistance. The best example of this is with sulfonamides and TMP. SMX/TMP works by inhibiting folic acid synthesis by inhibiting the dihydropteroate synthetase and dihydrofolate reductase enzymes, respectively. These enzymes are required for bacterial folic acid synthesis. Excess production of these two enzymes in some strains of bacteria can render the antibiotic ineffective.

A specific area of interest in antimicrobial development is targeting the prevention or overcoming drug resistance.

TABLE 8.22

Antimicrobial Resistance

Antibiotic/Antibiotic Class	Bacterial Enzyme Production	Decreased Membrane Permeability	Promotion of Antibiotic Efflux	Altered Target Sites/Protection of Target Site	Altered Target Enzymes	Overproduction of Target
Penicillins	✓	✓	✓		✓	
Cephalosporins	✓	✓	✓		✓	
Monobactams	✓	✓				
Carbapenems	✓	✓	✓			
Fluoroquinolones		✓	✓	✓	✓	
Macrolides	✓		✓	✓		
Aminoglycosides	✓			✓		
Tetracyclines	✓		✓	✓		
Sulfamethoxazole/trimethoprim					✓	✓
Glycopeptides				✓		
Oxazolidinones				✓		
Streptogramins	✓		✓	✓		
Clindamycin	✓			✓		
Metronidazole		✓			✓	
Chloramphenicol	✓	✓				
Rifampin				✓		
Nitrofurantoin					✓	

CASE STUDY*

M.T., a 62-year-old woman, is started on linezolid for MRSA vertebral osteomyelitis. Her medications include warfarin, atorvastatin, and citalopram.

1. Which of the following is true for linezolid?
   a. It is effective against MRSA but not VRE.
   b. It works by disrupting bacterial cell wall synthesis.
   c. She can be converted to oral treatment as soon as her white blood cells return to normal.
   d. Thrombocytopenia occurs in a small percentage of patients.
2. A few days later, M.T. exhibits signs of confusion, high blood pressure, and tremor. Which of the following is a probable reason for these signs/symptoms?

a. Linezolid is known for increasing blood pressure in elderly patients.
b. Linezolid is a mild monoamine oxidase inhibitor and is creating increased interacting with citalopram to created increase levels of serotonin.
c. M.T.'s infection is getting worse and the linezolid needs to be changed to a more wide-spectrum antibiotic.
d. Atorvastatin is interacting with the linezolid creating a rhabdomyolysis-like syndrome.
e. After several weeks, M.T.'s infection improves.

* Answers can be found online.

ANTIMICROBIAL STEWARDSHIP

Overuse of antibiotics is well documented and has led to increased resistance to various strains of bacteria worldwide. Some examples of drug-resistant bacteria include extended-spectrum beta-lactamases against *E. coli* and *Klebsiella*, carbapenem-resistant *Klebsiella*, FQ-resistant gonococcus, MRSA, and vancomycin-intermediate *S. aureus*. Given the slow development of new antibiotics for the treatment of resistant pathogens, appropriate antibiotic use is crucial. The Infectious Diseases Society of America has developed antibiotic stewardship guidelines. These guidelines recommend a multidisciplinary approach to improving antibiotic use, particularly in the hospital setting. A few ways to improve antibiotic use include formulary restrictions, evidence-based prescribing, dose optimization, antibiotic streamlining, and de-escalation. To minimize resistance, all prescribers must make an effort to ensure appropriate antibiotic use.

Bibliography

Andes, D. R., & Craig, W. A. (2015). Cephalosporins. In G. L. Mandell, J. E. Bennett, & R. Dolin (Eds.), *Principles and practice of infectious diseases* (8th ed.). Philadelphia, PA: Churchill Livingstone.
Bolon, M. K. (2009). The newer fluoroquinolones. *Infectious Disease Clinics of North America, 23*, 1027–1051.
Calfee, D. P. (2015). Rifamycins. In G. L. Mandell, J. E. Bennett, & R. Dolin (Eds.), *Principles and practice of infectious diseases* (8th ed.). Philadelphia, PA: Churchill Livingstone.
Chambers, H. F. (2015). Penicillins. In G. L. Mandell, J. E. Bennett, & R. Dolin (Eds.), *Principles and practice of infectious diseases* (8th ed.). Philadelphia, PA: Churchill Livingstone.
Chambers, H. F. (2015). Other beta-lactam antibiotics. In G. L. Mandell, J. E. Bennett, & R. Dolin (Eds.), *Principles and practice of infectious diseases* (8th ed.). Philadelphia, PA: Churchill Livingstone.
Huckell, V. F. (2011). Infective endocarditis. In R. S. Porter, & J. L. Kaplan (Eds.), *The Merck manual of diagnosis and therapy* (19th ed.). Whitehouse Station, NJ: Merck Sharpe & Dohme Corp.
Leibovici, L., Vidal, L., & Paul, M. (2009). Aminoglycoside drugs in clinical practice: An evidence-based approach. *Journal of Antimicrobial Chemotherapy, 63*, 246–251.
Levison, M. E. (2004). Pharmacodynamics of antimicrobial drugs. *Infectious Disease Clinics of North America, 184*, 51–65.
Matthews, S. J., & Lancaster, J. W. (2009). Doripenem monohydrate, a broad-spectrum carbapenem antibiotic. *Clinical Therapeutics, 31*(1), 42–63.
Meyers, B., & Salvatore, M. (2015). Tetracyclines and chloramphenicol. In G. L. Mandell, J. E. Bennett, & R. Dolin (Eds.), *Principles and practice of infectious diseases* (8th ed.). Philadelphia, PA: Churchill Livingstone.
Opal, S. M., & Pop-Vicas, A. (2015). Molecular mechanisms of antibiotic resistance in bacteria. In G. L. Mandell, J. E. Bennett, & R. Dolin (Eds.), *Principles and practice of infectious diseases* (8th ed.). Philadelphia, PA: Churchill Livingstone.
Paterson, D. L., & DePestel, D. D. (2009). Doripenem. *Clinical Infectious Diseases, 49*, 291–298.
Rice, L. B. (2009). The clinical consequences of antimicrobial resistance. *Current Opinion in Microbiology, 12*(5), 476–481.
Rybak, M. J., Lomaestro, B., Rotschafer, J. C., et al. (2009). Therapeutic monitoring of vancomycin in adult patients: A consensus review of the American Society of Health-System Pharmacists, the Infectious Diseases Society of America, and the Society of Infectious Diseases Pharmacists. *American Journal of Health-System Pharmacy, 66*, 82–98.
Salvatore, M., & Meyers, B. (2005). Metronidazole. In G. L. Mandell, J. E. Bennett, & R. Dolin (Eds.), *Principles and practice of infectious diseases* (8th ed.). Philadelphia, PA: Churchill Livingstone.
Saravolatz, L. D., Stein, G. E., & Johnson, L. B. (2009). Telavancin: A novel lipoglycopeptide. *Clinical Infectious Diseases, 49*(15), 1908–1914.
Society for Healthcare Epidemiology of America; Infectious Diseases Society of America; Pediatric Infectious Diseases Society. (2012). Policy statement on antimicrobial stewardship by the Society for Healthcare Epidemiology of America (SHEA), the Infectious Diseases Society of America (IDSA), and the Pediatric Infectious Diseases Society (PIDS). *Infection Control and Hospital Epidemiology, 33*(4, Special Topic Issue: Antimicrobial Stewardship (April 2012)), 322–327.
Stahlmann, R., & Lode, H. (2010). Safety considerations of fluoroquinolones in the elderly. *Drugs and Aging, 27*(3), 193–209.
Wilcox, M. H. (2005). Update on linezolid: The first oxazolidinone antibiotic. *Expert Opinion on Pharmacotherapy, 6*(13), 2315–2326.
Zuckerman, J. M., Qamar, F., & Bono, B. R. (2009). Macrolides, ketolides, and glycylcyclines: Azithromycin, clarithromycin, telithromycin, tigecycline. *Infectious Disease Clinics of North America, 23*, 997–1026.

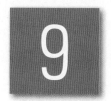

9

Complementary and Alternative Medicine

Virginia P. Arcangelo

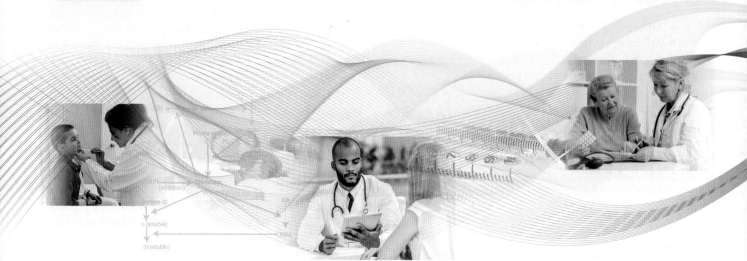

There has been a tremendous growth in the use of complementary and alternative medicine (CAM) in the United States in recent years. *Complementary medicine* is defined as that used together with conventional medicine. *Alternative medicine* is that used in place of conventional medicine. In 1995, the National Institute of Health's Office of Alternative Medicine defined CAM as the "broad domain of healing resources that encompasses all health systems, modalities, and practices and their accompanying theories and beliefs other than those intrinsic to the politically dominant health system of a particular society or culture in a given historical period. CAM includes all such practices and ideas self-defined by their users as preventing or treating illness or promoting health and well-being." There has also been an increase in the use of integrative medicine by practitioners. *Integrative medicine* is the combination of mainstream medicine and CAM.

In 2012, 33.2% of adults and 11.6% of children in the Unites States used complementary approaches to health care. The most frequent users of CAM are between 45 and 64 years of age with a higher education and income level. Women use CAM more frequently than men (Clarke et al., 2015).

People use CAM because they want more control over their medical care, they feel an affinity for a holistic or "natural" approach, they are dissatisfied with the attitudes of their health care providers, they are discouraged with the increased cost of traditional medical care, or conventional medicine fails to meet their needs (**Box 9.1**). Most patients do not communicate the use of CAM with their providers unless specifically questioned about this.

DOMAINS OF CAM

There are five domains of CAM (**Box 9.2**): alternative medicine system, mind/body interventions, biologically based therapy, manipulation and body-based methods, and energy therapies. Alternative medicine systems are based on complete systems of theory and practice. Mind/body interventions incorporate a variety of techniques to enhance the mind's capacity to affect bodily function; a common practice is biofeedback. Biologically based therapy is treatment with substances found in nature. Manipulation and body-based methods are based on manipulation or movement of body parts; an example is chiropractic manipulation. Energy therapies involve the use of energy fields such as magnets.

NATIONAL CENTER FOR COMPLEMENTARY AND INTEGRATIVE HEALTH

Today, the National Center for Complementary and Integrative Health (NCCIH) is the federal government's agency responsible for scientific research on health interventions, practices, products, and disciplines that are not within the realm of mainstream medicine. It is the successor of the National Center for Complementary and Alternative Medicine (NCCAM), the predecessor to NCCIH, that was established in 1998 by congressional mandate. The stated mission of NCCAM was to define, through rigorous

- Advertising
- Affinity to the natural approach
- Deterioration of patient–provider relationship
- Desire to have control over treatment
- Ineffective treatment of chronic disease
- Dissatisfaction with prescription drugs
- High cost of traditional medical care, use of technology, and drugs
- Perceived effectiveness
- Perceived safety
- Rejection of established medical practices

REGULATION

Dietary supplements, which are defined as products taken orally that contain a "dietary product" intended to supplement the diet, are estimated to be used by one half to two thirds of the U.S. population (Bailey et al., 2011). These may include vitamins, minerals, herbs, amino acids, other botanicals, or substances such as enzymes, organ tissues, and metabolites. The products may be in the form of powder, capsules, tablets, gelcaps, or liquids. The increasing use of dietary supplements reflects the increased interest in "natural" medicine, fitness, health, and disease prevention. Also, consumers want to avoid the high cost of traditional drugs and the side effects of these drugs.

Manufacturers of dietary supplements are not required to perform clinical tests on new ingredients. The FDA can only stop a company from making a product when that product poses a significant risk to health. On the other hand, prescription drugs are put through rigorous clinical testing to determine there is no harm to the patient before they can be put on the market. The patient usually does not report bad side effects experienced, so adverse reactions are more slowly determined. More than 500 herbs are marketed in the United States; indeed, about 25% of the current pharmacopoeia is derived from botanicals. The cardiac glycoside digoxin comes from the foxglove plant. Aspirin comes from willow bark, oral contraceptives from Mexican yam, warfarin from sweet clover, and capsaicin from the red pepper plant.

In March 2003, the U.S. Food and Drug Administration (FDA) published new guidelines for dietary supplements that would prevent contamination with other herbs, pesticides, heavy metals, or prescription drugs. Manufacturers do not have to prove the supplement's quality but must meet certain FDA standards. The FDA can take action only if it finds that a product is unsafe once it is on the market. Each product

scientific investigation, the usefulness and safety of complementary and integrative health interventions and their roles in improving health and health care. It was dedicated to explore complementary and alternative healing practices in the context of rigorous science and to serve as an information clearinghouse and facilitate research and training programs, funded by the federal government. The mission of the NCCIH is to define, through rigorous scientific investigation, the usefulness and safety of complementary and integrative health interventions and their roles in improving health and health care (https://nccih.nih.gov/about/ataglance).

NCCIH identifies CAM practitioners. It also publishes alerts and advisories for specific products and practices, lists clinical trials of CAM, and provides treatment information.

Alternative Medicine Systems—These are built upon complete systems of theory and practice and have often evolved apart from and earlier than the conventional medical approach popular in the United States. Examples are homeopathic and naturopathic medicine and traditional Chinese medicine.

Mind/Body Interventions—This incorporates a variety of techniques designed to enhance the mind's capacity to affect bodily function and symptoms. This includes biofeedback, meditation, dance therapy, and art therapy.

Biologically Based Therapy—This is treatment with substances found in nature, including dietary supplements, herbal supplements, and "natural" but scientifically unproved treatment.

Manipulation and Body-Based Methods—These are based on manipulation or movement of body parts. Examples include chiropractic manipulation and massage therapy.

Energy Therapies—This is the use of energy fields. Biofield therapy affects the energy fields that purportedly surround and penetrate the human body and includes Reiki and Therapeutic Touch. Bioelectromagnetic therapy is based on treatment involving the unconventional use of electromagnetic fields. An example is magnet therapy.

BOX 9.3 — Label Requirements for Herbal Preparations

- Name
- Quantity of contents
- Ingredients and amounts
- Disclaimer: "This statement has not been evaluated by the FDA. This product is not intended to diagnose, treat, cure, or prevent disease."
- Supplemental facts panel:
  - Serving size
  - Amount
  - Active ingredients
- Other ingredients such as herbs for which no daily values exist
- Name and address of manufacturer, packer, or distributor

must have a label accurately listing the product's ingredients. **Box 9.3** lists label requirements for herbal preparations.

Products also have a "Supplemental Facts" panel that lists the appropriate serving size. Natural remedies cannot be patented, so the manufacturer does not need to take the time and money to conduct necessary tests.

Nutrition Labeling and Education Act

The Nutrition Labeling and Education Act (NLEA) was enacted by Congress in 1990 to provide a clear relationship of nutrition to disease. The purpose of the act was to educate consumers. Information required on the label includes nutritional information, in an easy-to-read format, with the amount of ingredient per serving, the percentage of daily values of the ingredients, and the standard serving size. The act also established that disease-related health claims could be used on labeling of nutritional products, provided there is agreement among qualified scientists that the claim is valid.

Dietary Supplement Health and Education Act

The Dietary Supplement Health and Education Act (DSHEA), passed in 1994, restricted the FDA's control over dietary supplements. It defined herbal products as dietary supplements, which are considered foods. Before this, products had to be proven safe by the FDA; those introduced after the act's passage had to be proven safe by the manufacturer. The manufacturer of a herbal preparation is responsible for the truthfulness of the claims made on a label and must have evidence supporting the claims; however, there is no standard for this evidence or does the manufacturer need to submit it to the FDA. The manufacturer may claim that the product affects the structure or function of the body as long as there is no claim of effectiveness in the prevention or treatment of a specific disease. A disclaimer must be provided stating that

the FDA has not evaluated the product. Since health claims are not preapproved, the statement "This statement has not been evaluated by the Food and Drug Administration. This product is not intended to diagnose, treat, cure or prevent any disease" must be on the label. Information regarding therapeutic claims for herbal products can be disseminated as long as the information is not misleading or product specific, is physically separated from the product, and has no product stickers affixed to it.

In 2000, the FDA allowed "structure and function" statements to be made. For example, cranberry products could say that the product supports urinary health but not that it treats urinary tract infections. It allowed for claims that do not relate to disease but are health maintenance claims ("maintains a healthy circulatory system"), nondisease claims ("helps you relax"), and claims for minor symptoms associated with life stages ("for common symptoms of premenstrual syndrome"). Anything that uses words such as "prevents," "treats," "cures," "mitigates," or "diagnoses disease" is subject to drug requirements. This act led to enormous growth in the dietary supplement industry, which today grosses over $18 billion annually.

RISKS

Many herbs and alternative medicines have not been studied adequately and may in fact be toxic. The fact that plants are "natural" does not make the use of agents from that plant free of risks! Adverse reactions can result from direct exposure to the component of the plant or from poor manufacturing process. The law does not require that adverse events resulting from the use of dietary supplements be reported to the FDA. Research studies of safety in people are not required because, as noted above, these agents are considered dietary supplements, not drugs. There is inappropriate dissemination of information and weak regulation in the industry. **Box 9.4** lists the dangers of herbal preparations.

BOX 9.4 — Dangers of Herbal Products

- Many herbs and alternative medicines have not been studied adequately and may be toxic.
- Research studies of safety in people are not required.
- Natural remedies cannot be patented, so the manufacturer does not take the time and money to conduct necessary tests.
- There may be unlisted ingredients in the product.
- There is inappropriate dissemination of information and weak regulation in the industry.
- Dosages can vary by manufacturer.
- Herbal supplements can be bought by anyone.
- There can be herb–drug interactions.

One example of an adverse reaction that has brought about governmental action is ephedra. Ephedra, a common ingredient in weight-loss products, can cause an increase in blood pressure, tremors, arrhythmia, seizures, strokes, myocardial infarction, and death. In April 2004, the FDA banned its sale.

There is no check on the ingredients in preparation. Analyses of herbal supplements have found differences between what is on the label and what is actually in the bottle. There may be less or more of the supplement than the label indicates. When tested, some supplements have been shown to contain an ingredient that is not on the label or even to contain contaminants. Some have been shown not to contain any of the herb listed on the label. Some may even contain prescription medications.

Herbal medicines can be purchased and consumed by anyone. They are less expensive than prescription drugs but can still be costly.

HERB–DRUG INTERACTIONS

Interactions between dietary supplements and drugs can be pharmacokinetic or pharmacodynamic. Pharmacokinetic interactions can be a change in the amount of active compounds available and are the consequence of alteration in absorption, distribution, metabolism, or excretion. For example, senna, a common ingredient in weight-loss products, has a laxative effect that can affect drug transit time and reduce absorption. Zinc lozenges, often used to relieve cold symptoms, may chelate fluoroquinolones and tetracyclines, decreasing serum levels of these antibiotics.

Pharmacodynamic interactions occur at the site of action and may be additive or antagonistic to prescribed drugs or other herbal preparations. Vitamin E doses of greater than 1,000 units per day can increase the anticoagulant effect of warfarin. Ephedra has additive effects with caffeine and at high doses can cause death.

There can be an effect on drug metabolism. Herbal products can affect cytochrome P450 (CYP) isoenzymes. For example, St. John's wort is a potent herbal inducer of CYP3A4.

PATIENT EDUCATION

The practitioner must question each patient about the use of CAM since most don't report usage. Patients must be aware that herbal preparations have pharmacologic properties. There are interactions with many prescription and over-the-counter (OTC) medications. All products should be purchased from a reliable source. The more ambitious the claim, the more suspicious the consumer should be of the product. The consumer can request professional health information from the company such as the nature of the company, testing procedures, quality control standards, and so forth.

Consumers should avoid excessive dosing. Taking higher than the recommended dosage can increase the possibility of adverse effects. All supplements should be discontinued during pregnancy and lactation and avoided in children under age 12.

Dietary supplements should not be used for serious health conditions without the advice and supervision of a qualified health professional. Most dietary supplements are meant to treat mild, short-term disorders. Combination products should be avoided. Combining more than two or three ingredients in one product is not good because it is impossible to tell which ingredient is causing side effects if they develop. Multivitamins are the exception.

All side effects should be reported to a health professional. The side effects may be due to the dietary supplement or from interaction with a prescribed drug.

Consumers can obtain information about CAM from many Web sites (**Box 9.5**).

COMMONLY USED HERBS

The following section reviews some commonly used dietary supplements (herbs). **Table 9.1** lists them by use for various organ systems. People use CAM for an array of diseases and conditions. American adults are most likely to use CAM for musculoskeletal problems such as back, neck, or joint pain. The supplements most commonly used are fish oil/omega-3s, glucosamine, echinacea, probiotics, and flaxseed oil.

Black Cohosh

Action and Proof of Efficacy

Black cohosh has vascular and estrogenic activity. Some studies have shown that black cohosh binds to estrogen receptors.

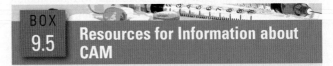

BOX 9.5   Resources for Information about CAM

https://nccih.nih.gov—National Center for Complementary and Integrative Health.
www.cancer.gov/cancertopics/cam.
www.biomedcentral.com/bmccomplementaltmed.
www.drugfacts.com—a free database to check interactions.
www.cfsan.fda.gov (1-888-723-3366)—provides information on safety of supplements. Adverse effects from a supplement can be reported at www.fda.gov/medwatch (1-800-FDA-1088).
www.naturalstandard.com/NaturalMedicines—the authority on integrative medicine and on dietary supplements, *natural medicines*, and *complementary alternative* and integrative therapies. The best and most authoritative Web site available on herbal *medicines*.

TABLE 9.1

Common Herbal Preparations

Suggested System	Name/Dosage	Use	Selected Adverse Events	Contraindications/Interactions	Special Considerations
Gastrointestinal (GI)	Acidophilus 10 colony-forming organisms per day	Restore normal oral, GI, and vaginal flora altered by antibiotics or *Candida* and bacterial infections	Flatulence	Warfarin—may decrease efficacy	
Health promotion	Black cohosh 40–200 PO mg/d	Relief of menstrual and menopausal symptoms	Increased perspiration, dizziness, nausea/vomiting, visual disturbances, reduced pulse	Anesthetics, antihypertensives, sedatives—may increase hypotensive effect Not for use in patients with estrogen-dependent tumors	
	Flaxseed 1 tablespoon bid to tid	Protection against prostate, colon, and breast cancers	Flatulence, stomach	May increase hypoglycemic effect of diabetic meds	
	Oil 15–30 mL daily	Lowers triglycerides	Pain, constipation, potential lowering of blood sugar	May increase clotting time with anticoagulants	
Respiratory disorders	Echinacea 50–1,000 mg/d	Shorten duration of symptoms of URI, wound healing	Nausea, rash	Those who are immunocompromised (may suppress T cells) Human immunodeficiency virus Tuberculosis Multiple sclerosis	May increase effects of estrogen supplements
Cardiovascular disorders	Garlic 600–800 mg/d, 1 clove of garlic daily	Lower cholesterol, prevent clot formation	Dizziness, irritation of mouth and esophagus, nausea, flatulence, malodorous breath and body, sweating	Warfarin (increased risk of bleeding)	Only taken for 8 wk
Neurologic/ psychological	Ginkgo biloba 40–80 mg/d in 2 or 3 divided doses	Peripheral vascular insufficiency, memory loss	Headache, dizziness, heart palpitations	Aspirin (increased risk of bleeding) Nifedipine (elevated nifedipine levels) Trazodone (increased sedation) Warfarin (increased risk of bleeding) Hypoglycemic agents (facilitates clearance to elevate blood sugar) Thiazide diuretics (increases blood pressure when combined)	The preparation must contain allicin, the active ingredient in garlic
Musculoskeletal	Glucosamine 500 mg PO tid	Antiarthritic	Potential to alter blood glucose levels, heartburn, diarrhea, nausea, abdominal pain	Sulfa allergy	
Neurologic/ psychological	Kava 100 mg three times per day	Depression	Headaches, disturbance in visual accommodation	Alcohol (increases activity) Alprazolam (may induce coma) Central nervous system (CNS) depressants (additive sedative effects) Levodopa (increases parkinsonian symptoms)	

(Continued)

TABLE 9.1

Common Herbal Preparations (*Continued*)

Suggested System	Name/Dosage	Use	Selected Adverse Events	Contraindications/Interactions	Special Considerations
Neurologic/psychological	Melatonin 5 mg PO hs Jet lag: 5 mg/d for 3 d before departure and ending 3 d after departure	Insomnia Jet lag	Headache, depression, drowsiness, confusion, hypothermia	Nifedipine (interferes with antihypertensive effect) Increased anxiolytic action with benzodiazepines	Drowsiness may occur within 30 min, so avoid operating machinery
Neurologic/psychological	St. John's wort 320 mg PO daily	Depression, anxiety, neuralgic pain	Dizziness, restlessness, sleep disturbances, dry mouth, constipation, GI distress, photosensitivity	Oral contraceptives (decreased efficacy) Cyclosporine (decreased levels) Digoxin (decreased levels) Nifedipine (decreased levels) Tricyclic antidepressants (decreased levels) Selective serotonin reuptake inhibitors (increased sedative effects and serotonin syndrome) Simvastatin (decreased cholesterol-lowering effect) Theophylline (decreased levels) Warfarin (decreased anticoagulant effect) Alcohol Monoamine oxide (MAO) inhibitors	Considered an MAO inhibitor
Neurologic/psychological	Valerian 200–500 mg PO HS for insomnia 200–300 mg PO bid for anxiety	Sleep disorders, anxiety	Excitability Blurred vision, nausea	Additive effects with alcohol and CNS depressants	
Respiratory	Zinc	Cold symptoms, wound healing	Nausea, bad taste, diarrhea, vomiting, mouth irritation		
Genitourinary disorders	Saw palmetto 320 mg/d PO	Benign prostatic hyperplasia	GI side effects, decreased libido, headache, back pain	Warfarin (increased risk of bleeding)	
Cardiovascular disease	Omega-3s 1–6 g/d	Decrease triglyceride levels, slow growth of atherosclerotic patches	GI upset	Blood thinners, antihypertensives	

Uses and Dosage

The action of estrogen-receptor binding is thought to mimic natural estrogen activity. Therefore, black cohosh is used for dysmenorrhea and vasomotor menopausal symptoms. The recommended dosage is 20 to 160 mg daily.

Adverse Reactions and Drug Interactions

Black cohosh can cause nausea, dizziness, increased perspiration, and bradycardia. It interacts with several classes of drugs, such as anesthetics and sedatives. It may increase the hypotensive effect of many antihypertensive agents. It also may increase the effects of estrogen supplements. Black cohosh is contraindicated in patients with estrogen-dependent tumors. Black cohosh also has salicylates.

Coenzyme Q10

Action and Proof of Efficacy

CoQ10 has antioxidant properties, is a membrane stabilizer, and is a cofactor in many metabolic pathways. It is produced by the human body and is necessary for the basic functioning of cells. CoQ10 levels are reported to decrease with age and to be low in patients with some chronic diseases such as heart conditions, muscular dystrophies, Parkinson disease, cancer, diabetes, and human immunodeficiency virus/acquired immunodeficiency syndrome. Some prescription drugs may also lower CoQ10 levels.

Uses and Dosage

CoQ10 is used in patients with hypertension, congestive heart failure, and migraines. There are studies being conducted to determine the role of CoQ10 in many other diseases. The recommended dose is 100 to 1,200 mg/d.

Adverse Reactions and Drug Interactions

Reactions may include nausea, vomiting, stomach upset, heartburn, diarrhea, loss of appetite, rash, insomnia, headache, dizziness, itching, irritability, increased light sensitivity of the eyes, fatigue, or flulike symptoms. It may reduce the effectiveness of warfarin or may add to the effects of other blood pressure-lowering drugs. It may affect thyroid hormone levels and alter the effects of thyroid drugs, such as levothyroxine, and may also interact with antiretroviral or antiviral drugs.

Echinacea

Action and Proof of Efficacy

Echinacea stimulates phagocytosis and increases respiratory cellular activity and mobility of leukocytes. A review of 19 German-controlled studies in treatment of the common cold showed that there may be some effect on the immune system, but a recent study showed no effect on children ages 2 to 11 (Karsch-Völk et al., 2014).

Uses and Dosage

Echinacea is used to help heal abscesses, burns, eczema, and skin wounds and to treat the common cold. The recommended dose is 50 to 1,000 mg/d.

Adverse Reactions and Drug Interactions

Echinacea may cause a rash. It should not be taken by immunocompromised patients. Long-term use may suppress T cells. There are no reported drug interactions.

Flaxseed

Action and Proof of Efficacy

Flaxseed is rich in lignans, one of the major classes of phytoestrogens. They are estrogen-like chemical compounds with antioxidant qualities, able to scavenge free radicals in the body. They are also rich in soluble and insoluble fiber. They are also rich ion omega-3 fatty acids.

Uses and Dosages

Consuming flaxseed may help protect against prostate, colon, and breast cancers. Flaxseed is thought to prevent the growth of cancerous cells because its omega-3 fatty acids disrupt malignant cells from clinging onto other body cells. In addition, the lignans in flaxseed have antiangiogenic properties—they stop tumors from forming new blood vessels. It helps with constipation. It also has the potential for lowering cholesterol, preventing hot flashes, and improving blood sugar.

The dosage for seed is 1 tablespoon two to three times a day and oil is 15 to 30 mL daily.

Adverse Reactions and Drug Interactions

Flaxseed can cause flatulence, stomach pains, nausea, constipation, diarrhea, and bloating.

Pregnant women should avoid consuming flaxseed because of its estrogen-like properties, which affect pregnancy outcome. People with a bowel obstruction should avoid flaxseed because of its high fiber content.

Since flaxseed may lower blood sugar, diabetics must monitor blood sugar closely. It may slow blood clotting so patients taking any medication that effects blood clotting should use it with caution, since it may increase the chance of bleeding.

Garlic

Action and Proof of Efficacy

Garlic has lipid-lowering and antithrombotic properties. Results from clinical studies are varied. Cholesterol-lowering effects, if any, have been shown to be small.

Uses and Dosage

Garlic is used to treat hyperlipidemia and to prevent clot formation. The product must contain allicin, the active ingredient in garlic. Fresh garlic is the most effective (one clove a day). The recommended dose is 600 to 800 mg/d.

Adverse Reactions and Drug Interactions

Garlic can cause dizziness, irritation of the mouth and esophagus, nausea, flatulence, malodorous breath and body odor, and sweating. Garlic increases the risk of bleeding when taking with anticoagulants. Garlic oil can reduce CYP2E1 activity by almost 40%, causing elevated serum levels of drugs whose major metabolic pathway includes CYP2E1, such as alcohol.

Ginkgo Biloba

Action and Proof of Efficacy

Ginkgo biloba promotes arterial and venous vascular changes that increase tissue perfusion and cerebral blood flow. It is also considered an antioxidant. Results from clinical trials are varied. Cholesterol-lowering effects, if any, have been shown to be small.

Uses and Dosage

Ginkgo biloba is used to treat peripheral vascular insufficiency and dementia. The recommended dose is 40 to 80 mg/d.

Adverse Reactions and Drug Interactions

Ginkgo biloba can cause headache, diarrhea, flatulence, nausea, and dermatitis. It interacts with anticoagulants and antiplatelets by affecting platelet activity. When taken with insulin and oral hypoglycemic agents, it causes increased clearance of insulin and oral hypoglycemic agents, resulting in elevated blood glucose levels. When taken with thiazide diuretics, it increases blood pressure.

Glucosamine

Action and Proof of Efficacy

Glucosamine stimulates the production of cartilage components and allow rebuilding of damaged cartilage. Studies have proven its safety and effectiveness in the treatment of osteoarthritis.

Uses and Dosage

Glucosamine is used for osteoarthritis and other joint diseases. The recommended dosage is 1,500 mg/d. It may take 2 weeks to realize the positive effect.

Adverse Reactions and Drug Interactions

Glucosamine can cause drowsiness, headache, abdominal pain, constipation, diarrhea, epigastric discomfort, and nausea. There are no known drug interactions. Glucosamine contains sodium, so care needs to be used in a patient with sodium restrictions.

Kava

Action and Proof of Efficacy

Kava inhibits the limbic system, suppressing emotional excitability and mood enhancement. Randomized, controlled clinical trials of kava use with anxiety provide some reasonable support for its use, but there are no clinical comparison trials with existing anxiolytics.

Uses and Dosage

Kava has been used to treat anxiety disorders. The recommended dosage is 100 mg three times per day.

Adverse Reactions and Drug Interactions

Kava can cause headaches, dizziness, and disturbances in visual accommodation. Alcohol can increase kava's activity. Central nervous system (CNS) depressants can cause an additive sedative effect. Taken together, levodopa and kava can cause an increase in parkinsonian symptoms. Absorption of kava is increased if it is taken with food. Kava increases the effects of alcohol.

Melatonin

Action and Proof of Efficacy

Melatonin release corresponds to periods of sleep. Studies have proven melatonin to be safe and effective for the short-term prevention of jet lag.

Uses and Dosage

Melatonin is used to prevent and treat jet lag and sleeping disturbances. The recommended dosage for sleeping disturbances is 5 mg at bedtime. The recommended dosage for jet lag is 5 mg/d for 3 days before departure and ending 3 days after departure.

Adverse Reactions and Interactions

Melatonin can cause altered sleep patterns, confusion, headache, hypothermia, sedation, tachycardia, hypertension, hyperglycemia, and pruritus. Interactions include increased anxiolytic action when taken with benzodiazepines.

Omega-3s/Fish Oil

Action and Proof of Efficacy

Omega-3s promote the relaxation and contraction of muscles, blood clotting, digestion, cell division, and the growth and movement of calcium and other substances in and out of cells. It also decreases inflammation and platelet aggregation.

Uses and Dosages

Omega-3s are primarily used to decrease triglyceride levels and slow the growth of atherosclerotic plaques. There is research being done to look at the effect of omega-3s on diabetes mellitus, rheumatoid arthritis, systemic lupus erythematosus, and osteoporosis. The recommended dosage is 1 to 6 g/d.

Adverse Reactions and Interactions

Omega-3s can cause gastrointestinal (GI) upset, including diarrhea, heartburn, and abdominal bloating. In high doses, they can interfere with blood thinners and antihypertensives.

Probiotics

Action and Proof of Efficacy

Probiotics are nonpathologic bacteria that reside in the GI tract. They help maintain a healthy balance of organisms in the intestines, promote binding of enterocytes within the GI tract, and prevent harmful bacteria from attaching to these cells.

Uses and Dosage

Probiotics are commonly used to restore normal oral, GI, and vaginal flora. They treat diarrhea, urinary tract infections, vaginitis, and irritable bowel syndrome. They may be used to manage atopic dermatitis in children. They are potentially useful in patients taking antibiotics because the normal flora may be disturbed by the bactericidal or bacteriostatic activity of the drug. Further, patients with *Candida* and bacterial infections may have an imbalance of normal flora. The recommended dosage is 1 capsule of 10 colony-forming units per day.

Adverse Reactions

Adverse reactions are GI related, primarily flatulence. Warfarin's efficacy may be reduced because acidophilus may enhance the intestinal absorption of vitamin K.

Saw Palmetto

Action and Proof of Efficacy

Saw palmetto inhibits the production of enzymes responsible for converting testosterone to more reactive dihydrotestosterone (DHT). Saw palmetto blocks the binding of DHT to prostate cells, inhibiting enlargement. Studies have shown a decrease in symptoms in patients with noncancerous enlargement of the prostate. Saw palmetto also increases urine flow and improves emptying of the bladder.

Uses and Dosage

Saw palmetto is used to treat benign prostatic hyperplasia (BPH). (See Chapter 33 for more information on BPH.) The recommended dosage is 320 mg daily.

Adverse Reactions and Drug Interactions

Adverse reactions include headache, hypertension, constipation, diarrhea, decreased libido, and back pain. There are no known drug interactions.

St. John's Wort

Actions and Proof of Efficacy

St. John's wort is a monoamine oxidase (MAO) inhibitor. It inhibits reuptake of serotonin, noradrenaline, adrenaline, and dopamine. Numerous studies of St. John's wort in patients with depressive disorders have shown that it is more effective than placebo and as effective as antidepressants; however, these studies had many flaws, and more studies need to be done.

Uses and Dosage

St. John's wort is used to treat depression, anxiety, and neuralgic pain. The recommended dosage is 100 to 500 mg daily.

Adverse Reactions and Drug Interactions

St. John's wort can cause dizziness, restlessness, sleep disturbances, dry mouth, constipation, GI distress, and photosensitivity. Drug interactions include an increase in MAO inhibition activity when taken with alcohol, MAO inhibitors, narcotics, and OTC cold and flu medicines. There is a decrease in levels of digoxin and cyclosporine. Serotonin syndrome may develop when used concurrently with amphetamines, selective serotonin reuptake inhibitors, trazodone, and tricyclic antidepressants.

Valerian

Actions and Proof of Efficacy

Valerian binds to gamma-aminobutyric acid alpha-receptor sites in the brain and CNS. It acts in a competitive action with any benzodiazepine. In nine randomized, placebo-controlled, double-blind studies in which valerian was used as a treatment for sleep disorders, some studies showed effectiveness but others showed none (Hadley & Petry, 2003).

Uses and Dosage

Valerian is used for insomnia, anxiety, and stress. The recommended dosages are 200 to 500 mg at bedtime for insomnia and 200 to 300 mg two times per day for anxiety.

Adverse Reactions and Drug Interactions

Valerian can cause excitability, blurred vision, and nausea. There are additive effects with alcohol and CNS depressants.

RECOMMENDING DIETARY SUPPLEMENTS

When recommending dietary supplements, the practitioner must be aware of several key points. The patient must be educated on the use of alternative therapies. Discussions and recommendations must be documented. The provider and patient must be aware of potential interactions.

INCREASING AWARENESS

Since the use of CAM is increasing, health care providers must be aware of the different modalities. At each visit, the patient should be asked about the use of OTC medications, vitamins, and supplements. The health care provider should check whether there are any interactions between medications and supplements.

Patients who choose to use CAM can be directed to reliable providers and reliable dietary supplements. NCCAM is an excellent source of information for both the patient and provider and can be accessed on the Internet (www.nccam.nih.gov) or by phone (1-888-644-6226).

CASE STUDY*

L.L. is a 67-year-old male who has been diagnosed with BPH. He is having difficulty with urination. He is currently on Cozaar 100 mg for HTN and his BP is well controlled. He is taking no other medications. The doctor has recommended medication for his BPH, but he would like to try a herbal supplement before taking a prescription medication.

1. What herbal supplement would he take?
2. What is the recommended dosage?
3. What are possible side effects of the herbal supplement?
4. What warnings should you give L.L. before he starts the herbal supplement.

* Answers can be found online.

Bibliography

Starred references are cited in the text

*Bailey, R. L., Gahche, J. J., Lentino, C. V., et al. (2011) Dietary supplement use in the United States, 2003–2006. *Journal of Nutrition, 141*(2), 261–266.

Black, L. I., Clarke, T. C., Barnes, P. M., et al. (2015). Use of complementary health approaches among children aged 4–17 years in the United States: National Health Interview Survey, 2007–2012. *National Health Statistics Report: No. 78.* Hyattsville, MD: National Center for Health Statistics.

Charlson, M. (2012). Complementary and alternative medicine. In L. Goldman (Ed.), *Goldman's Cecil medicine* (24th ed.). Philadelphia, PA: Saunders Elsevier.

*Clarke, T. C., Black, L. I., Stussman, B. J., et al. (2015). Trends in the use of complementary health approaches among adults: United States 2002–2012. *National Health Statistics Report: No. 78.* Hyattsville, MD: National Center for Health Statistics.

DerMarderosian, A., Liberti, L., Beutler, J. A., et al. (Eds.). (2008). *The review of natural products* (5th ed.). St. Louis, MO: Wolters Kluwer Health.

Gilmour, J., Harrison, C., Cohen, M. H., et al. (2011). Pediatric use of complementary and alternative medicine: Legal, ethical, and clinical issues in decision-making. *Pediatrics, 128*(Suppl. 4), S149–S154.

*Hadley, S., & Petry, J. J. (2003). Valerian. *American Family Physician, 67*(8), 1755–1758.

Hutchins, A. M., Brown, B. D., Cunnane, S. C., et al. (2013). Daily flaxseed consumption improves glycemic control in obese men and women with pre-diabetes: A randomized study. *Nutrition Research, 33*(5), 367–375.

*Karsch-Völk, M., Barrett, B., Kiefer, D., et al. (2014). Echinacea for preventing and treating the common cold. *Cochrane Database of Systematic Reviews, 2*(13), 1–90.

Loverr, E., & Ganta, N. (2010). Herbs and nutraceuticals: Tips for primary care providers. *Primary Care: Clinics in Office Practice, 37*(1), 13–30.

10 Pharmacogenomics

Isabelle Mercier ▪ Andrew M. Peterson ▪ Amalia M. Issa

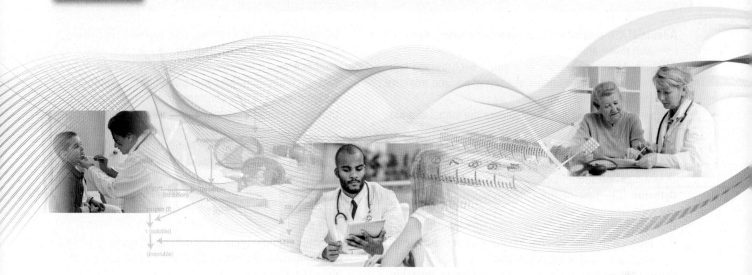

PHARMACOGENOMICS AND PERSONALIZED MEDICINE

Interpatient variability in drug therapy response is a well-known pharmacotherapeutic concept. Indeed, as far back as 1892, William Osler is reputed to have said "if it were not for the great variability among individuals, medicine might be a science and not an art" (Golden, 2004). In addition to factors such as age, sex, drug–drug interactions, and comorbidities, genetics also is known to play a role in interpatient variability of drug response.

The ability of genetic variability (inherited differences) to influence therapeutic drug response is the basis of pharmacogenetics and pharmacogenomics. Generally, **pharmacogenetics** refers to single or a few gene variations (called polymorphisms), whereas **pharmacogenomics** refers more broadly to the genome-wide (or an individual's entire DNA sequence) effects on drug therapy. **Personalized medicine** is a more recently coined term that includes pharmacogenetics/pharmacogenomics and refers to "an emerging practice of medicine that uses an individual's genetic profile to guide decisions made in regard to the prevention, diagnosis, and treatment of disease" (National Human Genome Research Institute, 2015) according to the National Institutes of Health (NIH). This term is now evolving to be "precision medicine."

We can think of pharmacogenomics as the basic science of personalized medicine, and indeed, much of the progress that has been made in the field of personalized medicine to date has been largely focused on pharmacogenomics.

This chapter is geared toward future clinicians, particularly nurse practitioners and physician assistants, to provide them with an overview of pharmacogenomics, the current state of the science, including some pertinent examples, some relevant applications, and promises, pitfalls, and policy implications.

BASIC CONCEPTS

Because pharmacogenomics is rooted in genetics, it is helpful to review some basic genetic concepts. Several of the definitions of key terms that are associated with genetics and pharmacogenomics can be found in **Box 10.1**.

The human genome is the underpinning to every human's individuality. With the exception of identical twins, the genome is different for every individual, though in the grand scheme of things there are only small differences among people's DNA that make us unique. The human genome consists of approximately 3 billion base pairs, 99.9% of which are the same among all humans with only 0.1% variation among individuals. The variations that occur with DNA (**polymorphisms**), along with environmental and dietary factors, create a patient's individuality, susceptibility to disease, and response to treatments. Included in this individuality is a person's ability to absorb, distribute, metabolize, and excrete drugs. Understanding the genetic components affecting these pharmacokinetic processes can help the clinician tailor treatment for a patient.

Each human has 23 pairs of **chromosomes**—22 are autosomal and look the same in males and females, and 1 pair is the sex chromosome, in which females have two X chromosomes and males have an X and a Y chromosome (**Figure 10.1**). These chromosomes reside in the nucleus of a cell (**Figure 10.2**). Each chromosome is composed of DNA, which carries the genetic information for the individual. Each chromosome can have hundreds or thousands of genes; it is estimated that there are more than 25,000 genes on the human genome. However, genes only make up about 1% of the total DNA found in humans.

Genes function to produce proteins involved in the millions of biological processes that support the function of

BOX 10.1 Definitions

Adenine (A)—One of the four nucleotide bases. Pairs with thymine

Alleles—Multiple versions of a gene. Each person typically inherits two alleles of each gene, one from the mother and one from the father.

Biomarkers—Molecules that indicate the status of a biological process

Chromosome—The organized structure of DNA and proteins, the "double helix." It contains genes and nucleotide sequences.

Cytosine (C)—One of the four nucleotide bases. Pairs with guanine

DNA (deoxyribonucleic acid)—A nucleic acid that contains genetic information and/or instructions used in the function of living organisms

Exon is the portion of a gene that codes for amino acids

Gene—A sequence of DNA that codes for a type of protein or RNA, serving a particular function in a cell

Genome—All of the genetic material in chromosomes of an organism

Guanine (G)—One of the four nucleotide bases. Pairs with cytosine

Haplotype—A combination of alleles. A haplotype may be a single locus of alleles, multiple loci, or even an entire chromosome.

Nucleotide—Molecules that make up the structural units of DNA and RNA. The four DNA nucleotides are adenine, cytosine, guanine, and thymine. For RNA, uracil is substituted for thymine.

Personalized medicine—A more recently coined term that includes pharmacogenetics/pharmacogenomics and refers to "an emerging practice of medicine that uses an individual's genetic profile to guide decisions made in regard to the prevention, diagnosis, and treatment of disease" (National Human Genome Research Institute, 2015).

Pharmacogenetics refers to the study of inherited differences in single gene variations (called polymorphisms) or a few genes, in drug metabolism and response.

Pharmacogenomics refers to the effects of genome-wide (or an individual's entire DNA sequence) effects on drug therapy.

Polymorphism—DNA sequence variation

RNA (ribonucleic acid)—A nucleic acid that carries genetic information and produces proteins used in the function of living organisms

SNPs (single nucleotide polymorphism)—A DNA sequence variation occurring when a single nucleotide differs between members of a species

Thymine (T)—One of the four nucleotide bases. Pairs with adenine

Wild type—The normal, as opposed to the mutant, gene, or allele

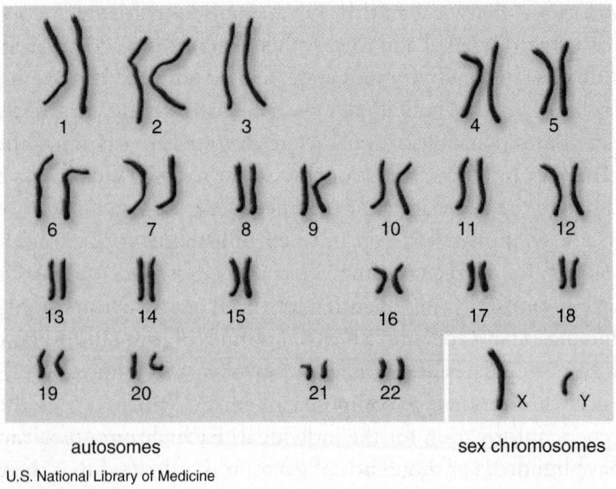

autosomes   sex chromosomes

U.S. National Library of Medicine

FIGURE 10.1   Human chromosomes. (Source: Genetics Home Reference [Internet] National Library of Medicine 2010. Retrieved from http://ghr.nlm.nih.gov/handbook/basics/howmanychromosomes. Cited December 30, 2010.)

the body every day. Genes that mutate or malfunction can have profound effects on the body. In the case in which a single gene mutates or malfunctions, the result is a monogenic disease, such as sickle cell anemia or cystic fibrosis. In most cases, however, there are multiple genes involved in the disease process. These are referred to as polygenic disorders.

Polygenic disorders may appear as a single clinical disorder but at the molecular level have multiple **biomarkers**. Biomarkers are molecules that indicate the status of a biological process. Examples of biomarkers include prostate-specific antigen (PSA) for prostate cancer or blood glucose level for diabetes. Genetic biomarkers, specific DNA sequences, are also being discovered.

The building blocks of DNA are the four **nucleotide** bases, including the two purines—**adenine** (A) and **guanine** (G)—and the two pyrimidines—**thymine** (T) and **cytosine** (C). DNA strands are linked through base pairing of the pyrimidines with the purines (A with T, G with C), conceptually forming the well-known double helix (see **Figure 10.2**). The arrangement of these base pairs along each chromosome is

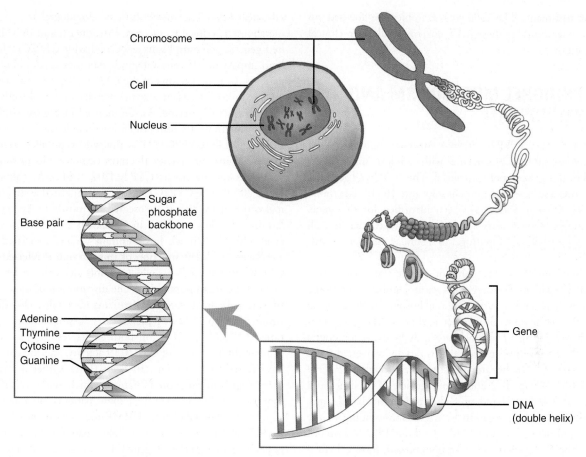

FIGURE 10.2   Relationship among human cell, chromosome, genes, and DNA.

called the *DNA sequence*. Variations in the base pairings range from **single nucleotide polymorphisms**, insertions or deletions of a nucleotide base, to changes in the number of copies of genes. These variations can alter the production or function of proteins, thus creating the variation in the expression of a disease or the response to drug therapy.

Single Nucleotide Polymorphisms

An SNP is a variation in the DNA sequence that differs between members of a species or paired chromosomes in an individual. For example, the following are two sequenced DNA fragments from different individuals: AAGCTA and AAGTTA. Note the only difference between these sequences is the substitution of thymidine (T) for cytosine (C). In this case, there are two versions (or **alleles**) of this gene. Each person typically inherits two alleles of each gene: one from the mother and one from the father. There can be up to 10 million SNPs in humans, but only those SNPs on coding regions of the gene or the area of the DNA responsible for turning genes on or off have an effect on humans. This concept of SNPs and differing alleles is important in the study of pharmacogenomics, as many of the genes responsible for drug activity and metabolism (e.g., cytochrome P-450 [CYP]) have different alleles on the same gene, producing different metabolic effects.

CLINICAL APPLICATIONS OF PHARMACOGENOMICS

A major current issue in medical care is that many therapies given to patients to treat their diseases (e.g., cardiovascular, cancer, diabetes) are misaligned with the patient's genetic makeup. There are two main consequences that directly result from this lack of molecular knowledge at the time of drug treatment: (1) patients can be given a therapy that inefficiently treats the underlying cause of the disease (lack of therapeutic effect) and (2) patients can be given a medication that can lead to adverse drug reactions (ADRs) that can be harmful or even fatal due to a difference in their genetic makeup. Clinicians and health care professionals must understand and acknowledge that some patients could be genetically predisposed to respond differently to a given drug. This genetic information should then be utilized to assure tailored therapy and safety.

The main organ involved in detoxification/metabolism of drugs is the liver. The cytochrome P-450 (CYP) superfamilies of liver enzymes are key players in drug metabolism as they are directly involved in the modification and processing of approximately 75% of all medications taken (Di, 2014; Guengerich, 2004). The impact of genetic modifications in these CYP enzymes has therefore an important impact on patient treatment. The following examples are focused on genetic alterations in these CYP enzymes and their clinical implications.

CLOPIDOGREL METABOLISM AND POLYMORPHISM

The P-450 2C19 (CYP2C19) liver enzyme is one of the best characterized P-450 isoenzyme with clinical implications linked to this genetic polymorphism. The *CYP2C19* gene has nine **exons** and is situated on chromosome 10. To date, more than 30 different SNPs have been identified for this gene. Interestingly, several years ago, reports emerged that not all patients metabolized clopidrogel in a similar manner, regardless of their age or weight.

Clopidogrel is a very common medication that is prescribed to patients undergoing acute coronary syndrome (ACS). When patients arrive at the hospital with a partial coronary obstruction, antiplatelet agents are the gold standard in preventing irreversible cardiac ischemia. Clopidogrel is given as an inactive prodrug that is rapidly converted to its active metabolite via hepatic bioactivation through CYP2C19 enzymes (see Chapters 2 and 3 for a review of prodrugs and biotransformation). Clopidogrel inhibits ADP-mediated platelet activation and aggregation by irreversibly binding to the platelet purinergic receptor P2RY12. About 15% of clopidogrel is modified into an active compound and 85% is hydrolyzed to inactive forms to be excreted.

Due to its potent nature, a timely intervention with these pharmacological agents is essential in preventing further blockage and death making dosage key in attaining efficacious and safe treatment. The metabolism of clopidogrel to its active metabolite is critical to successful treatment, and thus, inherited genetic polymorphisms associated with *CYP2C19* have a high impact on the physiological responses to clopidogrel in patients. Genetic variants of the *CYP2C19* gene result in normal, reduced, or absent enzyme activity or can directly lead to an overactive enzyme. As summarized in **Figure 10.3**, different mutations are responsible for these levels of enzymatic activity. While CYP2C19*1 is the **wild-type** allele resulting in normal enzyme activity, the most common loss-of-function variant is referred to as CYP2C19*2 (681G>A) (Shuldiner et al., 2009). The CYP2C19*2 allele is inherited as an autosomal codominant trait that cosegregates mostly to Asian population and is less common in Caucasian and Africans (Scott et al., 2011). A much less common variant associated with a reduced or absent function of this enzyme is referred to as CYP2C19*3 (636G>A), which is only detected in less than 10% of the Asian population. The distribution of these mutations in patients dictates how patients metabolize clopidogrel. Around 2% to 15% of patients carry loss-of-function mutations (*2/*2,*2/*3,*3/*3) on both alleles resulting in significantly reduced or lack of CYP2C19 activity, and these patients are referred to as poor metabolizers (PM). Other individuals carry a gain-of-function mutation, which makes CYP2C19 more active (*1/*17,*17/*17); these patients are referred to as ultrarapid metabolizers (URM) and consist of about 5% to 30% of patient populations. Most patients, however, have either a normal *CYP2C19* gene (*1/*1) without any mutations called extensive metabolizers (EM) or those with only one loss-of-function allele (*1/*2,*1/*3) are referred to as intermediate metabolizers (IM). Both EMs and IMs consist of 35% to 50% and 18% to 45% of a given population, respectively.

FIGURE 10.3 Clopidogrel therapy and CYP2C19.

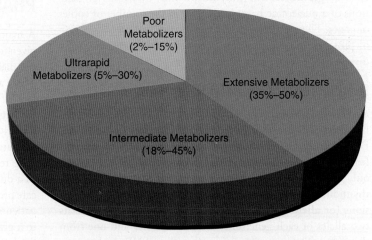

■ Normal Enzyme Activity: *1/*1 (wild-type alleles) no detected mutations

■ Intermediate Enzyme Activity: *1/*2 or *1/*3 one wild-type allele (*1) paired with an allele with decreased activity *2 (681G>A) or *3 (636G>A)

■ Normal or Increased Enzyme Activity: *1/*17 or *17/*17 enhanced activity allele *17 (−806C>T) with or without a wild-type allele *1

▥ Low or Absent Enzyme Activity: Combination of mutated alleles *2/*2, *2/*3 or *3/*3 resulting in a poor metabolizer phenotype

Warfarin Metabolism and Polymorphism

Warfarin is a commonly prescribed blood thinner used to prevent atrial fibrillation–induced strokes, as well as permanent damage following the onset of venous thromboembolism or pulmonary embolism. Warfarin exists as a racemic mixture of R-warfarin and S-warfarin (Qayyum et al., 2015). S-warfarin possesses the most anticoagulant properties through its action as a vitamin K antagonist. Vitamin K plays a crucial role in the coagulation cascade as its reduced form acts as a cofactor of γ-glutamyl carboxylase, an important enzyme that renders the coagulation factors II, VII, IX, and X functional through postribosomal synthesis (**Figure 10.4**). Importantly, in order for the coagulation cascade to be fully active, vitamin K needs to be in its reduced form. This is accomplished by an upstream enzyme called vitamin K epoxide reductase complex, subunit 1 (VKORC1). VKORC1 is the therapeutic target of warfarin and its inhibition results in decreased amounts of reduced vitamin K preventing coagulation factors from being activated (**Figure 10.4**) (Pan et al., 2015). Once its therapeutic window is achieved, S-warfarin is rapidly metabolized through the P-450 liver enzyme CYP2C9 to its inactive oxidized form (7-hydroxy warfarin). The rate at which S-warfarin is metabolized is highly dependent on the enzymatic activity of CYP2C9. As one might expect, a less efficient metabolism and clearance of warfarin could lead to accumulation of its active form systemically leading to sustained anticoagulation effects. Indeed, several incidents have been reported where accidental deaths have occurred due to excessive bleeding following warfarin

treatment. It was later discovered that some patients do not have a fully functional CYP2C9 enzyme due to alleles containing mutations, preventing the proper inactivation of the potent S-warfarin. There are two main CYP2C9 SNPs found in patients, *2 (R144C) and *3 (I359L), and *1 is referred to as the wild-type allele without mutations. The CYP2C9*1 individuals possess normal enzyme activity while CYP2C9*2 carriers exhibit a 30% decrease in activity and CYP2C9*3 patients have as much as 90% decrease in their enzymatic activity. Patients can carry two normal copies *1/*1, a normal copy and a polymorphic *1/*2, or could have both copies with polymorphism *2/*3. Clinical implication will be discussed below. The target enzyme VKORC1 has also shown the presence of inactivating mutation, the most common being -1639G>A.

Genetic Testing

The active metabolite of clopidogrel dictates its therapeutic efficacy. Therefore, the extent to which patients are capable of effectively producing these active metabolites through their liver CYP2C19 enzymes is directly linked to their treatment success and recovery from an ACS. In the case of clopidogrel, the PM are those who could benefit the most from genetic testing prior to therapy, as stated on package inserts and as suggested by the U.S. Food and Drug Administration (FDA). These PM are incapable of producing the active metabolite of clopidogrel and would suffer from an unsuccessful treatment of their coronary blockage. The Clinical Pharmacogenetics Implementation Consortium (CPIC) also recommends

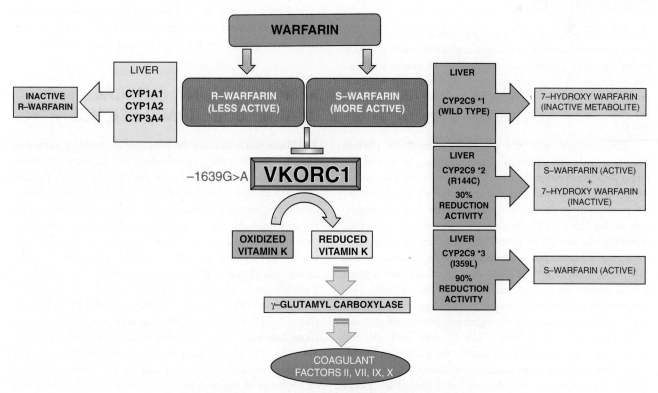

FIGURE 10.4 Warfarin therapy and VKORC1/CYP2C9 polymorphism.

special attention be given to URM and that alternative therapies be used in PM to treat their coronary obstruction (Scott et al., 2011). In addition, IM are also challenging to treat with clopidogrel as these patients have a higher number of residual platelets, which could lead to adverse cardiovascular outcomes (Shirasaka et al., 2015) and might also benefit from other forms of therapy.

For patients receiving warfarin treatment, genetic testing is recommended in order to predict which patients are carrying these mutations who would be at higher risk of bleeding (Maluso, 2015). For example, those that carry the VKORC1 mutation 1639 G>A produce less VKORC1 (referred to as A haplotype) than those with the regular G allele (G haplotype). Consequently, the A haplotype individual would require less warfarin to inhibit VKORC1 to produce similar anticoagulant effects. The same is true for patients that carry CYP2C9 *2 and *3 where the active form of warfarin does not go through clearance normally leading to immediate excessive bleeding. As a consequence, the therapeutic index of this blood thinner is extremely narrow and needs to be carefully assessed. Genetic testing is thus highly suggested to assess those patients that are genetically predisposed to metabolize clopidogrel and warfarin differently. Genetic testing offers a knowledge of this genetic information ahead of time to predict the efficacy of these life-saving drugs and guide the therapeutic window toward more successful therapy.

PROMISES, PITFALLS, AND POLICY IMPLICATIONS

In addition to pharmacogenomics, progress is being made with newer technologies such as next-generation sequencing (NGS) including whole genome sequencing (WGS), exome sequencing, and targeted RNA sequencing. Collectively, the rapid scientific developments are leading to a number of implications for policy, including both opportunities and challenges (Issa, 2015).

Pharmacogenomics and personalized medicine provide both economic opportunities and challenges. The cost of different pharmacogenomic tests continues to decline and there is increasing evidence for cost-effectiveness of pharmacogenomics, particularly its potential to reduce ADRs. It is also important to consider how pharmacogenomics might increase costs, including the storage of genetic samples, resources for computational analysis, and interpretation of the findings. While electronic health records (EHRs) and clinical decision support (CDS) systems are getting better and more user-friendly, they are generally not yet well equipped for the large amount of data that are being generated by the increasing amount of genomic information, particularly from WGS. In order for EHRs and CDS systems to become more useful for the greater implementation of pharmacogenomics and personalized medicine, a substantive investment in computational and clinical laboratory infrastructure has to be made at a national level.

Biobanks and handling of DNA samples present both scientific opportunities and policy challenges for regulatory agencies worldwide. Efforts to establish best practices and address regulation of processing, storage, and uses of samples are being undertaken by a number of national and international regulatory agencies including the FDA, the European Medicines Agency (EMA), Japan's Pharmaceuticals and Medical Devices Agency (PMDA), and Health Canada. One promising opportunity is that these agencies are working toward global harmonization of standards for the use of pharmacogenomic tests and targeted therapeutics.

Another area that is broadly presenting policy challenges involves ethical, legal, and social issues (ELSI) such as patient privacy and protection of data and genetic samples, return of results obtained within the context of research studies to patients, and decisions related to the use of genomic information and insurance coverage. Aimed at protecting Americans from future genetic discrimination, the *Genetic Information Nondiscrimination Act* (GINA) was passed in 2008 (GINA, 2008). However, a number of ELSI issues related to privacy and protection of genetic data remain to be addressed by legislators and policymakers. Issues surrounding education of health care providers and other stakeholders are also increasingly presenting barriers and challenges to the full implementation of pharmacogenomics. A number of studies have concluded that there remains a serious lack of knowledge of genetics and genomics on the part of clinicians. Steps are increasingly being taken to address the educational needs of current and future health care providers. Pharmacogenomics is being incorporated in the curricula of medical and pharmacy schools. Guidelines for clinical competencies in genetics and genomics have been proposed for physician assistants (Rackover et al., 2007) and PA students and others would benefit from reviewing the guidelines.

KEEPING UP WITH CLINICAL PHARMACOGENOMIC SCIENCE

The above discussion on the educational needs for future clinicians, including nurse practitioners and physician assistants, brings us to discuss how nurse practitioner or PA students can keep up with the state of science and clinical practice in pharmacogenomics. Although this is a rapidly evolving and fast-moving field, there are some resources that students and clinicians should be aware of and consult on a regular basis. Currently, there are over 150 U.S. FDA–approved drugs that incorporate pharmacogenomic information in the label (http://www.fda.gov/drugs/scienceresearch/researchareas/pharmacogenetics/ucm083378.htm). In addition to the FDA Web site and the FDA's "Table of Pharmacogenomic Biomarkers in Drug Labeling," there are other useful Web sites. For example, the DailyMed project (http://dailymed.nlm.nih.gov/dailymed/index.cfm), administered by the National Library of Medicine of the National Institutes of Health (NIH), provides detailed information about "package inserts" of many

CASE STUDY*

J.T. suffers from an irregular heart beat called atrial fibril-lation. On a Sunday afternoon, his wife noticed as J.T. was watching the football game on television that his face started to droop and his speech seemed abnormal. She asked him to smile and his smile was all of sudden very uneven. After he arrives at the hospital, it is determined he is having a stroke as a consequence of his atrial fibrillation.

1. The therapy of choice for J.T. in this particular case is warfarin. However, following a few hours of warfa-rin therapy, J.T.' wife noticed several bruises appear-ing under his skin that seemed to be coming out of nowhere. From a genetic standpoint, what could be happening to J.T.?
   a. He could have a mutation in his liver CYP2C19 enzyme causing a 90% decrease in warfarin clear-ance leaving more S-warfarin in his blood causing excessive bleeding.
   b. He could have a mutation in his liver CYP2C9 enzyme causing a 90% decrease in warfarin clear-ance leaving more S-warfarin in his blood causing excessive bleeding.
   c. He could have a mutation in his liver CYP2C9 enzyme causing a 90% decrease in warfarin clearance leaving more R-warfarin in his blood causing excessive bleeding.
   d. He could have a mutation in his liver CYP1A1 enzyme causing a 90% decrease in warfarin clear-ance leaving more S-warfarin in his blood causing excessive bleeding.

2. Following genetic testing, it was discovered that J.T. can metabolize warfarin perfectly through his liver as all his CYP enzymes came back normal (no mutations). Which of the following options could thus explain his excessive bleeding?
   a. J.T. is A haplotype for VKORC1.
   b. J.T. is G haplotype for VKORC1.
   c. J.T. is T haplotype for VKORC1.
   d. J.T. is C haplotype for VKORC1.

3. Knowing J.T. genetic testing results, what should be done concerning the dose of warfarin?
   a. A lower dose should be given.
   b. A higher dose should be given.
   c. No change in the dosage is necessary.
   d. No warfarin should be given to J.T. in the first place.

* Answers can be found online.

prescription drugs, including pharmacogenomic information. The DailyMed Web site is user-friendly and has a powerful search engine, making it easy to navigate (National Library of Medicine, Daily Med Project).

The NIH also maintains the clinicaltrials.gov (National Library of Medicine, 2000) Web site, which is a mandatory listing of all clinical trials being conducted and this Web site includes information on the purpose of the clinical trial, the study's eligibility requirements, sites where the clinical study is being conducted, the status of patient recruitment and enroll-ment, and contact information for the investigators. Although clinicaltrials.gov is not restricted to pharmacogenomics and includes all ongoing trials, it is possible to search for pharma-cogenomic studies, thereby allowing clinicians opportunities to learn more about the latest in clinical pharmacogenomic research, and possibly provide their patients with opportuni-ties to enroll in specific trials.

CONCLUSION

In summary, among the most promising applications of phar-macogenomics is the potential to minimize or prevent ADRs. Progress has been made in the clinical implementation of phar-macogenomics, with several molecular companion diagnostics paired with targeted therapeutics. Many other biomarkers are currently being tested to predict response to therapies.

However, to date, the implementation of pharmacogenomics into clinical practice has presented with various ELSI and pol-icy challenges.

Bibliography

*Starred references are cited in the text.
*ClinicalTrials.gov. Bethesda, MD: National Library of Medicine (US). (2000). Retrieved from clinicaltrials.gov on April 22, 2015.
*Di, L. (2014). The role of drug metabolizing enzymes in clearance. *Expert Opinion on Drug Metabolism & Toxicology, 10*(3), 379–393.
*Genetic Information Nondiscrimination Act of 2008, Public Law 110–233, Stat. 122 (2008).
*Golden, R. (2004). A history of William Osler's The principles and practice of medicine. Osler Library studies in the history of medicine. No. 8. Montreal: McGill University.
*Guengerich, F. P. (2004). Cytochrome P450: What have we learned and what are the future issues? *Drug Metabolism Reviews, 36*(2), 159–197.
*Issa, A. M. (2015). Ten years of personalizing medicine: How the incorpora-tion of genomic information is changing practice and policy. *Personalized Medicine, 12*(1): 1–3.
*Maluso, A. (2015). Pharmacogenomic Testing and Warfarin Management. *Oncology Nursing Forum, 42*(5), 563–565.
*National Human Genome Research Institute. "All About The Human Genome Project (HGP)". Retrieved from http://www.genome.gov/Education/ on April 22, 2015.
*National Library of Medicine (US). Daily Med project. Retrieved from http://dailymed.nlm.nih.gov/dailymed/index.cfm on April 22, 2015.
National Library of Medicine (US). (2013). Genetics Home Reference. Bethesda, MD: The Library. Retrieved from http://ghr.nlm.nih.gov/ on April 22, 2015.

*Pan, Y., Cheng, R., Li, Z., et al. (2015). PGWD: Integrating personal genome for warfarin dosing. *Interdisciplinary Sciences* [Epub ahead of print].

*Qayyum, A., Najmi, M. H., Khan, A. M., et al. (2015). Determination of S- and R-warfarin enantiomers by using modified HPLC method. *Pakistan Journal Pharmaceutical Science*, *28*(4), 1315–1321.

*Rackover, M., Goldgar, C., Wolpert, C., et al. (2007). Establishing essential physician assistant clinical competencies guidelines for genetics and genomics. *Journal of Physician Assistant Education*, *18*(2), 47–48.

*Scott, S. A., Sangkuhl, K., Gardner, E. E., et al. (2011). Clinical Pharmacogenetics Implementation Consortium guidelines for cytochrome P450-2C19 (CYP2C19) genotype and clopidogrel therapy. *Clinical Pharmacology Therapeutics*, *90*(2), 328–332. doi: 10.1038/clpt.2011.132.

*Shirasaka, Y., Chaudhry, A. S., McDonald, M., et al. (2015). Interindividual variability of CYP2C19-catalyzed drug metabolism due to differences in gene diplotypes and cytochrome P450 oxidoreductase content. *Pharmacogenomics Journal*. doi: 10.1038/tpj.2015.58 [Epub ahead of print].

*Shuldiner, A. R., O'Connell, J. R., Bliden, K. P., et al. (2009). Association of cytochrome P450 2C19 genotype with the antiplatelet effect and clinical efficacy of clopidogrel therapy. *The Journal of the American Medical Association*, *302*(8), 849–857. doi: 10.1001/jama.2009.1232.

*US Food and Drug Administration Table of Pharmacogenomic Biomarkers in Drug Labels. Retrieved from http://www.fda.gov/Drugs/ScienceResearch/ResearchAreas/Pharmacogenetics/ucm083378.htm on April 22, 2015.

UNIT 2

Pharmacotherapy for Skin Disorders

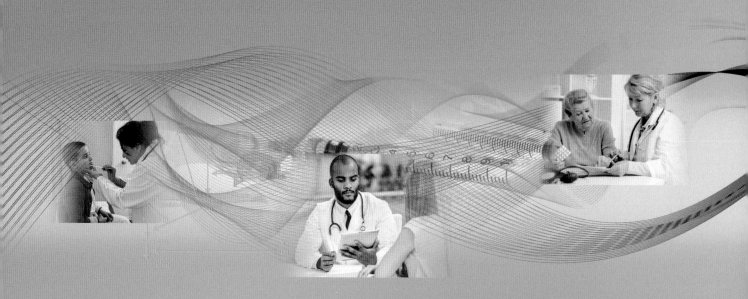

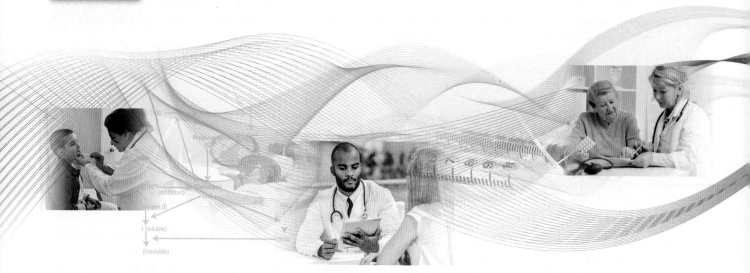

11 Contact Dermatitis

Virginia P. Arcangelo

Dermatitis is an alteration in skin reactivity caused by exposure to an external agent. It is a combination of genetic and environmental factors. It can occur after a single exposure or multiple exposures to an agent or in response to an allergen. The resulting dermatitis usually appears as an inflammatory process. According to the American Academy of Dermatology, contact dermatitis is a common problem and results in approximately 5.7 million visits to health care providers each year. Almost any substance can be a potential irritant. Diaper dermatitis (sometimes called *diaper rash*) is the most common form of irritant contact dermatitis (ICD) in childhood.

CAUSES

Two types of contact dermatitis are irritant and allergic dermatitis. ICD results from exposure to any agent that has a toxic effect on the skin. *Allergic* contact dermatitis (ACD) results from exposure to an antigen that causes an immunologic response. Atopic dermatitis (eczema), a form of allergic dermatitis characterized as a pruritic, chronic inflammatory condition, affects between 5% and 10% of the population in the United States (Goodheart, 2008). It most often begins in childhood.

PATHOPHYSIOLOGY

ICD is not an allergic response. It is a result of damage to the water–protein–lipid matrix of the outer layer of skin. It appears as an erythematous, scaly eruption resulting from friction, exposure to a chemical, or a thermal injury. The severity of the reaction depends on the condition of the skin, the concentration

and the toxicity of the irritant, and the length of exposure. The reaction appears only in the area exposed to the irritant.

ACD (e.g., poison ivy) is an immunologically mediated response to an allergen (antigen). During the initial sensitization phase, the host is immunized to the allergen. After reexposure, a more rapid and potent secondary immune response occurs. The second phase manifests in ACD, and T cells are key mediators of the reaction. On activation, T cells release cytokines, chemokines, and cytotoxins, causing stimulation of local blood vessels; recruitment of immune cells, such as macrophages and eosinophils; and subsequent amplification of the sensitization response. Within 5 to 7 days after sensitization, there is visual evidence of the response. On subsequent exposures, however, dermatitis may develop within 6 to 18 hours. Hypersensitivity can occur after one exposure or after years of repeated exposures. Contact dermatitis may spread extensively beyond the area of contact.

In atopic dermatitis, there are high concentrations of serum immunoglobulin (Ig) E, decreased numbers of immunoregulatory T cells, defective antibody-dependent cellular cytotoxicity, and decreased cell-mediated immunity. The pathogenesis of atopic dermatitis involves genetic factors, skin barrier defects, and immune dysregulation. The genetics of atopic dermatitis is an area of intense research and plays a significant role in IgE production and allergic sensitization. More recently, the association of atopic dermatitis with filaggrin (FLG) gene mutations suggests the role of skin barrier defects in the pathogenesis of atopic dermatitis. FLG is a protein essential to the normal barrier function of the skin. Deficiency in FLG may contribute to the physical barrier defects in atopic dermatitis and predispose patients to increased transepidermal water loss, infection, and inflammation associated with the exposure of cutaneous immune cells to allergens.

155

PHARMACOGENOMICS

A genetic basis for atopic dermatitis has long been recognized with a family history of disease as a risk factor. Before characterization of the human genome, heritability studies combined with family-based linkage studies supported the definition of atopic dermatitis as a complex trait in which interactions between genes and environmental factors and the interplay between multiple genes contribute to disease manifestation. The gene encoding FLG has been most consistently replicated as associated with atopic dermatitis. Most gene studies to date have focused on adaptive and innate immune response genes, but there is increasing interest in skin barrier dysfunction genes (Barnes, 2010).

DIAGNOSTIC CRITERIA

ICD and ACD appear as linear streaks of papules, vesicles, and blisters that are very pruritic. In ICD, the lesions are found only in the area of exposure to the irritant. In ACD, the lesions are usually more diffuse, and they may present over an underlying area of edema.

Lesions in atopic dermatitis include papules, erythema, excoriations, and lichenification. In infants, the face, chest, legs, and arms are the most commonly involved areas; lesions are scaly and red and may be crusted patches and plaques. In children, the most common sites are the antecubital and popliteal fossae, the neck, wrists, ankles, eyelids, scalp, and behind the ears. Lesions are usually lichenified because of constant scratching. In adults, the neck, antecubital and popliteal fossae, face, wrist, and forearms are the most commonly involved areas. Lesions may appear as poorly defined, pruritic, erythematous papules and plaques. This may present specific therapeutic opportunities; however, at this time, maintaining a normal epidermal barrier is key.

INITIATING DRUG THERAPY

The most effective form of treatment for contact dermatitis is prevention. The patient must become aware of the causes or triggers and plan ways to avoid them. Before initiating therapy, the practitioner first needs to determine the severity of the problem. If the symptoms are mild, cool compresses may offer relief, and baths with colloidal oatmeal may offer relief from pruritus. Compresses of Burow solution are effective for drying the vesicles and bullae that may be associated with contact dermatitis. If these treatments fail or if the dermatitis is more extensive, drug therapy is initiated.

Before initiating drug therapy, delivery of the drug to the skin, protection/barrier function, and cosmetic acceptability must be considered. Ointment and gels offer the best delivery and protection barrier. Creams are less greasy but less effective. Lotions are dilute creams. Solutions are alcohol-based liquids and are useful for treating the scalp because they do not coat the hair.

Moisturizers used generously and frequently increase skin hydration, and their lipid component improves the damaged skin barrier. Lipid-rich moisturizers both prevent and treat ICD.

Barrier creams containing dimethicone or perfluoropolyethers, cotton liners, and softened fabrics help to prevent ICD.

Goals of Drug Therapy

The goals of drug therapy for dermatitis are as follows:

- Restoration of a normal epidermal barrier
- Treatment of inflammation of skin
- Control of itching

The mainstays of therapy for contact dermatitis are topical corticosteroids. There are also topical immunosuppressives available. Systemic corticosteroids are recommended for widespread symptoms, and antihistamines are used for relieving intense pruritus.

For mild or moderate localized dermatitis, topical corticosteroids applied twice daily are usually effective within a few days and should be continued for 2 weeks. Lower-potency agents should be applied to the face and intertriginous areas, and higher-potency steroids should be reserved for the extremities and torso. Topical calcineurin inhibitors (e.g., tacrolimus or pimecrolimus) may be used as an alternative to low-potency topical corticosteroids in chronic ICD.

Emollients or occlusive dressings may improve barrier repair in dry, lichenified skin. Traditional petrolatum-based emollients are accessible and inexpensive, and they have been shown to be as effective as an emollient containing skin-related lipids. To relieve pruritus, a lotion of camphor, menthol, and hydrocortisone (Sarnol-HC) is soothing, drying, and antipruritic. Pramoxine, a topical anesthetic in a lotion base (Prax), can also relieve pruritus.

Topical Corticosteroids

Topical steroidal therapy is safer than systemic steroidal therapy. Steroidal agents are effective for smaller outbreaks. Because of their anti-inflammatory and antimitotic actions, they reduce inflammation and the buildup of scale.

Topical corticosteroids are classified according to potency (**Table 11.1**), with the fluorinated agents being more potent. Ideally, the least potent topical corticosteroid should be used for the shortest possible time in treating dermatitis. Topical corticosteroids should be avoided if there are additional bacterial, viral, or fungal skin infections, and they are not recommended for prophylaxis.

Dosage

Treatment may be initiated with an intermediate- or high-potency topical corticosteroid. A lower-potency corticosteroid may be used after the symptoms subside. As a rule, short-term therapy with more potent topical corticosteroids is preferred to longer-term therapy with less potent corticosteroids. Low-potency corticosteroids should be used in the facial and intertriginous regions because fluorinated and high-potency

TABLE 11.1

Classification of Topical Corticosteroids by Potency

Low Potency	Intermediate Potency	High Potency	Very High Potency
alclometasone dipropionate 0.05% (Aclovate—c, o)	betamethasone valerate 0.12% (Luxiq foam)	amcinonide 0.1% (Cyclocort—c, l, o)	betamethasone dipropionate augmented 0.05% (Diprolene—o, g)
fluocinolone acetonide 0.01% (Synalar—s)	desonide 0.05% (DesOwen—c, l, o, Tridesilon—c, o)	betamethasone dipropionate augmented 0.05% (Diprolene AF—emollient cream, Diprolene—lotion)	clobetasol propionate 0.05% (Temovate—c, g, o, scalp preparation, Temovate-E—emollient cream, Clobex, Cormax, Olux)
hydrocortisone base or acetate 0.5% (Cortisporin—c, Mantadil—c)	desoximetasone 0.05% (Topicort LP—emollient cream)	desoximetasone 0.05% (Topicort—g)	
hydrocortisone base or acetate 1% (Cortisporin—o, Hytone [1% or 2.5%]—c, l, o, Proctocort—c, Vytone—c)	fluocinolone acetonide 0.025% (Synalar—c, o)	desoximetasone 0.25% (Topicort—emollient cream, o)	diflorasone diacetate 0.05% (Psorcon—o)
	flurandrenolide 0.025% or 0.05% (Cordran SP—c, Cordran—o)	diflorasone diacetate 0.05% (Florone—o, Psorcon—c)	fluocinonide 0.1% (Vanos—c)
triamcinolone acetonide 0.025% (Aristocort—c, Aristocort A—c, Kenalog—c, l, o)	fluticasone propionate 0.005% or 0.05% (Cutivate—o 0.005%, c 0.05%)	fluocinonide 0.05% (Lidex—c, g, o, s, Lidex-E—emollient cream)	flurandrenolide 4 mcg/sq c (Cordran tape)
	hydrocortisone butyrate 0.1% (Pandel—c)	halcinonide 0.1% (Halog—c, o, s, Halog-E—emollient cream)	halobetasol propionate 0.05% (Ultravate—c, o)
	hydrocortisone butyrate 0.1% (Locoid—c, o, s)	triamcinolone acetonide 0.5% (Aristocort—c, o, Aristocort A—c, Kenalog—c)	
	hydrocortisone valerate 0.2% (Westcort—c, o)		
	mometasone furoate 0.1% (Elocon—c, o, l)		
	prednicarbate 0.1% (Dermatop—emollient cream)		
	triamcinolone acetonide 0.1% (Aristocort—c, o, Aristocort A—c, o, Kenalog—c, o)		
	triamcinolone acetonide 0.2% (Kenalog—aerosol)		

c, cream; l, lotion; o, ointment; g, gel; s, solution.

corticosteroids applied to the face may cause atrophy of the tissue or trigger steroidal rosacea. If it is necessary to use either type of agent, use should be limited to a very brief time. The maximum recommended length of treatment with topical corticosteroids is 2 weeks for adults and 1 week for children.

Preparations

Topical corticosteroids are available in creams, ointments, lotions, gels, solutions, or sprays. Creams are the most desirable because they are not as obvious when applied. They are, however, water based, which causes more skin drying. Ointments and gels are the most potent and the most lubricating, and they have occlusive properties. In areas with large amounts of hair or widespread dermatitis, lotions, gels, spray products, and solutions are easiest to apply. Occlusion by a dressing of an area of a topical corticosteroid application increases hydration and hence penetration, thereby enhancing efficacy.

Correct Usage

Tolerance to a topical corticosteroid is common. To prevent this, chronic use is not recommended. Using the topical corticosteroid preparation only in the case of recurrence of contact

dermatitis, and not prophylactically, or prescribing intermittent dosing (e.g., every 4 days) may be effective methods of controlling tolerance.

Application

Penetration of a topical corticosteroid is enhanced when the skin is hydrated. This can be accomplished by moistening the skin before application or by using an occlusive dressing constructed from a material such as a plastic shower cap (for the scalp), gloves (for hands), or plastic wrap or a sock (on other extremities).

Adverse Events

Although topical corticosteroids are relatively safe to use, some adverse events may occur (**Table 11.2**). The prolonged use of fluorinated corticosteroids on the face can cause atrophy and acne-like eruptions. This usually is seen after therapy stops and may last for several months. With prolonged use, ecchymoses may develop on the arms in elderly patients. Moreover, epidermal atrophy, manifested by striae; shiny, thin skin; or telangiectases, can occur with prolonged use, or a hypersensitivity reaction may occur, usually in response to the vehicle in which the medication is delivered. Frequent and prolonged

TABLE 11.2

Topical Corticosteroids Used for Contact Dermatitis: Selected Adverse Events and Special Considerations

	Selected Adverse Events	Special Considerations
See Table 11.1 for listing of topical corticosteroids by potency.	Skin irritation Acneiform lesions Striae Skin atrophy Burning Irritation Pruritus Erythema Folliculitis	Applying to moist skin and covering with occlusive dressing increase efficacy except with very high–potency topical corticosteroids Can cause or intensify cataracts or glaucoma if used near eyes Use lowest potency on thin/atrophic skin and children. Pregnancy category C

Topical Immunosuppressants
pimecrolimus (Elidel) 1%
tacrolimus (Protopic) 0.03%, 0.1%
    Apply a light layer BID
    For use in children age 2 years and older
	Skin burning
	Pruritus
	Flu-like symptoms
	Erythema
		Do not use with occlusive dressing.
		Apply for 1 week after clearing.
		Pregnancy category C
		Not recommended for children under age 2

use of topical corticosteroids in fold areas can cause atrophy, telangiectasia, or striae, and their use on the face can also cause steroid rosacea. Topical corticosteroids can potentiate or cause cataract formation or glaucoma when used around the eyes for prolonged periods.

Systemic Corticosteroids

If the dermatitis is widespread or resistant to treatment with topical steroidal preparations, oral corticosteroids may be used. Systemic corticosteroids inhibit cytokine and mediator release, attenuate mucus secretion, upregulate beta-adrenergic receptors, inhibit IgE synthesis, decrease microvascular permeability, and suppress the influx of inflammatory cells and the inflammatory process.

Systemic corticosteroids are prescribed in a tapering dose schedule. The starting dose of 1 mg/kg is decreased by 5 mg every 2 days for 2 to 3 weeks. The entire dose of steroids can be taken at the same time in the morning. This will minimize sleep disturbances. Taking the corticosteroids for less than 2 weeks may cause rebound dermatitis, especially with poison ivy. If dermatitis flares up during the tapering, the dosage can be increased and tapered again.

Although these medications are readily absorbed when taken orally, peak plasma concentrations are not achieved for 1 to 2 hours. For more information about systemic corticosteroids, refer to Chapter 25.

Contraindications

Because they suppress the immune response, systemic corticosteroids are contraindicated in patients with systemic mycoses and in patients receiving a vaccination. These drugs also should be used cautiously in people with tuberculosis, hypothyroidism, cirrhosis, renal insufficiency, hypertension, osteoporosis, and diabetes mellitus.

Adverse Events

Systemic corticosteroids mask infection. In short-term use, they may cause gastrointestinal upset. Mood changes (hyperactivity, anxiety, depression) may be evident and sleep disturbances may occur, especially if medication is taken late in the day. The effects of systemic corticosteroids may be decreased if they are administered with barbiturates, hydantoins, or rifampin.

Topical Immunosuppressives

Topical immunosuppressives act on T cells by suppressing cytokine transcription. These agents are used in patients with moderate to severe atopic dermatitis who cannot tolerate topical steroids or are not responsive to other treatments or where there is a concern for topical steroid–induced atrophy. Because they do not cause skin atrophy, these medications are especially useful for the treatment of atopic dermatitis involving the face, including the periocular and perioral areas.

Tacrolimus and pimecrolimus are the preparations currently available. They are applied twice a day until the lesions clear and then for an additional 7 days. The skin is dried before application.

Contraindications

Care should be used when administering these drugs with drugs in the CYP3A family. The drugs should not be used under occlusive dressings.

Adverse Effects

There can be transient burning and pruritus, which disappear with continued use. The concomitant ingestion of alcohol can cause redness and flushing. Sun protection is recommended.

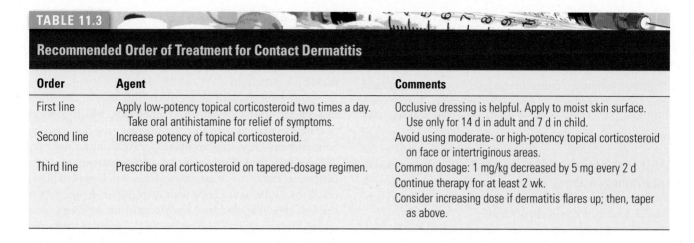

TABLE 11.3

Recommended Order of Treatment for Contact Dermatitis

Order	Agent	Comments
First line	Apply low-potency topical corticosteroid two times a day. Take oral antihistamine for relief of symptoms.	Occlusive dressing is helpful. Apply to moist skin surface. Use only for 14 d in adult and 7 d in child.
Second line	Increase potency of topical corticosteroid.	Avoid using moderate- or high-potency topical corticosteroid on face or intertriginous areas.
Third line	Prescribe oral corticosteroid on tapered-dosage regimen.	Common dosage: 1 mg/kg decreased by 5 mg every 2 d. Continue therapy for at least 2 wk. Consider increasing dose if dermatitis flares up; then, taper as above.

Antihistamines

Antihistamines are used to relieve pruritus associated with contact dermatitis. The best time to use them is before bed to promote sleep because the main side effect is drowsiness. Antihistamines are discussed in Chapter 47.

Selecting the Most Appropriate Agent

In contact and atopic dermatitis, topical corticosteroids are the first line of therapy (see **Table 11.1**). These agents are for short-term use. The recommended treatment order is listed in **Table 11.3**.

First-Line Therapy

A topical corticosteroid preparation with low to intermediate potency applied twice a day is the appropriate first-line therapy. If improvement does not occur, a higher-potency topical corticosteroid may be tried rather than increasing the time of administration of the lower-potency agent. Occlusive dressings and application to moist skin may be efficacious in treating the acute phase. Low-potency topical corticosteroids are used on the face and intertriginous areas. Oral antihistamines are used to relieve pruritus and reduce the response to the cause.

Second-Line Therapy

Second-line therapy calls for a more potent topical corticosteroid. Topical immunosuppressants are another consideration for second-line therapy.

Third-Line Therapy

Systemic corticosteroids are useful for treating widespread dermatitis. They are given on a tapered-dose schedule. The recommended dose is 1 mg/kg, with the dose decreased every 2 days for at least 2 weeks and up to 3 weeks. If a flare-up occurs during the tapering, the dosage can be increased again. When treating severe poison ivy, for example, oral corticosteroids are continued for 2 to 3 weeks to prevent rebound dermatitis, which may occur if therapy is discontinued before that time.

Figure 11.1 provides an algorithm of contact dermatitis treatment.

Special Populations

Pediatric

Topical corticosteroids should be used for only 7 days in children younger than age 6 and at the lowest potency. Topical corticosteroids can cause atrophy of the skin. Topical immunosuppressants

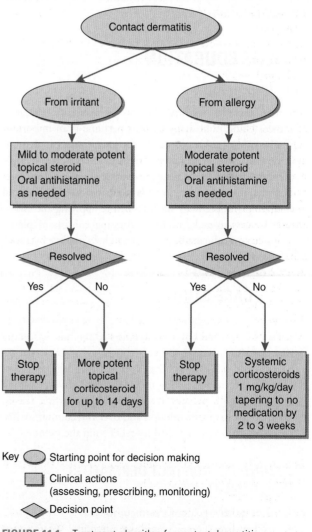

FIGURE 11.1 Treatment algorithm for contact dermatitis.

are considered only for patients age 2 and older. Topical immunosuppressants will not cause atrophy of the skin.

Geriatric

The most common causes of contact dermatitis in elderly patients are topical medications (e.g., neomycin [Myciguent]) and the bases of other topical medications. The adhesives on adhesive patches may also cause contact dermatitis. The rash of contact dermatitis does not present in a classic pattern in the elderly. Instead of vesicles or inflammation, the area exposed to the irritant may simply become scaly. Topical corticosteroids can cause atrophy of the skin in elderly people, which is a problem because their skin is already friable.

MONITORING PATIENT RESPONSE

The response to therapy is monitored by visual examination of the affected parts of the anatomy and the reported resolution of symptoms. The patient should return for follow-up evaluation within 2 or 3 days of initiation of therapy. If a bacterial infection recurs secondary to contact dermatitis, it may be treated as discussed in Chapter 14.

PATIENT EDUCATION

Drug Information

Education includes teaching patients to avoid the causative substance. Using mild soaps without perfume is an important preventive measure. As appropriate, the practitioner can demonstrate how to apply topical preparations to moist skin and apply an occlusive dressing to increase the efficacy of topical corticosteroids. Penetration of topical steroids is enhanced 10- to 100-fold by hydrating (moistening) the area before applying the medication. An easy-to-make occlusive dressing consists of plastic wrap applied over the medicated area and held in place by a sock or tape. On the hands, a glove can act as an occlusive dressing. On the head area, a shower cap can be used.

Occlusive dressings should not be used with topical immunosuppressants. The patient should avoid alcohol and should use sunscreen.

Most patients with atopic dermatitis require hydration through the liberal use of bland emollients, which serve to hydrate the stratum corneum and maintain the lipid barrier. Sufficient emollients applied liberally several times a day may be enough to significantly reduce the disease activity of atopic dermatitis. Parents of infants and toddlers should apply a bland emollient to the entire body with each diaper change. Older children should apply bland emollients in the morning, after school, and at bedtime. Bathing should be limited to brief, cool showers once daily. Soap, which dries and irritates the skin, should be avoided, but gentle lipid-free cleansers are beneficial.

Skin hydration is best accomplished through daily soaking baths for 10 to 20 minutes. It is important to remind patients and caregivers to apply a topical medication or moisturizer immediately after bathing. This is to seal in the water that has been absorbed into the skin and to prevent evaporation that can lead to further drying of the skin.

Complementary and Alternative Medicine

Some supplements are thought to be helpful in atopic dermatitis. Ginkgo biloba antagonizes platelet-aggregating factors, a key chemical mediator in atopic dermatitis. Zinc can be used at a dosage of 50 mg/day until the condition clears. Use of fish oil supplements incorporates omega-3 fatty acids into the membrane phospholipid pools.

Recommendations for supplements are as follows:

- Vitamin A 50,000 international units daily
- Vitamin E 400 international units daily
- Zinc 50 mg daily, to be decreased as the condition clears
- EPA 540 mg and DHA 360 mg daily or flaxseed oil 10 g daily
- Evening primrose oil 3,000 mg daily

CASE STUDY*

J. F., a 15-year-old boy who weighs 110 pounds, is seeking treatment for a very itchy rash consisting of linear streaks of papules, vesicles, and blisters on his arms, legs, and face. He tells you he was hiking in the woods 2 days ago along trails lined with patches of shiny weeds with three leaves. He tried using calamine lotion and over-the-counter hydrocortisone cream but has had no relief from the itching.

DIAGNOSIS: CONTACT DERMATITIS (POISON IVY)

1. List specific goals of treatment for J. F.
2. What drug therapy would you prescribe? Why?
3. What are the parameters for monitoring the success of the therapy?
4. Discuss specific patient education based on the prescribed therapy.
5. List one or two adverse reactions for the selected agent that would cause you to change therapy.
6. What would be the choice for second-line therapy?
7. What over-the-counter and alternative medications would be appropriate for J. F.?
8. What lifestyle changes would you recommend to J. F.?
9. Describe one or two drug–drug or drug–food interactions for the selected agent.

* Answers can be found online.

Bibliography

Starred references are cited in the text.

Baeck, M., & Goossens, A. Systemic contact dermatitis to corticosteroids. *Allergy, 67*(12), 1580–1585.

*Barnes, K. (2010). Update on genetics of atopic dermatitis: Scratching the surface in 2009. *Journal of Allergy and Clinical Immunology, 125*(1), 16–29.

Friedman, P. S., Sanchez-Elsner, T., & Schnuch, A. (2015). Genetic factors in susceptibility to contact sensitivity. *Contact Dermatitis, 72*(5), 263–274.

Fyhrquist-Vanni, N., Alenius, H., & Lauerma, A. (2007). Contact dermatitis. *Dermatology Clinics, 25*(4), 613–623.

*Goodheart, H. P. (2008). *A photoguide of common skin disorders: Diagnosis and management* (3rd ed.). Philadelphia, PA: Lippincott Williams & Wilkins.

Jung, T., & Stingl, G. (2008). Atopic dermatitis: Therapeutic concepts evolving from new pathophysiological insights. *Journal of Allergy and Clinical Immunology, 122*(6), 1074–1081.

Lee, J., & Bielory, A. (2010). Complementary and alternative interventions in atopic dermatitis. *Immunology and Allergy Clinics of North America, 30*(3), 411–424.

Ong, P., & Baguniewicz, M. (2008). Atopic dermatitis. *Primary Care: Clinics in Office Practice, 35*(1), 105–107.

Peroni, A., Colato, C., Schena, D., et al. (2010). Urticarial lesions: If not urticarial what else? The differential diagnosis of urticaria. *Journal of the American Academy of Dermatology, 62*(4), 541–555.

Piliang, M. (2009). Atopic dermatitis. In W. Carey (Ed.), *Cleveland Clinics: Current clinical medicine*. Philadelphia, PA: Saunders Elsevier.

Scalf, L. (2007). Contact dermatitis: Diagnosing and treating skin conditions in the elderly. *Geriatrics, 62*(6), 14–19.

Taylor, J., & Amado, A. (2009). Contact dermatitis and related conditions. In W. Carey (Ed.), *Cleveland Clinics: Current clinical medicine*. Philadelphia, PA: Saunders Elsevier.

12

Fungal Infections of the Skin

Virginia P. Arcangelo

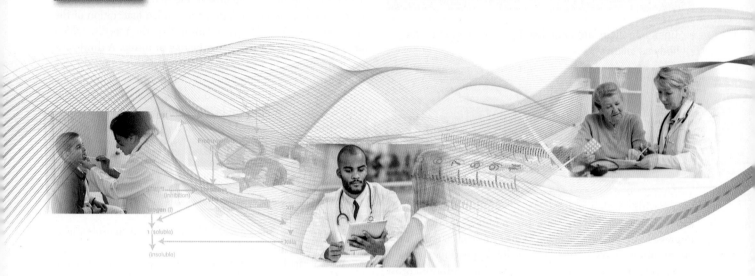

Fungi live in the dead, horny outer layer of the skin. The organisms penetrate only the stratum corneum—the surface layer of the skin—and infect the skin, hair, and nails. They cause tinea, tinea versicolor, and candidiasis.

TINEA

Dermatophytes are a group of fungi that infect nonviable keratinized cutaneous tissues. Dermatophytosis, more commonly called *tinea*, is a condition caused by dermatophytes. Tinea is further classified by the location of the infection (**Box 12.1**).

Tinea capitis primarily affects children ages 3 to 9. This age group may also be infected with tinea corporis. *Tinea pedis* most commonly affects the adolescent population and young adults. Immunocompromised patients have an increased incidence and more intractable dermatophytosis. *Tinea unguium*, infection of the nails, is also called *onychomycosis*. It is caused by various yeast, fungi, and molds.

CAUSES

General factors that predispose to fungal infections include warm, moist, occluded environments, family history, and a compromised immune system. Infection is spread from person to person by animals, especially cats and dogs, and by inanimate objects.

PATHOPHYSIOLOGY

Dermatophytes grow only on or within keratinized structures. Most infections result from five specific species of fungus: *Trichophyton rubrum*, *Trichophyton tonsurans*, *Trichophyton*

mentagrophytes, *Microsporum canis*, and *Epidermophyton floccosum*. These can be found on humans, on animals, and in the soil. They produce enzymes (keratinases) that allow them to digest keratin, causing epidermal scale; thickened, crumbly nails; or hair loss.

DIAGNOSTIC CRITERIA

General symptoms of fungal infections in hair and skin include pruritus, burning, and stinging of the scalp or skin. An inflammatory dermal reaction may cause erythema and vesicles. Diagnosis is confirmed by several mechanisms. One mechanism is microscopic evaluation of the stratum corneum with 10% potassium hydroxide (KOH) preparation. At the margin of the lesion, scale is scraped with a No. 15 knife blade and placed on a slide. KOH is then added and the slide inspected under the microscope. Fungi appear as rod-shaped filaments with branching.

Another mechanism for diagnosis is the fungal culture. A specimen of infected tissue is applied to a dermatophyte test medium on an agar plate. If the infecting organism is a fungus, the plate will change color—from yellow to pink or red—in approximately 2 weeks.

A third diagnostic method involves using a Wood lamp, which produces a bright green fluorescence in the presence of a tinea infection caused by *Microsporum* species. A major disadvantage of this test is that other fungal infections may be undiagnosed because the Wood lamp test identifies only *Microsporum*.

Tinea Capitis

Presentation of tinea capitis varies widely. There may be generalized, diffuse seborrheic dermatitis-like scalp scaling, although more common signs and symptoms include impetigo-like

Tinea infections are identified by their location on the body as follows:

- Head: tinea capitis
- Body: tinea corporis
- Hand: tinea manus
- Foot: tinea pedis
- Groin: tinea cruris
- Nails: tinea unguium (onychomycosis)

lesions with crusting and redness, areas of hair loss with broken hairs, and possibly inflammatory nodules. Although often impressive, cervical lymphadenitis does not correlate with the extent of scalp inflammation. Finally, approximately 15% of patients have a cross-infection with tinea corporis. Most cases of tinea capitis are found in prepubertal children, with a disproportionate amount in African Americans. It is very contagious.

Most cases (90%) are caused by *T. tonsurans*. *Microsporum audouinii*, spread from human to human, and *M. canis*, spread from animals, are other organisms.

Tinea capitis presents in several ways:

- Inflamed, scaly, alopecic patches, especially in infants
- Diffuse scaling with multiple round areas with alopecia secondary to broken hair shafts, leaving residual black stumps
- "Gray patch" type with round, scaly plaques of alopecia in which the hair shaft is broken off close to the surface
- Tender, pustular nodules

Tinea Corporis

Tinea corporis is called "ringworm" when it affects the face, limbs, or trunk, but not the groin, hands, or feet. The typical presentation of tinea corporis is a ring-shaped lesion with well-demarcated margins, central clearing, and a scaly, erythematous border. It is caused by contact with infected animals, by human-to-human transmission, and from infected mats in wrestling. The organisms responsible are *M. canis*, *T. rubrum*, and *T. mentagrophytes*.

Tinea Cruris

Tinea cruris is often referred to as *jock itch*. A fungal infection of the groin and inguinal folds, tinea cruris spares the scrotum. The most common causes are *T. rubrum* or *E. floccosum*. Typically, the lesion borders are well demarcated and peripherally spreading. The lesions are large, erythematous, and macular, with a central clearing. A hallmark of tinea cruris is pruritus or a burning sensation. There is often an accompanying fungal infection of the feet.

Tinea Pedis

Interdigital tinea pedis, commonly called *athlete's foot*, is characterized by scaling and itching in the web spaces between the toes and sometimes denudation and sodden maceration of the skin. Another variation is inflammatory tinea pedis, which presents with vesicles involving the toes or instep. A third variety is the moccasin style, which presents with itching, chronic noninflammatory scaling, and thickness and cracking of the epidermis on the sole, heel, and often up the side of the foot. This is a common problem in young men.

Most cases are caused by *T. rubrum*, which evokes a minimal inflammatory response. The *T. mentagrophytes* organism produces vesicles and bullae.

There are three types of tinea pedis:

- Interdigital, which presents as scaling, maceration, and fissures between the toes
- Plantar, which presents as diffuse scaling of the soles, usually on the entire plantar surface
- Acute vesicular, which presents as vesicles and bullae on the sole of the foot, the great toe, and the instep

Tinea Manus

Tinea manus is a dermatophyte infection of the hand. This is always associated with tinea pedis and is usually unilateral. The lesions are marked by mild, diffuse scaling of the palmar skin, and vesicles may be grouped on the palms or fingernails involved.

Tinea Unguium

Tinea unguium (onychomycosis) is a fungal infection of the nail. Typically affected are the toenails, which become thick and scaly with subungual debris. Onycholysis, a separation of the nail from the nail bed, may be seen. The infection usually begins distally at the tip of the toe and moves proximally and through the nail plate, producing a yellowish discoloration and striations in the actual nail. Under the nail, a hyperkeratotic substance accumulates that lifts the nail up. If untreated, the nail thickens and turns yellowish brown. Onychomycosis is usually asymptomatic but can act as a portal of entry for a more serious bacterial infection.

Organisms causing onychomycosis include dermatophytes, *E. floccosum*, *T. rubrum*, *T. mentagrophytes*, *Candida albicans*, *Aspergillus*, *Fusarium*, and *Scopulariopsis*.

Some health insurance plans refuse to reimburse for drug therapy without confirmation of the diagnosis. Tests that verify the diagnosis include the KOH test and culture.

INITIATING DRUG THERAPY

Fungal infections can be prevented by applying powder containing miconazole (Monistat) or tolnaftate (Tinactin) to areas prone to fungal infections after bathing. The areas can be dried completely with a hair dryer on low heat.

Goals of Drug Therapy

Pharmacologic therapy is directed against the offending fungus and the site of infection. Therapy is topical or systemic, depending on the location of the lesion. Topical therapy is used for most skin infections. The exceptions are tinea capitis and tinea unguium (onychomycosis).

Topical Azole Antifungals

Topical azoles (**Table 12.1**) impair the synthesis of ergosterol, the main sterol of fungal cell membranes. This allows for increased permeability and leakage of cellular components and results in cell death. Topical azoles are fungicides that are effective against tinea corporis, tinea cruris, and tinea pedis as well as cutaneous candidiasis. They should be applied once or twice a day for 2 to 4 weeks. Therapy should continue for 1 week after the lesions clear. However, therapy is not recommended during pregnancy or lactation and is administered cautiously in hepatocellular failure. Ketoconazole (Nizoral), in particular, should be avoided in patients with sulfite sensitivity. Adverse effects include pruritus, irritation, and stinging.

Topical Allylamine Antifungals

These agents are effective against dermatophyte infections but have limited effectiveness against yeast. Patients treated with these agents may undergo a shorter treatment period with less likelihood of relapse. Topical allylamines are applied twice daily. Potential side effects include burning and irritation.

TABLE 12.1

Overview of Antifungal Medications

Generic (Trade) Name and Dosage	Selected Adverse Events	Contraindications	Special Considerations
Topical Agents			
clotrimazole ointment (Lotrimin), powder (Desenex). Gently massage ointment into affected and surrounding skin areas bid × 4 wk; powder as needed.	Erythema, irritation, stinging, pruritus	Pregnancy or lactation Use cautiously in patients with hepatocellular failure	May be purchased OTC
miconazole (Micatin, Monistat Derm). Cover affected areas with cream lotion or powder bid for 2–4 wk.	Irritation, maceration	Pregnancy or lactation	Avoid applying near eyes.
ketoconazole (Nizoral). Apply to affected and surrounding areas once daily for 2–4 wk.	Irritation, stinging, pruritus	Asthma Not administered to people who are sensitive to sulfites Pregnancy or lactation	Not recommended in children
oxiconazole (Oxistat). Apply to affected and surrounding areas one to two times daily for 2–4 wk.	Pruritus, burning	Pregnancy or lactation	Avoid applying near eyes or mucous membranes.
sulconazole (Exelderm). Apply to affected and surrounding areas bid × 4 wk.	Pruritus, burning sensation, erythema	Pregnancy or lactation	Not recommended in children Avoid contact with eyes.
ciclopirox (Loprox). Apply to affected area bid × 4 wk.	Pruritus, burning sensation		Not recommended in children younger than age 10 Lotion formulation good for nails Avoid occlusive dressing.
naftifine (Naftin). Apply to affected area once daily × 4 wk	Burning, stinging, dryness, erythema, itching		Not recommended in children Avoid occlusive dressings. Avoid contact with mucous membranes.
terbinafine (Lamisil). Apply to affected area bid × 4 wk.	Burning, irritation, skin exfoliation, dryness		Not recommended in children Avoid occlusive dressings. Avoid contact with mucous membranes.
tolnaftate (Tinactin). Apply small amount bid × 4 wk.	Stinging, burning, irritation		Not recommended in children younger than age 2
selenium sulfide (Selsun) 1% (OTC), 2.5%. Massage into affected area, rest 15 min, and rinse thoroughly	Irritation, hair loss		
nystatin (Mycostatin) 100,000 units/mL. Infants: 1 mL each side of mouth Adults: 2–3 mL each side of mouth	GI upset, oral irritation		Continue use for at least 48 h after clinical cure. Keep in mouth as long as possible before swallowing.

(Continued)

TABLE 12.1

Overview of Antifungal Medications (*Continued*)

Generic (Trade) Name and Dosage	Selected Adverse Events	Contraindications	Special Considerations
Oral Agents			

griseofulvin (Grifulvin V)
    Microsize:
    Adult 500–1,000 mg
    Child 10–15 mg/kg/d
    Ultramicrosize:
    Adult: 330–660 mg
    Child: 10 g/kg/d
	Headaches, nausea, vomiting, diarrhea, photosensitivity	Pregnancy
		Patients with porphyria or hepatic failure
			Ultramicrosize particle increases absorption.
			Prescribe with caution to patients who are sensitive to penicillin.
			Drug is most effective when taken with a high-fat meal.
			Drug is well tolerated in young children.
			Monitor complete blood count and LFT with long-term use. Drug use may aggravate lupus erythematosus.
			Use with alcohol produces antabuse-like effects.
			Drug interactions: antagonizes oral contraceptives and warfarin and is antagonized by barbiturates

ketoconazole (Nizoral) 200 mg/d	Nausea, vomiting, abdominal pain, urticaria, pruritus	Do not use with other drugs metabolized by CYP3A.	Not recommended in children
itraconazole (Sporanox) 200 mg/d	GI upset, rash, fatigue, headache, dizziness, edema	Do not use with other drugs metabolized by CYP3A	Not recommended in children May use pulse dosing Remains in nails for 4–5 mo Ingestion of food increases absorption.
terbinafine (Lamisil) 62.5–250 mg/d	GI disturbance, LFT abnormalities, urticaria, pruritus	Liver or renal disease	Not recommended in children

fluconazole (Diflucan)
    Adults: 100–200 mg/d
    Children: 3–6 mg/kg/d
	GI disturbance, headache, rash, hepatotoxicity		Decrease dose if creatinine clearance <50 mL/min.
			Drug interactions: potentiates warfarin, theophylline, oral hypoglycemics.
			May increase serum levels of phenytoin, cyclosporine.
			Thiazides increase fluconazole levels.
			May decrease effect of oral contraceptives

CYP3A, cytochrome P-450 enzyme 3A; GI, gastrointestinal; LFT, liver function tests; OTC, over the counter.

Griseofulvin

Mechanism of Action

Griseofulvin is a fungistatic that deposits in keratin precursor cells, increasing new keratin resistance to fungal invasion.

Adverse Events

Adverse effects include nausea, vomiting, diarrhea, headache, or photosensitivity. Evaluation of renal, hepatic, and hematopoietic systems is recommended before initiating therapy, particularly because this drug may aggravate lupus erythematosus.

Interactions

Griseofulvin increases levels of warfarin (Coumadin) and decreases levels of barbiturates and cyclosporine (Sandimmune). It may decrease the efficacy of oral contraceptives and may cause a serious and unpleasant reaction with alcohol. Patients should be advised not to drink beverages or any other preparation containing alcohol while taking the drug.

Systemic Allylamine Antifungals

Terbinafine (Lamisil) is a synthetic allylamine derivative that inhibits squalene epoxidase, a key enzyme in fungal biosynthesis. This causes a deficiency of ergosterol causing fungal cell death. It is used in the treatment of onychomycosis.

Dosage

For fingernail onychomycosis, the dose is 250 mg/d for 6 weeks; toenail onychomycosis requires 250 mg/d for 12 weeks.

Adverse Events

Adverse events include diarrhea, dyspepsia, rash, increase in liver enzymes, and headache. Evaluation of alanine aminotransferase (ALT) and aspartate aminotransferase (AST) levels is recommended before starting therapy and at 6 to 8 weeks into therapy if it is long-term because it can cause liver failure, although this is rare.

Interactions

Terbinafine is potentiated by cimetidine (Tagamet) and antagonized by rifampin (Rifadin). Cyclosporine levels should be monitored when the patient is taking both cyclosporine and terbinafine.

Systemic Azole Antifungals

Systemic azoles inhibit cytochrome P-450 (CYP) enzymes and fungal 14-α-demethylase, inhibiting synthesis of ergosterol. Systemic therapy is required for tinea capitis and tinea unguium. Itraconazole (Sporanox), a systemic azole, has a high affinity for keratin and is lipophilic, which causes high levels to accumulate in the hair and nail. It has a long half-life, so pulse dosing, in which periods of drug therapy are alternated with periods without therapy, is feasible.

Dosage

The dosage of itraconazole is 200 mg once daily for 12 weeks for toenail infection. For fingernail infection, the dose is 200 mg twice daily for 1 week, then 3 weeks off, and repeat dosing with 200 mg twice daily for 1 week. The drug is not recommended for children, and ingestion of food increases absorption.

The dosage of fluconazole is usually 200 mg on the first day and then 100 mg each day for at least 2 weeks. For children, it is 6 mg/kg/d on day 1 and then 3 mg/kg/d.

Contraindications

A systemic azole should not be given with drugs metabolized by the CYP3A enzyme, including β-hydroxy-β-methylglutaryl coenzyme A (HMG-CoA) reductase inhibitors such as quinidine (Quinidex) or others. The azole antifungals should not be used in pregnancy.

Adverse Events

Adverse effects associated with systemic azole therapy include gastrointestinal upset, rash, fatigue, hepatic dysfunction, edema, and hypokalemia.

Interactions

Severe hypoglycemia may occur with hypoglycemic drugs. In addition, systemic azole therapy may potentiate triazolam (Halcion), midazolam (Versed), and warfarin. Fluconazole (Diflucan) levels are increased with use of hydrochlorothiazide (HydroDIURIL). Anticholinergics, histamine-2 blockers, and antacids should be avoided within 2 hours of taking an oral azole so that absorption is not compromised.

Selecting the Most Appropriate Agent

Topical agents work well for most tineas but not for tinea capitis and tinea unguium. If tinea capitis is especially severe and painful in a child, prednisone (Deltasone) 1 mg/kg/d can be given for 3 to 4 days as adjunct therapy. To be effective, all therapy must be adequate in dose and duration. If a pet carries the fungus, the pet must be treated. For more information, see **Figure 12.1**.

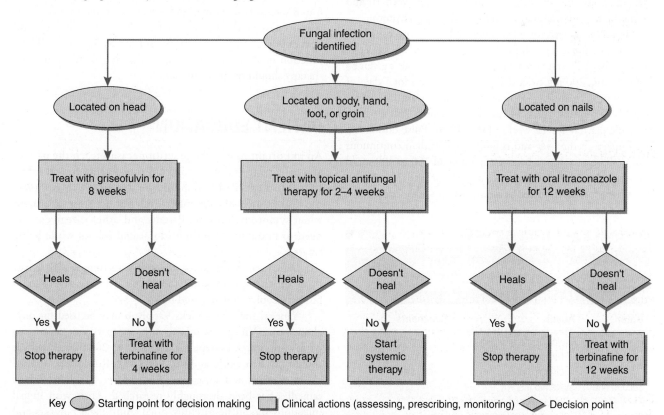

FIGURE 12.1   Treatment options for fungal skin infections.

TABLE 12.2

Recommended Order of Treatment for Tinea Capitis

Order	Agent	Comments
First line	griseofulvin (Grifulvin V)	Treatment lasts a minimum of 8 wk. Take medication with a high-fat meal.
Second line	terbinafine (Lamisil) or itraconazole (Sporanox)	Treatment lasts 4 wk.

When selecting an oral agent to treat onychomycosis, consideration must be given to cost of the agent, patient motivation and compliance, the age and health of the patient, and drug interactions and side effects of the medications.

First-Line Therapy

Topical therapy is recommended for cases of tinea corporis, pedis, cruris, or manus when the infection affects a limited area. The topical antifungal is applied 3 cm beyond the margin of the lesion. Therapy should continue for at least 2 weeks and for 1 week after the lesion clears (**Table 12.2**).

First-line therapy for tinea capitis is microsize griseofulvin (**Table 12.3**) administered with milk or food to promote absorption. Treatment is for 8 weeks. The adult dose is 500 mg daily, and the pediatric dose ranges between 10 and 20 mg/kg/d. Children may attend school during therapy.

First-line therapy for tinea unguium (onychomycosis) consists of systemic agents. Topical preparations are not effective because they penetrate the nails poorly. Itraconazole is given by pulse dosing, 200 mg twice daily with a full meal for 7 days of each month. Treatment for fingernails lasts 3 months and for toenails, 4 months. Also effective for toenails is 200 mg itraconazole per day for 12 weeks (**Table 12.4**). Pulse dosing has less impact on the liver and is more popular than continuous dosing. Fluconazole can be given at a dose of 150 to 400 mg/d for 1 to 4 weeks or 150 mg once a week for 9 to 10 months. Treatment for onychomycosis is only 40% to 50% effective.

TABLE 12.3

Recommended Order of Treatment for Tinea Corporis, Tinea Cruris, and Tinea Pedis

Order	Agent	Comments
First line	Topical azole antifungals for 2–4 wk (1 wk past clinical cure)	Use medications for 2 wk even after the rash is gone.
Second line	Systemic therapy: terbinafine (Lamisil) or fluconazole (Diflucan)	

TABLE 12.4

Recommended Order of Treatment for Onychomycosis

Order	Agent	Comments
First line	itraconazole (Sporanox) or terbinafine (Lamisil)	Take with food. Treatment lasts 12 wk. Not recommended for children

Second-Line Therapy

Second-line therapy for tinea corporis, pedis, cruris, or manus is needed if the infection fails to respond to topical therapy, if there are multiple lesions, or if treatment areas are repeatedly shaved. Second-line therapy consists of terbinafine 250 mg/d for 2 to 6 weeks or fluconazole 150 mg/wk for 2 to 4 weeks.

Second-line therapy for tinea capitis involves using itraconazole, terbinafine, or fluconazole if treatment failure occurs with griseofulvin despite adequate dosage and time.

MONITORING PATIENT RESPONSE

When patients use terbinafine or itraconazole, the AST/ALT levels and white blood cell counts need to be monitored at 6 to 8 weeks. Follow-up evaluations need to monitor both the effectiveness of the therapy and results of liver, kidney, and hematopoietic diagnostic studies. If tests disclose elevated liver function or if creatinine clearance exceeds 40 mL/min, drug therapy should be discontinued.

PATIENT EDUCATION

An important role of the practitioner is to teach the patient about hygiene and ways to avoid transferring fungal infection to others. Patients should be instructed to complete the full course of treatment and not to stop treatment when symptoms subside. Parents and other caregivers also need to know that children can attend school while being treated.

Patients may dry areas susceptible to fungus with a hair dryer after bathing to ensure full drying. The hair dryer should be set to cool or low to avoid burns.

Vinegar soaks and Vicks VapoRub may be used for onychomycosis. Vinegar is mixed with one part vinegar to two parts warm water. Feet are soaked for 15 to 20 minutes daily. It should not be used long term. Vicks VapoRub can be applied to the toenails and socks put over the feet. Neither of these remedies has been thoroughly researched. Areas with fungal infections should be carefully dried. Antifungal powders and sprays can be used for prophylaxis.

TINEA VERSICOLOR

Tinea versicolor, also called pityriasis versicolor, is an opportunistic superficial yeast infection. It is a chronic, asymptomatic infection characterized by well-demarcated, scaling patches of varied coloration, from whitish to pink, tan, or brown.

CAUSES

An overgrowth of the hyphal form of *Pityrosporum ovale* causes tinea versicolor, which is most common in young adults (older than age 15). The fungal infection occurs mostly in subtropical and tropical areas. In temperate zones, it is more common in the summer months but is seen in physically active people year-round. Moist skin surfaces predispose to tinea versicolor. The infection rarely causes symptoms other than discoloration, and patients usually seek treatment for cosmetic purposes.

PATHOPHYSIOLOGY

Pityrosporum ovale has an enzyme that oxidizes fatty acids in the skin surface lipids, forming dicarboxylic acids, which inhibit tyrosinase in epidermal melanocytes and cause hypomelanosis (loss of pigmentation).

DIAGNOSTIC CRITERIA

Skin lesions of tinea versicolor are well-defined, round or oval macules with an overlay of scales that may coalesce to form larger patches. They most often form on the trunk, upper arms, and neck. There may be mild itching. The diagnosis is confirmed by positive KOH test findings, which reveal budding yeast and hyphae.

INITIATING DRUG THERAPY

Topical agents for treating tinea versicolor include selenium sulfide lotion or shampoo and azole creams. The treatment may be repeated in 3 to 4 weeks and before the next warm season or travel to a tropical area. For widespread or stubborn disease, systemic itraconazole or fluconazole may be prescribed for 7 to 10 days.

Goals of Therapy

The goal of therapy for tinea versicolor is resolution of lesions. Therapy lasts for 3 to 4 weeks. Because the lesions may recur in warm weather, prophylaxis consists of applying selenium sulfide lotion or shampoo twice a month.

Selenium Sulfide

Selenium sulfide, the drug of choice for tinea versicolor, has antifungal properties (**Table 12.5**). It is applied once a day to the affected skin for 15 minutes and then rinsed off.

TABLE 12.5		
Recommended Order of Treatment for Tinea Versicolor		
Order	**Agent**	**Comments**
First line	selenium sulfide solution 1% or 2.5% topical azole cream or spray	Topical therapy is used for localized lesions. Use if lesions are resistant or widespread.
Second line	itraconazole (Sporanox)	

Contraindicated during pregnancy and lactation, it can be used with caution in instances of acute inflammation or exudation. Skin folds and genitalia are carefully rinsed. Selenium sulfide must be kept away from eyes. Potential adverse effects include irritation and increased hair loss.

Selecting the Most Appropriate Agent

Lesions may reappear because the infection is a result of microorganisms that normally inhabit the skin, so twice-monthly application of selenium sulfide is suggested as prophylaxis.

First-Line Therapy

Selenium sulfide solution (2.5%) as a lotion or shampoo (Selsun) is applied once a day. Pyrithione zinc (Head and Shoulders shampoo) can also be used. An antifungal topical agent is used. Choices include terbinafine cream or spray, ketoconazole, or sulconazole nitrate (Exelderm) for 3 to 4 weeks. The treatment can be repeated before the next warm season.

Second-Line Therapy

For resistant or widespread tinea versicolor, systemic therapy with itraconazole (200 mg for 5 days) may be prescribed.

PATIENT EDUCATION

It may take several months for the discoloration to disappear. Prophylactic application of ketoconazole cream or shampoo one to two times a week can prevent recurrence. The treatment can be repeated before the next exposure to warm weather.

CANDIDIASIS

Cutaneous candidiasis is a superficial fungal infection of the skin and mucous membranes. It is commonly found in the diaper area, oral cavity, intertriginous areas, nails, vagina, and male genitalia. It can occur at any age and in both sexes. It is classified by its location on the body (**Box 12.2**).

BOX 12.2   Varieties of Candidiasis

Candidal infections are identified by their location on the body as follows:

- Axillae, under pendulous breasts, groin, intergluteal folds: intertrigo
- Glans penis: balanitis
- Follicular pustules: candidal folliculitis
- Nail folds: candidal paronychia
- Mouth and tongue: oral candidiasis (thrush)
- Area included under diaper: diaper dermatitis

CAUSES

Cutaneous candidiasis, which is caused by *C. albicans*, a yeast-like fungus, occurs on moist cutaneous sites. Predisposing factors include infection, diabetes, use of systemic and topical corticosteroids, and immunosuppression. It is commonly found in people who immerse their hands in water. It thrives in occluded sites.

PATHOPHYSIOLOGY

Normally found on the skin and mucous membranes, *C. albicans* invades the epidermis when warm, moist conditions prevail or when there is a break in the skin that allows overgrowth.

DIAGNOSTIC CRITERIA

Candidiasis has several classifications. Intertrigo presents as red, moist papules or pustules. It is found in the axillae, inframammary areas, groin, and between fingers and toes.

Diaper dermatitis presents as erythema and edema with papular and pustular lesions, erosion, and oozing. Scaling may be evident at the margin of the lesions.

Interdigital candidiasis is an erythematous eroded area with surrounding maceration between the fingers and toes, whereas balanitis presents as multiple discrete pustules on the glans penis and preputial sac. Balanitis that involves the scrotum can be painful. It is most common in uncircumcised men.

Paronychia and onychia present as redness and swelling of the nail folds. Swelling lifts the wall from the nail plate, causing purulent infection.

Follicular candidiasis appears as small, discrete pustules in the ostia of hair follicles, and oral candidiasis (thrush) presents as white plaques on an erythematous base. It is found mostly in infants and immunocompromised patients. The tongue is usually involved.

INITIATING DRUG THERAPY

Candidiasis can be prevented by keeping intertriginous areas dry when possible. Also, washing with benzoyl peroxide and applying powder containing miconazole may be beneficial.

Goals of Therapy

The goal of therapy is restoration of the mucous membranes to normal.

Nystatin

Nystatin (Mycostatin) is a fungicide that binds to sterols in the cell membrane of the fungus, causing a change in the membrane's permeability. This allows intracellular components to leak, thereby causing cell death.

Used to treat thrush in infants and adults, nystatin is placed in each side of the mouth three times daily (see **Table 12.1**). The solution is kept in the mouth as long as possible and then swallowed. Therapy continues for 10 to 14 days and at least 48 hours after clinical clearing. Adverse effects include GI upset and oral irritation.

Selecting the Most Appropriate Agent

First-Line Therapy

For cutaneous candidiasis, cool wet soaks with Burow solution can be applied two to three times daily in macerated areas. Intertriginous areas are kept dry by powdering (e.g., with Zeasorb AF Powder), by exposing them to air, or by drying with a hair dryer after bathing. Antifungal creams (clotrimazole [Lotrimin], ketoconazole) can be applied once or twice a day for 10 days (**Table 12.6**).

TABLE 12.6   Recommended Order of Treatment for Candidiasis

Order	Cutaneous Agent	Oral Agent	Comments
First line	Cool soaks with Burow solution; Topical azole	Oral nystatin (Mycostatin)	Burow solution is used in macerated areas. Topical azole is used for 10 d. Systemic therapy is used if no response to topical therapy.
Second line	itraconazole (Sporanox) or fluconazole (Diflucan)	itraconazole or fluconazole	NA

For oral candidiasis, oral nystatin is used for 10 to 14 days, or one clotrimazole troche is given orally five times a day for 2 weeks.

Second-Line Therapy

For failure to respond to treatment, patients have the option of second-line therapy. Systemic itraconazole may be prescribed to adults only for cutaneous or oral candidiasis. For children and adults, oral fluconazole may be prescribed.

MONITORING PATIENT RESPONSE

Response to therapy should be evaluated in 2 weeks. Follow-up for patients receiving long-term systemic therapy (2 weeks; not necessary for pulse therapy) is recommended every month to monitor liver function. Patients undergoing pulse therapy do not need monitoring as regularly. Human immunodeficiency virus infection and diabetes mellitus should be ruled out in patients who have recurring problems with candidiasis.

Complementary and Alternative Medicine

There are several over-the-counter remedies that may be helpful in treating fungal infections. One is apple cider vinegar taken orally. This has antimicrobial properties and helps kill the fungus. It can also promote a faster recovery. Two tablespoons of apple cider vinegar are mixed in one cup of warm water and drunk two times a day. It can also be applied externally when mixed with equal parts vinegar and water.

The application of plain yogurt is another remedy. The probiotics present in plain yogurt can keep the growth of fungi in check by producing lactic acid.

Tea tree oil has natural antifungal compounds that help kill the fungi that cause fungal infections. Plus, its antiseptic qualities inhibit the spread of the infection to other body parts.

Tea is another remedy for fungal infections. The tannins in tea can help kill the fungi responsible for fungal infections. Plus, tea has antibiotic and astringent properties that help get rid of the symptoms of a fungal infection like the burning sensation, swelling, and skin irritation. Tea bags are steeped and then cooled and applied to the affected area.

CASE STUDY*

M.B. is a 42-year-old diabetic woman who presents with thickened, yellow toenails that are painful when she wears dress shoes. Her blood sugar level is well controlled. She is taking the following medications: metformin 500 mg tid, cimetidine 300 mg qid, and Accupril 10 mg daily. A toenail culture comes back positive for fungus.

1. List specific goals of treatment for M.B.
2. What drug therapy would you prescribe? Why?
3. What are the parameters for monitoring success of the therapy?
4. Discuss specific patient education based on the prescribed therapy.
5. List one or two adverse reactions for the selected agent that would cause you to change therapy.
6. What would be the choice for second-line therapy?
7. What over-the-counter and/or alternative medications would be appropriate for M.B.?
8. What lifestyle changes would you recommend to M.B.?
9. Describe one or two drug–drug or drug–food interactions for the selected agent.

* Answers can be found online.

Bibliography

Alberta-Wszolek, L., Two, A. M., Li, C., et al. (2014). Fungal infections. In K. A. Arndt, J. T. S. Hsu, M. Alam, et al. (Eds.), *Manual of dermatologic therapeutics* (8th ed., pp. 124–135). Philadelphia, PA: Wolters Kluwer.

Al-Waili, N. S. (2014). An alternative treatment for pityriasis versicolor, tinea cruris, tinea corporis and tinea faciei with topical application of honey, olive oil and beeswax mixture: An open pilot study. *Complementary Therapeutic Medicine, 12*(1), 45–47.

Chussil, J. T. (2015). Superficial fungal infections. In M. Bobonich, & M. Nolen (Eds.), *Dermatology for advanced practice clinicians* (pp. 181–195). Philadelphia, PA: Wolters Kluwer.

13

Viral Infections of the Skin

Virginia P. Arcangelo

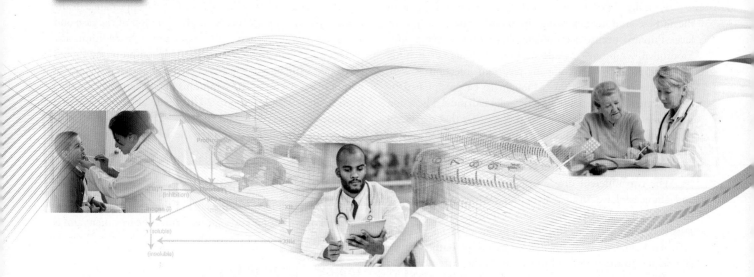

Viruses producing skin lesions may be categorized into three groups: herpes viruses, papillomaviruses, and pox viruses. Herpes and papillomaviruses each affect approximately 20% of the adult population in the United States, with an even distribution between the sexes.

Viruses are further classified by family—either the ribonucleic acid family or the deoxyribonucleic acid (DNA) family. Herpes viruses, papillomaviruses, and pox viruses are members of the DNA family.

Viruses are obligate intracellular parasites that consist of a nucleic acid core surrounded by one or more proteins. A host cell is required for viral replication. Several mechanisms exist for viral replication, and different DNA viruses replicate by their own specific mechanism. Pox viruses replicate entirely in the cytoplasm. Herpes viruses replicate their own polymerase, along with several of their own enzymes. Papillomavirus proteins contribute to the initiation of DNA replication.

HERPES VIRUS INFECTIONS

CAUSES

Seven types of herpes viruses are associated with human illness: herpes simplex virus type 1 (HSV-1), herpes simplex virus type 2 (HSV-2), varicella-zoster virus (VZV), Epstein-Barr virus, cytomegalovirus, human herpes virus type 6 (HHV-6), and human herpes virus type 8 (HHV-8).

HSV-1 infection usually involves the face and skin above the waist. HSV-2 is most commonly associated with the genitalia and the skin below the waist. A life-threatening neonatal infection is associated with HSV-2 in a baby whose mother is infected with the virus; the infection is transmitted during vaginal birth.

Herpes zoster (shingles) and varicella (chickenpox) are the result of VZV infection. The overall incidence of herpes zoster is 3.2 per 1,000 (Htwe et al., 2007). Risk factors include aging, female gender, recent transplant, human immunodeficiency virus (HIV) infection, and cancer. Infectious mononucleosis is a result of Epstein-Barr virus infection. HHV-6 is associated with a mild childhood illness called roseola. HHV-8 is associated with Kaposi sarcoma, especially in patients with HIV infection. HSV-1 and VZV are discussed in this chapter; HSV-2 is discussed in Chapter 35.

PATHOPHYSIOLOGY

Herpes viruses replicate their own polymerase along with several of their own enzymes. HSV is highly contagious. It is spread by direct contact with skin or mucous membrane. After the primary infection, the virus retreats to the dorsal root ganglion, where it remains latent until it is reactivated by triggers such as stress, viral infections, or sunlight.

Those who have had varicella virus infection are most prone to herpes zoster. After the primary infection resolves, the virus retreats to the dorsal root ganglion, where it remains dormant. Herpes zoster is caused by reactivation of the virus, most often with no apparent cause. There is a migration of virions through the axon to the skin of one or several adjacent axons. In immunocompetent patients, recurrent episodes are uncommon.

DIAGNOSTIC CRITERIA

Infection with HSV-1 and HSV-2 causes vesicular eruptions that are painful and often recurrent. The common incubation period of 4 to 10 days is followed by the eruption of clustered vesicles on an erythematous base. Distribution of the virus into autonomic and sensory nerve endings allows the virus to remain latent.

Typically, HSV-1 causes oral or facial infections, with the most common sites being the mouth, pharynx, lips, or face. Primary occurrences usually have intense symptoms. Prodromal symptoms include burning, tingling, or itching; these symptoms may accompany recurrent infection as well. Recurrence of the infection is thought to be precipitated by fatigue, stress, trauma, fever, or ultraviolet radiation. The lesion presents as a single vesicle or group of vesicles that overlie an erythematous base. They become pustules and become crusted or erode. Lesions recur at the site innervated by the dorsal root ganglion inhabited by the virus.

The two different diseases caused by VZV (chickenpox and shingles) have similar symptoms. After an incubation period of 10 to 20 days, chickenpox (primary varicella) manifests with fever and malaise followed by the outbreak of itchy, vesicular lesions on an erythematous base. The outbreak usually begins on the trunk and progresses to the extremities and face. Primary varicella occurs most often in children. Adults infected with primary varicella tend to have more systemic effects, especially if they have preexisting medical conditions.

A reactivation of VZV in the nerve root ganglion is referred to as herpes zoster, or shingles. The infection characteristically begins with neuralgia in the affected dermatome, followed by an outbreak of grouped vesicles on an erythematous base, clustered in a unilateral pattern of the dermatome. In two thirds of infections, the lesions are on the trunk. Additional symptoms include fever, myalgia, and increasing localized pain. The most common presentation of herpes virus infection in the elderly is VZV in the form of herpes zoster. Three fourths of all cases of shingles occur in patients older than age 50. A significant complication of herpes zoster is postherpetic neuralgia, pain in the dermatome site that lasts longer than 6 weeks after resolution of the infection.

INITIATING DRUG THERAPY

Although nonpharmacologic interventions, such as soaks with Burow's solution, help to relieve symptoms, HSV-1 infection is treated primarily with other topical agents. In the case of severe infection in an immunocompromised patient, treatment may be with systemic drug therapy, which shortens the duration of symptoms; however, there is no treatment to prevent recurrence.

For oral HSV-1 infections (oral herpes), symptoms may or may not respond to viscous lidocaine (Xylocaine) 2% applied to the lesion. A solution of diphenhydramine (Benadryl) elixir and aluminum hydroxide/magnesium hydroxide (Maalox) mixed in a 1:1 proportion can be used as an oral rinse four times a day. Sucking on popsicles also can provide temporary relief.

For primary VZV infections that manifest as chickenpox, systemic therapy is used only in special cases and is not recommended for uncomplicated disease. For VZV infections that manifest as herpes zoster, antiviral agents may help relieve symptoms. Patients should be treated if the rash has been present for fewer than 72 hours or if new lesions are still developing. If therapy starts within 72 hours of the appearance of the lesion, systemic therapy decreases the duration of the rash and the acute pain associated with herpes zoster. In addition, any patient older than age 50 who is immunocompromised should be treated with antiviral agents. The use of antiviral therapy in herpes zoster decreases the symptoms of postherpetic neuralgia from 62 days with placebo to 20 days with acyclovir. Antiviral agents used are acyclovir, famciclovir, and valacyclovir. All antiviral agents have shown to shorten the duration of postherpetic neuralgia, but none prevent it.

Goals of Drug Therapy

In herpes virus infections, the goal of therapy is to reduce the duration of symptoms and suppress pain. The treatment aim is to stop reproduction of the virus.

Topical Antiviral Agents

Two topical agents—acyclovir 5% and penciclovir (Denavir)—are available to treat herpes infections. These agents work by inhibiting viral DNA synthesis (**Table 13.1**). They may decrease healing time.

Patients usually apply topical acyclovir every 3 hours, six times per day, for 7 days. Penciclovir is applied every 2 hours, during waking hours, for 4 days. Adverse effects include mild skin irritation and pruritus.

Systemic Antiviral Agents

The three first-line systemic agents are acyclovir (Zovirax), famciclovir (Famvir), and valacyclovir (Valtrex), although famciclovir and valacyclovir are more bioavailable than acyclovir. Systemic antivirals are highly effective against herpes virus. In general, antiviral therapy is recommended for adolescents, adults, and high-risk patients, but not usually for healthy children younger than age 12 (see **Table 13.1**).

Contraindications

Caution should be used in patients with renal disease because antivirals are excreted by the renal system. They are also contraindicated in patients with congestive heart failure and in lactation. Dosage adjustments are made for patients with a creatinine clearance rate less than 25 mL/min.

Adverse Events

Adverse effects include headaches, vertigo, depression, and tremors. Patients may also experience gastrointestinal symptoms and rashes.

Interactions

The effect of antiviral agents is increased in patients taking probenecid, and patients taking zidovudine (Retrovir) may experience drowsiness.

TABLE 13.1

Overview of Antiviral Agents for Herpes Virus Infections

Generic (Trade) Name and Dosage	Selected Adverse Events	Contraindications	Special Considerations
Topical Therapy			
acyclovir 5% (Zovirax) Apply every 3 h, six times per day for 7 d	Pruritus, pain on application	Do not use on mucous membranes or near eyes.	Must use glove or finger cot for application
penciclovir 1% (Denavir) Apply every 2 h for 4 d while awake	Headache, mild skin irritation	Renal impairment	Begin using drug at earliest sign or symptom.
Systemic Therapy			
acyclovir (Zovirax) *For HSV-1* 200 mg five times per day for 10 d for initial outbreak; 200 mg five times a day for 5 d for recurrence *For VZV infection* Children: 20 mg/kg qid for 5 d Adults: 800 mg five times a day for 7 d	Nausea, vomiting, headache, CNS disturbance, rash, malaise	Renal impairment	Do not exceed maximum dose. Least effective antiviral Reserved for use in children
famciclovir (Famvir) *For HSV-1* 250 mg tid for 10 d for initial outbreak; 125 mg tid for recurrence or 1,000 mg bid for 1 day *For VZV infection* 500 mg tid for 7 d	Headache, GI disturbance, paresthesias	Renal dysfunction	May be affected by drugs metabolized by aldehyde oxidase
valacyclovir (Valtrex) *For HSV-1* 1 g bid for 10 d *For VZV infection* 1 g tid for 7 d *For recurrent HSV* 2,000 mg bid for 1 d	GI upset, headache, dizziness, abdominal pain	Renal impairment HIV	Be alert for renal or CNS toxicity with nephrotoxic drugs.

HSV, herpes simplex virus; VZV, varicella-zoster virus.

Acyclovir

The prototypical antiviral agent acyclovir acts by inhibiting viral DNA replication. The drug works only in cells infected by HSV. A disadvantage of oral acyclovir is its low bioavailability of 10% to 20%.

The recommended acyclovir dosage for an initial episode of HSV disease in an immunocompetent host is 200 mg orally five times per day for 7 to 10 days (see **Table 13.1**). The recommended dosage for recurrent episodes is 200 mg five times per day for 5 days. For patients with recurrent infections, treatment prophylaxis is recommended with 400 mg twice daily. For an immunocompromised patient, the recommended treatment is 400 mg five times per day for 7 to 10 days. For suppression therapy, 400 mg twice a day is the dosage. The children's dosage of acyclovir is 5 mg/kg/d in five divided doses for 7 days.

The recommended dosage for treating VZV infections in children is 20 mg/kg four times per day for 5 days. Adult dosing is 800 mg five times per day for 7 to 10 days.

Famciclovir

Famciclovir is the diacetyl ester prodrug of penciclovir. It is an acyclic guanosine analog. After first-pass metabolism, it is well absorbed and converted to penciclovir. The oral bioavailability of famciclovir ranges from 5% to 75%.

The dosage of famciclovir is 250 mg three times per day for 7 to 10 days for an initial episode of illness; for recurrent episodes, the dose is 1,000 mg twice daily for 1 day and 250 mg twice a day for suppression therapy.

Valacyclovir

Valacyclovir is a prodrug of acyclovir and is converted rapidly. First-pass metabolism converts valacyclovir to acyclovir with 50% bioavailability.

The dosage of valacyclovir is 1,000 mg three times a day for 7 to 10 days for initial infection, 2,000 mg two times a day for 1 day for recurrent infections, and 1,000 mg daily for suppression therapy.

Selecting the Most Appropriate Agent

Of the various antiviral agents available, which is most effective for which disorder? Which agents are used when the first choice fails?

First-Line Therapy: Herpes Simplex Virus Type 1

First-line therapy for HSV-1 is topical acyclovir 5% every 3 hours six times a day for 7 days or penciclovir cream 1% every 2 hours during waking hours for 4 days in immunocompetent patients. Acyclovir is usually the first choice because it is less expensive than valacyclovir or famciclovir. Immunocompromised patients may need oral acyclovir 200 mg five times a day for 7 days, valacyclovir 500 mg twice a day for 5 days, or famciclovir 500 mg twice a day for 7 days (**Figure 13.1** and **Table 13.2**).

TABLE 13.2

Recommended Order of Treatment for HSV-1 Infection

Order	Agent	Comments
First line	Topical therapy with acyclovir 5% (Zovirax) or penciclovir 1% (Denavir)	Begin treatment at earliest sign of outbreak.
Second line	Systemic therapy with acyclovir (Zovirax), famciclovir (Famvir), or valacyclovir (Valtrex)	

First-Line Therapy: Varicella-Zoster Virus

Systemic therapy is used only in patients with complicated disease or in children with pulmonary disease or taking steroids and not for uncomplicated disease. It is prescribed only if the

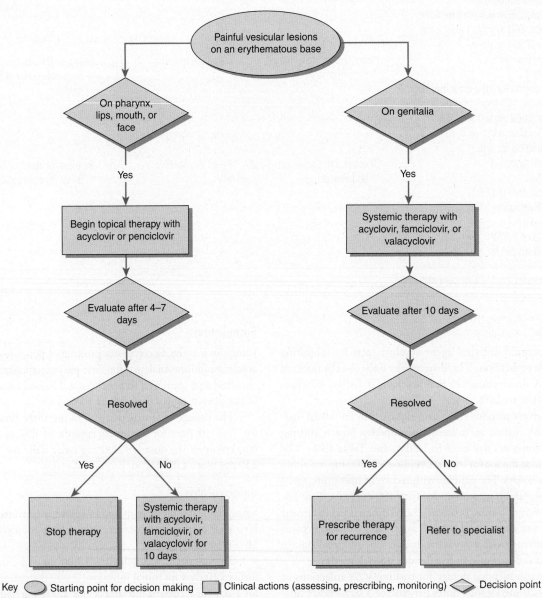

FIGURE 13.1   Treatment recommendations **(left)** for outbreaks of herpes simplex virus type 1 (HSV-1) and **(right)** for HSV-2.

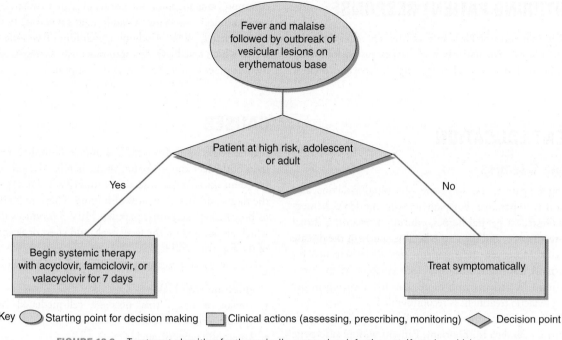

FIGURE 13.2   Treatment algorithm for the varicella-zoster virus infection manifested as chickenpox.

rash has been present for less than 24 hours. Acyclovir is used at a dosage of 20 mg/kg four times a day for 5 days (**Figure 13.2** and **Table 13.3**).

First-Line Therapy: Herpes Zoster

Systemic antiviral therapy can be started if the herpes zoster outbreak is less than 72 hours in duration or longer than 72 hours but with new lesions appearing, the patient is older than age 50, or the patient is immunosuppressed. Therapy consists of acyclovir 800 mg five times a day for 7 to 10 days, valacyclovir 1 g three times a day, or famciclovir 500 mg three times a day for 7 days (**Figure 13.3**). Cost is a driving force in prescribing acyclovir before valacyclovir and famciclovir because it is less expensive.

Oral analgesics, such as acetaminophen, aspirin, and nonsteroidal anti-inflammatory drugs, are helpful in pain control.

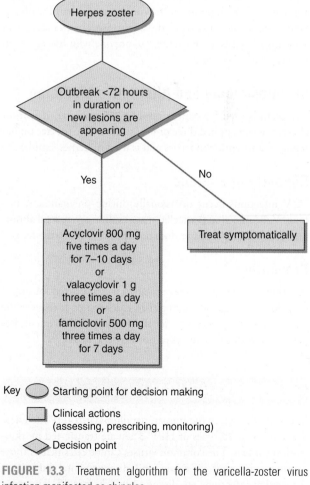

FIGURE 13.3   Treatment algorithm for the varicella-zoster virus infection manifested as shingles.

TABLE 13.3

Recommended Order of Treatment for Varicella-Zoster Virus Infection

Order	Agents	Comments
First line	acyclovir (Zovirax), famciclovir (Famvir), valacyclovir (Valtrex)	For children, the maximum dose is 800 mg qid. Acyclovir is the only approved agent for primary varicella. Antiviral therapy for primary varicella is recommended for adolescents, adults, and high-risk patients, but not for healthy children.

MONITORING PATIENT RESPONSE

Follow-up evaluation of HSV infection is not required if the symptoms resolve. For patients with herpes zoster, follow-up is recommended at 3 days after starting therapy and then at 1 week.

PATIENT EDUCATION

Lifestyle Changes

Educating the patient about hygiene, precipitating factors, and prevention is imperative. For patients with the HSV-2 infection manifested as genital herpes, education regarding sexual activity, recurrence, and the unpredictable course of the disease is necessary. Moreover, these patients should be screened for other sexually transmitted diseases. (See Chapter 35 for more information.) In patients with more than five recurrences per year, prophylactic treatment is recommended.

In patients with herpes zoster, follow-up monitoring for postherpetic neuralgia is important. Patients with postherpetic neuralgia should understand that pain management is the goal of therapy.

Because the herpes virus is spread by skin contact, patients need to recognize the importance of wearing gloves when applying medications and of thorough, careful hand washing. Skin-to-skin contact is avoided. Patients with herpes zoster can transmit the virus as chickenpox to anyone who has not been infected with the virus.

Complementary and Alternative Medicine

Capsaicin is used for pain control in herpes zoster. It is most effective when applied three or four times a day. Tea tree oil has reported antiseptic properties and is used in herpes simplex.

Special Populations

VZV infections occur occasionally during pregnancy. A primary VZV infection (varicella) may result in severe fetal abnormalities, but herpes zoster does not appear to harm the fetus.

Prevention

A vaccine, Zostavax, is now available. It is approved for everyone older than age 60 who has had chickenpox. It reduces the risk of developing herpes zoster and results in less frequent, less painful, and shorter courses of postherpetic neuralgia.

WARTS (VERRUCAE)

Warts are caused by the human papillomavirus (HPV). There are more than 80 types of HPV. They are transferred by skin-to-skin contact. The common viruses can be classified as those causing anogenital infections and nonanogenital infections. Anogenital infections are discussed in Chapter 35. The most common nonanogenital infections present as warts. These are very common, especially in children: at some time in their life, approximately 20% of school-age children have one or more warts, which usually regress spontaneously. Categories of warts include plantar, filiform, flat, and common.

CAUSES

Plantar warts result from HPV-1 and commonly occur on the soles of the feet and the palms of the hands. *Verruca vulgaris*—common warts—is an infection with HPV-2. These present on the fingers or toes or at sites of trauma. They are flesh-colored to brown, hyperkeratotic papules. HPV-3 produces flat warts, which are located on the face, neck, and chest or flexor regions of the forearms and legs.

Factors that predispose to HPV include the following:

- Infection with HIV
- Intake of drugs that decrease cell-mediated immunity (prednisone, cyclosporin)
- Chemotherapeutic agents
- Pregnancy (may cause proliferation)
- Handling raw meat, fish, or other animal matter

PATHOPHYSIOLOGY

HPV proteins contribute to the initiation of DNA replication. Plantar warts are most commonly caused by HPV-1, HPV-2, HPV-4, HPV-31, and HPV-32. The virus enters through skin abrasions and infects the cells of the basal layers of the skin. There is no diffusion to the deep tissues. Viral replication is slow and is closely dependent on the differentiation of the host cells. Viral DNA is present in the basal cells, but the viral antigens and the infecting virus are produced only when the cells start to become squamous and keratinized once they reach the surface. The incubation period is usually 4 to 6 months, with transmission by direct contact or by fomite.

DIAGNOSTIC CRITERIA

Warts are papillomatous, corrugated, hyperkeratotic growths found only on the epidermis, especially in areas subjected to repeated trauma. They can be solitary, multiple, or clustered. Warts are named based on their clinical appearance, location, or both.

Filiform warts are found primarily on the face and neck and present as tan, finger-like projections. Plantar warts (verruca plantaris) are found on the metatarsal areas, heels, and toes. Common warts (V. vulgaris) occur most often on the hands and fingers, knees, and elbows and have an asymmetric distribution. Flat warts (Verruca plana) are found mostly on the forehead, chin, cheeks, arms, and dorsa of the hands.

They are flat and well defined and may be flesh colored or darker brown. Flat warts can be spread by shaving and are found in the beard area in men and on the legs in women. These HPV infections are rarely associated with malignancy. Typically, the incubation period is 2 to 6 months.

INITIATING DRUG THERAPY

The natural history of cutaneous HPV infection is spontaneous resolution in months or a few years, so aggressive therapy may not be needed unless the patient reports pain. If treatment is initiated, the choice of medication depends on age of the patient, whether pain is involved, and the location of the wart. Filiform and flat warts are removed by a dermatologist. Topical treatment with salicylic acid (DuoFilm) is usually the starting point for all other warts. It is easier to treat small verrucae rather than waiting until they are large.

Goals of Therapy

The goal of therapy is eradication of the virus and lesion, although there is no way to actually kill HPV.

Salicylic Acid

Salicylic acid is a keratolytic (peeling) agent. It is available in a variety of strengths for specific types or sites of verrucae. It comes in liquid, gel, and patches. Usually, 17% salicylic acid is used to treat small lesions. Mediplast is a patch product that is 40% salicylic acid plaster; it is useful for large lesions and can be cut to fit the wart.

Dosage

The solution is left on overnight. The patch is applied and left on for 5 to 6 days. Treatment continues for up to 12 weeks. The patient is instructed to soak the area in water for 5 minutes and dry the area before applying the topical preparation.

Contraindications

Topical therapy is contraindicated in patients with diabetes mellitus or impaired circulation and on moles, birthmarks, or unusual warts with hair growth. The most common adverse effect is skin irritation.

Selecting the Most Appropriate Agent

Since the immune system seems to play the most important role in HPV, treatment stimulates the immune system to deal more effectively with the virus. Most warts cure themselves over time, especially in the immunocompetent host.

First-Line Therapy

Filiform or flat warts are removed by a dermatologist. For common warts, topical salicylic acid in a 17% concentration is used; it is applied at bedtime for approximately 8 weeks

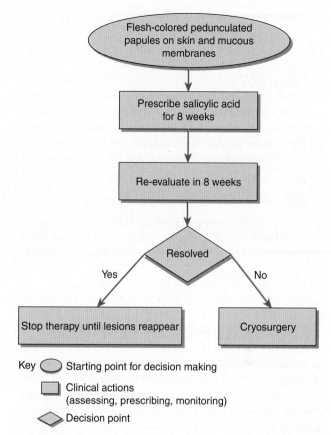

FIGURE 13.4 Treatment algorithm for nonanogenital human papillomavirus infection.

or until the wart is gone. For plantar warts, a 40% salicylic acid preparation is used in plaster or patch form that is cut to the size of the wart and applied at bedtime. The preparation remains in place for 24 to 48 hours. When removed, the area is rubbed with a pumice stone to remove dead white keratin. This is repeated for approximately 8 weeks or until the wart is gone (**Figure 13.4** and **Table 13.4**).

Second-Line Therapy

If patient-applied therapy fails, cryosurgery, electrotherapy, or carbon dioxide laser surgery can be performed.

TABLE 13.4

Recommended Order of Treatment for Nonanogenital Infection with Human Papillomavirus

Order	Agent	Comments
First line	Salicylic acid	Used as first-line agent to treat all types of verrucae
Second line	Cryosurgery, electrosurgery, or carbon dioxide laser surgery	Refer patient to specialist.

CASE STUDY*

B.H. is a 72-year-old man who presents for evaluation of several painful red bumps on his left side. The pain radiates around to his chest. The rash resembles blisters that are just forming. He noticed them yesterday, and more are forming. His wife is receiving chemotherapy for breast cancer. His laboratory results are all normal, and his creatinine is 1.2.

DIAGNOSIS: HERPES ZOSTER

1. List specific treatment goals for **B.H.**
2. What, if any, drug therapy would you prescribe? Why?
3. What are the parameters for monitoring the success of the therapy?
4. Discuss specific patient education based on his history and the therapy.
5. List one or two adverse effects he may get from the prescribed therapy.
6. What over-the-counter medications and/or alternative therapy might you recommend?
7. What lifestyle changes might you recommend for **B.H.**?
8. Describe one or two drug–drug or drug–food interactions for the selected agent.

* Answers can be found online.

MONITORING PATIENT RESPONSE

In nonanogenital HPV infections, multiple treatments may be necessary. Patients should understand the importance of follow-up beyond the initial wart removal, because the virus may remain. Patients may need weekly treatment until the wart is eradicated.

PATIENT EDUCATION

Patients need to be informed that viral warts may recur.

Bibliography

Starred references are cited in the text.

Bader, M. S. (2013). Herpes zoster: Diagnostic, therapeutic, and preventive approaches. *Postgraduate Medicine, 125*(5), 78–91.

Decker, C. (2010). Skin and soft tissue infections in athletes. *Disease-a-Month, 56*(7), 414–421.

Elston, D. (2009). Update on cutaneous manifestations of infectious diseases. *Medical Clinics of North America, 93*(6), 1283–1290.

*Htwe, T., Mushtag, A., Robinson, S., et al. (2007). Infections in the elderly. *Infectious Disease Clinics of North America, 21*(3), 711–743.

Melancon, J. M. (2014a). Herpes simplex. In K. A. Arndt, T. S. Hsu, M. Alam, et al. (Eds.), *Manual of dermatologic therapeutics* (8th ed., pp. 150–160). Philadelphia, PA: Wolters Kluwer.

Melancon, J. M. (2014b). Herpes zoster and varicella. In K. A. Arndt, T. S. Hsu, M. Alam, et al. (Eds.), *Manual of dermatologic therapeutics* (8th ed., pp. 161–172). Philadelphia, PA: Wolters Kluwer.

Morrison, V. A., Oxman, M. N., Levin, M. J., et al. (2013). Safety of zoster vaccine in elderly adults following documented herpes zoster. *Journal of Infectious Diseases, 208*(4), 559–563.

Noska, K. (2015). Viral infections. In M. Bobonich, & M. Nolen (Eds.), *Dermatology for advanced practice clinicians* (pp. 147–164). Philadelphia, PA: Wolters Kluwer.

Plesacher, M., & Dexter, W. (2007). Cutaneous fungal and viral infections in athletes. *Medical Clinics of North America, 93*(6), 1283–1290.

Ruocco, E., Donnarumma, G., Barone, A., et al. (2007). Bacterial and viral skin diseases. *Dermatologic Clinics, 25*(4), 663–676.

Zhang, J., Xie, F., Delzell, E., et al. (2012). Association between vaccination for herpes zoster and risk of herpes zoster infection among older patients with selected immune-mediated diseases. *Journal of the American Medical Association, 308*(1), 43–49.

14 Bacterial Infections of the Skin

Jason J. Schafer ▪ Maria C. Foy

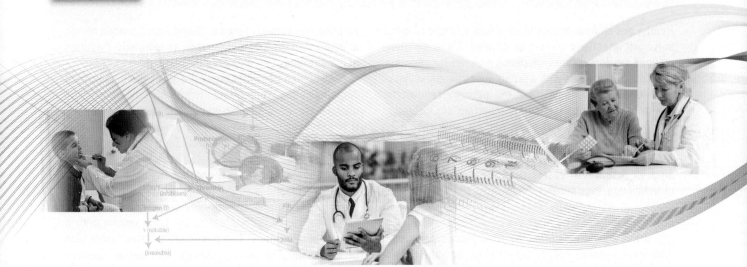

Bacterial skin infections range from those that are minor and heal without consequence to those that are more severe and may be disfiguring or even life threatening. Minor infections are quite common and are often self-treated by patients without formal medical care. The majority of wounds seen in health care practice are easily managed with appropriate wound care and antibiotic therapy, if indicated.

Common primary skin infections resulting from bacteria include impetigo, bullous impetigo, folliculitis, felons, paronychias, and cellulitis. (See **Box 14.1** for information about associated problems.) These are discussed in this chapter, along with the less common infections erysipelas, ecthyma, furuncles, and carbuncles. This chapter also contains a brief discussion of necrotizing fasciitis, a very serious infection treated in an inpatient setting by specialists. See the accompanying color plates for an illustration of some of these infections.

CAUSES

The bacterial organisms most commonly responsible for causing skin infections are *Staphylococcus aureus* and beta-hemolytic forms of streptococci such as *Streptococcus pyogenes* (group A *Streptococcus* or GAS) and *Streptococcus agalactiae* (group B *Streptococcus*) (**Tables 14.1 and 14.2**).

Impetigo and Ecthyma

In the past, superficial skin infections, such as impetigo, a common infection characterized by scattered vesicular lesions, were caused by GAS. However, a shift in normal skin flora has occurred in the United States, and now impetigo is due primarily to *S. aureus* alone or less commonly in combination with GAS. Bullous impetigo, a variation of impetigo, is caused primarily by *S. aureus*.

Ecthyma is a chronic form of impetigo that affects deeper layers of the skin. Usually the causes are the same as those of impetigo; however, gram-negative organisms, such as *Pseudomonas aeruginosa*, or fungal organisms may also play a role. This is especially true in diabetic or immunocompromised patients. Ecthyma can develop from minor wounds, scabies, insect bites, or any condition that causes itching, scratching, and excoriation.

Impetigo is more common in children but can also be seen in adults. It is most often diagnosed during hot, humid weather when bacterial colonization of the skin occurs more easily. Both impetigo and ecthyma are communicable and can be transmitted through person-to-person contact, often in schools or day care centers. Poor hygiene and crowded living conditions are other factors that can contribute to the development of these infections (Gorbach, 2004).

Cellulitis and Erysipelas

Cellulitis is an infection involving the skin and subcutaneous layers. It has the potential to spread systemically and cause serious illness. It can develop in any type of wound, ranging from a minor break in the skin to more serious laceration, puncture, or burn. Other common precipitants include stasis dermatitis, stasis ulcers, edema of the lower extremity, venous insufficiency, and obesity (Odell, 2003). In intravenous (IV) drug users, cellulitis typically develops at injection sites. The characteristics of infection depend on many factors, including the type of wound, the organisms involved, and the patient.

Most cases of cellulitis are caused by GAS or *S. aureus*. Patients with certain predisposing factors, however, may be at risk for infections caused by other organisms, including

BOX 14.1   Danger: Bites and Other Puncture Wounds

Human and animal bites and puncture wounds of other sorts are infections waiting to develop. Because these wounds are associated with such a high risk for infection, antibiotic prophylaxis with a broad-spectrum penicillin or quinolone usually begins with the patient's request for health care. Tetanus is also an important consideration in puncture wounds and bites, and patients should be immunized as needed.

If the wound was created by a clean object and is in an area that is well vascularized, treatment, in addition to antibiotics, may consist simply of washing thoroughly; soaking in warm, soapy water several times a day; and observing the site for a few days.

If the wound was made by an object contaminated with fecal material, soil, or other debris, or if the patient is diabetic or has a compromised circulation, broad-spectrum antibiotics are required based on the probable causative organism.

Care for bite wounds depends on several factors, including whether the biter was a human or an animal, the location of the wound, and whether the wound is primarily a puncture or a laceration. All bite wounds should be cleaned thoroughly with soap and water. Puncture bites should be irrigated with normal saline solution. Extensive

wounds may require surgical debridement, tendon repair, or suturing. If the bite is located on an extremity, elevation of the extremity will help prevent swelling.

All human bites that break the skin should be treated with antibiotics. Appropriate choices include amoxicillin–clavulanate or ampicillin–sulbactam for IV treatment. Oral doxycycline can be used for patients who are allergic to penicillin. Treatment should be given for a full 7 to 10 days.

Minor animal bites may not require antibiotic therapy unless the wound is on the hand, foot, or face. However, the infection rate in animal bites can range from 2% to 20%, and it may be prudent to treat the wound with a course of antibiotics. The possibility of rabies must also be addressed. The same agents used for human bites are also appropriate for animal bites.

Although most puncture wounds heal without incident, patients should be instructed to observe for signs of infection, including inflammation, persistent pain, swelling, or purulent drainage. If a puncture wound becomes infected, further systemic antibiotic therapy is required and should be based on Gram stain and culture results. A follow-up visit should be scheduled within days to ensure that the wound is healing without further infection.

Escherichia coli, *P. aeruginosa*, and *Klebsiella* species (**Table 14.2**). *Pasteurella multocida* is the primary cause of cellulitis from animal bites and scratches, although *S. aureus* and GAS may also be present. **Table 14.2** lists additional causes.

Staphylococcus aureus organisms that are resistant to commonly used antibiotics have recently emerged as a major cause of community-acquired skin infections. These organisms are resistant to all penicillins and cephalosporin agents and are

referred to as community-associated methicillin-resistant *S. aureus* (CA-MRSA) (DeLeo et al., 2010). Infections resulting from these organisms can be particularly challenging to manage because of their resistance to commonly used antibiotics. Also, as opposed to other skin infections, CA-MRSA infections may occur in otherwise healthy individuals but are most common among patients with close contact with others colonized or infected with CA-MRSA. Transmission of this pathogen

TABLE 14.1

Selected Organisms That Cause Skin Infections

	Impetigo and Ecthyma	Bullous Impetigo	Erysipelas	Folliculitis, Furuncles, and Carbuncles	Paronychias
Gram-Positive Organisms					
Staphylococcus aureus	X	X	X (very few)	X	X
Group A *Streptococcus*	X		X		X
Group B *Streptococcus*	X (newborn impetigo)		X (newborn)		
Gram-Negative Organisms					
Proteus mirabilis				X (facial) (folliculitis)	
Pseudomonas aeruginosa	X (occasionally ecthyma)			X (hot tub folliculitis)	X
Klebsiella species				X (folliculitis)	
Enterobacter species				X (occasionally folliculitis)	

TABLE 14.2

Organisms That Cause Cellulitis

Organism	Condition
Staphylococcus aureus	Common
Group A Streptococcus	Common
Haemophilus influenzae B	Children (periorbital cellulitis*)
Streptococcus pneumoniae	Children
Escherichia coli	Opportunistic in compromised patients
Pseudomonas aeruginosa	Folliculitis from underchlorinated hot tubs
Klebsiella species	Opportunistic in compromised patients
Enterobacter species	Opportunistic in compromised patients
Pasteurella multocida	Animal bites and scratches
Anaerobic organisms	Diabetes, ulcers, trauma, crush wounds
Erysipelothrix rhusiopathiae	Fish handlers, usually on the hand
Aeromonas hydrophila	Freshwater-related injury, immunosuppressed patients
Vibrio species	Seawater-related injuries

*Uncommon now because of the use of HIB vaccine.

appears to occur most commonly when there are crowded living conditions (e.g., military bases, prisons) or close physical contact between individuals, particularly when injury to the skin is common (e.g., athletes).

Erysipelas, predominantly caused by *S. pyogenes*, is a superficial form of cellulitis and is seen more often in children, especially infants, and the elderly. Also known as *St. Anthony's fire*, it is an acute condition that can spread rapidly through the skin and lymphatics, causing significant mortality (up to 5%) if left untreated.

Pustular Infections

Pustular infections include folliculitis, furunculosis, and carbunculosis. Folliculitis is a superficial infection of the hair follicle commonly caused by *S. aureus*. Patients who have been taking prolonged antibiotic therapy for acne, however, may acquire folliculitis from gram-negative organisms such as *Klebsiella, Enterobacter*, or *Proteus* species. Lesions associated with folliculitis are usually found on the cheek or chin, under the nose, or on the central facial areas (Trent et al., 2001). *Pseudomonas aeruginosa* can also cause folliculitis, particularly in those who frequently use hot tubs, as a result of inadequate chlorination.

Furunculosis (furuncles) and carbunculosis (carbuncles) are also pustular infections usually caused by *S. aureus*. Both conditions involve deeper areas of the skin and can develop from unresolved cases of folliculitis.

Irritation from shaving, plucking, and waxing of hair may contribute to folliculitis. Other predisposing factors include humid conditions, tight clothing, diabetes, occlusion of the hair follicles from cosmetics or sunscreens, poor hygiene, and occupational exposure to heavy grease or solvents.

Other common skin infections, such as paronychia (an infection surrounding a nail bed) and a felon (an infection affecting the tip of a digit), are usually caused by *S. aureus*, *S. pyogenes*, or *Pseudomonas* species and occasionally other gram-negative bacilli.

Necrotizing Fasciitis

Necrotizing fasciitis is an extremely serious infection of the subcutaneous tissues that can be life threatening if not diagnosed early and treated appropriately. Management often requires emergent surgical interventions to remove infected tissue in combination with antibiotic therapy. It is most likely to occur in middle-aged, elderly, or seriously debilitated patients (Sadick, 1997). The mortality rate is typically 20% to 30% but can approach up to 50% in patients with underlying vascular disease. Often, the initial lesion is minor, such as an insect bite or boil; it is rarely associated with Bartholin gland or perianal abscesses (Gorbach, 2004). However, 20% of cases have no visible lesions (Gorbach, 2004). Patients with diabetes and alcoholism may have no evidence of trauma (Odell, 2003).

Necrotizing fasciitis is often a polymicrobial infection caused by combinations of pathogens that include *S. pyogenes*, *S. aureus*, and anaerobic bacteria such as *Bacteroides fragilis* and Peptostreptococci. GAS and *S. aureus* can also cause necrotizing fasciitis alone as a monomicrobial infection. *Clostridium perfringens*, an anaerobic bacterium commonly found in soil, can cause "gas gangrene," a type of necrotizing fasciitis that can occur following deep penetrating trauma injuries (Ustin & Malangoni, 2011). Varicella infection is often considered a risk factor for invasive skin infections, including necrotizing fasciitis (Wilhelm & Edson, 2001).

Patients with necrotizing fasciitis are very ill and require intensive care. Surgical debridement of infected areas and IV antibiotic therapy are also commonly indicated. Patients who are elderly or debilitated or who have predisposing medical conditions, such as diabetes, advanced atherosclerotic disease, and lesions starting in an extremity and progressing into the back, chest wall, or buttock muscles, have a poor prognosis (Gorbach, 2004).

PATHOPHYSIOLOGY

The skin is composed of three layers. The outer layer is the epidermis, the first line of defense against infection. Nail tissue is part of the epidermis. Underneath is the dermis, which contains connective tissue, blood vessels, nerves, hair follicles, sweat glands, and sebaceous glands. The innermost layer is composed of subcutaneous tissue. Skin infections may be classified according to the depth of penetration and the layer and skin structure affected.

BOX 14.2 Predisposing Factors in Skin Infections

Chronic carriers of *Staphylococcus aureus*
Diabetes mellitus
Peripheral vascular disease
Venous stasis
Alcoholism (malnutrition)
Immune deficiency
Corticosteroid therapy
Obesity
Trauma or burns
Poor hygiene
Warm, humid conditions
Topical irritants
Tight clothing

Under normal circumstances, bacteria present on the skin as normal flora cause no harm. However, a break in the skin can allow these organisms to penetrate and proliferate, resulting in a skin infection. Some people are persistent carriers of *S. aureus* in the nasal, perineal, or axillary areas. These individuals may be more prone to developing skin infections and more likely to experience recurrences.

Patients with predisposing medical conditions (**Box 14.2**), such as diabetes, immune system disorders, and malnutrition from alcoholism or other causes, are more prone to skin infection because of poor wound healing. Also at a higher risk for skin infection are those with circulatory compromise of the arterial, venous, or lymphatic systems. Wound infections in patients with these conditions have the potential to become more serious and invasive, requiring IV antibiotic therapy, hospitalization, or referral to a specialist. Wound infections can also become more serious when treatment is delayed. The practitioner must be alert for these situations and act promptly.

In addition, many organisms aside from GAS or *S. aureus* may cause skin infections in patients with chronic conditions like diabetes. These organisms include *E. coli*, *Klebsiella* species, and *P. aeruginosa*. Infections in these patients are often more difficult to manage clinically and have the tendency to become chronic. Infections that do resolve with appropriate therapy have a high risk of recurrence. A common example of this scenario is a diabetic foot infection.

DIAGNOSTIC CRITERIA

Impetigo and Ecthyma

Impetigo, a highly contagious, common primary skin infection in children, is most frequently found on the face, scalp, or extremities. It begins as scattered, discrete macules that itch and are spread by scratching. These macules then develop into vesicles and pustules on an erythematous base that eventually rupture, oozing a purulent liquid. Once dried, the lesions appear thick, with a characteristic honey-colored crust on the surface. Once healed, scarring is rare. Regional lymphadenopathy may be present, and lesions may itch; however, fever or other systemic complaints are uncommon. The infection is diagnosed clinically by the appearance of hallmark honey-colored crusts. A Gram stain of the vesicular fluid can confirm the diagnosis if there is clinical uncertainty.

Impetigo may also present with bullous lesions and can be referred to as bullous impetigo. Found on the face, scalp, extremities, trunk, and intertriginous areas, it affects primarily newborns and children ages 3 to 5 (Wilhelm & Edson, 2001). Bullous impetigo is characterized by the formation of superficial, flaccid bullae on the skin. The brownish-gray lesions are sometimes crusted or have an erythematous halo. They also appear to be smooth and shiny, as if they were coated with lacquer.

In the most severe form of bullous impetigo, exfoliation of large areas of the skin can occur in what is called "scalded skin" syndrome. This presentation is most common in infants but can also occur in those who are immunosuppressed. It is thought to occur more often in patients who are sensitive to toxins produced by staphylococcal organisms (Barg et al., 1998). Such cases carry a greater risk for more invasive infection because of the loss of large amounts of the skin, the body's protective barrier.

Ecthyma occurs when a case of impetigo worsens and spreads deeply to the dermis. Much less common than impetigo, ecthyma usually affects debilitated individuals and the elderly (Odell, 2003). Signs of ecthyma are usually found on the lower extremities, beginning with the formation of vesicles that then develop into shallow ulcerations. The ulcerations enlarge over several days and are surrounded by an erythematous halo. Because the infection affects the deeper layers of the skin, scarring is often seen after ulcerations heal (Wilhelm & Edson, 2001). Lesions are usually painful and may persist for weeks to months.

Cellulitis and Erysipelas

Cellulitis is a potentially serious infection involving the skin and subcutaneous tissue. In adults, it most commonly affects the lower extremities and begins with a skin break resulting from a localized trauma that may not be apparent. In children, cellulitis usually results from an insect bite or wound. The disease can spread through the superficial layers of skin and cause painful erythema, with the affected area warm and tender to the touch. Pitting edema can also be present, and the skin may be shiny and have an "orange peel" appearance. The margins of cellulitis are diffuse, not sharply demarcated, and the affected area is flat and usually edematous. In open wounds, purulent drainage and necrosis may be present. Red streaks may develop proximal to the area of infection, indicating lymphatic spread or lymphangitis. Crepitus may be present, suggesting involvement of anaerobic organisms. Systemic symptoms of fever, chills, and malaise and regional adenitis are also common and can indicate bacteremia. In fact, these symptoms may be present before cellulitis is clearly evident.

Cellulitis due to CA-MRSA may be accompanied by the presence of an abscess or a furuncle that contains a necrotic center (DeLeo et al., 2010). These infections may progress rapidly and cause local tissue destruction, possibly leading to systemic infection. In addition to painful erythema, the abscess present may spontaneously drain but often will require an incision and drainage procedure for proper management.

Erysipelas, a type of cellulitis limited to the superficial layers of the skin, is most common in children, especially infants and the elderly, but it can occur in healthy individuals who have sustained only minor wounds. Other patients who are at risk include those with venous insufficiency or underlying skin ulcers, diabetics, alcoholics, or those with nephritic syndrome. Erysipelas is most commonly found on the lower extremities but can also be present on the face and scalp. Erysipelas begins as an area of sharply demarcated erythema that spreads rapidly over a period of minutes to hours. The affected area is slightly raised, firm, warm, and tender to the touch. Erythema spreads along local lymphatic channels, which gives the skin a typical "orange peel" appearance due to lymphatic obstruction.

Common systemic symptoms include pain, malaise, chills, and fever. In more serious cases, patients may appear seriously ill. Erysipelas occurring on the face often follows a respiratory infection; this presentation can be particularly serious due to the potential occurrence of cavernous sinus thrombosis (Odell, 2003). Erysipelas can recur, usually in the same area as a previous infection, especially in patients with venous insufficiency or lymphedema (Wilhelm & Edson, 2001).

Pustular Infections

Folliculitis is usually superficial and occurs on hairy areas of the skin, especially the bearded parts of the face and the intertriginous areas. Early lesions appear as erythematous papules that turn into small pustules within approximately 48 hours. As a result, it is common to see various lesions at different stages of development. These lesions may itch initially and then rupture and form crusts. Folliculitis is often recurrent and can represent over months or even years.

A furuncle, which develops from folliculitis, is a painful, pus-filled nodule that encircles a hair follicle. The condition is most commonly found in adolescents or in those with predisposing conditions such as diabetes, immunodeficiency, or poor hygiene. A carbuncle is a confluence of several furuncles that form deep within the dermis. They are often found on the upper back or the thick skin at the back of the neck, especially in men over age 40.

Furuncles and carbuncles are found in hairy areas or in areas of friction. Common sites are the neck, face, axillae, forearms, upper back, groin, buttocks, and thighs. A lesion begins with pruritus and tenderness. It becomes fluctuant in several days as the collection of pus enlarges. Ranging in size from 0.5 to 3 cm, it appears as a pointed, yellow lesion on the skin. As the lesion enlarges, tenderness increases and the lesion often ruptures spontaneously. Systemic manifestations are not usually seen with furuncles, but carbuncles are frequently accompanied by systemic signs such as fever, malaise, and headache.

A paronychia is an infection of the tissue surrounding a nail bed. It is associated with nail biting, hangnails, or finger sucking; it may occur in people who have their hands in water frequently. Diabetic patients are also at a higher risk. A paronychia involving the toenail most often results from an ingrown nail. The infected area appears red and swollen and is painful. Pus, which may accumulate, may sometimes be expressed with gentle pressure; this usually relieves the discomfort. Systemic symptoms are uncommon.

A felon, which may follow a fingertip wound, is an infection that involves the pulp space in the tip of a digit. It is potentially more serious than a paronychia because it is confined in a closed space. The affected digit is erythematous, edematous, and exquisitely tender. The edema has the potential to compromise the arterial supply of the digit. If left untreated, abscess and tissue necrosis can occur. An additional danger is the possibility of bony or joint involvement, which can lead to loss of function.

Necrotizing Fasciitis

Patients with necrotizing fasciitis are extremely ill, requiring intensive care and treatment by specialists. The infection may initially appear similar to cellulitis, although severe pain, erythema, and edema are commonly present. Necrotizing fasciitis may be differentiated from cellulitis by its rapid spread, tissue destruction, and lack of response to usual antibiotic therapy. The subcutaneous tissue will have a wooden-hard feel, as compared to cellulitis and erysipelas, where this tissue is usually yielding and can be palpated. Other symptoms that distinguish necrotizing fasciitis from cellulitis are high fever (102°F to 105°F [38.9°C to 40.6°C]), intense pain and tenderness at the site, and swelling of the affected extremity. Drainage is also usually present and is described as "dishwater pus" (Sadick, 1997). As this infection progresses and tissue destruction spreads, pain may be replaced by anesthesia, and patients may show signs of sepsis, including hemodynamic instability and multiorgan dysfunction.

INITIATING DRUG THERAPY

An increasing challenge in treating skin infections is the problem of antibiotic-resistant organisms. Choosing the appropriate agent is not as simple as it once was, and prescribers must be aware of resistance, as well as regional variations in the prevalence and susceptibility of infecting organisms.

Because warm, humid conditions and poor hygiene may play a role in skin infections, especially impetigo, treatment begins with good hygiene (**Box 14.3**), avoidance of irritants, and meticulous wound care as appropriate. For some very minor infections, these measures along with a topical agent may be sufficient. Adjunctive treatment for most skin infections (e.g., bullous impetigo and erysipelas) includes warm soaks and elevation of the affected area if the infection involves an extremity. However, most bacterial skin infections require treatment with systemic antibiotics.

BOX 14.3 Strategies to Prevent Skin Infections

Wash hands frequently to prevent spread of infecting organisms.

Clean skin twice daily with soap and water or antibacterial soap (e.g., Hibiclens, Lever 2000).

Avoid scratching.

Use warm soaks to promote drainage of pustular matter.

Avoid irritants, including tight clothing, shaving, sunscreens, and occlusive cosmetics and deodorants.

The majority of infections are treated in the outpatient setting with oral antibiotic agents. Patients with more serious infections, however, may require hospitalization and IV medications or referral to a specialist. Treatment decisions are based on the practitioner's knowledge of the patient's predisposing conditions, the patient's present state of health, and the type and stage of the infection.

In many cases, systemic antibiotic therapy (**Table 14.3**) is prescribed empirically based on knowledge of the organisms commonly responsible for specific skin infections, such as *S. aureus* and GAS. With potentially serious infections such as a felon or cellulitis, a specimen of wound drainage should be obtained for culture and sensitivity testing. Empiric therapy will be initiated pending the results.

In the case of puncture or bite wounds that are not initially infected, antibiotics are prescribed as prophylaxis

TABLE 14.3

Overview of Selected Antibiotics for Skin Infections

Generic (Trade) Name and Dosage	Selected Adverse Events	Contraindications	Special Considerations
Broad-Spectrum Penicillins			
amoxicillin–clavulanate (Augmentin) Adults: 500–875 mg q12h or 250–500 mg q8h PO Children: 22.5 mg/kg q12h PO or 13.3 mg/kg q8h PO	Nausea, vomiting, diarrhea, rash, allergic reactions, fungal infection **Serious:** pseudomembranous colitis, seizures (high doses)	Allergy to penicillin Use with caution in severe renal disease, less severe allergy to cephalosporins.	Take with or without food. Food may decrease GI symptoms. Interactions: warfarin, oral contraceptives Safe for young children.
dicloxacillin (Dynapen) Adults: 125–250 mg 6h PO Children: 3.125–6.25 mg/kg q6h PO	Same as amoxicillin–clavulanate Drug-induced hepatitis	Penicillin allergy Use with caution in severe renal or hepatic disease, pregnancy, lactation.	Take on empty stomach for best absorption. Interactions: warfarin.
First-Generation Cephalosporins			
cephalexin (Keflex) Adults: 500 mg q12h PO Children: 12.5–25 mg/kg q12h PO	Nausea, vomiting, diarrhea, rash, allergic reactions, fungal infections **Serious:** pseudomembranous colitis, seizures (high doses) Stevens-Johnson syndrome, hemolytic anemia	Serious penicillin allergy, allergy to cephalosporins Use with caution in renal disease, pregnancy, lactation.	Take with or without food. Food may decrease GI symptoms.
cefazolin (Ancef) Adults: 500 mg q12h PO or 1 g q6–8h IV Children: 25–50 mg/kg divided into 3 or 4 equal doses PO	Same as cephalexin	Same as cephalexin.	Same as cephalexin.
Second-Generation Cephalosporins			
cefaclor (Ceclor) Adults: 250–500 mg q8h or 375–500 mg q12h PO (extended release) Children: 6.7–13.3 mg/kg q8h not to exceed 1 g/d	Same as cephalexin	Same as cephalexin.	Same as cephalexin.
cefprozil (Cefzil) Adults: 250–500 mg q12h PO or 500 mg q24h PO Children: 20 mg/kg q24h	Same as cephalexin	Same as cephalexin.	Same as cephalexin.
cefuroxime (Ceftin, Zinacef) Adults: 250–500 mg q12h PO Children: 15 mg/kg q12h PO	Same as cephalexin	Same as cephalexin.	Same as cephalexin; swallow whole because of bitter taste.

TABLE 14.3

Overview of Selected Antibiotics for Skin Infections (*Continued*)

Generic (Trade) Name and Dosage	Selected Adverse Events	Contraindications	Special Considerations
Third-Generation Cephalosporins			
cefpodoxime (Vantin) Adults: 400 mg q12h PO	Same as cephalexin	Same as cephalexin.	Same as cephalexin.
ceftriaxone (Rocephin) Adults: 0.5–1.0 g q12h IM or IV or 1–2 g q24h IM or IV Children: 50–75 mg/kg q24h IM or IV not to exceed 2 g	Same as cephalexin and also pseudolithiasis	Same as cephalexin.	No known interactions IM: dilute with lidocaine to reduce pain at injection site.
Fluoroquinolones			
ciprofloxacin (Cipro) Adults: 500–750 mg q12h PO Children: not approved	Nausea, diarrhea, altered taste, dizziness, drowsiness, headache, insomnia, agitation, confusion **Serious:** pseudomembranous colitis, Stevens-Johnson syndrome	Allergy to fluoroquinolone. Children younger than age 18, pregnancy. Use with caution in renal disease, central nervous system disease, elderly, lactation (safety not established).	Food slows absorption. Interactions: antacids, zinc, sucralfate, iron, theophylline, warfarin, probenecid, foscarnet, glucocorticoids, didanosine.
levofloxacin (Levaquin) Adults: 500–750 mg qd PO Children: not approved	Same as ciprofloxacin		
moxifloxacin (Avelox) Adults: 400 mg qd PO	Same as ciprofloxacin		
Miscellaneous			
clindamycin (Cleocin) Adults: 150–450 mg q6h PO Children: 2–5 mg/kg q6h PO or 2.7–6.7 mg/kg q8h	Nausea, vomiting, diarrhea, rash, allergic reaction, fungal infections **Serious:** pseudomembranous colitis	Allergy, previous pseudomembranous colitis, severe hepatic disease Use with caution in pregnancy and lactation.	Take with or without food with full glass of water. Interactions include kaolin (decreases absorption).
daptomycin (Cubicin) Adults: 4 mg/kg IV daily Children: not approved	Creatine phosphokinase (CPK) elevation with or without myopathy (reversible)	Allergy to daptomycin, children younger than age 18.	Monitor for CPK elevations, especially in patients receiving HMG-CoA reductase inhibitors.
linezolid (Zyvox) Adults: 600 mg IV or PO q12h Children: 10 mg/kg q8h	Bone marrow suppression, rare optic neuritis, or peripheral neuropathy with long-term use	Allergy, uncontrolled hypertension, and concurrent use of monoamine oxidase (MAO) inhibitors.	Interaction with selective serotonin reuptake inhibitors and MAO inhibitors.
tigecycline (Tygacil) Adults: 100 mg × 1 dose, then 50 mg q12h Children: not approved	Nausea (26%) and vomiting (18%) are common	Allergy to tigecycline; also use caution in patients with allergies to tetracyclines.	Dosage adjustment is necessary for severe hepatic impairment.
trimethoprim/sulfamethoxazole (Bactrim) Adults: 1–2 double-strength tablets q12h Children: 8 mg/kg trimethoprim component/day orally divided q12h	Bone marrow suppression, rash, nausea, and vomiting	Allergy to sulfonamides or trimethoprim, pregnant patients at term, nursing mothers.	Should not be used to treat infections due to group A *Streptococcus*.
vancomycin (Vancocin) Adults: 15 mg/kg IV q12h Children: 10 mg/kg IV q6h	Infusion-related reactions, phlebitis, renal impairment	Allergy to vancomycin.	Monitor serum concentrations.

because of the high risk of infection associated with these wounds.

Topical medications, such as mupirocin (Bactroban) ointment, can be occasionally used as primary therapy for minor infections (e.g., impetigo) or alternatively used in combination with systemic agents for more serious infections. In some patients thought to be chronic carriers of *S. aureus*, infections may be recurrent. Topical mupirocin ointment applied to the nares or perineal or axillary areas may be used prophylactically as an attempt to eliminate this chronic carrier state and prevent recurrent infections (Fitzpatrick et al., 1997).

Several other adjunctive measures may also be used in combination with drug therapy. Bedside warm soaks and incision and drainage procedures may help resolve pustular lesions. Sterile saline dressings and cool Burow's compresses may be used to decrease the pain associated with cellulitis (Rose, 2004). Patients with a paronychia may need to have the nail bed decompressed to relieve the pressure, and deeper and more invasive infections almost always require incision and drainage.

Goals of Drug Therapy

The goals in treating bacterial skin infections are to cure the infection, prevent worsening, minimize scarring, and prevent recurrence. Many minor infections resolve within 10 to 14 days. If resolution does not occur, alternative agents may be prescribed. The prescriber must decide when it is appropriate to initiate treatment with an alternative agent or whether a referral to a specialist for more definitive diagnosis and treatment is indicated.

Antibiotics

Several classes of antibiotic agents are useful for treating bacterial skin infections. For information on specific agents, refer to **Table 14.3.** In certain circumstances, a combination of antibiotics may be necessary to treat an infection because of multiple pathogens (i.e., a polymicrobial infection). Agents may be administered topically, orally, intramuscularly, or intravenously, depending on the specific infection and the condition of the patient.

The most common adverse effects occurring with most antibiotics are nausea, vomiting, diarrhea, rashes, allergic reactions, and urticaria. Also, patients taking antibiotic therapy, especially prolonged therapy, can develop fungal infections such as vaginal candidiasis or thrush.

A less common but potentially life-threatening adverse effect of antibiotic therapy is pseudomembranous colitis. This causes severe diarrhea and is the result of overgrowth of the bacterium *Clostridium difficile*. Anaphylaxis and seizures (especially when high doses of antibiotics are used) may also occur. To minimize the risk of these events, a thorough patient history is essential before prescribing these drugs. There are also many interactions between antibiotics and other medications a patient might be taking. For information on selected drug interactions, see **Table 14.3.**

Broad-Spectrum Penicillins

Most skin infections are caused by GAS and *S. aureus*. In the past, therapy with penicillin was usually effective in treating these infections. With the growing problem of antibiotic resistance, however, it is now necessary to choose a broad-spectrum agent. For example, many strains of *S. aureus* produce the enzyme penicillinase, which can inactivate penicillin. In this case, the provider should choose an agent that is penicillinase resistant. Useful agents in this class for treating specific skin infections include amoxicillin–clavulanate (Augmentin) or dicloxacillin (Dynapen).

Amoxicillin–clavulanate has bactericidal action against many organisms, including beta-hemolytic streptococci, *S. aureus*, *E. coli*, and *P. mirabilis*. The clavulanate portion of the drug is a beta-lactamase inhibitor which allows amoxicillin to remain active in the presence of certain beta-lactamase enzymes such as the penicillinase produced by *S. aureus*. Amoxicillin–clavulanate is well absorbed orally and is more resistant to acid inactivation than other penicillins.

Common side effects are nausea, vomiting, diarrhea, rash, and urticaria. Patients who are allergic to penicillin should not be given this agent, and it should be used with caution in patients with severe renal impairment.

Dicloxacillin has bactericidal activity against penicillinase-producing strains of *S. aureus*. It is administered orally, and the adverse effect profile is similar to that of amoxicillin–clavulanate. In addition, dicloxacillin should be used with caution in patients with severe renal and hepatic impairment (see **Table 14.3**).

First-Generation Cephalosporins

In this class, commonly used drugs for treating skin infections are cephalexin (Keflex) and cefazolin (Ancef). These agents have bactericidal activity against many organisms, including GAS and penicillinase-producing *S. aureus*. They also have limited activity against *Klebsiella pneumoniae*, *P. mirabilis*, and *E. coli*.

Cephalexin is administered orally and has excellent bioavailability, while cefazolin is administered intravenously. Their adverse effect profiles are similar to that of the broad-spectrum penicillins. These drugs should not be used in patients with a severe penicillin allergy, and dosage adjustments are necessary in patients with renal insufficiency (see **Table 14.3**).

Second-Generation Cephalosporins

Second-generation cephalosporins that are useful for skin infections include cefaclor (Ceclor), cefuroxime (Ceftin, Zinacef), and cefprozil (Cefzil). They are effective against the same organisms as first-generation cephalosporins but have additional activity against certain gram-negative organisms, including *H. influenzae*, *E. coli*, *K. pneumoniae*, and *Proteus* organisms. These agents are all well absorbed orally and their adverse effect profiles are similar to that of the first-generation cephalosporins. They should not be given to patients who have a severe allergy to penicillin or an allergy to other cephalosporins. Dosage adjustments are necessary in patients with renal insufficiency (see **Table 14.3**).

Third-Generation Cephalosporins

Useful third-generation cephalosporins for treating skin infections include cefpodoxime (Vantin), ceftriaxone (Rocephin), and ceftazidime (Fortaz). These drugs are usually reserved for more serious infections and are not typically chosen as first-line agents. In addition, ceftriaxone and ceftazidime are not available as oral agents. Ceftriaxone is administered either intramuscularly or intravenously, and ceftazidime can only be administered intravenously. Cefpodoxime is available only as an oral agent.

The spectrum of antibacterial activity for these agents is similar to that of the second-generation cephalosporins. However, they are less effective against *S. aureus* and more effective against certain gram-negative organisms, including *Enterobacter, H. influenzae, E. coli, K. pneumoniae,* and *Proteus* species. Ceftazidime is the only agent in this group that can be recommended for infections caused by *P. aeruginosa*. Ceftriaxone is absorbed intramuscularly, but this route of administration may be painful. Cefpodoxime is well absorbed orally.

The adverse effect profile for these agents is similar to that of the other cephalosporins and broad-spectrum penicillins. Care should be taken in prescribing them in the presence of severe renal or hepatic impairment, and these agents cannot be administered to patients with severe penicillin or cephalosporin allergies. Rarely, ceftriaxone may cause pseudolithiasis (see **Table 14.3**).

Clindamycin

Clindamycin (Cleocin) is an alternative agent that can be considered for treating bacterial skin infections due to *S. aureus* and GAS when patients are allergic to penicillins and cephalosporins. It also may retain activity against CA-MRSA strains of bacteria, but susceptibility testing should be performed prior to use, especially in geographic regions where activity for CA-MRSA is inconsistent. In addition, clindamycin may be considered when anaerobic bacterial coverage is necessary for polymicrobial infections.

Clindamycin is available for oral or IV administration and is generally well tolerated. Common side effects include diarrhea, nausea, and abdominal pain. Also, this agent has been more commonly associated with *C. difficile*–associated pseudomembranous colitis.

Fluoroquinolones

Levofloxacin (Levaquin), moxifloxacin (Avelox), and ciprofloxacin (Cipro) are the fluoroquinolone antibiotics used in the treatment of skin and skin structure infections. They are useful for serious infections in patients with penicillin allergies that have infections caused by gram-negative organisms. Their spectrum of activity includes many gram-negative bacteria, such as *E. coli, Klebsiella,* and *Enterobacter* species. In addition,

levofloxacin and ciprofloxacin are often active against *P. aeruginosa*. Each fluoroquinolone agent is available IV and orally and each has excellent bioavailability.

Common adverse effects are diarrhea, nausea, abdominal pain, dizziness, drowsiness, headache, and insomnia. Uncommon but severe events include Stevens-Johnson syndrome, seizures, Achilles tendon rupture, and pseudomembranous colitis. These agents also have several drug interactions (see **Table 14.3**).

Fluoroquinolone antibiotics are not recommended in children younger than age 18 or during pregnancy and lactation. They are also contraindicated in patients allergic to other fluoroquinolones. These medications should be used cautiously in elderly patients and patients with central nervous system diseases, seizure disorders, or renal impairment.

Vancomycin, Daptomycin, Telavancin, Dalbavancin, Oritavancin, Linezolid, Tedizolid, and Tigecycline

These agents have consistent antibacterial activity against drug-resistant, gram-positive pathogens including MRSA. Vancomycin remains the drug of choice for bacterial skin infections due to MRSA when parenteral therapy is necessary; however, daptomycin, telavancin, dalbavancin, oritavancin, linezolid, tedizolid, and tigecycline are also effective but are more expensive options. Dalbavancin and oritavancin are unique due to their very long half-lives. As a result, treatment with dalbavancin requires only two doses given one week apart, while oritavancin is indicated to treat bacterial skin infections using only a single IV dose. Linezolid and tedizolid are the only agents in this group that are available orally, which provides an option for clinicians to switch from IV to oral therapy when patients are clinically stable but require additional treatment.

Despite their activity against MRSA, each agent has significant side effects and the potential for drug–drug interactions should be considered prior to initiating therapy.

Trimethoprim/Sulfamethoxazole

Trimethoprim/sulfamethoxazole is another useful agent for the treatment of CA-MRSA infections that can be managed with oral therapy. It is important, however, to remember that this agent does not have reliable activity for infections caused by GAS. Therefore, the diagnosis of CA-MRSA should be certain prior to treatment.

Adverse effects associated with trimethoprim/sulfamethoxazole include GI intolerance, rash, pruritus, and hyperkalemia. In addition, this agent may cause photosensitivity, and patients should be counseled to wear sun protection during therapy.

Topical Agents

Topical agents may be used as first-line treatment or adjunctively in bacterial skin infections. Mupirocin ointment is effective against *S. aureus* and some streptococcal infections. It is also used over the long term to eliminate nasal, axillary, or groin carriage of *S. aureus*, which is thought to contribute to recurrent infections in some patients.

Mupirocin ointment is minimally absorbed systemically. It is metabolized by the skin and usually well tolerated. Adverse effects are few but include headache, cough, rhinitis, pharyngitis, upper respiratory tract congestion, and taste perversion with nasal use. Burning, stinging, rash, erythema, or itching can occur when applied topically. Mupirocin should not be used in patients with an allergy to the drug and should not be used with other nasal products. It should be used with caution in patients with impaired renal function due to possible absorption of polyethylene glycol through an open wound (*Drug Facts and Comparisons*, 2004).

The topical preparation of gentamicin is available in a cream or an ointment. It is a powerful topical agent and is effective against many organisms, including GAS, *S. aureus*, and *Pseudomonas* species. Topical gentamicin can be used for a variety of primary and secondary skin infections. It is safe for children older than age 12 months. It is usually well tolerated, although irritation may occur. Occasionally, fungal infection or overgrowth of nonsusceptible bacteria may occur at the site of use.

Selecting the Most Appropriate Agent

Practice guidelines are available to assist clinicians in the management of skin infections including the selection of appropriate antimicrobial therapy (Stevens et al., 2014). Most bacterial skin conditions are treated empirically based on the prescriber's knowledge of the organisms most likely to cause a particular infection (**Table 14.4**). When the organism is not known, the potential for serious infection is present, or the patient is already extremely ill, the prescriber needs to confirm the diagnosis and organism either by skin biopsy or wound culture. In such cases, empiric treatment begins with a broad-spectrum agent until organism susceptibility is available and a diagnosis is made.

Other important factors in choosing an antibiotic agent include patient allergies, pregnancy status, renal and hepatic function, and age. Practical concerns that affect compliance include the taste of the medication (especially in treating children), its adverse effect profile, how frequently it must be taken,

and how much it costs. An antibiotic agent may be changed if the condition does not improve or if intolerable effects impede compliance or pose a danger to the patient. **Figures 14.1 and 14.2** give an overview of the drug selection process.

First-Line Therapy: Impetigo and Ecthyma

For minor cases of impetigo, topical mupirocin ointment applied three times daily for 7 to 10 days may be sufficient treatment (Fitzpatrick et al., 1997). Some practitioners advocate debriding the crusts to promote topical absorption, but debridement is painful and often unnecessary. Mupirocin is less effective in the bullous form of impetigo (Gorbach, 2004).

In most cases, an oral antibiotic is prescribed for 7 to 10 days. A broad-spectrum penicillin (e.g., amoxicillin–clavulanate or dicloxacillin) or a first-generation cephalosporin (e.g., cephalexin) is a good first choice. In cases of penicillin allergy, clindamycin is a good alternative, but in many communities, *S. aureus* has become resistant to this agent. In patients suspected of being chronic carriers of *S. aureus*, topical mupirocin ointment may be applied to the nares to eradicate the organisms and prevent recurrence (Fitzpatrick et al., 1997).

Oral agents, such as dicloxacillin or cephalexin, are usually required for the treatment of ecthyma. Because of the chronicity of this condition, antibiotics are often given for a 2- to 3-week period; IV antibiotics may be required (Swartz, 2000). The same agents used to treat impetigo are effective for ecthyma unless the practitioner suspects infection due to *P. aeruginosa*. In these cases, a medication that provides appropriate coverage, such as ciprofloxacin, may be prescribed. Because of the depth of ulceration and chronic nature of ecthyma, healing may take weeks to months, and scarring is probable (Fitzpatrick et al., 1997). Debridement is not recommended due to the increased chance of bacteremia.

Second-Line Therapy: Impetigo and Ecthyma

Although bullous impetigo is treated initially with the same agents used for impetigo (**Table 14.4**), severe cases, or cases of scalded skin syndrome, may need to be treated intravenously with a drug such as nafcillin (Swartz, 2000).

TABLE 14.4			
Recommended Order of Treatment for Bacterial Skin Infections			
Infection	**First-Line Therapy**	**Second-Line Therapy**	**Third-Line Therapy**
Impetigo, bullous impetigo, and ecthyma	Oral antibiotic for 7–10 d	Alternate oral antibiotic for 7–10 d or refer	
Cellulitis	Oral antibiotic for 7–10 d	Admit for IV antibiotic treatment or refer	
Erysipelas	Oral antibiotic for 7–10 d	Admit for IV antibiotic treatment or refer	
Furuncles and carbuncles	Oral antibiotic for 7–10 d or refer	Alternate oral antibiotic for 7–10 d or refer	
Paronychias	Tetanus prophylaxis, as appropriate, and oral antibiotic for 7–10 d	Alternate oral antibiotic for 7–10 d or refer	
Felon and puncture wound	Tetanus prophylaxis, as appropriate, and oral antibiotic for 7–10 d	Continue oral antibiotic if infection continues	Alternate oral antibiotic for 7–10 d or refer

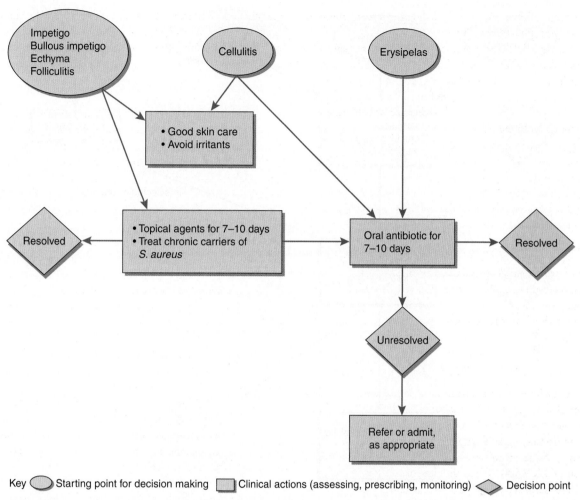

FIGURE 14.1 Treatment algorithm for impetigo, cellulitis, erysipelas, and other bacterial skin infections. *Note:* If the patient has necrotizing fasciitis, admit to hospital and refer to specialist.

First-Line Therapy: Cellulitis and Erysipelas

Treatment for mild cellulitis should begin promptly and usually on an outpatient basis with oral antibiotic therapy. Those who are more seriously ill require parenteral therapy and possibly hospitalization. Systemic treatment is always required for cellulitis.

In addition to severity, current guidelines suggest evaluation skin infections for the presence of purulence to assist clinicians in their antibiotic decision making (Stevens et al., 2014). For example, patients with mild-to-moderate cellulitis without systemic signs of infection or the presence of purulence should receive antibiotic therapy directed against GAS. Penicillin VK, amoxicillin/clavulanate, or dicloxacillin would be acceptable options. In contrast, purulent infections (furuncles, carbuncles, and abscesses) should be managed with incision and drainage procedures often in combination with empiric antibiotic therapy directed against *S. aureus* including CA-MRSA. Patients with infection due to CA-MRSA cannot be effectively treated with cephalosporins or penicillins. These patients will require antibiotics with CA-MRSA activity, including trimethoprim-sulfamethoxazole, minocycline, clindamycin, or linezolid. Patients with serious CA-MRSA infections requiring

parenteral therapy can be treated with vancomycin, linezolid, or daptomycin (DeLeo et al., 2010).

Erysipelas is treated aggressively because it has the potential to spread so rapidly. A good first choice is an oral agent such as oral penicillin V or amoxicillin–clavulanate or a cephalosporin such as cephalexin. In patients who are seriously ill, hospitalization and IV antibiotic therapy are required. Even in serious cases, improvement usually occurs rapidly within the first 48 hours.

Second-Line Therapy: Cellulitis and Erysipelas

If the infection does not respond to the initial course of treatment, patients should be promptly referred or admitted for IV therapy. Wounds that become secondarily infected may require debridement, with frequent cleansing and dressing changes. Surgical debridement may be necessary.

First-Line Therapy: Pustular Infections

Systemic therapy may not be needed for folliculitis; warm compresses can be used to facilitate drainage. Topical treatments may be helpful and include mupirocin, gentamicin,

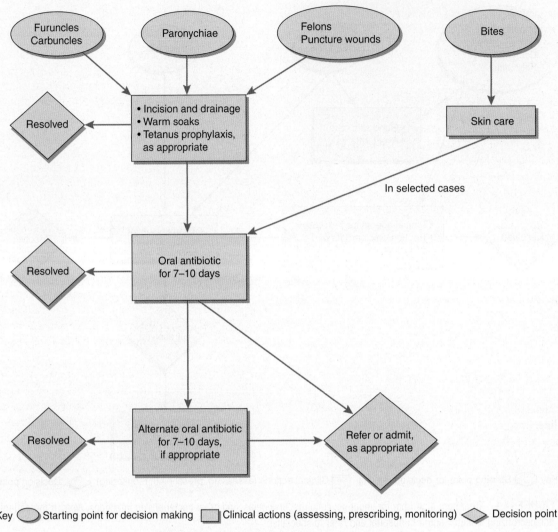

FIGURE 14.2   Treatment algorithm for pustular infections.

or bacitracin. However, if folliculitis is deep, with extensive involvement, systemic therapy may be started empirically with an oral antistaphylococcal agent. *P. aeruginosa* folliculitis may be treated with an antipseudomonal penicillin, a cephalosporin, or a fluoroquinolone if it is persistent or severe (Rose, 2004).

Moist heat applications are usually adequate for the treatment of mild furunculosis. However, if drainage is performed, if the furuncle is located above midface, or if the furuncle is surrounded by an area of cellulitis, oral antistaphylococcal antibiotics (dicloxacillin, cephalexin, or clindamycin) may be indicated. Treatment is continued for up to 2 weeks until the area of acute inflammation has improved. IV antibiotics may be indicated in patients who are systemically ill.

For patients with a paronychia, systemic antibiotics are necessary if the infection does not resolve on its own or after surgical drainage. Topical preparations do not penetrate the nail bed well and generally are not indicated for treatment (Hacker & Roaten, 1999). Effective agents include amoxicillin–clavulanate, cephalexin, dicloxacillin, or erythromycin. This condition is often recurrent.

After surgical drainage, a felon is treated with antibiotic therapy based on culture and Gram stain results. Tetanus prophylaxis is given as needed.

Second-Line Therapy: Pustular Infections

Folliculitis and furuncles may recur in patients who are chronic carriers of *S. aureus*. Topical mupirocin applied to the nostrils, perineum, or axillae may be needed to eradicate the organism and prevent recurrence. Very severe cases of furunculosis or carbunculosis may require parenteral therapy.

First-Line Therapy: Necrotizing Fasciitis

Aggressive surgical intervention is usually needed for the treatment of necrotizing fasciitis. Empiric antibiotic therapy usually includes combination therapy to cover for the variety of pathogens that are possible causes of infection. Examples of antibiotic combinations for necrotizing fasciitis include piperacillin–tazobactam, clindamycin, and vancomycin or linezolid; imipenem–cilastatin and vancomycin or linezolid;

ceftazidime, clindamycin, and vancomycin or linezolid. Once culture results are available, antibiotic therapy can be tailored appropriately.

SPECIAL CONSIDERATIONS

When choosing topical or systemic therapy in a pregnant patient, a drug in category B should be chosen over a drug in category C whenever possible. Below is a list of commonly used medications for skin and skin structure infections and their associated categories. Of particular note, tigecycline, a derivative of tetracycline, is a category D medication and should be avoided during pregnancy.

Amoxicillin–clavulanate: category B
Cephalexin and other cephalosporins: category B
Clarithromycin: category C
Clindamycin: category B
Daptomycin: category B
Dicloxacillin: category B
Erythromycin and azithromycin: category B
Fluoroquinolones: category C
Gentamicin topical: category C
Linezolid: category C
Mupirocin: category C
Tigecycline: category D
Trimethoprim/sulfamethoxazole: category C
Vancomycin: category C

MONITORING PATIENT RESPONSE

The therapy for bacterial skin conditions is monitored by follow-up visits (see **Figures 14.1 and 14.2**). Most cases of impetigo heal rapidly without scarring or other adverse effects. These patients may not need to be seen again unless the condition does not resolve. However, untreated lesions may last for weeks and develop into ecthyma, which is the more chronic and severe form of impetigo. These patients should continue to be followed. Folliculitis, although not serious, is often recurrent or chronic. Emphasis should be placed on controlling aggravating factors and promoting good hygiene measures. Follow-up or referral is required if the condition spreads or does not resolve.

Secondary infection such as osteomyelitis or endocarditis is a risk in carbunculosis. For this reason, systemic antibiotics are always given after lesions are drained. These patients also may require parenteral therapy. In recurrent cases of carbunculosis, the patient should be tested for human immunodeficiency virus. Close follow-up is important.

Patients with cellulitis and erysipelas should be followed closely because of the potential for a serious systemic infection. It is sometimes necessary to change antibiotic agents or increase the duration of treatment if the patient fails to improve. Follow-up or referral may be necessary for paronychia, which often recurs.

PATIENT EDUCATION

Drug Information

Patients treated with systemic antibiotic therapy must be taught to take their medication around the clock to sustain the proper blood level. They also must understand the importance of taking the medication for the prescribed length of time and not to discontinue their medication even if they feel their infection is resolved.

There are common side effects with most antibiotics, such as nausea, vomiting, diarrhea, and rash. Some medications must be taken with or without food. These instructions should be emphasized to the patient. Some medications may cause dizziness, drowsiness, or photosensitivity, and patients should be advised accordingly.

Antibiotics can predispose a patient to fungal infections such as vaginal candidiasis or oral thrush. Patients should be told to report these symptoms so that appropriate treatment can be implemented. Some antibiotics may cause a decreased effectiveness of oral contraceptives, so patients should be told to use an alternate form of contraception while on their medication until their next menstrual cycle. They should also be told if their medication is not safe to use during pregnancy or lactation if applicable. Alternate medication should be prescribed in those cases or if there is any uncertainty about their pregnancy status.

Patients should be told to report signs of allergic reaction, fever, or severe diarrhea, especially if it contains blood, mucus, or pus. Unusual bleeding or bruising should also be reported. These adverse effects may be signs of a serious medication reaction.

Most topical medications are relatively well tolerated. However, some are in an alcohol base and are flammable. Patients should avoid smoking while and shortly after applying their medication. Other topical agents, such as clindamycin, may be absorbed systemically even when used in the topical form, putting the patient at risk for adverse effects.

Nutrition/Lifestyle Changes

Patients need to learn proper methods of hygiene (**Box 14.3**) to prevent the spread of infection, secondary infection, or recurrence. Patients with paronychia must be instructed to keep their hands dry as much as possible. An antifungal cream may be useful when indicated to prevent superinfection.

In cases where there are open wounds, wound care instruction is essential. Some infections, such as impetigo, present a risk to others. Patients with impetigo should avoid contact with infants, small children, the elderly, or those who are debilitated due to the highly contagious nature of the illness.

Although most bacterial skin infections are self-limiting and resolve quickly with treatment, some have the potential to become much more serious. Patients should be taught to report symptoms such as fever, increased erythema or streaking, chills, or malaise that may indicate a worsening of their condition. Also, the chronic nature of some skin infections, such as folliculitis, should be emphasized so that patients understand that treatment may be long term and recurrent.

CASE STUDY*

M.R. is a 66-year-old woman with diabetes mellitus. She is obese and has difficulty caring for herself. She presents with a nonpurulent erythematous area on her left lower leg that began 2 weeks ago as an insect bite. The area was itchy but not painful. She has had an intermittent, low-grade fever for the past week but otherwise feels well. She states that the redness has gotten worse and there is now mild swelling in her lower leg near the lesion. Her only medication is insulin, and she has no allergies.

DIAGNOSIS: CELLULITIS

1. List specific goals of treatment for M.R.
2. What drug therapy would you prescribe? Why?

3. What are the parameters for monitoring success of therapy?
4. Discuss specific patient education based on the prescribed therapy.
5. List one or two adverse reactions for the selected agent that would cause you to change therapy.
6. What would be the choice for second-line therapy?
7. What over-the-counter or alternative medications would be appropriate for M.R.?
8. What lifestyle changes would you recommended for M.R.?
9. Describe one or two drug–drug or drug–food interactions for the selected agent.

* Answers can be found online.

Complementary and Alternative Medicine

Topical magnesium and iodine topical solutions are likely to be effective for the treatment of skin infections. Magnesium can speed the healing of wounds in patients with skin ulcers, boils, and carbuncles. However, if treatment is prolonged, damage can occur to the skin around the area of treatment (Natural Medicines Comprehensive Database, 2004). Iodine is an effective antiseptic agent; a 2% solution is recommended. Skin irritation, stains, and sensitization have been associated with its use.

Topical trypsin is possibly effective for wound cleansing and wound healing. Trypsin is contained in some U.S. Food and Drug Administration–approved products for wound debridement such as Granulex and Dermuspray (Natural Medicines Comprehensive Database, 2004). Pain and burning may occur with its use.

Other complementary therapies have been tried for wound healing, but most have insufficient data regarding their effectiveness. Some of these therapies include aloe, gotu kola, hyaluronic acid, goldenseal, bee propolis, and cartilage.

Bibliography

Starred references are cited in the text.
Abyad, A. (2004). Cellulitis. In M. R. Dambro (Ed.), *Griffith 5-minute clinical consult* (12th ed.). New York, NY: Lippincott Williams & Wilkins. Retrieved from http://online.statref.com on August 1, 2004.
*Barg, N., Gantz, N., Jarvis, W., et al. (1998). Common and potentially fatal *Staph* infections. *Patient Care, 32*(6), 26–49.
Billica, W. H. (2004). Impetigo. In M. R. Dambro (Ed.), *Griffith 5-minute clinical consult* (12th ed.). New York, NY: Lippincott Williams & Wilkins. Retrieved from http://online.statref.com on August 1, 2004.
*DeLeo, F. R., Otto, M., Kreiswirth, B. N., et al. (2010). Community associated methicillin-resistant *Staphylococcus aureus*. *Lancet, 375*, 1557–1568.
Drug Facts and Comparisons. (2004). St. Louis, MO: Facts and Comparisons.
*Fitzpatrick, T. B., Johnson, R. A., Wolff, K., et al. (1997). Cutaneous bacterial infections. In *Color atlas and synopsis of clinical dermatology:*

Common and serious diseases (3rd ed., pp. 604–621). New York, NY: McGraw-Hill.
*Gorbach, S. L. (2004). Skin and soft tissue infections. In S. L. Gorbach, J. Q. Bartlett, & N. R. Blacklow (Eds.), *Infectious disease* (3rd ed.). New York, NY: Lippincott Williams & Wilkins.
*Hacker, S. M., & Roaten, S. P. (1999). Strategies for managing bacterial skin infections. *Patient Care, 33*(2), 53–71.
Kincaid, S. A. (2004). Erysipelas. In M. R. Dambro (Ed.), *Griffith 5-minute clinical consult* (12th ed.). New York, NY: Lippincott Williams & Wilkins. Retrieved from http://online.statref.com on August 1, 2004.
Kravetz, J. D., & Federman, D. G. (2004). Treatment of mammalian bites. In J. D. Kravetz, editorial consultant. *ACP's PIER: The physicians' information and education resource.* Philadelphia, PA: American College of Physicians. Retrieved from http://online.statref.com on August 1, 2004.
Mancini, A. J. (2002). Skin infections and exanthems. In A. M. Rudolph, & C. D. Rudolph (Eds.), *Rudolph's pediatrics* (21st ed.). New York, NY: McGraw-Hill Medical Publishing Division. Retrieved from http://online. statref.com on August 1, 2004.
Micromedex Healthcare Series: Thomson Micromedex, Greenwood Village, Colorado Edition, expires September 2004.
Millikan, L. (2004). Paronychia. In M. R. Dambro (Ed.), *Griffith 5-minute clinical consult* (12th ed.). New York, NY: Lippincott Williams & Wilkins. Retrieved from http://online.statref.com on August 1, 2004.
*Natural Medicines Comprehensive Database online. Retrieved August 6, 2004, through Doylestown Hospital's Web site. http://www.naturaldatabase.com
The Natural Pharmacist, Consumer Edition on-line. Retrieved August 9, 2004, through Gadsden Regional Medical Center's Web site: http://www. gadsdenregional.com
*Odell, M. L. (2003). Skin infections and infestations. In A. K. David, T. A. Johnson, M. Phillips, & J. E. Scherger (Eds.), *Family medicine: Principles and practice* (6th ed.). New York, NY: Springer-Verlag. Retrieved from http://online.statref.com on August 1, 2004.
Pierce, N. F. (1995). Bacterial infections of the skin. In L. R. Barker, J. R. Burton, & P. D. Zieve (Eds.), *Principles of ambulatory medicine* (4th ed., pp. 300–306). Baltimore, MD: Lippincott Williams & Wilkins.
*Rose, L. C. (2004). Folliculitis. In M. R. Dambro (Ed.), *Griffith 5-minute clinical consult* (12th ed.). New York, NY: Lippincott Williams & Wilkins. Retrieved from http://online.statref.com on August 1, 2004.
*Sadick, N. S. (1997). Current aspects of bacterial infections of the skin. *Dermatology Clinics, 15*, 341–349.
Stevens, D. L. (2004). In D. L. Stevens, editorial consultant. *ACP's PIER: The physicians' information and education resource. Cellulitis and soft tis-*

sue infections. Philadelphia, PA: American College of Physicians. Retrieved from http://online.statref.com on August 1, 2004.

*Stevens, D. L., Bisno, A. L., Chambers, H. F., et al. (2014). Practice guidelines for the diagnosis and management of skin and soft tissue infections: 2014 update by the Infectious Diseases Society of America. *Clinical Infectious Disease, 59*(2), e10–e52.

*Swartz, M. (2000). Cellulitis and subcutaneous tissue infections. In G. L. Mandell, J. E. Bennett, & R. Dolin (Eds.), *Mandell, Douglas, and Bennett's principles and practices in infectious disease* (5th ed.). New York, NY: Churchill Livingstone.

*Trent, J. T., Federman, D., & Kirsner, R. S. (2001). Common bacterial skin infections. *Ostomy Wound Management, 47*(8), 30–34.

*Ustin, J. S., & Malangoni, M. A. (2011). Necrotizing soft-tissue infections. *Critical Care Medicine, 39*(9), 2156–2162.

*Wilhelm, M. P., & Edson, R. S. (2001). Clinical syndromes 13: Skin and soft tissue infections. In W. R. Wilson, & M. A. Sande (Eds.), *Current diagnosis and treatment of infectious diseases, section II*. New York, NY: Lange Medical Books/McGraw-Hill Medical Publishing Division. Retrieved from http://online.statref.com on August 1, 2004.

15 Psoriasis

Shelly Schneider

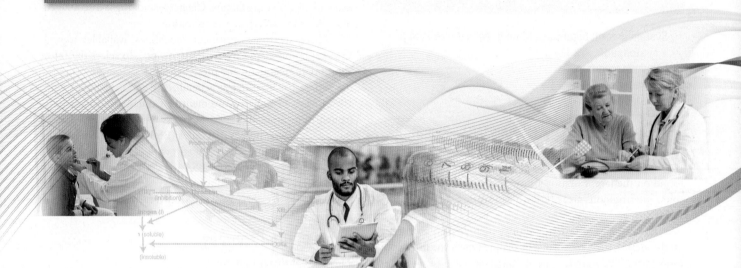

Psoriasis is a debilitating disease characterized by recurrent exacerbations and remissions. It affects between 2% and 3% of the U.S. population, with a higher incidence in whites and an equal distribution between the sexes. Approximately 36% of patients with psoriasis have a positive family history. The cost of outpatient treatment for psoriasis averages $1.6 to $3.2 billion annually.

There appear to be two peak ages of onset: between ages 16 and 22 and between ages 57 and 60. Psoriasis has an element of physical discomfort, with pain, itching, stinging, cracking, and bleeding of the lesions. In approximately 10% of patients with psoriasis, the disease develops into psoriatic arthritis.

Psoriasis affects almost all aspects of life, including sexual relationships and emotional well-being. In addition, patients with psoriasis spend 1 or more hours a day caring for their skin. Of a survey group of patients with psoriasis, up to 25% felt at some point in their life that they would rather be dead than alive with psoriasis.

Psoriasis affects approximately 2.5% of Whites and 1.3% of Blacks in the United States, with approximately 150,000 newly diagnosed cases every year. The incidence of psoriasis is somewhat lower in Asians (0.4%). Generally, it is more common in individuals living at higher latitudes or in colder locales and less common in individuals who have greater sun exposure. There seems to be a genetic factor associated with psoriasis. Based on population studies, the risk of psoriasis in children is estimated to be 41% if both parents are affected, 14% if one parent is affected, and 6% if one sibling is affected, and a family history can be found in 5% to 10% of patients who have psoriasis.

CAUSES

A definitive cause for psoriasis is unknown, although there are several possible etiologic factors: abnormal epidermal cell cycle, hereditary factors, and trigger factors, including trauma, infection, endocrine imbalance, climate, and emotional stress.

Physical trauma, such as rubbing, scratching, or sunburn, is a major exacerbating factor in psoriasis, and this is referred to as *Koebner phenomenon*. A precipitating event, in some cases of guttate psoriasis, is a streptococcal infection. Stress plays a role in as many as 40% of psoriasis flares in adults and children. Exacerbations of psoriasis may develop from the use of certain drugs (**Box 15.1**).

PATHOPHYSIOLOGY

Psoriasis is an autoimmune-mediated process driven by abnormally activated helper T cells. Activation of these T cells can occur through specific interactions with antigen-presenting cells (APCs) or via nonspecific superantigen interactions (i.e., guttate psoriasis is triggered by streptococcal antigens). APC activation requires costimulatory signals. Once activated, psoriatic T cells produce a type 1 helper T cell–dominant cytokine profile that includes interleukin-2 (IL-2), tumor necrosis factor-alpha (TNF-α), interferon-γ, and IL-8. These cytokines act to attract and activate neutrophils, which are responsible for much of the inflammation seen in psoriasis. Other factors leading to neutrophil recruitment and activation are complement split products and leukotrienes (arachidonic acid metabolites from the 5-lipoxygenase pathway).

DIAGNOSTIC CRITERIA

Psoriasis is diagnosed by observation of characteristic, well-demarcated, erythematous papules or plaques surrounded by silvery or whitish scales. The lesions are symmetric and usually

BOX 15.1 Drugs Known to Exacerbate Psoriasis

Systemic corticosteroids (when dose is decreased or stopped)
Lithium carbonate
Antimalarials
Beta-blockers
Systemic interferon
Alcohol

found on the face, extensor joints, anogenital area, palms and soles, intertriginous areas (known as inverse psoriasis), trunk, scalp, ears, and nails.

The varieties of psoriatic disease include plaque, guttate, erythrodermic, and pustular. The plaque type is the most common form. The guttate type is characterized by small, scattered, teardrop-shaped papules and plaques. In many cases, psoriasis begins as the guttate form. The erythrodermic form is characterized by generalized intense erythema and shedding of scales. Finally, the pustular type has three additional forms: generalized, localized, and palmar–plantar. All share a similar characteristic: 2- to 3-mm sterile pustules on specific body regions.

Clinical presentation of the plaque type of psoriasis consists of sharply demarcated, erythematous papules and plaques with marked silvery-white scales. Bleeding may follow removal of the scales (Auspitz sign). The elbows, knees, and scalp are the most common areas for psoriatic plaques. Pitting and discoloration of the nails also characterizes psoriasis. In some cases, the nail may separate from the nail bed—referred to as onycholysis.

INITIATING DRUG THERAPY

Before beginning drug therapy, the patient is usually counseled to avoid precipitating factors. Cigarette smoking is discouraged since this can exacerbate the condition.

There are three treatment modalities available: topical agents, phototherapy, and systemic agents. To select the most appropriate treatment, the prescriber must determine whether the patient has localized or generalized psoriasis. Patients with 10% or less of body involvement can usually be successfully treated in a primary care setting with topical agents, whereas those with greater body surface area (BSA) involvement usually require treatment by a dermatologist with phototherapy or systemic therapy. In estimating BSA involvement, the prescriber keeps in mind that the palm represents 1% BSA; this can be used as a tool to estimate total BSA involvement.

Goals of Drug Therapy

The goals of therapy are to:

- Decrease the size and thickness of the plaques
- Decrease pruritus
- Improve emotional well-being and quality of life
- Put the patient in remission
- Have minimal side effects from treatment

It is imperative to use a management strategy that has the least possible toxicity and that is acceptable to the patient. Sequential therapy is thought to be effective because psoriasis is a chronic disease requiring long-term maintenance therapy and treatment of exacerbations. The three phases of sequential therapy are the clearing, transitional, and maintenance phases. **Table 15.1** identifies topical and systemic preparations used in psoriasis treatment.

TABLE 15.1

Overview of Selected Agents for Psoriasis

Generic (Trade) Name and Dosage	Selected Adverse Events	Contraindications	Special Considerations
Topical Agents			
Emollients (Eucerin, Lubriderm, Moisturel, CeraVe, Cetaphil) Apply to affected skin three or four times daily.	Folliculitis, maceration, miliaria		Avoid applying near eyes.
Tar Preparations Coal tar Apply at bedtime and allow to remain on skin. Emulsion: 15–25 mL dissolved in bath water Shampoo	Irritation, photoreactions, unpleasant odor, folliculitis	Open or infected lesions	Preparation may stain skin and clothing. With emulsion, immerse affected area for 10 to 20 min three to seven times a week. Shampoo should be massaged into wet scalp and rinsed, then applied a second time and left on for 5 min.

TABLE 15.1

Overview of Selected Agents for Psoriasis (*Continued*)

Generic (Trade) Name and Dosage	Selected Adverse Events	Contraindications	Special Considerations
Antipsoriatics anthralin (Drithocreme, Micanol) Apply for 30–60 min, and then remove.	Irritation	Renal disease, acute psoriasis	Preparation may stain skin, towels, sinks, and tubs. Avoid applying near eyes and mucous membranes. Irritation can be avoided by applying emollients to unaffected skin.
Vitamin D Analogs calcipotriene (Dovonex) Apply bid.	Burning and stinging, skin peeling, rash	Hypercalcemia, vitamin D toxicity	Do not use on face.
Vitamin A Derivatives tazarotene (Tazorac) Once a day at bedtime	Pruritus, erythema		Avoid vitamin A.
Topical Corticosteroids hydrocortisone (Cortisporin)	Burning, folliculitis, hypothalamic–pituitary–adrenal axis suppression	Primary bacterial infections or fungal infections	Use lowest effective dose. Avoid prolonged use. Use occlusive dressing.
Systemic Agents apremilast (Otezla)	GI upset, diarrhea	Known hypersensitivity	Starter kit to minimize side effects.
cyclosporine (Cyclosporine A, Sandimmune) Maximum dose 2–5 mg/kg/d	Tremor, gingival hyperplasia, GI upset, hypertension, renal dysfunction, acne	Pregnancy and lactation; caution in impaired renal and hepatic function	Increased risk of digoxin toxicity. Interacts with lovastatin, diltiazem, ketoconazole. Decreased therapeutic effect with use of hydantoins, rifampin, sulfonamides.
etretinate (Acitretin) 25–50 mg daily	Elevation in lipid levels, abnormal liver function, alopecia, rash, dry skin, pruritus	Alcohol use, pregnancy, and lactation	Perform pretreatment lipid and liver function tests. Advise female patients not to become pregnant while taking this medication. Take with meals.
methotrexate (MTX, Rheumatrex) 12.5–25 mg/kg/wk	Headache, blurred vision, fatigue, malaise, GI distress, gingivitis, hepatotoxicity, chills, bone marrow depression, rash alopecia, fever	Pregnancy and lactation; caution inpatients with renal and hepatic compromise, leukopenia	Drug decreases the level of digoxin. Increased risk of toxicity with salicylates, phenytoin, sulfonamides. Take folic acid 1 mg on nontreatment days.
Biologics adalimumab (Humira) 80 mg subcutaneously initially then 40 mg every other week	Headache, nausea, rash, reaction at injection site	Concurrent live vaccine, active infection; caution in pregnancy	Used for psoriatic arthritis.
etanercept (Enbrel) 50 mg twice a week for 3 mo, then 50 mg weekly by subcutaneous injection	Infection, injection site pain, localized erythema, rash, upper respiratory infection, abdominal pain, vomiting	Concurrent live vaccine, active infection; caution in pregnancy, impaired renal function, asthma, blood dyscrasia, central nervous system demyelinating disease, history of recurrent infections	A maximum of 25 mg can be given in each site, requiring two injections. It is given subcutaneously. Not to be given with live vaccines.
infliximab (Remicade) IV 5 mg/kg	GI upset, headache, fatigue, cough, congestive heart failure	Severe congestive heart failure	Not to be given with live vaccines.
Secukinumab (Cosentyx) 150–300 mg	Nasopharyngitis, upper respiratory infection	Infection	
Ustekinumab (Stelara)	Infection	Malignancy, infection	

Emollients

Emollients are useful for all cases of psoriasis as an adjunct therapy. These agents hydrate the stratum corneum, decrease water evaporation, and soften the scales of the plaques. They are available in lotions, creams, and ointments. The thicker the preparation, the more effective it is. Commercially available agents include Eucerin cream/lotion, Lubriderm, and Moisturel. In addition to preserving moisture, emollients have a mild antipruritic effect. Newer products include CeraVe and Cetaphil.

Topical Corticosteroids

The foundation of topical treatment is topical corticosteroids. They play an important role in treating psoriasis by decreasing erythema, pruritus, and scaling. They promote vasoconstriction. They are fast acting but not intended for long-term use. Topical corticosteroids are classified into several categories based on potency and vasoconstrictive properties. Low-potency corticosteroids are safer for long-term use and for use at thin-skinned sites such as the face and groin. The most effective topical treatment is a medium- or high-potent agent used for a limited time, followed by a less potent agent for maintenance. Occlusion of the area where the topical steroid is applied is recommended. Saran wrap can be used, or Cordran tape is also effective. This method increases the absorption (hence the potency) of the topical preparation.

Topical corticosteroids may be used for longer periods on thicker skin because thicker skin does not absorb medication as well as thinner skin. Topical corticosteroids have a rapid onset of action. They decrease erythema, inflammation, and pruritus. For more information on topical corticosteroids, see Chapter 11.

Coal Tars

Coal tar (Cutar) contains polycyclic hydrocarbon compounds formed from bituminous coal. It depresses deoxyribonucleic acid (DNA) synthesis and has anti-inflammatory and antipruritic properties. Several preparations are available, including an ointment, a gel preparation, a bath preparation, and shampoo. Coal tar can be used as an initial therapy, usually with adjunct topical corticosteroids.

Coal tar is applied overnight and at home because of the offensive odor. The emulsion is dissolved in bath water (15 to 25 mL), and the patient immerses the affected area in the water for 10 to 20 minutes. It is used for 30 to 45 days, three to seven times a week. The shampoo preparation is massaged into a wet scalp and rinsed. It is applied a second time and left on the scalp for 5 minutes.

Efficacy of the ointment or gel is based on the amount of time that the medication is on the body. There is a slow response to coal tar therapy, and it is not used for acute exacerbations or on open or infected lesions.

Some disadvantages of coal tar include the unpleasant odor, staining of clothes, skin and fiberglass (even with the clear preparation), and photosensitivity. These disadvantages tend to lead to poor compliance. In addition, folliculitis commonly occurs, especially in areas with dense hair follicles. This requires discontinuing the medication.

Anthralin

Anthralin (Drithocreme, Micanol) is another topical treatment for psoriasis. It is a coal tar derivative.

Mechanism of Action

There are two possible mechanisms of action: inhibition of DNA synthesis and a decrease in epidermal proliferation. Anthralin is a good therapy if the patient has a limited number of lesions, but its use is time consuming.

Dosage

Anthralin is applied for 30 minutes to 1 hour and then removed. It should be applied only to the lesion, not to unaffected skin. Treatment starts with a low strength that is gradually increased. Staining of the psoriasis plaques signifies that treatment is decreasing cellular proliferation. Treatment is time consuming but short term.

Time Frame for Response

There is a slow onset of action, and response is slow as well.

Contraindications

Anthralin therapy is contraindicated in acute psoriasis and inflammation.

Adverse Events

Anthralin therapy may be limited by irritation of the unaffected skin. Irritation can be prevented by applying emollients to the normal skin. The medication stains clothing a brownish-purple and permanently stains towels, tubs, and sinks.

Vitamin D Analogs

Calcipotriene (Dovonex) and Calcipotriol are vitamin D analogs for treating mild to moderate psoriasis. They are supplied in creams, ointments, and topical foam.

Mechanism of Action

Its mechanism of action is a reduction of cell proliferation by binding to receptors in epidermal keratinocytes. The drug is also thought to have an anti-inflammatory effect. It is effective for long-term use and maintenance therapy and is often used as rotational therapy with topical steroids.

Dosage

A thin layer is applied twice a day to affected skin for 6 to 8 weeks. It is also used as rotational therapy or by pulse dosing (off-and-on therapy), in which the patient follows the therapeutic regimen for 2 weeks, followed by 1 week off. Use with a potent topical corticosteroid is most effective. The patient must be cautioned not to use more than 100 g/wk.

Time Frame for Response

Some improvement is usually seen in 2 to 4 weeks, although therapy is recommended for 6 to 8 weeks. An advantage of calcipotriene is its similar efficacy to that of medium- to high-potency topical corticosteroids. Unlike corticosteroids, however, calcipotriene does not cause skin atrophy or hypo-thalamic–pituitary–adrenal axis suppression. However, it is an irritant and therefore should not be used on the face. It is contraindicated in patients with hypercalcemia and vitamin D toxicity.

Adverse Events

The most common adverse effects of calcipotriene are mild and include dry skin, peeling, and rash. Hypercalcemia may be caused by vitamin D ingestion but is rare if the patient uses less than 100 g of calcipotriene per week.

Retinoid (Vitamin A Derivative)

Tazarotene (Tazorac) is a topical retinoid used for mild to moderate psoriasis.

Mechanism of Action

This drug normalizes epidermal differentiation, decreases hyperproliferation, and diminishes inflammation of the cells in the skin. Use of tazarotene promotes longer remission of psoriasis.

Dosage

It comes in a clear, nonstaining gel and cream (0.05% and 0.1%) and is applied in a thin layer once a day at bedtime. Skin must be air dried and the area left unoccluded. The preparation can be used for the body, scalp, hairline, and face but not on the genitalia or intertriginous areas or around the eyes.

Time Frame for Response

After 1 week of therapy, diminished scaling is noted. Clearing is seen in approximately 8 weeks.

Contraindications

Tazarotene can cause fetal harm, so it is started in menstruating women during menses; these women should ensure that they do not become pregnant during therapy.

Adverse Events

Adverse effects of tazarotene include pruritus, erythema of the skin, and mild to moderate burning. The use of topical corticosteroids counteracts these effects. The patient must be warned that the psoriasis may get worse before it improves.

Interactions

Vitamin A ingestion is to be avoided, and tazarotene is used with caution with other photosensitizers such as tetracyclines and with other topical irritants such as abrasives, depilatories, or permanent wave solutions.

Systemic Retinoids

Acitretin (Soriatane) is a systemic retinoid used for long-term psoriasis therapy.

Mechanism of Action

Acitretin normalizes epidermal differentiation and diminishes hyperproliferation and inflammation of cells in the skin.

Dosage

Initially, acitretin starts at 25 mg a day and then can be increased to a 25- to 50-mg dose given once a day with the main meal until the lesions clear, which occurs gradually.

Contraindications

Acitretin is contraindicated in pregnancy and lactation and with the use of alcohol. It cannot be used in patients with severe renal impairment and increased lipid levels. The patient cannot donate blood for 3 years after therapy. Caution is used if there is a history of depression, obesity, or alcohol abuse.

Adverse Events

Adverse effects include lipid elevations, abnormal liver function, alopecia, skin peeling, pruritus, dry skin, dry mouth, epistaxis, paresthesia, paronychia, and pseudotumor cerebri.

Interactions

Drug interactions occur with methotrexate (MTX, Rheumatrex), alcohol, and progestin-only contraceptives. Women must not ingest alcohol during therapy or for 2 months afterward because alcohol prolongs the teratogenic potential of the drug.

Methotrexate

Methotrexate is used to treat generalized psoriasis.

Mechanism of Action

Methotrexate inhibits folic acid reductase, resulting in the inhibition of cellular replication and selection of the most rapidly dividing cells.

Dosage

The initial dose is 2.5 mg a week administered in three doses over a 24-hour period. It is then titrated to a dose of 12.5 to 25 mg a week. With improvement in the disease, the dose is reduced and other agents are used. Folic acid, 1 mg daily, should be taken on nontreatment days.

Contraindications

Methotrexate is contraindicated in pregnancy and lactation, and the drug is used with caution in patients with renal and hepatic disorders and leukopenia.

Adverse Events

Common adverse effects include headache, blurred vision, fatigue, malaise, gastrointestinal (GI) distress, gingivitis, hepatic toxicity, bone marrow depression, rash, alopecia, and chills and fevers.

Interactions

There is an increased risk of toxicity if the patient is taking other medications, such as salicylates, phenytoin (Dilantin), and sulfonamides. Use of methotrexate also decreases the serum level of digoxin (Lanoxin).

Cyclosporine

Mechanism of Action

Cyclosporine suppresses cell-mediated immune reactions and humoral immunity. It inhibits production of IL-2, which is responsible for producing T-cell proliferation. Cyclosporine promotes rapid remission for severe psoriasis. It is usually used for short-term treatment of severe exacerbations.

Dosage

The maximum dose for use in psoriasis is 2 to 5 mg/kg/d. Maintenance therapy is at lower doses.

Contraindications

Cyclosporine is contraindicated in pregnancy and lactation and must be used cautiously in patients with impaired renal function and malabsorption.

Adverse Events

Adverse effects include tremor, gingival hyperplasia, GI upset, hypertension, nephrotoxicity, hirsutism, and acne. Lesions can recur within days to weeks after treatment, and rebounds with worse symptoms are not uncommon.

Interactions

Cyclosporine use increases the risk for nephrotoxicity if the patient uses other nephrotoxic agents, and it also increases the risk for digoxin toxicity. Cyclosporine interacts with lovastatin (Mevacor), diltiazem (Cardizem), and ketoconazole (Nizoral), and its therapeutic effect is decreased with concomitant hydantoin (Dilantin), rifampin (Rifadin), and sulfonamide use.

PHOSPHODIESTERASE 4 INHIBITORS

Apremilast (Otezla)

Mechanism of Action

Apremilast is an oral small molecule specific to cyclic adenosine monophosphate (cAMP).

The specific mechanism is not well understood.

Dosage

A starter pack is designed to allow for titration and then progress up to 30 mg twice daily.

Contraindications

Patients with a known hypersensitivity to apremilast or to other ingredients.

Adverse Events

The most common adverse event is GI distress and diarrhea which may be self-limiting.

Interactions

Apremilast exposure is decreased when Otezla is coadministered with strong CYP450 inducers (i.e., rifampin) and may decrease efficacy.

The "Biologics"

The "biologics" interact with specific targets in the T cell–mediated inflammatory process. They have an anti-inflammatory effect through the inhibition of cytokine release, prevention of T-cell activation, depletion of pathologic T cells, and blocking the interactions that lead to T-cell activation or migration into the tissue. They also alter the balance of the T-cell types and inhibit key inflammatory cytokines, such as tumor necrosis factor (TNF).

Etanercept

Etanercept (Enbrel) contains human TNF receptor.

Mechanism of Action

It binds and inhibits TNF, the cytokine that helps regulate the body's immune response to inflammation. It is used in moderate to severe psoriasis.

Dosage

The dose of etanercept in psoriasis is 50 mg subcutaneously twice a week initially for 3 months. Maintenance dose is 50 mg sq weekly, with a maximum of 25 mg given at one site. It requires two injections in separate sites. A purified protein derivative test must be negative before treatment starts.

Contraindications

Contraindications include a concurrent live vaccine and an active infection. Caution is recommended in pregnant patients (although it is a category B drug) and patients with impaired renal function, asthma, a history of blood dyscrasias, central nervous system demyelinating disease, and a history of chronic recurrent infections.

Adverse Events

Adverse events include infection, injection site pain, localized erythema, rash, upper respiratory infections, abdominal pain, and vomiting.

Interactions

There is an increased chance of infection with immunosuppressants. Live vaccines should be given 2 weeks before or 1 month after therapy to ensure adequate immunization.

Infliximab

Mechanism of Action

Infliximab (Remicade) is a monoclonal antibody that targets TNF-α and inhibits its activity.

Dosage

Infliximab is given by intravenous infusion over at least 2 hours. The dose is 5 mg/kg at week 0, week 2, and week 6 and then once every 8 weeks. Patients must be tested for tuberculosis (TB) before administration.

Contraindications

It is contraindicated in moderate to severe congestive heart failure. It should not be given in conjunction with live vaccines.

Adverse Events

Adverse events include infection, headache, GI upset, fatigue, cough, pruritus, and congestive heart failure.

Interactions

Immunosuppressants increase the risk of infection.

Adalimumab

Mechanism of Action

Adalimumab (Humira) is a recombinant humanized immunoglobulin G1 monoclonal antibody that binds to TNF-α. It reduces signs and symptoms of active arthritis and psoriatic arthritis.

Dosage

Adalimumab is given subcutaneously into the thigh or abdomen. The dose is initially 80 mg followed by 40 mg every other week starting the week after the initial dose and is rapid acting. Patients must be tested for TB before administration.

Contraindications

It should not be given in conjunction with live vaccines.

Adverse Events

Adverse events include headache, injection site reactions, nausea, and rash.

Interactions

Immunosuppressants increase the risk of infection.

Ustekinumab

Mechanism of Action

Ustekinumab (Stelara) is a human interleukin-12 and interleukin-23 antagonist.

Dosage

Administered subcutaneously, two weight-based doses are available, 45 mg for patients weighing less than 100 kg (220 lb) and 90 mg for patients weighing greater than 100 kg (220 lb) four times a year.

Contraindications

Ustekinumab is not recommended for patients with a sensitivity to any of the excipients.

Adverse events

May include nasopharyngitis and upper respiratory tract infections. Serious infections and malignancies may occur.

Interactions

Live vaccines should not be given to patients taking ustekinumab.

Secukinumab

Mechanism of Action

Secukinumab (Cosentyx) is a monoclonal antibody that binds to interleukin-17 blocking the cytokine interaction with its receptor.

Dosing

Three hundred milligrams administered subcutaneously (in divided doses of 150 each) every week for 5 weeks and then once every month.

Contraindications

Similar to all other biologic agents.

Adverse Events

Similar to all other biologic agents.

Interactions

No live vaccines.

Selecting the Most Appropriate Agent

Selection of therapy depends on the patient's age, type of lesion, site and involvement, and previous treatments. Mild to relatively moderate psoriasis (less than 10% BSA) can be treated by a primary care provider. Topical treatment of psoriasis is the first step and is usually effective for mild disease. Patients with more generalized disease are referred to a dermatologist for treatment and phototherapy, and systemic agents are used (Table 15.2 and Figure 15.1).

It appears that combination therapy with systemic agents and other modalities has synergistic value. In combination therapy, the dose can often be reduced, causing less toxicity from the drugs. Systemic therapy with phototherapy is also effective.

First-Line Therapy

First-line therapy includes moisturizers and topical steroids. For 2 weeks, a high-potency or very high–potency topical steroid is applied twice a day and covered by an occlusive dressing of plastic wrap. A low-potency preparation is used on the face and intertriginous areas. An ointment is recommended because it provides the most moisture. An emollient also is used to keep the area moist.

TABLE 15.2

Recommended Order of Treatment for Psoriasis

Order	Therapy	Comments
First line	High-potency topical corticosteroids applied to moist skin and use of occlusive dressing twice a day for 2 wk. Use emollients as adjunct therapy.	Use when <10% of body surface area is affected.
Second line	If the patient responded well to first-line therapy, provide a 1-wk rest from the topical corticosteroids and initiate another 2 wk of therapy with the same agent for two more times. OR Taper the high-potency topical corticosteroid to once or twice a week and add a vitamin D analog twice a day.	If there is remission, applying the topical steroids once or twice a week may maintain remission.
Third line	Refer to dermatologist for systemic therapy.	For use with >20% body surface area, PUVA is used with coal tar or anthralin; PUVB is used with psoralens.

PUVA (B), psoralens with ultraviolet A (B).

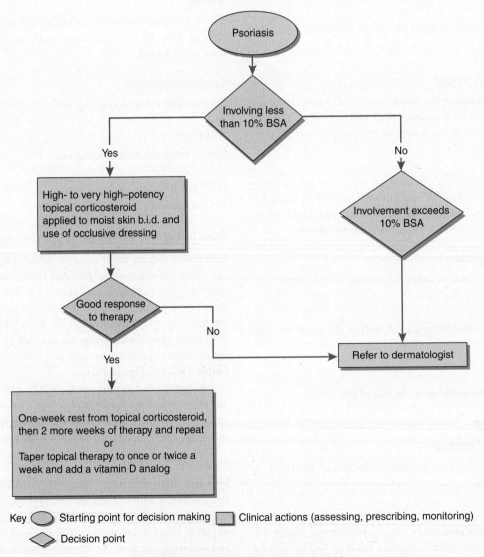

FIGURE 15.1 Treatment algorithm for psoriasis.

Second-Line Therapy

If the patient's response to first-line therapy is not optimal, several second-line choices are available. If the patient had a good response to first-line therapy, therapy may consist of a 1-week rest from the topical corticosteroids and then another 2 weeks of therapy with the same agent for two more times. If the psoriasis goes into remission, applying the topical steroids once or twice a week may maintain the remission.

Another option is to taper the high-potency topical corticosteroid use to once or twice a week and add a vitamin D analog twice a day to the regimen. This produces a better result than either drug used alone. The topical corticosteroid helps clear the plaques and reduces irritation from the vitamin D preparation.

Third-Line Therapy

If first- and second-line treatments fail, a patient is referred to a dermatologist, who may use ultraviolet B light treatments, antimetabolites, etanercept, or psoralens plus ultraviolet A light therapy.

MONITORING PATIENT RESPONSE

The goal of chronic topical corticosteroid therapy is to use the lowest effective potency to control symptoms. Follow-up initially may need to be monthly and then may progress to every 2 to 3 months. In addition, referral for counseling, if desired, may help address related emotional issues.

PATIENT EDUCATION

Drug Information

In patients with psoriasis, education regarding stress monitoring and control is important, as is education regarding the disease process and treatment goals. The patient should understand that psoriasis is not contagious.

Patients may also benefit from information and support from groups such as the National Psoriasis Foundation (1-800-723-9166, www.psoriasis.org).

Showing the patient how to apply topical steroids is an important aspect of care, particularly if the medications are to be used only twice a day and applied lightly on moist skin.

Lifestyle Changes

Symptom control, rather than cure, is the goal of therapy. Patients may help control symptoms by exposing their skin to the sun. This should be accomplished by gradually increasing the length of exposure. Emphasis should be placed on the importance of using sunscreen and avoiding sunburn. To prevent infection, patients must take care not to cut the lesions when shaving (if there are lesions in the area).

Psoriasis can be triggered by infections, stress, and changes in climate that can dry skin. These should be avoided when possible.

Complementary and Alternative Medicine

Fish oil is thought to alter the immune response and in small quantities can relieve itching and scaling. It has an effect on chronic plaque psoriasis in doses of 6 to 15 g daily. An alternative is to eat fish three times a week. Aloe vera was shown to be effective in treatment of psoriasis. In a 16-week study, there was 82.8% clearing of psoriatic plaque using 0.5% hydrophilic aloe vera cream three times a day. Glucosamine has been shown to relieve some of the pain of arthritis from psoriasis.

CASE STUDY*

P.B. is a 58-year-old woman with a history of hypertension. She seeks treatment for scattered plaques with a silvery-white scale on her elbows, forearms, and knees. The BSA affected is approximately 8%. She is very self-conscious about the lesions: "I just want them to go away." Her medications include propranolol 40 mg tid and furosemide 40 mg daily. She has a positive family history of psoriasis and reports high levels of stress in her job and life. She smokes a pack of cigarettes per day.

DIAGNOSIS: PSORIASIS

1. List specific goals for treatment for **P.B.**
2. What drug therapy would you prescribe? Why?
3. What are the parameters for monitoring the success of the therapy?
4. Discuss specific patient education based on the prescribed therapy.
5. List one or two adverse reactions for the selected agent that would cause you to change therapy.
6. What would be the choice for second-line therapy?
7. What OTC or alternative medications would be appropriate for **P.B.**?
8. What lifestyle changes would you recommend to **P.B.**?
9. Describe one or two drug–drug or drug–food interactions for the selected agent.

* Answers can be found online.

Bibliography

Bos, J. (2007). Psoriasis, innate immunity, and gene pools. *Journal of the American Academy of Dermatology, 56*(3), 468–471.

Busard, C., Zweegers, J., Limpens, J., et al. (2014). Combined Use of Systemic Agents for Psoriasis: A Systematic Review. *JAMA Dermatology, 150*(11), 1213–1220.

Feldman, S. (2014). Five factors for choosing the right biologic treatment. *The Dermatologist, 22*(9), 26–29.

Feldman, S., Horn, E., Balkreshnan, R., et al. (2008). Psoriasis: Improving adherence to topical therapy. *Journal of the American Academy of Dermatology, 59*(6), 1009–1016.

Gaspari, A. (2006). Innate and adaptive immunity and pathophysiology of psoriasis. *Journal of the American Academy of Dermatology, 54*(3, Suppl. 2), S67–S80.

Lam, J., Palifka, J., & Dohil, M. (2008). Safety of dermatological drugs used in pregnant patients with psoriasis and other inflammatory skin diseases. *Journal of the American Academy of Dermatology, 59*(2), 295–315.

Levin, D., & Gottlieb, A. (2009). Evaluation and management of psoriasis: An internist's guide. *Medical Clinics of North America, 93*(6), 1291–1303.

Menter, A., Korman, N., Elmets, C., et al. (2010). Guidelines of care for management of psoriasis and psoriatic arthritis. *Journal of the American Academy of Dermatology, 62*(1), 114–135.

Yamauchi, P. S., & Bagel, J. (2015). Next generation biologics in the management of plaque psoriasis: A literature review of IL-17 inhibition. *Journal of Drugs in Dermatology, 14*(3), 244–250.

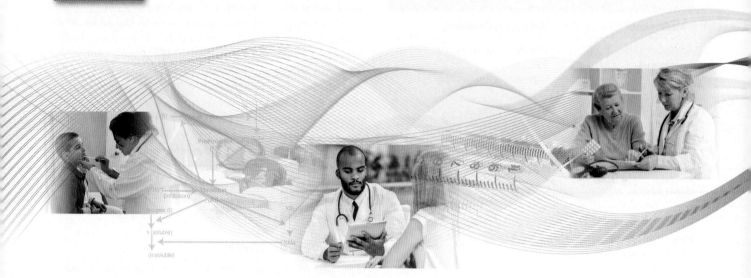

16   Acne Vulgaris and Rosacea

Virginia P. Arcangelo

ACNE VULGARIS

Acne vulgaris is viewed by many as a rite of passage during the adolescent years. Up to 90% of all teenagers report having some form of acne. Adults suffer from the effects of acne as well: between 30% and 50% of adult women report experiencing acne. Consumers spend millions of dollars annually on prescription and over-the-counter (OTC) acne preparations.

The psychosocial costs of acne are great. Adolescents are particularly affected by physical defects, no matter how minor they appear to others. The health care practitioner must be particularly sensitive to the perceived seriousness of the acne in addition to the clinical picture. What may seem inconsequential to the practitioner may be devastating to the patient. No matter how minor the acne may appear to the provider, it is important to ask patients if they are concerned about their acne and whether they would like treatment.

CAUSES

Historically, numerous theories of the cause of acne vulgaris have been proposed, yet the exact cause remains unknown. Foods, stress, and dirt, although not causative, may exacerbate existing acne, which is why it is important to obtain a complete health history to ascertain precipitating factors. For example, a variety of drugs, physical occlusants, and conditions may exacerbate acne. Certain drugs used to treat tuberculosis, seizure disorders, or steroid-dependent chronic illness or depression may cause a drug-induced acneiform rash (**Table 16.1**). Drug-induced acne should be suspected when all lesions are in the same stage (e.g., the lesions are uniformly

all pustules or all open comedones), covering the face, chest, trunk, arms, and legs.

Acne may be exacerbated in teenagers and adults whose skin is exposed to oily agents, such as makeup, oil-based sunscreen, and oil-based hair products that come in contact with the forehead and temporal regions of the face (referred to as *pomade acne*). Friction acne from tight-fitting clothes, such as football helmets and hatbands, is found over the skin rubbed by the clothes. Exposure to animal-, vegetable-, and petroleum-based oils used in workplaces such as fast food restaurants and automotive garages may also exacerbate acne. Thus, although eating French fries may not cause acne, cooking them may make the acne worse. Emotional stress may contribute to acne exacerbations in persons prone to breakouts, but studies have not consistently proven the correlation.

Women with a history of menstrual irregularities, hirsutism, and treatment-resistant acne should be evaluated for androgen excess associated with polycystic ovarian disease.

PATHOPHYSIOLOGY

Acne usually begins 1 to 2 years before the onset of puberty, when androgen production increases. Excess androgen causes increased sebum production. For unknown reasons, abnormal keratinization causes retention of sebum in the pilosebaceous follicle. This produces open comedones (blackheads) and closed comedones (whiteheads).

When closed comedones continue to produce keratin and sebum, the pilosebaceous follicle ruptures and inflames the surrounding tissue. If the inflammation is close to the surface, a papule forms. If it is deeper in the dermis, a larger papule or nodule forms. These deeper, nodular acne cysts cause permanent scars.

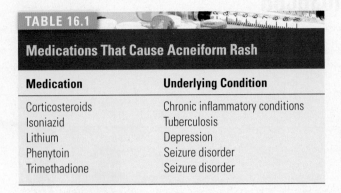

TABLE 16.1

Medications That Cause Acneiform Rash

Medication	Underlying Condition
Corticosteroids	Chronic inflammatory conditions
Isoniazid	Tuberculosis
Lithium	Depression
Phenytoin	Seizure disorder
Trimethadione	Seizure disorder

Although *Propionibacterium acnes*, an anaerobic gram-positive bacterium, is present as normal flora in the pilosebaceous follicle, acne vulgaris is not an infectious entity. Rather, it is believed that *P. acnes* produces lipolytic enzymes that in turn produce biologically active extracellular products. These in turn attract polymorphonuclear leukocytes and monocytes, which increase inflammation.

DIAGNOSTIC CRITERIA

Acne vulgaris is diagnosed from the clinical presentation of the patient's skin. It is classified and subsequently treated depending on its severity.

The mildest form of acne is comedonal. Both open and closed comedones may be present. Mild inflammatory acne is manifested by papules. Moderate inflammatory acne consists of pustules and some cysts. Severe cystic acne consists of cysts, nodules, and scarring (**Table 16.2**).

INITIATING DRUG THERAPY

Skin care is the most important nonpharmacologic tool in the management of acne vulgaris. The patient should be instructed to wash the face gently two or three times a day with a mild soap such as Basis, Cetaphil, Neutrogena, or Purpose. Care should be taken to avoid harsh, drying cleansers. Washing should be gentle because scrubbing the skin may exacerbate the acne. Comedo removal, although therapeutic, should be

TABLE 16.2

Classification of Acne Vulgaris

Classification	Physical Findings
Comedonal acne	Open comedones (blackheads), closed comedones (whiteheads)
Mild inflammatory acne	Papules
Moderate inflammatory acne	Pustules, cysts
Severe cystic acne	Cysts, nodules, "ice-pick" scarring

undertaken only by someone skilled in the proper technique. Picking or popping pimples may increase tissue damage and infection. The health care provider should advise the patient to avoid manipulating the acne with the fingers.

In general, use of personal care products should be minimized. Moisturizers and cosmetics should be water based, noncomedogenic, and fragrance free. If hair preparations are used, they should also be water based. The patient should be instructed to apply hair products so that they do not come in contact with facial skin.

The practitioner also needs to stress that ingestion of specific foods, such as chocolate, greasy foods, colas, and iodide-containing foods, does not cause acne. Elimination diets are not considered therapeutic unless the patient reports an exacerbation associated with a certain food. In that case, the food must be avoided for 4 to 6 weeks and then gradually reintroduced to see what effect that food has on the acne.

Goals of Drug Therapy

The goal of pharmacotherapy is to minimize the number and severity of new lesions, prevent scarring, and improve the patient's appearance. The patient must be counseled that improvement of acne vulgaris takes time—usually 4 to 6 weeks. Some form of therapy will probably need to be continued throughout adolescence and even into young adulthood.

Pharmacotherapy choices are based on the severity of the acne. Currently, successful therapy usually relies on a combination of medications. The synergistic effect of two or more drugs from different classes produces the best results. See **Table 16.3** for a summary of acne medications.

Comedolytics

Retinoic Acid (Tretinoin)

Marketed under the trade names Retin-A and Avita, retinoic acid is the acid form of vitamin A. When applied topically, retinoic acid acts on the epidermis with little systemic absorption to decrease cohesion between epidermal cells and increase epidermal cell turnover. The result is expulsion of open comedones and the conversion of closed comedones to open ones.

When used properly, retinoic acid causes mild erythema and peeling of the skin. Some patients cannot tolerate daily use or prolonged contact at the initiation of therapy. For example, fair-skinned patients should be advised to start out using the product every other day. Alternatively, the patient may be instructed to apply retinoic acid to the face for 15 to 30 minutes each night and then wash off the medication. Gradually, the length of time the medication remains on the face is increased until it can be tolerated overnight. It is best to apply the medication on clean, thoroughly dry skin to avoid excessive irritation. Side effects of retinoic acid include erythema, local skin irritation, and photosensitivity. Patients should be advised to avoid prolonged exposure to the sun or to wear a noncomedogenic sunscreen formulated specifically for use on the face.

TABLE 16.3

Overview of Topical and Oral Acne Preparations

Generic (Trade) Name and Dosage	Selected Adverse Events	Contraindications	Special Considerations
Topical Medications			
tretinoin (Retin-A, Avita) 0.025%, 0.05% cream, gel 0.04%, 0.1% microspheres Apply once daily; increase strength as tolerated.	Erythema, local skin irritation, photosensitivity	Eczema, sunburn	Apply to dry skin for short periods or on alternate nights until better tolerated. Avoid products with high concentrations of alcohol, astringents, spices, lime. Pregnancy category C
benzoyl peroxide (many) 2.5%–5.0% once a day; increase to two or three times daily.	Irritation	Sunscreens containing para-aminobenzoic acid (PABA) may cause transient skin discoloration.	Product may bleach fabrics. Apply at different time from other topical medications.
azelaic acid (Azelex) 20% cream Apply twice a day.	Pruritus, irritation		Darker-pigmented people may have hypopigmentation. Exacerbation of asthma.
clindamycin (Cleocin T) Apply to skin twice a day.	Burning; stinging of eyes; possibly pseudomembranous colitis		Discontinue use if diarrhea develops. Pseudomembranous colitis may develop. Drug may potentiate neuromuscular blocking agents.
erythromycin (many) 2%–3% topical Apply twice daily.	Irritation	Allergy to erythromycin	None
tazarotene (Tazorac) 0.05%, 0.1% gel, cream Apply once daily.	Irritation, photosensitivity	Pregnancy category X	Obtain negative pregnancy test and use reliable contraception during medication use.
Oral Medications			
tetracycline (many) 500–1,000 mg daily divided bid/qid Taper to 250 mg/d after improvement; attempt to discontinue after 4–6 mo of therapy.	Photosensitivity, gastric irritation, decreased effectiveness of oral contraceptives	Age younger than 12 y Pregnancy category D	Drug may increase serum digoxin levels. Drug absorption is reduced if taken with antacids, iron, zinc, dairy products. Drug use may increase blood urea nitrogen values if renal system is impaired.
erythromycin (many) 500–1,000 mg/d divided bid/qid	Nausea, vomiting, diarrhea, rash, allergic reactions, fungal infection, hepatitis, ototoxicity	Allergy to erythromycin or macrolide Not recommended for children younger than age 2 mo	Take on an empty stomach for better absorption 1 h before or 2 h after a meal. Enteric-coated form can be taken with or without food. Interactions: warfarin, theophylline, cisapride, digoxin, and others
isotretinoin (Accutane, generic) 0.5–1.0 mg/kg bid	Increased cholesterol and triglyceride levels; dry skin and mucous membranes; depression; aggressive, violent behaviors; back pain; arthralgias in pediatric patients	Adolescents before cessation of growth Pregnancy category X	Prescriber must be registered in SMART program. Female patients of childbearing age must have two negative pregnancy tests prior to therapy initiation and monthly negative pregnancy test while on therapy. Monitor cholesterol and triglyceride levels, complete blood count, liver function tests before therapy, at 4 wk, and as indicated
ethinyl estradiol with norgestimate (Ortho Tri-Cyclen, Tri-Sprintec) 1 tablet daily		Premenarchal girls, male patients	Women who smoke should avoid use of oral contraceptives.

Retinoic acid is available in cream (0.025%, 0.05%, and 0.1%), gel (0.01% and 0.025%), liquid (0.05%), and microsphere (0.04% and 0.1%) formulations. The microsphere formulation encapsulates the active ingredient in microspheres, which act as a reservoir that slowly releases the retinoic acid. Although the microsphere product contains a higher percentage of medication, the slow-release formulation produces less irritation, making it one of the mildest dosage forms.

Adapalene Gel

Adapalene (Differin), a topical medication for treating noninflammatory acne, is a derivative of naphthoic acid, which binds to retinoid receptors. It is considered less irritating than retinoic acid. Up to 40% of patients report irritation, but it subsides during the first month of treatment. Adapalene is applied in the same way as retinoic acid. A small amount is applied either every other day or for short periods in the evening until the drug can be tolerated overnight. Side effects of adapalene include hyperpigmentation and photosensitivity.

Tazarotene Gel

A retinoid prodrug, tazarotene gel (Tazorac) is effective against both comedonal and inflammatory acne as well as psoriasis. Despite being a topical drug, tazarotene is considered teratogenic (pregnancy category X) and should be used only by women who take systemic contraceptives and who have a negative pregnancy test.

Care should be taken when using the medication with tetracycline because it potentiates the photosensitivity reaction. Other side effects include dry skin, erythema, and pruritus.

Comedolytic Bactericidals

Benzoyl Peroxide

Benzoyl peroxide is both a comedolytic and bactericidal agent specific to *P. acnes*. It has a role in inflammatory acne because of its antibacterial qualities. By decreasing *P. acnes* levels, it decreases the inflammation caused by leukocytic and monocytic attraction to the pilosebaceous follicle.

The major side effect of benzoyl peroxide is irritation. Like all comedolytics, benzoyl peroxide is applied initially in a low-percentage formulation in a nonirritating base. The patient increases the dosage strength and frequency. Because benzoyl peroxide may bleach colored items, the patient should be instructed not to let the product come in contact with brightly colored towels, pillowcases, or clothing. If used with retinoic acid, benzoyl peroxide should be applied in the morning and retinoic acid before bedtime.

Benzoyl peroxide is available in various strengths and bases, both OTC and by prescription. Gel formulations, which are considered more effective, are available in 2.5%, 4%, 5%, 10%, and 20% strengths. Lotions (5%, 10%, and 20%) and creams (5% and 10%) are also available.

Before using prescription-strength benzoyl peroxide, the patient should be instructed to discontinue any washes or lotions containing benzoyl peroxide that he or she may already be using. Inadvertent use of the two products may increase irritation.

Azelaic Acid

Azelaic acid (Azelex) is believed to interfere with the deoxyribonucleic acid synthesis of acne-causing bacteria. The drug is considered as effective as topical macrolide antibiotics in treating papulopustular acne. Azelaic acid is supplied as a 20% cream and is applied topically twice a day. In dark-pigmented people, hypopigmentation may develop from use.

Topical Antibiotics

Topical antibiotics may be prescribed when comedolytic antibacterials are either not effective or not tolerated and systemic antibiotics are not desired. Topical antibiotics inhibit the growth of *P. acnes* and decrease the number of comedones, papules, and pustules. Clindamycin 2% (Cleocin T) or erythromycin 2% or 3% (many brands) is supplied in solutions, saturated pads, lotions, and gels. Rarely, topical clindamycin has been implicated in pseudomembranous colitis and regional enteritis. The practitioner should advise patients to discontinue therapy if diarrhea develops.

Oral Antibiotics

When improvement cannot be achieved with topical therapy, oral antibiotics may be considered. Oral antibiotics are indicated for inflammatory acne because they suppress *P. acnes* as well as inhibit bacterial lipases, neutrophil chemotaxis, and follicular inflammation. There is no indication for their use in noninflammatory acne.

Tetracycline

Tetracycline is the most commonly used oral antibiotic for treating inflammatory acne. Doses begin at 500 to 1,000 mg/d and are tapered to 250 mg/d after improvement occurs. Clinical improvement takes at least 3 to 4 weeks.

Tetracycline permanently stains the teeth in children, so it should not be prescribed for patients younger than 12 years of age. Moreover, the drug is a teratogen. It may also decrease the effectiveness of oral contraceptives. Therefore, caution should be used when prescribing it for sexually active female patients. Patient education should include directions to avoid concurrent ingestion of milk products, iron preparations, and antacids, which decrease absorption. Ideally, the medication should be taken on an empty stomach.

Side effects of tetracycline include photosensitivity, gastric irritation, blood dyscrasias, and pseudotumor cerebri (benign intracranial hypertension). Caution should be used in treating patients who have renal failure or who are concurrently taking digoxin because tetracycline may increase serum digoxin levels.

Erythromycin

Erythromycin and its derivatives are good alternatives when tetracycline fails or is not tolerated. They can also be used when the patient is younger than age 10 or pregnant. A common side effect is gastrointestinal upset. There are drug interactions with digoxin, theophylline, and cyclosporine.

Other Systemic Drugs

Given in doses between 500 and 1,000 mg/d, erythromycin is as effective as tetracycline. It is helpful in treating people with tetracycline allergy. Minocycline and doxycycline have also been used, but there is no advantage over tetracycline or erythromycin. Minocycline is considerably more expensive.

Retinoic Acid Derivatives: Isotretinoin

Isotretinoin (Accutane) has changed the management of acne therapy. It is reserved for patients with severe nodulocystic acne when other treatments fail. Isotretinoin is a retinoic acid derivative. Although the exact mechanism is unknown, it decreases sebum production, follicular obstruction, and the number of skin bacteria. It also has an anti-inflammatory action.

Dosage

Isotretinoin is given at a dose of 0.5 to 1 mg/kg/d. Therapy continues for 15 to 20 weeks unless significant improvement occurs sooner. If therapy needs to be repeated, 2 months should elapse before restarting the drug.

Contraindications

Because isotretinoin, a teratogen, is associated with serious birth defects, only prescribers registered in the SMART (System to Manage Accutane-Related Teratogenicity) program (Roche Laboratory) may prescribe Accutane. Similar programs are in place for generic isotretinoin. The SMART program requires prescribers to study Roche's Guide to Best Practices and sign and return a letter of understanding that details the risks of pregnancy while on Accutane. The letter of understanding is an agreement to follow the recommendations of the SMART program, which includes obtaining two negative pregnancy tests prior to initiation of the drug and obtaining monthly pregnancy tests during therapy for all female patients. A yellow self-adhesive Accutane qualification sticker is to be placed on every prescription written, regardless of the gender of the patient. Only 30 days of drug can be prescribed at one time. Female patients able to bear children should be counseled to use two forms of contraception (Roche Laboratories, 2002). It is recommended that this drug be prescribed by a dermatologist.

Before initiating therapy, a baseline complete blood count and chemistry profile and fasting triglyceride and cholesterol levels should be obtained. A complete blood count and a chemistry profile should then be obtained 1 month after the start of therapy. Pregnancy should be avoided for 1 month after therapy is discontinued.

Adverse Events

The most significant adverse effect of isotretinoin is teratogenicity. A 25-fold increase in fetal abnormalities has been documented. Even without external abnormalities, approximately 50% of children exposed to isotretinoin in utero have subnormal intelligence.

Approximately 25% of patients experience cholesterol and triglyceride elevations. Pseudomotor cerebri has been reported when isotretinoin therapy is combined with tetracycline. Almost all patients report dry skin and mucous membranes, including cheilitis, severe dry skin, and difficulty wearing contact lenses. Other side effects include musculoskeletal aches and corneal opacities. Therapy should not be initiated in adolescents who have not finished growing because the drug may cause premature closure of the epiphyses.

A "black box" warning was added in 2002, warning of an increase in aggressive or violent behaviors in patients as well as back pain in children: 29% of children developed back pain and 22% experienced arthralgias (FDA MedWatch, 2002).

Other Medications

Topical Antibiotic–Benzoyl Peroxide Combinations

Marketed as Benzamycin, the combination of erythromycin 3% and benzoyl peroxide 5% in a gel base may increase compliance when a topical antibiotic is needed in addition to one or more other topical medications. The gel is applied once or twice a day. Although the product requires refrigeration, small quantities may be transferred to another container for up to 10 days, which tends to promote therapeutic adherence. Benzamycin is also marketed in pouches (Benzamycin Pak) that are mixed by the patient and therefore do not require refrigeration. The pack holds the two active ingredients in separate chambers, and they can be mixed as needed.

Similarly, a combination of clindamycin 1% and benzoyl peroxide 5% gel (BenzaClin Gel, Duac Gel) is available. Unlike Benzamycin, these products have a shelf life of 3 months at room temperature and do not require refrigeration.

Hormonal Therapy

Oral contraceptives can be used in women when conventional topical and systemic therapies have failed. Oral contraceptives will be discussed in Chapter 55. Oral contraceptives that contain ethinyl estradiol, levonorgestrel, and norgestimate or drospirenone are effective in the treatment of acne. Some other oral contraceptives may exacerbate acne. Relative to other therapies, oral contraceptives are inexpensive. They reduce both comedonal and inflammatory acnes and are worth considering for women who are already taking or considering taking systemic contraceptives.

Selecting the Most Appropriate Agent

The most important consideration in selecting a therapeutic regimen is matching the severity of the acne to the appropriate pharmacologic agent (**Figure 16.1** and **Table 16.4**).

First-Line Therapy

The first line of therapy for comedonal acne is topical medication. Topical comedolytics encourage faster turnover of the surface skin. The addition of bactericidals or topical antibiotics enhances results for patients with closed comedones and pustules.

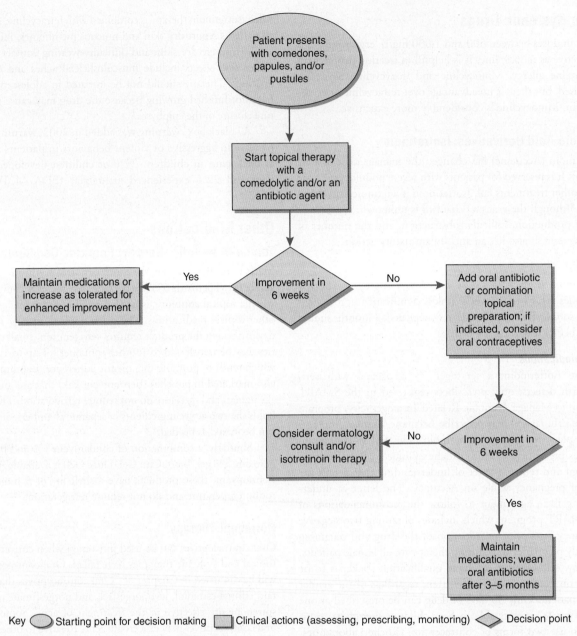

FIGURE 16.1 Treatment algorithm for acne.

TABLE 16.4		
Recommended Order of Treatment for Acne		
Order	**Agent**	**Comments**
First line	Topical therapy	Improvement takes ~6 wk.
Second line	Oral medications	Monitor in 6 wk.
Third line	Isotretinoin or refer to dermatologist	Prescribe with caution to women of childbearing age. Pregnancy category X

Second-Line Therapy

Patients whose acne does not respond to topical therapy may need oral medications. The practitioner may initiate treatment with oral antibiotics in addition to topical medications for more severe papulocystic acne. Oral contraceptives are a useful and cost-effective alternative for sexually active women.

Third-Line Therapy

Isotretinoin is reserved for the most severe forms of nodulocystic acne. Special care must be taken when prescribing this agent for women who can become pregnant. Practitioners who are not registered with the SMART program or who cannot comply with the necessary monitoring and follow-up may feel more comfortable referring the patient to a dermatologist for evaluation and treatment.

SPECIAL POPULATION CONSIDERATIONS

Pediatric

Because of the risk of dental enamel defects and bone growth retardation, the use of tetracycline is contraindicated in children younger than age 12. Growth retardation in children who have not reached adult height is associated with isotretinoin use. Children may also experience increased arthralgias and back pain with the use of isotretinoin.

Women of Childbearing Age

Women of childbearing age who are using isotretinoin or tazarotene gel must not become pregnant because of the teratogenicity of the products. Practitioners may suggest that a long-acting contraceptive, such as Depo-Provera, be used. If pregnancy occurs, the patient must be counseled accordingly. Tetracycline, also considered teratogenic, may decrease the effectiveness of oral contraceptives. Women taking this antibiotic should rely on a long-acting contraceptive or a barrier method to prevent pregnancy. Retinoic acid is labeled pregnancy category C and is not recommended for use in pregnant women or nursing mothers.

Ethnic

Azelaic acid may cause hypopigmentation in patients with dark skin.

MONITORING PATIENT RESPONSE

Follow-up should be scheduled monthly to monitor the patient's response to therapy, provide reassurance, and encourage adherence to therapy. Monthly visits provide the opportunity to adjust medications and dosages as the patient's acne responds to treatment. The ideal management is long-term topical therapy. If isotretinoin is prescribed, laboratory tests should be obtained before therapy and 1 month into therapy, as described previously.

PATIENT EDUCATION

Drug Information

The practitioner may show the patient how to apply topical preparations correctly to prevent excessive irritation (**Box 16.1**). An important consideration in prescribing topical therapy is that many gels and solutions contain significant amounts of alcohol. If a patient is sensitive to alcohol-based preparations or is experiencing significant dryness despite low

---

BOX 16.1   General Principles for Applying Topical Acne Preparations

- Initiate therapy with a lower concentration of active ingredient and then work up to a higher concentration as tolerated.
- Choose a product with a lower percentage of alcohol for people with sensitive skin.
- Apply the product to clean, dry skin. Allow at least 20 minutes to elapse between washing the face and applying the medication.
- Use the smallest amount of medication necessary for coverage.
- Apply in "dots" over the desired area and then rub into skin.
- Apply one drying agent in the morning and another in the evening to avoid excessive irritation.

---

concentrations of active ingredients, the practitioner may consider switching to a preparation that does not contain alcohol, such as a cream or aqueous gel.

Nutritional factors play an important role in the pathogenesis of acne. A diet with a low glycemic load, higher in protein than carbohydrates and fats, can decrease lesion counts in acne vulgaris. A low glycemic–load diet has also been associated with a reduction in calorie intake, body mass index, and insulin resistance. Improved insulin sensitivity leads to a decrease in androgen production and a concordant improvement in the symptoms of acne vulgaris.

Patients should be cautioned to avoid using excessive amounts of topical medications in the hope that it will speed improvement. Instead, irritation will most likely be the result, and that may discourage continuation of therapy.

Patience is the key to resolution of acne. Adolescents looking for a quick cure may be disappointed. All forms of acne therapy require a minimum of 4 to 6 weeks before results are seen. It is important to provide appropriate follow-up and encouragement and to have the patient return for evaluation and refinement of the treatment program.

Patient-Oriented Information Sources

The Web sites www.acne.org and www.nih.gov/medlineplus/acne.html (a site from the National Institutes of Health) provide information about acne and treatment.

COMPLIMENTARY AND ALTERNATIVE MEDICINE

Brewer's yeast has been use in Western Europe as a treatment for acne. It contains chromium which decreases insulin resistance. In one study of 139 subjects with acne, over 80%

showed significant improvement in symptoms (Weber et al., 1989). The recommended dose is 2 g three times a day.

Zinc is involved in the maintenance of skin health and immune function, local hormone activation, and production of retinol-binding protein. It has shown some bacteriostatic action against *P. acnes* and inhibitory action on the production of retinol-binding protein.

Another product that has shown to improve acne severity is tea tree oil. It has less skin irritation that benzoyl peroxide. A solution of 5% to 15% is applied once a day.

ROSACEA

Occasionally mistaken for acne vulgaris, rosacea is an acne-iform disorder that begins in midlife (ages 30 to 50). It is estimated that rosacea affects over 16 million people by the National Rosacea Society. The rash is symmetric and limited to the central part of the face. Fair-skinned people with a tendency to blush are more often affected. Although rosacea is more likely to develop in women, men who are affected may have a more severe form of the disorder. Rosacea is not frequently seen in skin of color.

CAUSES

Rosacea does not have a clear cause. Various theories suggest bacterial infection, fungal infection, hair follicle mite (*Demodex folliculorum*) infestation, menopausal changes, and, more recently, *Helicobacter pylori* infection. Sun exposure, excessive face washing, and irritating cosmetics may exacerbate rosacea.

PATHOPHYSIOLOGY

Early vascular rosacea consists of simple erythema in response to cold exposure. Extravascular fluid accumulates. As a result, blood flow to the superficial dermis increases. Persistent telangiectasia occurs late in the vascular stage of the disorder. During this period, ocular involvement may develop, consisting of mild conjunctivitis, dry eyes, burning, blepharitis, and occasionally keratitis and corneal ulceration.

The second stage of rosacea represents lymphatic failure. It results in epidermal epithelial hyperplasia and pilosebaceous gland hyperplasia with fibrosis, inflammation, and telangiectasia. Clinical changes include persistent erythema, telangiectases, papules, and pustules. Rhinophyma, the characteristic deep inflammation and connective tissue hypertrophy of the nose, may begin to develop during this stage. Rhinophyma is almost exclusively seen in men older than age 40 and is treatable only by surgery.

Late-stage rosacea is recognized by persistent deep erythema, dense telangiectases, papules, pustules, nodules, and persistent edema of the central part of the face.

DIAGNOSTIC CRITERIA

The diagnosis of rosacea is based on the history and clinical presentation. Fixed telangiectasia is the hallmark of this disorder. In patients younger than age 30, acne should be ruled out. In patients with systemic symptoms, systemic lupus erythematosus should be ruled out. Bacterial cultures should be performed to rule out *Staphylococcus aureus* folliculitis and gram-negative folliculitis. Patients who do not respond to systemic antibiotics should be evaluated for *D. folliculorum* infestation.

Approximately 50% of patients report ocular involvement, so any ocular symptoms should be investigated. Referral to an ophthalmologist should be considered if the practitioner suspects corneal ulceration or keratitis.

INITIATING DRUG THERAPY

The goal of therapy is to minimize the disfiguring effects of rosacea and prevent further tissue damage. As with acne, the patient's concerns with regard to appearance must be considered. Patients with rosacea may feel stigmatized. Treatment during the early phase (vasodilation) is difficult. Patients may not respond to treatment until the condition progresses to the inflammatory stage.

Topical Antibacterials

Metronidazole

Topical metronidazole (MetroGel, Noritate) has anti-inflammatory properties (**Table 16.5**). It is available in 0.75% and 1% strengths and is applied twice a day in a thin layer on the face, avoiding the eyes. Adverse events include burning, skin irritation, transient erythema, mild dryness, and pruritus. Metronidazole is available in cream, gel, and lotion. Initial results should be seen in approximately 3 weeks and the full effect in approximately 9 weeks. Patients are then maintained on the agent indefinitely. Patients who receive concurrent anticoagulant therapy should be monitored closely for an enhanced anticoagulation effect.

Combination Medications

Sodium sulfacetamide 10% with sulfur 5% (Sulfacet-R, Novacet, Clenia) also has anti-inflammatory properties when used to treat rosacea. It is applied one to three times a day. It is contraindicated in patients with kidney disease and in those sensitive to sulfa drugs. Application to eyes and areas of denuded skin is to be avoided. Adverse events include local irritation and allergic dermatitis.

TABLE 16.5

Overview of Topical Agents for Rosacea

Generic (Trade) Name and Dosage	Selected Adverse Events	Contraindications	Special Considerations
metronidazole 0.75% gel, cream, lotion (MetroGel, etc.) 1.0% cream (Noritate)	Burning sensation, irritation, erythema (transient), mild dryness, pruritus	Children Breast-feeding mothers	Avoid eyes. With anticoagulant therapy, monitor closely for enhanced anticoagulation.
sodium sulfacetamide 10% with sulfa 5% (Sulfacet-R, Novacet) sodium sulfacetamide 10% with sulfa 5% and urea 10% (Rosula) One to three times a day in thin layer	Local irritation, allergic dermatitis	Kidney disease Breast-feeding mothers Sulfa allergy	Avoid eyes and denuded skin. Pregnancy category C
azelaic acid 15% (Finacea) Apply thin film two times daily.	Burning, stinging, pruritus	Children	Hypopigmentation in patients with dark complexions

Rosula is a combination of sulfacetamide 10%, sulfur 5%, and urea 10%. The addition of urea helps to soothe and relieve redness and inflammation.

Azelaic Acid

Azelaic acid (Finacea), also indicated for acne, has been shown to be effective in treating papules and pustules associated with rosacea. Supplied as a 15% gel, it is indicated for the topical treatment of inflammatory papules and pustules of mild to moderate rosacea. Patients with dark complexions may experience hypopigmentation.

Oral Antibiotics

When topical agents have not improved the patient's condition, oral antibiotic agents may be considered. Antibiotics are used for their anti-inflammatory effect rather than their antibiotic properties. Oral antibiotics are indicated for patients with ocular symptoms.

Tetracycline

Tetracycline is the antibiotic of choice for treating rosacea. Tetracycline is prescribed in doses of 500 mg twice a day to initiate remission. After 2 weeks, the dose can be lowered to 250 mg twice a day for an additional 4 weeks. If no inflammatory lesions are present at 6 weeks, the dose may be lowered to 250 mg once a day. After 3 to 5 months, the practitioner may consider discontinuing the oral antibacterial while continuing topical metronidazole therapy.

Doxycycline

Doxycycline (Vibramycin, Monodox, Doryx), a tetracycline derivative, is sometimes more effective than tetracycline. It is given in doses of 100 mg twice daily and then tapered after 2 weeks to 50 mg twice daily. After improvement occurs, the dose may be lowered to 50 mg/d and then stopped after 3 to 5 months while maintaining metronidazole cream. Patients should be cautioned to avoid sun exposure while taking doxycycline.

Erythromycin

Erythromycin (E-mycin, Ery-Tab) is a useful agent when tetracycline is contraindicated. Dosages and tapering regimens are identical to those used for tetracycline.

Trimethoprim/Sulfamethoxazole

Trimethoprim/sulfamethoxazole has been used successfully in patients with acne refractory to other antibiotics and in gram-negative acne.

Isotretinoin

Isotretinoin (Accutane) may be prescribed for patients who do not respond to oral and topical antibiotics. It is given in doses of 0.5 to 1.0 mg/kg/d for up to 8 months. Precautions and laboratory follow-up as described in the section on acne should be maintained.

Selecting the Most Appropriate Agent

Initial drug therapy choices should include a topical agent. Cases that involve ocular symptoms should be treated with oral antibiotics.

First-Line Therapy

The first-line treatment of rosacea consists of topical therapy. If no improvement is seen after 6 weeks, second-line therapy begins.

Second-Line Therapy

Second-line treatment consists of adding an oral antibiotic. After 2 weeks, the dose is reduced by 50%, and then, after

TABLE 16.6

Recommended Order of Treatment for Rosacea

Order	Agent	Comments
First line	Topical medication	Improvement takes 6 wk.
Second line	Oral antibiotics	Improvement takes 6 wk.
Third line	Oral isotretinoin; consider referral to dermatologist.	Pregnancy category X

6 weeks, the oral antibiotic is discontinued altogether and the topical treatment continues indefinitely.

Third-Line Therapy

Third-line treatment consists of oral isotretinoin or referral to a dermatologist. **Table 16.6** lists the lines of therapy for rosacea, and **Figure 16.2** outlines rosacea treatment.

MONITORING PATIENT RESPONSE

As discussed throughout this chapter, the patient's response is monitored regularly by observation and follow-up visits to adjust medications and provide support and encouragement during therapy.

PATIENT EDUCATION

Patients with rosacea need to recognize what triggers the condition. The goal of management is to avoid flare-ups. Although each patient responds differently to triggers, common triggers are sun exposure, strong winds, cold weather, warm environment, strenuous exercise, alcoholic beverages, spicy foods, hot foods and beverages, and stress.

It is important that a broad-spectrum UVA/UVB sunscreen be used and applied frequently.

Patients may be advised to avoid harsh cleansers, rough washcloths, and pulling or tugging at the skin. Cosmetic foundations with a green tint may camouflage redness. Additional information and consumer education may be obtained through the National Rosacea Society (1-888-NO BLUSH, http://www.rosacea.org).

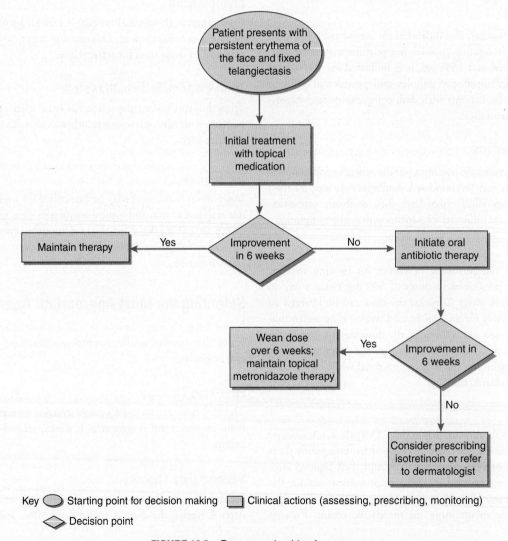

Key   ◯ Starting point for decision making   ▭ Clinical actions (assessing, prescribing, monitoring)

◇ Decision point

FIGURE 16.2   Treatment algorithm for rosacea.

CASE STUDY*

J.S., age 16, comes to your office for a routine physical examination. You notice that she has facial acne that she is hiding with heavy makeup. She has tried Clearasil inconsistently without relief. She works at a fast food restaurant as a cook after school and on the weekends. Her mother has made her stop eating chocolates and greasy foods, but that has not seemed to help her. She is concerned because her prom is in 6 weeks and she wants her face clear. On physical examination, there are open and closed comedones as well as papules on her face and back. No scarring is evident. **J.S.** confides that she has recently become sexually active.

DIAGNOSIS: ACNE VULGARIS

1. List specific treatment goals for **J.S.**
2. What drug therapy would you prescribe? Why?
3. What are the parameters for monitoring the success of the therapy?
4. Describe specific patient education based on the prescribed therapy.
5. List one or two adverse reactions for the selected agent that would cause you to change therapy.
6. What would be the choice for second-line therapy?
7. What over-the-counter or dietary supplement would you recommend to **J.S.**?
8. What dietary and lifestyle changes should be recommended for **J.S.**?
9. Describe one or two drug–drug or drug–food interactions for the selected agent.

* Answers can be found online.

Bibliography

Starred references are cited in the text.

Burris, J., Rietkerk, W., & Woolf, K. (2013). Acne: The role of medical nutrition therapy. *Journal of the Academy of Nutrition and Dietetics, 113*(3), 416–430.

DelRossi, J., & Kim, G. (2009). Optimizing the use of oral antibiotics in acne vulgaris. *Dermatologic Clinics, 27*(1), 33–42.

Goldgar, C., Keahey, D., & Houchens, J. (2009). Treatment options for acne rosacea. *American Family Physician, 80*(5), 461–468.

Grove, G., Zerweck, C., & Gwazdauskas, J. (2013). Tolerability and irritation potential of four topical acne regimens in healthy subjects. *Journal of Drugs in Dermatology, 12*(6), 644–649.

Leyden, J., DelRossi, J, & Webster, G. (2009). Clinical considerations in the treatment of acne vulgaris and other inflammatory skin disorders. *Dermatologic Clinics, 27*(1), 1–15.

Mechcatie, E. (2004). Pregnancies lead to more isotretinoin restrictions. *Pediatric News, 56*(4), 651–663.

*Roche Laboratories. (2002). *Accutane (isotretinoin) capsules complete product information*. Nutley, NJ: Author.

Snyder, S., Crandell, I., Davis, S. A., et al. (2014). Medical adherence to acne therapy: A systematic review. *American Journal of Clinical Dermatology, 15*(2), 87–94

*U.S. Food and Drug Administration. (2002). MedWatch 2002 Safety Alert– Accutane (isotretinoin) Dear Accutane Prescriber letter. Rockville, MD: Author. Retrieved from http://www.fda.gov/medwatch/SAFETY/2002/accutane_deardoe_10-2002.htm on September 6, 2004.

*Weber, G., Adamczyk, A., & Fretag, S. (1989). Treatment of acne with a yeast preparation. *Fortschritte der Medizin, 107*(26), 563–566.

Webster, G. (2009). Rosacea. *Medical Clinics of North America, 93*(6), 1183–1194.

Pharmacotherapy for Eye and Ear Disorders

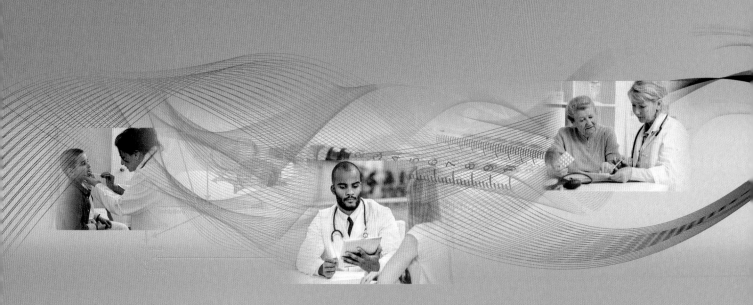

Ophthalmic Disorders

Joshua J. Spooner

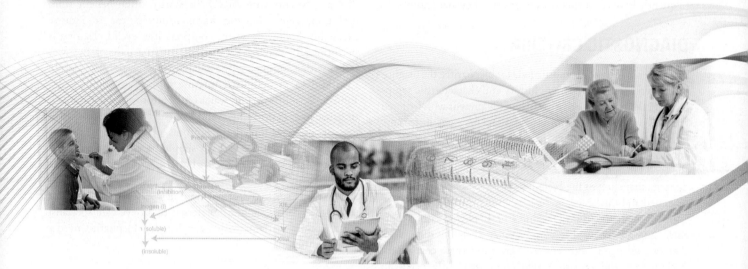

There are many conditions and disorders of the eye, but only a few, such as blepharitis and conjunctivitis, should be diagnosed and treated by a primary care provider. The remaining ocular conditions are usually treated by eye care specialists. Nonetheless, prescribers should be familiar with drug therapy for the more common ophthalmic conditions (glaucoma, keratoconjunctivitis sicca), as they are likely to encounter patients being treated for these disorders.

EYELID MARGIN INFECTIONS: BLEPHARITIS

The eye is well protected externally by the eyebrow, eyelashes, and eyelids. If these protective mechanisms are compromised, the eye becomes predisposed to disease. Externally, the eyelid structures are composed of skin with a high degree of elasticity, muscles that elevate the upper eyelid and close the eyelids, and the tarsal plate, which contains the meibomian glands. Through frequent blinking, the eyelids maintain an even flow of tears over the cornea. Internally, the eyelid structure is lined by the palpebral conjunctiva, which folds upon itself and then covers the sclera of the eyeball up to the corneoscleral junction. Located at the lid margins are the openings to the long sebaceous meibomian glands; these glands secrete the oily film that prevents tears from evaporating. At the base of the eyelash, hair follicles are the superficial modified sebaceous glands of Zeis and the sweat glands of Moll. Any of these glands may become functionally disrupted.

Blepharitis is an inflammation of the eyelid margin. Although it is a common eye disorder in the United States, epidemiologic information on its incidence or prevalence is not robust.

CAUSES

Blepharitis can be caused by a bacterial infection (staphylococcal blepharitis), inflammation or hypersecretion of the sebaceous glands (seborrheic blepharitis), meibomian gland dysfunction (MGD blepharitis), or a combination of these (American Academy of Ophthalmology [AAO], 2013a). Staphylococcal and seborrheic blepharitis primarily involve the anterior eyelid; both have also been referred to as anterior blepharitis.

PATHOPHYSIOLOGY

Although the gram-positive organisms *Staphylococcus epidermidis* and *Staphylococcus aureus* are found on the eyelids of a high proportion of healthy subjects, *S. aureus* is observed more frequently among patients with staphylococcal blepharitis. While *S. epidermidis* and *S. aureus* are thought to play a role in the development of staphylococcal blepharitis, their role in disease production remains unclear. Toxin production, immunologic mechanisms, *Demodex folliculorum* mite infestation, and antigen-induced inflammatory reactions have all been reported with blepharitis (AAO, 2013a; Zhao et al., 2012).

Seborrheic blepharitis typically occurs as part of the more comprehensive condition of seborrheic dermatitis, with dandruff of the scalp, eyebrows, eyelashes, nasolabial folds, and external ears. Seborrheic blepharitis is more commonly found in the geriatric population because of its association with rosacea.

Manifestations of MGD blepharitis include thickening of the eyelid margin, plugging of the meibomian orifices, prominent blood vessels crossing the mucocutaneous junction, and formation of chalazia (painless firm lumps on the eyelid). These changes may lead to atrophy of the meibomian glands (AAO, 2013a). Compared to healthy patients, meibomian gland secretions are more turbid among patients with MGD blepharitis. These secretions block the gland orifices and become a growth medium for bacteria. Patients with MGD blepharitis frequently have coexisting rosacea or seborrheic dermatitis.

DIAGNOSTIC CRITERIA

There are no specific diagnostic tests for blepharitis; the diagnosis is often based upon patient history and characteristic symptoms. Patients with blepharitis frequently present with irritated red eyes and report a burning sensation. Increases in tearing, blinking, and photophobia are frequently reported, as is eyelid sticking and contact lens intolerance. Upon close inspection, the eyelid margins appear red, greasy, and crusted, with eyelid deposits that cling to the eyelashes. The eyelid margins may be ulcerated and thickened, and eyelashes may be missing.

Although the clinical features of staphylococcal, seborrheic, and MGD blepharitis are similar, there are differences that can aid in the differential diagnosis of these conditions. Eyelash loss and eyelash misdirection frequently occur in staphylococcal blepharitis but are rare in seborrheic blepharitis. The eyelid deposits are matted and scaly in staphylococcal blepharitis, oily or greasy in seborrheic blepharitis, and fatty and possibly foamy in MGD blepharitis. Chalazia are most likely to occur in MGD blepharitis.

INITIATING DRUG THERAPY

The underlying cause of the blepharitis must be treated, particularly if it is due to seborrheic dermatitis or rosacea. Treatment for all types of blepharitis includes strict eyelid hygiene and warm compresses. The use of warm compresses with a clean washcloth can soften adherent encrustations; once-daily use of compresses is generally sufficient (AAO, 2013a). Patients with MGD blepharitis often benefit from eyelid massage following warm compress use to remove excess oil. Following warm compress use, eyelid cleaning is performed by having the patient rub the base of the eyelashes with a commercially available eyelid cleaner (EyeScrub, OCuSOFT) or a diluted mixture of baby shampoo (e.g., Johnson & Johnson) and water on a cotton swab, cotton ball, or gauze pad. Performing eyelid hygiene daily or several times a week often blunts the symptoms of chronic blepharitis (Guillon et al., 2012). Patients should be advised that eyelid hygiene may be required for life because symptoms frequently recur if eyelid hygiene is discontinued.

Patients suspected of having a new case of seborrheic or MGD blepharitis should be referred to an eye care specialist for a workup. Patients with staphylococcal blepharitis need a topical antibiotic.

Goals of Drug Therapy

The goals of drug therapy are to eradicate the pathogens causing the blepharitis and to reduce the signs and symptoms of blepharitis.

Topical Ophthalmic Antimicrobials

Topical ophthalmic antimicrobials are used for the treatment of and prophylaxis against external bacterial infections (**Table 17.1**). They kill the offending pathogen and other susceptible organisms.

TABLE 17.1

Overview of Antimicrobial Ophthalmic Agents

Generic (Trade) Name and Dosage	Selected Adverse Events	Contraindications	Special Considerations
Single-Agent Products			
sulfacetamide sodium 10% solution (Bleph-10) Dosing Solution: 1–2 drops every 2–3 h initially according to the severity of infection Dosing may be tapered as the condition responds. Usual duration of therapy is 7–10 d.	Local irritation, itching, stinging, burning, periorbital edema	Allergy to sulfa drugs Do not use in infants less than age 2 mo.	A significant percentage of *Staphylococcus* species are resistant to sulfa drugs. Do not use in patients with purulent exudates.
bacitracin 500 units/g ointment Dosing: apply one to three times a day	Blurred vision, redness, burning, eyelid edema		Ointments may blur vision and retard corneal wound healing.
erythromycin 0.5% ointment Dosing: apply up to 1 cm to the affected eye(s) up to six times a day	Redness, ocular irritation		Ointments may blur vision and retard corneal wound healing.
gentamicin 0.3% solution or ointment (Gentak) Dosing Solution: 1–2 drops in the affected eye(s) every 4 h Ointment: ½ inch to the affected eye two or three times a day	Ocular burning and irritation, nonspecific conjunctivitis, conjunctival epithelial defects, conjunctival hyperemia, bacterial and fungal corneal ulcers		In severe infections, dosage of the solution may be increased to as much as 2 drops every hour. Ointments may blur vision and retard corneal wound healing.

TABLE 17.1

Overview of Antimicrobial Ophthalmic Agents (*Continued*)

Generic (Trade) Name and Dosage	Selected Adverse Events	Contraindications	Special Considerations
tobramycin 0.3% solution or ointment (Tobrex) Dosing Solution: 1–2 drops into the infected eye every 4 h Ointment: ½ inch every 8–12 h	Lid itching, lid swelling, conjunctival hyperemia, nonspecific conjunctivitis, bacterial and fungal corneal ulcers		Ointments may blur vision and retard corneal wound healing. For more severe infections, the initial dose may be increased to 2 drops every 60 min (solution) or 1 inch every 3–4 h (ointment).
besifloxacin 0.6% suspension (Besivance) Dosing: 1 drop in the affected eye(s) three times a day for 7 d	Conjunctival redness, blurred vision, eye irritation, eye pain, pruritus		
ciprofloxacin 0.3% solution or ointment (Ciloxan) Dosing Solution: 1–2 drops every 2 h while awake for 2 d and then 1–2 drops every 4 h while awake for 5 d Ointment: ½ inch three times a day for 2 d and then ½ inch twice a day for 5 d	Local burning and discomfort, white crystalline precipitate formation, conjunctival hyperemia, altered taste		Ointments may blur vision and retard corneal wound healing. This is the only ophthalmic fluoroquinolone available as an ointment.
gatifloxacin 0.3% solution (Zymaxid) Dosing: 1 drop in the affected eye every 2 h while awake for 1 d and then 1 drop in the affected eye up to four times daily while awake for 6 d	Conjunctival irritation, tearing, papillary conjunctivitis, eyelid edema, ocular itching, dry eye		
levofloxacin 0.5% solution (Quixin) Dosing: 1 drop in the affected eye every 2 h while awake for 2 d and then 1 drop in the affected eye up to four times daily while awake for 5 d	Temporarily decreased or blurred vision, eye irritation, itching, dry eye		
moxifloxacin 0.5% solution (Moxeza, Vigamox) Dosing: Moxeza: 1 drop in the affected eye two times a day for 7 d Vigamox: 1 drop in the affected eye three times a day for 7 d	Decreased visual acuity, dry eye, ocular itching and discomfort, ocular hyperemia		
ofloxacin 0.3% solution (Ocuflox) Dosing: 1–2 drops in the affected eye every 2–4 h for 2 d and then 1–2 drops four times a day	Ocular burning and stinging, itching, redness, edema, blurred vision, photophobia		Rare reports of dizziness and nausea with use
azithromycin 1% solution (AzaSite) Dosing: 1 drop in affected eye(s) twice daily for 2 d and then 1 drop once daily for 5 d	Eye irritation, dry eye, ocular discharge		Refrigerate bottle; once opened, discard after 14 d.
Combination Products			
polymyxin B sulfate, bacitracin ointment Dosing: apply every 3–4 h for 7–10 d, depending upon the severity of infection.	Local irritation (burning, stinging, itching, redness), lid edema, tearing, rash		Ointments may blur vision and retard corneal wound healing.
polymyxin B sulfate, trimethoprim sulfate solution (Polytrim) Dosing: 1 drop in the affected eye(s) every 3 h (maximum six doses a day) for 7–10 d	Local irritation (burning, stinging, itching, redness), lid edema, tearing, rash		
polymyxin B sulfate, gramicidin, neomycin solution (Neosporin) Dosing: 1–2 drops into the affected eye(s) every 4 h for 7–10 d	Itching, swelling, conjunctival erythema, local irritation		Dosage of the solution may be increased to as much as 2 drops every hour for severe infections.
polymyxin B sulfate, bacitracin zinc, and neomycin ointment Dosage: apply every 3–4 h for 7–10 d, depending upon the severity of infection.	Itching, swelling, conjunctival erythema, local irritation		Acute infections may require dosing every 30 min. Ointments may blur vision and retard corneal wound healing.

TABLE 17.2

Recommended Order of Treatment for Blepharitis

Order	Agent	Comments
First line	Erythromycin 0.5% ophthalmic ointment	Ointments tend to cause a greater degree of blurry vision than solutions.
	or	
	Bacitracin 500 units/g ointment	Erythromycin and bacitracin are available as inexpensive generic products.
	or	
	An ophthalmic fluoroquinolone solution (besifloxacin, gatifloxacin, levofloxacin, or moxifloxacin)	The remaining ophthalmic fluoroquinolones do not provide good staphylococcal coverage.
Second line	Referral to an ophthalmologist	

Selecting the Most Appropriate Agent

Topical antimicrobials that are effective against staphylococci are listed in **Table 17.2**.

First-Line Therapy

Topical antibiotics such as bacitracin ointment or erythromycin 0.5% ophthalmic ointment are used first line for staphylococcal blepharitis and should be applied to the eyelid margins one or more times daily or at bedtime for a few weeks. Therapy selection is based on allergies and patient preference for ointment or solution (drops). Ointments tend to cause a greater degree of blurry vision than the solutions; if a patient prefers a solution, a fluoroquinolone (besifloxacin, gatifloxacin, levofloxacin, or moxifloxacin) would be suitable. The AAO (2013a) recommends that the frequency and duration of treatment should be guided by the severity of the condition and the response to treatment.

Second-Line Therapy

If the blepharitis fails to respond to the first-line therapy after several weeks or the condition appears to worsen at any time (including any vision loss or corneal involvement), the patient should be referred to an ophthalmologist for a complete evaluation.

PATIENT EDUCATION

Patients should be educated about the chronic nature of blepharitis. While chronic blepharitis is rarely cured, improved eyelid hygiene, warm massages, and occasional antibiotic use (for staphylococcal blepharitis) can improve symptoms. Counsel contact lens wearers to refrain from wearing contact lenses during an acute case of blepharitis, especially if antibiotic therapy has been initiated. Contact lens wearers with chronic blepharitis should consult with their eye care professional to determine whether contact lens use is safe.

EXTERNAL SURFACE OCULAR INFECTIONS: CONJUNCTIVITIS

Conjunctivitis is the most common cause of a red, painful eye in the United States (Horton, 2015). Conjunctivitis is an inflammation of the bulbar conjunctiva (the clear membrane that covers the white part of the eye) or the palpebral conjunctiva (the lining of the inner surfaces of the eyelids). Conjunctivitis is commonly referred to as *pink eye*.

CAUSES

The most common organisms seen in acute bacterial conjunctivitis are the gram-positive *Staphylococcus* and *Streptococcus* species and the gram-negative *Moraxella* and *Haemophilus* species; less common organisms include *Neisseria gonorrhoeae* and *Chlamydia trachomatis* (CDC, 2014). In children, up to 50% of conjunctivitis cases are of bacterial origin. The most common pathogens in neonates are *N. gonorrhoeae* and *C. trachomatis*, while *S. aureus*, *Haemophilus influenzae*, *Streptococcus pneumoniae*, and *Pseudomonas aeruginosa* are the most commonly isolated organisms in children with bacterial conjunctivitis (Sethuraman & Kamat, 2009).

Viruses account for the majority of conjunctivitis cases in adults. The most common viral etiology is adenovirus infection (Horton, 2015); conjunctivitis due to an adenovirus is highly contagious. Other viruses associated with conjunctivitis include the herpes simplex virus, the varicella-zoster virus, and molluscum contagiosum (AAO, 2013b).

Allergic conjunctivitis is fairly common and is frequently mistaken for bacterial conjunctivitis. There are three common types of allergic conjunctivitis: seasonal (hay fever) conjunctivitis, due to seasonal release of plant allergens; vernal conjunctivitis, which is of unknown origin but is thought to be due to seasonal airborne antigens; and atopic conjunctivitis, which occurs in people with atopic dermatitis or asthma.

Conjunctivitis can also be caused by mechanical or chemical irritants. A foreign body on the eye (typically a contact lens) can lead to giant papillary conjunctivitis.

PATHOPHYSIOLOGY

General mechanisms of infection are at work in bacterial and viral conjunctivitis. In bacterial conjunctivitis, the infecting organism is obtained via contact with an infected individual and transmitted to the eye by fingertips. Neonates with conjunctivitis may have become inoculated during childbirth by their infected mother. Transmission of viral conjunctivitis is usually through direct contact with infected persons, contact with contaminated surfaces, or contaminated swimming pool water (Cronau et al., 2010; Wong & Anninger, 2014). In both bacterial and viral conjunctivitis, the infectious agent causes the inflammation of the conjunctiva. Mechanical and chemical irritants that cause conjunctivitis operate in the same manner.

In allergic conjunctivitis, symptoms are caused by the immunoglobulin (Ig)E-mediated release of mast cells in the conjunctiva (Kari & Saari, 2012).

DIAGNOSTIC CRITERIA

In addition to the hallmark red or pink eye, classic patient complaints that occur in conjunctivitis include itching or burning sensations of the eyes, ocular discharge ("leaky eye"), eyelids that are stuck together in the morning, and a sensation that a foreign body is lodged in the eye. Patients may also report a feeling of fullness around the eye. Moderate to severe pain and light sensitivity are not typical features of a primary conjunctival inflammatory process (Azari & Barney, 2013). If these symptoms are present, or if the patient reports blurred vision that does not improve with blinking, the patient should be referred to an eye care professional, as a more serious ocular disease process (such as a corneal abrasion or keratoconjunctivitis) may be occurring. Neonates with signs of conjunctivitis should be referred to an eye care professional for immediate examination, as bacterial conjunctivitis due to *C. trachomatis* or *N. gonorrhoeae* can lead to serious eye damage.

Although many symptoms of conjunctivitis are nonspecific (tearing, irritation, stinging, burning, and conjunctival swelling), inspection and patient history can help determine the cause of illness. Patients who report that their eyelids were stuck together upon awakening most likely have bacterial conjunctivitis (Deibel et al., 2013); this sticking is caused by a purulent ocular discharge. Because gonococcal conjunctivitis produces a copiously purulent discharge, the cause of any copiously purulent conjunctivitis should be suspected as *N. gonorrhoeae* until Gram-stain testing proves otherwise. Bacterial conjunctivitis usually starts in one eye and can become bilateral a few days later.

Viral conjunctivitis produces a profuse watery discharge. Similar to bacterial conjunctivitis, viral conjunctivitis usually starts in one eye and can become bilateral within a few days. While unlikely, photophobia and a foreign body sensation may be reported. Examination may reveal a tender preauricular node. A rapid, in-office immunodiagnostic test with high sensitivity and specificity for adenovirus is available (Sambursky et al., 2013).

In allergic conjunctivitis, itching is the hallmark symptom; it can be mild to severe and may manifest as excessive blinking. A history of recurrent itching or a personal or family history of hay fever, asthma, atopic dermatitis, or allergic rhinitis is suggestive of allergic conjunctivitis. In general, a patient with conjunctivitis who does not report an itchy eye does not have allergic conjunctivitis. Unlike bacterial or viral conjunctivitis, allergic conjunctivitis usually presents with bilateral symptoms. An ocular discharge may or may not be present; if present, it may be watery or mucoid. Aggressive forms of allergic conjunctivitis are vernal conjunctivitis in children and atopic conjunctivitis in adults. Atopic and vernal conjunctivitis are associated with shield corneal ulcers and perilimbal

accumulation of eosinophils (Horner-Trantas dots) (Nijm et al., 2011). Atopic conjunctivitis is associated with eyelid thickening, conjunctival scarring, blepharitis, and corneal scarring (AAO, 2013b).

Giant papillary conjunctivitis occurs mainly in contact lens wearers. These patients report excessive itching, mucus production and discharge, and increasing intolerance to contact lens use. Upon examination, the upper tarsal conjunctiva may show inflammation and papillae greater than 0.3 mm (Donshik et al., 2008). Ptosis may occur in severe cases (AAO, 2013b).

INITIATING DRUG THERAPY

Before drug therapy is prescribed, both the patient and the practitioner should be aware that bacterial and viral conjunctivitis are highly contagious and are spread by contact. Therefore, good hand-washing and instrument-cleansing techniques are imperative. The etiology of illness should be determined, as treatment is different for bacterial, viral, and allergic conjunctivitis.

Goals of Drug Therapy

The goals of drug therapy are to eradicate the offending organism (for bacterial conjunctivitis), to relieve symptoms and to quicken the resolution of the disease. A patient with bacterial conjunctivitis should experience improvement in symptoms a few days after the start of antibiotic therapy; the organisms remain active (and contagious) for 24 to 48 hours after therapy begins. With viral conjunctivitis, the disease is contagious for at least 7 days after symptoms appear; it may be contagious for up to 14 days.

Antibiotics

Although bacterial conjunctivitis caused by typical pathogens (*Staphylococcus*, *Streptococcus*, *Pneumococcus*, *Moraxella*, and *Haemophilus* species) is usually self-limiting, antibiotic therapy is justified because it can shorten the course of the disease, which reduces person-to-person spread, and lowers the risk of sight-threatening complications. The choice of antibiotic is usually empirical. Five to seven days of therapy with agents such as erythromycin ointment or bacitracin–polymyxin B ointment or solution is usually effective. While well tolerated, sulfacetamide has weak to moderate activity against many organisms. The aminoglycosides have good gram-negative coverage but incomplete coverage of *Streptococcus* and *Staphylococcus* species and a relatively high incidence of corneal toxicity. The fluoroquinolones also have good gram-negative coverage; the older fluoroquinolones (ciprofloxacin, norfloxacin, and ofloxacin) have poor coverage of *Streptococcus* species, while the newer fluoroquinolones (besifloxacin, gatifloxacin, levofloxacin, and moxifloxacin) offer improved gram-positive coverage.

Because gonococcal infection is serious, immediate treatment of conjunctivitis due to *N. gonorrhoeae* with a 250-mg intramuscular (IM) injection of ceftriaxone (Rocephin) plus a single 1-g dose of oral azithromycin is recommended for adults and children who weigh at least 45 kg. Children who weigh less than 45 kg should receive a single 125-mg IM injection of ceftriaxone, while 25 to 50 mg/kg of ceftriaxone intravenous or IM (not to exceed 125 mg) is the appropriate dose for neonates. Cephalosporin-allergic patients should be referred to an infectious disease specialist. Topical antibiotic therapy is not necessary but is often initiated to prevent secondary infection (AAO, 2013b).

As *C. trachomatis* is now the most common cause of conjunctivitis in neonates in the United States, the long-time standard prophylactic agent for neonates, topical 1% silver nitrate solution, is no longer recommended or commercially available in the United States. Topical treatment of neonatal chlamydial conjunctivitis is ineffective and unnecessary (American Academy of Pediatrics, 2012). In adults and children at least 8 years old, *C. trachomatis* infection is treated with a single 1-g dose of azithromycin or 7 days of therapy with doxycycline 100 mg twice daily. Children who weigh at least 45 kg but are less than 8 years old should receive the single dose of azithromycin 1 g. Neonates and children who weigh less than 45 kg should receive 50 mg/kg/d of erythromycin base or erythromycin ethylsuccinate, divided into four doses a day for 14 days (AAO, 2013b). Identification of either *Chlamydia* or *N. gonorrhoeae*

conjunctivitis requires that the patient's sexual partner also be treated.

Antihistamines

The ophthalmic antihistamines alcaftadine and emedastine prevent the histamine response in blood vessels by preventing histamine from binding with its receptor site and are useful in reducing the symptoms of allergic conjunctivitis. Ocular adverse events with these agents include transient stinging or burning upon instillation, dry eyes, red eyes, and blurred vision. Oral antihistamines can also help to relieve symptoms in many patients (see **Table 17.3**).

Mast Cell Stabilizers

The mast cell stabilizers (bepotastine, cromolyn, lodoxamide, and nedocromil) inhibit hypersensitivity reactions and prevent the increase in cutaneous vascular permeability that accompanies allergic reactions. These agents may be helpful for patients with allergic conjunctivitis. Ocular adverse events include transient burning, stinging or discomfort, pruritus, blurred vision, dry eyes, taste alteration, and foreign body sensation (see **Table 17.3**).

TABLE 17.3

Overview of Antiallergy Ophthalmic Agents

Generic (Trade) Name and Dosage	Selected Adverse Events	Contraindications	Special Considerations
Antihistamines			
alcaftadine 0.25% solution (Lastacaft) Dosing: 1 drop in the affected eye once daily	Eye irritation, burning and stinging, itching		Labeling: wait 10 min following administration before inserting contact lenses.
emedastine 0.05% solution (Emadine) Dosing: 1 drop in the affected eye up to four times a day	Blurred vision, burning and stinging, dry eyes, foreign body sensation, hyperemia, itching		Labeling: wait 10 min following administration before inserting contact lenses.
Mast Cell Stabilizers			
bepotastine 1.5% solution (Bepreve) Dosing: 1 drop into the affected eye(s) twice daily	Mild taste following instillation, eye irritation		Labeling: refrain from contact lens use while exhibiting signs and symptoms of allergic conjunctivitis. Labeling: wait 10 min following administration before inserting contact lenses.
cromolyn 4% solution (Crolom) Dosing: 1–2 drops in each eye four to six times a day at regular intervals	Burning and stinging, conjunctival injection, watery eyes, itching, dry eye, styes		Labeling: refrain from contact lens use while under treatment.
lodoxamide 0.1% solution (Alomide) Dosing: 1–2 drops in each eye four times a day	Burning and stinging, ocular itching, blurred vision, dry eye, tearing, hyperemia, foreign body sensation		Labeling: refrain from contact lens use while under treatment.
nedocromil 2% solution (Alocril) Dosing: 1–2 drops in each eye twice a day	Ocular burning and stinging, unpleasant taste, redness, photophobia		Labeling: refrain from contact lens use while exhibiting the signs and symptoms of allergic conjunctivitis.

TABLE 17.3

Overview of Antiallergy Ophthalmic Agents (*Continued*)

Generic (Trade) Name and Dosage	Selected Adverse Events	Contraindications	Special Considerations
Antihistamine/Mast Cell Stabilizer			
azelastine 0.05% solution (Optivar) Dosing: 1 drop into each affected eye twice daily	Ocular burning and stinging, headache, bitter taste, eye pain, blurred vision		Labeling: wait 10 min following administration before inserting contact lenses.
epinastine 0.05% solution (Elestat) Dosing: 1 drop in each eye twice a day	Burning sensation, folliculosis (hair follicle inflammation), hyperemia, itching		Labeling: wait 10 min following administration before inserting contact lenses.
ketotifen 0.025% solution (Alaway, Zaditor, Thera Tears Allergy) Dosing: 1 drop in the affected eye(s) every 8–12 h, no more than twice daily	Conjunctival injection, burning and stinging, conjunctivitis, dry eye, itching, photophobia		Labeling: wait 10 min following administration before inserting contact lenses.

olopatadine 0.1% (Patanol), 0.2% (Pataday), or 0.7% (Pazeo) solution
  Dosing
  0.1%: 1–2 drops in each affected eye twice daily
  0.2%, 0.7%: 1 drop in the affected eye(s) once daily
	Ocular burning and stinging, dry eye, headache, foreign body sensation, hyperemia, lid edema, itching		Labeling: wait 10 min following administration before inserting contact lenses.

Nonsteroidal Anti-inflammatory Drugs			
ketorolac 0.5% solution (Acular) Dosing: 1 drop four times a day	Stinging and burning, corneal edema, iritis, ocular irritation or inflammation		Use with caution in patients with aspirin sensitivities and patients with bleeding disorders or those receiving anticoagulant therapy. Labeling: do not administer while wearing contact lenses.
Vasoconstrictors (Decongestants)			
naphazoline 0.012% or 0.03% solutions (Clear Eyes), 0.02% solution (VasoClear), and 0.1% solution (AK-Con) Dosing: 1–2 drops in the affected eye(s) every 3–4 h, up to four times a day	Stinging, blurred vision, mydriasis, redness, punctate keratitis, increased IOP	Narrow-angle glaucoma Narrow-angle without glaucoma	Use should be limited to 72 h. Contains benzalkonium chloride; use with contact lenses not addressed in labeling
oxymetazoline 0.025% solution (Visine L.R.) Dosing: 1–2 drops in the affected eye(s) every 6 h	Stinging, blurred vision, mydriasis, redness, punctate keratitis, increased IOP	Narrow-angle glaucoma Narrow-angle without glaucoma	Use should be limited to 72 h. Contains benzalkonium chloride; use with contact lenses not addressed in labeling
tetrahydrozoline 0.05% solution (Visine, Murine for Red Eyes, Clear Eyes Triple Action) Dosing: 1–2 drops up to four times a day	Stinging, blurred vision, mydriasis, redness, punctate keratitis, increased IOP	Narrow-angle glaucoma Narrow-angle without glaucoma	Use should be limited to 72 h. Contains benzalkonium chloride; use with contact lenses not addressed in labeling
Topical Corticosteroids			

dexamethasone 0.1% solution (AK-Dex, Decadron) or 0.1% suspension (Maxidex)
  Dosing
  Solution: 1–2 drops every hour during the day and every 2 h at night initially, reduced to 1 drop every 4 h with favorable response
  Suspension: 1–2 drops less than four to six times a day in mild disease; hourly in severe disease
	IOP elevation, loss of visual acuity, cataract formation, secondary ocular infection, globe perforation, stinging and burning	Dendritic keratitis
		Fungal disease
		Viral disease of the cornea and conjunctiva
		Mycobacterial eye infection
			Labeling: wait 15 min following administration before inserting contact lenses.

(*Continued*)

TABLE 17.3

Overview of Antiallergy Ophthalmic Agents (*Continued*)

Generic (Trade) Name and Dosage	Selected Adverse Events	Contraindications	Special Considerations
fluorometholone 0.1% ointment or suspension (FML, Flarex) or 0.25% suspension (FML Forte) Dosing Ointment: ½ inch ribbon one to three times daily; during initial 24–48 h, dosing may be increased to every 4 h. Suspension: 1 drop two to four times daily; during initial 24–48 h, dosing may be increased to every 4 h.	IOP elevation, glaucoma, posterior subcapsular cataract formation, delayed wound healing	Dendritic keratitis Vaccinia and varicella Fungal disease Viral disease of the cornea and conjunctiva Mycobacterial eye infection	
loteprednol 0.2% or 0.5% suspension (Alrex, Lotemax) Dosing 0.2% solution: 1 drop in the affected eye(s) four times a day 0.5% solution: 1–2 drops in the affected eye(s) four times a day	IOP elevation, loss of visual acuity, cataract formation, secondary ocular infection, globe perforation, stinging and burning, dry eye, itching, photophobia	Dendritic keratitis Fungal disease Viral disease of the cornea and conjunctiva Mycobacterial eye infection	If needed, dosing of the 0.5% solution can be increased to 1 drop every hour during the first week of therapy. Labeling: wait 10 min following administration before inserting contact lenses.
prednisolone 0.12% or 1% suspension (Pred Mild, Omnipred, Pred Forte) or 1% solution Dosing Solution: 2 drops four times a day Suspension: 1–2 drops two to four times a day; dose may be increased during the initial 24–48 h	IOP elevation, cataract formation, delayed wound healing, secondary ocular infection, acute uveitis, globe perforation, stinging and burning, conjunctivitis	Dendritic keratitis Fungal disease Viral disease of the cornea and conjunctiva Mycobacterial eye infection Acute, purulent, untreated eye infections	Labeling: wait 15 min following administration before inserting contact lenses.

Antihistamine/Mast Cell Stabilizer

Several products (azelastine, epinastine, ketotifen, and olopatadine) have the combined properties of an antihistamine and a mast cell stabilizer, providing immediate relief of itching and long-term suppression of histamine release. Ketotifen is available without a prescription. These agents are given one or three times a day and have a side effect profile similar to the antihistamines and mast cell stabilizers (see **Table 17.3**).

Nonsteroidal Anti-Inflammatory Ophthalmic Drugs

The ophthalmic nonsteroidal anti-inflammatory (NSAID) ketorolac may be useful for treating the itch associated with allergic conjunctivitis. The NSAIDs inhibit the biosynthesis of prostaglandin by decreasing the activity of the enzyme cyclooxygenase. Ketorolac is administered 1 drop four times a day into the affected eye. It should be used with caution in patients with aspirin sensitivities and patients who have bleeding disorders or are receiving anticoagulant therapy because ophthalmic NSAIDs are absorbed systemically. Adverse events include transient stinging and burning, irritation and inflammation, corneal edema, and iritis (see **Table 17.3**).

Vasoconstrictors (Decongestants)

Vasoconstrictor eye drops (naphazoline, oxymetazoline, and tetrahydrozoline) may offer relief to patients with allergic conjunctivitis. With the exception of the higher-strength (0.1%) naphazoline solution, these agents are available without a prescription. Side effects include stinging, blurred vision, mydriasis, and increased redness; punctate keratitis and increased intraocular pressure (IOP) may also occur. These agents are contraindicated in patients with narrow-angle glaucoma or a narrow angle without glaucoma. Rebound congestion may occur with frequent or extended use of these agents; use should be limited to a maximum of 72 hours (see **Table 17.3**).

Topical Corticosteroids

Topical corticosteroids have been shown to reduce inflammation in allergic conjunctivitis. Low-dose corticosteroid therapy can be used at infrequent intervals for short-term periods (1 to 2 weeks) (AAO, 2013b). Long-term use of topical corticosteroids is associated with severe side effects, including ocular infection, cataract formation, and glaucoma (Bowling & Russell, 2011) (see **Table 17.3**).

Selecting the Most Appropriate Agent

Treatment of bacterial conjunctivitis is aimed at eradicating the offending organism. Cultures are not indicated unless the infection does not resolve with first-line therapy (**Table 17.4** and **Fig. 17.1**).

There is conflicting information about the use of soft contact lenses while taking ophthalmic medications that contain the preservative benzalkonium chloride. This preservative, which is in many of the ophthalmic antihistamines, mast cell stabilizers, NSAIDs, vasoconstrictors, and topical steroids reviewed in this section, may be absorbed by contact lenses. While no products identify contact lens use as an absolute contraindication to therapy, some (e.g., cromolyn, lodoxamide, and nedocromil) have warnings advising against the use of

---

TABLE 17.4

Recommended Order of Treatment for Conjunctivitis

Order	Agent	Comments
Bacterial Conjunctivitis (nongonococcal, nonchlamydial)		
First line	Erythromycin ointment *or* Bacitracin–polymyxin B ointment or solution	Ointments tend to cause a greater degree of blurry vision than solutions.
Second line	Ophthalmic fluoroquinolones (besifloxacin, gatifloxacin, levofloxacin, or moxifloxacin)	The remaining ophthalmic fluoroquinolones do not provide good staphylococcal coverage.
Seasonal (Hay Fever) Conjunctivitis		
First line	Topical antihistamine (alcaftadine or emedastine)	Minimization of exposure to the offending allergen, cool compresses, and artificial tears may also be helpful.
Second line	Addition of a brief course of low-potency topical corticosteroid to the first-line agent *or* For recurrent or persistent disease: a product with antihistamine/mast cell stabilizer properties	Use of the topical corticosteroids should not exceed 2 wk.
Third line	Ophthalmic ketorolac	
Vernal/Atopic Conjunctivitis		
First line	Topical antihistamine or oral antihistamine or mast cell stabilizer	Minimization of exposure to the offending allergen, cool compresses, and artificial tears may also be helpful.
Second line	For acute exacerbations: addition of a brief course of low-potency topical corticosteroid to the first-line agent	
Viral Conjunctivitis		
First line	Topical antihistamines *or* Artificial tears *or* Cold compresses	There is no effective treatment for viral conjunctivitis; treatment is for symptom mitigation.
Second line	In severe cases: a low-potency topical corticosteroid	Use of the topical corticosteroids should not exceed 2 wk.
Giant Papillary Conjunctivitis		
Mild disease	One or more of the following: replace contact lenses more frequently, decrease contact lens wearing time, increase the frequency of enzyme treatment, use preservative-free lens care systems, switch to disposable lenses, administer mast cell stabilizer, change the contact lens polymer	
Moderate or severe disease	Same as mild disease *and* Discontinuation of contact lens wear for several weeks or a brief course of topical corticosteroid treatment	

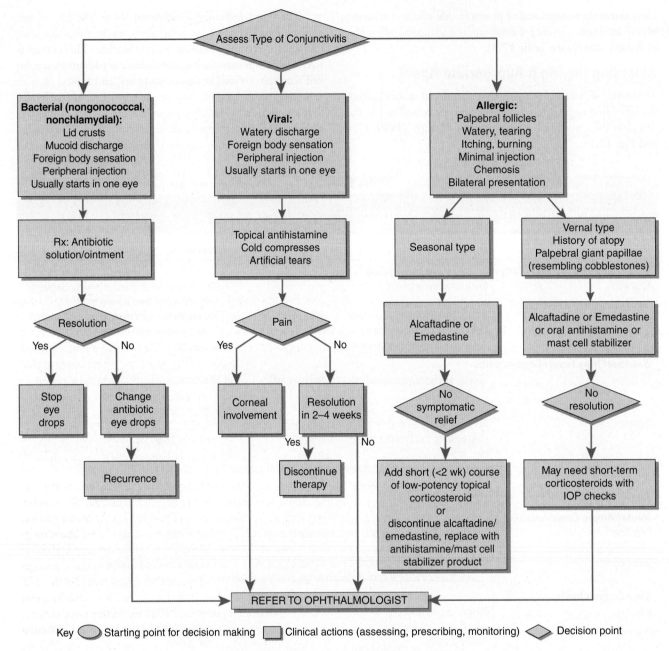

FIGURE 17.1   Treatment algorithm for conjunctivitis.

contact lenses during therapy; others advise patients to wait 10 to 15 minutes after administering the medication before reinserting contact lenses (see **Table 17.3**). Regardless of the etiology, contact lens wearers should refrain from wearing contact lenses during an acute case of conjunctivitis.

Bacterial Conjunctivitis

The treatment of bacterial conjunctivitis is aimed at the organisms *S. aureus*, *S. pneumoniae*, and *H. influenzae*. First-line treatments include 7 to 10 days of therapy with erythromycin ointment (two or three times a day) or polymyxin B–trimethoprim solution (1 drop every 3 to 4 hours). Therapy selection can be based on patient preference for ointment or

solution. If bacterial conjunctivitis does not resolve with first-line therapy, the patient should be referred to an eye care professional so that cultures may be taken to rule out *C. trachomatis*. The ophthalmic fluoroquinolones with improved gram-positive organism coverage (besifloxacin, gatifloxacin, levofloxacin, or moxifloxacin) can be used as second-line therapy.

Gonococcal infection requires immediate treatment. Ceftriaxone plus azithromycin is recommended for adults and children who weigh at least 45 kg; children who weigh less than 45 kg and neonates should receive a reduced dose of ceftriaxone. In adults and children at least 8 years old, *C. trachomatis* infection is treated with azithromycin or doxycycline. Azithromycin should be used in children who weigh at least

45 kg but are less than 8 years old, while neonates and children who weigh less than 45 kg should receive erythromycin base or erythromycin ethylsuccinate.

Seasonal (Hay Fever) Conjunctivitis

Steps should be taken to minimize exposure to the offending allergen. The ophthalmic antihistamines alcaftadine or emedastine can be used as first-line therapy for mild seasonal conjunctivitis. If symptom control is inadequate, a brief course (1 to 2 weeks) of a low-potency topical corticosteroid can be added to the regimen. If the condition is persistent, a mast cell stabilizer or, preferably, an agent with antihistamine and mast cell stabilizer properties (azelastine, epinastine, ketotifen, or olopatadine) can be used. The ophthalmic NSAID ketorolac should be reserved for third-line therapy. Patients may also benefit from the use of cool compresses and artificial tears (which dilute allergens and help manage coexisting tear deficiency).

Vernal/Atopic Conjunctivitis

Similar to seasonal conjunctivitis, general treatment measures for vernal/atopic conjunctivitis include minimizing exposure to the offending allergen and use of cool compresses and artificial tears. The topical antihistamines (alcaftadine or emedastine), oral antihistamines, or mast cell stabilizers (bepotastine, cromolyn, lodoxamide, or nedocromil) can be used as first-line agents for the treatment of vernal or atopic conjunctivitis. For patients with acute exacerbations, a topical corticosteroid can be added to the first-line agent for control of severe symptoms.

Viral Conjunctivitis

There is no effective treatment for viral conjunctivitis; patients should be informed of the risk of spreading the infection to the other eye (in unilateral infection) or to other people. Topical antihistamines, artificial tears, or cool compresses can be used to relieve symptoms. In severe cases of adenoviral keratoconjunctivitis with marked chemosis or lid swelling, epithelial sloughing, or membranous conjunctivitis, topical corticosteroids can be helpful in reducing symptoms and preventing scarring.

Giant Papillary Conjunctivitis

Management of giant papillary conjunctivitis centers around identifying and modifying the causative entity. Treatment of mild giant papillary conjunctivitis due to contact lens use can consist of one or more of the following: more frequent replacement of contact lenses, reduction in contact lens wearing time, increase in the frequency of enzyme treatment, use of preservative-free lens care systems, switching to disposable lenses, administration of a mast cell stabilizer, and change of the contact lens polymer (AAO, 2013b). In moderate or severe giant papillary conjunctivitis due to contact lens use, discontinuation of contact lens use for several weeks or a brief course of topical corticosteroid therapy may be necessary.

MONITORING PATIENT RESPONSE

If symptoms begin to improve within 48 hours, no follow-up is needed. If there is no improvement, the patient should be referred to an eye care professional for evaluation.

PATIENT EDUCATION

It is important to instruct patients with bacterial or viral conjunctivitis to wash their hands carefully to prevent spreading infection. Organisms in bacterial conjunctivitis remain active (and contagious) for 24 to 48 hours after therapy begins, while patients with viral conjunctivitis can remain contagious for up to 14 days. Patients should be taught how to apply the medication in the inner aspect of the lower eyelid. The tip of the container should not touch the eyelashes, as it may contaminate the medication and result in therapy failure or reinfection. Patients should not share eye medications because this can spread the infection. To improve the effectiveness of an ophthalmic antibiotic, crusted eyelids should be gently cleansed before instilling medication. Regardless of the etiology, contact lens wearers should refrain from wearing contact lenses during an acute case of conjunctivitis.

DRY EYE SYNDROME: KERATOCONJUNCTIVITIS SICCA

Keratoconjunctivitis sicca, commonly referred to as dry eye syndrome (DES), is a common ophthalmologic abnormality involving bilateral disruption of tear film on the ocular surface. Estimates of the prevalence of dry eye in the United States range from 10% to 20%, with the prevalence markedly higher for individuals over the age of 80 years compared to those younger than 60 years of age (19.0% vs. 8.4%) (Moss et al., 2000). DES can occur intermittently or as a chronic condition that becomes a self-perpetuating syndrome. While the majority of patients with DES experience non–sight-threatening ocular irritation and intermittently blurred vision, patients with severe DES are at risk for severe vision loss due to ocular surface keratinization, corneal scarring, and corneal ulceration (AAO, 2013c).

CAUSES

DES is a multifactorial disease. It can be the result of decreased tear production, increased tear evaporation, or a combination of these factors (Akpek & Smith, 2013). In addition, decreased tear secretion and clearance initiate an inflammatory response on the ocular surface, and research suggests that this inflammation plays a role in the pathogenesis of DES (Schaumberg et al., 2011).

Risk factors for DES include advanced age, female gender, and a history of LASIK surgery. Individuals with concomitant inflammatory conditions (allergies, asthma, or rheumatoid arthritis), infectious diseases (hepatitis C, human immunodeficiency virus/acquired immunodeficiency syndrome, or Epstein-Barr virus), or conditions such as Sjögren syndrome, Parkinson disease, or Bell palsy are also at increased risk for DES. Symptoms caused by dry eye may be exacerbated by environmental factors such as wind, reduced humidity, cigarette smoke, and heating and air conditioning. Systemic medications such as antihistamines, diuretics, anticholinergics, antidepressants, beta-blockers, antipsychotics, postmenopausal estrogens, and isotretinoin can also exacerbate dry eye symptoms (AAO, 2013c).

PATHOPHYSIOLOGY

Tears are composed of three layers: a mucus layer that coats the cornea, allowing the tear to adhere to the eye; a middle aqueous layer, which provides moisture and supplies oxygen and nutrients to the cornea; and an outer lipid film layer that seals the tear film on the eye and prevents evaporation. The outer lipid film layer is replenished by eyelid blinking, which relubricates and redistributes the lipid layer across the ocular surface. The ocular surface and tear-secreting glands function as an integrated unit to maintain the tear supply and to clear used tears. Aging, ocular surface diseases (such as herpes simplex virus keratitis), or surgeries that disrupt the trigeminal afferent sensory nerves, systemic inflammatory diseases, and systemic diseases and medications that disrupt the efferent cholinergic nerves that stimulate tear secretion can disrupt this functional unit and result in an unstable and poorly maintained tear film (Rocha et al., 2008; AAO, 2013c). Decreased tear secretion and clearance leads to an inflammatory response on the ocular surface, which is also believed to play a role in DES.

DIAGNOSTIC CRITERIA

Family practitioners should always refer patients reporting dry eye to an ophthalmologist if there is moderate to severe pain, vision loss, corneal infiltration or ulceration, or no response to therapy (AAO, 2013c). Making the diagnosis of DES, particularly the mild form, can be difficult because of the unpredictable correlation between reported symptoms and clinical signs and the relatively poor sensitivity/specificity of existing diagnostic tests (AAO, 2013c). Because most dry eye conditions are chronic, repeat observation will allow a more accurate clinical diagnosis of DES.

Signs and symptoms of DES include a dry eye sensation, ocular irritation, redness, burning, and stinging, a foreign body or gritty sensation, blurred vision, contact lens intolerance, an increased frequency of blinking, and, paradoxically, increased tearing (AAO, 2013c; National Eye Institute [NEI], 2010). The inability to cry under emotional distress has also been reported among DES patients (NEI, 2010). DES symptoms tend to worsen in dry climates, in the wind, during air travel, with prolonged visual efforts, and toward the end of the day (AAO, 2013c).

A physical examination (including a test of visual acuity, an external examination, and slit-lamp biomicroscopy) should be performed to document the signs of DES; to assess the quality, quantity, and stability of the tear film; and to rule out other causes of ocular irritation (AAO, 2013c). Additional tests can be used to lend some objectivity to the diagnosis. Tear breakup time testing can be useful for patients with mild symptoms. For patients with moderate to severe aqueous tear deficiency, the diagnosis can be made with one or more of the following tests (performed in this sequence): tear breakup time, ocular surface dye staining (rose bengal, fluorescein, or lissamine green), or the Schirmer wetting test (AAO, 2013c). Individuals with moderate to severe dry eye who have a family history of autoimmune disorders and/or signs and symptoms of an autoimmune disorder should be evaluated for an underlying autoimmune disorder.

INITIATING DRUG THERAPY

Before starting drug therapy, the patient should try nonpharmacologic interventions such as environmental control (increasing air humidity, avoiding drafts and cigarette smoke) and scheduling regular breaks during computer use and reading. Unfortunately, these interventions result in limited effectiveness and produce few lasting improvements in DES symptoms. Exogenous medical factors that can cause DES (i.e., blepharitis, meibomianitis) should be addressed, and prescription medications that can exacerbate DES symptoms should be discontinued when possible.

If the nonpharmacologic interventions fail to eliminate DES symptoms, drug therapy is appropriate. **Table 17.5** gives information about the drugs used to treat DES.

Goals of Drug Therapy

The goals of therapy in DES are to relieve discomfort, maintain and improve visual function, and reduce or prevent structural damage (AAO, 2013c). Therapy should attempt to normalize tear volume and composition so that the eye tissues are properly lubricated, nourished, and protected, resulting in improved patient satisfaction and clinical outcomes.

Artificial Tears and Lubricants

Artificial tears and lubricants can be used as palliative therapies to relieve DES symptoms. Designed to mimic the composition of natural tears, artificial tears contain lipids, water with dissolved salts and proteins, and mucin. Artificial tears and lubricants are over-the-counter products, available in a variety of formulations (solutions, gels, ointments). Ointments and gels may make the eyelids sticky and blur vision, and are often used only at bedtime.

For patients with mild DES, use of artificial tears four times daily plus a lubricating ointment at bedtime may be useful. As the severity of dry eye increases, administration of artificial tears can increase to hourly. Preservative-free preparations should be used if the patient applies tears more than four times a day (AAO, 2013c).

TABLE 17.5

Overview of Dry Eye Syndrome Agents

Generic (Trade) Name and Dosage	Selected Adverse Events	Contraindications	Special Considerations
Artificial Tear Substitutes			
Solutions containing preservatives: 20/20, Blink Tears, Clear Eyes, Comfort Tears, Fresh Kote, HypoTears, Isopto Tears, Murine, Natural Balance Nu-Tears, OptiZen, Puralube Tears, Refresh Liquigel, Refresh Tears, Soothe Hydration, Soothe XP, Systane, Tearisol, Tears Again, Tears Plus, Tears Naturale, Visine Tears	Stinging, blurred vision		Should not be used more than four to six times per day (except for in severe disease); if use in excess of four times a day is necessary, use a preservative-free preparation.
Preservative-free solutions: Bion Tears, Blink Tears PF, Moisture Eyes PF, Refresh Classic, Refresh Celluvisc, Refresh Optive, Refresh Plus, Soothe PF, Tears Naturale Free, Visine Tears PF, Viva-Drops	Stinging, blurred vision		
Ocular Lubricants			
Ointments containing preservatives: GenTeal PM, Puralube, Refresh Lacri-Lube, Stye, Tears Again, Lacri-Lube S.O.P.	Blurred vision		
Gels containing preservatives: Blink Gel Tears, Tears Again Night & Day	Blurred vision		
Preservative-free ointments: Dry Eyes, Duratears Naturale, HypoTears, Lacri-Lube NP, LubriFresh PM, Refresh PM, Soothe Night Time, Systane Nighttime, Tears Naturale PM	Blurred vision		
Preservative-free gels: GenTeal Severe Eye Relief	Blurred vision		
Cholinergic			
cevimeline 30-mg tablets (Evoxac) Dosing: 1 tablet three times a day	Excessive sweating, nausea, rhinitis, excessive salivation, asthenia	Uncontrolled asthma Acute iritis Narrow-angle glaucoma	Dehydration may develop from excessive sweating. Visual disturbances may impair the ability to drive, especially at night.
pilocarpine 5-mg tablets (Salagen) Dosing: 1 tablet four times a day	Excessive sweating, headache, urinary frequency, nausea, flushing, dyspepsia	Uncontrolled asthma Acute iritis Narrow-angle glaucoma	Dehydration may develop from excessive sweating. Visual disturbances may impair the ability to drive, especially at night.
Anti-inflammatory			
cyclosporine 0.05% emulsion (Restasis) Dosing: 1 drop in each eye twice a day, approximately 12 h apart	Ocular burning, blurred vision, conjunctival hyperemia, discharge, eye pain, foreign body sensation, pruritus, stinging		Use the emulsion from a single-use vial immediately after opening; discard the remaining contents.

Cholinergic Agonists

The cholinergic agonists pilocarpine and cevimeline are indicated for the treatment of dry mouth in patients with Sjögren syndrome. These agents bind to muscarinic receptors, stimulating secretion of the salivary and sweat glands and improving tear function. However, these agents are more effective for treating dry mouth compared to dry eye. The main adverse event with these agents is excessive sweating, reported in 18% to 40% of patients. The use of these agents is contraindicated in patients with uncontrolled asthma and when miosis is undesirable (acute iritis, narrow-angle glaucoma).

Topical Cyclosporine

Cyclosporine ophthalmic emulsion has been reported to increase aqueous tear production and decrease ocular irritation symptoms in patients with DES. It prevents T cells from

TABLE 17.6

Recommended Order of Treatment for Dry Eye

Order	Agent	Comments
First line	Mild DES: artificial tear substitute four times a day *or* Moderate to severe DES: preservative-free artificial tear substitute, administered up to hourly	If the patient has underlying Sjögren syndrome, administer pilocarpine tablets 5 mg four times a day or cevimeline tablets 30 mg three times a day.
Second line	Cyclosporine 0.05% ophthalmic emulsion twice a day	Ophthalmic corticosteroid therapy may be useful for the short-term (2-wk) suppression of irritation secondary to inflammation.

activating and releasing cytokines that incite the inflammatory component of dry eye. Side effects include ocular burning, conjunctival hyperemia, discharge, itching, and blurred vision.

Topical Corticosteroids

Topical corticosteroids have been shown to reduce inflammation in DES by reducing cytokine levels in the conjunctival epithelium. Low-dose corticosteroid therapy can be used at infrequent intervals for short-term (2 weeks) suppression of irritation secondary to inflammation (AAO, 2013c). Long-term use of topical corticosteroids is associated with severe side effects, including ocular infection, cataract formation, and glaucoma (Bowling & Russell, 2011).

Selecting the Most Appropriate Agent

Agent selection is determined by the severity of DES and the underlying pathophysiology (**Table 17.6**).

First-Line Therapy

For patients with mild DES, the use of a tear substitute four times a day is appropriate. For moderate or severe DES, artificial tears can be used as often as hourly, although administration that frequently may be cumbersome. Preservative-free preparations should be used if the patient uses tears more than four times a day. A lubricating ointment applied at bedtime may also be useful.

A patient with DES and underlying Sjögren syndrome may benefit from therapy with oral pilocarpine 5 mg four times daily or oral cevimeline 30 mg three times daily.

Second-Line Therapy

Patients with moderate to severe DES who fail to experience any improvement in symptoms with artificial tears may benefit from therapy with 0.05% cyclosporine ophthalmic emulsion 1 drop in each eye twice a day. Due to the side effect profile, corticosteroid therapy is limited to second-line therapy for short-term (2 weeks) suppression of irritation secondary to inflammation.

Third-Line Therapy

Patients with severe DES that fails to respond to drug therapy are candidates for permanent punctal occlusion or tarsorrhaphy.

MONITORING PATIENT RESPONSE

The frequency and extent of follow-up will depend upon the severity of DES and the therapeutic approach selected. Patients with mild DES can be seen once or twice per year for follow-up if symptoms are controlled by therapy. Patients with sterile corneal ulceration associated with DES require careful, sometimes daily, monitoring (AAO, 2013c).

PATIENT EDUCATION

Patients with DES should be educated about the chronic nature of the disease and given specific instructions about their therapeutic regimens. Patients with moderate to severe DES are at an elevated risk for contact lens intolerance.

GLAUCOMA (PRIMARY OPEN-ANGLE GLAUCOMA)

Glaucoma is a group of eye diseases involving optic neuropathy characterized by irreversible damage to the optic nerve and retinal ganglion cells (**Fig. 17.2**). Over time, this deterioration results in the loss of visual sensitivity and field, which frequently goes unnoticed until a significant amount of damage has occurred. Glaucoma is the leading cause of irreversible blindness in the world (Pascolini & Mariotti, 2012). There are numerous types of glaucoma, including primary open-angle glaucoma (POAG), acute closed-angle glaucoma, normal-tension glaucoma, and narrow-angle glaucoma. POAG accounts for up to 70% of glaucoma cases in the United States and afflicts 2.2 million Americans (AAO, 2015; King et al., 2013); as such, this section will specifically review POAG.

CAUSES

Several studies have shown that the prevalence of POAG increases with increasing IOP (Gordon et al., 2002; Leske et al., 2003). The median IOP in large populations is 15.5 ± 2.5 mm Hg. Previously, it was thought that increased IOP was the sole cause of POAG, but it is now recognized that IOP is one of

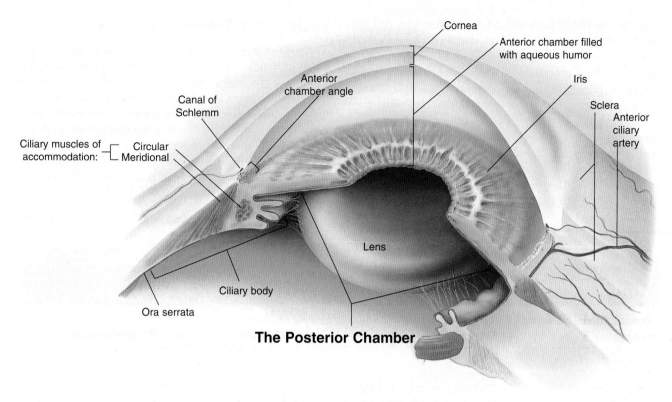

FIGURE 17.2 Anatomy of the eye.

several factors associated with the development of POAG, and an increased IOP is not required for the diagnosis of POAG.

Additional risk factors for the development of POAG include increasing age, black race (three times greater than whites), a family history of glaucoma, a thin central cornea, and type 2 diabetes mellitus (AAO, 2015).

PATHOPHYSIOLOGY

The pathophysiology of glaucoma-induced vision loss is not well understood. Aqueous humor is produced by the ciliary body and secreted into the posterior chamber of the eye. A pressure gradient in the posterior chamber forces the aqueous humor between the iris and lens and through the pupil into the anterior chamber. Aqueous humor in the anterior chamber leaves the eye through two methods: filtration through the trabecular meshwork to Schlemm canal (80% to 85%) or traversal of the anterior face of the iris and absorption into iris blood vessels (uveoscleral outflow). In POAG, the increase in IOP is a result of degenerative changes in the trabecular meshwork and Schlemm canal that result in a decrease in the outflow of the aqueous humor (Abel & Sorensen, 2013).

DIAGNOSTIC CRITERIA

Symptoms of POAG do not manifest until substantial damage has already occurred. The diagnosis of any glaucoma should be made by an eye care professional. Any patients reporting

visual field loss should be referred to an eye care professional for prompt evaluation.

During the physical examination, IOP is measured in each eye, preferably with a Goldmann-type applanation tonometer, before gonioscopy or dilation of the pupil (AAO, 2015). Unfortunately, the measurement of IOP is not an effective method for screening populations for glaucoma. At an IOP cutoff of 21 mmHg, the sensitivity for the diagnosis of POAG by tonometry was 47.1% (Tielsch et al., 1991), and half of all individuals with POAG are measured with an IOP of less than 22 mm Hg at a single screening (Leske et al., 2003). As such, the AAO recommends, in addition to the measurement of IOP, that a physical examination include the following elements: patient history, test of pupil reactivity, slit-lamp biomicroscopy of the anterior segment, determination of central corneal thickness, gonioscopy, evaluation of the optic nerve head and retinal nerve fiber layer, documentation of the optic nerve head appearance, evaluation of the fundus, and evaluation of the visual field (AAO, 2015).

INITIATING DRUG THERAPY

The goals of therapy for POAG are to control IOP, to stabilize the status of the optic nerve and retinal fiber layer, and to stabilize the visual field (AAO, 2015). Most cases of glaucoma can be controlled and vision loss prevented with early detection and treatment. Treatment of POAG entails decreasing aqueous humor production, increasing aqueous outflow, or a combination of both.

Over the past 20 years, glaucoma management has changed significantly, primarily due to the introduction of pharmaceutical agents that have shown clinical effectiveness (**Table 17.7**). These agents have been associated with a significant reduction in surgery rates among glaucoma patients (Fraser & Wormald, 2006).

Once a target IOP has been determined, treatment may include drug therapy, laser therapy, or surgery. Topical medication is, in most cases, indicated as first-line therapy. Several trials have clearly shown that reducing IOP by treatment with ocular hypotensive medication can prevent or reduce the risk of progression of glaucoma. Further, the more IOP is reduced, the risk of glaucomatous eye damage decreases.

Goals of Drug Therapy

The goals of drug therapy for POAG are to reduce IOP to a target level and to prevent or slow the progression of vision loss. In patients with POAG, the initial IOP target should be 20% to 30% lower than baseline. Additional IOP lowering may be justified, based upon the severity of the existing optic nerve damage, the speed at which the damage occurred, and the presence of other risk factors such as family history and age (AAO, 2015). Visual fields and optic nerve status should be monitored for signs of change; if progression is detected, the IOP target should be lowered.

TABLE 17.7

Overview of Glaucoma Agents

Generic (Trade) Name and Dosage	Selected Adverse Events	Contraindications	Special Considerations
Beta-blockers			
betaxolol 0.25% suspension or 0.5% solution (Betoptic S) Dosing: 1–2 drops in the affected eye(s) twice daily	Discomfort on instillation, tearing, allergic reactions, decreased corneal sensitivity, edema, bradycardia, hypotension, dizziness	Cardiogenic shock Second- or third-degree AV block Sinus bradycardia Overt cardiac failure	A cardioselective (beta-1) blocker; it has fewer effects on pulmonary and cardiovascular parameters.
carteolol 1% solution Dosing: 1 drop in the affected eye(s) twice daily	Transient eye irritation, burning, tearing, conjunctival hyperemia, edema, bradycardia, hypotension, arrhythmia, palpitations	Bronchial asthma or severe COPD Sinus bradycardia Second- or third-degree AV block Overt cardiac failure Cardiogenic shock	May be absorbed systemically; the same adverse reactions seen with oral beta-blockers may occur. May mask the symptoms of acute hypoglycemia or hyperthyroidism
levobunolol 0.25% or 0.5% solution (Betagan) Dosing: 1–2 drops in the affected eye(s) once daily (0.5%) or twice daily (0.25%)	Burning and stinging, blepharoconjunctivitis, urticaria, ataxia, bradycardia, arrhythmia, hypotension, syncope, heart block	Bronchial asthma or severe COPD Sinus bradycardia Second- or third-degree AV block Overt cardiac failure Cardiogenic shock	May be absorbed systemically; the same adverse reactions seen with oral beta-blockers may occur. May mask the symptoms of acute hypoglycemia or hyperthyroidism
metipranolol 0.3% solution (OptiPranolol) Dosing: 1 drop in the affected eye(s) twice a day	Transient local discomfort, conjunctivitis, eyelid dermatitis, blepharitis, blurred vision, headache, asthenia, angina, palpitation, bradycardia	Bronchial asthma or severe COPD Symptomatic sinus bradycardia Second- or third-degree AV block Overt cardiac failure Cardiogenic shock	May be absorbed systemically; the same adverse reactions seen with oral beta-blockers may occur. May mask the symptoms of acute hypoglycemia or hyperthyroidism
timolol 0.25% or 0.5% solution (Timoptic, Betimol, Istalol) or gel-forming solution (Timoptic-XE) Dosing: Solution: 1 drop in the affected eye(s) twice daily Gel-forming solution: 1 drop in the affected eye(s) once daily	Ocular irritation, decreased corneal sensitivity, visual disturbances, conjunctivitis, tearing, headache, dizziness, bradycardia, arrhythmia	Bronchial asthma or severe COPD Sinus bradycardia Second- or third-degree AV block Overt cardiac failure Cardiogenic shock	May be absorbed systemically; the same adverse reactions seen with oral beta-blockers may occur. May mask the symptoms of acute hypoglycemia or hyperthyroidism. Other ophthalmic medications should be administered 10 min before the gel-forming solution.

TABLE 17.7

Overview of Glaucoma Agents (*Continued*)

Generic (Trade) Name and Dosage	Selected Adverse Events	Contraindications	Special Considerations
Carbonic Anhydrase Inhibitors			
brinzolamide 1% suspension (Azopt) Dosing: 1 drop in the affected eye(s) three times a day	Blurred vision, bitter taste, blepharitis, dermatitis, dry eye, headache, hyperemia ocular pain, pruritus	Sulfa allergy	
dorzolamide 1% solution (Trusopt) Dosing: 1 drop in the affected eye(s) three times a day	Ocular burning and stinging, bitter taste, keratitis, ocular allergy, blurred vision, tearing, photophobia	Sulfa allergy	
Prostaglandins			
bimatoprost 0.03% solution (Lumigan) Dosing: 1 drop in the affected eye(s) once daily in the evening	Conjunctival hyperemia, growth of eyelashes, ocular pruritus, dry eye, iris discoloration, visual disturbance, eye pain, pigmentation of the periocular skin, foreign body sensation		Iris discoloration is irreversible; incidence less than with latanoprost.
latanoprost 0.005% solution (Xalatan) Dosing: 1 drop in the affected eye(s) once daily in the evening	Iris discoloration, blurred vision, burning and stinging, conjunctival hyperemia, itching, eyelash changes, eyelid skin darkening		Iris discoloration is irreversible. Requires refrigeration until dispensed.
tafluprost 0.0015% solution (Zioptan) Dosing: 1 drop in the affected eye(s) once daily in the evening	Conjunctival hyperemia, ocular stinging, headache, ocular pruritus, dry eye, growth of eyelashes, iris discoloration, pigmentation of the periocular skin		Iris discoloration is irreversible.
travoprost 0.004% solution (Travatan Z) Dosing: 1 drop in the affected eye(s) once daily in the evening	Ocular hyperemia, decreased visual acuity, eye discomfort, foreign body sensation, eye pain, pruritus		Iris discoloration is irreversible. May interfere in pregnancy; should not be used during pregnancy or by those attempting to become pregnant
Adrenergic Agonists			
apraclonidine 0.5% solution (Iopidine) Dosing: 1–2 drops in the affected eye(s) three times a day	Hyperemia, tearing, pruritus, lid edema, dry mouth, foreign body sensation, eyelid retraction	Hypersensitivity to clonidine Patients receiving MAO inhibitors	For short-term use only A 1% solution is available for prevention of postsurgical elevations in IOP.
brimonidine 0.1%, 0.15%, or 0.2% solution (Alphagan P) Dosing: 1 drop in the affected eye(s) three times a day, approximately 8 h apart	Ocular hyperemia, ocular pruritus, visual disturbance, somnolence, headache, fatigue, drowsiness, dry mouth	Patients receiving MAO inhibitors	Not recommended in children less than age 2
Cholinergic Agonists			
pilocarpine 1%, 2%, or 4% solution (Isopto Carpine) Dosing: 1–2 drops three or four times a day	Stinging and burning, tearing, ciliary spasm, blurred vision, brow ache, hypertension, tachycardia, bronchospasm, salivation	Acute iritis or other conditions where papillary constriction is undesirable	
Combination Products			
brimonidine and timolol 0.2%–0.5% solution (Combigan) Dosing: 1 drop in the affected eye(s) every 12 h	See individual components.	See individual components.	Combined effect results in greater IOP lowering than either agent alone, but not as great as brimonidine three times a day and timolol two times a day administered concomitantly.

(Continued)

TABLE 17.7

Overview of Glaucoma Agents (*Continued*)

Generic (Trade) Name and Dosage	Selected Adverse Events	Contraindications	Special Considerations
dorzolamide and timolol 2%–0.5% solution (Cosopt) Dosing: 1 drop into the affected eye(s) two times a day	See individual components.	See individual components.	Combined effect results in greater IOP lowering than either agent alone, but not as great as dorzolamide three times a day and timolol two times a day administered concomitantly.
brinzolamide and brimonidine 1%–0.2% solution (Simbrinza) Dosing: 1 drop into the affected eye(s) three times a day	See individual components.	See individual components.	

AV, atrioventricular mode; COPD, chronic obstructive pulmonary disease; MAO, monoamine oxidase.

Beta-Blockers

Beta-blockers are the benchmark against which other IOP-lowering medications are measured. Beta-blockers reduce adenylyl cyclase activity, which in turn reduces the production of aqueous humor in the ciliary body. Beta-blockers lower IOP an average of 20% to 25%. There are five ophthalmic beta-blockers available in the United States: timolol, levobunolol, carteolol, and metipranolol are nonselective beta-blockers, while betaxolol is a beta$_1$-selective agent. Although nonselective beta-blockers may be more efficacious in lowering IOP, selective beta-blockers appear to be better tolerated systemically, particularly in patients with chronic obstructive pulmonary disease.

The ophthalmic beta-blockers are typically applied twice daily. Timolol is available in a solution that forms a gel upon application, allowing once-daily dosing. Side effects include stinging, burning, dry eye, and blurred vision. Topical beta-blockers can be absorbed systemically and may cause bradycardia, reduced blood pressure, aggravation of congestive heart failure, heart block, bronchospasm in asthma patients, and central nervous system (CNS) side effects such as hallucinations and depression. Betaxolol is less likely to cause these systemic side effects, but a risk still exists. All of the ophthalmic beta-blockers are contraindicated in patients with sinus bradycardia, second- or third-degree atrioventricular node block, overt cardiac failure, and cardiogenic shock, and all except betaxolol are contraindicated in patients with bronchial asthma or severe chronic obstructive pulmonary disease.

Prostaglandins

The prostaglandin F$_{2\alpha}$ analogs bimatoprost, latanoprost, tafluprost, and travoprost reduce IOP by improving the uveoscleral outflow of aqueous humor. Given once a day, the prostaglandin F$_{2\alpha}$ analogs reduce IOP by 25% to 33%. Studies of bimatoprost, latanoprost, and travoprost found no statistical difference in IOP lowering between agents (Li et al., 2006).

These agents are more effective when given at bedtime rather than in the morning. Latanoprost requires refrigeration until dispensed; latanoprost and travoprost should be discarded within 6 weeks of the time the package is opened. Tafluprost is supplied in single-use containers packaged within a foil pouch; unused single-use containers should be discarded 28 days after opening the pouch. Side effects of the prostaglandins include ocular hyperemia, blurred vision, pruritus, dry eye, lengthening and thickening of the eyelashes, and conjunctival hyperemia. These agents are also associated with irreversible iris discoloration, most often affecting patients with mixed-color irises. Iris discoloration is reported by 7% to 12% of latanoprost users, with discoloration starting between 18 and 26 weeks after commencement of therapy. Compared to latanoprost, the incidence of iris discoloration is lower for bimatoprost and travoprost. In addition, darkening of the eyelid skin (periocular hyperpigmentation) can occur with these agents; therapy discontinuation often results in reversal of periocular hyperpigmentation 3 to 6 months after therapy discontinuation.

Carbonic Anhydrase Inhibitors

The topical carbonic anhydrase inhibitors (CAIs) brinzolamide and dorzolamide work through the reversible and competitive binding of carbonic anhydrase. Carbonic anhydrase acts as a catalyst for the reversible hydration of carbonic acid, which plays a role in fluid transport in various cell systems. By decreasing bicarbonate formation, the movement of bicarbonate, sodium, and fluid into the posterior chamber of the eye declines, and less aqueous fluid is generated, reducing IOP (Abel & Sorensen, 2013). While the topical CAIs reduce IOP to a lesser extent (15% to 26%) than beta-blockers, prostaglandins, or systemic CAIs, they are rarely associated with systemic side effects.

The topical CAIs are given three times a day. Side effects include ocular burning and stinging, bitter taste, blurred vision, itching, tearing, and keratitis. The topical CAIs are contraindicated in patients with hypersensitivity to sulfonamides and are not recommended for use in patients with severe renal impairment, respiratory acidosis, and electrolyte disorders.

The systemic CAIs (acetazolamide, methazolamide, and dichlorphenamide) are the most potent agents for reducing IOP, producing a 25% to 40% decrease in IOP. However, these agents produce severe side effects such as paresthesias, gastrointestinal disturbances (anorexia, nausea, and weight loss), metallic taste, CNS effects (lethargy, malaise, and depression), electrolyte disturbances, and renal calculi, which limit their use in the elderly population (Swenson, 2014).

Adrenergic Agonists

The adrenergic agonists apraclonidine and brimonidine activate the presynaptic alpha-2 receptors, inhibiting the release of norepinephrine. As less norepinephrine is available for activation of postsynaptic beta receptors on the ciliary epithelium, the formation of aqueous humor is reduced.

Apraclonidine and brimonidine reduce IOP by 18% to 27%. Brimonidine is a highly selective alpha-2 agonist, causing little or no alpha-1 activity. In addition to decreasing aqueous humor, it increases uveoscleral outflow. Side effects include dry mouth, fatigue, ocular hyperemia, somnolence, and headache. Apraclonidine is a relatively selective alpha-2 agonist; it is associated with some alpha-1 activity, which can lead to mydriasis, conjunctival bleeding, and eyelid retraction. Apraclonidine is primarily indicated for short-term adjunctive therapy, as the efficacy of apraclonidine diminishes over time; the benefit for most patients lasts less than 1 to 2 months. Both agents are contraindicated in patients taking monoamine oxidase inhibitors. In addition, brimonidine has been associated with respiratory and cardiac depression in infants and should be used with caution in children under age 2.

The nonselective ophthalmic adrenergic agonists epinephrine and dipivefrin (epinephrine prodrug) are no longer available in the United States. These agents provided lackluster IOP control and were associated with adverse reactions such as stinging and tearing, brow ache, and the formation of black conjunctival spots and conjunctival deposits.

Cholinergic Agonists

Pilocarpine is a direct-acting cholinergic agonist. Pilocarpine stimulates the parasympathetic muscarinic receptor site to increase aqueous outflow through the trabecular meshwork. While effective in lowering IOP by 20% to 30%, pilocarpine usually needs to be given four times a day. Side effects include eye pain, brow ache, blurred vision, and accommodative spasms. It can also provoke miotic responses such as papillary constriction, which can decrease night vision. The intense dosing regimen and the side effect profile make adherence difficult.

Combination Products

Combination products simplify administration and can promote adherence to therapy. Solutions of timolol 0.5% in combination with dorzolamide 2% or brimonidine 0.2%

are available, as is a combination of brimonidine 0.2% and brinzolamide 1%. The combined effect results in additional IOP reduction compared to either agent alone, but the result is often less than each agent administered separately.

Selecting the Most Appropriate Agent

The AAO does not recommend a specific agent as first-line therapy. When the first-line agent drug fails to reduce IOP, the AAO recommends that it be discontinued in favor of another therapy before the original agent is supplanted by other medications. If a first-line agent lowers IOP but fails to lower IOP to the target level, combination therapy and discontinuation of therapy in favor of another agent are appropriate options. When selecting the first-line therapy for glaucoma, factors such as efficacy, side effects, cost, and dosing frequency should all be considered. **Table 17.8** lists the recommended order of treatment for these agents.

First-Line Therapy

The prostaglandins are often utilized as first-line therapy for POAG because they possess the best balance between efficacy, safety, and ease of dosing regimen.

Second-Line Therapy

If the prostaglandin fails to decrease IOP to a significant extent, the patient should be switched to a different class of medicine. Beta-blockers are recommended because of their efficacy, tolerability, and ease of dosing. If the IOP decreases with a prostaglandin but fails to reach the target IOP, an additional medication from a different class (such as a beta-blocker) should be added.

TABLE 17.8

Recommended Order of Treatment for Glaucoma

Order	Agent	Comments
First line	Prostaglandin ophthalmic solution (bimatoprost, latanoprost, tafluprost, or travoprost)	An ophthalmic beta-blocker may be substituted if the patient cannot afford the prostaglandins.
Second line	Substitution of an ophthalmic beta-blocker (if failure to decrease IOP to a significant extent) *or* Addition of an ophthalmic beta-blocker (if IOP is significantly decreased but not to goal)	
Third line	Addition of an ophthalmic carbonic anhydrase inhibitor *or* addition of brimonidine	Dorzolamide is available in a combination product with timolol.

CASE STUDY*

V.S., age 12, presents with a feeling that there is sand in his eye. He had a cold a week ago and woke up this morning with his left eye crusted with yellowish drainage. On physical examination, he has injected conjunctiva on the left side, no adenopathy, and no vision changes. His vision is 20/20. Fluorescein staining reveals no abrasion. He is allergic to sulfa.

DIAGNOSIS: CONJUNCTIVITIS

1. List specific goals of treatment for **V.S.**
2. What drug therapy would you prescribe? Why?
3. What are the parameters for monitoring the success of the therapy?

4. Discuss the education you would give to the parents regarding drug therapy.
5. List one or two adverse reactions for the selected agent that would cause you to change therapy.
6. What would be the choice for second-line therapy?
7. What over-the-counter or alternative medications would be appropriate for **V.S.**?
8. What dietary and lifestyle changes should be recommended for **V.S.**?
9. Describe one or two drug–drug or drug–food interactions for the selected agent.

* Answers can be found online.

Third-Line Therapy

If a patient fails to reach the target IOP with the first-line and second-line therapies, a topical CAI (usually the fixed combination of timolol and dorzolamide to keep the dosing regimen simple) can be added. If this fails, dorzolamide should be discontinued in favor of brimonidine.

MONITORING PATIENT RESPONSE

Patients with POAG should receive follow-up evaluations and care from their eye care professional to determine the effectiveness of therapy. In addition to a recent history, a physical examination including a slit-lamp biomicroscopy and tests of visual acuity and IOP in each eye should be performed (AAO, 2015). The practitioner must distinguish between the impact of a prescribed agent on IOP and ordinary background fluctuations of IOP.

PATIENT EDUCATION

Patients should wash their hands before administering glaucoma medications. Patients should be taught how to apply the medication in the inner aspect of the lower eyelid. The tip of the container should not touch the eyelashes or any part of the eye because this may contaminate the medication. Contact lenses should be removed prior to administration, and patients should separate administration of different glaucoma medications by at least 10 minutes.

Bibliography

Starred references are cited in the text.

*Abel, S. R., & Sorensen, S. J. (2013). Eye disorders. In B. K. Alldredge, et al. (Eds.), *Applied therapeutics: The clinical use of drugs* (10th ed., pp. 1301–1322). Philadelphia, PA: Wolters Kluwer.

*Akpek, E. K., & Smith, R. A. (2013). Overview of age-related ocular conditions. *American Journal of Managed Care Pharmacy, 19*, S67–S75.

Akpek, E. K., Lindsley, K. B., Adyanthaya, R. S., et al. (2011). Treatment of Sjogren's syndrome-associated dry eye: An evidence based review. *Ophthalmology, 118*, 1242–1252.

Alves, M., Carrana Fonseca, E., Alves, M. F., et al. (2013). Dry eye disease treatment: A systematic review of published trials and a critical appraisal of therapeutic strategies. *The Ocular Surface, 11*, 181–192.

*American Academy of Ophthalmology Cornea/External Disease Panel, Preferred Practice Guidelines Committee. (2015). *Primary open-angle glaucoma.* San Francisco, CA: AAO.

*American Academy of Ophthalmology Cornea/External Disease Panel, Preferred Practice Guidelines Committee. (2013a). *Blepharitis.* San Francisco, CA: AAO.

*American Academy of Ophthalmology Cornea/External Disease Panel, Preferred Practice Guidelines Committee. (2013b). *Conjunctivitis.* San Francisco, CA: AAO.

*American Academy of Ophthalmology Cornea/External Disease Panel, Preferred Practice Guidelines Committee. (2013c). *Dry eye syndrome.* San Francisco, CA: AAO.

*American Academy of Pediatrics. (2012). *Chlamydia trachomatis.* In L. K. Pickering (Ed.), *Red book: Report of the Committee on Infectious Diseases* (29th ed., pp. 276–281). Elk Grove Village, IL: American Academy of Pediatrics.

*Azari, A. A., & Barney, N. P. (2013). Conjunctivitis: A systematic review of diagnosis and treatment. *Journal of the American Medical Association, 310*(16), 1721–1729.

*Bowling, E., & Russell, G. E. (2011). Topical steroids in the treatment of dry eye. *Review of Cornea and Contact Lenses, 3*(March).

*Centers for Disease Control and Prevention. (2014). *Conjunctivitis (pink eye) for clinicians.* Atlanta, GA: National Center for Immunization and Respiratory Diseases.

*Cronau, H., Kankanala, R. R., & Mauger, T. (2010). Diagnosis and management of red eye in primary care. *American Family Physician, 81*, 137–144.

*Deibel, J. P., & Cowling, K. (2013). Ocular inflammation and infection. *Emergency Medicine Clinics of North America, 31*(2), 387–397.

*Donshik, P. C., Ehlers, W. H., & Ballow, M. (2008). Giant papillary conjunctivitis. *Immunology and Allergy Clinics of North America, 28*, 83–103.

Emanuel, M. E., & Gedde, S. J. (2014). Indications for a systemic work up in glaucoma. *Canadian Journal of Ophthalmology, 49*, 506–511.

*Fraser, S. G., & Wormald, R. L. P. (2006). Hospital episode statistics and changing trends in glaucoma surgery. *Eye, 22*, 3–7.

*Gordon, M. O., Beiser, J. A., Brandt, J. D., et al. (2002). The Ocular Hypertension Treatment Study: Baseline factors that predict the onset of primary open-angle glaucoma. *Archives of Ophthalmology, 120*, 714–720.

*Guillon, M., Maissa, C., & Wong, S. (2012). Symptomatic relief associated with eyelid hygiene in anterior blepharitis and MGD. *Eye and Contact Lens, 38*(5), 306–312.

*Horton, J. C. (2015). Disorders of the eye. In D. L. Kasper et al. (Ed.), *Harrison's principles of internal medicine* (19th ed.). New York, NY: McGraw-Hill.

*Kari, O., & Saari, K. M. (2012). Diagnostics and new developments in the treatment of ocular allergies. *Current Allergy and Asthma Reports, 12*, 232–239.

King, A., Azuara-Blanco, A., & Tuulonen, A. (2013). Glaucoma. *British Medical Journal, 346*, f3518.

Lee, S. H., Oh, D. H., Jung, J. Y., et al. (2012). Comparative ocular microbial communities in humans with and without blepharitis. *Investigative Ophthalmology and Vision Science, 53*(9), 5585–5593.

*Leske, M. C., Heijl, A., Hussein, M., et al. (2003). Factors for glaucoma progression and the effect of treatment: The Early Manifest Glaucoma Trial. *Archives of Ophthalmology, 121*, 48–56.

Levesy, M. E., & DeFlorio, P. (2010). Ophthalmologic conditions. In K. J. Knoop et al. (Ed.), *The atlas of emergency medicine* (3rd ed.). New York, NY: McGraw-Hill.

*Li, N., Chen, X. M., Zhou, Y., et al. (2006). Travoprost compared to other prostaglandin analogues or timolol in patients with open angle glaucoma or ocular hypertension: Meta-analysis of randomized, controlled trials. *Clinical and Experimental Ophthalmology, 34*, 755–764.

Lindsley, K., Matsumura, S., Hatef, E., et al. (2012). Interventions for chronic blepharitis. *Cochrane Database of Systematic Reviews*, (5), CD005556.

McCulley, J. P., Uchiyama, E., Aranowicz, J. D., et al. (2006). Impact of evaporation on aqueous tear loss. *Transactions of the American Ophthalmological Society, 104*, 121–128.

*Moss, S. E., Klein, R., & Klein, B. E. (2000). Prevalence and risk factors for dry eye syndrome. *Archives of Ophthalmology, 118*, 1264–1268.

*National Eye Institute. (2010). *Facts about dry eye*. Bethesda, MD: Author.

*Nijm, L. M., Garcia-Ferrer, F. J., Schwab, I. R., et al. (2011). Conjunctiva and tears. In P. Riordan-Eva, et al. (Eds.), *Vaughan & Asbury's general ophthalmology* (18th ed.). New York, NY: McGraw-Hill.

*Pascolini, D., & Mariotti, S. P. M. (2012). *Global data on visual impairments 2010*. Geneva, Switzerland: World Health Organization.

*Rocha, E. M., Alves, M., Rios, J. D., et al. (2008). The aging lacrimal gland: Changes in structure and function. *The Ocular Surface, 6*, 162–174.

*Sambursky, R., Tauber, S., Schirra, F., et al. (2013). Sensitivity and specificity of the AdenoPlus test for diagnosing adenoviral conjunctivitis. *JAMA Ophthalmology, 131*, 17–21.

*Schaumberg, D. A., Nichols, J. J., Papas, E. B., et al. (2011). The international workshop on meibomian gland dysfunction: Report of the subcommittee on the epidemiology of, and associated risk factors for, MGD. *Investigative Ophthalmology and Visual Science, 52*, 1994–2005.

Schwartz, K., & Budenz, D. (2004). Current management of glaucoma. *Current Opinion in Ophthalmology, 15*, 119–126.

*Sethuraman, U., & Kamat, D. (2009). The red eye: Evaluation and management. *Clinical Pediatrics, 48*, 588–600.

*Swenson, E. R. (2014). Safety of carbonic anhydrase inhibitors. *Expert Opinion on Drug Safety, 13*, 459–472.

Tanna, A. P., & Lin, A. B. (2015). Medical therapy: What to add after a prostaglandin analog? *Current Opinion in Ophthalmology, 26*, 116–120.

*Tielsch, J. M., Katz, J., Singh, K., et al. (1991). A population-based evaluation of glaucoma screening: The Baltimore Eye Survey. *American Journal of Epidemiology, 134*, 1102–1110.

Turnbull, A. M., & Mayfield, M. P. (2012). Blepharitis. *British Medical Journal, 344*, e3328.

Vivino, F. B., Al-Hashimi, I., Khan, Z., et al. (1999). Pilocarpine tablets for the treatment of dry mouth and dry eye symptoms in patients with Sjögren syndrome. *Archives of Internal Medicine, 159*, 174–181.

Wong, T. Y., & Hyman, L. (2008). Population-based studies in ophthalmology. *American Journal of Ophthalmology, 146*, 656–663.

*Wong, M. M., & Anninger, W. (2014). The pediatric red eye. *Pediatric Clinics of North America, 61*, 591–606.

*Zhao, Y. E., Wu, L. P., Hu, L., et al. (2012) Association of blepharitis with Demodex: A meta-analysis. *Ophthalmic Epidemiology, 19*(2), 95–102.

18 Otitis Media and Otitis Externa

Laura L. Bio

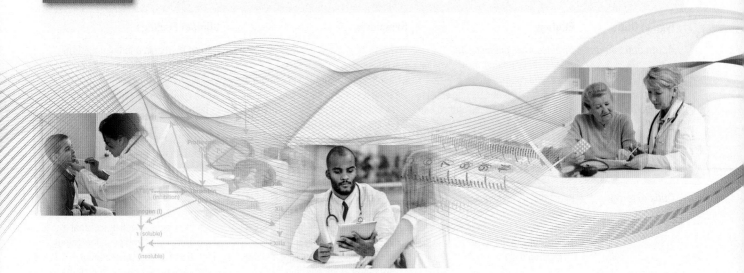

Infections of the ear are a common problem in children due to anatomical predisposition, but they can also affect adults. Acute otitis media (AOM), otitis media with effusion (OME), and otitis externa (OE; also known as *swimmer's ear*) are the most common infection or inflammatory conditions of the ear. Although antibiotics and vaccination programs have decreased the frequency of infections, identification, diagnosis, and management of these infections are essential to prevent permanent hearing loss, chronic or recurrent ear infections, mastoiditis, meningitis, and speech or language delay.

OTITIS MEDIA AND OTITIS EXTERNA

Otitis media (OM) may manifest as AOM or chronic OME (Lieberthal et al., 2013). OM has historically posed a major social and economic burden, occurring at an alarming rate of 19 million cases per year. It continues to impact antibiotic expenditures because it is the most common infection for which antibiotics are prescribed for children. In spite of the strict 2004 American Academy of Pediatrics (AAP) AOM guideline, the rate of antibiotic prescribing for OM has remained constant. The recent 2013 AAP AOM guideline and clinical reports emphasize the need for judicious antibiotic prescribing for upper respiratory infections (URIs) to reduce the risk of antibiotic resistance and adverse effects (Hersh et al., 2013).

AOM is defined as an acute onset of signs and symptoms of a middle ear infection and inflammation, such as middle ear effusion and erythema, respectively (**Table 18.1**). AOM is the most common bacterial respiratory tract infection in children and predominantly effects infants and children age 6 months

to 2 years. During the year 2006, 11.8% of all children under age 18 years were diagnosed with OM (8.8 million cases) (Soni, 2006). Meanwhile, OME is inflammation of the middle ear with fluid collection behind the TM, but signs and symptoms of an acute infection are absent (Pelton, 2012). OME typically precedes or follows AOM (Pichichero, 2013).

Otitis externa (OE) may present in acute and chronic forms. OE is defined as an inflammation of the outer ear and ear canal. Acute OE roughly affects 1 in 123 persons in the United States based on the 2.4 million visits to ambulatory care centers and emergency departments in 2007 (CDC, 2011). Children 5 to 14 years of age account for approximately half of all visits. OE is most often associated with swimming, local trauma, use of hearing aids, and high, humid temperatures (**Table 18.1**). Unlike AOM, in which the mainstay of treatment is systemic antibiotics, topical antibiotic therapy is usually adequate for the treatment of OE. Oral antibiotics may be recommended for patients with acute OE infections extending outside the ear canal or certain host factors such as diabetes, immune deficiency, or inability to effectively deliver topic therapy. Systemic antibiotics should also be considered for patients with recurrent episodes of OE or clinical signs of necrotizing (i.e., malignant) OE, which is a serious and potentially life-threatening complication of the infection extending to the mastoid or temporal bone. Immunocompromised patients, including the elderly with diabetes and human immunodeficiency virus, are at the highest risk of necrotizing OE. Chronic OE is a single episode lasting longer than 3 months or four or more episodes in 1 year and often the result of allergies, chronic dermatologic conditions, or inadequately treated acute OE (Rosenfeld et al., 2004; Schaefer & Baugh, 2012).

TABLE 18.1

Comparing Types of Otitis

Type of Otitis	Etiology	Symptoms	Clinical Findings
Acute otitis media	Streptococcus pneumoniae Haemophilus influenzae nontypable Moraxella catarrhalis	Otalgia Ear pulling Upper respiratory infection symptoms	Diffuse erythema and bulging of the TM Decreased mobility of the TM
Otitis media with effusion	Eustachian tube obstruction causing sterile effusion in the middle ear	Hearing loss that may be manifested by delayed language development in young children or decreased school performance in older children Feeling of ear fullness Popping sensation with swallowing, yawning, or blowing the nose	Clear, yellowish, or bluish-gray fluid behind the TM, with or without air bubbles TM may be retracted with decreased movement
Otitis externa	Infectious: Pseudomonas aeruginosa, Staphylococcus aureus, Streptococcus species Necrotizing (malignant): P. aeruginosa	Infectious: erythema and swelling of the external canal with otalgia and itching, muffled hearing, watery or thick discharge from the ear Necrotizing: persistent foul-smelling discharge, deep ear pain	Infectious: pain with movement of tragus, raised area of induration on the tragus, swollen external auditory canal, red pustular lesions Necrotizing: progressive cranial nerve palsies, granulations in the external ear canal

TM, tympanic membrane.

CAUSES

Acute Otitis Media and Otitis Media with Effusion

The most frequently isolated bacteria from middle ear fluid are *Streptococcus pneumoniae*, nontypable *Haemophilus influenzae*, and *Moraxella catarrhalis*, followed by the less common group A *Streptococcus* and *Staphylococcus aureus*. The precise frequency for each AOM pathogen has changed over time due to changes in vaccination coverage. Historically, *S. pneumoniae* dominated AOM etiology, but after implementation of the 13-serotype conjugate vaccine, beta-lactamase producing *H. influenzae* and *M. catarrhalis* has emerged as more common (Pichichero, 2013).

Although many cases are caused by bacterial pathogens, viruses play a significant role in the pathogenesis and course of treatment. Viral pathogens, such as respiratory syncytial virus, influenza A and B, parainfluenza, enterovirus, and rhinovirus, have all been isolated in nasopharyngeal secretion of children with URI (Pichichero, 2013). Most cases of AOM follow viral URI since it facilitates bacterial AOM by enhancing the bacteria's ability to ascend the nasopharynx and infect the middle ear (Pelton, 2012). Single virus isolates are recovered from 2% to 20% of AOM tympanocenteses.

Otitis Externa

Ninety-eight percent of OE cases in the United States are caused by bacteria, most commonly *Pseudomonas aeruginosa* and *S. aureus* (Schaefer & Baugh, 2012). The etiology of OE is different than that of OM because the flora of the external auditory canal is similar to that of the skin including *Staphylococcus epidermidis*, *S. aureus*, *Corynebacteria* species, and *Propionibacterium acnes*. Fungi, predominantly *Aspergillus* and *Candida* species, cause less than 5% of OE in the United States but may be more common in subtropical or tropical climates (Boyce, 2012). Fungal OE, otomycosis, may also occur in cases in which prolonged antibiotic courses are given for bacterial OE, causing an alteration in ear canal skin flora. Chronic OE may be noninfectious but caused by inflammatory skin disorders and allergic reactions (Schaefer & Baugh, 2012). Necrotizing (malignant) OE is caused by *P. aeruginosa*.

PATHOPHYSIOLOGY

Otitis Media

AOM frequently follows a URI (usually of viral etiology) in which the eustachian tube closes secondary to inflamed mucous membranes (Lieberthal et al., 2013). The pathophysiology of AOM is multifactorial but is mainly the result of eustachian tube dysfunction. The eustachian tube protects the middle ear from nasopharyngeal secretions, provides drainage of secretions produced in the middle ear into the nasopharynx, and permits equilibration of air pressure to atmospheric pressure in the middle ear. The structure of a child's eustachian tube differs from that of an adult's. The adult eustachian tube lies at 45 degrees to the horizontal plane and allows for secretions to drain from the middle ear to the nasopharynx. The child's eustachian tube, however, is short and horizontal. When a child develops mild inflammation or edema of the eustachian tube, the ear has difficulty clearing secretions due to the almost horizontal placement of the eustachian tube. Persistent secretions, incomplete drainage, and the absence of aeration breed an environment for bacterial growth within the middle ear, resulting in AOM (Pelton, 2012). The incidence of AOM is highest during winter months, which coincide with the seasonal peak of URIs. Risk factors for AOM include congenital defects such as cleft palate and Down syndrome, young age (highest incidence in children below age 2), family history, and children who attend day care or are relatives of children in day care. The following risk factors have also been associated, however inconsistently, with an increased risk of AOM: male sex, exposure to secondhand smoke, allergies, and lack of exclusive breast-feeding for the first 6 months of life (Hoberman et al., 2002).

OME is thought to result from prolonged blockage of the eustachian tube, which in turn causes negative pressure within the middle ear that allows fluid to accumulate and persist, and may result in conductive hearing loss (Pelton, 2012). The presence of effusion does not always correlate to the presence of an infection. In fact, bacterial pathogens are reported in only 20% to 30% of middle ear effusions (Pelton, 2012).

Otitis Externa

OE is a cellulitis of the ear canal skin and subdermis with or without infection (Rosenfeld et al., 2013). Children, adolescents, and adults are all at risk for developing this infection. This condition may occur as a result of many different factors. The most common predisposing factor is swimming, especially in freshwater. Additional OE risk factors include eczema or seborrhea resulting in excessive itching, trauma from cerumen removal, use of hearing aids, chronic otorrhea, and immunocompromised states such as diabetes (Schaefer & Baugh, 2012). Disruption of the ear canal homeostasis from prolonged periods of water exposure (head immersion), loss of protective cerumen barrier, and disruption of the epithelium all result in varied pH and compromised local immune defenses, which allows bacteria and other pathogens to harbor infection.

Resistance

The increasing rates of antimicrobial resistance are a major cause and concern for treatment failure of AOM. The increasing incidence warrants the judicious use of antibiotics. Mechanisms of resistance include alteration of drug binding sites and the production of antibiotic inactivating enzymes, for example, beta-lactamases. Organisms such as *H. influenzae* and *M. catarrhalis* can produce these enzymes, which essentially render many beta-lactam antibiotics useless. It is for this reason that antibiotics that remain stable in the presence of beta-lactamase–producing enzymes must be chosen to ensure treatment success. A detailed discussion of treatment options is discussed in the management section of this chapter.

Drug-resistant *S. pneumoniae* (DRSP) remains a threat in the treatment of AOM. Penicillin, historically, has been the mainstay of treatment against *S. pneumoniae*. However, the increasing prevalence of penicillin-intermediate and penicillin-resistant strains has discouraged the use of penicillin and its derivatives. Furthermore, penicillin-resistant strains may also confer resistance to other antibiotics such as macrolides, trimethoprim–sulfamethoxazole, and clindamycin. The mechanism of penicillin-resistant *S. pneumoniae* is the alteration of the penicillin-binding site resulting in elevated minimum inhibitory concentration (MIC). This may be overcome by administering high-dose amoxicillin if deemed intermediate susceptibility based on the MIC. It should be noted that infections caused by penicillin-resistant *S. pneumoniae* have mostly been reported in children younger than age 2.

Beta-lactamase production is the mechanism by which organisms such as *H. influenzae* and *M. catarrhalis* develop resistance. Beta-lactamase inhibitors in combination with beta-lactam therapy, such as amoxicillin–clavulanic acid or beta-lactamase stable cephalosporins (i.e., cefixime, cefpodoxime), can overcome this mechanism of resistance. Therefore, these agents should be recommended for treatment if these organisms are suspected, specifically in the setting of treatment failure or recurrent infection.

DIAGNOSTIC CRITERIA AND CLINICAL PRESENTATION

Acute Otitis Media

The presentation of AOM includes abrupt onset of symptoms such as fever, otalgia, irritability, and tugging on the affected ear; the tympanic membrane (TM) appears bulging, erythematous, and immobile to pneumatic otoscopy upon inspection indicating middle ear effusion. The averbal infant may express otalgia by tugging, rubbing, or holding the affected ear, excessive crying, fever, or changes in sleep or behavior pattern. The diagnosis of AOM requires abrupt onset of symptoms (less than 48 hours), presence of middle ear effusion, and signs or symptoms of middle ear inflammation, including erythema of the TM, hearing loss, and otalgia (Lieberthal et al., 2013). Otorrhea may also be present and will affect management (**Table 18.2**).

TABLE 18.2

Diagnostic Criteria for Acute Otitis Media

1. History of acute onset of signs/symptoms
2. Presence of middle ear effusion (indicated by one of the following)
   a. Bulging of TM
   b. Limited or absent TM mobility
   c. Otorrhea
   d. Air–fluid level behind TM
3. Signs and symptoms of middle ear inflammation
   a. Erythema of TM
   b. Otalgia

The absence of acute inflammatory signs and symptoms presumes a diagnosis of OME. Patients with OME are usually asymptomatic but may complain of a full sensation in the ear and hearing loss. Upon examination, the TM may not appear bulging, but air–fluid levels may be apparent. AOM and OME require differentiation since OME should not be treated with antibiotics due to probable viral etiology or result of AOM resolution.

Tympanocentesis, the process by which fluid is drained from the middle ear, is recommended for recurrent treatment failure to ensure proper diagnosis of the causative organism and determine the presence of bacterial resistance. This process relieves pressure in the middle ear cavity and promotes drainage, but it is reserved for treatment failures due to the potential risk of permanent hearing loss and facial paralysis.

INITIATING DRUG THERAPY

Goals of Drug Therapy

The goals of therapy for AOM include symptomatic pain relief, appropriate use of antibiotics to prevent complications, and judicious use of antibiotics to prevent future antimicrobial resistance. Symptomatic pain relief can be achieved with the use of acetaminophen or a nonsteroidal anti-inflammatory drug (NSAID) such as ibuprofen. Antibiotics are utilized to eradicate the infecting organism and prevent complications such as mastoiditis and hearing impairment. Antibiotic use is not without concerns, such as resistance and adverse effects. For these reasons, clinicians should avoid unnecessary use of antibiotics.

Over-the-Counter Therapy

Acetaminophen and NSAIDs should be offered early to relieve pain regardless of antibiotic use, unless hypersensitivity exists. Local topical anesthetics containing benzocaine or procaine may provide brief additional pain relief for children over 5 years of age.

Observational Therapy

The decision to manage AOM with antibiotics is based on patient-specific characteristics such as age, bilateral involvement, presence of otorrhea, and severity of illness (Lieberthal et al., 2013). All patients with suspected AOM who are younger than age 6 months should receive antibiotics. For patients with nonsevere, unilateral AOM without otorrhea who are older than age 6 months, the role of antibiotics is unclear, and the decision to provide symptomatic relief with close observation can be made. The decision to observe and withhold antibiotics is based on the high rate of spontaneous resolution (approximately 80%) and overlap of nonspecific AOM symptoms with viral URIs (Hersh et al., 2013). In addition, judicious antibiotic prescribing reduces the risk of resistance and reduces common adverse effects associated with antibiotic therapy.

Patients with otorrhea or severe symptoms (i.e., toxic-appearing child, persistent otalgia more than 48 hours, temperature ≥102.2°F in the past 48 hours, or uncertain access to follow-up after visit) require antibiotic therapy regardless of age. Bilateral AOM requires antibiotic therapy only if the patient is less than 2 years of age. Patients 2 years old or greater with bilateral AOM without otorrhea or severe symptoms may initially be managed with observation therapy after a discussion with the child's family to understand the decision. Observation therapy requires implementation of follow-up within 48 to 72 hours to ensure antibiotics can be initiated if the child's condition worsens or fails to improve. The technique for observational therapy is controversial: observe with or without a prescription with instructions to fill after 2 to 3 days if symptoms persist (Chao et al., 2008). This decision should be based on the prescriber's discussion with the caregiver and assessment of likelihood to adhere to the plan.

Penicillins

First-line therapy for AOM is high-dose amoxicillin for adequate middle ear penetration and to overcome intermediate-resistant *S. pneumoniae* (Lieberthal et al., 2013; **Figure 18.1**; **Table 18.3**). If the child has received amoxicillin in the past 30 days and has concurrent purulent conjunctivitis or allergy to penicillin, amoxicillin may not be appropriate. Recent receipt of amoxicillin or failure to improve while on amoxicillin raises concern of resistant organisms causing the infection, such as *M. catarrhalis* and *H. influenzae*. Therefore, the addition of beta-lactamase inhibitor to beta-lactam is necessary. Amoxicillin–clavulanate is a combination product commercially available in the United States in various concentrations of the oral suspension, chewables, tablets, and extended-release tablets. The major difference among these formulations is the ratio of clavulanate to amoxicillin and therefore may not be interchanged. The most common adverse effect of amoxicillin–clavulanate is diarrhea, which is dependent on the dosage of clavulanate (Block et al., 2006). Since high-dose amoxicillin is recommended for AOM treatment, use of amoxicillin–clavulanate standard ratio (clavulanate to amoxicillin, 1:7) would result in excess exposure of clavulanate and diarrhea. Therefore, the ES formulation for oral suspension (ratio 1:14) or XR formulation for tablets (ratio 1:16) should be recommended to limit excess exposure to clavulanate and therefore reduce the incidence of diarrhea.

Cephalosporins

If the presence of a penicillin allergy is elicited from the patient or caregiver, the type of reaction should be assessed. Fortunately, the cross-reactivity between penicillins and most second-generation and third-generation cephalosporins is low due to distinct chemical structures (Pichichero, 2005). Therefore, oral formulations of cefdinir and cefpodoxime, which are third-generation cephalosporins, and cefuroxime, which is a second-generation cephalosporin, are recommended

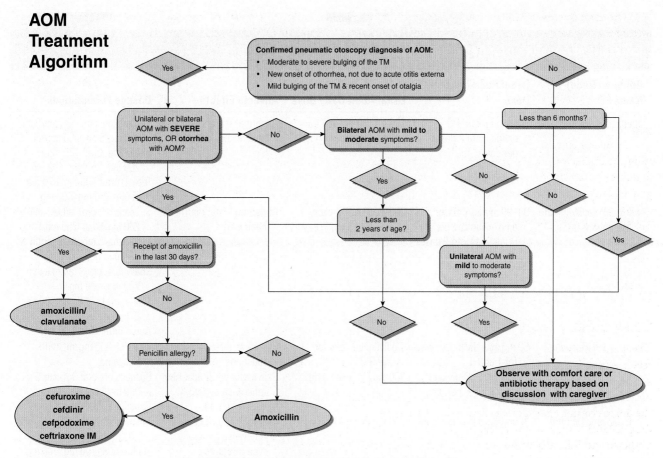

FIGURE 18.1   Treatment algorithm for acute otitis media.

for penicillin-allergic patients, regardless of reaction type (both anaphylactic and urticarial reaction) (**Table 18.3**).

Patients who are persistently vomiting or cannot tolerate oral medication for other reasons, ceftriaxone, a third-generation cephalosporin, administered as intramuscular injection, is an option for initial or repeat antibiotic treatment due to treatment failure.

Macrolides

Historically, macrolides including azithromycin and erythromycin were recommended for patients with a history of anaphylactic reaction to penicillins. Due to limited macrolide efficacy against both *S. pneumoniae* and *H. influenzae* and lower rate of cross-sensitivity to cephalosporins among penicillin-allergic patients than previously reported, macrolides are no longer recommended by the AAP (Lieberthal et al., 2013).

Clindamycin

Similar to macrolides, clindamycin historically was an option for patients who had an anaphylactic to penicillin. But again, due to concerns of clindamycin's lack of activity against *H. influenzae* or *M. catarrhalis*, it is no longer recommended. Clindamycin may be used for suspected penicillin-resistant *S. pneumoniae*, but it may not be effective against multi–drug-resistant strains, such as serotype 19A (Kaplan et al., 2015).

Selecting the Most Appropriate Agent

Figure 18.1 outlines the process for selecting the most appropriate agent.

First-Line Therapy

Amoxicillin is considered the first-line treatment for AOM in patients who have severe symptoms and who have not had a course of amoxicillin in the past 30 days. For those patients who had a course of amoxicillin in the recent past, treatment with the combination amoxicillin–clavulanate is indicated. In patients with a penicillin allergy, one of the cephalosporins is indicated as the first-line treatment.

Second-Line Therapy

After 48 to 72 hours of persistent patient's symptoms under observation therapy, antibiotic therapy should be initiated. Upon the decision to initiate antibiotic therapy, the same antibiotic decision algorithm applies as discussed earlier (**Figure 18.1**). Patients who received antibiotics for more than 72 hours and severe symptoms persist are deemed treatment failure. Treatment failure may be due to the presence of a resistant organism, a viral infection, which is unresponsive to antibiotic therapy, inadequate concentration of antibiotic in the middle ear, or noncompliance with the prescribed regimen. Treatment failure requires

TABLE 18.3

Overview of Antibiotics for Acute Otitis Media

Generic (Trade) Name	Usual Pediatric Daily Dose	Usual Adult Daily Dose	Adverse Effects	Dosage Formulations
amoxicillin (various)	80–90 mg/kg/d PO divided into 2 doses per day	2–3 g/d PO divided into 2 to 3 doses per day	Abnormal taste, diarrhea, headache, skin rash	Suspension, oral: 125 mg/5 mL, 250 mg/5 mL, 400 mg/mL Chewable, oral: 125 mg, 200 mg, 250 mg, 400 mg Tablet, oral: 500 mg, 875 mg Capsule: 250 mg, 500 mg
amoxicillin–clavulanate (Augmentin)	80–90 mg/kg/d based on amoxicillin component PO divided into 2 doses per day	250–500 mg PO every 8 h; or 875 mg PO every 12 h	Abnormal taste, diarrhea, headache	Suspension, oral: amoxicillin* 200 mg/5 mL, 250 mg/5 mL, 400 mg/5 mL; Augmentin ES-600†: 600 mg/5 mL Chewable, oral:* amoxicillin 200 mg, 400 mg Tablet, oral:‡ 250 mg, 500 mg, 875 mg Augmentin XR§ 1,000 mg
ceftriaxone (Rocephin)	50 mg/kg/d IM once daily for 1 or 3 d	1 g IM once daily for 1 or 3 d	Skin rash, injection site reactions	IM: 250–350 mg/mL with lidocaine
cefdinir (Omnicef)	14 mg/kg/d PO divided into 2 doses per day	300 mg PO twice a day	Skin rash and GI upset but otherwise generally well tolerated	Suspension, oral: 125 mg/5 mL, 250 mg/5 mL Capsule, oral: 300 mg
cefpodoxime (Vantin)	10 mg/kg/d PO once daily	200 mg PO twice a day	Skin rash and GI upset but otherwise generally well tolerated	Suspension, oral: 50 mg/5 mL, 100 mg/5 mL Tablet, oral: 100 mg, 200 mg
cefuroxime (Ceftin)	30 mg/kg/d PO divided into 2 doses per day	250–500 mg PO twice a day	Skin rash and GI upset but otherwise generally well tolerated	Suspension, oral: 125 mg/5 mL, 250 mg/5 mL Tablet, oral: 250 mg, 500 mg
clindamycin (various)	30 mg/kg/d PO divided into 3 doses per day	300–450 mg PO every 6–8 h	Diarrhea, *C. difficile*–associated diarrhea, rash	Suspension, oral: 75 mg/5 mL Capsule, oral: 75 mg, 150 mg, 300 mg

*Standard ratio of clavulanate to amoxicillin of 1:7.
†ES ratio of clavulanate to amoxicillin of 1:14.
‡Standard 125 mg of clavulanate per tablet.
§XR ratio of clavulanate to amoxicillin of 1:16.

escalation to the next step in management and is highly dependent on the initial therapy. If the patient does not improve with high-dose amoxicillin treatment, therapy should be switched to amoxicillin–clavulanate. If a patient fails amoxicillin–clavulanate, an oral cephalosporin (i.e., cefpodoxime, cefuroxime, cefdinir), or 1-dose ceftriaxone intramuscular injection should receive a 3-day course of intravenous ceftriaxone (Leibovitz et al., 2000). Tympanocentesis is an option for patients who have repeatedly failed therapy for bacteriologic diagnosis. The effusion is sent for Gram stain, culture, and antibiotic susceptibility testing to tailor therapy to the causative organism.

Monitoring Patient Response

The standard duration of antibiotic therapy is 10 days for patients younger than 2 years of age or to manage severe AOM. Patients 2 years old or greater should be treated with a 7-day

course of antibiotics. Patients age 6 years and older may benefit from a shorter, 5-day course of therapy (Lieberthal et al., 2013). Symptoms of AOM should improve within 2 to 3 days, and the patient should achieve complete resolution of symptoms after 7 days, although asymptomatic MEE may persist if inspected by pneumatic otoscope. The patient or caregiver must be counseled to continue antibiotic therapy even if symptoms resolve before completion of the entire therapy course to prevent recurrence.

RECURRENT ACUTE OTITIS MEDIA

Recurrent AOM is defined as more than three episodes within 6 months or four episodes within 12 months, with one episode in the preceding 6 months. Recurrence is most commonly due to relapse (infection with the same organism) or reinfection

(infection with a different organism). Management of recurrent AOM remains controversial. Antibiotic prophylaxis is no longer recommended due to risk outweighing the benefit, as mentioned below, and evidence supporting placement of tympanostomy tubes is limited. The American Academy of Otolaryngology: Head and Neck Surgery Foundation published guidelines state tympanostomy should be ordered to children with bilateral OME for 3 months or longer with documented hearing difficulties (Rosenfeld et al., 2013). An additional indication is for children at increased risk of speech, language, or learning problems from OME due to baseline sensory, physical, cognitive, or behavioral factors. Hearing assessment in infants and children requires varying tools depending on age to detect hearing loss (mean response greater than 20 dB), including evoked optoacoustic emissions, auditory brainstem response, visual reinforcement audiometry, play audiometry, or conventional audiometry (Harlor et al., 2009). Myringotomy and insertion of tympanostomy tubes improve AOM symptoms by allowing drainage of the effusion. These tubes maintain a disease-free state typically in the first 6 months after insertion; however, the benefit thereafter is unknown (McDonald et al., 2008). Complications of tube placement include otorrhea, myringosclerosis, perforation, and tissue granulation as seen on otoscopic examination (Vlastarakos et al., 2007).

Prophylaxis and/or Prevention

Use of antibiotic prophylaxis for recurrent AOM is controversial due to lack of supporting evidence. Cost, adverse effects, and contribution to bacterial resistance emergence do not outweigh the small reduction in frequency of AOM with long-term antibiotic prophylaxis. Therefore, antibiotic prophylaxis is no longer recommended for children with recurrent AOM (Leach & Morris, 2006).

The Centers for Disease Control and Prevention's (CDC) recommended schedule for vaccines should be followed to reduce preventable diseases. The vaccines pertinent to the prevention of AOM are the pneumococcal, *H. influenzae* type B, and influenza vaccine. Please refer to the prevention section of this chapter for a detailed discussion on target vaccine groups and current recommendations.

OTITIS EXTERNA

DIAGNOSTIC CRITERIA AND CLINICAL PRESENTATION

OE presents with symptoms of ear canal inflammation such as ear pain, itching, or fullness; signs of ear canal inflammation such as tenderness of tragus and/or pinna; and erythematous ear canal with occasional otorrhea. Hearing is usually unaffected unless pressure and fullness in the ear exist, producing occasional conductive or sensorineural hearing loss. Jaw pain may also be present. Acute OE diagnosis requires rapid onset of signs and symptoms within 48 hours in the past 3 weeks.

Differentiation from other possible causes of otalgia, otorrhea, and inflammation of the ear canal, such as AOM, is important due to overlapping pathologies that require alteration in treatment.

Patient evaluation should include history of symptoms, water exposure, local trauma, past medical history of inflammatory skin disorders or diabetes, and history of ear surgeries or local radiotherapy. Otoscopic examination of the ear canal and TM may require cerumen or debris removal for visualization. If the TM is bulging or erythematous, the patient should be worked up for OM. Examination of pinna and adjacent skin for regional lymphadenitis and cellulitis is included as well. Otomycosis, fungal OE, presents with intense pruritus, aural fullness, clear otorrhea, and fluffy, cotton-like debris in the external ear canal upon examination (Kesser, 2011). Necrotizing OE diagnosis is confirmed with a raised erythrocyte sedimentation rate and abnormal computed tomography or magnetic resonance imaging scan to detect a skull base osteomyelitis (Rosenfeld et al., 2013).

INITIATING DRUG THERAPY

Goals of Drug Therapy

The goals of OE treatment are similar to OM, which are eradicating the causative organisms and decreasing the accompanying pain. This can be accomplished with direct ototopical application of antimicrobial agents and systemic analgesic and/or anti-inflammatory drugs.

Management of OE begins with clearing any obstructing debris or excess cerumen from the canal (i.e., aural toilet) and checking the integrity of the TM to determine if extension beyond the ear canal is present. Topical therapy is the mainstay of OE treatment (i.e., antibiotics, steroids, or combination treatments). Topical antimicrobials are preferred over systemic administration to achieve high concentration at the site of infection while reducing systemic adverse effects to the patient. Selection of the appropriate product must include evaluation of the patient's infection, predisposing factors, adherence, and medication costs (Boyce, 2012).

Pain relief can be achieved with orally administered acetaminophen or NSAIDs given alone or in combination with an opioid for mild to moderate pain (Rosenfeld et al., 2013). Topical anesthetic drops, such as benzocaine otic solution, are not recommended due to potential masking of underlying disease states and lack of FDA approval for OE indication.

Antibiotic Therapy

If edema prevents application of the drops, a compressed cellulose ear wick can be placed into the ear to facilitate drug delivery. The medication should be applied to the wick until inflammation subsides and the wick falls out or is removed as instructed by a clinician (usually within 24 to 48 hours). Ototopical antimicrobials for OE include aminoglycosides, polymyxin B, and quinolones. Ototopical selection is based on several factors including TM condition (e.g., perforation, tympanostomy tubes), risk of adverse effect, adherence issues, cost, patient preference, and physician experience/preference (**Table 18.4**). Systemic antimicrobials are not recommended for uncomplicated, acute OE, but for infections extending beyond the ear canal or when certain factors are present such as uncontrolled diabetes, immunocompromised, history of radiotherapy, or inability to deliver topical antibiotics. Otomycosis requires debridement and topical antifungal therapy, such as a powdered mixture of Chloromycetin, sulfanilamide, Fungizone, and hydrocortisone (Kesser, 2011). Necrotizing OE is managed with surgical debridement and systemic, prolonged antipseudomonal and antistaphylococcal antibiotics.

Fluoroquinolones

The fluoroquinolone antibiotics, that is, ciprofloxacin and ofloxacin, are often used to treat infections associated with OE, due to its ideal antipseudomonal activity. Higher bacteriologic and clinical cure rates have been observed with quinolone-containing otic drops compared to nonquinolone therapy (Mösges et al., 2011). In addition, these agents may be more tolerable compared to neomycin/polymyxin B due to frequent administration, less adverse effects (e.g., stinging), and lower risk of hypersensitivity. This information must be balanced with the high cost of quinolone otic preparations. Ciprofloxacin 0.3%/dexamethasone 0.1% (Ciprodex) and ofloxacin (Floxin Otic) are commercially available fluoroquinolone formulations. (See **Table 18.4** for dosage and adverse effect information.) The addition of a corticosteroid to the antibiotic formulation is controversial. The anti-inflammatory effects potentially include reduced pain, swelling, and itching. Dohar (2003) reported on a controlled study suggesting that the addition of hydrocortisone decreases the duration of pain by about 1 day. However, additional studies have not been conducted to confirm this point. The risk of local immunosuppression and potential hypersensitivity reactions should be studied in light of potential benefits. Of note, the Floxin Otic preparation does not contain a corticosteroid.

Aminoglycoside Antibiotics

The combination product neomycin sulfate/polymyxin B/hydrocortisone acetate (Cortisporin) has historically been used for OE. The combination of the gram-positive coverage of the aminoglycoside neomycin and the antipseudomonal activity of polymyxin has made this combination the gold standard of treatment in the past. The same controversy regarding the addition of a corticosteroid exists with this combination. Concerns associated with the side effect profile, particularly the hypersensitivity reactions related to neomycin (and possibly the preservative), and frequency of dose administration must be weighed against the low cost for the generic product. Furthermore, otomycosis with neomycin has been reported, although the number of reports is low and the data are speculative. Due to concerns of ototoxicity, aminoglycosides should not be used if the TM is not intact since the risk of injury outweighs the benefit and efficacious, nonototoxic antibiotics are available (i.e., quinolones) (Haynes et al., 2007).

Selecting the Most Appropriate Agent

First-Line Therapy

OE with intact or nonintact TM is treated initially with a fluoroquinolone antibiotic. The selection of ciprofloxacin versus ofloxacin depends on the formulary status of the agents as well as the clinician's experience with added corticosteroids (**Table 18.5**).

Second-Line Therapy

Neomycin/polymyxin B combinations are considered second-line agents, primarily due to their side effect profile and precaution against use for nonintact TM OE. The lower cost of these agents, however, warrants consideration, particularly in patients without insurance or other means of paying for the more expensive fluoroquinolones.

TABLE 18.4

Overview of Treatment for Otitis Externa

Generic (Trade) Name and Dosage	Selected Adverse Events	Contraindications	Special Considerations
polymyxin B sulfate, neomycin, and hydrocortisone Children: 3 drops into ear canal three to four times daily for maximum of 10 d Adults: 4 drops into ear canal three to four times daily for maximum of 10 d	Superinfection, contact dermatitis, ototoxicity with prolonged use	Herpes simplex, fungal, tubercular, or viral otic infections Perforated eardrum Prescribe with caution in pregnancy (category C drug) and in breast-feeding patients	Use otic drops for a maximum of 10 d
ofloxacin (Floxin) Children 1–12 y: 5 drops into ear canal bid for 10 d Children >12 y and adults: 10 drops bid for 10 d	Pruritus, site reaction, dizziness, earache, vertigo, taste perversion, paresthesia, rash	Not recommended for patients <1 y, perforated eardrum Prescribe with caution in pregnancy (category C drug) and in breast-feeding patients	Use otic drops for a maximum of 10 d

TABLE 18.5		
Recommended Order of Treatment for Otitis Externa		
Order	**Agents**	**Comments**
First line	Fluoroquinolone drops	Floxin is not recommended for patients <1 y Use all otic drops for a maximum of 10 d
Second line	Combination neomycin/polymyxin B drops	Vosol is not recommended for patients <3 y All drops are contraindicated in cases of perforated eardrum
Third line	Antifungal drops Systemic antipseudomonal or antistaphylococcal agent	Considered if a patient fails to respond to initial topical antibiotic therapy Consider if ear canal obstruction cannot be relieved or if infection extends beyond the ear canal

Third-Line Therapy

Antifungals can be considered if a patient fails to respond to initial topical antibiotic therapy (e.g., clotrimazole, miconazole, bifonazole, ciclopirox olamine, tolnaftate) (Vennewald et al., 2010). Systemic antibiotic therapy with *P. aeruginosa* and *S. aureus* coverage is recommended if ear canal obstruction cannot be relieved or if infection extends beyond the ear canal.

Special Population Considerations

Children with tympanostomy tubes placed within 1 year of an acute OE episode are assumed to have nonintact TM and therefore should not receive an ototoxic antibiotic. Historical concerns of fluoroquinolone use in children are not relevant due to the minimal systemic absorption and small dose administered ototopically.

MONITORING PATIENT RESPONSE

Symptom improvement should occur within 48 to 72 hours after appropriate treatment initiation, but complete symptom resolution may take up to 2 weeks. Reassessment of patients who fail initial therapy may include addressing patient adherence with therapy, re-examination of the ear canal and TM, a culture of the ear canal to identify causes of infection and target therapy, and consideration of underlying dermatologic disorders.

PREVENTION

Prevention is the key and plays a significant role in reducing the overall burden of illness (e.g., office visits, antibiotic expenditures, severity of illness). Vaccination programs have been shown to have a favorable outcome on decreasing the overall incidence of the AOM, namely, those caused by *S. pneumoniae*, influenza virus, and *H. influenzae*.

The introduction of the heptavalent pneumococcal polysaccharide conjugate vaccine (PCV-7, Prevnar-7; serotypes 4, 6B, 9V, 14, 18C, 19F, and 23F) decreased the overall

incidence of invasive pneumococcal disease by 69% in children younger than age 2 from 1998 to 1999 and 2001 (Pichichero & Casey, 2007). Specifically, reductions in OM office visits and severity of illness have been observed since the introduction of the vaccine (Black et al., 2000). The serotypes in the 7-valent vaccine when brought to the market in 2000 represented approximately 70% of the serotypes found in AOM. Unfortunately, after PCV-7 introduction, otopathogenic *S. pneumoniae* serotype 19A had been identified as resistant to all FDA-approved antibiotics for children with AOM (Pichichero & Casey, 2007). A 13-valent pneumococcal conjugate vaccine (PCV-13, Prevnar-13; serotypes 1, 3, 4, 5, 6A, 6B, 7F, 19A, in addition to the 7 serotypes of PCV-7) approved by the U.S. FDA in 2010 contains the 6 serotypes responsible for 63% of invasive pneumococcal disease and has replaced PCV-7 in the childhood vaccination schedule (CDC, 2015).

Pneumococcal vaccination includes two formulations: PCV and polysaccharide (PPSV) for infants younger than age 2 and children older than age 2 with comorbidities, respectively. PPSV contains 23 pneumococcal serotypes indicated for children age 2 and older with chronic disease such as chronic lung disease or congenital heart disease and not indicated in infants younger than age 2 due to poor immunogenicity (Committee on Infectious Disease, 2010).

Administration of the influenza and *H. influenzae* type B (HiB) vaccines are also routinely recommended in children to decrease potential infections caused by them. The HiB vaccine is a polysaccharide, conjugated protein carrier indicated for infants age 6 weeks and older. The influenza vaccine is recommended for all children ages 6 months to 18 years, but the selection of the correct formulation is dependent on the age of the patient. Influenza vaccine is available as a trivalent inactivated IM injection and live attenuated vaccine as an intranasal administration, which is indicated in infants older than age 6 months and children older than age 2 who are not immunocompromised or pregnant or have exacerbative pulmonary diseases, respectively (CDC, 2015).

For up-to-date Advisory Committee on Immunization Practices (ACIP) vaccine administration schedules, check the CDC Web site at www.cdc.gov/vaccines (CDC, 2015).

CASE STUDY*

C.J., age 17, is on his high school swim team. He presents with sudden onset of right ear pain that worsens at night. He says that the pain intensifies when he touches his ear and that he has a feeling of fullness in the ear. On examination, the auditory canal is edematous and erythematous, with yellow crusting. His temperature is 97.8°F, and his TM is pearly gray with landmarks intact.

DIAGNOSIS: OTITIS EXTERNA

1. What drug therapy would you prescribe? Why?
2. What are the parameters for monitoring success of the therapy?

3. Discuss specific patient education based on the prescribed therapy.
4. List one or two adverse reactions for the selected agent that would cause you to change therapy.
5. What would be the choice for second-line therapy?
6. What over-the-counter and/or alternative medications would be appropriate for **C.J.**?
7. What lifestyle changes would you recommend to **C.J.**?
8. Describe one or two drug–drug or drug–food interaction for the selected agent.

* Answers can be found online.

PATIENT EDUCATION

Drug Information

Administration of ototopical products requires patient education and potentially an assistant to administer the drops for them as self-administration may be difficult. Ototopicals should be warmed to body temperature before instillation to avoid dizziness. To warm the otic solution, the patient should hold or roll the bottle in the hand for 1 to 2 minutes. To instill drops, the patient should lie with the affected ear upward, administer enough drops to fill the ear canal (or saturate the ear wick if in place), gently tug the auricle to help expel trapped air and assist drug delivery, and remain in this position for about 5 minutes to help the solution penetrate into the ear canal.

Nutrition/Lifestyle Changes

The use of hypoallergenic ear canal molds when swimming or showering is controversial for the prevention of OE. Drying the ears with a cool hair dryer to aid removal of fluid after swimming may be beneficial. The patient should avoid trying to remove ear wax mechanically with cotton-tipped swabs to prevent trauma. It is important for the patient to avoid water in the ear until the infection clears (usually 5 to 7 days) and for 4 to 6 weeks afterward. To accomplish this, hair can be washed in a sink instead of a shower or tub, and the patient can use a shower cap when bathing.

Complementary and Alternative Medications

"Home remedies" of a 1:1 solution of white vinegar and rubbing alcohol have never been evaluated or substantiated and therefore are not recommended for OE. In addition, ear candles are not efficacious and may be harmful (e.g., hearing loss).

Bibliography

Starred references are cited in the text.

*Black, S. L., Shinefield, H., Fireman, B., et al. (2000). Efficacy, safety and immunogenicity of heptavalent pneumococcal conjugate vaccine in children. Northern California Kaiser Permanente Vaccine Study Center Group. *Pediatric Infectious Disease Journal, 19*(3), 187–195.

*Block, S. L., Schmier, J. K., Notario, G. F., et al. (2006). Efficacy, tolerability, and parent-reported outcomes for cefdinir vs. high-dose amoxicillin/clavulanate oral suspension for acute otitis media in young children. *Current Medical Research and Opinion, 22*(9), 1839–1847.

*Boyce, T. G. (2012). Otitis externa and necrotizing otitis externa. In S. Long (Ed.), *Principles and practices of pediatric infectious diseases* (4th ed.). Edinburgh, UK: Saunders.

*Centers for Disease Control and Prevention. (2011). Estimated burden of acute otitis externa—United States, 2003–2007. *MMWR Morbidity and Mortality Weekly Report, 60*, 605–609.

*Centers for Disease Control and Prevention. (2015). Immunization schedules. Retrieved from http://www.cdc.gov/vaccines/schedules/

*Chao, J. H., Kunkov, S., Reyes, L. B., et al. (2008). Comparison of two approaches to observation therapy for acute otitis media in the emergency department. *Pediatrics, 121*(5), e1352–e1356.

*Committee on Infectious Disease. (2010). Recommendations for the prevention of *Streptococcus pneumoniae* infections in pneumococcal polysaccharide vaccine (PPSV23) infants and children: Use of 13-valent pneumococcal conjugate vaccine. *Pediatrics, 126*, 186–190.

*Dohar, J. E. (2003). Evolution of management approaches for otitis externa. *Pediatric Infectious Disease Journal, 22*(4), 299–308.

*Harlor, A. D., Bower, C., Committee on Practice and Ambulatory Medicine, & the Section on Otolaryngology–Head and Neck Surgery. (2009). Hearing assessment in infants and children: Recommendations beyond neonatal screening. *Pediatrics, 124*, 1252–1263.

*Haynes, D. S., Rutka, J., & Hawke, M. (2007). Ototoxicity of ototopical drops—an update. *Otolaryngologic Clinics of North America, 40*, 669–683.

*Hersh, A. L., Jackson, M. A., Hicks, L. A., et al. (2013). Principles of judicious antibiotic prescribing for bacterial upper respiratory tract infections in pediatrics. *Pediatrics, 132*, 1146–1154.

*Hoberman, A., Marchant, C. D., Kaplan, S., et al. (2002). Treatment of acute otitis media consensus recommendations. *Clinical Pediatrics, 41*, 373–390.

*Kaplan, S. L., Center, K. J., Barson, W. J., et al. (2015). Multicenter surveillance of *Streptococcus pneumoniae* isolates from middle ear and mastoid cultures in the 13-valent pneumococcal conjugate vaccine era. *Clinical Infectious Diseases, 60*(9), 1339–1345.

*Kesser, B. W. (2011). Assessment and management of chronic otitis media. *Current Opinion in Otolaryngology & Head and Neck Surgery, 19*, 341–347.

*Leach, A. J., & Morris, P. S. (2006). Antibiotics for the prevention of acute and chronic suppurative otitis media in children. *Cochrane Database of Systematic Reviews*, (4), CD004401.

*Leibovitz, E., Piglansky, L., Raiz, S., et al. (2000). Bacteriologic and clinical efficacy of one day vs. three day intramuscular ceftriaxone for treatment of nonresponsive acute otitis media in children. *The Pediatric Infectious Diseases Journal, 19*(11), 1040–1045.

*Lieberthal, A. S., Carroll, A. E., Chonmaitree, T., et al. (2013). The diagnosis and management of acute otitis media: Clinical practice guideline. *Pediatrics, 113*, e964–e999.

*McDonald, S., Langton Hewer, C. D., & Nunez, D. A. (2008). Grommets (ventilation tubes) for recurrent acute otitis media in children. *Cochrane Database of Systematic Reviews*, (4), CD004741.

*Mösges, R., Nematian-Samani, M., Hellmich, M., et al. (2011). A meta-analysis of the efficacy of quinolone containing otics in comparison to antibiotic-steroid combination drugs in the local treatment of otitis externa. *Current Medical Research and Opinion, 27*(10), 2053–2060.

*Pelton, S. (2012). Otitis media. In S. Long (Ed.), *Principles and practices of pediatric infectious diseases* (4th ed.). Edinburgh, UK: Saunders.

*Pichichero, M. E. (2005). A review of evidence supporting the AAP recommendation for prescribing cephalosporin antibiotics for penicillin-allergic patients. *Pediatrics, 115*, 1048–1057.

*Pichichero, M. E. (2013). Otitis media. *Pediatric Clinics of North America, 60*, 391–407.

*Pichichero, M. E., & Casey, J. R. (2007). Emergence of a multiresistant serotype 19a pneumococcal strain not included in the 7-valent conjugate vaccine as an otopathogen in children. *Journal of the American Medical Association, 298*(15), 1772–1778.

Prevnar. (2011). *Pneumococcal 13-valent Conjugate Vaccine package insert.* Philadelphia, PA: Wyeth Pharmaceuticals.

*Rosenfeld, R. M., Culpepper, L., Doyle, K. J., et al. (2004). Clinical practice guideline: Otitis media with effusion. *Otolaryngology—Head and Neck Surgery, 130*, s95–s118.

*Rosenfeld, R. M., Schwartz, S. R., Pynnonen, M. A., et al. (2013). Clinical practice guideline: Tympanostomy tubes in children. *Otolaryngology—Head and Neck Surgery, 149*, S1–S35.

*Schaefer, P., & Baugh, R. F. (2012). Acute otitis externa: An update. *American Family Physician, 86*(11), 1055–1061.

Seely, D. R., Quigley, S. M., & Langman, A. W. 1996. Ear candles—efficacy and safety. *Laryngoscope, 106*(10), 1226–1229.

*Soni, A. (2008). Ear infections (otitis media) in children (0–17): Use and expenditures. Statistical Brief No. 228. Agency for Healthcare Research and Quality. Retrieved from http://www.meps.ahrq.gov/mepsweb/data_files/publications/st228/stat228.pdf on June 28, 2015.

*Vennewald, I., Nat, D. R., & Klemm, E. (2010). Otomycosis: Diagnosis and treatment. *Clinics in Dermatology, 28*, 202–211.

*Vlastarakos, P. V., Nikolopoulos, T. P., Korres, S., et al. (2007). Grommets in otitis media with effusion: The most frequent operation in children. But is it associated with significant complications? *European Journal of Pediatrics, 166*(5), 385–391.

Wang, C. Y., Lu, C. Y., Hsieh, Y. C., et al. (2004). Intramuscular ceftriaxone in comparison with oral amoxicillin-clavulanate for the treatment of acute otitis media in infants and children. *Journal of Microbiology, Immunology and Infection, 37*(1), 57–62.

UNIT 4

Pharmacotherapy for Cardiovascular Disorders

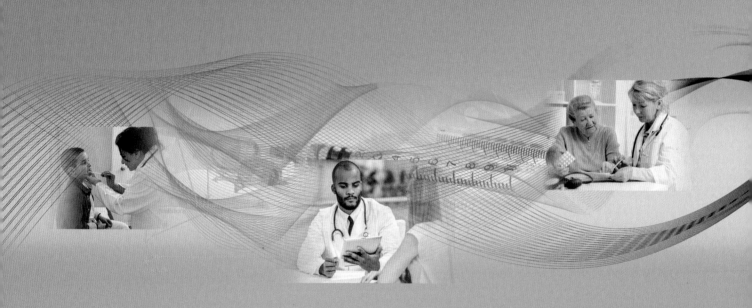

19 Hypertension

Kelly Barranger ■ Diane E. Hadley

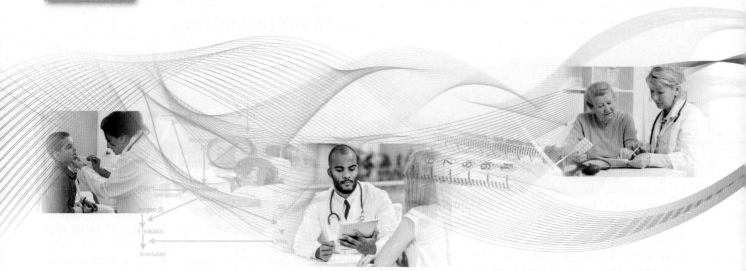

Hypertension or high blood pressure (BP) is one of the common chronic conditions managed by primary care providers and other health practitioners. It increases the risk for cardiovascular disease and chronic kidney disease (CKD). Heart disease is a prevalent cause of death in the United States, thus making management of a patient's BP crucial. Approximately, 70 million Americans or one out of three adults in the United States has hypertension. The total costs associated with hypertension in 2011 in the United States were approximately $46 billion in health care services, medications, and missed days of work (Mozzafarian et al., 2015). Despite these alarming numbers, many people are unaware that they have hypertension because the disease can be asymptomatic; therefore, the disease is appropriately nicknamed "the silent killer."

The prevalence of hypertension continues to grow due to the increasing age of our population, obesity, and high dietary salt intake. According to the Centers for Disease Control and Prevention (CDC), approximately 69% of adults 20 years and older are overweight and 35% of adults age 20 years and older are obese. Obesity, impaired renal function, and diabetes mellitus are all associated with resistant hypertension (Vongpatanasin, 2014).

Hypertension increases with age and affects all ethnic groups. However, blacks suffer disproportionately from hypertension and its effects, leading to high rates of cardiovascular morbidity and mortality. Hypertension in blacks occurs at an earlier age, is more severe, and results in organ damage such as coronary heart disease, stroke, and end-stage renal disease more often than it does in whites.

CAUSES

Hypertension is classified as primary or essential, secondary, or idiopathic when there is no identifiable cause for elevation in BP. Approximately 95% of adults have primary or essential hypertension, and the exact cause of primary hypertension is not known. Environmental factors (excess salt, obesity, and sedentary lifestyle) and genetic factors (inappropriately high activity of the renin–angiotensin–aldosterone system [RAAS] and the sympathetic nervous system) are hypothesized contributing factors and are being studied. An additional cause of hypertension is secondary to aorta artery stiffening secondary to increasing age. This is referred to as isolated or predominant systolic hypertension. It is characterized by high systolic blood pressure (SBP) with normal diastolic blood pressure (DBP) and is found primarily in elderly people.

Secondary hypertension, where the cause of high BP can be identified, accounts for 5% of all hypertensions. The main types of secondary hypertension are CKD (anemia, low GFR, small kidney), renovascular hypertension (abdominal bruit, elevated plasma renin activity, greater than 30% elevation of creatinine with starting BP-lowering agents), hypothyroidism (elevated TSH), hyperparathyroidism (elevated calcium), pheochromocytoma, sleep apnea, and primary aldosteronism (hypokalemia, ratio serum aldosterone/plasma renin activity greater than 25:30).

Furthermore, medications can serve as a factor that may increase BP. Examples include oral contraceptives, nicotine, steroids, appetite suppressants, tricyclic antidepressants, the antidepressant venlafaxine (Effexor), cyclosporine (Sandimmune), nonsteroidal anti-inflammatory drugs (NSAIDs), and some nasal decongestants (which include over-the-counter preparations). Herbal products that affect BP include capsicum, goldenseal, licorice root, ma huang (Ephedra), Scotch broom, witch hazel, and yohimbine.

PATHOPHYSIOLOGY

Role of the Nervous System

The central and autonomic nervous systems play a key dual role in regulating BP. Centrally located presynaptic beta receptors stimulate the release of norepinephrine, while alpha-2 receptors inhibit norepinephrine release. Receptors located in the periphery also regulate BP. These receptors are located on effector cells that are innervated by sympathetic neurons. Stimulation of alpha-1 receptors located on arterioles and venules causes vasoconstriction, while activation of the beta-2 receptors on these vessels produces vasodilation. Beta-1 receptors, which are located in the heart and kidneys, regulate heart rate and contractility, which ultimately impacts cardiac output. Because BP is the product of cardiac output and peripheral resistance, any reduction in cardiac output results in a decrease in BP. Therefore, blockade of beta-1 receptors decreases cardiac output, peripheral resistance, and BP.

Baroreceptors, which are nerve endings located in large arteries such as the aortic arch and carotids, additionally play a significant role in regulating BP. These receptors are sensitive to changes in BP. When BP drops drastically, the baroreceptors send an impulse to the brain stem, which results in vasoconstriction and increased heart rate and contractility. In contrast, elevation in BP increases baroreceptor activity, which results in vasodilation and decreased heart rate and contractility.

Peripheral autoregulatory components also play a role in controlling BP. Normally, rises in BP result in sodium and water elimination by the kidney. In turn, plasma volume, cardiac output, and BP decrease. Dysfunction of this mechanism can raise plasma volume and BP.

Role of the Renal System

RAAS regulates sodium, potassium, and fluid balance in the body. Renin, an enzyme secreted by the juxtaglomerular cells on the afferent arterioles of the kidney, is released in response to changes in BP caused by reduced renal perfusion, decreased intravascular volume, or increased circulation of catecholamines. Renin catalyses the conversion of angiotensinogen to angiotensin I. Angiotensin I is converted to the potent vasoconstrictor angiotensin II by angiotensin-converting enzyme (ACE). Angiotensin II causes direct vasoconstriction and stimulation of the sympathetic nervous system. Angiotensin II also stimulates release of aldosterone from the adrenal gland, which results in the retention of sodium and water. In normal physiology, angiotensin II directly inhibits further release of renin through a negative feedback system. If the negative feedback system fails, BP rises. Hyperinsulinemia is another

contributing factor to hypertension by causing sodium retention and stimulating the sympathetic nervous system.

DIAGNOSTIC CRITERIA

Hypertension is defined as an elevation in SBP and/or DBP. As suggested by the 2014 Eighth Report of the Joint National Committee (JNC 8) guidelines, hypertension is defined as a BP of 150/90 mm Hg or higher in adults 60 years and older. The guidelines also highlights that a BP of 140/90 or higher in adults younger than 60 is defined as hypertension. Two studies within the primary literature, SHEP and Syst-EUR, used placebo-controlled approaches to evaluate people over the age of 60 with systolic hypertension and the HYVET study evaluated patients over the age of 80. The JNC 8 panel could not recommend a lower threshold value for those over 60 since no evidence existed that less than 140 mm Hg was better than less than 150 mm Hg for protecting patients from harm. Additionally, the ASH (American Society of Hypertension) and ISH (International Society of Hypertension) recommend an SBP of less than 150 (as opposed to less than 140 mm Hg) be used only in those over 80 years of age.

The biggest difference between JNC 7 and JNC 8 were the defined BP treatment goals. Additionally, another difference between JNC 7 and JNC 8 is that prehypertension was not addressed in JNC 8. This was well defined in JNC 7 as SBP ranging from 120 to 139 mm Hg and DBP ranging from 80 to 89 mm Hg and therefore remains valid. Another distinct difference was the use of very specific compelling indications within JNC 7 while JNC 8 used broader compelling indications. Finally, JNC 8 guidelines are more evidence based utilizing randomized controlled trials and have clear target ranges.

Hypertension is not diagnosed on an initial reading; rather, it is confirmed after three readings at least 1 week apart. BP measurements should be obtained after the patient has had time to relax for at least 5 minutes. Patients should be seated in a chair, back supported, rather than on an examination table, with feet on the floor, uncrossed, and arm supported at heart level. Patients should avoid smoking cigarettes 30 minutes before the reading, should not exercise heavily immediately before the reading, should not drink caffeine during the hour preceding the reading, and should avoid adrenergic stimulants, such as phenylephrine. For an accurate reading, the appropriate-size sphygmomanometer cuff should be used. The cuff should encompass 80% of the arm, and the width of the cuff should be at least 40% of the length of the upper arm (Screening for high blood pressure, 2007). At the initial evaluation, BP should be measured in both arms. If the readings are different, the arm with the higher reading should be used for measurements thereafter. It is preferable to take two readings, 1 to 2 minutes apart and use the average of these measurements. In older people, it is useful to obtain standing BP, after 1 minute and again after 3 minutes, to check for postural effects.

The diagnosis of hypertension should be confirmed at an additional patient visit, usually 1 to 4 weeks after the first measurement. On both occasions, the SBP and DBP should be higher than recommendations listed above per age. The U.S. Preventive Services Task Force (USPSTF) recommends BP monitoring in adult patients over the age of eighteen. If the BP is very high (SBP greater than 180), initiate the appropriate triage and treatment should occur. If available resources are not adequate to permit a convenient second visit, the initial diagnosis can be made and treatment can be started.

Ambulatory BP monitoring (ABPM) is recommended for patients with suspected variable BP. Contributing factors can include "white coat hypertension," episodic hypertension, hypertension resistant to increasing medication regimens, hypotensive symptoms while taking antihypertensive medications, and autonomic dysfunction. Patients with "white coat hypertension" have a persistently elevated BP in the doctor's office but a persistently normal BP at other times. ABPM readings correlate better with target organ damage than clinical measurements. ABPM also identifies patients in whom BP does not drop significantly during sleep. More aggressive treatment may be necessary for these patients, who are known to be at higher cardiovascular risk. An elevated systolic BP is a more potent cardiovascular risk factor than an elevated diastolic BP.

Physical Examination

A thorough examination should be performed including a personal history, first-degree family history of cardiovascular disease, poor dietary habits, and a history of prescription medications, smoking/tobacco product use, daily caffeine intake (if applicable), ETOH consumption, over-the-counter medications, and herbal products. For patients with documented hypertension, lifestyle should be evaluated and other cardiovascular risk factors or concomitant disorders should be identified to determine the extent of target organ damage and to assess the patient's overall cardiovascular risk status. Most prevalent target damage concern is concentrated to the cardio, cerebral, and renal tissue.

Physical examination includes two or more measured seated BP readings with verification in the contralateral arm; weight and height; body mass index (BMI) (calculated as weight in kilograms divided by the square of height in meters); waist circumference; muscle strength; funduscopy exam; auscultation for carotid, abdominal, and femoral bruits; palpation of the thyroid gland; thorough examination of the heart and lungs; examination of the abdomen for enlarged kidneys, enlarged liver, masses, and abnormal aortic pulsation; palpation of the lower extremities for edema and pulses; and neurologic assessment for sign of previous stroke.

Diagnostic Tests

The following laboratory tests should be routinely performed: electrocardiogram, blood glucose, hemoglobin, hematocrit, complete urinalysis, and complete chemistry panel especially serum potassium, creatinine, estimated glomerular filtration rate, liver function tests, calcium and magnesium, glycosylated hemoglobin (hemoglobin A1c), and fasting lipid panel

(9- to 12-hour fast), which includes total cholesterol, low-density lipoprotein (LDL) cholesterol, high-density lipoprotein (HDL) cholesterol, and triglycerides. Further testing should be performed based on clinical findings.

INITIATING THERAPY
Goals of Drug Therapy

Treatment guidelines are cumbersome due to the different classifications of hypertensive patients with or without comorbidities of diabetes and/or CKD and also elderly versus nonelderly patients. Per JNC 8 guidelines, treatment should be initiated when BP is 140/90 or higher in adults younger than 60 and treated to a goal of less than 140/90 mm Hg. Similarly, the National Institute for Health and Care Excellence (NICE) 2013 guidelines support the same BP goal; however, they recommend this for patients 80 and younger. In adult patients with hypertension and diabetes, pharmacologic treatment should be initiated when BP is 140/90 mm Hg or higher, regardless of age, per the JNC 8 guidelines and the American Diabetes Association (ADA) 2015 Standards of Medical Care in Diabetes guidelines. The JNC 8 goal for diabetic patients, regardless of race, is less than 140/90 mm Hg. The ADA guidelines state as a caveat, however, that younger patients can be considered for a more aggressive BP target of ≤130/80 mm Hg if this can be achieved without side effects. The American College of Cardiology (ACC), American Heart Association (AHA), and the CDC also recommend a BP goal of less than 140/90 mm Hg for diabetic patients (Go et al., 2014).

Furthermore, the National Kidney Foundation (KDOQI) 2012 commentary on the 2012 KDIGO clinical practice guidelines for nondiabetic patients with hypertension and CKD with normal to mild albuminuria states the BP goal is ≤140/90 mm Hg. However, for severe albuminuria patients, the BP goal is ≤130/80 mm Hg. Thus, BP treatment per the KDOQI guidelines would be initiated at the respective targets listed above (Taler et al., 2013). The current 2014 JNC 8 guidelines recommend treatment in adult CKD patients with BP of 140/90 mm Hg or higher and their goal is a BP less than 140/90 mm Hg. Lastly, for elderly patients, JNC 8 recommends treatment for BP of 150/90 mm Hg or higher in adults 60 years and older to aim at a BP goal of less than 150/90 mm Hg. In contrast, the NICE guidelines from 2013 state that for patients above the age of 80 years old, their BP goal is less than 150/90 mm Hg.

The goal of antihypertensive therapy is to manage hypertension and reduce cardiovascular disease (including lipid disorders, glucose intolerance or diabetes, obesity, and smoking) and renal disease. The treatment goal of SBP is less than 140 mm Hg and DBP less than 90 mm Hg with special note of higher goals for elderly patients as listed above. In the past, guidelines have recommended treatment values of less than 130/80 mm Hg for patient with diabetes, CKD, and coronary artery disease. However, evidence to support this lower target is lacking and recent guidelines, such as JNC 8, have increased the BP target goal. For instance, the ACCORD trial, BP trial arm, demonstrated that aggressive reduction of BP target (less than 120/80 mm Hg) in type 2 DM patients did not reduce combined cardiovascular and renal outcomes compared with usual care (target BP less than 140/90 mm Hg) (Cushman et al., 2010). Among secondary outcomes, strokes were reduced by the lower BP goals but at the expense of twice as many serious side effects. Several meta-analyses have demonstrated that lowering BP to below 130 mm Hg systolic does not reduce mortality rates or most cardiovascular outcomes (Mancia et al., 2013). It is important to inform patients that the treatment of hypertension is usually expected to be a lifelong commitment

and can be dangerous for them to terminate treatment without first consulting their provider.

Figure 19.1 summarizes widely used guidelines for hypertension treatment.

Nonpharmacological Antihypertensive Treatment

All patients diagnosed with hypertension should be counseled about the benefits and a way to implement a combination of dietary and lifestyle modifications for BP reduction. Patients are encouraged to maintain appropriate body weight (BMI

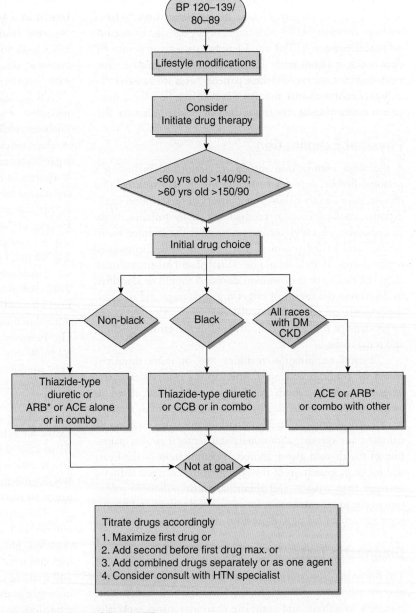

FIGURE 19.1 Modified JNC VIII Treatment for hypertension. (CKD, chronic kidney disease.) (Adapted from James, P., Oparil, S., Carter, B., et al. (2014). 2014 Evidence-based guideline for the management of high blood pressure in adults. Report from the panel members appointed to the Eighth Joint National Committee (JNC 8). *Journal of the American Medical Association, 311,* 507–520; Pharmacist's Letter. (2014). Treatment of hypertension: JNC 8 and more. *Pharmacist's Letter/Prescriber's Letter,* Feb. 2014, Detail-Document #300201.)

of 19.5 to 24.9) and adopt the Dietary Approaches to Stop Hypertension (DASH) diet, USDA Food Pattern diet, or the AHA diet. These diets focus on a high quantity of fruits, vegetables, and low-fat dairy products. They specifically focus on reduction of saturated and total fat. Other recommended lifestyle modifications include restriction of dietary sodium to less than 2.4 g daily, encouragement of physical activity (at least 120 minutes/week of aerobic activity), and reduction in alcohol consumption (Eckel et al., 2014). Patients classified as prehypertensive are ideal candidate for aggressive dietary and lifestyle changes to lower BP and prevent onset of overt hypertension. All patients diagnosed with hypertension should be utilizing lifestyle modifications as a backbone to treatment.

Overview of Pharmacological Antihypertensive Agents

Diuretics

There are five classes of diuretics: carbonic anhydrase inhibitors (which are not used for hypertension because of their weak antihypertensive effects), thiazides, thiazide-like diuretics, loop diuretics, and potassium-sparing diuretics. Diuretics decrease BP by causing diuresis, which results in decreased plasma volume, stroke volume, and cardiac output (see **Table 19.1**). During chronic therapy, their major hemodynamic effect is reduction of peripheral vascular resistance. As a result of drug-induced diuresis, adverse effects of hypokalemia and hypomagnesemia may lead to cardiac arrhythmias. Patients at greatest risk are those receiving digitalis therapy, those with LVH, and those with ischemic heart disease.

Thiazide Diuretics

Mechanism of Action

Thiazide diuretics work by increasing the urinary excretion of sodium and chloride in equal amounts (see **Table 19.1**). They inhibit the reabsorption of sodium and chloride in the thick ascending limb of the loop of Henle and the early distal tubules. The antihypertensive action requires several days to produce effects. The duration of action of the thiazides requires a single daily dose to control BP. Thiazide diuretics cause an increase potassium and bicarbonate excretion and decrease calcium excretion. Additionally, they cause uric acid retention; therefore, caution should be used in patients with a history of gout. Diuretic-induced hyperuricemia may produce gouty arthritis or uric acid stones.

Contraindications

Thiazide diuretics are not recommended in patients with a creatinine clearance of less than 30 mL/min and are contraindicated in those who have renal decompensation or are hypersensitive to thiazides or sulfonamides.

Adverse Events

Side effects include hypokalemia, hypomagnesemia, hypercalcemia, hyperuricemia, and hyperglycemia. As a result of drug-induced diuresis, hypokalemia occurs in 15% to 20% of patients taking low-dose thiazide diuretics; therefore, potassium supplements can be utilized by some patients. Combination therapy with thiazide and potassium-sparing diuretics (e.g., hydrochlorothiazide [Microzide] and triamterene [Dyrenium]) may be prudent when potassium levels are less than 4.0 mEq/L and the patient is taking a thiazide diuretic or when a low potassium level may potentiate drug toxicity, as in patients concurrently taking digoxin (Lanoxin). Other side effects include tinnitus, paresthesia, abdominal cramps, nausea, vomiting, diarrhea, muscle cramps, weakness, and sexual dysfunction.

Loop Diuretics

Mechanism of Action

Loop diuretics are indicated in the presence of edema associated with congestive heart failure, hepatic cirrhosis, and renal disease (see **Table 19.1**). This class of drug is useful when greater diuresis is desired compared to thiazide diuretics. In general, loop diuretics should be reserved for hypertensive patients with chronic renal insufficiency and/or need more severe diuresis.

Furosemide and ethacrynic acid inhibit the reabsorption of sodium and chloride, not only in proximal and distal tubules but also in the loop of Henle. In contrast, bumetanide is more chloruretic than natriuretic and may have an additional action in the proximal tubule.

Contraindications

Loop diuretics are contraindicated in patients who are anuric, in patients hypersensitive to these compounds or to sulfonylureas, and in patients with hepatic coma or in states of severe electrolyte depletion. Ethacrynic acid is contraindicated in infants.

Adverse Events

Loop diuretics may cause the same side effects as thiazides, although the effects on serum lipids and glucose are not as significant, and hypocalcemia may occur instead (see **Table 19.1**). The metabolic abnormalities, such as hyperlipidemia and hyperglycemia, usually occur with high doses of diuretics and can be avoided by using low doses of the drug. Loop diuretics may lead to electrolyte and volume depletion more readily than thiazides; they have a short duration of action, but the thiazide diuretics are more effective than loop diuretics in reducing BP in patients with normal renal function. Therefore, loop diuretics should be reserved for hypertensive patients with renal dysfunction (serum creatinine of more than 2.5).

Potassium-Sparing Diuretics

In the kidney, potassium is filtered at the glomerulus and then absorbed parallel to sodium throughout the proximal tubule and thick ascending limb of the loop of Henle, so that only minor amounts reach the distal convoluted tubule. As a result, potassium appearing in urine is secreted at the distal tubule and collecting duct. The potassium-sparing diuretics interfere with sodium reabsorption at the distal tubule, thus decreasing potassium secretion (see **Table 19.1**). This drug can be used

TABLE 19.1

Overview of Selected Antihypertensive Agents

Generic (Trade) Name and Dosage	Selected Adverse Events	Contraindications	Special Considerations
Selected Diuretics			
THIAZIDE AND THIAZIDE-LIKE			
chlorthalidone 12.5–100 mg qd	Hyperuricemia, hypokalemia, hypomagnesemia, hyperglycemia, hyponatremia, hypercalcemia, hypercholesterolemia, hypertriglyceridemia, rashes, and other allergic reactions	High doses are relatively contraindicated in patients with hyperlipidemia, gout, and diabetes.	Preferred in patients with creatinine clearance >30 mL/min
hydrochlorothiazide (Microzide) 12.5–25 mg qd	Same as chlorthalidone	Same as chlorthalidone	Same as chlorthalidone
indapamide (Lozol) 1.25–5 mg qd	Same as chlorthalidone	Same as chlorthalidone	Same as chlorthalidone
metolazone (Zaroxolyn) 2.5–5 mg qd	Less or no hypercholesterolemia		
LOOP DIURETICS			
bumetanide (Bumex) 0.5–5 mg bid–tid	Dehydration, circulatory collapse, hypokalemia, hyponatremia, hypomagnesemia, hyperglycemia, metabolic alkalosis, and hyperuricemia (short duration of action, no hypercalcemia)	High doses are relatively contraindicated in patients with hyperlipidemia, gout, and diabetes.	Effective in patients with creatinine clearance <30 mL/min
ethacrynic acid (Edecrin) 25–100 mg bid–tid	Same as bumetanide (only nonsulfonamide diuretic, ototoxicity)	Same as bumetanide	Same as bumetanide
furosemide (Lasix) 20–320 mg qd	Same as bumetanide	Same as bumetanide	Same as bumetanide
torsemide (Demadex) 5–20 mg qd	Short duration of action and no hypercalcemia	Same as bumetanide	Same as bumetanide
POTASSIUM-SPARING DIURETICS			
amiloride (Midamor) 5–10 mg qd–bid	Hyperkalemia, GI disturbances, and rash	High doses are relatively contraindicated in patients with hyperlipidemia, gout, and diabetes.	Effective in patients with creatinine clearance <30 mL/min
spironolactone (Aldactone) 12.5–100 mg qd–bid**	Hyperkalemia, GI disturbances, rash, gynecomastia, hirsutism, and menstrual irregularities	Same as amiloride	Ideal in patients with heart failure; in GFR < 30, use is not recommended.
eplerenone (Inspra) 50 mg qd to 50 mg bid**	Hyperkalemia, GI disturbances, rash, gynecomastia, hirsutism, and menstrual irregularities	Same as amiloride	Not recommended in CrCl < 30 mL/min
triamterene (Dyrenium) 50–150 mg qd–bid	Hyperkalemia, GI disturbances, and nephrolithiasis	Same as amiloride	Effective in patients with creatinine clearance <30 mL/min

** Also known as an aldosterone receptor antagonist

Generic (Trade) Name and Dosage	Selected Adverse Events	Contraindications	Special Considerations
Beta-Adrenergic Blocking Agents			
SELECTED BETA-BLOCKERS			
atenolol (Tenormin) 25–100 mg qd	Fatigue, depression, bradycardia, decreased exercise tolerance, congestive heart failure, aggravates peripheral arterial insufficiency, bronchospasm, masks signs and symptoms of hypoglycemia, Raynaud phenomenon, insomnia, vivid dreams or hallucinations, acute mental disorder, and impotence; sudden withdrawal can lead to exacerbation of angina and MI.	Contraindicated in first trimester of pregnancy and heart failure (except carvedilol, bisoprolol, and metoprolol succinate); relatively use in caution with patients with asthma (prefer low-dose cardioselective agents).	Abrupt cessation should be avoided; taper the dose of beta-blocker over a 2-wk period. Advantageous in patients with angina, tachycardia, and acute MI; hypertensive patients with left ventricular hypertrophy

TABLE 19.1

Overview of Selected Antihypertensive Agents (*Continued*)

Generic (Trade) Name and Dosage	Selected Adverse Events	Contraindications	Special Considerations
bisoprolol (Zebeta) 2.5–10 mg qd	Same as atenolol	Same as atenolol	Same as atenolol
metoprolol tartrate (Lopressor) 50–100 qd–bid	Same as atenolol	Same as atenolol	Same as atenolol
nadolol (Corgard) 40–120 mg qd	Same as atenolol	Same as atenolol	Same as atenolol
propranolol (Inderal, Inderal LA) 40–160 mg bid and 60–180 mg bid	Same as atenolol	Same as atenolol	Same as atenolol
metoprolol succinate (Toprol-XL) 50–100 mg qd–bid	Same as atenolol	Same as atenolol	Same as atenolol; one of the agents recommended for heart failure patients
pindolol (Visken) 10–40 mg bid	Same as atenolol, but with less resting bradycardia and lipid changes	Same as atenolol	Same as atenolol
acebutolol (Sectral) 200–600 mg bid	Same as atenolol, but with less resting bradycardia and lipid changes; positive antinuclear antibody test and occasional drug-induced lupus	Same as atenolol	Same as atenolol
ALPHA- AND BETA-BLOCKERS			
carvedilol (Coreg) 12.5–50 mg bid	Similar to atenolol but more postural hypotension and bronchospasm	Same as atenolol	Same as atenolol; one of the agents recommended for heart failure patients
labetalol (Trandate) 200–800 mg bid	Hepatotoxicity	Same as atenolol	Same as atenolol; does not affect serum lipids
Angiotensin-Converting Enzyme (ACE) Inhibitors			
SELECTED ANGIOTENSIN-CONVERTING ENZYME (ACE) INHIBITORS			
benazepril (Lotensin) 10–40 mg qd–bid	Common: cough; hypotension, particularly with a diuretic or volume depletion; hyperkalemia; rash; loss of taste; leukopenia; angioedema; neutropenia; and agranulocytosis in <1% of patients	Contraindicated in pregnancy; avoid in patients with bilateral renal artery stenosis or unilateral stenosis.	First line in hypertensive diabetic patients with proteinuria; congestive heart failure patients with systolic dysfunction
captopril (Capoten) 25–100 mg bid–tid	Same as benazepril; rash in 10% of patients; loss of taste	Same as benazepril	Same as benazepril
enalapril maleate (Vasotec) 2.5–40 mg qd–bid	Same as benazepril	Same as benazepril	Same as benazepril
fosinopril (Monopril) 10–40 mg qd	Same as benazepril	Same as benazepril	Same as benazepril
lisinopril (Prinivil, Zestril) 10–40 mg qd	Same as benazepril	Same as benazepril	Same as benazepril
moexipril (Univasc) 7.5–30 mg qd	Same as benazepril	Same as benazepril	Same as benazepril
quinapril (Accupril) 10–80 mg qd	Same as benazepril	Same as benazepril	Same as benazepril
ramipril (Altace) 2.5–20 mg qd	Same as benazepril	Same as benazepril	Same as benazepril
trandolapril (Mavik) 1–4 mg qd	Same as benazepril	Same as benazepril	Same as benazepril

(Continued)

TABLE 19.1

Overview of Selected Antihypertensive Agents (*Continued*)

Generic (Trade) Name and Dosage	Selected Adverse Events	Contraindications	Special Considerations
Angiotensin II Receptor Blockers **Selected agents are listed.*			
losartan (Cozaar) 25–100 mg qd–bid	Similar to ACE inhibitors but causes cough rarely; angioedema (very rare) and hyperkalemia		
valsartan (Diovan) 80–320 mg qd			
candesartan cilexetil (Atacand) 8–32 mg qd			
irbesartan (Avapro) 150–300 mg qd			
telmisartan (Micardis) 20–80 mg qd			
eprosartan (Teveten) 400–800 mg qd–bid			
olmesartan (Benicar) 20–40 mg qd			
Calcium Channel Blocking Agents **Selected agents are listed.* NONDIHYDROPYRIDINES			
diltiazem HC1 (Cardizem SR, Cardizem CD, Dilacor XR, Tiazac) 180–420 mg qd and (Diltia XR) 120–480 mg qd	Dizziness, headache, edema, and constipation (especially verapamil); lupus-like rash with diltiazem; conduction defects, worsening of systolic dysfunction, and gingival hyperplasia (nausea, headache)	Avoid in patients with AV node dysfunction (second- or third-degree heart block) or left ventricular (systolic) dysfunction.	Swallow whole; do not chew, divide, or crush.
verapamil HC1 (Isoptin SR, Calan SR, Verelan) 120–480 mg qd DIHYDROPYRIDINES	Constipation	Same as diltiazem	Swallow whole; do not chew, divide, or crush.
amlodipine (Norvasc) 2.5–10 mg qd	Dizziness, headache, rash, peripheral edema, flushing, headache, and gingival hypertrophy		Swallow whole; do not chew, divide, or crush. Elderly patients with isolated systolic hypertension
felodipine (Plendil) 2.5–20 mg qd	Same as amlodipine		Swallow whole; do not chew, divide, or crush.
isradipine (DynaCirc) 2.5–10 mg bid and (DynaCirc CR) 5–10 mg bid	Same as amlodipine		Swallow whole; do not chew, divide, or crush.
nicardipine (Cardene SR) 60–120 mg bid	Same as amlodipine		Swallow whole; do not chew, divide, or crush.
nifedipine (Procardia XL) 30–60 mg qd	Same as amlodipine		Swallow whole; do not chew, divide, or crush. Do not use sublingually.
nisoldipine (Sular) 10–40 mg qd	Same as amlodipine		Swallow whole; do not chew, divide, or crush.
Alpha-Blockers			
doxazosin (Cardura) 1–16 mg qd	First-dose phenomenon, postural hypotension, lassitude, vivid dreams, depression, headache, palpitations, fluid retention, weakness, priapism, and drowsiness		Administer initially at bedtime; start with low dose and titrate slowly. Ideal for hypertensive patients with benign prostatic hypertrophy

TABLE 19.1

Overview of Selected Antihypertensive Agents (*Continued*)

Generic (Trade) Name and Dosage	Selected Adverse Events	Contraindications	Special Considerations
prazosin (Minipress) 2–20 mg bid–tid	Same as doxazosin		Same as doxazosin
terazosin (Hytrin) 1–20 mg qd–bid	Same as doxazosin		Same as doxazosin
Central Agonists			
clonidine (Catapres) 0.1–0.8 mg bid–tid	Sedation, dry mouth, bradycardia, withdrawal hypertension, bradycardia, and heart block	Avoid prescribing for noncompliant patients.	Do not stop therapy abruptly without consulting health-care provider first.
transdermal (Catapres TTS) one patch weekly (0.1–0.3 mg/d)			
guanabenz (Wytensin) 4–64 mg bid	Similar to clonidine	Similar to clonidine	Tolerance of alcohol may decrease.
guanfacine (Tenex) 0.5–2.0 mg qd	Similar to clonidine	Similar to clonidine	Take at bedtime.
methyldopa (Aldomet) 250–1000 mg bid	Drowsiness, sedation, fatigue, depression, dry mouth, orthostatic hypotension, bradycardia, heart block, and autoimmune disorders, including colitis; hepatitis and hemolytic anemia <1% of patients		Urine may darken after voiding when exposed to air.
Direct Vasodilators			
hydralazine (Apresoline) 25–100 mg bid	Tachycardia, aggravation of angina, headache, dizziness, fluid retention, lupus-like syndrome, dermatitis, drug fever, hepatitis, and peripheral neuropathy		Beneficial use in black patients with heart failure
minoxidil (Loniten) 2.5–80 mg qd–bid	Tachycardia, aggravation of angina, dizziness, fluid retention, and hypertrichosis	Avoid in patients taking nitrates.	Restrict to patients with refractory hypertension.
Adrenergic Antagonists			
guanadrel (Hylorel) 10–75 mg bid	Postural hypotension, exercise hypotension, diarrhea, weight gain, syncope, and retrograde ejaculation		Restrict to patients with refractory hypertension.
guanethidine (Ismelin) 10–50 mg qd	Similar to guanadrel, but greater incidence of diarrhea	Relatively contraindicated in depression	Maximal effect not seen for 2–4 wk. Avoid doses above 0.25 mg daily in patients with depression.
reserpine (Serpasil) 0.5–0.25–0.1 mg qd	Nasal stuffiness, drowsiness, GI disturbances, bradycardia, and nightmares with high doses		

as a possible agent for HTN; however, its true benefit is indicated within heart failure. Secondary to the Randomized Spironolactone Evaluation Study (RALES), in 1999, showed the benefits of low-dose spironolactone (Aldactone) to improve morbidity and mortality rates in patients with severe heart failure (Pitt et al., 1999). Potassium-sparing diuretics have the potential for causing hyperkalemia and hyponatremia, especially in patients with renal insufficiency or diabetes and in patients receiving concurrent treatment with an ACE inhibitor (ACEI), NSAIDs, or potassium supplements.

Contraindications

Contraindications are the same as for the diuretic class. Additionally, aldosterone antagonists and potassium-sparing diuretics can cause hyperkalemia and hyponatremia and should be avoided in patients with serum potassium levels of more than 5 mEq/L.

Adverse Events

Side effects include gynecomastia, hirsutism, and menstrual irregularities.

Beta-Adrenergic Blockers

Mechanism of Action

Beta-1 receptors, located predominantly in the heart and kidney, regulate heart rate, renin release, and cardiac contractility (see **Table 19.1**). Beta-2 receptors, located in the lungs, liver, pancreas, and arteriolar smooth muscle, regulate bronchodilation and vasodilation. Beta-blockers reduce BP by blocking central and peripheral beta receptors, which results in decreased cardiac output and sympathetic outflow.

Despite several pharmacologic differences in the available beta-blockers, they are all effective in treating hypertension. Beta-blockers that mostly bind to beta-1 receptors are referred to as *cardioselective* because they do not significantly block beta-2 receptors. These agents include metoprolol tartrate (Lopressor), metoprolol succinate (Toprol-XL), atenolol (Tenormin), nebivolol (Bystolic), and bisoprolol (Zebeta) and may be safer than nonselective beta-blockers for patients with asthma, chronic obstructive pulmonary disease, and peripheral vascular disease. At higher doses, however, selective beta-blockers lose cardioselectivity and may aggravate a pre-existing condition.

Some beta-blockers possess intrinsic sympathomimetic activity (ISA); these agents are partial beta-receptor agonists that reduce heart rate and contractility during excessive sympathetic outflow. In resting states, heart rate and contractility are maintained. Typical medications include pindolol (Visken) and acebutolol (Sectral).

Studies suggest that beta-blockers may decrease sympathetic activity involved with the progression of heart failure (see Chapter 22, Heart Failure). For example, carvedilol (Coreg) and metoprolol succinate (Toprol-XL) decreased mortality rates in patients with heart failure and decreased ventricular remodeling (which results in LVH). Beta-blockers should be used only in patients with stable congestive heart failure and be temporarily discontinued if the patient has an acute decompensation. Practitioners should refer any patient with heart failure to a cardiologist for evaluation of therapy.

Patients should be cautioned not to discontinue therapy abruptly. The dose of beta-blockers should be tapered gradually over 14 days to prevent withdrawal symptoms, which include unstable angina, myocardial infarction (MI), or even death in patients with underlying cardiovascular disease. Patients without coronary artery disease may experience sinus tachycardia, palpations, increased sweating, and fatigue.

Contraindications

Beta-blockers should be avoided in patients who have sinus bradycardia, asthma (if needed, low-dose cardioselective beta-blockers are preferred), chronic obstructive pulmonary disease, second- or third-degree heart block, or overt cardiac failure. Non-ISA beta-blockers are the preferred agents for treating hypertension in patients with coexisting coronary artery disease and especially in patients after MI. Beta-blockers should be used cautiously, but not avoided, in patients with resting ischemia or severe claudication secondary to peripheral vascular disease, reactive airway disease, systolic congestive heart failure, diabetes mellitus, or depression.

Adverse Events

The most common side effects of beta-blockers are fatigue, drowsiness, dizziness, bronchospasm, nausea, and vomiting. Serious side effects include bradycardia, atrioventricular (AV) conduction abnormalities, and the development of congestive heart failure. In diabetic patients beta-blockers can mask all of the symptoms of hypoglycemia (low blood sugar) with the exception of sweating.

ACE Inhibitors

Mechanism of Action

ACEIs such as captopril (Capoten), enalapril (Vasotec), and lisinopril (Zestril, Prinivil) exert an antihypertensive effect by the inhibiting ACE enzyme, which converts angiotensin I to angiotensin II, which is a potent vasoconstrictor (see **Table 19.1**). ACEIs also inhibit the degradation of bradykinin and increase the synthesis of vasodilating prostaglandins. ACEIs decrease morbidity and mortality rates in patients with congestive heart failure, post-MI, and systolic dysfunction.

Contraindications

ACEIs should be avoided in patients with bilateral renal artery stenosis or unilateral stenosis because of the risk of acute renal failure. They are not recommended to be used in combination with an angiotensin II receptor blocker (ARB) or a renin inhibitor due to all of these agents working on the RAAS system and increasing the incidence of side effects. They are also contraindicated in patients who have experienced angioedema and during pregnancy because of their teratogenic effects.

Adverse Events

The most common side effects associated with ACEIs include chronic dry cough, rashes (most common with captopril [Capoten]), and dizziness. Hyperkalemia can occur but is at a higher risk in patients with renal disease or diabetes. Angioedema is a rare but dangerous side effect that occurs most frequently in blacks; it is reversible on discontinuation of the agent. Laryngeal edema, another rare adverse effect, is life-threatening and requires immediate medical attention.

Angiotensin II Receptor Blockers

Mechanism of Action

ARBs block the vasoconstriction and aldosterone-secreting effects of angiotensin II by selectively blocking the binding of angiotensin II to the angiotensin II receptor found in many tissues (see **Table 19.1**). They are indicated for patients with hypertension, nephropathy in type 2 diabetes, and heart failure and those who cannot tolerate the side effects associated with ACEIs.

The results of the Losartan Intervention For Endpoint reduction in hypertension study (LIFE), from 2002, suggest that losartan is more effective than atenolol in reducing cardiovascular morbidity and mortality in diabetic patients with hypertension and left ventricular hypertrophy (Dahlöf et al., 2002). Available ARBs are losartan (Cozaar), valsartan (Diovan), candesartan (Atacand), telmisartan (Micardis), eprosartan (Teveten), olmesartan (Benicar), and irbesartan (Avapro). The incidence of cough and hyperkalemia associated with this class of drugs is lower than with ACEIs but still may occur.

Contraindications

Caution should be used in patients with renal and hepatic function impairment. Angioedema can also be seen with ARB therapy, but with much less frequency than with ACEIs. There should be some justification (heart failure or proteinuric nephropathy) for the use of ARBs in patients having experienced ACEI–related angioedema. Like ACEIs, ARBs are contraindicated in pregnancy. Combination with ACEI and/or renin inhibitors is not recommended.

Adverse Events

Adverse reactions include dizziness, upper respiratory tract infections, cough, viral infection, fatigue, diarrhea, pain, sinusitis, pharyngitis, and rhinitis. Angioedema is less likely; however, it can occur with these agents. There is some cross-reactivity between ACEIs and ARBs; therefore, if angioedema occurs in a patient on an ACEI, the risk is still present with an ARB.

Renin Inhibitors

Mechanism of Action

Renin inhibitors block the conversion of angiotensinogen to angiotensin I. Angiotensin I suppression decreases the formation of angiotensin II (see **Table 19.1**). Angiotensin II functions within the RAAS as a negative inhibitory feedback mediator within the renal parenchyma to supress the further release of renin. The reduction in angiotensin II levels suppresses this feedback loop, leading to further increased plasma renin concentrations and subsequent low plasma renin activity. The first effective oral direct renin inhibitor, aliskiren (Tekturna), was approved by the U.S. Food and Drug Administration in March 2007. Aliskiren lowers BP to a degree comparable to most other agents. There are no clinical trial data of aliskiren on outcomes in hypertension, diabetes, or CVD.

Contraindications

This drug is not recommended in combination with ACEI and ARB therapy due to similar mechanisms of action. This medication should be avoided during pregnancy secondary to directly acting on the renin–angiotensin system can cause fetal and neonatal morbidity.

Adverse Events

Significant adverse events include diarrhea and angioedema (rare).

Calcium Channel Blockers

Mechanism of action

Calcium channel blockers (CCBs) share the the movement of calcium ions across the cell (see **Table 19.1**). The effect on the cardiovascular system is muscle relaxation and vasodilation. Nondihydropyridines, such as verapamil (Calan) and diltiazem (Cardizem), decrease heart rate and slow cardiac conduction at the AV node. The dihydropyridines (amlodipine [Norvasc], felodipine [Plendil], nifedipine [Procardia XL], nicardipine [Cardene SR], nisoldipine [Sular], and isradipine [DynaCirc]) are potent vasodilators. CCBs are effective as monotherapy and are especially effective in black patients. CCBs are indicated for treating hypertension associated with ischemic heart disease. CCBs are similar in antihypertensive effectiveness but differ in other pharmacodynamic effects. In addition, for use in HTN, these agents are recommended specifically for Prinzmetal angina treatment.

Contraindications

First-generation CCBs such as verapamil and diltiazem may accelerate the progression of congestive heart failure in a patient with cardiac dysfunction; therefore, these agents are not first line.

Diltiazem and verapamil should also be avoided in patients with AV node dysfunction (second- or third-degree heart block) or left ventricular (systolic) dysfunction when the ejection fraction measures less than 45%. Short-acting nifedipine should not be used for treating essential hypertension or hypertensive emergencies because of its association with causing inconsistent fluctuations in BP and reflex tachycardia.

Adverse Events

The dihydropyridine agents (nifedipine, nicardipine, isradipine, felodipine, nisoldipine, and amlodipine) produce symptoms of vasodilation, such as headache, flushing, palpations, and peripheral edema. Other side effects of nifedipine include dizziness, gingival hyperplasia, mood changes, and various gastrointestinal (GI) complaints. Nifedipine may cause reflex tachycardia as a result of stimulating the baroreceptors in response to an acute drop in BP. Diltiazem and verapamil can cause GI upset, peripheral edema, and hypotension. Rare side effects include bradycardia, AV block, and congestive heart failure. Verapamil can cause constipation in the elderly.

Peripheral Alpha-1 Receptor Blockers

Mechanism of Action

Doxazosin (Cardura), prazosin (Minipress), and terazosin (Hytrin) are selective alpha-1 receptor blockers that are effective in patients with benign prostatic hypertrophy and not usually prescribed solely for HTN treatment (see **Table 19.1**). Peripheral alpha-1 receptor blockers act peripherally by dilating both arterioles and veins, causing relaxation of smooth muscle.

Contraindications

In the presence of cardiovascular disease, alpha-1 receptor blockers should be avoided, as the Antihypertensive and Lipid-Lowering Treatment to Prevent Heart Attack (ALLHAT) study, in 2003, showed that these patients had an increase in mortality (Papademetriou et al., 2003). The use of tadalafil (Cialis), sildenafil (Viagra), and vardenafil (Levitra) is not recommended to be taken concurrently with alpha-1 receptor blockers due to an increased risk of symptomatic hypotension. If both agents are prescribed, a washout window of at least 4 to 6 hours is recommended.

Adverse Events

The most common side effect associated with this class of antihypertensive medications is the first-dose phenomenon, which consists of dizziness or faintness, palpitations, or syncope. These agents should be administered initially at bedtime and the dosage should be adjusted slowly. With chronic administration, even at low doses, fluid and sodium accumulate, requiring concurrent diuretic therapy. Other side effects include vivid dreams and depression.

Central Alpha-2 Receptor Agonists

Mechanism of Action

Central alpha-2 agonists stimulate alpha-2 adrenergic receptors in the brain, resulting in decreased sympathetic outflow, cardiac output, and peripheral resistance (see **Table 19.1**). These agents may cause fluid retention, and in most cases, combination with a diuretic can be considered. Clonidine (Catapres), methyldopa (Aldomet), guanabenz (Wytensin), and guanfacine (Tenex) should not be used as initial monotherapy. Abrupt cessation of alpha-2 agonist therapy may result in a compensatory increase in the norepinephrine level, therefore increasing BP.

Contraindications

Central agonists should be used cautiously in patient with severe coronary insufficiency, conduction disturbances, recent MI, cerebrovascular disease, and renal failure. Abrupt cessation should be avoided.

Adverse Events

These agents may cause fluid retention, sedation, and dry mouth. Also, the first-dose effect of dizziness and syncope is possible.

Direct Vasodilators

Mechanism of Action

The direct vasodilators hydralazine (Apresoline) and minoxidil (Loniten) cause arteriolar smooth muscle relaxation, resulting in BP reduction (see **Table 19.1**). Direct vasodilators should be reserved for patients with essential or severe hypertension. Both hydralazine and minoxidil may cause fluid retention and reflex tachycardia, which can be treated with a concurrent diuretic and a beta-blocker or other agent (clonidine, diltiazem, or verapamil) that slows the heart rate.

Contraindications

Hydralazine should be used with caution in patients with coronary artery disease and mitral valvular rheumatic heart disease. Minoxidil is contraindicated in patients with pheochromocytoma, acute MI, and dissecting aortic aneurysm.

Adverse Events

Hydralazine is associated with a lupus-like syndrome that is dose related at dosages greater than 300 mg/d. Other adverse reactions include dermatitis, drug fever, and peripheral neuropathy. Minoxidil may cause a drug-induced hirsutism, which is unfavorable to most female patients.

Adrenergic Antagonists

Mechanism of Action

Reserpine (Serpasil), guanethidine (Ismelin), and guanadrel (Hylorel) inhibit the sympathetic system by depleting norepinephrine stores in the central nervous system (see **Table 19.1**). This results in a decrease in peripheral vascular resistance and a reduction in BP. In patients who use these agents, depression may result from decreased catecholamine and serotonin levels in the central nervous system.

Adverse Effects

Reserpine's use is limited because of its side effect profile, which includes depression, impotence, diarrhea, bradycardia, drowsiness, and nasal stuffiness. Guanadrel and guanethidine also produce numerous adverse effects, such as diarrhea, impotence, orthostatic hypotension, and syncope. They should be used with caution.

SELECTING THE MOST APPROPRIATE AGENT

First-line therapy should be influenced by the age, ethnicity/race, and other conditions (diabetes, coronary disease, etc.). Long-acting drugs that need to be taken once daily are preferred to shorter acting drugs because this will reduce nonadherence. For this reason, when more than one drug is prescribed, combination products can simplify treatment. However, combination products can be more expensive.

According to the JNC 8 guidelines, for black patients with hypertension, with or without diabetes, CCB or thiazide diuretics are recommended. For all other ethnicities, according to JNC 8, HTN treatment options include ACEIs or ARB, thiazide diuretics, or CCB. Additionally, per the JNC 8 guidelines, all adult CKD patients regardless of having diabetes are recommended either an ACEI or an ARB for hypertension therapy. This is in contrast to JNC 7, which recommended using diuretics as monotherapy in preference of other antihypertensive agents.

If a diuretic is chosen, the longer acting and more potent agent chlorthalidone should be considered as first-line treatment given that it has the highest level of clinical trial evidence supporting its use. Recent data support that monotherapy with a β-blocker (in particular atenolol because of excess risks of strokes) or an α-blocker (caused by excess risks of CHF events by doxazosin in the ALLHAT study) should be discouraged because they are less effective than most other agents (Law et al., 2009), although β-blockers might be effective in the secondary prevention of ischemic heart disease and meta-analyses suggest that β-blockers are inferior in the prevention of strokes (Bangalore et al., 2007).

Studies have shown that isolated systolic hypertension (SBP greater than 160 mm Hg with DBP less than 90 mm Hg) is a potent risk factor for strokes and CVD. Among patients older than 50 years, SBP levels are more strongly related to CVD and renal disease than DBP. Treatment of isolated systolic hypertension leads to improved CVD outcomes regardless of achieved DBP. Although there have been long-standing concern and debate about the risks of the "J-curve," whereby excessive reductions in DBP may lead to increased risk for CHD events, the overall evidence supports that this effect is limited to high-risk patients with established CAD. Treatment-induced reduction in SBP to less than 140 mm Hg provides a greater overall event reduction and is offset by any adverse effect of excessive lowering of DBP (Mancia et al., 2013). Nevertheless, careful monitoring of certain individuals in this scenario is warranted, including those older than 80 years, patients with active angina worsened by BP lowering, and people with excessively low DBP (less than 65 mm Hg) or orthostatic hypotension.

Additionally, the Avoiding Cardiovascular events through Combination therapy in Patients Living with Systolic Hypertension (ACCOMPLISH) trial demonstrated a significant 20% reduction in combined cardiovascular events in patients treated with a combination of an ACEI plus CCB (benazepril + amlodipine) compared with patients treated with an ACEI plus a thiazide diuretic (benazepril + hydrochlorothiazide) (Jamerson et al., 2008). Furthermore, the Ongoing Telmisartan Alone and in Combination with Ramipril Global Endpoint Trial (ONTARGET) study demonstrated that combined ACEI + ARB therapy did not prevent cardiovascular events more than monotherapy. In fact, it showed that renal outcomes were worsened by this combination and higher risk of adverse events (Yusuf et al., 2008).

If the patient is not at goal, the ACC/AHA/CDC recommends that physicians increase the dose of the medications and/or add a drug from a different class. Similarly, JNC 8 states if the target BP is not reached within one month after initiating pharmacologic therapy, the dose of the initial medication should be increased or a second medication should be added. If the BP goal is not reached using two drugs, it is recommended adding a third drug. Should the patient still not be at goal, physicians should question patient adherence, request readings from home, or consider secondary causes of hypertension. A hypertension specialist should be considered if the patient still fails to get to goal, after being on multiple medications, since the patient may have resistant hypertension.

For select individuals, it was concluded that some alternative treatments, notably resistance and isometric exercise, device-guided slow breathing, and certain meditation techniques, can serve as effective and helpful adjuvants to lower BP. Whether or not patients are able to adhere to these nonpharmacologic lifestyle treatments to control BP over several years remains uncertain.

Special Population Considerations
Pediatric Patient Population

The current JNC 8 guidelines address adult BP goals not pediatric BP goals. Instead, hypertension diagnosis and treatment of hypertension is managed by the fourth report from the National High Blood Pressure Education Working Group for Hypertension Management Children and Adolescents. This guideline highlights diagnosis based on the child's age and goal ranges of the SBP and/or DBP falls into percentiles. Treatment regimens are recommended to be individualized and starting doses of antihypertensive agents between adults and children are not equivalent.

Geriatric Patient Population

The Trial of Nonpharmacological Interventions in the Elderly (TONE) showed that in older patients with hypertension, BP can be reduced by low-sodium diets and weight loss. In some instances, patients could discontinue their antihypertensive medications or reduce the number of medications required to remain normotensive (Sander, 2002).

Elderly patients are very sensitive to medications that cause sympathetic inhibition and are at greater risk of becoming volume depleted than their younger patients. Decreased renal and hepatic function complicates hypertension treatment and increases the risk of adverse events in this population. Antihypertensive medications should be started at low doses and titrated slowly. If choosing to use beta-blockers in the elderly, it is prudent to use the newer beta-blockers such as nebivolol and carvedilol as they may provide a better safety profile and better morbidity and mortality outcome (Kaiser et al., 2014). According to the SHEP trial, patients with isolated systolic hypertension should start hypertensive therapy with a diuretic due to decrease in stroke incidence unless there is a compelling reason to avoid its use. The long-acting dihydropyridine CCBs are also effective and are an alternative in these patients. Clinical trials have demonstrated that in older patients with isolated systolic hypertension, low diastolic BP was associated with a higher mortality rate for any given level of systolic BP. Postural hypotension should also be closely monitored in this population.

Women Patient Population

There are no significant differences in BP response between genders. Women taking oral contraceptives may have an increase in BP, and the risk of hypertension may increase with the duration of oral contraceptive use. If hypertension develops as a result of oral contraceptive use, an alternate contraception method should be used. Because of the risk of stroke associated with oral contraceptive use and cigarette smoking, women taking oral contraceptives should be encouraged not to smoke cigarettes, and women older than age 35 should not take oral contraceptives if they continue to smoke.

Women diagnosed with hypertension before pregnancy should continue taking antihypertensive agents throughout pregnancy. Few are safe for use, however, during pregnancy. ACEIs, rennin inhibitors, and ARBs should be avoided during pregnancy because they are teratogenic. Beta-blockers should also be avoided during early pregnancy because of the risk of fetal growth retardation. Methyldopa is recommended for women who are diagnosed with hypertension during pregnancy. Consultation with a woman's OB-GYN specialty practitioner regarding an antihypertensive recommendation should occur in all cases.

Black Patient Population

The incidence of hypertension and hypertension-related complications is believed to be higher in blacks than in any ethnic group. Some blacks experience hypertension before age 10, which was attributed to two major risk factors: obesity and inactivity. Other risk factors include a diet high in sodium and low in potassium. This has resulted in the greatest incidence of stroke, end-stage renal disease, cardiovascular disease, and death in this population. Blacks who are diagnosed and treated have a lower incidence of complications.

Blacks have physiologic characteristics that contribute to this risk, including low circulating renin levels with excessive levels of angiotensin II, endothelial dysfunction as a result of reduced bradykinin and nitric oxide, abnormal sympathetic nervous system activation, and higher levels of intracellular calcium stores. Blacks are more responsive to monotherapy with diuretics. Results from the ALLHAT found that chlorthalidone and amlodipine were superior to ACEIs in treating blacks (Papademetriou et al., 2003). Alpha-blockers should not be used as initial monotherapy per the conclusions of this trial (Papademetriou et al., 2003). ACEIs may induce angioedema, which occurs two to four times more frequently in blacks.

Diabetic Patient Population

The coexistence of hypertension and diabetes mellitus is very common. Hypertension increases cardiovascular risks in diabetic patients. Current guidelines recommend lowering BP to less than 140/90. This is a consensus among the following guidelines: the American Heart Association/American College of Cardiology, the American Society of Hypertension/International Society of Hypertension, the American Diabetes Association (ADA) 2015 standards of care guidelines, and the Eighth Joint National Committee. The American Diabetes Association, 2015 standard of care guidelines recommend that hypertensive diabetic patients be treated if they have a DBP greater than 80 or an SBP greater than 140 with a target BP of less than 140/80.

All patients should be encouraged to modify their lifestyle, to limit sodium intake, lose weight, and exercise for 150 minutes/week. All major antihypertensive drug classes, RAAS blockers, beta blockers, diuretics, and calcium blockers are useful in diabetic patients. ACEI and ARBs are considered the cornerstone of therapy. Studies have shown these classes to be beneficial in reducing overall cardiovascular risk, nephropathy, renal failure, and retinopathy. Combination therapy consisting of two RAAS blockers or the use of ACEI and an ARB in combination is not recommended because of the risk of causing renal impairment, hypotension, and hyperkalemia.

HYPERTENSIVE EMERGENCY/ HYPERTENSIVE URGENCY

Hypertensive crisis or malignant hypertension is defined as an extremely high SBP and/or DBP according to JNC 7. Hypertensive emergency was not addressed by JNC 8 guidelines. Hypertensive crisis is further divided into two categories based upon evidence of target organ damage. If end organ damage is present, the condition is classified as hypertensive emergency. Hypertensive crisis without evidence of organ damage is classified as hypertensive urgency. In hypertensive emergencies, the therapeutic goal is to protect remaining end organ function, reduce risk of complications, and improve outcomes. BP reduction should be made in a controlled fashion and not aimed at normalizing the BP quickly as this can exacerbate target organ damage. The BP itself may not be as important as the rate of elevation. Patients with a chronic history of hypertension can tolerate high levels than that of a normotensive patient. Hypertensive urgencies are severe elevation of BP with no target organ dysfunction. A majority of these patients present as a result of noncompliance or inadequate treatment.

In hypertensive emergencies, presenting symptoms may include chest pain, dyspnea, and neurologic deficits. The physical examination must include serial BP measurements in both arms, lung and heart auscultation, renal artery auscultation, neurologic evaluation, and funduscopic evaluation. Imaging studies should be obtained if the patient presents with chest or back pain and unequal pulses in the upper extremities. Electrocardiogram and cardiac enzymes are part of the initial workup for shortness of breath or chest pain and echocardiogram is useful if heart failure is suspected.

Immediate treatment with an intravenous antihypertensive agent(s) is needed to salvage viable tissue. The marked elevation in BP results in arteriolar fibrinoid necrosis, endothelial damage, platelet and fibrin deposition in the media of smooth muscle, and loss of autoregulatory function. This results in end organ ischemia such as encephalopathy, MI, unstable angina, pulmonary edema, eclampsia, stroke, intracranial hemorrhage, life-threatening arterial bleeding, or aortic dissection. These patients require hospitalization and parenteral drug therapy.

The drug of choice to treat hypertensive emergencies depends on the clinical situation. BP control can be achieved over several hours (24 to 48 hours) with either IV or oral medications depending on the urgency of the situation. Commonly used medications include direct vasodilators (hydralazine), nitrates (sodium nitroprusside, nitroglycerin), CCBs (nicardipine, clevidipine), sympathoplegic agents (labetalol, esmolol), alpha-I blockers (phentolamine), and ACEIs (enalaprilat). After the BP is lowered, the patient's drug regimen should be assessed to determine possible causes of the hypertensive emergency/urgency such as medication nonadherence, adverse effects that interfere with the patient's lifestyle, and/or a complex medication regimen that could be simplified.

MONITORING PATIENT RESPONSE

Follow-Up and Monitoring

BP should be measured at every routine visit. The patients' efforts and lifestyle modifications should be discussed at each visit. Referral to a hypertension specialist may be indicated if the BP goal is not achieved despite several medications, if resistant hypertension is suspected, or if clinical consultation is needed for the more complicated patients. Serum creatinine and potassium levels should be monitored once or twice a year in patients taking antihypertensive medications once the levels have proven to be stable. When initially adding medication or increasing doses of drugs that have electrolyte abnormalities as an adverse effect, frequent monitoring is warranted.

The importance of adhering to the drug regimen cannot be overemphasized. The practitioner needs to be alert for signs of nonadherence and should ask patients about their experiences or problems with adhering to the drug regimen. Side effects should be discussed, and changes in medications may or may not be considered at each visit.

PATIENT EDUCATION

Patient education is a vital part of hypertension treatment. Because most patients are free of symptoms, they must be educated about the disease, the importance of adhering to therapy, and the consequences of uncontrolled hypertension. Patient education booklets are available from most well-known organizations such as the AHA, which may be used to reinforce the information provided by the practitioner.

Because each antihypertensive medication has some side effects, the patient needs to be informed about what they are, what actions to take to relieve minor side effects, and what to do about intolerable or dangerous side effects. Adherence to hypertensive medication regimen should be assessed at each office encounter. Since the objective of drug therapy is to

CASE STUDY*

R.S., a 65-year-old black man, was referred to the hypertension clinic for evaluation of high BP noted on an initial screening. He reports having headaches and nocturia. He states that he has gained 8 pounds over the last year.

Past medical history
  Appendectomy 30 years ago
  Peptic ulcer disease 10 years ago
  Type 2 diabetes mellitus for 10 years
  Gout
Family history
  Father had hypertension; died of myocardial infarction
    at age 55
  Mother had diabetes mellitus and hypertension; died
    of cerebrovascular accident at age 60
Physical examination
  Height 69 in, weight 90 kg
  BP: 140/89 mm Hg (left arm), 138/82 mm Hg (right arm)
  Pulse: 84 beats/minute, regular
  Funduscopic examination: mild arterial narrowing,
    sharp discs, no exudates or hemorrhages
Laboratory findings
  Blood urea nitrogen: 24 mg/dL
  Serum creatinine: 1.1 mg/dL
  Glucose: 95 mg/dL
  Potassium: 4.0 mEq/L
  Total cholesterol: 201 mg/dL

High-density lipoprotein cholesterol: 30 mg/dL
Triglycerides: 167 mg/dL
Urinalysis: within normal limit (no proteinuria)
Electrocardiogram and chest radiograph: mild left ventricular hypertrophy
Social history
  Tobacco: 35 pack years
  Alcohol: 1 pint of vodka/week
  Coffee: 2 cups/day

DIAGNOSIS: STAGE 1 HYPERTENSION

1. List specific goals for treating **R.S.'s** hypertension.
2. What drug therapy would you prescribe? Why?
3. What are the parameters for monitoring success of the therapy?
4. Discuss specific patient education based on the prescribed therapy.
5. List one or two adverse reactions for the selected agent that would cause you to change therapy.
6. What would be the choice for second-line therapy?
7. What over-the-counter and/or alternative medications would be appropriate for **R.S.**?
8. What lifestyle changes would you recommend to **R.S.**?
9. Describe one or two drug–drug or drug–food interaction for the selected agent.

* Answers can be found online.

lower BP without intolerable effects, the patient needs to know which adverse reactions should be reported to the practitioner and which ones may be relieved by switching to an alternative drug in a different class. The patient also needs to know that several different agents may be tried before finding the one that best controls his or her BP with minimal or no side effects. Other important teaching involves information about lifestyle changes and the consequences of uncontrolled hypertension.

Nutrition/Lifestyle Changes

As described above, it is important to remind hypertensive patients about the key role of a lifestyle effects on BP. Patients should follow a healthy diet, restrict sodium, and quit smoking (if applicable) and alcohol consumption. Patients should also be reminded to maintain a healthy weight and get regular exercise for better control of BP.

Complementary and Alternative Medications

To date, there is no evidence that alternative medications reduce BP.

CONCLUSION

As you can see, hypertension is a complex chronic disease in terms of both pathophysiology and treatment. Successful treatment of high pressure can help prevent several negative outcomes.

Bibliography

*Starred references are cited in the text.

*American Diabetes Association. (2015). Standards of medical care in diabetes 2015—Section 8: Cardiovascular disease and risk management. *Diabetes Care, 38*(Suppl. 1), S49–S57.

*Bangalore, S., Parkar, S., Grossman, E., et al. (2007). A meta-analysis of 94,492 patients with hypertension treated with beta blockers to determine the risk of new onset diabetes mellitus. *American Journal of Cardiology, 100*, 1254–1262.

Basile, J. (2010). One size does not fit all: The role of vasodilating β-blockers in controlling hypertension as a means of reducing cardiovascular and stroke risk. *The American Journal of Medicine, 123*, S9–S15.

Bloch, M. J. (2003). The diagnosis and management of renovascular disease: A primary care perspective. *Journal of Clinical Hypertension, 5*, 210–218.

Brown, N. J., Ray, W. A., Snowden, M., et al. (1996). Black Americans have an increased rate of angiotensin-converting enzyme inhibition associated angioedema. *Clinical Pharmacology and Therapeutics, 60*, 8–13.

Burkhart, G. A., Brown, N. J., Griffin, M. R., et al. (1996). Angiotensin-converting enzyme inhibitor-associated angioedema: Higher risk in blacks than whites. *Pharmacoepidemiology and Drug Safety, 5*, 149–154.

CAPRICORN Investigators. (2001). Effects of carvedilol on outcome after myocardial infarction in patients with left-ventricular dysfunction: The CAPRICORN randomised trial. *Lancet, 357*, 1385–1390.

Chobanian, A. (2008). Does it matter how hypertension is controlled? *New England Journal of Medicine, 359*, 2485–2488.

*Cushman, W., Evans, G., Byington, R., et al. (2010). Effects of intensive blood-pressure control in type 2 diabetes mellitus. *New England Journal of Medicine, 362*, 1575–1585.

*Dahlöf, B., Devereux, R., Kjeldsen, S, et al. (2002). Cardiovascular morbidity and mortality in the Losartan Intervention For Endpoint reduction in hypertension study (LIFE): A randomised trial against atenolol. *Lancet, 359*, 995–1003.

*Eckel, R., Jakicic, J., Ard, J. D., et al. (2014). 2013 AHA/ACC guideline on lifestyle management to reduce cardiovascular risk: A report of the American College of Cardiology/American Heart Association Task Force on practice guidelines. *Circulation, 129*, S76–S99.

Eknoyan, G., Lameire, N., et al. (2012). KDIGO clinical practice guideline for the management of blood pressure in chronic kidney disease. *Kidney International Supplements, 2*, 341–342.

Escobar, C., & Barrios, V. (2009). Combined therapy in the treatment of hypertension. *Fundamental & Clinical Pharmacology, 24*, 3–8.

Forman, J., & Brenner, B. (2006). Hypertension and microalbuminuria: The bell tolls for thee. *Kidney International, 69*, 22–28.

Garcia-Donaire, J., & Ruilope, L. (2009). Multiple action fixed combinations. Present or future? *Fundamental & Clinical Pharmacology, 24*, 37–42.

Go, A., Bauman, M., Coleman, S., et al. (2014). An effective approach to high blood pressure control. *Hypertension, 63*, 878–885.

Go, A., Mozaffarian, D., Roger, V., et al. (2014). Heart disease and stroke statistics—2014 update: A report from the American Heart Association, *Circulation, 129*(3), e28–e292. doi:10.1161/01.cir.0000441139.02102.80.

Grossman, Y., Shlomai, G., & Grossman, E. (2014). Treating hypertension in type 2 diabetes. *Expert Opinion on Pharmacotherapy, 15*, 2131–2140.

He, J., Klag, M. J., Appek, L. J., et al. (1999). The renin–angiotensin system and BP: Differences between blacks and whites. *American Journal of Hypertension, 12*(6), 555–562.

Head, G. (2014). Ambulatory blood pressure monitoring is ready to replace clinic blood pressure in the diagnosis of hypertension. Pro side of the argument. *Hypertension, 64*, 1175–1181.

*Jamerson, K., Weber, M., Bakris, G., et al. (2008). Benazepril plus amlodipine or hydrochlorothiazide for hypertension in high-risk patients (ACCOMPLISH). *New England Journal of Medicine, 359*(23), 2417–2428.

*James, P., Oparil, S., Carter, B., et al. (2014). 2014 Evidence-based guideline for the management of high blood pressure in adults. Report from the panel members appointed to the eighth Joint National Committee (JNC_8). *Journal of the American Medical Association, 311*, 507–520.

Joint National Committee on Prevention, Detection, Evaluation, and Treatment of High BP. (2003). Seventh report of the Joint National Committee on Prevention, Detection, Evaluation, and Treatment of High BP (JNC VII). *Journal of the American Medical Association, 289*, 2560–2572.

Jordan, J., & Grassi, G. (2010). Belly fat and resistant hypertension. *Journal of Hypertension, 28*, 1131–1133.

*Kaiser, E., Lotze, U., Schafer, H. (2014). Increasing complexity: Which drug class to choose for treatment of hypertension in the elderly? *Clinical Interventions in Aging, 9*, 459–475.

*Law, M., Morris, J., Wald, N. (2009). Use of blood pressure lowering drugs in the prevention of cardiovascular disease: Meta-analysis of 147 randomised trials in the context of expectation from perspective epidemiological studies. *British Medical Journal, 338*, b1665.

Lee, M. (2014). Erectile dysfunction. In J. T. DiPiro, R. L. Talbert, G. C. Yee, et al. (Eds.), *Pharmacotherapy: A pathophysiologic approach* (9th ed., p. 1349). New York, NY: McGraw-Hill.

Mancia, G., De Backer, G., Dominiczak, A., et al. (2007). 2007 Guidelines for the management of arterial hypertension: The task force for the management of arterial hypertension of the European Society of *Hypertension* (ESH) and of the European Society of Cardiology (ESC). *Journal of Hypertension, 25*, 1105–1187.

*Mancia, G., Fagard, R., Narkiewicz, K., et al. (2013). 2013 ESH/ESC guidelines for the management of arterial hypertension: The task force for the management of arterial hypertension of the European Society of Hypertension (ESH) and of the European Society of Cardiology (ESC). *Journal of Hypertension, 31*, 1281–1357.

Messerli, F., & Panjrath, G. (2009). The J-curve between blood pressure and coronary artery disease or essential hypertension: Exactly how essential? *Journal of the American College of Cardiology, 20*, 1827–1834.

*Mozzafarian, D., Benjamin, E., Go, A., et al. (2015). Heart disease and stroke statistics—2015 update: A report from the American Heart Association. *Circulation, 131*(4), e29–e322.

National High Blood Pressure Education Program [NHBPEP] Working Group. (1994). National High Blood Pressure Education Program Working Group report on hypertension in diabetes. *Hypertension, 23*, 145–158, 555–576.

National High Blood Pressure Education Working Group on High Blood Pressure in Children and Adolescents. (2004). Fourth report on the diagnosis, evaluation, and treatment of high blood pressure in children and adolescents. *Pediatrics, 114*, 555–576.

National Institute for Health Care Excellence (NICE). (2013). Quality statement 4—Blood pressure targets. Retrieved from https://www.nice.org.uk/guidance/qs28 on June 18, 2015.

Nwanko, T., Yoon, S. S., Burt, V., et al. (2013). *Hypertension among adults in the US: National Health and Nutrition Examination Survey, 2011–2012.* NCHS Data Brief, No. 133. Hyattsville, MD: Nation Center for Health Statistics, Centers for Disease Control and Prevention, U.S. Department of Health and Human Services.

Ong, K., Cheung, B., Man, Y., et al. (2006). Prevalence, awareness, treatment, and control of hypertension among United States adults. *Journal of Clinical Hypertension, 49*, 69–75.

Ostchega, Y., Dillon, C., & Hughes, J. (2007). Trends in hypertension prevalence, awareness, treatment, and control in older U.S. adults: Data from the national health and nutrition examination survey 1988 to 2004. *Journal of the American Geriatrics Society, 55*, 1056–1065.

*Papademetriou, V., Piller, L., Ford, C., et al. (2003). Characteristics and lipid distribution of a large, high-risk, hypertension population: The lipid-lowering component of the antihypertensive and lipid-lowering treatment to prevent heart attack trail (ALLHAT). *Journal of Clinical Hypertension, 5*, 377–385.

Piper, M. A., Evans, C. V., Burda, B. U., et al. (2014). *Screening for high blood pressure in adults: A systematic evidence review for the U.S. Preventive Services Task Force.* Evidence Synthesis No. 121. AHRQ Publication No. 13-05194-EF-1. Rockville, MD: Agency for Healthcare Research and Quality.

*Pitt, B., Remme, W., Cody, R., et al. (1999). The effect of spironolactone on morbidity and mortality in patients with severe health failure (RALES). *New England Journal of Medicine, 341*(10), 709–717.

Poole-Wilson, P., Swedberg, K., Cleland, J., et al. (2003). Comparison of carvedilol and metoprolol on clinical outcomes in patients with chronic heart failure in the Carvedilol Or Metoprolol European Trial (COMET): Randomised controlled trial. *Lancet, 362*, 7–13.

Rakel, R., & Rakel, D. (2013). *Textbook of family medicine. Cardiovascular disease* (9th ed.). Philadelphia, PA: Elsevier.

Ramos, A., & Varon, J. (2014). Current and newer agents for hypertensive emergencies. *Current Hypertension Reports, 16*, 450.

Redon, J., & Lurbe, E. (2014). Ambulatory blood pressure monitoring is ready to replace clinic blood pressure in diagnosis of hypertension. Con side of the argument. *Hypertension, 64*, 1169–1174.

*Sander, G. (2002). High blood pressure in the geriatric population: Treatment considerations. *American Journal of Geriatric Cardiology, 11*, 223–232.

Saseen J. J., & MacLaughlin E. J. (2014). Hypertension. In: DiPiro, J. T., Talbert, R. L., Yee, G. C., et al. (Eds.), *Pharmacotherapy: A pathophysiologic approach* (9th ed., pp. 49–84). New York, NY: McGraw-Hill.

*U.S. Preventive Services Task Force. (2007). Screening for high blood pressure: U.S. Preventive Services Task Force reaffirmation recommendation statement. *Annals of Internal Medicine, 147*, 783–787.

SHEP Cooperative Research Group. (1991). Prevention of stroke by antihypertensive drug treatment in older persons with isolated systolic hypertension. *Journal of the American Medical Association, 265*, 3255–3264.

Sica, D. (2002). ACE inhibitors and stroke: New considerations. *Journal of Clinical Hypertension, 4*, 126–129.

Sica, D., & Black, H. (2002). ACE inhibitor-related angioedema: Can angiotensin-receptor blockers be safely used? *Journal of Clinical Hypertension, 4*(5), 375–380.

*Taler, S., Agarwal, R., Bakris, G., et al. (2013). KDOQI US Commentary on the 2012 KDIGO clinical practice guideline for management of blood pressure in CKD. *American Journal of Kidney Diseases, 62*, 201–213.

Taylor, A., & Bakris, G. (2010). The role of vasodilating B-blockers in patients with hypertension and the cardiometabolic syndrome. *The American Journal of Medicine, 123*, S21–S26.

Tierney, L., McPhee, S., & Papadakis, M. (2004). *Current medical diagnosis and treatment.* New York, NY: McGraw-Hill.

Ungar, A., Pepe, G., Lambertucci, L., et al. (2009). Low diastolic ambulatory blood pressure is associated with greater all-cause mortality in older patients with hypertension. *Journal of the American Geriatrics Society, 57*, 291–296.

U.S. Preventive Services Task Force. (2007). Screening for high blood pressure: U.S. Preventive Force Reaffirmation Recommendation Statement. *Annals of Internal Medicine, 147*, 783–786.

*Vongpatanasin, W. (2014). Resistant hypertension. A review of diagnosis and management. *Journal of the American Medical Association, 311*, 2216–2224.

Yancy, C., Fowler M., Colucci, W., et al. (2001). Race and the response to adrenergic blockade with carvedilol in patients with chronic heart failure. *New England Journal of Medicine, 344*, 1358–1365.

*Yusuf, S., Teo, K., Pogue, J., et al. (2008). Telmisartan, ramipril, or both in patients at high risk for vascular events. *New England Journal of Medicine, 358*, 1547–1559.

Weber, M., Schiffrin, E., White, W., et al. (2014). Clinical practice guidelines for the management of hypertension in the community. A statement by the American Society of Hypertension and the International Society of Hypertension. *Journal of Hypertension, 32*, 1–13.

Wright, J., Jamerson, K., & Ferdinand, K. (2007). The management of hypertension in African Americans. *Journal of Clinical Hypertension, 9*, 468–475.

20 Hyperlipidemia

John Barron ■ Vincent J. Willey

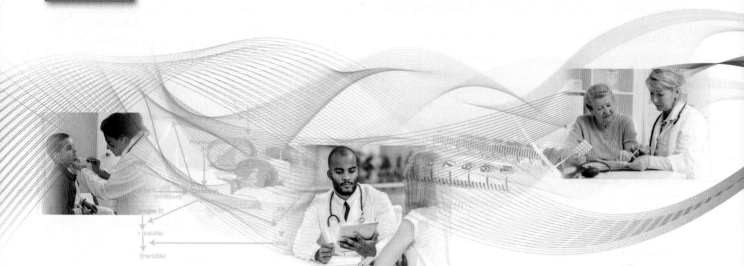

Hyperlipidemia is a blood disorder characterized by elevations in blood cholesterol levels. The term is often used synonymously with *dyslipidemia* and *hypercholesterolemia*. Hyperlipidemia is one of the major contributing risk factors in the development of coronary heart disease (CHD). It is estimated that approximately 15.5 million people in the United States have CHD, with approximately 375,000 deaths each year (American Heart Association, 2015). In addition, approximately $215 billion is spent each year on direct and indirect costs from CHD.

Informed estimates indicate that approximately greater than 100 million adults aged 20 and older had total cholesterol levels above 200 mg/dL using data from 2009 to 2012, representing approximately 47% of adults in the United States (American Heart Association, 2015). However, data from the National Health and Nutrition Examination Survey (NHANES) suggest that the percentage of patients with elevated cholesterol may be decreasing.

Numerous large studies have shown that reducing elevated cholesterol levels reduces morbidity and mortality rates in patients with and without existing CHD (Downs et al., 1998; Frick et al., 1987; Heart Protection Study Collaborative Group, 2002; Lewis et al., 1998; Long-Term Intervention With Pravastatin in Ischaemic Disease [LIPID] Study Group, 1998; Ridker et al., 2008; Scandinavian Simvastatin Survival Study Group, 1994; Shepherd et al., 1995). Although these and other trials have clearly shown the benefits of treating high cholesterol levels and other preventive measures, including the use of aspirin, beta-blockers, and angiotensin-converting enzyme inhibitors in the treatment of patients with coronary artery disease, long-term use of these medications across the population is still suboptimal (Newby et al., 2006).

CAUSES

In hyperlipidemia, serum cholesterol levels may be elevated as a result of an increased level of any of the lipoproteins. (See the section on Pathophysiology: Lipoproteins and Lipid Metabolism.) The mechanisms for hyperlipidemia appear to be genetic (primary) and environmental (secondary). In fact, the most common cause of hyperlipidemia (95% of all those with hyperlipidemia) is a combination of genetic and environmental factors.

Some individuals are genetically predisposed to elevated cholesterol levels. They may inherit defective genes that lead to abnormalities in the synthesis or breakdown of cholesterol. These may include abnormalities in low-density lipoprotein (LDL) receptors and mutations in apolipoproteins that lead to increased production of cholesterol or decreased clearance of cholesterol from the bloodstream. (See the section on Pathophysiology: Lipoproteins and Lipid Metabolism.)

Secondary factors may include medications (e.g., beta-blockers and oral contraceptives), concomitant disease states or other conditions (e.g., diabetes mellitus and pregnancy), diets high in fat and cholesterol, lack of exercise, obesity, and smoking (**Box 20.1**).

PATHOPHYSIOLOGY

The major plasma lipids are cholesterol, triglycerides, and phospholipids. Cholesterol is a naturally occurring substance that is required by the body to synthesize bile acids and steroid hormones and to maintain the integrity of cell membranes. Although cholesterol is found predominantly

BOX 20.1 Secondary Causes of Hyperlipidemia

Disease States	Drugs
Acute hepatitis	Alcohol
Diabetes mellitus	Beta-blockers
Hypothyroidism	Glucocorticoids
Nephrotic syndrome	Oral contraceptives
Primary biliary cirrhosis	Progestins
Systemic lupus erythematosus	Thiazide diuretics
Uremia	

in the cells, approximately 7% circulates in the serum. It is this serum cholesterol that is implicated in atherosclerosis. Triglycerides are made up of free fatty acids and glycerol and serve as an important source of stored energy. Phospholipids are essential for cell function and lipid transport. Because these lipids are insoluble in plasma, they are surrounded by special fat-carrying proteins, called *lipoproteins*, for transport in the blood.

Lipoproteins are produced in the liver and intestines, but endogenous production of lipoproteins occurs primarily in the liver. Lipoproteins consist of a hydrophobic (water-insoluble) inner core made of cholesterol and triglycerides and a hydrophilic (water-soluble) outer surface composed of apolipoproteins and phospholipids. Apolipoproteins are specialized proteins that identify specific receptors to which the lipoprotein will bind. They are thought to play a role in the development or prevention of hyperlipidemia because they control the interaction and metabolism of the lipoproteins.

Lipoproteins and Lipid Metabolism

The major lipoproteins are named according to their density. They include chylomicrons, very–low-density lipoproteins (VLDLs), intermediate-density lipoproteins (IDLs), LDLs, and high-density lipoproteins (HDLs).

Chylomicrons

Chylomicrons, the largest lipoproteins, are composed primarily of triglycerides. Chylomicrons are produced in the gut from dietary fat and cholesterol that has been solubilized by bile acids (exogenous pathway). Chylomicrons normally are not present in the blood after a 12- to 14-hour fast.

Very–Low-Density Lipoproteins

VLDLs are primarily composed of cholesterol and triglycerides and are the major carrier of endogenous triglycerides. On secretion into the bloodstream, lipoprotein lipase and hepatic lipase hydrolyze the triglyceride core by a mechanism similar to that which occurs with chylomicrons. As the triglyceride content decreases, the lipoprotein becomes progressively smaller with a

higher percentage of cholesterol; it is now referred to as an IDL. IDL is a short-lived lipoprotein that is converted to LDL or is taken up by LDL receptors on the liver. LDL, the final product of the metabolism of VLDL, contains the most cholesterol by weight of all the lipoproteins. It is estimated that 60% to 75% of the total cholesterol is contained in LDLs (Talbert, 1997).

Approximately 50% of LDL is taken up by the liver, and the remaining 50% is taken up by peripheral cells. Increased levels of LDL cholesterol are directly related to the probability that atherosclerosis will develop. Thus, LDL cholesterol is usually referred to as "bad" cholesterol.

High-Density Lipoproteins

HDL particles are produced in the liver and intestine. The primary function of HDL cholesterol is to remove LDL cholesterol from the peripheral cells and to remove triglycerides that result from the degradation of chylomicrons and VLDL particles. The HDL then transports these particles to the liver for metabolism. This process is termed *reverse cholesterol transport*. For this reason, HDL is often referred to as "good" cholesterol.

Pathogenesis of Atherosclerosis

Atherosclerosis is characterized by the development of lesions resulting from accumulations of cholesterol in the blood vessel wall. Atherosclerosis primarily affects the larger arteries, including the coronary arteries.

The atherogenic process begins with the accumulation of LDL cholesterol under the endothelial lining of the innermost arterial layer, the intima. As LDLs accumulate, circulating monocytes attach to the endothelial lining and penetrate between the endothelial cells into the subendothelial space. On entry into the subendothelial space, the monocytes form into macrophages, which then ingest the LDLs. Macrophages, in particular, have a high affinity for modified (oxidized) LDL. As the macrophages ingest the modified LDL, they are converted into foam cells and form the *fatty streak*, which is the initial lesion in the atherogenic process. These lesions commonly affect the coronary arteries. Formation begins in the midteens, and the lesions grow as the person ages.

Once the fatty streak forms, the oxidized LDL and macrophages act in other ways that promote the progression of the atherogenic lesion. Oxidized LDL appears to act as a chemotactic agent, recruiting other circulating monocytes and preventing macrophages from leaving the subendothelial space. Macrophages also produce chemotactic factors as well as growth factors. The growth factors cause proliferation of smooth muscle cells from the media into the fatty streak, leading to the formation of a fibrous plaque (Ross & Glomset, 1976). Fibrous plaques are usually raised and protrude into the lumen of the artery, thereby compromising blood flow.

As the foam cells grow, the endothelium stretches and may become damaged. This leads to platelet aggregation and clot formation. In many instances, these fissures heal and incorporate the thrombi inside the plaque. This process may occur dozens of times and eventually may produce a complicated lesion. The formation of complicated lesions is the major cause of acute cardiovascular (CV) events. However, in some instances, rupture of a small, unstable plaque may also cause the formation of a single large clot that totally occludes the vessel. The fibrous plaques that are most likely to rupture are those that have large lipid cores and a thin fibrous cap, a layer of smooth muscle cells directly over the lipid core. Large plaques with a strong fibrous cap may be more stable and less likely to rupture (Cooke & Bhatnagar, 1997; McKenney & Hawkins, 1995).

The primary symptom associated with atherosclerosis is chest pain known as *angina*. Symptoms occur when the lesion compromises blood flow in the vessel lumen. A lesion that occludes approximately 50% of the lumen usually causes symptoms when more blood flow is required (i.e., exercise-induced angina). As the lesions grow and occlude more than 70% of the vessel, anginal symptoms may occur even when the person is resting (Cooke & Bhatnagar, 1997).

RISK ASSESSMENT

In 2013, the American College of Cardiology and the American Heart Association released guidelines on the assessment of CV risk (2013 ACC/AHA CV risk guidelines). While these guidelines encompass more than just assessment based on lipid levels, lipids are still an important part of the overall CV risk assessment for a patient. The workgroup echoed a well-established but important framework that the intensity of an intervention should be proportional to the individual's absolute risk for having a future atherosclerotic cardiovascular disease (ASCVD) event (**Box 20.2**). Health care practitioners can then utilize this framework by assessing a patient's ASCVD risk, discussing benefits and risks associated with potential therapies, and reviewing the patient's goals and preferences for treatment.

The 2013 ACC/AHA CV risk guidelines recommend assessment of traditional ASCVD risk factors in patients age 20

BOX 20.2 Atherosclerotic Vascular Disease (ASCVD)

Coronary Heart Disease (CHD)
Myocardial infarction
Significant myocardial ischemia (angina pectoris)
History of coronary artery bypass graft
History of coronary angioplasty
Angiographic evidence of lesions

Peripheral Vascular Disease
Claudication

Carotid Artery Disease
Thrombotic stroke
Transient ischemic attack

to 79 without a history of CVD every 4 to 6 years. In addition to lipid levels, these traditional risk factors include age, gender, systolic blood pressure, antihypertensive therapy use, presence of diabetes, and smoking status. While for the estimation of 10-year risk for ASCVD only total and HDL cholesterol levels are required, a full lipid panel, which also contains LDL cholesterol and triglycerides, should be obtained to fully evaluate a patient's ASCVD risk. A past medical history should also be obtained to determine if the patient has already had an ASCVD event such as an MI or thromboembolic stroke. Those patients with a past medical history of ASCVD, labeled as secondary prevention patients, are at a higher risk for a future ASCVD event than are those without a history of ASCVD, labeled as primary prevention.

To quantify the ASCVD risk in a primary prevention patient, the 2013 ACC/AHA CV risk guidelines recommend the use of the Pooled Cohort Equations that are race and gender specific. This risk assessment tool estimates the 10-year ASCVD risk for patients 40 to 79 years of age and the lifetime ASCVD risk for patients 20 to 59 years of age. The Pooled Cohort Equations are based off of multiple studies beyond the original Framingham study and were hoped to be an improvement on the Framingham risk calculator because the equations were developed in a broader population, including African Americans, and a fuller definition of ASCVD was utilized (CHD death, nonfatal MI, and fatal/nonfatal stroke). Patients with a 10-year ASCVD risk ≥7.5% are considered at elevated risk for a future ASCVD event. Some individuals have criticized the accuracy of the results the Pooled Cohort Equations generate for some patients and the use of a cut point for elevated risk of ≥7.5%. In order to potentially improve the ASCVD risk assessment in patients with borderline risk based on the traditional risk factors and to help inform treatment decisions, the 2013 ACC/AHA CV risk guidelines also addressed the use of several novel risk markers. Although the workgroup responsible for the development of these guidelines reviewed multiple novel risk markers, they identified the following four that were considered to show promise for clinical utility: family history of CVD, high-sensitivity C-reactive protein (hs-CRP), coronary artery calcium (CAC) score, and ankle–brachial index (ABI). hs-CRP is a marker for inflammation, and levels ≥2 mg/L have been associated with an increased risk of ASCVD.

Lifestyle Modification

In 2013, the American College of Cardiology and the American Heart Association also released guidelines on lifestyle management to reduce CV risk (2013 ACC/AHA lifestyle guidelines). These guidelines focused primarily on dietary therapy, exercise, weight loss, moderation of alcohol intake, and smoking cessation.

Diet

The guidelines recommend a diet that is high in fruits, vegetables, whole grains, low-fat dairy products, poultry, fish, legumes, nontropical vegetable oils, and nuts. It also recommends limiting sweets, sugar-sweetened beverages, and red meats. Individuals should try to limit caloric intake of saturated fat to no more that 5% to 6% of total calories. Additionally, it is recommended to limit intake of trans fats. Diets that are recommended include the Dietary Approaches to Stop Hypertension (DASH) dietary pattern, the USDA Food Pattern, or the AHA Diet.

In addition, overweight patients should attempt to lose weight. The ability to lose weight depends on the amount of calories consumed and the amount of calories burned. The goal for overweight patients should be a realistic, gradual, and steady loss of weight. Once an ideal weight is achieved, caloric intake is adjusted to maintain that weight.

Exercise

Regular physical exercise may provide several benefits in patients with hyperlipidemia.

The guidelines encourage individuals to participate in aerobic physical activity three to four times a week, with each session averaging about 40 minutes. As mentioned, it should be used along with dietary therapy to promote weight loss. Exercise may benefit the lipid profile by reducing triglycerides and raising HDL levels. Exercise may also improve control of diabetes and coronary blood flow.

Moderation of Alcohol Intake and Smoking Cessation

Excessive alcohol intake may elevate serum lipid levels, specifically triglyceride levels, but in moderation (no more than one drink per day for women and two drinks per day for men), alcohol may improve HDL levels and has been associated with lower ASCVD rates (Brien et al., 2011). Despite these benefits, alcohol should not be recommended for ASCVD prevention because the consequences associated with excessive alcohol use outweigh any benefits.

Cigarette smoking is an independent risk factor in the development of ASCVD (Huxley & Woodward, 2011). Although smoking minimally affects cholesterol levels, it contributes to the development of ASCVD by damaging the vascular endothelium and promoting platelet aggregation, which results in increased risk of clot formation. Smoking cessation can reduce this risk and should be encouraged by all health care professionals. The risk of developing ASCVD decreases by approximately 50% within 1 to 2 years of smoking cessation.

INITIATING DRUG THERAPY

The 2013 ACC/AHA treatment guidelines recommend use of HMG-CoA reductase inhibitors (statins) for ASCVD prevention in four groups of patients, termed "statin benefit groups." The statin benefit groups include individuals who are (1) ≥21 years of age and have clinical ASCVD or (2) do not have ASCVD but have LDL-C values ≥190 mg/dL or (3) are 40 to

TABLE 20.1
Four Major Statin Benefit Groups

Statin Benefit Group	Statin Dose Intensity
1. Have clinical ASCVD	High intensity ages ≤75 Moderate intensity >75 y
2. No ASCVD but have LDL-C values ≥190 mg/dL	High intensity unless contraindicated or unable to tolerate
3. No ASCVD and 40–75 y old with type 1 or type 2 diabetes mellitus and have LDL-C values of 70–189 mg/dL	Moderate-intensity statin if 10-year ASCVD risk is <7.5% High-intensity statin if 10-year ASCVD risk is ≥7.5%
4. No ASCVD or diabetes mellitus and are 40–75 y old with LDL-C values of 70–189 mg/dL and have a 10-year risk of ASCVD of ≥7.5%	Moderate-intensity statin if 10-year ASCVD risk is ≥7.5%.

75 years old with type 1 or type 2 diabetes mellitus and have LDL-C values of 70 to 189 mg/dL, or (4) are 40 to 75 years old with LDL-C values of 70 to 189 mg/dL and have a 10-year risk of ASCVD of ≥7.5% (**Table 20.1**).

The recommended statin and dose to use are based upon the expected reduction in LDL-C levels. High-intensity statins are those that can lower LDL-C by 50% or more, on average. Moderate-intensity statins reduce LDL-C by about 30% to 49%, and low-intensity statins typically reduce LDL-C by less than 30%. Specific medications and doses for each category are listed in **Table 20.2**.

In individuals with clinical ASCVD, a high-intensity statin is recommended in those ≤75 years of age, unless contraindicated (known hypersensitivity, active liver disease, women who are pregnant or may become pregnant, or nursing mothers) or unable to tolerate dose, in which a moderate-intensity statin should be used. For individuals with ASCVD who are greater than 75 years of age, a moderate-dose statin is recommended.

TABLE 20.2
Statin Dose Intensity (Daily Dose)

Generic Name (Trade Name)	High Intensity	Moderate Intensity	Low Intensity
atorvastatin (Lipitor)	40–80 mg	10–20 mg	NA
rosuvastatin (Crestor)	20–40 mg	5–10 mg	NA
simvastatin (Zocor)	NA	20–40 mg	10 mg
lovastatin (Mevacor)	NA	40 mg	20 mg
pravastatin (Pravachol)	NA	40–80 mg	10–20 mg
fluvastatin (Lescol)	NA	80 mg	20–40 mg
pitavastatin (Livalo)	NA	2–4 mg	1 mg

Individuals who do not have ASCVD but whose LDL-C is ≥190 mg/dL should receive high-intensity statin, unless contraindicated or unable to tolerate high-intensity statin.

A moderate-intensity statin is recommended for individuals aged 40 to 75 years old who have diabetes mellitus and have LDL-C between 70 and 189 mg/dL. High-intensity statin is recommended for patients meeting these criteria whose 10-year ASCVD risk is ≥7.5%. For diabetic patients aged less than 40 or greater than 75 years old, it is recommended to evaluate 10-year ASCVD risk to determine whether or not statin therapy should be considered.

For patients aged 40 to 75 years old without ASCVD, without diabetes mellitus, and whose LDL-C is between 70 and 189 mg/dL, treatment with a moderate-intensity statin is indicated when 10-year ASCVD risk is ≥7.5%.

Goals of Statin Therapy and Monitoring

The 2013 guidelines do not provide a specific recommendation on target cholesterol levels. However, they do recommend obtaining a fasting lipid panel within 1 to 3 months after initiating treatment for the purpose of evaluating medication adherence. For individuals whose response is less than expected, providers should assess reasons for nonadherence, including intolerance to the statin. Inadequate response would include an LDL-C reduction of less than 50% for those on high-intensity statin, and less than 30% LDL-C reduction in those on moderate-intensity statin. If intolerance to the statin is not an issue, providers should reinforce the need for adherence. For individuals who do have the expected response, they should be monitored every 3 to 12 months for continued assessment. If response continues to be lower than expected, then consider adding a nonstatin medication. Decreasing the statin dose could also be recommended in patients whose LDL-C decreases to less than 40 mg/dL.

Statin Intolerance

The statins are well tolerated by most patients and long-term therapy does not appear to have any serious risks. The most common complaint with statin use is muscle-related symptoms, including pain, tenderness, weakness, and fatigue. These symptoms combined with a creatine phosphokinase (CPK) level 10 times above the upper normal limits are consistent with a diagnosis of myopathy. If severe symptoms occur, the patient should be evaluated for rhabdomyolysis, a severe breakdown of muscle cells that leak into the urine and can result in renal failure. If suspected, the statin should be discontinued and should have creatinine kinase, serum creatinine, and urinalysis performed.

If individuals develop mild to moderate muscle-related symptoms, it is reasonable to discontinue the statin and see if the symptoms resolve. If symptoms resolve after discontinuation, and patient has no other contraindications, it is recommended to restart the same statin at a lower dose or start a different statin at a lower intensity dose. If patient is able to tolerate the lower dose statin, the dose can gradually be increased

to recommended dose as tolerated. Individuals who are unable to achieve recommended statin dose or tolerate statins all together should consider use of nonstatin medications.

HMG-CoA Reductase Inhibitors (Statins)

Statins primarily block the conversion of HMG-CoA to mevalonate, which is the rate-limiting step in the production of cholesterol in the liver. Blocking the production of cholesterol in the liver leads to an increase in the number of LDL cholesterol receptors on the liver. As a result, a larger amount of LDL cholesterol is taken up by the liver, thereby decreasing the amount of LDL cholesterol in the bloodstream (**Figure 20.1**).

LDL receptors are also involved with the uptake of VLDL and IDL, thus leading to a decrease in triglyceride levels. In addition, modest increases in HDL tend to occur. Despite having the same mechanism of action, there are differences between the agents, including the magnitude of their cholesterol lowering (**Table 20.2**). For example, fluvastatin (Lescol) can lower LDL cholesterol levels up to approximately 36% with the maximum dose, whereas atorvastatin (Lipitor) and rosuvastatin (Crestor) can lower LDL cholesterol levels up to 60% at maximum doses.

Maximum effects usually are seen after 4 to 6 weeks of therapy. For this reason, dosage adjustments should not be made more frequently than every 4 weeks.

Contraindications

There are several instances when statins are contraindicated or should be used with caution. Although no studies have been conducted in pregnant women, lovastatin causes skeletal malformations in rats, so statins are contraindicated during pregnancy. These agents should be used with extreme caution in women who are breast-feeding because they may be excreted in breast milk.

Statins are also contraindicated in patients with active liver disease or with unexplained elevated aminotransferase levels. They should be used with caution in patients who consume large amounts of alcohol or have a history of liver disease.

Adverse Events

The statins are well tolerated by most patients and long-term therapy does not appear to have any serious risks, although statin intolerance is still an important issue. As mentioned previously, the most common cause of statin intolerance is due to myopathies. Gastrointestinal (GI) complaints and headache are typically among the most commonly reported adverse events, but they are usually mild and transient. Asymptomatic elevations in liver function test (LFT) values may also occur. Traditionally, LFTs were recommended to be monitored at baseline (before starting therapy), at 6 and 12 weeks after starting or titrating therapy, and periodically thereafter. However, after decades of use and data from numerous clinical trials, these monitoring parameters have been relaxed. The 2013 ACC/AHA cholesterol treatment guidelines recommend that transaminase (ALT) levels should be performed before initiating statin therapy and

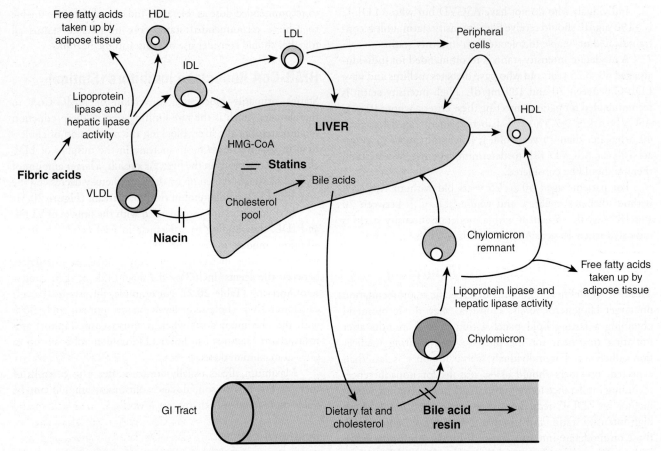

FIGURE 20.1 How lipid-lowering drugs work. The statins work in the liver by blocking the conversion of HMG-CoA to mevalonate, which is involved in producing cholesterol. The bile acid resins bind bile acid in the intestines for excretion in the feces so that lipids are not absorbed by the intestinal tract and returned to the liver. Niacin works to decrease circulating triglyceride and LDL cholesterol and fibric acid derivatives appear to lower triglyceride levels and stimulate lipoprotein lipase, which enhances the breakdown of VLDL to LDL cholesterol.

during therapy only as clinically indicated if hepatotoxic symptoms present. This approach is consistent with most of the package insert recommendations for the statins.

Interactions

The risk of myopathy is most common when using statins at high doses or in combination with drugs that can also cause myopathy (including other lipid-lowering agents) or that can affect the metabolism of the statins (e.g., cyclosporine, erythromycin, azole antifungals). Moreover, myopathy may occur at any time during therapy. Patients should be instructed to report any unusual muscle pain or weakness during therapy.

The practitioner should encourage the patient to take the statins in the evening or at bedtime because a significant amount of cholesterol production seems to occur during sleep. By taking the medication before bedtime, peak concentrations of medication occur during sleep. Exceptions are lovastatin, which has an increased bioavailability when taken with food and is usually taken with the evening meal, and atorvastatin and rosuvastatin, which can be taken at any time during the day because of their long half-lives.

Cholesterol Absorption Inhibitors

Currently, there is only one cholesterol absorption inhibitor on the market, ezetimibe (Zetia). Ezetimibe appears to act at the brush border of the small intestine and inhibits the absorption of cholesterol, leading to a decrease in the delivery of intestinal cholesterol to the liver. This causes a reduction of hepatic cholesterol stores and an increase in clearance of cholesterol from the blood; this distinct mechanism is complementary to that of HMG-CoA reductase inhibitors.

Zetia, introduced in April 2003, is indicated for use as monotherapy or as combination therapy with a statin. LDL cholesterol levels are reduced by up to 18% with monotherapy and up to an additional 25% when added to ongoing statin therapy. Together with a statin, LDL cholesterol reductions of more than 50% have been noted. The recommended dosage of ezetimibe is 10 mg daily. If taken with a bile acid sequestrant, ezetimibe should be taken 2 hours before or 4 hours after the bile acid (**Table 20.3**).

The Ezetimibe and Simvastatin Hypercholesterolemia Enhances Atherosclerosis Regression (ENHANCE) trial, which

TABLE 20.3

Doses and Lipid-Lowering Ability of Other Available Agents

Class	Generic Name (Trade Name)	Usual Daily Dose	LDL*	HDL*	Triglycerides*
Bile acid resins	cholestyramine (Questran, Questran Light, Prevalite)	4–16 g	↓13%–32%	↑3%–5%	↑0%–15%
	colesevelam (Welchol)	3.75 g	↓15%–18%	↑3%	↑9%–10%
Cholesterol absorption inhibitors	ezetimibe (Zetia)†	10 mg	↓16%–19%	↑3%–4%	↓5%
			↓33%–60%	↑8%–11%	↓19%–40%
Niacin‡	niacin (various)	1.5–3.0 g	↓12%–21%	↑18%–30%	↓15%–44%
Fibric acid derivatives	gemfibrozil (Lopid)	600 mg bid	0	↑6%	↓31%
	fenofibrate (various)	48–200 mg qd	↓20%	↑11%	↓38%
Combination products	lovastatin/niacin	20/500 to 40/2,000 mg	↓30%–42%	↑20%–30%	↓32%–44%
simvastatin/ezetimibe		10/10 to 80/10 mg	↓45%–60%	↑6%–10%	↓23%–31%

*Effects on lipid levels are dose dependent.
†Results in first line are those seen when used as monotherapy (Bays et al., 2001). Second results are those seen when used with statin therapy (Kerzner et al., 2003 [lovastatin]; Davidson et al., 2002 [simvastatin]; Ballantyne et al., 2003 [atorvastatin]).
‡Dose must be titrated slowly (usually weekly) to avoid side effects.

evaluated the impact of adding ezetimibe to simvastatin, found no significant change in carotid artery intima–media thickness (a marker for atherosclerosis progression) despite significant decreases in LDL cholesterol and CRP levels (Kastelein et al., 2008). However, the more recent Improved Reduction in Outcomes: Vytorin Efficacy International Trial (IMPROVE-IT) showed that the addition of ezetimibe 10 mg to simvastatin 40 mg reduced CV events compared to simvastatin alone. While the magnitude of the results were not large (5.8% relative risk reduction, 2.0% absolute risk reduction—both statistically significant), they were very important in that it was the first trial to demonstrate incremental benefit in ASCVD event reduction with a nonstatin added to a statin compared to the statin alone.

Contraindications

Ezetimibe is contraindicated in patients who have a hypersensitivity to any component of the medication. The combination of ezetimibe with an HMG-CoA reductase inhibitor is contraindicated in patients with active liver disease or unexplained persistent elevations in serum transaminases. There are no adequate, controlled studies of ezetimibe in pregnant women, so use during pregnancy is indicated only if the potential benefit outweighs any potential risk to the fetus.

Adverse Events

Adverse events with ezetimibe are minimal. Adverse events noted in clinical trials include headache, diarrhea, and abdominal pain. In addition, myopathy and rhabdomyolysis have been noted when given in combination with statins. The incidence of elevated liver enzymes was similar to placebo.

Bile Acid Resins

Bile acid resins decrease cholesterol absorption through the exogenous pathway. These agents are not absorbed from the GI tract. They act to bind bile acids in the intestines, forming an insoluble complex that is excreted in the feces. This decreases the return of cholesterol to the liver. The body responds to this by increasing LDL receptors on the liver, which in turn increases the amount of LDL cholesterol taken up by the liver and thus decreases LDL cholesterol levels in the bloodstream (see **Figure 20.1**). Unfortunately, this process also leads to increased production of VLDL particles. As a result, triglyceride levels rise, especially in patients with elevated baseline triglyceride levels. Bile acid resins can decrease LDL cholesterol levels by 15% to 30%, increase HDL levels by approximately 3%, and increase triglyceride levels by up to 15% (**Table 20.3**). As with the statins, these effects are dose related.

Maximum effects of cholesterol lowering are seen in approximately 3 weeks. Bile acid resins are indicated as adjunct therapy for patients who do not respond to dietary therapy alone. Because of their safety with long-term use, they are extremely useful in young adult men and premenopausal women who are at relatively low CV risk. These agents are contraindicated in patients with biliary obstruction or chronic constipation.

Contraindications

Bile acid resins should not be used in patients whose fasting triglyceride levels are ≥ 300 mg/dL, as it may lead to a severe increase in triglyceride levels. They can be used with caution in patients whose baseline triglycerides are between 250 and 299 mg/dL, with monitoring every 4 to 6 weeks.

Adverse Events

Bile acid resins are not absorbed, and therefore, systemic adverse events are minimal. Monitoring for abnormal LFT values is not required. The most common adverse events are GI related and include flatulence, bloating, abdominal pain, heartburn, and constipation. For these reasons, some patients, such as elderly patients, may not be good candidates for bile acid resins.

Interactions

Because bile acid resins block the absorption of cholesterol from the GI tract, they should be taken with meals to maximize effectiveness. These agents are usually administered once or twice daily but can be taken up to four times a day. If taken once a day, a bile acid resin should be taken with the largest meal. The two major agents in this class are cholestyramine (Questran, Questran Light, Prevalite) and colesevelam (Welchol).

Cholestyramine is available as a powder and colestipol is available as granules or tablets. The powder and granules should be mixed with water, noncarbonated beverages, soups, or pulpy fruits such as applesauce. The tablets should be swallowed whole with water or other fluids. These agents should not be taken dry because they can cause esophageal distress. Patients should avoid taking these agents with carbonated beverages because it may result in increased GI discomfort. Medications taken concomitantly, such as thyroid hormones, antibiotics, and fat-soluble vitamins, should be taken at least 1 hour before or 4 hours after the bile acid resin because of their potential to bind to other medications and decrease their bioavailability.

Niacin

Niacin (nicotinic acid) is a naturally occurring B vitamin that can improve cholesterol levels when used at doses 100 to 300 times the recommended daily allowance as a vitamin. Niacin's mechanism of action is uncertain, but the substance appears to decrease VLDL synthesis in the liver, inhibit lipolysis in adipose tissue, and increase lipoprotein lipase activity. This results in decreased triglyceride and LDL cholesterol levels in the bloodstream (see **Figure 20.1**). LDL cholesterol levels can be decreased by 15% to 25% and triglycerides by up to 50%, whereas HDL cholesterol levels may be increased by up to 35% (see **Table 20.3**). Although niacin is one of the most effective agents in improving cholesterol levels, most patients cannot tolerate the adverse events associated with its use (see Adverse Events). Additionally, there is very little evidence to suggest that it can reduce ASCVD events further when added to statin therapy.

Dosage

Doses of immediate release products are at least 1.5 g niacin daily are usually required to achieve beneficial effects on lipid levels. However, to minimize adverse events, dosages need to be titrated gradually. The usual starting dose for immediate release products is 50 to 100 mg two or three times a day. The dose can be increased every 1 to 2 weeks until a dosage of 1.0 to 1.5 g daily is reached; this should take approximately 4 to 5 weeks. This dosage range provides significant increases (15% to 30%) in HDL cholesterol levels and decreases (20% to 30%) in triglyceride levels. However, for maximal LDL cholesterol lowering, dosages of 3 g/d or more may be necessary. Niacin is available in both immediate-release and sustained-release formulations. Maximum effects usually are

seen after 4 to 6 weeks of therapy on the aforementioned dosages.

Contraindications

Niacin is contraindicated in patients with hepatic dysfunction, severe hypotension, persistent hyperglycemia, acute gout, new-onset atrial fibrillation, or active peptic ulcers. In addition, niacin can elevate uric acid levels and worsen glucose control. Therefore, niacin is not a first-line treatment agent in patients with gout or diabetes mellitus, and it should be used cautiously in these populations.

Adverse Events

Niacin use has been limited primarily because of its extensive adverse events. Although it is one of the most effective agents for improving lipid profiles, many patients cannot tolerate the adverse events. The most common adverse events are attributed to an increase in prostaglandin activity and include pruritus and flushing of the face and neck. A dose of aspirin, 325 mg, taken 30 minutes before the niacin dose may decrease the severity. As mentioned earlier, niacin can also increase uric acid levels and worsen glucose control and should be used cautiously, if at all, in patients with a history of gout or diabetes mellitus. Baseline glucose and uric acid levels should be checked in all patients starting niacin therapy.

Other adverse events include GI side effects (it is contraindicated in patients with an active peptic ulcer), rash, hepatotoxicity, and, rarely, acanthosis nigricans (hyperpigmentation of the skin, usually in the axilla, neck, or groin). Unlike statins, LFTs are still recommended to be monitored at 6 and 12 weeks after initiating or titrating therapy and periodically thereafter.

Fibric Acid Derivatives

Fibric acid derivatives class of lipid-lowering drugs mainly affects triglyceride and HDL cholesterol levels. The exact mechanism of action of fibric acid derivatives is unclear, but the principal effect of triglyceride lowering appears to result from the stimulation of lipoprotein lipase, which enhances the breakdown of VLDL to LDL cholesterol (see **Figure 20.1**).

These agents may also inhibit hepatic VLDL production, and they lower triglyceride levels up to 60% and increase HDL cholesterol by up to 30%. Although gemfibrozil and clofibrate (Atromid-S) have minimal effects on LDL cholesterol lowering, fenofibrate (TriCor) has been shown to decrease LDL cholesterol by up to 20%. Fibric acid derivatives are primarily indicated in patients who have severely elevated triglyceride levels and who have not responded to dietary therapy (see **Table 20.3**).

Gemfibrozil and fenofibrate are the currently available fibric acid derivatives.

Dosage

Gemfibrozil is given in 600-mg doses twice daily with breakfast and dinner. No titration of dose is necessary, although some patients may respond at lower doses. Fenofibrate therapy is initiated at 43 to 67 mg/d (depending upon formulation). The dosage can be increased to a maximum of 200 mg/d. Because its absorption is increased when taken with food, fenofibrate should be taken with meals.

Contraindications

Fibric acid derivatives are contraindicated in patients with a history of gallstones and in those with severe hepatic or renal dysfunction. No studies have been conducted in pregnant women, so therefore, these agents should be used only if the benefits clearly outweigh any risks to the fetus.

Adverse Events

The fibric acid derivatives usually are well tolerated. The most common adverse events are GI related and include epigastric pain, nausea and vomiting, dyspepsia, flatulence, and constipation. Myopathy may occur and the incidence is increased when fibric acid derivatives are used with lovastatin and simvastatin and, to a lesser degree, other statins and niacin. As with the other systemic lipid-lowering agents, hepatotoxicity can occur, and LFTs should be monitored at 6 and 12 weeks and periodically thereafter. If LFT values increase to more than three times the upper normal limits, the fibric acid derivative should be discontinued. Other adverse events include rhabdomyolysis, cholestatic jaundice, gallstones, and, rarely, leukopenia, anemia, and thrombocytopenia.

Interactions

As mentioned previously, the incidence of myopathy is increased when fibric acids, especially gemfibrozil, are used in combination with lovastatin and simvastatin and, to a lesser degree, other statins and niacin. In fact, the combination of gemfibrozil and simvastatin is contraindicated. Fenofibrate should be used with caution in patients taking anticoagulant therapy because it can increase the effects of the anticoagulant. Doses of the anticoagulant should be lowered and levels monitored closely if fenofibrate therapy is initiated.

Omega-3 Fatty Acids

Similar to fibric acids, omega-3 fatty acids are not considered a major class of lipid-lowering drugs due to a lack of LDL cholesterol lowering. In some cases, omega-3 fatty acids may increase LDL cholesterol levels. Additionally, there have been no studies showing reduced CV morbidity and mortality. There are numerous over-the-counter dietary supplements that contain omega-3 fatty acids, and omega-3-acid ethyl esters by prescription. These agents are all indicated as an adjunct to diet for the treatment of severe hypertriglyceridemia. Patients should be on a lipid-lowering diet before treatment with any omega 3 fatty acids or omega-3-acid ethyl esters is initiated.

Dosage

All prescription Omega 3 products are given as a once- or twice-daily dose. Patients can take either 4 g (four capsules) daily or 2 g (two capsules) twice daily. There is no dose titration.

Contraindications

Any omega 3 fatty acids is contraindicated in patients with a known hypersensitivity to the drug. To date, there is no evidence to suggest that patients who have fish allergies are at an increased risk for an allergic reaction with these agents. There are no studies that have included pregnant women, so it should only be used if the benefits outweigh any potential risks to the fetus.

Adverse Events

Omega-3 fatty acids are generally well tolerated. Some of the side effects noted in clinical trials include flulike symptoms, belching, taste changes, upset stomach, and back pain.

Interactions

There has been some evidence to suggest that omega-3 fatty acids prolong bleeding time, but no studies have been performed to determine if there is an interaction with concomitant use of anticoagulants.

Medications for Familial Homozygous Hypercholesterolemia

Familial homozygous hypercholesterolemia (FH) is a rare genetic disorder characterized by dysfunctional LDL cholesterol receptors on the liver, which leads to severely elevated cholesterol levels (LDL cholesterol levels greater than 600 mg/dL) and ASCVD at an early age. Due to the lack of function of the LDL cholesterol receptors, many lipid-modifying agents including statins show significantly reduced effects on LDL cholesterol reduction in this clinical setting. In 2013, mipomersen and lomitapide were approved in the United States for the treatment of FH. Mipomersen (Kynamro) and lomitapide (Juxtapid) have been shown to reduce LDL cholesterol levels by 25% and 40%, respectively, on top of what had been achieved with maximum tolerated statin doses. Due to the extremely small overall patient population affected by FH, ASVCD event reduction studies will not be possible. Severe liver toxicity is associated with these agents. Due to this, specific FDA-mandated training is required before prescribing these medications, which should only be used in patients with FH.

Two new medications, alirocumab (Praulent) and evolocumab (Repatha), which are monoclonal antibodies that target proprotein convertase subtilisin/kexin type 9 (PCSK9) were approved by the FDA in late 2015. These agents, which are injectables, provide LDL-C lowering of up to 60% or more when used alone or when added on to statin therapy, though no studies have been completed to date to determine if these reductions in cholesterol result in fewer CV events. Initial indications for use are adjunct to maximally tolerated statin therapy in adults with heterozygous and/or homozygous familial hypercholesterolemia or clinical ASCVD.

Combination Therapy

In the past, it was thought that it would be beneficial for patients to be prescribed combination lipid-lowering therapy to achieve desired cholesterol levels, particularly those with severe hypertriglyceridemia or severely elevated LDL cholesterol levels who do not respond adequately to a statin alone or are intolerant to statin doses needed to attain desired LDL-C reduction. Statin/niacin and statin/gemfibrozil have been used together for patients with severely elevated LDL cholesterol, low HDL cholesterol, and hypertriglyceridemia. Currently, there are two products available that include a statin and niacin in a single formulation: lovastatin/niacin (Advicor) and simvastatin/niacin (Simcor). However, to date, there have been no studies showing an increased benefit in reducing CV morbidity and mortality from either of these combinations. Combining statins with a cholesterol absorption inhibitor has shown added benefits in reducing both LDL cholesterol and ASCVD event rates. As previously mentioned, this is the only lipid medication combined with a statin to show incremental benefits in ASCVD event rates. Bile acid resins can be used safely and effectively with statins, niacin, and fibric acid derivatives to enhance LDL cholesterol lowering. The only concern with using bile acid resins in combination is ensuring that the concomitant medications are taken at least 1 hour before or 4 hours after the resin to ensure adequate GI absorption.

Alternative Therapy

Antioxidant therapy has been a major focus of studies on preventing ASCVD, but its preventive benefits have yet to be determined. In theory, antioxidants block the conversion of LDL cholesterol to a modified (oxidized) LDL in the vascular endothelium. As mentioned previously, modified LDL cholesterol appears to be more atherogenic than nonoxidized LDL cholesterol. Thus, blocking the production of oxidized LDL cholesterol may slow the atherogenic process. The major antioxidants that have been studied include vitamin E, vitamin C, and beta carotene, a precursor of vitamin A. Most of the beneficial evidence has been seen with the use of vitamin E, but there is no strong evidence to support vitamin E use.

Other alternatives include garlic, vinegar, and fish oils. Although some evidence suggests that these may be beneficial, no conclusive evidence exists to support their use.

SELECTING THE MOST APPROPRIATE THERAPY

Choosing which drug to use in which order is individualized and based on the patient's clinical status, the impact on heart health by the surrogate marker of cholesterol lowering, and an assessment of patient compliance. Factors that affect compliance include side effects, cost of therapy, health beliefs supporting the need to lower cholesterol levels, and the understanding that this is a lifelong treatment. In a study by Wei et al. (2013), the primary reasons for discontinuation of statins are muscle pain (60%), cost of therapy (16%), and perceived lack of efficacy (13%). Further, the Statin Intolerance Panel (2014) recommends that a patient-centered approach is important to reduce statin intolerance; true intolerance is estimated at a rate of approximately 10%. See **Table 20.4** and **Figure 20.2** for further guidance in drug selection.

Special Population Considerations
Pediatric

Pharmacologic therapy may be considered in children older than age 10 if lifestyle modifications cannot adequately lower cholesterol levels. Use in children younger than age 10 usually is not recommended because atherosclerotic lesions are not

---

TABLE 20.4

Selecting the Most Appropriate Agent

	Agents	Comments
First line	Statins	Most experts agree that the benefits of treatment with statins are a class-wide effect. Choice of agent and dose is dependent upon the statin benefit group that an individual is classified.
Second line	Cholesterol absorption inhibitors	Cholesterol absorption inhibitors can be used alone or in combination with statins. When used in combination, LDL cholesterol lowering of ~60% has been shown, resulting in fewer ASCVD events.
	Niacin and bile acid resins	Niacin has beneficial effects on each of the lipoproteins, but most patients cannot tolerate the side effects of the drug.
		Bile acids are not systemically absorbed and can be used in patients who cannot tolerate the effects of statins or in combination with statins for patients who are unable to reach LDL goal on a statin alone.
Third line	Fibric acid derivatives	Fibric acid derivatives are reserved for patients with very high triglyceride levels (>1,000 mg/dL) who do not respond to dietary interventions or in combination with other agents for patients with elevated triglyceride levels that cannot be controlled with other agents.

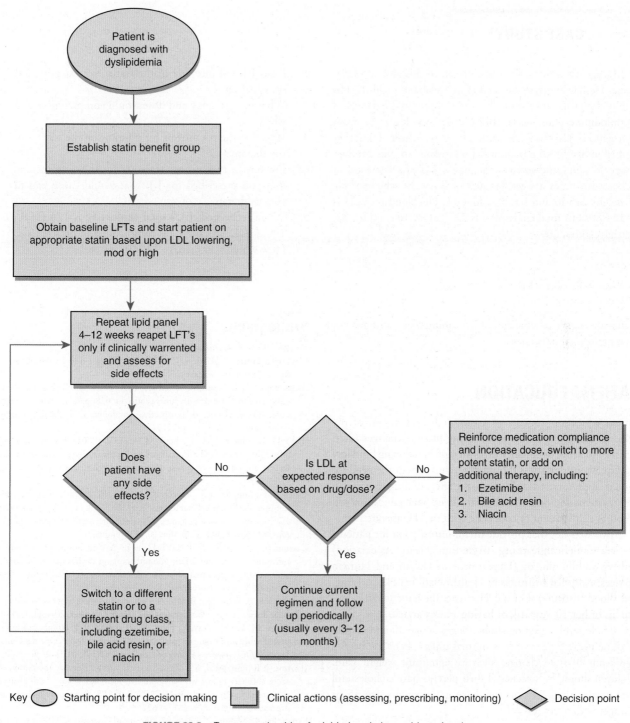

Key ⬭ Starting point for decision making   ▭ Clinical actions (assessing, prescribing, monitoring)   ⬦ Decision point

FIGURE 20.2   Treatment algorithm for initiating cholesterol-lowering therapy.

thought to develop before this age. A consultation with a lipid specialist is recommended for any child with elevated cholesterol levels.

Geriatric

Though there have not been a large number of patients over the age of 75 included in most randomized clinical trials, evidence does support continuation of use of

statins in individuals who have been taking them. If statins are used, it is recommended to use a moderate-intensity statin.

Women

Statins are classified as category X by the U.S. Food and Drug Administration and should not be used by pregnant women because of the potential for fetal abnormalities. Most other

CASE STUDY*

J.J., age 55 white male, has come in for his annual physical. He has hypertension and type 2 diabetes mellitus. His blood pressure is controlled with lisinopril 20 mg daily and amlodipine 5 mg daily (BP 132/82 mm Hg). His most recent HbA1c was 7.2% while taking metformin. His father died at age 55 of a myocardial infarction, and his brother, age 57, just underwent angioplasty. **J.J.** eats fast food at least five times a week because of his work schedule. He weighs 245 lb and stands 5-foot-11. His blood pressure is 134/80. His total cholesterol is 237 (LDL, 162; HDL, 35; triglycerides, 200).

1. Does **J.J.** fall into any of the statin risk categories? If so, which one?
2. What drug therapy and dose would you prescribe, and why?
3. What are the parameters for monitoring the success of the therapy?
4. List one or two adverse reactions for the drug therapy that you prescribed for **J.J.** that would cause you to change therapy.
5. When rechecked, **J.J.'s** total cholesterol is 174 (LDL, 100; HDL, 38), but he is complaining of muscle pain. How would you manage **J.J.'s** treatment?

* Answers can be found online.

agents are classified as category C, meaning that tests have not been performed in humans.

PATIENT EDUCATION

Patient education consists of a thorough explanation of the value of modifying habits and making lifestyle changes (diet, exercise) to avoid or enhance drug therapy in reducing lipid levels. Equally important is thorough teaching about the need for regular laboratory tests to evaluate the effect of drug therapy on body systems and organs, such as the liver. Such education will encourage the patient to cooperate with the therapeutic plan.

Two websites that provide useful information for patients are www.americanheart.org (American Heart Association) and www.nhlbi.nih.gov (Department of Health and Human Services, National Institutes of Health, National Heart, Lung, and Blood Institute). On the latter site, the patient can calculate his or her 10-year risk of having a heart attack.

Cholesterol screening should begin at age 20 and should be done every 5 years if it is normal unless there has been a significant lifestyle change, such as significant weight gain. Children should be screened if their parents have a cholesterol level greater than 240 or they have grandparents age 55 or younger with overt ASCVD.

Drug Information

Grapefruit juice may increase the potency of all statins except pravastatin. Patients taking statins should report any new muscle pain, since these drugs can cause myopathy and, rarely, rhabdomyolysis.

Nutrition

The patient should eat a diet low in saturated fats and cholesterol. The diet can include up to 35% daily fats, but no more than 7% saturated fats.

Bibliography

*Starred references are cited in the text.
*American Heart Association. (2015). Heart disease and stroke statistics. Retrieved from www.americanheart.org
*Ballantyne, C. M., Houri, J., Notarbartolo, A., et al. (2003). Effect of ezetimibe coadministered with atorvastatin in 628 patients with primary hypercholesterolemia: A prospective, randomized, double-blind trial. Circulation, 107(19), 2409–2415.
*Bays, H. E., Moore, P. B., Drehobl, M. A., et al. (2001). Effectiveness and tolerability of ezetimibe in patients with primary hypercholesterolemia: Pooled analysis of two phase II studies. Clinical Therapeutics, 23(8), 1209–1230.
*Brien, S. E., Ronksley, P. E., Turner, B. J., et al. (2011). Effect of alcohol consumption on biological markers associated with risk of coronary heart disease: Systematic review and meta-analysis of interventional studies. British Medical Journal, 342, d636. doi: 10.1136/bmj.d636.
Cannon, C. P. (2014). IMPROVE-IT trial: A comparison of ezetimibe/simvastatin versus simvastatin monotherapy on cardiovascular outcomes after acute coronary syndromes. American Heart Association 2014 Scientific Sessions, November 17, 2014. Chicago, IL.
*Cooke, J. P., & Bhatnagar, R. (1997). Pathophysiology of atherosclerotic vascular disease. Disease Management and Health Outcomes, 2(Suppl. 1), 1–8.
*Davidson, M. H., McGarry, T., Bettis, R., et al. (2002). Ezetimibe coadministered with simvastatin in patients with primary hypercholesterolemia. Journal of the American College of Cardiology, 40(12), 2125–2134.
*Downs, J. R., Clearfield, M., Weis, S., et al. (1998). Primary prevention of acute coronary events with lovastatin in men and women with average cholesterol levels: Results of AFCAPS/TexCAPS. Journal of the American Medical Association, 279, 1615–1622.
Expert Panel, National Cholesterol Education Program. (2001). Executive summary of the third report of the National Cholesterol Education Program (NCEP) Expert Panel on Detection, Evaluation and Treatment of High Blood Cholesterol in Adults (Adult Treatment Panel III). Journal of the American Medical Association, 285, 2486–2497.
*Frick, H., Elo, O., Kaapa, K., et al. (1987). Helsinki Heart Study: Primary prevention trial with gemfibrozil in middle-aged men with dyslipidemia. New England Journal of Medicine, 257, 3233–3240.
Genest, J., McPherson, R., Frohlich, J., et al. (2009). Canadian Cardiovascular Society/Canadian guidelines for the diagnosis and treatment of dyslipidemia and prevention of cardiovascular disease in the adult—2009 recommendations. Canadian Journal of Cardiology, 25, 567–579.
Guyton, J., Bays, H., Grundy, S., et al. (2014). An assessment by the Statin Intolerance Panel: 2014 update. Journal of Clinical Lipidology, 8(3), S72–S81. doi: 10.1016/j.jacl.2014.03.002

*Heart Protection Study Collaborative Group. (2002). MRC/BHF Heart Protection Study of cholesterol lowering with simvastatin in 20,536 high-risk individuals: A randomised placebo-controlled trial. *Lancet, 360,* 7–22.

*Huxley, R., & Woodward, M. (2011). Cigarette smoking as a risk factor for coronary heart disease in women compared with men: A systematic review and meta-analysis of prospective cohort studies. *Lancet, 378*(9799), 1297–1305.

*Kastelein, J. J., Akdim, F., Stroes, E. S., et al.; For the ENHANCE Investigators. (2008). Simvastatin with or without ezetimibe in familial hypercholesterolemia. *New England Journal of Medicine, 358,* 1431–1443.

*Kerzner, B., Corbelli, J., Sharp, S., et al. (2003). Efficacy and safety of ezetimibe coadministered with lovastatin in primary hypercholesterolemia. *American Journal of Cardiology, 91*(4), 418–424.

*Lewis, S. J., Moye, L. A., Sacks, F. M., et al. (1998). Effect of pravastatin on cardiovascular events in older patients with myocardial infarction and cholesterol levels in the average range: Results of the Cholesterol and Recurrent Events (CARE) Trial. *Annals of Internal Medicine, 129,* 681–689.

*Long-Term Intervention With Pravastatin in Ischaemic Disease (LIPID) Study Group. (1998). Prevention of cardiovascular events and death with pravastatin in patients with coronary heart disease and a broad range of initial cholesterol levels. *New England Journal of Medicine, 339,* 1349–1357.

*McKenney, J. M., & Hawkins, D. W. (1995). *Handbook on the management of lipid disorders.* Springfield, NJ: National Pharmacy Cholesterol Council/Scientific Therapeutics Information, Inc.

McKenney, J. M., Jones, P. H., Adamczyk, M. A., et al. (2003). Comparison of efficacy of rosuvastatin vs. atorvastatin, simvastatin and pravastatin in achieving lipid goals. Results from STELLAR trial. *Current Medical Research and Opinion, 19*(8), 689–698.

Mozaffarian, D., Benjamin, E., Go, A., et al. (2015). Executive summary: Heart disease and stroke statistics—2015 update. A report from the American Heart Association. *Circulation, 131,* 434–441. doi: 10.1161/CIR. 0000000000000157

National Heart, Lung and Blood Institute. (2002). *Morbidity and mortality: 2002 chartbook on cardiovascular, lung and blood disease.* Bethesda, MD: U.S. Department of Health and Human Services, Public Health Service.

*Newby, L. K., LaPointe, N. M., Chen, A. Y., et al. (2006). Long-term adherence to evidence-base secondary prevention therapies in coronary artery disease. *Circulation, 113,* 203–212.

Pearson, T. A., Mensah, G. A., Alexander, R. W., et al. (2003). Markers of inflammation and cardiovascular disease: Application to clinical and public health practice: A statement for healthcare professionals from the centers for disease control and prevention and the American Heart Association. *Circulation, 107,* 499–511.

*Ridker, P. M., Danielson, E., Fonseca, F. A., et al. (2008). Rosuvastatin to prevent vascular events in men and women with elevated C-reactive protein. *New England Journal of Medicine, 359,* 2195–2207.

Ridker, P. M., Hennekens, C. H., Buring, J. E., et al. (2000). C-reactive protein and other markers of inflammation in the prediction of cardiovascular disease in women. *New England Journal of Medicine, 342,* 836–884.

*Ross, R., & Glomset, J. A. (1976). The pathogenesis of atherosclerosis (first of two parts). *New England Journal of Medicine, 295,* 369–377.

Rubins, H. B., Robins, S. J., Collins, D., et al. (1999). Gemfibrozil for the secondary prevention of coronary heart disease in men with low levels of high-density lipoprotein cholesterol. *New England Journal of Medicine, 341,* 410–418.

Sacks, F. M., Pfeffer, M. A., Moye, L. A., et al. (1996). The effect of pravastatin on coronary events after myocardial infarction in patients with average cholesterol levels: The Cholesterol and Recurrent Events Trial. *New England Journal of Medicine, 335,* 1001–1009.

*Scandinavian Simvastatin Survival Study Group. (1994). Randomized trial of cholesterol lowering in 4,444 patients with coronary heart disease: The Scandinavian Simvastatin Survival Study (4S). *Lancet, 344,* 1383–1389.

*Shepherd, J., Cobb, S. M., Ford, I., et al. (1995). Prevention of coronary heart disease with pravastatin in men with hypercholesterolemia: The West of Scotland Coronary Prevention Study. *New England Journal of Medicine, 333,* 1301–1307.

*Talbert, R. L. (1997). Hyperlipidemia. In J. T. Dipiro, R. L. Talbert, G. C. Yee, G. R. Matzke, B. G. Wells, & L. M. Posey (Eds.), *Pharmacotherapy: A pathophysiologic approach* (3rd ed., pp. 459–489). Stamford, CT: Appleton & Lange.

*Wei, M., Ito, M., Cohen, J., et al. (2013). Predictors of statin adherence, switching, and discontinuation in the USAGE survey: Understanding the use of statins in America and gaps in patient education. *Journal of Clinical Lipidology, 7*(5). 472–483. doi: 10.1016/j.jacl.2013.03.001

Weinberger, Y. & Han, B. (2015). Statin treatment for older adults: The impact of the 2013 ACC/AHA cholesterol guidelines. *Drugs and Aging, 32,* 87–93. doi: 10.1007/s40266-014-0238-5

21 Chronic Stable Angina

Andrew M. Peterson ◼ Christopher C. Roe

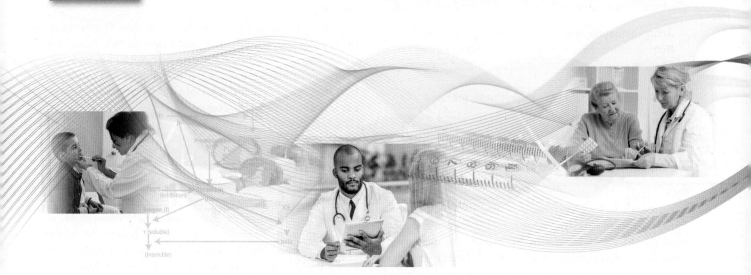

Cardiovascular disease was responsible for nearly 40.6% of deaths recorded in 2014, making it the leading cause of death in the United States (Go et al., 2014). Angina is a clinical syndrome caused by coronary heart disease (CHD) and affects nearly 10.2 million Americans. In 2010, the cost of cardiovascular disease was estimated to be nearly $315.4 billion (Go et al., 2014).

Fortunately, the overall mortality rate from CHD has been declining. The reason for this decline is the improved treatments for cardiovascular disease, including angina. Despite this hopeful note, angina remains a significant challenge for primary care management. Successful management depends on an in-depth understanding of the pathologic process, diagnosis, and treatment of this symptom complex.

Angina is a syndrome—a constellation of symptoms—that results from myocardial oxygen demand being greater than the oxygen supply (myocardial ischemia). By definition, angina is associated with reversible ischemia, so it does not result in permanent myocardial damage. Myocardial infarction (MI) is the result of irreversible ischemia when myocardial tissue is permanently damaged.

Patients with angina may report left-sided chest pain, discomfort, heaviness, or pressure, and the sensation may radiate to the back, neck, jaw, and throat or arms. Usually, these sensations last 1 to 15 minutes. Patients may also experience shortness of breath or fatigue. It is important to note, however, that not all patients present with "angina" in a typical fashion. For example, dyspnea on exertion may be the only presenting symptom. If a patient presents with unique symptoms, his or her group of symptoms associated with identified ischemia is called that patient's "anginal equivalent." **Box 21.1** lists common and unique terms used to describe angina.

Angina is called *stable* when the paroxysmal chest pain or discomfort is provoked by physical exertion or emotional stress and is relieved by rest and/or nitroglycerin (NTG). Stable angina exists when the stimulating factors or activities and the degree and duration of discomfort have not changed for the past 60 days.

Anginal episodes that increase in frequency, duration, or severity are referred to as *unstable*. Unstable angina is experienced when the patient is at rest or if the episode is prolonged or progressive. Unstable angina has also been called *preinfarction angina*, *crescendo angina*, or *intermittent coronary syndrome*. It is differentiated from stable angina by the fact that symptoms may be triggered by minimal physical exertion or may be present at rest. Patients who experience unstable angina are at high risk for developing an MI.

Other types of angina include variant (or Prinzmetal) angina, nocturnal angina, angina decubitus, and postinfarction angina. Stable angina is frequently managed in the primary care setting and is the focus of this chapter.

CAUSES

The development of angina is directly related to the risk factors that have been identified for CHD. Nonmodifiable risk factors for CHD cannot be altered or improved by the patient; they include age, family history, and gender. Modifiable risk factors may be controlled or treated by lifestyle modifications or pharmacologic therapy to reduce the risk of morbidity or mortality from CHD. Modifiable risk factors include cigarette smoking, hypertension, dyslipidemia, diabetes, obesity, and physical inactivity. **Box 21.2** lists the risk factors for chronic stable angina.

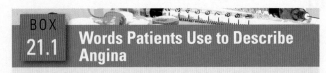

BOX 21.1 Words Patients Use to Describe Angina

Ache, toothache-like, dull
Burning, heartburn, soreness, bursting, searing indigestion
Choking, strangling, compressing, constricting, tightness, viselike
Discomfort, fullness, swelling, heaviness, pressure, weight, uncomfortable

Nonmodifiable Risk Factors

Age

It is uncommon for men younger than age 40 and premenopausal women to have symptomatic CHD, but the incidence increases with age and is increased in women after menopause. More than 80% of patients who die of CHD are over age 65 (American Heart Association, 2010). This increasing incidence of CHD with age is likely linked to age-related changes in the vasculature and the higher prevalence of other CHD risk factors among older persons.

Heredity

A family history of premature CHD in a first-degree relative (i.e., mother, father, sister, or brother) is a strong predictor for CHD in an individual. Premature CHD is defined as occurring in a man younger than age 55 or in a woman younger than age 65. The strong association between family history and the development of CHD has been consistently demonstrated in several studies. Furthermore, race has been shown to be a factor. Data show that 44% of African Americans have high blood pressure versus 27.4% of Whites, thus increasing their risk of a cardiovascular event (Go et al., 2014). Therefore, individuals

BOX 21.2 Risk Factors for Chronic Stable Angina

NONMODIFIABLE RISK FACTORS

Age
Heredity
Gender

MODIFIABLE RISK FACTORS

Cigarette smoking
Hypertension
Dyslipidemia
Diabetes
Obesity
Physical inactivity

with a family history of CHD should be carefully screened for other CHD risk factors and managed appropriately.

Gender

In general, the risk of CHD is higher for men than women. Male gender is considered a nonmodifiable risk factor for CHD. Differences for CHD susceptibility diminish, however, when comparing postmenopausal women and older men. In fact, after age 65, the incidence of CHD increases in women, but it does not reach that of men.

Modifiable Risk Factors

Cigarette Smoking

Cigarette smoking increases the risk of CHD by at least twofold to threefold. Smoking increases the incidence of atherosclerosis by a mechanism that is not clearly understood. It is thought to increase the release of catecholamines, which leads to elevated blood pressure due to an increased workload of the heart caused by an increase in the heart rate and peripheral vascular constriction. Catecholamines also increase the release of free fatty acids, which increases the amount of lipids in the blood. Smoking lowers high-density lipoprotein (HDL) levels and increases low-density lipoprotein (LDL) levels, and is thought to promote platelet activation, which increases the risk of clot formation in the arteries. All patients with CHD risk factors or established disease should be instructed to stop smoking. See Chapter 53 for a more detailed discussion of smoking cessation.

Hypertension

It is estimated that over 77.9 million Americans have elevated blood pressure (Go et al., 2014). Hypertension is a major risk factor for CHD and can lead to vascular complications that increase morbidity and mortality. Additionally, the higher the blood pressure, the higher the risk of MI and other cardiovascular events.

Atherosclerotic changes in the vasculature are exacerbated by increased pressure. Increased blood pressure alone also causes injury to the inner lining of the arteries, resulting in atherosclerotic changes and thrombus formation. As the arteries become stiff and narrow, the blood flow that normally increases during physical activity is restricted to a greater degree, resulting in ischemic symptoms. Chapter 19 provides further discussion of drug therapy for hypertension.

Dyslipidemia

Nearly half of the American population has high cholesterol (American Heart Association, 2010). Cholesterol plays a substantial role in the pathophysiology of atherosclerosis and CHD. High levels of LDL cholesterol and low levels of HDL cholesterol are associated with an increased risk of cardiovascular disease and occurrence of MI or other poor cardiovascular outcomes. Treatment of dyslipidemia in patients with CHD using pharmacologic and nonpharmacologic means has been shown in multiple large-scale studies to reduce the risk of cardiovascular death. In 2014, a new guideline was released outlining the diagnosis and treatment of dyslipidemia in adults. See Chapter 20 for more detailed information on the treatment of dyslipidemia.

Diabetes

Cardiovascular disease is the most common cause of death in patients with diabetes. In fact, patients with diabetes have the same risk of having an MI as a patient who already has a history of an MI. Although data have not shown a clear or conclusive link between glucose control and cardiovascular risk reduction, an effort should be made to prevent or treat diabetes in these patients. For a complete discussion of diabetes treatment, see Chapter 45.

Obesity

In the United States, 68.2% of the population is considered overweight or obese (Go et al., 2014). The increasing incidence of obesity has been attributed to poorer nutrition and a more sedentary lifestyle.

Obesity is a risk factor for CHD in both men and women. Hypertension, dyslipidemia, and diabetes are more common in patients who are obese, but obesity also increases cardiovascular risk independent of these other risk factors by a mechanism that is not well understood. Even modest weight loss can improve blood pressure, hypertension, and insulin resistance and reduce cardiovascular risk. Weight loss is discussed in Chapter 54.

Physical Inactivity

A sedentary lifestyle predisposes patients to CHD. Regular physical exercise reduces blood pressure, maintains a healthy weight, and improves dyslipidemia, but it also reduces the risk of CHD independent of these changes. Patients should be carefully screened and counseled before beginning an exercise program. Exercise may include walking, running, cycling, or formalized aerobic exercise routines. It is recommended that patients get 30 to 60 minutes of aerobic exercise every day at least 5 days per week. Resistance training on 2 day/week may also be of benefit.

PATHOPHYSIOLOGY

Angina is a symptomatic manifestation of reversible myocardial ischemia, which occurs when demand for oxygen in the myocardium exceeds available supply. This imbalance between oxygen supply and demand is caused by limited blood supply due to narrowing of the blood vessels that supply the heart muscle. The most common cause of this narrowing of the coronary arteries is atherosclerotic disease. Rarely, vasospasm of the coronary arteries narrows the arteries, thereby limiting the blood supply to the heart muscle. Other even more uncommon sources of anginal symptoms are thrombosis, aortic stenosis, primary pulmonary hypertension, and severe hypertension.

Atherosclerotic Disease

The pathophysiology of angina involves atherosclerosis, a disorder of lipid metabolism resulting in the deposit of cholesterol in the blood vessel. Over time, this causes a reactive endothelial injury that eventually results in a narrowing of the vessels by episodes of acute thrombosis. The narrow arteries impair the ability of oxygen and nutrients to reach the myocardium. This reduction in blood supply, or ischemia, impairs myocardial metabolism. The myocardial cells remain alive but cannot function normally. Once the blood supply is restored, cardiac function returns to normal. If the ischemia is caused by complete occlusion of the coronary artery, an MI (cell death) occurs.

Regardless of the risk factors that cause the development of atherosclerosis and resulting restriction of coronary blood supply, the pathophysiologic process is essentially the same. The three layers of the arterial wall—intima, media, and adventitia—are affected by structural changes that lead to CHD. The intima is a single layer of endothelial cells, constituting the innermost surface of the artery. It is impermeable to the substances in the blood. The media is the middle layer of the artery and is made up almost entirely of smooth muscle. The outer layer, or adventitia, consists mainly of smooth muscle cells, fibroblasts (which are normally only in this layer), and loose connective tissue. Atherosclerotic changes in the artery occur in stages. Normally, the intima is thin and contains only an occasional muscle cell. As a person ages, the intima slowly increases in thickness and muscle cells proliferate.

Atherosclerosis primarily affects the intima of the arterial wall. It normally takes years to develop, and clinical manifestations do not occur until the disorder is well advanced. CHD progresses through three developments—the fatty streak, the fibrous plaque, and the complicated lesion.

The Fatty Streak

Thought to begin in childhood, the fatty streak is caused by the development of fatty, lipid-rich lesions that result from macrophages adhering to the intact endothelial surface. The macrophages take in lipids, which leads to a thickening of the intimal layer. Smooth muscle cells migrate to the intima and become lipid laden. The lesions at this stage do not obstruct the artery. However, on examination, fatty streaks appear in the coronary arteries as early as age 15. They continue to enlarge through the third decade of life and appear to be a precursor to plaque formation, although the process is not clearly understood.

The Fibrous Plaque

The raised fibrous plaque is a white, elevated area on the surface of the artery. It signals the beginning of progressive changes in the arterial wall, including protrusion of the lesion into the lumen of the artery. These more advanced lesions begin to develop at approximately age 30 in most patients. The major change in the arterial intima during this phase is the migration and proliferation of smooth muscle cells and the formation of a fibrous cap over a deeper deposit of extracellular lipid and cell debris. The lipid accumulation directly or indirectly reduces the blood supply. The decrease in blood supply is permanent and results in cell necrosis and cell debris.

The Complicated Lesion

A complicated lesion contains a fibrous plaque, calcium deposits, and a thrombus formed by hemorrhage into the plaque. The complicated lesion results from continuing cell degeneration. As the complicated lesion, with its lipid, necrotic center, becomes larger, it calcifies. The intimal surface may develop open or ruptured areas that degenerate into an ulcer. The damage is most likely to occur in areas where blood flow creates the greatest amount of stress in the vessel, such as at branches and bifurcations. The damaged surface allows blood from the artery lumen to enter the lipid core. Then, platelets adhere and thrombus formation begins. The thrombus expands and distorts the plaque, which becomes larger and begins to block the lumen of the artery. The blockage impedes the blood flow needed to supply extra oxygen and nutrients to meet the increased workload of the heart. The result is cardiac ischemia and anginal symptoms. These symptoms are relieved when either the workload of the heart is decreased or administration of vasodilating drugs increases blood flow to the myocardium. Complete blockage can cause permanent myocardial death because the cells are entirely deprived of oxygen and blood flow cannot be restored in time to revive the cardiac cells, resulting in an MI.

Coronary Artery Vasospasm

A less common cause of restricted coronary blood supply may be coronary vasospasm, a narrowing of the coronary artery lumen. This narrowing is produced by an arterial muscle spasm and limits the blood supply to the myocardium. The exact cause is unknown, but it is thought to occur when the smooth muscles of the coronary arteries contract in response to neurogenic stimulation. Cigarette smoking and hyperlipidemia appear to play a role in this type of angina because they interfere with normal neurogenic control of the arterial intima.

Spasm is suspected of playing a role in acute MI, as well as in triggering anginal episodes. Coronary artery spasm also can occur with abrupt nitrate withdrawal, cocaine use, and direct mechanical irritation from cardiac catheterization. However, the exact mechanisms leading to spasm are still unclear.

Activation of Ischemic Episodes

Regardless of the existing pathophysiologic process, ischemic episodes that result in anginal pain are usually activated by two situations occurring simultaneously or independently: (1) ambient factors that increase myocardial oxygen demand and (2) circumstances that decrease oxygen supply. For example, the person with atherosclerosis (noncompliant arteries) climbs a flight of stairs. The activity increases the workload of the heart, and the myocardium needs more oxygen. The damaged arteries are unable to meet this demand. In some situations,

the arteries may be so constricted that they are unable to deliver an adequate amount of oxygen even if the person is in a resting state. Therapy is directed at resolution or control of these situations so that the heart can receive the oxygen it needs to meet the physical demands of the body. Control of the blood flow to the heart by increasing it when necessary prevents the pathophysiologic process responsible for the myocardial ischemia.

DIAGNOSTIC CRITERIA

Health History

The health history is an important part of the diagnosis and management of angina. The chief complaint for most patients is usually chest pain or discomfort, but other symptoms may predominate, such as neck or jaw pain or shortness of breath. The patient should be asked to describe the duration, quality, location, severity, and radiation of the pain. Additionally, the practitioner should inquire about potential triggers of the pain and any accompanying symptoms, such as dyspnea, diaphoresis, nausea, or palpitations. The practitioner also should explore what interventions relieved the patient's pain or symptoms, such as rest or NTG.

For all patients with angina, an assessment of CHD risk factors should be performed to determine an individual patient's risk for CHD and to better target pharmacologic and nonpharmacologic management. Practitioners should ask patients about both nonmodifiable and modifiable risk factors, including family history, cigarette smoking, hypertension, dyslipidemia, diabetes, and physical inactivity. A past history of cerebrovascular disease or the presence of peripheral vascular disease also increases a patient's risk of CHD.

Physical Findings

Most commonly, practitioners will not have the opportunity to examine a patient during an acute anginal episode. In that case, the physical examination should focus on the assessment of risk factors and the cardiovascular system as a whole. For example, the practitioner should assess a patient for obesity during the physical examination. Additionally, the vasculature may be evaluated by looking for funduscopic changes or decreased peripheral pulses. Hypertension may be evident from taking the patient's blood pressure, and clinical signs and symptoms of heart failure may include murmurs, gallops, changes in the heart sounds, edema, rales, or organomegaly. Patients with dyslipidemia may exhibit xanthomas or cholesterol nodules.

If a physical exam is performed during an episode of anginal pain, a variety of findings may be present. These may include extra heart sounds, mild hypertension, tachycardia, or tachypnea. A paradoxical split of S_2 may indicate altered left ventricular (LV) heart function associated with the ischemic discomfort.

Diagnostic Tests

Before therapy for angina can be properly prescribed, diagnostic testing is necessary to identify a cardiac cause of the patient's chest pain. Diagnostic testing includes electrocardiography, echocardiography, exercise tolerance testing, radioisotope imaging, and coronary artery angiography.

Patients with new, current, or recent chest pain should have an electrocardiogram (ECG) to detect signs of cardiac ischemia. During an acute anginal episode, ST segment depressions with or without symmetric T-wave inversions may be noted in the leads that correspond to the myocardium affected. During pain-free intervals, however, the ECG reverts to baseline. ECG changes that may be present in the patient with chronic CHD include evidence of a prior MI, LV hypertrophy, and repolarization abnormalities.

Echocardiography is recommended if valvular disease or heart failure is suspected, if the patient has a history of MI, or if the patient experiences ventricular arrhythmias. Most patients with intermittent episodes of chest pain should undergo an exercise tolerance test with ECG monitoring (also called a *stress test*) to evaluate the risk of future cardiac events. Those suspected of having coronary ischemia based on the presence of anginal symptoms should undergo testing within 72 hours of symptoms (Fihn et al., 2012). One notable exception would be patients with a high probability of CHD, such as a patient with known coronary disease and classical angina symptoms; these patients should be referred to a specialist for potential advanced interventional therapies. Further testing with radioisotope perfusion testing or coronary artery angiography may be indicated for subgroups of patients. If diagnostic testing confirms cardiac ischemia as the cause of anginal symptoms, drug therapy is warranted.

INITIATING DRUG THERAPY

The treatment goals for the management of angina include relieving the acute anginal episode, preventing additional anginal episodes, preventing progression of CHD, reducing the risk of MI, improving functional capacity, and prolonging survival. These goals should be accomplished while maintaining the patient's quality of life and avoiding adverse events associated with therapy.

Nonpharmacologic therapy is the cornerstone of treatment for patients with angina. The practitioner must assess the patient's modifiable risk factors and work with him or her to reduce the risk for CHD. Practitioners should counsel patients on smoking cessation at each clinic visit and provide support and access to pharmacologic treatment if necessary. Patients should be instructed to maintain a normal weight by consuming a low-fat, low-cholesterol diet, and practitioners should provide dietary counseling and refer interested patients to dietitians for further support. Finally, practitioners should encourage patients to engage in regular aerobic exercise.

Further details on these lifestyle modifications are provided in Chapters 19, 20, 53, and 54.

The practitioner should emphasize to the patient that nonpharmacologic therapy and lifestyle modifications supplement drug therapy and should continue indefinitely.

Goals of Drug Therapy

After the patient has been properly instructed on nonpharmacologic therapy for angina, appropriate drug therapy may be initiated. A summary of selected agents is provided in **Table 21.1**. Several classes of medications are used to treat angina, including angiotensin-converting enzyme (ACE) inhibitors, nitrates, beta-blockers, calcium channel blockers, and antiplatelet agents.

Angiotensin-Converting Enzyme Inhibitors and Angiotensin Receptor Blockers

The 2012 Guideline for the Diagnosis and Management of Patients with Stable Ischemic Heart Disease recommends that patients with ejection fractions of less than 40% or those with hypertension, diabetes, or kidney disease be placed on an ACE inhibitor unless contraindicated (Fihn et al., 2012). When patients cannot take an ACE inhibitor, an angiotensin receptor blocker (ARB) may be used (Fihn et al., 2012). ACE inhibitors include captopril (Capoten), ramipril (Altace), enalapril (Vasotec), quinapril (Accupril), benazepril (Lotensin), perindopril (Aceon), and lisinopril (Prinivil, Zestril). ARBs include losartan (Cozaar), valsartan (Diovan), candesartan (Atacand), telmisartan (Micardis), eprosartan (Teveten), olmesartan (Benicar), and irbesartan (Avapro).

Mechanism of Action

ACE inhibitors affect the enzyme responsible for the conversion of angiotensin I to angiotensin II. ARBs block the vasoconstriction and aldosterone-secreting effects of angiotensin II by selectively blocking angiotensin II from binding to angiotensin II receptors found in many tissues. Angiotensin II is a potent vasoconstrictor and also stimulates aldosterone secretion. Blocking the production of angiotensin II results in reduced vasoconstriction and sodium and water retention, thus reducing preload, afterload, and ejection fraction. These benefits are helpful in chronic stable angina, heart failure (Chapter 22), and hypertension (Chapter 19).

Dosage

ACE inhibitors and ARBs should be initiated at low doses and followed by gradual dosage increases if the lower doses are well tolerated. Renal function and serum potassium should be assessed within 1 to 2 weeks of starting therapy and periodically thereafter, especially in patients with preexisting diabetes or those receiving potassium supplementation. **Table 21.1** shows the doses of some common ACE inhibitors and ARBs when used to treat chronic stable angina.

TABLE 21.1

Overview of Agents Used to Treat Chronic Stable Angina

Generic (Trade) Name and Dosage	Selected Adverse Events	Contraindications	Special Considerations
Selected Angiotensin-Converting Enzyme Inhibitors			
captopril (Capoten) Start: 6.25 mg or 12.5 mg tid Therapeutic range: 25–100 mg tid	Common: cough; hypotension, particularly with a diuretic or volume depletion; hyperkalemia, loss of taste, and leukopenia; angioedema, neutropenia, and agranulocytosis in <1% of patients; rash in >10% of patients	Contraindicated in pregnancy; avoid in patients with bilateral renal artery stenosis or unilateral stenosis	Renal impairment related to ACE inhibitors is seen as an increase in serum creatinine and azotemia, usually in the beginning of therapy. Monitor BUN, creatinine, and K levels when starting.
enalapril (Vasotec) Start: 2.5 mg qd or bid Range: 5–20 mg qd or bid daily	Same as above	Same as above	Same as above Use only 2.5 mg/d in patient with impaired renal function or hyponatremia.
fosinopril (Monopril) Start: 10 mg qd Range: 10–40 mg qd	Same as above	Same as above	Same as above Use only 5 mg/d in patient with impaired renal function or hyponatremia.
lisinopril (Zestril, Prinivil) Start: 5 mg qd Range: 5–20 mg qd	Same as above	Same as above	Same as above Use only 2.5 mg/d in patient with impaired renal function or hyponatremia.
quinapril (Accupril) Start: 5 mg bid Range: 20–40 bid	Same as above	Same as above	Same as above Use only 2.5 mg/d in patient with impaired renal function or hyponatremia.
ramipril (Altace) Start: 1.25 mg twice daily Range: 1.25–5 mg twice daily	Same as above	Same as above	Same as above
Selected Angiotensin Receptor Blockers (ARBs)			
losartan (Cozaar) Start: 12.5 mg/d Range: 50–100 mg/d	Dyspnea, hypotension, hyperkalemia	Angioedema secondary to ACE inhibition	May be used in patients experiencing cough due to ACE inhibitor
valsartan (Diovan) Start: 80 mg/d Range: 80–160 mg twice daily	Same as above	Same as above	Same as above
Short-Acting Nitrates			
nitroglycerin (Nitrostat, NitroQuick) 0.4 mg SL prn	Headache, dizziness, tachycardia, hypotension, edema	Combination with phosphodiesterase-5 inhibitors (e.g., sildenafil, vardenafil, and tadalafil)	For acute treatment of anginal episodes
isosorbide dinitrate (ISDN; Isordil, Sorbitrate) 5 mg SL prn	Above notes also apply	Above notes also apply	Above notes also apply
Long-Acting Nitrates			
nitroglycerin Topical ointment (Nitro-Bid) ½–1 in bid–tid	Above notes also apply Local irritation and erythema with topical application	Above notes also apply	For chronic prevention of anginal episodes Use nitrate-free interval to reduce risk of nitrate tolerance.

Drug (dose)	Adverse Effects	Contraindications/Cautions	Notes
Transdermal patch (Minitran, Nitro-Dur, Nitrol, Transderm-Nitro) 0.2–0.8 mg/h		Above notes also apply	Potential hypotensive effect with vasodilators. Tapering is recommended after long-term use. Onset of action with transdermal application is ~60 min.
isosorbide mononitrate (ISMN) Immediate release (Ismo, Monoket) 5–20 mg bid; Extended release (Imdur) 30–120 mg bid	Above notes also apply	Above notes also apply	Above notes also apply. Extended-release formulations should be swallowed whole.
Beta-Blockers			
propranolol Immediate release (Inderal) 40–160 mg bid; Extended release (Inderal LA) 80–240 mg qd	Fatigue, dizziness, decreased exercise tolerance, bradycardia, hypotension, dyspnea	Use with caution in patients with reactive airway disease. Bradycardia (heart rate <45 beats per minute). Acutely decompensated heart failure	Abrupt cessation of beta-blocker therapy should be avoided. Extended-release formulations should be swallowed whole.
atenolol (Tenormin) 25–100 mg qd	Above notes also apply	Above notes also apply	Above notes also apply. Dose adjustment needed in chronic kidney disease
metoprolol Immediate release (metoprolol tartrate, Lopressor) 25–200 mg tid; Extended release (metoprolol succinate, Toprol-XL) 50–100 mg qd	Above notes also apply	Above notes also apply	Toprol-XL tablets may be split, but should not be chewed or crushed.
Calcium Channel Blockers			
amlodipine (Norvasc) 2.5–10 mg qd	Headache, dizziness, flushing, edema, gingival hyperplasia	Severe conduction abnormalities. Use with caution in patients with preexisting bradycardia or CHF.	Useful for patients with isolated systolic hypertension
nifedipine (extended release, Adalat CC, Procardia XL) 30–60 mg qd	Above notes also apply	Above notes also apply	Should be swallowed whole
diltiazem (extended release, Cardizem CD, Dilacor XR, Tiazac) 180–420 mg qd	Headache, nausea, conduction abnormalities, gingival hyperplasia	Above notes also apply	Should be swallowed whole
verapamil Immediate release (Calan, Isoptin) 80–320 mg bid; Extended release (Calan SR, Isoptin SR) 120–480 mg qd	Above notes also apply Constipation	Above notes also apply	Extended-release formulations should be swallowed whole.
Antiplatelet Agents			
aspirin 81–325 mg qd	Nausea, dyspepsia	Allergy to aspirin; Bleeding disorders	For primary and secondary prevention of cardiovascular events
clopidogrel (Plavix) 75 mg qd	Nausea	Allergy to clopidogrel; Bleeding disorders	Alternative antiplatelet agent for aspirin-intolerant or aspirin-allergic patients
Ranolazine			
ranolazine (Ranexa) 500–1,000 mg qd	Dizziness, nausea, constipation	Patients taking strong inhibitors of CYP3A4 and/or severe hepatic impairment	Should be swallowed whole

Contraindications

ACE inhibitors are contraindicated in pregnancy and should be avoided in patients with bilateral renal artery stenosis or unilateral stenosis.

Adverse Effects

Side effects of ACE inhibitors are uncommon but may include an irritating cough and excessive drops in blood pressure, particularly in hypovolemic patients or those already on diuretics. Hyperkalemia may also occur; however, the incidence is less with ARBs than with ACE inhibitors. A serious adverse effect with ACE inhibitors is angioedema, which usually occurs early in treatment. Angioedema secondary to an ACE inhibitor is a contraindication to further ACE inhibitor use, but an ARB may be used cautiously in its place. Other adverse effects include rash, loss of taste, neutropenia, and agranulocytosis.

Interactions

Due to the effects on angiotensin II and aldosterone, ACE inhibitors contribute to potassium retention as sodium is preferentially excreted. This raises the possibility of a hyperkalemia state for the patient and must be monitored routinely. Similarly, patients taking lithium are at increased risk for lithium toxicity due to its decreased renal excretion. Other important ACE inhibitor interactions can be found in Chapter 19, **Table 22.3.**

Nitrates

The nitrates are one of the original medications used for controlling angina, and they are still commonly used to halt an acute anginal attack, to prevent predictable episodes, and for chronic treatment to prevent anginal episodes.

Mechanism of Action

Nitrates and their analogs are potent agents and have profound effects on vascular smooth muscle. The nitrates cause dilation throughout the vasculature—in the peripheral arteries and veins as well as the coronary arteries. When dilated, the veins return less blood to the heart, thereby reducing LV filling volume and pressure (preload). This decreases the workload of the heart. Another primary effect of the nitrates is coronary arterial dilation, which results in increased blood flow and oxygen supply to the myocardium. Nitrates do not directly influence the chronotropic or inotropic actions of the heart, so their administration does not affect or alter cardiac function but rather decreases the work of the heart and increases myocardial oxygenation. Nitrates are moderately effective in lessening coronary vasospasm.

Rapid-Acting Nitrates

The sublingual forms of NTG are rapid acting. (See **Table 21.1.**) These medications are used for acute attacks of angina. Short-acting nitrates are also used for prophylaxis of angina in situations when an anginal episode can be reasonably predicted by the patient, such as during walking, climbing stairs, or sexual activity. To be effective, NTG must be administered sublingually to avoid hepatic first-pass metabolism, which would inactivate the medication.

Sublingual NTG (Nitrol, Isordil, others) remains the first-line therapy for managing acute angina episodes. NTG may be adequate treatment for patients who experience angina no more frequently than once a week. NTG usually relieves anginal symptoms within 1 to 5 minutes and provides short-term (up to 30 minutes) relief. NTG tablets or spray (0.3 to 0.6 mg) is used sublingually for immediate symptomatic treatment of anginal episodes. The practitioner instructs the patient to rest at the time of pain, take a single dose, repeat the dose if the pain does not resolve within 5 minutes, and call emergency medical services if the pain is not relieved with three doses.

Patients should be instructed to mark the date they open a bottle of NTG tablets or first use an NTG spray canister. Tablets in an opened glass bottle of NTG retain efficacy for only 1 year and should be discarded after that time period. NTG canisters retain their efficacy for up to 3 years.

The main advantage of rapid-acting nitrates is their ability to halt an episode of angina once it has begun. Generally, the adverse effects of short-acting nitrates are related to their vasodilatory effects; however, patients may also experience burning under the tongue with sublingual preparations.

Long-Acting Nitrates

Due to their short duration of action, short-acting nitrates such as sublingual NTG are not suitable for maintenance therapy; long-acting nitrates must be used for chronic prophylaxis of anginal episodes. Long-acting nitrates act to maintain vasodilation, thereby continuously decreasing the workload of the heart and maintaining blood flow to the heart. The most prescribed long-acting nitrates are isosorbide dinitrate (ISDN; oral [Cedocard SR, Isordil, others]), isosorbide mononitrate (ISMN; oral [Imdur, Ismo, Monoket, others]), and long-acting transdermal NTG preparations (transdermal [Minitran, Nitro-Dur, Transderm-Nitro, others], topical [Nitro-Bid, others]).

Isosorbide Dinitrate (Oral)

Single oral doses of 20 to 40 mg significantly improve hemodynamic parameters and exercise tolerance, and the effect continues for several hours. The starting dose should be low (e.g., ISDN 5 mg three times a day) and the dosage should be advanced slowly in small increments every 1 to 2 weeks to minimize side effects. The dose is increased until control is obtained, side effects become intolerable, systolic blood pressure falls to 100 mm Hg or below, resting heart rate increases more than 10 beats per minute, or postural hypotension occurs.

Intestinal absorption with ISDN is unpredictable, especially when taken with food, so oral nitrates should be taken on an empty stomach, 1 hour before or 2 hours after food intake. A drawback to ISDN products is the short half-life (approximately 2 to 4 hours) and duration of action, which necessitates multiple doses during the day.

Isosorbide Mononitrate (Oral)

ISMN is a long-acting metabolite derivative of ISDN. Formulated in extended-release tablets, ISMN can be administered in fewer doses (Imdur, once daily; other products, twice daily). A common twice-daily starting regimen is 20 mg (immediate release) orally at 7 AM and 3 PM, allowing for a nitrate-free period to reduce the risk of nitrate tolerance. A starting dose using extended-release ISMN (Imdur) is 30 to 60 mg orally in the morning. Like ISDN, ISMN should also be taken on an empty stomach. Extended-release formulations of ISMN must be taken whole, without crushing or chewing the tablet.

Nitroglycerin (Transdermal)

Transdermal NTG is long-acting and effective for treating and preventing anginal pain. Two percent (2%) NTG ointment may be applied to the skin as an adjunct to isosorbide therapy for nocturnal pain or, with repeated daily dosing, used alone for anginal treatment. One half to one inch of the ointment is applied to a clean, hairless area of the torso before bed. Alternatively, the ointment may be applied every 4 to 6 hours while awake, allowing for an 8- to 12-hour nitrate-free interval. Measurement guides are provided with the product to assist in dosing. The dose is increased by a half inch at a time until pain relief is achieved.

Transdermal NTG patches may also be used as a long-acting nitrate. Therapy is typically initiated with a 5-mg (0.2 mg/h) or 10-mg (0.4 mg/h) patch, which should be left in place for 12 to 14 hours and then removed to prevent nitrate tolerance. Nitrate patches should be applied to the torso intact, since cutting a patch destroys the drug delivery system. Care should be taken to ensure that a previously applied patch is removed before applying a new patch.

Nitrate Tolerance

A drawback to the use of nitrates to treat angina is the potential for the development of nitrate tolerance. Nitrate tolerance refers to the loss of ability of the smooth muscles to respond to the action of the nitrates. Tolerance develops to both the peripheral and coronary vasodilator effects of nitrates. This phenomenon occurs with continuous nitrate use over prolonged periods. Tolerance is both dose and time dependent. Nitrate tolerance can be seen after as few as 7 to 10 days of continuous administration. Nitrate tolerance may also develop with frequent sublingual administration of nitrates, if the oral tablets are given four times daily in evenly spaced intervals or if the transdermal patches are left on the skin for 24-hour periods.

Prevention of nitrate tolerance is based on a treatment plan that provides for rapid changes in blood nitrate levels over a given time, usually 24 hours. To prevent nitrate tolerance, one 10- to 12-hour nitrate-free interval per day is necessary. In this manner, the intervals between doses need not be equal. For example, the patch can be applied in the morning and removed in the evening. The same schedule can be developed for patients taking oral medications. The medication is given three times during the day when the patient is awake.

The patient does not receive any medication during the night to minimize the risk of nitrate tolerance. Combination antianginal therapy (e.g., a beta-blocker plus a long-acting nitrate) should be used for patients whose anginal symptoms are not controlled during the nitrate-free interval.

Adverse Events

The common side effects of the nitrates are related to their vasodilatory effects: headache, flushing, dizziness, weakness, and orthostatic hypotension. Additionally, since all segments of the vascular system relax in response to nitrates, reflex tachycardia often results as the heart compensates for the blood pressure drop to maintain cardiac output. Transdermal nitrate products may also cause irritation of the skin at the site of application.

Most of the side effects associated with nitrates abate or disappear with continuation of therapy. By starting therapy at a low dose and slowing titrating the dose upward, side effects are minimized and may not present at all. However, starting with a high dose can produce severe side effects (especially headache), and if side effects are intolerable, the patient may self-discontinue the medication.

If a patient has been receiving nitrate therapy long term, it should not be abruptly discontinued because of the risk of rebound hypertension and angina. If discontinuation of nitrate therapy is required, it should be done by tapering the dose over a period of time.

Caution should be exercised when using nitrates in combination with vasodilators due to additive hypotensive effects. Concurrent use of nitrates and phosphodiesterase-5 inhibitors such as sildenafil (Viagra), vardenafil (Levitra), or tadalafil (Cialis) is contraindicated due to the potential for severe hypotension.

Beta-Blockers

Beta-blockers are very effective in managing angina. They reduce the workload of the heart and decrease overall myocardial oxygen demand and consumption through antagonism of adrenergic receptors. This is accomplished by a reduction in the heart rate and myocardial contractility, both at rest and during periods of normal exercise. As such, they are particularly beneficial for treating exertional angina.

Nitrates and beta-blockers have complementary effects on myocardial oxygen supply and demand and therefore are often used together. Because beta-blockers reduce the heart rate, they can be used to control the reflex tachycardia that sometimes occurs with the administration of nitrates. This reduction in heart rate also allows more time for coronary artery filling and therefore myocardial perfusion during diastole.

Mechanism of Action

Beta-blockers can be categorized according to their cardioselectivity, that is, the degree of preferential affinity for $beta_1$ receptors, which predominate in the heart and are the principal target of these medications. Beta antagonists that block only $beta_1$ receptors are considered *cardioselective* beta-blockers. Those that block both $beta_1$ and $beta_2$ receptors are *nonselective*.

There are many beta-blockers available, all of which block beta$_1$ receptors. However, many agents also block beta$_2$ receptors, which predominate in the lungs.

Beta$_1$-receptor blockade is desirable in a patient with angina because it causes a slowing of the heart rate and a reduction in myocardial contractility. These effects reduce myocardial oxygen demand and therefore improve and prevent anginal symptoms.

Blockage of beta$_2$ receptors can lead to bronchoconstriction; therefore, nonselective beta-blockers should be used with caution in patients with uncontrolled or unstable reactive airway disease. At low to intermediate doses, cardioselectivity is demonstrated by atenolol (Tenormin) and metoprolol (Lopressor). Propranolol (Inderal) is an example of a nonselective beta-blocker. However, even cardioselective beta-blockers show nonselective action at high doses.

Propranolol is a nonselective beta-blocker with a short half-life (4 to 6 hours). Immediate-release formulations of propranolol must be dosed multiple times per day, but sustained-release preparations for once-daily dosing are also available. Other nonselective beta-blockers include nadolol and timolol.

Atenolol and metoprolol are selective beta$_1$ antagonists. These drugs, which preferentially block beta$_1$ receptors, were developed to eliminate the unwanted bronchoconstriction effect of the agents that also block beta$_2$ receptors. These agents may be a better choice for patients with severe or uncontrolled asthma or chronic obstructive pulmonary disease (COPD). However, when these agents are prescribed at high dosage levels, they lose their cardioselective properties. Atenolol has a long duration of action and therefore may be dosed once daily. Atenolol is renally cleared; therefore, dose adjustments must be made based on the patient's eGFR. Immediate-release metoprolol tartrate (Lopressor) must be given two to three times daily, but extended-release metoprolol succinate (Toprol-XL) is given only once daily. Both atenolol and metoprolol tartrate are available in generic forms and are relatively inexpensive. A generic form of metoprolol succinate is now available; however, it remains expensive when compared to the immediate-release preparation.

Pindolol and acebutolol are beta-blockers that also possess some agonist activity. They are not completely blockers in that they have the ability also to stimulate weakly both beta$_1$ and beta$_2$ receptors, possessing so-called *intrinsic sympathomimetic activity* (ISA). Drugs possessing ISA can stimulate the beta receptor to which they are bound, yet, as antagonists, they block the activation of the receptor by the more potent endogenous catecholamines, epinephrine and norepinephrine. Because of the agonist action, there is a diminished effect on cardiac rate and cardiac output. Patients who cannot tolerate the other beta-blockers because of preexisting bradycardia or heart block may tolerate these agents.

Contraindications

Beta-blockers are relatively contraindicated and therefore should be used cautiously in patients with preexisting bradycardia because beta blockade may lower the heart rate further. Additionally, beta-blockers should not be used if a patient is experiencing an acute episode of decompensated heart failure. The addition of a beta-blocker in this situation has the potential to negatively impact the patient by further reducing heart rate and contractility. Finally, as discussed above, beta-blockers should be used with caution in patients with reactive airway disease. In patients with stable or controlled asthma or COPD, a selective beta-blocker may be a better choice to minimize the risk of bronchospasm.

Adverse Events

Beta-blockers have the potential to adversely affect cardiac function. These effects include slowing the sinoatrial node and atrioventricular (AV) conduction, leading to symptomatic bradycardia and heart block. Sinus arrest is possible. If the patient has preexisting cardiac conduction system disease, a preparation with some intrinsic beta-agonist activity may be chosen to minimize these adverse events. These patients require close and frequent monitoring to ensure that early conduction system disease is managed promptly. Beta-blockers should not be given to patients with a slow heart rate at baseline due to the potential for severe bradycardia.

Since beta-blockers attenuate the "fight or flight" response, the clinical manifestations of hypoglycemia may be masked. Therefore, patients with diabetes should be instructed to more closely monitor their serum glucose to avoid severe hypoglycemic reactions. Typical symptoms of hypoglycemia, including tachycardia, tremor, or sweating, may be decreased or absent when these patients are taking a beta-blocker.

Abrupt withdrawal of beta-blockers can precipitate an acute withdrawal syndrome that may be manifested by tachycardia, hypertensive crises, angina exacerbation, acute coronary insufficiency, or even MI (Antman & Sabatine, 2013). For this reason, beta-blocker therapy should always be tapered. Withdrawal is of particular concern in the anginal patient on large doses of beta-blockers who is faced with an emergency situation that makes it impossible to continue taking the prescribed beta-blocker for more than 48 hours.

Beta-blockers may also cause adverse central nervous system effects, including drowsiness and depression. These effects may occur more frequently in the elderly or in patients with preexisting depression or psychiatric disorders. In these patients, careful monitoring of mood, sleep pattern, and sexual and cognitive functioning is necessary.

Calcium Channel Blockers

Calcium channel blockers are effective in managing angina because they exert vasodilatory effects on the coronary and peripheral vessels. Depending on the specific agent, they have the potential to depress cardiac contractility, heart rate, and conduction, which may mediate their antianginal effects. These drugs are effective in relieving coronary constriction associated with vasospastic angina.

Mechanism of Action

Calcium plays a major role in the electrical excitation and contraction of cardiac and vascular smooth muscle cells. The calcium channel blockers inhibit the entrance of calcium into smooth muscle cells of the coronary and systemic arterial vessels, which inhibits muscular contraction and therefore causes vasodilation. These vasodilatory effects are more pronounced on arteries than veins because of the relatively large amount of smooth muscle found in the arteries. Because calcium channel blockers do not cause substantial venous dilation, they do not reduce preload. Nondihydropyridine calcium channel blockers reduce heart rate by slowing conduction through the sinoatrial and AV nodes, and they depress cardiac contractility.

Two major groups of calcium channel blockers are available: the dihydropyridines and the nondihydropyridines.

Dihydropyridines

The dihydropyridine calcium channel blockers are potent dilators of the coronary and peripheral arteries. Due to the vasodilatory effect of these agents, they may cause reflex tachycardia due to a reduction in systemic blood pressure. Since dihydropyridines do not alter conduction, they do not slow the sinus rate.

There are many dihydropyridine calcium channel blockers available. Nifedipine is an example of a first-generation dihydropyridine; nicardipine, felodipine, isradipine, and amlodipine are second-generation dihydropyridines. In general, the second-generation agents are better tolerated than the first-generation agents.

All of these agents are administered orally, and they have relatively short half-lives. Doses should be titrated upward slowly to minimize orthostasis or other adverse events. Several dihydropyridines (e.g., nifedipine, nicardipine) must be administered as multiple daily doses unless the sustained formulations are used. Amlodipine is administered once daily.

Nondihydropyridines

Although diltiazem and verapamil are both nondihydropyridine calcium channel blockers, they display different effects on the cardiovascular system. Verapamil has a pronounced effect on cardiac conduction, reducing the rate of electrical conduction through the AV node. Verapamil also exerts negative inotropic and chronotropic effects, suppressing contractility, reducing heart rate, and therefore causing a reduction in oxygen demand. However, due to this effect, verapamil should be used with caution in those patients with depressed cardiac function or AV conduction abnormalities. Immediate-release formulations of verapamil must be administered as divided doses, but sustained-release products are administered once daily.

Like verapamil, diltiazem reduces the heart rate but to a lesser extent. Diltiazem also has a less potent effect than verapamil on conduction and contractility, but it is a more potent vasodilator. Diltiazem has immediate- and sustained-release formulations. The immediate-release formulation usually is taken four times a day before meals; the sustained-release formulation is taken daily on an empty stomach.

Contraindications

Before a calcium channel blocker can be selected for treating angina, a careful assessment must be done to determine a patient's LV and conduction system function. Nondihydropyridine calcium channel blockers with negative inotropic properties may worsen preexisting LV dysfunction. Patients with conduction system disease are poor candidates for nondihydropyridine calcium channel blocker therapy because of the risk of bradyarrhythmias.

The nondihydropyridine calcium channel blockers are contraindicated in patients with heart block because of the significant depression of AV node conduction. Additionally, calcium channel blockers should be used with caution in patients with sick sinus syndrome and hypotension.

Adverse Events

In general, adverse events accompanying the dihydropyridine calcium channel blockers are more common with the first-generation than the second-generation agents. Leg edema, a common problem, results from vasodilation, which causes fluid to pool in the legs. In some cases, the edema may be so severe that new-onset heart failure may be suspected. In this situation, dosage reduction or drug discontinuation may be considered. Other common side effects of the calcium channel blockers include fatigue, dizziness, headache, flushing, and gingival hyperplasia. Verapamil is associated with constipation much more often than the other calcium channel blockers.

Antiplatelet Therapy

Antiplatelet drugs inhibit platelet aggregation through a variety of mechanisms. Aspirin inhibits platelet activation through irreversible enzyme antagonism to block prostaglandin synthesis, and clopidogrel reduces ADP-induced platelet activation. Aggregation is a normal process that causes disease when the platelets adhere to vessel walls, causing thrombus formation. Antiplatelet therapy limits the formation of the thrombus, thereby decreasing the risk of progressive CHD. When antiplatelet medications are used to treat patients with angina, the chances of having an MI are reduced.

In patients with stable angina, the risk of MI can be lowered with daily aspirin therapy. Aspirin acts by blocking prostaglandin synthesis, which prevents formation of the platelet-aggregating substance thromboxane A_2. Current angina recommendations suggest that all patients with acute or chronic ischemic heart disease receive aspirin 75 to 162 mg daily as primary or secondary prevention of cardiovascular disease (Fihn et al., 2012). Doses of aspirin greater than 162 mg have been shown to increase the risk of adverse events without any enhanced benefit.

Adverse events associated with aspirin use include dyspepsia, bruising, and bleeding. Enteric-coated aspirin may be prescribed to minimize gastrointestinal symptoms. Aspirin is contraindicated in patients with a known aspirin hypersensitivity.

Clopidogrel is another antiplatelet agent that may be used in patients with angina. It reduces ADP-induced platelet activation by antagonizing the platelet ADP receptors. Clopidogrel is recommended for prevention of MI in angina patients who have contraindications to aspirin. Like aspirin, clopidogrel has been shown to reduce the incidence of morbidity and mortality in patients with established cardiovascular disease.

The dose of clopidogrel is 75 mg daily. Bleeding events associated with clopidogrel are similar to aspirin, although it typically exhibits better gastrointestinal tolerance. However, clopidogrel is metabolized to its active component, in part by the CYP2C19 system, which in certain patients shows significant genetic variation. Data have shown that this genetic variation may play a role in the effectiveness of this agent, particularly in those who have a slow metabolism. For further discussion of antiplatelet agents, refer to Chapter 49.

Ranolazine

Ranolazine (Ranexa) is a unique antianginal agent that can be used alone or in combination with nitrates, beta-blockers, calcium channel blockers, or ACE inhibitors. Currently, its primary role is as an adjunctive agent for patients who are not achieving adequate symptom relief with other agents.

Mechanism of Action

The mechanism of action of ranolazine is not well understood, but it is thought to block late-phase sodium channels, which often remain open during hypoxic or ischemic events. An increase in intracellular sodium during late phase affects sodium-dependent calcium channels, thus increasing the amount of calcium entering the cell and causing a calcium overload. This overload can lead to further or continued contraction of the myocardium, increasing oxygen demand. By blocking late-phase sodium channels, ranolazine decreases calcium overload and breaks the cycle of ischemia.

Dosage

Ranolazine is taken orally at 500 mg twice daily and can be titrated up to a maximum of 1,000 mg twice daily. Ranexa tablets should be swallowed whole, not crushed or split. There may need to be a dose reduction in patients taking CYP3A4 inhibitors, such as diltiazem and verapamil.

Contraindications

Ranolazine is contraindicated in patients taking ketoconazole, itraconazole, clarithromycin, and other strong CYP3A4 inhibitors.

Adverse Events

Ranolazine prolongs the QTc interval in a dose-related manner; however, in long-term studies, there has been no association with an increased risk of proarrhythmia or sudden death. Regardless, caution should still be used because there is little experience with doses greater than 1,000 mg twice daily. Dose-related dizziness, headache, constipation, and nausea are common adverse effects. Other adverse events include palpitations, vertigo, dry mouth, peripheral edema, hypotension, and, less commonly, angioedema and renal failure.

Interactions

As noted earlier, patients taking potent CYP3A4 inhibitors should not take ranolazine, and less potent inhibitors warrant monitoring. Conversely, agents that induce the CYP3A4 system, such as rifampin, carbamazepine, phenytoin, and St. John's wort, may decrease plasma concentrations of ranolazine. Ranolazine, through the P-glycoprotein system, may increase digoxin levels.

Selecting the Most Appropriate Antianginal Therapy

Choosing the appropriate medications for treating a patient with angina can be challenging. The primary goal is to design a regimen that will reduce the frequency and severity of anginal episodes. Subsequent adjustments are made empirically based on the patient's response to treatment, disease progression, risk factor modification, and patient satisfaction and adherence (**Figure 21.1**).

Acute Treatment of Anginal Episodes

All patients with angina should be provided a short-acting nitrate for acute treatment of anginal episodes. Additionally, patients with infrequent episodes of angina can be managed effectively with short-acting nitrates alone. They are a good choice for the patient who has infrequent attacks or predictable pain on exertion.

Chronic Prevention of Anginal Episodes

Patients with repeated episodes of angina should receive long-acting therapy for chronic prophylaxis. All patients should be receiving aspirin. In addition, there are three classes of agents that may be used for chronic antianginal therapy: beta-blockers, calcium channel blockers, and long-acting nitrates. The initial choice of an antianginal agent should be based on the patient's specific characteristics, such as physical exam findings and coexisting medical conditions. Treatment with a single agent is generally used for initial antianginal therapy, whereas combination therapy is instituted for patients who fail monotherapy.

First-Line Therapy

In the absence of contraindications, beta-blockers are the agents of choice for prevention of acute anginal episodes in patients with or without a history of MI. Beta-blockers reduce the frequency and likelihood of anginal episodes and reduce CHD-related morbidity and mortality. Additionally, beta-blockers are useful as antihypertensive and antiarrhythmic agents. Beta-blockers are particularly useful in patients whose anginal symptoms are related to physical exertion.

For patients whose anginal symptoms have been linked to coronary vasospasm, a calcium channel blocker may be considered for initial treatment. See **Table 21.2** for more information.

Second-Line Therapy

For patients who do not respond sufficiently to therapy with a single antianginal agent, combination therapy should be attempted. When initial treatment with a beta-blocker is not successful, either a calcium channel blocker or a long-acting nitrate may be added to beta-blocker therapy.

A long-acting nitrate/beta-blocker regimen is safe, effective, and low in cost. Nitrates and beta-blockers are well

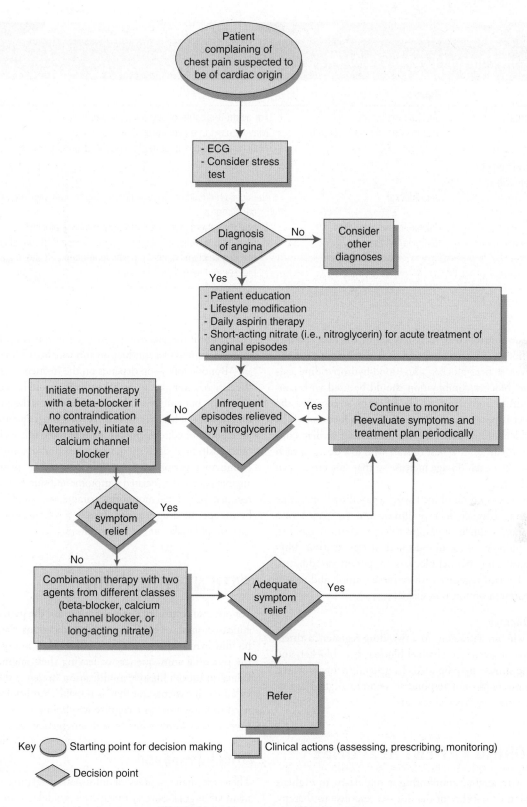

FIGURE 21.1 Treatment algorithm for angina.

tolerated, and their effects are complementary. Reflex tachycardia caused by nitrates is blunted by a beta-blocker. The control of reflex tachycardia is beneficial because a decrease in heart rate lowers myocardial oxygen demand. The combination of

nitrates and beta-blockers is an accepted treatment of angina, and they are often used together.

A beta-blocker plus a calcium channel blocker is another typical combination. Patients who have anginal symptoms

TABLE 21.2

Recommended Order of Treatment for Angina

Order	Agents	Comments
For all patients	Short-acting nitrate aspirin (if not contraindicated)	For acute treatment of anginal episodes May be used to prevent predictable episodes May be used alone in patients with infrequent episodes
Chronic prevention of anginal episodes		
First line	Beta-blocker	Reduces workload of heart by decreasing overall myocardial oxygen consumption
	Calcium channel blocker	Useful for patients who cannot tolerate a beta-blocker
Second line	Combination therapy	If monotherapy fails, add another agent from a different class: beta-blocker, calcium channel blocker, long-acting nitrate (e.g., beta-blocker and long-acting nitrate)

that cannot be controlled by beta-blocker or calcium channel blocker monotherapy often respond to a combination of the two. However, a beta-blocker plus nondihydropyridine calcium channel blocker combination should be used with caution. When drugs from these two classes are given together, the additive effect is potent suppression of AV conduction, which may be problematic in patients with preexisting cardiac conduction abnormalities. It is best to start with low doses of each drug and monitor each dosage increase so that side effects can be identified early.

Nitrates are often combined with a nondihydropyridine calcium channel blocker, such as diltiazem or verapamil, or a second-generation dihydropyridine calcium channel blocker, such as amlodipine. Since nitrates and first-generation dihydropyridine calcium channel blockers are potent vasodilators, they should be used together with extreme caution and only if no other treatment option is available.

Third-Line Therapy

In patients who are refractory to a two-drug regimen, a three-drug regimen of a calcium channel blocker, beta-blocker, and a long-acting nitrate may be used. In general, patients whose anginal symptoms do not respond to two antianginal agents should be referred to a specialist's care.

MONITORING PATIENT RESPONSE

In patients with angina, monitoring is important to evaluate for progression or stability of the disease, response to therapy, and presence or absence of adverse events.

Patient monitoring begins when a stress test is performed to confirm the diagnosis of angina. Once the diagnosis is made, stress tests may be repeated if there is a change in the pattern of anginal symptoms. Additionally, patients with stable angina should have an ECG if the history or physical examination

changes or if the practitioner suspects new myocardial ischemia or development of a conduction abnormality (Fihn et al., 2012).

Routine follow-up depends on the frequency and severity of the patient's complaints. Stable patients should be seen every 2 to 6 months, but visits should be more frequent if the patient's symptoms change or become more severe or more frequent. Medication initiation and adjustment also require more office visits. At each office visit, vital signs should be taken and a complete physical examination performed. The patient should be questioned about anginal pain and associated symptoms and side effects of the drug regimen. Additional monitoring parameters should be determined by the specific drug regimen. Ideally, a patient's antianginal regimen should make him or her symptom-free.

PATIENT EDUCATION

For optimal control of anginal symptoms, the patient should be educated on his or her disease and medications. Patients should be informed of the seriousness of coronary artery disease and the potential consequences of leaving their angina untreated. Education about lifestyle modification strategies should be provided to all patients as often as possible. Additionally, patients need to know how to recognize worsening or escalating symptoms so they know when to seek emergency care.

Drug Information

There are many sources of information relating to the treatment of angina. Several therapeutic guidelines are available to the practitioner, including those from the American College of Cardiology and American Heart Association, the American College of Chest Physicians, the European Society of Cardiology, and many other organizations. Specific questions relating to pharmacologic agents used in the treatment of angina may be addressed using the *Physician's Desk Reference, Drug Facts and*

CASE STUDY*

E.H. is a 45-year-old African American man who recently moved to the community from another state. He requests renewal of a prescription for a calcium channel blocker, prescribed by a physician in the former state. He is unemployed and lives with a woman, their son, and the woman's 2 children. His past medical history is remarkable for asthma and six "heart attacks" that he claims occurred because of a 25-year history of drug use (primarily cocaine). He states that he used drugs as recently as 2 weeks ago. He does not have any prior medical records with him. He claims that he has been having occasional periods of chest pain. He is unable to report the duration or pattern of the pain.

Before proceeding, explore the following questions: What further information would you need to diagnose angina (substantiate your answer)? What is the connection between cocaine use and angina? Identify at least three tests that you would order to diagnose angina.

DIAGNOSIS: ANGINA

1. List specific goals of treatment for E.H.
2. What dietary and lifestyle changes should be recommended for this patient?
3. What drug therapy would you prescribe for E.H. and why?
4. How would you monitor for success in E.H.?
5. Describe one or two drug–drug or drug–food interactions for the selected agent.
6. List one or two adverse reactions for the selected agent that would cause you to change therapy.
7. What would be the choice for the second-line therapy?
8. Discuss specific patient education based on the prescribed first-line therapy.
9. What over-the-counter and/or alternative medications would be appropriate for E.H.?

* Answers can be found online.

Comparisons, Epocrates, or another drug reference. Finally, information regarding ongoing clinical trials for angina and other conditions may be obtained from a Web site provided by the National Institutes of Health (www.clinicaltrials.gov).

Patient-Oriented Information Sources

Practitioners may provide disease- and treatment-related information to patients with information from a variety of sources. The Web site for the American Heart Association (www.americanheart.org) has many resources available to explain cardiovascular disease and angina in a fashion that patients will understand. Also, the American Academy of Family Physicians (www.familydoctor.org) provides on its Web site a variety of resources under the heading of "Patient Ed." Finally, the National Heart, Lung, and Blood Institute describes for patients the disease of angina, its causes, and appropriate treatments under the "Diseases and Conditions Index" (http://www.nhlbi.nih.gov/health/dci/Diseases/Angina/Angina_WhatIs.html).

Complementary and Alternative Medications

Although there are a variety of complementary medications, such as Coenzyme Q10 and vitamin E, that allege to provide symptom relief for patients with angina, no herbal or supplement medication has been shown to have efficacy similar to that of the traditional agents described above. Chelation therapy also has anecdotal reports of anginal symptom improvement, but there are no randomized controlled trials that support its use (Fihn et al., 2012). If at all possible, practitioners should counsel patients to adhere to treatment regimens that have shown efficacy in the treatment of angina.

Patients should be educated on each of the medications they are provided. They should know the importance of taking their medications as prescribed. They should be informed of each medication's indication and possible side effects, and what to do if they miss one or more doses of a scheduled medication, such as a long-acting nitrate. Additionally, practitioners should educate patients about the proper storage of all medications.

Bibliography

Starred references are cited in the text.

Alaeddini, J. (2015). Angina pectoris. Retrieved from http://emedicine.medscape.com/article/150215-overview on August 20, 2015.

*Antman, E., & Sabatine, M. (2013). *Cardiovascular therapeutics: A companion to Braunwald's heart disease.* New York, NY: Elsevier Health Sciences.

*American Heart Association. (2010). *Heart and stroke facts: 2004 update.* Dallas, TX: American Heart Association.

*Fihn, S. D., Gardin, J. M., Abrams, J., et al. (2012). 2012 ACCF, AHA, ACP, AATS, PCNA, SCAI, STS guideline for the diagnosis and management of stable ischemic heart disease. *Journal of the American College of Cardiology, 60,* e44–e164.

*Go, A. S., Mozaffarian, D., Roger, V. L., et al. (2014). AHA statistical update: Heart disease and stroke statistics—2014 update: A report from the American Heart Association. *Circulation, 129,* e28–e292.

Jneid, H., Anderson, J. L., Wright, R., et al. (2012). 2012 ACCF/AHA focused update of the guideline for the management of patients with unstable angina/non–ST-elevation myocardial infarction (updating the 2007 guideline and replacing the 2011 focused update): A report of the American College of Cardiology Foundation/American Heart Association Task Force on practice guidelines. *Journal of the American College of Cardiology, 60*(7), 645–681. doi: 10.1016/j.jacc.2012.06.004.

Katzung, B., & Chatterjee, M. (1998). Vasodilators and the treatment of angina pectoris. In B. Katzung (Ed.), *Basic and clinical pharmacology* (7th ed.). Stamford, CT: Appleton & Lange.

Kones, R. (2010). Recent advances in the management of chronic stable angina I: Approach to the patient, diagnosis, pathophysiology, risk stratification, and gender disparities. *Vascular Health and Risk Management, 6,* 635–656.

Lanza, G. A., Careri, G., & Crea, F. (2012). Contemporary reviews in cardiovascular medicine: Mechanisms of coronary artery spasm. *Circulation*, *124*, 1774–1782. doi: 10.1161/Circulationsaha.222.037283.

Libby, P., Ridken, P., & Hansson, G. (2011). Progress and challenges in translating the biology of atherosclerosis. *Nature*, *473*, 317–325. doi: 10.1038/nature10146.

Maron, D. J., Grundy, S. M., Ridler, P. M., et al (2004). Dyslipidemia, other risk factors, and the prevention of coronary heart disease. In V. Fuster, R. W. Alexander, & R. A. O'Rourke (Eds.), *Hurst's the heart* (11th ed., pp. 1093–1122). New York, NY: McGraw-Hill.

O'Rourke, R. A., O'Gara, P., & Douglas, J. S. (2004). Diagnosis and management of patients with chronic ischemic heart disease. In V. Fuster, R. W. Alexander, & R. A. O'Rourke (Eds.), *Hurst's the heart* (11th ed., pp. 1465–1494). New York, NY: McGraw-Hill.

Palaniswamy, C., & Aronow, W. (2011). Treatment of stable angina pectoris. *American Journal of Therapeutics*, *18*(5), e138–e152. doi: 10.1097/MJT.0b013e3181f2ab9d.

Patrano, C., Coller, B., FitzGerald, G. A., et al. (2004). Platelet-active drugs: The relationships among dose, effectiveness, and side effects: The seventh ACCP conference on antithrombotic and thrombolytic therapy. *Chest*, *126*(3, Suppl.), 234S–264S.

Ross, R. (1998). Factors influencing atherogenesis. In R. Alexander, R. Schant, & V. Fuster (Eds.), *Hurst's the heart* (9th ed., pp. 1139–1160). New York, NY: McGraw-Hill.

Sitia, S., Tomasoni, L., Atzeni, F., et al. (2010). From endothelial dysfunction to atherosclerosis. *Autoimmunity Reviews*, *9*(12), 830–834. doi: 10.1016/j.autrev.2010.07.016.

Stone, N. J., Robinson, J. G., Lichtenstein, A. H., et al. (2014). 2013 ACC/AHA guideline on the treatment of blood cholesterol to reduce atherosclerotic cardiovascular risk in adults. *Journal of the American College of Cardiology*, *63*, 2889–2934.

Tarkin, J., & Kaski, J. (2013). Pharmacological treatment of chronic stable angina pectoris. *Clinical Medicine*, *13*(1), 63–70.

Walker, B. F. (2004). Nonatherosclerotic coronary heart disease. In V. Fuster, R. W. Alexander, & R. A. O'Rourke (Eds.), *Hurst's the heart* (11th ed., pp. 1173–1214). New York, NY: McGraw-Hill.

22 Heart Failure

Andrew M. Peterson ■ Melody D. Randle ■ Troy L. Randle

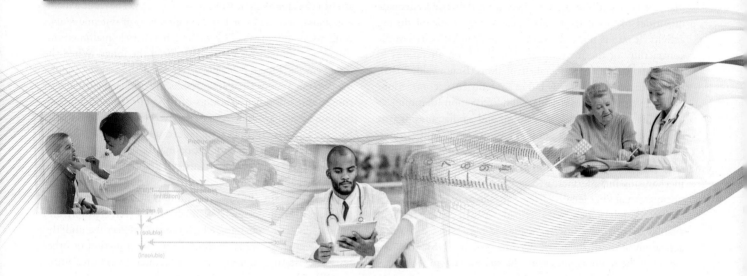

Heart failure (HF), one of the most serious consequences of cardiovascular disease, has rapidly become one of the most important health problems in cardiovascular medicine. Nearly 5 million Americans have HF today, with an incidence approaching 20 per 1,000 among persons older than age 65 (Go et al., 2013). At age 40, the lifetime risk of developing HF for both men and women is 1 in 5. The incidence of HF increases with age (Go et al., 2013). HF is more common in men than in women, due to the higher incidence of ischemic heart disease in men. Approximately 75% of all ambulatory patients with HF are age 60 or older (Go et al., 2013). As the population is aging, the number of people with HF will significantly increase in the future. In people diagnosed with HF, the mortality rates remain approximately 50% within 5 years of diagnosis (Go et al., 2013). Health care disparities place African Americans at highest risk for HF (Bahrami et al., 2008).

In the United States, HF incidence has largely remained stable over the past several decades, with more than 650,000 new HF cases diagnosed annually. HF incidence increases with age, rising from approximately 20 per 1,000 individuals 65 to 69 years of age to greater than 80 per 1,000 individuals among those 85 years of age or older. Approximately 5.1 million persons in the United States have clinically manifest HF, and the prevalence continues to rise, and 7% of all cardiac deaths are due to HF.

The economic impact of HF also is significant. The large number and often high complexity of hospitalizations for HF make this diagnosis very costly. The total cost of HF hospitalizations in the United States has been estimated at $8 billion. After hypertension, HF is the second most common indication for physician office visits. The estimated direct and indirect cost of HF in the United States for 2009 was $37.2 billion (Go et al., 2013). Consequently, improved quality of life is considered a worthy health care goal, and the therapeutic

approach to HF is directed toward increasing the patient's ability to maintain a positive quality of life with symptom-free activity and to enhance survival. Vasodilator therapy, especially with the angiotensin-converting enzyme (ACE) inhibitors, has made significant contributions toward achieving this goal.

CAUSES

The development of HF may be related to many etiologic variables. Coronary artery disease, hypertension, and idiopathic cardiomyopathy are the most frequently cited risk factors for HF. Acute conditions that may result in HF include acute myocardial infarction (MI), arrhythmias, pulmonary embolism, sepsis, and acute myocardial ischemia. Gradual development of HF may be caused by liver or renal disease, primary cardiomyopathy, cardiac valve disease, anemia, bacterial endocarditis, viral myocarditis, thyrotoxicosis, chemotherapy, excessive dietary sodium intake, and ethanol abuse.

Drugs also can worsen HF. Drugs that may cause fluid retention, such as nonsteroidal anti-inflammatory drugs (NSAIDs), steroids, hormones, antihypertensives (e.g., hydralazine [Apresoline], nifedipine [Procardia XL]), sodium-containing drugs (e.g., carbenicillin disodium [Geopen]), and lithium (Eskalith, others), may cause congestion. Beta-blockers, antiarrhythmics (e.g., disopyramide [Norpace], flecainide [Tambocor], amiodarone [Cordarone], sotalol [Betapace]), tricyclic antidepressants, and certain calcium channel blockers (e.g., diltiazem [Cardizem], nifedipine, verapamil [Calan]) have negative inotropic effects and further decrease contractility in an already depressed heart. Direct cardiac toxins (e.g., amphetamines, cocaine, daunorubicin [DaunoXome], doxorubicin [Adriamycin], and ethanol) also can worsen or induce HF.

PATHOPHYSIOLOGY

HF is a pathophysiologic state in which abnormal myocardial function inhibits the ventricles from delivering adequate quantities of blood to metabolizing tissues at rest or during activity. It results not only from a decrease in intrinsic systolic contractility of the myocardium but also from alterations in the pulmonary and peripheral circulations (Braunwald, 2015). The cardiac dysfunction is either in ventricular contraction/ejection (systolic) or ventricular filling/relaxation (diastolic).

When the heart fails as a pump and cardiac output (the volume of blood pumped out of the ventricle per unit of time) decreases, a complex scheme of compensatory mechanisms to raise and maintain cardiac output occurs. These compensatory mechanisms include increased preload (volume and pressure or myocardial fiber length of the ventricle prior to contraction [end of diastole]), increased afterload (vascular resistance), ventricular hypertrophy (increased muscle mass), and dilatation, activation of the sympathetic nervous system (SNS), and activation of the renin–angiotensin–aldosterone system (RAAS).

Although initially beneficial for increasing cardiac output, these compensatory mechanisms are ultimately associated with further pump dysfunction. In effect, the consequence of activating the compensatory systems is worsening HF. This is often referred to as the *vicious cycle of HF* (**Figure 22.1**). Without therapeutic intervention, some of the compensatory mechanisms continue to be activated, ultimately resulting in a reduced cardiac output and a worsening of the patient's symptoms. An understanding of the compensatory mechanisms makes it clear why one goal in treating HF is to interrupt this vicious cycle and why various drugs are used in managing patients with HF.

DIAGNOSTIC CRITERIA

The signs and symptoms of HF are useful in diagnosing and assessing a patient's clinical response to therapy. The clinical manifestations of HF are in part due to pulmonary or systemic venous congestion and edema. When the left ventricle malfunctions, congestion initially occurs proximally in the lungs. When the right ventricle functions inadequately, congestion in the supplying systemic venous circulation results in peripheral edema, liver congestion, and other indicators of right HF (**Box 22.1**). Both pulmonary and systemic congestion eventually develop in most patients with left HF. In fact, the chief cause of right HF is left HF.

Depressed ventricular function may be confirmed by echocardiography, radionuclide ventriculography, magnetic resonance imaging, or cardiac catheterization. Abnormalities in the electrocardiogram (ECG) are common and include arrhythmias, conduction delays, left ventricular (LV) hypertrophy, and nonspecific ST–T changes, which typically reflect the underlying etiology. Laboratory findings from liver function or other tests disclose such abnormalities as elevated blood urea nitrogen (BUN) and creatinine levels, hyponatremia, and elevated serum enzymes of hepatic origin. The circumstances in which the symptoms of HF occur are also particularly important in determining the severity of disease in a particular patient.

The New York Heart Association (NYHA) classifies the functional incapacity of patients with cardiac disease into four levels depending on the degree of effort needed to elicit symptoms (**Table 22.1**):

* *Class I:* Patients may have symptoms of HF only at levels that would produce symptoms in normal people.

FIGURE 22.1 Vicious circle of heart failure.

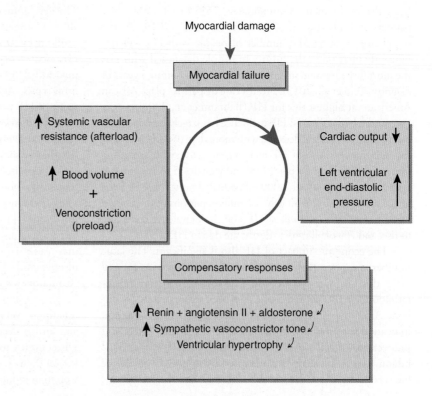

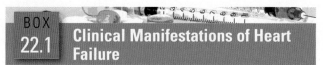

BOX 22.1 Clinical Manifestations of Heart Failure

Left Ventricular Failure—Pulmonary Congestion

Symptoms: Cough, dyspnea, dyspnea on exertion, orthopnea, paroxysmal nocturnal dyspnea, nocturia

Signs: Cardiomegaly, S_3 heart sound, bibasilar rales, signs of pulmonary edema, tachycardia, increased respiratory rate

Right Ventricular Failure—Systemic Congestion

Symptoms: Peripheral pitting edema, abdominal pain, anorexia, bloating, constipation, nausea, vomiting

Signs: Hepatomegaly, distention of the jugular veins, hepatojugular reflex, signs of portal hypertension, ascites, splenomegaly

Decreased Cardiac Output

Peripheral cyanosis, fatigue, decreased tissue perfusion, decrease in metabolism and renal elimination of drugs, decreased appetite, angina, increased risk for thromboembolism

TABLE 22.1
NYHA Functional Classification/ACCF/AHA Stages of HF

Class	Definition	Class	Definition
None		A	At high risk for HF without structural heart disease or symptoms of HF
I	No limitation of physical activity. Ordinary physical activity does not cause undue fatigue or dyspnea.	B	Structural heart disease but without signs or symptoms of HF
II	Slight limitation of physical activity. Comfortable at rest, but ordinary physical activity results in fatigue or dyspnea.	C	Structural heart disease with prior or current symptoms of HF
III	Marked limitation of physical activity. Comfortable at rest, but less than ordinary activity causes fatigue or dyspnea		
IV	Unable to carry on any physical activity without symptoms. Symptoms are present even at rest. If any physical activity is undertaken, symptoms are increased.	D	Refractory HF requiring specialized interventions

- *Class II:* Patients may have symptoms of HF on ordinary exertion.
- *Class III:* Patients may have symptoms of HF on less than ordinary exertion.
- *Class IV:* Patients may have symptoms of HF at rest.

The American College of Cardiology/American Heart Association (ACC/AHA) has developed a classification system that categorizes the progression of HF and is intended to complement the NYHA classification (**Table 22.1**):

- *Stage A:* Patients who are at high risk for developing HF but have no structural heart disease
- *Stage B:* Patients with structural heart disease who have never had symptoms of HF
- *Stage C:* Patients with past or current symptoms of HF associated with underlying structural heart disease
- *Stage D:* Patients with end-stage disease who require specialized treatment strategies, such as mechanical circulatory support, continuous IV inotrope infusions, cardiac transplantation, or hospice care

INITIATING DRUG THERAPY

In the past, digitalis, glycosides, and diuretics were the mainstays of therapy for HF. However, the concept of HF has changed dramatically from a narrow focus on the weakened heart to a broadened view of the systemic pathophysiologic state, with peripheral as well as myocardial factors playing important roles. Individualization of pharmacologic therapy is a cornerstone of care and now based on the stage of HF. The goals of therapy are to improve the quality of life, decrease mortality, and reduce the compensatory mechanisms causing the symptoms. Three general approaches are used:

1. An underlying cause of HF is treated if possible (e.g., surgical correction of structural abnormalities/valvular heart disease or medical treatment of conditions such as hypertension, diabetes mellitus, or dyslipidemia).
2. Precipitating factors that produce or worsen HF are identified and minimized (e.g., fever, anemia, arrhythmias, medication noncompliance, or drugs).
3. After these two steps, drug therapy to control the HF and improve survival becomes important.

Nonpharmacologic management techniques should be used along with pharmacologic therapy in patients with HF. In the past, reduced activities and bed rest were considered a standard part of the care of patients with HF. However, it has been determined that short periods of bed rest result in reduced exercise tolerance and aerobic capacity. There is insufficient evidence to recommend a specific type of training program or the routine use of supervised rehabilitation programs. Although most patients should not participate in heavy labor or exhausting sports, aerobic activity should be encouraged (except during periods of acute decompensation). For example, according to the Agency for Healthcare Research and Quality (AHRQ), regular exercise (e.g., walking or cycling) is recommended for patients with stable class I to III disease.

Goals of Drug Therapy

Pharmacologic management of patients with HF is critical in reducing symptoms and decreasing mortality. In most cases, drug therapy is long term and consists of ACE inhibitors and beta blockers for class I indications. Diuretics, aldosterone antagonists, hydralazine, nitrates, digoxin (Lanoxin), and others medications are also used. **Table 22.2** provides an overview of drugs used to treat HF.

In patients with a history and reduced ejection fraction (EF), ACE inhibitors (ACE-I) or angiotensin receptor blockers (ARBs) should be used to prevent HF. In patients with an MI and reduced EF, beta-blockers should be used to prevent HF and a statin also given.

Angiotensin-Converting Enzyme Inhibitors (ACE-I)

Patients who have HF resulting from LV systolic dysfunction and who have an LV EF less than 35% to 40% should be given a trial of ACE inhibitors, unless they cannot tolerate treatment with these drugs. The ACE inhibitors may be considered therapy in the subset of patients who present with fatigue or mild dyspnea on exertion and who do not have any other signs or symptoms of volume overload. In patients with evidence for, or a prior history of, fluid retention, ACE inhibitors are usually used together with diuretics. (See section on Selecting the Most Appropriate Agent.) ACE inhibitors are also recommended for use in patients with LV systolic dysfunction who have no symptoms of HF. The clinical and mortality benefits of the ACE inhibitors have been shown in numerous uncontrolled and controlled, randomized clinical trials.

ACE inhibitors (ACE-I) have a positive effect on cardiac function (i.e., reduced preload and afterload, increased cardiac index, and EF) and the signs and symptoms of HF (e.g., dyspnea, fatigue, orthopnea, and peripheral edema). As a result, exercise capacity is increased, NYHA functional classification is significantly improved, and morbidity and mortality rates in patients with HF, including those who have suffered an MI, are reduced because these drugs can attenuate ventricular dilation and remodeling.

Captopril (Capoten), enalapril (Vasotec), fosinopril (Monopril), lisinopril (Zestril), quinapril (Accupril), trandolapril (Mavik), ramipril (Altace), and perindopril (Aceon) are the ACE inhibitors currently indicated for treating HF (see **Table 22.2**). The ACE inhibitors that are approved for use in patients with LV dysfunction, and have been shown to prolong survival, are enalapril, captopril, and lisinopril. Quinapril and fosinopril are labeled for symptom reduction in HF, but data are lacking as to their effect on mortality rates.

Mechanism of Action

"Balanced" vasodilators, including the ACE inhibitors and angiotensin II receptor blockers, cause vasodilation on both the venous and arterial sides of the heart and therefore provide the hemodynamic and clinical benefits of both preload and afterload reduction.

Activation of the RAAS is an important compensatory mechanism in HF (**Figure 22.2**). ACE catalyzes the conversion of angiotensin I to angiotensin II, a potent vasoconstrictor and stimulant of aldosterone secretion. ACE inhibitors are uniquely effective in managing HF by interrupting stimulation of the RAAS, inhibiting the contributions of this system to the downward spiral of HF. The pharmacodynamic properties of ACE inhibitors involve specific competitive binding to the active site of ACE.

Angiotensin II interacts with at least two known membrane receptors, type 1 and type 2 (AT_1 and AT_2). By blocking formation of angiotensin II, ACE inhibitors indirectly produce vasodilation and a decrease in systemic vascular resistance (LV afterload). In addition, because angiotensin II stimulates aldosterone secretion by the adrenal cortex and provides negative feedback for plasma renin, inhibition of angiotensin II may lead to decreased aldosterone and increased renin activity. This prevents aldosterone-mediated sodium and water retention and may produce a small increase in serum potassium levels. The reduction in volume expansion due to ACE inhibition decreases ventricular end-diastolic volume (i.e., preload). Because ACE (kininase II) is involved in the breakdown of bradykinin, a vasodilator, a decrease in kininase II activity by an ACE inhibitor could increase bradykinin as well as prostaglandin production, either of which can lead to vasodilation.

ACE inhibitors produce vasodilation, inhibit fluid accumulation, and increase blood flow to vital organs, such as the brain, kidney, and heart, without precipitating reflex tachycardia. The hemodynamic effects of ACE inhibitors in HF include decreased preload, afterload, and mean arterial pressure, as well as increased cardiac output. EF is also improved. Clinical benefits to patients with HF include improvement in exercise duration, NYHA functional class, dyspnea/fatigue focal index, and signs and symptoms of HF, as well as increased survival.

Dosage

ACE inhibitors should be initiated at low doses followed by gradual dosage increases if the lower doses have been well tolerated. Renal function and serum potassium should be assessed within 1 to 2 weeks of starting therapy and periodically thereafter, especially in patients with preexisting hypotension, hyponatremia, diabetes, or azotemia, or if they are receiving potassium supplementation. Doses should be titrated as tolerated by the patient to the target doses shown in clinical trials to decrease morbidity and mortality (e.g., 150 mg/d in divided doses of captopril; 20 mg/d of enalapril or lisinopril). The doses of ACE inhibitors can be increased to these effective doses unless the patient cannot tolerate high doses. The practitioner should provide the following information to patients taking ACE inhibitors:

- Adverse effects may occur early in therapy but do not usually prevent long-term use of the drug.
- Symptomatic improvement may not be seen for several weeks or months.

TABLE 22.2

Overview of Selected Agents Used to Treat Heart Failure

Generic (Trade) Name and Dosage	Selected Adverse Events	Contraindications	Special Considerations
Selected Angiotensin-Converting Enzyme Inhibitors			
captopril (Capoten) Start: 6.25 mg or 12.5 mg tid Therapeutic range: 25–100 mg tid	Common: cough; hypotension, particularly with a diuretic or volume depletion; hyperkalemia, loss of taste, leukopenia; angioedema, neutropenia, and agranulocytosis in <1% of patients; rash in >10% of patients	Contraindicated in pregnancy Avoid in patients with bilateral renal artery stenosis or unilateral stenosis.	Renal impairment related to ACE inhibitors is seen as an increase in serum creatinine and azotemia, usually in the beginning of therapy. Monitor BUN, creatinine, and K levels when starting.
enalapril (Vasotec) Start: 2.5 mg qd or bid Range: 5–20 mg qd or bid daily	Same as above	Same as above	Same as above Use only 2.5 mg/d in patient with impaired renal function or hyponatremia.
fosinopril (Monopril) Start: 10 mg qd Range: 10–40 mg qd	Same as above	Same as above	Same as above Use only 5 mg/d in patient with impaired renal function or hyponatremia.
lisinopril (Zestril, Prinivil) Start: 5 mg qd Range: 5–20 mg qd	Same as above	Same as above	Same as above Use only 2.5 mg/d in patient with impaired renal function or hyponatremia.
quinapril (Accupril) Start: 5 mg bid Range: 20–40 bid	Same as above	Same as above	Same as above Use only 2.5 mg/d in patient with impaired renal function or hyponatremia.
ramipril (Altace) Start: 1.25 mg twice daily Range: 1.25–5 mg twice daily	Same as above	Same as above	Same as above
trandolapril (Mavik) Start: 0.5–1 mg daily Target dose: 4 mg	Same as above	Same as above	Same as above
Selected Thiazide and Thiazide-like Diuretics			
chlorthalidone (Hygroton) 12.5–50 mg qd	Hyperuricemia, hypokalemia, hypomagnesemia, hyperglycemia, hyponatremia, hypercalcemia, hypercholesterolemia, hypertriglyceridemia, pancreatitis, rashes and other allergic reactions	High doses are relatively contraindicated in patients with hyperlipidemia, gout, and diabetes.	Thiazide diuretics preferred in patients with CrCl >30 mL/min
hydrochlorothiazide (HydroDIURIL, Microzide) 12.5–50 mg qd	Same as chlorthalidone	Same as chlorthalidone	Same as chlorthalidone
metolazone (Zaroxolyn) 2.5–10 mg qd	Less or no hypercholesterolemia	Same as chlorthalidone	Same as chlorthalidone
Loop Diuretics			
bumetanide (Bumex) 0.5–5 mg qd–bid	Dehydration, circulatory collapse, hypokalemia, hyponatremia, hypomagnesemia, hyperglycemia, metabolic alkalosis, hyperuricemia (short duration of action, no hypercalcemia)	High doses are relatively contraindicated in patients with hyperlipidemia, gout, and diabetes.	Effective in patients with CrCl <30 mL/min Monitor BUN, creatinine, and K levels when starting and with dosage changes.
ethacrynic acid (Edecrin) 25–100 mg bid–tid	Same as bumetanide (only nonsulfonamide diuretic, ototoxicity)	Same as bumetanide	Same as bumetanide

(Continued)

TABLE 22.2

Overview of Selected Agents Used to Treat Heart Failure (*Continued*)

Generic (Trade) Name and Dosage	Selected Adverse Events	Contraindications	Special Considerations
furosemide (Lasix) 20–320 mg bid–tid	Same as bumetanide	Same as bumetanide	Same as bumetanide
torsemide (Demadex) 5–20 mg qd–bid	Short duration of action, no hypercalcemia	Same as bumetanide	Same as bumetanide
Potassium-Sparing Diuretics			
amiloride (Midamor) 5–20 mg qd–bid	Hyperkalemia, GI disturbances, rash	High doses are relatively contraindicated in patients with hyperlipidemia, gout, and diabetes.	Same as bumetanide
spironolactone (Aldactone) 12.5–100 mg qd–bid	Hyperkalemia, GI disturbances, rash, gynecomastia	Same as amiloride	Spironolactone ideal in patients with heart failure
triamterene (Dyrenium) 50–150 mg qd–bid	Hyperkalemia, GI disturbances, nephrolithiasis	Same as amiloride	Same as bumetanide
Other Agents			
digitalis/digoxin (Lanoxin) 0.25 mg qd	Ventricular tachycardia, paroxysmal atrial tachycardia, fatigue, anorexia, nausea	Allergy, ventricular tachycardia, ventricular fibrillation, heart block, sick sinus syndrome, idiopathic hypertrophic sub-aortic stenosis, acute MI, renal insufficiency, electrolyte abnormalities Use with caution in pregnancy and lactation.	Check potassium levels before starting. Check serum levels once a year.
hydralazine (Apresoline) 25–75 mg tid	Postural hypotension, tachycardia	Coronary artery disease, aortic stenosis	Advise patient to avoid rapid changes in position. Patient can be started on 10 mg tid if elderly, with severe heart failure, or hypotensive.
isosorbide dinitrate (ISDN) (Isordil) 10–40 mg tid	Headache, dizziness, tachycardia, retrosternal discomfort, blurred vision, rash, flushing	Hypersensitivity to nitrates, closed-angle glaucoma, early MI, head trauma, pregnancy (category C)	Advise patient to avoid rapid changes in position.
Beta-Blockers			
bisoprolol (Zebeta) Start: 5 mg daily Range: 5–20 mg daily	Bradycardia, congestive heart failure, atrioventricular block, postural hypotension, vertigo, fatigue, depression, broncho-spasm, impotence, insomnia, decreased exercise tolerance, impaired peripheral circulation, generalized edema, sinusitis	Sinus bradycardia, second- or third-degree heart block, asthma, liver abnormalities	Advise patient to avoid abrupt cessation of therapy. Observe for signs of dizziness for 1 h when dose is increased.
carvedilol (Coreg) 3.125–50 mg bid	Same as above	Same as above	Same as above
metoprolol Start: 6.25 mg 2–3 times daily Range: 50–100 mg 2–3 times daily	Same as above	Same as above	Same as above

TABLE 22.2

Overview of Selected Agents Used to Treat Heart Failure (*Continued*)

Generic (Trade) Name and Dosage	Selected Adverse Events	Contraindications	Special Considerations
Selected Angiotensin Receptor Blockers			
losartan (Cozaar) Start: 12.5 mg/d Range: 50–100 mg/d	Dyspnea, hypotension, hyperkalemia	Angioedema secondary to ACE inhibition	May be used in patients experiencing cough due to ACE inhibitor
valsartan (Diovan) Start: 80 mg/d Range: 80–160 mg twice daily	Same as above	Same as above	Same as above
Other Agents			
dobutamine (Dobutrex) 2–5 mcg/kg/min intravenously	Elevated blood pressure, increased heart rate, angina, hypotension	Idiopathic hypertrophic sub-aortic stenosis	May increase insulin requirements
ivabradine (Corlanor) 2.5–7.5 mg bid	Bradycardia, HTN, atrial fibrillation, visual disturbances	Severe hepatic impairment, sick sinus syndrome, SA block without pacemaker, resting HR <60, atrial fibrillation, BP <90/50	Avoid grapefruit.

- ACE inhibitors may reduce the risk of disease progression even if the patient's symptoms have not responded favorably to treatment (Savarese et al., 2013).

Captopril, lisinopril, ramipril, and trandolapril have been shown to reduce mortality rates in patients who have had an MI and who have HF symptoms. The indications for these ACE inhibitors in this population vary slightly, and the dosing in patients after MI differs from the dosing for patients with chronic HF. Captopril is indicated to improve survival after MI in clinically stable patients with LV dysfunction manifested as an EF of 40% or less and to reduce the incidence of overt HF and subsequent hospitalizations for HF. Captopril may be

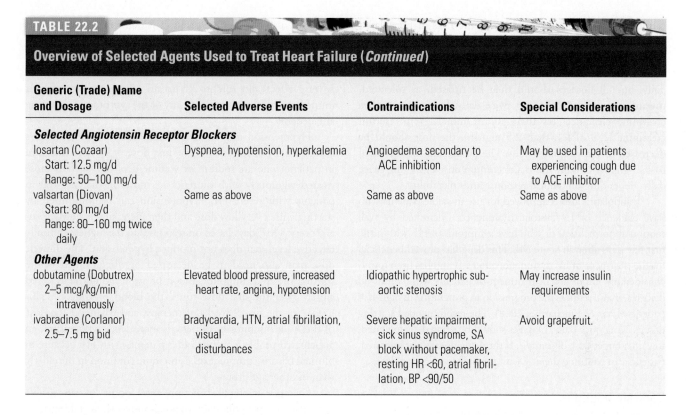

FIGURE 22.2 The renin–angiotensin–aldosterone (RAA) syndrome.

initiated with a single dose of 6.25 mg. If the patient tolerates this dose, the dose should be titrated in increments to a maximum of 50 mg three times a day as long as tolerated (systolic blood pressure greater than 100 mm Hg). Other post-MI therapies (e.g., thrombolytics, aspirin, and beta-blockers) may be used concurrently.

Lisinopril has been shown to decrease mortality rates in both acute and post-MI patients. Lisinopril also is indicated for treating hemodynamically stable patients within 24 hours of an acute MI to improve survival. Patients should receive, as appropriate, the standard recommended treatments, such as thrombolytics, aspirin, and beta-blockers. The first 2.5-mg dose of lisinopril may be given to hemodynamically stable patients within 24 hours of the onset of symptoms of acute MI. The dose of lisinopril should be titrated as tolerated to a dose of 10 mg daily. Dosing should be continued for 6 weeks. At that time, the patient should be assessed for signs and symptoms of HF, and therapy should be continued if necessary. The dose should be decreased to 2.5 mg in patients with a low systolic blood pressure (below 120 mm Hg) when treatment is started or during the first 3 days after the MI. If hypotension occurs (systolic blood pressure below 100 mm Hg), a daily maintenance dose of 5 mg may be given with temporary reductions to 2.5 mg if needed. If prolonged hypotension occurs (systolic blood pressure below 90 mm Hg for at least 1 hour), lisinopril therapy should be discontinued. Patients who develop symptoms of HF should receive the usual effective dose of lisinopril for HF, with a goal of 20 mg/d.

Ramipril has also been approved for stable patients who have shown clinical signs of HF within the first few days after an acute MI. It is used to decrease the risk of death (principally cardiovascular death) and to decrease the risks of HF-related hospitalization and progression to severe or resistant HF. The starting dose is 2.5 mg twice daily. A patient who becomes hypotensive at this dose may be switched to 1.25 mg twice daily, but all dosages should then be titrated, as tolerated, toward a target dose of 5 mg twice daily. In patients with a creatinine clearance less than 40 mL/min/1.73 m^2 (serum creatinine level of less than 2.5 mg/dL), the dose should be decreased to 1.25 mg once daily. The dosage may be increased to 1.25 mg twice daily up to a maximum dose of 2.5 mg twice daily, depending on clinical response and tolerability.

Trandolapril also is approved for use in stable patients who have evidence of LV systolic dysfunction (identified by wall motion abnormalities) or who have symptoms of HF within the first few days after an acute MI. This drug has proved beneficial for the treatment of LV dysfunction after MI and has been found considerably important in treatment of patients with comorbid diabetes. It also reduces the progression to proteinuria in high-risk patients (Diaz & Ducharme, 2008). The recommended starting dose is 1 mg once daily. Dosages should be titrated, as tolerated, toward a target dose of 4 mg/d. If the 4-mg dose is not tolerated, patients can continue therapy with the highest tolerated dose.

Contraindications

Patients should not receive an ACE inhibitor if they have experienced life-threatening adverse effects (e.g., angioedema or anuric renal failure) during previous exposure or if they are pregnant. Angioedema is a potentially fatal allergic reaction that may cause sudden difficulty in breathing, speaking, and swallowing accompanied by obvious swelling of the lips, face, and neck. Patients should receive an ACE inhibitor with caution if they have any of the following:

- Very low systemic blood pressure (systolic blood pressure less than 80 mm Hg)
- Markedly increased serum creatinine levels (above 3 mg/dL)
- Bilateral renal artery stenosis (previously considered a contraindication)
- Elevated serum potassium levels (above 5.5 mmol/L)

In addition, ACE inhibitors should not be given to hypotensive patients who are at immediate risk for cardiogenic shock and who require intravenous (IV) pressor support (e.g., dobutamine [Dobutrex] or epinephrine [Adrenalin, others]). These patients should receive treatment for their pump failure first; then, once they are stabilized, the HF should be reevaluated.

When taken by pregnant women during the second and third trimesters, ACE inhibitors can cause injury and even death to the fetus. When pregnancy is detected, the ACE inhibitor should be discontinued immediately due to the teratogenic effects.

Adverse Events

The most common adverse reactions of ACE inhibitors are dizziness, headache, fatigue, diarrhea, cough, and hypotension. Angioedema of the face, extremities, lips, tongue, glottis,

or larynx also has been reported in patients treated with ACE inhibitors. Angioedema associated with throat or laryngeal edema may be fatal because of airway blockage, which causes suffocation. Patients should be advised about this possible adverse effect and told to go to an emergency department immediately if they experience any of the symptoms suggesting angioedema.

Hypotension may occur with any of the ACE inhibitors and is usually observed after the first dose. It is more common in patients who are sodium or volume depleted, such as those treated vigorously with diuretics or those on dialysis, and in patients with severe HF. Hypotension can be minimized by starting with a very low dose and then increasing it slowly (usually every 3 to 7 days based on response) to the highest clinically effective level that does not produce hypotension. The diuretic dose may also need to be decreased or discontinued before starting the ACE inhibitor. Blood pressure should be followed closely after the first dose (until the blood pressure is stabilized), for the first 2 weeks of therapy, and whenever the dose of the ACE inhibitor or diuretic is increased. Hypotension, an anticipated problem among older patients with HF because of blunted baroreceptor reflexes, is no more common in the elderly than in other age groups.

Changes in renal function may occur in susceptible patients (i.e., patients with hyponatremia; those taking high doses of diuretics; those with low cardiac output, diabetes mellitus, severe HF, or preexisting renal impairment) because of inhibition of the RAAS. Patients with bilateral or unilateral renal artery stenosis should receive ACE inhibitors with extreme caution and should be monitored closely because renal failure may occur. The increases in serum creatinine and BUN that may occur are usually reversible by adjusting the dose of the ACE inhibitor, diuretic, or both. Furthermore, an increase in serum creatinine not exceeding 30% of the basal value is now being viewed as an indicator that the drug is working (i.e., there is adequate ACE inhibition) and not that it has caused renal failure and the drug may be continued in these patients. However, the initial dose of an ACE inhibitor should be reduced with increasing severity of HF, and the titration period should be monitored carefully. Age-related declines in renal function may slow the elimination of ACE inhibitors and thus increase the level and duration of their effects. Therefore, it may be necessary to reduce the initial dose of ACE inhibitors in the elderly or in patients with a serum creatinine level of 2.5 mg/dL or more. These patients may not tolerate as high a dose as other patients with HF but should be titrated to the highest possible dose.

Diuretic-induced potassium loss (hypokalemia) may be reduced when an ACE inhibitor is used in combination with a diuretic. However, hyperkalemia may occur in patients with renal impairment or in those receiving a potassium-sparing diuretic, a potassium supplement, or potassium-containing salt substitutes. ACE inhibitors should be administered cautiously if hypokalemia exists and discontinued if hyperkalemia exists. Frequent monitoring of serum potassium levels should be performed.

A cough is a common adverse event associated with ACE inhibitor therapy, occurring in 5% to 20% of patients. It is thought to be due to increased production of bradykinins or substance P, both of which lower the cough reflex. The cough is described as an annoying, ticklish, dry cough that is reversible on discontinuation of the ACE inhibitor. In patients with HF, cough is rarely severe enough to require discontinuation of therapy. Patients who experience cough should be questioned to determine whether this symptom is due to the ACE inhibitor or to pulmonary edema. The ACE inhibitor should be implicated only after other causes have been excluded. In most cases, the patient and family can be advised that if the cough is bothersome but not intolerable, the benefits of ACE inhibitor therapy outweigh this adverse effect. However, if the cough is persistent and troublesome, the clinician can suggest withdrawing the ACE inhibitor and trying alternative medications (e.g., an ARB or a combination of hydralazine and isosorbide dinitrate [HYD/ISDN]).

Because HF is common among the elderly and increases in prevalence with age, safety and efficacy in this population are important. When ACE inhibitors first became available, many experts believed that because elderly patients tend to have low plasma renin activity, these agents would be relatively ineffective. Furthermore, the physiologic consequences of aging may alter the absorption, distribution, and elimination of drugs, as well as the sensitivity of the patient to drugs. Thus, it was recognized that safety and efficacy studies should be conducted in this important patient population. A number of studies have been completed, and they document that ACE inhibitors are well tolerated and effective for elderly patients with HF. Studies have not yet identified differences in response between the elderly and younger patients. However, greater sensitivity of some older patients cannot be ruled out. Older patients receiving ACE inhibitors do not experience more adverse effects than do younger patients (Masoudi et al., 2004).

Interactions

The ACE inhibitors have been associated with very few significant drug–drug interactions. One or all of the ACE inhibitors have been used in combination with digoxin, methyldopa (Aldomet), prazosin (Minipress), hydralazine, beta-blockers, nitrates, and calcium channel blockers. The drug interactions that should be kept in mind are listed in **Table 22.3**.

Diuretics

During initial evaluation, the clinician should determine whether the patient manifests symptoms (e.g., orthopnea, paroxysmal nocturnal dyspnea, or dyspnea on exertion) or signs (e.g., pulmonary rales, a third heart sound, or jugular venous distention) of volume overload. Patients with HF and significant volume overload should be started immediately on a diuretic in conjunction with an ACE inhibitor and a beta-blocker (see **Table 22.2**).

TABLE 22.3

Drug Interactions Associated with the Angiotensin-Converting Enzyme Inhibitors

Interacting Agent	Potential Effect
antacids	Decrease the bioavailability of captopril; therefore, separate administration times by 2 h.
aspirin	Decreases hemodynamic response of ACE inhibitor
capsaicin	Triggers or exacerbates the coughing that is associated with ACE inhibitor treatment
lithium	In combination with ACE inhibitor, causes increased serum lithium levels and symptoms of lithium toxicity
nonsteroidal anti-inflammatory drugs	In combination with ACE inhibitor, promotes sodium and water retention and diminishes control of hypertension and heart failure
potassium supplements/ potassium-sparing diuretics/salt substitutes	In combination with ACE inhibitor, increases risk of hyperkalemia
rifampin	Reduces the pharmacologic effects of enalapril
tetracycline	In combination with quinapril, tetracycline undergoes decreased absorption (28%–37%), possibly from the high magnesium content in quinapril.

Mechanism of Action

Diuretics cause an increase in sodium and water excretion by the kidney by inhibiting the reabsorption of sodium or chloride. Thiazide diuretics work at the distal tubule of the kidney. Loop diuretics (bumetanide, furosemide, or torsemide) exert their effect at the loop of Henle as well as the proximal and distal tubules. Thus, loop diuretics are more potent in inhibiting sodium, chloride, and water excretion. Diuretics decrease preload by reducing the volume overload. An immediate effect (extrarenal) is an increase in venous capacity, with resultant redistribution of venous blood away from the lungs toward the periphery, which results in a decrease in pulmonary capillary pressure.

Dosage

Therapy is commonly initiated with low doses of a diuretic (e.g., furosemide [Lasix] 20 to 40 mg/d), and the dose is increased until urine output increases and weight decreases, usually by 0.5 to 1.0 kg daily. Increases in the dose of the diuretic may be required to sustain the loss of weight. The goal is to reduce symptoms as well as eliminate physical signs of fluid retention by restoring jugular venous pressures toward normal, by eliminating edema, or both. Patients with persistent volume overload despite initial medical management may require one of the following:

- More aggressive administration of the current diuretic (e.g., IV administration)
- A combination of diuretics (e.g., loop diuretic and metolazone [Zaroxolyn])
- Short-term use of drugs that increase renal blood flow (e.g., dopamine [Intropin])

Although patients are commonly prescribed a fixed dose of diuretic, the dose of these drugs should be adjusted ideally on a daily basis. This can be accomplished in most cases by having the patient record his or her weight daily and allowing the patient or an appropriately trained health professional to adjust the dosage if the weight increases or decreases beyond a specified range for that patient. Thus, the most useful approach for practitioners to select the dose of, and monitor the response to, diuretic therapy is by measuring body weight, preferably on a daily basis. Practitioners should educate patients on the importance of weighing themselves and contacting a health care professional when weight increases or symptoms return. This may help to avoid hospitalization of the patient with HF.

Patients with pulmonary edema or with marked volume overload should be given an IV loop diuretic initially. Diuretics should then be titrated to achieve resolution or improvement of signs and symptoms of volume overload. There is no standard target dose. Excessive diuresis should be avoided before starting an ACE inhibitor. Volume depletion may lead to hypotension or renal insufficiency when ACE inhibitors are started.

Spironolactone (Aldactone) has taken a larger, but controversial, role in the treatment of HF. In the Randomized Aldactone Evaluation Study (RALES), study of spironolactone use in HF revealed a decrease in morbidity and mortality (Pitt et al., 1999). A more recent global study of spironolactone did not support the findings of RALES supported (Pitt et al., 2014). Spironolactone lacked efficacy within patient subgroups who also had comorbid problems of blood pressure and diabetes. The researchers speculated this variance could be explained by different treatments around the world. However, in the absence of any other similar drug, cardiology experts still support the use of spironolactone. Spironolactone acts to competitively bind at the aldosterone receptor site of the distal convoluted renal tubules, which causes increased amounts of water and sodium to be excreted. Therefore, low doses (25 to 50 mg/d) of spironolactone merit consideration in patients with recent or current NYHA class IV symptoms. The efficacy and safety of aldosterone antagonists in patients with mild or moderate HF remain unknown.

Adverse Events

Potassium depletion commonly occurs when patients are treated chronically with diuretics, except with the use of spironolactone. However, ACE inhibitors decrease renal potassium losses and raise serum potassium levels, so many patients with HF who are treated with both agents may not have potassium depletion. Concomitant administration of ACE inhibitors alone or in combination with potassium-sparing agents (e.g., spironolactone) can prevent electrolyte depletion in most patients with HF. Diuretics may also cause magnesium depletion, which often accompanies potassium depletion. If high doses of diuretics are used, magnesium levels should be followed and oral supplementation given when needed (Mg 1.5 mEq/L).

Interactions

NSAIDs (including aspirin) may blunt the natriuretic effect of diuretics. Therefore, patients receiving daily therapy with NSAIDs may need an increase in the dose of the diuretic to compensate for fluid retention. Diuretics may decrease lithium clearance, which may raise lithium levels into the toxic range. Lithium levels should be monitored in patients receiving both drugs. Patients may be at an increased risk of ototoxicity when high doses of loop diuretics and other ototoxic drugs (e.g., aminoglycosides) are used concomitantly.

Angiotensin II Type 1 Receptor Blockers (ARBs)

These antagonists were developed to offer the advantages of increased selectivity and specificity and to maintain blockade of the circulating and tissue RAAS at the AT_1 receptor level, without the adverse reactions associated with ACE inhibitors. ARBs do not block the degradation of vasoactive substances (e.g., bradykinin, enkephalins, and substance P) and may not cause the adverse effects, such as cough, related to ACE inhibitor–induced bradykinin accumulation.

Of the currently approved ARBs, losartan (Cozaar) has been the most extensively studied in patients with HF. Losartan lowers blood pressure, systemic vascular resistance, pulmonary capillary wedge pressure, and heart rate and raises the cardiac index. Dyspnea on exertion and HF exacerbation decrease with losartan. Compared with the ACE inhibitor enalapril, losartan shows no significant difference in terms of altered exercise capacity (6-minute walk test), clinical status (dyspnea–fatigue index), neurohumoral activation (norepinephrine, N-terminal atrial natriuretic factor), laboratory evaluation, or incidence of adverse effects. Comparisons with another ACE inhibitor, captopril, show that losartan has the same incidence of persistent renal dysfunction and no difference in the incidence of death or HF hospital admissions. Further studies with other ACE inhibitors in various patient populations are needed to determine whether losartan reduces morbidity and mortality to a greater degree than the ACE inhibitors. The initial studies of losartan for treating HF seem promising. In addition, studies of the combination of ARBs and ACE inhibitors are also being conducted. Although combination therapy with an ACE inhibitor and ARB has been shown to be of benefit in the Val-HeFT and CHARM trials, there is hesitancy in clinical practice due to effects on renal function. It is reasonable to prescribe ARBs instead of ACE inhibitors only in patients who cannot tolerate ACE inhibitors because of angioedema or intractable cough. Even though the pathways are different, ARBs should be used cautiously (if at all) in patients that developed angioedema with ACE inhibitors.

Mechanism of Action

ARBs block the physiologic effects of angiotensin II by inhibiting receptor stimulation. The currently marketed ARBs—candesartan (Atacand), eprosartan (Teveten), losartan (Cozaar), olmesartan (Benicar), telmisartan (Micardis), valsartan (Diovan), and irbesartan (Avapro)—are approved by the US Food and Drug Administration (FDA) for the management of hypertension. These antagonists were developed to offer the advantages of increased selectivity and specificity and to maintain blockade of the circulating and tissue RAAS at the AT_1 receptor level, without the adverse reactions associated with ACE inhibitors. ARBs do not block the degradation of vasoactive substances (e.g., bradykinin, enkephalins, and substance P) and may not cause the adverse effects, such as cough, related to ACE inhibitor–induced bradykinin accumulation.

When ARBs were introduced into practice, there was a theoretical consideration that reducing the production of angiotensin II with an ACE inhibitor and blocking the remaining angiotensin II with an ARB would be better than either therapy alone. However, the Val-HeFT study showed that adding an ARB to ACE inhibitor therapy is not beneficial.

Dosage

The doses of these agents vary. **Table 22.2** lists selected ARBs and their doses, but a more complete review of these agents can be found in Chapter 19. Regardless of which agent is selected, the practitioner should monitor the patient's renal function and blood pressure.

Adverse Events

ARB therapy may be associated with hypotension. This usually occurs with the first dose but may also occur during upward titration or when clinical status worsens. This situation is most common among patients with hyponatremia, hypovolemia, low baseline blood pressure, renal impairment, and high baseline levels of renin or aldosterone. Potentiation of the vasodilator effects of bradykinin and prostaglandins appears to contribute to this hypotension. Theoretically, ARBs, which do not interfere with the degradation of these peptides, should result in fewer episodes of first-dose hypotension. However, this beneficial effect remains to be proven in clinical trials. In addition, specific ARBs could block the deleterious effects of angiotensin II produced by non–ACE-dependent pathways that are not blocked by ACE inhibitors.

The most common adverse events with losartan include dyspnea, worsening of HF, hypotension, dizziness, cough, and upper respiratory tract infection. The ARBs appear as likely as the ACE inhibitors to produce hypotension, worsening renal function, and hyperkalemia. Also, like ACE inhibitors, these agents are contraindicated in pregnancy, especially during the second and third trimesters.

Beta-blockers

Historically, beta-blockers have been contraindicated for treating HF. The negative inotropic effect, bradycardic effect, and peripheral constriction of the beta-blockers can all exacerbate HF. However, observations from experimental studies and controlled clinical trials indicate that prolonged activation of the SNS can accelerate the progression of HF. The studies also determined that the risks of such progression can be substantially decreased through the use of pharmacologic agents that interfere with the actions of the SNS on the heart and peripheral blood vessels. Thus, the use of beta-blockers is gaining acceptance as a treatment for HF.

The new recommendations strongly advocate using beta-blockers for treating patients with HF. As stated previously, the recommendations state that all patients with stable NYHA class II to class IV HF due to LV systolic dysfunction should receive a beta-blocker unless they have a contraindication to its use or have shown to be unable to tolerate treatment with the drug. Beta-blockers should not be used in unstable patients or in acutely ill patients ("rescue" therapy), including those who are in the intensive care unit with refractory HF requiring IV support. Beta-blockers can be initiated once patients are clinically compensated. Also, if a patient is already on a beta-blocker, it can be continued as long as the patient is hemodynamically stable. Beta-blockers are recommended to improve symptoms and clinical status and to decrease the risk of death and hospitalization in patients with mild to moderate (NYHA class II) or moderate to severe (NYHA class III) HF who have an LV EF of less than 35% to 40%. Beta-blockers should be added to preexisting treatment with diuretics and an ACE inhibitor and may be used together with digitalis or vasodilators.

Carvedilol, a nonselective beta-adrenergic receptor blocker with vasodilating action (through alpha-adrenergic blocking action) previously approved for the management of essential hypertension, has become the first beta-blocker approved in the United States for treating HF. It is intended to reduce the progression of disease as evidenced by cardiovascular death, cardiovascular hospitalization, or the need to adjust other HF medications. Similarly, the extended-release formulation of metoprolol, metoprolol succinate, was shown to be superior to placebo in decreasing mortality in HF patients. Bisoprolol (Zebeta) is also a beta-blocker used in the treatment of HF that decreases mortality.

Mechanism of Action

Catecholamines can cause peripheral vasoconstriction that can exacerbate loading conditions in the failing heart and may precipitate myocardial ischemia and ventricular arrhythmias. In addition, activation of the SNS can increase heart rate, which may adversely affect the relation between myocardial supply and demand and more importantly may exacerbate the abnormal force–frequency relation that exists in HF. In addition, catecholamines activate cellular pathways that can lead to the loss of myocardial cells by a process of programmed cell death (apoptosis), which has been implicated in the progression of HF.

In experimental models of HF, pharmacologic interference with the SNS can favorably alter the natural history of the disease, similar to the manner in which antagonism of the RAAS by ACE inhibitors can modify the course of HF. Extensive research implicating the target mechanism, increased adrenergic drive, as being unfavorable to the natural history of systolic dysfunction and the HF clinical syndrome has been done. This has led to the conclusion that the primary mechanism of action of beta-blockers in chronic HF is to prevent and reverse adrenergically mediated intrinsic myocardial dysfunction and remodeling. This occurs through a time-dependent, biologic effect involving inhibition of beta-adrenergic mechanisms directly or indirectly responsible for the development of cellular contractile dysfunction and remodeling (Doughty et al., 2004). In addition, one of the beta-blockers used in patients with HF, carvedilol, has direct antioxidant effects that may decrease the role played by apoptosis in the progression of HF (Dandona, 2007).

Studies have shown that carvedilol and metoprolol improve LV function, hemodynamic parameters, and various symptoms of HF. Carvedilol also improves submaximal exercise tolerance and NYHA classification. In multicenter clinical trials, carvedilol was associated with a highly significant 65% reduction in the risk of death versus placebo (all patients received conventional therapy in addition to carvedilol or placebo). This was due to a decrease in both death due to pump failure and sudden death. In addition, carvedilol decreases the risk of hospitalization for cardiovascular causes and the combined risk of all-cause mortality and cardiovascular hospitalization (Pasternak et al., 2014).

Dosage

Adverse effects with carvedilol usually occur early in therapy and are more frequent and severe with higher doses. Because of this, the starting dose of carvedilol is 3.125 mg twice daily, and each dose titration should be done slowly over a 2-week period, doubling the dose each time. At initiation of each new dosage, the patient should be observed for 1 hour for signs of dizziness or light-headedness. In addition, blood pressure should be monitored. The maximum recommended dosage is 25 mg twice daily in patients weighing less than 85 kg and 50 mg twice daily in patients weighing 85 kg or greater. In addition, patients should be seen in the office during titration and evaluated for symptoms of worsening HF, vasodilation (i.e., dizziness, light-headedness, and symptomatic hypotension), or bradycardia to determine their tolerance for carvedilol. Treatment with metoprolol starts at 6.25 mg two or three times daily, and the dose is titrated slowly up to a target of 100 mg two or three times daily.

Initiation of therapy with a beta-blocker may produce fluid retention, which may be severe enough to cause pulmonary or peripheral congestion and worsening symptoms of HF. Increases in body weight may occur after 3 to 5 days of starting treatment and if untreated may lead to worsening symptoms within 1 to 2 weeks. For this reason, practitioners should ask patients to weigh themselves daily. The amount of weight gain then guides the practitioner in prescribing an increase in the diuretic dosage until the patient's weight is restored to pretreatment levels. The dose of carvedilol may also have to be decreased; occasionally, the drug must be temporarily discontinued.

Excessive vasodilation may occur with initiation of therapy. It is usually asymptomatic but may be accompanied by dizziness, light-headedness, or blurred vision. Vasodilatory adverse effects are usually seen within 24 to 48 hours of the first dose or increments in dose but usually subside with repeated dosing without any change in the dose of carvedilol or other medications. The risk of hypotension may be minimized by taking the beta-blocker, ACE inhibitor, or vasodilator (if used) at different times during the day. Practitioners can work with patients to develop a regimen that is convenient and minimizes adverse effects. The practitioner may need to reduce the dose of the ACE inhibitor or vasodilator if hypotension is excessive. If the patient's heart rate decreases to less than 50 beats per minute or second- or third-degree heart block occurs, the patient should contact the practitioner, who may then decrease the dose of the beta-blocker. Practitioners should evaluate the patient's concomitant medications for drug interactions that also may decrease heart rate or cause heart block (e.g., diltiazem or flecainide).

Contraindications

Beta-blockers should not be used in patients with bronchospastic disease, symptomatic bradycardia, or advanced heart block (unless treated with a pacemaker). Patients should receive a beta-blocker with caution if they have asymptomatic bradycardia (heart rate below 60 beats per minute). Despite concerns that beta blockade may mask some of the signs of hypoglycemia, patients with diabetes mellitus may be particularly likely to experience a reduction in morbidity and mortality with beta-blocker therapy. The GEMINI trial showed that carvedilol improved insulin resistance, maintained glycemic control, and reduced progression to microalbuminuria.

Adverse Events

The adverse effect profile of beta-blockers in patients with HF is consistent with the pharmacology of the drug and the health status of the patient. The most common adverse effects are dizziness, fatigue, and worsening of HF. Other adverse reactions that occur less frequently include bradycardia, hypotension, generalized edema, dependent edema, sinusitis, and bronchitis. Rare cases of liver function abnormalities have been reported in patients receiving carvedilol, but no deaths due to these abnormalities have been reported. Mild hepatic injury related to carvedilol has been reversible and has occurred after short- and long-term therapy. Carvedilol should be discontinued if a patient has laboratory evidence of liver function abnormalities or jaundice.

Practitioners should advise patients receiving therapy with carvedilol or other beta-blockers of the following:

- Adverse effects may occur early in therapy but usually do not prevent long-term use of the drug.
- Symptomatic improvement may not be seen for 2 to 3 months.
- Beta blockade may reduce the risk of disease progression even if the patient's symptoms have not responded favorably to treatment.

Digoxin

Digoxin can prevent clinical deterioration in patients with HF due to LV systolic dysfunction and can improve these patients' symptoms. However, it does not decrease the mortality rate. The latest large trial, the Digitalis Investigation Group (DIG) study, showed that survival was not changed by use of digoxin (0.125 to 0.5 mg) in NYHA class II and III patients with HF who were taking diuretics and ACE inhibitors. However, digoxin significantly decreased the number of hospitalizations compared with placebo. This effect seemed to be more pronounced in patients with the lowest EFs and the most enlarged hearts. However, digoxin increased the risk of non-HF causes of cardiac death from presumed arrhythmia or MI (Digitalis Investigation Group, 1997).

The ACTION HF organization recommends digoxin to improve the clinical status of patients with HF due to LV systolic dysfunction and recommends that it should be used in conjunction with diuretics, an ACE inhibitor, and a beta-blocker. In addition, digoxin is recommended in patients with HF who have rapid atrial fibrillation, even though beta-blockers may be more effective in controlling the ventricular response during exercise. If a patient is receiving digoxin but not an ACE inhibitor or a beta-blocker, treatment with digoxin should not be withdrawn, but appropriate therapy with the neurohormonal antagonists should be instituted. Patients should not receive digoxin if they have significant sinus or atrioventricular (AV) block, unless the block has been treated with a permanent pacemaker. Digoxin should be used cautiously in patients receiving other drugs that can depress sinus or AV nodal function (e.g., amiodarone or a beta-blocker), although these patients usually tolerate digoxin without difficulty. In addition, digoxin is not indicated for the stabilization of patients with acutely decompensated HF (unless they have rapid atrial fibrillation). There are no data to recommend using digoxin in patients with asymptomatic LV dysfunction (NYHA class I).

Mechanism of Action

Digoxin produces a mild inotropic effect by inhibiting cell membrane sodium–potassium adenosine triphosphatase activity and thereby enhancing calcium entry into the cell. Calcium enhances contractile protein activity, allowing for a greater force and velocity of contraction.

Dosage

Loading doses of digoxin usually are not needed in patients with HF. The typical dosage of 0.25 mg daily may be initiated if there is no evidence of renal dysfunction. Patients who have reduced renal function, who have baseline conduction abnormality, or who are small or elderly should be started on 0.125 mg daily or lower (such as every other day). Levels of 0.9 to 1.2 ng/mL are considered therapeutic, but levels as high as 2.5 ng/mL may be tolerated. It is not clear whether the beneficial effects of digoxin are greater at higher serum levels. Although it has been suggested that serum levels

may be used to guide the selection of an appropriate dose of digoxin, there is no evidence to support this approach (Packer & Cohn, 1999).

Steady state is reached in approximately 1 week in patients with normal renal function, although 2 to 3 weeks may be required in patients with renal impairment. When steady state is achieved, the patient should be evaluated for symptoms of toxicity. In addition, an ECG, serum digoxin level, serum electrolytes, BUN, and creatinine should be obtained. It is not clear whether regular serum digoxin monitoring is necessary, but levels should be checked once a year after a steady state is achieved. In addition, levels should be checked if HF status worsens, renal function deteriorates, signs of toxicity develop (e.g., confusion, nausea, anorexia, visual disturbances, arrhythmias), or additional medications are added that could affect the digoxin level.

Adverse Events

Signs of digoxin toxicity develop in approximately 20% of patients, and up to 18% of digoxin-toxic patients die from the arrhythmias that occur. Noncardiac symptoms are related to the central nervous system (CNS) and gastrointestinal (GI) tract. Anorexia is often an early manifestation, with nausea and vomiting following. The CNS adverse effects include headache, fatigue, malaise, disorientation, confusion, delirium, seizures, and visual disturbances. The noncardiac symptoms do not always precede the cardiac symptoms. Cardiac toxicity manifested by arrhythmias can take the form of almost every known rhythm disturbance (e.g., ectopic and re-entrant cardiac rhythms and heart block).

Digoxin should be discontinued (often with consideration of reinstitution at a lower dose after 2 to 3 days if the patient is benefiting from therapy) if any of the following is noted:

- Elevated digoxin level
- Substantial reduction in renal function
- Symptoms of toxicity
- Significant conduction abnormality (e.g., symptomatic bradycardia due to second- or third-degree AV block or high-degree AV block in atrial fibrillation)
- An increase in ventricular arrhythmias

Practitioners should counsel patients about the potential adverse effects of digoxin. They also should stress the importance of taking digoxin exactly as it is prescribed to avoid toxicity or a subtherapeutic effect.

Interactions

The medications that most often cause an increase in digoxin levels are quinidine (Cardioquin, others), amiodarone, flecainide, propafenone (Rythmol), spironolactone, and verapamil. It may be necessary to decrease the dose of digoxin when treatment with these drugs is initiated. Antibiotics may decrease gut flora and prevent bacterial inactivation of digoxin, and anticholinergic agents may decrease intestinal motility. Both of these drug classes also may increase digoxin levels. Antacids, cholestyramine (Questran), neomycin (Mycifradin Sulfate), and kaolin–pectin (Kaopectate) may inhibit the absorption of digoxin and decrease digoxin levels. Patients should be advised to take digoxin at least 2 hours before these medications. Diuretics can enhance digoxin toxicity by decreasing renal clearance of digoxin and by causing electrolyte changes, including hypokalemia, hypomagnesemia, and hypercalcemia (thiazides). Before any new medications are added to a patient's regimen, the prescriber should determine whether the medication interacts with digoxin.

Hydralazine/Isosorbide Dinitrate

The HYD/ISDN combination of vasodilators is an appropriate alternative in African American patients with contraindications to or intolerance of ACE inhibitors. The combination should not be used for treating HF in patients who have not tried ACE inhibitors and should not be substituted for ACE inhibitors in patients who are tolerating ACE inhibitors without difficulty. No studies have specifically addressed the use of HYD/ISDN for patients who cannot take or tolerate ACE inhibitors, and the FDA has not approved HYD/ISDN for use in patients with HF. Isosorbide mononitrate also is not approved for HF and has not been studied for treating HF. HYD/ISDN is not as beneficial as the ACE inhibitor enalapril in reducing mortality rates during the first 2 years of treatment. However, this combination has been shown to achieve an absolute reduction in mortality rates compared with placebo during the first 3 years of treatment. The combination increases exercise capacity as much as enalapril, but adverse effects are a significant problem.

Mechanism of Action

Vasodilators may be classified by their mechanism of action or their site of action (venodilators, arteriolar dilators, or "balanced" vasodilators). ISDN is a venodilator that redistributes blood volume to the venous side of the heart to the systemic circulation, away from the lungs, which decreases the ventricular blood volume (preload). Hydralazine, along with prazosin and minoxidil (Loniten), which are not used for treating HF, is an arteriolar dilator. Hydralazine decreases the resistance the heart encounters during contraction (afterload), which allows for increased stroke volume (volume of blood leaving the heart) and increased cardiac output. Balanced vasodilators, including the ACE inhibitors and ARBs, cause vasodilation on both the venous and arterial sides of the heart and therefore provide the hemodynamic and clinical benefits of both preload and afterload reduction (as discussed in other sections).

Dosage

Isosorbide dinitrate usually should be initiated at 10 mg three times a day and increased weekly to 40 mg three times a day as tolerated (up to 160 mg/d). Hydralazine should be initiated at 25 mg three times a day and increased weekly to 75 mg three or four times a day (up to 300 mg/d). Patients with low blood pressure, severe HF, or advanced age can be started on 10 mg three times a day for both agents.

Adverse Events

Adverse events include reflex tachycardia, headache, flushing, nausea, dizziness, syncope, nitrate tolerance, and sodium and water retention. Nitrate tolerance can be avoided by providing a nitrate-free period of 10 to 14 hours.

Interactions

Other drugs that lower blood pressure, including diuretics, may cause additive hypotension, and blood pressure should be monitored.

Other Agents

Amiodarone

Amiodarone is approved in the United States for treating refractory life-threatening ventricular arrhythmias. Amiodarone has been studied in patients with HF with ventricular arrhythmias to assess whether it reduces mortality rates. Some studies demonstrated that low-dose amiodarone (300 mg/d) reduced mortality rates, whereas others found no improvement (Doval et al., 1994; Singh et al., 1995). A meta-analysis of 13 randomized, controlled trials of prophylactic amiodarone in patients with recent MI (8 trials) or HF (5 trials) found that amiodarone reduced the rate of arrhythmic/sudden death in high-risk patients with recent MI or HF (Amiodarone Trials Meta-Analysis Investigators, 1997).

The FDA has not approved amiodarone for treating HF. According to the most recent HF guidelines (Yancy et al., 2013), amiodarone is the only antiarrhythmic to have neutral effects on mortality from HF. Further studies are needed to determine whether it is useful for routine prophylactic treatment of patients with ventricular arrhythmias and non-ischemic HF. It may be beneficial in patients at high risk for arrhythmic/sudden death, patients with primary cardiomyopathy, or patients with both (Amiodarone Trials Meta-Analysis Investigators, 1997; Gheorghiade et al., 1998). The recommendations suggest that some class III antiarrhythmic agents (e.g., amiodarone) do not appear to increase the risk of death in patients with chronic HF. Such drugs are preferred over class I agents when used for treating atrial fibrillation in patients with LV systolic dysfunction. Because of its known toxicity and equivocal evidence for efficacy, amiodarone is not recommended for general use to prevent death (or sudden death) in patients with HF already treated with drugs that reduce mortality rates (e.g., ACE inhibitors or beta-blockers).

Mechanism of Action

Amiodarone is classified as a Vaughn-Williams class III (potassium channel blocking) antiarrhythmic drug, but it also possesses class I (sodium blocking), class II (beta blocking), and class IV (calcium channel blocking) antiarrhythmic effects. It also has vasodilatory properties. The therapeutic benefit of amiodarone may be due to its beta-blocking effects and not to an antiarrhythmic effect.

Dosage

Before treatment with amiodarone starts, the practitioner should make sure the patient does not have hyperthyroidism or advanced liver disease. In addition, pulmonary function tests, chest radiography, ophthalmologic examination, and neurologic assessment are recommended before initiating therapy. The maintenance dosage should be 200 to 300 mg/d. High doses of amiodarone may cause initial cardiac decompensation with abnormal hemodynamics; therefore, use of high loading doses in patients with very severe forms of HF should be avoided.

Interactions

Amiodarone interacts with warfarin (Coumadin; increases the international normalized ratio) and digoxin (increases digoxin levels).

Corlanor (Ivabradine)

Corlanor is a relatively new drug in the treatment of HF to reduced risk of hospitalization. It is indicated for patients with stable, symptomatic chronic HF with LVEF ≤35% and in sinus rhythm with resting heart rate greater than or equal to 70 bpm, and taking beta-blockers at the highest dose they can tolerate, or are not taking beta-blockers because there is a medical reason to avoid the use of β-blockers.

Mechanism of Action

Corlanor (ivabradine) is a hyperpolarization-activated cyclic nucleotide-gated channel blocker that reduces the spontaneous pacemaker activity of the cardiac sinus node by selectively inhibiting the I_f current (I_f), resulting in heart rate reduction with no effect on ventricular repolarization and no effects on myocardial contractility.

Dosage

The initial dose is 5 mg orally twice a day with meals, and the maximum dose is 7.5 mg orally twice a day. Dosing is adjusted based on keeping the heart rate between 50 and 60 bpm and the overall tolerability of the drug. In patients who have a resting heart rate greater than 60 bpm, dosing should be increased by 2.5 mg up to the maximum of 7.5 mg twice a day. For patients with resting heart rates between 50 and 60 bpm, the dose should be maintained. Finally, if the resting heart rate is less than 50 bpm, the dose should be decreased by 2.5 mg and tolerability reassessed. If the dose is already 2.5 mg twice a day, then discontinue the drug.

Interaction

Because Corlanor is metabolized by the CYP3A4 pathway of the P450 concomitant, use of CYP3A4 inhibitors will increase the concentration of ivabradine and use of CYP3A4 inducers will decrease the concentration. With increased plasma concentrations, bradycardia and conduction disturbance may be exacerbated. Examples of strong CYPA4 inhibitors include azole antifungals (e.g., ketoconazole, itraconazole), macrolide antibiotics (e.g., clarithromycin), and HIV protease inhibitors. Examples of moderate CYPA4 inhibitors include diltiazem, verapamil, and grape juice. Finally, examples of strong CYPA4 inducers include St. John's wort, rifampicin, barbiturates, and phenytoin.

Contraindications

Corlanor is contraindicated in sick sinus syndrome or AV block (unless a pacemaker is inserted), severe liver disease, worsened HF symptoms, resting heart rate of less than 60, and blood pressure less than 90/50. Corlanor is also contraindicated in COPD, hypotension, or asthma and concomitant use of strong cytochrome P450 3A4 (CYP3A4) inhibitors.

Adverse Events

The most common adverse events in Corlanor are bradycardia, hypertension, atrial fibrillation and phosphenes, and visual brightness. Postmarketing reports of additional reactions include hypotension, angioedema, rash, pruritus, urticaria, vertigo, and diplopia.

Selecting the Most Appropriate Agent

The 2013 ACCF/AHA clinical practice guidelines changed the approach to the management of patients with HF. Instead of digoxin, an ACE inhibitor is now the drug of first choice. **Table 22.4** and **Figure 22.3** summarize therapeutic regimens. In patients with a history of MI and reduced EF, ACE inhibitors (ACE-I) or ARB should be used to prevent HF. In patients with an MI and reduced EF, beta-blockers should be used to prevent HF and a statin also given.

First-Line Therapy

The ACE inhibitors are now considered the first-line choice for routine use in patients with HF. ACE inhibitors may also be considered for treatment of those who are stage A as classified by the ACC/AHA (Yancy et al., 2013). According to the clinical practice guidelines, patients with systolic dysfunction should receive a trial of an ACE inhibitor unless contraindications are present. (See discussion of ACE inhibitors.) The ACE inhibitors may be considered sole therapy in HF patients who have fatigue or mild dyspnea on exertion and who do not have any other signs or symptoms of volume overload. However, if

TABLE 22.4

Recommended Order of Treatment for Heart Failure

Order	Agents	Comments
First line	ACE-I (or ARB) with or without a diuretic (depends on fluid retention)	Monitor patient's response carefully.
Second line	ACE-I (or ARB) and beta-blocker with a diuretic	In patient with mild heart failure, use a potassium-sparing diuretic when serum potassium level is <4.0 mEq/L.
Third line	ARB, beta-blocker, aldosterone agonist, diuretic, and digoxin	

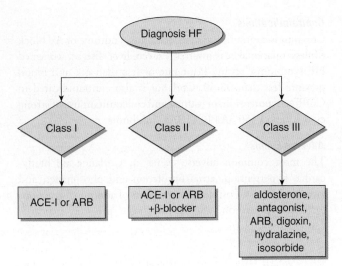

FIGURE 22.3 Treatment algorithm for chronic heart failure. (Adapted with permission from Yancy, C. W., Jessup, M., Bozkurt, B., et al. (2013). 2013 ACCF/AHA guideline for the management of heart failure. *Journal of the American College of Cardiology, 62*(16), e147–e239. Copyright © 2013 American College of Cardiology Foundation and the American Heart Association, Inc. Published by Elsevier Inc. All rights reserved.)

these symptoms persist after the target dose of the ACE inhibitor is reached, a diuretic should be added. (See Second-Line Therapy.) Thus, ACE inhibitor therapy is appropriate for patients in NYHA class I as a means of preventing HF and in patients in NYHA class II to IV with symptoms to decrease mortality rates. (See discussion of ACE inhibitors.) They may be used in conjunction with beta-blockers, which are also considered first-line therapy.

If the patient is unable to tolerate an ACE inhibitor, an ARB can be used.

Beta-blockers with vasodilating action have been approved for treating HF. (See discussion of beta-blockers.) Beta-blockers are initial therapy.

The recommendations state that all patients with stable NYHA class II or III HF due to LV systolic dysfunction should receive a beta-blocker unless the drug is contraindicated or cannot be tolerated. Beta-blockers should be used with diuretics and ACE inhibitors. Blockers should not be used in unstable patients or in acutely ill patients (rescue therapy), including those who are in the intensive care unit with refractory HF requiring IV support. Studies of beta-blocker therapy in various types of patients with HF are continuing to define their role.

Second-Line Therapy

Diuretics are used to increase sodium and water excretion, correct volume overload (which manifests as dyspnea on exertion), and maintain sodium and water balance. Patients with HF and signs of significant volume overload should be started immediately on a diuretic in addition to an ACE inhibitor. Patients with mild HF or concomitant hypertension may be managed

adequately on thiazide diuretics. However, a loop diuretic is preferred in most patients, particularly those with renal impairment or marked fluid retention. A potassium-sparing diuretic or potassium supplement should be used for patients with serum potassium concentrations less than 4.0 mEq/L. Patients with persistent volume overload despite initial medical management may require more aggressive administration of the current diuretic (e.g., IV administration), more potent diuretics, or a combination of diuretics (e.g., furosemide and metolazone, or furosemide and spironolactone).

Third-Line Therapy

The AHRQ clinical practice guidelines state that digoxin should be used in patients with severe HF and should be added to the medical regimen of patients with mild or moderate failure who remain symptomatic after optimal management with ACE inhibitors and diuretics. The ACTION HF recommendations state that digoxin is recommended to improve the clinical status of patients with HF due to LV systolic dysfunction and should be used with diuretics, an ACE inhibitor, and a beta-blocker. Both groups suggest that digoxin may be beneficial in patients with HF when there is a second indication for digoxin therapy (e.g., a supraventricular arrhythmia for which digoxin is specifically indicated). However, there remains a question of whether the benefits of digoxin therapy outweigh its risks.

Fourth-Line Therapy

Fourth-line therapy consists of ARBs, such as losartan, the HYD/ISDN combination of vasodilators, or an aldosterone antagonist, such as spironolactone. A new drug, Corlanor, can be added to the regime.

According to the AHRQ guidelines and the ACTION HF recommendations, the HYD/ISDN combination is an appropriate alternative in African American patients with contraindications to or intolerance of ACE inhibitors; although, some practitioners continue to use it in all patient populations. There is little evidence to support using nitrates alone or hydralazine alone in treating HF. Spironolactone at a low dosage of 12.5 to 25 mg once daily should be considered for patients who are receiving standard therapy and who have severe HF (with recent or current NYHA class IV standing) caused by LV systolic dysfunction. Patients should have a normal serum potassium level (5.0 mmol/L) and adequate renal function (serum creatinine 2.5 mg/dL).

Special Populations
Pediatric

Children with HF usually have maturational differences in contractile function or congenital structural or genetic heart dysfunction. Drug data for children with HF are not well established. In general, treatment for class I acute HF includes IV inotropes (excluding digoxin) and IV diuretics. For class II failure, digoxin may be added, and for class III, oxygen may be administered. Drug therapy in children is highly individualized according to the child's condition and setting and is usually managed by a specialist in pediatric cardiology.

Geriatric

Because of age-related reductions in renal function, elderly patients may be particularly susceptible to drug-induced decreases in blood pressure, making careful monitoring essential not only at baseline but also when dosage or drug adjustments are instituted. Blood pressure, renal function, and potassium levels should be monitored regularly. Changes in renal function may also affect the elimination of digoxin, and patients should be monitored for digoxin toxicity and educated to recognize its signs and symptoms.

An important issue in drug therapy for elderly patients with HF is therapeutic compliance. In one study, investigators identified the primary reason for hospitalization of elderly patients with HF as noncompliance with diet and medication therapy; moreover, the investigators concluded that up to 40% of readmissions could be prevented by therapeutic compliance and appropriate discharge planning, follow-up, and adequate patient and caregiver education (SOLVD Investigators, 1991).

Women

In pregnant women, ACE inhibitor therapy may pose the risk of congenital birth defects. The same is true for ARB therapy. Corlanor (ivabradine) also has potential for fetal toxicity and appropriate birth control is necessary. For both ACE or ARB inhibitors, and Corlanor if a woman becomes pregnant, the drug should be stopped immediately.

MONITORING PATIENT RESPONSE

A careful history and a physical examination guide outcomes and direct therapy. The patient's symptoms and activities should be explored; any worsening suggests the need to adjust therapy. Although ECG exercise testing is not recommended, repeated testing may be ordered if the patient has a new heart murmur or a new MI or suddenly deteriorates despite compliance with the medication regimen. Serum electrolyte levels, renal function, blood pressure, and diuretic use should be monitored regularly, particularly in patients taking ACE inhibitors. Within 2 weeks of initial ACE inhibitor therapy, serum potassium, creatinine, and BUN measurements should be repeated. If values are stable, monitoring can occur at 3-month intervals or within 1 week of a change in dosage of the ACE inhibitor or diuretic drug.

Response to initial ACE inhibitor therapy should be monitored by blood pressure measurements at 1 to 2 hours (captopril) and 4 to 6 hours for long-acting drugs (enalapril or lisinopril). Blood pressure and heart rate should be monitored for 1 hour after initiating carvedilol to assess tolerance to the drug; clinical reevaluation should occur at each increase in dose and with any worsening of symptoms (increasing fatigue, decreased exercise tolerance, weight gain).

Patients taking spironolactone should have their serum potassium level measured after the first week of therapy, at regular intervals thereafter, and after any change in dose or concomitant medications that may affect potassium balance.

PATIENT EDUCATION

Practitioners must take an active role in patient education to enhance compliance and help prevent medication errors and adverse effects. Patients taking ACE inhibitors, such as captopril and moexipril (Univasc), should take them at least 1 hour before meals. They should also be advised of potential adverse effects, particularly the effects that signal a dangerous reaction: sore throat, fever, swelling of hands or feet, irregular heartbeat, chest pains, and signs of angioedema (swelling of the face, eyes, lips, or tongue; difficulty swallowing or breathing; hoarseness). If these occur, the patient should notify the health care professional at once.

Patients taking diuretics need to know that they can take the medication with food or milk to prevent GI upset and they can schedule administration so that the need to urinate does not interrupt sleep. Because some diuretics cause photosensitivity, patients should use sunblock or avoid extensive exposure to sunlight. The practitioner can show the patient how to rise slowly from a lying or sitting position to avoid orthostatic hypotension.

Patients need to understand how to monitor their symptoms and weight fluctuations, restrict their sodium intake, take their medications as prescribed, and stay physically active.

Patients taking digoxin should understand that discontinuing the medication can be dangerous and that they should consult their health care provider before doing so. They should avoid taking over-the-counter medications, such as antacids, cold and allergy products, and diet drugs. Reportable signs and symptoms are loss of appetite, low stomach pain, nausea, vomiting, diarrhea, unusual fatigue or weakness, headache, blurred or yellow vision, rash or hives, or mental depression.

Women of childbearing age need to know that ACE inhibitors and ARBs should be avoided if pregnancy is a possibility. Patients taking spironolactone should know the signs and symptoms to report (muscle weakness or cramps and fatigue).

Nutrition/Lifestyle Changes

Dietary sodium intake should be limited to 2 or 3 g daily. Although a 2-g daily sodium intake is preferred, patient compliance may be poor because most patients find such a diet unpalatable. Patients with mild or moderate (NYHA class II or III) HF may tolerate 3 g daily. Alcohol decreases myocardial contractility, and therefore, consumption of alcoholic beverages should be discouraged or limited to one drink (i.e., a glass of beer or wine or a cocktail containing 1 ounce or less of alcohol) per day. Patients with HF should avoid excessive fluid intake, but fluid restriction is not advisable unless hyponatremia develops.

Patients should stop smoking because cigarettes cause cardiac injury. In addition to pharmacology therapy and lifestyle, revascularization may be necessitated. Some patients with HF experience severe limitation or repeated hospitalizations despite aggressive drug therapy and intervention; thereby, cardiac transplantation may be a reasonable option.

CASE STUDY*

I.W., aged 62, is a male who is new to your practice. He is reporting shortness of breath on exertion, especially after climbing steps or walking three to four blocks. His symptoms clear with rest. He also has difficulty sleeping at night (he tells you he needs two pillows to be comfortable).

He tells you that 2 years ago, he suddenly became short of breath after hurrying for an airplane. He was admitted to a hospital and treated for acute pulmonary edema. Three days before the episode of pulmonary edema, he had an upper respiratory tract infection with fever and mild cough. After the episode of pulmonary edema, his blood pressure has been consistently elevated. His previous physician started him on a sustained-release preparation of diltiazem 180 mg/d. His medical history includes moderate prostatic hypertrophy for 5 years, adult-onset diabetes mellitus for 10 years, hypertension for 10 years, and degenerative joint disease for 5 years. His medication history includes hydrochlorothiazide (HydroDIURIL) 50 mg/d, atenolol (Tenormin) 100 mg/d, controlled-delivery diltiazem 180 mg/d, glyburide (DiaBeta) 5 mg/d, and indomethacin (Indocin) 25 to 50 mg three times a day as needed for pain. While reviewing his medical records, you see that

his last physical examination revealed a blood pressure of 160/95 mm Hg, a pulse of 95 bpm, a respiratory rate of 18, normal peripheral pulses, mild edema bilaterally in his feet, a prominent S3 and S4, neck vein distention, and an enlarged liver.

DIAGNOSIS: HEART FAILURE CLASS II

1. List specific goals of treatment for I.W.
2. What drug(s) would you prescribe? Why?
3. What are the parameters for monitoring the success of your selected therapy?
4. Discuss specific patient education based on the prescribed therapy.
5. Describe one or two drug–drug or drug–food interactions for the selected agent(s).
6. List one or two adverse reactions for the selected agent(s) that would cause you to change therapy.
7. What would be the choice for the second-line therapy?
8. What over-the-counter or alternative medications would be appropriate for this patient?
9. What dietary and lifestyle changes should be recommended for I.W.?

* Answers can be found online.

Bibliography

Starred references are cited in the text.

Ahmed, A., & Dell'Italia, L. J. (2004). Use of beta-blockers in older adults with chronic heart failure. *American Journal of the Medical Sciences, 328*(2), 100–111.

*Amiodarone Trials Meta-Analysis Investigators. (1997). Effect of prophylactic amiodarone on mortality after acute myocardial infarction and in congestive heart failure: Meta-analysis of individual data from 6500 patients in randomized trials. *Lancet, 350*, 1417–1424.

Anderson, J., Jacobs, A., Albert, N., et al. (2013). 2013 ACCF/AHA guideline for the management of heart failure. *Journal of the American College of Cardiology, 62*(16), 147–239. doi: 10.1016/j.jacc.2013.05.019.

*Bahrami, H., Kronmal, R., Bluemke, D. A., et al. (2008). Differences in the incidence of congestive heart failure by ethnicity: The multi-ethnic study of atherosclerosis. *Archives of Internal Medicine, 168*(19), 2138–2145. doi: 10.1001/archinte.168.19.2138.

*Braunwald, E. (2015). Clinical manifestations of heart failure. In E. Braunwald (Ed.), *Heart disease* (pp. 471–484). Philadelphia, PA: W.B. Saunders.

*Dandona, P., Ghanim, H., & Brooks, D. P. (2007). Antioxidant activity of carvedilol in cardiovascular disease. *Journal of Hypertension, 25*, 731–741.

*Diaz, A., & Ducharme, A. (2008). Update on the use of trandolapril in the management of cardiovascular disorders. *Vascular Health and Risk Management, 4*(6), 1147–1158.

*Digitalis Investigation Group. (1997). The effect of digoxin on mortality and morbidity in patients with heart failure. *New England Journal of Medicine, 336*, 525–533.

*Doughty, R. N., Whalley, G. A., Walsh, H. A., et al. (2004). CAPRICORN Echo Substudy Investigators. Effects of carvedilol on left ventricular

remodeling after acute myocardial infarction: The CAPRICORN Echo Substudy. *Circulation, 109*, 201–206.

*Doval, H. C., Nul, D. R., Grancelli, H. O., et al. (1994). Randomized trial of low-dose amiodarone in severe congestive heart failure. *Lancet, 344*, 493–498.

*Gheorghiade, M., Cody, R. J., Francis, G. S., et al. (1998). Current medical therapy for advanced heart failure. *American Heart Journal, 135*, S2231–S2248.

*Go, A. S., Mozaffarian, D., Roger, V. L., et al. (2013). Heart disease and stroke statistics—2013 update: A report from the American Heart Association. *Circulation, 127*(1), e6–e245.

Gottlieb, S. S., Dickstein, K., Fleck, E., et al. (1993). Hemodynamic and neurohormonal effects of the angiotensin II antagonist losartan in patients with congestive heart failure. *Circulation, 88*, 1602–1609.

Kober, L., Torp-Pedersen, C., Carlsen, J. E., et al. (1995). A clinical trial of the angiotensin-converting-enzyme inhibitor trandolapril in patients with left ventricular dysfunction after myocardial infarction. *New England Journal of Medicine, 333*, 1670–1676.

Konstam, M. A., Neaton, J. D., Dickstein K., et al. (2009). Effects of high-dose versus low-dose losartan on clinical outcomes in patients with heart failure (HEAAL study): A randomised, double-blind trial. *Lancet, 374*, 1840–1848.

Krum, H., & Teerlink, J. (2011). Heart failure 2: Medical therapy for chronic heart failure. *Lancet, 378*, 713–721.

Margo, K. Luttermoser, G., & Shaugnessy, A. (2001). Spironolactone in left-sided heart failure: How does it fit in? *American Family Physician, 64*(8), 1393–1398, 1399.

*Masoudi, F., Rathore, S., Wang, Y., et al. (2004). National patterns of use and effectiveness of angiotensin-converting enzyme inhibitors in older patients with heart failure and left ventricular systolic dysfunction. *Circulation, 110*, 724–731. doi: 10.1161/01.CIR.0000138934.28340.ED.

Nair, A., Timoh, T., & Fuster, V. (2012). Contemporary medical management of systolic heart failure. *Circulation, 76*, 268–277.

*Packer, M., & Cohn, J. N., on behalf of the Steering Committee and Membership of the Advisory Council to Improve Outcomes Nationwide in Heart Failure. (1999). Consensus recommendations for the management of chronic heart failure. *American Journal of Cardiology, 83*, 1A–38A.

Packer, M., O'Connor, C. M., Ghali, J. K., et al., for the Prospective Randomized Amlodipine Survival Evaluation Study Group. (1996). Effect of amlodipine on morbidity and mortality in severe chronic heart failure. *New England Journal of Medicine, 335*, 1107–1114.

*Pasternak, B., Svanström, H., Melbye, M., et al. (2014). Association of treatment with carvedilol vs metoprolol succinate and mortality in patients with heart failure. *JAMA Internal Medicine, 174*(10), 1597–1604. doi: 10.1001/jamainternmed.2014.3258.

Pitt, B., Pfeffer, M., Assmann, S., et al. (2014). Spironolactone for heart failure with preserved ejection fraction. *New England Journal of Medicine, 370*(15), 1383–1392. doi: 10.1056/NEJMoa1313731.

Pitt, B., Segal, R., Martinez, F. A., et al. (1997). Randomised trial of losartan versus captopril in patients over 65 with heart failure (Evaluation of Losartan in the Elderly Study, ELITE). *Lancet, 349*, 747–752.

*Pitt, B., Zannad, F., Remme, W. J., et al. (1999). The effect of spironolactone on morbidity and mortality in patients with severe heart failure. *New England Journal of Medicine, 341*(10), 709–717.

Pressler S. J., Subramanian U., Kareken D., et al. (2010). Cognitive deficits and health-related quality of life in chronic heart failure. *Journal of Cardiovascular Nursing, 25*(3), 189–198.

*Savarese, G., Costanzo, P., Cleland, J. G., et al. (2013). A meta-analysis reporting effects of angiotensin-converting enzyme inhibitors and angiotension receptor blockers in patients without heart failure. *Journal American College of Cardiology, 61*(3), 131–142. doi: 10.1016/j.jacc.2012.10.011. Epub 2012 Dec 5.

*Singh, S. N., Fletcher, R. D., Fischer, S. G., et al. (1995). Amiodarone in patients with congestive heart failure and symptomatic ventricular arrhythmias. *New England Journal of Medicine, 333*, 77–82.

Smith, T. W., Braunwald, E., & Kelly, R. A. (2015). The management of heart failure. In E. Braunwald (Ed.), *Heart disease* (pp. 485–543). Philadelphia, PA: W.B. Saunders.

*SOLVD Investigators. (1991). Effect of enalapril on survival in patients with reduced left ventricular ejection fractions and HF. *New England Journal of Medicine, 3325*, 303–310.

*Yancy, C. W., Jessup, M., Bozkurt, B., et al. (2013). 2013 ACCF/AHA guideline for the management of heart failure. *Journal of the American College of Cardiology, 62*(16), e147–e239.

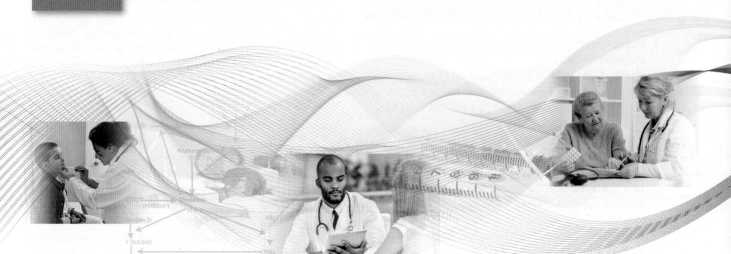

23

Arrhythmias

Cynthia A. Sanoski ■ Andrew M. Peterson

Cardiac arrhythmias are abnormal cardiac rhythms, including tachyarrhythmias (an increase in heart rate) and bradyarrhythmias (a decrease in heart rate). Arrhythmias may be asymptomatic or symptomatic, causing palpitations, weakness, loss of consciousness, heart failure (HF), and sudden death. Searching for a reversible cause of the arrhythmia is the first step in patient care. However, in many cases, antiarrhythmic drugs (AADs) are necessary to permit stabilization until the underlying condition is normalized. Many patients require chronic drug therapy for an arrhythmia due to an underlying disease condition that makes them chronically susceptible to cardiac arrhythmias that are associated with high morbidity and mortality rates.

CAUSES

Arrhythmias may result from structural or electrical/conduction system changes in the heart that may compromise cardiac function and cardiac output. Conditions that give rise to arrhythmias include myocardial ischemia, chronic HF, hypertension, valvular heart disease, hypoxemia, thyroid abnormalities, electrolyte disturbances, drug toxicity, excessive caffeine or ethanol ingestion, anxiety, and exercise. Some of these conditions are reversible, and some cause structural changes that are not reversible.

PATHOPHYSIOLOGY

Basic Electrophysiology

Electrically active myocardial cells (non–pacemaker-type cells) at rest maintain a potential difference between their intracellular fluid and the extracellular fluid. When excited, these cells

manifest a characteristic sequence of transmembrane potential changes called the *action potential*. The resting membrane potential is –90 mV with respect to the extracellular fluid. The activity of the sodium–potassium pump and the permeability of the membrane to sodium, potassium, and calcium ions determine the membrane potential of a cardiac cell at any given time. Permeability is defined by the diffusion of ions across the membrane through various ion-selective channels. The phases of the action potential correspond to the excitation state of a myocardial cell (**Box 23.1**).

Arrhythmias can result from disorders of impulse formation and/or impulse conduction. Several factors are believed to be involved in precipitating arrhythmias. There may be a defect in the normal mechanism of spontaneous phase 4 depolarization or an increased automaticity of pacemaker cells. In addition, ectopic pacemakers in normally quiescent tissue are responsible for arrhythmias originating from disorders of impulse formation. Impulse conduction defects occur when the impulse is slowed or blocked because of functional unidirectional block, a change in conduction velocity, or a change in the refractory period. Furthermore, simultaneous abnormalities of impulse formation and conduction may occur.

AADs are used to treat abnormal electrical activity of the heart. The drugs outlined in this chapter are used to treat, suppress, or prevent two major mechanisms of arrhythmias—an abnormality in impulse formation (i.e., increased automaticity) or an abnormality in impulse conduction (i.e., reentry).

Automaticity

Automaticity refers to the ability of the cardiac cells to depolarize spontaneously. Three factors determine automaticity: maximum diastolic depolarization, the rate of depolarization,

- **Phase 0** is when rapid depolarization occurs due to the rapid influx of Na^+.
- **Phase 1** is a brief initial repolarization period. Inactivation of the inward Na^+ current and activation of the outward K^+ current cause this brief but rapid phase of repolarization.
- **Phase 2** is a plateau period during which there is little change in membrane potential. The outward K^+ current and the influx of Ca^{2+} through calcium channels typify the plateau period. The offsetting effect of these currents creates only a small net change in potential, thus creating a plateau.
- **Phase 3** is a period of repolarization that is characterized primarily by K^+ efflux.
- **Phase 4** is a gradual depolarization of the cell, with Na^+ gradually leaking into the intracellular space, balanced by decreasing efflux of K^+. As the cell is slowly depolarized during this phase, an increase in Na^+ permeability occurs, which again leads to phase 0.

and the level of the threshold potential. Arrhythmias resulting from abnormal automaticity include sinus tachycardia and junctional tachycardia. The sinoatrial (SA) node has the most rapid rate of depolarization during diastole and reaches threshold first. Cells of the atrioventricular (AV) node and His–Purkinje system have automaticity but a slower rate of phase 4 depolarization. The primary role of the SA node is as the pacemaker of the heart. The SA node is sensitive to alterations in autonomic nervous system output and in its biochemical surroundings. Catecholamine stimulation leads to a shorter action potential duration and increases the spontaneous rate of depolarization. Vagal stimulus and endogenous purines such as adenosine increase outward potassium currents, thus inhibiting depolarization. Increased adrenergic innervation produces major changes in ionic current activity in the SA node.

Another mechanism for arrhythmias due to abnormal impulse formation is intracellular calcium overload, called *after-depolarization*. If after-depolarizations reach threshold, a new action potential is generated and propagated in adjacent cells. After-depolarizations may occur in response to hypothermia, electrolyte imbalance, catecholamine excess, or stretch. Late after-depolarizations may also be of particular importance in some of the arrhythmias caused by digoxin toxicity.

Reentry

Reentry involves indefinite propagation of the impulse and continued activation of previously refractory tissue. Reentrant foci occur if there are two pathways for impulse

conduction, an area of unidirectional block (prolonged refractoriness) in one of these pathways, and slow conduction in the other pathway. A refractory period occurs when the cell cannot be activated after having already fired. Excitability determines the strength of a stimulus required to initiate a new action potential at any given point during the action potential cycle.

Types of Arrhythmias

Arrhythmias evolve either above or below the ventricles and can be regular or irregular. *Supraventricular arrhythmias* evolve above the ventricles in the atria, SA node, or AV node. These arrhythmias may present with either tachycardia or bradycardia or with regularity or irregularity. *AV nodal arrhythmias* originate at or within the AV node and are caused by delayed or absent SA node conduction to the AV node. Supraventricular and AV nodal arrhythmias are not usually life threatening; however, they may become troublesome and lead to reduced cardiac output related to decreased ventricular filling.

Ventricular arrhythmias originate in the ventricles or the bundle of His. These types of arrhythmias are usually symptomatic and may cause loss of consciousness or death. Therefore, arrhythmias in this category require immediate intervention. Underlying clinical conditions that usually give rise to these arrhythmias are myocardial ischemia/infarction, dilated and hypertrophic cardiomyopathies, electrolyte disorders, hypoxia, hyperthyroidism, valvular diseases, and drug toxicity. **Box 23.2** lists arrhythmias by category.

DIAGNOSTIC CRITERIA

The practitioner must first assess the patient via a thorough and sometimes urgent history and physical examination. There may be no symptoms, or the patient may present with symptoms such as chest pain, shortness of breath, decreased level of consciousness, syncope, confusion, diaphoresis, weakness, and palpitations. The practitioner should ask when the symptoms started, how long they have lasted, their frequency, and how the patient tolerated the symptoms.

It also is important to assess the patient's risk factors for development of arrhythmias, such as previous coronary artery disease (CAD), myocardial infarction (MI), dilated or hypertrophic cardiomyopathy, hypertension, valvular heart disease, alcohol or drug abuse, or prescription drug use (e.g., digoxin, AADs). The practitioner should focus the physical examination on heart rate and blood pressure; presence of extra, irregular, or skipped beats; rate, rhythm, amplitude, and symmetry of peripheral pulses; and response to exercise.

Laboratory and diagnostic studies also are vital in diagnosing arrhythmias. The practitioner should examine the 12-lead electrocardiogram (ECG) for evidence of myocardial ischemia; calculation of the PR interval, QRS interval, and QT interval; presence of premature atrial or ventricular contractions;

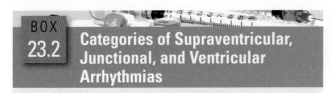

Categories of Supraventricular, Junctional, and Ventricular Arrhythmias

SUPRAVENTRICULAR ARRHYTHMIAS

Sinus tachycardia
PSVT (originates above or within the AV node and conducts to the His–Purkinje system) (e.g., AV nodal reentrant tachycardia, AV reentrant tachycardia)
Sinus bradycardia
AF
AFl
Atrial tachycardia
Premature atrial contractions
WPW syndrome

JUNCTIONAL ARRHYTHMIAS

Nonparoxysmal AV junctional tachycardia (heart rate > 60 beats/min)
Junctional escape rhythm (heart rate 40–60 beats/min)
Premature AV junctional complexes
AV dissociation
First-degree heart block
Second-degree heart block (Mobitz type I [Wenckebach], Mobitz type II)
Third-degree (complete) heart block

VENTRICULAR ARRHYTHMIAS

Premature ventricular contractions
VT
VF
TdP (a rapid form of polymorphic VT associated with a long QT interval)

characteristics of Wolff-Parkinson-White (WPW) syndrome; presence or absence of P waves; and relationship between P waves and QRS complexes. Continuous cardiac monitoring is needed for patients who have episodes of life-threatening arrhythmias so that electrical cardioversion and/or AADs can be administered as immediate interventions.

A complete blood count, basic metabolic profile (to assess electrolyte concentrations), thyroid function tests, and a digoxin level should be performed as necessary to determine any underlying causes of the arrhythmia. In addition, an echocardiogram should be performed to assess left ventricular (LV) function. If myocardial ischemia is suspected as a cause of the arrhythmia, the patient should undergo further evaluation with measurement of cardiac enzymes, performance of cardiac stress testing, and, possibly, cardiac catheterization.

INITIATING DRUG THERAPY

During the past several decades, the treatment approach for both atrial and ventricular arrhythmias has been gradually shifting away from the use of AADs toward the use of various nonpharmacological therapies. Several factors have likely contributed to the decline in AAD use over the years. The negative results of the Cardiac Arrhythmia Suppression Trial (CAST) likely had a significant influence on the downward prescribing patterns of class I AADs. In addition, increasing clinical evidence to support the use of nonpharmacological strategies for the treatment of both supraventricular and ventricular arrhythmias has likely contributed to the decline in the use of AADs as a whole. Numerous studies establishing that a rhythm-control regimen does not confer any benefit over a rate-control regimen in patients with persistent atrial fibrillation (AF) may have also contributed to this decline in AAD use.

Treatable conditions may cause the arrhythmia. Identification of treatable causes before administering an AAD is a priority. Conditions that may cause arrhythmias are electrolyte imbalances (e.g., hypokalemia, hypomagnesemia), drug overdose, drug interactions with other medications or herbal supplements, renal failure, thyroid disorders, metabolic acidosis, hypovolemia, MI, pulmonary embolism, cardiac tamponade, tension pneumothorax, dissecting aortic aneurysm, hypoxemia, and valvular or congenital defects in the heart.

Nonpharmacological therapies, such as radiofrequency catheter ablation and implantable cardioverter–defibrillators (ICDs), are also available to treat various arrhythmias. ICDs are used in the management of ventricular arrhythmias, and their benefits have been demonstrated in several clinical trials (Antiarrhythmics Versus Implantable Defibrillators [AVID] Investigators, 1997; Bardy et al., 2005; Buxton et al., 1999; Connolly et al., 2000; Kuck et al., 2000; Moss et al., 1996, 2002). Radiofrequency catheter ablation permanently terminates the arrhythmia by ablating the focal area where the arrhythmia occurs. This procedure can be used for AF, atrial flutter (AFl), and symptomatic drug-refractory ventricular tachycardia (VT).

Goals of AAD Therapy

The overall goals of AAD therapy are to relieve the acute episode of irregular rhythm, establish sinus rhythm (SR), and prevent further episodes of the arrhythmia. Typical agents used to treat arrhythmias include AADs (classes I through IV), digoxin, adenosine, and atropine (**Table 23.1**).

Drug Classification

AADs are organized into four classes, I (Ia, Ib, Ic), II, III, and IV (Vaughan Williams, 1984). Although the Vaughan Williams classification system is the most widely used method for grouping AADs based on their electrophysiologic actions, using this classification system requires some points of exception to be made. This system is somewhat incomplete, and it excludes certain drugs including digoxin, adenosine, and

TABLE 23.1

Overview of Selected Antiarrhythmic Agents

Generic (Trade) Name and Dosage	Selected Adverse Effects	Contraindications	Special Considerations
adenosine (Adenocard) Adult: 6 mg IV push over 1–2 s; repeat with 12 mg IV push if sinus rhythm not obtained within 1–2 min after first dose; may repeat 12-mg dose a second time if no response in 1–2 min	Headache, chest pain, light-headedness, dizziness, nausea, flushing, dyspnea, blurred vision	2nd-/3rd-degree heart block or sick sinus syndrome in the absence of a pacemaker	Monitor ECG during administration. Use cautiously in patients with asthma (bronchoconstriction may occur). Each dose should be immediately followed with a 10-mL saline flush.
amiodarone (Cordarone, Nexterone, Pacerone) *AF* Adult IV: 5 mg/kg over 30 min, then continuous infusion of 1 mg/min for 6 h, then 0.5 mg/min; convert to PO when hemodynamically stable and able to take PO medications Adult PO: 400 mg bid–tid for 1 wk, until patient receives ~10 g total, then 200 mg PO daily *Pulseless VT/VF* Adult IV: 300 mg IV push/IO; can give additional 150 mg IV push/IO if persistent VT/VF; if stable rhythm achieved, initiate continuous infusion at 1 mg/min for 6 h, then 0.5 mg/min; convert to PO when hemodynamically stable and able to take PO medications (see PO dose under stable VT) *Stable VT (with a pulse)* Adult IV: 150 mg (diluted in 100 mL of D5W or saline) over 10 min; may repeat dose every 10 min, if necessary for breakthrough VT; if stable rhythm achieved, initiate continuous infusion at 1 mg/min for 6 h, then 0.5 mg/min; convert to PO when hemodynamically stable and able to take PO medications Adult PO: 1,200–1,600 mg/d in 2 or 3 divided doses for 1 wk, until patient receives ~15 g total, then 300–400 mg PO daily	IV: hypotension, bradycardia, heart block, phlebitis PO: corneal microdeposits, optic neuritis, nausea, vomiting, anorexia, pulmonary fibrosis, bradycardia, tremor, ataxia, paresthesias, insomnia, constipation, abnormal liver function tests, hypothyroidism, hyperthyroidism, blue-gray discoloration of skin, photosensitivity	2nd-/3rd-degree heart block or sick sinus syndrome in the absence of a pacemaker	Advise patient to apply sunscreen and to minimize areas of exposure to sun. Patients should have chest x-ray performed annually. Liver function and thyroid function tests should be performed every 6 mo. Pulmonary function tests and ophthalmologic exam should be performed if patient becomes symptomatic. A chest x-ray, pulmonary function tests, liver function tests, and thyroid function tests should also be performed at baseline. An ophthalmologic exam should be performed at baseline if the patient has significant visual abnormalities. Monitor for drug interactions (CYP3A4 substrate; CYP3A4, 2C9, 2D6, and P-gp inhibitor).
atropine Adult: 0.5 mg IV every 3–5 min; not to exceed 3 mg total dose	Palpitations, tachycardia, dry mouth, dizziness	Acute angle-closure glaucoma, obstructive uropathy, tachycardia, obstructive disease of GI tract	Administer IV over 1 min. Monitor ECG during administration.

TABLE 23.1

Overview of Selected Antiarrhythmic Agents (*Continued*)

Generic (Trade) Name and Dosage	Selected Adverse Effects	Contraindications	Special Considerations
digoxin (Lanoxin) Adult LD (IV or PO): 0.25–0.5 mg over 2 min; may give 0.125–0.25 mg q6h for 2 more doses for a total dose of 1 mg or 10–15 mcg/kg Adult MD: 0.125–0.25 mg IV or PO daily in normal renal function	Anorexia, nausea, vomiting, diarrhea, headache, dizziness, vertigo, visual disturbances (yellow-green halos), confusion, hallucinations, arrhythmias, AV conduction disturbances (heart block, AV junctional rhythm, bradycardia)	2nd-/3rd-degree heart block or sick sinus syndrome in the absence of a pacemaker	Teach patient how to take pulse. Dose adjustment required in renal impairment. Monitor for drug interactions (P-gp substrate).
diltiazem (Cardizem) Adult IV: 0.25 mg/kg over 2 min; if ventricular rate remains uncontrolled after 15 min, can repeat with 0.35 mg/kg over 2 min; then initiate continuous infusion of 5–15 mg/h Adult PO: Start with 30 mg four times daily and ↑ to 180–480 mg/d in divided doses (SR can be given once daily)	Dizziness, headache, edema, heart block, bradycardia, HF exacerbation, hypotension	2nd-/3rd-degree heart block or sick sinus syndrome in the absence of a pacemaker, LVSD	Teach patient how to take pulse and blood pressure. Monitor for drug interactions (CYP3A4 substrate and inhibitor).
disopyramide (Norpace) Adult (<50 kg): IR: 100 mg PO q6h; SR: 200 mg PO q12h Adult (>50 kg): IR: 150 mg PO q6h; SR: 300 mg PO q12h; may ↑ up to 800 mg/d	Hypotension, HF exacerbation, nausea, anorexia, dry mouth, urinary retention, blurred vision, constipation, TdP	2nd-/3rd-degree heart block or sick sinus syndrome in the absence of a pacemaker, LVSD	Dose adjustment required in renal impairment (CrCl ≤ 40 mL/min; SR form not recommended when CrCl ≤40 mL/min). Monitor for drug interactions (CYP3A4 substrate).
dofetilide (Tikosyn) Adult: 125–500 mcg PO bid	Chest pain, headache, dizziness, insomnia, nausea, diarrhea, dyspnea, TdP	CrCl < 20 mL/min, QT interval >440 msec, concomitant use of cimetidine, dolutegravir, hydrochlorothiazide, ketoconazole, megestrol, prochlorperazine, QTc-prolonging drugs, trimethoprim/sulfamethoxazole, or verapamil	Patients must be hospitalized for ≥3 days for therapy initiation. Dose adjustment required in renal impairment (CrCl ≤60 mL/min). Dose must also be adjusted based on QT interval. Monitor for drug interactions.
dronedarone (Multaq) Adult: 400 mg PO bid (with meals)	Nausea, vomiting, diarrhea, HF exacerbation, hepatic impairment, pulmonary toxicity, renal impairment/failure	Permanent AF, NYHA class IV HF, NYHA class II–III HF with recent hospitalization for decompensated HF, 2nd-/3rd-degree heart block or sick sinus syndrome in the absence of a pacemaker, heart rate <50 beats/min, concurrent use of potent CYP3A4 inhibitors or QTc-prolonging drugs, QT interval ≥500 msec, PR interval >280 msec, severe hepatic impairment, history of amiodarone-induced hepatic or pulmonary toxicity	Instruct patient to report adverse reactions or any signs/symptoms of HF immediately. Monitor for drug interactions (CYP3A4 substrate; CYP2D6, CYP3A4, and P-gp inhibitor).

(*Continued*)

TABLE 23.1

Overview of Selected Antiarrhythmic Agents (*Continued*)

Generic (Trade) Name and Dosage	Selected Adverse Effects	Contraindications	Special Considerations
esmolol (Brevibloc) Adult: 500 mcg/kg/min IV for 1 min, then maintenance infusion of 50 mcg/kg/min; if inadequate response, rebolus with 500 mcg/kg/min for 1 min and ↑ infusion rate by 50 mcg/kg/min; repeat this process until desired response achieved or maximum infusion rate of 300 mcg/kg/min is reached	Hypotension, wheezing, bronchospasm, heart block, bradycardia, HF exacerbation	2nd-/3rd-degree heart block in the absence of a pacemaker, decompensated HF, sinus bradycardia	Use with caution in patients with LVSD.
flecainide Adult: 50 mg PO q12h up to a maximum of 300 mg/d	Dizziness, headache, lightheadedness, syncope, blurred vision or other visual disturbances, dyspnea, HF exacerbation, arrhythmias	2nd-/3rd-degree heart block in the absence of a pacemaker, recent MI, ischemic heart disease, cardiogenic shock, HF	Dose adjustment required in renal impairment (CrCl ≤ 50 mL/min). Monitor for drug interactions (CYP2D6 substrate).
ibutilide (Corvert) Adult (<60 kg): 0.01 mg/kg IV over 10 min; can repeat with another dose if AF/AFl does not terminate within 10 min after end of initial dose Adult (≥60 kg): 1 mg IV over 10 min; can repeat with another dose if AF/AFl does not terminate within 10 min after end of initial dose	TdP, hypotension, heart block, headache, nausea	Preexisting hypokalemia or hypomagnesemia, QT interval >440 msec	Monitor ECG during administration. Stop infusion if QT interval prolongation or ventricular arrhythmias occur. Correct electrolyte abnormalities before administering.
lidocaine (Xylocaine) *Pulseless VT/VF* Adult: 1–1.5 mg/kg IV push/IO; may give additional 0.5–0.75 mg/kg IV push/IO every 5–10 min, if persistent VT/VF (maximum cumulative dose = 3 mg/kg); if stable rhythm achieved, initiate continuous infusion of 1–4 mg/min *Stable VT (with a pulse)* Adult: 1–1.5 mg/kg IV push; may give additional 0.5–0.75 mg/kg IV push every 5–10 min, if persistent VT (maximum cumulative dose = 3 mg/kg); if stable rhythm achieved, initiate continuous infusion of 1–4 mg/min	Seizures, confusion, stupor, dizziness, bradycardia, respiratory depression, slurred speech, blurred vision, muscle twitching, tinnitus	Hypersensitivity to amide local anesthetics, 2nd-/3rd-degree heart block in the absence of a pacemaker	A lower infusion rate (1–2 mg/min) should be used in older adults or patients with HF or hepatic disease. Monitor for drug interactions (CYP1A2 and CYP3A4 substrate)

TABLE 23.1

Overview of Selected Antiarrhythmic Agents (*Continued*)

Generic (Trade) Name and Dosage	Selected Adverse Effects	Contraindications	Special Considerations
metoprolol (Lopressor) Adult IV: 2.5–5 mg over 2 min; can repeat every 5 min (maximum cumulative dose = 15 mg over 10- to 15-min period) Adult PO: IR: 25 mg bid; SR: 50 mg daily; may ↑ up to 400 mg/d	Bradycardia, HF exacerbation, heart block, bronchospasm, fatigue, ↓ exercise tolerance, dizziness, hypotension	2nd-/3rd-degree heart block in the absence of a pacemaker, decompensated HF, heart rate <45 beats/min	Use IV with caution in patients with LVSD. Teach patient how to take pulse and blood pressure. Instruct patient to not discontinue drug abruptly (may lead to hypertensive crises, angina, or MI). Use metoprolol succinate (SR) when initiating PO therapy in patients with LVSD.
mexiletine Adult: 200 mg PO q8h; may ↑ up to 400 mg PO q8h	Dizziness, drowsiness, paresthesias, blurred vision, tremor, seizures, confusion, arrhythmias, nausea, vomiting	2nd-/3rd-degree heart block in the absence of a pacemaker, cardiogenic shock	Monitor for drug interactions (CYP1A2 and CYP2D6 substrate).
procainamide Adult: 15–18 mg/kg IV over 60 min, then continuous infusion of 1–4 mg/min	Bradycardia, heart block, hypotension, HF exacerbation, TdP	Hypersensitivity to procaine, 2nd-/3rd-degree heart block in the absence of a pacemaker	Monitor ECG during administration. Stop infusion if QT interval prolongation or ventricular arrhythmias occur. Use with caution, if at all, in renal impairment.
propafenone (Rythmol) Adult: IR: 150 mg PO q8h (up to a maximum of 300 mg PO q8h); SR: 225 mg PO q12h (up to a maximum of 425 mg PO q12h)	Dizziness, drowsiness, HF exacerbation, blurred vision, arrhythmias, heart block, bradycardia, taste disturbances, bronchospasm	2nd-/3rd-degree heart block in the absence of a pacemaker, bradycardia, cardiogenic shock, HF, bronchospastic disorders	Teach patient how to take pulse and blood pressure. Instruct patient to not discontinue drug abruptly (may lead to hypertensive crises, angina, or MI).
propranolol Adult IV: 1 mg over 1 min; may repeat every 5 min up to a total dose of 5 mg Adult PO: 10–20 mg q6–8h; can ↑ to 80–240 mg/d in 2–4 divided doses	Bradycardia, HF exacerbation, heart block, bronchospasm, fatigue, ↓ exercise tolerance, dizziness, hypotension	2nd-/3rd-degree heart block or sick sinus syndrome in the absence of a pacemaker, LVSD Relatively contraindicated in asthma	Teach patient how to take pulse and blood pressure. Instruct patient to not discontinue drug abruptly (may lead to hypertensive crises, angina, or MI).
quinidine Adult: Sulfate: 200–400 mg PO q6h, up to a maximum of 600 mg PO q6h Gluconate: 324 mg PO q8–12h, up to a maximum of 972 mg PO q8–12h	TdP, heart block, hypotension, tinnitus, diarrhea, nausea, vomiting, fever, HF exacerbation, thrombocytopenia	Allergy or sensitivity to quinidine or cinchona derivatives, long QT syndrome (may predispose to TdP)	Instruct patient to take drug with food if GI distress occurs. Monitor for drug interactions (CYP3A4 substrate; CYP2D6 inhibitor).
sotalol (Betapace, Betapace AF) *AF (Betapace AF)* Adult: 80 mg PO bid, up to a maximum of 160 mg PO bid *Ventricular Arrhythmias (Betapace)* Adult: 80 mg PO bid, up to a maximum of 320 mg PO bid	Bradycardia, heart block, HF exacerbation, TdP, bronchospasm	2nd-/3rd-degree heart block in the absence of a pacemaker, bradycardia, HF, asthma, long QT syndrome (may predispose to TdP)	Patients must be hospitalized for ≥3 days for therapy initiation. Teach patient how to take pulse and blood pressure. Dose adjustment required in renal impairment (CrCl ≤ 60 mL/min) Instruct patient to not discontinue drug abruptly (may lead to hypertensive crises, angina, or MI).

(*Continued*)

TABLE 23.1			
Overview of Selected Antiarrhythmic Agents (*Continued*)			
Generic (Trade) Name and Dosage	**Selected Adverse Effects**	**Contraindications**	**Special Considerations**
verapamil (Calan) Adult IV: 2.5–5 mg over 2 min; if ventricular rate remains uncontrolled after 15–30 min, can double initial dose and administer over 2 min; then initiate continuous infusion of 5–10 mg/h Adult PO: 240–360 mg/d in 3 divided doses (SR can be given once daily)	Constipation, bradycardia, heart block, HF exacerbation, hypotension, dizziness, peripheral edema	2nd-/3rd-degree heart block or sick sinus syndrome in the absence of a pacemaker, LVSD	Encourage patient to ↑ fluid and fiber intake to combat constipation. Teach patient how to take pulse and blood pressure. Monitor for drug interactions (CYP3A4 substrate and inhibitor).

AF, atrial fibrillation; AFl, atrial flutter; AV, atrioventricular; bid, twice daily; CrCl; creatinine clearance; CYP, cytochrome P-450, D5W, 5% dextrose in water; ECG, electrocardiogram; GI, gastrointestinal; HF, heart failure; IO, intraosseous; IR, immediate-release; IV, intravenous; LD, loading dose; LVSD, left ventricular systolic dysfunction; MD, maintenance dose; MI, myocardial infarction; NYHA, New York Heart Association; P-gp, P-glycoprotein; PO, oral; SR, sustained release; TdP, torsades de pointes; tid, 3 times daily; VF, ventricular fibrillation; VT, ventricular tachycardia.

atropine. In addition, the classification is not pure, and there is some overlapping of drugs into more than one category. For instance, amiodarone and dronedarone have electrophysiologic properties of all four Vaughan Williams classes. Furthermore, this system does not take into account that the active metabolites of AADs may have different electrophysiologic effects than their parent drugs. For example, *N*-acetyl procainamide (NAPA), the major active metabolite of procainamide, blocks outward potassium channels and therefore can be considered a class III AAD. Although procainamide blocks outward potassium channels, it also primarily blocks inward sodium currents, thereby making it a class Ia AAD. Therefore, the overall electrophysiologic effect produced by procainamide depends upon the relative concentrations of procainamide and NAPA that are present in the body, which can vary based on several clinical factors. The Vaughan Williams classification scheme (**Box 23.3**) identifies drugs that block sodium channels (class Ia, Ib, and Ic), those that are β-blockers (class II), those that block potassium channels (class III), and those that are nondihydropyridine calcium channel blockers (CCBs) (class IV).

Class I AADs

This class of drugs, known as the sodium channel blockers, may be subdivided into classes Ia, Ib, and Ic according to the rate of sodium channel dissociation. These agents vary in the rate at which they bind and then dissociate from the sodium channel receptor. Class Ib AADs bind to and dissociate from the sodium channel receptor quickly ("fast on–off"), while class Ic AADs slowly bind to and dissociate from this receptor ("slow on–off"). The binding kinetics of the class Ia AADs are intermediate between those of the class Ib and Ic agents. In addition, class I AADs possess rate dependence, whereby sodium channel blockade is greatest at fast heart rates (i.e., tachycardia) and least during slower heart rates (i.e., bradycardia) (see **Table 23.1**).

Class Ia Drugs
Quinidine
Quinidine is a broad-spectrum AAD that may be used to treat supraventricular and ventricular arrhythmias. This drug slows conduction velocity (phase 0), prolongs refractoriness (phase 3), and decreases automaticity (phase 4). Quinidine widens the QRS complex, prolongs the QT interval, and slightly prolongs the PR interval on the ECG. Quinidine has been used in the management of AF, AFl, AV nodal reentrant tachycardia, and VT.

Quinidine has potent anticholinergic properties that affect the SA and AV nodes. Therefore, quinidine can increase the SA nodal discharge rate and AV nodal conduction. Consequently, in patients with AF or AFl, these anticholinergic effects may lead to a more rapid ventricular rate. Therefore, the AV node should be adequately inhibited with the use of an AV nodal blocking drug, such as a β-blocker, nondihydropyridine CCB (e.g., diltiazem or verapamil), or digoxin prior to administering quinidine in these patients. Quinidine also blocks α₁-receptors, which can lead to vasodilation and subsequent dose-related hypotension, especially when administered intravenously.

The most common adverse effects associated with quinidine are gastrointestinal (GI) (nausea, vomiting, and diarrhea). As with other class Ia drugs, quinidine can cause

Classification of Antiarrhythmic Drugs

CLASS I—SODIUM CHANNEL BLOCKERS

Ia (intermediate onset/offset)
  disopyramide
  procainamide
  quinidine
Ib (fast onset/offset)
  lidocaine
  mexiletine
Ic (slow onset/offset)
  flecainide
  propafenone*

CLASS II—β-BLOCKERS

atenolol
esmolol
metoprolol
propranolol

CLASS III—POTASSIUM CHANNEL BLOCKERS

amiodarone†
dofetilide
dronedarone†
ibutilide
sotalol*

CLASS IV—CALCIUM CHANNEL BLOCKERS

diltiazem
verapamil

---

*Also has β-blocking properties (class II)
†Also has sodium channel blocking (class I), β-blocking (class II), and calcium channel blocking (class IV) properties

proarrhythmia, specifically torsades de pointes (TdP). Other adverse effects associated with quinidine include thrombocytopenia, hepatitis, cinchonism (tinnitus, blurred vision, headache), worsening of underlying HF, and hemolytic anemia.

Quinidine is a substrate of the cytochrome P-450 (CYP) 3A4 isoenzyme and an inhibitor of the CYP2D6 isoenzyme. Therefore, quinidine can interact with any drug that inhibits or induces CYP3A4 (e.g., inhibitors: ketoconazole, erythromycin, amiodarone, verapamil, diltiazem; inducers: rifampin, phenobarbital, phenytoin) or is a substrate of CYP2D6 (e.g., β-blockers). Quinidine can also significantly increase serum digoxin concentrations.

Procainamide

Procainamide has basically the same electrophysiologic effects as those of quinidine, except that procainamide does not have the anticholinergic activity of quinidine. Procainamide slows conduction velocity (phase 0), prolongs refractoriness (phase 3), and decreases automaticity (phase 4). Procainamide widens the QRS complex, prolongs the QT interval, and slightly prolongs the PR interval on the ECG. NAPA, the major metabolite of procainamide, blocks outward potassium currents and thereby has class III electrophysiologic properties. NAPA prolongs the QT interval. Procainamide is a broad-spectrum AAD and has been used to treat supraventricular and ventricular arrhythmias.

Procainamide is only available in the intravenous (IV) formulation; all of its oral formulations have been discontinued. Therefore, adverse effects that would most likely occur with chronic therapy (e.g., systemic lupus erythematosus, agranulocytosis) should no longer be a concern. Most of the adverse effects associated with IV administration of procainamide include bradycardia, AV block, hypotension, worsening of underlying HF, and TdP.

Procainamide and NAPA can accumulate in patients with renal impairment. Therefore, serum concentrations must be monitored regularly to assess for efficacy and toxicity. The therapeutic ranges of procainamide and NAPA are 4 to 10 mcg/mL and 15 to 25 mcg/mL, respectively.

Disopyramide

Disopyramide slows conduction velocity (phase 0), prolongs refractoriness (phase 3), and decreases automaticity (phase 4). These effects are manifested as a prolonged QT interval and a slightly prolonged QRS complex on the ECG. Disopyramide has direct and indirect effects on the heart rate similar to those of quinidine. Disopyramide is a broad-spectrum AAD and has been used to treat supraventricular and ventricular arrhythmias. However, the clinical use of this agent is limited because of its potent anticholinergic and negative inotropic effects. If disopyramide is used to treat AF or AFl, the practitioner should give an AV nodal blocking agent (e.g., β-blocker, diltiazem, verapamil, or digoxin) to minimize its vagolytic effect.

The primary adverse effects associated with disopyramide are precipitation of HF and anticholinergic effects (e.g., dry mouth, urinary retention, constipation, blurred vision). Disopyramide is contraindicated in patients with HF with reduced ejection fraction (HFrEF) (left ventricular ejection fraction [LVEF] of 40% or less) because it can cause significant depression of myocardial contractility. Disopyramide can also cause TdP.

Class Ib Drugs

The class Ib AADs include lidocaine and mexiletine. These agents decrease automaticity and conduction velocity and shorten refractoriness. These AADs primarily exert their electrophysiologic effects on the ventricular myocardium since they have little or no effect on atrial tissue.

Lidocaine

Lidocaine is categorized as a class Ib AAD; however, its electrophysiologic effects are different in that it is selective to ischemic tissue, and especially to active fast sodium channels in the bundle of His, Purkinje fibers, and ventricular myocardium. Thus, lidocaine has little effect on conduction in nonischemic tissue and the atrial myocardium. Lidocaine also has very little effect on the automaticity of the SA node. However, lidocaine does suppress the automaticity of ectopic ventricular pacemakers and Purkinje fibers. In normal tissues, the action potential duration is shortened and conduction velocity shows little change with lidocaine. However, in depolarized fibers or in fibers damaged by ischemia, lidocaine prolongs the action potential and slows conduction.

Lidocaine is primarily effective in treating ventricular arrhythmias, especially those associated with acute MI. Prophylactic administration in patients with acute MI demonstrated a decreased incidence of ventricular fibrillation (VF) but no difference in prehospital treatment outcomes of acute MI and no improvement or even higher mortality rates in hospitalized patients. Selective administration of lidocaine to patients with VF associated with MI or cardiac arrest also demonstrated no improvement in survival rates (Wyse et al., 1988). The use of lidocaine as prophylaxis against VT or VF in patients with MI is not warranted. Its use should be reserved for the treatment of ventricular arrhythmias.

Lidocaine is not effective in the treatment of supraventricular arrhythmias such as AF or AFl. However, lidocaine can be used for the treatment of digoxin-induced arrhythmias (atrial and ventricular) because of its selectivity for depolarized myocardium.

Lidocaine is eliminated primarily by hepatic metabolism, with the metabolic rate being proportional to hepatic blood flow. In patients with HFrEF, the volume of distribution in the central compartment is decreased and hepatic blood flow may be reduced if cardiac output is depressed. Hepatic impairment slows lidocaine's clearance rate but does not affect its volume of distribution.

The principal adverse effects associated with lidocaine are central nervous system (CNS) effects (i.e., dizziness, paresthesia, disorientation, tremor, agitation). At higher concentrations, seizures and respiratory arrest may occur with the use of lidocaine. Lidocaine's adverse effects are more frequent in the elderly, in patients with HFrEF or hepatic disease, and during prolonged administration (more than 24 hours). Therefore, these patients should be closely monitored for signs and symptoms of lidocaine toxicity. Lidocaine concentrations should also be closely monitored in these patients. The therapeutic range of lidocaine is 1.5 to 6 mg/L. Lidocaine toxicity is most commonly observed at concentrations greater than 5 mg/L.

Mexiletine

Mexiletine is a structurally related oral analog of and has similar electrophysiologic effects, antiarrhythmic effects, and adverse events to lidocaine. Mexiletine decreases conduction velocity (phase 0) preferentially in ischemic tissue.

Mexiletine is effective in the treatment of VT. Combining mexiletine with a second AAD (class IA or III) is more effective than mexiletine monotherapy for the treatment of refractory VT. However, its clinical use is limited by a high incidence of GI reactions such as nausea and vomiting. CNS adverse effects such as dizziness, confusion, ataxia, and speech disturbances may lead the practitioner to discontinue treatment with this drug. Mexiletine can also cause proarrhythmia, although the incidence is lower when compared to other AADs.

Class Ic Drugs

Flecainide

Flecainide is a potent blocker of sodium channels during phase 0 of the action potential, thereby slowing conduction velocity in the Purkinje fibers and AV node and diminishing automaticity in the Purkinje fibers. Because of the slowed cardiac conduction, increases in the PR interval and QRS duration may be seen on the ECG.

Flecainide is most commonly used in clinical practice for the treatment of supraventricular arrhythmias, such as AF and AFl. Flecainide has very good efficacy in terms of restoring and maintaining SR in patients with AF (Camm et al., 2012; Slavik et al., 2001). Flecainide has been shown to restore SR in 75% to 90% of patients with AF at 8 hours (with single, oral loading doses of 300 mg) as well as maintain SR in up to 77% of patients at 1 year. Although flecainide is approved by the U.S. Food and Drug Administration (FDA) for the treatment of life-threatening sustained VT, it is rarely, if ever, used for this indication, primarily due to its suboptimal efficacy and the potential for proarrhythmic events (Anderson et al., 1983). There may be a resurgence in the use of flecainide for the use of ventricular arrhythmias, as this AAD has been more recently shown to be effective in suppressing exercise-induced ventricular arrhythmias in patients with catecholaminergic polymorphic VT that is refractory to β-blocker therapy (Van der Werf et al., 2011).

The CAST was conducted to determine if suppression of asymptomatic or mildly symptomatic premature ventricular contractions (PVCs) with the class Ic AADs, flecainide, encainide, or moricizine would reduce the incidence of death from arrhythmia in post-MI patients (CAST Investigators, 1989). Despite adequate suppression of ventricular arrhythmias, flecainide significantly increased mortality from arrhythmia or cardiac arrest (presumably due to proarrhythmia) and significantly increased total mortality. Overall, the results of this trial demonstrated that the use of AADs to suppress asymptomatic PVCs in post-MI patients does not improve survival and is most likely detrimental. The use of flecainide should be avoided in patients with any form of structural heart disease (SHD), which includes CAD, HF, or LV hypertrophy.

Adverse effects associated with flecainide include blurred vision, dizziness, headache, tremor, nausea, vomiting, conduction disturbances, and ventricular arrhythmias (sustained VT) that can be quite resistant to cardioversion. Flecainide also has potent negative inotropic effects that may lead to worsening HF.

Propafenone

Propafenone has the same ability to block sodium channels, slow conduction velocity, and diminish automaticity in the AV node and Purkinje fibers as flecainide. However, propafenone also has a mild, nonselective β-blocking effect. Although propafenone is FDA approved for the treatment of life-threatening ventricular arrhythmias, its use in clinical practice has been limited to the management of supraventricular arrhythmias such as AF. Propafenone has been shown to be effective for restoring and maintaining SR in patients with AF (Miller et al., 2000; Roy et al., 2000). The use of single, oral loading doses of propafenone (450 to 600 mg) in patients with recent-onset AF has been associated with conversion rates of 72% to 76% at 8 hours (Slavik et al., 2001). Although propafenone was not evaluated in the CAST and has not been associated with increased mortality in other trials, there still tends to be an overall negative perception of this drug's safety in patients with SHD. Until the safety of propafenone can be demonstrated conclusively in a large, randomized, prospective trial in patients with SHD, its use should be avoided in this population.

Adverse effects associated with propafenone include blurred vision, dizziness, headache, nausea, vomiting, fatigue, bronchospasm, taste disturbances (metallic taste), conduction disturbances (bradycardia, heart block, QRS prolongation), and ventricular arrhythmias (sustained VT) that can be quite resistant to cardioversion. Propafenone also has potent negative inotropic effects that may lead to worsening HF.

Class II AADs

β-Blockers are useful in suppressing ventricular arrhythmias. They also are used for treating many supraventricular arrhythmias because of their ability to block receptor sites in the conduction system and subsequently slow AV nodal conduction and the SA nodal rate, which in turn slows the ventricular rate. Furthermore, β-blockers are helpful when used in combination with other AADs or in treating the underlying cause of some arrhythmias (ischemia, catecholamine excess) (see **Table 23.1**).

β-Blockers decrease automaticity (decrease the slope of phase 4 depolarization in the sinus node and in the Purkinje fibers) and conduction velocity (phase 0) and prolong refractoriness (phase 3). Changes in the ECG caused by β-blockers are a sinus bradycardia, consisting of a normal or slightly prolonged PR interval and occasional shortening of the QT interval. In addition to being negative chronotropic drugs (decrease AV nodal conduction), β-blockers are also negative inotropic agents (decrease cardiac contractility). Both of these properties enable β-blockers to decrease myocardial oxygen consumption, which is useful especially in patients with underlying CAD. Patients with sinus node dysfunction or AV conduction system defects may have significant sinus bradycardia when a β-blocker is initiated.

In general, β-blockers lower the heart rate and blood pressure, decrease myocardial contractility, decrease oxygen consumption in the myocardium, and lower cardiac output. β-Blockers have a diverse range of uses, including paroxysmal

supraventricular tachycardia (PSVT), AF, AFl, and arrhythmias caused by catecholamine excess, ischemia, mitral valve prolapse, hypertrophic cardiomyopathy, and MI. β-Blockers also reduce complex ventricular arrhythmias, including VT. The VF threshold is increased with the use of β-blockers in animal models, and β-blockers have been found to decrease VF in patients with acute MI. β-Blockers reduce myocardial ischemia, which may reduce the likelihood of VF. All β-blockers (without intrinsic sympathomimetic activity) are relatively similar in efficacy for the treatment of supraventricular and ventricular arrhythmias. Selection of a particular β-blocker is usually based on the safety profile of the individual agent.

The adverse effects associated with β-blockers depend on their selectivity for β_1 or β_2 receptors. Bronchospasm may be seen in patients with asthma and chronic obstructive pulmonary disease; this adverse effect is not eliminated by the use of selective β_1-blockers since these agents gradually become nonselective as the dose is increased. HF, hypotension, bradycardia, and depression also are common adverse effects of β-blockers. In addition, patients receiving β-blockers often report fatigue and impotence.

Class III AADs

Class III AADs include amiodarone, dofetilide, dronedarone, ibutilide, and sotalol. Ibutilide and dofetilide are used to treat AF and AFl. Amiodarone and sotalol can be used to treat both supraventricular and ventricular arrhythmias. Dronedarone is FDA approved to reduce the risk of hospitalization from cardiovascular (CV) causes in patients in SR with a history of paroxysmal or persistent AF.

Patients receiving class III AADs should be monitored closely for ECG changes such as increased ventricular ectopy and changes in PR interval, QRS duration, and QT interval. Practitioners should avoid using class III AADs concomitantly with other drugs that can prolong the QT interval to minimize the risk of TdP (see **Table 23.1**).

Amiodarone

Amiodarone is a unique drug in that it possesses electrophysiologic characteristics of all four Vaughan Williams classes of AADs. While amiodarone is primarily a potassium channel blocker (blocks the rapid and slow components of the delayed rectifier potassium current), it also blocks sodium channels, has nonselective β-blocking activity, and has weak calcium channel blocking properties. As a result, amiodarone reduces automaticity (phase 4) and conduction velocity (phase 0) and prolongs refractoriness (phase 3). When administered intravenously, amiodarone's β-blocking and calcium channel blocking activities are more predominant. Amiodarone has minimal to no negative inotropic effects, which makes it one of the few AADs that can be safely used in patients with HFrEF.

Amiodarone is approved by the FDA for the management of life-threatening recurrent ventricular arrhythmias. However, its off-label use for AF has increased over the past decade not only because of its increased efficacy in maintaining

SR as compared to other AADs but also because of it is one of the few AADs proven to be safe in patients with concomitant SHD. Amiodarone is often given IV for the acute treatment of life-threatening ventricular arrhythmias, such as VT or VF. IV amiodarone can also be used to terminate AF acutely. Even though ICDs now play a primary role in the chronic management of ventricular arrhythmias, amiodarone is still used in patients who refuse or are not candidates for these devices. Also, amiodarone (with a β-blocker) can also be used as adjunctive therapy in these patients if frequent ICD discharges occur (Connolly et al., 2006).

Because of amiodarone's poor oral bioavailability, large volume of distribution, and long half-life, its onset of action may not be apparent for several months. To achieve efficacy more quickly, loading doses of oral amiodarone must be initially used to saturate the myocardial stores. Once the patient is appropriately loaded with oral amiodarone, the dose should be reduced to the recommended maintenance dose to minimize the incidence of adverse events.

Because of its extremely large volume of distribution and high lipophilicity, amiodarone has the potential to accumulate and cause adverse effects in numerous organs with chronic use, with the lungs, thyroid, eyes, heart, liver, skin, GI tract, and CNS being most notably affected. Unlike other amiodarone-induced adverse effects, pulmonary toxicity can be life threatening. Pulmonary toxicity can develop in up to 15% of patients receiving amiodarone (Range et al., 2013). Definitive diagnosis of amiodarone-induced pulmonary toxicity is difficult, since many of the subjective and objective findings are nonspecific. Patients may present with cough, dyspnea, or fever. The chest radiograph may reveal diffuse infiltrates, and pulmonary function tests may demonstrate a reduction in the diffusion capacity. If pulmonary toxicity is detected, amiodarone should be immediately discontinued. Corticosteroids may be needed to treat the pulmonary inflammation. To screen for pulmonary toxicity in patients receiving amiodarone, pulmonary function tests and a chest radiograph should be obtained at baseline. Subsequently, a chest radiograph should be obtained on an annual basis, while pulmonary function tests can be repeated if symptoms develop (Goldschlager et al., 2007).

Because it contains approximately 38% iodine by weight, amiodarone may also cause thyroid abnormalities that can manifest as either hypothyroidism or hyperthyroidism (Bogazzi et al., 2012). Hypothyroidism is the more common form of amiodarone-induced thyroid dysfunction. Although patients often report increased lethargy, the diagnosis of amiodarone-induced hypothyroidism is made upon detection of elevated levels of thyroid-stimulating hormone (TSH). Patients developing amiodarone-induced hypothyroidism can usually be treated with thyroid hormone supplementation (i.e., levothyroxine). The diagnosis of amiodarone-induced hyperthyroidism should be suspected if patients present with new or recurrent arrhythmias. Patients developing hyperthyroidism have abnormally low TSH levels and can usually be treated with antithyroid medications (i.e., methimazole, propylthiouracil). To screen for thyroid dysfunction in patients receiving amiodarone, thyroid function tests should be performed at baseline and then every 6 months throughout therapy (Goldschlager et al., 2007).

Ocular complications induced by amiodarone often manifest as corneal microdeposits, which occur in virtually every patient (Passman et al., 2012). Although these opacities rarely produce visual disturbances, photophobia, halos, and blurred vision have been reported. Because of their relatively benign nature, these opacities do not require routine monitoring or discontinuation of amiodarone when they develop. Chronic amiodarone therapy has also been associated with optic neuritis and optic neuropathy. Since these ocular disturbances are vision threatening, amiodarone must be discontinued once the diagnosis is confirmed. To screen for these complications, ophthalmologic examinations should be performed at baseline only if patients have significant visual abnormalities and then later only if symptoms develop (Goldschlager et al., 2007).

GI adverse effects are relatively common and occur most frequently when amiodarone-loading doses are administered. Typically, patients report nausea, vomiting, loss of appetite, and abdominal pain. Constipation can also occur during long-term therapy. These GI disturbances can be minimized by dividing the total daily dose into 2 to 3 doses and by taking the drug with food. Liver function test abnormalities can also develop. Although elevations in aspartate aminotransferase and alanine aminotransferase levels are relatively common with amiodarone therapy, overt hepatotoxicity rarely occurs (Babatin et al., 2008). Liver enzyme levels usually return to baseline following reduction of the amiodarone dose or discontinuation of the drug. To screen for these hepatic abnormalities, liver function tests should be performed at baseline and then every 6 months throughout therapy (Goldschlager et al., 2007).

Although laboratory tests cannot detect amiodarone-induced CV, neurologic, and dermatologic toxicities, patients should still be clinically evaluated for these adverse effects on a routine basis. Compared with other AADs, amiodarone produces fewer CV adverse effects. The bradycardia and heart block that can develop merely represent an accentuation of amiodarone's pharmacologic and electrophysiologic properties. Additionally, even though amiodarone markedly prolongs the QT interval, TdP is rare. Neurologic toxicities associated with amiodarone occur frequently and may include tremors, ataxia, peripheral neuropathy, fatigue, and insomnia. The most common dermatologic reactions observed during amiodarone therapy are photosensitivity and a blue-gray skin discoloration (Jaworski et al., 2014). Photosensitivity reactions can range from extremely tanned areas to sunburned areas with erythema and edema. Blue-gray skin discoloration, which often appears on the patient's face and hands, may be related to the cumulative dose and duration of therapy. To prevent these dermatologic toxicities, patients receiving amiodarone should use opaque sunscreens such as zinc oxide while outdoors.

Patients receiving amiodarone also need to be monitored for drug interactions. Amiodarone is a substrate of the CYP3A4 isoenzyme, a potent inhibitor of the CYP3A4, 2C9, and 2D6 isoenzymes and an inhibitor of P-glycoprotein. Amiodarone significantly interacts with digoxin and warfarin, which are commonly used in patients with AF. Amiodarone potentiates the anticoagulant effects of warfarin, which results in an increased international normalized ratio (INR) and an increased risk of bleeding (Sanoski & Bauman, 2002). When amiodarone and warfarin are initiated concurrently or when warfarin is initiated in a patient already receiving amiodarone, warfarin should be started at a dose of 2.5 mg daily. When amiodarone is initiated in a patient already receiving warfarin, the warfarin dose should be empirically reduced by approximately 30% (Sanoski & Bauman, 2002). Amiodarone can also double serum digoxin concentrations. Therefore, the digoxin dose should be empirically reduced by 50% when amiodarone is initiated. Furthermore, to minimize the risk of myopathy or rhabdomyolysis, the doses of simvastatin and lovastatin should not exceed 20 mg/d and 40 mg/d, respectively, when coadministered with amiodarone.

Dronedarone

Like amiodarone, dronedarone is primarily considered a class III AAD, but it exhibits electrophysiological properties of all four Vaughan Williams classes. Although structurally related to amiodarone, dronedarone's structure has been modified through the addition of a methylsulfonyl group and the removal of iodine to potentially limit the risk of toxicity. Dronedarone also has a considerably shorter half-life (24 hours) when compared with amiodarone (greater than 50 days), which allows for steady state to be achieved in 5 to 7 days without the need for loading doses.

The efficacy and safety of dronedarone have been evaluated in several clinical trials. Dronedarone has been shown to be more effective than placebo in maintaining SR in patients with paroxysmal AF or AFl (Singh et al., 2007). In another trial, the use of dronedarone was associated with a significant reduction in the incidence of hospitalization due to CV events or death when compared to placebo in patients with persistent or paroxysmal AF and at least one additional risk factor for death (Hohnloser et al., 2009). A trial that evaluated the efficacy and safety of dronedarone in patients with New York Heart Association (NYHA) class III or IV HF (LVEF of 35% or less) was terminated prematurely after significantly more patients in the dronedarone group died (primarily because of worsening HF) compared with the placebo group (Køber et al., 2008). Based on the results of this particular trial, dronedarone is contraindicated in patients with advanced HF (NYHA class IV or NYHA class II or III with a recent hospitalization for decompensated HF). Dronedarone has also been shown to be significantly less effective than amiodarone in reducing AF recurrences (Le Heuzey et al., 2010). Another trial that enrolled older adult patients with permanent AF and risk factors for major vascular events was terminated prematurely after significantly more patients in the dronedarone group died (primarily from CV causes), were hospitalized for HF, and suffered a stroke when compared with the placebo group (Connolly et al., 2011). Based on the results of this trial, dronedarone is contraindicated in patients with permanent AF (i.e., those who cannot be restored to SR).

Dronedarone is a substrate of the CYP3A isoenzyme, a moderate inhibitor of the CYP3A and CYP2D6 isoenzymes, and an inhibitor of P-glycoprotein. Because of the potential for significantly increasing dronedarone concentrations, concomitant use of potent CYP3A inhibitors (i.e., ketoconazole, itraconazole, voriconazole, cyclosporine, clarithromycin, and ritonavir) or inducers (e.g., rifampin, phenobarbital, phenytoin, carbamazepine, and St. John's wort) should be avoided. No significant interaction has been observed between dronedarone and warfarin. Dronedarone may significantly increase serum digoxin concentrations by about 2.5-fold. Therefore, when concomitantly using dronedarone with digoxin, the digoxin dose should be empirically reduced by 50%. Dronedarone can also significantly increase dabigatran concentrations. The dose of dabigatran should be reduced to 75 mg twice daily in patients with AF who have a creatinine clearance (CrCl) of 30 to 50 mL/min. Concomitant use with dabigatran should be avoided in patients with AF who have a CrCl less than 30 mL/min. To minimize the risk of myopathy or rhabdomyolysis, the doses of simvastatin and lovastatin should not exceed 10 mg/d when administered concomitantly with dronedarone.

The most common adverse effects associated with dronedarone in the clinical trials were GI disturbances, including nausea, vomiting, and diarrhea. However, postmarketing reports have suggested that more significant organ toxicities, including severe hepatic injury, interstitial lung disease (i.e., pneumonitis, pulmonary fibrosis), and acute kidney injury, may also be associated with this AAD. Although a prolonged QT interval can occur with dronedarone, TdP is rare.

Sotalol

Sotalol is a class III AAD that also has nonselective β-blocking properties. Sotalol blocks the rapid component of the delayed rectifier potassium current, which prolongs atrial and ventricular refractoriness. Sotalol exhibits reverse-use dependence, whereby its action potential–prolonging effects are lessened at higher heart rates and increased at lower heart rates. Sotalol increases the QT interval by prolonging ventricular repolarization and may give rise to TdP. The QT interval prolongation with sotalol is a dose-dependent effect. The QT interval should be closely monitored during treatment. Sotalol should be discontinued if the QT interval exceeds 550 msec. The practitioner should avoid combining sotalol with other drugs that increase the QT interval.

Sotalol is effective for the treatment of supraventricular and ventricular arrhythmias. Although sotalol is not effective for conversion of AF, it is an effective agent for maintaining SR in patients with AF (Roy et al., 2000). Several trials have been conducted to compare the efficacy of sotalol and amiodarone in patients with AF (Roy et al., 2000; Singh et al., 2005). The results of these trials suggest that amiodarone is more effective than sotalol in restoring SR in patients with AF. Amiodarone is also more effective than sotalol in maintaining patients in SR, except for in those patients with CAD, where the efficacy of these AADs appears to be similar. In patients with an ICD, sotalol has also been shown to significantly reduce arrhythmia recurrence and discharge from the ICD (Pacifico et al., 1999).

Because sotalol is eliminated primarily by the kidneys, the initial dosing regimen must be based on the patient's CrCl. The practitioner should routinely monitor the patient's renal function throughout therapy to determine if any dosing adjustments are necessary. Sotalol should not be used to treat AF if the patient's CrCl is less than 40 mL/min. The practitioner should also routinely monitor electrolytes, especially if the patient is concomitantly receiving diuretics, since hypokalemia and hypomagnesemia can increase the risk of TdP. Because of concern about TdP when initiating therapy with sotalol, patients must be hospitalized and placed on telemetry for at least 3 days.

Most of the adverse effects associated with sotalol can be attributed to its β-blocking activity (e.g., bradycardia, fatigue, dyspnea). The β-blocking effect of sotalol may decrease cardiac contractility; therefore, this drug should be avoided in patients with HFrEF.

Dofetilide

Dofetilide acts as a selective potassium channel blocker, affecting the rapid component of the delayed rectifier potassium current. This results in a prolonged action potential and QT interval. Dofetilide affects the atria more than the ventricles. It also exhibits reverse-use dependence.

Dofetilide is approved for the conversion of AF or AFl to SR and for the maintenance of SR in patients with permanent AF or AFl. In a study comparing the efficacy and safety of dofetilide with those of placebo, patients randomized to dofetilide were more likely to convert to SR with ascending doses (Singh et al., 2000). At 1 year, slightly more than 50% of patients in the group taking 500 mcg of dofetilide remained in SR. Like amiodarone, dofetilide also has been proven to be safe to use in patients with underlying HFrEF (Køber et al., 2000; Torp-Pedersen et al., 1999).

As with other AADs, the main concern with dofetilide is the dose-dependent onset of TdP and other ventricular arrhythmias. Other adverse effects associated with dofetilide include headache and dizziness.

Dofetilide has a number of important drug interactions. The concomitant use of cimetidine, dolutegravir, ketoconazole, hydrochlorothiazide, megestrol, prochlorperazine, trimethoprim–sulfamethoxazole, or verapamil with dofetilide is contraindicated since these drugs can significantly increase plasma concentrations of dofetilide. Additionally, drugs that prolong the QT interval should not be used concomitantly with dofetilide because of the increased risk of a prolonged QT interval and TdP.

Because dofetilide is eliminated primarily by the kidneys, the initial dosage must be based on the patient's CrCl. The dosage of dofetilide should be decreased in patients with renal impairment (CrCl of less than 60 mL/min). The drug should not be given to patients with a CrCl of less than 20 mL/min or a QT interval greater than 440 msec at baseline. Because of concern about TdP when initiating therapy with dofetilide, patients must be hospitalized and placed on telemetry for at least 3 days.

Ibutilide

Ibutilide is structurally related to L-sotalol, but it has no β-blocking activity. It prolongs the action potential by increasing the slow inward sodium current and blocking the rapid component of the delayed rectifier potassium current, which prolongs atrial and ventricular refractoriness. Ibutilide is available only in IV form. It is indicated only for the acute termination of AF or AFl.

Ibutilide restores SR in approximately 50% of patients with AF or AFl. However, it is more effective for restoring SR in patients with AFl than in those with AF (Stambler et al., 1996). Ibutilide also appears to be effective for facilitating direct-current cardioversion (DCC) of AF (Oral et al., 1999). The major adverse effect associated with ibutilide is TdP. Patients with HFrEF or electrolyte abnormalities (e.g., hypokalemia or hypomagnesemia) are especially at risk for developing proarrhythmia with ibutilide.

Class IV AADs

The class IV AADs, verapamil and diltiazem, are nondihydropyridine CCBs used to treat supraventricular arrhythmias, including PSVT, AF, and AFl. By inhibiting the inward movement of calcium through calcium channels located in cell membranes, these drugs slow conduction, prolong refractoriness, and decrease automaticity in the SA and AV nodes. In AF or AFl, these drugs slow conduction through the AV node and thereby slow the ventricular rate. Their cardiac effects are vascular relaxation, a negative inotropic effect, and a negative chronotropic effect. Verapamil has more potent negative inotropic effects than diltiazem.

Because of their potent negative inotropic effects, both verapamil and diltiazem should be avoided in patients with HFrEF because they are likely to precipitate worsening HF symptoms. These drugs also should not be used in patients with an accessory pathway or WPW syndrome because they can shorten the refractory period of the accessory pathway and subsequently increase the ventricular rate, which may lead to VF.

Bradycardia, heart block, headache, flushing, dizziness, and peripheral edema are the most common adverse effects of diltiazem and verapamil. Verapamil can also cause constipation. The practitioner should use caution when using IV verapamil because significant hypotension can occur (Phillips et al., 1997).

The practitioner should be cautious when administering these agents concomitantly with β-blockers, digoxin, or clonidine because of the increased risk of bradycardia and heart block. Since diltiazem and verapamil are substrates and inhibitors of the CYP3A4 isoenzyme, the practitioner should also use caution when concomitantly administering either of these drugs with other agents that are also metabolized by this isoenzyme.

Other AADs

Several other AADs are commonly used to treat abnormal cardiac impulse formation or conduction. Digoxin, adenosine, and atropine are used in the treatment of various cardiac arrhythmias (see **Table 23.1**).

Digoxin

Digoxin's predominant antiarrhythmic effect is on the AV node of the conduction system. Digoxin affects the autonomic nervous system by stimulating the parasympathetic division, which increases vagal tone. This vagal effect slows conduction through the AV node and prolongs the AV nodal refractory period.

Digoxin is commonly used to slow electrical impulse conduction through the AV node, thus slowing the ventricular rate in supraventricular arrhythmias such as AF or AFl. Digoxin is not effective for converting AF or AFl to SR. Although digoxin is frequently used to control the ventricular rate in patients with HFrEF and concomitant AF or AFl, its use tends to be limited by its relatively slow onset of action and its inability to control the ventricular rate during exercise. Even after an appropriate loading dose is administered, digoxin's peak onset of effect is delayed for up to 6 to 8 hours. Achievement of steady-state concentrations may take up to a week in patients with normal renal function, or even longer in patients with renal impairment. The increased sympathetic tone generated during exercise tends to offset the vagal effects of digoxin, which limits its efficacy under these conditions. In patients with HFrEF and concomitant AF or AFl, digoxin can provide effective ventricular rate control without increasing the risk of worsening HF symptoms because of its additional positive inotropic effects.

Digoxin toxicity can be precipitated by declining renal function, electrolyte disturbances, and drug interactions. Because digoxin is primarily excreted unchanged by the kidneys, a decline in the CrCl can predispose a patient to digoxin toxicity. Hypokalemia, hypomagnesemia, and hypercalcemia can also predispose the myocardium to the toxic effects of digoxin. Concomitant drug therapy with agents such as amiodarone, dronedarone, or verapamil can also increase serum digoxin concentrations. Potential signs and symptoms of digoxin toxicity include heart block, ventricular arrhythmias, visual disturbances (e.g., blurred vision, yellow/green halos), dizziness, weakness, nausea, vomiting, diarrhea, and anorexia. Digoxin has a narrow therapeutic index. The therapeutic range for digoxin in patients with AF and normal LV systolic function (LVEF >40%) is 0.8 to 2 ng/mL. Because of the potential risk of increased mortality with higher serum concentrations, the therapeutic range for digoxin in patients with AF and concomitant HFrEF (LVEF of 40% or less) is 0.5 to 0.9 ng/mL.

Adenosine

Adenosine is an AAD used for converting PSVT to SR. It activates potassium channels and, by increasing the outward potassium current, hyperpolarizes the membrane potential, decreasing spontaneous SA nodal depolarization. Adenosine may also decrease the inward calcium current by blocking adenylate cyclase, which normally increases the inward calcium current. Automaticity (phase 4) and conduction (phase 0) are inhibited in the SA and AV nodes. The most common

adverse effects of adenosine include chest discomfort, dyspnea, flushing, and headache. Sinus arrest can also occur. However, because of adenosine's short half-life of 10 seconds, these adverse effects are short-lived. Adenosine is administered IV because of its short half-life.

Atropine

Atropine is a parasympatholytic drug that enhances both sinus nodal automaticity and AV nodal conduction through direct vagolytic action. Atropine blocks acetylcholine at parasympathetic neuroeffector sites. Atropine is used almost exclusively in the monitored clinical setting for the treatment of symptomatic bradycardia.

Patients who do not experience signs or symptoms of hemodynamic compromise, ischemia, or frequent ventricular ectopy do not require atropine in bradycardic events. Atropine has been reported to be harmful in some patients with AV block at the His–Purkinje level (type II AV block and third-degree AV block with a new wide QRS complex). Atropine can be used in these situations, but the practitioner must monitor the patient closely for paradoxical slowing of the heart rate.

Atropine may induce tachycardia, which may result in poor outcomes in patients with myocardial ischemia or an MI. Therefore, atropine should be used cautiously in these patients.

Selecting the Most Appropriate Agent

Determining the cause and type of the arrhythmia is essential to selecting the most appropriate drug therapy. **Figures 23.1** to **23.5**, as well as **Table 23.1**, guide the practitioner in the initial assessment of which drug to use for patients with various types of arrhythmias.

The first main question to ask when selecting drug therapy is whether the slow or fast rate of the arrhythmia makes the patient ill or symptomatic. A symptomatic patient is one with an arrhythmia characterized by low blood pressure, shock, chest pain, shortness of breath, decreased level of consciousness, pulmonary congestion, HF, or acute MI. These patients may require more urgent treatment, perhaps even with nonpharmacological interventions (e.g., DCC, defibrillation) to immediately terminate the arrhythmia. The practitioner should not make clinical decisions based only on the rhythm displayed on the monitor. The practitioner needs to assess the patient's symptoms to determine how urgent the situation is and how quickly treatment needs to be initiated. Treatment of various arrhythmias is discussed in the first-line and second-line therapy sections. **Table 23.2** consolidates the various treatment regimens.

Second, the practitioner must think of treatable conditions that might be causing the arrhythmia. The patient's medical history and laboratory values are important to assess whenever patients present with arrhythmias. Some possible causes of arrhythmias are electrolyte imbalances (i.e., hypokalemia, hypomagnesemia), drug overdose/toxicity, drug interactions, renal failure, hyperthyroidism, metabolic acidosis,

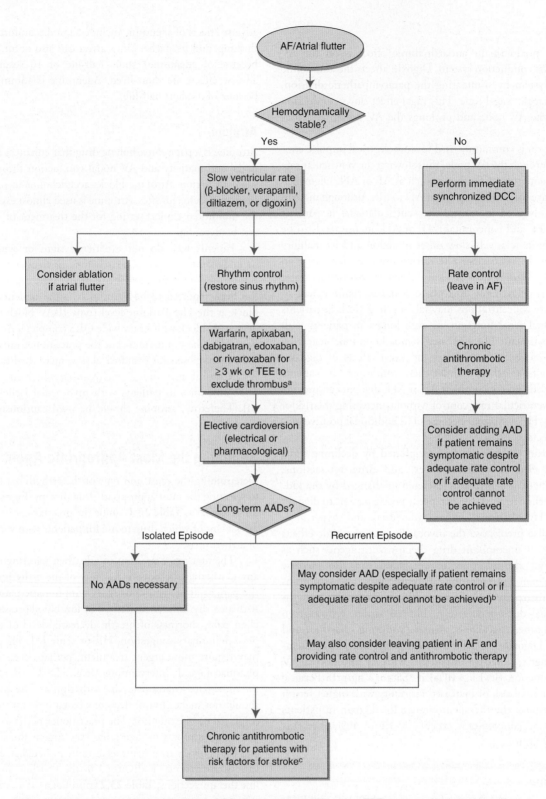

AAD, antiarrhythmic drug; AF, atrial fibrillation; DCC, direct current cardioversion; TEE, transesophageal echocardiogram
a If AF <48 h, 3 wk of anticoagulation prior to cardioversion is unnecessary in patients at high risk for stroke; initiate
  unfractionated heparin, a low-molecular weight heparin, apixaban, dabigatran, edoxaban, or rivaroxaban
  as soon as possible either before or after cardioversion.
b Radiofrequency ablation may be considered for patients who fail or do not tolerate ≥1 AAD.
c Chronic antithrombotic therapy should be considered in all patients with AF and risk factors for stroke regardless of
  whether they remain in sinus rhythm.

FIGURE 23.1   Treatment algorithm for AF and AFl.

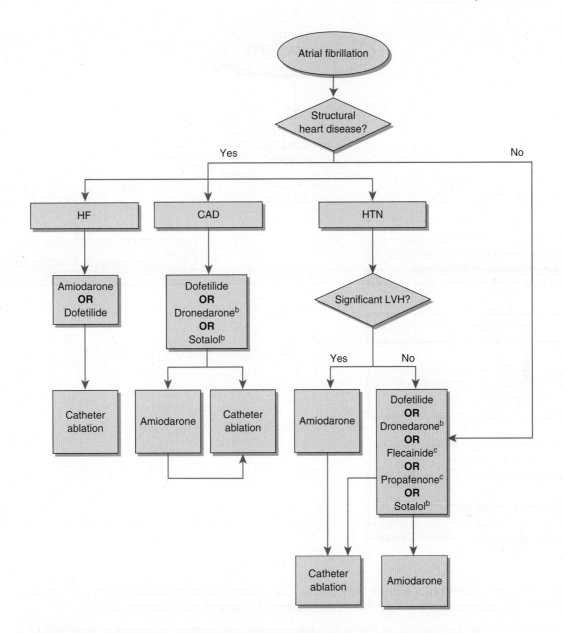

[a] Within each of the boxes, the drugs are listed alphabetically and not in order of suggested use. However, the sequence of the boxes does imply the order of suggested use.
[b] Should only be used if patient has normal left ventricular systolic function.
[c] Should only be used if patient has no other form of structural heart disease.
CAD, coronary artery disease; HF, heart failure; HTN, hypertension; LVH, left ventricular hypertrophy.

FIGURE 23.2 Treatment algorithm for selecting AAD therapy for maintenance of SR in patients with recurrent paroxysmal or persistent AF[a]. (Adapted from January, C. T., Wann, L. S., Alpert, J. S., et al. (2014). 2014 AHA/ACC/HRS guideline for the management of patients with atrial fibrillation: a report of the American College of Cardiology/American Heart Association Task Force on Practice Guidelines and the Heart Rhythm Society. *Circulation, 130,* e199–e267.)

hypovolemia, MI, pulmonary embolism, cardiac tamponade, tension pneumothorax, dissecting aortic aneurysm, and hypoxia related to pulmonary disorders, or structural defects in the heart itself. The practitioner may have to correct the cause of the arrhythmia before initiating drug therapy, especially if the patient is asymptomatic. However, time may be a critical factor when treating symptomatic arrhythmias.

Initial vagal maneuvers may serve as both diagnostic and therapeutic purposes for certain arrhythmias. For example, carotid sinus massage may make the flutter waves in AFl more apparent. Appearance of flutter waves allows the practitioner to differentiate AFl from AF, PSVT, or other tachycardias. Examples of vagal maneuvers include unilateral carotid sinus massage, breath holding, facial immersion in ice water,

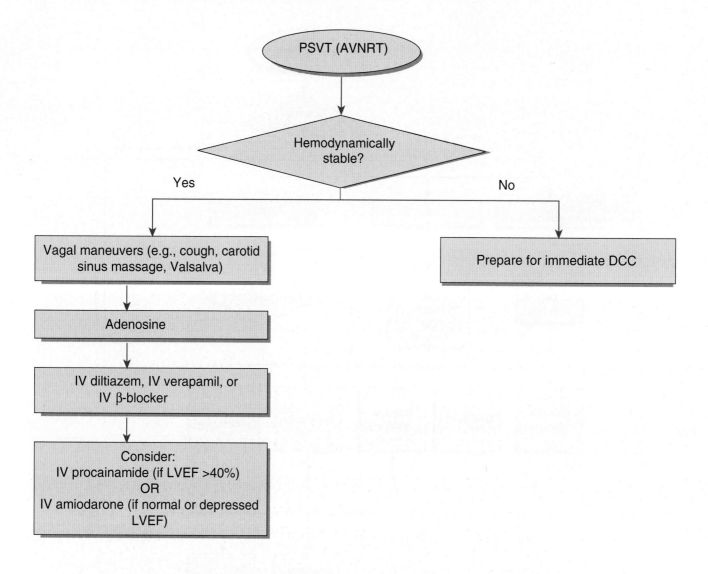

AVNRT, atrioventricular nodal reentrant tachycardia; DCC, direct current cardiversion; IV, intravenous; LVEF, left ventricular ejection fraction; PSVT, paroxysmal supraventricular tachycardia.

FIGURE 23.3 Treatment algorithm for PSVT (due to atrioventricular nodal reentrant tachycardia). (Adapted from Neumar, R. W., Otto, C. W., Link, M. S., et al. (2010). Part 8: Adult advanced cardiovascular support: 2010 American Heart Association Guidelines for Cardiopulmonary Resuscitation and Emergency Cardiovascular Care. *Circulation, 122*(Suppl. 3), S729–S767.)

coughing, nasogastric tube placement, gag reflex stimulation by tongue blade or fingers, eyeball massage, squatting, digital sweep of the anus, and bearing down as during a bowel movement. Many patients who have recurrent PSVT with disorders such as mitral valve prolapse often learn how to do these maneuvers to terminate the arrhythmia themselves. It is important to note that eyeball massage should never be taught, encouraged, or performed because it may cause retinal detachment. Unilateral carotid sinus massage (firm massage of the carotid sinus that never lasts for more than 5 to 10 seconds) should be performed only with continuous ECG monitoring and an IV line in place. The procedure should be avoided in

older adult patients and should not be performed on patients with carotid bruits because it may occlude already impaired circulation to the brain. Likewise, the practitioner should avoid ice water facial immersion in patients with CAD because of the potential for inducing ischemia.

AF/AFI

AF and AFl may be stable or unstable. Patients presenting with severe hypotension, syncope, HF, or angina would be considered to be hemodynamically unstable and would require more urgent treatment. When the patient is hemodynamically stable,

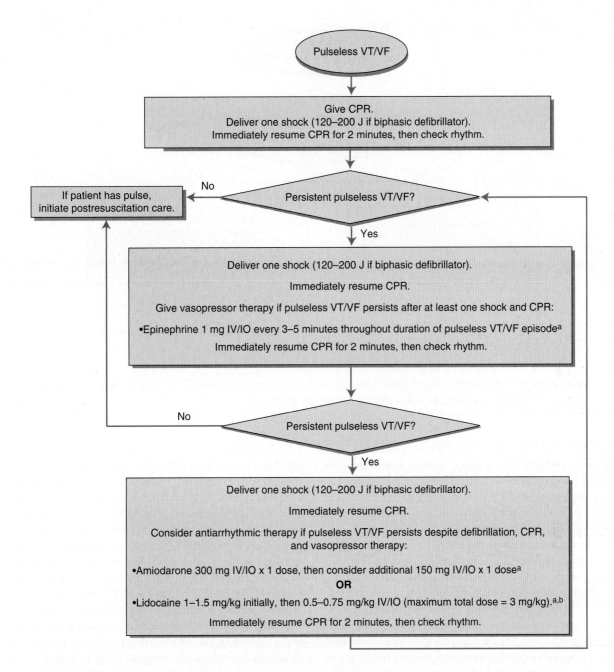

a If IV or IO access cannot be established, epinephrine, and lidocaine may be administered by the endotracheal route. Because of the potential risk of pulmonary toxicity, IV amiodarone should not be administered down an endotracheal tube.

b Lidocaine can be used as alternative to IV amiodarone.

CPR = cardiopulmonary resuscitation; IO = intraosseous; IV = intravenous; J = joules; VF = ventricular fibrillation; VT = ventricular tachycardia;

FIGURE 23.4 Treatment algorithm for pulseless VT/VF. (Adapted from Link, M. S., Berkow, L. C., & Kudenchuk, P. J., et al. (2010). Part 7: Adult advanced cardiovascular life support: 2015 American Heart Association Guidelines Update for Cardiopulmonary Resuscitation and Emergency Cardiovascular Care. *Circulation, 132*(Suppl. 2), S444–S464.)

the practitioner should consider conditions that may be causing the AF or AFl. Such conditions include acute MI, hypoxia, pulmonary embolism, electrolyte imbalance (i.e., hypokalemia, hypomagnesemia), drug toxicity (especially digoxin or sympathomimetic agents), thyrotoxicosis, and alcohol intoxication.

Since new-onset AF can be due to acute MI, the practitioner should look for ischemic changes on the 12-lead ECG. If acute ischemic changes appear, admission of the patient to the hospital in a monitored bed may be needed. Obviously, treatment and correction of acute causes of AF or AFl should be a priority.

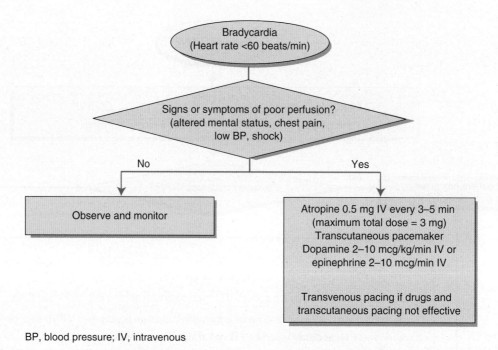

BP, blood pressure; IV, intravenous

FIGURE 23.5 Treatment algorithm for bradycardia. (Adapted from Neumar, R. W., Otto, C. W., Link, M. S., et al. (2010). Part 8: Adult advanced cardiovascular support: 2010 American Heart Association Guidelines for Cardiopulmonary Resuscitation and Emergency Cardiovascular Care. *Circulation, 122*(Suppl. 3), S729–S767.

If untreated, AF and AFl can lead to serious hemodynamic and thromboembolic consequences. A rapid ventricular rate can induce angina in patients with underlying CAD or worsening signs and symptoms of HF in patients with HFrEF. A persistently rapid ventricular rate may lead to the development of a tachycardia-induced cardiomyopathy. Loss of synchronized atrial contraction can lead to a significant reduction in cardiac output, which can especially affect patients with underlying HF. In addition, loss of coordinated atrial contraction can lead to the pooling of blood and subsequent thrombus formation. Therefore, AF and AFl can lead to serious thromboembolic complications, particularly ischemic stroke. Overall, the treatment goals for AF and AFl are controlling the ventricular rate, preventing thromboembolic events, and possibly restoring and maintaining SR. **Figure 23.1** illustrates an algorithm for the management of AF and AFl.

First-Line Therapy

If the patient presenting with AF or AFl is hemodynamically unstable (i.e., severe hypotension, syncope, HF, or angina), immediate DCC is first-line therapy. If the patient is hemodynamically stable and has a rapid ventricular rate, the first priority is to control the ventricular rate. In the acute treatment of AF, the selection of a drug to control the ventricular rate depends on the patient's LV systolic function (January et al., 2014). In patients with normal LV systolic function (LVEF > 40%), IV diltiazem, IV verapamil, or an IV β-blocker is preferred over digoxin because of their relatively quick onset. β-Blockers are especially useful in high adrenergic states (i.e., postoperative patients, hyperthyroidism). The use of digoxin

is limited by its relatively slow onset of action and its inability to control heart rate in high adrenergic states (i.e., exercise). In patients with HFrEF (LVEF of 40% or less), an IV β-blocker or IV digoxin is preferred, since these agents also are used to treat HFrEF. Diltiazem or verapamil should be avoided in these patients because their potent negative inotropic effects may precipitate worsening HF symptoms. β-Blockers should be avoided in patients who are exhibiting signs and/or symptoms of decompensated HF. In those patients who are having worsening HF symptoms, IV digoxin or IV amiodarone is recommended as first-line therapy for controlling the ventricular rate. IV amiodarone can also be used for ventricular rate control in any patient with AF who is refractory to or has contraindications to β-blockers, diltiazem, or verapamil. Since amiodarone is a class III AAD, the practitioner should be aware that the patient may convert to SR when using this agent. Patients with AF that has persisted for longer than 48 hours are at risk for thromboembolic events if conversion to SR occurs in the absence of therapeutic anticoagulation. Therefore, in these patients who have not been therapeutically anticoagulated, IV amiodarone should be avoided.

Second-Line Therapy

Once the ventricular rate is acutely controlled, patients should be evaluated for the possibility of restoring SR if AF persists. The results of six landmark clinical trials (Pharmacological Intervention in Atrial Fibrillation [PIAF], Rate Control versus Electrical Cardioversion for Persistent Atrial Fibrillation [RACE], Atrial Fibrillation Follow-up Investigation of Rhythm Management [AFFIRM], Strategies of Treatment

TABLE 23.2

Recommended Order of Treatment for Arrhythmias

Order	Agents	Comments
AF/AFI		
First line	Hemodynamically unstable patient: synchronized DCC. Start with 100 J and proceed to 200, 300, and 360 J if not successful in the preceding cardioversions. Hemodynamically stable patient with rapid ventricular rate: • LVEF > 40%: IV diltiazem, IV verapamil, or IV β-blocker • LVEF ≤ 40%: IV β-blocker or IV digoxin	Start with 50 J in patients with AFI. Premedicate whenever possible when performing DCC. IV amiodarone can be used for ventricular rate control in any patient with AF/AFI who is refractory to or has contraindications to β-blockers, diltiazem, or verapamil; avoid using for ventricular rate control if the AF/AFI has been present >48 h as these patients may be at risk for thromboembolic events induced by conversion to SR.
Second line	Patients with 1st episode of arrhythmia (if likely to convert to and remain in SR): Electrical or pharmacological cardioversion can be considered once ventricular rate acutely controlled. For pharmacological cardioversion, the AAD used depends on the presence of SHD. Decision of whether to proceed acutely with cardioversion depends on the duration of the arrhythmia: • <48 h: May proceed with cardioversion without prolonged period of anticoagulation. If patient at high risk of stroke, IV unfractionated heparin, a low molecular weight heparin (subcutaneously at treatment doses), apixaban, dabigatran, edoxaban, or rivaroxaban should be initiated as soon as possible either before or after cardioversion. Anticoagulate with warfarin (INR target range 2.0–3.0), apixaban, dabigatran, edoxaban, or rivaroxaban for ≥4 wk following successful cardioversion in these high-risk patients. While these anticoagulants can also be initiated immediately before or after cardioversion in patients at low risk for stroke, it is also reasonable to not initiate antithrombotic therapy in these patients. Decisions regarding long-term antithrombotic therapy after this time period should be primarily based on the patient's risk for stroke and not on whether he/she is in SR. • >48 h or unknown duration: Anticoagulate with warfarin (INR target range 2.0–3.0), apixaban, dabigatran, edoxaban, or rivaroxaban for ≥3 weeks before proceeding with cardioversion. Anticoagulate with warfarin (INR target range 2.0–3.0), apixaban, dabigatran, edoxaban, or rivaroxaban for ≥4 wk following successful cardioversion. Decisions regarding long-term antithrombotic therapy after this time period should be primarily based on the patient's risk for stroke and not on whether he/she is in SR. For patients with persistent or recurrent AF, a strategy of ventricular rate control and anticoagulation is a reasonable alternative to rhythm control. Selection of PO drug for ventricular rate control (diltiazem, verapamil, β-blocker, or digoxin) depends on patient's LV function. Antithrombotic therapy should be based on the patient's CHA$_2$DS$_2$-VASc risk score.	A TEE can be performed in patients with AF >48 h or unknown duration to exclude the presence of thrombi and to facilitate cardioversion. IV unfractionated heparin or subcutaneous low molecular weight heparin (at treatment doses) should be started at the time the TEE will be performed. If a thrombus is detected, cardioversion should not be performed and the patient should be anticoagulated indefinitely. If no thrombus is detected, cardioversion can be performed within 24 h without the need for the initial 3-wk period of anticoagulation. These patients will still require anticoagulation after cardioversion for ≥4 wk. Decisions regarding long-term antithrombotic therapy after this time period should be primarily based on the patient's risk for stroke and not on whether he/she is in SR. For AADs to be used for acute pharmacologic cardioversion, see **Figure 22.2.** Goal heart rate is based on patient's LV systolic function: • LVEF > 40% and no or acceptable symptoms of AF: <110 beats/min (at rest) • LVEF ≤ 40%: <80 beats/min (at rest) PO agents for ventricular rate control: • LVEF > 40%: diltiazem, verapamil, or β-blocker • LVEF ≤ 40%: β-blocker (i.e., carvedilol, metoprolol succinate, or bisoprolol) or digoxin

(Continued)

TABLE 23.2

Recommended Order of Treatment for Arrhythmias (*Continued*)

Order	Agents	Comments
Third line	Chronic AAD therapy can be considered for patients who remain symptomatic despite having adequate ventricular rate control or for those in whom adequate ventricular rate control cannot be achieved. The AAD used depends on patient's LV function and the type of SHD that may be present. For patients with permanent AF, a strategy of ventricular rate control and anticoagulation should be considered. Selection of PO drug for ventricular rate control (diltiazem, verapamil, β-blocker, or digoxin) depends on patient's LV function. Antithrombotic therapy should be based on the patient's CHA_2DS_2-VASc risk score. Radiofrequency catheter ablation may be considered in patients with symptomatic episodes of recurrent AF who fail or do not tolerate at least one class I or class III AAD.	PO AADs for chronic rhythm control: • No SHD: dofetilide, dronedarone, flecainide, propafenone, or sotalol; amiodarone is considered alternative if patient fails or does not tolerate one of the initial AADs. • LVEF ≤ 40%: amiodarone or dofetilide • CAD: dofetilide, dronedarone, or sotalol; amiodarone is considered alternative if patient fails or does not tolerate one of the initial AADs • Significant LV hypertrophy: amiodarone Avoid flecainide and propafenone in patients with *any* form of SHD.
PSVT (due to AVNRT) First line	Hemodynamically unstable patient: synchronized DCC (50–100 J, biphasic). Hemodynamically stable patient: vagal maneuvers	Premedicate whenever possible when performing DCC. Examples of vagal maneuvers include unilateral carotid sinus massage, Valsalva maneuver, facial immersion in ice water, and coughing. Carotid sinus massage should be avoided in patients with carotid bruits or history of cerebrovascular disease.
Second line	IV adenosine If persistent PSVT, use IV diltiazem, IV verapamil, or IV β-blocker; if PSVT remains persistent, can use IV procainamide (if LVEF > 40%) or IV amiodarone (for normal or depressed LVEF)	
Third line	If patient continues to have frequent episodes of PSVT or infrequent episodes accompanied by severe symptoms, refer for possible radiofrequency catheter ablation. If patient is not a candidate for or refuses radiofrequency catheter ablation, PO diltiazem, verapamil, β-blocker, or digoxin can be used for chronic therapy.	If PSVT is infrequent and/or accompanied by only mild symptoms, no chronic therapy is needed.
Nonsustained VT First line	No SHD: • Asymptomatic or minimal symptoms: No drug therapy • Symptomatic: PO β-blocker Post-MI patients: • LVEF > 40%: PO β-blocker regardless of the presence of symptoms • LVEF ≤ 40%: EP testing; if sustained VT/VF, ICD should be placed; if sustained VT/VF noninducible, PO β-blocker or amiodarone may be used.	Correct reversible causes. Post-MI patients with normal LV systolic function should receive a β-blocker even if they have no or minimal symptoms associated with the nonsustained VT to ↓ mortality associated with the MI. If frequent shocks occur in patients with an ICD, PO amiodarone and β-blocker combination therapy or sotalol monotherapy can be used.
Sustained VT First line	Hemodynamically unstable patient: synchronized DCC (100 J, biphasic). Hemodynamically stable patient: IV procainamide, IV amiodarone, or IV sotalol	Premedicate whenever possible when performing DCC. Correct reversible causes.
Second line	Hemodynamically stable patient: IV lidocaine; synchronized DCC should be considered if AAD therapy fails. Once arrhythmia acutely terminated, patient should be considered for ICD placement. If patient refuses or is not a candidate for an ICD, PO amiodarone can be considered.	If frequent shocks occur in patients with an ICD, PO amiodarone and β-blocker combination therapy or sotalol monotherapy can be used.

TABLE 23.2

Recommended Order of Treatment for Arrhythmias (*Continued*)

Order	Agents	Comments
Pulseless VT/VF		
First line	Start CPR, establish an airway, and deliver one shock (biphasic defibrillator: 120–200 J); immediately resume CPR for 2 min, then check rhythm.	Correct reversible causes.
Second line	If patient remains in pulseless VT/VF, deliver one shock and then immediately resume CPR; if pulseless VT/VF persists after at least one shock and CPR, give vasopressor therapy (epinephrine 1 mg IV push/IO every 3–5 min through pulseless VT/VF episode) (give drug during CPR; do not interrupt CPR to give drug); immediately resume CPR for 2 min, then check pulse.	
Third line	If patient remains in pulseless VT/VF, deliver one shock and then immediately resume CPR; if pulseless VT/VF persists despite defibrillation, CPR, and vasopressor therapy, consider AAD therapy (IV amiodarone; lidocaine may be used as alternative) (give drugs during CPR; do not interrupt CPR to give drugs); immediately resume CPR for 2 min; then check pulse.	
Bradycardia		
First line	Stable: Close observation Signs/symptoms of poor perfusion (e.g., altered mental status, chest pain, hypotension, shock): Immediately administer IV atropine (0.5 mg every 3–5 min, up to 3 mg total dose). If ineffective, transcutaneous pacing or sympathomimetic continuous infusion (dopamine or epinephrine) should be initiated.	Correct reversible causes.
Second line	If drug therapy and transcutaneous pacing are ineffective, transvenous pacing should be utilized.	

AAD, antiarrhythmic drug; AF, atrial fibrillation; AFl, atrial flutter; AVNRT, atrioventricular nodal reentrant tachycardia; CAD, coronary artery disease; CPR, cardiopulmonary resuscitation; DCC, direct-current cardioversion; ICD, implantable cardioverter–defibrillator; INR, international normalized ratio; IV, intravenous; J, joules; LV, left ventricular; LVEF, left ventricular ejection fraction; MI, myocardial infarction; PO, oral; PSVT, paroxysmal supraventricular tachycardia; SHD, structural heart disease; SR, sinus rhythm; TEE, transesophageal echocardiogram; VF, ventricular fibrillation; VT, ventricular tachycardia.

of Atrial Fibrillation [STAF], How to Treat Chronic Atrial Fibrillation [HOT-CAFE], and Atrial Fibrillation and Congestive Heart Failure [AF-CHF]) have provided practitioners with significant insight into the comparative efficacy of rate control (controlling ventricular rate; patient remains in AF) and rhythm control (restoring and maintaining SR) treatment strategies in patients with AF (Carlsson et al., 2004; Hohnloser et al., 2000; Opolski et al., 2004; Roy et al., 2008; Van Gelder et al., 2002; Wyse et al., 2002). The results of all of these trials essentially demonstrated that there were no significant differences in outcomes between patients who received a rate-control strategy and those who received a rhythm-control strategy. Therefore, based on these findings, a rate-control strategy appears to be a viable alternative to a rhythm-control strategy in patients with persistent or recurrent AF. Consequently, considering the potential toxicities of AADs, it is reasonable to initially consider a rate-control strategy in these patients, including those with concomitant

HF. However, a rhythm-control strategy should be considered for those patients who remain symptomatic despite having adequate ventricular rate control or for those in whom adequate ventricular rate control cannot be achieved. The results of the above clinical trials do not necessarily apply to patients experiencing their first episode of AF. If these particular patients are likely to convert to and remain in SR, a rhythm-control strategy may be considered.

If the decision is made to restore SR in hemodynamically stable patients with AF, either electrical (i.e., DCC) or pharmacological (i.e., AADs) cardioversion may be used. The decision to use either of these methods is often based on the practitioner's or patient's preference. DCC is associated with higher success rates than pharmacological cardioversion. However, this method requires sedation or anesthesia and may be rarely associated with complications such as sinus arrest or ventricular arrhythmias. Pharmacological cardioversion is associated with adverse effects (e.g., TdP) and drug interactions.

In those patients in whom it is decided to restore SR, it is important to note that the process of cardioverting the patient from AF to SR may place the patient at risk for a thromboembolic event. Restoration to SR may dislodge thrombi in the atria. This risk is present regardless of whether an electrical or pharmacological method is used to restore SR. In patients undergoing DCC or pharmacological cardioversion, it is imperative to determine how long the patient has been in AF because the risk of thrombus formation increases if the AF duration exceeds 48 hours. If AF has been present for more than 48 hours or for an unknown duration, cardioversion should not be performed acutely because of the risk of thromboembolism. These patients should be therapeutically anticoagulated with warfarin (INR target range 2.0 to 3.0) or one of the target-specific oral anticoagulants (e.g., apixaban, dabigatran, edoxaban, or rivaroxaban) for at least 3 weeks (January et al., 2014). After that time, the patient can undergo DCC or pharmacological cardioversion, which should be followed by therapeutic anticoagulation with warfarin (INR target range 2.0 to 3.0), apixaban, dabigatran, edoxaban, or rivaroxaban for at least 4 weeks. If the 3 weeks of oral anticoagulant therapy prior to cardioversion is not feasible, the patient may alternatively undergo a transesophageal echocardiogram (TEE) prior to cardioversion to look for any thrombi that may be present in the atria or ventricles. If no thrombus is observed on TEE, the patient can undergo cardioversion. In these patients, anticoagulant therapy with either IV unfractionated heparin (target activated partial thromboplastin time 60 seconds; acceptable range 50 to 70 seconds) or low molecular weight heparin (subcutaneously at treatment doses) should be initiated at the time the TEE will be performed (You et al., 2012). Cardioversion should then be performed within 24 hours of the TEE. Alternatively, warfarin therapy (INR target range of 2.0 to 3.0) may be used for at least 5 days prior to the TEE and cardioversion. If cardioversion is successful, therapeutic warfarin (INR target range 2.0 to 3.0), apixaban, dabigatran, edoxaban, or rivaroxaban should be continued for at least 4 weeks regardless of the patient's baseline risk of stroke (January et al., 2014). Decisions regarding long-term antithrombotic therapy after this 4-week time period should be primarily based on the patient's risk for stroke and not on whether he/she is in SR. If a thrombus is seen on TEE, cardioversion should not be performed, and the patient should be anticoagulated indefinitely. If cardioversion is considered in these patients at a later time, a TEE should again be performed.

When the duration of AF is definitively known to be less than 48 hours, a prolonged period of anticoagulation is not necessary prior to proceeding with electrical or pharmacological cardioversion because the risk of thromboembolism is deemed to be low. In those patients who are at high risk for stroke, IV unfractionated heparin (target activated partial thromboplastin time 60 seconds; acceptable range 50 to 70 seconds), a low molecular weight heparin (subcutaneously at treatment doses), apixaban, dabigatran, edoxaban, or rivaroxaban should be initiated as soon as possible either before or after cardioversion (January et al., 2014). If cardioversion is successful in these high-risk patients, therapeutic anticoagulation with warfarin (INR target range 2.0 to 3.0), apixaban, dabigatran, edoxaban,

or rivaroxaban should be continued for at least 4 weeks. While the above anticoagulants can also be initiated immediately before or after cardioversion in patients at low risk for stroke, it is also reasonable to not initiate antithrombotic therapy in these patients. Decisions regarding long-term antithrombotic therapy after this 4-week time period should be primarily based on the patient's risk for stroke and not on whether he/she is in SR.

If the practitioner decides to proceed with pharmacological cardioversion as the initial therapy, the selection of drug is primarily based on the presence of SHD (i.e., CAD, HF, LV hypertrophy). Pharmacological cardioversion is most effective when initiated within 7 days of the onset of AF. The AADs with proven efficacy during this time frame include dofetilide, flecainide, ibutilide, propafenone, or amiodarone (oral or IV). The class Ia AADs, disopyramide, procainamide, and quinidine, have limited efficacy or have been incompletely studied for this purpose. Sotalol is not effective for converting AF to SR. Although the use of single, oral loading doses of propafenone or flecainide is effective in restoring SR, these drugs should only be used in patients without underlying SHD. Ibutilide may also be considered in patients without underlying SHD. When utilizing the approach of administering single, oral loading doses of flecainide or propafenone for AF conversion for the first time, patients must be hospitalized to monitor for the development of proarrhythmic adverse effects. If no adverse arrhythmic events occur during this hospitalization, then patients will be educated to self-administer an oral loading dose of flecainide or propafenone at the onset of AF symptoms (e.g., palpitations) in the future. A patient's ventricular rate should be adequately controlled with AV nodal-blocking drugs prior to administering a class Ic (or class Ia) AAD for cardioversion since these AADs can precipitate an increased ventricular response as a result of their vagolytic effects. In patients with SHD, propafenone, flecainide, and ibutilide should be avoided because of the increased risk of proarrhythmia. Instead, amiodarone or dofetilide should be primarily used in this patient population (January et al., 2014).

If the practitioner does not wish to proceed with cardioversion, an initial management strategy of ventricular rate control and anticoagulation is also reasonable. As previously stated, this strategy, whereby the patient is left in AF, has been shown to be an acceptable alternative to rhythm control for the chronic management of AF. The selection of an oral drug for chronic ventricular rate control is primarily based on the patient's LV systolic function. In patients with normal LV systolic function (LVEF > 40%), an oral β-blocker, diltiazem, or verapamil is preferred over digoxin (January et al., 2014). Digoxin can be added if adequate ventricular rate control cannot be achieved with one of these drugs. In patients with HFrEF (LVEF of 40% or less), an oral β-blocker, or digoxin is preferred because these drugs can also concomitantly be used to treat chronic HF. The nondihydropyridine CCBs should be avoided in patients with HFrEF because of their potent negative inotropic effects. In patients with AF and stable HF symptoms (NYHA class II or III), the β-blockers, carvedilol, metoprolol succinate, or bisoprolol should be used as first-line therapy because of their documented survival benefits in patients with HFrEF. Other β-blockers should be avoided in these patients because their effects on survival in HF are unknown. Digoxin should be used as first-line therapy in patients with AF and decompensated HFrEF (NYHA class IV) because β-blocker therapy may exacerbate HF symptoms. Oral amiodarone may also be considered if adequate ventricular rate control cannot be achieved with or the patient has contraindications to β-blockers or nondihydropyridine CCBs (January et al., 2014). In patients with persistent AF who have no or acceptable symptoms and stable LV systolic function (LVEF greater than 40%), the goal heart rate should be less than 110 beats/min at rest (January et al. 2014; Van Gelder et al., 2010). In patients with LVSD (LVEF of 40% or less), a stricter heart rate goal (less than 80 beats/min) should be considered to minimize the potential harmful effects of a rapid heart rate response on ventricular function.

Assessing the patient's risk of stroke becomes important for selecting the most appropriate antithrombotic regimen. The most recent guidelines for the treatment of AF have recommended the CHA_2DS_2-VASc scoring system for stroke risk stratification in patients with AF (January et al., 2014). With this risk index, patients with AF are given 2 points each if they have a history of a previous stroke, transient ischemic attack, or thromboembolism or if they are at least 75 years old. Patients are given one point each for being at least 65 to 74 years old, having hypertension, having diabetes, having congestive HF, having vascular disease (e.g., MI, peripheral arterial disease, or aortic plaque), or being female. (CHA_2DS_2-VASc is an acronym for each of these risk factors.) The points are added up, and the total score is then used to determine the most appropriate antithrombotic therapy for the patient. Patients with a CHA_2DS_2-VASc score of 2 or higher are considered to be at high risk for stroke. In these patients, oral anticoagulant therapy with warfarin (target INR, 2.5; range, 2.0 to 3.0), apixaban, dabigatran, edoxaban, or rivaroxaban is preferred over aspirin. Patients with a CHA_2DS_2-VASc score of 1 are considered to be at intermediate risk for stroke. In these patients, oral anticoagulant therapy (warfarin [target INR: 2.5; range: 2.0 to 3.0], apixaban, dabigatran, edoxaban, or rivaroxaban), aspirin 75 to 325 mg/d, or no antithrombotic therapy can be selected. Patients with a CHA_2DS_2-VASc score of 0 are considered to be at low risk for stroke. The guidelines state that it is reasonable to not give any antithrombotic therapy to patients who are considered to be at low risk for stroke. Please refer to Chapter 50 for a further discussion of anticoagulation in AF.

The need for antithrombotic therapy should be assessed in all patients with AF regardless of whether a rate-control or rhythm-control strategy is initiated. In addition, if patients are considered candidates for antithrombotic therapy, this regimen should be continued if SR is restored because of the potential for patients to have episodes of recurrent AF.

Third-Line Therapy

For those patients who remain symptomatic despite having adequate ventricular rate control or for those patients in whom adequate ventricular rate control cannot be achieved, it is reasonable to consider AAD therapy to maintain SR once they have been converted to SR. The selection of an AAD to maintain SR is primarily based on the presence of SHD

(January et al., 2014) (see **Figure 23.2**). In patients without SHD, dofetilide, dronedarone, flecainide, propafenone, or sotalol should be considered initially, since these AADs have the best long-term safety profile. Amiodarone can be used as alternative therapy if the patient fails or does not tolerate one of these initial AADs. In patients with any type of SHD, the class Ic AADs, flecainide and propafenone, should be avoided. In these patients, the selection of AAD therapy is based upon the type of SHD present. In patients with LVSD (LVEF of 40% or less), either oral amiodarone or dofetilide can be used. Both dronedarone and sotalol should be avoided in patients with LVSD because of the risk of increased mortality (dronedarone) or worsening HF (sotalol). In patients with CAD, dofetilide, dronedarone, or sotalol can be used as initial therapy. In these patients, sotalol and dronedarone should only be used if their LV systolic function is normal. Amiodarone can be considered as an alternative therapy in these patients if these AADs are not tolerated. In patients with significant LV hypertrophy, amiodarone is the drug of choice. Patients with symptomatic episodes of recurrent AF who fail or do not tolerate at least one class I or III AAD may also be considered for radiofrequency catheter ablation (January et al., 2014).

PSVT (Due to AV Nodal Reentrant Tachycardia)

First-Line Therapy

Hemodynamically unstable PSVT requires first-line therapy of synchronized DCC to restore SR and correct hemodynamic compromise. Unless contraindicated, patients with mild to moderate symptoms can be initially managed with vagal maneuvers (e.g., unilateral carotid sinus massage, Valsalva maneuver, facial immersion in ice water, and coughing). **Figure 23.3** illustrates an algorithm for the management of PSVT due to AV nodal reentrant tachycardia.

Second-Line Therapy

If vagal maneuvers are unsuccessful or if PSVT recurs after successful vagal maneuvers, second-line therapy is AADs. The drug of choice for PSVT is adenosine (Neumar et al., 2010). Clinical studies have shown that adenosine is as effective as IV verapamil in initial conversion of PSVT. Adenosine does not produce hypotension to the degree that verapamil does, and it has a shorter half-life. If a total of 30 mg of adenosine does not successfully terminate PSVT, further doses of this agent are unlikely to be effective. Therefore, in patients with persistent PSVT, other AADs will need to be used. In these patients, IV diltiazem, verapamil, or a β-blocker can be used. If PSVT continues despite these treatment measures, the use of IV procainamide (LVEF > 40%) or amiodarone (normal or depressed LVEF) can also be considered.

Third-Line Therapy

Third-line therapy focuses on the management of chronic PSVT. Chronic preventive therapy is usually necessary if the patient has either frequent episodes of PSVT that require therapeutic intervention or infrequent episodes of PSVT that are accompanied by severe symptoms. Radiofrequency catheter ablation is considered first-line therapy for most of these patients because of its effectiveness in preventing recurrence of PSVT and its relatively low complication rate. Drug therapy with oral diltiazem, verapamil, β-blockers, or digoxin can also be considered if the patient is not a candidate for or refuses to undergo radiofrequency catheter ablation.

Nonsustained VT

VT that spontaneously terminates within 30 seconds is known as nonsustained VT. Given the poor survival of patients who experience cardiac arrest, it is essential to identify the most effective treatment strategies to prevent the initial episode of sustained VT or sudden cardiac death from occurring.

The presence of nonsustained VT in patients without SHD is not associated with an increased risk of sudden cardiac death. Therefore, drug therapy is not necessary in these patients if they are asymptomatic. However, if these patients do become symptomatic, treatment options include a β-blocker, nondihydropyridine CCB, class Ic AAD, or catheter ablation (depending on the underlying etiology) (Pedersen et al., 2014). Post-MI patients (especially those with LVSD) who develop nonsustained VT are at increased risk for sudden cardiac death. For these patients, the selection of therapy is based on the patient's LV systolic function. In patients who experience nonsustained VT due to prior MI, and have an LVEF greater than 40%, drug therapy is not necessary to treat the arrhythmia if they are asymptomatic. However, these patients should still chronically receive a β-blocker specifically to reduce mortality associated with the MI. β-Blockers are also effective if these patients develop significant symptoms associated with the nonsustained VT. In patients who experience nonsustained VT due to prior MI, and have an LVEF of 40% or less, electrophysiologic testing is often performed when asymptomatic nonsustained VT occurs (Pedersen et al., 2014). If sustained VT or VF is induced, an ICD is then recommended (Epstein et al., 2013). If sustained VT or VF is not induced, a β-blocker or amiodarone can be initiated.

Sustained VT

VT that persists for at least 30 seconds or that requires electrical or pharmacological termination because of hemodynamic instability is known as sustained VT. Since sustained VT can degenerate into VF, the treatment goals are to terminate the VT acutely and then prevent recurrence of the arrhythmia.

First-Line Therapy

If the patient is hemodynamically unstable (i.e., severe hypotension, syncope, HF, or angina), immediate synchronized DCC is first-line therapy. If the patient is hemodynamically stable, IV amiodarone, IV procainamide, or IV sotalol can be considered (Neumar et al., 2010). Lidocaine can be used as alternative therapy. Synchronized DCC should be considered if AAD therapy fails.

Second-Line Therapy

Once the acute episode is terminated, measures should be taken to prevent recurrent episodes of VT. Based on the results of several trials, ICDs are clearly indicated as first-line therapy in patients with a history of sustained VT or VF (Epstein et al., 2013). If the patient with an ICD experiences frequent discharges because of recurrent ventricular arrhythmias or new-onset supraventricular arrhythmias (e.g., AF), either amiodarone and a β-blocker or sotalol monotherapy can be used. For the patient who refuses or is not a candidate for an ICD, oral amiodarone should be used as an alternative therapy.

Pulseless VT/VF

The majority of cases of sudden cardiac death can be attributed to VF. Sustained VT usually precedes VF and most commonly occurs in patients with CAD. VF is usually not preceded by any symptoms and always results in a loss of consciousness and eventually death if not treated. Immediate treatment is essential in patients who develop VF or pulseless VT, since survival is reduced by 10% for every minute that the patient remains in the arrhythmia. It is imperative to identify and correct any potential reversible causes for the arrhythmia.

For administration of drug therapy during an episode of pulseless VT/VF, while IV access is preferred, the guidelines recommend the intraosseous (IO) route as an alternative if IV access cannot be established (Neumar et al., 2010). IO access can be used not only for administration of drugs and fluids but also for obtaining blood for laboratory monitoring. If neither IV nor IO access can be established, the endotracheal route can then be used for the administration of only certain agents (i.e., atropine, lidocaine, epinephrine, and vasopressin). **Figure 23.4** illustrates an algorithm for the management of pulseless VT/VF.

First-Line Therapy

In patients with pulseless VT/VF, high-quality cardiopulmonary resuscitation (CPR) should be immediately initiated until a defibrillator or automated external defibrillator (AED) arrives (Kleinman et al., 2015). High-quality CPR is composed of the following components: minimizing interruptions in chest compressions (i.e., providing chest compressions for at least 80% of the time that the patient is in cardiac arrest), delivering 100 to 120 chest compressions per minute, delivering chest compressions at a depth of at least 2 inches (but avoiding a depth of greater than 2.4 inches), minimizing leaning over the patient's chest (leaning can result in a reduction in venous return and cardiac output), and providing a ventilation rate of 10 breaths per minute. Each cycle of CPR involves delivering 30 chest compressions followed by two breaths. If a defibrillator or AED is not readily available, hands-only CPR (compressions only; no ventilations) should be provided if the bystander possesses no CPR training or is trained but lacks confidence in providing effective CPR with rescue breaths. If the bystander possesses CPR training and is confident in their ability to provide effective CPR with rescue breaths, conventional cycles of CPR (30 chest compressions followed by two breaths) should be delivered until a defibrillator or AED becomes available. Once an advanced airway (e.g., endotracheal tube) is placed, chest compressions should be delivered continuously at a rate of 100 to 120 compressions per minute without pausing for ventilation (should be provided by a separate individual at a rate of one breath every 6 seconds). Once a defibrillator or AED arrives, defibrillation should be administered immediately.

With regard to defibrillation, delivery of only one shock at a time is recommended in patients with pulseless VT/VF to minimize interruptions in chest compressions (Link et al., 2015). For biphasic defibrillators, the dose of the shock is device specific (usually 120 to 200 J); the maximum dose available can be used for the initial shock if the effective dose range of the defibrillator is unknown. This dose or a higher dose can then be used for any subsequent shocks that may be needed. After delivery of the initial shock in patients with pulseless VT/VF, CPR should be immediately resumed and continued for 2 minutes, after which the patient's pulse and rhythm should be checked. Delaying pulse and rhythm checks until after this period of CPR is administered is intended to minimize interruptions in chest compressions and increase the potential for success with defibrillation. If pulseless VT/VF persists, another shock should be delivered at the appropriate dose, followed by 2 minutes of CPR. This general sequence of resuscitation and defibrillation should be followed for as long as the patient remains in pulseless VT/VF.

Second-Line Therapy

If pulseless VT/VF persists after delivery of at least one shock and CPR, vasopressor therapy with epinephrine should be initiated (Link et al., 2015). Although vasopressin had previously been recommended in the 2010 guidelines as an alternative vasopressor to epinephrine, this drug is no longer recommended in the pulseless VT/VF treatment algorithm in the recently updated guidelines. The recommended dosage of epinephrine for pulseless VT/VF is 1 mg given IV push/IO every 3 to 5 minutes throughout the duration of the pulseless VT/VF episode.

Third-Line Therapy

If pulseless VT/VF persists despite the use of defibrillation, CPR, and vasopressor therapy, AAD therapy can be considered. IV amiodarone is recommended as first-line AAD therapy for the treatment of pulseless VT/VF (Link et al., 2015). This agent has been shown to be safe and effective in the management of both in-hospital and out-of-hospital pulseless VT/VF (Dorian et al., 2002; Kudenchuck et al., 1999). Compared to lidocaine, IV amiodarone has been associated with a significantly higher rate of survival to hospital admission in patients with out-of-hospital cardiac arrest due to VF (Dorian et al., 2002). Lidocaine may be considered as an alternative to IV amiodarone for pulseless VT/VF that persists despite the use of defibrillation, CPR, and vasopressor therapy (Link et al., 2015).

IV procainamide is no longer recommended for pulseless VT/VF. The routine use of IV magnesium sulfate in patients with pulseless VT/VF is not recommended.

If the patient is resuscitated from the pulseless VT/VF episode, measures should be taken to prevent recurrent episodes of cardiac arrest. Based on the results of several trials, ICDs are clearly indicated as first-line therapy in patients with a history of sustained VT or VF (Epstein et al., 2013). If patients with an ICD experience frequent discharges because of recurrent ventricular arrhythmias or new-onset supraventricular arrhythmias (e.g., AF), either amiodarone and a β-blocker or sotalol monotherapy can be used. For patients who refuse or are not candidates for an ICD, oral amiodarone should be used as an alternative therapy.

Bradycardia

If patients with bradycardia present with signs and symptoms of adequate perfusion, only close observation is required. If patients with bradycardia develop signs or symptoms of poor perfusion (e.g., altered mental status, chest pain, hypotension, shock), IV atropine (0.5 mg every 3 to 5 minutes, up to 3 mg total dose) should be immediately administered (Neumar et al., 2010). If atropine is not effective, either transcutaneous pacing or a continuous infusion of a sympathomimetic agent, such as dopamine (2 to 10 mcg/kg/min) or epinephrine (2 to 10 mcg/min) (i.e., dopamine or epinephrine), should be initiated. If symptomatic bradycardia persists despite any of these measures, transvenous pacing should be utilized. **Figure 23.5** illustrates an algorithm for the management of bradycardia.

Special Population Considerations
Pediatric

The epidemiology of arrhythmias is different between adults and children. Adults have arrhythmias primarily of a cardiac origin, whereas children have arrhythmias primarily of a respiratory origin.

Tachyarrhythmias occasionally compromise infants and young children. PSVT is the most common arrhythmia in young children. It typically occurs during infancy or in children with congenital heart disease. PSVT with ventricular rates exceeding 180 to 220 beats/min can produce signs of shock. If signs of shock appear, synchronized cardioversion or administration of adenosine can be done in an emergency. Common causes of PSVT in young children and infants are congenital heart disease (preoperative) such as Ebstein's anomaly, transposition of the great arteries, or a single ventricle. Postoperative PSVT also can occur after atrial surgery for correction of congenital defects of the heart. Other common causes of PSVT in children are drugs such as sympathomimetics (cold medications, theophylline, β-agonists). WPW syndrome and hyperthyroidism also can cause PSVT. Common causes of AF and AFl in children are intra-atrial surgery, Ebstein's anomaly, heart disease with dilated atria (aortic valve regurgitation), cardiomyopathy, WPW syndrome, sick sinus syndrome, and myocarditis.

Bradycardia is a common arrhythmia in seriously ill infants or children. It is usually associated with a reduction in cardiac output and is an ominous sign, suggesting that cardiac arrest is imminent. The first-line therapy for this arrhythmia in infants and young children is administration of oxygen, support respiration, epinephrine, and, possibly, atropine.

Pulseless VT and VF are treated much the same way as in adults (de Caen et al., 2015). The recommended dose of epinephrine for a child with pulseless VT/VF is 0.01 mg/kg IV/IO, administered as 0.1 mL/kg of a 1:10,000 concentration every 3 to 5 minutes throughout the duration of the pulseless VT/VF episode. If IV/IO access cannot be established, epinephrine can be administered endotracheally (0.1 mg/kg administered as 0.1 mL/kg of a 1:1,000 concentration).

Geriatric

With aging, body fat increases, lean body tissue decreases, and hepatic and renal system changes set the stage for potential overdosage and toxicity, particularly in the case of AADs. Similarly, declining organ function affects the amount and dosage of the drug prescribed as well as the occurrence of adverse effects. Cardiac disease and chronic conditions such as HF exacerbate the decline in organ function. Together, these factors can increase the risk of an adverse effect from the AADs the practitioner prescribes.

For example, digoxin toxicity is relatively common in older adult patients who are not receiving a reduced dosage to accommodate for the reduced renal function. It is imperative for the practitioner to assess the patient's baseline renal and hepatic function to determine whether certain AADs are safe to use and the most appropriate dosage to use in this patient.

Signs and symptoms of adverse effects of many drugs are confusion, weakness, and lethargy. These signs and symptoms are often attributed to senility or disease. Therefore, it is important for the practitioner to take a thorough drug history and to document accurately the dosages and frequencies prescribed in the patient record. If the practitioner merely attributes confusion to old age, the patient may continue to receive the drug while actually experiencing drug toxicity. Furthermore, the practitioner may add another drug to treat the complications caused by the original AAD, compounding the issue of polypharmacy and excessive medication.

AADs sometimes require accurate and timely dosing. If an older adult patient forgets to take a dose or cannot remember when he or she took the last dose, undermedication or overmedication may occur. This can be dangerous when AADs are prescribed. Many older adults have multiple prescriptions, even for the same medication, and therefore take an overdose of the drug. Consequently, it is essential to review medications with older adult patients and make sure they understand and can follow a safe drug therapy regimen.

MONITORING PATIENT RESPONSE

The goals of AAD therapy are to restore SR and prevent recurrences of the original arrhythmia or development of new arrhythmias. Evaluating the outcomes of AAD therapy requires the practitioner to schedule regular follow-up visits after initial treatment of the arrhythmia. The outcomes to be closely monitored include impulse generation and conduction from the SA node to the AV node, time interval for conduction, heart rate within a normal range that is age specific, and patterns of AV and ventricular conduction.

Data to be monitored to evaluate therapeutic outcomes vary from the simple to complex. The patient may monitor some of them and needs to be taught the signs and symptoms to look for and the expectations from the therapeutic regimen. Patients with arrhythmias may be monitored on a regular or periodic basis with 12-lead ECGs, 24-hour Holter monitors, blood pressure, heart rate, echocardiograms, electrolytes, and serum drug levels (when applicable).

In addition, the patient needs to self-monitor for symptoms such as lightheadedness, dizziness, syncopal episodes, palpitations, chest pain, shortness of breath, or weight gain. Other clinical outcomes to be monitored are those that affect quality of life, such as activity tolerance, organ perfusion, cognitive function, fear, anxiety, and depression.

PATIENT EDUCATION

Drug Information

Included in the therapeutic plan for arrhythmias is patient education. Learning outcomes can be evaluated by monitoring compliance with the medication regimen, recurrences of arrhythmia, adverse effects, weight gain, blood pressure, heart rate, and emergency department visits or hospitalizations.

AADs have narrow therapeutic windows. Toxicity is common at normal dosages. Consequently, patient education is essential for providing maximal benefits and avoiding adverse effects and accidental overdosing or underdosing.

The patient, family, and significant others should be taught the basics, such as the name of the drug (both the generic and trade name), the dose, the frequency and timing of the dose, and the reason the drug is needed. This may avoid duplicate prescribing and administration of AADs. The patient should communicate, either verbally or in writing, the names and dosages of these drugs to all other health care providers and should wear a medical identification device listing all medications. In addition, the patient should inform his or her health care provider when any new prescription, over-the-counter, or complementary or alternative medications are started so that potential drug interactions can be minimized or avoided.

The practitioner should provide written instructions for the medication regimen. Providing instructions in large print and simple language may be helpful to patients who have difficulty with memory, hearing, or vision. Instructions should include what to do when the patient misses a dose of medication, has an adverse response to the medication, or wants to stop taking the drug. If β-blockers are prescribed, the patient should be warned that abrupt discontinuation may result in rebound angina, an increased heart rate, and hypertension.

The symptoms associated with these adverse effects also should be identified.

The practitioner can also teach the patient or caregiver how to take blood pressure and pulse readings, how to interpret the readings, and how to recognize and respond to signs and symptoms of hypotension, dizziness, chest pain, shortness of breath, peripheral edema, or palpitations. The patient should take his or her weight each day and call the practitioner if weight gain of over 2 lb occurs. If the patient has difficulty learning these monitoring techniques or cannot perform them, he or she may need to schedule regular follow-up appointments for monitoring. Patients with AF or AFl should know the signs and symptoms of a stroke.

In today's health care environment, the insurance plan's pharmacy provider sometimes makes substitutions with generics or less expensive brands of medications. To prevent harmful drug effects, the patient needs to be aware of this practice and should be cautioned not to change brands of the prescribed AAD or anticoagulant without the approval of the practitioner.

An important teaching point from an ethical and legal perspective is to warn the patient to avoid hazardous activities such as driving, using electrical tools, climbing ladders, or any activity that would put the patient or others in harm's way until the effects of the drug are demonstrated. Patients with an ICD should refrain from driving for at least 6 months after the last arrhythmic event (for devices implanted for secondary prevention) or for at least 7 days following implantation of the ICD (for devices implanted for primary prevention). Documentation of patient teaching on risks, benefits, lifestyle modification, and safety issues with AAD treatment should always be entered in the patient's medical record.

Nutrition

Clear instructions should be given to avoid alcohol, excessive salt intake, and caffeine during treatment for arrhythmias.

Many AADs may cause periods of hypotension resulting in dizziness, or the dose of the drug may need to be regulated, especially in the initial weeks.

Complementary and Alternative Medications

The practitioner must emphasize to the patient the importance of reporting the use of any of these agents so that interactions with AAD therapy can be minimized or avoided. While the information regarding potential interactions between AADs and specific complementary and alternative medications is relatively sparse, there are a few notable interactions of which practitioners should be aware. Patients taking AADs should avoid licorice root. Licorice has mineralocorticoid effects, which can promote hypokalemia. In patients taking digoxin, the presence of hypokalemia may predispose the patient to digoxin toxicity. In patients taking other AADs, the presence of hypokalemia may promote the development of atrial or ventricular arrhythmias. In addition, certain licorice preparations have been shown to cause a prolonged QT interval, which may increase the risk for TdP in patients receiving class III AADs. The use of Siberian ginseng or oleander should also be avoided in patients receiving digoxin, as digoxin toxicity may result. The use of St. John's wort may decrease digoxin concentrations; therefore, digoxin concentrations should be closely monitored when concomitant therapy is used. St. John's wort may also decrease plasma concentrations of amiodarone and dronedarone, which may predispose the patient to arrhythmia recurrence. Consequently, the use of St. John's wort in patients receiving amiodarone or dronedarone should be avoided. Patients with a history of atrial or ventricular arrhythmias should also be instructed to avoid the use of any medication containing ephedra (e.g., Ma Huang) because it can promote the development of arrhythmias.

CASE STUDY*

H.T. is a 66-year-old man with HFrEF (NYHA class III) who presents to the emergency department with shortness of breath and palpitations. An ECG reveals AF with a heart rate of 130 beats/min. He states that these symptoms have been occurring for the past 5 days. **H.T.** has a past medical history of diabetes (A1C 12.2%) and chronic kidney disease requiring hemodialysis. His current medications include insulin glargine 40 units subcut every evening, insulin lispro 12 units subcut before meals, metoprolol succinate 100 mg PO daily, and lisinopril 5 mg PO daily. His vitals are BP 145/95 mm Hg and HR 130 beats/min.

DIAGNOSIS: ATRIAL FIBRILLATION

1. Which of the following would be the most appropriate treatment to acutely manage this patient's symptoms?
   a. Metoprolol IV
   b. Diltiazem IV
   c. Digoxin IV
   d. Amiodarone IV
2. What additional therapy, if any, should be recommended for this patient to prevent thromboembolic complications?
   a. No antithrombotic therapy is necessary because his CHA_2DS_2-VASc score is 0.
   b. Dabigatran because his CHA_2DS_2-VASc score is 1.
   c. Apixaban because his CHA_2DS_2-VASc score is 2.
   d. Warfarin because his CHA_2DS_2-VASc score is 3.

*Answers can be found online.

Bibliography

Starred references are cited in the text.

*Anderson, J. L., Lutz, J. R., & Allison, S. B. (1983). Electrophysiologic and antiarrhythmic effects of oral flecainide in patients with inducible ventricular tachycardia. *Journal of the American College of Cardiology, 2,* 105–114.

*Antiarrhythmics Versus Implantable Defibrillators (AVID) Investigators. (1997). A comparison of antiarrhythmic-drug therapy with implantable defibrillators in patients resuscitated from near-fatal ventricular arrhythmias. *New England Journal of Medicine, 337,* 1576–1583.

*Babatin, M., Lee, S. S., & Pollak, P. T. (2008). Amiodarone hepatotoxicity. *Current Vascular Pharmacology, 6,* 228–236.

*Bardy, G. H., Lee, K. L., Mark, D. B., et al. (2005). Amiodarone or an implantable cardioverter-defibrillator for congestive heart failure. *New England Journal of Medicine, 352,* 225–237.

*Bogazzi, F., Tomisiti, L., Bartalena, L., et al. (2012). Amiodarone and the thyroid: A 2012 update. *Journal of Endocrinological Investigation, 35,* 340–348.

*Buxton, A. E., Lee, K. L., Fisher, J. D., et al. (1999). A randomized study of the prevention of sudden death in patients with coronary artery disease. *New England Journal of Medicine, 341,* 1882–1890.

Cairns, J. A., Connolly, S. J., & Roberts, R. (1997). Randomized trial of outcome after myocardial infarction in patients with frequent or repetitive ventricular premature depolarizations: CAMIAT. *Lancet, 349,* 675–682.

*Camm, A. J., Camm, C. F., & Savelieva, I. (2012). Medical treatment of atrial fibrillation. *Journal of Cardiovascular Medicine, 13,* 97–107.

*Cardiac Arrhythmia Suppression Trial Investigators. (1989). Preliminary report: Effect of encainide and flecainide on mortality in a randomized trial of arrhythmia suppression after myocardial infarction. *New England Journal of Medicine, 321,* 406–412.

*Carlsson, J., Miketic, S., Windeler, J., et al. (2004). Randomized trial of rate-control versus rhythm-control in persistent atrial fibrillation: The Strategies of Treatment of Atrial Fibrillation (STAF) study. *Journal of the American College of Cardiology, 41,* 1690–1696.

*Connolly, S. J., Camm, A. J., Halperin, J. L., et al. (2011). Dronedarone in high-risk atrial fibrillation. *New England Journal of Medicine, 365,* 2268–2276.

*Connolly, S., Gent, M., Roberts, R. S., et al. (2000). Canadian Implantable Defibrillator Study (CIDS): A randomized trial of the implantable cardioverter defibrillator versus amiodarone. *Circulation, 101,* 1297–1302.

*Connolly, S. J., Dorian, P., Roberts, R. S., et al. (2006). Comparison of beta-blockers, amiodarone plus beta-blockers, or sotalol for prevention of shocks from implantable cardioverter defibrillators: The OPTIC study. *Journal of the American Medical Association, 295,* 165–171.

Dager, W. E., Sanoski, C. A., Wiggins, B. S., et al. (2006). Pharmacotherapy considerations in advanced cardiac life support. *Pharmacotherapy, 26,* 1703–1729.

*de Caen, A. R., Berg, M. D., Chameides, L., et al. (2015). Part 12: Pediatric advanced life support: 2015 American Heart Association Guidelines Update for Cardiopulmonary Resuscitation and Emergency Cardiovascular Care. *Circulation, 132*(Suppl. 2), S526–S542.

*Dorian, P., Cass, D., & Schwartz, B., et al. (2002). Amiodarone as compared with lidocaine for shock-resistant ventricular fibrillation. *New England Journal of Medicine, 346,* 884–890.

*Epstein, A. E., DiMarco, J. P., Ellenbogen, K. A., et al. (2013). 2012 ACCF/AHA/HRS focused update incorporated into the ACCF/AHA/HRS 2008 guidelines for device-based therapy of cardiac rhythm abnormalities: A report of the American College of Cardiology/American Heart Association Task Force on Practice Guidelines and the Heart Rhythm Society. *Journal of the American College of Cardiology, 61,* e6–e75.

*Goldschlager, N., Epstein, A. E., Naccarelli, G., et al. (2007). A practical guide for clinicians who treat patients with amiodarone. *Heart Rhythm, 4,* 1250–1259.

*Hohnloser, S. H., Crijns, H. J., van Eickels, M., et al. (2009). Effect of dronedarone on cardiovascular events in atrial fibrillation. *New England Journal of Medicine, 360,* 668–678.

*Hohnloser, S. H., Kuck, K. H., & Lilienthal, J. (2000). Rhythm or rate control in atrial fibrillation—Pharmacological Intervention in Atrial Fibrillation (PIAF): A randomised trial. *Lancet, 356,* 1789–1794.

*January, C. T., Wann, L. S., Alpert, J. S., et al. (2014). 2014 AHA/ACC/HRS guideline for the management of patients with atrial fibrillation: A report of the American College of Cardiology/American Heart Association Task Force on Practice Guidelines and the Heart Rhythm Society. *Circulation, 130,* e199–e267.

*Jaworski, K., Walecka, I., Rudnicka, L., et al. (2014). Cutaneous adverse reactions of amiodarone. *Medical Science Monitor, 20,* 2369–2372.

*Kleinman, M. E., Brennan, E. E., Goldberger, Z. D., et al. (2015). Part 5: Adult basic life support and cardiopulmonary resuscitation quality: 2015 American Heart Association Guidelines Update for Cardiopulmonary Resuscitation and Emergency Cardiovascular Care. *Circulation, 132*(Suppl. 2), S414–S435.

*Køber, L., Bloch-Thomsen, P. E., Møller, M., et al. (2000). Danish Investigations of Arrhythmia and Mortality on Dofetilide (DIAMOND) Study Group. Effect of dofetilide in patients with recent myocardial infarction and left-ventricular dysfunction: A randomised trial. *Lancet, 356,* 2052–2058.

*Køber, L., Torp-Pedersen, C., McMurray, J. J., et al. (2008). Increased mortality after dronedarone therapy or severe heart failure. *New England Journal of Medicine, 358,* 2678–2687.

*Kuck, K. H., Cappato, R., Siebels, J., et al. (2000). Randomized comparison of antiarrhythmic drug therapy with implantable defibrillators in patients resuscitated from cardiac arrest: The Cardiac Arrest Study Hamburg (CASH). *Circulation, 102,* 748–754.

*Kudenchuck, P. J., Cobb, L. A., Copass, M. K., et al. (1999). Amiodarone for resuscitation after out-of-hospital cardiac arrest due to ventricular fibrillation. *New England Journal of Medicine, 341,* 871–879.

*Le Heuzey, J. Y., De Ferrari, G. M., Radzik, D., et al. (2010). A short-term, randomized, double-blind, parallel-group study to evaluate the efficacy and safety of dronedarone versus amiodarone in patients with persistent atrial fibrillation: The DIONYSOS study. *Journal of Cardiovascular Electrophysiology, 21,* 597–605.

*Link, M. S., Berkow, L. C., Kudenchuk, P. J., et al. (2015). Part 7: Adult advanced cardiovascular life support: 2015 American Heart Association Guidelines Update for Cardiopulmonary Resuscitation and Emergency Cardiovascular Care. *Circulation, 132*(Suppl. 2), S444–S464.

*Miller, M. R., McNamara, R. L., Segal, J. B., et al. (2000). Efficacy of agents for pharmacological conversion of atrial fibrillation and subsequent maintenance of sinus rhythm: A meta-analysis of clinical trials. *Journal of Family Practice, 49,* 1033–1046.

*Moss, A. J., Hall, W. J., Cannom, D. S., et al. (1996). Improved survival with an implanted defibrillator in patients with coronary disease at high risk for ventricular arrhythmia. *New England Journal of Medicine, 335,* 1933–1940.

*Moss, A. J., Zareba, W., Hall, W. J., et al. (2002). Prophylactic implantation of a defibrillator in patients with myocardial infarction and reduced ejection fraction. *New England Journal of Medicine, 346,* 877–883.

*Neumar, R. W., Otto, C. W., Link, M. S., et al. (2010). Part 8: Adult advanced cardiovascular support: 2010 American Heart Association Guidelines for Cardiopulmonary Resuscitation and Emergency Cardiovascular Care. *Circulation, 122*(Suppl. 3), S729–S767.

*Opolski, G., Torbicki, A., Kosior, D. A., et al. (2004). Rate control vs. rhythm control in patients with nonvalvular persistent atrial fibrillation: The results of the Polish How to Treat Chronic Atrial Fibrillation (HOT CAFE) Study. *Chest, 126,* 476–486.

*Oral, H., Souza, J. J., Michaud, G. F., et al. (1999). Facilitating transthoracic cardioversion of atrial fibrillation with ibutilide pretreatment. *New England Journal of Medicine, 340,* 1849–1854.

*Pacifico, A., Hohnloser, S. H., Williams, J. H., et al. (1999). Prevention of implantable-defibrillator shocks by treatment with sotalol: Sotalol Implantable Cardioverter-Defibrillator Study Group. *New England Journal of Medicine, 340,* 1855–1862.

*Passman, R. S., Bennett, C. L., Purpura, J. M., et al. (2012). Amiodarone-associated optic neuropathy: A critical review. *American Journal of Medicine, 125,* 447–453.

*Pedersen, T. P., Kay, G. N., Kalman, J., et al. (2014). EHRA/HRS/APHRS expert consensus on ventricular arrhythmias. *Heart Rhythm, 11,* e166-e196.

*Phillips, B. G., Gandhi, A. J., Sanoski, C. A., et al. (1997). Comparison of intravenous diltiazem and verapamil for the acute treatment of atrial fibrillation and flutter. *Pharmacotherapy, 17,* 1238–1245.

*Range, F. T., Hilker, E., Breithardt, G., et al. (2013). Amiodarone-induced pulmonary toxicity: A fatal case report and review of the literature. *Cardiovascular Drugs and Therapy, 27,* 247–254.

*Roy, D., Talajic, M., Dorian, P., et al. (2000). Amiodarone to prevent recurrence of atrial fibrillation. *New England Journal of Medicine, 342,* 913–920.

*Roy, D., Talajic, M., Nattel, S., et al. (2008). Rhythm control versus rate control for atrial fibrillation and heart failure. *New England Journal of Medicine, 358,* 2667–2677.

*Sanoski, C. A., & Bauman, J. L. (2002). Clinical observations with the amiodarone/warfarin interaction: Dosing relationships with long-term therapy. *Chest, 121,* 19–23.

*Singh, B. N., Connolly, S. J., Crijns, H. J., et al. (2007). Dronedarone for maintenance of sinus rhythm in atrial fibrillation or flutter. *New England Journal of Medicine, 357,* 987–999.

*Singh, S. N., Singh, B. N., Reda, D. J., et al. (2005). Amiodarone versus sotalol for atrial fibrillation. *New England Journal of Medicine, 352,* 1861–1872.

*Singh, S., Zoble, R. G., Yellen, L., et al. (2000). Efficacy and safety of oral dofetilide in converting to and maintaining sinus rhythm in patients with chronic atrial fibrillation or atrial flutter: The Symptomatic Atrial Fibrillation Investigative Research on Dofetilide (SAFIRE-D) Study. *Circulation, 102,* 2385–2390.

*Slavik, R. S., Tisdale, J. E., & Borzak, S. (2001). Pharmacological conversion of atrial fibrillation: A systematic review of available evidence. *Progress in Cardiovascular Diseases, 44,* 121–152.

*Stambler, B. S., Wood, M. A., Ellenbogen, K. A., et al. (1996). Efficacy and safety of repeated intravenous doses of ibutilide for rapid conversion of atrial flutter or fibrillation. *Circulation, 94,* 1613–1621.

*Torp-Pedersen, C., Moller, M., Bloch-Thomson, P. E., et al. (1999). Dofetilide in patients with congestive heart failure and left ventricular dysfunction. Danish Investigations of Arrhythmia and Mortality on Dofetilide Study Group. *New England Journal of Medicine, 341,* 857–865.

*Van der Werf, C., Kannankeril, P. J., Sacher, F., et al. (2011). Flecainide therapy reduces exercise-induced ventricular arrhythmias in patients with catecholaminergic polymorphic ventricular tachycardia. *Journal of the American College of Cardiology, 57,* 2244–2254.

*Van Gelder, I. C., Groenveld, H. F., Crijns, H. J. G. M., et al. (2010). Lenient versus strict rate control in patients with atrial fibrillation. *New England Journal of Medicine, 362,* 1363–1373.

*Van Gelder, I. C., Hagens, V. E., Bosker, H. A., et al. (2002). The Rate Control Versus Electrical Cardioversion for Persistent Atrial Fibrillation Study Group. A comparison of rate control and rhythm control in patients with recurrent persistent atrial fibrillation. *New England Journal of Medicine, 347,* 1834–1840.

*Vaughan Williams, E. M. (1984). A classification of antiarrhythmic actions reassessed after a decade of new drugs. *Journal of Clinical Pharmacology, 24,* 129–147.

*Wyse, D. G., Kellen, J., Rademaker, A. W. (1988). Prophylactic versus selective lidocaine for early ventricular arrhythmias of myocardial infarction. *Journal of the American College of Cardiology, 12,* 507–513.

*Wyse, D. G., Waldo, A. L., DiMarco, J. P., et al. (2002). A comparison of rate control and rhythm control in patients with atrial fibrillation. *New England Journal of Medicine, 347,* 1825–1833.

*You, J. J., Singer, D. E., Howard, P. A., et al. (2012). Antithrombotic therapy for atrial fibrillation: Antithrombotic therapy and prevention of thrombosis, 9th ed: American College of Chest Physicians Evidence-Based Clinical Practice Guidelines. *Chest, 141,* e531S–e575S.

UNIT 5

Pharmacotherapy for Respiratory Disorders

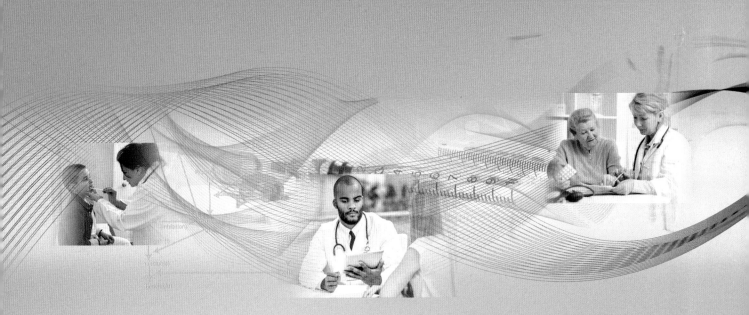

24 Upper Respiratory Infections

Karleen Melody ▪ Anisha B. Grover

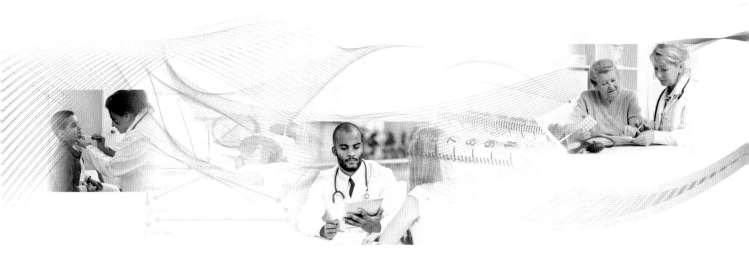

Upper respiratory tract infections (URIs), including the common cold and rhinosinusitis, are some of the most common problems seen in primary care. URIs are usually self-limiting, minor illnesses that account for half or more of all acute illnesses. It is difficult to differentiate the common cold from rhinosinusitis or allergic rhinitis (see Chapter 48). URIs commonly involve rhinitis, which refers to irritation and inflammation of the intranasal mucous membrane and is characterized by nasal congestion, nasal discharge, sneezing, and postnasal drip. Other common URI symptoms include tenderness over the sinuses, fever, headache, malaise, sore throat, myalgias, a full feeling around the eyes and ears, and coughing. Symptoms may present individually or in combination, and it can be difficult to determine whether the cause is viral or bacterial.

URIs can progress to involve acute or chronic complications. In children especially, URIs may progress to otitis media. In a small percentage of cases, the viral or bacterial cause may travel, causing rhinosinusitis and bronchitis. Acute respiratory infections have been projected to kill approximately 3.9 million people annually and represent a leading cause of mortality in children living in developing countries who are less than 5 years of age (Liu et al., 2012). There also is an enormous economic burden associated with URIs.

COMMON COLD

Acute infectious rhinitis, also known as the common cold, nasopharyngitis, rhinopharyngitis, or acute coryza, is caused by one of more than 200 viral types and most commonly involves rhinovirus. It is one of the most common infections and is usually minor and self-limiting. Coryza is an acute inflammation of the mucous membranes of the respiratory passages, particularly of the nose, sinuses, and throat, and is characterized by sneezing, rhinorrhea (watery nasal discharge), and coughing.

In 2012, the U.S. Attitudes of Consumers Toward Health, Cough, and Cold (ACHOO) survey was developed to collect information regarding participant demographics, basic knowledge of cough and cold symptoms, treatment choices, and treatment preferences (Blaiss et al., 2015). Of the 2,505 survey participants, 84.6% had experienced at least one cold in the past year and lasted approximately 1 to 7 days. Cough was the most common cold symptom, affecting 73.1% of participants, and this symptom, along with nasal congestion, was reported as the most bothersome symptom. A subsequent publication examined the data from this study in order to assess the impact of cough and cold on daily activity, productivity, and absenteeism (Dicpinigaitis et al., 2015). Fifty-two percent of participants described the impact on daily life as a "fair amount" to "a lot" for the duration of the illness (Dicpinigaitis et al., 2015). During the time of a cold, participants reported a decrease in productivity by a mean of 26.4%. Almost half of respondents reported absenteeism from work or school lasting 1 to 2 days (Dicpinigaitis et al., 2015). A survey published in 2002 reported an approximate $2 billion spent in the United States annually on over-the-counter (OTC) preparations to relieve cold symptoms, predominantly in children (West, 2002). Another survey published in 2003 estimated that noninfluenza viral respiratory infections result in an annual $40 billion in costs. This includes costs related to cold-related absenteeism, including 70 million missed workdays, 186 million missed school days, and 126 million missed workdays among caregivers of children suffering from colds (Fendrick et al., 2003).

CAUSES

The pathogen most frequently associated with common colds is human rhinovirus (HRV), a single-stranded ribonucleic acid accounting for one half to two thirds of common colds (Jacobs et al., 2013). The coronavirus, respiratory syncytial virus, influenza virus, human parainfluenza virus, human metapneumovirus, and adenovirus can also contribute to cold-like symptoms, but HRVs are the single most pervasive cause of colds and in some cases can increase the susceptibility to bacterial infection within the upper and lower airway epithelial cells (Jacobs et al., 2013).

Predisposition to viral infections can be attributed to many factors, including frequent exposure to viral infectious agents; in children, the age of the child; and the inability to resist invading organisms because of allergies, malnutrition, immune deficiencies, physical abnormalities, or other comorbid conditions. Some experts propose a relationship between the host response to the virus and the production of cold symptoms. Studies show that common colds are more frequent or more severe in those under increased stress, probably as a result of stress weakening the immune system.

PATHOPHYSIOLOGY

If there is a breakdown or failure in the protective barriers of the URI (i.e., cough, gag, and sneeze reflexes, lymph nodes, immunoglobulin [Ig] A antibodies, and rich vasculature), viral pathogens trigger an acute inflammatory reaction with release of vasoactive mediators and increased parasympathetic stimuli. This produces congestion and rhinorrhea. Viral URI also produces inflammatory mediators that increase the sensitivity of afferent sensory nerves in the airway, which may contribute to the cough typically associated with the common cold.

Bradykinin and lysyl-bradykinin contribute to the pathogenesis of HRV infections. An increase in kinin levels is associated with increased permeability of the vasculature. However, histamine levels remain unchanged, indicating the lack of involvement of mast cells and basophils (Jacobs et al., 2013). The involvement of prostaglandins can be elucidated by the demonstrated effectiveness of cyclooxygenase inhibitors in reducing headache, malaise, myalgias, and cough during HRV infection.

Transmission of HRV occurs predominantly by intranasal or conjunctival inoculation and has been attributed to three methods: airborne transmission by small particles (droplets), airborne transmission by large particles, and direct contact. Large particle transmission is not efficient and requires prolonged exposure. Direct contact involves donor nose-to-hand contact, which is then transmitted to the hand of a recipient. From there, transmission occurs primarily when the infected hand makes contact with the eyes or nose. Although conjunctival cells are not thought to harbor HRV, it probably can be passed through the tear duct into the nose. HRVs can survive indoors for a range of hours to days at room temperature

(Jacobs et al., 2013). Rhinoviruses grow in the upper airway and attach and gain entry to host cells by binding to an intracellular adhesion molecule. Infection begins in the adenoidal area and spreads to the ciliated epithelium in the nose. HRVs remain infectious for at least 3 hours after drying on hard surfaces such as telephones or countertops, but they do not last as long on porous surfaces, such as tissues.

DIAGNOSTIC CRITERIA

The expansion in the availability of laboratory diagnostics includes the collection and processing of specimens, detection and serology of antigens, conventional and rapid virus culture, and many other technologies; however, diagnostic tests are not recommended (Jacobs et al., 2013). In order to evaluate specimens, collection would have to occur as soon as possible after symptom onset, since HRV titers are most elevated during the first 2 days of clinical presentation. The short duration of most colds results in an impractical window of appropriate timing, and there are inaccuracies involved in the diagnostic process, making the testing process unreasonable.

The most commonly used method of diagnosis involves symptom evaluation. Onset of common cold signs and symptoms occurs 1 to 2 days after viral infection and peaks in approximately 2 to 4 days. A cough may persist following the resolution of other symptoms. Symptoms consist primarily of clear nasal discharge, sneezing, nasal congestion, cough, low-grade fever (below 102°F [38.9°C]), scratchy or sore throat, mild aches, chills, headache, watery eyes, tenderness around the eyes, full feeling in the ears, and fatigue. In children, the presentation could also include fever with seizures, anorexia, vomiting, diarrhea, and abdominal pain. Symptoms usually resolve in approximately 1 week, but they may linger for up to 2 weeks.

INITIATING DRUG THERAPY

Improper treatment of the common cold by clinicians is common for several reasons. It is often difficult to determine whether the cause is viral or bacterial. There is no cure for the common cold; therefore, treatment strategies are supportive in nature and consist primarily of symptom relief.

Nonpharmacologic alternatives to treating the common cold are the first line of treatment. Rest allows the body to gain strength. An alternative to decongestants and expectorants involves increasing water or juice intake, which assists in liquefying tenacious secretions, making expectoration easier, soothing scratchy, sore throats, and relieving dry skin and lips. Saline gargles also are effective for soothing sore throats. Saline nasal flushes and irrigation may have slight benefit in clearing nasal passages without the risk for rebound congestion; however, evidence remains limited (Fokkens et al., 2012).

Coughing caused by chest congestion can cause a muscular chest pain. Menthol rubs can soothe this ache and open airways for some congestion relief. Menthol lozenges also have been effective in soothing scratchy throats and clearing nasal passages. Petrolatum-based ointments for raw and macerated skin around the nose and upper lip ease the drying effects of dehydration and the use of multiple tissues. Inhalation of steam has not demonstrated benefit in the drainage of mucus or the destruction of the cold virus and is therefore not recommended (Fokkens et al., 2012).

Goals of Drug Therapy

The main goals of treatment for the common cold are relief of symptoms, reduction of the risk for complications, and prevention of spread to others.

Decongestants

Decongestants come in topical or oral preparations and can be somewhat effective for the short-term relief of cold symptoms (Fashner et al., 2012). Topical decongestants, such as oxymetazoline hydrochloride (Afrin) and phenylephrine hydrochloride (Afrin Childrens, Little Remedies, Neo-synephrine), are available in nasal spray and pump mist preparations. Oral decongestants, such as pseudoephedrine (Sudafed) and phenylephrine (Sudafed PE), are also available. Decongestants are typically available OTC. Preparations containing pseudoephedrine can be obtained without a prescription but are available behind the counter and must be purchased from a pharmacy.

Mechanism of Action

Decongestants are sympathomimetic agents that stimulate alpha- and beta-adrenergic receptors, causing vasoconstriction in the respiratory tract mucosa and thereby improving ventilation. Topical decongestants have little systemic absorption but work locally by slowing ciliary motility and mucociliary clearance. Oral agents have the same mechanism of action and assist in the clearance of nasal mucus and obstruction. Their use may help to prevent rhinosinusitis and eustachian tube blockage in patients susceptible to these conditions.

Dosage

Oxymetazoline hydrochloride 0.05% nasal spray and pump mists can be used in patients who are at least 6 years old at a dosage of 2 to 3 sprays in each nostril not more often than every 10 to 12 hours. Patients should not exceed 2 doses of oxymetazoline in a 24-hour time period. Phenylephrine nasal sprays are available as 0.125%, 0.25%, 0.5%, and 1% preparations. For specific dosing recommendations, please see **Table 24.1**. Despite the ability to use the spray every 4 hours, it should generally not be used more than two to three times daily. Topical decongestants should not be used for more than 3 days because prolonged use can cause rhinitis medicamentosa (rebound congestion), which is characterized by severe nasal edema, rebound congestion, and increased discharge due to decreased receptor sensitivity. Rebound congestion interferes with ciliary action and dries the nasal mucosa.

TABLE 24.1

Overview of Agents for Upper Respiratory Infections

Generic (Trade) Name and Dosage	Selected Adverse Events	Contraindications	Special Considerations
Decongestants			
oxymetazoline hydrochloride (Afrin, Mucinex Sinus, Neo-Synephrine, Vicks Sinex) Nasal spray and pump mists (0.05%) ≥6 y: 2–3 sprays per nostril q10–12h	Palpitations, headaches	Hypersensitivity	These drugs may cause rebound congestion. Use only 2–3 d, then switch to oral decongestants.
phenylephrine hydrochloride (Neo-Synephrine, Sudafed PE, Afrin Childrens) Nasal spray (0.125%) 2–5 y: 2–3 sprays per nostril q4h Mild nasal spray (0.25%) 6–12 y: 2–3 sprays per nostril q4h Regular nasal spray (0.5%) ≥12 y: 2–3 sprays per nostril q4h Extra strength nasal spray (1%) ≥12 y: 2–3 sprays per nostril q4h Tablet, oral (10 mg) ≥12 y: 10 mg q4h	Palpitations, headaches	Hypersensitivity, urinary retention, severe uncontrolled hypertension, coronary artery disease, MAO inhibitor use within 14 d	These drugs may cause rebound congestion. Use only 2–3 d, then switch to oral decongestants.

(Continued)

TABLE 24.1

Overview of Agents for Upper Respiratory Infections (*Continued*)

Generic (Trade) Name and Dosage	Selected Adverse Events	Contraindications	Special Considerations
pseudoephedrine (Sudafed) IR tablet, oral (30 mg) ≥12 y: 60 mg q4–6h 6–11 y: 30 mg q4–6h 12-hour tablet, oral (120 mg) ≥12 y: 120 mg q12h ER tablet, oral (240 mg) ≥12 y: 240 mg q24h	Palpitations, headaches, increased blood pressure, dizziness, GI upset, tremor, insomnia	Hypersensitivity, narrow-angle glaucoma, severe uncontrolled hypertension, coronary artery disease, MAO inhibitor use within 14 d	Give at least 2 h before bedtime. Do not crush, break, or chew tablets.
Expectorants			
guaifenesin (Antitussin, Mucinex, Robitussin, Uni-Tussin) Liquid, oral (100–200 mg/5 mL) Solution, oral (100 mg/5 mL) Syrup, oral (100 mg/ 5 mL) Packet, oral (50 mg, 100 mg) 6 mo–12 y: 25–50 mg q4h 2–5 y: 50–100 mg q4h 6–12 y: 100–200 mg q4h ≥12 y: 200–400 mg q4h IR tablet, oral (200 or 400 mg) ≥12 y: 200–400 mg q4h ER tablet, oral (600 mg) ≥12 y: 600–1,200 mg q12h	Drowsiness, headache, dizziness, GI upset	Hypersensitivity	Not given for prolonged time if cough persists or accompanied by high fever Oral packet may be swallowed whole or opened and sprinkled on soft food.
Antitussives			
dextromethorphan (Delsym) Lozenge, oral (5 mg) Capsule, oral, 15 mg Sublingual strip, oral (7.5 mg) Gel, oral (7.5 mg/5 mL) Syrup, oral (varying strengths) IR liquid, oral (varying strengths) 4–6 y: 2.5–7.5 mg q4–8h 6–12 y: 5–10 mg q4h ≥12 y: 10–20 mg q4h or 30 mg q6–8h ER liquid, oral (30 mg/5 mL) 4–6 y: 15 mg q12h 6–12 y: 15 mg q6–8h ≥12 y: 60 mg q12h	Dizziness, nausea, drowsiness	Hypersensitivity, MAO inhibitor use within 14 d	None
benzonatate (Tessalon Perles) Capsule, oral (100 or 200 mg) ≥10 y: 100–200 mg q8h	Constipation, drowsiness, headache, GI upset, confusion	Hypersensitivity	
Anti-inflammatories			
naproxen sodium (Naprosyn, Aleve) Tablet, oral (220 mg) ≥12 y: 220 mg q8–12h	Dizziness, drowsiness, headache, edema, abdominal pain, constipation, nausea, heartburn	Hypersensitivity	Take on full stomach to reduce GI upset.
Anticholinergics			
ipratropium bromide (Atrovent) Nasal spray (0.06%) ≥12 y: 2 sprays per nostril bid–qid 5–11 y: 2 sprays per nostril tid	Headache, epistaxis, pharyngitis, nasal dryness	Hypersensitivity to atropine Use caution in patients with narrow-angle glaucoma, BPH, bladder neck obstruction, pregnancy, and lactation	Safety and efficacy not established beyond 4 d

TABLE 24.1

Overview of Agents for Upper Respiratory Infections (*Continued*)

Generic (Trade) Name and Dosage	Selected Adverse Events	Contraindications	Special Considerations
Antihistamines			
diphenhydramine (Benadryl) Tablet, oral (25 mg) $\geq$12 y: 25–50 mg q4–6h	Confusion, dizziness, drowsiness, fatigue, paradoxical excitability, nervousness, headache, sedation, blurred vision, dry mouth, hallucinations, tachycardia, urinary retention	Hypersensitivity, patients who are breast-feeding, neonates, premature infants	Caution in elderly, as it may increase fall risk.
chlorpheniramine (Chlor-Trimeton) IR tablet, oral (4 mg) $\geq$12 y: 4 mg q4–6h ER tablet, oral (12 mg) $\geq$12 y: 12 mg q12h	Headache, fatigue, nervousness, dizziness, nausea, dry mouth, GI upset, urinary retention, blurred vision	Hypersensitivity, narrow-angle glaucoma, bladder neck obstruction, symptomatic prostate hypertrophy, during acute asthma attacks, stenosing peptic ulcer, pyloro-duodenal obstruction	Caution in elderly, as it may increase fall risk.
amoxicillin with clavulanic acid (Augmentin) Adults or children >40 kg: 500 mg q8h Children 3 mo to adolescence who are $\leq$40 kg: 20 mg/kg/d q8h or 25 mg/kg/d q12h Children <3 mo: 30 mg/kg/d every 12 h Children with severe ABRS: 40 mg/kg/d q8h or 45 mg/kg/d q12h CrCl 10–30 mL/min: 250–500 mg q12h CrCl < 10 mL/min: 250–500 mg q24h	Common: GI upset, rash, vaginal infections, photosensitivity Rare: Stevens-Johnson syndrome, seizures	Hypersensitivity or allergy to penicillin or cephalosporins Do not use ER formulation in patients with CrCl < 30 mL/min	"High dose" (2 g q12h) is reserved for patients with risk for antibiotic resistance.*
Doxycycline (Oracea) Adults and children >8 y of age weighing >45 kg: 200 mg daily in 1–2 divided doses	Common: GI upset, rash, vaginal infections, headache Rare: Stevens-Johnson syndrome, hepatotoxicity	Hypersensitivity or allergy to tetracyclines	Not recommended for children $\leq$8 y of age Take on an empty stomach if tolerated.
levofloxacin (Levaquin) Adults: 500–750 mg q24h Children: 10–20 mg/kg/d q12–24h CrCl 20–49 mL/min: 500 mg × 1 followed by 250 mg q24h or 500 mg × 1 followed by 750 mg q48h	Common: GI upset, rash, dyspepsia, headache, chest pain, decreased blood glucose, edema, photosensitivity, vaginal infections Black box warning for tendon inflammation and rupture	Hypersensitivity or allergy to fluoroquinolones	Avoid in patients with myasthenia gravis. Can prolong QTc interval. Avoid concurrent use with other medications that prolong the QTc interval. Avoid taking with corticosteroids due to increased risk of ruptured Achilles tendon.
moxifloxacin (Avelox) Adults: 400 mg q24h	Same as above	Same as above	Same as above
clindamycin (Cleocin) Children: 30–40 mg/kg/d divided q8h	Common: GI upset	Hypersensitivity or allergy to lincosamides	Must be taken with third-generation cephalosporins.
cefpodoxime (Vantin) Children >2 mo and <12 y: 5 mg/kg q12h Children $\geq$12 y: 200 mg q12h	Common: GI upset headache	Caution with penicillin allergy	Interacts with antacids, H2 antagonists.
cefixime (Suprax) Children >6 mo and <12 y: 4 mg/kg q12h Children $\geq$12 y: 400 mg divided every 12–24 h	Same as above	Same as above	Same as above.

*Patients with ABRS from regions with high endemic rates of resistant *S. pneumoniae*, those with severe infection, children in daycare, ages <2 or >65, immunosuppressed or those with a recent hospitalization or antibiotic use within the past month.

Oral pseudoephedrine is available in 30-mg tablets in preparations that vary with regard to duration of action. Adults greater than 12 years of age can take a short-acting preparation at a dose of 60 mg every 4 to 6 hours or a long-acting preparation at a dose of 120 mg every 12 hours. All-day preparations are also available at a dosage of 240 mg and should not be taken more than once in a 24-hour time period. Children who are 4 to 5 years of age can take a 15-mg dose every 4 to 6 hours to a maximum daily dose of 60 mg. Children aged 6 to 12 should take 30 mg every 4 to 6 hours and should not exceed 120 mg within 24 hours. Oral preparations should be given at least 2 hours before bedtime, and extended-release (ER) formulations should not be crushed, broken, or chewed. Oral phenylephrine has not demonstrated consistent benefit and should not be recommended.

Time Frame for Response

Topical decongestants have a rapid onset of action and can begin to work within several minutes. Oral decongestants have a slower onset of action of approximately 30 minutes.

Contraindications

Decongestants are contraindicated in patients with hypersensitivity to any component of the formulation, narrow-angle glaucoma, severe uncontrolled hypertension, and coronary artery disease and in patients who have been treated with a monoamine oxidase (MAO) inhibitor within 14 days. Caution is recommended in patients with hypertension, cardiovascular disease, renal impairment, hyperthyroidism, diabetes, prostatic hypertrophy, and urinary incontinence.

Adverse Events

Adverse drug events (ADEs) include increased blood pressure and heart rate, palpitations, headache, dizziness, gastrointestinal (GI) distress, insomnia, and tremor. These reactions are especially seen at doses above 210 mg. In patients with controlled hypertension, products can be taken for a short course and with frequent monitoring.

Interactions

Decongestants interact with appetite suppressants, MAO inhibitors (hypertensive crisis), and beta-adrenergic agents (bradycardia and hypertension). Decongestants are less effective when taken with drugs that acidify the urine and more effective when taken with drugs that alkalize the urine.

Expectorants

One of the most important nondrug considerations in treating coughs involves an exploration of the etiology, because the prolonged use of OTC expectorants or other cough products may mask symptoms of a serious underlying disorder. This drug should not be used for more than 1 week. If the cough persists, additional measures should be investigated. The most commonly available expectorant is guaifenesin (Antitussin, Mucinex, Robitussin). Some studies have shown this product to have limited advantage over increased fluid intake, and evidence regarding benefit is generally controversial (Fashner et al., 2012).

Mechanism of Action

Expectorants, including water, increase the output of respiratory tract fluid by decreasing the adhesiveness and surface tension of the respiratory tract and by facilitating the removal of viscous mucous.

Dosage

Guaifenesin is available in both liquid and tablet oral preparations. Some preparations are available in the form of oral sprinkles, which may be swallowed whole or sprinkled on soft food, such as applesauce. The recommended dose for adults over the age of 12 is 200 to 400 mg every 4 hours to a maximum daily dose of 2.4 grams (g). ER tablets can be taken at a dosage of 600 to 1,200 mg every 12 hours, with the same maximum daily dose as the immediate-release (IR) preparations. For children less than 4 years of age, a physician or pharmacist should be consulted prior to treatment with expectorants. If recommended by a health care professional, children aged 6 months to 2 years can be given a dose of 25 to 50 mg every 4 hours to a maximum of 300 mg/d. Children aged 2 to 5 can take a dose of 50 to 100 mg every 4 hours, not to exceed 500 mg/d. Children who are 6 to 12 years of age can be given a dose of 100 to 200 mg every 4 hours to a maximum of 1.2 mg/d.

Time Frame for Response

Expectorants have an onset of action of approximately 1 to 2 hours.

Contraindications

Expectorants are contraindicated in patients with hypersensitivity to any component of the formulation.

Adverse Events

ADEs include drowsiness, headache, dizziness, and GI upset.

Interactions

There are no known drug interactions.

Antitussives

Cough suppressants, such as dextromethorphan (Delsym) and benzonatate (Tessalon Perles), are available in oral preparations, including liquids, gels, capsules, lozenges, and sublingual strips, but studies have shown minimal benefit with the common cold (Fashner et al., 2012). For some patients, these agents may reduce cough frequency and help achieve sleep; however, consistent benefit has not been demonstrated. There is little evidence to support the use of narcotic antitussives, such as codeine and hydrocodone, to relieve cough. Many practitioners believe that cough suppressants are ineffective in children.

Mechanism of Action

Antitussives may diminish the cough reflex by direct inhibition of the cough center in the medulla.

Dosage

Patients over the age of 12 years can take IR preparations of dextromethorphan at a dose of 10 to 20 mg every 4 hours or 30 mg every 6 to 8 hours. ER products can be taken at a dose of 60 mg twice daily. Adult patients should not exceed a dose of 120 mg within a 24-hour time period. Dextromethorphan is not recommended for children less than 4 years of age. Children who are 4 to 6 years of age may take an IR preparation at a dose of 2.5 to 7.5 mg every 4 to 8 hours or an ER preparation at a dose of 15 mg twice daily to a maximum of 30 mg/d. Children aged 6 to 12 years may take IR preparations at a dose of 5 to 10 mg every 4 hours or 15 mg every 6 to 8 hours. ER preparations can be taken at a dose of 30 mg twice daily. The maximum dose of dextromethorphan for this age range is 60 mg per 24-hour time period.

Benzonatate can be taken by patients greater than 10 years of age at a dose of 100 to 200 mg three times daily, as needed with total daily doses not to exceed 600 mg.

Time Frame for Response

Onset of action is noted within 15 to 30 minutes.

Contraindications

Antitussives are contraindicated in a patient who has a hypersensitivity to these agents or in a patient who has taken an MAO inhibitor within 2 weeks.

Adverse Events

Adverse events include dizziness, nausea, and drowsiness.

Interactions

Drug–drug interactions occur with concomitant use of amiodarone (Cordarone), MAO inhibitors, quinidine, and proserotonergic drugs, such as selective serotonin reuptake inhibitors, serotonin norepinephrine reuptake inhibitors, or triptans. Caution should also be used with other antidepressants.

Anti-inflammatories and Analgesics

Mechanism of Action

Cyclooxygenase inhibitors, such as nonsteroidal anti-inflammatory drugs (NSAIDs), inhibit prostaglandin secretions, which can reduce headache, malaise, myalgias, cough, and even sneezing. Naproxen (Naprosyn, Aleve) is available as an oral tablet or suspension and is the NSAID of choice in the American College of Clinical Pharmacy (ACCP) guidelines because it does not impact viral shedding (Jacobs et al., 2013).

Dosage

Naproxen available in an OTC preparation can be taken by patients who are 12 years of age or older at a dose of 220 mg every 8 to 12 hours. Total daily dosage should not exceed 600 mg. NSAIDs should be taken with food to avoid GI upset.

Time Frame for Response

Effects are noted within 1 to 2 hours.

Contraindications

Contraindications include hypersensitivity to any component of the formulation. Caution should be used for patients with active peptic ulcers or GI bleeds, bleeding disorders, asthma, severe hepatic impairment, severe renal impairment involving a creatinine clearance (CrCl) of less than 30 milliliters per minute (mL/min), severe uncontrolled heart failure, and hyperkalemia, or who are in their third trimester or are breastfeeding. Aspirin, a common NSAID, should not be used in children because of the secondary risk of Reye syndrome. Patients should also refrain from taking acetaminophen (Tylenol) and ibuprofen (Motrin, Advil) because these drugs are believed to shed the virus. NSAIDs are discussed in greater detail in Chapter 7.

Adverse Events

Adverse events include dizziness, drowsiness, headache, edema, abdominal pain, constipation, nausea, and heartburn.

Interactions

Naproxen may increase the action of antiplatelet agents, anticoagulants, lithium, methotrexate, haloperidol, potassium-sparing diuretics, quinolone antibiotics, salicylates, tacrolimus, tenofovir, vitamin K antagonists, and several other drugs. The levels of naproxen may be increased by angiotensin-converting enzyme (ACE) inhibitors, angiotensin II receptor blockers (ARBs), tricyclic antidepressants, cyclosporine, ketorolac, omega-3 fatty acids, proserotonergic agents, and several other drugs.

Anticholinergic Agents

Ipratropium bromide (Atrovent) nasal spray is available at concentrations of 0.03% and 0.06% and has been recommended for rhinorrhea associated with the common cold. This agent has not shown consistent benefit for the alleviation of nasal congestion or sneezing (Fokkens et al., 2012).

Mechanism of Action

Local application of anticholinergic agents to the nasal mucosa inhibits vagally mediated reflexes by antagonizing the action of acetylcholine at the cholinergic receptor, thereby inhibiting secretions from the serous and seromucous glands lining the nasal mucosa. The result is a decrease in nasal discharge and rhinorrhea.

Dosage

Adults greater than 12 years of age should use the ipratropium bromide 0.06% nasal spray at a dose of 2 sprays per nostril three to four times daily. Children who are 5 to 11 years of age can use the 0.06% solution at a dose of 2 sprays in each nostril three times daily. The safety and efficacy of use beyond 4 days for patients with the common cold has not been established.

Time Frame for Response

The onset of action for these products is 30 to 60 minutes.

Contraindications

Ipratropium bromide is contraindicated in patients with hypersensitivity to any component of the formulation, including atropine or its derivatives. Caution should be used in patients with narrow-angle glaucoma, prostatic hyperplasia, or bladder neck obstruction.

Adverse Events

Adverse effects include headache, epistaxis, pharyngitis, and nasal dryness.

Interactions

There are no known drug interactions.

Antihistamines

Antihistamines should not be recommended as monotherapy for the treatment of cough and other cold symptoms, as they are ineffective. Antihistamine-induced dryness may even exacerbate symptoms of congestion and cause upper airway obstruction by impairing the flow of mucus. For symptoms of rhinorrhea and a feeling of fullness in the ears, first-generation antihistamines, such as diphenhydramine and chlorpheniramine, may be effective when combined with decongestants. See commentary below on combination treatments. Treatment of cough with second-generation, nonsedating antihistamines, such as loratadine (Claritin) and cetirizine (Zyrtec), is ineffective and should not be recommended (Pratter, 2006). Antihistamines are discussed further in Chapter 48.

Mechanism of Action

Antihistamines are theorized to block the release of histamine from mast cells and basophils in the nasal passageways that is activated by cold virus inoculation. This release of histamine may result in the sneezing symptom that affects patients during the course of a common cold. Antihistamines competitively antagonize histamine at the H1 receptor, and first-generation antihistamines also competitively antagonize acetylcholine activity at the neuronal muscarinic receptors.

Dosage

Antihistamines are not recommended for symptoms of the common cold in children less than 12 years of age. Diphenhydramine can be given at a dose of 25 to 50 mg every 4 to 6 hours, to a maximum of 300 mg daily. IR preparations of chlorpheniramine can be given at a dose of 4 mg every 4 to 6 hours, and ER preparations can be given at a dose of 12 mg every 12 hours. The total daily dose of chlorpheniramine should not exceed 24 mg.

Time Frame for Response

The onset of action for first-generation antihistamines is typically 30 to 60 minutes.

Contraindications

Diphenhydramine should not be used in patients with hypersensitivity, in patients who are breast-feeding, and in neonates or premature infants. Caution should be used in patients with asthma, cardiovascular disease, increased intraocular pressure, prostatic hyperplasia, bladder neck obstruction, and thyroid dysfunction.

Chlorpheniramine is contraindicated in patients with hypersensitivity, narrow-angle glaucoma, bladder neck obstruction, symptomatic prostate hypertrophy, during acute asthma attacks, stenosing peptic ulcer, and pyloroduodenal obstruction. Use should also be avoided in newborns due to possible association with sudden infant death syndrome.

Neither first-generation antihistamine listed in this section should be used as a sedative to help a child sleep. Additionally, these agents should be used with caution in elderly patients, due to the increased risk for confusion, constipation, and dizziness.

Adverse Events

The ability of first-generation antihistamines to pass the blood–brain barrier and the impact on acetylcholine contributes to a higher incidence of anticholinergic and central nervous system ADEs, as compared to the second-generation products. These can include confusion, dizziness, drowsiness, fatigue, paradoxical excitability, nervousness, headache, sedation, blurred vision, dry mouth, hallucinations, tachycardia, and urinary retention.

Interactions

First-generation antihistamines may potentiate the effects of other sedative drugs or alcohol.

Combination Treatments

A limitless selection of combination products is available for the alleviation of cough and cold symptoms. These products can often be difficult to recommend, as they contain multiple active ingredients, each associated with unique ADEs. If recommending one of these products, it is important to ensure that there is an indication for each active ingredient, to avoid overmedicating the patient. Additionally, individual symptoms may last for varying durations; therefore, even if the patient initially presented with symptoms matching each ingredient, they may be overmedicating at some point during the course of their illness if some symptoms persist longer than others. For example, congestion may predominate in the first few days, but a cough may last for up to 2 weeks. If a patient purchases products that each contain only one active ingredient, they have increased flexibility in medicating specific symptoms for the appropriate amount of time.

For sneezing, rhinorrhea, acute cough, and postnasal drip, a combination of decongestant and first-generation antihistamine may be effective in adult or adolescent patients. Evidence for this combination treatment is generally limited and of poor quality; therefore, clinically significant benefits are difficult to conclude. The benefit of symptomatic relief should be weighed against the risk for adverse effects. This combination has not proven effective in children under the age of 12 (Fokkens et al., 2012).

Several products also combine expectorants and antitussives. This combination is not recommended, as the ingredients are associated with opposing mechanisms. As stated previously, expectorants increase respiratory tract fluid output, while antitussives diminish the cough reflex.

Selecting the Most Appropriate Agent

Because symptoms of a cold are manifested individually or in combination, not everyone will present with the same signs and symptoms. Therefore, the therapeutic approach involves treatment of symptoms as specifically as possible (**Figure 24.1**).

First-Line Therapy

Initial therapy consists of symptom relief. For nasal obstruction and rhinorrhea, which are caused by secretions and increased vascular permeability with leakage of serum into the nasal mucosa, topical decongestants, such as oxymetazoline hydrochloride (Afrin) or phenylephrine hydrochloride (Neo-Synephrine), are often used for the first 3 days, when the patient feels the worst. If other symptoms are diminished but nasal obstruction remains a problem, the use of an oral decongestant, such as pseudoephedrine, or a combination decongestant and antihistamine, or an antihistamine alone may relieve symptoms and help prevent complications such as

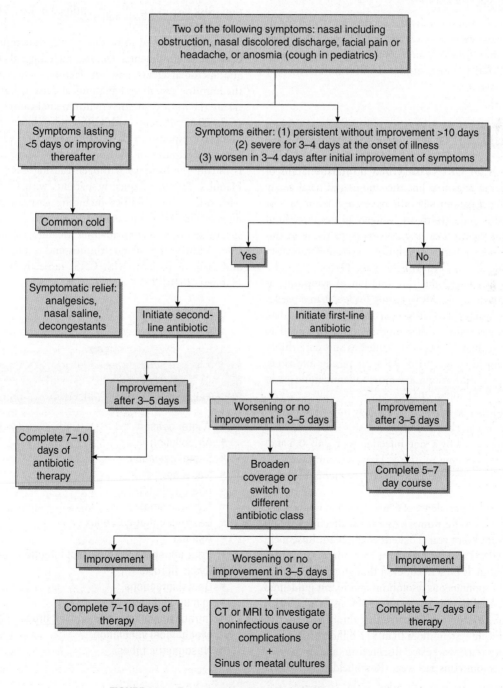

FIGURE 24.1   Treatment algorithm for the URIs: cold and sinusitis.

sinusitis and eustachian tube blockage. Anti-inflammatories, such as naproxen, may be recommended to relieve aches and discomfort.

Second-Line Therapy

Second-line therapy may be instituted if first-line therapy fails to relieve symptoms or if complications, such as secondary infection (ear infections, sinusitis, bronchitis, or pneumonia), develop. The therapy should be specific to the disorder.

MONITORING PATIENT RESPONSE

Patient response is monitored by the decrease of symptoms. If symptoms decrease without onset of complications, then therapy was successful. If the common cold does not improve in 8 to 10 days, a bacterial cause is suspected and antibiotic therapy should be considered.

RHINOSINUSITIS

Rhinosinusitis is an URI characterized by inflammation of the mucous membranes that line the sinuses and nasal cavity causing nasal blockage, purulent discharge, and facial pain or pressure. Sinusitis and rhinitis are unlikely to occur without inflammation of the nasal cavity membranes, so the term rhinosinusitis provides a better description of the inflammatory disease involving the URI (Rosenfield et al., 2015).

Rhinosinusitis is classified by duration of symptoms as either acute rhinosinusitis (ARS), lasting for less than 4 weeks, or chronic rhinosinusitis (CRS), persisting for more than 12 weeks. Rhinosinusitis with symptoms lasting more than 4 weeks and less than 12 weeks is defined as subacute rhinosinusitis (Rosenfield et al., 2015). ARS is typically infectious, whereas CRS is less infectious and more inflammatory mediated (Dykewicz & Hamilas, 2010).

ARS can further be stratified by etiology into viral rhinosinusitis (AVRS) or acute bacterial rhinosinusitis (ABRS). ARS is more frequently caused by a viral infection with only 0.5% to 2% of AVRS transitioning to ABRS. However, antibiotics are prescribed in 85% to 98% of ARS cases (Dykewicz & Hamilas, 2010).

ARS has a global prevalence of 6% to 15% and is one of the most common reasons for primary care visits, affecting over 30 million Americans every year (Fokkens et al., 2014; Rosenfield et al., 2015). ARS is also the fifth most common diagnosis for which an antibiotic is prescribed, even though there is consistent evidence of spontaneous resolutions and recent guidelines recommend restricting antibiotic use (Fokkens et al., 2014; Rosenfield et al., 2015). It is estimated that rhinosinusitis costs the U.S. health care system more than $11 billion on medications, laboratory tests, workplace absenteeism, and outpatient and emergency room visits each year (Rosenfield et al., 2015).

CAUSES

Most cases of AVRS can be attributed to respiratory viruses including rhinovirus, influenza, and parainfluenza virus. The most common pathogens involved in ABRS include *Streptococcus pneumoniae*, *Haemophilus influenzae*, and *Moraxella catarrhalis*, with the latter being the most common pathogen in pediatric cases (Dykewicz & Hamilas, 2010). Most healthy persons harbor bacteria in their URIs with no problems until the bodily defenses are weakened or drainage from the sinuses is blocked by a cold or other viral infection. Then, bacteria that may have been living harmlessly in the nose can multiply and invade the sinuses, causing a secondary infection. Risk factors for ARS are outlined in **Box 24.1** (Anselmo-Lima & Sakana, 2015).

CRS is believed to be due to a dysfunctional interaction between environmental factors, including allergens, toxins, and microbial agents, and host factors, such as a deficiency of the immune system and anatomical defects. Fungi and bacteria are the most common environmental causes of CRS (Lam et al., 2015). Patients with CRS tend to have a higher immunological response to the *Alternaria* species, which is a fungi commonly found in the sinus mucus. *Staphylococcus aureus* is usually the bacterial pathogen causing CRS (Dykewicz & Hamilas, 2010). Frequently, patients with CRS will present with other comorbidities including gastroesophageal reflux disease, defects in mucociliary clearance (as in cystic fibrosis), or anatomical abnormalities including nasal septal deviation. Additionally, allergic rhinitis and asthma occur in 60% and 20% of patients with CRS, respectively (Dykewicz & Hamilas, 2010).

> **BOX 24.1** **Selected Risk Factors for ARS**
>
> - Winter season
> - Air pollution
> - Septal deviation
> - Nasal polyps
> - Allergic rhinitis
> - Tobacco smoke
> - Gastroesophageal reflux
> - Asthma
> - Prior upper respiratory tract infection
> - Cystic fibrosis
> - Dental infections
> - Immunodeficiency
> - Intranasal medications or illicit drugs
> - Mechanical ventilation
> - Nasogastric tubes

PATHOPHYSIOLOGY

There are four paired, air-filled cavities that make up the sinuses. Small tubular openings called the sinus ostia connect the sinus cavities and facilitate drainage of the sinuses into the nasal cavity using ciliated cells. Proper sinus functioning requires motile cilia, unobstructed ostia, and mucus of a low viscosity that allows transport (Dykewicz & Hamilas, 2010). The nose reacts to the viral invasion by increasing production of mucus and sending white blood cells to the lining of the nasal passage, which causes inflammation. This inflammation results in dysfunctional cilia, obstruction of the ostia, or both. Blocked sinuses provide an ideal environment for bacterial growth, which can lead to a secondary bacterial infection. Air trapped within a blocked sinus, along with pus or other secretions, can increase pressure on the sinus wall. The result is sinus pain, which can sometimes be intense. Similarly, when a swollen membrane prevents air from entering a paranasal sinus cavity, a vacuum can form, causing additional pain.

DIAGNOSTIC CRITERIA

The diagnosis of ARS in adults at primary health care levels is based on the presence of two or more of the following hallmark symptoms: nasal congestion, nasal discharge, facial pain or headache, and anosmia (loss of smell). For pediatric patients, cough replaces decreased sense of smell as one of the four hallmark symptoms. Additionally, a patient may present with painful swallowing, cough, ear pressure, fever, and fatigue (Anselmo-Lima & Sakana, 2015). The clinical presentation of AVRS and ABRS is very similar and therefore difficult to differentiate based on symptoms alone. Therefore, practitioners need to rely on symptom severity, duration, and nature to differentiate between AVRS and ABRS (Fokkens et al., 2014). The European Respiratory Society/European Academy of Allergy and Clinical Immunology rhinosinusitis guidelines characterize ABRS if three of the hallmark symptoms previously mentioned are present (Fokkens et al., 2012). The Infectious Disease Society of America (IDSA) has identified three clinical features to distinguish patients who have ABRS versus AVRS: (1) symptoms persistent greater than 10 days from onset without any clinical improvement, (2) severe symptoms or an elevated temperature (≥102°F) and either facial pain or purulent nasal discharge lasting for 3 to 4 consecutive days at the onset of illness, and (3) symptoms worsen (fever, headache, or increased nasal discharge) following a typical viral URI that lasted 5 to 6 days after an initial improvement of symptoms (Chow, 2012). Radiographic imaging in ARS is not recommended (Rosenfield et al., 2015).

Diagnostic tests such as nasal endoscopy or computerized tomography (CT) scan should be used to diagnose CRS. However, diagnosis in most patients is based on the presence of two or more hallmark symptoms lasting longer than 12 weeks.

INITIATING DRUG THERAPY

Primarily specialists manage CRS; therefore, ARS will be the focus of this section. Before initiating drug therapy, it is critical to determine the etiology of ARS because antibiotic therapy is inappropriate to prescribe for patients with AVRS. For both AVRS and ABRS, it is recommended to provide the patient with symptomatic relief including analgesics, topical intranasal steroids, and/or nasal saline irrigation. For patients meeting diagnosis criteria for ABRS as previously described, practitioners should either offer watchful waiting or treat with antibiotics.

While weighing these choices, the practitioner should consider a few points. The first is the ability for the patient to follow up when choosing the watchful waiting option (Rosenfield et al., 2015). Another consideration when deciding whether or not to initiate antibiotics is that systematic reviews have demonstrated that antibiotics did not provide benefits in uncomplicated ARS and only reduced length of disease by less than half a day (Fokkens et al., 2014). This evidence should be weighed against the risk of adverse effects with antibiotics and antibiotic resistance before prescribing antibiotics for ABRS. The need for a specialist referral should also be contemplated when considering drug therapy. Reasons to refer may include mental status changes, visual disturbances, immunosuppressive illness, anatomic defects, unilateral findings, recurrent URI, or a history of antibiotic resistance (Chow et al., 2012).

The recommended length of therapy for uncomplicated ABRS in adults is 5 to 7 days, whereas treatment duration in children should be 10 to 14 days (Chow et al., 2012).

Goals of Drug Therapy

The primary treatment goal is to restore sinuses to health. Other goals include decreasing the duration and severity of symptoms, promoting appropriate use of antibiotic treatment, preventing complications and the progression from acute illness to chronic disease, and preventing the transmission of illness to other people.

Antibiotics

Obtaining cultures is only recommended for patients who do not respond to first- or second-line treatment; therefore, management strategies will focus on the empiric treatment of ABRS. Guidelines no longer recommend the regular use of macrolides, third-generation cephalosporins, or trimethoprim–sulfamethoxazole (Bactrim) for empiric treatment due to their high resistance rates with *S. pneumoniae*.

Amoxicillin and Amoxicillin–Clavulanate
Mechanism of Action

Amoxicillin, a beta-lactam antibiotic, inhibits synthesis of the bacterial cell wall by binding to one or more of the penicillin-binding proteins causing the bacteria to lyse. Adding clavulanate to amoxicillin expands its spectrum of activity by inhibiting beta-lactamases that inactivate amoxicillin.

Dosage

Amoxicillin–clavulanate (Augmentin) is dosed based on the amoxicillin component and is available in 250-, 500-, or 875-mg IR oral tablets and 1,000-mg ER tablets. Amoxicillin–clavulanate is also available in a 125, 250, 200 or 400 mg/5 mL suspension and 200- or 400-mg chewable tablets. For adults or adolescents weighing greater than 40 kg, a dose of 500 mg every 8 hours or 875 mg every 12 hours should be given. Infants less than 3 months old should be given 30 mg/kg/d every 12 hours. Children aged 3 months to adolescents weighing less than 40 kg should be given 20 mg/kg/d every 8 hours or 25 mg/kg/d every 12 hours for mild infections. For severe infections in this pediatric population, a dose of 40 mg/kg/d every 8 hours or 45 mg/kg/d every 12 hours should be prescribed. "High-dose" amoxicillin consists of 2,000 mg every 12 hours and should be reserved for children and adults with ABRS from regions with high endemic rates of resistant *S. pneumoniae*, those with severe infection, children in daycare, patients of ages less than 2 or greater than 65, immunosuppressed individuals, and those with a recent hospitalization or antibiotic use within the past month. For patients with a CrCl of 10 to 30 mL/min or less than 10 mL/min, the recommended dose is 250 to 500 mg every 12 hours and 250 to 500 mg every 24 hours, respectively. No dose adjustments are required in hepatic impairment.

Contraindications

Amoxicillin is contraindicated in patients who have a history of an allergic reaction to beta-lactam antibiotics or any component of the formulation (e.g., penicillins, cephalosporins), cholestatic jaundice, or hepatic dysfunction. The ER formulation of amoxicillin–clavulanate has an additional contraindication for use in patients with a CrCl of less than 30 mL/min or those on hemodialysis.

Adverse Events

Diarrhea is the most frequent ADE that patients experience while taking amoxicillin. Other common ADEs include rash or hives, nausea, vomiting, photosensitivity, and vaginal infections.

Interactions

Amoxicillin may increase levels of methotrexate and warfarin and can decrease the effects of mycophenolate and the typhoid vaccine, and therefore, patients should be monitored accordingly. Concurrent use of probenecid and amoxicillin should be avoided as probenecid may increase the levels of amoxicillin. Tetracyclines may reduce the effect of amoxicillin and should also be avoided. Additionally, caution is warranted in patients taking allopurinol because they may have an increased risk of allergic reaction to amoxicillin.

Doxycycline

Mechanism of Action

Doxycycline (Oracea, Vibramycin), a tetracycline antibiotic, binds with the 30S and possibly the 50S ribosomal subunit(s) of the bacteria, which inhibits protein synthesis resulting in bacteriostatic effects.

Dosage

Doxycycline has an off-label use to treat ABRS at a dose of 200 mg daily in one to two divided doses for adults and children older than 8 years of age and weighing greater than 45 kg. It is available in 50-, 75-, 100-, or 150-mg capsules or tablets; 40-mg delayed-release capsules; and 25 or 50 mg/5 mL suspensions. In children older than 8 years of age weighing less than or equal to 45 kg, the dose is 2 to 5 mg/kg/d in one to two divided doses. Doxycycline is not recommended for children 8 years and younger. No dose adjustments are necessary in hepatic or renal impairment.

Contraindications

The only contraindication is a hypersensitivity to tetracyclines or any component of the formulation.

Adverse Events

Although GI ADEs such as nausea, vomiting, diarrhea, and abdominal pain are common ADEs of doxycycline, diarrhea occurs less frequently than with amoxicillin. Other common ADEs include vaginal infections, headache, and rash. Stevens-Johnson syndrome and hepatotoxicity are rare but serious ADEs associated with doxycycline.

Interactions

Antacids, lanthanum, bismuth subsalicylate, sucralfate, bile acid sequestrants, calcium, multivitamins, and quinapril can lower the absorption or concentration of tetracyclines and should be given 2 hours prior or 6 hours after doxycycline. Iron salts may decrease the levels of doxycycline and vice versa, so therapy can be modified to ferrous gluconate, which does not have this interaction. The following medications should be used with caution because of their effect on reducing doxycycline levels: barbiturates, carbamazepine, fosphenytoin, phenytoin, and rifampin. Doxycycline should be avoided in patients on retinoic acid derivatives due to increased risk of ADEs and toxicity as well as neuromuscular blocking agents due to enhanced neuromuscular blocking effects. Furthermore, chronic alcohol consumption and food or milk reduce the serum levels of doxycycline. Patients on warfarin should be monitored closely while on tetracyclines as they may increase the risk of bleeding.

Levofloxacin and Moxifloxacin

Mechanism of Action

Fluoroquinolone antibiotics such as levofloxacin (Levaquin) and moxifloxacin (Avelox) inhibit topoisomerase IV and DNA gyrase, which are essential enzymes that maintain the superhelical structure of DNA and are required for DNA replication and transcription, repair, recombination, and transposition.

Dosage

Levofloxacin is available in the following oral preparations: 25 mg/mL suspension and 250-, 500-, or 750-mg tablets. Recommended dosing of levofloxacin in adults is 500 to 750 mg every 24 hours for 5 to 7 days. Levofloxacin can be used off-label for pediatrics and should be dosed 10 to 20 mg/kg/d every 12 to 24 hours. Patients with a CrCl of 20 to 49 mL/min should be prescribed a 500-mg loading dose followed by 250 mg every 24 hours or 750 mg every 48 hours. Patients with a CrCl of 10 to 19 mL/min or on hemodialysis should be prescribed a 500-mg loading dose followed by 250 mg every 48 hours or a loading dose of 750 mg followed by 500 mg every 48 hours. Hepatic dosing adjustments are not required. Moxifloxacin is recommended for adults at a dose of 400 mg every 24 hours and should not be used in children. It is available in the following oral formulations: 400 mg/250 mL solution or 400-mg tablet.

Contraindications

The only contraindication is a hypersensitivity to quinolones or any component of the formulation.

Adverse Events

The most common ADEs with fluoroquinolones are GI disturbances such as nausea, diarrhea, constipation, abdominal pain, vomiting, and dyspepsia. Less common ADEs such as rash, headache, chest pain, decreased blood glucose, edema, photosensitivity, and vaginal infections can occur. A rare but serious ADE of fluoroquinolones involves exacerbations of myasthenia gravis; therefore, this medication should be avoided in patients with this disease. Fluoroquinolones also have a black box warning for tendon inflammation and rupture, so they should be avoided in patients older than 60 years of age, who are taking concurrent corticosteroids, or have had a solid organ transplant.

Interactions

Antacids, lanthanum, sucralfate, calcium, sevelamer, didanosine, multivitamins, quinapril, and magnesium, iron, and zinc salts can lower the absorption or concentration of fluoroquinolones and should be given 2 hours prior or 6 hours after doxycycline. Fluoroquinolones may also prolong the QTc interval; therefore, caution should be used with other medications that can prolong the QTc interval. Fluoroquinolones can also interact with antidiabetic agents resulting in poor blood glucose control. The use of corticosteroids and fluoroquinolones is not recommended due to the increased risk of ruptured Achilles tendon. Patients on warfarin should be monitored closely while on fluoroquinolones as they may increase the risk of bleeding.

Clindamycin

Mechanism of Action

Clindamycin (Cleocin), a lincosamide antibiotic, reversibly binds to 50S ribosomal subunits preventing the formation of a peptide bond, which in turn inhibits bacterial protein synthesis. Depending upon drug concentration, infection site, and organism, this action results in bacteriostatic or bactericidal effects.

Dosage

Since the use of clindamycin is only recommended in pediatric patients after failing initial therapy or in those with an increased risk of antibiotic resistance, only pediatric dosing will be discussed. Clindamycin is available in 75- or 150-mg oral capsules and 75 mg/5 mL solution and should be dosed at 30 to 40 mg/kg/d divided every 8 hours. Clindamycin is only recommended with concomitant use of cefpodoxime or cefixime for 10 to 14 days (Chow et al., 2012).

Contraindications

The only contraindication is a hypersensitivity to lincosamide antibiotics or any component of the formulation.

Adverse Events

Common ADEs include diarrhea, nausea, vomiting, and abdominal pain.

Interactions

Lincosamide antibiotics may enhance the neuromuscular-blocking effects of neuromuscular-blocking agents and should be avoided.

Cefpodoxime and Cefixime

Mechanism of Action

Cefpodoxime (Vantin) and cefixime (Suprax), third-generation cephalosporin antibiotics, inhibit synthesis of the bacterial cell wall by binding to one or more of the penicillin-binding proteins, causing the bacteria to lyse.

Dosage

Since the use of third-generation cephalosporins is only recommended in pediatric patients after failing initial therapy or in those with an increased risk of antibiotic resistance, only pediatric dosing will be discussed. Recommended dosing of cefpodoxime for children older than 2 months but less than 12 years of age is 5 mg/kg/d and 200 mg every 12 hours for children 12 years and older. Cefpodoxime is available in 50 or 100 mg/5 mL suspensions or 100- or 200-mg oral tablets. Recommended dosing of cefixime for children older than 6 months but less than 12 years of age is 8 mg/kg/d divided every 12 hours and 400 mg divided every 12 to 24 hours for children 12 years and older. Cefixime is available in 400-mg oral capsules and tablets, 100- or 200-mg chewable tablets, as well as in 100, 200, and 500 mg/5 mL suspensions. Both agents must be used in combination with clindamycin for 10 to 14 days (Chow et al., 2012).

Contraindications

The only contraindication is a hypersensitivity to cephalosporins or any component of the formulation.

Adverse Events

Diaper rash and diarrhea are the most common ADEs associated with third-generation cephalosporins. Other common ADEs include nausea, vomiting, abdominal pain, and headache.

Interactions

Cephalosporins may increase the nephrotoxic effect of aminoglycosides and should be monitored with concurrent use. Antacids and histamine-2 receptor antagonists may decrease the absorption of cephalosporins and therefore their dosing should be separated by 2 hours. Additionally, effects of warfarin may be enhanced when taken concurrently with cephalosporins, so patients should be monitored more carefully.

Symptomatic Therapy

Nonpharmacologic therapies include the following: adequate rest and hydration, elevating the head of the bed while sleeping, use of a humidifier, and avoidance of environmental factors such as allergens, cigarette smoke, and pollution (Peters et al., 2014). Unlike the common cold, topical or oral decongestants or antihistamines should not be used as adjunctive treatment in ABRS (Chow et al., 2012). Intranasal corticosteroids are recommended as adjunctive treatment, particularly in patients with a history of allergic rhinitis (see Chapter 48) (Chow et al., 2012). Even though there is minimal clinical evidence supporting the benefit of nasal lavage in rhinosinusitis to improve ciliary function and reduce inflammation, it is a generally recommended treatment strategy. Surgical intervention is to be avoided in ARS and should be individualized in patients with CRS. A lack of randomized controlled trials has resulted in the absence of a gold standard technique (Anselmo-Lima & Sakana, 2015).

Selecting the Most Appropriate Agent

Due to the increasing levels of antimicrobial resistance worldwide, clinicians must re-evaluate their approaches to treating ARS by using evidence-based methods of diagnosis and treatment. As mentioned previously, it is imperative to differentiate AVRS from ABRS. When ABRS pathogen is suspected or diagnosed, antibiotics may not always be the optimal choice; therefore, patients need to be educated regarding the appropriate initial treatment regimens. When prescribing antibiotics, the provider should consider cost, formulation, whether the patient is at risk for resistant bacteria (**Box 24.2**), and if the patient can be compliant with the selected regimen.

First-Line Therapy

Amoxicillin–clavulanate is preferred over amoxicillin for ABRS in adults and children. For penicillin-allergic adults, doxycycline, levofloxacin, or moxifloxacin should be used. Levofloxacin is the antibiotic of choice in children with a penicillin allergy.

> **BOX 24.2   Risk Factors for Antibiotic Resistance**
>
> - Age <2 or >65
> - Child in daycare
> - Prior antibiotics in the past month
> - Comorbidities
> - Immunocompromised

Second-Line Therapy

Second-line agents for patients include doxycycline (not recommended for most children), levofloxacin, or moxifloxacin. Combination therapy with clindamycin and a third-generation oral cephalosporin such as cefixime or cefpodoxime is an alternative treatment for children with a penicillin allergy.

MONITORING PATIENT RESPONSE

Patients should notice relief within 48 to 72 hours. If there is no relief of symptoms in 3 to 5 days or symptoms worsen after 48 to 72 hours of treatment, an alternative antibiotic should be selected. It is recommended that patients who fail to respond to first- or second-line treatment should have cultures collected via direct sinus aspiration rather than nasopharyngeal swab. Alternatively, endoscopically guided cultures of the middle meatus could be taken in adults; however, the integrity of this option in pediatric patients has not been established. CT, which is preferred over magnetic resonance imaging, may also be necessary to investigate noninfectious causes (Chow et al., 2012). Once an uncomplicated episode of ARS resolves, there is no further evaluation required (Peters et al., 2014).

PATIENT EDUCATION

The role of the practitioner is to make the patient aware not only of appropriate symptom management but also of prevention. It is essential that patients understand that symptoms of viral and bacterial URIs are similar, that viral URIs and allergies are more prevalent than bacterial URIs, and that antibiotics are not appropriate to treat viral URIs. Education about the importance of completing the full course of antibiotics, should they be prescribed, despite symptoms subsiding in 48 to 72 hours is also imperative. The patient also needs to know how to recognize and respond to ADEs of antibiotic therapy, especially because allergic reactions are more prevalent with these drugs than other drug classes.

Education needs to begin before cold and flu season so that patients can take steps to prevent disease and to make educated decisions on whether a health care visit is needed or whether the symptoms are likely to be self-limiting. Progress toward the development of vaccines to prevent viral URIs has been difficult due to the abundance of existing viral serotypes (Jacobs et al., 2013). Approved prophylactic antiviral therapies do not currently exist; therefore, prevention consists of behavioral modifications.

Drug Information

The ACCP published an evidence-based clinical practice guideline on cough and the common cold (Irwin et al., 2006). The National Institute for Health and Clinical Excellence (NICE) published a guideline using evidence from randomized placebo-controlled trials in 2008 regarding the prescribing of antibiotics for self-limiting respiratory tract infections in adults and children in primary care (Centre for Clinical Practice, 2008). This document describes evidence from randomized placebo-controlled trials that demonstrate the limited efficacy of antibiotics in the treatment of most respiratory tract infections, including acute otitis media (AOM), acute cough/ bronchitis, acute sore throat/pharyngitis/tonsillitis, ARS, and the common cold. In 2012, the Infectious Disease Society of America published a Clinical Practice Guideline for Acute Bacterial Rhinosinusitis in Children and Adults (Chow et al., 2012). Additionally in 2012, there was a European Position Paper on Rhinosinusitis and Nasal Polyps (Fokkens et al., 2012). A common theme found in all of these guidelines was to use caution regarding the inappropriate prescribing of antibiotics, which may contribute to drug-related adverse events and an increase in antibiotic-resistant organisms.

Patient-Oriented Information Sources

The American Academy of Family Physicians, American Rhinologic Society, Cleveland Clinic, Mayo Clinic, and Centers for Disease Control and Prevention are organizations that provide patient-oriented information on their Web sites. Another helpful Web site for patient-oriented information resources is www.medicine.net.

Lifestyle Changes

The most important aspect of patient education is to prevent contraction of the virus by practicing good hygiene, such as frequent hand washing, getting adequate sleep and exercise, and avoiding contact with infected people. One study found hand sanitizers containing ethanol to be significantly more effective than hand washing with soap and water (Turner et al., 2010). It is important to consider that hand washing by any method is effective, even without antiseptic. Social distancing can involve avoidance of crowded public spaces or the temporary closing of schools or day cares. Since these strategies can be difficult to execute, utilization of surgical respiratory masks may be a more feasible approach, particularly in health care settings. Another important aspect of patient education is teaching patients to prevent spreading the virus through correct tissue disposal, hand washing, covering the mouth when coughing, and so on.

For persons prone to ARS, it may be uncomfortable to swim in pools treated with chlorine, because it irritates the lining of the nose and sinuses. Divers often get sinus congestion and infection when water is forced into the sinuses from the nasal passages. Air travel may also pose a problem for persons with ARS or CRS. As the air pressure in a plane is reduced, pressure can build up in the head, blocking sinuses or eustachian tubes. The patient may feel discomfort in the sinus or middle ear during ascent or descent of the airplane.

Alternative Therapies

There is a growing interest in alternative or complementary therapies for treating the common cold. A review of complementary and alternative medicine for the prevention and

treatment of the common cold was published in *Canadian Family Physician* in 2011 (Nahas & Balla, 2011). *Echinacea angustifolia*, *Echinacea pallida*, and *Echinacea purpurea* have all been studied, but *E. purpurea* is associated with the most evidence. These products have been investigated for their effects in increasing and enhancing many immune processes, including macrophage activation, cytokine production, phagocytosis, natural killer cell activity, lymphocyte and monocyte production, and antibody response. Among conducted studies, there is a high degree of variability in the species, plant parts, and method of extraction that have been used. Therefore, despite a moderate level of evidence supporting the use of *E. purpurea* for the treatment of the common cold, it is challenging to recommend specific product formulations or doses. The use of these products for the prevention of cold symptoms has not shown benefit. *Echinacea* products are available in a variety of preparations, including a crude extract at a daily dose of 2,000 to 3,000 mg, a pressed juice at a daily dose of 6 to 9 mL, and a tincture at a daily dose of 0.75 to 1.5 mL. Use should be avoided in patients who are allergic to *Echinacea* or members of the Asteraceae or Compositae families, including chrysanthemums, daisies, marigolds, and ragweed. Caution should also be used in patients with asthma and seasonal allergies, as they may have a higher risk of experiencing allergic reactions. Adverse effects include hives, rash, itching, GI upset, and headache. There are no known drug interactions.

Panax ginseng (Asian ginseng) and *Panax quinquefolius* (North American ginseng) have been studied for the stimulation of macrophages, natural killer cells, and lymphocytes, as well as for increased production of cytokines and antibodies. Data to support the use of ginseng for the prevention or treatment of the common cold are limited and conflicting; therefore, use of these products is not recommended. Side effects include headache, GI upset, anxiety, and insomnia. Drug interactions include phenelzine, involving the induction of mania; warfarin, involving an increase in international normalized ratio (INR); and alcohol, involving increased blood clearance. These products should not be used by pregnant or breast-feeding patients, due to the risk of estrogenic effects and teratogenicity.

Vitamin C has been a focus of several studies related to the common cold, due to its antioxidant properties, its impact on glutathione regeneration, and its theoretical ability to activate neutrophils and monocytes. Studies have implemented a wide range of doses and have explored the use of this product in both the prevention and treatment of the common cold. An interesting finding involves the potential reduction of colds in study participants who were exposed to subarctic cold or intense physical activity. Patients taking doses of 200 to 2,000 mg daily of vitamin C had half as many colds as those taking placebo, according to a small group of trials studying a total of 642 patients (Nahas & Balla, 2011). Based on the review of many studies, vitamin C can be recommended at a dose of at least 1 g/d for the prevention of colds and may also reduce the duration of symptoms by 1 to 2 days.

Allium sativum, or allicin, is found in garlic and is activated upon chopping or chewing. It is inactivated when cooked. It has been studied for its antiviral properties against HRVs. Evidence supporting the use of this product for the prevention of the common cold is limited, but it can be recommended at a dose of 180 mg of allicin. The use of fresh garlic is not reasonable, as each clove contains approximately 5 to 9 mg of allicin. Odor-free formulations are ineffective, as these do not contain allicin. The most common ADE is malodorous belching. Evidence does not support the use of this product for treatment.

Probiotics have been investigated for their role in the improvement of mucosal barrier function, GI microflora, and gut-associated lymphoid tissue. They may also interfere with toxin and cell binding sites. Current literature does not support the use of these products for the prevention or treatment of the common cold.

Several trials have studied zinc, due to a proposed mechanism involving the interference with rhinovirus protein cleavage or the disruption of capsid binding to adhesion molecules in the epithelium of the nasal passageways. Results have been variable, but several studies have demonstrated the potential for these products to shorten the duration and severity of cold symptoms. The difficulty exists in selecting the appropriate dose and proper formulation. Lozenges that contain at least 13 mg of elemental zinc can be recommended for use every 2 hours at the immediate onset of cold symptoms. ADEs include bitter taste and nausea. Intranasal zinc should not be used due to its potential association with anosmia. Use of zinc for 6 to 8 weeks may contribute to copper deficiency.

In ARS and CRS, complementary or alternative medicines have also been considerably utilized. Similarly to the common cold, evidence-based recommendations are difficult to suggest due to the scarcity of randomized controlled trials. One study that included 102 patients with ARS examined the use of *Pelargonium sidoides* (*P. sidoides*) extract, a common root plant from South Africa. This study concluded that *P. sidoides* may be effective in relieving symptoms; however, some doubt exists because of a poor quality of evidence (Fokkens et al., 2012).

Myrtol, an essential oil derived from pine, lime, and eucalyptus, showed a statistically significant difference in the improvement of sinusitis symptom scores and reduced the need for an antibiotic after treatment with myrtol (Fokkens et al., 2012).

CASE STUDY*

J.M. is a 45-year-old female with past medical history of controlled hypertension, controlled asthma, and eczema. She has a 4-day history of nasal congestion, headache, sore throat, sneezing, and productive cough. She denies fever, nausea, vomiting, and myalgias. She has three children who recently went back to school following a summer vacation. No one else in her household is currently presenting with similar symptoms. She has no known drug allergies but is allergic to mums and ragweed. She calls her primary care provider's office requesting a medication to treat her illness.

She takes several medications, including the following:

- Mometasone 220 mcg—1 puff daily for asthma
- Albuterol 90 mcg—1 to 2 puffs q4–6 hours as needed for shortness of breath
- Lisinopril 10 mg—one tablet by mouth daily for hypertension
- Oxymetazoline hydrochloride 0.05% nasal spray—2 sprays per nostril bid × 3 days

1. Which of the following is the MOST appropriate drug to recommend?
   a. Oxymetazoline hydrochloride 0.05% nasal spray—2 sprays per nostril bid until symptoms resolve
   b. Naproxen 220 mg—one tablet by mouth every 12 hours as needed until symptoms resolve
   c. Dextromethorphan ER oral liquid—60 mg every 12 hours until symptoms resolve
   d. Amoxicillin–clavulanic acid 500 mg every 8 hours for 7 days
2. Which of the following nonpharmacological therapies is NOT recommended?
   a. Steam inhalation
   b. Increased water intake
   c. Menthol lozenges
   d. Saline gargle
3. **J.M.** is insistent on taking a complementary therapy to help treat her symptoms. What is the MOST appropriate recommendation?
   a. *Echinacea purpurea* tincture—0.75 mL
   b. Fresh garlic—3 cloves
   c. Acidophilus probiotic—1 tablet daily
   d. Vitamin C—1 g

* Answers can be found online.

Bibliography

Starred references are cited in the text.

*Anselmo-Lima, W., & Sakana, E. (2015). Rhinosinusitis: Evidence and experience. *Brazilian Journal of Otorhinolaryngology, 81*, S1–S49.

*Blaiss, M. S., Dicpinigaitis, P. V., Eccles, R., et al. (2015). Consumer attitudes on cough and cold: US (ACHOO) survey results. *Current Medical Research and Opinion*, 1–12 (e-publication ahead of print).

Centre for Clinical Practice. (2008). *Respiratory tract infections—Antibiotic prescribing. Prescribing of antibiotics for self-limiting respiratory tract infections in adults and children in primary care.* London, UK: National Institute for Health and Clinical Excellence, NICE Clinical Guideline 69, 1–121.

*Chow, A. W., Benninger, M. S., Brook, I., et al. (2012). ISDA Clinical Practice Guideline for acute bacterial rhinosinusitis in children and adults. *Clinical Infectious Diseases, 54*(8), 1041–1045.

*Dicpinigaitis, P. V., Eccles, R., Blaiss, M. S., et al. (2015). Impact of cough and common cold on productivity, absenteeism, and daily life in the United States: ACHOO Survey. *Current Medical Research and Opinion*, 1–7 (e-publication ahead of print).

*Dykewicz, M., & Hamilas, D. (2010). Rhinitis and sinusitis. *Journal of Allergy and Clinical Immunology, 125*(2), S103–S115.

*Fashner, J., Ericson, K., & Werner, S. (2012). Treatment of the common cold in children and adults. *American Family Physician, 86*(2), 153–159.

*Fendrick, A. M., Monto, A. S., Nightengale, B., et al. (2003). The economic burden of non-influenza-related viral respiratory tract infection in the United States. *Archives of Internal Medicine, 163*(4), 487–494.

*Fokkens, W. J., Lund, V. J., Mullol, J., et al. (2012). European position paper on rhinosinusitis and nasal polyps 2012. *Rhinology*, Suppl. 23, 1–298.

*Fokkens, W. J., Hoffmans, R., & Thomas, M. (2014). Avoid prescribing antibiotics in acute rhinosinusitis. *British Medical Journal, 349*, 1–3.

Irwin, R. S., Baumann, M. H., Bolser, D. C., et al. (2006). Diagnosis and management of cough: ACCP evidence-based clinical practice guidelines. *Chest, 129*(Suppl. 1), 1S–23S.

*Jacobs, S. E., Lamson, D. M., St. George, K., et al. (2013). Human rhinoviruses. *Clinical Microbiology Reviews, 26*(1), 135–162.

*Lam, K., Schleimer, R., & Kern, R. (2015). The etiology and pathogenesis of chronic rhinosinusitis: A review of current hypotheses. *Current Allergy and Asthma Reports, 15*(7), 540.

*Liu, L., Johnson, H. L., Cousens, S., et al. (2012). Global, regional, and national causes of child mortality: An updated systematic analysis for 2010 with time trends since 2000. *Lancet, 379*(9832), 2151–2161.

*Nahas, R., & Balla, A. (2011). Complementary and alternative medicine for prevention and treatment of the common cold. *Canadian Family Physician, 57*(1), 31–36.

*Peters, A. T., Spector, S., Hsu, J., et.al. (2014). Diagnosis and management of rhinosinusitis: A practice parameter update. *Annals of Allergy, Asthma & Immunology, 113*, 347–385.

*Pratter, M. R. (2006). Cough and the common cold: ACCP evidence-based clinical practice guidelines. *Chest, 129*(Suppl. 1), 72S–74S.

*Rosenfield, R. M., Piccirillo, J. F., Chandrasekhar, S. S., et al. (2015). Clinical practice guideline (update): Adult sinusitis executive summary. *Otolaryngology-Head and Neck Surgery, 152*(4), 598–609.

Tam, T., Little, P., & Stokes, T. (2008). Antibiotic prescribing for self-limiting respiratory tract infections in primary care: Summary of NICE guidance. *British Medical Journal, 337*, a437.

*Turner, R. B., Fuls, J. L., & Rodgers, N. D. (2010). Effectiveness of hand sanitizers with and without organic acids for removal of rhinovirus from hands. *Antimicrobial Agents and Chemotherapy, 54*(3), 1363–1664.

*West, J. V. (2002). Acute upper airway infections. *British Medical Bulletin, 61*, 215–230.

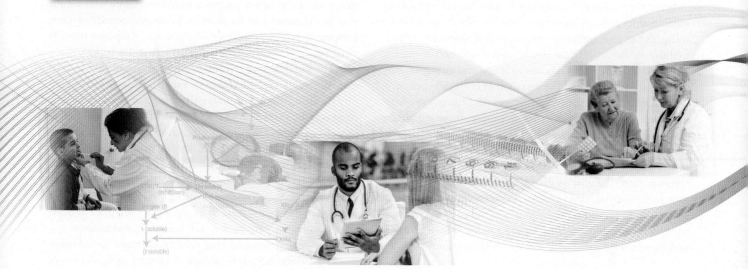

25 Asthma

Karen J. Tietze

Approximately 25.7 million people in the United States have asthma, with a prevalence of 9.5% and 7.7% in children 0 to 17 years and adults 18+ years, respectively (Moorman et al., 2012). Asthma is more common in persons below 100% of the federal poverty rate and in persons living in the northeast United States (Moorman et al., 2012). Asthma prevalence is greater in blacks than in whites (11.2% vs. 7.7%), in boys than in girls (11.1% vs. 7.8%), and in women than in men (9.7% vs. 5.7%) (Moorman et al., 2012). In 2009, asthma accounted for 10.6 million office visits, 2.1 million emergency department visits, and 479,300 hospitalizations (Moorman et al., 2012). The cost of asthma in the United States is approximately $56 billion per year (Centers for Disease Control and Prevention [CDC], 2013b). The noneconomic costs of asthma are high. Nine persons with asthma die from asthma every day and nearly one in three adults and one in two children miss 1 day or more of work or school for asthma-related reasons (CDC, 2013b).

The current National Asthma Education and Prevention Program (NAEPP) guidelines for the diagnosis and management of asthma were released in 2007 (NAEPP, 2007). The guidelines, originally developed in 1997 by an expert panel commissioned by the NAEPP Coordinating Committee of the National Heart, Lung, and Blood Institute (NHLBI) of the National Institutes of Health (NIH), were updated in 2002 and 2007. The 1993 Global Initiative for Asthma (GINA) Global Strategy for Asthma Management and Prevention report, an international collaboration of the NHLBI and the World Health Organization, is updated annually (GINA, 2014).

CAUSES

Asthma is a heterogeneous chronic inflammatory medical condition of unknown etiology. The hygiene hypothesis theorizes that a lack of exposure to a variety of microbiological agents at a young age creates a predominant T helper cell type-2 (Th2) lymphocyte immune response that is associated with allergy (Brown et al., 2013). Some genetic associations have been identified. For example, although there is no single "asthma gene," more than 100 single nucleotide polymorphisms (SNPs) of the gene that encodes the ADAM metallopeptidase domain 33 gene (ADAM33) have been identified. Smooth muscle, fibroblasts, and myofibroblasts express ADAM-related proteins with a variety of signaling, adhesion, and fusion functions that influence the epithelial–mesenchymal unit (EMTU). Additionally, more than 25 polymorphic genes expressed in the EMTU have been identified.

Common asthma phenotypes include allergic asthma, nonallergic asthma, late-onset asthma, asthma with fixed airflow limitation, and asthma with obesity. Symptom triggers include upper respiratory tract viral infections, allergens, exercise, changes in the weather, laughter, exposure to inhaled irritants (e.g., smoke, vehicle exhaust fumes, strong smells), gastroesophageal reflux disease (GERD), aspirin (in individuals sensitive to aspirin), stress, and exposure to sulfites. Hormonal changes during a woman's menstrual cycle or during pregnancy may trigger or worsen asthma symptoms.

PATHOPHYSIOLOGY

Asthma is characterized by airway narrowing and airway hyperresponsiveness. The chronic airway inflammation and structural airway changes characteristic of asthma are the result of interactions between the activated EMTU and inflammatory mediators (Holgate, 2008). Key cellular mediators include chemokines, cysteinyl leukotrienes, cytokines, histamine, nitric oxide, and prostaglandins. Sources of these mediators include airway epithelial cells, mast cells, eosinophils, and T lymphocytes. In the presence of these cellular mediators, airway smooth muscle cells proliferate, hypertrophy, and express inflammatory proteins; endothelial cells recruit circulatory inflammatory cells; and fibroblasts and myofibroblasts produce collagens and proteoglycans (components of connective tissue). Cellular mediators activate airway cholinergic nerves causing bronchoconstriction and mucous secretion and airway sensory nerves causing cough and the sensation of chest tightness.

Chronic airway structural changes, including subepithelial fibrosis, increased airway smooth muscle, increased airway wall blood vessels, increased airway epithelium goblet cells, and submucosal gland hypertrophy, are the result of airway inflammation and other mechanisms independent of airway inflammation. The airways narrow as a result of airway smooth muscle contraction, airway edema, airway wall thickening from structural changes, and mucus plugging. Airway hyperresponsiveness is caused by excessive airway smooth muscle contraction, airway wall thickening, and sensory nerve stimulation.

DIAGNOSTIC CRITERIA

The diagnosis of asthma is based on the presence of symptoms consistent with asthma and the presence of variable airflow limitation. Typical asthma symptoms include wheeze, shortness of breath, cough, and chest tightness. These symptoms are not exclusive to asthma; persons with a variety of upper and lower respiratory tract (e.g., inhaled foreign body, vocal cord dysfunction,

bronchopulmonary dysplasia, cystic fibrosis, chronic obstructive pulmonary disease) and cardiovascular (e.g., pulmonary emboli, heart failure) medical conditions have the same symptoms. Asthma symptoms and symptom severity are variable. Persons with asthma may be symptom free for short or prolonged periods of time. Symptom intensity varies from mild to severe; symptoms typically worsen at night or early morning, often waking the patient.

The physical examination is nonspecific and may be normal. Wheezing may be absent or range from soft end-expiratory wheezing to loud inspiratory and expiratory wheezing; the chest may be silent during a severe exacerbation. Nasal polyps or signs of allergic rhinitis or other atopic medical conditions such as eczema may be present. Persons with a severe asthma exacerbation may present with hunched shoulders, a preference for sitting upright, cyanosis, use of accessory respiratory muscles (abdominal, sternocleidomastoid), elevated or decreased blood pressure, tachycardia or bradycardia, tachypnea or bradypnea, an inability to speak in full sentences, and anxiety.

Spirometry measures lung volumes during a forced maximal exhalation. Airflow limitation is assessed using the forced expiratory volume in the first second (FEV_1), the total volume of exhaled air (forced vital capacity, FVC), and the FEV_1/FVC ratio. Airflow obstruction is present when the FEV_1/FVC is less than 0.70. Bronchoprovocation testing with methacholine or histamine may be performed in patients with suspected asthma who have normal baseline airflow. The current NAEPP guidelines categorize asthma severity in children older than 4 years of age and adults according to nonspirometric and spirometric criteria (**Tables 25.1** and **25.2**). Children 0 to 4 years of age are

---

TABLE 25.1

Asthma Severity—Chronic Disease Classification (Age 12 Years and Older)

Severity Components	Intermittent Step 1	Mild Persistent Step 2	Moderate Persistent Step 3 and Step 4	Severe Persistent Step 5 and Step 6
Symptoms	2 or fewer days per week	More than 2 days per week but not daily	Daily	Throughout the day
Nighttime awakenings	2 or fewer nights per month	3 to 4 nights per month	More than 1 night per week but not nightly	Often 7 nights per week
Short-acting beta$_2$-adrenergic agonist use for symptom control	2 or fewer days per week	More than 2 days per week but not more than one time per day	Daily	Several times per day
Interference with normal activity	None	Minor limitation	Some limitation	Extremely limited
Exacerbations requiring systemic corticosteroids	0–1 per year	2 or more per year	2 or more per year	2 or more per year
Lung function Normal FEV_1/FVC: 8–19 y: 85% 20–39 y: 75% 40–59 y: 75% 60–80 y: 70%	Normal FEV_1 between exacerbations $FEV_1 \geq 80\%$ predicted FEV_1/FVC normal	$FEV_1 \geq 80\%$ predicted FEV_1/FVC normal	$FEV_1 > 60\%$ but $< 80\%$ predicted FEV_1/FVC reduced 5%	$FEV_1 < 60\%$ predicted FEV_1/FVC reduced $> 5\%$

Severity is determined by the most severe category for any feature.
FEV_1, forced expiratory volume in 1 second; FVC, forced vital capacity.
From National Asthma Education and Prevention Program, National Heart, Lung and Blood Institute, National Institutes of Health. 2007 *Expert Panel Report III: Guidelines for the diagnosis and management of asthma.* Bethesda, MD: U.S. Department of Health and Human Services. Originally published July 2007. Revised 2002, August 2007. NIH Publication No. 07-4051. Retrieved from http://www.nhlbi.nih.gov/files/docs/guidelines/asthgdln.pdf

TABLE 25.2

Asthma Severity—Chronic Disease Classification (Children 5–11 Years of Age)

Severity Components	Intermittent	Mild Persistent	Moderate Persistent	Severe Persistent
Symptoms	2 or fewer days per week	More than 2 days per week but not daily	Daily	Throughout the day
Nighttime awakenings	2 or fewer nights per month	3 to 4 nights per month	More than 1 night per week but not nightly	Often 7 times per week
Short-acting beta$_2$-adrenergic agonist use for symptom control	2 or fewer days per week	More than 2 days per week but not daily	Daily	Several times per day
Interference with normal activity	None	Minor limitation	Some limitation	Extremely limited
Exacerbations requiring systemic corticosteroids	0 to 1 per year	2 or more per year	2 or more per year	2 or more per year
Lung function	Normal FEV$_1$ between exacerbations FEV$_1$ ≥ 80% predicted FEV$_1$/FVC > 85%	FEV$_1$ ≥ 80% predicted FEV$_1$/FVC > 80%	FEV$_1$ 60%–80% predicted FEV$_1$/FVC = 75–80%	FEV$_1$ < 60% predicted FEV$_1$/FVC < 75%

Severity is determined by the most severe category for any feature.

FEV$_1$, forced expiratory volume in 1 second; FVC, forced vital capacity.

From National Asthma Education and Prevention Program, National Heart, Lung and Blood Institute, National Institutes of Health. 2007 *Expert Panel Report III: Guidelines for the diagnosis and management of asthma*. Bethesda, MD: U.S. Department of Health and Human Services. Originally published July 2007. Revised 2002, August 2007. NIH Publication No. 07-4051. Retrieved from http://www.nhlbi.nih.gov/files/docs/guidelines/asthgdln.pdf

classified according to nonspirometric criteria (**Table 25.3**). A reduced peak expiratory flow (PEF) is consistent with airway obstruction but is not diagnostic of asthma. PEF is commonly used for self-monitoring and assessment of airway obstruction reversibility following inhalation of a short-acting bronchodilator. Spirometry is performed at baseline (prior to starting treatment), after 3 to 6 months of treatment, then repeated annually or more frequently if indicated.

Airflow obstruction reversibility, an important parameter for the diagnosis of asthma, is documented by comparing baseline FEV$_1$ to postbronchodilator FEV$_1$ 10 to 15 minutes following the administration of 2 to 4 puffs of a short-acting

TABLE 25.3

Asthma Severity—Chronic Disease Classification (Children 0 to 4 Years of Age)

Severity Components	Intermittent	Mild Persistent	Moderate Persistent	Severe Persistent
Symptoms	2 or fewer days per week	More than 2 days per week but not daily	Daily	Throughout the day
Nighttime awakenings	0	1 to 2 nights per month	3–4 nights per month	More than 1 night per week
Short-acting beta$_2$-adrenergic agonist use for symptom control	2 or fewer days per week	More than 2 days per week but not daily	Daily	Several times per day
Interference with normal activity	None	Minor limitation	Some limitation	Extremely limited
Exacerbations requiring systemic corticosteroids	0 to 1 per year	≥2 in 6 mo or ≥4 wheezing episodes per 1 y lasting >1 day AND risk factors for persistent asthma		

Severity is determined by the most severe category for any feature.

FEV$_1$, forced expiratory volume in 1 second; FVC, forced vital capacity.

From National Asthma Education and Prevention Program, National Heart, Lung and Blood Institute, National Institutes of Health. 2007 *Expert Panel Report III: Guidelines for the diagnosis and management of asthma*. Bethesda, MD: U.S. Department of Health and Human Services. Originally published July 2007. Revised 2002, August 2007. NIH Publication No. 07-4051. Retrieved from http://www.nhlbi.nih.gov/files/docs/guidelines/asthgdln.pdf

TABLE 25.4

Asthma Control Assessment

	Well Controlled	Not Well Controlled	Very Poorly Controlled
Symptoms	2 or fewer days per week	More than 2 days per week	Throughout the day
Nighttime awakenings	2 or fewer nights per month	1 to 3 nights per week	4 or more nights per week
Interference with normal activities	None	Some limitations	Extremely limited
Short-acting beta$_2$-adrenergic agonist use for symptom control	2 or fewer days per week	More than 2 days per week	Several times per day
FEV$_1$ or PEF	>80% predicted or personal best	60%–80% predicted or personal best	<60% predicted or personal best
Validated questionnaire	ATAQ™ 0 ACT™ ≥ 20	ATAQ™ 1–2 ACT™ 16–19	ATAQ™ 3–4 ACT™ ≤ 15
Exacerbations	0 to 1 per year	≥2 per year	≥2 per year
Recommended action*	• Maintain current step • Regular follow-up every 1–6 mo • Consider stepping down if well controlled for at least 3 mo	• Step up one step • Reevaluate in 2–6 weeks	• Consider short-course oral CS • Step up 1–2 steps • Reevaluate in 2 weeks

*If medication-related side effects, consider alternate treatment options.
From National Asthma Education and Prevention Program, National Heart, Lung and Blood Institute, National Institutes of Health. 2007 *Expert Panel Report III: Guidelines for the diagnosis and management of asthma.* Bethesda, MD: U.S. Department of Health and Human Services. Originally published July 2007. Revised 2002, August 2007. NIH Publication No. 07-4051. Retrieved from http://www.nhlbi.nih.gov/files/docs/guidelines/asthgdln.pdf

beta-adrenergic drug. The NAEPP guidelines define airflow obstruction reversibility as an increase in FEV$_1$ of at least 12% and an absolute increase in FEV$_1$ of at least 200 mL (NAEPP, 2007).

INITIATING DRUG THERAPY

Drug therapy is initiated according to the age-specific NAEPP chronic disease recommendations (**Tables 25.4 to 25.6**). All persons with asthma, regardless of the severity of asthma, require a short-acting beta$_2$-adrenergic agonist (SABA) bronchodilator for quick relief of acute symptoms. Long-term control medication is added according to the severity of disease. The GINA guidelines recommend reassessing 1 to 3 months after starting treatment and then every 3 to 12 months (GINA, 2015).

Treatment can be stepped down to a less intensive regimen if asthma symptoms have been well controlled for 3 months. Stepping down treatment is done systematically with close monitoring of asthma control. Oral corticosteroids are reduced

TABLE 25.5

Stepwise Approach for Managing Asthma (Children ≥12 Y of Age and Adults)

Step 1 Intermittent	Step 2 Mild Persistent	Step 3 Moderate Persistent	Step 4 Moderate Persistent	Step 5 Severe Persistent	Step 6 Severe Persistent
Preferred: SABA PRN	Preferred: Low-dose ICS Alternative: Cromolyn, LTRA, or theophylline	Preferred: Low-dose ICS + LABA OR Medium-dose ICS Alternative: Low-dose ICS + either LTRA, theophylline, or zileuton	Preferred: Medium-dose ICS + LABA Alternative: Medium-dose ICS + either LTRA, theophylline, or zileuton	Preferred: High-dose ICS + LABA AND Consider omalizumab for patients who have allergies	Preferred: High-dose ICS + LABA + oral CS AND Consider omalizumab for patients who have allergies

Patient education and environmental control at each step
Quick-relief medication for all patients

SABA, inhaled short-acting beta$_2$ agonist; ICS, inhaled corticosteroid; LABA, inhaled long-acting beta$_2$ agonist; CS, corticosteroid.
From National Asthma Education and Prevention Program, National Heart, Lung and Blood Institute, National Institutes of Health. 2007 *Expert Panel Report III: Guidelines for the diagnosis and management of asthma.* Bethesda, MD: U.S. Department of Health and Human Services. Originally published July 2007. Revised 2002, August 2007. NIH Publication No. 07-4051. Retrieved from http://www.nhlbi.nih.gov/files/docs/guidelines/asthgdln.pdf

TABLE 25.6

Stepwise Approach for Managing Asthma (Children 5–11 y of Age)

Step 1 Intermittent	Step 2 Mild Persistent	Step 3 Moderate Persistent	Step 4 Moderate Persistent	Step 5 Severe Persistent	Step 6 Severe Persistent
Preferred:SABA PRN	Preferred: Low-dose ICS Alternative: Cromolyn, LTRA, or theophylline	Preferred: EITHER: Low-dose ICS + either LABA, LTRA, or theophylline OR Medium-dose ICS	Preferred: Medium-dose ICS + LABA Alternative: Medium-dose ICS + either LTRA or theophylline	Preferred: High-dose ICS + LABA Alternative: High-dose ICS + either LTRA or theophylline	Preferred: High-dose ICS + LABA + oral systemic CS Alternative: High-dose ICS + either LTRA or theophylline + oral systemic corticosteroid

Patient education and environmental control at each step
Quick-relief medication for all patients

SABA, inhaled short-acting beta$_2$ agonist; ICS, inhaled corticosteroid; LABA, inhaled long-acting beta$_2$ agonist; CS, corticosteroid.
From National Asthma Education and Prevention Program, National Heart, Lung and Blood Institute, National Institutes of Health. 2007 *Expert Panel Report III: Guidelines for the diagnosis and management of asthma*. Bethesda, MD: U.S. Department of Health and Human Services. Originally published July 2007. Revised 2002, August 2007. NIH Publication No. 07-4051. Retrieved from http://www.nhlbi.nih.gov/files/docs/guidelines/asthgdln.pdf

and then discontinued first. The dose of inhaled corticosteroid (ICS) may then be reduced by 50%. Further reductions in therapy can be made by reducing the dose of the ICS/long-acting bronchodilator regimen to once daily. The long-term control regimen may be stopped if the person with asthma has been free of symptoms for 6 to 12 months and has no risk factors for exacerbations (GINA, 2015).

Treatment is stepped up if persons with asthma are not well controlled despite 2 to 3 months of treatment with long-term control medication. Medication adherence, inhaler drug delivery technique, environmental exposures, and concurrent medications must be assessed and any issues addressed before stepping up to a more intensive medication regimen. Alternate treatment should be stopped and the preferred treatment regimen tried before stepping up therapy.

Goals of Drug Therapy

The NAEPP goals of asthma therapy are to reduce impairment and reduce risk (NAEPP, 2007). Impairment may be reduced by preventing chronic and/or problematic symptoms and maintaining near "normal" pulmonary function. The patient and family should be satisfied and their expectations met. Indicators of reduced impairment include the ability to maintain normal activities (e.g., work, school) and the infrequent use (2 days or fewer per week) of short-acting "rescue" bronchodilators.

Asthma control and the presence of risk factors for exacerbations should be assessed and documented during each patient encounter (NAEPP, 2007). The NAEPP levels of asthma control include well controlled, not well controlled, and very poorly controlled (**Table 25.7**). Assessment

TABLE 25.7

Stepwise Approach for Managing Asthma (Children 0–4 Years of Age)

Step 1 Intermittent	Step 2 Mild Persistent	Step 3 Moderate Persistent	Step 4 Moderate Persistent	Step 5 Severe Persistent	Step 6 Severe Persistent
Preferred: SABA PRN	Preferred: Low-dose ICS Alternative: Cromolyn or montelukast	Preferred: Medium-dose ICS	Preferred: Medium-dose ICS + either LABA or montelukast	Preferred: High-dose ICS + either LABA or montelukast	Preferred: High-dose ICS + either LABA or montelukast AND Oral systemic CS

Patient education and environmental control at each step
Quick-relief medication for all patients

SABA, inhaled short-acting beta$_2$ agonist; ICS, inhaled corticosteroid; LABA, inhaled long-acting beta$_2$ agonist; CS, corticosteroid.
From National Asthma Education and Prevention Program, National Heart, Lung and Blood Institute, National Institutes of Health. 2007 *Expert Panel Report III: Guidelines for the diagnosis and management of asthma*. Bethesda, MD: U.S. Department of Health and Human Services. Originally published July 2007. Revised 2002, August 2007. NIH Publication No. 07-4051. Retrieved from http://www.nhlbi.nih.gov/files/docs/guidelines/asthgdln.pdf

of the level of control over the previous 2 to 4 weeks is based on information from the patient, including self-assessment using validated questionnaires, pulmonary function (FEV_1 or PEF), and the number of asthma exacerbations in the preceding year. The two self-assessment questionnaires incorporated in the NAEPP asthma control assessment include the Asthma Therapy Assessment Questionnaire™ (ATAQ) and the Asthma Control Test™ (ACT); age-appropriate versions are available. The ATAQ™ consists of four questions with a maximum score of 4 points; a score of 3 to 4 points indicates very poorly controlled asthma. The ACT™ consists of five questions with a maximum score of 25 points; a score of 19 points or less indicates asthma is not as controlled as it could be.

Risk may be reduced by preventing exacerbations and optimizing drug therapy. The presence of one or more of the following factors increases the risk for an asthma exacerbation (GINA, 2015):

- Uncontrolled asthma symptoms
- Use of more than one 200-dose short-acting bronchodilator canisters per month
- Inadequate ICS
- Low FEV_1, especially if less than 60% of predicted

- Important psychological or socioeconomic problems
- Inhaled irritant exposures (e.g., smoke, allergens)
- Comorbidities that trigger and/or worsen asthma (e.g., rhinosinusitis, allergies, obesity)
- Eosinophilia
- Pregnancy
- History of one or more asthma exacerbations in the last 12 months
- History of intubation or intensive care unit admission for asthma

Risks for developing fixed airflow obstruction include chronic exposure to inhaled irritants (e.g., tobacco smoke, chemicals), lack of treatment with ICS, a low FEV_1 at the time of diagnosis, chronic mucus hypersecretion, sputum eosinophilia, and blood eosinophilia. Risks for medication-related adverse effects include a prior history of allergy or adverse reaction to a similar medication, addition of medications that interact with asthma medications, and altered hepatic or renal function from concurrent medical conditions or advanced age.

Drugs used to treat asthma include beta$_2$-adrenergic agonists, corticosteroids, leukotriene modifiers, mast cell stabilizers, methylxanthines, and monoclonal antibodies (**Table 25.8**).

TABLE 25.8

Overview of Selected Agents Used to Treat Asthma

Generic (Trade) Name and Adult Dosage	Selected Adverse Events	Contraindications	Special Considerations
Short-Acting Beta$_2$-Adrenergic Agonists albuterol (Proventil HFA, Ventolin HFA, ProAir HFA) MDI 90 mcg/inhalation; 1–2 inhalations q4–q6 h as needed albuterol (ProAir) DPI 117 mcg/inhalation 1–2 inhalations q4–q6 h as needed albuterol (Accuneb) 0.083% (2.5 mg/3 mL), 0.5% (2.5 mg/0.5 mL) solution for nebulization; 2.5 mg three to four times a day as needed	Tachycardia, skeletal muscle tremor, nervousness, dizziness, hypokalemia, hyperglycemia	Hypersensitivity to beta$_2$-adrenergic agonists Hypersensitivity to lactose or milk proteins (dry powder formulations; product specific)	Fewer systemic effects with inhaled therapy Use with caution in patients with cardiovascular disease, diabetes mellitus, glaucoma, hyperthyroidism, or seizure disorders Beta-adrenergic blockers diminish the bronchodilator effects Concurrent sympathomimetic drugs, monoamine oxidase inhibitors, or tricyclic antidepressants enhance the risk of adverse effects
Inhaled Corticosteroids beclomethasone aerosol for inhalation 40 mcg/inhalation and 80 mcg/inhalation (Qvar) budesonide aerosol powder 90 mcg/actuation and 180 mcg/actuation; suspension 0.25 mg/2 mL, 0.5 mg/2 mL, 1 mg/2 mL (Pulmicort) ciclesonide aerosol solution for inhalation 80 mcg/actuation and 160 mcg/actuation (Alvesco)	Oral candidiasis, hoarseness	Hypersensitivity to corticosteroids Hypersensitivity to lactose or milk proteins (dry powder formulations; product specific)	Dosage depends on asthma severity, prior use of bronchodilators, inhaled corticosteroids, and oral corticosteroids Dosing interval depends on specific product: beclomethasone, budesonide, and ciclesonide are given twice daily; fluticasone and mometasone may be given daily or twice daily depending on the dosage formulation and prior history

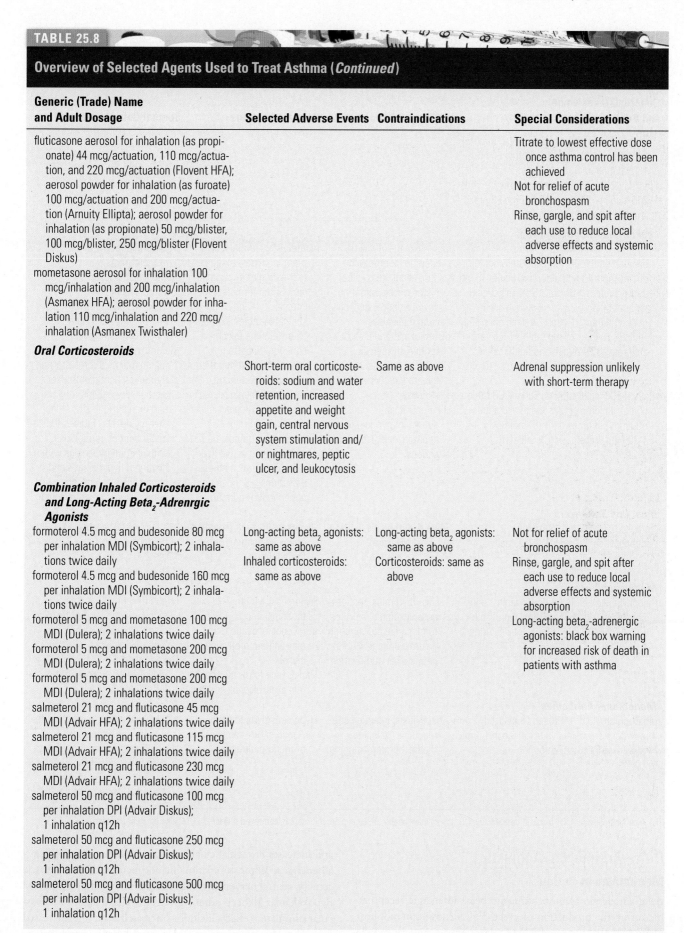

TABLE 25.8

Overview of Selected Agents Used to Treat Asthma (*Continued*)

Generic (Trade) Name and Adult Dosage	Selected Adverse Events	Contraindications	Special Considerations
fluticasone aerosol for inhalation (as propionate) 44 mcg/actuation, 110 mcg/actuation, and 220 mcg/actuation (Flovent HFA); aerosol powder for inhalation (as furoate) 100 mcg/actuation and 200 mcg/actuation (Arnuity Ellipta); aerosol powder for inhalation (as propionate) 50 mcg/blister, 100 mcg/blister, 250 mcg/blister (Flovent Diskus) mometasone aerosol for inhalation 100 mcg/inhalation and 200 mcg/inhalation (Asmanex HFA); aerosol powder for inhalation 110 mcg/inhalation and 220 mcg/inhalation (Asmanex Twisthaler)			Titrate to lowest effective dose once asthma control has been achieved Not for relief of acute bronchospasm Rinse, gargle, and spit after each use to reduce local adverse effects and systemic absorption
Oral Corticosteroids	Short-term oral corticosteroids: sodium and water retention, increased appetite and weight gain, central nervous system stimulation and/or nightmares, peptic ulcer, and leukocytosis	Same as above	Adrenal suppression unlikely with short-term therapy
Combination Inhaled Corticosteroids and Long-Acting Beta$_2$-Adrenrgic Agonists formoterol 4.5 mcg and budesonide 80 mcg per inhalation MDI (Symbicort); 2 inhalations twice daily formoterol 4.5 mcg and budesonide 160 mcg per inhalation MDI (Symbicort); 2 inhalations twice daily formoterol 5 mcg and mometasone 100 mcg MDI (Dulera); 2 inhalations twice daily formoterol 5 mcg and mometasone 200 mcg MDI (Dulera); 2 inhalations twice daily formoterol 5 mcg and mometasone 200 mcg MDI (Dulera); 2 inhalations twice daily salmeterol 21 mcg and fluticasone 45 mcg MDI (Advair HFA); 2 inhalations twice daily salmeterol 21 mcg and fluticasone 115 mcg MDI (Advair HFA); 2 inhalations twice daily salmeterol 21 mcg and fluticasone 230 mcg MDI (Advair HFA); 2 inhalations twice daily salmeterol 50 mcg and fluticasone 100 mcg per inhalation DPI (Advair Diskus); 1 inhalation q12h salmeterol 50 mcg and fluticasone 250 mcg per inhalation DPI (Advair Diskus); 1 inhalation q12h salmeterol 50 mcg and fluticasone 500 mcg per inhalation DPI (Advair Diskus); 1 inhalation q12h	Long-acting beta$_2$ agonists: same as above Inhaled corticosteroids: same as above	Long-acting beta$_2$ agonists: same as above Corticosteroids: same as above	Not for relief of acute bronchospasm Rinse, gargle, and spit after each use to reduce local adverse effects and systemic absorption Long-acting beta$_2$-adrenergic agonists: black box warning for increased risk of death in patients with asthma

(*Continued*)

TABLE 25.8

Overview of Selected Agents Used to Treat Asthma (*Continued*)

Generic (Trade) Name and Adult Dosage	Selected Adverse Events	Contraindications	Special Considerations
vilanterol 25 mcg and fluticasone (as furoate) 100 mcg per inhalation DPI (Breo Ellipta); 1 inhalation q24h vilanterol 25 mcg and fluticasone (as furoate) 200 mcg per inhalation DPI (Breo Ellipta); 1 inhalation q24h			
Leukotriene-Modifying Drugs montelukast 10-mg tablets, 4-mg, and 5-mg chewable tablets, 4-mg packet (Singulair); adolescents 15 and older and adults 10 mg daily, children ≥6 y to <15 y 5 mg once daily, children ≥2 y to <6 y 4 mg once daily, children ≥1 y to <2 y 4 mg once daily zafirlukast 10- and 20-mg tablets (Accolate); children ≥12 y of age and adults 20 mg twice daily; children 5–11 y of age 10 mg twice daily zileuton 600 mg IR tablets, 600 mg CR tablets (Zyflo); children ≥12 y of age and adults 600 mg four times daily (IR tablets) or 1,200 mg twice daily (CR tablets)	montelukast, zafirlukast, zileuton: neuropsychiatric events (e.g., sleep disturbances, agitation, anxiety, depression, suicidal thinking) montelukast: headache, fatigue, dyspepsia zafirlukast: headache, hepatotoxicity (rare but serious) zileuton: sinusitis, nausea, pharyngolaryngeal pain, hepatotoxicity (rare but serious)	montelukast, zafirlukast, zileuton: hypersensitivity to the drug or any component of the formulation montelukast 4- and 5-mg chewable tablets contain phenylalanine (a component of aspartame); contraindicated in patients with phenylketonuria. zafirlukast is contraindicated in persons with hepatic impairment including cirrhosis. zileuton is contraindicated in persons with active liver disease or transaminase elevations ≥3 times the upper limit of normal.	Not for relief of acute asthma exacerbations. montelukast is taken once daily in the evening zafirlukast: consider liver function testing; early detection may increase recovery zileuton: obtain baseline liver function tests prior to starting therapy; repeat monthly for 3 mo, every 2–3 mo for 9 mo and then periodically; stop therapy if ALT > 5 times the upper limit of normal; use with caution in persons with a history of liver disease and/or in persons who consume substantial quantities of alcohol
Mast Cell Stabilizers cromolyn 20 mg/2 mL solution for nebulization; 20 mg four times daily	Taste disturbances, nausea Anaphylaxis (rare)	Hypersensitivity of cromolyn or any component of the formulation	Not for relief of acute bronchospasm Takes 2–6 weeks for full response to treatment
Methylxanthines theophylline extended–release tablets and capsules, elixir (80 mg/15 mL), oral solution (80 mg/15 mL), intravenous solution	Tachyarrhythmias, restlessness, insomnia, seizures, tremor, nausea, vomiting, gastroesophageal reflux, peptic ulcer aggravation	Hypersensitivity to theophylline. Intravenous dosage forms may contain propylene glycol. Oral dosage forms may contain dyes, alcohol, or sugar.	Use with caution in patients with tachyarrhythmias, peptic ulcer disease, seizure disorders, hyperthyroidism Dose to therapeutic theophylline plasma serum concentration (10–20 mg/L)
Monoclonal Antibodies omalizumab (Xolair); 150 mg lyophilized powder per vial (delivers 150 mg in 1.4 mL sterile water for injection)	Anaphylaxis, injection site reactions (pain, erythema, burning, stinging)	Hypersensitivity to omalizumab or any component of the formulation	Black box warning for risk of life-threatening anaphylaxis Dose depends on serum IgE and patient weight; dosing interval (every 2 weeks or every 4 weeks) depends on the dose

HFA, hydrofluoroalkane; MDI, metered-dose inhaler; DPI, dry powder inhaler; IR, immediate release; CR, controlled release; ALT, alanine aminotransferase.

Beta$_2$-Adrenergic Agonists

Mechanism of Action

Beta$_2$-adrenergic agonists stimulate beta$_2$-adrenergic receptors, increasing the production of cyclic 3′5′ adenosine monophosphate (cAMP). Increased cAMP relaxes airway smooth muscle and increases bronchial ciliary activity. Adverse effects of beta$_2$-adrenergic receptor stimulation include increased skeletal muscle activity, central nervous system stimulation, hyperglycemia, and hypokalemia. All beta$_2$-adrenergic agonists have slight cardiovascular stimulatory effects including increased heart rate, increased force of cardiac contractility, and increased cardiac conductivity.

Dosage and Time Frame for Response

The SABAs (e.g., albuterol, levalbuterol) have a quick onset (peak effect 10 minutes) and a short duration of action (3 to 4 hours). Salmeterol, the first long-acting beta$_2$-adrenergic agonist (LABA), has an onset of action of about 2 hours and a 12-hour duration of action. Formoterol has an onset of action of 3 minutes and a 12-hour duration of action. Vilanterol has an onset of action of about 15 minutes and a 24-hour duration of action. Arformoterol, the R-enantiomer of formoterol, and other ultra-long-acting beta$_2$-adrenergic agonists (ULABAs) indacaterol and olodaterol are not FDA approved for the management of asthma. Oral (e.g., albuterol syrup and tablets; terbutaline tablets) and parenteral (e.g., terbutaline) dosage forms are available but have limited clinical use due to the quick onset of action, ease of administration, beta$_2$-adrenergic specificity, and minimal systemic exposure with the inhaled route of administration. SABAs are indicated for the relief of acute asthma symptoms. LABAs are indicated for chronic maintenance therapy.

Contraindications

Beta$_2$-adrenergic agonists are contraindicated in persons with a history of hypersensitivity to beta-adrenergic agonists or any component of the formulation. Beta$_2$-adrenergic agonists should be used with caution in patients with known cardiovascular disease, diabetes mellitus, glaucoma, hyperthyroidism, or seizure disorders.

Adverse Effects

LABAs are associated with an increased risk of asthma-related deaths; product package inserts contain a black box warning of this risk. In addition, manufacturers of LABAs must participate in a Risk Evaluation and Mitigation Strategy (REMS) program that requires a patient medication guide and health care professional education. In 2010, the FDA released new safety requirements for LABAs when used in the treatment of asthma (FDA, 2010). LABAs must be used in combination with an asthma controller medication such as an ICS. LABAs must be used for the shortest duration of time and then discontinued if possible. Combination products containing the LABA plus an ICS are recommended for pediatric and adolescent persons with asthma.

Common adverse effects with SABA and LABA include tachycardia, skeletal muscle tremor commonly seen as a fine hand tremor, nervousness, dizziness, hypokalemia, and hyperglycemia. Adverse effects are more common with high doses of inhaled drug and systemic administration (oral, parenteral).

Interactions

Other sympathomimetic drugs (e.g., catecholamines, catecholamine analogs, and amphetamines) increase the risk for beta$_2$-adrenergic agonist adverse effects and toxicities. Nonselective and higher doses of beta$_1$-selective adrenergic blocking drugs diminish the bronchodilator effects of the beta$_2$-adrenergic agonists; the risk-to-benefit ratio must be considered before prescribing beta-adrenergic blocking drugs. Concurrent administration of beta-adrenergic agonists and monoamine oxidase inhibitors (MAOIs) or tricyclic antidepressants (TCAs) increases blood pressure and the risk of stroke.

MAOIs and TCAs must be discontinued at least 14 days prior to initiating beta$_2$-adrenergic agonists. Thiazide (e.g., hydrochlorothiazide) and loop diuretics (e.g., furosemide) enhance the hypokalemic effect of beta$_2$-adrenergic agonists. The oxazolidinones (e.g., linezolid, tedizolid) enhance the hypertensive effect of beta$_2$-adrenergic agonists. Atomoxetine, a selective norepinephrine reuptake inhibitor indicated for the management of attention deficit hyperactivity disorder, may increase the tachycardic effect of beta$_2$-adrenergic agonists.

Corticosteroids

Mechanism of Action

Corticosteroids reduce airway inflammation by inhibiting or inducing the production of end-effector proteins. An activated intracellular drug–receptor complex binds to glucocorticoid-responsive elements in the gene promoter regions of DNA, stimulating or inhibiting protein transcription. End-effector proteins alter vascular tone, vascular permeability, and body water distribution; stimulate lipolysis, gluconeogenesis, and glycogen secretion; increase responsiveness of beta-adrenergic receptors; mobilize amino acids from muscles; impair leukocyte migration; and inhibit nuclear factor-kappa, which regulates production of proinflammatory proteins such as cytokines, interleukins, interferons, and chemokines.

Dosage and Time Frame for Response

ICS are indicated for all persons with persistent asthma. The dosage of the ICS depends on the severity of asthma. Low-dose ICS are indicated for persons with mild persistent asthma (Step 2). Medium-dose ICS are indicated for persons with moderate persistent asthma (Steps 3 and 4). High-dose ICS are indicated for persons with severe persistent asthma (Steps 5 and 6). ICS differ in terms of oral bioavailability, pulmonary deposition, on-site activation, receptor binding affinity, lipophilicity, protein binding, and pharmacokinetics.

A short course of oral corticosteroids (e.g., a 5- to 10-day course of therapy with prednisone 40 to 60 mg/day in one or two divided doses per day with rapid dose reduction) is indicated for the treatment of an acute asthma exacerbation.

The onset of action of systemic and ICS (hours to days) is delayed due to the time it takes for the drug to influence protein expression. It takes several hours for lung function to improve in response to systemic (oral or intravenous) corticosteroids. The response to ICS typically begins during the first week of therapy and continues to increase for weeks to months with continued treatment.

Contraindications

Corticosteroids are contraindicated in persons with a history of hypersensitivity to corticosteroids or any component of the formulation.

Adverse Events

Common adverse events with ICS include oral candidiasis and dysphonia. Patients should be counseled to rinse their mouth, gargle, and spit out the water after each dose. Common adverse effects with short-term oral corticosteroids include sodium and water retention (peripheral edema, increased blood pressure, exacerbation of congestive heart failure), hyperglycemia, increased appetite and weight gain, CNS stimulation and/or nightmares, peptic ulcer, and leukocytosis.

Common adverse effects with long-term (more than 14 days) high doses (typically greater than 7.5 mg/d of prednisone or equivalent) include adrenal suppression, muscle wasting, myopathy, decreased bone mineral density, posterior subcapsular cataracts, dermal thinning, ecchymosis, and peptic ulcer. Persons taking high-dose ICS are at risk of the same adverse effects.

Interactions

Corticosteroids are metabolized by the hepatic cytochrome P-450 isoenzyme CYP3A4. Corticosteroids induce CYP2C19 and CYP3A4. The prescriber should check for potential drug interactions before prescribing corticosteroids and counsel persons with COPD to check with the prescriber before starting or stopping any nonprescription, prescription, or complementary medication.

Concurrent use of ICS and strong inhibitors of CYP3A4 (e.g., ritonavir, clarithromycin, itraconazole, ketoconazole, telithromycin) increases the risk of systemic corticosteroid adverse effects and is not recommended.

Systemic corticosteroids decrease the response to skin tests, enhance adverse effects from live vaccines, and decrease the response to oral antidiabetic drugs. Antacids decrease the oral bioavailability of oral corticosteroids; counsel the patient to wait at least 2 hours between doses of an antacid and oral corticosteroid.

Leukotriene Modifier Drugs

Mechanism of Action

There are two types of leukotriene modifiers: the 5-lipoxygenase (5-LO) inhibitors and the leukotriene receptor antagonists. Zileuton inhibits 5-lipoxygenase (5-LO), preventing the first and second steps in the conversion of arachidonic acid to the bronchoconstrictor and proinflammatory cysteinyl leukotrienes (LTC4, LTD4, and LTE4). Montelukast and zafirlukast bind to cysteinyl leukotriene receptors on eosinophils and other proinflammatory cells, preventing LTC4, LTD4, and LTE4 from binding to the receptors and the subsequent bronchoconstrictor and proinflammatory responses.

Dosage and Time Frame for Response

Leukotriene modifiers, less effective than inhaled glucocorticoids or beta$_2$-adrenergic agonists, are indicated as alternate medications for the long-term control of mild persistent asthma and for the long-term control of moderate persistent asthma when used in combination with ICS. The montelukast dose for adolescents ≥15 years of age and adults is 10 mg daily in the evening; dosages for children 1 year of age to less than 15 years of age depend on the child's age. The zafirlukast dose for adolescents ≥12 years and adults is 20 mg twice daily; the dose for children 5 to 11 years of age is 10 mg twice daily. The zileuton dose for adolescents

≥12 years of age and adults is 600 mg four times daily (immediate-release formulation) or 1,200 mg twice daily (extended-release formulation).

Response to treatment with leukotriene modifiers is gradual, with improved symptoms and lung function observed during the first week of therapy and continued improvement over the following weeks of continued treatment. Heterogeneity in response to treatment with leukotriene modifiers has been observed and may be associated with genetic variations in the leukotriene metabolic pathway and bioavailability of the drugs (Tantisira and Drazen, 2009).

Contraindications

All leukotriene modifiers are contraindicated in persons with a history of hypersensitivity to the leukotriene modifier or any component of the formulation. The montelukast chewable tablet contains phenylalanine and is contraindicated in persons with phenylketonuria. Zafirlukast and zileuton are contraindicated in persons with hepatic impairment. Zileuton is contraindicated in persons with active liver disease and in persons with transaminase elevations ≥3 times the upper limit of normal. Baseline liver function tests should be obtained prior to starting zileuton therapy, monthly for 3 months, every 2 to 3 months for 9 months, and then periodically thereafter; zileuton should be discontinued if the serum ALT is greater than five times the upper limit of normal.

Adverse Events

Headache is a common adverse event reported with leukotriene modifiers. Churg-Strauss syndrome, a systemic vasculitis, is a rare but potentially serious immune-mediated idiosyncratic reaction reported with leukotriene modifiers. Neuropsychiatric events (behavioral changes and sleep disturbances) were identified postmarketing (FDA, 2009).

Interactions

Significant drug interactions are reported for the leukotriene modifiers. Montelukast is CYP2C8, CYP2C9, and CYP4A4 substrate; medications such as carbamazepine, phenytoin, phenobarbital, and rifampin induce montelukast metabolism resulting in decreased montelukast drug concentrations and effectiveness. Zafirlukast is a CYP2C9 and CYP2C8 substrate; a weak inhibitor of CYP1A2, CYP2C19, CYP2D6, and CYP3A4; and a moderate inhibitor of CYP2C8/9; medications such as erythromycin and theophylline decrease zafirlukast drug concentrations and effectiveness. Zileuton is a minor CYP1A2, CYP2C9, and CYP3A3/4 substrate and a weak inhibitor of CYP1A2. Zileuton decreases theophylline metabolism doubling the theophylline drug concentration. Zileuton decreases warfarin metabolism, increasing warfarin activity.

Mast Cell Stabilizers

Mechanism of Action

Mast cells, present in body tissues that interact with the environment (e.g., lungs, skin, gastrointestinal tract), release preformed proinflammatory mediators and stimulate the synthesis of newly formed proinflammatory mediators when activated by antigens. Mast cell stabilizers prevent the release and synthesis of proinflammatory mediators by inhibiting the influx of calcium into activated mast cells. Preformed mediators (e.g., histamine, proteases, proteoglycans, and cytokines) are responsible for the acute allergy response. Newly synthesized mediators (e.g., prostaglandins, cysteinyl leukotrienes, platelet activating factor) are potent mediators of inflammation. Mast cell-derived cytokines and chemokines (e.g., interleukin-4, interleukin-5, tumor necrosis factor alpha) recruit and activate additional inflammatory cells, extending the inflammatory response.

Dosage and Time Frame for Response

Cromolyn is marketed as a solution for nebulization (20 mg/2 mL). The initial dose is 20 mg four times a day. Once asthma symptoms are controlled, the dose may be tapered to the lowest effective dose (e.g., 20 mg three to four times a day). It takes 2 to 4 weeks of regular treatment to achieve maximum benefit. Less than 10% of the administered dose reaches the airways. Cromolyn absorbed from the lungs is rapidly eliminated unchanged in the urine and bile.

Contraindications

Cromolyn is contraindicated in persons with a history of hypersensitivity to cromolyn or any component of the formulation.

Adverse Events

Adverse events reported with cromolyn include a bad taste in the mouth and nausea. Rare cases of IgE-mediated allergic responses including anaphylaxis and rash have been reported. Anaphylaxis usually appears within minutes of drug administration. A rash may appear hours to days following drug administration.

Interactions

Significant drug interactions have not been identified for cromolyn.

Methylxanthines

Mechanism of Action

Methylxanthine bronchodilators (theophylline, aminophylline) relax bronchial smooth muscle, enhance diaphragmatic contractility, and have a slight anti-inflammatory effect; the exact mechanisms of action are not known. Methylxanthines, nonselective phosphodiesterase inhibitors, increase cAMP by inhibiting phosphodiesterase 1, 2, 3, 4, and 7. Increased cAMP relaxes airway smooth muscle and increases bronchial ciliary activity. The enhanced diaphragmatic contractility is probably mediated by weak adenosine antagonism. The slight anti-inflammatory effect is mediated by other molecular mechanisms.

Dosage and Time Frame for Response

Theophylline and aminophylline, the ethylenediamine salt of theophylline, are dosed to a target serum drug concentration. Aminophylline is approximately 80% theophylline. Although the therapeutic theophylline serum drug concentration range is generally accepted to be 10 to 20 mg/L, persons with asthma may do well with lower serum drug concentrations or experience unacceptable adverse effects with plasma drug concentrations within the therapeutic range. The half-life of theophylline is short (approximately 8 hours in nonsmokers); sustained-release dosage formulations (q12h and q24h) are recommended to improve patient adherence. Theophylline is metabolized in the liver; many medical conditions and drugs induce or inhibit theophylline metabolism. It is therefore important to monitor the serum drug concentrations and individualize the dosage based upon patient response, concurrent medical conditions, and drug interactions.

Contraindications

Theophylline and aminophylline are contraindicated in persons with a history of hypersensitivity to theophylline or any component of the formulation. Patients with a history of allergy to aminophylline are most likely allergic to the ethylenediamine component of the medication, not theophylline. Methylxanthines should be used with caution in patients with a history of tachyarrhythmias, peptic ulcer disease, seizure disorders, or hyperthyroidism. Intravenous dosage forms may contain propylene glycol, which can accumulate in persons with renal dysfunction. Large amounts of propylene glycol may cause lactic acidosis, hyperosmolality, seizures, and respiratory depression. Oral dosage forms may contain dyes, alcohol, or sugar.

Adverse Events

Common adverse events with methylxanthines include tachyarrhythmias, restlessness, insomnia, tremor, nausea, vomiting, gastroesophageal reflux, seizures, and peptic ulcer aggravation. Tachycardia and potentially life-threatening cardiac arrhythmias may occur at therapeutic concentrations. Seizures usually occur with serum theophylline concentrations above 35 mg/L but may occur at lower concentrations.

Interactions

Theophylline is primarily metabolized by the hepatic cytochrome P-450 isoenzymes CYP1A2, CYP2E1, and CYP3A4; theophylline is a minor substrate of CYP2C9 and CYP2D6. Hepatic metabolism can be induced or inhibited by hundreds of drugs and by medical conditions that affect hepatic function. The prescriber should check for potential drug interactions before prescribing theophylline and counsel persons with asthma to check with the prescriber before starting or stopping any nonprescription, prescription, or complementary medication.

Examples of commonly used drugs that inhibit theophylline metabolism (increase theophylline serum concentration) include ciprofloxacin, cimetidine, erythromycin, and allopurinol. Examples of commonly used drugs that induce theophylline metabolism (decrease theophylline serum concentration) include phenobarbital, diphenylhydantoin, and rifampin. The prescriber should check for potential drug interactions before prescribing theophylline and counsel persons with asthma to check with the prescriber before starting or stopping any non-prescription, prescription, or complementary medication.

Smoking induces theophylline metabolism, lowering the serum drug concentration. Caffeine and sympathomimetic drugs have similar adverse effects as the methylxanthines; concurrent use increases the risk of adverse effects. Theophylline may antagonize the sedating and anxiolytic effect of benzodiazepines.

Omalizumab

Mechanism of Action

Omalizumab, a recombinant humanized monoclonal anti-IgG antibody, selectively binds to circulating IgE forming immune complexes that prevent IgE from binding to high-affinity IgE receptors on the surface of mast cells and basophils and the subsequent release of histamine and other mediators of allergy. Omalizumab also decreases the number of high-affinity receptors on basophils.

Dosage and Time Frame for Response

Omalizumab is indicated for treatment of persons with severe persistent allergic asthma with total serum IgE levels from 30 to 700 IU/mL. The dose is based on the total serum IgE and patient weight. The dosing interval depends on the dose. Persons needing more than 300 mg every 4 weeks are dosed on an every 2-week schedule to minimize the number of injections per dose.

The peak omalizumab serum concentration is achieved in about a week. The half-life of omalizumab is long (approximately 20 days), providing a long duration of effect (4 to 6 weeks). Individual responses are highly variable. The response to treatment should be assessed after 16 weeks of therapy. The optimal duration of therapy is not known. Circulating IgE increases rapidly after therapy is stopped with a return of symptoms. However, omalizumab may induce a long-term remission.

Contraindications

Omalizumab is contraindicated in persons with a history of hypersensitivity to omalizumab or any component of the formulation.

Adverse Events

Omalizumab is associated with a high risk of anaphylaxis; product package inserts contain a black box warning of this risk. Signs and symptoms of anaphylaxis include bronchospasm, angioedema of the throat or tongue, hypotension, and syncope. Anaphylaxis may occur with the first dose or after multiple doses. Anaphylaxis may occur within the first hour after treatment or be delayed for several days. Most anaphylactic reactions have occurred in the first 2 hours after the first 3 doses. Patients should be observed closely for 2 hours after the first 3 doses and for 30 minutes after following doses and should be given an epinephrine autoinjector for home administration (Pelaia et al., 2011).

Injection site reactions are common. Nearly half (45%) of persons experience an injection site reaction, including bruising, redness, warmth, burning, stinging, itching, pain, induration, and inflammation. The injection site reactions appear within an hour of injection and persist for about a week.

Less common adverse events (less than 10%) include dizziness, fatigue, arthralgias, and dermatitis.

Interactions

Omalizumab may increase the toxicity of belimumab, a monoclonal antibody indicated for the management of systemic lupus erythematosus.

Selecting the Most Appropriate Drug

Initial drug therapy selection depends on patient age and asthma severity (**Tables 25.4** to **25.6**) (NAEPP, 2007).

First-Line Therapy

A short-acting rescue bronchodilator to be used as needed is required for all persons with asthma, regardless of asthma severity. Chronic maintenance therapy with an asthma controller medication is indicated for persons with persistent asthma. Mild intermittent asthma (Step 1) is managed with a short-acting rescue bronchodilator. The preferred therapy for adults with Step 2 mild persistent asthma is low-dose ICS. The preferred therapy for adults with moderate persistent asthma (Step 3 and Step 4) is low- to medium-dose ICS plus a LABA bronchodilator or medium-dose ICS. Adults with Step 5 and Step 6 severe persistent asthma are treated with high-dose ICS plus a LABA bronchodilator; omalizumab may be added for adults with confirmed allergic asthma.

Alternative Therapy

Alternative therapies to low-dose ICS for persons with Step 2 mild persistent asthma include cromolyn, a leukotriene modifier, or theophylline. Alternative therapies to the combination of a low-dose ICS and a LABA bronchodilator for persons with Step 3 moderate persistent asthma include a combination of low-dose ICS plus a leukotriene modifier or theophylline. Alternative therapies to the combination of medium-dose ICS plus a long-acting beta$_2$-adrenergic agonist for persons with Step 4 moderate persistent asthma include a combination of medium-dose ICS plus a leukotriene modifier or theophylline.

Special Considerations

All persons with asthma should receive an annual influenza vaccine. The Center for Disease Control Advisory Committee on Immunization Practices recommends that immunocompetent children with asthma aged 6 to 18 years and adults with asthma 19 years of age and older receive the 23-valent pneumococcal polysaccharide vaccine (PPSV23) (CDC, 2012; CDC, 2013a). The 13-valent pneumococcal conjugate vaccine (PCV13) is recommended for persons receiving long-term systemic corticosteroids.

Pediatric

Not all asthma medications are indicated for use in children. For example, omalizumab is FDA approved for use in adults and children 12 years of age and older. Even within the same class of medication, age-related indications may differ. Among the leukotriene modifiers, montelukast is FDA approved for children ≥1 year of age, zafirlukast is FDA approved for children ≥5 years of age, and zileuton is FDA approved for children ≥12 years of age.

Parents and adolescents may express concerns about the effect of ICS on adult height. A small (mean 1.2 cm) decrease in adult height is reported with ICS (Kelly et al., 2012). The effect appears to be the greatest with drug administration during the prepubertal years and with larger daily doses. Use of the lowest effective dose may reduce the risk.

Pulmonary function testing is indicated for children 5 years of age and older. Pulmonary function testing in younger children is unreliable.

Use of some respiratory drug delivery devices is limited to older children; younger children may not be able to reliably generate an adequate inspiratory flow rate to disperse the medication (GINA, 2015). Older children (greater than 8 years of age) can effectively use a pressurized metered-dose inhaler. The combination of a pressurized metered-dose inhaler plus a spacer device is appropriate for younger children, including infants. Drug delivery with a nebulizer is effective for all ages. The RespiClick dry powder inhaler is FDA approved for adults and children 12 years of age and older.

Geriatric

Elderly persons with asthma are diagnosed and managed the same as younger persons. However, there are several unique age-related issues that must be considered (Reed, 2010). Recognition of asthma-related symptoms is delayed due to reduced activity levels and a tendency to regard symptoms as part of normal aging. Diagnosis of asthma in elderly persons may be difficult due to the presence of medical conditions with similar signs and symptoms (e.g., other cardiopulmonary conditions such as congestive heart failure). Elderly persons with asthma are more likely to be taking multiple other medications, increasing the likelihood of drug–drug and drug–medical condition interactions. Kinesthetic motor skills, visual acuity, and inspiratory flow may decline with aging making it difficult for patients to prepare and self-administer medication with respiratory drug delivery devices.

Women

Women with asthma may be concerned about the use of medications during and after pregnancy. There are fewer risks to the fetus from treating with standard asthma medications than from uncontrolled asthma during pregnancy (NAEPP, 2005). For most women, asthma is more difficult to control during pregnancy; the current guidelines recommend monthly assessments with baseline spirometry and then PEF monitoring with a peak flow meter.

The NAEPP guidelines provide specific recommendations for preferred and alternate medications to be used during pregnancy (NAEPP, 2007). Albuterol is the preferred short-acting bronchodilator. Low-dose ICS are the preferred therapy for Step 2 mild persistent asthma; alternatives include cromolyn, leukotriene receptor antagonists, and theophylline. A combination of low-dose ICS plus a long-acting inhaled beta₂-adrenergic agonist or medium-dose ICS are the preferred therapy for Step 3 moderate persistent asthma. The guidelines recommend high-dose ICS for severe persistent asthma;

budesonide is preferred. Systemic corticosteroids may be indicated for management of severe uncontrolled asthma in which the risk to the life of the mother and fetus is greater than the risk of systemic corticosteroids.

Ethnic

Culturally specific beliefs regarding cause of disease, acceptance of acute or chronic medications, medication color, dosage formulation, and route of administration may influence a person's acceptance and adherence to the prescribed drug and nondrug therapy. Persons with asthma may seek care from healers and may use natural remedies. It is important to ask about, respect, and integrate these beliefs into the asthma management plan.

Genomics

There are no gene-specific therapeutic recommendations for managing asthma.

ACUTE EXACERBATION

Persons with mild or persistent asthma may experience an acute exacerbation of any severity (NAEPP, 2007). An asthma exacerbation is characterized by an acute or subacute episode of any combination of symptoms, including chest tightness, wheezing, cough, and worsening shortness of breath. Mild exacerbations may be self-managed at home; moderate or severe exacerbations are managed in an urgent office visit or emergency department or may require hospital admission.

A mild exacerbation is characterized by dyspnea with activity and an initial PEF 70% or better than predicted or personal best. A moderate exacerbation is characterized by dyspnea that interferes with or limits usual activity and an initial PEF 40% to 69% of predicted or personal best. A severe exacerbation is characterized by dyspnea at rest that interferes with conversation and a PEF less than 25% of predicted or personal best. During a life-threatening exacerbation, the person may be too dyspneic to speak, may have a silent chest, and may have a PEF less than 25% of predicted or personal best.

Initial self-care for an asthma exacerbation consists of 2 to 6 puffs of the quick-relief SABA inhaler albuterol; the dose may be repeated in 20 minutes and then every 3 to 4 hours for the next 24 to 48 hours or until the patient's symptoms and PEF are stable (NAEPP, 2007). Depending on the response to the initial SABA doses, additional therapy, such as a short course of oral corticosteroid, may be added. Persons with marked wheezing and dyspnea and PEF less than 50% predicted or personal best that continues after the initial albuterol doses should repeat the albuterol dose and seek emergency care.

Emergency department and hospital-based management of asthma depend on exacerbation severity (NAEPP, 2007). All patients are treated with oxygen to achieve S₃O₂ of 90% or greater and repetitive (up to 3 doses in the first hour) or continuous high-dose short-acting inhaled beta₂-adrenergic bronchodilator; most patients need systemic corticosteroids. The NAEPP guidelines recommend adding repetitive high doses (0.5 mg nebulizer solution or 8 puffs by MDI) of the short-acting anticholinergic bronchodilator ipratropium bromide to the short-acting beta$_2$-adrenergic bronchodilator when treating patients with severe exacerbations (NAEPP, 2007). Subsequent treatment depends on the exacerbation severity and patient response.

MONITORING PATIENT RESPONSE

It takes approximately 3 to 4 months to achieve maximal benefit with most asthma controller medications. The GINA guidelines recommend that persons with asthma be assessed 1 to 3 months after initiation of therapy and then every 3 to 12 months thereafter depending on the clinical urgency; persons with asthma should be seen within one week of an acute asthma exacerbation (GINA, 2015). The NAEPP guidelines recommend that persons with mild or moderate persistent asthma controlled for 3 months or longer be seen every 6 months; persons with more severe asthma should be seen more frequently (NAEPP, 2007). Spirometry is performed at baseline (prior to starting treatment), after 3 to 6 months of treatment, than repeated annually or more frequently if indicated.

The control of asthma, risk factors, response to treatment (including review of the peak flow diary if part of the self-monitoring plan), adherence, drug delivery techniques, exacerbation history, and occurrence of medication-related adverse effects should be assessed and documented at every patient interaction. The NAEPP guidelines recommend that spirometry be performed at the time of initial assessment, once symptoms and PEF have stabilized in response to initial treatment, when asthma is out of control, and at least every 1 to 2 years (NAEPP, 2007).

PATIENT EDUCATION

Exercise-Induced Bronchospasm

Exercise-induced bronchospasm (EIB), acute airway narrowing in response to exercise, is a common asthma trigger but may occur in persons without an asthma diagnosis. Environmental exposures associated with EIB include exposure to cold air, dry air, high ozone air, high allergen environments, and airborne particulates. Symptoms are variable and nonspecific but may include chest tightness, cough, wheezing, and dyspnea; symptoms may be mild to severe. Symptoms typically appear within a few minutes after exercise begins and continue for 10 to 15 minutes after exercise stops.

Nonpharmacologic management includes warming up before exercise or breathing through a face mask or scarf to prewarm and humidify inspired air; dietary modifications (e.g., low-salt diet, dietary supplementation with fish oils) have been proposed (Parsons, 2013). A short-acting beta$_2$-adrenergic agonist is administered 15 minutes before exercise to prevent EIB. A mast cell–stabilizing drug (e.g., cromolyn) or short-acting anticholinergic drug (e.g., ipratropium bromide) may be considered if an SABA is ineffective. Controller medications (e.g., daily ICS with or without a LABA and/or a leukotriene

receptor antagonist) are indicated if preventive therapy is needed daily or more frequently (Parsons, 2013).

Environmental Control

Common environmental allergens include house dust mites, cockroaches, furred animals, indoor and outdoor molds, and pollens. House dust mites live on human skin cells found in dust; the allergen is found in fecal pellets and body fragments. Environmental control consists of removal of items that collect dust (e.g., carpets, curtains, stuffed animals), encasement of mattresses and bedding in mite-impermeable covers, and keeping the environment dust-free. Maintaining household humidity at ≤50% and the household temperature at 70°F may reduce the dust mite population. Cockroaches are controlled by encasing food supplies, removing waste food from the environment, preventing access to water, repairing cracks and openings around pipes, and use of insecticide bait traps. Ideally, furred animals should be removed from the home and contact with furred animals outside the home discouraged. Minimally, furred animals should be kept out of the bedroom of the person with asthma. Persons with outdoor mold allergies should avoid decaying vegetation. Indoor mold exposure avoidance strategies include ventilating high humidity areas, lowering the household humidity to less than 50%, removing carpets on concrete slabs, and sealing structural defects to prevent water from entering the home. Pollen avoidance strategies include staying indoors as much as possible, especially in the evenings, and keeping car and house windows closed.

Self-Monitoring

The current NAEPP asthma guidelines encourage all persons with moderate or severe persistent asthma, a history of severe exacerbations, or poorly controlled asthma to have a written asthma action plan. The written asthma action plan includes a daily management plan and how to recognize and manage worsening asthma. The asthma action plan is individualized based on symptoms, PEF, or both symptoms and PEF. An asthma action plan based on PEF is recommended for patients who have poor perceptions of worsening asthma.

A written asthma action plan is organized around three zones: green zone (doing well; PEF 80% or more of personal best), yellow zone (worsening asthma; PEF 50% to 79% of personal best), and red zone (medical alert; PEF less than 50% of personal best). Template asthma action plans for children and adults are available from the National Institute of Health and several professional organizations. A green zone plan includes instructions for preventing asthma symptoms (e.g., long-term control medication regimen, medications to prevent exercise-induced bronchoconstriction, and avoidance strategies for environmental triggers). The yellow zone plan includes a list of symptoms suggestive of worsening asthma and instructions for managing the worsening lung function (e.g., add a medication, increase the dose of a current medication, whom to call for help, how to monitor the response). The red zone plan includes symptoms that indicate a medical alert and instructions for managing the worsening lung function (e.g., add a medication, whom to call, and when to seek emergency help).

Respiratory Drug Delivery Systems

Device-specific patient education regarding the correct use of the specific expiratory drug delivery system is essential. Multiple types of respiratory drug delivery devices are marketed, each with unique drug administration techniques. Respiratory drug delivery systems include metered-dose inhalers, holding chambers (valved and nonvalved), dry powder inhalers (single-dose inhalers, premetered blisters, and reservoir style), soft mist inhaler, and small volume nebulizers (jet nebulizers and ultrasonic nebulizers). Each type of device has advantages and disadvantages; device selection depends on product availability, patient age, patient ability, cost, and patient preference. General drug delivery device administration techniques are listed in **Table 25.9**; refer to the product package inserts for device-specific drug administration information.

Drug Information

The NAEPP and GINA guidelines contain pharmacologic class and product-specific drug information. Drug information is available on professional organization (e.g., the American Academy of Allergy, Asthma, and Immunology [AAAAI]), nonprofit organization (e.g., The American Lung Association [ALA]), and government (e.g., NIH) Web sites. Pharmaceutical company websites often include links to respiratory drug delivery device videos. Pharmacy therapeutics and medical pulmonary textbooks provide more in-depth drug information.

Patient-Oriented Information Sources

Many national, state, and local government websites (e.g., National Heart, Lung, Blood Institute, Center for Disease Control; NHLBI) contain information and links to other resources for persons with asthma. Professional organizations such as the AAAAI, the American Academy of Family Physicians, (AAFP), and the American Academy of Pediatrics (AAP) provide information for persons with asthma on their websites. Other organizations such as the ALA and the Asthma and Allergy Foundation of America (AAFA) provide patient information on their websites. Websites for the NAEPP and the GINA contain patient-oriented information.

Nutrition/Lifestyle Changes

There is no "asthma diet" though good nutrition is important to maintain overall health. Physical activity is important; persons with asthma should be encouraged to remain physically active.

Complementary and Alternative Medications

More than 20 types of complementary and alternative medical treatments are used for the management of asthma, including many types of herbal remedies, homeopathic medications, acupuncture, chiropractic therapy, breathing techniques, relaxation techniques, and yoga. The current NAEPP guidelines do not recommend any complementary and alternative medical therapies (NAEPP, 2007). Clinicians should ask persons with asthma about the use of these therapies, especially herbal and other products, to identify potential disease and drug interactions.

TABLE 25.9

Drug Delivery Device Techniques

Device	General Technique
Pressurized metered-dose inhalers	1. Remove dust cap 2. Inspect for debris 3. Shake vigorously for 5 s 4. Hold the device upright (mouthpiece down) 5. Position mouthpiece; do not block with the tongue 6. Press down on the canister and breathe in at the same time (midinspiration actuation is more effective but is very difficult to perform) 7. Continue to inhale to the end of a quiet breath (about 4–6 s) 8. Hold breath for 10 s 9. Exhale slowly 10. Replace dust cap Wait at least 1 min between puffs for SABAs and 15–30 s for all other drugs
Spacers and valved holding chambers	1. Visually check for debris 2. Prepare metered-dose inhaler 3. Insert metered-dose inhaler in spacer 4. Hold the spacer/valved holding chamber level 5. Gently exhale to end of a quiet breath 6. Press the canister once 7. Immediately inspire slowly and deeply 8. Remove spacer from the mouth 9. Hold breath for 10 s 10. Exhale slowly

(Continued)

TABLE 25.9

Drug Delivery Device Techniques (*Continued*)

Device	General Technique
Dry powder inhalers	1. Remove cover 2. Prepare dose 3. Exhale softly *away* from device 4. Seal lips around mouthpiece 5. Inhale rapidly and forcefully 6. Remove device from the mouth 7. Hold breath for 10 s 8. Exhale softly *away* from device 9. Replace cover
Small volume nebulizers	1. Place the equipment on a stable surface 2. Connect the tubing to the compressor 3. Hold the medication chamber upright; add the premixed drug solution or measure and add drug and saline 4. Place the lid on the medication chamber 5. Connect the tubing to the medication chamber 6. Turn on the air compressor 7. Check for the generation of a fine mist 8. Sit up comfortably straight 9. Seal lips around the mouthpiece; do not block with the tongue 10. Holding the medication chamber upright, breathe in and out normally; take a deeper breath and hold it for a few seconds every minute or so 11. Continue until the medication chamber begins to sputter 12. Turn off the compressor 13. Disconnect the medication chamber and tubing

CASE STUDY*

S.C. is a 21-year-old college student. She presents with intermittent wheezing. She has a history of asthma as a child but had been free of symptoms until this year. She has symptoms 1 to 2 days/week but denies nocturnal wheezing. Her symptoms do not interfere with her normal activities. She has never taken systemic corticosteroids and has never been hospitalized for asthma. On physical exam, you observe soft end-expiratory wheezing at the bases bilaterally. Pulmonary function tests today show an FEV_1/FVC of 80% with an FEV_1 90% of predicted. She has no other medical conditions and is not taking any nonprescription, prescription, or complementary alternative medicines. She has no known environmental or drug allergies.

DIAGNOSIS: ASTHMA

1. List specific goals for treatment for **S.C.**
2. What drug therapy would you prescribe? Why?
3. What are the parameters for monitoring success of the therapy?
4. Discuss specific patient education based on the prescribed therapy.
5. List one or two adverse reactions for the selected agent that would cause you to change therapy.
6. What would be the choice for second-line therapy?
7. What over-the-counter and/or alternative medications would be appropriate for **S.C.**?
8. What lifestyle changes would you recommend for **S.C.**?
9. Describe one or two drug–drug or drug–food interactions for the selected agent.

* Answers can be found online.

Bibliography

Starred references are cited in the text.

*Brown, E. M., Arrieta, M.-C., & Finlay, B. B. (2013). A fresh look at the hygiene hypothesis: How intestinal microbial exposure drives immune effector responses in atopic disease. *Seminars in Immunology, 25,* 378–387.

*Centers for Disease Control and Prevention. (2012). Use of 13-valent pneumococcal conjugate vaccine and 23-valent pneumococcal polysaccharide vaccine for adults with immunocompromising conditions: Recommendations of the Advisory Committee on Immunization Practices (ACIP). *Morbidity and Mortality Weekly Report, 61,* 816–819.

*Centers for Disease Control and Prevention. (2013a). Use of 13-valent pneumococcal conjugate vaccine and 23-valent pneumococcal polysaccharide vaccine among children aged 6-18 years with immunocompromising conditions: Recommendations of the Advisory Committee on Immunization Practices (ACIP). *Morbidity and Mortality Weekly Report, 62,* 521–524.

*Center for Disease Control and Prevention. (2013b). Asthma's Impact on the Nation. Retrieved from http://www.cdc.gov/asthma/impacts_nation/infographic.htm#readtext

*Food and Drug Administration (FDA). (2009). Updated information on leukotriene inhibitors: Montelukast (marketed as Singulair), zafirlukast (marketed as Accolate), and zileuton (marketed as Zyflo and Zyflo CR). Retrieved from http://www.fda.gov/drugs/drugsafety/postmarketdrugsafetyinformationforpatientsandproviders/drugsafetyinformationforhealthcareprofessionals/ucm165489.htm on August 28, 2009.

*Food and Drug Administration (FDA). (2010). Drug safety communication: New safety requirements for long-acting inhaled asthma medications called long-acting beta agonists (LABAs). Retrieved from http://www.fda.gov/Drugs/DrugSafety/PostmarketDrugSafetyInformationforPatientsandProviders/ucm200776.htm on February 18, 2010.

*Global Initiative for Asthma (GINA). (2015). Global strategy for asthma management and prevention. Retrieved from http://www.ginasthma.org/

*Holgate, S. T. (2008). The airway epithelium is central to the pathogenesis of asthma. *Allergology International, 67,* 1–10.

*Kelly, H. W., Sternberg, A. L., Lescher, R., et al. (2012). Effect of inhaled glucocorticoids in childhood on adult height. *New England Journal of Medicine, 367,* 904–912.

*Moorman, J. E., Akinbami, L. J., Bailey, C. M., et al. (2012). National Surveillance of Asthma: United States, 2001–2010. National Center for Health Statistics. *Vital and Health Statistics, 3*(35), 1–59.

*National Asthma Education and Prevention Program, National Heart, Lung and Blood Institute, National Institutes of Health. 2005. *Expert panel report: Managing asthma during pregnancy: Recommendations for pharmacology treatment— 2004 update.* U.S. Department of Health and Human Services. Revised January 2005. NIH Publication No. 05-5246. Retrieved from http://www.nhlbi.nih.gov/gov/files/docs/resources/lung/astpreg_full.pdf

*National Asthma Education and Prevention Program, National Heart, Lung and Blood Institute, National Institutes of Health. 2007 *Expert Panel Report III: Guidelines for the diagnosis and management of asthma.* Bethesda, MD: U.S. Department of Health and Human Services. Originally published July 2007. Revised 2002, August 2007. NIH Publication No. 07-4051. Retrieved from http://www.nhlbi.nih.gov/files/docs/guidelines/asthgdln.pdf

*Parsons, J. P., Hallstrand, T. S., Mastronarde, J. G., et al. (2013). An official American Thoracic Society clinical practice guideline: Exercise-induced bronchoconstriction. *American Journal of Respiratory and Critical Care Medicine, 187,* 1016–1027.

*Pelaia, G., Gallelli, L., Renda, T., et al. (2011). Update on optimal use of omalizumab in management of asthma. *Journal of Asthma and Allergy, 4,* 49–59.

*Reed, C. E. (2010). Asthma in the elderly: Diagnosis and management. *Journal of Allergy and Clinical Immunology, 126,* 681–687.

*Tantisira, K. G., Drazen, J. M. (2009). Genetics and pharmacogenetics of the leukotriene pathway. *Journal of Allergy and Clinical Immunology, 124,* 422–427.

26 Chronic Obstructive Pulmonary Dise...

Karen J. Tietze

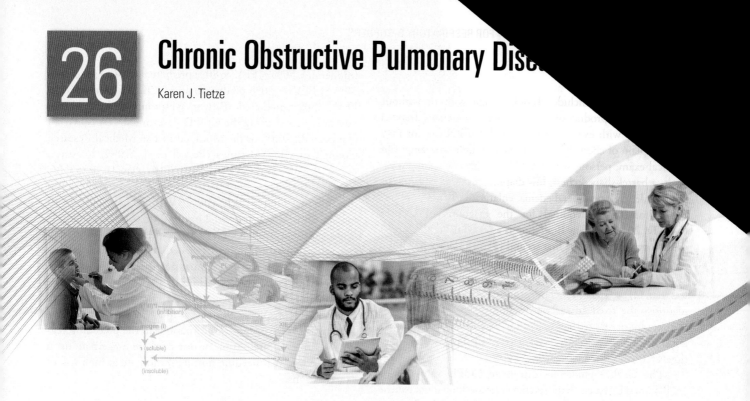

Chronic obstructive pulmonary disease (COPD) is characterized by chronic progressive airflow limitation. COPD typically is thought of as chronic bronchitis and/or emphysema. However, chronic bronchitis, defined clinically as cough and sputum production for at least 3 months of the year in at least two consecutive years, occurs independently of COPD and may not be associated with fixed airflow limitation. Emphysema refers to alveolar destruction, one of several structural abnormalities in COPD. The current Global Obstructive Lung Disease (GOLD) guidelines do not include either term in the definition of COPD (GOLD, 2016).

In the United States, COPD affects 6.8 million noninstitutionalized adults (Schiller et al., 2012) and 10.8% of institutionalized residents (NSRCF, 2010). COPD is the third leading cause of death in the United States accounting for 138,080 deaths in 2010 (Schiller et al., 2012). In 2010, the cost of COPD in the United States was estimated to be nearly $50 billion, including nearly $30 billion in direct health care expenditures (ALA, 2015).

Historically identified with older men, COPD demographics have shifted. In 2009, COPD prevalence was highest in women of all age groups, except for the oldest age groups (75 and older) in which the prevalence among men and women was the same (Akinbami & Liu, 2011). COPD prevalence increases with age (Akinbami & Liu, 2011). For women, the highest prevalence is among women aged 65 to 74. For men, the highest prevalence is among men aged 75 to 84. In men and women aged 45 to 64 and women aged 65 and older, the prevalence of COPD is higher in whites than in blacks (NHLBI, 2012). One of the challenges identifying persons with COPD is that people are asymptomatic during the early stages of the disease; by the time symptoms appear, the disease has progressed significantly.

CAUSES

Tobacco smoking is the most common risk factor for COPD (U.S. DHHS, 2014). Although most persons with COPD have smoked tobacco, not all tobacco smokers develop COPD. Other risk factors for COPD include exposure to air pollutants in the home and the workplace, a history of severe respiratory infections as a child, and hereditary alpha-1 antitrypsin deficiency.

PATHOPHYSIOLOGY

In susceptible persons, chronic exposure to inhaled noxious particles results in lung inflammation. Inflammatory cells (neutrophils, macrophages, and CD8+ T lymphocytes) produce a variety of proinflammatory mediators (interleukins, tumor necrosis factor, leukotrienes, and growth factors), proteases (oxidants), and oxidants (nitrogen species) (GOLD, 2016; MacNee, 2006). The imbalances between proteases and antiproteases and oxidants and antioxidants lead to irreversible changes in the peripheral airways (i.e., squamous metaplasia, mucous metaplasia, small airway fibrosis), lung parenchyma (i.e., parenchymal destruction), and pulmonary blood vessels (i.e., pulmonary vascular remodeling). These changes result in airflow obstruction, hyperinflation, mucous hypersecretion, ciliary dysfunction, and gas exchange abnormalities (GOLD, 2016; MacNee, 2006). Inflammation most likely is the common link between COPD and the extrapulmonary medical conditions associated with COPD including systemic venous thromboembolism, anemia, metabolic syndrome, sleep disturbances, osteoporosis, obesity, anxiety, and depression (Cavailles et al., 2013).

...with or without
...ogressive dyspnea
...OPD may or may
...lible wheezing. On
...nave wheezing, cya-
...,ms, and signs of cor
...ged heart).

...diagnosis of COPD
...sessed using the forced
...FEV$_1$), the total volume
of exhale...   ...VC), and the FEV$_1$/FVC
ratio. Airflow obstruc...   ...when the FEV$_1$/FVC is
less than 0.70. A postbronchodilato. FEV$_1$/FVC less than 70%
identifies the fixed airway obstruction of COPD. Although
peak expiratory flow (the highest flow rate during forced exhalation) is sensitive, it lacks specificity and is not used to diagnose COPD.

The GOLD guidelines categorize COPD into groups
(A, B, C, and D) based on the severity of airflow limitation, patient
symptoms, and exacerbation risk (**Table 26.1**). GOLD group
A is characterized as low risk, less symptoms. GOLD group B
is characterized as low risk, more symptoms. GOLD group C
is characterized as high risk, less symptoms. GOLD group D is
characterized as high risk, more symptoms.

Severity of airflow limitation is based on postbronchodilator FEV$_1$. The four GOLD spirometric levels of severity
include GOLD 1 (mild), FEV$_1$ ≥ 80% of predicted; GOLD 2

(moderate), 50% ≤ FEV$_1$ < 80% predicted; GOLD 3 (severe),
30% ≤ FEV$_1$ < 50% predicted; and GOLD 4 (very severe),
FEV$_1$ <30% predicted. Patient symptoms and breathlessness are assessed using the COPD Assessment Test (CAT™)
(Jones et al., 2009) or the Modified British Medical Research
Council (mMRC) dyspnea (Bestall et al., 1999) questionnaires. Persons with CAT™ scores of less than 10 or mMRC
scores of 0 to 1 are considered to have less symptoms and
breathlessness, respectively. Persons with CAT™ scores of 10
or more or mMRC scores of 2 or more are considered to have
more symptoms and breathlessness, respectively. Exacerbation
risk is based on the number of exacerbations in the preceding
year not needing hospitalization and needing hospitalization.
Persons with 0 to 1 exacerbations in the preceding year not
needing hospitalization or no exacerbations in the preceding
year needing hospitalization are at low risk of exacerbations.
Persons with two or more exacerbations in the preceding year
not needing hospitalization or one or more exacerbations in
the preceding year needing hospitalization are at high risk of
exacerbations.

INITIATING DRUG THERAPY

The current GOLD guidelines recommend drug therapy based
on the COPD group (**Table 26.2**). Nondrug therapy includes
tobacco cessation, avoidance of environmental and occupational irritants, and energy conservation. A variety of drug and

TABLE 26.1

COPD Categories

Group	Symptoms	GOLD Spirometric Risk	Exacerbations in Preceding Year NOT NEEDING Hospitalization	Exacerbations in Preceding Year NEEDING Hospitalization
A Low Risk, Less Symptoms	mMRC 0–1 CAT™ < 10	Grade 1: Mild, FEV$_1$/FVC < 70%, and FEV$_1$ ≥ 80% predicted Grade 2: Moderate, FEV$_1$/FVC < 70%, and FEV$_1$ ≥ 50% to < 80% predicted	0–1	0
B Low risk, More Symptoms	mMRC ≥ 2 CAT™ ≥ 10	Grade 1: Mild, FEV$_1$/FVC < 70%, and FEV$_1$ ≥ 80% predicted Grade 2: Moderate, FEV$_1$/FVC < 70%, and FEV$_1$ ≥ 50% to < 80% predicted	0–1	0
C High Risk, Less Symptoms	mMRC 0–1 CAT™ < 10	Grade 3: Severe, FEV$_1$/FVC < 70%, and FEV$_1$ ≥ 30% to < 50% predicted Grade 4: Very severe, FEV$_1$/FVC < 70%, and FEV$_1$ < 30% predicted	≥2	≥1
D High Risk, More Symptoms	mMRC ≥ 2 CAT™ ≥ 10	Grade 3: Severe, FEV$_1$/FVC < 70%, and FEV$_1$ ≥ 30% to < 50% predicted Grade 4: Very severe, FEV$_1$/FVC < 70%, and FEV$_1$ < 30% predicted	≥2	≥1

From Global Strategy for the Diagnosis, Management, and Prevention of Chronic Obstructive Pulmonary Disease. (2016). Global initiative for chronic obstructive lung disease.
Retrieved from www.goldcopd.org

TABLE 26.2

Initial Treatment of COPD

Group	As Needed Medication	First Choice Maintenance Medication	Second Choice Maintenance Medication	Comments
A	SABA or SAMA	Not indicated	LAMA or LABA or SABA + SAMA	One short-acting bronchodilator; SABA if on LAMA
B	SABA, SAMA, or SABA plus SAMA	LAMA or LABA	LAMA + LABA	One or two short-acting bronchodilators; SABA if on LAMA
C	SABA, SAMA, or SABA plus SAMA	ICS + LAMA or ICS + LABA	LAMA + LABA or LAMA + PDE4I or LABA + PDE4I	One or two short-acting bronchodilators; SABA if on LAMA
D	SABA, SAMA, or SABA plus SAMA	ICS + LAMA or ICS + LABA	ICS + LAMA + LABA or ICS + LABA + PDE4I or LABA + LAMA or LAMA + PDE4I	One or two short-acting bronchodilators; SABA if on LAMA

SABA, short-acting beta$_2$ agonist; SAMA, short-acting anticholinergic; LABA, long-acting beta$_2$ agonist; LAMA, long-acting anticholinergic; ICS, inhaled corticosteroid; PDE4I, phosphodiesterase 4 inhibitor.
From Global Strategy for the Diagnosis, Management, and Prevention of Chronic Obstructive Pulmonary Disease. (2016). Global initiative for chronic obstructive lung disease. Retrieved from www.goldcopd.org

nondrug therapies are available for tobacco cessation. All health care professionals should ask every patient at every encounter about tobacco smoking and then advise, assess, assist, and arrange for smoking cessation interventions as appropriate. Outdoor exercise and exertion should be avoided when pollution levels are high or temperatures are extreme. Maintaining physical activity is recommended for all persons with COPD. Persons with group B or D COPD may benefit from pulmonary rehabilitation and energy conservation techniques.

Goals of Drug Therapy

COPD is an irreversible but treatable medical condition; the goals of therapy are to reduce symptoms and reduce risk (GOLD, 2016). Medications, improving exercise tolerance, and improving overall health status may reduce symptoms and improve quality of life. Risk may be reduced by delaying disease progression and preventing and treating exacerbations. Drugs used to treat COPD include beta$_2$-adrenergic agonists, anticholinergics, corticosteroids, methylxanthines, and phosphodiesterase 4 inhibitors (**Table 26.3**).

Beta$_2$-Adrenergic Agonists

Mechanism of Action

Beta$_2$-adrenergic agonists stimulate beta$_2$-adrenergic receptors, increasing the production of cyclic 3'5' adenosine monophosphate (cAMP). Increased cAMP relaxes airway smooth muscle and increases bronchial ciliary activity. Adverse effects of beta$_2$-adrenergic receptor stimulation include increased skeletal muscle activity, central nervous system stimulation, hyperglycemia, and hypokalemia. All beta$_2$-adrenergic agonists have slight cardiovascular stimulatory effects including increased heart rate,

increased force of cardiac contractility, and increased cardiac conductivity.

Dosage and Time Frame for Response

The short-acting inhaled beta$_2$-adrenergic agonists (SABAs) (e.g., albuterol, levalbuterol) have a quick onset (peak effect 10 minutes) and a short duration of action (3 to 4 hours). Salmeterol, the first long-acting beta$_2$-adrenergic agonist (LABA), has an onset of action of about 2 hours and a 12-hour duration of action. Formoterol and arformoterol have an onset of action of 3 minutes and 7 to 20 minutes, respectively, and a 12-hour duration of action. The newer LABAs indacaterol, vilanterol, and olodaterol, sometimes called ultra-long–acting beta$_2$-adrenergic agonists (ULABAs), have an onset of action of several minutes and a 24-hour duration of action. Oral (e.g., albuterol syrup and tablets, terbutaline tablets) and parenteral (e.g., terbutaline) dosage forms are available but have limited clinical use due to the quick onset of action, ease of administration, beta$_2$-adrenergic agonist specificity, and minimal systemic exposure with inhaled beta$_2$-adrenergic agonists. SABAs are indicated for the relief of acute COPD symptoms. LABAs are indicated for chronic maintenance therapy.

Contraindications

Beta-adrenergic agonists are contraindicated in persons with a history of hypersensitivity to beta-adrenergic agonists or any component of the formulation. Beta$_2$-adrenergic agonists should be used with caution in patients with known cardiovascular disease, diabetes mellitus, glaucoma, hyperthyroidism, or seizure disorders.

TABLE 26.3

Overview of Selected Agents Used to Treat COPD

Generic (Trade) Name and Adult Dosage	Selected Adverse Events	Contraindications	Special Considerations
Short-Acting Beta$_2$-Agonists albuterol (Proventil HFA, Ventolin HFA, ProAir HFA) MDI 90 mcg/inhalation 1–2 inhalations q4–q6 hours as needed albuterol (ProAir) DPI 117 mcg/inhalation 1–2 inhalations q4–q6 hours as needed albuterol (AccuNeb) 0.083% (2.5 mg/3 mL), 0.5% (2.5 mg/0.5 mL) solution for nebulization 2.5 mg three to four times a day as needed	Tachycardia, skeletal muscle tremor, nervousness, dizziness, hypokalemia, hyperglycemia	Hypersensitivity to beta$_2$-adrenergic agonists Hypersensitivity to lactose or milk protein (dry powder formulations, product specific)	Fewer systemic effects with inhaled therapy Use with caution in patients with cardiovascular disease, diabetes mellitus, glaucoma, hyperthyroidism, or seizure disorders Beta-adrenergic blockers diminish the bronchodilator effects Concurrent sympathomimetic drugs, monoamine oxidase inhibitors, or tricyclic antidepressants enhance the risk of adverse effects
Short-Acting Anticholinergics ipratropium bromide (Atrovent) MDI 17 mcg/inhalation; 34 mcg four times daily ipratropium bromide (Atrovent) solution for nebulization 0.02%; 500 mcg (2.5 mL) three to four times per day	Cough, dry mouth, dry throat, throat irritation, blurred vision, mydriasis, dyspepsia	None	Use with caution in patients with narrow-angle glaucoma, myasthenia gravis, prostatic hyperplasia, or bladder neck obstruction
Combination Short-Acting Anticholinergic and Short-Acting Beta$_2$-adrenergic Agonist ipratropium bromide plus albuterol (DuoNeb) solution for nebulization 500 mcg ipratropium bromide plus 2.5 mg albuterol per 3 mL/3 mL every 4–6 h ipratropium bromide plus albuterol (Combivent Respimat) SMI 20 mcg ipratropium bromide plus 100 mcg albuterol per inhalation; 1 inhalation four times daily	Same as above	Same as above	Same as above
Long-Acting Beta$_2$-agonists arformoterol (Brovana) 15 mcg/2 mL solution for nebulization; 15 mcg twice daily formoterol (Perforomist) 20 mcg/2 mL solution for nebulization; 20 mcg q12h formoterol (Foradil Aerolizer) DPI 12 mcg/inhalation; 12 mcg q12h indacaterol (Arcapta Breezhaler) DPI 75 mcg/inhalation; 75 mcg once daily olodaterol (Striverdi Respimat) SMI 2.5 mcg/actuation; 5 mcg once daily salmeterol (Serevent Diskus) DPI 50 mcg/inhalation; 50 mcg q12h	Same as above	Same as above	Same as above Not for relief of acute bronchospasm
Long-Acting Anticholinergics tiotropium bromide (Spiriva HandiHaler) DPI 18 mcg; 18 mcg once daily tiotropium bromide (Spiriva Respimat) SMI 2.5 mcg/inhalation; 5 mcg once daily aclidinium bromide (Tudorza Pressair) DPI 400 mcg/actuation; 400 mcg twice daily umeclidinium bromide (Incruse Ellipta) DPI 62.5 mcg/inhalation; 62.5 mcg once daily	Same as above	Same as above	Same as above Not for relief of acute bronchospasm

TABLE 26.3

Overview of Selected Agents Used to Treat COPD (*Continued*)

Generic (Trade) Name and Adult Dosage	Selected Adverse Events	Contraindications	Special Considerations
Combination Long-Acting Anticholinergic and Long-Acting Beta$_2$-agonists			
tiotropium 2.5 mcg and olodaterol 2.5 mcg per inhalation SMI (Stiolto Respimat); two inhalations once daily	Long-acting anticholinergics: same as above Long-acting beta$_2$-agonists: same as above	Long-acting anticholinergics: same as above Long-acting beta$_2$-agonists: same as above	Not for relief of acute bronchospasm
Combination Long-Acting Beta$_2$-agonists and Corticosteroids			
formoterol 4.5 mcg and budesonide 160 mcg per inhalation MDI (Symbicort); 2 inhalations twice daily salmeterol 50 mcg and fluticasone 250 mcg per inhalation DPI (Advair Diskus); 1 inhalation q12h vilanterol 25 mcg and fluticasone 100 mcg per inhalation DPI (Breo Ellipta); 1 inhalation daily	Long-acting beta$_2$-agonists: same as above Inhaled corticosteroids: oral candidiasis, hoarseness	Long-acting beta$_2$-agonists: same as above Corticosteroids: hypersensitivity to corticosteroids	Not for relief of acute bronchospasm Rinse, gargle, and spit after each use to reduce local adverse effects and systemic absorption Inhaled corticosteroids increase the risk of pneumonia; indicated for patients with grades C and D COPD
Oral Corticosteroids			
	Short-term oral corticosteroids: sodium and water retention, increased appetite and weight gain, CNS stimulation and/or nightmares, peptic ulcer, and leukocytosis	Same as above	Adrenal suppression unlikely with short-term therapy
Methylxanthines			
theophylline extended-release tablets and capsules, elixir (80 mg/15 mL), oral solution (80 mg/15 mL), intravenous solution	Tachyarrhythmias, restlessness, insomnia, seizures, tremor, nausea, vomiting, gastroesophageal reflux, peptic ulcer aggravation	Hypersensitivity to theophylline Intravenous dosage forms may contain propylene glycol Oral dosage forms may contain dyes, alcohol, or sugar	Use with caution in patients with tachyarrhythmias, peptic ulcer disease, seizure disorders, hyperthyroidism Dose to therapeutic theophylline serum concentration (10–20 mg/L)
Phosphodiesterase 4 Inhibitors			
roflumilast (Daliresp) 500 mcg tablet 500 mcg once daily	Supraventricular tachyarrhythmias, weight loss, diarrhea, anxiety, depression including suicidal behavior/ideation and completed suicide	Hypersensitivity to roflumilast Contraindicated in patients with moderate to severe hepatic impairment (Child-Pugh class B or C)	Adjunctive therapy with bronchodilators Not for relief of acute bronchospasm

MDI, metered-dose inhaler; DPI, dry powder inhaler; SMI, soft mist inhaler; CNS, central nervous system.

Adverse Effects

Common adverse effects with beta$_2$-adrenergic agonists include tachycardia, skeletal muscle tremor commonly seen as a fine hand tremor, nervousness, dizziness, hypokalemia, and hyperglycemia. Adverse effects are more common with high doses of inhaled drug and systemic administration (oral, parenteral).

Interactions

Other sympathomimetic drugs (e.g., catecholamines, catecholamine analogs, and amphetamines) increase the risk for beta$_2$-adrenergic agonist adverse effects and toxicities. Nonselective and higher doses of beta$_1$-selective adrenergic blocking drugs diminish the bronchodilator effects of the beta$_2$-adrenergic agonists; the risk to benefit ratio must be considered before prescribing beta-adrenergic blocking drugs. Concurrent administration of beta-adrenergic agonists and monoamine oxidase inhibitors (MAOIs) or tricyclic antidepressants (TCAs) increases blood pressure and the risk of stroke. MAOIs and TCAs must be discontinued at least 14 days prior to initiating beta$_2$-adrenergic agonists. Thiazide (e.g., hydrochlorothiazide) and loop diuretics (e.g., furosemide) enhance the hypokalemic effect of beta$_2$-adrenergic agonists. The oxazolidinones (e.g., linezolid, tedizolid) enhance the hypertensive effect of beta$_2$-adrenergic agonists. Atomoxetine, a selective norepinephrine reuptake inhibitor indicated for the management of attention deficit hyperactivity disorder, may increase the tachycardic effect of beta$_2$-adrenergic agonists.

Anticholinergics

Mechanism of Action

Anticholinergic drugs competitively block acetylcholine at muscarinic receptors, decreasing cGMP. The decreased cGMP results in a relatively higher proportion of cAMP. Increased cAMP relaxes airway smooth muscle and increases bronchial ciliary activity. Anticholinergic drugs also decrease mucus secretion, dilate the pupil, and prevent acetylcholine-induced release of allergenic mediators from mast cells. Although atropine, the classic anticholinergic, crosses the blood–brain barrier and stimulates the central nervous system, the drugs used to manage COPD are quaternary amines. Quaternary amines are poorly absorbed after oral administration and unable to cross the blood–brain barrier.

Dosage and Time Frame for Response

The short-acting anticholinergic (SAMA) ipratropium bromide has an onset of action within 15 minutes, a peak effect within 1 to 2 hours, and a duration of action of 2 to 5 hours. The long-acting anticholinergics (LAMAs) tiotropium bromide, aclidinium bromide, and umeclidinium bromide have a duration of action of 24 hours or more.

Contraindications

Anticholinergics are contraindicated in persons with a history of hypersensitivity to anticholinergics or any component of the formulation. Anticholinergics should be used with caution in patients with narrow-angle glaucoma, myasthenia gravis, prostatic hyperplasia, or bladder neck obstruction.

Adverse Effects

The most common adverse effects with inhaled anticholinergics are dry mouth, cough, and, if the medication gets in the eyes, blurred vision. Due to poor absorption after oral administration, systemic side effects are uncommon but may include restlessness, dizziness, gastrointestinal distress, and urinary obstruction. Paradoxical bronchospasm may occur after administration of inhaled anticholinergics.

Interactions

Concurrent administration of drugs with anticholinergic properties (e.g., first-generation antihistamines) increases the risk of anticholinergic adverse effects.

Corticosteroids

Mechanism of Action

Corticosteroids reduce airway inflammation by inhibiting or inducing the production of end-effector proteins. An activated intracellular drug–receptor complex binds to glucocorticoid responsive elements in the gene promoter regions of DNA, stimulating or inhibiting protein transcription. End-effector proteins alter vascular tone, vascular permeability, and body water distribution; stimulate lipolysis, gluconeogenesis, and glycogen secretion; increase responsiveness of beta-adrenergic receptors; mobilize amino acids from muscles; impair leukocyte migration; and inhibit nuclear factor-kappa, which regulates production of proinflammatory proteins such as cytokines, interleukins, interferons, and chemokines.

Dosage and Time Frame for Response

Moderate to high doses of inhaled corticosteroids are indicated as a component of the chronic maintenance regimen for patients with GOLD groups C and D. Inhaled corticosteroids are used in combination with long-acting bronchodilators to reduce the risk of exacerbations in persons with COPD at high risk of exacerbations. There is no evidence for lower doses or for benefit in persons at lower exacerbation risk.

A short-course of oral corticosteroids (e.g., prednisone 40 mg daily for 5 days) is indicated for the treatment of an acute COPD exacerbation. The dose is lower and the duration of therapy is shorter than for patients with asthma exacerbations.

The onset of action of systemic and inhaled corticosteroids (hours to days) is delayed due to the time it takes for the drug to influence protein expression. It takes several hours for lung function to improve in response to systemic (oral or intravenous) corticosteroids. The response to inhaled corticosteroid typically begins during the first week of therapy and continues to increase for weeks to months with continued treatment.

Contraindications

Corticosteroids are contraindicated in persons with a history of hypersensitivity to corticosteroids or any component of the formulation.

Adverse Events

Common adverse events with inhaled corticosteroids include oral candidiasis and dysphonia. Patients should be counseled to rinse their mouth, gargle, and spit out the water after each dose. Common adverse effects with short-term oral corticosteroids include sodium and water retention (peripheral edema, increased blood pressure, exacerbation of congestive heart failure), hyperglycemia, increased appetite and weight gain, CNS stimulation and/or nightmares, peptic ulcer, and leukocytosis.

Common adverse effects with long-term (more than 14 days) high doses (typically greater than 7.5 mg/d of prednisone or equivalent) include adrenal suppression, muscle wasting, myopathy, decreased bone mineral density, posterior subcapsular cataracts, dermal thinning, ecchymosis, and peptic ulcer. Persons taking high-dose inhaled corticosteroids are at risk of the same adverse effects.

Interactions

Corticosteroids are metabolized by the hepatic cytochrome P-450 isoenzyme CYP3A4. Corticosteroids induce CYP2C19 and CYP3A4. The prescriber should check for potential drug interactions before prescribing corticosteroids and counsel persons with COPD to check with the prescriber before starting or stopping any nonprescription, prescription, or complementary medication.

Concurrent use of inhaled corticosteroids and strong inhibitors of CYP3A4 (e.g., ritonavir, clarithromycin, itraconazole, ketoconazole, telithromycin) increases the risk of systemic corticosteroid adverse effects and is not recommended.

Systemic corticosteroids decrease the response to skin tests, enhance adverse effects from live vaccines, and decrease the response to oral antidiabetic drugs. Antacids decrease the oral bioavailability of oral corticosteroids; counsel the patient to wait at least 2 hours between doses of an antacid and oral corticosteroid.

Methylxanthines

Mechanism of Action

Methylxanthine bronchodilators (theophylline, aminophylline) relax bronchial smooth muscle, enhance diaphragmatic contractility, and have a slight anti-inflammatory effect; the exact mechanisms of action are not known. Methylxanthines, nonselective phosphodiesterase inhibitors, increase cAMP by inhibiting phosphodiesterase 1, 2, 3, 4, and 7. Increased cAMP relaxes airway smooth muscle and increases bronchial ciliary activity. The enhanced diaphragmatic contractility is probably mediated by weak adenosine antagonism. The slight anti-inflammatory effect is mediated by other molecular mechanisms.

Dosage and Time Frame for Response

Theophylline and aminophylline, the ethylenediamine salt of theophylline, are dosed to a target serum drug concentration. Aminophylline is about 80% theophylline. Although the therapeutic serum drug concentration range is generally accepted to be 10 mg to 20 mg/L, persons with COPD may do well with lower serum drug concentrations or experience unacceptable adverse effects with serum drug concentrations within the therapeutic range. The half-life of theophylline is short (approximately 8 hours in nonsmokers); sustained-release dosage formulations (q12h and q24h) are recommended to improve patient adherence. Theophylline is metabolized in the liver; many medical conditions and drugs induce or inhibit theophylline metabolism. It is therefore important to monitor the serum drug concentrations and individualize the dosage based upon patient response, concurrent medical conditions, and drug interactions.

Contraindications

Theophylline and aminophylline are contraindicated in persons with a history of hypersensitivity to theophylline or any component of the formulation. Patients with a history of allergy to aminophylline are most likely allergic to the ethylenediamine component of the medication, not theophylline. Methylxanthines should be used with caution in patients with a history of tachyarrhythmia, peptic ulcer disease, seizure disorders, or hyperthyroidism. Intravenous dosage forms may contain propylene glycol, which can accumulate in persons with renal dysfunction. Large amounts of propylene glycol may cause lactic acidosis, hyperosmolality, seizures, and respiratory depression. Oral dosage forms may contain dyes, alcohol, or sugar.

Adverse Events

Common adverse events with methylxanthines include tachyarrhythmias, restlessness, insomnia, tremor, nausea, vomiting, gastroesophageal reflux, seizures, and peptic ulcer aggravation. Tachycardia and potentially life-threatening cardiac arrhythmias may occur at therapeutic concentrations. Seizures usually occur with serum theophylline concentrations above 35 mg/L but may occur at lower concentrations.

Interactions

Theophylline is primarily metabolized by the hepatic cytochrome P-450 isoenzymes CYP1A2, CYP2E1, and CYP3A4; theophylline is a minor substrate of CYP2C9 and CYP2D6. Hepatic metabolism can be induced or inhibited by hundreds of drugs and by medical conditions that affect hepatic function. The prescriber should check for potential drug interactions before prescribing theophylline and counsel persons with COPD to check with the prescriber before starting or stopping any nonprescription, prescription, or complementary medication.

Examples of commonly used drugs that inhibit theophylline metabolism (increase theophylline serum concentration) include ciprofloxacin, cimetidine, erythromycin, and allopurinol. Examples of commonly used drugs that induce theophylline metabolism (decrease theophylline serum concentration) include phenobarbital, diphenylhydantoin, and rifampin. The prescriber should check for potential drug interactions before prescribing theophylline and counsel persons with COPD to check with the prescriber before starting or stopping any nonprescription, prescription, or complementary medication.

Smoking induces theophylline metabolism, lowering the serum drug concentration. Caffeine and sympathomimetic drugs have similar adverse effects as the methylxanthines; concurrent use increases the risk of adverse effects. Theophylline may antagonize the sedating and anxiolytic effect of benzodiazepines.

Phosphodiesterase 4 Inhibitors

Mechanism of Action

Roflumilast inhibits phosphodiesterase 4, an enzyme commonly found in respiratory inflammatory cells (e.g., neutrophils, monocytes, macrophages, CD4$^+$ and CD8$^+$ T lymphocytes) and structural cells (e.g., endothelial cells, epithelial cells, smooth muscle cells, and fibroblasts). Phosphodiesterase 4 inhibition increases intracellular cAMP, modifying the inflammatory response in these respiratory cells and structures.

Dosage and Time Frame for Response

Roflumilast is an alternative maintenance medication for patients with GOLD groups C and D COPD. The dose is 500 mcg daily. Although roflumilast increases FEV_1 slightly, the increase may not be clinically significant. Roflumilast is used to reduce the risk of exacerbations in persons at high risk for exacerbations.

Contraindications

Roflumilast is contraindicated in persons with a history of hypersensitivity to roflumilast or any component of the formulation. Roflumilast undergoes hepatic metabolism. Given the risk for serious and potentially life-threatening adverse events, roflumilast is contraindicated in persons with Child-Pugh B or C moderate to severe liver impairment.

Adverse Events

Roflumilast increases the risk of suicide even in persons with no history of suicidal ideation; several completed suicides were reported during preapproval trials. Patients and their families must be counseled to report new or worsening insomnia, anxiety, depression, suicidal thoughts, or changes in mood. Weight loss has been reported with roflumilast. Patient weight must be monitored regularly. Roflumilast should be discontinued if persons with COPD experience significant weight loss while taking the drug.

Interactions

Roflumilast is metabolized by the hepatic cytochrome P-450 isoenzymes CYP3A4 and CYP1A2. CYP3A4 inhibitors and dual CYP3A4 and CYP1A2 inhibitors impair roflumilast hepatic metabolism, increasing the serum concentration of roflumilast and increasing the risk for clinically significant adverse events, and should only be used with caution. The concurrent administration of strong CYP3A4 inducers such as rifampicin, phenobarbital, carbamazepine, and phenytoin is not recommended.

Immunizations

All persons with COPD should receive an annual influenza vaccine. The Center for Disease Control Advisory Committee on Immunization Practices recommends that immunocompetent and adults with COPD receive the 23-valent pneumococcal polysaccharide vaccine (PPSV23) (CDC, 2012, 2013). The 13-valent pneumococcal conjugate vaccine (PCV13) is recommended for persons receiving long-term systemic corticosteroids.

Oxygen

Chronic oxygen therapy (greater than 15 hours/d) is indicated for persons with COPD if twice over a 3-week period of disease stability the resting P_aO_2 is ≤55 mm Hg or the S_aO_2 is 88% or less with or without hypercapnia (Stoller et al., 2010). For persons with COPD and pulmonary hypertension, congestive heart failure, or polycythemia (hematocrit greater than 55%), chronic oxygen therapy is indicated if the P_aO_2 is 55 to 60 mm Hg or the S_aO_2 is 88% or less.

Antibiotics

Respiratory infections (viral or bacterial) are common causes of COPD exacerbations. A 5- to 10-day course of antibiotics is indicated if all three cardinal symptoms of an acute exacerbation (i.e., increased dyspnea, increased sputum volume, purulent sputum) are present or purulent sputum and one other cardinal symptom are present or if the person requires mechanical ventilation (GOLD, 2016). The most common bacterial pathogens associated with COPD exacerbations are *Haemophilus influenzae*, *Streptococcus pneumoniae*, and *Moraxella catarrhalis*; persons with a history of frequent exacerbations are at risk for infections with *Pseudomonas aeruginosa* (Sethi & Murphy, 2008). Local antibiotic sensitivity and resistance patterns must be considered when selecting the antibiotic.

Selecting the Most Appropriate Drug

Initial drug therapy selection depends on COPD severity, symptoms, and exacerbation risk (**Table 26.2**).

First-Line Therapy

All persons with COPD need at least one short-acting bronchodilator for self-management of acute symptoms. Either the short-acting beta$_2$-adrenergic agonist albuterol or the SAMA ipratropium bromide is indicated; a SABA is preferred for persons taking a LAMA for maintenance therapy. The combination SABA plus SAMA is an option for persons with GOLD group B, C, or D COPD.

Maintenance therapy is not indicated as first-line therapy for persons with GOLD group A COPD. The first-line maintenance therapy for persons with GOLD group B COPD is a LAMA or a LABA. The first-line maintenance therapy for persons with GOLD groups C and D is an inhaled corticosteroid plus a LAMA or LABA.

Second-Line Therapy

The second-line maintenance therapy for persons with GOLD group A is a LAMA, LABA, or the combination of a SABA plus a SAMA. The combination of a LAMA plus a LABA is second-line therapy for persons with GOLD groups B, C, and D. The combination of the phosphodiesterase 4 inhibitor roflumilast plus a LAMA or LABA is another second-line option for persons with GOLD groups C and D COPD. Other second-line therapy options for persons with GOLD group D include triple therapy (inhaled corticosteroid plus a LAMA plus a LABA) or quadruple therapy (inhaled corticosteroid plus LAMA plus LABA plus roflumilast).

Other Options

Theophylline, alone or in combination with first-line or second-line regimens for GOLD groups A, B, C, and D, is an option. A SABA, SAMA, or the combination of a SABA plus a SAMA may be used alone or in combination with first-line or second-line regimens for GOLD groups B, C, and D.

Special Considerations

Geriatric

Older persons with COPD at risk of cardiovascular disease or with known cardiovascular disease may be at risk from the cardiovascular stimulatory effects of beta$_2$-adrenergic agonists, especially with higher doses; inhaled anticholinergics may be better tolerated. Theophylline clearance may be decreased in older persons with COPD increasing the risk of theophylline cardiovascular stimulatory adverse effects. Theophylline dosing must be individualized and serum drug concentrations monitored closely. Elderly persons are more likely to be taking multiple other medications, increasing the likelihood of drug–drug and drug–medical condition interactions. Kinesthetic motor skills, visual acuity, and inspiratory flow may decline with aging making it difficult for patients to prepare and self-administer medications using respiratory drug delivery devices. Higher doses of inhaled corticosteroids and repeated doses of oral corticosteroids may increase the risk of osteoporosis. Women and men with known osteopenia or osteoporosis should be advised to take supplemental calcium (1,000 to 1,500 mg calcium) and vitamin D (400 units) per day.

Women

There are no gender-specific recommendations for managing COPD.

Ethnic

Culturally specific beliefs regarding cause of disease, acceptance of acute or chronic medications, medication color, dosage formulation, and route of administration may influence a person's acceptance and adherence to the prescribed drug and nondrug therapy. Persons with COPD may seek care from healers and may be using natural remedies. It is important to ask about, respect, and integrate these beliefs into the COPD management plan.

Genomics

There are no gene-specific therapeutic recommendations for managing COPD.

ACUTE EXACERBATIONS

COPD exacerbations are common; a frequent exacerbator experiences two or more exacerbations per year. Viral or bacterial respiratory infections are common causes of acute exacerbations though the cause may not be identifiable. The GOLD guidelines define a COPD exacerbation as "An acute event characterized by a worsening of the patient's respiratory symptoms that is beyond normal day-to-day variation and leads to a change in medication" (GOLD, 2016). Exacerbations are characterized by an acute change in one or more of the following symptoms: cough (increased frequency and severity), sputum (increased volume or change in appearance), and dyspnea (increased). The decision to hospitalize a person for management of an acute COPD exacerbation often is difficult. Indicators for hospitalization include severe baseline COPD, presence of significant comorbidities, older age, inadequate home support, new cardiopulmonary signs on physical exam (e.g., cyanosis), and failure of drug therapy to resolve the exacerbation (GOLD, 2016). Discharge may be considered when the person has been clinically stable for 12 to 24 hours and needs the short-acting bronchodilator no more frequently than every 4 hours.

Management of an acute COPD exacerbation includes increasing the dose and/or frequency of the short-acting bronchodilator (SABA or SAMA); adding a 5-day course of oral corticosteroids (e.g., prednisone 40 mg daily) if the FEV$_1$ is less than 50% of predicted; adding a 5- to 10-day course of antibiotics if all three cardinal COPD exacerbation symptoms, are present (increased dyspnea, increased sputum volume, and purulent sputum), the person has purulent sputum plus one other cardinal or the person required endotracheal intubation and mechanical ventilation; and supplemental oxygen to maintain the P$_a$O$_2$ 55 mm Hg or more (GOLD, 2015).

MONITORING PATIENT RESPONSE

Routine follow-up appointments should be scheduled every 2 to 3 months. Self-assessment questionnaires should be completed at each visit. Assess trends in patient symptoms, including cough, sputum, breathlessness, and fatigue, and determine if the person smokes tobacco or is exposed to environmental inhaled toxins. Encourage and support smoking cessation. Identify exacerbations and discuss modifiable factors. Assess medication adherence and identify any medication-related adverse effects. Evaluate respiratory drug administration techniques to ensure adequate drug delivery. Assess serum theophylline concentrations before adjusting the dose and no sooner than 48 hours after a change in dose. For persons on a stable theophylline regimen, assess the serum theophylline concentration at least annually. Perform the physical exam, monitoring lung function and any comorbidities. The GOLD 2016 guidelines recommend that spirometry be performed at least annually (GOLD, 2016).

PATIENT EDUCATION

Patient education includes counseling about medications, including indications, dosing, mechanisms of action, potential side effects, and drug delivery techniques. Advise persons with COPD to avoid medications that suppress the respiratory system, including first-generation antihistamines, cough suppressants, narcotics, and tranquilizers. Encourage all persons with COPD to check with a health care professional before starting any nonprescription, prescription, or complementary alternative medication.

Drug Information

The GOLD guidelines contain pharmacologic class and product-specific drug information. Drug information is available on professional organization (e.g., the American College of Chest Physicians), nonprofit organization (e.g., the American Lung Association), and government (e.g., National Institutes of Health) Web sites. Pharmaceutical company Web sites often include links to respiratory drug delivery device videos. Pharmacy therapeutics and medical pulmonary textbooks provide more in-depth drug information.

Patient-Oriented Information Sources

Patient-oriented information about COPD is available from many resources. Local support groups, often affiliated with local hospitals, provide ongoing multidisciplinary support for patients and their families. Many Web sites provide patient-oriented information. Sources of noncommercial information include the National Heart, Lung, and Blood Institute Web site (www.nhlbi.nih.gov), the American Lung Association Web site (www.lungusa.org), and the American College of Chest Physicians Web site (www.chest.net.orgeducaton/patient/guide/copd).

Nutrition/Lifestyle Changes

Weight loss frequently occurs in persons with COPD; as many as one third to one half of persons with COPD are undernourished. Low body weight in persons with COPD is associated with impaired pulmonary status, reduced diaphragmatic mass, lower exercise capacity, and a higher mortality rate. Weight loss occurs because of increased energy requirements; metabolic and mechanical inefficiency contribute to the increased energy expenditure. An imbalance between protein synthesis and protein breakdown may cause a disproportionate depletion of fat-free mass. Persons with COPD need to be on an appropriate diet; supplemental nutrition may be necessary.

Complementary and Alternative Medications

The current GOLD guidelines do not recommend any complementary and alternative medical therapies (GOLD, 2016). Clinicians should ask persons with COPD about the use of these therapies, especially herbal and other products, to identify potential disease and drug interactions.

Respiratory Devices

Patient education regarding inhaled drug administration is essential (**Table 26.4**). Respiratory drug delivery systems include metered-dose inhalers, dry powder inhalers, soft mist inhalers, and nebulizers. Each device has unique characteristics, requiring different dose preparation and inhalation steps. This can be very confusing, especially for older persons with COPD using multiple different respiratory drug delivery systems.

TABLE 26.4

Drug Delivery Device Techniques

Device	General Technique
Pressurized metered-dose inhalers	1. Remove dust cap. 2. Inspect for debris. 3. Shake vigorously for 5 s. 4. Hold the device upright (mouthpiece down). 5. Position mouthpiece; do not block with tongue. 6. Press down on the canister and breathe in at the same 7. time (midinspiration actuation is more effective but is very difficult to perform). 8. Continue to inhale to the end of a quiet breath (about 4–6 s). 9. Hold breath for 10 s. 10. Exhale slowly. 11. Replace dust cap. 12. Wait at least 1 min between puffs for short-acting beta$_2$-adrenergic agonists and 15–30 s for all other drugs.

TABLE 26.4

Drug Delivery Device Techniques (*Continued*)

Device	General Technique
Spacers and valved holding chambers	1. Visually check for debris. 2. Prepare metered-dose inhaler. 3. Insert metered-dose inhaler in spacer. 4. Hold the spacer/valved holding chamber level. 5. Gently exhale to end of a quiet breath. 6. Press the canister once. 7. Immediately inspire slowly and deeply. 8. Remove spacer from mouth. 9. Hold breath for 10 s. 10. Exhale slowly.
Dry powder inhalers	1. Remove cover. 2. Prepare dose. 3. Exhale softly *away* from device. 4. Seal lips around mouthpiece. 5. Inhale rapidly and forcefully. 6. Remove device from mouth. 7. Hold breath for 10 s. 8. Exhale softly *away* from device. 9. Replace cover.
Soft mist inhaler	Priming: Prime for first use (different priming instructions if not used for more than 3 d and if not used for more than 21 d). 1. Hold upright with cap closed. 2. Turn clear base in the direction of the white arrows until it clicks (half a turn). 3. Flip open cap. 4. Breathe out slowly and fully. 5. Close lips around the end of the mouthpiece. 6. Point the inhaler to the back of throat. 7. While taking a slow deep breath, press the dose-release button. 8. Continue to breathe in slowly for as long as possible. 9. Remove inhaler from mouth. 10. Hold breath for 10 s. 11. Exhale slowly.
Small-volume nebulizers	1. Place the equipment on a stable surface. 2. Connect the tubing to the compressor. 3. Hold the medication chamber upright; add the premixed drug solution or measure and add drug and saline. 4. Place the lid on the medication chamber. 5. Connect the tubing to the medication chamber. 6. Turn on the air compressor. 7. Check for the generation of a fine mist. 8. Sit up comfortably straight. 9. Seal lips around the mouthpiece; do not block with tongue. 10. Holding the medication chamber upright, breathe in and out normally; take a deeper breath and hold it for a few seconds every minute or so. 11. Continue until the medication chamber begins to sputter. 12. Turn off the compressor. 13. Disconnect the medication chamber and tubing.

CASE STUDY*

M.V. is a 53-year-old accountant who smoked a pack of cigarettes a day for 30 years. He quit smoking 6 months ago. He presents with shortness of breath while hurrying on level ground or walking up a slight hill but is not limited doing any activities at home. He complains of a chronic productive morning cough. He was treated at home for one respiratory infection last year. On physical exam, you observe wheezing throughout all lung fields, hyperresonance on percussion of the lungs, and low flat diaphragms. He has no cyanosis, clubbing, or edema. His mMRC dyspnea score is 1. His CAT™ score is 6. Pulmonary function studies show an FEV_1/FVC less than 70% with an FEV_1 72% of predicted. He has no other medical conditions and is not taking any nonprescription, prescription, or complementary alternative medicine. He has no known drug allergies.

DIAGNOSIS: CHRONIC OBSTRUCTIVE PULMONARY DISEASE

1. List specific goals for treatment for M.V.
2. What drug therapy would you prescribe? Why?
3. What are the parameters for monitoring success of the therapy?
4. Discuss specific patient education based on the prescribed therapy.
5. List one or two adverse reactions for the selected agent that would cause you to change therapy.
6. What would be the choice for second-line therapy?
7. What over-the-counter and/or alternative medications would be appropriate for M.V.?
8. What lifestyle changes would you recommend to M.V.?
9. Describe one or two drug–drug or drug–food interactions for the selected agent.

* Answers can be found online.

Bibliography

Starred references are cited in the text.

*Akinbami, L. J., & Liu, X. (2011, June). Chronic obstructive pulmonary disease among adults ages 18 and over in the United States, 1998–2009. NCHD Data Brief No. 63.

*American Lung Association. Chronic Obstructive Pulmonary Disease (COPD) Fact Sheet. (2015). Retrieved from http://www.lung.org/lung-disease/copd/resources/facts-figures/COPD-Fact-Sheet-html

*Bestall, J. C., Paual, E. A., Garrod, R., et al. (1999). Usefulness of the Medical Research Council (MRC) dyspnoea scale as a measure of disability in patients with chronic obstructive pulmonary disease. *Thorax, 54,* 581–586.

*Cavailles, A., Brinchault-Rabin, G., Dixmier, A., et al. (2013). Comorbidities of COPD. *European Respiratory Reviews, 22,* 454–475.

*Center for Disease Control. (2012). Use of 13-valent pneumococcal conjugate vaccine and 23-valent pneumococcal polysaccharide vaccine for adults with immunocompromising conditions: Recommendations of the Advisory Committee on Immunization Practices (ACIP). *Morbidity and Mortality Weekly Report, 61,* 816–819.

*Center for Disease Control. (2013). Use of 13-valent pneumococcal conjugate vaccine and 23-valent pneumococcal polysaccharide vaccine among children aged 6–18 years with immunocompromising conditions: Recommendations of the Advisory Committee on Immunization Practices (ACIP). *Morbidity and Mortality Weekly Report, 62,* 521–524.

*Global Strategy for the Diagnosis, Management, and Prevention of Chronic Obstructive Pulmonary Disease. (2016). Global initiative for chronic obstructive lung disease. Retrieved from www.goldcopd.org

*Jones, P. W., Harding, G., Berry, P., et al. (2009). Development and first validation of the COPD Assessment Test. *European Respiratory Journal, 34,* 648–654.

*MacNee, W. (2006). Pathology, pathogenesis, and pathophysiology. *British Medical Journal, 332,* 1202–1204.

*National Center for Health Statistics. (2010). Health care use: Assisted living and other residential care. 2010 National Survey of Residential Care Facilities (NSRCF) Data Dictionary: Resident public-use file. Washington, DC: National Center for Health Statistics, Centers for Disease Control and Prevention, U.S. Department of Health and Human Services. Retrieved from ftp://ftp.cdc.gov/pub/Health_Statistics/NCHS/Dataset_Documentation/NSRCF/2010/2010NSRCF_ResidentPublicUseFileDataDictionary.pdf

*National Institutes of Health. National Heart, Lung, and Blood Institute. (2012). Morbidity & Mortality: 2012 Chart Book on Cardiovascular, Lung, and Blood Diseases. Retrieved from www.nhlbi.nih.gov/files/docs/research/2012_ChartBook.pdf

*Schiller, J. S., Lucas, J. W., Ward, B. W., et al. (2012). Summary health statistics for U.S. adults: National Health Interview Survey, 2010. National Center for Health Statistics. *Vital and Health Statistics, 10*(252).

*Sethi, S., & Murphy, T. F. (2008). Infection in the pathogenesis and course of chronic obstructive pulmonary disease. *New England Journal of Medicine, 359,* 2355–2365.

*Stoller, J. K., Panos, R. J., Krachman, S., et al. (2010). Oxygen therapy for patients with COPD: Current evidence and the long-term oxygen treatment trial. *Chest, 138,* 179–187.

*U.S. Department of Health and Human Services. (2014). The health consequences of smoking—50 years of progress: A report of the surgeon general. Atlanta, GA: U.S. Department of Health and Human Services, Centers for Disease Control and Prevention, National Center for Chronic Disease Prevention and Health Promotion, Office on Smoking and Health. Retrieved from http://www.surgeongeneral.gov/library/reports/50-years-of-progress/exec-summary.pdf

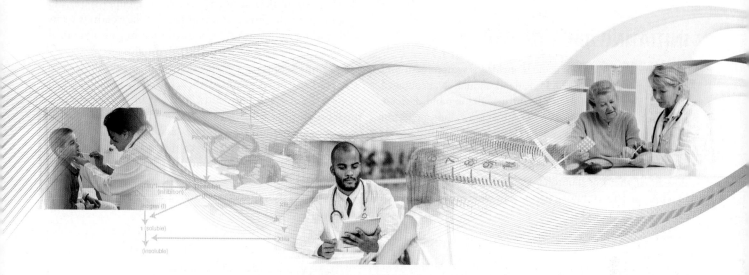

27 Bronchitis and Pneumonia

Andrew J. Grimone ■ Virginia P. Arcangelo ■ Eric T. Wittbrodt

ACUTE BRONCHITIS

In the United States, acute bronchitis is diagnosed in 5% of adults and accounts for over 10 million outpatient office visits annually (Liapikou & Torres, 2014). The disease is a reversible inflammatory condition of the tracheobronchial tree that occurs in all age groups and is usually self-limiting. Typically, acute bronchitis occurs during the winter months. Predisposing factors for acute bronchitis include cold air, damp climates, fatigue, malnutrition, and inhalation of irritating substances, such as polluted air and cigarette smoke.

CAUSES

Viral infections cause over 90% of acute bronchitis episodes; the most common respiratory viruses associated with acute bronchitis are rhinovirus, coronavirus, influenza virus A and B, parainfluenza virus, adenovirus, and respiratory syncytial virus (RSV). Bacterial infections cause less than 10% of acute bronchitis (Liapikou & Torres, 2014). The only bacterial microorganisms implicated in the pathogenesis of uncomplicated acute bronchitis are *Bordetella pertussis*, *Chlamydophila pneumoniae*, and *Mycoplasma pneumoniae*. Limited evidence indicates that other common respiratory tract pathogens such as *Streptococcus pneumoniae* can contribute to acute bronchitis.

PATHOPHYSIOLOGY

Acute bronchitis is characterized by infection of the tracheobronchial tree. This infection results in hyperemic and edematous mucous membranes, yielding an increase in bronchial secretions. Destruction of the respiratory epithelial lining and reduced mucociliary function result from these changes. This process is usually transient and resolves after the infection clears.

DIAGNOSTIC CRITERIA

Signs and symptoms of acute bronchitis are preceded by manifestations of an upper respiratory tract infection such as coryza, malaise, chills, back and muscle pain, headache, and sore throat. If fever is present, it rarely exceeds 102.2°F (39°C) and lasts for 3 to 5 days. Fever is more commonly seen with adenovirus, influenza virus, and *M. pneumoniae* infection. The hallmark of acute bronchitis is a cough that is initially dry and nonproductive; however, as the production of bronchial secretions increases, the cough becomes more abundant and mucoid. The cough usually lasts for 7 to 10 days, although in some patients, it can persist for weeks to months. Patients also present with phlegm, hoarseness, and wheezing.

Pulmonary examination may reveal signs of coarse, moist bilateral crackles, rhonchi, and wheezing. The chest x-ray typically reveals no active disease; thus, a chest x-ray is not indicated unless pneumonia is suspected. The usefulness of cultures to identify the causative microorganisms is limited because most cases of acute bronchitis are viral in origin, and cultures usually are negative or grow normal nasopharyngeal flora. Laboratory tests may reveal a normal or slightly elevated white blood cell (WBC) count.

The high reported incidence of acute bronchitis can be correlated with the absence of definitive diagnostic signs or laboratory tests. Thus, the diagnosis is based purely on the patient's risk factors and signs and symptoms. In many patients, an upper respiratory tract infection (sinusitis or allergic rhinitis) may be misdiagnosed as acute bronchitis.

INITIATING DRUG THERAPY

The general treatment for acute bronchitis is symptomatic and supportive care (**Figure 27.1**). Patients should be encouraged to drink plenty of fluids to prevent dehydration and decrease the viscosity of bronchial secretions. Bed rest is indicated until fever subsides. Mild analgesic/antipyretic therapy is effective for relief of fever and musculoskeletal pains. Aspirin or acetaminophen (Tylenol; 650 mg in adults or 10 to 15 mg/kg per dose in children) or ibuprofen (Advil, others; 200 to 400 mg in adults or 5 to 10 mg/kg per dose in children) administered

every 4 to 6 hours can be used as analgesic/antipyretic therapy. Acetaminophen is the agent of choice because aspirin should be avoided in children, given the correlation of aspirin and the development of Reye syndrome in this age group. Aspirin and ibuprofen should also be used cautiously in the elderly, patients with a history of peptic ulcer disease or recent gastrointestinal (GI) bleeding, and patients with renal insufficiency.

Nonprescription cough and cold medications (see Chapter 24) often are used to help reduce the signs and symptoms of acute bronchitis. The use of nonprescription medications that contain various combinations of antihistamines, sympathomimetic agents, and antitussives can result in dehydration of bronchial secretions. This could lead to further aggravation of symptoms, which prolongs the recovery process. Cough that is associated with acute bronchitis can become bothersome. Dextromethorphan, an antitussive

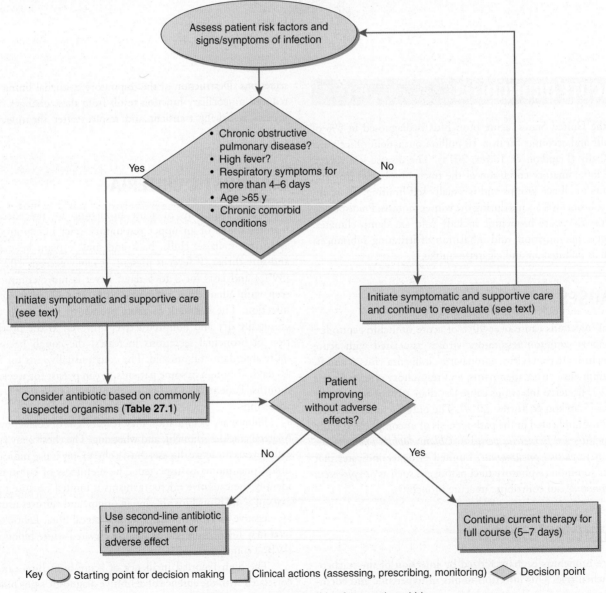

FIGURE 27.1 Treatment algorithm for acute bronchitis.

agent, is recommended to help treat mild, persistent cough. Severe cough may require a more potent cough medication that contains codeine or hydrocodone.

In patients with fever and a productive cough persisting beyond 4 to 6 days, treatment with antibiotics may be indicated to treat bacterial coinfection, especially in patients with underlying pulmonary disease.

Goals of Drug Therapy

The goals of pharmacotherapy include providing the patient with comfort and, in severe cases, treating associated dehydration and respiratory compromise. If antibiotics are administered, minimizing side effects is also a goal.

Antibiotics

Antibiotics are often prescribed for patients with acute bronchitis; however, in otherwise healthy patients, they offer little relief from the respiratory symptoms of the disease and do not shorten the course of the illness. Therefore, routine use of antibiotics for acute bronchitis is discouraged. Despite this, studies have shown that approximately two thirds of patients diagnosed with acute bronchitis in the United States are prescribed antibiotic therapy. Part of the reason for antibiotic overprescribing is lack of patient and caregiver education on the causes of acute bronchitis. Surveys suggest that over 50% of patients believe that antibiotics are effective in treating viral upper respiratory tract infections. Patient education on appropriate treatment is crucial to prevent inappropriate antibiotic use. One educational method useful in teaching patients and caregivers about this illness is selection of descriptive words such as "chest cold" or "viral upper respiratory tract infection" instead of using the term "acute bronchitis."

Antibiotics are indicated if the patient has concomitant chronic obstructive pulmonary disease (COPD), high fevers, purulent sputum, or respiratory symptoms for more than 4 to 6 days. Additionally, antibiotics may be considered in patients over 65 years of age or those with chronic diseases such as heart failure, diabetes mellitus, or serious neurological disorders. Empiric antibiotic therapy should be directed against the microorganisms commonly suspected to cause acute bronchitis.

Selecting the Most Appropriate Agent

Table 27.1 lists the antibiotics that are commonly used to treat acute bronchitis caused by bacteria. Aminopenicillins such as amoxicillin (Amoxil) are effective against infections caused by *S. pneumoniae* and *Haemophilus influenzae*.

For microorganisms that produce beta-lactamase, such as *Moraxella catarrhalis* and *H. influenzae*, aminopenicillins given in combination with a beta-lactamase inhibitor, such as amoxicillin–clavulanate (Augmentin), or a second- or third-generation cephalosporin should be administered.

For acute bronchitis due to atypical bacteria such as *M. pneumoniae* and *Chlamydophila* species, macrolides (e.g., erythromycin [Eryc], clarithromycin [Biaxin], or azithromycin [Zithromax]) or doxycycline (Vibramycin) are effective. Doxycycline should not be used in children younger than age 8.

TABLE 27.1

Acute Bronchitis: Drug Therapy for Selected Microorganisms

Microorganism	Treatment
H. influenzae	aminopenicillin (amoxicillin)
M. catarrhalis, H. influenzae (beta-lactamase producing)	amoxicillin + clavulanate (Augmentin)
M. pneumoniae, Chlamydophila pneumoniae	macrolide (erythromycin, clarithromycin, or azithromycin) or doxycycline
B. pertussis	macrolide (erythromycin, clarithromycin, or azithromycin)
Influenza A	oseltamivir or zanamivir
Influenza B	oseltamivir or zanamivir

In this population, the agent of choice is a macrolide. If *B. pertussis* is the likely microorganism, erythromycin or another macrolide is the drug of choice.

During epidemics caused by influenza A or B virus, oseltamivir (Tamiflu) and zanamivir (Relenza Diskhaler) may be administered early in the course of the illness to minimize symptoms of influenza in adults and pediatrics who have been symptomatic for no longer than 2 days. For more information about antibiotic/antimicrobial therapy, refer to Chapter 8.

CHRONIC BRONCHITIS

Chronic bronchitis is a component of COPD, which is one of the five leading causes of death in the United States. (See Chapter 26 for a discussion of COPD.) The standard description/definition of chronic bronchitis is productive cough and sputum production for 3 months per year for at least two consecutive years. An acute exacerbation of chronic bronchitis is defined as worsening of respiratory symptoms such as increased cough, sputum, and dyspnea that warrants a change in medications. Chronic bronchitis primarily affects adults and occurs more commonly in men than in women. Over 10% of the adult population in the United States aged 40 or older is afflicted with chronic bronchitis, which accounts for a large amount of health care expenditures and lost wages (Kim & Criner, 2013). Patients with chronic bronchitis are more likely to have frequent and severe episodes of acute bacterial bronchitis. Exacerbations of COPD account for more than 50% of the overall cost related to the treatment of COPD (Qureshi et al., 2014). Because many infections are untreated, the exact morbidity of acute exacerbations of chronic bronchitis is unknown.

CAUSES

Several factors are implicated in the pathogenesis of chronic bronchitis, leading to chronic inflammation and sputum production. The predominant factor in chronic bronchitis is cigarette smoke, a well-known respiratory irritant, and most patients with chronic bronchitis have a history of cigarette smoking. However, chronic bronchitis has been noted in 4% to 22% of patients who never smoked (Kim & Criner, 2013), suggesting other causative factors. Occupational dust, fumes, and environmental pollution are some additional risk factors that contribute to the etiology of the disease. The presence of gastroesophageal reflux and hypersecretion of mucus in patients with asthma has also been shown to yield symptoms of chronic bronchitis. Evidence suggests that recurrent respiratory infections may predispose a person to development of chronic bronchitis, although the exact reason for this is unclear.

Colonization of the lower airways with bacteria such as *H. influenzae*, *M. catarrhalis*, and *S. pneumoniae* has been frequently detected in patients with chronic bronchitis. Up to 25% of patients with stable COPD have been found to be colonized with these bacteria. These and other microorganisms harbored in the bronchial epithelium act as reservoirs for infection when patient host defenses become compromised. In patients with acute exacerbations of COPD, 70% to 80% of cases are triggered by bacterial or viral infections (Liapikou & Torres, 2014). Viral infections account for nearly one third of acute exacerbations. Other bacteria such as *Pseudomonas aeruginosa* and Enterobacteriaceae are more likely to be associated with acute exacerbations in patients with frequent exacerbations and advanced stages of COPD. Exposures to environmental pollution or unknown factors contribute to the remainder of acute exacerbations. The frequency and severity of exacerbations of chronic bronchitis are more frequent and severe with increasing stages of COPD.

PATHOPHYSIOLOGY

Several physiologic abnormalities of the bronchial mucosa may lead to chronic bronchitis. It has been suggested that patients with chronic bronchitis are predisposed to respiratory infections because of overproduction and hypersecretion of mucus from goblet cells and impaired mucociliary clearance due to chronic inhalation of irritating substances. A factor leading to impaired mucociliary clearance is the replacement of ciliated epithelium with nonciliated metaplastic cells. This leads to the inability of the bronchi to clear the profuse, thick, sticky secretions present in patients with chronic bronchitis. In addition, inhalation of toxic irritants results in bronchial obstruction because of stimulation of cholinergic activity and increased bronchomotor tone.

DIAGNOSTIC CRITERIA

As with acute bronchitis, cough is the hallmark of chronic bronchitis. Cough, with sputum production, can be mild or severe and may be stimulated by simple conversation. Many patients with chronic bronchitis expectorate a large quantity of white to yellow tenacious sputum in the morning. Because of the characteristics of sputum, many patients complain of a foul taste in the mouth.

Clinical assessment and the patient's medical history contribute to the diagnosis of chronic bronchitis. Other diseases such as bronchiectasis, cardiac failure, cystic fibrosis, tuberculosis, pulmonary emboli, and lung carcinoma must be excluded before diagnosing a patient with chronic bronchitis or an acute exacerbation of chronic bronchitis. Patients with chronic bronchitis must have a cough with sputum production for at least 3 consecutive months for 2 consecutive years.

Physical examination of patients with chronic bronchitis is usually unremarkable except that chest auscultation reveals inspiratory and expiratory rales, rhonchi, and mild wheezing; normal breath sounds are diminished. As the severity of the disease progresses, an increase in the anteroposterior diameter of the thoracic cage (barrel chest appearance), hyperresonance on percussion, and limited mobility of the diaphragm are observed. Pulmonary function tests demonstrate a decrease in vital capacity and prolongation of expiratory flow. Other features of disease progression include clubbing of the fingers, cor pulmonale, hepatomegaly, and edema of the lower extremities.

The diagnosis of an acute exacerbation of chronic bronchitis relies on the clinical presentation of an acute change in symptoms. Since an acute exacerbation of chronic bronchitis is defined as worsening of respiratory symptoms that warrants a change in medications, diagnosis focuses on early changes in symptoms such as an increase in frequency and severity of cough. Other symptoms include increased sputum production, purulent sputum, hemoptysis, chest congestion and discomfort, increased dyspnea, and wheezing. Malaise, loss of appetite, and fever may also be present. True chills (rigors) and high-grade fever suggest pneumonia rather than an acute exacerbation of chronic bronchitis. This finding requires a chest x-ray for diagnosis. The duration of worsening or new symptoms, number and frequency of previous exacerbations, severity of underlying disease, comorbidities, and current treatment regimen for COPD are helpful in assessing a patient who presents with an acute exacerbation of chronic bronchitis. In these patients, pulse oximetry is useful for tracking and/or adjusting supplemental oxygen therapy. An electrocardiogram (ECG) may help in the diagnosis of or to rule out cardiac problems. A complete blood count (CBC) will help to identify leukocytosis.

To determine the need for hospitalization during an acute exacerbation of chronic bronchitis, the presence of severe symptoms including use of accessory muscles, worsening or new cyanosis, development of peripheral edema, hemodynamic instability, or deterioration in mental status needs to be assessed. A sputum gram stain can assist in empiric antibiotic prescribing. Sputum culture and susceptibility testing may guide the clinician in choosing appropriate antibiotic therapy. In outpatients, sputum cultures are not often feasible or practical, as they take too long to return and frequently do not provide reliable results (i.e., more than 4 hours often elapses between expectoration of sputum and analysis in the laboratory). However, a sputum culture should be considered, especially in patients with frequent exacerbations requiring

TABLE 27.2

Classification of Chronic Bronchitis and Treatment Options for Acute Exacerbations

Clinical Status	Risk Factors	Microorganisms	Treatment
Simple chronic bronchitis	Increased sputum production and purulence, no major risk factors, less than 3 exacerbations/year	*S. pneumoniae, H. influenzae,* and *M. catarrhalis* (low risk for antibiotic resistance)	First-line: amoxicillin, doxycycline, macrolide, or sulfamethoxazole/trimethoprim Second-line: amoxicillin–clavulanate (Augmentin); second- or third-generation cephalosporin
Complicated chronic bronchitis	FEV$_1$ < 50% of predicted value, advanced age (over 65 y of age), significant comorbidity (e.g., cardiac disease, diabetes, renal or hepatic insufficiency), home oxygen use, antibiotic use in the past 3 mo, and/or 3 or more exacerbations/year	*S. pneumoniae, H. influenzae, M. catarrhalis,* (resistance to beta-lactam antibiotics common)	First-line: amoxicillin–clavulanate (Augmentin XR); second- or third-generation oral cephalosporin; doxycycline Second-line: macrolide; fluoroquinolone (levofloxacin, moxifloxacin, gemifloxacin)
Severe complicated chronic bronchitis	FEV$_1$ < 35% of predicted value with risk factors for *P. aeruginosa* (frequent or recent antibiotic use, chronic corticosteroid use, advanced disease, and/or history of bronchiectasis)	The above microorganisms and Enterobacteriaceae, *P. aeruginosa* (more likely to have antibiotic-resistant bacteria)	levofloxacin or ciprofloxacin

Data from Global Initiative for Chronic Obstructive Lung Disease (GOLD). (2015). Retrieved from www.goldcopd on July 10, 2015.

antibiotic use, failing current antibiotic therapy, known or suspected resistant pathogens, severe airflow limitation, and/or exacerbations requiring mechanical ventilation. Additionally, procalcitonin, a biomarker specific for bacterial infections, can be obtained to help in determining the presence of active infection. However, this test is currently reserved for patients in acute care settings, given the cost, lack of widespread availability, and delayed turnaround time for results.

A classification system for patients with chronic bronchitis is frequently used to identify high-risk patients and select the appropriate antimicrobial therapy for acute exacerbations according to the suspected microorganism. **Table 27.2** outlines the classification system and treatment options, taking into consideration the baseline clinical status, risk factors, and common pathogens.

Patients with uncomplicated chronic bronchitis have little or no lung impairment and no major risk factors for antibiotic resistance. The most common pathogens include *H. influenzae, M. catarrhalis,* and *S. pneumoniae.* Viral infections should be considered before bacterial infections in this patient category. Although antibiotic resistance is less common in this group, over 50% of *H. influenza* and *M. catarrhalis* produce beta-lactamase, making amoxicillin ineffective. This should be considered especially in patients who fail amoxicillin therapy.

Patients with complicated chronic bronchitis include those with moderate to severe (FEV$_1$ 50% less than predicted) lung impairment, those who are elderly (over 65 years of age), those who have frequent exacerbations, and those who have

comorbid illnesses such as congestive heart failure, diabetes mellitus, chronic renal failure, or chronic liver disease. The most common pathogens isolated in severe chronic bronchitis are *H. influenzae, S. pneumoniae,* and *M. catarrhalis.* Frequent exacerbations in this population increase the likelihood of antibiotic use and the risk for antibiotic resistance, including penicillin-resistant *S. pneumoniae.*

Patients with severe complicated chronic bronchitis have characteristics similar to those in the previous group, but they have severe airflow obstruction and often have constant purulent sputum production. The same microorganisms found in the other groups should be considered in these patients; however, gram-negative microorganisms such as *P. aeruginosa* and Enterobacteriaceae should also be suspected.

INITIATING DRUG THERAPY

A complete assessment of the patient's occupational and environmental history should be performed to treat chronic bronchitis properly. Patients should reduce or eliminate cigarette smoking and their exposure to second-hand smoke. This can be accomplished by counseling sessions and the use of nicotine replacement therapy. Also, exposure to inhaled irritants at work or home should be reduced or eliminated. Pharmacologic treatment should be optimized to prevent or control symptoms, reduce the frequency of exacerbations, and improve quality of life. (See Chapter 26 for a discussion of COPD.)

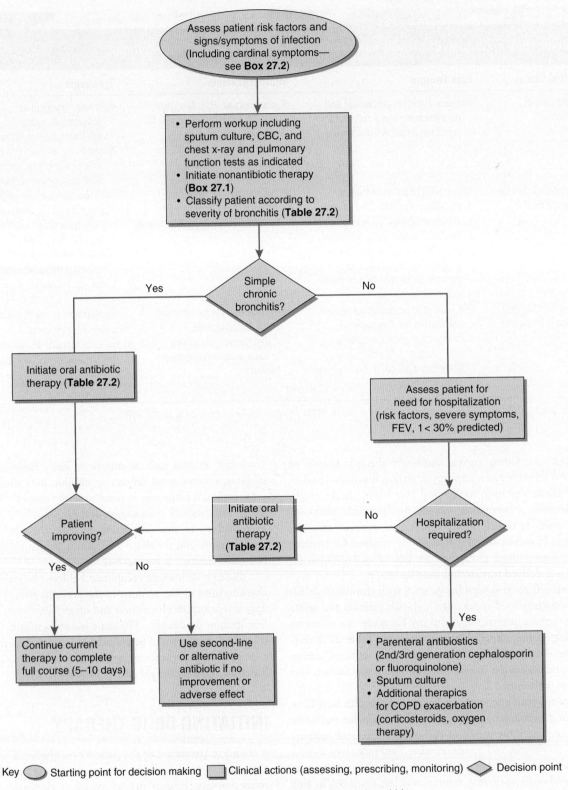

FIGURE 27.2 Treatment algorithm for chronic bronchitis.

The approach to treatment of acute exacerbations of chronic bronchitis is multifactorial (**Figure 27.2**). The therapies listed in **Box 27.1** should be initiated. Antibiotics should be initiated in patients with the three "cardinal symptoms" (**Box 27.2**) (or at least two cardinal symptoms if increased purulence of sputum is one of the two symptoms) or in hospitalized patients who require mechanical ventilation. Fever alone is not an indication for antibiotic therapy.

- Stop smoking
- Avoid inhalation of polluted air
- Increase ingestion of fluids (nonalcoholic)
- Humidify atmosphere
- Use short-acting bronchodilators
- Treat any associated asthma

Data from Global Initiative for Chronic Obstructive Lung Disease (GOLD). (2015). Retrieved from www.goldcopd on July 10, 2015.

Goals of Drug Therapy

There are two goals for the treatment of exacerbations of chronic bronchitis: to minimize the impact of the current exacerbation and to prevent the development of subsequent exacerbations with prolonged infection-free intervals. Depending on the severity of the exacerbation and the underlying disease, exacerbations can be managed in the outpatient or inpatient setting. More than 80% of exacerbations can be managed on an outpatient basis (Global Initiative for Chronic Obstructive Lung Disease [GOLD], 2015).

Antimicrobial Therapy

Among the antimicrobial agents used to treat acute exacerbations of chronic bronchitis are the aminopenicillins (amoxicillin) with or without clavulanic acid, cephalosporins, tetracyclines, macrolides, and fluoroquinolones. **Table 27.3** reviews antibiotic agents used for patients with chronic bronchitis and pneumonia.

Aminopenicillins

Aminopenicillins, such as amoxicillin, inhibit the final step of bacterial cell wall synthesis by binding to one or more of the penicillin-binding proteins. They are safe for use in children, adults, and pregnant women. **Table 27.3** reviews the dose of amoxicillin for acute exacerbations of chronic bronchitis.

BOX
27.2
Cardinal Symptoms Associated with Exacerbations of COPD

- Increase in dyspnea (shortness of breath)
- Increase in sputum volume
- Increase in or presence of sputum purulence

Contraindications

Aminopenicillins should not be administered to patients with severe hypersensitivity reactions to these agents.

Adverse Events

Hypersensitivity reactions to aminopenicillins manifest as eosinophilia or rash (urticarial, erythematous, morbilliform). Angioedema, exfoliative dermatitis, and erythema multiforme have also been reported as hypersensitivity reactions to aminopenicillins. These reactions occur less frequently than does eosinophilia or rash. Rarely, Stevens-Johnson syndrome has been reported as a hypersensitivity reaction to aminopenicillins.

Nausea, vomiting, and diarrhea, however, are the most common adverse effects that occur with aminopenicillins. Diarrhea is more common with amoxicillin–clavulanate. Pseudomembranous colitis may occur during or after the antibiotic treatment.

Interactions

Aminopenicillins may interrupt the enterohepatic circulation of estrogen by reducing the bacterial hydrolysis of conjugated estrogen in the GI tract. Therefore, the efficacy of oral contraceptives is decreased. Probenecid may increase the effects of aminopenicillins by competing with renal tubular secretion. An increased risk for rash occurs with the coadministration of allopurinol (Zyloprim) and aminopenicillins; the exact mechanism of this interaction has not been established.

Cephalosporins

Cephalosporins consist of several agents, including cephalexin (Keflex), cefaclor (Ceclor), cefuroxime axetil (Ceftin), cefpodoxime (Vantin), cefdinir (Omnicef), and others that are frequently used for the treatment of acute exacerbations of chronic bronchitis. Like penicillins, cephalosporins inhibit bacterial cell wall synthesis by binding to one or more of the penicillin-binding proteins. These drugs are safe for use by children and adults. The dosages of cephalosporins are listed in **Table 27.3**.

Contraindications

Cephalosporins are contraindicated in patients who have had hypersensitivity reactions to any member of the cephalosporin class of antimicrobial agents. There is a 5% to 7% cross-sensitivity reaction between cephalosporins and penicillins, and therefore, cephalosporins should be avoided in patients who have had an anaphylactic reaction to penicillins.

Adverse Events

Nausea, diarrhea, and vomiting are common adverse effects with cephalosporins. Fungal infections and pseudomembranous colitis can also occur with the administration of cephalosporins.

Interactions

Probenecid increases the serum concentrations of cephalosporins by reducing their renal clearance.

TABLE 27.3

Overview of Selected Antibiotics for Bronchitis and Pneumonia

Generic (Trade) Name and Dosage	Selected Adverse Events	Contraindications	Special Considerations
Aminopenicillins			
amoxicillin (Amoxil, Trimox) Adults: 500 mg q8h or 875–1,000 mg q12h Children: 40 mg/kg/d in divided doses q8h–12 h (high-dose regimen 80–90 mg/kg/d in divided doses q12h)	Nausea, vomiting, diarrhea, gastritis, rash, hypersensitivity reactions	Hypersensitivity reactions to penicillin derivatives Pregnancy category B	High incidence of development of rash in patients with infectious mononucleosis. Amoxicillin should be used with extreme caution in this patient population. Take with or without food. Food may decrease GI symptoms. Interacts with warfarin and oral contraceptives; probenecid decreases renal excretion, and allopurinol increases the risk of rash. Safe for young children
amoxicillin–clavulanate Adults: Augmentin 500 mg/125 mg q8h or 875/125 mg q12h Augmentin XR 2000 mg/125 mg q12h Children: Same as for amoxicillin Augmentin ES 90 mg/kg/d in divided doses q12h	Nausea, vomiting, diarrhea, gastritis, hypersensitivity reactions, Stevens-Johnson syndrome, seizures (high doses)	Hypersensitivity reactions to penicillin, clavulanic acid Pregnancy category B	High incidence of development of rash in patients with infectious mononucleosis. Amoxicillin clavulanate should be used with extreme caution in this patient population. Take with or without food. Food may decrease GI symptoms. Interacts with warfarin and oral contraceptives; probenecid decreases renal excretion, and allopurinol increases the risk of rash. Safe for young children
Cephalosporins			
cephalexin (Keflex) Adults: 500 mg q6h Children: 25–100 mg/kg/d in divided doses q6h to q8h; not to exceed 4,000 mg/d	Nausea, vomiting, diarrhea, rash, hypersensitivity reactions, fungal infections Serious: pseudomembranous colitis, seizures (high doses)	Hypersensitivity or allergy to cephalosporin antibiotics Not recommended in children <1 mo Pregnancy category B	Avoid cephalosporins for patients who have had an anaphylactic hypersensitivity reaction to other beta-lactam antibiotics. Use with caution in patients with a delayed type of reaction to other beta-lactam antibiotics. Take with or without food. Food may decrease GI symptoms. Probenecid decreases renal excretion.
cefaclor (Ceclor) Adults: 250–500 mg q8h Children: 20–40 mg/kg/d in divided doses q8–12 h	Nausea, vomiting, diarrhea, rash, hypersensitivity reactions, fungal infections Serious: Pseudomembranous colitis	Hypersensitivity to cephalosporin Not recommended in children <1 mo Pregnancy category B	Avoid cephalosporins for patients who have had an anaphylactic hypersensitivity reaction to other beta-lactam antibiotics. Use with caution in patients with a delayed type of reaction to other beta-lactam antibiotics. Take with or without food. Food may decrease GI symptoms. Probenecid decreases renal excretion.
cefuroxime axetil (Ceftin) Adults: 250–500 mg q12h Children: 20–30 mg/kg/d in divided doses q12h	Same as above	Same as above	Same as above
cefpodoxime (Vantin) Adults: 200 mg q12h Children: 10 mg/kg/d in divided doses q12h; not to exceed 400 mg/d	Same as above	Same as above	Same as above

TABLE 27.3

Overview of Selected Antibiotics for Bronchitis and Pneumonia (*Continued*)

Generic (Trade) Name and Dosage	Selected Adverse Events	Contraindications	Special Considerations
cefdinir (Omnicef) Adults: 300 mg q12h Children: 14 mg/kg/d once daily or in divided doses q12h; not to exceed 600 mg/d	Same as above	Same as above	Same as above
Tetracyclines			
doxycycline (Vibramycin, Doryx, Vibra-Tab, Monodox) Adults: 100 mg q12h or 200 mg q24h Children: Not recommended for use in children less than 8 y of age	GI upset (nausea, vomiting, diarrhea, bulky, loose stools, anorexia), hypersensitivity reactions, photosensitivity reactions, superinfection, enterocolitis, rash, blood dyscrasias, hepatotoxicity	Hypersensitivity reactions to any tetracycline Pregnancy category D, breast-feeding Not recommended in children. Use of drug during tooth development may cause dental discoloration.	Capsules or tablets should be administered with adequate amounts of fluid. Capsules or tablets should not be given to patients with esophageal obstruction. Antacids containing aluminum, calcium, or magnesium should be given 1–2 h before. Avoid sunlight or ultraviolet light.
Sulfonamides			
trimethoprim–sulfamethoxazole (Bactrim) Adults: 800 mg sulfamethoxazole/160 mg trimethoprim (TMP) q12h (for PCP: 15–20 mg TMP/kg/d in divided doses q6–8 h) Children >2 mo: 8 mg TMP/kg/d in divided doses q12h (for PCP: 15–20 mg TMP/kg/d in divided doses q6–8 h)	Nausea, vomiting, rash, pruritus, urticaria, photosensitivity, Stevens-Johnson syndrome, toxic epidermal necrolysis	Allergy to sulfa Pregnancy category C (D at term)	Preferred agent in the treatment of pneumonia secondary to Pneumocystis jiroveci pneumonia (PCP) in patients with HIV/AIDS or other immunosuppression
Macrolides			
erythromycin (Eryc, PCE) Adults: 250–500 mg q6h Children: 30–50 mg/kg/d in divided doses q6h (not to exceed 4,000 mg/d)	Abdominal pain and cramping, nausea, vomiting, diarrhea, hepatic dysfunction, QTc prolongation, urticaria, fungal infection, skin eruptions, rash, ototoxicity	Allergy to erythromycin, hypersensitivity to macrolides, hepatic dysfunction, or preexisting liver disease Pregnancy category B	Erythromycin is a potent inhibitor of CYP450 3A4 isoenzymes. Screen medication list for potential drug–drug interactions prior to initiating erythromycin. Avoid in patients with known prolongation of QTc intervals and in patients receiving class IA (quinidine, procainamide) or class III (dofetilide, amiodarone, sotalol) antiarrhythmic agents. Take on empty stomach for better absorption 1 h before or 2 h after a meal.
clarithromycin (Biaxin) Adults: 500 mg q12h or 1,000 mg q24h Children >6 mo: 15 mg/kg/d in divided doses q12h	Diarrhea, nausea, abnormal taste, dyspepsia, abdominal discomfort, fungal infection, pseudomembranous colitis, hepatic dysfunction, QTc prolongation, headache, mild urticaria, mild skin eruptions	Hypersensitivity to macrolides, hepatic dysfunction or preexisting liver or renal disease, pregnancy, or breast-feeding Pregnancy category C	Clarithromycin is a potent inhibitor of CYP450 3A4 isoenzymes. Screen medication list for potential drug–drug interactions prior to initiating clarithromycin. Avoid in patients with known prolongation of QTc intervals and in patients receiving class IA (quinidine, procainamide) or class III (dofetilide, amiodarone, sotalol) antiarrhythmic agents. Tablets and oral suspension can be taken with or without food. Extended-release tablets should be taken with food.

(Continued)

TABLE 27.3

Overview of Selected Antibiotics for Bronchitis and Pneumonia (*Continued*)

Generic (Trade) Name and Dosage	Selected Adverse Events	Contraindications	Special Considerations
azithromycin (Zithromax) Bronchitis: Adults: 500 mg once daily for 3 d or 500 mg for 1 d and then 250 once daily for 4 additional days CAP: 500 mg once daily for 5–7 d Children >6 mo: 10 mg/kg for 1 d and then 5 mg/kg once daily for 4 additional days	Diarrhea, loose stools, nausea, abdominal pain, dizziness, headache, rash photosensitivity, fungal infection, dizziness, fatigue, palpitations, QTc prolongation	Hypersensitivity to macrolides Use with caution in hepatic disease. Pregnancy category B	Prolongation of QTc intervals has been reported in patients receiving azithromycin. Use with caution in patients with a history of QTc prolongation or in patients receiving class IA (quinidine, procainamide) or class III (dofetilide, amiodarone, sotalol) antiarrhythmic agents. Administer the suspension 1 h before or 2 h after a meal. Use of antacids with aluminum or magnesium decreases peak serum levels.
Fluoroquinolones			
levofloxacin (Levaquin) 500–750 mg once daily Not recommended for use in children less than 18 y of age	Nausea, diarrhea, vomiting, abdominal pain or discomfort, hypersensitivity reactions, photosensitivity, confusion, dizziness, hallucinations, pseudomembranous colitis	Hypersensitivity to quinolone antibiotics Pregnancy category C	All fluoroquinolones are associated with an increased risk of tendinitis and tendon rupture. The risk is higher in older patients over 60 y of age, in patients taking corticosteroids, and in patients with kidney, heart, or lung transplants. Antacids, sucralfate, iron, or multivitamins with zinc should be administered 2 h before or 2 h after taking levofloxacin as these agents may interfere with the GI absorption of levofloxacin.
moxifloxacin (Avelox) 400 mg once daily Not recommended for use in children less than 18 y of age	Same as above	Same as above	Same as above. Moxifloxacin should be administered 4 h before or 8 h after taking antacids, sucralfate, iron, or multivitamins with zinc as these agents may interfere with the GI absorption of moxifloxacin.
gemifloxacin (Factive) 320 mg once a day Not recommended for use in children less than 18 y of age	Same as above	Same as above	Same as above. Antacids, sucralfate, iron, or multivitamins with zinc should be administered 2 h before or 3 h after taking gemifloxacin as these agents may interfere with the GI absorption of gemifloxacin

Doxycycline

Doxycycline inhibits protein synthesis by binding with the 30S ribosomal subunit of susceptible microorganisms. The dosage of doxycycline is listed in **Table 27.3**.

Contraindications

Doxycycline is contraindicated in patients with severe hypersensitivity reactions to doxycycline or tetracycline. The drug should not be administered to children younger than 8 years of age; its use in infants has resulted in retardation of bone growth. Doxycycline can localize in the enamel of developing teeth, resulting in enamel hypoplasia and permanent yellow-gray to brown tooth discoloration. Doxycycline is a pregnancy category D drug and should not be administered to pregnant or lactating women.

Adverse Events

GI adverse effects such as nausea, vomiting, diarrhea, and bulky, loose stools commonly occur with the administration of doxycycline. Superinfection, enterocolitis, blood dyscrasias, and hepatotoxicity have also been reported to occur with the administration of doxycycline.

Interactions

The administration of antacids, iron, and bismuth subsalicylate (Pepto-Bismol), which contain divalent or trivalent cations, reduces the efficacy of doxycycline by impairing its absorption because of chelation of the cation by doxycycline. Barbiturates, phenytoin (Dilantin), and carbamazepine (Tegretol) can reduce the serum concentration of doxycycline by induction of hepatic metabolism. The effects of warfarin (Coumadin) can be potentiated when administered with doxycycline.

Doxycycline can decrease vitamin K production by GI bacteria. The significance of this interaction is unknown, but patients should be monitored for signs of bleeding when anticoagulant drugs are used concomitantly with doxycycline.

Macrolides

The three macrolides—erythromycin, clarithromycin, and azithromycin—work by inhibiting ribonucleic acid–dependent protein synthesis by binding to the 50S ribosomal subunit. The dosage regimens of the macrolides are listed in **Table 27.3**.

Contraindications

Macrolides are contraindicated in patients with known hypersensitivity reactions to erythromycin, clarithromycin, or azithromycin, and these products should not be administered to patients with hepatic impairment or preexisting liver disease. Clarithromycin and some formulations of erythromycin should not be administered to pregnant and lactating women because the safety of these agents has not been fully established.

Adverse Events

Abdominal pain, cramping, nausea, vomiting, diarrhea, and hepatic dysfunction commonly occur with the administration of macrolides. Skin rashes and pseudomembranous colitis have also been reported.

Interactions

Erythromycin and clarithromycin are inhibitors of the hepatic cytochrome P-450 microsomal enzyme system (CYP3A4) and P-glycoproteins (Pgp). Elevations of carbamazepine (Tegretol), cyclosporine (Sandimmune), theophylline (Slo-Phyllin), zidovudine (Retrovir), ritonavir (Norvir), midazolam (Versed), sildenafil (Viagra), digoxin, and warfarin can occur when these agents are administered concomitantly with erythromycin or clarithromycin. There are many interactions with erythromycin and clarithromycin, so a complete drug interaction assessment should be done prior to initiating either of these antibiotics. Antacids should not be administered simultaneously with azithromycin as they may inhibit azithromycin absorption.

Fluoroquinolones

Levofloxacin (Levaquin), moxifloxacin (Avelox), and gemifloxacin (Factive) (the so-called antipneumococcal or respiratory fluoroquinolones) inhibit deoxyribonucleic acid gyrase and topoisomerase IV in susceptible microorganisms, thereby interfering with bacterial replication. The dosing regimens of the fluoroquinolones are listed in **Table 27.3**.

Contraindications

Fluoroquinolones are contraindicated in patients with known hypersensitivity reactions to any member of the fluoroquinolone class. Fluoroquinolones generally should not be administered to patients younger than age 18. Limited data are available for use in pregnant or lactating women; thus, these medications should only be used when the benefit outweighs the risk. Gemifloxacin, levofloxacin, and moxifloxacin should be used cautiously in patients with known prolongation of the QT interval, in patients with uncorrected hypokalemia, and in those receiving class IA (e.g., quinidine, procainamide) or class III (e.g., amiodarone, sotalol) antiarrhythmic agents. These agents should also be used cautiously in patients who are receiving other agents known to prolong the QT interval, such as erythromycin, antipsychotics, and tricyclic antidepressants.

Gemifloxacin and levofloxacin are eliminated through the kidneys; therefore, dosage adjustments are necessary in patients with renal impairment. Moxifloxacin is metabolized primarily through sulfate and glucuronide conjugation. Moxifloxacin should be administered with caution to patients with hepatic insufficiency due to the risk for QT prolongation.

Adverse Events

GI adverse effects (e.g., nausea, diarrhea, vomiting, and abdominal pain) have commonly been reported with the administration of fluoroquinolones. Central nervous system adverse effects such as headache, agitation, confusion, and restlessness have occurred after the administration of fluoroquinolones. Photosensitivity has been reported with the administration of some fluoroquinolones.

Interactions

Fluoroquinolones should not be administered concomitantly with antacids, calcium products, sucralfate (Carafate), iron, and multivitamins. These products should be spaced at least 2 to 4 hours apart from the fluoroquinolone. The manufacturers of moxifloxacin recommend spacing at least 4 hours before or 8 hours after the administration of iron- or zinc-containing multivitamins, magnesium, calcium, or aluminum products or sucralfate.

Selecting the Most Appropriate Agent

For simple chronic bronchitis, treatment with an aminopenicillin (amoxicillin) or doxycycline is sufficient. In patients with complicated chronic bronchitis, therapy with amoxicillin–clavulanate, a second- or third-generation cephalosporin, a macrolide, or fluoroquinolone is effective. Fluoroquinolones should be reserved for patients who fail alternative antibiotics, those with allergies or contraindications to alternative antibiotics, or patients with resistant pathogens. Overuse of this class of medications has led to increased resistance among certain bacteria. For severe complicated chronic bronchitis, a fluoroquinolone (such as levofloxacin) is the agent of choice because gram-negative microorganisms, such as *Pseudomonas* species, need to be considered as potential pathogens. (**Table 27.2** and **Figure 27.2** provide more information about treatment choices.) In addition to antibiotic therapy, use of short-acting bronchodilators, short courses of corticosteroids (e.g., prednisone for 5 to 10 days), and oxygen supplementation are used in the treatment of acute exacerbations of chronic bronchitis.

Special Population Considerations

Pediatric

Antimicrobials related to the tetracyclines (e.g., doxycycline) may discolor dental enamel in fetuses and children while teeth are developing and should be avoided in children less than 8 years of age.

Women

Women who take antibiotics, especially the aminopenicillins, may experience secondary symptoms, such as vaginitis, that require treatment.

MONITORING PATIENT RESPONSE

Signs and symptoms of infection should improve within days of drug administration. If patients fail to improve, sputum culture and susceptibility should be performed to evaluate the possibility of resistance. Additionally, if fever with chills develops, additional workup (e.g., chest x-ray) should be considered to rule out pneumonia.

The recommended duration of antimicrobial therapy for acute exacerbation of chronic bronchitis is 5 to 10 days. This decreases morbidity and increases the posttherapy infection-free period in patients. Some patients may require a longer duration of therapy or hospitalization for parenteral antibiotic therapy. Because patients with chronic bronchitis are predisposed to recurrent infections, antimicrobial agents that were previously successful in eradicating the infection should be readministered. However, frequent use of antibiotics increases the risk of resistance; thus, patients should be monitored for response. In patients who fail to respond, bacterial resistance should be considered.

Measures to prevent exacerbations of chronic bronchitis should be initiated, as recurrent exacerbations are associated with accelerated decline in lung function. Frequent exacerbations are associated with reduced physical activity, poor quality of life, and increased risk of death. One method to prevent exacerbations is annual administration of an influenza vaccine. This reduces the rate and severity of infections with the influenza virus in some patients with chronic bronchitis. Patients should also receive the pneumococcal vaccine. Sufficient data do not exist to support the theory that the pneumococcal vaccine may reduce the frequency or severity of exacerbations in patients with chronic bronchitis. However, this vaccine may potentially reduce the frequency of pneumococcal pneumonia. The use of long-term antibiotics to prevent acute exacerbations is generally discouraged. However, azithromycin 250 mg orally once daily for a year has been shown to reduce the frequency of exacerbations and improve quality of life in patients with COPD (Albert et al., 2011). The mechanism is thought to be related to anti-inflammatory properties of azithromycin and not antibacterial activity. The use of azithromycin for this purpose is generally limited to select patients with moderate to severe underlying COPD.

PATIENT EDUCATION

Drug Information

The patient needs to understand that the entire course of antimicrobial therapy should be finished to ensure eradication of the causative microorganisms. Moreover, the patient should be cautioned to report adverse effects, such as diarrhea, immediately to the health care provider for further evaluation. Other adverse effects may include photosensitivity, and the patient needs to be advised to protect the skin from excessive exposure to sunlight or ultraviolet light, particularly when taking doxycycline. If sunburn-like reactions or skin eruptions occur, the patient should contact the prescriber immediately.

Additional patient counseling includes whether to take the drug with food or on an empty stomach. Storage instructions include whether the drug needs refrigeration, as does the oral suspension of amoxicillin, which is stable for only 7 days at room temperature but for 14 days under refrigeration. The reconstituted oral suspension of amoxicillin–clavulanate should be kept in the refrigerator, as should most oral cephalosporin suspensions.

Patients should be encouraged to take the macrolides with food to lessen the GI adverse effects, except for the oral suspension of azithromycin, which must be taken on an empty stomach. Most oral suspensions of erythromycin should be refrigerated, but the oral suspension of clarithromycin should not be refrigerated because it is more palatable when taken at room temperature. The oral suspension of azithromycin can be refrigerated if the patient so desires.

Because fluoroquinolones may cause dizziness and light-headedness, patients need to be aware of this when operating an automobile or other potentially dangerous machinery or engaging in activities requiring mental alertness or coordination.

COMMUNITY-ACQUIRED PNEUMONIA

Pneumonia is an infection of the lungs that leads to consolidation of the usually air-filled alveoli. It occurs in all age groups and can be caused by various pathogens, including viruses, bacteria, mycobacteria, mycoplasma, and fungi. Systemic viral infections such as influenza A or B in adults and measles or varicella in children can also lead to pneumonia.

Pneumonia occurs in about 3 to 4 million people each year in the United States, with over one million patients requiring hospitalization (Remington & Sligl, 2014). The symptoms of pneumonia include cough, chills, shortness of breath, sputum production, and chest pain. Physical examination includes fever in most, tachycardia, and tachypnea, with decreased breath sounds and crackles on auscultation in about 80% of cases. Pneumonia is classified by where it was acquired: community-acquired pneumonia (CAP), health care–associated pneumonia (HCAP), and hospital-acquired pneumonia (HAP). The latter two types of pneumonia occur in patients with exposure to the hospital and/or health care settings that predispose them to different pathogens than seen in CAP. This chapter focuses on the diagnosis and treatment of CAP.

Pneumonia carries an age-adjusted mortality rate of up to 22%. CAP is an acute infection of the lower respiratory tract that is usually associated with:

- symptoms of acute infection and acute infiltrates detected by chest x-ray OR
- auscultatory findings consistent with pneumonia on physical examination

Elderly individuals and those with other coexistent illnesses such as COPD, diabetes mellitus, renal insufficiency, congestive heart failure, and chronic liver disease are at a high risk for acquiring pneumonia compared with other patient populations. Additionally, individuals with immunosuppression related to malignancy, chronic corticosteroid use or other myelosuppressive medications, or history of HIV infection have an increased risk for developing pneumonia. New microorganisms as a cause of CAP and the emergence of antimicrobial-resistant organisms require broader antimicrobial coverage in treating CAP, as compared to bronchitis.

CAUSES

Although several pathogens are identified in CAP, the etiology is only established in about 40% of cases. *S. pneumoniae* is the most commonly isolated pathogen. Up to 65% of all diagnosed CAP cases can be attributed to *S. pneumoniae* (Remington & Sligl, 2014). However, widespread use of the pneumococcal vaccine has reduced the incidence of *S. pneumoniae* as a causative pathogen. Other pathogens that have been commonly isolated in patients with CAP are *H. influenzae* (12%), *S. aureus* (2%), and gram-negative bacilli (1%). Less common pathogens that have been implicated in CAP are *M. catarrhalis*, *Streptococcus pyogenes*, *Chlamydia psittaci*, and *Neisseria meningitidis*. Atypical microorganisms, such as *Legionella* species, *M. pneumoniae*, and *C. pneumoniae*, account for 10% to 20% of cases. Between 2% and 15% of CAP cases are due to viral infections (Remington & Sligl, 2014). The most common virus known to be associated with CAP is the influenza virus; however, parainfluenza virus, RSV, and adenovirus also have been isolated as CAP pathogens. Methicillin-resistant *S. aureus* (MRSA) has emerged as the most common pathogen isolated in community-acquired skin and soft tissue infections and is increasingly recognized as a cause of CAP.

PATHOPHYSIOLOGY

Microorganisms gain access to the lower respiratory tract by inhalation as airborne particles, by way of the bloodstream to the lung from an extrapulmonary site of infection or, most commonly, through aspiration of oropharyngeal contents. This is a common method of transmission of microorganisms into the lower respiratory tract for both healthy and ill people.

DIAGNOSTIC CRITERIA

Patients with pneumonia typically present with cough, fever, dyspnea, malaise, pleuritic chest pain, and/or sputum production. It is difficult to distinguish other respiratory tract infections such as bronchitis from pneumonia based on signs and symptoms alone (**Figure 27.3**). A chest x-ray plays a critical role in differentiating pneumonia from other infections and can also indicate whether coexisting conditions, such as COPD, heart failure, and/or pleural effusions, are present.

The presence of infiltrates on chest x-ray usually indicates pneumonia, which necessitates antibiotic treatment. In general, chest x-rays cannot distinguish between bacterial and nonbacterial microorganisms. The patterns found on chest x-ray in patients with pneumonia are not helpful in making a specific etiologic diagnosis; however, certain findings on the chest x-ray can guide the practitioner to a diagnosis. The severity of illness can also be detected by an x-ray; multilobar involvement typically indicates severe illness. A Gram stain of the sputum specimen is useful in the initial evaluation of patients with pneumonia, as it can assist with empiric antibiotic prescribing. However, 40% to 60% of patients do not produce sputum, and in those who do, poor sampling reveals oropharyngeal colonization in nearly half of all culture results. Therefore, obtaining a sputum culture in outpatients is not necessary (Mandell et al., 2007). However, sputum cultures should be obtained in patients requiring hospitalization and when resistant microorganisms are suspected. Blood cultures should be obtained in patients with severe CAP requiring hospitalization. Urinary antigen tests are used to detect *S. Pneumoniae* or *Legionella pneumophila* as a cause of pneumonia. The urinary antigen tests may reveal positive results even after initiation of antibiotic therapy. Limitations of urinary antigen tests include the potential for false-negative results due to poor sensitivity and false-positive *S. pneumoniae* urinary antigen results in children colonized with *S. pneumoniae*. Additionally, the urinary Legionella antigen test only detects one serogroup of *L. pneumophila*, although it is the most common type that causes Legionella pneumonia. Due to the need to obtain a urine specimen and added cost of testing, urinary antigen tests may not be practical for use in the outpatient setting. Invasive diagnostic techniques such as transtracheal aspiration, bronchoscopy, bronchoalveolar lavage, and direct needle aspiration may be useful in patients with severe CAP.

It can be difficult to determine when an outpatient needs hospitalization for closer observation. There are severity scoring tools [Pneumonia Scoring Index (PSI), CURB-65, and

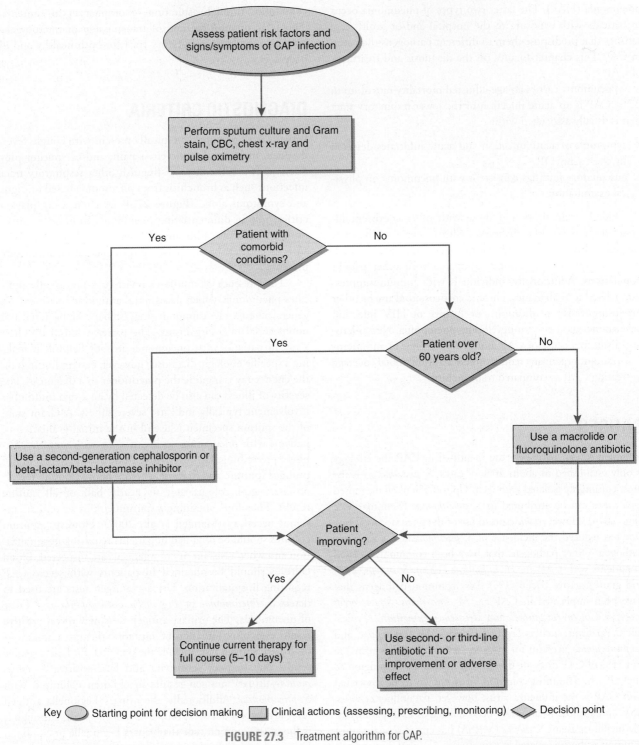

FIGURE 27.3   Treatment algorithm for CAP.

SMART-COP] available online to assess adult patients and assist in determining the risk of morbidity and mortality associated with pneumonia and the need for hospitalization. **Box 27.3** lists some objective findings of severe CAP that suggest the need for hospitalization. Once patients are hospitalized, several routine tests must be performed to determine the severity of illness, possible complications, the status of underlying conditions, and the most appropriate treatment choices. A WBC count is not useful for distinguishing between the various causative microorganisms; however, a WBC count greater than 12,000 cells/mm³ typically suggests bacterial infection. Pulse oximetry can help reflect the severity of the disease. An arterial oxygen saturation of less than 90% on room air is a standard criterion for hospital admission.

BOX 27.3 Indications for Hospitalization Secondary to Pneumonia

- Severe vital sign abnormality: pulse >140/min, systolic blood pressure <90 mm Hg, and respiratory rate >30/min
- Altered mental status (newly diagnosed): disorientation to person, place, or time and stupor or coma
- Arterial hypoxemia: Arterial oxygen saturation <90% or a P_aO_2 <60 mm Hg
- Suppurative pneumonia-related infection: empyema, septic arthritis, meningitis, and endocarditis
- Inability to tolerate oral medications
- Severe electrolyte, hematologic, and metabolic laboratory value not known to be chronic
- Lack of adequate outpatient support services for follow-up treatment

Data from Mandell, L. A., Wunderink, R. G., Anzueto, A., et al. (2007). Infectious Diseases Society of America/American Thoracic Society consensus guidelines on the management of community acquired pneumonia in adults. *Clinical Infectious Diseases, 44*, S27–S72.

INITIATING DRUG THERAPY

General treatment approaches for pneumonia consist of providing adequate hydration (replacement of loss of water that may occur because of fever, poor intake, or vomiting),

providing bronchodilators for dyspnea, and controlling fever with acetaminophen, ibuprofen, or aspirin. Additionally, in severe cases of CAP with hypoxia, supplemental oxygen may be needed until symptoms improve. Early identification of the causative microorganism is optimal for proper management of CAP. However, diagnostic tests cannot always identify all potential pathogens and no single antimicrobial regimen covers all possible causes; therefore, empiric therapy is common.

Goals of Drug Therapy

The goals of pharmacotherapy for pneumonia include eradicating the offending microorganism through the selection of appropriate antibiotic therapy, complete clinical cure, preventing complications from pneumonia (e.g., respiratory failure, sepsis, empyema), and minimizing adverse effects of medications.

Unless diagnostic tests can determine a specific etiology upon diagnosis, which is not commonly the case, empiric antibiotics should be initiated for CAP. Empiric antibiotic treatment for pneumonia should always be active against *S. pneumoniae* because this pathogen is the most common pathogen identified as a cause of bacterial pneumonia. For adults treated as outpatients without recent antibiotic use or existing comorbidities (e.g., COPD, diabetes, renal insufficiency), treatment with a macrolide (clarithromycin or azithromycin) or doxycycline is recommended (**Table 27.4**). In adult outpatients with an increased risk for poor outcomes (comorbidities and/or recent antibiotic use), a beta-lactam (high-dose amoxicillin, amoxicillin–clavulanate, or a second- or third-generation cephalosporin)

TABLE 27.4 Recommended Outpatient Antimicrobial Treatment for CAP in Adults

Category	Preferred Agents
Previously healthy; no recent antibiotic use; no risk factors for DRSP infection*	A macrolide (azithromycin or clarithromycin) or doxycycline
Presence of comorbidities (chronic heart, lung, liver, or renal disease; diabetes mellitus; alcoholism; malignancy; asplenia; immunosuppressing conditions or use of immunosuppressing drugs), use of antimicrobials within the previous 3 mo (in which case an alternative from a different class should be selected), or other risk factors for DRSP*	B-lactam [high-dose amoxicillin (e.g., 1 g three times daily) or amoxicillin–clavulanate (2 g twice a day)] is preferred; alternatives include cefpodoxime, cefdinir, and cefuroxime + a macrolide (azithromycin, clarithromycin, or erythromycin)[†].
Geographic region with a high rate (>25%) of macrolide-resistant *S. pneumoniae* (for any patient, including those without comorbidities)	Fluoroquinolone (moxifloxacin, gemifloxacin, or levofloxacin) alone Consider the use of alternative agents such as high-dose amoxicillin, amoxicillin–clavulanate + a macrolide (if atypical organisms suspected) Fluoroquinolone (moxifloxacin, gemifloxacin, or levofloxacin [750 mg]) alone
Suspected aspiration	Amoxicillin–clavulanate or clindamycin
Influenza pneumonia	Oseltamivir 75 mg PO twice daily for 5 d or zanamivir 10 mg (two inhalations) twice daily for 5 d. Begin within 2 d of signs or symptoms.

*Risks for drug-resistant *S. pneumoniae* (DRSP) include age >65 y, beta-lactam therapy within the previous 3 mo, alcoholism, immunosuppressive therapy, and exposure to a child in day care.
[†]Doxycycline may be used as an alternative in patients with an intolerance or allergy to macrolides.
Data from Mandell, L. A., Wunderink, R. G., Anzueto, A., et al. (2007). Infectious Diseases Society of America/American Thoracic Society consensus guidelines on the management of community acquired pneumonia in adults. *Clinical Infectious Diseases, 44*, S27–S72.

plus a macrolide or an antipneumococcal fluoroquinolone (e.g., levofloxacin, moxifloxacin, gemifloxacin) alone is recommended (**Table 27.4**). Doxycycline may be used as an alternative in patients intolerant or allergic to azithromycin. Ciprofloxacin should not be used for treating CAP because of the high level of resistance that *S. pneumoniae* exhibits to this drug.

Community-acquired MRSA (CA-MRSA) is a common pathogen isolated in community-acquired skin and soft tissue infections and is increasingly recognized as a cause of CAP. CA-MRSA pneumonia typically presents as a severe, rapidly progressing pneumonia with sepsis, often in children or healthy young adults. Antimicrobial agents with consistent in vitro activity against CA-MRSA isolates include vancomycin, clindamycin, sulfamethoxazole/trimethoprim, linezolid, and ceftaroline. Although it is not necessary to provide empiric coverage of MRSA for all pneumonia cases, it should be strongly considered for patients with severe pneumonia associated with sepsis, especially persons with concurrent influenza, contact with someone infected with MRSA, or radiographic evidence of necrotizing pneumonia. Patients infected with CA-MRSA pneumonia frequently require hospitalization due to the severity of symptoms.

Differences among antibiotic agents were discussed previously in the chronic bronchitis section and must be considered when choosing antimicrobial therapy for CAP. Resistance patterns also should be considered when choosing an antibiotic. Because 15% to 30% of *S. pneumoniae* isolates in the United States are resistant to doxycycline and macrolides, caution should be used in prescribing these medications as first-line agents in areas where resistance is more prevalent. Aminopenicillins, such as amoxicillin, have excellent activity against *S. pneumoniae* and remain the drug of choice to treat *S. pneumoniae*; however, amoxicillin does not have activity against beta-lactamase producing strains of *H. influenzae* and *M. catarrhalis*. Adding a beta-lactamase inhibitor to amoxicillin (e.g., amoxicillin–clavulanate) provides activity against these beta-lactamase–producing organisms and may be an option in place of macrolides or doxycycline. If beta-lactam antibiotics are used and a patient fails therapy, atypical pathogens (*L. pneumophila*, *C. pneumoniae*, and *M. pneumoniae*) should be considered, as beta-lactam antibiotics do not cover these pathogens. Macrolides, fluoroquinolones, and doxycycline have activity against the atypical pathogens that can cause pneumonia. If Legionella pneumonia is suspected, a macrolide or fluoroquinolone is preferred. If aspiration pneumonia is suspected, the antibiotic of choice is amoxicillin–clavulanate. Clindamycin is an alternative for aspiration pneumonia in patients with an allergy to penicillins.

Adult hospitalized patients should receive a beta-lactam, such as cefotaxime (Claforan) or ceftriaxone (Rocephin) in combination with a macrolide (azithromycin or clarithromycin) or a fluoroquinolone with activity against *S. pneumoniae* (**Table 27.5**). Patients hospitalized in the intensive care unit for pneumonia should receive the same therapy as do other

---

TABLE 27.5	
Recommended Antimicrobial Treatment for CAP in Adults Requiring Hospitalization	

Category	Preferred Agents
General inpatient medical ward	Parenteral beta-lactam antibiotic (ceftriaxone, cefotaxime, ampicillin/sulbactam, ertapenem) + a macrolide (azithromycin or clarithromycin)*
	Fluoroquinolone (moxifloxacin, gemifloxacin, or levofloxacin) alone
Intensive care/critically ill	Same as above
Intensive care with risk for pseudomonas	Antipseudomonal beta-lactam (piperacillin/tazobactam, cefepime, imipenem, or meropenem) + either ciprofloxacin or levofloxacin
	Antipseudomonal beta-lactam (piperacillin/tazobactam, cefepime, imipenem, or meropenem) + an aminoglycoside + azithromycin
	Antipseudomonal beta-lactam (piperacillin/tazobactam, cefepime, imipenem or meropenem) and an antipneumococcal fluoroquinolone (moxifloxacin or levofloxacin)
	If CA-MRSA suspected, add vancomycin or linezolid†
Influenza pneumonia‡	Oseltamivir 75 mg PO twice daily for 5 d (longer courses may be required in severely ill patients). Treatment of any person with confirmed or suspected influenza who requires hospitalization is recommended, even if the patient presents more than 48 h after illness onset.
Influenza with bacterial superinfection‡	Ceftriaxone, cefotaxime, or fluoroquinolone (levofloxacin or moxifloxacin) + vancomycin or linezolid
Suspected aspiration	Ampicillin/sulbactam, piperacillin/tazobactam, or clindamycin

*Doxycycline may be considered as an alternative in patients with an intolerance or allergy to macrolides.
†Risk factors for CA-MRSA infection include preceding influenza, previous infection/colonization with MRSA, cavitary infiltrates, and/or suspected necrotizing pneumonia.
‡Refer to Chapters 8 and 24 for additional information on antimicrobial therapy and treatment guidelines.
Data from Mandell, L. A., Wunderink, R. G., Anzueto, A., et al. (2007). Infectious Diseases Society of America/American Thoracic Society consensus guidelines on the management of community acquired pneumonia in adults. *Clinical Infectious Diseases, 44,* S27–S72.

hospitalized patients, unless *P. aeruginosa* is a concern. In these cases, antibiotics with broader gram-negative coverage (e.g., piperacillin–tazobactam, cefepime, or a carbapenem) should be added.

Selecting the Most Appropriate Agent

Identification of the likely microorganism simplifies treatment for pneumonia. The reader is referred to the comprehensive references for appropriate antimicrobial agents that are commonly used once pathogens have been identified (see **Figure 27.3**).

Special Population Considerations

Pediatric

Antimicrobial therapy is not routinely required for preschool-aged children with CAP, because viral pathogens are responsible for the majority of clinical disease. For mild to moderate CAP of bacterial origin treated in the outpatient setting, amoxicillin should be used as first-line therapy for previously healthy, appropriately immunized infants and preschool children through adolescent age (**Table 27.6**). Amoxicillin

provides appropriate coverage for *S. pneumoniae*, the most prominent pathogen in children. If atypical organisms, such as *M. pneumoniae* or *C. pneumoniae*, are suspected, a macrolide antibiotic should be prescribed. Antiviral therapy for influenza (oseltamivir or zanamivir) should be administered as soon as possible to children with moderate to severe CAP consistent with influenza virus. Treatment after 48 hours of symptomatic infection may still provide clinical benefit to those with more severe disease.

For children requiring hospitalization, ampicillin or penicillin G should be administered to fully immunized infants or school-aged children in areas without local high-level penicillin resistance against *S. pneumoniae*. Empiric therapy with a third-generation parenteral cephalosporin (ceftriaxone or cefotaxime) should be prescribed for hospitalized infants and children who are not fully immunized, in regions where local epidemiology of documented high-level penicillin resistance against *S. pneumoniae*, or for infants and children with life-threatening infection. Empiric combination therapy with a macrolide, in addition to a beta-lactam antibiotic, should be prescribed for hospitalized children when *M. pneumonia* and *C. pneumoniae*

TABLE 27.6

Recommended Antimicrobial Treatment of CAP in Children

	First-Line Therapy	Alternative Therapy
Treatment for Outpatient Therapy in Children		
Suspected bacterial infection in preschool age children (<5 y of age) (preschool)	amoxicillin 90 mg/kg/d in two divided doses	amoxicillin–clavulanate 90 mg/kg/d based on amoxicillin component in two divided doses. If atypical organisms suspected: azithromycin 10 mg/kg on day 1, followed by 5 mg/kg/d once daily on days 2–5 or clarithromycin 15 mg/kg/d in two divided doses
Suspected bacterial infection in children ≥5 y of age	amoxicillin 90 mg/kg/d in two divided doses; amoxicillin–clavulanate 90 mg/kg/d (based on amoxicillin component) in two divided doses	Same as above. In children >7 y of age, doxycycline may be used.
Influenza suspected or influenza widespread in the community	oseltamivir (refer to product information for weight-based dosing) for 5 d; zanamivir (children ≥7 y of age) 2 inhalations (10 mg total per dose) in two divided doses for 5 d	
Treatment for Hospitalized Children		
All ages (fully immunized)*; local penicillin resistance rates against *S. pneumoniae* is low.	ampicillin or penicillin G plus azithromycin (if atypical pathogens considered). Add clindamycin or vancomycin if CA-MRSA suspected.	Alternatives to ampicillin and penicillin G include ceftriaxone or cefotaxime. Alternatives to azithromycin include clarithromycin or erythromycin. In children >7 y of age, doxycycline may be used
All ages (not fully immunized or unknown)*; local penicillin resistance rates against *S. pneumoniae* is high or unknown.	ceftriaxone or cefotaxime + azithromycin if atypical pathogens considered. Add clindamycin or vancomycin if CA-MRSA suspected	Alternatives to azithromycin include clarithromycin or erythromycin. In children >7 y of age, doxycycline may be used.

*Childhood immunizations include conjugate vaccines for *H. influenzae* type b and *S. pneumoniae*.
Data from Bradley, J. S. Byington, C. L., Shah, S. S., et al. (2011). The management of community-acquired pneumonia in infants and children older than 3 months of age: Clinical practice guidelines by the Pediatric Infectious Diseases Society and the Infectious Diseases Society of America. *Clinical Infectious Diseases, 53*(7), e25–e76.

are significant considerations. Vancomycin or clindamycin should be provided in addition to beta-lactam therapy if *S. aureus* (particularly CA-MRSA) is suspected.

MONITORING PATIENT RESPONSE

The patient's response to therapy must be evaluated carefully. Response to treatment should be based on clinical illness, pathogen isolated, severity of illness, host factors, and chest x-ray findings. Subjective symptoms usually respond within 3 to 5 days of initiating therapy. Objective findings such as fever, leukocytosis, and chest x-ray abnormalities resolve at different times. Fever lasts for 2 to 4 days in most cases of CAP; however, defervescence occurs more quickly with *S. pneumoniae* infection. Leukocytosis usually resolves by the 4th day of initiation of antimicrobial therapy. Chest x-rays indicate that signs of pneumonia last longer than symptoms. Of course, this depends on many factors, such as the causative microorganism and underlying illness. The overall suggested chest x-ray follow-up is 7 to 12 weeks after initiation of therapy. In clinical practice, patients who develop clinical cure may not require a follow-up chest x-ray.

Duration of therapy for treating CAP depends on the severity of the illness, response to therapy, and the antimicrobial agent used to treat the infection. The standard treatment duration for CAP is 7 to 10 days for most patients; however, shorter courses of therapy are effective, especially in those with mild pneumonia. Because the half-life of azithromycin is around 68 hours, it remains in the tissues longer than erythromycin or clarithromycin. Five days of azithromycin therapy is sufficient to treat mild CAP. Additionally, 5 days of levofloxacin (750 mg once daily) is recommended. Patients with a poor response to therapy or those with Legionella pneumonia who are immunocompetent typically receive 14 days of treatment. Patients with complications from pneumonia, such as empyema, may require longer courses lasting 2 to 4 weeks.

PATIENT EDUCATION

The patient must take the full course of medication even though he or she may feel better within days of initiation of antibiotics. Early discontinuation of therapy can result in reinfection or the development of resistant microorganisms. If the patient continues to worsen despite several days of therapy, he or she should contact the prescriber immediately. The organism causing infection in the patient could be resistant to the antibiotic originally prescribed. Refer to the chronic bronchitis section for further information on drug therapy and specific patient education.

CASE STUDY*

G.G., a 59-year-old male, presents to the clinic with complaints of cough, shortness of breath, and increased sputum production. His past medical history is significant for COPD with chronic bronchitis, hypertension, diabetes, and hyperlipidemia. He reports that his sputum has increased in consistency and amount over the past few days. His last exacerbation was about 6 months ago, for which he received amoxicillin. This is his third exacerbation in the past year. He has a 40-pack year history of cigarette smoking and quit smoking 3 years ago. He does not take chronic steroids. Physical exam reveals rhonchi and expiratory wheezes. His vital signs are blood pressure 140/83 mm Hg, pulse rate 80 beats/min, respiration rate 20 breaths/min, and temperature 98.8°F. He has no known drug allergies. A sputum Gram stain in the office reveals purulent sputum (presence of WBCs). Chest x-ray findings are negative for pneumonia.

DIAGNOSIS: ACUTE EXACERBATION OF CHRONIC BRONCHITIS

1. Which of the following would suggest the need for antibiotic therapy in **G.G.**?
    a. Cough, history of smoking, and expiratory wheezes on physical examination
    b. Elevated respiratory rate and shortness of breath
    c. Increased dyspnea, increased sputum production, and increased sputum purulence
    d. History of previous COPD exacerbations, cough, and fever
2. What is a likely pathogen associated with an acute exacerbation of chronic bronchitis in **G.G.**?
    a. *Mycobacterium tuberculosis*
    b. *Pseudomonas aeruginosa*
    c. *Staphylococcus aureus*
    d. *Streptococcus pneumonia*
3. What antibiotic would be most appropriate to treat an acute exacerbation of chronic bronchitis in **G.G.**?
    a. Amoxicillin–clavulanate
    b. Azithromycin
    c. Linezolid
    d. Sulfamethoxazole/trimethoprim

* Answers can be found online.

Bibliography

Starred references are cited in the text.

*Albert, R. K., Connett, J., Bailey, W. C., et al. (2011). Azithromycin for prevention of exacerbations of COPD. *New England Journal of Medicine*, *365*(8), 689–698.

*Bradley, J. S., Byington, C. L., Shah, S. S., et al. (2011). The management of community-acquired pneumonia in infants and children older than 3 months of age: Clinical practice guidelines by the Pediatric Infectious Diseases Society and the Infectious Diseases Society of America. *Clinical Infectious Diseases*, *53*(7), e25–e76.

*Global Initiative for Chronic Obstructive Lung Disease (GOLD). (2015). Retrieved from www.goldcopd on July 10, 2015.

Ho, E. D. (2013). Community-acquired pneumonia in adults and children. *Primary Care: Clinics in Office Practice*, *40*, 655–669.

*Kim, V., & Criner, G. J. (2013). Chronic bronchitis and chronic obstructive pulmonary disease. *American Journal of Respiratory and Critical Care Medicine*, *187*(3), 228–237.

*Liapikou, A., & Torres, A. (2014). Pharmacotherapy for lower respiratory tract infections. *Expert Opinion on Pharmacotherapy*, *15*(16), 2307–2318.

*Mandell, L. A., Wunderink, R. G., Anzueto, A., et al. (2007). Infectious Diseases Society of America/American Thoracic Society consensus guidelines on the management of community acquired pneumonia in adults. *Clinical Infectious Diseases*, *44*, S27–S72.

Musher, D. M., & Thorner, A. R. (2014). Community-acquired pneumonia. *New England Journal of Medicine*, *371*(17), 1919–1928.

Pakhale, S., Mulpuru, S., Verheih, T. J. M., et al. (2014). Antibiotics for community-acquired pneumonia in adult outpatients (review). *Cochrane Database of Systematic Reviews*, *10*, CD002109.

*Qureshi, H., Sharafkhaneh, A., & Hanania N. A. (2014). Chronic obstructive pulmonary disease exacerbations: Latest evidence and clinical implications. *Therapeutic Advances in Chronic Disease*, *5*(5), 212–227.

*Remington, L. T., & Sligl, W. I. (2014). Community-acquired pneumonia. *Current Opinion in Pulmonary Medicine*, *20*, 215–224.

Wunderink, R. G., & Waterer, G. W. (2014). Community-acquired pneumonia. *New England Journal of Medicine*, *370*(6), 543–551.

Pharmacotherapy for Gastrointestinal Tract Disorders

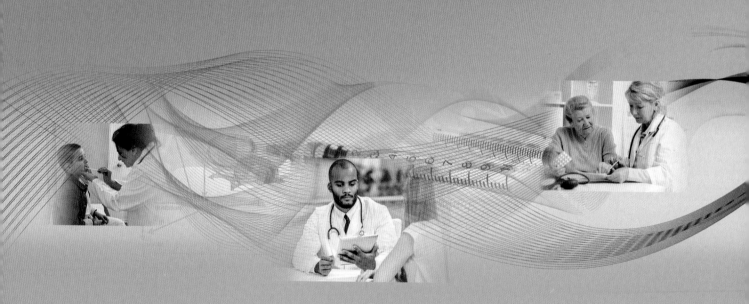

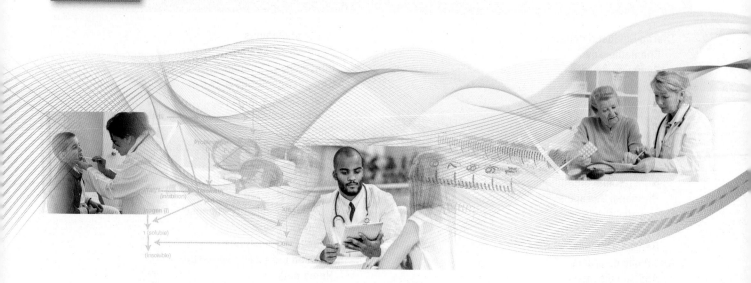

28 Nausea and Vomiting

Virginia P. Arcangelo ■ Veronica F. Wilbur

Nausea and vomiting are common complaints in humans. The severity of the event can range from a slight discomfort or queasiness to uncontrollable, forceful vomiting. Despite this range of symptoms, all are perceived to be uncomfortable and troublesome and should be treated in a proper and timely manner. Patients may refer to this experience by many different names: *upchuck, urp, queasy, throw up,* and *puke,* to name a few. There are many different causes of nausea and vomiting, such as motion sickness, pregnancy, and medications. Likewise, many treatment options can be used to manage this complication. People of all ages experience emesis, although the etiology may be related to age-specific factors. Drugs are most frequently used for the treatment of nausea and vomiting, but alterations of nondrug factors may decrease the severity of emesis. This chapter reviews the pathophysiology and pharmacotherapy of specific types of nausea and vomiting.

CAUSES

There are multiple causes for nausea and vomiting; however, some of the most common are from the ingestion or administration of substances or drugs, gastrointestinal (GI) disorders, neurologic processes, and metabolic disorders. The presence of noxious stimuli is frequently a cause of nausea and vomiting. Supratherapeutic digoxin (Lanoxin) and theophylline (Theo-Dur or Slo-Phyllin) are known to produce emesis. Nausea and vomiting occur more frequently with high-dose chemotherapy than with moderate doses of the same drugs. Erythromycin and some penicillin derivatives are acknowledged for inducing uncomfortable GI complications. Emesis can also result from excessive ethanol intake. It is well known that other sensory experiences, such as pungent odors or gruesome sights, can

induce nausea and vomiting. **Box 28.1** presents specific etiologies for nausea and vomiting.

Patient-specific factors that increase susceptibility to nausea and vomiting include age, previous nausea and vomiting experiences, and sex. Most of the research identifying these characteristics was done in patients receiving chemotherapy. Poor control of nausea and vomiting with previous surgeries or chemotherapy predisposes a patient to subsequent episodes of emesis, also referred to as *anticipatory nausea and vomiting.* This form of emesis is often difficult to treat with standard antiemetics drug therapy.

Patients who receive previously received chemotherapy have been noted to experience emesis compared to those who are chemotherapy naive. Additionally, younger female patients are noted to have a greater risk of emesis (Hesketh, 2008). Surprisingly, patients who have higher chronic ethanol intake exceeding 100 g/d (roughly 5 beers or mixed drinks per day) are associated with better emesis control and decreased incidence of vomiting. A history of motion sickness may increase the risks of nausea and vomiting in another situation, such as with chemotherapy or surgery. Children in general experience nausea and vomiting more frequently than do adults. Obesity and anxiety have also been associated with heightened emesis incidence (Hesketh, 2008).

The prevalence of nausea and vomiting may complicate 20% to 70% of surgical procedures (Gan, 2008). Prevalence is also increased by the use of certain inhalation agents (nitrous oxide, in particular) and by concomitant use of opiate medications; the use of propofol as an intravenous anesthetic agent lowers the risk of postoperative nausea and vomiting (PONV). PONV is more likely to occur after general than regional anesthesia, and its prevalence increases in parallel with the duration of surgery and anesthesia. PONV is especially common

Nausea and Vomiting

BOX 28.1   Etiologies of Nausea and Vomiting

Therapy-induced causes
    Chemotherapy
    Radiation therapy
    Opiates
    Anticonvulsants
    Ipecac
    Antibiotics
    Digitalis or digoxin toxicity
    Theophylline
    Nonsteroidal anti-inflammatory drugs
    Hormonal therapies
Drug withdrawal
    Opiates
    Benzodiazepines
Metabolic disorders
    Addison disease
    Water intoxication
    Volume depletion
    Diabetic ketoacidosis
    Hypercalcemia
    Renal dysfunction–uremia
Gastrointestinal mechanisms
    Mechanical gastric outlet obstruction
        Peptic ulcer disease
        Gastric carcinoma
        Pancreatic disease
    Motility disorders
    Gastroparesis
    Drug-induced gastric stasis
    Irritable bowel syndrome
    Postgastric surgery
    Idiopathic gastric stasis
    Intra-abdominal emergencies
        Acute pancreatitis
        Acute pyelonephritis
        Acute cholecystitis

        Acute cholangitis
        Acute viral hepatitis
        Intestinal obstruction
    Acute gastroenteritis
        Viral gastroenteritis
        Salmonellosis
        Shigellosis
        Staphylococcal gastroenteritis (enterotoxins)
Cardiovascular disease
    Acute myocardial infarction
    Congestive heart failure
    Shock and circulatory collapse
Neurologic processes
    Cerebellar hemorrhage
    Increased intracranial pressure
        Hematoma
        Subdural effusion
        Tumor (benign or malignant)
        Hydrocephalus
        Reye syndrome
    Headache
        Migraine
        Severe hypertension
    Head trauma
    Vestibular disorders
Psychogenic causes
    Anorexia nervosa
    Anticipatory
Miscellaneous causes
    Pregnancy
    Noxious odors
    Ingestion of an irritant
    Operative procedures
    Septicemia
    Nicotine

---

after gynecologic and middle ear surgery and also occurs more commonly with abdominal and orthopedic surgery than with laparoscopic or other extra-abdominal operations. PONV is also more likely in those with a history of PONV or motion sickness.

PATHOPHYSIOLOGY

The pathophysiology of nausea and vomiting is complex (**Figure 28.1**) and involves the modulation of medullary sites and neurotransmitters. Many sensory centers accept noxious stimuli from the body, including the chemoreceptor trigger zone (CTZ), visceral afferent nerves, cerebral cortex, limbic system, vestibular system, and midbrain intracranial pressure receptors.

Modulation of Nausea and Vomiting

These stimuli are transmitted to the *emetic complex* (EC), a loose group of organized neurons throughout the medulla, which coordinates the sensory inputs and the act of vomiting. The EC is the key component in the modulation of nausea and vomiting. Located in the lateral reticular formation

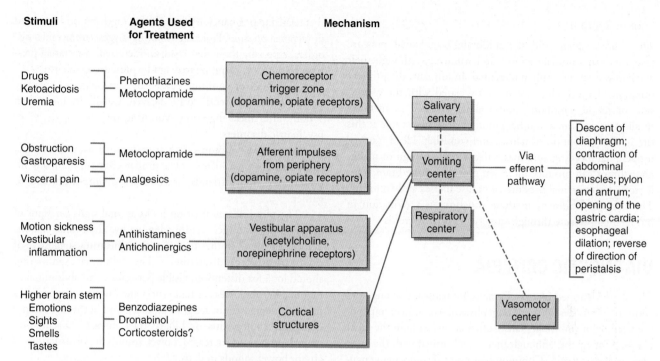

Stimuli	Agents Used for Treatment	Mechanism

FIGURE 28.1 Pathophysiology of nausea and vomiting. (Reprinted from Koda-Kimble, M. A., & Young, L. Y. (2012). Nausea and vomiting. In M. A. Koda-Kimble, L. Y. Young, & B. J. Guglielmo (Eds.), *Applied therapeutics: The clinical use of drugs* (10th ed.). Philadelphia, PA: Lippincott Williams & Wilkins, with permission.)

of the medulla, it receives afferent impulses from the aforementioned sensory centers. On activation of the EC, efferent impulses are sent to the nucleus tractus solitarius, an intertwined neural network that innervates the salivary, vasomotor, and respiratory centers and cranial nerves VIII and X. Efferent impulses are also sent to the stomach, abdominal muscles, diaphragm, and associated sphincters to execute the involuntary act of vomiting. Much like the sensory centers that stimulate it, the vomiting center is rich in dopamine, histamine, serotonin, and acetylcholine receptors and can also be affected by binding to opiate and benzodiazepine receptors. An intact EC is essential for coordination of the vomiting act or the emetic reflex.

Stimulatory Centers

The CTZ is one of the most important chemosensory organs responsible for the detection of noxious stimuli. It is uniquely located in the area postrema in the floor of the fourth ventricle of the (medulla) brain and is exposed to both blood and cerebrospinal fluid (CSF). Thus, toxins in both the blood and CSF can stimulate a response by the CTZ. These toxins may be drugs (chemotherapy, opiates, and digoxin), poisons, or substances found naturally in the body (excess calcium, hormones). The CTZ is rich in neurotransmitter receptors for dopamine, serotonin, histamine, and acetylcholine. Neurokinin 1 (NK) receptors found in the cerebral cortex/thalamus/limbic system also feed in the EC. An antiemetic effect is elicited when these receptors are blocked.

Gastrointestinal Tract

The GI tract and pharynx are sites of origin for the stimulation of nausea and vomiting. Visceral afferent nerves, also referred to as *splanchnic nerves*, from the pharynx and GI tract transmit impulses from local neuroreceptors along the vagus nerve to the vomiting center. The GI tract is rich in local dopamine, histamine, and serotonin receptors. The visceral afferent nerves are also responsible for transmitting stimuli from other peripheral sites such as the heart, lungs, and testes; hence, the vomiting response may occur when a person has been punched in the abdomen or kicked in the groin. Abdominal surgery is another example in which visceral afferent nerves are involved in nausea and vomiting.

Central Nervous System

Motion sickness is primarily a central nervous system (CNS) response mediated by the vestibular system. Acetylcholine and histamine receptors have been found in the vestibular center. Blockade of these receptors provides some degree of protection from emesis. The cerebral cortex, the largest portion of the brain, is responsible for the motor coordination of the body, sensory perception, learning, memory, and many other functions. Afferent impulses from specific sites of the cerebral cortex can result in emesis. The cerebellum is responsible for the regulation of balance, equilibrium, and coordination. Disruption of this portion of the brain can lead to temporary or chronic nausea and vomiting. These structures may also play a role in anticipatory emesis.

Limbic System

The limbic system and the midbrain intracranial pressure receptors can stimulate nausea and vomiting, although their mechanisms are not fully understood. In humans, the primary function of the limbic system is associated with the expression of mood, emotions, and feelings, as well as memory recall. Anxiety, fear, and other emotions may play a role at this site in the perception of nausea and vomiting. Head trauma, intracranial bleeding, and mass effect from a benign or malignant tumor can produce increased pressure in the brain. This increased intracranial pressure can cause nausea and vomiting. The optimal treatment in these situations is a reduction in intracranial pressure through surgery or corticosteroids.

DIAGNOSTIC CRITERIA

The three identified phases of emesis are nausea, retching, and vomiting. Nausea is the unpleasant physical sensation of impending retching or vomiting. Nausea often occurs without the other two steps of emesis, although they are all treated with the same pharmacologic agents. Common symptoms accompanying nausea are flushing, pallor, tachycardia, and hypersalivation. Gastric stasis, decreased pyloric tone, mucosal blood flow, and contractions of the duodenum with reflux into the stomach are physiologic responses to nausea. Retching, the second phase of emesis, is the involuntary synchronized labored movement of abdominal and thoracic muscles before vomiting. Vomiting is the coordinated contractions of the abdominal and thoracic muscles to expel the gastric contents. The lower esophageal sphincter contracts, allowing GI retroperistalsis. The actual expulsion of gastric contents differentiates vomiting from retching.

The acuteness of the symptomatology is based on history and physical examination. Several issues need to be addressed such as whether this is an acute emergency, such as mechanical obstruction, perforation, or peritonitis, clinical clues that the problem is likely to be self-limited, such as would be expected with viral gastroenteritis or a potentially offending medication. The goal is to determine whether empiric treatment with an antiemetic, a gastric acid-suppressing, or a prokinetic agent would be beneficial or whether the patient should be admitted to the hospital to correct fluid and electrolyte imbalance.

Acute nausea and vomiting differs considerably from that of chronic nausea and vomiting differing in symptom duration. Acute onset of nausea and vomiting suggests gastroenteritis, pancreatitis, cholecystitis, or a drug-related side effect. When nausea and vomiting are associated with diarrhea, headache, and myalgias, the cause is viral gastroenteritis; in this instance, symptoms should resolve spontaneously within 5 days. A more insidious onset of nausea without vomiting is suspicious of gastroparesis, a medication-related side effect, metabolic disorders, pregnancy, or even gastroesophageal reflux disease. Nausea and vomiting are considered chronic when their duration is longer than 1 month.

Timing and description of the vomiting are important. Vomiting that occurs in the morning before breakfast is typical of that related to pregnancy, uremia, alcohol ingestion, and increased intracranial pressure. Projectile vomiting suggests intracranial disorders, especially those that result in increased intracranial pressure. In this case, vomiting may not be preceded by nausea.

The onset of vomiting caused by gastroparesis or gastric outlet obstruction tends to be delayed, usually by more than 1 hour, after meal ingestion. Vomiting may be suggestive of psychiatric disorders.

Associated symptoms such as abdominal pain, fever, diarrhea, vertigo, or a history of a similar contemporaneous illness among family, friends, or associates are important data to gather.

The physical examination looks at vital signs for signs of dehydration. Jaundice, lymphadenopathy, abdominal masses, and occult blood in the stool may reveal features suggestive of thyrotoxicosis or Addison disease. The abdominal examination should look for distention, visible peristalsis, and abdominal or inguinal hernias. Areas of tenderness are important: tenderness in the midepigastrium suggests an ulcer, and in the right upper quadrant, cholecystitis or biliary tract disease. Auscultation may demonstrate increased bowel sounds in obstruction or absent bowel sounds in ileus.

INITIATING THERAPY

The treatment of nausea, retching, or vomiting in any patient begins with an evaluation and correction of possible causes. Most sources of nausea and vomiting may be reversed or palliated by surgery or medical interventions. Infectious causes should be promptly treated with antibiotics, and metabolic disorders require medical management. Some drug toxicities may be treated with antidotes, such as digoxin toxicity reversed with digoxin immune Fab (Digibind). The following section discusses medications used to treat nausea and vomiting. They should be used with definitive treatments when possible.

Alterations in a patient's daily activities may aid in managing nausea and vomiting and decrease the resources used to control the problem. Nonpharmacologic management of nausea and vomiting should be tailored to the presumed etiology.

Changes in a patient's diet may affect the frequency or severity of nausea and vomiting, such as avoidance of spicy foods and excessive grease or oil, and decreased caffeine intake. Professional counseling or group therapy may prove favorable for patients with psychogenic nausea and vomiting.

Hypnosis, behavior modification, and imagery are beneficial tools in controlling nausea and vomiting that has an anxiety component, such as chemotherapy-related anticipatory emesis. However, prevention of anticipatory nausea and vomiting is the optimal form of management.

Goals of Drug Therapy

The goals of drug therapy are simple: to alleviate the subjective feeling of nausea and the objective act of vomiting and their

BOX 28.2 Complications of Nausea and Vomiting

Metabolic abnormalities

- Dehydration
- Alkalosis
- Hypokalemia
- Hypomagnesemia
- Hyponatremia
- Hypochloremia
- Malnutrition

Structural damage

- Wound dehiscence
- Esophagogastric tears/Mallory-Weiss tears
- Increased bleeding under skin flaps
- Tension on suture lines

Patient dissatisfaction

- Noncompliance
- Poor oral intake; anticipatory nausea and vomiting
- Delayed ambulation after surgery/procedures
- Fatigue
- Depression

Increased use of resources

- Prolongation of hospital stay
- Unexpected hospital admission
- Alteration or additional therapy

Aspiration pneumonia
Venous hypertension

---

associated complications (**Box 28.2**). It is important to rely on the patient's subjective response when evaluating the efficacy of a specific therapy for nausea. Secondary goals are to minimize drug toxicity/adverse events and contain costs. The prevention of nausea and vomiting is the goal in the setting of chemotherapy and certain surgical procedures. Control or improvement in nausea and vomiting should occur within 5 to 60 minutes of a pharmacologic intervention. If this does not ensue, another method should be used promptly. **Table 28.1** reviews available antiemetic agents, dosages, comparable efficacy, and adverse effects. Pregnancy risk factors are included in the discussion of each drug class and in the pregnancy-related nausea and vomiting section.

Phenothiazines

Phenothiazines are a commonly used class of drugs to treat nausea and vomiting. Prochlorperazine (Compazine) and promethazine (Phenergan) are the most frequently used drugs in this class.

Mechanism of Action

Their mechanism of action presumably involves dopamine receptor blockade in the CTZ. Anticholinergic activity in the vomiting and vestibular centers of the brain may also contribute to the mechanism of action.

The phenothiazines may be used as monotherapy for mild to moderate nausea and vomiting or in combination with other antiemetics for more severe nausea and vomiting. A dose–response quality has been noted for this drug class; however, the incidence of adverse effects such as extrapyramidal effects and sedation can also be associated with higher doses. Promethazine has activities of an antihistamine antiemetic and could also be classified with the antihistamine–anticholinergic class of drugs. The phenothiazines are a viable and practical option for long-term treatment of nausea and vomiting. Products are available in oral, rectal, and injectable formulations. To improve tailoring of the drug regimen to the patient, oral preparations are available as tablets, sustained-release capsules, and liquids. Rectal suppositories are useful in patients who cannot retain oral medications and when intravenous (IV) access is not an option. Suppositories should be avoided in patients who are thrombocytopenic because of the increased risk of bleeding or hemorrhage.

Contraindications

Caution should be used in patients taking concomitant drugs that cause CNS depression, such as sedatives, hypnotics, and opiates, because further sedation may result. Phenothiazines may exacerbate the symptoms of Parkinson disease. The safety of phenothiazines during pregnancy is controversial; most studies find phenothiazines to be safe for the mother and fetus if used occasionally in low doses. Most phenothiazines are in pregnancy risk category C. Phenothiazines may decrease the seizure threshold and should be used cautiously in patients with seizure disorders.

The phenothiazines are relatively inexpensive in relation to most of the other drug classes, with the exception of the sustained-release phenothiazine preparations, which tend to be costly.

Adverse Events

The most common adverse event of phenothiazine use is drowsiness or sedation. Phenothiazines also have the ability to evoke extrapyramidal symptoms (EPSs) by blocking the central dopaminergic receptors involved in motor function, particularly at higher doses. EPSs may present as dystonic reactions, feelings of motor restlessness, and parkinsonian signs and symptoms. Masklike face, drooling, tremor, cogwheel rigidity, pill-rolling motion, lack of ability to initiate voluntary movement, and gait abnormalities are all severe examples of parkinsonian presentations. Dystonic reactions may include spasm of the neck muscles or torticollis, extensor rigidity of back muscles, mandibular tics, difficulty swallowing or talking, and perioral spasms, often with protrusion of the tongue. Motor restlessness may consist of agitation, jitteriness, tapping

TABLE 28.1

Overview of Selected Antiemetic Agents

Generic (Trade) Name and Dosage	Selected Adverse Events	Contraindications	Special Considerations
Phenothiazines			
chlorpromazine (Thorazine) 10–25 mg q4–6 h prn PO, 25–50 mg q4–6h prn IV, IM, 50–100 mg q6–8h prn rectal	Sedation or drowsiness EPSs: agitation, insomnia, motor restlessness, spasms of facial muscles, protrusion of tongue, and mandibular tics Anticholinergic effects: dry mouth, urinary retention, and blurred vision	Hypersensitivity Cautious use with other CNS depressants, Parkinson syndrome, poorly controlled seizure disorder, and severe hepatic dysfunction	Increased incidence of autonomic response with IV administration Higher incidence of EPSs
fluphenazine (Prolixin) 0.5–5 mg q6–8h prn PO, IM	Same as above	Same as above	
perphenazine (Trilafon) 2–6 mg q4–6h prn PO, 5–10 mg q6h prn IM	Same as above	Same as above	Higher incidence of EPSs compared with other phenothiazines
prochlorperazine (Compazine) 5–10 mg q4–6h prn PO, rectal, IM, IV 10–30 mg bid PO sustained-release capsule	Same as above	Same as above	Sustained-release capsule more expensive Higher incidence of EPSs compared with other phenothiazines
promethazine (Phenergan) 12.5–25 mg q4–6h prn PO, rectal, IM, IV	Same as above	Same as above	
Antihistamines and Anticholinergics			
benzquinamide (Emete-con) 50 mg q3–4h prn IM 25 mg q3–4h prn IV	Sedation or drowsiness, confusion Anticholinergic effects: dry mouth, tachycardia, blurred vision, urinary retention, constipation	Hypersensitivity Caution in narrow-angle glaucoma, asthma, prostatic hypertrophy	IV preparation not recommended
dimenhydrinate (Dramamine) 50–100 mg q4–6h prn PO, IM, IV	Same as above	Same as above	Do not exceed 200 mg/d
diphenhydramine (Benadryl) 25–50 mg q6–8h prn PO, 10–50 mg q2–4h prn IM, IV	Same as above	Same as above	Do not exceed 200 mg/d
hydroxyzine (Atarax, Vistaril) 25–100 mg q4–6h prn PO, IM	Same as above	Same as above	
meclizine (Antivert, Bonine) 25–50 mg q24h prn PO	Same as above	Same as above	
scopolamine (Transderm Scop) 1.5 mg q3d transdermal patch	Same as above	Same as above	
trimethobenzamide (Tigan) 250 mg q6–8h prn PO 200 mg q6–8h prn IM, rectal	Same as above	Same as above	
Benzodiazepines			
lorazepam (Ativan) 0.5–2 mg q4–8h prn PO, IM, IV	Drowsiness or fatigue, confusion, constipation	Same as above	Dose should be low in frail, elderly, or critically ill patients
diazepam (Valium) 2–5 mg bid–qid prn PO, IM, IV	Same as above	Same as above	Same as above

TABLE 28.1

Overview of Selected Antiemetic Agents (*Continued*)

Generic (Trade) Name and Dosage	Selected Adverse Events	Contraindications	Special Considerations
Serotonin Antagonists			
dolasetron (Anzemet) 100 mg PO 1 h before chemotherapy 100 mg IV 30 min before chemotherapy 12.5 mg IV 15 min before cessation of anesthesia 100 mg PO 2 h before surgery	Headache, diarrhea, ECG changes	Hypersensitivity Use with caution in patients with severe cardiac dysfunction	Very expensive (IV > PO) Use only when indicated
granisetron (Kytril) 10 µg/kg IV 30 min before chemotherapy 1 mg PO bid (q12h)—start before chemotherapy (Sancuso) patch—3.1 mg/24 h (1 patch)	Same as above	Same as above	Very expensive (IV > PO) Use only when indicated IV dose often rounded to 1- or 2-mg doses
ondansetron (Zofran) 0.15 mg/kg IV 30 min before chemotherapy and at 4 and 8 h Oral—tablet and melt 4 mg, 8 mg	Same as above	Same as above	Generic, less expensive than other in the class
NK1 Antagonist			
aprepitant (Emend) Oral—40, 80, 125 mg 3 h prior to induction of anesthesia, 1 h prior to chemotherapy	Heartburn, confusion, decreased urination, dizziness Dyspepsia, fatigue, constipation, erythema, skin allergic reactions	Hypersensitivity to product, contraindication with some chemotherapy agents Possible hypersensitivity to 5-HT3 component, serotonin syndrome	Interacts with contraceptives Extremely expensive Interactions with dexamethasone, midazolam, oral contraceptives
NK1/Serotonin Antagonist Combo			
netupitant/palonosetron (Akynzeo) 300 mg/0.5 mg			
Other Antiemetics			
dexamethasone (Decadron) 8–20 mg IV/PO before chemotherapy; 4–8 mg IV bid (delayed nausea and vomiting)	Hyperactivity, GI irritation, mood swings, depression, hyperglycemia, anxiety	Hypersensitivity Use with caution in diabetic patients, history of ulcers, young male patients	Give IV over 5–15 min Administer orally with food Avoid chronic administration
methylprednisolone (Solu-Medrol) 125–500 mg IV q6h	Same as above	Same as above	Same as above
dronabinol (Marinol) 5–15 mg/m^2 PO 1–3 h before chemotherapy and q4h × 6 2.5–10 mg PO bid	Sedation, confusion, dysphoria, increased appetite	Use with caution if patient is receiving other CNS depressants	Controlled substance
antacids 15–30 mL q2–4h prn	Diarrhea, constipation	Renal dysfunction	May decrease absorption of other drugs
metoclopramide (Reglan)	EPSs		Side effects are dose dependent
20–30 mg PO qid prn, 1–2 mg/kg IV before chemotherapy and q2–4h (high dose)	Diarrhea Drowsiness		EPS reversible with diphenhydramine
doxylamine/pyridoxine (Diclegis) 10 mg each drug	Drowsiness, dizziness, impaired coordination, headache, urinary retention	Caution with CV disease, hyperthyroid, HTN, COPD, lower resp. tract sx	Only drug approved for nausea and vomiting of pregnancy by FDA Doxylamine—first-generation antihistamine

of feet, and insomnia. Extrapyramidal reactions can be easily treated with the use of diphenhydramine (Benadryl) 25 mg orally or parenterally three to four times a day or benztropine (Cogentin) 1 to 4 mg orally or parenterally twice a day. Autonomic responses, such as hypotension and tachycardia, have been observed with IV phenothiazine use, particularly chlorpromazine. Hypotension and sedation are less likely to occur with prochlorperazine, thiethylperazine, and perphenazine, but these three agents are associated with a higher frequency of EPSs. Dry mouth, urinary retention, blurred vision, and other anticholinergic effects may occur with phenothiazine use. Reversible agranulocytosis is rarely associated (less than 1%) with phenothiazine therapy. This effect occurs more frequently in women and with chronic phenothiazine use. Cholestatic jaundice and photosensitivity are reactions that can occur rarely within the first few months of chronic phenothiazine use. These are more frequently observed in phenothiazine use for psychiatric conditions rather than emesis control.

Monitoring parameters include EPSs and parkinsonian symptoms. Doses may need to be decreased in severe hepatic dysfunction. Complete blood counts should be regularly monitored in chronic phenothiazine use (see **Table 28.1**).

Interactions

These drugs potentiate CNS depression with alcohol and other CNS depressants. They potentiate the action of α blockers and levels of the drug can be increased with propranolol. Anticonvulsant drug doses may have to be adjusted. They may antagonize oral anticoagulants.

Antihistamines–Anticholinergics

A plethora of agents are available in the antihistamine–anticholinergic drug class. These agents are most useful for mild nausea, such as motion sickness. Hydroxyzine (Vistaril, Atarax), meclizine (Bonine, Antivert), dimenhydrinate (Dramamine), and scopolamine (Transderm Scop) are some of the more common agents of this class. Unlike most of the other classes of agents discussed in this chapter, some of the antihistamine–anticholinergic agents are available without a prescription.

Mechanism of Action

The mechanism of action appears to be interruption of visceral afferent pathways that are responsible for stimulating nausea and vomiting. These drugs are most frequently administered orally, but some can be given IV, intramuscularly, transdermally, or rectally.

The antihistamines are particularly useful for the treatment and prevention of motion sickness. For this indication, it is recommended that a dose be taken at least 30 to 60 minutes before the event (e.g., boating, air flight, car ride) and then repeated at regular intervals several times a day. The scopolamine patch is a highly useful agent for the prevention of motion sickness. A patch should be applied to clean, dry skin 1 to 2 hours before the potentially emetogenic event, and a new patch may be reapplied every 3 days.

Many of the antihistamines and anticholinergics have been used for the treatment of nausea in pregnancy.

Contraindications

Precautions are recommended with asthma, glaucoma, and GI or urinary obstruction. Antihistamines–anticholinergics are not recommended for nursing mothers.

Adverse Events

Adverse effects limit the use of anticholinergics–antihistamines. Patients frequently experience sedation, drowsiness, or confusion. The anticholinergic effects are troublesome, including blurred vision, dry mouth, urinary retention, and tachycardia. These anticholinergic effects are also dose related and occur more frequently as the dose increases or the drug is given more often. Caution is warranted in patients with narrow-angle glaucoma, prostatic hypertrophy, and asthma because these patients are more prone to the anticholinergic effects of these drugs.

Anticholinergic effects may be managed by nondrug therapies. Chewing gum or sucking on ice chips or hard candy may refresh a dry mouth. The intake of a high-fiber diet and adequate daily fluid consumption may curb constipation.

Monitoring for anticholinergic effects is of paramount importance. Severe effects may warrant discontinuation of the drug. Symptoms of overdose may include dilated pupils, tachycardia, hypertension, CNS depression, flushed skin, or, more seriously, respiratory failure and circulatory collapse. Adverse effects occur more commonly in patients with renal or hepatic dysfunction.

Interactions

These drugs can potentiate CNS depression with alcohol, tranquilizers, and sedative–hypnotics.

Benzodiazepines

Often used for other indications, benzodiazepines offer useful qualities to the antiemetic armamentarium. Not only do these agents treat and prevent emesis, they can cause anxiolysis and amnesia. These latter effects are particularly beneficial in anticipatory nausea and vomiting associated with chemotherapy.

Lorazepam (Ativan) is the most frequently used benzodiazepine for nausea and vomiting. Its mechanism of action is not fully elucidated; however, it probably acts centrally to inhibit the vomiting center. Lorazepam has only moderate antiemetic properties and is usually used in combination with other agents to control chemotherapy-associated anticipatory nausea and vomiting and delayed chemotherapy-associated nausea and vomiting.

Dosage

Both oral and parenteral forms of lorazepam are available. Patient-specific variables should be considered when identifying an appropriate dose. Usual oral or IV doses range from 0.5 to 2 mg at least 30 minutes before start of chemotherapy. As-needed (prn) antiemetic doses range from 0.5 to 3 mg IV or orally every 4 to 6 hours. To prevent oversedation, patients with poor performance status, the elderly, or frail individuals require low initial doses of lorazepam. Patients with compromised pulmonary or poor cardiac function should receive IV lorazepam with caution and have close monitoring of respiratory and cardiac status.

Contraindications

Lorazepam is not recommended for use in patients with hepatic or renal failure. Several studies have indicated that diazepam (Valium) may also cause fetal toxicity when administered to pregnant women and thus should be avoided in this patient population. The benzodiazepines are in pregnancy risk category D.

Adverse Events

For benzodiazepines, CNS depression occurs most often, with drowsiness, fatigue, memory impairment, impaired coordination, and confusion occurring frequently. Lorazepam has an amnesic effect that for some patients is a benefit, whereas others may find it unacceptable. Paradoxical CNS stimulation resulting in restlessness, anxiety, nightmares, and increased muscle spasticity may occur. The drug should be discontinued if paradoxical stimulation occurs. Other adverse effects include constipation, headache, and increased or decreased appetite. Parenteral administration may cause hypotension, bradycardia, or apnea, particularly in the elderly and critically ill (see **Table 28.1**).

Monitoring parameters include cardiovascular and respiratory status for initial doses. Because the liver metabolizes the benzodiazepines, liver function tests should be assessed before dosing. The presence of adverse CNS effects should be evaluated with each clinic or hospital visit.

Interactions

These drugs potentiate CNS depression when used with other drugs that depress the CNS and alcohol.

Serotonin Antagonists

The serotonin antagonists are another class of antiemetics. Ondansetron (Zofran), granisetron (Kytril, Sancuso), palonosetron (Aloxi), and dolasetron (Anzemet) are available in the United States.

Mechanism of Action

These agents work by antagonizing the type 3 serotonin ($5HT_3$) receptors centrally in the CTZ and also peripherally at the vagal and splanchnic afferent fibers from the enterochromaffin cells in the upper GI tract. The serotonin antagonists were initially indicated for the treatment and prevention of chemotherapy-induced nausea and vomiting. They have changed the way nausea and vomiting are treated and have greatly improved the quality of life for patients receiving highly emetogenic chemotherapy regimens. Radiation-induced nausea and vomiting and PONV are two other areas where the serotonin antagonists have been studied. The unequivocal efficacy and lack of significant adverse effects make these agents ideal for select indications.

The serotonin antagonists are available orally as tablets and liquids and parenterally for IV use. Because these agents are used to prevent nausea and vomiting, oral administration in this situation is encouraged, even with highly emetogenic chemotherapy. There have been few data to support superior efficacy of one agent over another when used at recommended dosages (Barrett et al., 2011). While the cost of the serotonin antagonist preparations can be higher than other antiemetics, the recent advent of generic ondansetron (Zofran) has made this class more available for treatment of nausea and vomiting. However, this class of medication still needs to be used conservatively and appropriately. Many institutions have created antiemetic guidelines to identify the approved indications of serotonin antagonists to optimize care and resources. The appropriateness of these agents in specific circumstances is discussed later.

Contraindications

There are inadequate human data for use in pregnancy; however, animal studies do not reveal evidence of harm to the fetus. Two case reports cite the efficacy of ondansetron in the treatment of hyperemesis gravidarum, without adverse sequelae to the fetus. The serotonin antagonists are in pregnancy risk category B. The serotonin antagonists should be used with caution in breast-feeding mothers; once again, human data are lacking, but ondansetron is distributed into the milk of lactating rats.

Adverse Events

Mild to moderate headache can occur in patients receiving oral or parenteral serotonin antagonists, followed in frequency by diarrhea. A few patients experience severe headaches requiring discontinuation of the drug. Other adverse effects that occur in less than 10% of patients are abdominal or epigastric pain, increased serum hepatic enzyme levels on liver function tests, hypertension, malaise or fatigue, constipation, pruritus, and fever. Rare cardiovascular effects have been reported, although a definite causal relationship has not been established. All three of the agents can cause electrocardiographic (ECG) alterations (prolonged PR interval and QT interval and widened QRS complex). This is best documented in the studies of dolasetron, but these ECG changes were deemed to be clinically nonsignificant by the authors (Audhuy et al., 1996). Conservatively, in patients with severe cardiac dysfunctions such as arrhythmia and heart block, the serotonin antagonists should be used cautiously.

Important monitoring parameters for serotonin antagonists include baseline and follow-up liver function tests. Dosage reductions may be made for severe hepatic dysfunction. To avoid ECG-related complications, electrolyte assessment and correction of hypokalemia and hypomagnesemia are indicated (see **Table 28.1**).

Interactions

Caution is used when given with drugs that prolong cardiac conduction interval, diuretics, and cumulative high-dose anthracycline.

Metoclopramide and Other Antiemetics

Metoclopramide (Reglan) has been used to treat nausea and vomiting caused by several different stimuli. It is a highly useful agent in the treatment of diabetic gastric stasis, postsurgical gastric stasis, and gastroesophageal reflux, which may be associated with some degree of nausea.

Mechanism of Action

For these indications, metoclopramide enhances motility and gastric emptying by increasing the duration and extent of esophageal contractions, the resting tone of the lower esophageal sphincter, gastric contractions, and peristalsis of the duodenum and jejunum. Metoclopramide is also used in the prevention and treatment of chemotherapy-induced nausea and vomiting. Its mechanism of action is dopamine receptor inhibition in the CTZ. The central and peripheral actions of this agent make it efficacious in multiple clinical situations. Metoclopramide can be administered orally, IV, and intramuscularly. A sugar-free syrup exists for diabetic patients who cannot take the pills. Because metoclopramide is eliminated primarily by the kidneys, the dose of this drug should be decreased by 50% if the patient's creatinine clearance is less than 40 mL/min. Subsequent doses are based on the patient's clinical response. Periodic assessment of renal function is prudent. Patients should be informed of the sedative qualities of this agent and that use of other CNS depressants could potentiate this effect.

Adverse Events

The most clinically concerning adverse effects of metoclopramide are EPSs. Much like the effects seen with high doses of phenothiazines, facial spasms, rhythmic protrusions of the tongue, involuntary movements of limbs, motor restlessness, agitation, and other dystonic reactions can occur. These effects occur most commonly in children and young adults, in men more than women, and at high doses of metoclopramide. Twenty-five percent of adults ages 18 to 30 experience dystonic reactions after receiving high-dose metoclopramide for treatment of chemotherapy-induced emesis. EPSs occur within 24 to 48 hours of the initial dose and subside within 24 hours of drug discontinuation. High-dose metoclopramide is usually defined as 2 mg/kg per dose. EPSs can be prevented or treated with the addition of diphenhydramine 25 to 50 mg IV or orally. IV administration of diphenhydramine is preferred for serious presentations. Other reversal agents are benztropine and diazepam. Secondary to its actions in the intestinal tract, metoclopramide can cause diarrhea. Management of diarrhea includes discontinuation or dosage reduction of metoclopramide, increased fluid resuscitation, and electrolyte replacement. The use of metoclopramide may not be a prudent choice in a patient who already has diarrhea. Drowsiness and fatigue are noted in approximately 10% of patients. There are inadequate data for the use of metoclopramide in pregnancy; however, supratherapeutic doses in rats did not produce evidence of fetal harm. Metoclopramide is in pregnancy risk category B. Metoclopramide is known to be distributed into breast milk but does not appear to present a risk to the infant if the mother is taking 45 mg/d or less.

Interactions

A hypertensive crisis can occur when metoclopramide is used with monoamine oxidase inhibitors. Additive sedation can be seen when used with alcohol or other CNS depressants. These drugs are antagonized by anticholinergics and narcotics. They may diminish gastric and accelerate intestinal absorption of drugs and food.

Corticosteroids

Corticosteroids are usually reserved for chemotherapy-induced nausea and vomiting. Appreciation of the antiemetic properties of this class of agents occurred when clinicians observed decreased episodes of nausea and vomiting with Hodgkin disease protocols that included prednisone compared with protocols that did not include prednisone.

Mechanism of Action

The true mechanism of action in the relief of nausea and vomiting is unknown, but one postulated theory is the inhibition of prostaglandins. In nausea and vomiting secondary to increased intracranial pressure, corticosteroids provide relief by decreasing inflammation. Dexamethasone (Decadron) and methylprednisolone (Solu-Medrol) are the two most common corticosteroids used; however, the addition of prednisone (Deltasone) to lymphoma and leukemia chemotherapy regimens can provide heightened control of emesis. These corticosteroids are almost always used in combination with other agents in the control or prevention of emesis from highly emetogenic regimens.

Corticosteroids are available orally and parenterally. The oral form is beneficial for low doses or prolonged administration, but may cause significant GI toxicity. Patients should be encouraged to take oral corticosteroids with food to minimize GI irritation and complications. IV administration is ordinarily used in the prevention of nausea and vomiting, primarily to avoid GI complications. IV preparations should be infused over 5 to 15 minutes to prevent burning, flushing, and itching sensations associated with the phosphate salt dissociation. Of the corticosteroids studied, the utility of dexamethasone has been best defined. In clinical trials, single-agent dexamethasone was superior to prochlorperazine and comparable with high-dose metoclopramide when used for mildly to moderately emetogenic chemotherapy regimens. The combination of dexamethasone and high-dose metoclopramide was the standard of care for prevention of cisplatin-induced emesis until the introduction of the serotonin antagonists. IV doses of dexamethasone as a premedication range from 8 to 20 mg.

Corticosteroids should be used with caution in uncontrolled diabetic patients. Sliding-scale insulin or careful alterations of oral hypoglycemic agent regimens may be used for unacceptably high blood glucose levels.

Adverse Events

Although very useful, the corticosteroids are associated with many toxicities and adverse effects. Mental disturbances range from mood swings, depression, anxiety, and aggression to frank psychosis and personality changes. Men are particularly susceptible to this aggressive behavior. Headache, restlessness, and insomnia are not infrequent, particularly with higher doses of corticosteroids. Patients and family members and loved ones will benefit from knowing that these effects may occur with therapy. Sleep aids may be necessary for secondary insomnia. Temazepam (Restoril) or diphenhydramine are viable options. Variable increases in blood glucose and decreased glucose tolerance result from glucocorticoid use. Regular evaluation of blood glucose in diabetic patients is warranted. Glucocorticoids, especially in large or chronic doses, can increase the susceptibility to and mask the symptoms of infection, such as fever. Many consequences of long-term corticosteroid use can be detrimental. Muscle wasting, adrenocortical insufficiency, fluid and electrolyte disturbances, cataract formation, and atrophy of the protein matrix of bone resulting in osteoporosis, vertebral compression fractures, aseptic necrosis of femoral or humeral heads, and pathologic fractures are some of the most serious complications of chronic corticosteroid use. Whenever possible, chronic corticosteroid use should be curtailed.

Interactions

Glucocorticoids may decrease effects of barbiturates, hydantoins, rifampin, and ephedrine. Potassium levels should be monitored when glucocorticoids are used with potassium-depleting diuretics.

Cannabinoids

Cannabinoids are indicated only for nausea and vomiting associated with chemotherapy. In the 1970s, it was observed that patients on chemotherapy who smoked marijuana experienced a lower incidence of nausea and vomiting. Investigators then determined that tetrahydrocannabinol (THC) has antiemetic properties.

Mechanism of Action

The true mechanism of action of THC is unknown, but it is most likely related to effects on the vomiting center and the opiate receptors in the CNS and cerebral cortex but probably does not involve the CTZ. The agent available in the United States is dronabinol (Marinol).

The cannabinoids can be used to treat and prevent chemotherapy-induced nausea and vomiting. Because it is necessary to reach therapeutic blood levels of THC before chemotherapy administration to prevent emesis, administration of the cannabinoids should occur at least 6 to 12 hours before chemotherapy. Emesis can be controlled from mildly to moderately emetogenic chemotherapy regimens, and cannabinoids may provide some relief to patients where other agents have failed. When used with mildly to moderately emetogenic regimens, THC has been found to be superior to placebo, prochlorperazine, low-dose metoclopramide, and haloperidol. These agents are seldom front-line therapy because of their incidence and severity of adverse effects.

Patients should be cautioned about the deleterious CNS effects and told not to drive or operate machinery. Dosages can be reduced if the patient is experiencing CNS toxicities. Patients should avoid alcohol and other CNS depressants.

Adverse Events

Most of the adverse effects of the cannabinoids are CNS related and include sedation, ataxia, and dysphoria. Dysphoria may be expressed as confusion, hallucinations, anxiety, fear, memory loss, time distortion, and other undesired occurrences. Orthostatic hypotension, blurred vision, and tachycardia have been observed with the use of these drugs. With repeated doses, the patients usually become tolerant to most of the CNS adverse effects, but not to the antiemetic activity. There is a correlation between antiemetic response and a psychological "high." Younger patients and patients who have had previous experiences with recreational cannabinoids appreciate greater antiemetic efficacy from this drug class. The side effects of the cannabinoids occur more frequently than with many of the other agents and are particularly distressing to older adults. One potentially beneficial adverse effect is appetite stimulation, which may prove useful in hematology and oncology patients. The cannabinoids are in pregnancy risk category D and should be avoided in pregnancy or lactation.

Antacids

Over-the-counter (OTC) antacid preparations may provide relief to patients experiencing mild nausea and vomiting. The general mechanism by which these agents exhibit their effects is by coating the stomach and neutralizing gastric acid. Most preparations contain one or several of the following: calcium carbonate, magnesium hydroxide, aluminum hydroxide, or aluminum carbonate. Between 15 and 30 mL orally of an antacid preparation may provide relief. Patients should be encouraged to seek medical attention if they experience continued nausea and vomiting, and the patient may need medical workup for more serious GI diseases.

Toxicities from OTC antacids are infrequent, but they do exist. The agents containing magnesium may cause diarrhea; conversely, the agents containing aluminum or calcium may cause constipation. These adverse effects are dose dependent. Calcium-containing antacids can cause phosphate depletion. Caution should be used in patients with renal dysfunction because aluminum and magnesium may accumulate. Antacids, by coating the GI tract, can decrease the absorption of many oral medications such as digoxin, some antibiotics, corticosteroids, and allopurinol (Zyloprim), which may lead to decreased efficacy of therapy. (For additional information on antacids, see Chapter 29.)

Selecting the Most Appropriate Agent

Nausea and Vomiting Not Chemotherapy Induced

It is necessary for the practitioner to assess the etiology of the nausea and vomiting. If an organic cause can be determined, the cause should be corrected to alleviate the symptoms. For example, if the nausea and vomiting is a side effect of a medication, the medication is to be discontinued. If the cause is diabetic ketoacidosis, insulin is given. **Figure 28.2** shows the treatment algorithm.

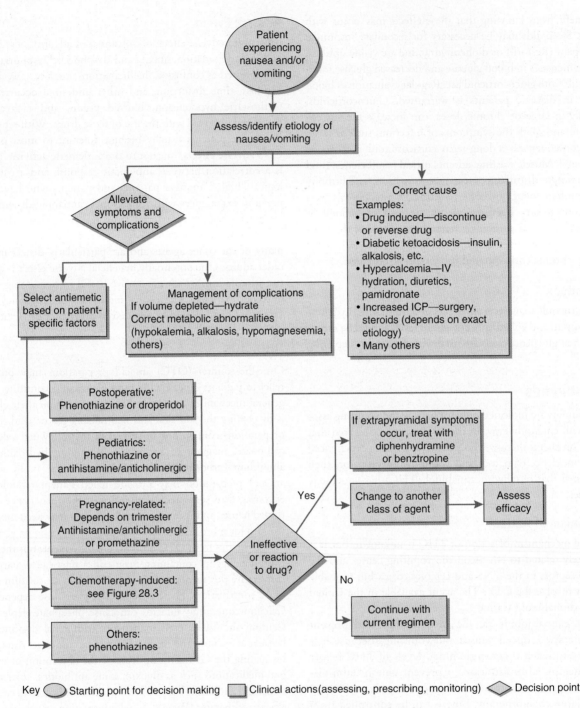

FIGURE 28.2   Treatment algorithm for nausea and vomiting.

First-Line Therapy

An antiemetic is selected based on patient-specific factors. Initially, a phenothiazine is used for mild to moderate nausea and vomiting. Promethazine and prochlorperazine are usually effective.

Second-Line Therapy

If the above treatment is not effective, an antihistamine or anticholinergic preparation can be used. These are usually not as effective as phenothiazines but may be useful in mild nausea.

Third-Line Therapy

If the first two therapies are not successful, the patient should be re-evaluated for a physiological cause that has not been treated and therapy based on patient data.

Table 28.2 lists the recommended order of treatment for nausea and vomiting.

Chemotherapy-Induced Nausea and Vomiting

Nausea and vomiting are two of the toxicities of chemotherapy that patients fear most. Although not usually a life-threatening

TABLE 28.2
Recommended Order of Treatment for Nausea and Vomiting*

Order	Agents	Comments
First line	Phenothiazines	Most frequently used for mild to moderate nausea and vomiting Promethazine, prochlorperazine usually effective
Second line	Antihistamine Anticholinergic preparation	Usually not as efficacious as phenothiazines, but may be useful in mild nausea
Third line	Depends on response to other antiemetics	Tailor to patient-specific factors

*Consider patient-specific factors when choosing an antiemetic agent.

BOX 28.3 Emetogenic Potential of Chemotherapy Agents

Highly emetogenic (>90%)
  Carmustine >250 mg/m²
  Cisplatin >50 mg/m²
  Cyclophosphamide >1,500 mg/m²
  Dacarbazine
  Lomustine
  Mechlorethamine
  Streptozocin
Moderately high (60%–90%)
  Carboplatin
  Carmustine ≤250 mg/m²
  Cisplatin ≤50 mg/m²
  Cyclophosphamide ≤1,500 mg/m² or >750 mg/m²
  Cytarabine >1,000 mg/m²
  Doxorubicin >60 mg/m²
  Methotrexate >1,000 mg/m²
  Procarbazine oral
Moderate (30%–60%)
  Cyclophosphamide ≤750 mg/m²
  Cyclophosphamide oral
  Doxorubicin 20–60 mg/m²
  Idarubicin
  Ifosfamide
  Methotrexate 250–1,000 mg/m²
  Mitoxantrone
  Topotecan
Moderately low (10%–30%)
  Docetaxel
  Etoposide
  5-fluorouracil
  Gemcitabine
  Methotrexate >50 mg/m² or <250 mg/m²
  Mitomycin
  Paclitaxel
Low (<10%)
  Bleomycin
  Busulfan
  Chlorambucil oral
  Cladribine
  Fludarabine
  Hydroxyurea
  Melphalan oral
  Thioguanine oral
  Vinblastine
  Vincristine
  Vinorelbine

complication, uncontrolled nausea or vomiting can greatly affect a patient's quality of life and attitude. Fortunately, new agents and combinations of agents make it possible to control emesis.

The severity of chemotherapy-induced emesis depends on numerous factors. Most significant is the intrinsic ability of the chemotherapy regimen to cause nausea and vomiting. Before the U.S. Food and Drug Administration approves a drug for use, phase 1 and 2 studies must be performed to prove efficacy and safety and identify adverse effects. The incidence and severity of nausea and vomiting are initially reported at this time, when the drug is given as a single agent. Each chemotherapy agent can be identified as having highly, moderately high, moderate, moderately low, and low emetogenic potential. Based on this information, antiemetic regimens can be tailored to the chemotherapy regimen to prevent emesis. Mechanisms to identify the emetogenicity of combination chemotherapy regimens are presented in this section. Other factors that may increase the incidence of chemotherapy-induced nausea and vomiting are previous exposure to chemotherapy, psychosocial factors such as anxiety and depression, poor performance status, and younger age (less than 30 years). A history of alcohol abuse and male sex may correlate with a decreased incidence or severity of nausea and vomiting. The classifications of chemotherapy-induced nausea and vomiting include acute, delayed, and anticipatory.

Acute Emesis

Acute emesis is vomiting occurring within 24 hours of treatment. The onset of acute emesis is usually within 1 to 2 hours after the start of chemotherapy. It peaks within 4 to 10 hours and resolves within 24 hours, but these factors vary from agent to agent. This most common type of chemotherapy-induced nausea and vomiting is associated with a higher frequency and severity than the other two classifications. Acute emesis is strongly related to the agent or agents administered and the doses given. (**Box 28.3** identifies the emetogenic potential of specific agents.)

By definition, highly emetogenic chemotherapy agents induce emesis in greater than 90% of patients receiving that drug without antiemetic premedication. Chemotherapy agents that have moderately high emetogenicity cause emesis in 60%

to 90% of patients receiving chemotherapy. Chemotherapy that is moderately emetogenic has an incidence of 30% to 60%, moderately low has a 10% to 30% incidence of emesis, and low emetogenicity is defined as an incidence of less than 10%.

All patients receiving single agents that are moderately to highly emetogenic should be adequately pretreated to prevent the incidence of nausea and vomiting for at least 24 hours or the expected duration of nausea or vomiting. The current standard of care of antiemetic prophylaxis is the combination of a serotonin antagonist and a corticosteroid, such as granisetron or ondansetron with dexamethasone, at least 30 minutes before chemotherapy administration. Repeated doses may need to be given to prevent and treat emesis for 24 hours, depending on the pharmacokinetics of the agents used. Some practitioners use once-daily administration of serotonin antagonists, claiming that once the receptors are blocked, duration of receptor binding is the functional component rather than the plasma half-life. Because the purpose of these agents is to prevent nausea and vomiting, and the patient is not actively experiencing these effects, it is often acceptable to administer antiemetics orally. Combination regimens containing drugs that are moderately to highly emetogenic are given prophylactically in similar fashion. Although the aforementioned antiemetic combination is not universally effective, an estimated 70% to 90% of patients experience sufficient control. Examples of difficult clinical situations that may prohibit the use of a corticosteroid include poorly controlled diabetes and uncontrolled hypertension.

Contraindications to serotonin antagonists include hypersensitivity or severe cardiac dysfunction. Alternative prophylactic antiemetics must be chosen for patients who have relative contraindications and are to receive emetogenic chemotherapy. High-dose metoclopramide with dexamethasone may be considered an option to a serotonin antagonist with dexamethasone because this was the gold standard for highly emetogenic regimens before the appearance of ondansetron. Once again, the antiemetic regimen should be tailored to the patient and the chemotherapy regimen.

Single-agent or combination chemotherapy regimens that are expected to be moderately low or low in emetogenic potential can be managed less aggressively. These drugs do not warrant the use of a serotonin antagonist. For some chemotherapy regimens and agents, such as the taxanes and fluorouracil, premedication frequently is not necessary; however, patients should be encouraged to use antiemetic medications as needed to control any nausea and vomiting after chemotherapy. Premedication with dexamethasone with or without a phenothiazine or metoclopramide may be used if a patient experiences nausea and vomiting from previous chemotherapy. All of these antiemetic drugs may be scheduled for a 24- to 36-hour period to prevent any nausea and vomiting. Patient-specific factors must be considered to identify an appropriate antiemetic regimen.

Regardless of the emetogenicity of a chemotherapy regimen or the use of premedications, antiemetics should be prescribed for prn or breakthrough use. Preferred prn antiemetics,

BOX 28.4 Basic Principles of Chemotherapy Antiemetic Therapy

- Consider emetogenic potential of chemotherapy regimen.
- Give appropriate antiemetics to prevent nausea and vomiting at least 30 minutes before emetogenic chemotherapy.
- Schedule antiemetics throughout anticipated period of nausea and vomiting risk.
- Always prescribe prn antiemetics for breakthrough nausea and vomiting between scheduled doses.
- Use antiemetic combinations with nonoverlapping mechanisms of action and adverse effects, when possible.
- Consider patient-specific variables when choosing a regimen (e.g., anxiety, performance status).
- Re-evaluate patients frequently during and between chemotherapy courses for efficacy and toxicity of antiemetic regimen.
- Consider nonpharmacologic interventions, especially in patients with anticipatory nausea and vomiting.

such as prochlorperazine or metoclopramide, are effective, inexpensive, and easily administered. These agents provide reliable, safe control of mild nausea. These agents may be used before meals to alleviate anorexia secondary to nausea. Patients should be counseled about the common adverse effects of these agents, and each patient should be encouraged to report ineffective control of nausea and vomiting. When adhered to, the basic principles of chemotherapy antiemetic therapy (**Box 28.4**) are tremendously effective.

Delayed Emesis

Delayed nausea and vomiting is defined as emesis that begins or persists more than 24 hours after completion of chemotherapy. Some investigators suggest that because there is a "peak" in incidence at 18 hours after cisplatin-based chemotherapy, a revised definition of delayed emesis should include this timetable. The new-found, reliable control of acute emesis from highly to moderately emetogenic chemotherapy regimens has unveiled delayed nausea and vomiting as a more vexing problem. Many chemotherapy agents produce mild delayed nausea and vomiting, but cyclophosphamide, cisplatin, and the anthracyclines are particularly noted for their delayed emesis.

Delayed emesis usually is not as frequent or severe as acute emesis. The mechanism of delayed emesis is believed to be different from that of acute emesis. It is believed that delayed emesis is mediated by neurotransmitters, although serotonin does not play a major role. Combination antiemetic regimens have proven to be more effective than single-agent therapies. Single-agent serotonin antagonists were found to be equally as

TABLE 28.3		
Order of Treatment for Chemotherapy-Induced Nausea and Vomiting		
Order	**Agents**	**Comments**
Acute Prophylaxis for High, Moderately High, and Moderately Emetogenic Regimens		
First line	Serotonin antagonist + dexamethasone	May add other agents as needed
Second line	High-dose metoclopramide + dexamethasone	Prophylaxis for EPSs with metoclopramide
Third line	Depends on response to other antiemetics	Tailor to patient-specific factors
Acute Prophylaxis for Moderately Low and Low Emetogenic Regimens		
First line	No premedication or phenothiazine ± dexamethasone	Depends on chemotherapy regimen
Second line	Metoclopramide ± dexamethasone	Use low-dose metoclopramide
Third line	Depends on response to other antiemetics	Tailor to patient-specific factors
Delayed Nausea and Vomiting		
First line	Metoclopramide + dexamethasone	Continue 3–4 d after chemotherapy
Second line	Long-acting phenothiazine + dexamethasone	Monitor for EPSs
Third line	Depends on response to other antiemetics	Tailor to patient-specific factors

effective as metoclopramide or placebo and less effective than dexamethasone, unlike their efficacy in preventing acute emesis. Regimens identified as most effective for delayed emesis include metoclopramide 0.5 mg/kg orally four times a day for 4 days with dexamethasone 8 mg orally twice a day for 2 days, followed by dexamethasone 4 mg orally twice a day for 2 days.

The use of scheduled phenothiazines (including long-acting phenothiazines) with dexamethasone is another effective option for the prevention of delayed nausea and vomiting. Addition of a benzodiazepine to the antiemetic regimen may prove useful for the control of emesis in anxious patients or patients with difficulty resting.

Anticipatory Emesis

Anticipatory nausea and vomiting occurs in up to 25% of patients receiving chemotherapy. It is usually associated with a history of uncontrolled nausea and vomiting with prior chemotherapy and is a conditioned response. Multiple factors can stimulate anticipatory nausea and vomiting, but most factors remind the patient of the previous unfavorable experience. For example, patients tell stories of becoming nauseated by the sight of their oncologist's office or by a smell that reminds them of receiving chemotherapy. Other triggers may be tastes, sounds, or thoughts of chemotherapy. Anticipatory nausea and vomiting most frequently occurs before the administration of chemotherapy, and it can lead to poorer control of nausea and vomiting with subsequent courses. The most effective treatment for delayed nausea and vomiting is prevention. It is crucial to premedicate adequately for highly to moderately emetogenic chemotherapy and to reassess control on a frequent and regular basis. This form of emesis is frequently refractory to standard antiemetic treatment; however, the benzodiazepines and butyrophenones may provide anxiolysis as well as antiemetogenicity. The addition of one of these agents is strongly encouraged for patients who have had previous unsatisfactory control of nausea and vomiting.

Many practice guidelines are available for the use of antiemetics in chemotherapy-induced nausea and vomiting. These guidelines are created by experts and are based on current literature (**Table 28.3** and **Figure 28.3**). To review treatment choices for other types of nausea and vomiting, see **Table 28.2** and **Figure 28.2**.

Special Population Considerations

Pediatric

The treatment of nausea and vomiting in children differs from that in adults. It is particularly important in the pediatric population to focus on treating the cause of the problem. The etiology of emesis can vary with age (**Box 28.5**). Because they are smaller, children are predisposed to dehydration and electrolyte abnormalities caused by emesis.

Pediatric patients experience more extrapyramidal or neuromuscular reactions to phenothiazines, particularly when the drugs are administered during an acute viral illness such as chickenpox, measles, or gastroenteritis. Because of its antihistamine quality, promethazine may be a viable phenothiazine option. Also, on a milligram-per-kilogram basis, children experience more extrapyramidal reactions from metoclopramide, even at IV doses as low as 0.5 mg/kg four times a day.

Most antiemetic agents are dosed according to milligram per kilogram of body weight or the age of the child, and many of the available agents are not recommended for use in patients younger than age 2 or 3. Some agents that are considered safe and effective in most situations are dimenhydrinate or oral or rectal trimethobenzamide (Tigan; IV not recommended). The phenothiazines are beneficial but should be used cautiously. For pediatric patients receiving chemotherapy, the prevention and treatment of emesis is similar to that in their adult counterparts, although specific pediatric dosing of the agents applies.

Women

Nausea and vomiting is experienced by more than 50% of pregnant women. A few women experience hyperemesis gravidarum, which can present as uncontrollable vomiting with

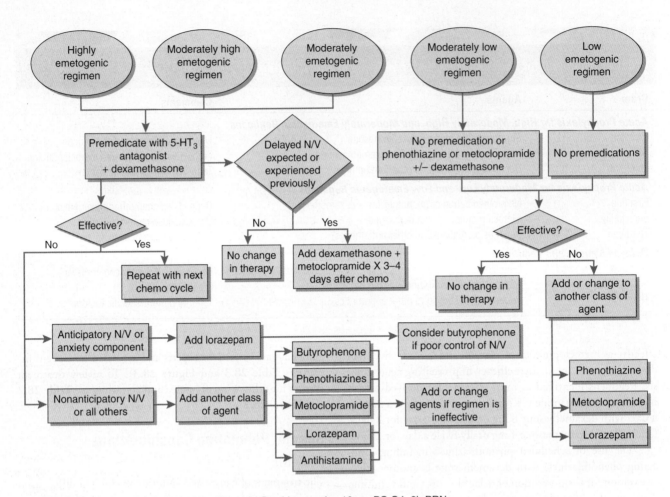

Prescribe PRN antiemetics for home use. Example: Prochlorperazine 10 mg PO Q4–6h PRN.
Antiemetic regimen should be continued for the duration of emetic potential of the agent(s).

Key ⬭ Starting point for decision making   ▢ Clinical actions(assessing, prescribing, monitoring)   ◇ Decision point

FIGURE 28.3   Treatment algorithm for chemotherapy-induced nausea and vomiting.

inability to tolerate oral intake. These symptoms are most common in the first trimester of gestation but can occur at any time during pregnancy. Pregnancy-related emesis is believed to be modulated by CTZ stimulation.

Teratogenicity is the paramount concern when evaluating the safety of an agent in pregnant women. The first trimester of the pregnancy is when drugs or other exogenous substances can most affect embryonal development. Many of the studies performed to study the teratogenic effects of drugs encounter several difficulties. Most fetal malformations occur rarely, and frequently, only a small sample size is obtained and reported. Mothers with underlying diseases, such as seizure disorder, hypertension, diabetes, and cancer, are known to have a higher incidence of infants with malformation. In these patient populations, the role of drugs versus the role of the disease in fetal abnormalities is unclear. Recall bias may play a factor in teratogenicity studies as well. Ultimately, current evidence-based information on the safety and risk of drugs during pregnancy should be used to make clinical decisions.

Most recently doxylamine–pyridoxine (Diclegis) combination pill was reintroduced as the only drug approved by the

FDA for treatment of nausea and vomiting from pregnancy and is considered first line for treatment (American College of Obstetricians and Gynecologists, 2015; Nuangchamnong & Niebyl, 2014). Other agents that are used for mild to moderate nausea and vomiting in pregnancy include the phenothiazines, antihistamine–anticholinergic agents, and metoclopramide. Antihistamine drugs are generally believed to be safe for the pregnant women and her fetus, although there are incidental findings of malformations in fetuses exposed to antihistamines. Anticholinergic drugs have been proven to cause neonatal meconium ileus. Conversely, some anticholinergic agents such as scopolamine have not been associated with consistent teratogenesis.

Phenothiazines readily cross the placenta, but the bulk of evidence indicates their use is safe in this population. Antacids, such as calcium carbonate, may provide safe and reliable relief from mild nausea. Antihistamines, phenothiazines, metoclopramide, haloperidol, droperidol, and ondansetron have all been used in hyperemesis gravidarum without adverse fetal sequelae. Drug classes that should be avoided in pregnant women are the benzodiazepines and cannabinoids. Increased rates of malformations and fetal complications have been

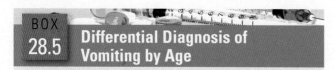

BOX 28.5 Differential Diagnosis of Vomiting by Age

NEWBORN

- Congenital obstructive GI malformations
  - Atresias or webs of esophagus or intestine
  - Meconium ileus or plug; Hirschsprung disease
- Inborn errors in metabolism

INFANT

- Acquired or milder obstructive lesions
  - Pyloric stenosis
  - Malrotation and volvulus
  - Intussusception
- Metabolic diseases, milder inborn errors of metabolism
- Nutrient intolerances
- Functional disorders: gastroesophageal reflux
- Psychosocial disorders: rumination, injury due to child abuse

CHILD OR ADOLESCENT

- Please refer to adult etiologies (**Box 28.1**).

associated with the use of these classes of agents; however, the use of other prescribed and illicit drugs by many of these mothers could cloud the picture. Corticosteroids are rarely used for the control of nausea and vomiting in pregnant women. The risks versus benefits of each drug and situation must be weighed carefully. Further studies to assess safety in this patient population are greatly needed.

MONITORING PATIENT RESPONSE

The best measure of nausea control is how the patient feels. To make evaluation of nausea more objective, nausea can be rated as none, mild, moderate, or severe. Another method is to ask the patient to rate the nausea on a scale from 0 to 10, with 0 equal to no nausea and 10 equal to severe nausea. These methods may help to compare nausea from day to day or week to week in the same patient. Vomiting is easily quantified by episodes per day and volume. If the volume of vomit exceeds 200 to 500 mL/d, the patient should be evaluated for electrolyte abnormalities.

PATIENT EDUCATION

It is pivotal to identify the cause of the nausea and vomiting and to educate the patient about actions that need to be taken. Many cases of mild nausea and vomiting can be alleviated without additional medications.

Drug Information

Some drugs may be taken with food to avoid GI discomfort, and dietary adjustments may prove to be helpful for some cases of nausea. This knowledge gives patients more control over their own well-being. Anxiety and mental illness are components of some occurrences of nausea and vomiting; therefore, counseling and education are the key components in the treatment of nausea and vomiting of this type. Patients can also be educated about the nonprescription drugs available. Realistic goals of nausea control should be set and discussed with the patient. For example, many women have morning sickness with pregnancy; however, medications should be used as infrequently as possible at the lowest dose possible.

With antiemetics, as with any other drug therapy, usual or serious toxicities should be reviewed with the patient. EPSs are frightening and uncomfortable; consequently, patients need to be aware of this potential effect and how to reverse it if necessary (diphenhydramine). Sedation and anticholinergic effects are common with many antiemetics. For most antiemetics, encourage caution when using machinery or driving. Proper administration of the medication should be reviewed. Will the patient take this on a schedule or only as needed? All of this information ensures that the patient has optimal benefit from the prescribed medication.

Nutritional and Lifestyle Changes

Maintenance of proper hydration during all forms of vomiting is important and should be emphasized to patients predisposed to nausea and vomiting (e.g., children, patients following surgery and chemotherapy, patients with GI disorders and infections). Rehydration with clear liquids is preferred over colas, milk, or caffeinated beverages. Patients should be educated on when to seek medical attention because of excessive vomiting or dehydration.

Complementary and Alternative Therapies

Patients suffering from nausea and vomiting of pregnancy (NVP) frequently do not receive therapy, in part because of fears of adverse effects of medications on the fetus. Several vitamin-based and herbal therapies have been shown to be effective and safe. Two randomized trials of vitamin B_6 have shown a benefit in reducing NVP. The recommended daily allowance is 1.3 to 2 mg/d. Women taking prenatal multivitamins are less likely to have severe NVP.

Ginger has been shown to reduce NVP. Ginger appears to work by inhibiting serotonin receptors in the GI tract and CNS. The dose of ginger for the powdered root form in motion sickness is 1 g up to 4 hours before an inciting event; in NVP, 250 mg four times a day; for chemotherapy-induced nausea and vomiting, 2 to 4 g daily; and for PONV, 1 g 1 hour before anesthesia induction.

Vitamin B_1 (thiamine) deficiency can lead to Wernicke encephalopathy in women with severe NVP. Replacement is needed for all women with vomiting of more than 3 weeks' duration. Prophylaxis with multivitamins and therapy with B_6, with or without doxylamine, are safe and effective therapies for NVP.

CASE STUDY*

S.B. is a 57-year-old African American man with newly diagnosed late-stage small cell lung cancer. He has undergone radiation therapy to the brain for his metastases and is to start chemotherapy next week. His past medical history includes hypertension. He has no known drug allergies. A combination chemotherapy regimen has been chosen: cisplatin 100 mg/m^2 for one dose on the first day and etoposide 100 mg/m^2 IV every day for 3 days. He has experienced nausea and vomiting.

DIAGNOSIS: CHEMOTHERAPY-INDUCED NAUSEA AND VOMITING

1. List specific goals for treatment for **S.B.**
2. What drug therapy would you prescribe? Why?

3. What are the parameters for monitoring success of the therapy?
4. Discuss specific patient education based on the prescribed therapy.
5. List one or two adverse reactions for the selected agent that would cause you to change therapy.
6. What would be the choice for the second-line therapy?
7. What OTC and/or alternative medications would be appropriate for this patient?
8. What dietary and lifestyle changes should be recommended for this patient?
9. Describe one or two drug–drug or drug–food interactions for the selected agent.

* Answers can be found online.

Bibliography

Starred references are cited in the text.

*American College of Obstetricians and Gynecologists. (2015). ACOG practice summary bulletin No. 153: Nausea and vomiting of pregnancy. *Obstetrics & Gynecology*, *126*(3), 687–688. doi: 10.1097/01.AOG.0000471177.80067.19.

American Gastroenterology Association. (2001). AGA medical position statement: Nausea and vomiting. *Gastroenterology*, *120*, 261–262. doi: 10.1053/gast.2001.20515.

*Audhuy, B., Cappelaure, P., Martin, M., et al. (1996). A double-blind, randomized comparison of the antiemetic efficacy of two intravenous doses of dolasetron mesylate and granisetron in patients receiving high-dose cisplatin chemotherapy. *European Journal of Cancer*, *32A*, 807–813.

*Barrett, T., DiPersio, D., Jenkins, C., et al. (2011). A randomized, placebo-controlled trial of ondansetron, metoclopramide, and promethazine in adults. *American Journal of Emergency Medicine*, *29*, 247–255. doi: 10.1016/j.ajem.2009.09.028.

Botrel, T., Clark, O., Clark, L., et al. (2011). Efficacy of palonosetron (PAL) compared to other serotonin inhibitors (5-HT3R) in preventing chemotherapy-induced nausea and vomiting (CINV) in patients receiving moderately or highly emetogenic (MoHE) treatment: Systematic review and meta-analysis. *Support Care Cancer*, *19*, 823–832. doi: 10.1007/s00520-010-0908-8.

Fresea, G., Klaussa, S., Herrmanna, K., et al. (2011). Nausea and vomiting as the reasons for encounter in general practice. *Journal of Clinical Medical Research*, *3*(1), 23–29. doi: 10.4021/jocmr410w.

*Gan, T. (2008). Postoperative nausea and vomiting-can it be eliminated? *Journal of American Medical Association*, *287*(10), 1233–1236. doi: 10.1001/jama.287.10.1233.

Gandara, D. R., Roila, F., Warr, D., et al. (1998). Consensus proposal for 5HT3 antagonists in the prevention of acute emesis related to highly emetogenic chemotherapy. *Supportive Care in Cancer*, *6*, 237–243.

Goodin, S., & Cunningham, R. (2002). 5-HT3-receptor antagonists for the treatment of nausea and vomiting: A reappraisal of their side-effect profile. *The Oncologist*, *7*, 424–436.

Hall, J., & Driscoll, P. (2005). The ABC of community emergency care: Nausea, vomiting and fever. *Emergency Medicine Journal*, *22*, 200–204. doi: 10.1136/emj.2004.022483.

Hasler, W., & Chey, W. (2003). Clinical management nausea and vomiting. *Gastroenterology*, *125*, 1860–1867. doi: 10.1053/j.gastro.2003.09.040.

*Hesketh, P. (2008). Chemotherapy-induced nausea and vomiting. *New England Journal of Medicine*, *358*, 2482–2494. doi: 10.1056/NEJMra0706547.

Lee, N. M., & Saha, S. (2011). Nausea and vomiting of pregnancy. *Gastroenterology Clinics of North America*, *40*(2), 309–vii. http://doi.org/10.1016/j.gtc.2011.03.009.

Michelfelder, A., Lee, K., & Boding, E. (2010). Integrative medicine and gastrointestinal disease. *Primary Care; Clinics in Office Practice*, *37*(2), 255–267.

Navair, R. (2007). Overview of updated antiemetic guidelines for chemotherapy-induced nausea and vomiting. *Community Oncology*, *4*(Suppl. 1), 3–11.

Navari, R. (2013). Management of chemotherapy-induced nausea and vomiting focus on newer agents and new uses for older agents. *Drugs*, *73*, 249–262. doi: 10.1007/s40265-013-0019-1.

Nolte, M. J., Berkery, R., Pizzo, B., et al. (1998). Assuring the optimal use of serotonin antagonist antiemetics: The process of development and implementation of institutional antiemetic guidelines at Memorial Sloan-Kettering Cancer Center. *Journal of Clinical Oncology*, *16*, 771–778.

*Nuangchamnong, N., & Niebyl, J. (2014). Doxylamine succinate–pyridoxine hydrochloride (Diclegis) for the management of nausea and vomiting in pregnancy: An overview. *International Journal of Women's Health*, *6*, 401–409. Retrieved from http://doi.org/10.2147/IJWH.S46653.

Ozgoli, G., Goli, M., & Simbar, M. (2009). Effects of ginger capsules on pregnancy, nausea, and vomiting. *The Journal of Alternative and Complementary Medicine*, *15*(3), 243–246. doi: 10.1089/acm.2008.0406.

Pantanwala, A., Amini, R., Hays, D., et al. (2009). Antiemetic therapy for nausea and vomiting in the emergency department. *The Journal of Emergency Medicine*, *39*(3), 330–336. doi: 10.1016/j.jemermed.2009.08.060.

Santana, T., Trufelli, D., deMatos, L., et al. (2015). Meta-analysis of adjunctive non-NK1 receptor antagonist medications for the control of acute and delayed chemotherapy-induced nausea and vomiting. *Support Care Cancer*, *23*, 213–222. doi: 10.1007/s00520-014-2392-z.

Scorza, K., Williams, A., Phillips, J. D., et al. (2007). Evaluation of nausea and vomiting. *American Family Physician*, *76*(1), 76–84.

Smith, H. S., Smith, E. J., & Smith, A. R. (2012). Pathophysiology of nausea and vomiting in palliative medicine. *Annals of Palliative Medicine*, *1*(2), 87–93. doi: 10.3978/j.issn.2224-5820.2012.07.04.

Tarbell, S., Shaltout, H., Wagoner, A., et al. (2014). Relationship among nausea, anxiety, and orthostatic symptoms in pediatric patients with chronic unexplained nausea. *Experimental Brain Research*, *232*, 2645–2650. doi: 10.1007/s00221-014-3981-2.

Zick, S., Ruffin, J., Lee, J., et al. (2009). Phase II trial of encapsulated ginger as a treatment for chemotherapy-induced nausea and vomiting. *Support Care Cancer*, *17*, 563–572. doi: 10.1007/s00520-008-0528-8.

29 Gastroesophageal Reflux Disease and Peptic Ulcer Disease

Alice Lim

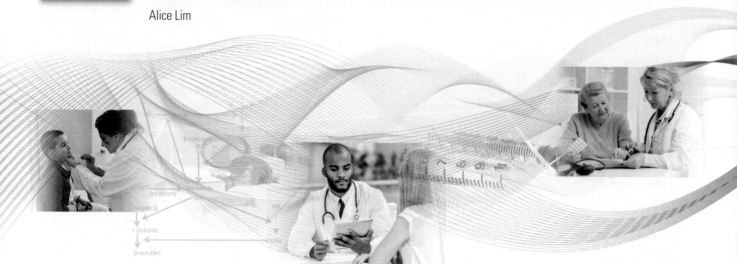

Gastroesophageal reflux disease (GERD) and peptic ulcer disease (PUD) are two disorders of the gastrointestinal (GI) tract that can cause tissue damage and unpleasant symptoms. They are both commonly encountered in the primary care and gastroenterology settings and can also significantly decrease a patient's health-related quality of life if left unmanaged.

GASTROESOPHAGEAL REFLUX DISEASE

GERD is defined as "troublesome symptoms and/or complications" resulting from the abnormal reflux of gastric contents into the esophagus or beyond, including the oral cavity or lungs. Troublesome symptoms are those that have a negative impact on the patient's well-being and quality of life.

Depending on how the patient presents, GERD syndromes may be classified into two categories: (1) symptoms present but without erosions seen on endoscopic exam or (2) those with esophageal tissue injury. Esophageal erosions occur as a result of repeated exposure to refluxed material for prolonged periods of time.

GERD may occur in all ages, but most commonly occurs in those older than 40 years of age. Patients with mild symptoms do not always seek medical treatment and instead self-treat with lifestyle changes or over-the-counter remedies. As a result, the true prevalence of the disease is difficult to assess. It is estimated that 18% to 28% of adults in the United States suffer GERD symptoms weekly. Prevalence seems to be increasing worldwide, with highest rates in Western countries and lowest rates found in East Asia.

CAUSES

Symptoms and/or tissue damage associated with GERD is caused by exposure of the esophagus to gastric contents. This happens as a result of relaxation of the lower esophageal sphincter (LES) due to increase in intra-abdominal pressure (e.g., obesity, pregnancy), delayed gastric emptying, hiatal hernia, or certain medications or foods as listed in **Table 29.1**. Additional risk factors include family history, smoking, alcohol consumption, respiratory diseases, obesity, and reclining or lying down after eating.

PATHOPHYSIOLOGY

Under normal circumstances, the LES serves as a barrier between the esophagus and stomach and, coupled with peristalsis, promotes the forward movement of food. Bicarbonate found in saliva and secreted by the esophageal mucosa buffers acid present in the esophagus. Problems with these normal defense mechanisms contribute to the development of GERD.

Lower Esophageal Sphincter

The LES is a 3- to 4-cm-long smooth muscle located at the distal end of the esophagus. It serves as a high-pressure barrier between the esophagus and stomach and acts to prevent retrograde passage of gastric contents into the esophagus. The LES relaxes on swallowing, allowing food to enter the stomach. A number of mechanisms can cause disruption of this barrier, such as transient LES relaxation (TLESR), increase in intra-abdominal pressure (e.g., pregnancy, obesity, bending over),

TABLE 29.1

Risk Factors for GERD

Causes of LES Relaxation

Foods	Drugs
Fatty foods	Anticholinergic agents
Chocolate	Benzodiazepines
Peppermint/Spearmint	Caffeine
Garlic	Calcium channel blockers (dihydropyridines)
Onions	Dopamine
Chili peppers	Estrogen/progesterone
Alcohol	Nicotine
Coffee/caffeinated drinks	Nitrates
	Theophylline
	Tricyclic antidepressants

Causes Direct Irritation of Esophageal Mucosa

Foods	Drugs
Spicy foods	Aspirin
Citrus juices	Bisphosphonates (e.g., alendronate)
Tomato products	Iron
Coffee	Nonsteroidal anti-inflammatory drugs (NSAIDs)
Tobacco chew	Potassium chloride

TABLE 29.2

Complications of GERD

Complication	Definition
Esophagitis	Inflammation of the lining of the esophagus
Erosive esophagitis	Erosion of the squamous epithelium of the esophagus
Peptic stricture development	Narrowing or tightening of the esophagus
Barrett's esophagus	Squamous epithelium of the esophagus is replaced by specialized columnar-type epithelium
Esophageal adenocarcinoma	Cancer of the esophagus

delayed gastric emptying, and hiatal hernia. Several foods and medications can also decrease LES tone as listed in **Table 29.1**.

TLESR is a normal physiological process that allows gas to escape the stomach and facilitate belching. This is typically accomplished without allowing liquids from escaping the stomach. In GERD, however, TLESR occurs more frequently and prolonged. TLESR is associated with more than half of the reflux episodes in patients with GERD.

Esophageal Clearance and Protection

The amount of time of exposure of gastric acid to the esophageal mucosa is an important determinant of GERD risk. Salivation and peristalsis contribute to the esophagus' ability to clear this content and minimize the duration of contact between the gastric contents and esophagus. Forty to fifty percent of patients with GERD have abnormal peristalsis. Swallowing saliva, which contains bicarbonate, helps to clear esophageal contents and neutralize acid present. However, certain patients have reduced salivary production, especially the elderly or those with Sjögren syndrome or xerostomia (dry mouth). Additionally, swallowing is hindered during sleep, leading to nocturnal GERD.

The esophageal mucosa contains mucus-secreting glands that act to protect the esophageal wall by secreting bicarbonate. However, repeated exposure to acid can compromise this defense system. Cellular damage results, leading to erosive esophagitis.

Gastric Emptying

Slow emptying of stomach contents can increase intragastric pressure, which consequently contributes to GERD. Factors that are associated with delayed emptying include smoking and high-fat meals. Medications that increase gastric emptying and motility can help.

Refluxate

The refluxate properties, acidity, and volume are important determinants of GERD risk. While the stomach can withstand very low pH levels and enzymatic activity of gastric secretions, the squamous cells lining the esophageal mucosa are more sensitive and readily damaged if exposed to this chemical environment. Gastric acid causes direct damage to the esophageal mucosa. Additionally, pepsin, which is a gastric enzyme responsible for the breakdown of food proteins, becomes activated in acidic environments, causing further injury to the esophageal lining.

Complications

Complications of GERD occur from repeated exposure to refluxed gastric contents for prolonged periods of time. These complications are outlined and defined in **Table 29.2**. Esophageal adenocarcinoma appears to occur more commonly in older white males with elevated body mass index (BMI). Since Barrett's esophagus is a risk factor for esophageal adenocarcinoma, screening for Barrett's esophagus is recommended in this particular group.

DIAGNOSTIC CRITERIA

Diagnosis is mainly dependent on patient report of symptoms and review of risk factors present. Symptoms are commonly classified as typical, atypical, and extraesophageal and are listed

TABLE 29.3

Symptoms of GERD

Typical Symptoms	Atypical Symptoms	Extraesophageal Symptoms
Acid regurgitation Heartburn	Epigastric fullness Epigastric pressure Epigastric pain Dyspepsia Nausea Bloating Belching	Chronic cough/ throat clearing Asthma/ bronchospasm Wheezing Hoarseness Sore throat Chronic laryngitis Dental erosions

in **Table 29.3**. They tend to occur after meals and may be aggravated by reclining or lying down. Typical symptoms occur more commonly and include acid regurgitation and heartburn. Generally, a diagnosis of GERD is assumed if patients respond to an empiric trial of acid suppression therapy. Diagnosis of patients who present with atypical symptoms is challenging, since their symptoms may be caused by other conditions, such as PUD and gastroparesis. For these patients, further diagnostic evaluation may be considered prior to empiric therapy. Similarly, those presenting with chest pain must be evaluated to rule out cardiac causes.

Extraesophageal reflux syndromes are associated with symptoms that occur in organs other than the esophagus. These symptoms should only be associated with GERD if they occur with other GERD symptoms or with evidence of tissue injury since these symptoms are nonspecific and have many other causes.

Diagnostic tests may be helpful in patients who do not respond to therapy or those presenting with extraesophageal syndrome to confirm GERD as a cause, or to detect complications of GERD. Endoscopy (with or without biopsy) may be used to assess mucosal injury or other complications like strictures. Biopsy is necessary to detect esophageal adenocarcinoma or Barrett's esophagus. Of note, normal endoscopy does not rule out GERD. On the other hand, tissue damage may not be specifically related to GERD. Other tests, such as ambulatory pH monitoring, can help to clarify diagnosis.

INITIATING DRUG THERAPY

Lifestyle modifications can alleviate GERD symptoms and should be encouraged in every patient. However, in many cases, patients will need to supplement lifestyle changes with medication therapy to control their symptoms.

Drug classes used to treat GERD and its symptoms include (1) antacids, (2) histamine-2 receptor antagonists (H_2RAs), and (3) proton pump inhibitors (PPIs). Generally, a trial of an H_2RA or PPI is given for 2 weeks to confirm the diagno-

sis of GERD. The dose is increased as needed until symptoms resolve. If the patient responds to therapy, it is continued for 4 to 16 weeks. Afterward, the drug is tapered over 1 month to the minimal dose that provides symptom relief if maintenance therapy is warranted. Repeating the initial effective medication is recommended if symptoms recur. Diagnostic testing is recommended if the patient does not respond to treatment.

Goals of Drug Therapy

The goals of pharmacologic therapy are to:

- relieve symptoms
- decrease the frequency and duration of reflux
- heal the esophageal mucosa
- prevent complications

PEPTIC ULCER DISEASE

Similar to GERD, PUD remains one of the most commonly encountered conditions and has high recurrence rates. As a result, PUD can result in significant impairment in quality of life.

CAUSES

There exist three common forms of PUD: *Helicobacter pylori*–positive ulcers, nonsteroidal anti-inflammatory drug (NSAID)-induced ulcers, and stress ulcers. *H. pylori* and NSAID-induced ulcers are chronic conditions that often recur in patients. Stress ulcers usually occur in critically ill patients or just following major trauma or serious illness. Management of stress ulcers is largely focused on prevention with PPIs or H_2RAs. Less commonly, peptic ulcers are also associated with Zollinger-Ellison syndrome (ZES), radiation, chemotherapy, vascular insufficiency, and other chronic diseases. These ulcers develop mostly in the stomach and duodenum, but may occasionally develop in the esophagus, jejunum, ileum, or colon.

An estimated 30% to 40% of the U.S. population is infected with *H. pylori*; however, this prevalence has been decreasing, possibly due to improved therapies and sanitation. *H. pylori* infection typically occurs in the first few years of life and is contracted through the fecal–oral route. Though *H. pylori* infection is common, only 15% of these cases eventually progress to ulcer formation. PUD occurs in 30% of patients chronically using NSAIDs and aspirin, and 1.5% of these patients experience GI bleeding or perforation. Risk factors for ulcers related to NSAID use are listed in **Table 29.4**.

PATHOPHYSIOLOGY

Under normal circumstances, the gastric and duodenal environments are able to maintain a state of homeostasis where food digestion can occur without compromising gastric tissue integrity. A number of defense mechanisms exist to prevent

TABLE 29.4

Risk Factors for NSAID-Related PUD (American College of Gastroenterology)

Level of Risk	Risk Factors
Low	No risk factors present
Moderate	Presence of 1–2 of the following: • Age > 65 y • High-dose NSAID use • History of uncomplicated ulcer • Multiple NSAID use • Concurrent use of aspirin, corticosteroids, or anticoagulants
High	More than 2 of the above risk factors History of complicated ulcer

tissue injury from acid and digestive functions of the GI tract. *H. pylori* and NSAIDs can disrupt these processes, leading to the formation of ulcers.

Gastric Acid

Hydrochloric acid (HCl) and pepsin are responsible for gastric mucosal damage found in PUD. Baseline acid production occurs during fasting states, whereas maximal acid production occurs following meals. Parietal cells are stimulated to release acid by histamine, acetylcholine, and gastrin. All of these stimuli are released by the sensation of food, including the sight, smell, and taste. After stimulation, acid is released through the proton pumps located on the parietal cells. In *H. pylori* infection, acid secretion is elevated above normal, while NSAIDs do not affect acid secretion.

Pepsin

In an acidic environment, pepsinogen is converted to active pepsin in the stomach. Pepsin is responsible for protein digestion, but also can contribute to gastric mucosal damage leading to PUD.

Mucosal Protection

The gastric lining contains a mucus layer that works to protect the underlying cells of the gastric wall against gastric acid. Bicarbonate secretion acts as a buffering agent and allows the epithelial lining to maintain a neutral pH despite the acidic levels found in the gastric lumen. Prostaglandins also provide mucosal protection by decreasing gastric acid production and increasing mucus production. Both *H. pylori* and NSAID use can impede these defenses.

Helicobacter pylori

A gram-negative spiral-shaped rod bacterium with flagella, *H. pylori* is found on the surface of gastric epithelium. Infection occurs when *H. pylori* penetrates the epithelial cells. The bacterium is able to survive in the acidic environment mainly due to its ability to hydrolyze urea into carbon dioxide and ammonia through the production of urease. *H. pylori* causes ulcer

formation by increasing acid production, increasing gastrin secretion, and releasing its own noxious enzymes and toxins. It is also a known carcinogen and if left untreated can lead to gastric mucosa–associated lymphoid tissue (MALT) lymphoma.

Nonsteroidal Anti-inflammatory Drugs (NSAIDs)

NSAIDs cause PUD through direct and indirect mechanisms. As weak acids, they are direct irritants against the mucosal wall. NSAIDs also have antiplatelet properties, further compounding the bleeding complications that can occur as a result of PUD.

NSAIDs that inhibit both cyclooxygenase (COX)-1 and COX-2, inhibit endogenous prostaglandin production. Inhibition of COX-1 in the stomach reduces the production of prostaglandin, whereas COX-2 is more associated with the processes that lead to fever and pain. Therefore, selective COX-2 inhibitors carry less risk for PUD compared to nonselective NSAIDs.

Complications

Complications of PUD include GI bleed (melena or hematemesis), perforation, penetration, or gastric outlet obstruction. Symptoms of PUD-related complications include changes in nature of the pain. Patients with perforation may complain of sharp sudden pains. Patients with gastric outlet obstruction may experience bloating, anorexia, nausea, vomiting, and weight loss.

DIAGNOSTIC CRITERIA

Though not all patients with PUD present with symptoms, the most common complaints include epigastric pain described as burning, fullness, discomfort, gnawing, cramping, or aching. The severity and frequency of the pain can fluctuate, with some patients reporting nocturnal pain. Often, heartburn, belching, and bloating accompany the pain. Symptom presentation is dependent on location of the ulcer. *H. pylori*–associated ulcers are more commonly found in the duodenum, while NSAID-associated ulcers are more commonly found in the stomach. Symptoms of duodenal ulcer typically occur about 1 to 3 hours following meals and are usually relieved by food intake. In gastric ulcer, nausea, vomiting, and anorexia are common symptoms, and food can precipitate ulcer pain.

More severe signs and symptoms are described as alarming features. These include prior history or family history of upper GI malignancy, unintentional weight loss, GI bleeding, iron deficiency anemia, dysphagia or odynophagia, early satiety, persistent vomiting, palpable mass, or lymphadenopathy.

Endoscopy with biopsy allows access to tissue for rapid urease tests and cultures to detect *H. pylori*. Endoscopy is considered the gold standard test and is appropriate for initial evaluation of patients older than 50 years of age who have new-onset dyspepsia or patients of any age who present with alarming features. It should also be considered in those who fail a trial of acid suppression therapy, though sensitivity of the rapid urease test may be diminished with use of medications that reduce urease activity, such as antibiotics or PPIs. Obtaining a culture can provide further guidance, especially if antibiotic-resistant strains are suspected. However, this method is time consuming and costly.

Less invasive tests are also available, and include serologic testing, urea breath test, and fecal antigen assays. These tests are more appropriate for patients younger than 50 who complain of dyspepsia but without alarming features. Serologic testing can be performed in the office with results returning in 15 minutes. However, it is less sensitive and specific compared to other tests. Moreover, it is not useful in confirming eradication of the bacteria, since patients can remain seropositive for a long period of time following treatment. Given its high specificity and short turnaround time, the urea breath test is the most common noninvasive diagnostic tool for PUD. Since medications can interfere with urease activity, bismuth-containing medications and antibiotics should be held for at least 28 days and PPIS for 7 to 14 days before testing. Therefore, it is most reliable for confirming eradication 6 to 8 weeks after therapy. Fecal antigen testing is also useful in both diagnosing infection before treatment and confirming eradication after treatment. Testing is less sensitive to the effects of medications. Still, the test should be withheld within 4 weeks of antibiotic use, 2 weeks of PPI use, and 24 hours of H_2RA use.

INITIATING DRUG THERAPY

Several pharmacologic agents are available for the treatment of PUD, and many overlap with the drugs used in the treatment of GERD. The choice in treatment depends on the etiology, presentation, and presence of complications.

For *H. pylori*–associated ulcers, a combination of antibiotics and acid suppression therapy can be prescribed. Relapses are common and can be prevented only by eradicating *H. pylori*; therefore, antibiotic therapy is indicated for all patients with *H. pylori*–induced ulcers. The empiric use of antisecretory agents for suspected PUD should be used with caution, since these can mask the symptoms of severe disease that warrants important diagnostic testing and long-term treatment. Thus, it is important to confirm *H. pylori* infection with serologic or urea breath testing prior to treatment.

Goals of Drug Therapy

The goals of pharmacologic therapy are to:

- relieve symptoms
- reduce acid secretion
- promote epithelial healing
- prevent recurrence
- prevent complications

For NSAID-induced PUD, an additional goal is to either identify an alternative for pain management or provide prophylaxis strategies to prevent ulcers if continued treatment with NSAIDs is necessary. Strategies include taking enteric-coated NSAIDs, taking with meals, adding misoprostol, or switching to a selective COX-2 inhibitor.

DRUG CLASSES FOR THE TREATMENT OF GERD AND PUD

The drugs used to treat GERD and PUD often overlap. Drug classes and their properties are described below and in **Table 29.5**.

TABLE 29.5

Drugs Used in the Management of GERD and PUD

Generic (Trade) Names	Selected Adverse Effects	Contraindications	Therapeutic Considerations
Antacids			
Calcium-, magnesium-, and aluminum-containing formulations	Rebound hyperacidity, diarrhea with magnesium-containing antacids, constipation with aluminum-containing antacids	None significant	Monitor for drug interactions Use magnesium–aluminum combination to avoid diarrhea or constipation
Histamine-2 Receptor Antagonists (H_2RAs)			
cimetidine (Tagamet) famotidine (Pepcid) nizatidine (Axid) ranitidine (Zantac)	Generally well tolerated, may experience headache, dizziness, confusion	Hypersensitivity to H_2RAs	Take without regard to meals Monitor for drug interactions Consider dose reduction in elderly and renal impairment May be scheduled or used on an as-needed basis

(Continued)

TABLE 29.5

Drugs Used in the Management of GERD and PUD (*Continued*)

Generic (Trade) Names	Selected Adverse Effects	Contraindications	Therapeutic Considerations
Proton Pump Inhibitors (PPIs) omeprazole (Prilosec, Zegerid) lansoprazole (Prevacid) pantoprazole (Protonix) esomeprazole (Nexium) dexlansoprazole (Dexilant) rabeprazole (AcipHex)	Diarrhea, constipation, abdominal pain, headache	Hypersensitivity to PPIs	Take 30–60 min before meals Do not crush, chew, or split delayed-release tablets
Antibiotics amoxicillin (Amoxil) clarithromycin (Biaxin) metronidazole (Flagyl) tetracycline	amoxicillin: diarrhea, nausea, vomiting clarithromycin: diarrhea, abnormal taste, nausea, vomiting metronidazole: headache, metallic taste, nausea, peripheral neuropathy tetracycline: GI upset, diarrhea, photosensitivity	amoxicillin: allergy to penicillin or other beta-lactams clarithromycin: allergy to macrolides, QT prolongation, use with astemizole, cisapride, pimozide, simvastatin, or lovastatin metoclopramide: allergy to metoclopramide tetracycline: allergy to tetracycline	Take without regard to meals, except tetracycline should be taken on empty stomach Avoid clarithromycin in retreatment for those who fail initial clarithromycin-containing regimen Avoid alcohol with metronidazole Avoid dairy, antacids, and iron products within 2 h of tetracycline administration
Misoprostol misoprostol (Cytotec)	Diarrhea, abdominal pain, cramping, nausea	Hypersensitivity to misoprostol, pregnancy	Take with food Reduce dose if diarrhea is intolerable Avoid in pregnancy
Sucralfate sucralfate (Carafate)	Constipation	Hypersensitivity to sucralfate	Take on empty stomach. Monitor for drug interactions.
Bismuth Subsalicylate bismuth subsalicylate (Pepto Bismol)	Black stools, darkened tongue, constipation, tinnitus	Hypersensitivity to salicylates	Avoid in pregnancy and lactation

Antacids

There are numerous antacids available over the counter. Common examples include calcium carbonate (e.g., Tums), magnesium salts, and aluminum salts. They may be used for mild, intermittent symptoms (less than two times per week) or as breakthrough for patients taking other acid suppression therapies.

Mechanism of Action

Antacids partially neutralize the HCl in the stomach. By increasing the pH level, the activation of pepsin is also inhibited. Another antacid product combined with alginic acid forms a viscous solution on the surface of gastric contents to serve as a barrier against reflux.

Dosage

Antacid dosage recommendations vary and can be administered on an as-needed basis.

Time Frame for Response

Antacids provide immediate symptom relief in mild GERD and thus are commonly used as self-treatment by patients. However, they have a short duration of action, warranting frequent administration in some patients. When used to treat chronic symptoms or PUD, the sole use of antacids should be avoided since they must be administered many times daily in large doses to achieve symptom relief. Additionally, antacids do not heal ulcers and instead may mask the symptoms of serious disease and prolong the initiation of other necessary interventions.

Contraindications

No significant contraindications exist for antacids.

Adverse Events

As antacids are minimally absorbed and work locally in the GI tract, the most frequent side effects are chalky taste, cramps, constipation (aluminum-containing products), or diarrhea (magnesium-containing products). Less commonly, calcium carbonate may cause hypercalcemia. Aluminum antacids should be used with caution in those with renal failure who are more susceptible to hyperaluminemia. Similarly, hypermagnesemia may result in hypotension, nausea, vomiting, and electrocardiographic changes and thus magnesium-containing antacids should also be avoided in those with renal impairment.

Drug Interactions

Antacids also have clinically significant drug interactions by altering the rate and extent of absorption of concomitantly administered drugs, such as iron, sulfonylureas, and tetracycline and quinolone antibiotics. It is recommended to take antacids 1 to 4 hours after other medications to avoid these interactions.

Histamine-2 Receptor Antagonists

H$_2$RAs are effective in mild GERD, ulcer healing, and *H. pylori* eradication when combined with other agents and may be used in the prevention of NSAID-related duodenal PUD. Like

antacids, these products are available over the counter. Because all H$_2$RAs are equipotent, the choice in therapy depends on adverse effect profile and drug interactions.

Mechanism of Action

H$_2$RAs reversibly inhibit the histamine-2 receptors on gastric parietal cells and thus decrease acid secretion and pepsin activation.

Dosage

Dosing recommendations vary by product and severity of symptoms (see **Table 29.6**). When used in anti-*H. pylori* regimens, they are used once or twice daily. Higher doses are required for prevention of NSAID-related ulcers.

Time Frame for Response

Onset of action is about 1 to 2 hours after administration. Therefore, H$_2$RAs may be used as needed or on an intermittent basis for mild heartburn. However, if there is lack of response

TABLE 29.6

Dosing and Administration for GERD Medications

Pharmacologic Agents	Dose	Administration Comments
Mild Symptomatic GERD		
Antacids	Varies depending on product	Use as needed, after meals, or at bedtime
Magnesium-, aluminum-, calcium-containing antacids	Dosing ranges from hourly to as needed	to control nocturnal symptoms
Histamine-2 Receptor Antagonists (Over the Counter)		
cimetidine (Tagamet HB)	200 mg once or twice daily	May be scheduled or used on an
famotidine (Pepcid AC)	10–20 mg once or twice daily	as-needed basis
nizatidine (Axid AR)	75 mg once or twice daily	
ranitidine (Zantac 75)	75 mg once or twice daily	
Proton Pump Inhibitors (Over the Counter)		
esomeprazole (Nexium 24H)	20 mg once daily	Take 30–60 min before breakfast or first
lansoprazole (Prevacid 24HR)	15 mg once daily	meal
omeprazole (Prilosec OTC)	20 mg once daily	
omeprazole/bicarbonate (Zegerid OTC)	20 mg/1,100 mg once daily	
Persistent Mild Symptomatic GERD, Moderate to Severe Symptomatic GERD		
Histamine-2 Receptor Antagonists (Prescription Strength)		
cimetidine (Tagamet)	400 mg twice daily	Duration of therapy: 6–12 wk
famotidine (Pepcid)	20 mg twice daily	Consider maintenance therapy if symp-
nizatidine (Axid)	150 mg twice daily	toms recur
ranitidine (Zantac)	150 mg twice daily	
Proton Pump Inhibitors (Prescription Strength)		
dexlansoprazole (Dexilant)	30 mg once daily	Take 30–60 min before breakfast or first
esomeprazole (Nexium)	20 mg once daily	meal (except dexlansoprazole)
lansoprazole (Prevacid)	15 mg once daily	Duration of therapy: 4–8 wk
omeprazole (Prilosec)	20 mg once daily	Consider maintenance therapy if symp-
omeprazole/bicarbonate (Zegerid)	20 mg once daily	toms recur
pantoprazole (Protonix)	20–40 mg once daily	
rabeprazole (AcipHex)	20 mg once daily	

(Continued)

TABLE 29.6

Drugs Used in the Management of GERD and PUD (*Continued*)

Pharmacologic Agents	Dose	Administration Comments
Persistent Moderate to Severe Symptomatic GERD, Healing of Erosive GERD, or Complications of GERD		
Histamine-2 Receptor Antagonists		
cimetidine (Tagamet)	400 mg four times daily or 800 mg twice daily	Duration of therapy: 8–12 wk Maintenance therapy recommended
famotidine (Pepcid)	20–40 mg twice daily	
nizatidine (Axid)	150 mg four times daily	
ranitidine (Zantac)	150 mg four times daily	
Proton Pump Inhibitors		
dexlansoprazole (Dexilant)	60 mg once daily	Take 30–60 min before breakfast or first meal (except dexlansoprazole)
esomeprazole (Nexium)	20–40 mg once daily	
lansoprazole (Prevacid)	30 mg twice daily	Duration of therapy: 4–16 wk
omeprazole (Prilosec)	20 mg twice daily	Maintenance therapy recommended
omeprazole/bicarbonate (Zegerid)	20 mg/1,100 mg twice daily	
pantoprazole (Protonix)	40 mg twice daily	
rabeprazole (AcipHex)	20 mg twice daily	

within 2 weeks, standard twice-daily dosing is reasonable. In standard dosing, symptomatic relief is achieved in 60% of patients after 12 weeks, and endoscopic esophageal healing occurs in 50% of patients after 12 weeks. Importantly, prolonged use may lead to reduced efficacy and tolerance.

Contraindications

These agents are contraindicated in hypersensitivity to H₂RAs.

Adverse Effects

H₂RAs are generally well tolerated. Patients may experience headache, fatigue, dizziness, and confusion. The risk of side effects increases in renal impairment, so dosages should be reduced in the elderly and in those with creatinine clearance less than 50 mL/min. Rarely, gynecomastia and impotence may occur with cimetidine use.

Drug Interactions

Many drug interactions exist, and a thorough review of concomitant medications must be made prior to initiation of H₂RAs. Drugs that are dependent on acid gastric environments for absorption may have decreased effects, such as ketoconazole and protease inhibitors. Cimetidine is a potent inhibitor of cytochrome P-450 (CYP-450) enzymes and may inhibit the metabolism of warfarin, phenytoin, theophylline, and other strong substrates of the CYP-450 system. Additionally, antacids may decrease the effect of H₂RAs and must be taken 1 to 2 hours after the H₂RA.

Proton Pump Inhibitors

As the most potent acid-suppressing agents available, PPIs are superior to H₂RAs in moderate to severe GERD, prevention of NSAID-induced PUD, and ulcer healing. They are given empirically in the management and diagnosis of GERD. For PUD, they are used in combination with anti–*H. pylori* regimens. Several are available in many dosage forms, including intravenous, powder, and orally disintegrating tablets. Currently, only omeprazole, omeprazole–bicarbonate, lansoprazole, and esomeprazole are available over the counter.

Mechanism of Action

PPIs inhibit gastric proton pumps located on the parietal cells, producing long-lasting suppression of acid secretion.

Dosage

When used empirically to treat GERD, once-daily dosing is recommended. If this is ineffective, the dose may be increased to twice-daily dosing. With the exception of omeprazole–bicarbonate and dexlansoprazole, they are most effective when taken in the morning, 30 to 60 minutes before the first meal. Omeprazole–bicarbonate is most effective in controlling nocturnal acid secretion when taken in the evening. The dual delayed-release action of dexlansoprazole allows for its efficacy when taken at any time during the day regardless of food intake. For those with nocturnal symptoms or those taking twice-daily doses, PPIs may be taken in the evening before dinner. As-needed dosing is not effective or recommended with PPIs.

Time Frame for Response

Sixty-six percent of reduction in acid secretion is seen by day 5 of PPI therapy. After 8 weeks of therapy, 83% of patients experience symptom relief, and endoscopic healing of esophageal tissue is seen in 78% of patients.

Contraindications

These agents are contraindicated in hypersensitivity to PPIs.

Adverse Effects

Side effects may include headache, diarrhea, constipation, and abdominal pain. Recently, PPIs have been evaluated for long-term adverse effects, including hypergastrinemia, fractures, infections (*Clostridium difficile* colitis and bacterial gastroenteritis), vitamin B_{12} deficiency, and hypomagnesemia. Data on the true risk of these outcomes with chronic PPI use are conflicting; however, the FDA advisory warns of the risk of osteoporosis and fractures in patients taking high-dose PPI therapy or if PPIs are used for more than 1 year, especially in those with other risk factors present. Generally, it is recommended to continue PPI therapy in patients with osteoporosis if indicated, but consideration of risk versus benefit must be given if the patient has additional risk factors for hip fracture. In the short term, PPIs may increase the risk of community-acquired pneumonia; however, this risk appears to disappear after long-term use.

Drug Interactions

Similar to H_2RAs, PPIs may decrease the efficacy of drugs that depend on an acidic gastric environment for adequate absorption. PPIs are also implicated in drug interactions involving the cytochrome (CYP) P-450 system. Omeprazole and lansoprazole are metabolized by CYP2C19, which is an enzyme necessary for the conversion of the antiplatelet drug clopidogrel to its active form. It has been suggested that inhibition of CYP2C19 by PPIs inhibits the efficacy of clopidogrel and may result in cardiovascular harm. The clinical significance of this interaction is not well understood, and reports demonstrate a lack of evidence of increased cardiac events when PPIs are used alongside clopidogrel. Decisions regarding concomitant use of these medications should consider both the benefits of acid-suppression therapy and the potential risk of cardiovascular complications. Omeprazole likely carries the highest risk for interaction, while pantoprazole has the least risk.

Antibiotics

Antibiotics are used in combination with acid-suppressing medications to eradicate *H. pylori*–induced PUD. They are ineffective when used as monotherapy due to high risk of resistance and should therefore be given with other antibiotics and acid suppression therapies. They do not have a role in GERD management.

Amoxicillin

Mechanism of Action
Amoxicillin is an aminopenicillin that kills bacteria by interfering with cell wall synthesis. It is most effective at neutral pH levels and therefore must be administered with an acid suppression agent such as a PPI or H_2RA.

Dosage
It is dosed at 1 g by mouth twice daily.

Time Frame for Response
A 10- to 14-day treatment duration is needed for maximal efficacy.

Contraindications
Amoxicillin must be avoided in those with allergy to penicillins or other beta-lactams.

Adverse Effects
The most common side effects associated with amoxicillin are diarrhea, nausea, and vomiting, which may be relieved by taking the medication with food. Patients should be monitored for hypersensitivity reactions.

Drug Interactions
Amoxicillin is not commonly implicated in drug interactions, though it may increase the anticoagulant effects of warfarin therapy.

Clarithromycin

Mechanism of Action
Clarithromycin is a macrolide antibiotic that inhibits bacterial protein synthesis. While highly effective against *H. pylori*, it is susceptible to resistance, so it should be avoided as retreatment if a clarithromycin-containing regimen fails.

Dosage
Clarithromycin is dosed 500 mg by mouth twice daily.

Time Frame for Response
A 10- to 14-day treatment course is needed for maximal efficacy.

Contraindications
Clarithromycin is contraindicated in known allergy to macrolide antibiotics, history of QT prolongation, and concomitant use with astemizole, cisapride, pimozide, simvastatin, or lovastatin.

Adverse Effects
The most common side effects associated with clarithromycin are diarrhea, abnormal taste, nausea, and vomiting, which may be relieved by taking the medication with food.

Drug Interactions
Clarithromycin is a strong CYP3A4 substrate and therefore should be used with caution when used concomitantly with strong CYP3A4 substrates, inducers, and inhibitors.

Metronidazole

Mechanism of Action
Metronidazole kills anaerobic bacteria and protozoa by interfering with DNA structure, causing inhibition of protein synthesis and subsequent cell death.

Dosage
Depending on the regimen, dosing ranges from 125 to 500 mg taken two to four times daily.

Time Frame for Response
A 10- to 14-day treatment course is needed for maximal efficacy.

Contraindications
Metronidazole is contraindicated in known allergy to metronidazole.

Adverse Effects
Metronidazole may cause headache, metallic taste, nausea, and peripheral neuropathy.

Drug Interactions

Alcohol consumption with metronidazole should be avoided to prevent disulfiram-like reactions. It may also increase the anticoagulant effect of warfarin.

Tetracycline

Mechanism of Action

Tetracycline inhibits bacterial protein synthesis and is effective against gram-positive and gram-negative bacteria.

Dosage

Tetracycline is dosed at 500 mg, two to four times daily depending on the regimen. It must be given either 2 hours before or 2 hours after food intake to optimize absorption.

Time Frame for Response

A 10- to 14-day treatment course is needed for maximal efficacy.

Contraindications

It is contraindicated in known allergy to tetracycline.

Adverse Effects

Side effects of tetracycline include GI upset, diarrhea, and photosensitivity.

Drug Interactions

Tetracycline is a major substrate and moderate inhibitor of CYP3A4. Antacids, dairy products, and iron may decrease the absorption of tetracycline.

Misoprostol

Misoprostol is used as prophylaxis against NSAID-induced ulcers in patients at high risk for gastric ulcers and its complications.

Mechanism of Action

Misoprostol is a synthetic prostaglandin E_1 analog that inhibits acid secretion and increases mucosal defenses.

Dosage

It is dosed at 200 mcg four times daily taken with food.

Time Frame for Response

Time to peak effect is between 6 and 22 minutes.

Contraindications

Misoprostol is contraindicated in hypersensitivity to prostaglandins and in pregnancy.

Adverse Effects

GI effects are common and include diarrhea, abdominal pain, flatulence, and nausea. A dose reduction to 100 mcg is warranted if diarrhea persists or is intolerable.

Drug Interactions

Antacids may increase the risk of adverse effects of misoprostol, especially those containing magnesium.

Sucralfate

Sucralfate is approved for the treatment and maintenance of duodenal ulcers. It is also used in stress ulcer prophylaxis. It is not effective in *H. pylori* eradication.

Mechanism of Action

Sucralfate forms a viscous, adhesive substance that attaches to and protects ulcers against noxious gastric content.

Dosage

Sucralfate is given 1 g by mouth four times daily.

Time Frame for Response

Paste formation and symptom improvement occurs in 1 to 2 hours after administration. Its short half-life necessitates frequent administration.

Contraindications

Sucralfate should not be used in known hypersensitivity to the drug.

Adverse Effects

The most common side effect is constipation. Systemic effects are not common since sucralfate is minimally absorbed from the GI tract. Because it contains aluminum, there is a possibility for aluminum toxicity, particularly in patients with impaired renal function.

Drug Interactions

Because sucralfate coats the GI mucosa, sucralfate may decrease the absorption and effect of many medications. Separating sucralfate by 2 hours before or 6 hours after administration of other drugs is prudent to avoid interactions.

Bismuth Subsalicylate

Bismuth subsalicylate is highly effective against *H. pylori* when used in combination with antibiotics. It is available both in chewable tablet and liquid form. It is also available as a combination with ranitidine for use with clarithromycin in the eradication of *H. pylori*.

Mechanism of Action

Bismuth subsalicylate has acid secretion suppressing effects. The bismuth component exhibits antimicrobial effects, preventing *H. pylori* adhesion to epithelial cells. The salicylate component may provide anti-inflammatory action as well.

Dosage

It is dosed at 525 mg by mouth four times daily.

Time Frame for Response

In *H. pylori* eradication regimens, it must be taken for 10 to 14 days to achieve maximal effects.

Contraindications

Bismuth subsalicylate should be avoided in sensitivity to salicylates.

Adverse Effects

Common side effects include black stools, darkened tongue, and constipation. At higher doses, tinnitus may be seen.

Drug Interactions

Due to the salicylate component, which acts similarly to aspirin, bismuth subsalicylate may increase bleeding risk when used with anticoagulants or antiplatelets.

SELECTING THE MOST APPROPRIATE AGENT FOR GERD

Initial treatment choice depends on the symptoms severity, symptom frequency, and whether complications are present or not (**Figure 29.1**).

First-Line Therapy

For patients with mild symptoms (typical symptoms fewer than three times a week), lifestyle changes should be initiated. Over-the-counter acid suppression therapies with antacids, H₂RAs, or PPIs can be added if lifestyle changes alone do not resolve symptoms. If symptoms are unrelieved after 2 weeks of lifestyle changes alongside acid suppression therapies, the patient should seek medical attention for advancement of pharmacologic therapy to an empiric acid suppression therapy or diagnostic testing as necessary.

For patients with moderate to severe symptomatic GERD or persistent mild GERD symptoms that are troublesome,

empiric prescription dosing of acid suppression therapy is first-line. There are two general approaches to therapy: step-up versus step-down. The step-up approach begins with lifestyle modifications and the gradual increase of pharmacologic intervention with an H₂RA, progressing to PPI therapy or surgery until symptom improvement. The step-down approach begins with PPI therapy, then stepping down to the lowest dose of either a PPI or H₂RA that is needed to control symptoms. PPIs are favored in moderate to severe GERD since they provide the most rapid relief of symptoms as well as the most optimal chance of tissue healing. Dosing of these agents is presented in **Table 29.6**. Combination therapy with H₂RAs plus PPIs has not been shown to be more effective and is generally not recommended.

Patients with evidence of erosive esophagitis will require high-dose acid suppression therapy for longer durations. Again, PPIs are preferred over H₂RAs due to its superiority in tissue healing.

After treatment with H₂RAs or PPIs, maintenance therapy should be considered to continue symptom control and to prevent complications. Patients with moderate-to-severe

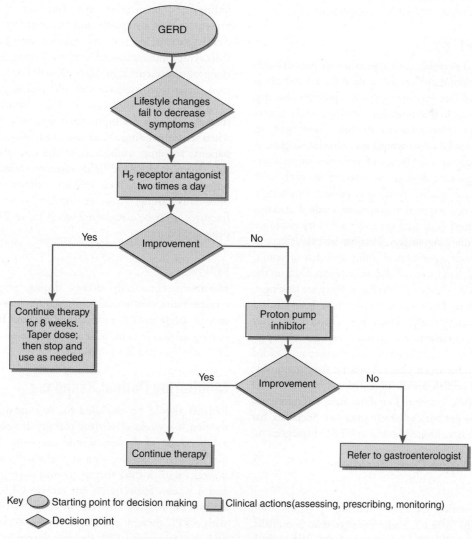

FIGURE 29.1   Treatment algorithm for GERD.

symptoms or erosive esophagitis are especially susceptible to rebound effects after treatment discontinuation, and often, PPI maintenance therapy is necessary for these patients. The treatment dose should be titrated down to the lowest most effective strength. Longstanding use of PPIs is limited by the potential for long-term adverse effects as discussed earlier.

Second-Line Therapy

For patients with incomplete response to acid suppression therapy, adding an H$_2$RA at bedtime may be beneficial in controlling overnight symptoms. H$_2$RAs are generally considered second-line after PPI therapy for erosive esophagitis and other complications of GERD due to weaker and slower tissue healing. For symptomatic GERD, if maximal doses have been reached with PPI therapy with partial or no response, once-daily PPI dosing may be increased to twice-daily dosing. Switching the PPI to another in the same class may be considered, but limited data support this practice.

Patients who do not respond to twice-daily PPI therapy, who present with atypical symptoms, or who present with alarming symptoms like dysphagia may need endoscopic testing to detect tissue injury and GERD complications.

Third-Line Therapy

Antireflux surgery is available as an alternative for patients who have atypical symptoms, refractory symptoms, or complications or cannot tolerate long-term acid suppression therapy. Fundoplication, the common procedure, attempts to reposition the LES to optimize intra-abdominal pressure. Ninety percent of patients report resolution of symptoms following surgery. A meta-analysis comparing the efficacy of antireflux surgery versus medical management showed more favorable effects with surgery in improving quality of life and patient satisfaction. Though fewer patients required maintenance medical management, a high proportion of patients still needed maintenance acid suppression following surgery. Possible adverse effects of the procedure include dysphagia, inability to belch or vomit, flatulence, bloating, and increased abdominal girth. Data on the long-term safety and efficacy of antireflux surgery are lacking.

Promotility drugs like metoclopramide have been studied for their use in treating GERD symptoms. Theoretically, they aim to target symptoms that arise as a result of slow gastric emptying. However, results of studies to date have not shown an added benefit to these agents when weighed against their many side effects. Similarly, baclofen has the potential to improve GERD symptoms, but owing to lack of long-term data and numerous adverse effects, it is not currently recommended. Sucralfate has also been shown to have limited benefit in GERD management.

Special Population Considerations
Pediatric

In infants, regurgitation known as "spitting up" is common and occurs daily in 50% of infants younger than 3 months. The cause is likely due to immaturity of the LES, which typically resolves by 12 to 14 months of age. These episodes usually do not cause discomfort or significant clinical consequences for the infant; however, children with chronic gastroesophageal reflux may exhibit poor growth, vomiting, hoarseness, coughing, and chronic sore throat. Management strategies include smaller more frequent meals and thickening the formula or breast milk with 1 to 2 tablespoons of rice cereal per 2 ounces of liquid. Keeping the infant upright for 30 minutes after feeding and raising the head of the crib may also help. If nonpharmacologic therapies fail, therapy with H$_2$RAs and PPIs may be indicated if the cause of symptoms is confirmed or likely to be GERD. Ranitidine is commonly used, but chronic use may lead to diminished efficacy over time. Overuse of ranitidine has been associated with infections and other adverse effects. PPIs have also been shown to be safe and effective in patients aged 1 to 17 years, although long-term safety is largely unknown.

Geriatric

Elderly patients are at higher risk for GERD due to their decreased ability to produce saliva and decreased gastric motility. Additionally, they are more likely to have comorbidities and medications that can further complicate the presentation of symptoms and treatment availability. Often, elderly patients do not seek medical care because they feel their symptoms are related to normal aging processes or their symptoms present atypically (dental erosions, chest pain, etc.). Even when they do seek pharmacologic management, drug interactions and adverse effects limit their choice in therapy. Due to declining renal function, exercise caution when recommending aluminum-containing antacids. Elderly patients are more vulnerable to the central nervous system side effects of H$_2$RAs. PPIs are often prescribed in this patient population due to their efficacy, relative tolerability, and once-daily dosing. However, the long-term effects on bone fractures must be considered when using PPI therapy for a prolonged duration.

Women

Heartburn commonly occurs during pregnancy due to increased intra-abdominal pressure. Over-the-counter antacids may be safely used in moderation. Sodium bicarbonate–containing medications must be avoided due to the risk of metabolic alkalosis and fluid overload.

Monitoring Patient Response

Patients should be evaluated for treatment response within the first few weeks of starting therapy. If symptoms decrease, a full course of therapy should continue. If symptoms do not completely resolve after 6 weeks with an H$_2$RA or after 4 weeks with a PPI, therapy continues for an additional 6 and 4 weeks, respectively. For erosive GERD, if symptoms do not improve by 8 weeks with an H$_2$RA or by 4 weeks with a PPI, therapy can extend to 12 weeks with an H$_2$RA and 16 weeks with a PPI. Patients should be monitored periodically for adverse effects accordingly. For patients who have persistent symptoms, consider endoscopy testing or referral to a gastroenterologist.

After remission is achieved, consider discontinuation of therapy. Most patients, however, will experience recurring symptoms and require retreatment. If recurrence is frequent, initiate maintenance therapy at the lowest effective dose after remission is achieved.

Patient Education

Drug Information

Patients should be educated on possible side effects and instructed to notify their health care providers if they become intolerable. Given the many potential drug–drug interactions, medication profiles must be reviewed and proper timing of administration of medications should be relayed to the patient.

Nutritional and Lifestyle Changes

Lifestyle changes should be incorporated into any GERD treatment plan. You should encourage weight loss, elevation of the head of the bed when sleeping, consuming smaller meals and avoiding causative foods, avoiding tight-fitting clothes, smoking cessation, moderation of alcohol, and avoiding recumbency for 3 hours after meals. Instead of making all of these changes

simultaneously, gradual approaches to lifestyle changes tend to be less overwhelming and more manageable for patients.

Complementary and Alternative Medicine

Peppermint is commonly used for the self-treatment of GERD. It is reported to accelerate gastric emptying and LES pressure. Patients with PUD, however, should avoid peppermint as it may potentiate ulcer formation. Acupuncture was shown to be effective in controlling regurgitation and heartburn in patients with persistent heartburn despite PPI therapy in one study. Electroacupuncture led to a decreased rate of TLESR in 14 healthy volunteers. Studies with larger sample sizes and longer durations are needed to confirm the benefit of this treatment modality for GERD.

SELECTING THE MOST APPROPRIATE AGENT FOR PUD

Choice in treatment depends on the etiology (*H. pylori* or NSAID induced), resistance patterns, and if complications are present. Because resistance patterns differ geographically, regimens that have been studied and validated in the United States are preferred (**Figure 29.2**).

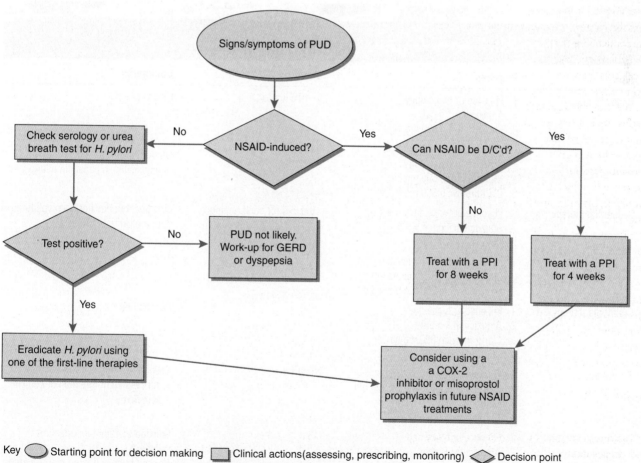

Key ⬭ Starting point for decision making   ▢ Clinical actions(assessing, prescribing, monitoring)   ◇ Decision point

FIGURE 29.2   Treatment algorithm for PUD.

First-Line Therapy

Recommended regimens are listed in **Table 29.7**. A PPI-based regimen with two antibiotics is commonly used. Amoxicillin is preferred since it is highly effective against *H. pylori* and resistance rates remain low. However, for patients with a penicillin allergy, metronidazole is a viable substitute for amoxicillin. Eradication rates with first-line regimens are between 70% and 85%, but rates have recently been declining due to a rise in clarithromycin resistance. Therefore, these regimens are not recommended where clarithromycin-resistant strains are prevalent. Longer, 14-day durations lead to higher eradication and lower resistance rates.

Sequential therapy, where the patient takes a PPI and amoxicillin for 5 days and follows that with triple therapy for another 5 days, has been shown to be just as effective as standard triple therapy in eradicating *H. pylori*. Though less costly compared to standard triple therapy, this regimen has not yet been validated in the United States.

In NSAID-induced ulcers, patients should be tested for *H. pylori* and treated with the above regimens if positive for infection. The NSAID should be discontinued, and a PPI, H₂RA, or sucralfate should be initiated (doses in **Table 29.8**). The NSAID could also be changed to a lower dose, acetaminophen, or a COX-2 inhibitor like celecoxib. If the NSAID must be continued, a PPI or misoprostol should be taken concomitantly with the NSAID to promote healing and prophylaxis of future ulcers. In cases where patients cannot discontinue the NSAID, H₂RAs are significantly less effective at healing ulcers. PPIs also appear to be more effective than misoprostol when NSAID therapy continues.

Successful eradication alone helps to prevent recurrence of *H. pylori*–induced ulcers; however, in patients who failed eradication therapy, have a history of ulcer-related complications, or have repeated recurrence of ulcers, maintenance therapy with a PPI or H₂RA should be considered.

Second-Line Therapy

For those who fail initial eradication therapy, a PPI-based regimen should be initiated using different antibiotics. Bismuth-based quadruple therapy is effective as salvage therapy for treatment failures. It is also preferred if cost is a major barrier to therapy. Emerging data on levofloxacin-based triple therapy support its efficacy and tolerability, but since this regimen has not been validated in the United States, and resistance rates are increasing, it should be reserved for salvage therapy only.

In areas with high rates of clarithromycin resistance, quadruple therapy with a PPI, amoxicillin, clarithromycin, and metronidazole has high eradication rates despite the regimen containing clarithromycin.

TABLE 29.7

Treatment for *H. pylori* Eradication

Type	Regimen	Duration	Comments
Triple therapy	1. PPI once or twice daily 2. Amoxicillin 1 g bid 3. Clarithromycin 500 mg bid	7–10 d (up to 14 d)	First line
	Or 1. PPI once or twice daily 2. Metronidazole 500 mg bid 3. Clarithromycin 500 mg bid	10–14 d	Metronidazole can substitute for amoxicillin in penicillin allergy.
Sequential therapy	1. PPI once or twice daily × 5 d 2. Amoxicillin 1 g bid × 5 d Followed by 1. PPI once or twice daily × 5 d 2. Clarithromycin 500 mg bid × 5 d 3. Metronidazole 500 mg bid × 5 d	10 d (5 d for each regimen)	First line, but has not been validated in the United States
Quadruple therapy	1. PPI once or twice daily 2. Amoxicillin 1 g bid 3. Clarithromycin 500 mg bid 4. Metronidazole 500 mg bid	10 d	Second line
Bismuth-based quadruple therapy	1. PPI twice daily 2. Bismuth subsalicylate 525 mg qid 3. Metronidazole 250 mg qid 4. Tetracycline 500 mg qid	10–14 d	Second line or as salvage therapy for persistent infection or penicillin allergy
Levofloxacin-based triple therapy	1. PPI once or twice daily 2. Amoxicillin 1 g bid 3. Levofloxacin 500 mg daily	10 d	Salvage therapy for persistent infection Has not been validated in the United States

TABLE 29.8

Dosing regimens for PUD management

Generic (Trade) Name	H. pylori Dose	NSAID-Induced Ulcer Prevention Dose	NSAID-Induced Ulcer Treatment Dose	Usual Range	Dose Adjustments
Proton Pump Inhibitor					
dexlansoprazole (Dexilant)	30–60 mg daily	30–60 mg daily	30–60 mg daily	30–60 mg/d	Dose adjustment for hepatic impairment
esomeprazole (Nexium)	40 mg daily or bid	20–40 mg daily	40 mg daily	20–40 mg/d	
omeprazole (Prilosec)	20–40 mg daily or bid	20 mg daily	20–40 mg daily	20–40 mg/d	
omeprazole/bicarbonate (Zegerid)					
pantoprazole (Protonix)	40 mg daily or bid	20 mg daily	40 mg daily	20–40 mg/d	
rabeprazole (AcipHex)	20 mg daily or bid	20 mg daily	20 mg daily	20 mg/d	
Histamine-2 Receptor Antagonists					
cimetidine (Tagamet)	400 mg bid	400 mg daily	300 mg qid or 400 mg bid or 800 mg qhs	800–1,600 mg/d in divided doses	Dose adjustment for renal and hepatic impairment
famotidine (Pepcid)	40 mg daily	20 mg daily	40 mg daily	20–40 mg/d	Dose adjustment for renal impairment
nizatidine (Axid)	150 mg bid	150 mg daily	150 mg bid or 300 mg daily	150–300 mg/d	
ranitidine (Zantac)	150 mg bid	150 mg daily	150 mg bid or 300 mg daily	150–300 mg/d	
Mucosal Protectants					
sucralfate (Carafate)	N/A	N/a	1 g qid	2–4 g/d	None
misoprostol (Cytotec)	N/A	200 mcg qid	200 mcg qid	400–800 mcg/d	None

H$_2$RA-based *H. pylori* eradication regimens are less preferred due to lower eradication rates.

Probiotics have a possible role in *H. pylori* infection when taken alongside eradication regimens. Preliminary data show increased eradication rates and decreased adverse effects, particularly diarrhea.

Third-Line Therapy

In the case of repeated *H. pylori* eradication treatment failures, or persistence of symptoms after 8 to 12 weeks of treatment, referral to a gastroenterologist for endoscopy and biopsy is warranted to establish diagnosis and exclude other causes.

Preventative Therapy in NSAID-Induced PUD

The risks of GI complications and cardiovascular safety must both be weighed when deciding the appropriate approach to prevention of PUD when NSAID therapy must be continued. Consequently, the American College of Gastroenterology provides guidance on choice of therapy when GI and cardiovascular risks are considered (**Table 29.9**). PPIs and misoprostol have both shown efficacy in preventing NSAID-induced ulcers, most of which are gastric ulcers. While PPIs are more commonly used due to its more tolerable side effect profile compared to misoprostol, large randomized controlled trials of PPI cotherapy are lacking. The trials available to date show promising results in preventing ulcers when taken with NSAIDs and even with COX-2 inhibitors. H$_2$RAs are not optimal since they are effective in preventing duodenal ulcers, not gastric ulcers. However, if H$_2$RAs must be used due to cost, high-dose regimens show greater efficacy compared to low doses. Of all NSAIDs, naproxen has the least cardiovascular risk associated and is preferred in patients with high risk for cardiovascular events.

Celecoxib is the only COX-2 inhibitor available in the United States and originally was thought to have less GI effects compared to nonselective NSAIDs. However, available evidence shows that it may have the same GI adverse effects compared to other NSAIDs, especially in patients taking concomitant aspirin. Additionally, there is a dose-dependent increase in cardiovascular events, particularly with higher doses and longer durations of treatment.

TABLE 29.9

Recommendations for Prevention of NSAID-Related Ulcers

Cardiovascular Risk	Gastrointestinal Risk	Recommendation
Low	Low (no risk factors)	NSAID alone
	Moderate (1–2 risk factors)	NSAID plus PPI or misoprostol
	High (>2 risk factors, history of complicated ulcer)	Alternative therapy, or COX-2 inhibitor plus PPI or misoprostol
High	Low (no risk factors)	Naproxen plus PPI or misoprostol
	Moderate (1–2 risk factors)	Naproxen plus PPI or misoprostol
	High (>2 risk factors, history of complicated ulcer)	Avoid NSAID and COX-2 inhibitor; seek alternative therapy

Special Population Considerations

Pediatric

H. pylori is most often contracted during childhood and has higher prevalence in communities with lower socioeconomic status and poorer sanitation conditions. In children with diagnosed *H. pylori*–associated PUD, pharmacologic eradication is recommended due to high relapse rates if left untreated. If *H. pylori* infection is confirmed in the absence of PUD or if an *H. pylori*–positive child has a first-degree relative with gastric cancer, consider treatment in these children. Triple therapy (PPI plus 2 antibiotics), sequential treatment, and bismuth-based therapy for 10 to 14 days are viable treatment options in children. Ideally, obtaining susceptibility data will guide therapy. Avoid tetracycline in children younger than 8 years of age due to risk for reduced bone growth and permanent tooth discoloration.

Geriatric

A number of factors put the elderly population at higher risk for PUD and its complications. Because older patients may not present with typical symptoms of *H. pylori* infection, diagnosis and treatment may be delayed. Comorbidities and concomitant medications, especially with NSAIDs, aspirin, bisphosphonates, and anticoagulants, further increase the risk of PUD. Additionally, mucosal defense mechanisms decline with age. Elderly patients have a higher potential for GI malignancies, and so endoscopy is the preferred method of diagnosis over noninvasive testing. *H. pylori* eradication regimens are similar for the adult population; however, older patients experience more treatment failures due to antibiotic resistance and problems with adherence. They are also more vulnerable to the adverse effects and drug interactions associated with treatment regimens. A treatment plan must be carefully individualized to each patient, and you should counsel patients on the importance of adherence to the entire treatment regimen.

Women

Women who are pregnant or planning to become pregnant should avoid misoprostol due to its abortifacient properties. Consider obtaining a negative pregnancy test in women of child-bearing age before initiating misoprostol.

Monitoring Patient Response

During treatment, patients should be assessed for resolution of symptoms, adverse effects, and adherence. Patients can expect resolution of symptoms within 7 days of antiulcer therapy and within a few days of discontinuing NSAIDs. If symptoms continue or recur after 14 days of treatment, this signifies treatment failure and a retreatment plan is necessary. In the case of treatment failures, patients should be assessed for adherence and proper administration of complex regimens.

Most patients with uncomplicated *H. pylori* infection will not need confirmation of eradication; however, consider confirming eradication with a urea breath test 6 to 8 weeks after the end of treatment in patients who are at risk for complications or have frequent recurrence of disease.

If patients continue NSAID therapy, monitor them closely for complications such as bleeding, obstruction, penetration, or perforation.

Patient Education

Drug Information

Nonadherence to treatment and prevention regimens is a significant cause of treatment failures. These regimens can be complex and costly and come with intolerable side effects. Additionally, since patients often feel better within several days of treatment initiation, they may feel compelled to discontinue their medications midtreatment. Counseling patients on the importance of full adherence to recommended therapies is essential in ensuring proper administration and maximal benefit of these therapies. Patients should also be informed of possible side effects to expect and how to appropriately manage them should they occur.

Nutritional and Lifestyle Changes

Encourage patients to avoid causative behaviors such as cigarette smoking and NSAID use (if possible). While no foods are known to increase the risk of PUD, some foods may exacerbate the symptoms and discomfort associated with PUD. Advise patients to avoid spicy foods, caffeine, and alcohol to aid in symptom relief. Stress reduction is also encouraged, as psychological stress is sometimes associated with worsening of symptoms.

CASE STUDY*

J.G. is a 42-year-old white man presenting with a 2-month history of intermittent midepigastric pain. The pain sometimes wakes him up at night and seems to get better after he eats a meal. **J.G.** informs you that his doctor told him that he had an infection in his stomach 6 months ago. He never followed up and has been taking over-the-counter Zantac 75 for 2 weeks without relief. He takes no other medications. He is concerned because the pain is continuing. He has no other significant history except he is a 20 pack-year smoker and he drinks 5 cups of coffee a day. He eats late at night and goes to bed about 30 minutes after dinner. He is allergic to penicillin.

DIAGNOSIS: PEPTIC ULCER DISEASE

1. List specific goals for treatment for **J.G.**
2. What drug therapy would you prescribe for **J.G.**? Why?

3. What are the parameters for monitoring success of the therapy?
4. Discuss specific patient education based on the prescribed therapy.
5. List one or two adverse reactions for the selected agent that would cause you to change therapy.
6. What would be the choice for second-line therapy?
7. What over-the-counter and/or alternative medications would be appropriate for **J.G.**?
8. What lifestyle changes would you recommend to **J.G.**?
9. Describe one or two drug–drug or drug–food interaction for the selected agent.

* Answers can be found online.

Complementary and Alternative Medicine

Few studies exist examining the effect of licorice and its ability to enhance gastric mucosal protective mechanisms. In a recent study, licorice appeared to be just as effective as bismuth when taken with amoxicillin, metronidazole, and omeprazole in the eradication of *H. pylori*. Given the small sample size and lack of data in the United States, more robust studies are needed to confirm its utility in the treatment and prevention of PUD. Adverse effects of licorice include hypertension and hypokalemia.

Bibliography

Badillo, R., & Francis, D. (2014). Diagnosis and treatment of gastroesophageal reflux disease. *World Journal of Gastrointestinal Pharmacology and Therapeutics, 5*(3), 105–112.

Becher, A., & El-Serag, H. (2011). Systematic review: The association between symptomatic response to proton pump inhibitors and health-related quality of life in patients with gastro-esophageal reflux disease. *Alimentary Pharmacology and Therapeutics, 34*, 618–627.

Chey, W. D., & Wong, B. C. Y.; Practice Parameters Committee of American College of Gastroenterology. (2007). Guideline on the management of *Helicobacter pylori* infection. *The American Journal of Gastroenterology, 102*, 1808–1825.

Chung, E. Y., & Yardley, J. (2013). Are there risks associated with empiric acid suppression treatment of infants and children suspected of having gastroesophageal reflux disease? *Hospital Pediatrics, 3*(1), 16–23.

Cizginer, S., Ordulu, Z., & Kadayifci, A. (2014). Approach to *Helicobacter pylori* infection in geriatric population. *World Journal of Gastrointestinal Pharmacology and Therapeutics, 5*(3), 139–147.

Dent, J., El-Serag, H. B., Wallander, M. A., et al. (2005). Epidemiology of gastro-esophageal reflux disease: A systematic review. *Gut, 54*, 710–717.

DeVault, K. R., & Castell, D. O. (2005). Updated guidelines for the diagnosis and treatment of gastroesophageal reflux disease. *The American Journal of Gastroenterology, 100*, 190–200.

Dickman, R., Schiff, E., Holland, A., et al. (2007). Clinical trial: Acupuncture vs. doubling the proton pump inhibitor dose in refractory heartburn. *Alimentary Pharmacology and Therapeutics, 26*, 1333–1344.

El-Serag, H. B., Sweet, S., Winchester, C. C., et al. (2014). Update on the epidemiology of gastro-esophageal reflux disease: A systematic review. *Gut, 63*(6), 871–880.

Fashner, J., & Gitu, A. C. (2015). Diagnosis and treatment of peptic ulcer disease and *H. pylori* infection. *American Family Physician, 91*(4), 236–242.

Gaude, G. S. (2009). Pulmonary manifestations of gastroesophageal reflux disease. *Annals of Thoracic Medicine, 4*(3), 115–123.

He, Y., Chan, E. W., Man, K. K., et al. (2014). Dosage effects of histamine-2 receptor antagonist on the primary prophylaxis of non-steroidal anti-inflammatory drug (NSAID)-associated peptic ulcers: A retrospective cohort study. *Drug Safety, 37*(9), 711–721.

Hassall, E. (2012). Over-prescription of acid-suppressing medications in infants: How it came about, why it's wrong, and what to do about it. *The Journal of Pediatrics, 160*(2), 193–198.

Hom, C., & Vaezi, M. F. (2013). Extra-esophageal manifestations of gastroesophageal reflux disease: Diagnosis and treatment. *Drugs, 73*, 1281–1295.

Kalach, N., Bontems, P., & Cadranel, S. (2015). Advances in the treatment of *Helicobacter pylori* infection in children. *Annals of Gastroenterology, 28*(1), 10–18.

Kim, D., & Velanovich, V. (2014). Surgical treatment of GERD: Where have we been and where are we going? *Gastroenterology Clinics of North America, 43*(1), 135–145.

Lagergren, J., Bergström, R., & Nyrén, O. (1999). Association between body mass and adenocarcinoma of the esophagus and gastric cardia. *Annals of Internal Medicine, 130*, 883–890.

Lanza, F. L., Chan, F. K. L., Quigley, E. M. M.; Practice Parameters Committee of the American College of Gastroenterology. (2009). Guidelines for the prevention of NSAID-related ulcer complications. *The American Journal of Gastroenterology, 104*, 728–738.

Momeni, A., Rahimian, G., Kiasi, A., et al. (2014). Effect of licorice versus bismuth on eradication of *Helicobacter pylori* in patients with peptic ulcer disease. *Pharmacology Research, 6*(4), 341–344.

O'Connor, A., Vaira, D., Gisbert, J. P., et al. (2014). Treatment of *Helicobacter pylori* infection 2014. *Helicobacter, 19*(Suppl. 1), 38–45.

Patrick, L. (2011). Gastroesophageal reflux disease (GERD): A review of conventional and alternative treatments. *Alternative Medicine Review, 16*(2), 116–133.

Peterson, W. L., Fendrick, A. M., Cave, D. R., et al. (2000). *Helicobacter pylori*-related disease: Guidelines for testing and treatment. *Archives of Internal Medicine, 160*, 1285–1291.

Rickenbacher, N., Kotter, T., Kochen, M. M., et al. (2014). Fundoplication versus management of gastroesophageal reflux disease: A systematic review and meta-analysis. *Surgical Endoscopy, 28*(1), 143–155.

Ryan, S. W. (2005). Management of dyspepsia and peptic ulcer disease. *Alternative Therapies in Health and Medicine, 11*(5), 26–29.

Scheiman, J. M. (2013). The use of proton pump inhibitors in treating and preventing NSAID-induced mucosal damage. *Arthritis Research and Therapy, 15*(Suppl. 3), S5.

Spechler, S. J., Sharma, P., Souza, R. F., et al. (2011). American Gastroenterological Association medical position statement on the management of Barrett's esophagus. *Gastroenterology, 140*, 1084–1091.

Vandenplas, Y., Rudolph, C. D., Di Lorenzo, C., et al. (2009). Pediatric gastroesophageal reflux clinical practice guidelines: Joint recommendations of the North American Society for Pediatric Gastroenterology, Hepatology, and Nutrition (NASPGHAN) and the European Society for Pediatric Gastroenterology, Hepatology, and Nutrition (ESPGHAN). *Journal of Pediatric Gastroenterology and Nutrition, 49*, 498–547.

Vakil, N., Veldhuyzen van Zanten, S., Kahrilas, P., et al. (2006). The Montreal definition and classification of gastro-esophageal reflux disease (GERD)—A global evidence-based consensus. *America Journal of Gastroenterology, 101*, 1900–1920.

Zou, D., Chen, W. H., Iwakiri, K., et al. (2005). Inhibition of transient lower esophageal sphincter relaxations by electrical acupoint stimulation. *American Journal of Physiology. Gastrointestinal and Liver Physiology, 289*(2), G197–G201.

30 Constipation, Diarrhea, and Irritable Bowel Syndrome

Veronica F. Wilbur

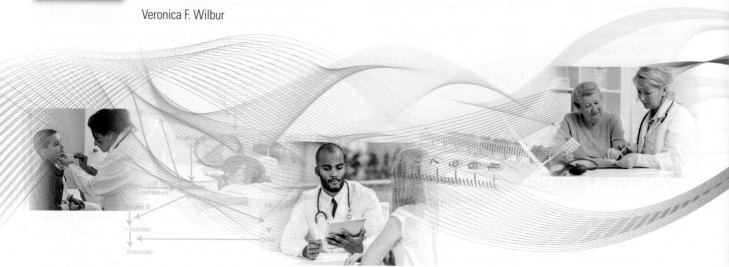

Functional bowel disorders of the lower gastrointestinal (GI) tract can include symptoms of hypogastric cramping, abdominal pain, diarrhea, or constipation. Constipation and diarrhea can be self-limiting or considered symptoms of possibly serious medical problems. Temporary dysfunctions of the bowel can include common GI upsets that can cause short-lived episodes of diarrhea or episodes of constipation. Irritable bowel syndrome (IBS) and chronic idiopathic constipation (CIC) are two of the most common GI complaints globally (Ford et al., 2014). Additionally, the increased prescribing of opiates and opioid narcotics has led to an increase in opioid-induced constipation (OIC) (Camerilli, 2011). IBS typically presents with vague, crampy hypogastric pain and can be accompanied by constipation, diarrhea, and/or alternating patterns, while CIC presents with issues of stool consistency and problems with defecation but without the presence of abdominal pain. Similar pharmacologic agents are used to treat the symptoms of IBS, CIC, OIC, or diarrhea, whether self-limited or chronic.

CONSTIPATION

Constipation is a common GI symptom that is defined as infrequent or difficult evacuation of stool. Every individual affected by constipation defines it differently, but normal defecation can vary from daily to three times a day or to every 3 days. Constipation can be a consequence of multiple factors, including diet, lifestyle, medications, and many disease states. In a systematic review of the epidemiology of constipation globally by Suares and Ford (2011), the mean prevalence of constipation in the general population was found to be 14%. Constipation affects 2.2 females to 1 male, and the incidence

increases with age, especially in those over age 65. Sommers et al. (2011) report a 41.5% increase of emergency room visits and ambulatory care visits for constipation between 2006 and 2011. The incidence of constipation in children is reported between 0.7% and 29% worldwide with prevalence equal between boys and girls (Rajindrajith & Devanarayana, 2011). Dietary and lifestyle modifications are the preferred therapy for constipation, but many patients use over-the-counter (OTC) laxatives for relief. Americans spend over $290 million billion for OTC and prescription laxatives and over $7.5 billion dollars annually for treatment (Pomeranz et al., 2013). Most of these laxatives are considered safe and effective, but overuse or abuse may have serious consequences.

CAUSES

Constipation is a diagnosis based on a thorough history and physical examination. If an identifiable cause is present, constipation is then classified as a secondary symptom. However, constipation may be a symptom of an underlying disease state (**Box 30.1**). The patient's lifestyle (e.g., diet, inactivity) or concomitant medications (**Box 30.2**) may also contribute to constipation. Chronic idiopathic constipation is usually caused by a reduction in the propulsive capacity of the colon (slow transit constipation) or a functional outlet. Another cause of constipation is from the use of opioid drugs and is classified as OIC. Although constipation is often a benign condition, it can be a symptom of a more serious problem. If left untreated in an elderly patient, constipation may lead to impaction, stercoral ulceration, anal fissures, megacolon, volvulus, and possibly carcinoma of the colon.

PATHOPHYSIOLOGY

The absorptive capacity and motility of the colon are major factors of bowel function. Approximately 9 L of fluid enters the small intestine daily from ingestion or intestinal secretions. The small intestine absorbs approximately 80% of this fluid load, which is approximately half of its capacity. The colon absorbs the remainder, with the exception of approximately 0.1 L of water that is passed in the stool. If absorption of the small intestine is reduced, the fluid load adds to the burden of the colon, which is capable of absorbing 4 to 5 L of fluid per day. Fluid in excess of this amount results in diarrhea. Likewise, excessive reabsorption of water results in constipation.

The colon can be divided into three distinctive functional areas: (1) the cecum and proximal colon, (2) the transverse colon, and (3) the distal colon and rectum. Each area performs different roles in preparing the chyme for expulsion. The variation in the neurogenic tone of each area affects the capacity of the colon to retain or release the fecal material.

The motility of the bowel is affected by the flow of chyme from the coloileal reflex, and its visceral hypersensitivity can contribute to the sense of urgency and tenesmus of proximal colonic transit. The neurogenic aspects of colon motility are poorly understood and need further study. Some of the stimuli thought to affect colonic activity are awakening from sleep or rest, ingestion of a high-calorie meal, and the sight or smell of food.

With OIC, the opioid receptors in the gut are mediated from the central nervous system (CNS) and reduce GI propulsion, thereby altering the autonomic outflow. Additionally, this reduces bowel tone and contractility, ultimately prolonging transit time of the stool. Other characteristics of OIC include increased anal sphincter tone and decreased response to anal distention resulting in difficulty with evacuation (Camerilli, 2011; Kumar et al., 2014).

DIAGNOSTIC CRITERIA

The definition of constipation varies widely between health care providers and patients. Constipation, as previously noted, can be idiopathic or caused by medications, or in rare cases organic. Therefore, a function definition is the infrequent bowel movements accompanied by straining with hard feces that lead to straining and a feeling of incomplete evacuation of the rectum. An important distinction between CIC and IBS is the absence of abdominal pain associated with the bowel pattern.

The diagnosis of constipation stems primarily from the history. A careful history (**Box 30.3**) can help the provider decide which diagnostic tests, if any, may be appropriate. Alarm symptoms include a sudden change in bowel habits after the age of 50 years, blood in stools, anemia, weight loss, and a family history of colon cancer (Bharucha et al., 2013) and require further workup.

INITIATING DRUG THERAPY

Lifestyle modifications are preferred over pharmacologic therapy for treating constipation. Diet, exercise, and bowel habit training are usually targeted. However, research is inconclusive as to the value of increasing fluid intake and exercise (Leung et al., 2011) and is controversial for the increased use of fiber (Ho et al., 2012). The recommendations for dietary fiber originated in 1971

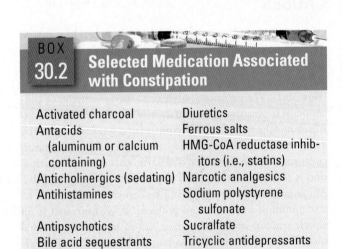

(Burkett, 1993) and gained widespread acceptance as necessary for a healthy diet and normal bowel movements; however, further study has not substantiated this premise. However, increasing fiber has not proven harmful, and according to the National Health Statistics Report (Clarke et al., 2015), Americans eat 5 to 14 g of fiber daily, far short of the most recent recommendations of 20 to 35 g by the American Dietetic Association (American Dietetic Association, 2008). Increased dietary fiber can be recommended for most patients without fear of colon obstruction. Fiber should be both soluble and insoluble in the form of fruits, vegetables, and whole grains, which cannot be digested by the body. Fiber should be slowly increased to 20 to 25 g/d over a 1- to 2-week period to improve compliance with therapy. Dietary fiber is still postulated to increase stool weight and shorten intestinal transit time. Fiber accelerates right colon transit, but there are few treatments for patients where the transit problem is the left colon. Fiber therapy may not be effective for all patients.

One additional lifestyle modification includes establishing a regular pattern for bathroom visits especially with the elderly. Patients should also be counseled not to ignore the urge to defecate, because this delay increases the time for absorption of fluid from the stool. Biofeedback, a method of retraining the pelvic floor muscles to relax during defecation, may be effective in selected patients.

Measures to treat patients with OIC currently mirror those of acute and chronic constipation; however, there is little research that supports this approach.

Goals of Drug Therapy

An adequate trial of lifestyle modification should be attempted first. If this fails, pharmacologic management with laxatives may be appropriate; however, there is little evidence that laxatives cause dependency and should be withheld from long-term treatment (Müller-Lissner et al., 2005; Wald, 2007).

The goal of therapy for constipation is to increase the water content of the feces and increase motility of the intestines to promote comfortable defecation, using the lowest effective dose of a laxative for the least amount of time possible. Only if a patient fails therapy for 3 to 6 months should the health care provider consider ordering colon transit studies to evaluate the transit time of stool in the intestine (Basson, 2015). Responses to laxatives vary and depend on the patient as well as the preparation. Several classes of laxatives are available for the symptomatic treatment of constipation: bulk-forming agents, saline laxatives, lubricant laxatives, surfactants (emollients), hyperosmotic laxatives, and stimulant laxatives. Proper selection of a laxative should be based on the individual clinical situation (**Table 30.1**).

TABLE 30.1			
Overview of Selected Laxatives and Atypical Agents			
Generic (Trade) Name and Dosage	**Selected Adverse Events**	**Contraindications**	**Special Considerations**
Bulk-Forming Laxatives			
methylcellulose (Citrucel) 2–6 g/d	Flatulence, stomach upset, fullness	GI obstruction	Take with plenty of water. Avoid in patients with GI ulceration.
psyllium (Metamucil) 3.4–10.2 g/d	Same as above	Same as above	Same as above Sugar-free formulation caution with phenylketonuria
polycarbophil (FiberCon) 1–6 g/d	Same as above	Same as above	Same as above Calcium content may interact with tetracycline or quinolone antibiotics.
malt soup extract (Maltsupex) 12–64 g/d	Same as above	Same as above	Same as above
wheat dextrin (Benefiber) Powder: 1 tbsp daily for age 6 and up chewables: Age 12—adult three tablets three times daily Ages 6–11 1½ tablets three times daily	Same as above	Same as above Not a good choice for those with possible celiac disease	Shelf life of 2 y Store in a cool environment. Less flatulence production than other bulking agents
Lubricants and Surfactants			
mineral oil 5–45 mL/d	Rectal seepage, irritation	Do not use with surfactants.	Impairs absorption of fat-soluble vitamins Caution in elderly and very young due to potential for development of lipid pneumonia
docusate sodium (Colace) 50–500 mg/d	Stomach upset	Do not use with mineral oil.	Most effective at preventing "straining" in high-risk patients (see text)

(Continued)

TABLE 30.1

Overview of Selected Laxatives and Atypical Agents (*Continued*)

Generic (Trade) Name and Dosage	Selected Adverse Events	Contraindications	Special Considerations
docusate calcium (Surfak) 50–240 mg	Same as above	Same as above	Same as above
docusate potassium (Dialose) 100–300 mg	Same as above	Same as above	Same as above
Saline Agents			
sodium phosphate enema (Fleet) 118 mL/d Only one enema in 24 h	Alterations in fluid/electrolyte balance, diarrhea	Caution in patients with congestive heart failure, hypertension, edema, and renal dysfunction.	Care should be taken in the elderly and those with existing electrolyte disturbances.
magnesium citrate 240 mL/d	GI upset, diarrhea	Caution in renal dysfunction.	Stagger administration times of tetracycline and quinolone antibiotics.
magnesium hydroxide (Phillips' milk of magnesia) 30–60 mL/d	GI upset, diarrhea	Same as above	Caution in renal dysfunction and the elderly. Stagger administration times of tetracycline and quinolone antibiotics.
magnesium sulfate (Epsom salt) 1–2 tsp in ½ glass water	GI upset, diarrhea	Same as above	Caution in renal dysfunction and the elderly. Stagger administration times of tetracycline and quinolone antibiotics.
Hyperosmotic Agents			
lactulose (Chronulac, Constilac, Duphalac) 15–60 mL	GI upset, diarrhea, flatulence	Caution in diabetic patients.	Use lactulose with caution in patients with diabetes.
sorbitol 130–150 mL	GI upset, diarrhea, flatulence	Same as above	Caution in diabetic patients.
Stimulants			
senna (Senokot) Tabs: 2–8/d Supp: 1 qhs Granules: 1–4 tsp/d	Griping, diarrhea, gas, discoloration of urine	GI obstruction	Caution for laxative abuse, cathartic colon.
bisacodyl (Dulcolax) Tabs: 1–3/d Supp: 1 pr qd	Griping, diarrhea, gas	GI obstruction	Do not crush or chew tablets. Avoid concomitant administration of antacids and pH-lowering agents.
castor oil 15–60 mL/d	Stomach upset, diarrhea, colic	GI obstruction	Too potent for routine use
Secretagogues—Chloride Channel Activators			
lubiprostone (Amitiza) 24-mcg capsule bid	Nausea is most common, diarrhea, abdominal pain, abdominal distention, and flatulence.	Known or suspected GI mechanical obstruction	Approved for both genders only for CIC/OIC Capsules must be taken whole and with food and water.
Guanylate Cyclase-C Agonist linaclotide (Linzess) 145 mg capsule daily	Diarrhea, abdominal pain, flatulence, and abdominal distention	Avoid in known or suspected mechanical obstruction.	Dose is different for IBS-C. Dose is different for IBS-C. Avoid in children <6 years old, but use with caution in 6–17 y.
Peripherally Acting Mu-Opioid Receptor Antagonist (PAMORA)			
naloxegol (Movantik) 12.5–25 mg tablet one daily	Abdominal pain, diarrhea, nausea, flatulence, vomiting headache, and hyperhidrosis	Same as above	Pregnancy Category C: can cause narcotic withdrawal for fetus Can cause narcotic withdrawal especially with methadone

Bulk-Forming Laxatives

Bulk-forming laxatives work by binding to the fecal contents and pulling water into the stool. This ultimately softens and lubricates the stool, eases its passage, and reduces straining. Water is reabsorbed from fecal masses that stay in the colon for extended periods, and the result is dry stools. Bulk-forming agents hold water in the stool or swell and increase stool bulk. The bulk stimulates the movement of the intestines and facilitates the passage of intestinal contents. These types of laxatives are not useful when constipation results from the use of opioid medications.

Bulk-forming laxatives generally consist of psyllium seed husk, methylcellulose, polycarbophil, and wheat dextrin, which are made of polysaccharides, cellulose derivatives, or wheat starch such as methylcellulose (Citrucel) or psyllium (Metamucil). Polycarbophil (FiberCon) and wheat dextrin (Benefiber) have significant water-absorptive properties and also are used as antidiarrheals. All bulk-forming agents used for constipation should be taken with plenty of fluid (8 ounces) to increase efficacy. Malt soup extract (Maltsupex) made from barley malt reduces fecal pH. This may contribute to its laxative effect. Traditionally, these products have been marketed only as powders, which must be dissolved in water. Now, many fiber products are available in powder, wafer, and Caplet forms. Patients may need to try several before finding one that works for them. Brand names include Metamucil, FiberCon, and Citrucel. Metamucil is the preferred agent because it is the safest and most physiologic. Sugar-free methylcellulose and psyllium products are available for patients with diabetes. Patients with celiac disease or gluten intolerance should avoid using wheat dextrin products.

Contraindications to the use of bulking agents are symptoms of an acute surgical abdomen, intestinal obstruction or perforation, or inability to drink an adequate amount of fluid.

Action for all agents may begin in 12 to 24 hours, but a full effect is not usually seen for up to 3 days.

A half-cup to one bowl daily of wheat bran can provide adequate fiber supplementation, but synthetic forms of fiber are often better absorbed than food. Other foods can also add fiber to the diet and should be reviewed with the patient. The patient should be encouraged to drink adequate amounts of fluid throughout the day; if not contraindicated, up to 2,500 mL is preferred. These agents are more likely to be used as preventive measures. However given, they can take effect within 12 to 24 hours, and some acute relief of symptoms is possible.

Adverse Events

Overall, these agents are usually well tolerated, but compliance can be a problem because the most common side effect is increased flatulence, and some bloating can occur. With severe constipation, all agents can cause abdominal fullness and cramping. If these agents are used excessively, nausea and vomiting may occur.

Contraindications

Because bulk-forming laxatives have the most physiologic effect and are not systemically absorbed, they are the preferred agents for symptomatic treatment of constipation. However, these agents are not completely benign and should be avoided in patients with strictures of the esophagus, GI ulcerations, or stenosis secondary to the possibility of obstruction from increased bulk of intestinal contents. In addition, some bulk-forming agents may contain as much as 20 g of carbohydrates per dose. Sugar-free bulk-forming agents are available and are recommended for diabetic patients.

Interactions

The sugar-free preparations may contain aspartame, which is metabolized to phenylalanine and should be used cautiously with patients who must restrict their phenylalanine intake. Wheat gluten is a by-product of extracting the gluten from wheat; however, complete extraction cannot be guaranteed and should be avoided in patients with gluten intolerance. Concomitant administration of calcium-containing bulk laxatives may reduce the effectiveness of quinolone or tetracycline, so patients should separate the administration time of these agents.

Hyperosmotic Laxatives

Lactulose (Cephulac), sorbitol, polyethylene glycol/electrolyte solution (PEG-ES, Colyte), and polyethylene glycol (PEG, MiraLAX) are examples of hyperosmotic laxatives. These agents serve as or are metabolized to solutes in the intestinal tract. The increased concentration of solutes creates osmotic pressure by drawing fluid from a less concentrated gradient to the more concentrated gradient inside the GI tract. This increase in osmotic pressure stimulates intestinal motility and propulsion of fecal contents. The PEG products do not degrade colonic bacteria and therefore produce less bloating. Glycerin (Colace Suppository, Fleet Glycerin Suppository, and Pedia-Lax Suppository) helps the stool to evacuate by similar mechanisms, but also provides local rectal stimulation.

In addition to its osmotic effect, glycerin also has a local irritant effect in the suppository form. The irritant action adds to the osmotic action to stimulate bowel movement.

Lactulose is a disaccharide analog that is metabolized by bacteria to acids that increase osmotic pressure and acidify the contents of the colon. The result is increased intestinal motility and secretion.

In addition to its use for the symptomatic treatment of constipation, sorbitol is also used to prevent constipation in combination with activated charcoal for poisoning. Sodium polystyrene sulfonate (Kayexalate), a cation exchange resin used for treating hyperkalemia, is often combined with sorbitol to reduce the potential for constipation from the resin.

PEG-ES is a nonabsorbable solution that acts as an osmotic agent. It is usually used to evacuate the bowel before a GI examination such as a flexible sigmoidoscopy or colonoscopy. The solution is reconstituted with 1 gallon of tap water and should be chilled before consumption to increase palatability. The patient should begin drinking the solution at 4 PM the day before the procedure. One glass (8 oz.) of the reconstituted solution should be consumed every 10 minutes over 3 hours until all 4 L are consumed. The patient should fast for 4 hours before ingesting the solution, and only clear liquids are allowed after ingestion.

Contraindications

Lactulose syrup should be used with caution in diabetic patients because it contains lactose and galactose. Lactose is also contraindicated in patients with appendicitis, acute surgical abdomen, fecal impaction, or intestinal obstruction. Caution must be used in diabetic patients because of sugar content.

Other osmotic agents such as magnesium hydroxide (milk of magnesia) or magnesium citrate (Citroma) can be used to promote defecation. Approximately 15% to 30% of the magnesium in these agents may be absorbed systemically; therefore, caution is needed in patients who have renal failure and decreased ability to excrete magnesium.

When taken appropriately, these agents are well tolerated. The most common adverse events are abdominal cramping and nausea. However, the use of these agents may be counterproductive in patients with changes in colonic transit time, IBS, or severe bloating and fullness (Wald, 2007).

In addition, sorbitol as a caloric sweetener has the potential to affect blood glucose levels and should be used with caution in diabetic patients. PEG-ES is not recommended in patients with gastric obstruction, bowel perforation, or colitis.

Adverse Reactions

Glycerin is among the safest laxative preparations available and is often used in infants and children. Rectal irritation is the most common side effect of glycerin suppositories. The most common side effects associated with lactulose and sorbitol include GI upset and diarrhea. PEG-ES rapidly cleanses the bowel and often causes nausea, abdominal fullness, cramps, and bloating.

Interactions

There are few documented interactions with the osmotic laxatives. However, because antacids may neutralize the acids produced from lactulose and interfere with its mechanism of action, concomitant administration of antacids should be avoided with lactulose. No other medications should be given within 1 hour of consumption of PEG-ES because the medication will likely be flushed from the GI tract.

Saline Laxatives

Like hyperosmotic laxatives, saline laxatives draw water into the intestine through osmosis. This creates an increase in intraluminal pressure and a resultant increase in intestinal motility. Magnesium citrate (citrate of magnesia), magnesium hydroxide (Phillips' milk of magnesia), magnesium sulfate (Epsom salt), sodium phosphate, and sodium biphosphate (Fleet enemas) are examples of saline laxatives (see **Table 30.1**). For treatment of constipation, the dose of sodium phosphate as an enema should not exceed the recommended volume or more than one dose in 24 hours. Magnesium citrate and sodium phosphate and biphosphate are used as bowel evacuants for endoscopic examinations such as flexible sigmoidoscopy or colonoscopy.

Contraindications

Oral sodium phosphate is no longer on the market due to concerns about severe electrolyte imbalances. However, the enema version still exists, but caution in administration should still be exercised. When prescribing sodium phosphate enemas, care should be exercised with individuals who are at higher risk for complications, including young children, individuals over 55 years of age, and those who are dehydrated, have kidney dysfunction or inflammation of the bowel, or are taking medications that can affect the kidneys. In addition, phosphates can accumulate in patients with renal dysfunction, leading to serious complications such as hyperphosphatemia, hypokalemia, hypocalcemia, hypernatremia, metabolic acidosis, and coma.

Magnesium hydroxide and magnesium sulfate are commonly used for the symptomatic treatment of constipation. Because the kidneys eliminate magnesium, magnesium-containing laxatives should be used with caution in the elderly and in patients with decreased renal function. Excessive magnesium levels can result in CNS depression (drowsiness), muscle weakness, decreased blood pressure, and electrocardiographic changes.

Adverse Events

Dehydration is a concern with the use of saline laxatives, and these agents must be used with caution in patients who cannot tolerate excessive fluid loss and dehydration.

Interactions

Because milk of magnesia also has antacid properties and can increase the pH of the intestines, it should not be administered at the same time with agents that require an acidic environment to be absorbed. The most common example of this type of interaction is with the antifungals itraconazole (Sporanox) and ketoconazole (Nizoral). Therefore, administration of any antacid should be separated from administration of ketoconazole or itraconazole by at least 2 hours. In addition, the magnesium found in magnesium hydroxide and magnesium sulfate can bind with tetracycline and quinolone antibiotics to form a nonabsorbable complex that may reduce the effectiveness of the antibiotics. Administration of quinolones and tetracyclines should be separated from administration of magnesium-containing compounds.

Stimulant Laxatives

These laxatives vary in effects but act by increasing peristalsis through direct effects on the smooth muscle of the intestines and simultaneously promoting fluid accumulation in the colon and small intestine. Because of the irritating effect of the agents on the musculature, these agents should be avoided in long-term treatment. Stimulant laxatives include bisacodyl (Dulcolax) and senna concentrates (Senokot, Senokot S).

Previously, long-term use of stimulant laxatives has been speculated to addictive and can create permanent injury to the colonic mucosa; however, the research does not support this premise (Kamm et al., 2011).

Contraindications

As with other laxatives, stimulants are contraindicated in patients with appendicitis, acute surgical abdomen, fecal impaction, or intestinal obstruction. Rectal fissures and hemorrhoids can be exacerbated by stimulation of defecation. Action begins 6 to 10 hours after oral administration and 15 minutes to 2 hours after rectal administration.

Adverse Events

These agents are not as well tolerated as the osmotic laxatives or bulking agents because of their side effects, which include nausea, vomiting, and abdominal cramping. These side effects can be more severe with cases of severe constipation. Long-term or excessive use can lead to laxative dependence.

Surfactant Laxatives

This class of laxatives reduces the surface tension of the liquid contents of the bowel. Ultimately, this promotes incorporation of additional liquid into the stool, forming a softer mass, and promotes easier defecation. However, stool softeners have insufficient data to support their efficacy, and fiber products may be superior to improve stool frequency (Brandt et al., 2005). Examples of this class include docusate sodium (Colace) and docusate calcium (Surfak). For patients who should not strain during defecation, this is the laxative of choice. Emollient laxatives only prevent constipation; they do not treat it. Combining these agents with fiber products helps promote defecation. Administration of emollient laxatives concomitantly with mineral oil is contraindicated because of increased absorption of the mineral oil. Action with these agents usually occurs between 1 and 3 days.

Contraindications

Docusate calcium or docusate potassium may be recommended for patients on sodium-restricted diets (e.g., hypertension, congestive heart failure). The sodium content of Colace (docusate sodium) is quite small (5.2 mg per capsule) and is likely insignificant.

Adverse Events

These agents are extremely well tolerated when used to prevent constipation. The most common side effect is stomach upset; other side effects, such as mild abdominal cramping, diarrhea, and throat irritation, are infrequent. Patients should take surfactants with plenty of water to improve effectiveness.

Interactions

Docusate, as a surfactant emollient laxative, may increase the absorption of mineral oil and potentially increase the risk for liver toxicity; therefore, this combination should be avoided.

Lubricant Laxatives

Mineral oil (liquid paraffin) coats and softens the stool and prevents reabsorption of water from the stool by the colon. Lubricant laxatives are effective at preventing straining in high-risk patients (e.g., rectal surgery, labor and delivery, stroke, hemorrhoids, hernia, myocardial infarction).

Contraindications

Mineral oil may be aspirated and cause lipid pneumonia when administered to young, elderly, or bedridden patients. With the availability of safer laxative preparations, mineral oil should probably be avoided in these populations. If mineral oil is chosen, it should not be administered to patients before bedtime or when they are reclining to prevent aspiration.

Adverse Events

Mineral oil has an unpleasant taste, and because it is not absorbed, large single doses can seep through the anal sphincter and cause irritation. Dividing doses may prevent this.

Interactions

Mineral oil can impair the absorption of fat-soluble vitamins A, D, E, and K. Because warfarin (Coumadin) interferes with the synthesis of vitamin K–dependent clotting factors, a reduction in absorption of vitamin K may increase the effects of the anticoagulant. Although no direct interactions with oral anticoagulants have been reported, prothrombin levels may decrease. The docusates, as surfactant emollient laxatives, may increase the absorption of mineral oil and potentially increase the risk for liver toxicity; therefore, this combination should be avoided.

Secretagogues

Chloride Channel Activators

There is only one drug in this class, lubiprostone (Amitiza), and it is a derivative from prostaglandin. While the entire mechanism is not understood, it appears to work by enhancing chloride-rich intestinal fluid without altering serum sodium and potassium concentrations. The activation of the chloride channel in the intestines pulls water into the lumen of the intestine. The drug is poorly absorbed systemically and appears to act locally on the intestines, improving stool consistency and motility. Lubiprostone is approved for treatment of adults, men and women with chronic constipation or OIC (see **Table 30.1**).

Contraindications

Lubiprostone is contraindicated in patients with potential mechanical obstruction, severe diarrhea, or hypersensitivity to components of the product. It is contraindicated in pregnant women and children.

Adverse Events

Nausea is the most common side effect of lubiprostone. The rate of nausea is dose dependent and was experienced by approximately 29% of patients. Other common GI side effects include diarrhea, abdominal pain, abdominal distention, and flatulence. The most commonly reported neurologic side effect is headache.

Interactions

No drug–drug interactions have been discovered with lubiprostone. In vitro studies showed the cytochrome P-450 isoenzymes are not inhibited by the drug.

Guanylate Cyclase-C Agonist

Linaclotide (Linzess) is the first of this class for the indications of CIC and IBS. The mechanism of action is topical rather than system, elevating intracellular cGMP, which stimulates secretion of chloride and bicarbonate into the intestinal lumen. Along with the increased fluid, stool transit time is accelerated. Linzess is approved for 18 years and older with CIC. The recommended dosage for CIC is 145 mcg orally once a day, 30 minutes prior to the first meal of the day.

Contraindications

Linaclotide is contraindicated for children less than 6 years old, and while it may be used off-label, the safety and efficacy between 6 and 17 years old has not been established. The drug should not be used if the patient has known or suspected mechanical obstruction.

Adverse Events

The most common side effect for linaclotide is diarrhea, reported by 20% of study participants. Other GI side effects include abdominal pain, flatulence, and abdominal distention. Some (4%) reported headache.

Interactions

Since linaclotide does not interact with the cytochrome P-450 system, no drug–drug interactions have been studied. Administration of recommended clinical doses is encouraged by the prescriber.

Peripherally Acting Mu-Opioid Receptor Antagonist (PAMORA)

This class acts as antagonist of opioid binding at the mu-opioid receptors. At the prescribed dose, this agent blocks in tissues such as the GI tract, therefore decreasing the constipating effects of opioids. Naloxegol (Movantik) is the only agent in this class. It is a PEGylated derivative of naloxone and a substrate for the P-glycoprotein transporter. This reduces the passive permeability across the blood–brain barrier and with recommended doses limits potential for interference with centrally mediated opioid analgesia.

The only indication for naloxegol is OIC, and the dose is 25 mg once daily, but if not tolerated can be reduced to 12.5 mg daily.

Contraindications

Naloxegol is contraindicated in patients with known or suspected GI obstruction or potential for GI perforation. Some patients can experience opioid withdrawal especially those who are receiving methadone. Naloxegol is pregnancy category C, and use in pregnancy may cause withdrawal for the unborn fetus.

Adverse Reactions

The most common reactions are related to the GI system and include abdominal pain, diarrhea, nausea, flatulence, vomiting, headache, and hyperhidrosis.

Interactions

Avoid concomitant use of moderate CYP3A4 inhibitors (e.g., diltiazem, erythromycin, verapamil) due to potential increased risk of adverse reactions. Use of strong CYP3A4 inducers (e.g., rifampin, carbamazepine, St. John's wort) is not recommended because they may decrease the efficacy of naloxegol. Avoid concomitant use of naloxegol with another opioid antagonist due to the increased risk of opioid withdrawal.

Selecting the Most Appropriate Agent

If lifestyle modification fails to reverse constipation, then selection of an appropriate laxative is necessary. The choice of laxative agent depends on several factors, including the type of constipation (acute, CIC, or OIC), medical history, goal of therapy, concomitant medications, and the potential for side effects, age, and personal preference. **Table 30.2** describes first-, second-, and third-line therapies (**Figure 30.1**).

First-Line Therapy

For all types of constipation, acute, CIC, and OIC, a bulk-forming laxative is recommended provided no contraindications exist. Bulk-forming laxatives are not systemically absorbed. In addition, their pharmacologic effect is the most physiologic, meaning they have an effect similar to that of the natural effect of fiber from food on the GI tract. Their side effects are usually mild, and if necessary, they can be administered safely for longer durations than other classes of laxatives such as the stimulants.

When hard or dry stools are the chief complaint or in situations where straining should be avoided (e.g., hernia, cardiovascular disease), a stool softener such as docusate is considered first-line therapy. Stool softeners also are not systemically absorbed, and their side effects are usually minimal.

Glycerin suppositories have a local irritant effect on the rectum and are probably the safest of all preparations. This is preferred as first-line therapy in infants.

Linaclotide (Linzess) and lubiprostone (Amitiza) can be considered as first-line therapy for constipation, especially if it is CIC. Both drugs can increase the incidence of diarrhea, but overall are very well tolerated and have no reported drug–drug interactions. These drugs have been proven to produce rapid and sustained improvement in bowel habits.

For OIC, naloxegol (Movantik) is considered first-line therapy along with bulk-forming laxatives and dietary approaches. Lubiprostone (Amitiza) also has the indication for OIC.

Second-Line Therapy

If a more rapid onset of action is desired, magnesium hydroxide may be chosen. Although it has a faster onset of action, dehydration from excessive use is a concern, particularly in patients unable to tolerate excessive fluid loss. In addition,

TABLE 30.2

Recommended Order of Treatment for Constipation

Order	Agents	Comments
First line	Bulk-forming agents (methylcellulose, psyllium, polycarbophil, malt soup extract, wheat dextrin)	Avoid in patients with GI obstruction or ulceration Take with plenty of water
	Docusate derivatives	Most effective at preventing straining at stool in high-risk patients (see text)
	Glycerin	Used most often in infants and small children
	naloxegol (Movantik)	Indication for OIC only
	linaclotide or lubiprostone	Consider for first or second line for CIC or OIC
Second line	Milk of magnesia, magnesium sulfate, lactulose, sorbitol	Caution in renal dysfunction and the elderly Use with caution in diabetic patients Caution: laxative abuse, cathartic colon
	linaclotide or lubiprostone	Add if not used as first line
Third line	Stimulant laxatives (senna, cascara sagrada, casanthranol, bisacodyl)	Impairs absorption of fat-soluble vitamins; use with caution in elderly and very young (lipid pneumonia)
	Mineral oil	Use with caution in congestive heart failure, hypertension, edema, and renal dysfunction
	Sodium biphosphates (only enema available)	
	Magnesium citrate	Used as a bowel evacuant for endoscopic examinations
	Castor oil	Too potent to be used routinely for constipation

magnesium-containing preparations should be avoided in patients with renal insufficiency or the elderly.

If the bulk-forming agents and magnesium hydroxide are ineffective or contraindicated, an osmotic laxative such as lactulose or sorbitol may be chosen. However, flatulence and the sweet taste limit compliance. In addition, lactulose and sorbitol should be used with caution in patients with diabetes.

If not used as first-line therapy, consider use of linaclotide (Linzess) and lubiprostone (Amitiza).

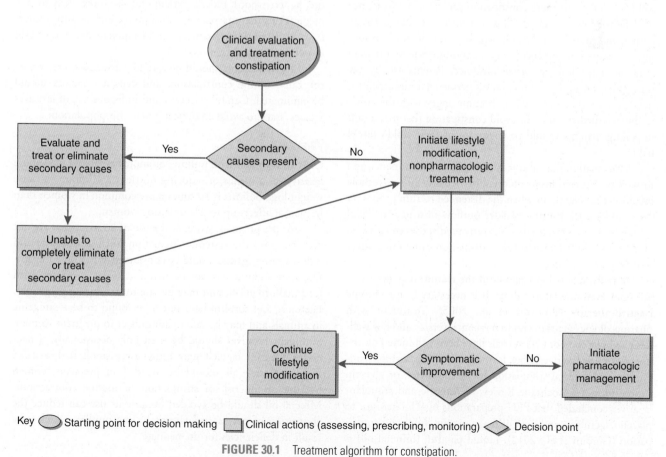

Key: ⬭ Starting point for decision making   ▭ Clinical actions (assessing, prescribing, monitoring)   ◇ Decision point

FIGURE 30.1   Treatment algorithm for constipation.

Third-Line Therapy

If bulk-forming or osmotic diuretics fail to work, a stimulant laxative may be chosen. Stimulant laxatives are very effective. Mineral oil is effective as a lubricant laxative and may be an option in patients who should avoid straining. However, although mineral oil would seem safe, its ability to impair absorption of necessary vitamins and to cause aspiration pneumonitis limits its use. In addition, seepage is an inconvenient side effect that likely limits compliance. If an agent is necessary to soften the stool to prevent straining, docusate is a safer alternative.

Sodium biphosphate as an enema is another option. These agents have the potential to cause fluid and electrolyte abnormalities and exacerbate concomitant disease states such as hypertension and congestive heart failure. Therefore, these agents should be used only after safer agents have failed. Because sodium biphosphate enemas and magnesium citrate solutions have a rapid onset of action, these agents are often preferred and are usually reserved for endoscopic procedures.

Castor oil is a potent cathartic that should not be used routinely for treating constipation.

Special Populations

Pediatric

Constipation can be distressing for children, particularly young children. Most children do not have an underlying pathophysiologic process. Stress over potty training or painful stools secondary to acute constipation can result in avoidance of defecation by the child. This in turn can result in larger, harder, and more painful stools, which eventually leads to soiling. Constipation and encopresis, a condition where soft stool is involuntarily lost, are often combined. Parents usually pay little attention to their child's bowel frequency unless incontinence occurs. The parents may become angry with the child, leading to further stress. To avoid constipation that may result in soiling, parents should be cognizant of their child's bowel habits.

Constipation may also result in urinary incontinence and urinary tract infections in children, particularly girls. Overflow incontinence may occur when the distended rectum presses on the bladder wall, causing bladder outflow obstruction. Fecal soiling in the external urethral opening predisposes constipated girls to infection. Treatment of constipation can reduce infection and incontinence.

Initially, manual evacuation of the rectum may be necessary; however, once this is done, it is necessary to use chronic laxative therapy (Borowitz et al., 2005). Treatment with pharmacologic agents in children is controversial, and few well-designed placebo-controlled trials have been conducted on the use of osmotic laxatives, fiber, formula-switching, sorbitol-containing juices, rectal stimulation by thermometer, or glycerin suppositories. A Cochrane Review of osmotic and stimulant laxatives concluded that PEG preparations may be superior to placebo, lactulose, and milk of magnesia for childhood constipation (Gordon et al., 2012). Liquid paraffin (mineral oil) is also a good alternative. The use of sodium phosphate enemas in children under 2 years of age has been associated with electrolyte disturbances, dehydration, and cardiac arrest.

For infants, malt soup extract or corn syrup (Karo) may be used at a dosage of 5 to 10 mL twice daily. For children older than 6 months, milk of magnesia, lactulose, or sorbitol at a dosage of 1 to 3 mL/kg/d given in one to two doses may be used. Senna syrup at a dosage of 5 to 10 mL/d for children ages 1 to 5 and 10 to 20 mL/d for children ages 5 to 15 is another option.

Geriatric

The choice of a laxative preparation may depend on the patient's attitude or beliefs about normal bowel habits. Normal bowel frequency can range from two or three bowel movements per day to two or three per week. However, many people think that less than one bowel movement per day is abnormal. These patients may seek an OTC laxative to keep them "regular." This concern about regular bowel movements is particularly common in the elderly. The self-reported incidence of constipation increases with advancing age, but the actual bowel movement frequency usually does not decline.

The overuse of laxatives in the elderly can be of particular concern because this population is more intolerant to the fluid and electrolyte abnormalities that accompany laxative abuse. In addition, many of the laxatives should be used with caution in elderly persons because they are more likely to have the disease states that some laxatives can exacerbate (e.g., heart failure, hypertension). Elderly patients are also more likely to take medications that may cause constipation, such as antipsychotics, tricyclic antidepressants, calcium supplements, and certain blood pressure medications.

Elderly patients should be carefully assessed to determine the cause of the constipation, and causative factors should be eliminated. Careful selection and judicious use of laxatives are necessary to avoid complications in this population.

Women

Girls and women with bulimia or anorexia nervosa may abuse laxatives as a means of reducing nutrient absorption to cause weight loss. Bulimia is 10 times more common in women than in men; it affects up to 3% of young women.

For the pregnant woman, the use of laxatives that are not absorbed into the systemic circulation, such as docusate and bulk-forming agents, should be considered as first-line therapy. Docusate sodium has not been found to be associated with fetal malformations and may be safe to use during pregnancy. Lactulose and sorbitol have not been found to be teratogenic in animals and may be safe to administer to pregnant women. Stimulant laxatives should be used only occasionally, if necessary. Cascara sagrada may cause loose stools in breast-fed infants. Castor oil should be avoided in pregnant women because of the risk of stimulation of uterine contractions. Mineral oil should be avoided because its use can reduce the absorption of necessary vitamins by the mother, which may result in deficiencies for the neonate.

MONITORING PATIENT RESPONSE

Monitoring the patient's response to laxative therapy usually is accomplished by asking the patient whether he or she has regained normal bowel patterns after using the laxative. Different patients have different perceptions of what "normal" bowel habits are. Depending on the factors affecting defecation, patients should be informed that the reason for treating with a laxative is not to increase the frequency of defecation but to promote comfortable defecation. Periodic use of laxatives can be safe as there is no substantial evidence of abuse potential.

PATIENT EDUCATION

In most cases, the occasional use of laxatives poses no major problems for the patient. Laxatives are relatively safe when used in moderation. However, the fact that many laxatives are available OTC may give consumers the false impression that constipation is a physiologic condition and there are no other alternatives for treatment. Understanding of constipation has expanded in recent years, and health care providers can provide other options for treatment.

Health care providers should work with patients who have constipation and guide them to the best treatment options. OTC laxatives carry a warning for the consumer not to use them for more than 7 days. For chronic constipation, use of a bulk-forming laxative may be a safer alternative, provided no contraindications exist. However, patients should be counseled that bulk-forming laxatives take time to work (up to 3 days). Because patients are usually looking for an immediate response, they may draw the conclusion that these agents are not effective if a bowel movement has not occurred within the first day.

Patient-Oriented Information Sources

Providing patients with information about constipation can help them understand constipation and their role in treatment. Patient education items are readily available on the Internet through the National Digestive Diseases Information Clearinghouse, which provides information to consumers on a wide variety of GI topics (see **Box 30.11**).

Nutrition/Lifestyle Changes

Patients should be educated on the lifestyle modifications discussed previously to reduce the need for a laxative. An increase in fluid intake improves the efficacy of most laxatives. Patients should also be educated on the potential for side effects of the laxative chosen as well as the appropriate method to administer the laxative.

Complementary and Alternative Medications

Little evidence exists that any specific herbal supplement or alternative treatment works to relieve constipation (Cherniak, 2013). However, probiotics found in yogurt and are relatively easy to obtain and worth trying.

DIARRHEA

True diarrhea is an increase in frequency of loose, watery stools (three or more daily), usually over a period of 24 to 48 hours. It is a relatively common disorder of the GI tract that is experienced occasionally by most people. The organisms that cause diarrhea are easily transferred from person to person through food and water. Globalization and industrialization of the world has increased the ability of these organisms to spread. Experts of infectious diseases estimate that 211 million people experience acute diarrhea every year; an average of 16 million seek medical attention, resulting in 1.2 million hospitalizations and >5,000 deaths (Bushen & Guerrant, 2003; Jones et al., 2007). Children, the elderly, and those who are immunocompromised are most susceptible to the complications of diarrhea, and serious dehydration can result from the disorder. Proper hydration and symptomatic treatment as well as elimination of causative factors are necessary to prevent these complications. Ultimately, diarrhea can have a profound impact on public health, and proper diagnosis and treatment can prevent an epidemic.

CAUSES

Diarrhea may be caused by a host of different medications (**Box 30.4**), infective organisms (**Box 30.5**), or disease states or procedures (**Box 30.6**). Prompt attention to causative factors, as well as rehydration, prevents complications.

Medications

Antibiotics may cause diarrhea by direct irritation of the intestinal tract or disruption of the normal intestinal flora. The poor absorption of erythromycin (E-mycin) lends itself to irritation of the GI tract. Clarithromycin (Biaxin) and azithromycin (Zithromax) may cause less diarrhea than erythromycin.

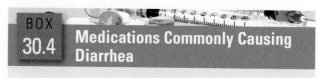

BOX 30.4 Medications Commonly Causing Diarrhea

Antacids (magnesium containing)
Antibiotics
Antidepressants (SSRIs)
Cholinergic agents
Colchicine
Digoxin
Gastrointestinal stimulants (metoclopramide)
Laxatives
Metformin
Prostaglandins (dinoprostone)
Prostaglandin analog (misoprostol)
Quinidine

Infective Organisms Associated with Diarrhea

Aeromonas species
Bacillus cereus
Campylobacter
Chlamydia trachomatis
Clostridium difficile
Cryptosporidium
Escherichia coli
Entamoeba histolytica
Giardia
Mycobacterium avium-intracellulare
Salmonella
Shigella
Staphylococcus aureus
Viral agents
Yersinia

The clavulanic acid component of the combination of amoxicillin–clavulanic acid (Augmentin) is also a GI irritant, and diarrhea is a common side effect. Tetracycline and ceftriaxone (Rocephin) cause diarrhea by disrupting the normal balance of the gut flora.

Clostridium difficile, a normal part of the flora of the colon in up to 20% of hospitalized patients, normally does not cause disease unless chemotherapeutic medications or antibiotics trigger its toxins. Only certain antibiotics have been implicated in *C. difficile*–associated diarrhea. Less common causes of *C. difficile* diarrhea are vancomycin (Vancocin), erythromycin, tetracyclines, trimethoprim–sulfamethoxazole (TMP-SMZ), quinolones, and aztreonam (Azactam). The antibiotics most likely to cause *C. difficile* diarrhea are beta-lactam antibiotics (penicillins, cephalosporins, and carbapenems) and clindamycin (Cleocin). **Box 30.7** gives more information.

Disorders and Procedures Associated with Diarrhea

Acquired immunodeficiency syndrome
Bowel resection
Colon cancer
Diverticulitis
Enteral feedings
Gastroenteritis
Hyperthyroidism
Inflammatory bowel disease
Irritable bowel syndrome
Lactose intolerance
Malabsorption
Pheochromocytoma

Treating *Clostridium difficile* Diarrhea

C. difficile diarrhea may occur weeks after stopping antimicrobial therapy. The diarrhea may progress to colitis if left untreated. While awaiting the results of *C. difficile* toxin assay of the stool specimen, empiric therapy with metronidazole (Flagyl) 500 mg PO tid Vancomycin therapy should not be empirically initiated unless there is no clinical improvement within 5 to 7 days.

Because routine use of vancomycin (Vancocin) may contribute to the emergence of vancomycin-resistant *Enterococcus* species, even though oral vancomycin is no longer costly and may be easily prescribed, it should be reserved for cases that fail to respond to oral metronidazole or for patients who are not able to tolerate oral metronidazole. Institute oral doses of vancomycin; start at 125 mg qid and increase to 500 mg qid for lack of response.

For *C. difficile* diarrhea advancing to colitis, the preferred agent is intravenous metronidazole 1 g every 24 hours with oral vancomycin at 500 mg qid, for 10 days or until colitis has resolved on computed tomography scan. Patients should not be given bowel antispasmodics because this may reduce the elimination of the toxins from the body.

Surawicz et al. (2013)

Infectious Organisms

Patients traveling to a developing region may contract diarrhea from bacterial organisms. *Giardia* should be suspected if the patient travels to mountainous areas, recreational waters, or Russia. Pathogens transmitted by the fecal-to-oral route should be suspected in homosexual men (*Shigella, Salmonella, Campylobacter,* and intestinal protozoa) and in patients exposed to day care centers (*Shigella, Giardia, Cryptosporidium*).

Traveler's diarrhea is usually a self-limiting, non–life-threatening illness affecting 20% to 50% of individuals who visit developing countries; however, it can become chronic disease process (Connor, 2013). The cause of travelers' diarrhea is ingestion of fecally contaminated food products or water. High-risk areas include Latin America, Africa, Asia, and the Middle East. The typical duration is 2 to 3 days; symptoms include nausea and vomiting, cramps, and bloody stools. The most common pathogen is *Escherichia coli*; *Salmonella, Shigella,* and *Campylobacter* are the culprits less frequently.

Dietary restrictions are the main prevention for travelers' diarrhea. Travelers should avoid foods and beverages that are not steaming hot, raw vegetables, unpeeled fruit, tap water, and ice.

PATHOPHYSIOLOGY

Diarrhea may be classified by duration and category. Acute diarrhea lasts 1 to 14 days and is considered self-limiting. Persistent diarrhea lasts longer than 14 days but less than 30 days, and chronic diarrhea last more than 30 days. Diarrhea may also be categorized as osmotic, secretory, or exudative (inflammatory), or the diarrhea may be related to altered intestinal motility (transit). Some diarrheal illnesses involve more than one of these mechanisms. Diarrhea may also be a defense mechanism against toxins and invading organisms.

Osmotic Diarrhea

Osmotic diarrhea occurs when nonabsorbed solutes are retained in the lumen of the intestinal tract. The result is a hyperosmolar state that pulls water and ions into the intestinal lumen. Poorly absorbed salts (magnesium sulfate), lactose (in lactase deficiency), and large amounts of sugar substitutes (sorbitol) found in candy or chewing gum, diet foods, and soft drinks draw fluid into the intestinal tract, resulting in an overload of the colon.

Secretory Diarrhea

In secretory diarrhea, colonic absorption of fluid is secondary to active transport of Na^+ through Na^+–K^+–adenosine triphosphatase activity in the colonic epithelium. The colon absorbs chloride by exchanging it for HCO_3^2 and by uptake of sodium chloride. Any agent that increases concentrations of cyclic adenosine 3, 5-monophosphate in the cells of the colon inhibits sodium chloride uptake and causes secretion of chloride. This results in secretion of fluid in the colon. Prostaglandins E2 and I2 and vasoactive intestinal peptide stimulate adenyl cyclase activity. Cholinergic agents and cholinesterase inhibitors cause secretion of sodium chloride and water. Secretory diarrhea can be classified as pure (e.g., cholera) or a part of a complex disease process (e.g., celiac disease, Crohn disease). Other stimuli that can cause secretory diarrhea include bacterial endotoxins, hormones from endocrine neoplasms, dihydroxy bile acids, hydroxylated fatty acids, and inflammatory mediators.

Exudative Diarrhea

Exudative (inflammatory) diarrhea may result from inflammatory diseases of the mucosa. Inflammation occurs due to the compromise of the tight junctions of the epithelial cells in the intestine. These diseases may cause an increase of blood, mucus, pus, and serum proteins that increase fluid and overload the colon, resulting in diarrhea. Enteritis, ulcerative colitis, and carcinoma are examples of inflammatory conditions that may result in exudative diarrhea.

Altered Intestinal Motility

Intestinal contents need to have sufficient time to be in contact with the lining of the intestinal tract for fluid, electrolytes, and nutrients to be absorbed adequately. Any factor that increases or decreases the motility of the intestinal tract may result in decreased absorption of fluid and electrolytes. Resection of the bowels, vagotomy, and certain agents (serotonin, laxatives, prostaglandins, prokinetic agents) can increase intestinal motility. Decreases in motility can result from autonomic injury or smooth muscle injury to the intestine and result in bacterial overgrowth, subsequently leading to diarrhea.

DIAGNOSTIC CRITERIA

A careful travel and social history is important to identify and treat specific causes, such as infection. Use of empiric antibiotic therapy is not recommended due to increasing resistance of many strains of bacteria. However, if a traveler is unable to comply with precautions, it may be prudent to prescribe a fluoroquinolone to hold in reserve. Selective testing of stool will be cost-effective while helping to guide the clinician in the use of specific therapy. According to the most recent guidelines of the Infectious Disease Society of America (Guerrant et al., 2001), diarrhea can be divided into three categories: community-acquired or traveler's diarrhea, nosocomial diarrhea, or persistent diarrhea. Each category can be specifically evaluated, leading to more precise therapy.

The fecal leukocyte, lactoferrin, or Hemoccult blood test is useful in patients with moderate to severe cases of acute infectious diarrhea because it supports the use of empiric antibiotic therapy in the febrile patient. However, measuring fecal leukocytes can be unreliable if specimens are transported, refrigerated, or frozen. Fecal lactoferrin, as a measure of polymorphonuclear neutrophils, has an advantage over fecal leukocytes as a highly sensitive and specific testing method for intestinal inflammation. Stool cultures have traditionally been used to identify the pathology of diarrhea, but the positive yields are very poor and incur high costs. Controversy exists regarding when to obtain stool cultures. The absence of vomiting with persistent diarrhea may also indicate the need for stool cultures. Hypotension, tachycardia, orthostasis, bloody stool, and abdominal pain and tenderness were not found to be good predictors of a positive stool culture.

Laboratory evaluation for ova and parasites should be performed in the following:

- A person not previously treated with empiric antiparasitic therapy
- A person with persistent diarrhea for more than 7 days
- A person who recently traveled to mountainous regions, Russia, or Nepal
- A person who was exposed to infants at day care centers or who was exposed through a community waterborne outbreak
- A person with bloody diarrhea with few or no fecal leukocytes
- Homosexual men or patients with acquired immunodeficiency syndrome (AIDS)

For food- or waterborne pathogens, the incubation period and clinical features can give clues as to the source of infection.

Diarrhea and vomiting 6 hours after exposure to a food item suggests exposure to *Staphylococcus aureus* or *Bacillus cereus*. An incubation period of 8 to 14 hours suggests *Clostridium perfringens*. With an incubation period greater than 14 hours, with vomiting as the predominant feature, viral agents are suspected. In patients with fever greater than 101.3°F (38.5°C) plus leukocyte-, lactoferrin-, or Hemoccult-positive stools, or acute dysentery (grossly bloody stools), the most common pathogens identified by normal stool culture are *Shigella*, *Salmonella*, *Campylobacter*, *Aeromonas*, and *Yersinia*. Additionally, patients with grossly bloody stools should be tested for *E. coli* O157 or HUS.

INITIATING DRUG THERAPY

Most cases of diarrhea are self-limiting and can be self-treated. However, patients with profuse, watery diarrhea with dehydration, passage of blood and mucus, and fever exceeding 101.3°F should be evaluated for an inflammation-producing pathogen. These patients may benefit from antimicrobial therapy. In addition, a good history helps to determine the cause of illness. In diarrhea caused by infectious organisms, the pathogen should be identified so that therapy may be initiated to eradicate the organism and to prevent exposure to unnecessary antibiotics.

For traveler's diarrhea (TD), prophylactic agents may be given to patients who should not, cannot, or will not comply with dietary restrictions. Chemoprophylaxis of TD is controversial and usually is not recommended for patients unless the patient has an underlying illness (AIDS, prior gastric surgery, other chronic disease process), the purpose of the trip is particularly important (politicians, honeymoon), or the patient cannot or will not comply with dietary restrictions. In such cases, the use of bismuth subsalicylate (BSS; Pepto-Bismol), 2 tablets four times daily, is recommended unless the reason for prophylaxis is a serious underlying illness. In these cases, a quinolone antibiotic or rifaximin should be used.

If prophylactic therapy is not prescribed, at the first symptoms of diarrhea, empiric therapy can be prescribed using a quinolone antibiotic, rifaximin, or azithromycin (**Table 30.3**). Patients should be properly hydrated, and BSS may be used to treat symptoms. Loperamide (Imodium) is a more effective option than BSS, but loperamide should be used with caution in the presence of fever or bloody stools because the antimotility effects of the drug may prolong disease by reducing the elimination of possible infectious pathogens. If an antidiarrheal medication is necessary, selection should be based on patient-specific variables, including potential side effects, convenience, efficacy, and the patient's symptoms. For patients with moderate or severe TD, empiric antimicrobial therapy with a quinolone antibiotic or rifaximin may be given (see **Table 30.3**). Patients with persistent diarrhea lasting 2 to 4 weeks without systemic symptoms or dysentery may be studied for the cause and treated or given metronidazole (Flagyl) for empiric anti-*Giardia* therapy.

Goals of Drug Therapy

The goals of drug therapy are to reduce the symptoms of diarrhea and to make the patient as comfortable as possible. Causative factors should be identified and eradicated. Fluid and electrolyte replacement is particularly important to avoid serious complications from dehydration. Rehydration is discussed later in this chapter.

Antidiarrheal Agents

Several types of drugs are used for the symptomatic relief of diarrhea; they include antimotility agents, adsorbents and absorbents, and the atypical antisecretory agent BSS. **Table 30.4** provides an overview of these drugs, and **Table 30.5** covers the recommended order of prescription.

Antimotility Agents

The antimotility agent loperamide is an opioid receptor agonist that acts on the µ-opioid receptors of the myenteric plexus of the large intestine, similar to the action of morphine without action on the CNS. This slows GI motility within the circular and longitudinal muscles of the intestines. Initially, this drug was classified as a controlled substance but in 1982 was declassified. It is not well absorbed and does not provide analgesic or euphoric effects.

Another similar agent is diphenoxylate with atropine (Lomotil). It is also chemically related to the narcotic meperidine. As with loperamide, it acts on decreasing GI motility. However, unlike loperamide, it can cross the blood–brain barrier and cause a euphoric effect. Combining diphenoxylate with atropine causes anticholinergic side effects if too much of the drug is ingested, decreasing the potential for abuse. Due to the potential for abuse, diphenoxylate with atropine is a controlled substance, Schedule V.

Contraindications

The antimotility effects may exacerbate infectious diarrhea by preventing the excretion of the infecting organism, allowing the organism more contact time in the intestines. Caution should be observed in using loperamide in patients with fever, bloody stools, or fecal leukocytes. In nondysenteric forms of diarrhea caused by invasive pathogens, loperamide can be used, provided antimicrobial therapy is administered.

Because loperamide undergoes extensive first-pass metabolism, caution should be used in patients with hepatic dysfunction because excessive side effects (CNS toxicity) may occur in these patients.

Because of the antimotility effects of diphenoxylate, it should be used with caution in patients with infectious diarrhea associated with fever or bloody stools. Diphenoxylate provides euphoric and analgesic effects at high doses but not at therapeutic doses. As previously stated for this reason, diphenoxylate is combined with atropine to discourage abuse. Diphenoxylate should be used with caution in patients with liver impairment because it is extensively metabolized by the liver.

TABLE 30.3

Indications for Empiric and Specific Antimicrobial Therapy in Infectious Diarrhea

Indication for Antimicrobial Therapy	Suggested Antimicrobial Therapy
Fever (oral temperature >101.3°F [38.5°C]) together with one of the following: dysentery (grossly bloody stools) or those with leukocyte-, lactoferrin-, or Hemoccult-positive stools	quinolone:*NF 400 mg, CF 500 mg (preferred), OF 300 mg bid for 3–5 d
Moderate to severe TD	quinolone:* CF 500 mg NF 400 mg, OF 300 mg bid for 1–5 d rifaximin 200 mg tid × 3 d if not complicated by above symptoms
Persistent diarrhea (possible *Giardia* infection)	metronidazole 250 mg qid for 7 d
Shigellosis	If acquired in the United States, give TMP-SMZ 160/800 mg bid for 3 d; if acquired during international travel, treat as febrile dysentery (above); check to be certain of susceptibility to drug used. If not from the United States, give third-generation cephalosporin.
Intestinal salmonellosis	If healthy host with mild or moderate symptoms, no therapy; for severe disease or that associated with fever and systemic toxicity or other important underlying conditions, use TMP-SMZ 160 mg/800 mg or quinolone:*NF 400 mg, CF 500 mg, OF mg bid for 5–7 d depending on speed of response
Campylobacteriosis	erythromycin stearate 500 mg bid for 5 d
Enteropathogenic *Escherichia coli* diarrhea (EPEC)	Treat as febrile dysentery
Enterotoxigenic *E. coli* diarrhea (ETEC)	Treat as moderate to severe TD
Enteroinvasive *E. coli* diarrhea (EIEC)	Treat as shigellosis
Enterohemorrhagic *E. coli* diarrhea (EHEC)	Antimicrobials are usually withheld except in particularly severe cases, in which usefulness of these drugs is uncertain.
Aeromonas diarrhea	Treat as febrile dysentery
Noncholera *Vibrio* diarrhea	Treat as febrile dysentery
Yersiniosis	For most cases, treat as febrile dysentery; for severe cases, give ceftriaxone 1 g qd IV for 5 d.
Giardiasis	metronidazole 250 mg qid for 7 d or (if available) tinidazole 2 g in a single dose or quinicine 100 mg tid for 7 d
Intestinal amebiasis	metronidazole 750 mg tid for 5–10 d plus a drug to treat cysts to prevent relapses: diiodohydroxyquin 650 mg tid for 20 d or paromomycin 500 mg tid for 10 d or diloxanide furoate 500 mg tid for 10 d
Cryptosporidium diarrhea	None; for severe cases, consider paromomycin 500 mg tid for 7 d
Isospora diarrhea	TMP-SMZ 160 mg/800 mg bid for 7 d
Cyclospora diarrhea	TMP-SMZ 160 mg/800 mg bid for 7 d

*Fluoroquinolones include norfloxacin (NF), ciprofloxacin (CF), and ofloxacin (OF).
TMP-SMZ, trimethoprim–sulfamethoxazole.
Reproduced by permission from American Journal of Gastroenterology. (1997). Commercially available oral rehydration solutions. *American Journal of Gastroenterology, 92,* 1962–1975. Copyright © 1997, Rights Managed by Nature Publishing Group.

Adverse Events

Adverse effects of loperamide include abdominal discomfort, constipation, and dry mouth. Although loperamide does not cross the blood–brain barrier, it may still induce drowsiness in some patients. Patients should be warned of the potential for drowsiness before driving or performing activities that require alertness. Although loperamide is usually well tolerated, it is not recommended in children younger than age 4 because shock, enterocolitis, fatal intestinal obstruction, and CNS toxicity have occurred.

Atropine has anticholinergic effects such as dry mouth, dry eyes, urinary retention, constipation, blurred vision, and tachycardia. Diphenoxylate may cause drowsiness or dizziness,

and patients should be warned of these effects and should avoid activities that require alertness. The liquid formulation is recommended in children because the dose needs to be carefully tailored to the child based on age and weight. Diphenoxylate with atropine can cause respiratory depression in infants and young children and should be avoided in children younger than age 4.

Interactions

Diphenoxylate may potentiate the action of depressants such as alcohol, barbiturates, or benzodiazepines. In addition, atropine may potentiate the effects of other agents with anticholinergic properties such as tricyclic antidepressants,

TABLE 30.4

Overview of Selected Antidiarrheals

Generic (Trade) Name and Dosage	Selected Adverse Events	Contraindications	Special Considerations
Antimotility Agents			
diphenoxylate/atropine (Lomotil) 2.5–5 mg qid	Dry mouth, dry eyes, urinary retention, blurred vision, drowsiness, dizziness	Caution in patients with liver disease, fever, bloody stool, or fecal leukocytes.	Drug Enforcement Administration Class V controlled substance
loperamide (Imodium) 4–16 mg/d in divided doses	Abdominal discomfort, constipation, drowsiness, dry mouth	Caution in patients with fever, bloody stools, or fecal leukocytes	May induce drowsiness; warn patients about driving or performing activities that require alertness.
Selected Antisecretory Agents			
bismuth subsalicylate (Pepto-Bismol) Start: two tablets or 30-mL range: two tablets or 30 mL every 30 min to 1 h up to eight doses	Black stools, darkening of tongue, tinnitus	Caution in patients who are aspirin sensitive or are taking medications that interact with warfarin.	Not recommended for children and adolescents due to the presence of salicylate component and potential Rye syndrome
polycarbophil (Fiber-Con) 1–6 g/d	Stomach upset, bloating, gas	Caution: Potential for drug interactions with tetracycline or quinolones	
kaolin and bismuth salicylate (Kaopectate) Start: 30–120 mL of liquid or two tablets after each bowel movement Range: Up to seven doses a day	Constipation, feeling of fullness, stomach bloating, gas	Do not use with children due to the salicylate component.	May adsorb nutrients and medications Separate administration time of adsorbents and other medications.
Semisynthetic Antibiotic			
rifaximin (Xifaxan) TD: 200 mg tablets tid × 3 d	Most common for TD—headache	Known hypersensitivity to rifaximin Bloody diarrhea	Discontinue for diarrhea that worsens or persists >48 h. Consider different antibiotics.

antipsychotics, and antihistamines. Diphenoxylate has a structure similar to that of meperidine, and when used concomitantly with monoamine oxidase inhibitors, it can induce a hypertensive crisis.

TABLE 30.5

Recommended Order of Treatment for Diarrhea

Order	Agents	Comments
First line	loperamide rifaximin (TD)	Easy to use, tablet or liquid Well tolerated, 3-day course
Second line	Adsorbents or antisecretory agent	Selection based on drug–drug interactions or allergies (e.g., aspirin sensitivity and BSS)
Third line	diphenoxylate	Side effect profile, especially with atropine added, lowers the utility of this agent

Atypical Antidiarrheals

Subsalicylate is the active ingredient found in Pepto-Bismol and Kaopectate. BSS includes the active ingredients bismuth, which stimulates prostaglandin, mucous, and bicarbonate secretion *in the stomach*, and salicylate inhibits prostaglandin and chloride secretion *in the large intestine*. The action of salicylic acid and bismuth on diarrhea is not well understood, but is thought to have anti-inflammatory action and antacid and mild antibiotic properties.

Kaopectate is now formulated with the active ingredients of subsalicylic acid and therefore has the same contraindications, adverse effects, and interactions. Further discussion of Kaopectate as an absorbent is found in the next section.

Contraindications

BSS and Kaopectate are broken down in the intestinal tract to salicylate; therefore, it should be used with caution in patients taking aspirin therapy or those hypersensitive to aspirin.

In addition, caution should be used in children and adolescents with the flu or chickenpox because this population is at risk for aspirin-induced Reye syndrome.

Adverse Effects

Side effects of BSS and Kaopectate with subsalicylate include black stools, darkening of the tongue, and tinnitus, which can be a potential sign of salicylate toxicity.

Interactions

Because BSS and Kaopectate with subsalicylate have a salicylate component, it may interact with other medications that interact with aspirin (e.g., warfarin).

Adsorbents and Absorbents

Mechanism of Action

Kaolinite is a naturally occurring magnesium aluminum silicate and is used in Kaopectate. Previous formulations of Kaopectate included a combination of kaolinite and attapulgite, which was removed from the formulation by the FDA and replaced by subsalicylate (Kim-Jung et al., 2004). Another adsorbent, pectin, has also been removed from the market. The current formulation of Kaopectate adsorbs water along with bacteria and toxins as well as helps to solidify loose stools. As an adsorbent, it is usually given after each bowel movement until diarrhea is relieved or a maximum dose is reached. The dose for adults is 30 mL every 30 to 60 minutes if needed or maximum of eight doses daily. Kaopectate is not approved for children due to the subsalicylate component.

Polycarbophil (FiberCon, Fiberall), an absorbent, absorbs water in the GI tract and is used as an antidiarrheal. Its fiber content also makes it useful as a bulk-forming laxative when taken with plenty of water.

Adverse Events

The most common side effects of the adsorbents are constipation and a feeling of fullness. Absorbents may also produce upset stomach, bloating, and gas. Adsorbents and absorbents are generally considered safe because the medication works locally and is not absorbed systemically. However, adsorbents may not be as effective as antimotility agents at reducing the symptoms of diarrhea.

Interactions

Adsorbents are not selective and may adsorb nutrients and medications. This interaction must be taken into consideration because several doses may be necessary each day. Separating administration times of adsorbents and other medications is advised. Polycarbophil contains calcium and may interact with fluoroquinolone and tetracycline antibiotics.

Semisynthetic antibiotic

Rifaximin

Rifaximin (Xifaxan) is a semisynthetic antibiotic that is only effective against noninvasive strains of *Escherichia coli*. The drug is a derivative of rifampin and acts to block transcription of the bacteria; therefore, it inhibits bacterial protein synthesis and growth. This acts to suppress diarrhea by altering the growth of the bacteria. The recommended dose for traveler's diarrhea is 200 mg three times daily for 3 days and may be administered with or without meals.

Contraindications

History of hypersensitivity to rifaximin, rifamycin antimicrobial agents, or any of the components of rifaximin

Adverse Effects

The most common side effects are peripheral edema, nausea, dizziness, fatigue, and muscle spasms. For TD, the most common side effect was headache. Additional postmarketing side effects include exfoliative dermatitis, rash, angioneurotic edema (swelling of the face and tongue and difficulty swallowing), urticaria, flushing, pruritus, and anaphylaxis.

Interactions

Rifaximin has a low risk of drug interactions because it is poorly absorbed into the bloodstream, and it does not significantly affect the cytochrome P-450 system. Coadministration with cyclosporine in healthy subjects resulted in the increased availability of rifaximin, but overall clinical significance is unknown.

Selecting the Most Appropriate Agent

The choice of antidiarrheal agent should be based on several factors, including the patient's history, potential side effects of the medication, potential for drug interactions, and efficacy of available agents (**Tables 30.3 and 30.5; Figure 30.2**).

First-Line Therapy

Although the adsorbents are not absorbed into the systemic circulation and are usually safe and well tolerated, they are not as effective at controlling diarrhea as loperamide. Therefore, loperamide may be considered as first-line therapy secondary to its efficacy. Loperamide is also reasonably well tolerated and has few drug interactions. However, patients should be warned about the potential for loperamide to cause drowsiness (particularly patients who must stay alert).

Because loperamide is an antimotility agent, it should be used with caution in patients with fever or bloody stools to avoid exacerbation of any type of infectious diarrhea. In addition, caution should be used in patients with liver failure.

Appropriate antibiotic therapy should be considered for infectious diarrhea. First line for travelers' diarrhea is ciprofloxacin or levofloxacin (see **Chapter 8 Antibiotics**). Rifaximin can also be considered as a first-line choice.

Second-Line Therapy

For patients who cannot tolerate loperamide or for those with contraindications, an adsorbent or antisecretory agent may be chosen.

Antisecretory agents such as BSS or Kaopectate should be used with caution in patients taking warfarin and should be avoided in children or adolescents with the flu. Antisecretory

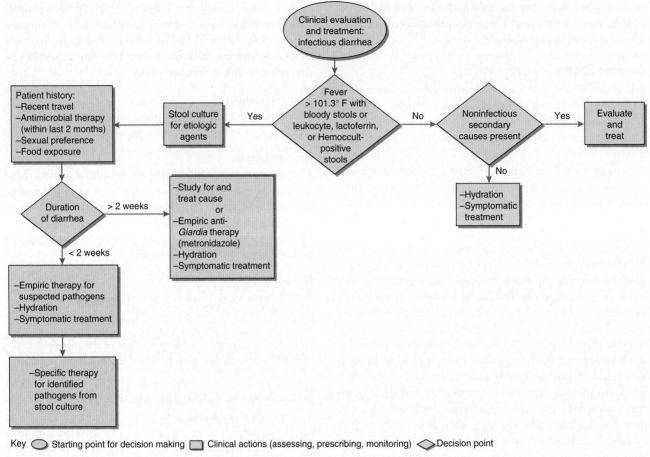

FIGURE 30.2   Treatment algorithm for diarrhea.

agents should also be avoided in patients with a documented hypersensitivity to salicylates. Black stools, darkening of the tongue, and tinnitus are side effects that may be disturbing to the patient. BSS may be useful for prophylaxis against TD and may be preferable over the adsorbents in a patient who also has indigestion or stomach upset that accompanies the diarrhea.

Although adsorbents may inhibit the absorption of nutrients from the diet and can cause some abdominal cramping, they are usually well tolerated.

Second-line antibiotic therapy is rifaximin, if the agent is known to be *Escherichia coli*, and has not responded to ciprofloxacin.

Third-Line Therapy

Although diphenoxylate with atropine is an effective agent for treating diarrhea, the atropine component can cause significant anticholinergic effects that may exacerbate certain conditions and interact with other agents with anticholinergic activity. In addition, diphenoxylate is a Drug Enforcement Administration Schedule V drug, and its potential for abuse limits this agent to third-line therapy. Third-line antibiotic therapy is azithromycin (see **Chapter 8**).

Special Populations

Pediatric

Recommendations for treatment of diarrhea in children have not changed since 1996 by the American Academy of Pediatrics, Provisional Committee on Quality Improvement, and Subcommittee on Acute Gastroenteritis. These recommendations apply to children ages 1 month to 5 years who have no previously diagnosed disorders. The main focus is on oral rehydration and zinc therapy (Lenters et al., 2013). Opiate and atropine combination drugs such as diphenoxylate with atropine should be avoided in acute diarrhea in children because of the potential for side effects and the limited scientific evidence for efficacy. Also, loperamide is not recommended based on limited scientific evidence, and BSS or Kaopectate is not appropriate due to the presence of subsalicylate. Adsorbents are also not recommended based on limited evidence. The committee recognized that major toxic effects from adsorbents are in general not a concern, but the potential for poor absorption of nutrients and antibiotics is a potential disadvantage. The final expert conclusion is that oral rehydration is the most important aspect of therapy, and routine use of antidiarrheal agents is not recommended based on lack of evidence or the potential for side effects.

If the health care provider still decides to choose diphenoxylate with atropine, the liquid formulation should be used because specific dosing is required based on the child's weight and age. In addition, diphenoxylate with atropine is contraindicated in children younger than age 2.

Geriatric

As with the pediatric population, rehydration is of paramount importance in the geriatric population. Elderly patients are likely to have multiple disease states that cause them to be intolerant of dehydration (e.g., congestive heart failure, diabetes, renal insufficiency). In addition, the antidiarrheal preparations may interact with agents that are commonly prescribed in the geriatric population. Diphenoxylate and loperamide may increase the sedative potential of benzodiazepines, antidepressants, anticholinergics, and antipsychotics. Adsorbents can reduce the absorption not only of important nutrients but also of other medications. BSS should be used with caution in elderly patients taking aspirin and agents that interact with aspirin.

Women

As with constipation, antidiarrheals such as the adsorbents that are not absorbed systemically should be considered as first-line therapy for pregnant women with diarrhea. However, adsorbents can inhibit the absorption of important nutrients. Iron supplementation may be particularly important in pregnant women taking adsorbents for diarrhea. Loperamide has not been shown to be teratogenic in animals but has been inadequately studied in humans; therefore, the routine use of loperamide is not recommended. Diphenoxylate with atropine should be avoided because it has been shown to be teratogenic in animals. In addition, malformations in infants after first trimester exposure have been reported. Both Lomotil and loperamide are excreted in breast milk. Salicylates have been shown to be teratogenic in animals. Therefore, use of BSS in the pregnant woman should be avoided.

MONITORING PATIENT RESPONSE

For most cases of diarrhea, the major concern is dehydration. Fluid and electrolyte depletion can lead to hypotension, tachycardia, and vascular collapse. Vascular collapse may occur quickly in the very old or the very young. Severe dehydration may result in decreased plasma volume and a decrease in perfusion, which may be of clinical significance, particularly in patients with congestive heart failure or chronic renal disease. Bicarbonate loss from excessive diarrhea may result in metabolic acidosis. This may be of particular concern in patients with type 1 diabetes mellitus who may be prone to ketoacidosis.

Patients should be monitored for signs of dehydration, such as orthostatic hypotension and poor skin turgor. The body weight of an infant is mostly water, and therefore, infants may be weighed to determine significant fluid loss and dehydration from severe diarrhea. Monitoring serum electrolytes as well as intake of fluid and output of stools benefits patients who are hospitalized secondary to dehydration.

As stated earlier, the goal of therapy is not only to prevent dehydration but also to make the patient as comfortable as possible. Monitoring the effectiveness of an antidiarrheal preparation requires interviewing the patient to ensure a decrease in stool frequency and improved formation. Frequency and formation of stools vary from patient to patient, and determination of relief is subjective on the patient's part.

PATIENT EDUCATION

To avoid complications, patients should be educated about appropriate rehydration. In most cases, simple replacement of fluid and electrolytes with soda crackers, broths, and soups is all that is necessary in the nondehydrated adult with diarrhea. Oral rehydration therapy (ORT) solutions should also be considered because most sports drinks do not have enough sodium to replace losses from diarrhea (Centers for Disease Control and Prevention, 2005); however, the palatability of ORT product makes them difficult to administer especially to children. Additionally, food and drink high in sugar content should be avoided because it may increase the osmotic load and worsen the diarrhea. In the elderly or immunocompromised patient, solutions with sodium content in the range of 45 to 75 mEq/L are recommended. Boiled potatoes, noodles, rice, cereals, crackers, bananas, yogurt, soup, and boiled vegetables are recommended during the acute phase of diarrhea. The diet may return to normal as stools become formed.

Infants and children are particularly susceptible to dehydration with diarrhea. Oral replacement therapy is the preferred treatment to replace fluids and electrolytes in children with mild to moderate dehydration because it is less expensive than intravenous therapy and can be administered in many settings, including the home. Oral glucose–electrolyte solutions available in the United States (**Table 30.6**) are based on physiologic principles and should be recommended over commonly used nonphysiologic solutions such as colas, apple juice, chicken broth, and sports beverages.

Currently, oral replacement solutions (ORSs) are recommended for children with mild to moderate diarrhea (CDC, 2003). In addition, age-appropriate feeding should be continued and fluids encouraged. For children with mild to moderate dehydration (3% to 5% loss of total body weight), 50 to 100 mL/kg of ORS is recommended plus 10 mL/kg for each loose stool to replace continuing fluid losses. Severe dehydration (loss of 10% total body weight) can result in shock and is a medical emergency requiring intravenous therapy with normal saline or lactated Ringer solution. In all situations, age-appropriate feeding should begin after dehydration is corrected.

Drug Information

Patients need to be aware of the potential side effects of antidiarrheal medications. Constipation can occur if these agents are taken for too long. Antidiarrheal agents taken in the setting

TABLE 30.6

Commercially Available Oral Rehydration Solutions

Product	Carbohydrate (g/L)	Na+ (mEq/L)	K+ (mEq/L)	Cl− (mEq/L)	Base (mEq/L)	Calories (kcal)
Infalyte* (Mead Johnson)	30 (rice syrup solids)	50	25	45	34 (citrate)	126
Pedialyte† (Ross Laboratories)	25 (dextrose)	45	20	35	30 (citrate)	100
Rehydralyte (Ross Laboratories)	25 (dextrose)	75†	20	65	30 (citrate)	100
WHO Solution§ (Ianas Bros. Packing Co.)	20 (glucose)	90†	20	80	10 (citrate)	80

*Available in hospitals as 6-ounce nursing bottle.

†Available in hospitals as 8-ounce nursing bottle.

‡The American Academy of Pediatrics recommends these solutions with sodium contents of 75–90 mEq/L for replacement of deficit during initial rehydration (*Pediatrics, 75,* 358, 1985).

§Must be mixed with 1 L of boiled or treated water; packets available in stores or pharmacies in all developing countries.

Source: Manufacturer's product information.

Reproduced by permission from American Journal of Gastroenterology. (1997). Commercially available oral rehydration solutions. *American Journal of Gastroenterology,* 92, 1962–1975. Copyright © 1997, Rights Managed by Nature Publishing Group.

of infectious diseases can prolong or worsen the disease. It is always best to contact a health care provider if diarrhea lasts more than 2 days.

Patient-Oriented Information Sources

Providing patients with information about acute diarrhea and what to expect can help them understand diarrhea and their role in the treatment. Patient education items are readily available on the Internet through the National Digestive Diseases Information Clearinghouse (NDDIC), which provides information to consumers on a wide variety of GI topics. The CDC also has a wide array of patient information about diarrhea (see **Box 30.11**).

Nutrition/Lifestyle Changes

It is not recommended to rest the gut. Oral intake and breast-feeding should continue to replace lost calories during illness. Early feeding will stimulate enterocyte renewal, ultimately promoting a quicker recovery of the gut. Additionally, feeding decreases the potential risk of malnutrition.

Complementary and Alternative Medications

Probiotics have shown some efficacy in the treatment of diarrhea. The presumed mechanism of action is to alter the composition of the intestinal microflora and act against enteric pathogens (Guarino, 2009). Yogurt is a source of probiotics; however, not all brands have the active ingredients. Acidophilus capsules can be used to treat diarrhea resulting from antibiotic use. It restores the natural flora to the bowel. One to 10 billion viable organisms per day in three or four divided doses are appropriate.

IRRITABLE BOWEL SYNDROME

IBS is a functional bowel disorder that presents with abdominal discomfort and an alteration in bowel pattern. The disorder is an international health problem that can be one of the most perplexing chronic abdominal complaints reported to primary care providers and gastroenterologists. Little has changed in the incidence of IBS with the rate continuing from 3% to 20% depending on the application of the Rome III criteria (Grundman & Yoon, 2010). Epidemiologic studies in North America suggest a prevalence of 10% to 15%, with a 4:1 female predominance, while 7% to 10% have IBS worldwide (Brandt et al., 2009; Lovell & Ford, 2012). Newer data also suggest that veterans of the Gulf War have a high prevalence of IBS compared to the general population, which increases the prevalence of IBS in men (Brandt et al., 2009). Work is currently being done on Rome IV criteria, but is not yet available. Future recommendations are going focusing on the use of evidence-based practice rather than consensus (http://www.romecriteria.org/romeiv_pub/romeiv_faqs.cfm).

Once thought to be associated primarily with psychological problems and stress, research is changing to an emphasis on motility of the gut, autonomic system imbalances, and increased visceral hypersensitivity (Akbar, 2009). A syndrome in childhood known as recurrent abdominal pain can be a hallmark of adult IBS. The majority of patients seeking care are ages 20 to 50, and symptoms can wax and wane over a lifetime.

CAUSES

For many years, the chief cause of IBS was thought to be primarily psychological. Now, however, research has identified physiologic but not pathologic causes that are accentuated by psychological stress. Symptoms generally are slow in onset, sometimes over weeks or months (Grundmann, 2010). Dysregulation occurs between the brain and the gut, leading to typical IBS symptoms. Commonly, the symptoms can be worse during times of physical and emotional stress, including sexual or physical abuse. In addition, some patients can identify foods that exacerbate the condition (e.g., lactose, caffeine, and fatty or spicy foods). Depending on the severity of the illness, pharmacotherapy may not be required and symptoms may respond solely to lifestyle changes. These lifestyle changes need to become incorporated into the patient's daily routines. Pharmacologic interventions may be required only intermittently to maintain symptom control.

PATHOPHYSIOLOGY

In general, the syndrome is believed to have the components of motility and sensory abnormalities. This leads to dysregulation of the bowel as modulated by the CNS. Many neuroimmune and neuroendocrine modulators, such as serotonin (5-HT), substance P, CCK, neurotensin, cytokines, and others, contribute to the increase in visceral sensitivity, central mechanisms controlling pain and dysregulation of the brain–gut axis. Local reflex mechanisms can also be responsible for mechanical distention of the gut in response to short-chain fatty acids, affecting the emptying rate of the proximal colon. The prevailing theory is that the emptying rate of the proximal colon may be the key determination of overall colon function. The GI tract is innervated intrinsically and extrinsically by various neurohormonal agents from local or distant sources. Intrinsic factors include the neurons found in the enteric nervous system, which function similarly to the CNS. Bowel motor dysfunction can be associated with inflammation as well as changes in neurotransmitters, such as 5-hydroxytryptamine (5-HT3; serotonin). This neurotransmitter is found in the GI tract, and blocking it pharmacologically can decrease visceral pain, colonic transit, and GI secretions. External factors that can alter colonic activity are eating and drinking, stress, and endogenous hormones. Increased motility and abnormal contractions of the intestinal tract can result in either diarrhea or constipation-predominant IBS, due to either accelerated whole-gut transit times or delays in colonic transit. The IBS patient's sensory perception of colonic activity in response to balloon dilatation is more sensitive than that of patients with normal colonic activity. Sensory perception is also accentuated by external factors that lead to enhanced sensations that differ from those of healthy patients. However, evidence is increasing that IBS is not a psychological illness. This is supported by the fact that IBS exists in about 12% to 20% of the general adult population.

DIAGNOSTIC CRITERIA

The hallmark symptom of IBS is abdominal pain associated with a change in the consistency of stools that is relieved by defecation. Symptoms are usually first noticed in young adulthood and can be persistent or intermittent. Weight loss, rectal bleeding, fever, acute onset, and onset after age 50 are unusual in IBS and should raise suspicion of organic causes, not IBS. Diagnosis can be predominantly based on symptoms and appropriate treatment initiated, with reassessment in 3 to 6 weeks.

In 1978, the original Manning criteria proposed identifying IBS based on the presence of four symptoms: abdominal distention, pain relief with bowel action, more frequent stools

> ### BOX 30.8 Rome III Criteria for Irritable Bowel Syndrome (2006)
>
> Diagnostic criterion must be fulfilled for the last 3 months with symptom onset at least 6 months prior to diagnosis.
> Recurrent abdominal pain or discomfort at least 3 days/month in the last 3 months associated with two of the following:
> - Improvement with defecation
> - Onset associated with change in frequency of stool
> - Onset associated with a change in form (appearance) of stool

with the onset of pain, and looser stools with the onset of pain. These criteria led to the establishment of an international group called the Multinational Working Teams for Diagnosis of Functional GI Disorders. This team identified key criteria for IBS, leading to the establishment of the Rome criteria (**Box 30.8**); the third revision focused on categorizing each type of IBS according to constipation, diarrhea, or mixed. However, the overall accuracy of the Rome criteria has led the American College of Gastroenterology (ACG) to simply define IBS as abdominal pain that occurs with altered bowel habits over a period of 3 months (Brandt et al., 2009). Therefore, for IBS to be considered as a diagnosis, the presenting clinical features may be sporadic, intermittent, or continuous but should be present for at least 3 months, as defined by the ACG. The Rome III criteria (**Box 30.8**) can be used to help verify the subtype, which can guide drug therapy.

The chief complaint most patients report is abdominal discomfort that can be relieved with defecation; however, symptom relief is often short-lived. Patients can also report abnormal bowel habits that alternate between diarrhea and constipation or are predominantly diarrhea or constipation; it is much more common to have bowel habits that are predominantly one type. Associated components can be abdominal distention, bloating, and gassiness. Extreme urgency after a meal can be common and can possibly result in an "explosive" bowel movement that relieves the overall discomfort.

Organic symptoms of abdominal pain that do not suggest IBS are those that awaken the patient from sleep, initial onset in the elderly years, a change in abdominal pain that is not associated with bowel movements, significant weight loss, rectal bleeding, steatorrhea, and fever. In addition, steadily worsening symptoms should be considered atypical. These symptoms would suggest the need for additional studies. However, compared to the general population, IBS patients are not more likely to have organic causes for disease.

A key component of IBS treatment is a thorough history of symptoms, psychosocial stress, medications (because of GI symptoms from many drugs), and dietary habits (to identify nutritional patterns, gaps, and intolerances). Even in the general population, stress can result in GI symptoms. However, in the patient with IBS, these symptoms can become more pronounced. The relationship between psychological distress and GI symptoms has been well researched. Chronic and acute life stresses, including a history of verbal or sexual abuse, especially in childhood, may preclude early symptoms of IBS. These chronic stresses can contribute later in life to IBS symptoms.

Physical examination findings are often normal except for a slight diffuse abdominal tenderness with palpation, especially in the left lower quadrant near the sigmoid colon. Mild abdominal distention may also be present.

In 2009, the ACG Task Force, in an evidence-based position paper on the management of IBS in North America, reinforced the recommendation that minimal, if any, testing is necessary. Current treatments were evaluated, and the conclusion was reached that care is often based on nonrandomized, non–placebo-controlled trials. The best available data show that only 1% of IBS patients have alarming symptoms signifying serious organic disease. Therefore, for patients without alarming features of IBS, routine diagnostic studies are not necessary. However, patients who are classified as IBS-D (diarrhea) or IBS-M (mixed) should be routinely tested for celiac sprue disease. Other studies such as abdominal ultrasound, flexible sigmoidoscopy, barium enema, or colonoscopy do not lead to any change in the proposed treatment and are therefore not recommended. Additional testing may be indicated for patients with the key symptoms previously identified or if the patient is older than age 50.

Types of IBS

Once identified according to the Rome III criteria (**Box 30.8**), patient definition of further subtypes of constipation (IBS-C), diarrhea (IBS-D), mixed (IBS-M), or unspecified (IBS-U) (**Box 30.9**) can further refine the diagnosis and focus for treatment. Symptoms can also be stratified as *mild, intermittent, or continuous* according to the predominant features of the patient's stool (Longstreth, 2006). While patients can stay predominately in one category, there is often overlap in symptomatology.

Mild IBS usually shows a sporadic pattern. Symptoms are worsened by stress and dietary factors. There is no alteration in the patient's daily activities because of the symptoms.

In *intermittent* IBS, the symptoms are worse and begin to affect the patient's daily life. It is more difficult to relate symptoms to specific precipitants, and a psychological component to the syndrome may be developing.

In *continuous* IBS, the symptoms affect every aspect of the patient's daily routines. An inability to pinpoint precipitants still exists, and there is a definite psychological component to the syndrome.

INITIATING DRUG THERAPY

Initial therapy is focused on establishing a therapeutic relationship and mapping out a long-term strategy. This provides the patient with knowledge regarding the disease process and lets the patient know that improvement may be a slow process, taking many months.

Patients with mild symptoms may be responsive to dietary and lifestyle changes (**Box 30.10**). Assessing the diet for potentially offending substances and removing those substances may improve symptoms. Hayes et al. (2014) found in a survey of patients with IBS that cereal products and spicy foods along with vegetables and fatty foods were a predominant cause of symptoms. These substances may be lactose, caffeine, beans, cabbage, fatty foods, or alcohol (Simren, 2001). In an earlier 1998 study, Versa and colleagues showed a positive correlation between IBS and lactose intolerance, female sex, and abdominal pain in childhood, and these early findings have been supported by additional research (Yang et al., 2014). A 2-week trial of a lactose-free diet is worth pursuing. Aspartame, an artificial sweetener found in many soft drinks and diet foods, may also provoke diarrhea. Trial elimination may also be worthwhile, especially in diarrhea-predominant IBS. However, with most IBS therapies, the placebo effect is often just as successful as the therapy itself.

Maintaining a daily diary of food intake, bowel patterns, and emotional stressors can be helpful in the treatment of IBS. It serves to identify factors that can be addressed and evaluates the effectiveness of treatment. Lifestyle modification requires the patient to understand the stressors in his or her life and the effect these stressors have on physiologic functions. Identifying ways to reduce stress can be critical to improving IBS symptoms. Biofeedback can be used to decrease gut sensitivity, along with

---

BOX 30.9 Subtyping of IBS by Predominant Stool Pattern

1. IBS with constipation (IBS-C)—hard or lumpy stools ≥25% and loose (mushy) or watery stools ≤25%
2. IBS with diarrhea (IBS-D)—loose (mushy) stools or watery stools ≥25% and hard or lumpy stools ≤25%
3. IBS mixed (IBS-M)—hard or lumpy stools ≥25% and loose (mushy) or watery stools ≥25%
4. IBS unclassified (IBS-U)—insufficient abnormality of stool, consistency to meet criteria for other classifications

---

BOX 30.10 Dietary and Lifestyle Changes

Avoid foods that exacerbate the symptoms (e.g., lactose, caffeine, fatty or spicy foods).
Incorporate routine exercise into daily activities.
Explore the life stressors that aggravate the symptoms.
Learn ways to deal with stress, such as meditation, counseling, and biofeedback.

relaxation tapes to decrease stressors. Daley et al. (2008) showed some benefit of regular exercise in reducing stress and improving bowel transit. However, as previously discussed in the section on constipation, exercise has little benefit on bowel transit time.

Goals of Drug Therapy

The pharmacologic agents used for IBS are the same as those discussed in the constipation and diarrhea sections of this chapter. The goal of pharmacotherapy for IBS is to alleviate or control the specific symptoms. Generally, clinical trials have

been inadequate to establish a definite link between administration of specific drugs and relief of symptoms. In patients with IBS, between 50% and 75% still have symptoms after 10 years (Canavan et al., 2014). In an open-label placebo trial, response rates to a placebo were as high as 53% (Kaptchuk et al., 2010).

Bulk-Forming Laxatives

Previously, administration of dietary fiber in the form of a bulking agent was commonly the first agent prescribed in IBS (**Table 30.7**). However, administration of fiber to patients

---

TABLE 30.7

Overview of Selected Agents Used to Treat Irritable Bowel Syndrome

Generic (Trade) Name and Dosage	Selected Adverse Events	Contraindications	Special Considerations
Selected Bulk-Forming Laxatives			
psyllium (Konsyl, Metamucil, Perdiem) Start: 1 tsp in 8 oz liquid bid–tid Range: 1–2 tsp in 8 oz liquid bid–tid	Abdominal fullness, increased flatus	Symptoms of acute surgical abdomen, intestinal obstruction, or perforation Inability to drink adequate amounts of water	Comes in granules, powder, or wafers Takes 12 h to 3 d to work
calcium polycarbophil (Equalactin, FiberCon, Mitrolan) Start: 500 mg tablets qd) Range: 500–1000 mg qid	Abdominal fullness, increased flatus	Same as above	Takes 12 h to 3 d to work
methylcellulose (Citrucel)) Start: 1 tsp in 8 oz liquid bid–tid) Range: 1–2 tsp in 8 oz liquid bid or tid	Nausea, abdominal cramps	Same as above	Takes 12 h to 3 d to work
Hyperosmotic Laxatives			
lactulose (Duphalac) syrup Start: 15–30 mL PO daily Range: 15–60 mg/d	Flatulence, intestinal cramps, diarrhea, nausea, vomiting, electrolyte imbalances	Galactose-restricted diets, appendicitis, acute surgical abdomen, fecal impaction, or intestinal obstruction Use with caution in diabetic patients.	
magnesium citrate (Citroma) oral solution Start: 5 oz qhs Range: 5–10 oz qhs magnesium hydroxide (Milk of Magnesia/MOM.)) Start: 15 mL qhs Range: 15–60 mL qhs	Abdominal cramping, nausea Abdominal cramping, nausea	End-stage renal disease End-stage renal disease	Can cause increased magnesium levels in patients with end-stage renal disease Same as above
Stimulant Laxatives			
bisacodyl (Dulcolax) Start: 10 mg PO in evening or before breakfast Range: 10–15 mg	Abdominal cramping, nausea, vomiting, burning sensation in rectum with suppositories		Oral: 6–8 h Rectal: 15–60 min
senna concentrates (Senokot) Start: 2 tabs or 1 level tsp at hs Range: 2–4 tabs or 1–2 tsp qhs	Abdominal cramping, nausea	Signs and symptoms of appendicitis, abdominal pain, nausea, vomiting	Elderly or debilitated, halve the dose
Surfactant Laxatives			
docusate calcium (Surfak) Start: 240 mg/d Range: 240 mg/d	None	None	May increase the systemic absorption of mineral oil
docusate sodium (Colace) Start: 50 mg/d Range: 50–200 mg/d	Bitter taste, throat irritation, nausea, rash	Signs and symptoms of appendicitis	Onset: 1–3 d Not to be used for acute relief of constipation

(Continued)

TABLE 30.7

Overview of Selected Agents Used to Treat Irritable Bowel Syndrome (*Continued*)

Generic (Trade) Name and Dosage	Selected Adverse Events	Contraindications	Special Considerations
Antidiarrheal Agents			
diphenoxylate HCl with atropine sulfate (Lomotil) Start: 5 mg qid Range: 5–10 mg qid; maintenance may be 10 mg qd	Sedation, dizziness, dry mouth, paralytic ileus	Pseudomembranous enterocolitis, obstructive jaundice, diarrhea caused by organisms that penetrate intestinal mucosa Under 2 y of age Pregnancy category C	Onset 45–60 min
loperamide HCl (Imodium) Start: 4 mg after first loose stool then 2 mg after each following stool Range: 4–16 mg/d	Constipation	Acute dysentery	Peak levels 2.5 h after liquid and 5 h after capsule
Selected Antispasmodics (Anticholinergic Agents)			
belladonna alkaloids (Donnatal) Start: 1 tab or capsule tid or qid Range: 1–2 tabs/capsules tid or qid	Drowsiness, anticholinergic effects, paradoxical excitement	Glaucoma, unstable coronary artery disease, GI or GU obstruction, paralytic ileus, severe ulcerative colitis	Antacids may inhibit absorption. Additive anticholinergic effects with other anticholinergics, antihistamines, narcotics, tricyclic antidepressants
dicyclomine HCl (Bentyl) Start: 20 mg qid Range: 20–40 mg qid if tolerated	Same as above	Same as above	Same as above
clidinium (Librax) Start: 1 capsule qid—ac and qhs Range: 1–2 capsules qid—ac and qhs	Drowsiness, anticholinergic effects, paradoxical excitement, ataxia, confusion, jaundice	Glaucoma, GI or GU obstruction	Same as above
hyoscyamine sulfate (Levsin, Levbid, Levsin SL) *Levsin* Start: 1 tab q4h prn Range: 1–2 tabs q4h prn; max 12 tabs/d *Levbid* Start: 1 tab q12h Range: 1–2 tabs q12h; max 4 tabs/d *Levsin SL* Start: 1 tab swallowed or chewed q4h prn Range: max 12 tabs/d	Same as above	Same as above	Same as above
Secretagogues—Chloride Channel Activators			
lubiprostone (Amitiza) IBS-C: 8 mcg capsules bid	Nausea, diarrhea, abdominal pain, dyspepsia	Known or suspected mechanical GI obstructions	Pregnancy category C Not approved for children For IBS only approved for women Must take medication with food and water, swallow whole
Semi-synthetic Antibiotic			
rifaximin (Xifaxan) IBS-D: 500 mg tablets tid × 14 d	Peripheral edema, nausea, dizziness, fatigue, and muscles spasms. Additional post-marketing side effects include exfoliative dermatitis, rash, angioneurotic edema (swelling of face and tongue and difficulty swallowing), urticaria, flushing, pruritus and anaphylaxis.	Known hypersensitivity to rifaximin Bloody diarrhea	If diarrhea continues consider evaluation for *C-Difficile* May repeat treatment up to two times for recurrent diarrhea at the same dose. Can be taken with or without food

with IBS has become controversial. While the hypothesis exists that fiber increases colonic transit time and therefore lessens colon wall tension and ultimately abdominal pain, clinical trials on the use of fiber in IBS have had small sample sizes and have been short in duration. Also, fiber can exacerbate the diarrhea and bloating component of IBS. This led the ACG Task Force to conclude that fiber is no more effective than placebo and is not recommended for the treatment of IBS.

Hyperosmotic Laxatives

When the patient requires a laxative, it is preferable to administer one that is osmotic (see **Table 30.7**). These agents can work either as a disaccharide sugar, which produces an osmotic effect in the colon, resulting in colonic distention and promotion of peristalsis, or by an osmotic effect in the small intestine, drawing water into the lumen and softening the stool. Lactulose or sorbitol, disaccharide sugars, can be used for patients with predominant constipation. PEG 3350 (MiraLAX) is a glycolated laxative that can be safely used for a long period without adverse pharmacologic effects.

Contraindications

The same contraindications exist as when using these agents to treat chronic constipation. Lactulose is contraindicated in patients who must restrict their galactose intake and in patients with appendicitis, acute surgical abdomen, fecal impaction, or intestinal obstruction. Caution must be used with administration to diabetic patients because of sugar content.

Other osmotic agents such as magnesium hydroxide (milk of magnesia) or magnesium citrate (Citroma) can be used to promote defecation. Approximately 15% to 30% of the magnesium in these agents may be absorbed systemically; therefore, caution needs to be used in patients who have renal failure and a decreased ability to excrete magnesium.

Adverse Events

When taken appropriately, these agents are well tolerated. The most common adverse events are abdominal cramping or nausea. Extensive, long-term use of these agents can lead to laxative dependence.

Stimulant Laxatives

These laxatives vary in effects but act by increasing peristalsis through a direct effect on the smooth muscle of the intestines and by simultaneously promoting fluid accumulation in the colon and small intestine. The recommendation is to use these agents intermittently due to the irritating effect of the agents on the musculature. Stimulant laxatives include bisacodyl (Dulcolax) and senna concentrates (Senokot, Senokot S). As with other laxatives, stimulants are contraindicated in patients with appendicitis, acute surgical abdomen, fecal impaction, or intestinal obstruction. Rectal fissures and hemorrhoids can be exacerbated by stimulation of defecation. Action begins 6 to 10 hours after oral administration and 15 minutes to 2 hours after rectal administration (see **Table 30.7**).

These agents are not as well tolerated as osmotic laxatives or bulking agents because of their side effects, which include nausea, vomiting, and abdominal cramping. These side effects can be more severe with cases of severe constipation. Several OTC products use the brand name of Dulcolax. One has the main ingredient of bisacodyl and another is docusate sodium, which is a stool softener. This could be important, especially when the patient has been instructed to use the drug as bowel preparation for a GI study.

Surfactant Laxatives

This class of laxatives reduces the surface tension of the liquid contents of the bowel. Ultimately, this promotes incorporation of additional liquid into the stool, forming a softer mass, and promotes easier defecation. Examples of this class include docusate sodium (Colace, Dulcolax) and docusate calcium (Surfak). This is the laxative of choice for patients who should not strain during defecation. However, emollient laxatives only prevent constipation; they do not treat it. Administration of emollient laxatives concomitantly with mineral oil is contraindicated because of increased absorption of the mineral oil. Action with these agents usually occurs in 1 to 3 days. The practitioner should consider this class for prevention purposes, not for acute treatment (see **Table 30.7**). These agents are extremely well tolerated when used to prevent constipation. Side effects include mild abdominal cramping, diarrhea, and throat irritation, but these are infrequent.

Antidiarrheal Agents

Antidiarrheal agents for patients with IBS with predominant diarrhea can be used on an occasional basis (see **Table 30.7**). Loperamide HCl (Imodium) inhibits peristaltic activity, thereby prolonging transit time, and it can increase anal sphincter tone. Approximately 40% of the drug is absorbed from the GI tract and 75% is metabolized in the hepatic system; excretion is primarily in the feces. As previously discussed, the drug does not cross the blood–brain barrier into the CNS. Because of these properties, it is the preferred agent for treating diarrhea. Conversely, diphenoxylate hydrochloride with atropine (Lomotil) is an opiate similar to meperidine that increases smooth muscle tone in the GI tract, inhibits motility and propulsion, and diminishes gut secretions. It is absorbed orally and extensively metabolized by the liver. It can affect the CNS, and atropine has been added to discourage abuse.

Neither of these antidiarrheal agents should be used in a patient suspected of having diarrhea from pseudomembranous colitis or ulcerative colitis or diarrhea resulting from poisoning or microbial infection. Diphenoxylate hydrochloride is contraindicated in patients who are hypersensitive to atropine or meperidine and patients with hepatic impairment. The atropine in Lomotil may aggravate glaucoma in patients with this disease. For additional discussion of contraindications and adverse events, see the diarrhea section.

Antispasmodic Agents

Treatment for patients with postprandial abdominal pain may require the use of antispasmodics (see **Table 30.7**). However, the efficacy of these medications remains unproven in controlled studies. The presumed desired action is by direct relaxation of the smooth muscle component of the GI tract. These agents competitively block the effects of acetylcholine at muscarinic cholinergic receptors that mediate the effects of parasympathetic postganglionic impulses. Examples of commonly used anticholinergics are dicyclomine hydrochloride (Bentyl) and hyoscyamine sulfate (Levbid, Levsin SL). Less commonly used are the belladonna alkaloids/phenobarbital (Donnatal) and clidinium/chlordiazepoxide (Librax); while both are still on the market, they can be difficult to find and expensive. These drugs are a combination of older benzodiazepines, antispasmodics, and/or antiepileptics. Dosing of the anticholinergics is variable, and general side effects are associated with the anticholinergic actions.

Contraindications

These agents are contraindicated in patients who have glaucoma, stenosing peptic ulcer, chronic obstructive pulmonary disease, cardiac arrhythmias, impaired liver or kidney function, and myasthenia gravis. Caution should be used in patients with hypertension, hyperthyroidism, and benign prostatic hyperplasia.

Adverse Events

Side effects include dry mouth, altered taste perception, nausea, vomiting, dysphagia, blurred vision, palpitations, and urinary hesitancy and retention. Anticholinergic side effects can be used as a measure of titration to achieve the desired pharmacologic end. It is important to monitor for signs of drug toxicity: CNS signs resembling psychosis, accompanied by peripheral effects that include dilated, nonreactive pupils; blurred vision; hot, dry, flushed skin; dry mucous membranes; dysphagia; decreased or absent bowel sounds; urinary retention; hyperthermia; tachycardia; hypertension; and increased respiration.

Antidepressants

Antidepressants as a class have also been used in the treatment of IBS. It is not clear whether these agents work by improving a concomitant depression or by improving the anxiety and stress often associated with IBS. Initial work was done with use of the tricyclic agents such as imipramine (Tofranil), desipramine (Norpramin), and amitriptyline (Elavil) in patients with severe symptoms. Careful monitoring is important when tricyclic antidepressants are given to patients with IBS in which constipation predominates, because these agents can cause constipation. Newer agents in the selective serotonin reuptake inhibitor (SSRI) class may also prove beneficial. It has been suggested based on current investigations that antidepressants alter perceived pain thresholds, which are often abnormal in patients with IBS. See Chapter 40 for further discussion of these drugs.

Serotonin-3 Receptor Antagonists

A newer class of drugs has evolved to address the brain–gut–neurotransmitter (5-HT3) connection with regard to colonic transit time. Currently, there is only one drug in this class.

In animal models, serotonin-3 receptor antagonist has been shown to decrease abdominal pain, slow colonic transit time, increase rectal compliance, and improve stool consistency. Indication for use of alosetron is for patients who have severe diarrhea and no constipation. The drug was first released in 1999, but later pulled from the market in 2000 due to concerns about ischemic colitis and severe constipation. In 2002, alosetron once again became available with special provisions by the FDA for provider education and distribution. The American Gastroenterology Association (2014) recommends *conditional* use of alosetron for IBS-D reflecting additional limitations based on FDA requirements.

Secretagogues

Chloride Channel Activators

As previously discussed in the constipation section, lubiprostone (Amitiza) is approved for CIC and OIC for both men and women; however, for treatment of IBS, it is only approved for use in women ≥ 18 years old. Lubiprostone is the only drug in this class. Lubiprostone became approved for IBS in 2008 and is prescribed at a lower strength starting at 0.5 mg twice a day.

Contraindications

Lubiprostone is contraindicated in patients with potential mechanical obstruction or hypersensitivity to components of the product.

Adverse Events

The side effect profile is similar to usage in chronic constipation; however, only GI effects are noted. Nausea is the most common side effect of lubiprostone. The rate of nausea is dose dependent and was experienced by approximately 8% of patients. Other common GI side effects include diarrhea, abdominal pain, and abdominal distention.

Interactions

No drug–drug interactions have been discovered with lubiprostone. In vitro studies showed the cytochrome P-450 isoenzymes are not inhibited by the drug.

Guanylate Cyclase-C Agonist

This class has been previously discussed in the constipation section. The mechanism of action for linaclotide (Linzess) is topical rather than systemic, elevating intracellular cGMP, which stimulates secretion of chloride and bicarbonate into the intestinal lumen. Along with the increased fluid, stool transit time is accelerated. Linzess is approved for 18 years and older with IBS. The recommended dosage for IBS is substantially increased to 290 mcg orally once a day, 30 minutes prior to the first meal of the day.

Semisynthetic antibiotic

Rifaximin

Rifaximin (Xifaxan) is a semisynthetic antibiotic also approved for treatment of IBS-D. It is only effective against noninvasive strains of *Escherichia coli*. The drug is a derivative of rifampin and acts to block transcription of the bacteria; therefore, it inhibits bacterial protein synthesis and growth. Additionally, rifaximin improves IBS-D symptoms of abdominal pain after a 10- to 14-day course of treatment. The recommended dose for IBS-D is 550 mg three times daily for 14 days; this differs from the TD administration. Rifaximin may be administered with or without meals. Patients with recurrent symptoms can be retreated up to two times with the same regime. If the diarrhea does not improve, providers should consider evaluation for *Clostridium difficile*.

Selecting the Most Appropriate Agent

The emphasis in the care of patients with IBS should be multidimensional. IBS can present in many stages: mild, moderate, or severe. In 2014, the American Gastroenterological Association (AGA) developed pharmacologic guidelines (Weinberg et al., 2014). These recommendations take into account the level of available data and analysis of risk/benefits for particular agents. As patient care evolves toward evidence-based medicine, the AGA notes that few comparative effectiveness studies exist of the various therapeutic alternatives for treatment of IBS. This fact continues to make prescribing for IBS a challenge for clinical care. Therefore, the standard is still the selection of the most appropriate drug therapy based on the presenting symptoms. Each case needs to be evaluated, and treatment should be individualized (**Figure 30.3** and **Table 30.8**).

First-Line Therapy

First-line therapy is selected based on the presenting symptoms. Qualitatively, patients often feel the burden of this disease but believe this is not appreciated by primary care providers and specialists. Pharmacologic agents need to be considered only when an exacerbation of the disease occurs. There is strong evidence that IBS-C should be treated with linaclotide or lubiprostone as a first-line therapy. Consider an osmotic laxative on a long-term basis for those who are adverse to the incidence of diarrhea with either linaclotide or lubiprostone. Antidiarrheal agents are conditionally recommended in patients with IBS-D. Loperamide is the preferred agent because it causes the least CNS activity and has the added benefit of improving anal sphincter tone.

With the additional problems of pain, gas, and abdominal bloating, a trial of an antispasmodic may relieve symptoms. Dicyclomine is the agent of first choice because of its shorter half-life, which may minimize the anticholinergic side effects of

the class. As with any chronic syndrome, use of low-level antidepressants may be helpful for symptom control. Psychological symptoms associated with IBS may be treated by antidepressants. Selection of an antidepressant should be based on the specific symptoms of depression, stress, or anxiety. The SSRIs are the most commonly selected agents because of their safety profile and efficacy.

Second-Line Therapy

Unresolved complaints of IBS-D can be treated with diphenoxylate hydrochloride, which has a longer duration of action but can be addictive because of its opioid properties and should be reserved for short-term use. Rifaximin should be tried for those whose diarrhea symptoms do not improve. For postprandial abdominal pain, gas, and abdominal bloating, longer-acting antispasmodics such as hyoscyamine sulfate can be considered. The second-line choice for psychological symptoms is the tricyclic antidepressants; these agents have more side effects than SSRIs.

Third-Line Therapy

The use of stimulant laxatives in cases of IBS-C should be reserved for more resistant cases, but these agents should be used with caution. They should not be used for long periods, and they can aggravate abdominal cramping. The older anticholinergics such as the belladonna alkaloids and clidinium should be used very sparingly for postprandial abdominal pain, gas, and abdominal bloating because they produce more intense anticholinergic side effects. In addition, both belladonna and clidinium are hard to find and can be expensive. Patients with IBS, no matter which subtype, need to have consistent evaluation and pharmacologic therapies changed as appropriate for their symptoms.

Special Considerations
Pediatric

Children with crampy abdominal pain, constipation, or diarrhea present a challenge to the practitioner. The approach to diagnosis follows the same parameters of adults; however, few if any of the pharmacologic agents are approved for pediatrics (Sandhu & Paul, 2014). Although these symptoms sound like IBS, there are no established criteria for children. As previously discussed, some experts think that these children may acquire IBS later in life. Treatment for these symptoms can include some of the same approaches of increasing fiber and use of antidiarrheal agents and the newer antispasmodics. Close follow-up is an important aspect of care.

Geriatric

Initial presentation of IBS in people older than age 50 is rare. Abdominal pain in older patients should be considered a more ominous symptom unless they have been previously diagnosed with IBS or spastic colon, a version of colitis. Older patients may report a long-standing history of bowel trouble with any of these diagnoses.

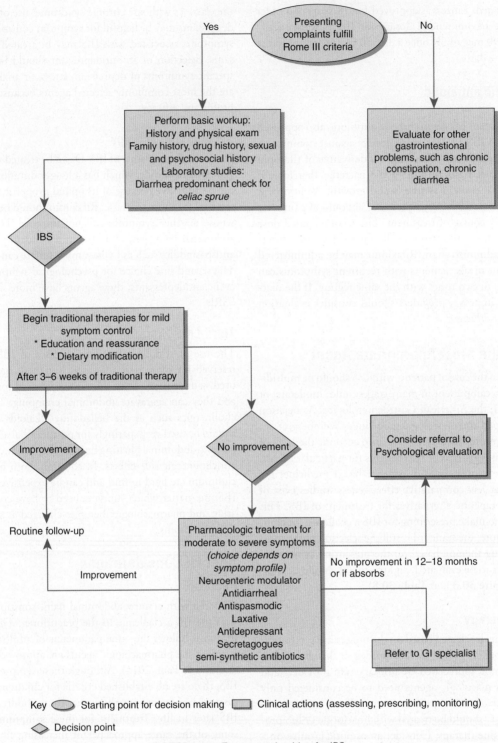

FIGURE 30.3 Treatment algorithm for IBS.

Women

In Western society, women are more likely to have IBS and to seek care. A history of verbal or sexual abuse may also contribute to IBS. Women have surgery more often when the origins of abdominal pains are unclear.

MONITORING PATIENT RESPONSE

Monitoring the patient's response to therapy should take place within 3 to 6 weeks of the initial evaluation. For patients with mild symptoms, the initial treatment includes

TABLE 30.8

Recommended Order for Treatment for Irritable Bowel Syndrome

Order	Agents	Comments
First Line		
Predominant constipation (IBS-C)	Osmotic laxative—lactulose syrup, magnesium citrate, magnesium hydroxide	Milk of magnesia is less expensive than citrate. Use magnesium products cautiously in patients with renal impairment. Use lactulose cautiously in diabetic patients.
	linaclotide or lubiprostone	Consider for first or second line for IBS-C
Predominant diarrhea (IBS-D)	Antidiarrheal—loperamide	May cause constipation
	hydrochloride (Imodium)	Caution about drowsiness; may have a dry mouth
	rifaximin	If diarrhea continues after a total of two treatments, consider *C. difficile.*
Abdominal bloating/gas	Antispasmodics—dicyclomine hydrochloride (Bentyl)	
Psychological symptoms	Antidepressants—SSRIs	Generally, as a class, these agents may be helpful with chronic syndromes. Cost may be an issue.
Second Line		Generalized CNS effects
Predominant constipation	Continue osmotic laxatives.	
	linaclotide or lubiprostone	If not used first line
Predominant diarrhea	Antidiarrheal—diphenoxylate hydrochloride (Lomotil)	Monitor for anticholinergic effects.
Abdominal bloating/gas	Antispasmodics—hyoscyamine sulfate (Levsin, Levbid, Levsin SL)	
Psychological symptoms	Antidepressants—tricyclic agents (imipramine, desipramine, amitriptyline) (Tofranil, Norpramin, Elavil)	Onset of action and steady states vary with each drug.
Third Line		
Predominant constipation	Laxatives—bisacodyl (Dulcolax), senna concentrates (Senokot), emollient laxatives, docusate sodium (Colace), docusate calcium (Surfak), alosetron (Lotronex)	Caution with cardiac patients. Can aggravate abdominal cramping. Use only as additive to keep stools soft. Only approved providers can prescribe alosetron.
Abdominal bloating/gas	Antispasmodics—belladonna alkaloids (Donnatal), clidinium (Librax)	More severe generalized anticholinergic effects

working with the patient regarding dietary and lifestyle changes, education about the disease process, and reassurance about lack of organic causes. Patients with intermittent symptoms require the same initial approach, but addition of pharmacologic therapy can prove helpful, if only for the placebo effect of the drugs. Psychological counseling may also be helpful with these patients. Severe IBS requires all of these interventions and the addition of intensive psychotherapy. Patients with mild to intermittent symptoms can easily be managed in the primary care office with close monitoring initially, every 3 to 6 weeks, and then more routine care.

IBS is a disease of exacerbations and remissions, but up to 70% of patients respond to treatment within 12 to 18 months. Those with a shorter duration of symptoms and fewer psychological symptoms have a better prognosis. Referral to a specialist should occur when there is no relief

with any therapies or when the patient has atypical symptomatology. Some patients do not respond. Continued symptoms rarely need a reappraisal of the diagnosis, but appropriate testing should be performed.

PATIENT EDUCATION

Patient education needs to cover dietary modifications, psychological stresses, and lifestyle changes. Begin by acknowledging the patient's fears and concerns, and show that you take them seriously. According to current evidence-based research, patients can be reassured of the absence of organic disease based on the history and physical examination. The patient should be informed that this is a chronic disease and that IBS does not lead to cancer, colitis, or an altered life expectancy. Making the necessary dietary changes can be crucial for symptom relief,

CASE STUDY*

C.J. is a 71-year-old woman who presents for follow-up. She complains of hard, dry stools over the past week. She remembers reading an educational brochure she picked up in her pharmacy that suggested increasing her fiber and fluid intake, but this has not alleviated her problem. **C.J.'s** past medical conditions include hypertension and chronic renal insufficiency. She had a stroke 1 year ago with little or no residual. Her medications include verapamil SR 240 mg daily, lisinopril 10 mg orally once daily, calcium carbonate 1,250 mg twice daily orally, and aspirin 325 mg orally once daily.

DIAGNOSIS: CONSTIPATION

1. List specific goals of treatment for this patient.
2. What drug therapy would you prescribe? Why?
3. What are the parameters for monitoring the success of the therapy?
4. Discuss specific patient education based on the prescribed therapy.
5. List one or two adverse reactions for the selected agent that would cause you to change therapy.
6. What would be the choice for second-line therapy?
7. What OTC or alternative medications would be appropriate for this patient?
8. What dietary and lifestyle changes should be recommended for this patient?
9. Describe one or two drug–drug or drug–food interactions for this patient.

* Answers can be found online.

especially with mild symptoms. A multidisciplinary approach is often the best method of care, using the services of a dietitian and psychological counselor.

Drug Information

A variety of drugs are available to help control symptoms, and most have minimal side effects. However, the drugs need to be used in conjunction with stress relief techniques, identification of influencing factors, and education about the disease to help provide an improved quality of life.

Patient-Oriented Information Sources

Many resources exist for patients with IBS. One of the most comprehensive resources is the ACG, which covers many topics on GI health. The International Foundation of Functional Bowel Disorders also has a comprehensive Web site with resources for both patients and health care providers (**Box 30.11**).

Nutrition/Lifestyle Changes

A major focus of caring for patients with IBS is helping them assess their diet, making adjustments as necessary. A trial of removing foods that trigger symptoms such as those containing

lactose and gluten from the diet poses no risks to the patient and may have a benefit if it relieves symptoms.

Bibliography

Starred references are cited in the text.
*Akbar, A. W. (2009). Visceral hypersensitivity in irritable bowel syndrome: Molecular mechanisms and therapeutic agents. *Alimentary Pharmacology and Therapeutics, 30,* 423–435.
Alajbegovic, S., Sanders, J., Atherly, D., et al. (2012). Effectiveness of rifaximin and fluoroquinolones in preventing travelers' diarrhea (TD): A systematic review and meta-analysis. *Systematic Reviews, 1,* 39. Retrieved from http://www.systematicreviewsjournal.com/content/1/1/39
American Academy of Pediatrics, Provisional Committee on Quality Improvement, Subcommittee on Acute Gastroenteritis. (1996). Practice parameter: The management of acute gastroenteritis in young children. *Pediatrics, 97*(3), 424–435.
*American Dietetic Association. (2008). Position of the American Dietetic Association: Health implication of dietary fiber. *Journal of the American Dietetic Association, 108,* 1716–1731.
Annelis, M., & Koch, T. (2003). Constipation and the preached trio: Diet, fluid, intake, exercise. *International Journal of Nursing Studies, 40,* 843. Abstract obtained from Medline.
Baig, M., Zhao, R., Woodhouse, S., et al. (2002). Variability in serotonin and enterochromaffin cells in patients with colonic inertia and idiopathic diarrhea as compared to normal controls. *Colorectal Disease, 4,* 348.
Barr, W., & Smith, A. (2014). Acute diarrhea in adults. *American Family Physician, 89*(3), 180–189.
*Basson, M. (2015). Constipation. *eMedicine Drugs & Diseases.* Retrieved from http://emedicine.medscape.com/article/184704-overview October 20, 2015.
Bertram, S., Kurland, M., Lydick, E., et al. (2001). The patient's perspective of irritable bowel syndrome. *Journal of Family Practice, 50*(6), 521.
Besedovsky, A., & Bu, L. (2004). Across the developmental continuum of irritable bowel syndrome: Clinical and pathophysiologic considerations. *Current Gastroenterology Reports, 6*(3), 247. Abstract obtained from Medline.
*Bharucha, A. E., Pemberton, J. H., & Locke, G. R. (2013). American gastroenterological association technical review on constipation. *Gastroenterology, 144*(1), 218–238. Retrieved from http://doi.org/10.1053/j.gastro.2012.10.028

BOX 30.11 Patient Resources for Irritable Bowel Syndrome

http://www.gastro.org/generalPublic.html
http://www.aboutibs.org/
http://www.iffgd.org/index.html
http://digestive.niddk.nih.gov/ddiseases/pubs/ibs/

*Borowitz, S., Cox, D., Kovatchev, B., et al. (2005). Treatment of childhood constipation by primary care physicians: Efficacy and predictors of outcome. *Pediatrics, 115*(4), 873–877.

Bouhnik, Y., Neut, C., Raskine, L., et al. (2004). Prospective randomized, parallel-group trial to evaluate the effects of lactulose and polyethylene glycol-4000 on colonic flora in chronic idiopathic constipation. *Alimentary Pharmacology and Therapeutics, 19*, 889. Abstract retrieved from http://ejournals.ebsoco.com on May 11, 2004.

*Brandt, L., Chey, W., Foxx–Orenstein, A., et al. American College of Gastroenterology Task Force on Irritable Bowel Syndrome. (2009). An evidence-based position statement on the management of irritable bowel syndrome. *American Journal of Gastroenterology*, S2.

*Brandt, L., Prather, C., Quigley, E., et al. (2005). Systematic review on the management of chronic constipation in North America. *American Journal of Gastroenterology, 100*(Suppl. 1), S5–S21.

Breesel, J., Marcus, R., Venezia, R., et al. (2012). The etiology of severe acute gastroenteritis among adults visiting emergency departments in the United States. *Journal of Infectious Disease, 205*, (9), 1374–1381. doi: 10.1093/infdis/jis206.

Bundeff, A., & Woodiss, CB. (2014). Selective serotonin reuptake inhibitors for the treatment of irritable bowel syndrome. *Annals of Pharmacotherapy, 48*(6), 777–784. doi: 10.1177/1060028011458151.

*Burkett, D. P. (1993). Epidemiology of cancer of the colon and rectum. 1971. *Diseases of the Colon and Rectum, 36*(11), 1071–1082.

*Bushen, O., & Guerrant, R. (2003). Acute infectious diarrhea: Approach and management in the emergency department. *Topics in Emergency Medicine, 25*, 139.

*Camerilli, M. (2011). Opioid-induced constipation: Challenges and therapeutic opportunities. *American Journal of Gastroenterology, 106*, 835–842. doi: 10.1038/ajg.2011.30.

Camerilli, M., Drossman, D., Becker, G., et al. (2014). Emerging treatments in neurogastroenterology: A multidisciplinary working group consensus statement on opioid-induced constipation. *Neurogastroenterology & Motility, 26*, 1386–1395. doi: 10.1111/nmo.12417.

*Canavan, C., West, J., & Card, T. (2014). The epidemiology of irritable bowel syndrome. *Clinical Epidemiology, 6*, 71–80. Retrieved from http://doi.org/10.2147/CLEP.S40245.

Centers for Disease Control and Prevention. (1992). The management of acute diarrhea in children: Oral rehydration, maintenance, and nutritional therapy. *Morbidity and Mortality Weekly Report, 41*(No. RR-16), 1–20.

*Centers for Disease Control and Prevention. (2003). *Managing acute gastroenteritis among children: Oral rehydration, maintenance and nutritional therapy.* Atlanta, GA: MMWR.

*Centers for Disease Control and Prevention. (2005). *Guidelines for the management of acute diarrhea.* Washington, DC: Department of Health and Human Services.

Chaussade, S., & Minic, M. (2003). Comparison of efficacy and safety of two doses of two different polyethylene glycol-based laxatives in the treatment of constipation. *Alimentary Pharmacologic and Therapeutics, 17*, 165.

*Cherniak, E. P. (2013). Use of complementary and alternative medicine to treat constipation in the elderly. *Geriatric Gerontology International, 13*, 533–538. doi: 10.1111/ggi.12023.

Chey, W., Webster, L., Sostek, M., et al. (2014). Naloxegol for opioid-induced constipation in patients with noncancer pain. *New England Journal of Medicine, 370*, 2378–2396. doi: 10.1056/NEJMoa1310246.

*Clarke, T., Black, L., Stussman, B., et al. (2015). *Trends in the use of complementary health approaches among adults: United States, 2002–2012. National Health Statistics Reports; No. 79.* Hyattsville, MD: National Center for Health Statistics.

Clave, P. (2011). Treatment of IBS-D with 5-HT3 receptor antagonists vs. spasmolytic agents: Similar therapeutical effects from heterogeneous pharmacological targets. *Neurogastroenterology & Motility, 23*, 1051–1055. doi: 10.1111/j.136-2982.2011.01808.x.

*Connor, B., (2013). Chronic diarrhea in travelers. *Current Infectious Disease Reports, 15*(3), 203–210. doi: 10.1007/s11908-013-0328-2.

*Daley, A., Grimett, C., Roberts, L., et al. (2008). The effects of exercise upon symptoms and quality of life in patients diagnosed with irritable bowel syndrome: A randomised control trial. *International Journal of Sports Medicine, 29*(9), 778–782.

De la Cabada Bauche, J., & DuPont, H. L. (2011). New developments in Traveler's diarrhea. *Gastroenterology & Hepatology, 7*(2), 88–95.

DePontini, F., & Tonini, M. (2001). Irritable bowel syndrome: New agents targeting serotonin receptor subtypes. *Drugs, 61*(3), 317.

DuPont, H., Ericsson, C., Farthing, M., et al. (2009). Expert review of the evidence base for prevention of travelers' diarrhea. *Journal of Travel Medicine, 16*(3), 149–160. doi: 10.1111/j.1708-8305.2009.00299.x.

DuPont, H. L., and the Practice Parameters Committee of the American College of Gastroenterology. (1997). Guidelines on acute infectious diarrhea in adults. *American Journal of Gastroenterology, 92*, 1962–1975.

Ellis, M., & Meadows, S. (2002). What is the best therapy for constipation in infants? *Journal of Family Practice, 51*, 708. Retrieved from http://www.jpoline.com/content/2002/08/jfp_0802_0708c.asp on June 30, 2004.

Engsbro, A., Simren, M., & Bytzer, P. (2012). Short-term stability of subtypes in the irritable bowel syndrome: Prospective evaluation using the Rome III classification. *Alimentary Pharmacology and Therapeutics, 35*, 350–359. doi: 10.111/j.1365-2036.2011.04948.x.

Faidon-Marios, L., Goodkin, O., Thoua, N., et al. (2015). Irritable bowel syndrome. *Motility and Functional Bowel Disease Medicine, 43*(5), 266–270.

FDA. (2002). *Postmarket drug safety for patients and providers: Lotronex (alosetron hydrochloride) information.* Retrieved from http://www.fda.gov/Drugs/DrugSafety/PostmarketDrugSafetyInformationforPatientsandProviders/ucm110450.htm

Field, M. (2003). Intestinal ion transport and the pathophysiology of diarrhea. *Journal of Clinical Investigation, 111*, 931.

*Ford, A., Moayyedi, P., Lacy, B., et al. (2014). American College of Gastroenterology monograph on the management of irritable bowel syndrome and chronic idiopathic constipation. *American Journal of Gastroenterology, 109*, S2–S26. doi: 10.1038/ajg.2014.187.

Gallagher, C. (2003). A guideline-based approach for managing acute gastroenteritis in children. *Journal for Specialist in Pediatric Nursing, 8*(3), 107.

*Gordon, M., Naidoo, K., Akobeng, A. K., et al. (2012). Osmotic and stimulant laxatives for the management of childhood constipation. *Cochrane Database of Systematic Reviews, 7*, Art.N.CD009118. doi: 10.1002/14651858.CD009118.pub2.

Grodzinsky, E., Walter, S., Viktorsson, L., et al. (2014). More negative self-esteem and inferior coping strategies among patients diagnosed with IBS compared with patients without IBS case-control study in primary care. *BioMed Central Family Practice, 16*, 6. doi: 10.1186/s1287-015-0225-x.

*Grundmann, O. (2010). Irritable bowel syndrome: Epidemiology, diagnosis and treatment: An update for health-care practitioners. *Journal of Gastroenterology and Hepatology, 25*(4), 691–699.

*Grundmann, O., & Yoon, S. (2010). Irritable bowel syndrome: Epidemiology, diagnosis and treatment: An update for health-care practitioners. *Journal Gastroenterology Hepatology, 25*(4), 691–699. doi: 10.1111/j.1440-1746.2009.06120.x. Epub 2010 Jan 13.

*Guarino, A. L. (2009). Probiotics as prevention and treatment for diarrhea. *Current Opinion in Gastroenterology, 25*(1), 18–23.

*Guerrant, R., Van Gilden, T., Steines, T., et al. (2001). Practice guidelines for the management of infectious diarrhea. *Clinical Infectious Disease, 32*, 331.

*Hayes, P., Corish, C., O'Mahony, E., et al. (2014). A dietary survey of patients with irritable bowel syndrome. *Journal of Human Nutrition and Dietetics, 27*(Suppl. 2), 36–47. doi: 10.1111/jhn.12114. Epub 2013 May 9.

*Ho, K., You Mei Tan, C., Ashik Mohd Daud, M., et al. (2012). Stopping or reducing dietary fiber intake reduces constipation and its associated symptoms. *World Journal of Gastroenterology, 18*(33), 4593–4506. doi: 10.3748/wjg.v18.i33.4593.

*Jones, T. F., McMillian, M. B., Scallan, E., et al. (2007). A population-based estimate of the substantial burden of diarrhoeal disease in the United States: FoodNet, 1996–2003. *Epidemiology and Infection, 135*(2), 293–301. doi: 10.1017/S0950268806006765.

*Kamm, M., Mueller-Lissner, S., Wald, A., et al. (2011). Oral bisacodyl is effective and well-tolerated in patients with chronic constipation. *Clinical Gastroenterology and Hepatology, 9*, 577–583. doi: 10.1016/j.cgh.2011.03.026.

*Kaptchuk, T. J., Friedlander, E., Kelley, J. M., et al. (2010). Placebos without Deception: A randomized controlled trial in irritable bowel syndrome. *PloS One, 5*(12), e15591. doi: 10.1371/journal.pone.0015591.

*Kim-Jung, L., Holquist, C., & Phillips, J. (2004). FDA drug safety: Kaopectate reformulation and upcoming labeling changes. *Drug Topics.* Retrieved from www.drugtopics.com on October 26, 2015.

*Kumar, L., Barker, C., & Emmanuel, A. (2014). Opioid-induced constipation: Pathophysiology, clinical consequences, and management. *Gastroenterology Research and Practice*, Article ID 141737, 1–6. doi: 10.1155/2014/141737.

Lacy, B. E., Levenick, J. M., & Crowell, M. D. (2012). Linaclotide: A novel therapy for chronic constipation and constipation-predominant irritable bowel syndrome. *Gastroenterology & Hepatology, 8*(10), 653–660.

*Lenters, L., Das, J., & Bhutta, Z. (2013). Systematic review of strategies to increase use of oral rehydration solution at the household level. *BioMed Central Public Health, 13*(Suppl. 3), S28. Retrieved from http://www.biomedcentral.com/1471-2458/13/S3/S28

Leonard, J., & Baker, D. (2015). Naloxegol: Treatment for opioid-induced constipation in chronic non- cancer pain. *Annals of Pharmacotherapy, 49*(3), 360–365. doi: 10.1177/1060028014560191.

*Leung, L., Riutta, T., Kotecha, J., et al. (2011). Chronic constipation: An evidence-based review. *Journal of American Board Family Medicine, 24*(4), 436–445. doi: 10.3122/jabfm.2011.04.100272.

Loening-Bauke, V., Miele, E., & Staiano, A. (2004). Fiber (glucomannan) is beneficial in the treatment of childhood constipation. *Pediatrics, 113*, 259.

*Longstreth, G. E. (2006). Functional bowel disorders. *Gastroenterology, 130*(5), 1480–1491.

*Lovell, R., & Ford, A. (2012). Global prevalence of and risk factors for irritable bowel syndrome. *Clinical Gastroenterology and Hepatology, 10*(7), 712–721.

Malek, M., Curns, A., Holmn, R., et al. (2006). Diarrhea- and rotavirus-associated hospitalizations among children less than 5 years of age: United States, 1997 and 2000. *Pediatrics, 117*(6), 1887–1892. doi: 10.1542/peds.2005-2351.

*Müller-Lissner, S., Kamm, M., Scarpignato, C., et al. (2005). Myths and misconceptions about chronic constipation. *American Journal Gastroenterology, 100*(1), 232–242.

National Digestive Diseases Information Clearinghouse. (2003). *What I need to know about constipation* [Brochure] (NIH publication No. 03-2754).

National Digestive Diseases Information Clearinghouse. (2004). *Constipation in children* [Brochure] (NIH publication No. 04-4633).

Occhipinti, K., & Smith, J. (2012). Irritable bowel syndrome: A review and update. *Colon-Rectal Surgery, 25*, 46–52. doi: 10.1055/s-0032-13011759.

Piescik-Lech, M., Shamir, R., Guarino, A., et al. (2013). Review article: The management of acute gastroenteritis in children. *Alimentary Pharmacology and Therapeutics, 37*(3), 289–303. Review article: The management of acute gastroenteritis in children.

Pimentel, M., Lembo, A., Chey, W., et al. (2011). Rifaximin therapy for patients with irritable bowel syndrome without constipation. *New England Journal of Medicine, 364*, 22–32.

*Pomeranz, J. L., Taylor, L. M., & Austin, S. B. (2013). Over-the-counter and out-of-control: Legal strategies to protect youths from abusing products for weight control. *American Journal of Public Health, 103*(2), 220–225. Retrieved from http://doi.org/10.2105/AJPH.2012.300962

*Rajindrajith, S., & Devanarayana, N. M. (2011). Constipation in children: Novel insight into epidemiology, pathophysiology and management. *Journal of Neurogastroenterology and Motility, 17*(1), 35–47. doi: 10.5056/jnm.2011.17.1.35.

Rao, S. S., & Go, J. T. (2010). Update on the management of constipation in the elderly: New treatment options. *Clinical Interventions in Aging, 5*, 163–171.

*Sandhu, B. K., & Paul, S. P. (2014). Irritable bowel syndrome in children: Pathogenesis, diagnosis and evidence-based treatment. *World Journal of Gastroenterology, 20*(20), 6013–6023. Retrieved from http://doi.org/10.3748/wjg.v20.i20.6013

Sayuk, G., & Gyawali, C.P. (2015). Irritable bowel syndrome: Modern concepts and management options. *The American Journal of Medicine, 128*(8), 817–827. doi: 10.1016/j.amjmed.2015.01.036.

Sbahi, H., & Cash, B. (2015). Chronic constipation: A review of current literature. *Current Gastroenterology Reports, 17*, 47. doi: 10.1007/s11894-015-0471-z.

Scallan, E., Griffin, P. M., Angulo, F. J., et al. (2011). Foodborne illness acquired in the united states—unspecified agents. *Emerging Infectious Diseases, 17*(1), 16–22. Retrieved from http://doi.org/10.3201/eid1701.P21101.

*Simren, M. E. (2001). Food related gastrointestinal symptoms in irritable bowel syndrome. *Digestion, 63*(2), 108–115.

Singh, E., & Redfield, D. (2009). Prophylaxis for travelers' diarrhea. *Current Gastroenterology Reports, 11*, 297–300.

Sloots, C. E., & Felt-Bersma, R. J. (2003). Rectal sensorimotor characteristics in female patients with idiopathic constipation with or without paradoxical sphincter contraction. *Neurogastrology and Motility, 15*, 187.

Smith, C., Hellebusch, S., & Mandel, K. (2002). Patient and physician evaluation of a new bulk fiber laxative tablet. *Gastroenterology Nursing, 26*, 31.

*Sommers, T., Corban, C., Sengupta, N., et al. (2015). Emergency department burden of constipation in the United States from 2006 to 2011. *American Journal of Gastroenterology, 110*, 572–579. doi: 10.1038/ajg.2015.64.

Steffen, R., DuPont, H., Heusser, R., et al. (1986). Prevention of diarrhea by the tablet form of bismuth subsalicylate. *Antimicrobial Agents and Chemotherapy, 29*, 625–627.

Stessman, M. (2003). Biofeedback: Its role in treatment of chronic constipation. *Gastroenterology Nursing, 26*, 251.

*Suares, N., & Ford, A., (2011). Prevalence of, and risk factors for chronic idiopathic constipation in the community systematic review a meta-analysis. *American Journal of Gastroenterology, 106*, 1582–1591. doi: 10.1038/ajg.2011.164; published online May 2, 2011.

*Surawicz, C., Brandt, L., Binion, D., et al. (2013). Guidelines for diagnosis, treatment, and prevention of *Clostridium difficile* infections. *American Journal of Gastroenterology, 108*, 478–498. doi: 10.1038/ajg.2013.4.

Talley, N. J., Jones, M., Nuyts, G., et al. (2003). Risk factors for chronic constipation. *American Journal of Gastroenterology, 98*(5), 1107. Abstract obtained from MedLine.

Thielman, N., & Guerrant, R. (2004). Acute infectious diarrhea. *New England Journal of Medicine, 350*, 38.

Toner, B., Emmott, S., Myran, D., et al. (1999). *Cognitive-behavioral treatment of irritable bowel syndrome: The brain-gut connection.* New York, NY: Guilford Press.

Verne, N., & Cerda, J. (1997). Irritable bowel syndrome: Streamlining the diagnosis. *Postgraduate Medicine, 102*(3), 197.

Versa, T., Seppo, L., Marteau, P., et al. (1998). Relief of irritable bowel syndrome in subjective lactose intolerance. *American Journal of Clinical Nutrition, 67*, 710–715.

Wald, A. (2006). Chronic constipation: Advances in management. *Neurogastroenterology and Motility, 19*(1), 4–10.

*Wald, A. (2007). Appropriate use of laxatives in management of constipation. *Current Gastroenterology Reports*, 410–414.

*Weinberg, D., Smalley, W., Heidelbaugh, J., et al. (2014). American Gastroenterological Association Institution guideline on the pharmacological management of irritable bowel syndrome. *Gastroenterology, 147*, 1146–1148. doi: 10.1053/j.gastro.2014.09.001.

*Yang, J., Fox, M., Cong, Y., et al. (2014). Lactose intolerance in irritable bowel syndrome patients with diarrhoea: The roles of anxiety, activation of the innate mucosal immune system and visceral sensitivity. *Alimentary Pharmacology and Therapeutics, 39*, 302–311. doi: 10.111/apt12582.

Yao, X., Yang, Y. S., Cui, L. H., et al. (2012). Subtypes of irritable bowel syndrome on Rome III criteria: A multicenter study. *Journal of Gastroenterology & Hepatology, 27*(4), 760–765. doi: 10.1111/j.1440-1746.2011.06930.x.

31 Inflammatory Bowel Disease

David Dinh

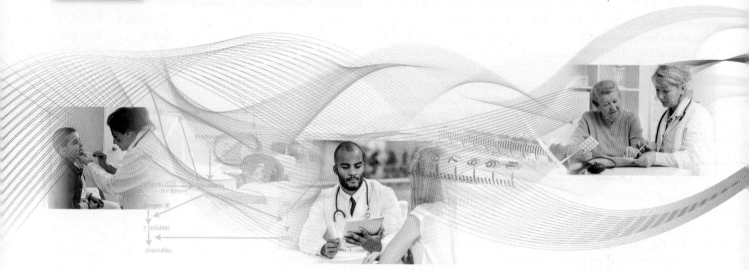

Inflammatory bowel disease (IBD) is a generic term used to describe two main chronic inflammatory conditions of the gastrointestinal (GI) tract: Crohn disease (CD) and ulcerative colitis (UC). Although these conditions are similar in clinical presentation, CD is a chronic inflammatory disease characterized by transmural lesions located at any point on the GI tract, whereas UC is a chronic disease consisting of mucosal inflammation limited to the rectum and colon. IBD affects approximately 1 million Americans. In 1998, the prevalence of CD was estimated to be approximately 359,000, and for UC, it is estimated to be 619,000 (National Institute of Diabetes and Digestive and Kidney Diseases, 2013). The incidence of UC has been relatively stable over the past five decades, whereas the incidence of CD is rising (Kornbluth & Sachar, 2010; Lichtenstein, Diamond, et al., 2009; Lichtenstein, Hanauer, et al., 2009). Both conditions are more common in Whites than in any other race, and those of Jewish descent have a three- to sixfold greater incidence than does the non-Jewish population. IBD shows no gender predilection and is usually first diagnosed in men or women between ages 15 and 25 (Kappelman et al., 2007). Although the mortality rate is low for the disease, it significantly affects the patient's overall mental status, physical health, and quality of life. The most common emotional issues surrounding uncontrolled IBD appear to be anger, frustration, depression, and low self-esteem. These issues usually stem from the patient's inability to participate in routine activities, leading to a decreased quality of life. The disease has a negative impact on social interactions and daily functional status, leading to decreased productivity and attendance at work or school, decreased social engagements, and loss of independence. Health-related issues mirror those related to poor GI absorption, including nutritional deficiencies, electrolyte

abnormalities, dehydration, cachexia, and iron deficiency anemia. Fatigue and lack of sleep are also common in patients with IBD. In addition, patients with long-standing CD may also be at risk for adenocarcinoma of the GI tract (Pederson et al., 2010). All of these may result in frequent hospitalizations, altered lifestyle, and poor general health. Overall, in 2004, IBD had an estimated financial burden of $328 million in indirect health care costs and over $1.8 billion dollars in direct costs (Everhart, 2008).

CAUSES

The etiology of CD and UC is related to the dysregulation of immunologic mechanisms. The inflammatory nature of the condition has led researchers to believe that an autoimmune mechanism may predispose patients to IBD. The development of IBD may be attributed to a defect in the GI mucosal barrier that results in enhanced permeability and increased uptake of proinflammatory molecules and infectious agents. Tissue biopsies of the GI mucosal lining from patients with IBD reveal a high proportion of immunologic cytokines, including tumor necrosis factor (TNF), leukotrienes, and interleukin-1 (IL-1). A few bacterial and viral organisms have been associated with disease progression, including *Mycobacterium paratuberculosis*, measles virus, and *Listeria monocytogenes*; however, none has been definitively correlated with IBD.

Much of the recent evidence suggests that IBD is a complex genetic disorder. The high incidence of IBD in the Jewish population supports a genetic component of the etiology of CD and UC. A study comparing relatives of patients with IBD with the general population found a 10-fold increase in risk of development of IBD in those with familial occurrence. In addition, studies in twins support the notion that the disease course and occurrence of CD is genetically influenced (Halfverson et al., 2007). Recently, the NOD2/CARD 15 gene has been associated with CD. Those who carry two copies of the risk alleles have been noted to be at higher risk for developing CD than others. The relationship between IBD and other genetic mutations and polymorphisms is currently being investigated. Until there are sufficient data to link a specific genetic mutation to IBD, the identification of genetic polymorphisms remains a research tool and not a clinical diagnostic tool.

Other factors, including psychological well-being and environmental triggers, may contribute to the exacerbation of IBD, although these factors do not have a predictable effect over a large population. Various studies have associated isolated mental instability or stressful events with IBD exacerbations, but a positive correlation between psychiatric illness and IBD is unsupported.

Environmental factors, including geographic location, dietary habits, drug-induced factors, and smoking status, are theorized to affect CD and UC exacerbations. IBD is more prevalent in the northern parts of the United States as well as in England and Scandinavian countries rather than the Mediterranean countries, suggesting that temperature or weather patterns may have an impact on CD or UC. Various dietary habits such as high sucrose consumption have been identified as exacerbating CD or UC, but no one particular food or group of foods seems to have a reliable effect in a large population. Oral contraceptive use and cigarette smoking have variable effects on CD versus UC; oral contraceptives and nicotine have been found to exacerbate CD, but not UC (Khalili et al., 2013). In addition, recently, the use of the antiacne product isotretinoin (Accutane) has been associated with the development of IBD, especially UC. The exact mechanism by which isotretinoin may cause IBD is unknown. However, isotretinoin does affect many immunologic mechanisms that may trigger IBD (Crockett et al., 2010; Reddy et al., 2006).

PATHOPHYSIOLOGY

Differentiating CD from UC is difficult because of their similar clinical presentations. Hallmark symptoms of IBD are bloody diarrhea, weight loss, and fever. Generally, CD can be distinguished from UC based only on endoscopic findings. The GI mucosal lining in CD is usually characterized by discontinuous, narrowed, thick, edematous, leathery patches with the presence of lesions, ulcerations, fissures, strictures, granulomas, and fibrosis. Fistulas and abscess formation occur most commonly in patients with deep transmural lesions. Granulomas and fistulas usually occur exclusively in patients with CD. UC usually affects the rectum and areas proximal, possibly extending throughout the entire large intestine with continuous, superficial uniform inflammation and ulceration. Other pathologic findings are rare in UC but may occur in patients with chronic, long-standing inflammation (**Table 31.1**).

TABLE 31.1

Common Signs and Symptoms of Crohn Disease versus Ulcerative Colitis

	Ulcerative Colitis	Crohn Disease
Signs		
Abdominal mass	0	++
Fistulas	+/−	++
Strictures	+	++
Small bowel involvement	+/−	++
Rectal involvement	++	+/++
Extraintestinal disease		
Arthritis/arthralgia	++	++
Erythema nodosum	+/−	+/−
Abnormal liver function test values	++	++
Iritis/uveitis	+/−	+/−
Ankylosing spondylitis	+	+
Growth retardation	+	+
Toxic megacolon	+	+/−
Recurrence after colectomy	0	+
Malignancy	+	+/−
Symptoms		
Fever	+	++
Diarrhea	++	++
Weight loss	++	++
Rectal bleeding	++	+
Abdominal pain	+	++

Key: +, common; ++, very common; +/−, possible; 0, rare.

Extraintestinal complications, including skin malformations, liver disease, joint deformities, and ocular manifestations, may also occur, although they are more common in CD than UC because of the more aggressive nature of CD, resulting in a higher probability of malabsorption of nutrients (see **Table 31.1**). Because the complications affect a variety of organ systems and result in nonspecific complaints, it is difficult to associate the complaints with CD or UC; however, it is important to be aware of the complications because their presence indicates poorly controlled disease.

DIAGNOSTIC CRITERIA

Because the clinical presentation of patients with CD or UC is nonspecific, definitive diagnosis relies on endoscopic or radiologic studies. Initial diagnosis of IBD must rule out other causes of bloody diarrhea such as infectious causes and other colitis conditions. Visualization techniques must be used to differentiate CD from UC because of their similar clinical presentations. Usually, endoscopic techniques are preferred over radiographs and radioactive isotopes because endoscopy permits direct visualization of the mucosal lining with increased specificity as to the extent of lesions, ulcerations, and inflammation as well as provides the opportunity to obtain mucosal specimens for biopsy and further evaluation. The risk of mucosal perforation, however, may limit the use of endoscopic technology in patients with severely active disease.

Sigmoidoscopy or colonoscopy is preferred as a first-line diagnostic procedure; however, for CD, an endogastroduodenoscopy may also be required to visualize the upper GI tract. Radiologic studies with contrast, including either an upper GI series or barium enema, may be preferred in patients with severely active symptoms to decrease the risk of mucosal perforation.

Antibody tests are sometimes helpful in determining the diagnosis of CD or UC. The perinuclear antineutrophil cytoplasmic antibody (pANCA) and/or the anti-*Saccharomyces cerevisiae* antibody (ASCA) tests may be positive in patients with IBD, but there is a significant rate of false-negative results, since only 60% to 70% of patients with CD or UC are actually antibody positive (Kornbluth & Sachar, 2010). The combination of a positive pANCA and a negative ASCA may indicate the presence of UC, whereas the opposite may indicate CD. However, the combined result still has a significant percentage of false negatives. Therefore, these tests are not used routinely to differentiate UC from CD.

INITIATING DRUG THERAPY

CD and UC share many clinical characteristics with pseudomembranous colitis, irritable bowel disease, peptic ulcer disease (PUD), traveler's diarrhea, colon cancer, and hemorrhoids. Evaluation of patients with suspected IBD must include a complete history focusing on recent use of antibiotics, recent international travel, diet history, use of laxatives or antidiarrheals, frequency and quality of daily bowel movements, history of PUD, and family history of IBD to rule out similar presenting conditions.

Physical examination should include assessment of vital signs and weight loss, a thorough abdominal examination, and special attention to extraintestinal complications. Guaiac testing and stool cultures may be helpful in ruling out PUD or infectious causes. Although there are no reliable surrogate laboratory markers that may indicate the presence of CD or UC, baseline laboratory studies, including electrolytes, liver panel, complete blood count (CBC), and hematology panel, are important in assessing the severity of the condition and patient well-being.

Initiation of proper drug therapy is based on the severity and extent of disease. CD may present as luminal or fistulizing disease. CD confined to the GI lumen can initially present as mild, moderate, or severe disease and is not predictable in its course. Fistulizing disease also has a varied clinical course, whereby certain patients may never experience a fistula and others may develop one early in the course of the disease. Treatment of fistulizing disease is typically more aggressive than that of luminal disease and may vary depending on the location of the fistula (bowel to bladder, bowel to skin, etc.). UC may be confined to the distal colon and rectum or may extend throughout

the colon. Due to the location of the disease, treatment options for distal UC are greater than for extensive disease. The Working Definitions of Crohn's Disease Activity or the Criteria for Severity of Ulcerative Colitis may be used as a guide to determine severity (**Tables 31.2** and **31.3**). Both scales are frequently used in clinical trials; however, they are modified for use in clinical practice. There are many validated scales used to assess the severity of UC; however, there is not one gold standard. Each scale highlights specific subjective and objective parameters that should be evaluated when assessing the progression of disease. Both scales highlight certain key features when predicting the severity of the condition, such as the frequency of stools per day and the presence of abdominal pain, fever, and anemia.

Treatment for IBD consists of aminosalicylates, corticosteroids, immunosuppressive agents, antibiotics, and biological agents. The decision to use one or a combination of these agents is based on the presence of CD versus UC, the severity of the disease, and whether treatment is targeted at active disease or maintenance of remission. In general, aminosalicylates are used for treating mild to moderate exacerbations of UC and CD

TABLE 31.2

Working Definitions of Crohn's Disease Activity

Mild to Moderate
- Ambulatory patients
- Able to tolerate oral alimentation
- No evidence of:
  - Dehydration
  - High fevers
  - Rigors
  - Prostration
  - Abdominal tenderness
  - Painful mass
  - Abdominal obstruction
- 10% weight loss

Moderate to Severe
- Failed treatment for mild to moderate disease OR
- Have
  - High fever
  - >10% weight loss
  - Abdominal pain/tenderness
  - Intermittent nausea or vomiting (without obstructive findings)
  - Significant anemia

Severe to Fulminant
- Persistent symptoms despite outpatient steroid therapy OR
- Have
  - High fever
  - Persistent vomiting
  - Intestinal obstruction
  - Rebound tenderness
  - Cachexia
  - Abscess

Remission
- Asymptomatic without inflammatory sequelae
- Not dependent on steroids

TABLE 31.3

Criteria for Severity of Ulcerative Colitis

Mild UC
- <4 stools daily (with or without blood)
- No presence of anemia, fever, or tachycardia
- Normal erythrocyte sedimentation rate (ESR)

Moderate UC
- >4 stools daily
- Minimal anemia, fever, or tachycardia

Severe UC
- >6 bloody stools daily
- Positive fever, tachycardia, anemia, or elevated ESR

Fulminant UC
- >10 stools daily
- Continuous bleeding
- Abdominal tenderness and distention
- Anemia requiring blood transfusion
- Colonic dilation

as well as for maintaining remission in IBD. Corticosteroids are used to treat acute exacerbations and should not be used chronically to maintain remission. Immunosuppressive agents are used for the purposes of maintaining remission in IBD, whereas intravenous (IV) cyclosporine is used in a limited population to treat severely active, steroid-refractory UC. Antibiotics are reserved for treating and maintaining remission in patients with mild CD. Biologic agents are typically reserved for inducing and maintaining remission in patients with steroid-refractory CD; however, the current recommendation is to use biologics in combination with thiopurines to induce remission in moderately severe CD (**Table 31.4**).

Goals of Drug Therapy

Because no pharmacologic cure is available for CD or UC, the goals of treatment focus on symptom management and quality-of-life issues. With proper treatment, the patient should be able to:

- resume normal daily activities
- restore general physical and mental well-being
- attain appropriate nutritional status
- maintain remission of disease
- decrease the number and frequency of exacerbations
- decrease side effects related to medications
- increase life expectancy

Ideally, patients should expect to recover from an acute exacerbation within 2 to 4 weeks, have minimal exacerbations throughout the year, and participate in any desired activity.

Aminosalicylates

Aminosalicylates remain the gold standard for the treatment of mild to moderate CD and UC. Although the exact mechanism of action is unknown, these drugs decrease inflammation in the GI tract by inhibiting prostaglandin synthesis, which results in a decrease in various immune mediators,

TABLE 31.4

Overview of Agents Used to Treat Inflammatory Bowel Disease

Generic (Trade) Name and Dosage	Selected Adverse Events	Contraindications	Special Considerations
Aminosalicylates			
sulfasalazine (Azulfidine, Azulfidine EN) Start: 500 mg twice daily Range: 1–8 g/d	Stevens-Johnson syndrome, rash, photosensitivity, nausea, vomiting, skin discoloration, agranulocytosis, crystalluria, hepatitis	Sulfa allergy, aspirin allergy, G6PD deficiency	Most efficacious at high doses Drug released in the proximal colon Available in enteric-coated tablets Dosage increases may occur as frequently as every other day.
oral mesalamine (Apriso, Asacol HD, Delzicol, Lialda, Pentasa) Start: depends on product Range: 1–4.8 g/d	Nausea, headache, malaise, abdominal pain, diarrhea	Aspirin allergy, G6PD deficiency	Products released differently in the GI tract May increase dose as frequently as every other day
rectal mesalamine (Rowasa Enema, Canasa suppository) Suppository Start: 1 g at bedtime Range: 1 g/d Enema Start: 4 g at bedtime Range: 1–4 g/d	Malaise, abdominal pain	Aspirin allergy, G6PD deficiency	Only for distal ulcerative colitis, proctitis Suppository is most effective in sigmoid colon, and enema may treat distal and sigmoid colon.

TABLE 31.4

Overview of Agents Used to Treat Inflammatory Bowel Disease (*Continued*)

Generic (Trade) Name and Dosage	Selected Adverse Events	Contraindications	Special Considerations

olsalazine (Dipentum)
  Start: 500 mg twice daily
  Range: 1–2 g
	Nausea, headache, malaise, abdominal pain, diarrhea	Aspirin allergy, G6PD deficiency	Drug released in proximal colon
			May increase dose as frequently as every other day
			Higher incidence of diarrhea

balsalazide (Colazide)
  Start: 1.5 g twice daily
  Range: 1.5–6.75 g
	Headache, abdominal pain, diarrhea	Aspirin allergy, G6PD deficiency	Only approved for treatment of mild to moderate ulcerative colitis

Selected Corticosteroids			

prednisone (Orasone, Deltasone)
  Start: 40–60 mg daily
  Range: 10–100 mg
	Hyperglycemia, increased appetite, insomnia, anxiety, tremors, hypertension, fluid retention, electrolyte imbalances	Active GI bleeding	Taper patient off steroids within 1–2 mo of initiation to decrease risk of long-term side effects.

oral methylprednisolone (Medrol)
  Start: 20–50 mg daily
  Range: 10–100 mg
	Same as above	Same as above	Same as above

IV methylprednisolone (Solu-Medrol)
  Start: 5–10 mg q6h
  Range: 10–50 mg
	Same as above	Same as above	IV treatment used for severe exacerbations
			Treatment duration should be a maximum of 7–14 d, then switch to oral therapy.

rectal hydrocortisone suppositories (Anusol-HC)
 	
  Start: 25 mg twice daily
  Range: 25–100 mg
	Same as above	Used only for distal ulcerative colitis treatment	

hydrocortisone enema (Cortenema)
  Start: 100 mg bedtime
  Range: 100 mg/d
	Enema is more effective than suppositories for distal colitis.		

IV hydrocortisone (Solu-Cortef)
  Start: 50–100 twice daily
  Range: 25–150 twice daily
	Same as above	Active GI bleeding	IV treatment used for severe exacerbations
			Treatment duration should be a maximum of 7–14 d, then switch to oral therapy.

dexamethasone (Decadron)
  Start: 5–15 mg daily
  Range: 2–20 mg/d
	Same as above	Same as above	Has longer onset of action than other agents

oral budesonide (Entocort EC)
  Start: 9 mg/day
  Maintenance: 6 mg/d for 3 mo
	Minimal nausea	Same as above	Minimal systemic absorption
			Taper after 8 wk of therapy.
			Effective for mild to moderately active luminal CD and maintenance

Selected Immunosuppressives			

azathioprine (Imuran)
  Start: 50 mg/d
  Range: 2–2.5 mg/kg
	Pancreatitis, fever, arthralgias, nausea, rash, agranulocytosis, diarrhea, malaise, hepatotoxicity	Pregnancy, active liver disease, bone marrow suppression	Decrease dose for patients with severe renal dysfunction

6-mercaptopurine (Purinethol)
  Start: 50 mg/d
  Range: 1–2.5 mg/kg
	Same as above	Same as above	Same as above

(*Continued*)

TABLE 31.4

Overview of Agents Used to Treat Inflammatory Bowel Disease (*Continued*)

Generic (Trade) Name and Dosage	Selected Adverse Events	Contraindications	Special Considerations

oral methotrexate (Rheumatrex)
    Start: 5 mg three times a week
    Range: 5–7.5 mg three times a week
	Hepatic cirrhosis and fibrosis, neutropenia, pneumonitis, skin rash, nausea, diarrhea	Same as above	Same as above

IV cyclosporine Start: 4–8 mg/kg/d	Hypertension, nephrotoxicity, superinfection, hypomagnesemia	Renal failure, hepatic failure	Only used for severely acute UC refractory to steroids; total duration of therapy 7–10 d; has many drug interactions

Selected Antibiotics
metronidazole (Flagyl)
    Start: 20 mg/kg/d
    Range: 10–20 mg/kg/d
	Nausea, diarrhea, disulfiram reaction, metallic taste, peripheral paresthesias, dizziness	Liver failure, renal failure, first trimester of pregnancy, uncontrolled seizure disorder	Should not be used with alcohol
			Most efficacious if used chronically >3 mo

ciprofloxacin (Cipro)
    Start: 500 mg twice daily
    Range: 500–2,000 mg/d
	Dizziness, nausea, diarrhea, photosensitivity	Children <12 y, pregnancy, uncontrolled seizure disorder	May cause arthropathies in patients <12 y
			Must be administered 2 h before or after divalent and trivalent cations

Tumor Necrosis Factor Inhibitors
IV infliximab (Remicade)
    Start: 5 mg/kg
    Range: 5–10 mg/kg
	Infusion reactions (urticaria, dyspnea, hypotension), TB, invasive fungal infections, lymphoma, lupus-like syndrome	Class III/IV heart failure, active TB, hepatitis B or other infections	For severe, refractory UC and luminal and fistulizing CD; administered over 2 h as a single infusion
			Induction regimen dosed at weeks 0, 2, and 6; maintenance regimen dosed every 8 wk

adalilimumab (Humira)
    Start: 160 mg SQ
    Maintenance: 40 mg every week or every other week
	Opportunistic infections (TB, fungal, bacterial, viral), lymphoma and other cancers, injection site reactions (erythema, pain, swelling)	Active TB, hepatitis B, or other infections	For luminal CD; induction regimen 160 mg initially and 80 mg at week 2

certolizumab pegol (Cimzia)
    Start: 400 mg at baseline, week 2, and week 4
    Maintenance: 400 mg every 4 wk
	Opportunistic infections (TB, fungal, bacterial, viral), lymphoma and other cancers, injection site reactions (erythema, pain, swelling)	Active TB, hepatitis B, or other infections	For luminal CD

Selective Adhesion Molecule Inhibitors IV natalizumab (Tysabri) 300 mg IV every 4 wk	Infusion reactions (urticaria, dyspnea, hypotension), opportunistic infections (TB, fungal, bacterial, viral) progressive multifocal leukoencephalopathy (PML), hepatotoxicity	Active TB, hepatitis B, or other infections, current or history of PML	Taper corticosteroid therapy according to clinical response; discontinue natalizumab if therapeutic benefit is not seen within first 12 wk of therapy.

IV vedolizumab (Entyvio)
    Start: 300 mg IV at baseline, week 2, and week 6
    Maintenance: 300 mg IV every 8 wk
	Infusion reactions (urticaria, dyspnea, hypotension), TB, invasive fungal infections, lymphoma, lupus-like syndrome	Active TB, hepatitis B, or other infections	Taper corticosteroid therapy off starting at week 6 of vedolizumab therapy.

G6PD, glucose-6-phosphate dehydrogenase.

including IL-1, cyclooxygenase, and thromboxane synthase. Therapy with these agents may improve symptoms within 1 week of initiating therapy or dosage adjustment. However, patients may need to take these agents long term to prevent exacerbations. Although they are safe for use in most patients, aminosalicylates are contraindicated in patients with aspirin allergy or glucose-6-phosphate dehydrogenase deficiency. Sulfasalazine is also contraindicated in patients who are hypersensitive to sulfa products (see **Table 31.4**). All of these agents must be used at maximum doses for maximum therapeutic benefit, although the incidence of side effects also increases with increased doses.

Sulfasalazine

Sulfasalazine (Azulfidine, Azulfidine EN) is efficacious and cost-effective for CD and UC therapy but has a limited role because of its unfavorable side effect profile. Sulfasalazine is a combination product that is cleaved in the proximal colon by bacterial azo-reductases to release sulfapyridine and mesalamine. The mesalamine compound is responsible for virtually all of the therapeutic effect, whereas sulfapyridine is responsible for many of the side effects associated with sulfasalazine. Sulfasalazine may be administered up to four times a day; the most effective and maximum daily dosage is 8 g daily.

Mesalamine

Mesalamine (Asacol, Rowasa, Pentasa, Lialda, Apriso, Canasa) is available in various formulations, including oral tablets, oral capsules, enemas, and rectal suppositories. Each formulation is released in various areas of the GI tract, allowing for targeted drug therapy; however, in clinical trials, the capsules and tablets had similar efficacy at equivalent doses. Asacol, which is one of the oral tablet products, is formulated with an acrylic resin coating that disintegrates at a pH of 7, allowing the active ingredient to be released in the distal ileum and colon. Similarly, Lialda, another oral tablet formulation, has a coating that disintegrates at a pH of 6 to 7, and the core of the tablet forms a matrix that is released across a pH of 6.8 to 7.2. Pentasa, which is a sustained-release capsule, has ethyl-cellulose-coated granules that allow for the slow release of the drug beginning in the proximal small intestine and continuing throughout the colon. This formulation has slightly different pharmacokinetics than Apriso, which is also a delayed-release capsule. Apriso capsules are enteric coated; they disintegrate at a pH above 6 and also contain granules that are formulated in a polymer matrix for extended release. Because each of the oral products has different pharmacokinetics, the dosing interval for the products ranges from once to four times a day (see **Table 31.4**). The rectal suppositories are used primarily for UC-associated proctitis, whereas the enema delivers mesalamine to the distal and sigmoid colon. The enema is typically given at bedtime to allow for direct contact of the drug with the mucosa for at least 8 hours. In patients with distal UC, a combination of oral and rectal mesalamine may

be an appropriate therapeutic option. Studies have shown that combination mesalamine therapy is more effective than either single mesalamine formulation.

Olsalazine

Olsalazine (Dipentum), the third aminosalicylate preparation, consists of two mesalamine molecules joined by an azo-bond. As with sulfasalazine, the azo-bond is cleaved by bacterial azo-reductases in the GI tract, allowing the drug to be released in the proximal colon. It is administered twice daily, with patients taking up to 8 capsules per day for a total dosage of 2 g/d. Although each tablet of olsalazine has twice as much active ingredient as do the mesalamine capsules, the efficacy is minimally enhanced.

Balsalazide

Balsalazide (Colazal) is a combination product consisting of 5-aminosalicylic acid (mesalamine), the therapeutically active portion of the molecule, and 4-aminobenzoyl-alanine, an inert moiety. The product is cleaved by bacterial azo-reductases in the colon to release the active compound. Each capsule contains granules of balsalazide that are insoluble in acid and designed to be delivered to the colon intact. It is administered three times a day, up to 9 capsules per day, for a total dosage of 6.75 g/d, equaling 2.4 g/d of pure mesalamine. Currently, it has been studied only for use in mild to moderate UC in both adults and children. Side effects and contraindications are similar to those of mesalamine.

Adverse Events

Mesalamine, olsalazine, and balsalazide are poorly absorbed from the GI tract and thus are considered primarily topical agents, with limited systemic side effects and drug interactions. The major side effects of mesalamine include headache, malaise, abdominal pain, and diarrhea. Olsalazine has a similar side effect profile but has a higher incidence of diarrhea than mesalamine. Initially, diarrhea may not be easily distinguished from an IBD exacerbation, and therefore, close monitoring of improvement of symptoms is essential. If the balsalazide capsules are opened and sprinkled in food, teeth staining may occur. In rare instances, mesalamine, olsalazine, and balsalazide have been associated with renal function impairment; therefore, renal function should be monitored during therapy. Sulfapyridine is absorbed systemically, accounting for many of the side effects and drug interactions incurred by sulfasalazine. Common adverse effects include nausea, vomiting, photosensitivity, oligospermia, and skin discoloration, which may be tolerable for most patients. Severe adverse reactions associated with sulfasalazine include Stevens-Johnson syndrome, agranulocytosis, crystalluria, pancreatitis, and hepatitis, which may necessitate discontinuation of therapy. Sulfasalazine is known to decrease folate levels; therefore, patients taking sulfasalazine should be supplemented with folic acid. Although drug interactions with sulfasalazine are limited, it may significantly decrease the effect of warfarin (Coumadin), and therefore, close monitoring of the international normalized ratio is essential.

Corticosteroids

Corticosteroids are used intermittently to treat acute IBD exacerbations only. Corticosteroids allow for immunosuppression and prostaglandin inhibition when the disease fails to respond to aminosalicylate therapy. Corticosteroids may be used in conjunction with aminosalicylates, immunosuppressants, or biologic agents or as monotherapy to treat acute exacerbations. Corticosteroids with relatively quick onset of action and high glucocorticoid activity, such as prednisone (Orasone, Deltasone) and methylprednisolone (Medrol), are desirable in the treatment of CD or UC. Controlled-release oral budesonide (Entocort EC) is a unique corticosteroid due to its long-acting formulation and limited potential for absorption from the GI tract, thus theoretically leading to a localized effect in the GI lumen with minimal systemic side effects. Oral budesonide has been used as the treatment of choice in patients with mild to moderate exacerbations of CD in combination with aminosalicylates or as monotherapy.

Dosage

Doses equivalent to oral prednisone 40 to 60 mg/d are initiated in patients with mild or moderate exacerbations of CD or UC. A beneficial effect is usually seen with 7 to 10 days of therapy. Patients with mild to moderate exacerbations of distal UC can be treated with oral or rectal corticosteroids for approximately 4 to 8 weeks, after which drug dosages are tapered. Hydrocortisone is the only rectal corticosteroid enema formulation available for use in distal UC exacerbations. There are many tapering regimens that have been studied. The most common is a 5- to 10-mg weekly taper until a daily dose of 20 mg is reached, at which time the dose is tapered by 2.5 mg/week. In severe exacerbations, patients should receive 3 to 10 days of IV corticosteroid therapy and then switch to oral corticosteroid therapy for the remainder of the treatment period (see **Table 31.4**).

Adverse Events

Short-term corticosteroid use (less than 3 months) is associated with increased glucose levels, increased appetite, insomnia, anxiety, tremors, and increased fluid retention, leading to increases in blood pressure and electrolyte imbalances. Although discontinuation of therapy as a result of these side effects is not recommended with short-term corticosteroid treatment, routine monitoring is necessary.

Long-term corticosteroid use is associated with decreased bone density, leading to osteoporosis; fat redistribution, leading to the characteristic "buffalo hump"; decreased prostaglandin synthesis, resulting in gastric and duodenal ulcers; hypertriglyceridemia; hypokalemia; cataracts; and hirsutism. Therefore, long-term treatment with corticosteroids is not

recommended. However, if patients are taking recurrent steroid therapy for recurrent exacerbations, monitoring for these side effects is imperative.

Interactions

Many corticosteroids are substrates of the cytochrome P-450 isoenzyme 3A4, including prednisone, prednisolone, methylprednisolone, and budesonide. Therefore, agents that inhibit or induce this enzyme system, such as ketoconazole, clarithromycin, phenytoin, and pioglitazone, may alter the efficacy of the corticosteroid. Budesonide requires an acidic environment (pH less than 5.5) to be released, so agents that inhibit acid production or neutralize acid in the GI tract (i.e., histamine-2 antagonists, proton pump inhibitors, antacids) may limit the effectiveness of budesonide. Corticosteroids may also decrease the effectiveness of antidiabetic and antihypertensive agents due to their ability to increase blood glucose levels and blood pressure.

Immunosuppressive Agents

Immunosuppressive agents are used in IBD as adjunctive treatment with aminosalicylates to induce and maintain remission if exacerbations occur while the patient is being tapered off corticosteroid therapy or if frequent exacerbations occur with maximum dosages of aminosalicylates. IV cyclosporine is an exception: it is solely used to treat severe, acute exacerbations of UC when the patient is refractory to corticosteroids.

Azathioprine and 6-Mercaptopurine

Azathioprine (Imuran) and 6-mercaptopurine (Purinethol) are antimetabolites that act as purine antagonists to inhibit the synthesis of protein, ribonucleic acid (RNA), and deoxyribonucleic acid (DNA). By doing so, azathioprine and 6-mercaptopurine decrease the production of various inflammatory mediators. Because 6-mercaptopurine is the active metabolite of azathioprine, these agents are similar in efficacy, side effect profile, and dosing frequency (see **Table 31.4**). Although these agents have a short plasma half-life of approximately 1 to 2 hours, both have active metabolites with long half-lives of 3 to 13 days, resulting in optimal therapeutic effects within 10 to 15 weeks of initiation of therapy. 6-Mercaptopurine is metabolized by the enzyme thiopurine methyltransferase (TPMT). The activity of this particular enzyme varies in patients based on a genetic polymorphism. Therefore, patients may be at a higher risk for certain side effects if they have low enzyme activity. TPMT testing is available to identify patients who may have low enzyme activity and, in turn, may experience more side effects.

These agents should be initiated during an acute exacerbation once the patient can tolerate oral medications to induce and maintain remission. Because of their slow onset of action, however, these agents are not effective for treating an acute exacerbation. The initial dosage of these agents is 50 mg/d in one dose; the dosage is increased every 2 weeks to a target dosage of 1 to 2 mg/kg/d for 6-mercaptopurine and 2 to 2.5 mg/kg/d for azathioprine. Because these agents are cleared by the renal system, dosages must be decreased in patients with creatinine clearance values under 50 mL/min. The dose for azathioprine and 6-mercaptopurine is usually decreased by 50% if the patient's creatinine clearance value falls below 50 mL/min to decrease the risk of accumulation and unwanted effects. Although these agents have the potential to cause significant adverse events, they are in general well tolerated. These agents should not be used in pregnancy or in patients with active liver disease.

Methotrexate

Methotrexate (Rheumatrex) has a therapeutic effect similar to that of azathioprine and 6-mercaptopurine; however, it inhibits intracellular dihydrofolate reductase, which results in inhibition of purine synthesis and suppression of IL-1 production. Both the intramuscular and oral preparations of methotrexate are efficacious in the induction and maintenance of CD remission, but similar efficacy has not been shown for UC. Doses of 25 mg/week injected intramuscularly or 5 mg orally three times a week have been effective in inducing remission in patients with steroid-dependent CD after 12 to 16 weeks of therapy. At low doses, methotrexate is nearly completely absorbed when administered orally; therefore, there is no foreseen benefit in using the intramuscular preparation over the oral formulation during normal GI function.

Methotrexate dosages must be adjusted based on renal function. Patients with creatinine clearance values less than 50 mL/min should receive 50% of the normal dose. Methotrexate should not be prescribed to patients with active liver disease or pregnant women.

Cyclosporine

Cyclosporine (Sandimmune, Neoral) is reserved for the acute treatment of severe, steroid-refractory exacerbations of UC in hospitalized patients. Cyclosporine is a lipophilic, fungus-derived polypeptide that suppresses cell-mediated immunity by predominantly inhibiting IL-2 synthesis and release. Therapeutic effect is correlated with appropriate dosing. IV infusion of cyclosporine has been found effective at dosages of 4 to 8 mg/kg/d for UC. The use of cyclosporine in acute CD exacerbations is reported to have variable results. Because of poor systemic absorption, oral cyclosporine should not be used. Improvement of symptoms with IV therapy usually occurs within 2 to 3 days, and the duration of therapy is usually 7 to 10 days.

Adverse Events

Although azathioprine and 6-mercaptopurine are usually well tolerated, significant side effects may occur. These agents are associated with both allergic- and nonallergic-type side effects. Allergic-type side effects include pancreatitis, fever, rash, arthralgias, malaise, nausea, and diarrhea, which may occur regardless of dose. The main nonallergic-type side effects include bone marrow suppression and hepatotoxicity, which appear to be dose dependent. Pancreatitis may occur at any point in therapy and warrants discontinuation of therapy. The development of pancreatitis precludes the use of either 6-mercaptopurine or azathioprine in the future. Leukopenia and hepatotoxicity usually occurs during the initiation phase of therapy and may be managed by decreasing the dose. If a patient experiences side effects with either of these agents, it is not beneficial to switch the patient to the other agent.

Side effects of methotrexate include hepatic cirrhosis and fibrosis, bone marrow suppression, pneumonitis, folic acid deficiency, and rash. Nausea and diarrhea are also reported, but they occur more frequently with the oral formulation. Bone marrow suppression and liver dysfunction are dose dependent, and doses should be decreased in patients with these disorders. Folic acid should be administered concomitantly to limit folic acid deficiency.

Cyclosporine is most associated with nephrotoxicity, hypomagnesemia, and hypertension. Risk factors for nephrotoxicity are high-dose treatment, long-term treatment, and advanced age. Discontinuation of cyclosporine may restore renal function within 2 weeks. Other side effects of cyclosporine include nausea, vomiting, opportunistic infections, paresthesias, tremor, and seizures. Opportunistic infections occur because of the drug's immunosuppressive effects and may be managed by appropriate antibiotic therapy.

Interactions

Cyclosporine significantly interacts with various agents because of its metabolism through the cytochrome P-450 3A4 isoenzyme system. Enzyme inhibitors, such as erythromycin (Eryc) and ketoconazole (Nizoral), increase blood levels of cyclosporine by inhibiting its metabolism, whereas enzyme inducers, such as phenytoin (Dilantin), carbamazepine (Tegretol), and rifampin (Rifadin), decrease cyclosporine blood levels. Grapefruit juice increases blood levels of cyclosporine, which may increase the incidence of side effects.

Antibiotics

The association between IBD and infectious causes has led to the use of antibiotics. Because the exact organism has not been isolated, it is difficult to determine which antibiotics are most appropriate for treatment. In general, an antibiotic that acts against gram-negative and *Mycobacterium* organisms with a low side effect profile and poor systemic absorption is desirable. Many agents have been studied, including broad-spectrum antibiotics, metronidazole (Flagyl), fluoroquinolones, antituberculars, and macrolides. However, based on the scarce published, controlled trials, mild to moderately active CD appears to respond only to metronidazole and ciprofloxacin (Cipro) (see **Table 31.4**). Beneficial effects of antibiotic therapy have not been replicated in patients with UC.

Metronidazole showed efficacy in treating perianal CD. Since then, however, a few studies have found beneficial effects of metronidazole in the treatment of mild to moderately active luminal and fistulizing CD when used in combination with aminosalicylates or alone. The mechanism by which metronidazole alone exerts its beneficial effects in CD is unknown, although it is thought that the immune-modulating effects are more prominent than the antibacterial effects.

The normal dosage for treatment of mild to moderately active CD is 20 mg/kg/d. Once remission is attained, the dosage is titrated to 10 mg/kg/d for maintenance. The usual duration of therapy is up to 12 months, although remission is usually attained within 1 to 2 months. Although exacerbations of CD have been reported with the discontinuation of metronidazole, long-term use is associated with significant side effects.

Ciprofloxacin has also been studied for perianal and luminal CD with mixed results. Ciprofloxacin covers gram-negative organisms and *Mycobacterium* species as well as some gram-positive organisms and is usually well tolerated. Along with inhibiting DNA gyrase, which is its main antibacterial mechanism of action, ciprofloxacin also is reported to have immunosuppressive properties. A dosage of oral ciprofloxacin of 500 mg, twice daily, is as efficacious as 4 g of mesalamine daily in preliminary trials. Remission is attained after approximately 6 weeks of therapy. Ciprofloxacin is contraindicated in children and pregnant women.

Adverse Events

Short-term metronidazole therapy is associated with fairly benign side effects, including dry mouth, metallic taste, nausea, and vomiting. Abdominal distress, including cramping and diarrhea, may also occur, but these effects are difficult to distinguish from IBD symptoms. Long-term use of metronidazole is associated with neurotoxic effects such as peripheral paresthesias, dizziness, pruritus, and vertigo that may warrant discontinuation of therapy.

Ciprofloxacin is usually well tolerated. The most common side effects include nausea, diarrhea, dizziness, and rashes secondary to photosensitivity. However, long-term treatment may result in tendinitis and tendon rupture.

Interactions

Metronidazole is associated with severe nausea and vomiting (disulfiram effect) if taken concurrently with alcohol. Ciprofloxacin inhibits theophylline (Slo-Phyllin) metabolism, so theophylline serum levels may need to be monitored with chronic ciprofloxacin use. Any divalent or trivalent cation, such as calcium or iron, may interfere with the absorption of ciprofloxacin; therefore, at least a 4-hour dosing interval should be maintained between these agents.

Biological Agents

Many biological agents are being investigated for the treatment of IBD, including TNF-α inhibitors, growth factors, lymphocyte inhibitors, and transcription inhibitors. Currently, there are two approved classes for the treatment of severe refractory luminal CD: TNF-α inhibitors [infliximab (Remicade), adalimumab (Humira), and certolizumab pegol (Cimzia)] and selective adhesion molecule inhibitors [natalizumab (Tysabri), vedolizumab (Entyvio)].

TNF-α inhibitors

Infliximab (Remicade) is indicated for maintaining remission in CD as well as treating UC and fistulizing CD. The GI mucosal tissues of patients with active CD are found to overexpress numerous immunologic cytokines, including TNF. Biological TNF-α is a proinflammatory cytokine that stimulates the expression of various immunologic cytokines, such as IL-8 and interferon-γ. The TNF-α inhibitor agents produce their effect by neutralizing soluble forms of TNF-α and competitively inhibit its binding to the TNF receptor. In addition, TNF-α inhibitors may also induce apoptosis of activated monocytes.

Infliximab is a synthetically derived immunoglobulin (Ig) G monoclonal antibody consisting of 25% murine antibodies and 75% human antibodies (see **Table 31.4**). Infliximab is available only as an IV solution, and it is administered at a dosage of 5 mg/kg over a minimum of 2 hours. A single infusion dose at baseline, week 2, and week 6 is administered for the treatment of an acute exacerbation; infusions every 8 weeks are used to maintain remission. The infusions may be delivered in an inpatient or a monitored outpatient setting. Repeated doses of the product may increase the risk of immunogenicity and infusion-related reactions due to the murine component of the product. Infliximab crosses the placenta and is detected in serum of infants for up to 6 months after in utero exposure and should be held after 30 weeks of gestation in pregnant women. Caution should be used when prescribing to patients with heart failure.

Adalimumab (Humira) is also a TNF-α inhibitor; however, it is a fully humanized IgG monoclonal antibody that binds specifically to human TNF. It is approved for maintaining remission of CD in adults and children and for treating and maintaining remission of UC in adults. In general, fully humanized monoclonal antibodies are associated with less immunogenicity and infusion-related reactions. Adalimumab is administered as a subcutaneous injection every 2 weeks and may be increased to once weekly if necessary (see **Table 31.4**). In addition to patients with CD who are naïve to TNF-α inhibitors, adalimumab is effective in patients with CD who may not have responded to infliximab.

Certolizumab pegol (Cimzia) is also a TNF-α inhibitor; however, it is not a full monoclonal antibody. Certolizumab pegol consists of only the fragment antigen-binding (FAB) fragment of human-derived IgG, which is attached to polyethylene glycol. Since certolizumab pegol does not contain certain regions of a full antibody, it cannot cause antibody-dependent cell cytotoxicity or induce apoptosis as with infliximab or adalimumab. The polyethylene glycol portion of the product allows for a longer duration of action and thus a longer duration between injections. Certolizumab pegol is administered in two subcutaneous injections initially and weeks 2 and 4. For those who elicit a clinical response, certolizumab pegol may be used every 4 weeks to maintain remission (see **Table 31.4**). Certolizumab pegol should not be used for the treatment of fistulizing CD, as it is no more effective than placebo. It has not been studied in the treatment of UC or in children.

Selective Adhesion Molecule Inhibitors

Selective adhesion molecule inhibitors should be reserved for patients who had an inadequate response or unable to tolerate conventional CD therapies and TNF-α inhibitors. Natalizumab is a humanized monoclonal antibody active against α_4 integrin subunit, which inhibits leukocyte adhesion and migration into inflamed tissue. Natalizumab (Tysabri) is indicated for the treatment of CD in adults and is administered intravenously as a 300-mg dose every 4 weeks and should be discontinued if there is no therapeutic benefit achieved within 12 weeks. When initiating natalizumab, patients should be tapered off of concomitant corticosteroid use according to clinical response. Antibody formation may occur with natalizumab and may result in infusion reactions, hypersensitivity reactions, and loss of efficacy. Natalizumab is not well studied in pregnant patients and should be enrolled into a pregnancy exposure registry if initiated.

Vedolizumab (Entyvio) is a humanized monoclonal antibody that targets $\alpha_4\beta_7$ integrin, preventing the migration of inflammatory lymphocytes into the gut mucosa. It is indicated for initiating and maintaining remission in adults for both CD and UC. Vedolizumab is administered intravenously as a dose of 300 mg at 0, 2, and 6 weeks, then every 8 weeks thereafter. In clinical trials, the glucocorticoid doses were left unaltered until week 6 and then tapered according to patient response. Therapy should be discontinued in patients who do not achieve a response within 14 weeks.

Other Agents

Ustekinumab (Stelara) is a human monoclonal antibody active against interleukin-12 and interleukin-23. It is approved for use in plaque psoriasis, but has been studied for inducing and maintaining remission in refractory CD in adults who were resistant to anti–TNF-α therapy. Patients had a significantly increased rate of inducing and maintaining clinical remission compared to placebo; however, the optimal dose remains unclear. Further studies are needed to determine the utility and role of ustekinumab for the treatment of CD.

Adverse Events

The primary side effects associated with TNF-α inhibitors are injection site–related reactions, which include erythema, itching, and swelling. Less common but significant side effects include the development of heart failure, tuberculosis (TB), hepatitis B reactivation, opportunistic infections, lymphoma and other malignancies, hepatotoxicity, vasculitis, and pancytopenia. Patients should be tested for latent TB and treated accordingly prior to treatment with TNF-α inhibitors. TNF-α inhibitors are contraindicated in patients with active TB and should be used cautiously in patients with heart failure.

Infliximab is also associated with infusion-related reactions, including transient hypersensitivity reactions, flushing,

headache, dyspnea, rash, and fever, possibly secondary to the murine component of the product. These side effects may be managed by pretreating patients with antihistamines, acetaminophen, and/or corticosteroids. In addition, mild to moderate infusion reactions may be managed by decreasing the infusion rate.

The primary side effects associated with selective adhesion molecule inhibitors are hypersensitivity and infusion reactions. Patients on natalizumab also have the potential to develop severe hepatotoxicity, and the drug carries a black box warning for increasing the risk of developing progressive multifocal leukoencephalopathy, particularly in patients with a history of John Cunningham (JC) virus.

Drug Interactions

Extensive drug interaction studies have not been performed to date, but due to their ability to alter the immunologic response, biologics should not be administered along with live vaccines. Commonly, TNF-α inhibitors are administered to patients who are also taking immunosuppressive agents. The administration of other immunosuppressant agents (e.g., azathioprine, methotrexate) with these agents has been shown to be beneficial by decreasing the risk of immunogenicity (development of autoantibodies) and decreasing infusion-related reactions (Lichtenstein, Diamond, et al., 2009; Lichtenstein, Hanauer, et al., 2009). No significant drug interactions have been reported when TNF-α inhibitors are given with conventional IBD therapy.

Selecting the Most Appropriate Agent

For many diseases and disorders, there are drug treatment protocols that make clear distinctions between first-line, second-line, and third-line therapies. However, in IBD, the decision to use one therapeutic modality over another is based on the location of the inflammation, the severity and extent of disease, the patient's tolerance of the therapy, patient compliance, and cost (**Table 31.5**). The American College of Gastroenterology has developed guidelines for managing CD and UC (Kornbluth & Sachar, 2010; Lichtenstein, Diamond, et al., 2009; Lichtenstein, Hanauer, et al., 2009).

Crohn Disease

Mild to moderately active luminal CD is typically treated with oral aminosalicylates alone or in combination with antibiotic therapy. However, monotherapy with budesonide has also been used with good results, especially in patients with ileal or right colonic disease. Oral agents are chosen over rectal agents because of the random presence of CD along the entire GI tract. Patients may be maintained on aminosalicylates or antibiotic therapy for months to years, but the goal is to taper the patient off the medication as soon as possible once remission is attained. Budesonide is indicated for 3 months to maintain remission in CD.

Treatment of moderate to severe CD usually consists of combination therapy with aminosalicylates and corticosteroids.

TABLE 31.5

Recommended Treatment Options for Crohn Disease and Ulcerative Colitis

Severity of Disease	Distal UC	Extensive UC	Luminal CD	Perianal/Fistulizing CD
Mild	Oral/rectal aminosalicylate OR Rectal corticosteroid	Oral aminosalicylate	Oral aminosalicylate WITH/WITHOUT Antibiotic therapy	Surgical drainage AND antibiotic therapy WITH/WITHOUT IV infliximab or SC adalimumab
Moderate	Oral aminosalicylate AND Rectal aminosalicylate Oral/rectal steroid	Oral aminosalicylate AND Oral steroid	Oral aminosalicylate AND Oral steroid (preferably budesonide)	
Severe	IV corticosteroid AND/OR IV cyclosporine	IV corticosteroid AND/OR IV cyclosporine	IV corticosteroid AND/OR biologics	
Fulminant	IV corticosteroids AND/OR IV cyclosporine, IV infliximab or SC adalimumab*	IV corticosteroid AND/OR IV cyclosporine, IV infliximab or SC adalimumab*	IV corticosteroid AND/OR biologics	
Remission	Oral/rectal aminosalicylate WITH/WITHOUT Oral immunosuppressive, IV infliximab or SC adalimumab*	Oral aminosalicylate WITH/WITHOUT Oral immunosuppressive, IV infliximab or SC adalimumab*	Oral aminosalicylate WITH/WITHOUT Oral immunosuppressive/ biologics	

*Consider selective adhesion-molecule inhibitors for inadequate response/failure with TNF-α inhibitors.

Corticosteroid therapy is used acutely on a short-term basis for patients with moderate to severe disease to attain remission. Because of their high side effect profile, steroids are not used chronically to maintain remission. Oral agents may be used for patients with moderate to severe disease. The typical duration of therapy is 4 to 12 weeks at the full dose, and then doses are tapered by 5 to 10 mg weekly until discontinued. If patients have had multiple exacerbations and are steroid refractory or have fistulizing disease, TNF inhibitors may be indicated. The 2013 American Gastroenterology Association guideline recommends using TNF-α inhibitors in combination with thiopurines over thiopurine monotherapy to induce remission in patients who have moderately severe CD.

Severe to fulminant disease requires definitive drug therapy in addition to substantial supportive care measures due to poor oral absorption and rapid GI transit time. Oral therapy, including aminosalicylates, should not be administered until the patient can tolerate oral alimentation. IV corticosteroids are indicated to decrease inflammation and induce immunosuppression. For patients with moderate to severe or severe to fulminant disease whose disease is refractory to corticosteroids (either oral or IV), biological agents are an option. Supportive care measures, such as IV fluids, bowel rest, and parenteral nutrition, should also be considered.

Therapy to maintain remission should be considered in patients who have frequent exacerbations or who are "steroid dependent." Immunosuppressive agents, including azathioprine, 6-mercaptopurine, methotrexate, and biologics, may be used with aminosalicylates to maintain remission in patients whose disease is refractory to aminosalicylate monotherapy. The immunosuppressant agents may take effect after 10 to 12 weeks. Therapeutic effect should be seen within 8 weeks of administration of biologics. Patients may be maintained on these agents for months to years, but the goal is to taper the patient off the medication as soon as possible due to the significant side effects. Antibiotics, specifically metronidazole and ciprofloxacin, have proved beneficial in maintaining remission of perianal and fistulizing CD with long-term use (**Figure 31.1**).

Ulcerative Colitis

For UC, guidelines specify various treatment approaches depending on the severity and location of disease. Distal colitis, identified as lesions below the splenic flexure, may be treated with oral, rectal, or IV agents depending on the severity of disease. Rectal agents should not be used in patients with extensive colitis due to the location of disease. The decision to use systemic or local preparations for distal colitis largely depends on patient preference; however, topical products allow for less systemic absorption, less frequent dosing, and a quicker onset of effect (**Figure 31.2**). Treatment of mild UC is best achieved with the use of aminosalicylates. The combination of oral and rectal aminosalicylates is more effective than either therapy alone. Corticosteroids may be used concurrently with aminosalicylates for moderate UC exacerbations. Depending on the severity of the exacerbation and the location of the lesions,

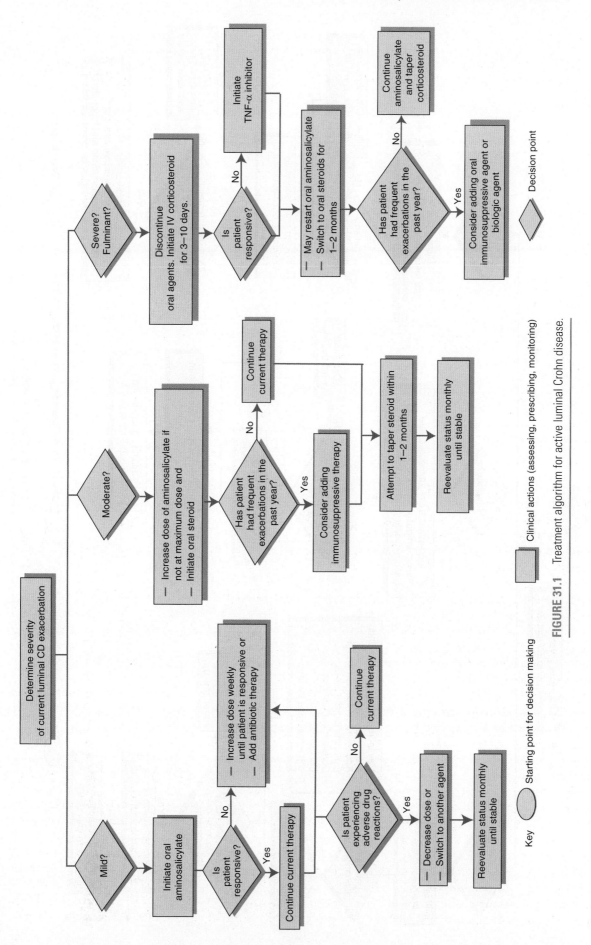

FIGURE 31.1 Treatment algorithm for active luminal Crohn disease.

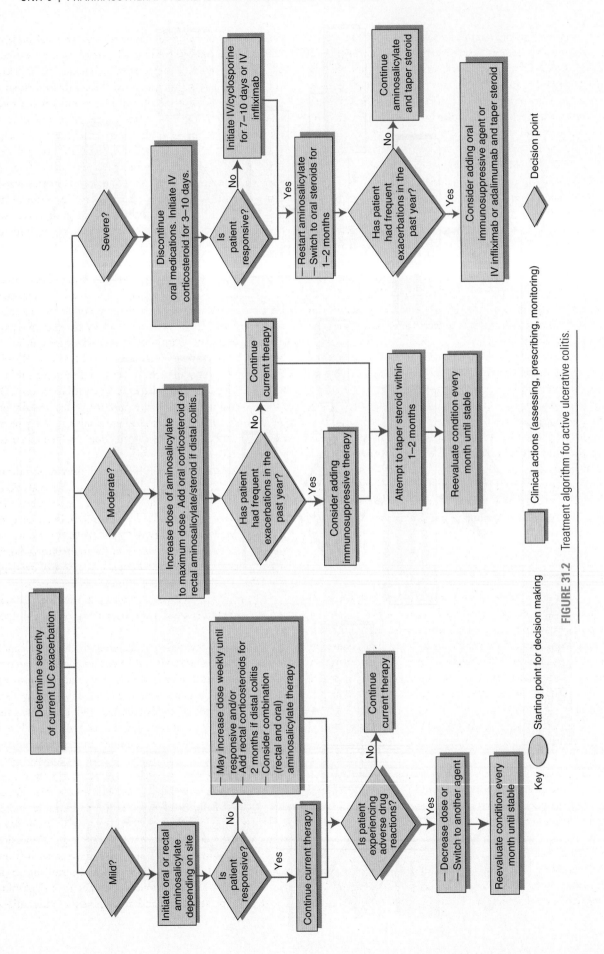

FIGURE 31.2   Treatment algorithm for active ulcerative colitis.

either rectal or oral preparations may be appropriate. Severe exacerbations may require hospitalization. Discontinuation of oral and topical therapy due to rapid GI transit time and the initiation of IV corticosteroid therapy are standard. If improvement in the condition is not seen in 7 to 10 days with IV corticosteroids, IV cyclosporine, IV infliximab, SC adalimumab, or IV vedolizumab may be considered. The use of IV cyclosporine is reserved for hospitalized patients who have not responded to IV steroids. Infliximab may be initiated in an outpatient or inpatient setting in patients with severe exacerbations after an adequate trial of steroids.

Surgery may be considered in patients whose disease fails to respond to drug therapy. The management of fulminant exacerbations is very similar to that of severe exacerbations, but the decision to perform a colectomy is considered at a much earlier stage for fulminant exacerbations. Along with definitive therapy, supportive measures including bowel rest, IV fluids, and adequate nutrition should be considered for those with severe and fulminant exacerbations. For those with frequent exacerbations or steroid dependence, immunosuppressive agents such as 6-mercaptopurine and azathioprine should be considered to induce and maintain remission. Typically, immunosuppressive agents are initiated after the patient can tolerate oral medications and are initiated along with aminosalicylate and corticosteroid therapy. The goal is to taper the corticosteroid and continue the aminosalicylate along with the immunosuppressive therapy for maintenance of remission.

Methotrexate has not been adequately studied in patients with UC and therefore is not recommended. Antibiotic therapy has not been shown to improve UC symptoms.

Drug Selection

Sulfasalazine was considered the first-line aminosalicylate because of its remarkable efficacy, low cost, and availability in oral liquid and tablet preparations; however, it must be taken four times a day and causes significant adverse drug reactions. For maximum therapeutic benefit, 4 to 8 g/d is necessary, so patients must take up to 16 tablets or 32 teaspoonfuls daily. In addition, immediate-release sulfasalazine has activity limited to the colon, making it less effective in conditions affecting the upper GI tract.

Mesalamine has emerged as the aminosalicylate of choice because of its availability in many formulations, dosing frequency, and its low side effect profile, but it is more expensive than sulfasalazine. Depending on the oral formulation and the severity of the disease, patients may need to take 6 to 16 pills daily to attain maximum therapeutic benefit. Normal dosages of oral mesalamine are 2 to 4.8 g/d. Olsalazine and balsalazide are not used as often because of their added cost without any significant clinical benefit.

The ideal corticosteroid for treating IBD would have high glucocorticoid activity, a low side effect profile, and targeted delivery to the diseased site and would be poorly absorbed from the GI tract, allowing for localized activity. Oral budesonide (Entocort) is approved specifically for the acute treatment of IBD due to its ideal characteristics, but due to its increased cost, other corticosteroids are used frequently to treat an acute exacerbation. The choice of steroid depends on the route of administration, onset of action, and glucocorticoid versus mineralocorticoid potency. In general, agents with more glucocorticoid activity are preferred over mineralocorticoid steroids because they have better anti-inflammatory action. Oral agents are used primarily in patients with localized or generalized disease with mild to moderate exacerbations, rectal formulations are reserved for patients with mild to moderate exacerbations of distal UC disease, and IV treatment may be initiated in patients with severe exacerbations of CD or UC.

The use of immunosuppressive agents varies based on the type of IBD and the severity of disease. Cyclosporine is reserved for the acute treatment of severe UC exacerbations because of the high cost of therapy and high incidence of severe side effects. Because of a lack of comparative trials of methotrexate and azathioprine or 6-mercaptopurine, it is difficult to determine which agent would be considered first line; however, there are more data to support the use of azathioprine or 6-mercaptopurine than methotrexate for CD and UC. Azathioprine and 6-mercaptopurine are equally efficacious, with similar pharmacokinetic, adverse drug reaction, and cost profiles, so no great distinction can be made between the two.

The main distinction between methotrexate and the other two agents is its availability as an intramuscular injection and its dosing schedule. The infrequent dosing schedule of oral and intramuscular methotrexate may promote either compliance or noncompliance with the medication, depending on the patient. Combining these agents for the induction and maintenance of remission is not recommended because of overlapping side effect profiles and lack of improved efficacy data.

If antibiotic therapy is warranted, metronidazole or ciprofloxacin is an acceptable agent, depending on patient-specific factors.

There are a few differences among the biologics that may make one agent more favorable in certain patients than others. Infliximab and adalimumab are the only products approved for the treatment of patients with severe, refractory UC or fistulizing CD. Therefore, it remains the best option in these patients at this time. For patients with luminal CD who are able to self-inject themselves, either adalimumab or certolizumab pegol may be an option. Adalimumab and certolizumab pegol are available as a prefilled syringe for convenience; however, adalimumab is administered subcutaneously as one injection every 2 weeks, whereas certolizumab pegol is administered subcutaneously as two injections every 4 weeks. Infliximab may also be used for luminal CD; however, since it is an IV infusion, it must be administered by a health care practitioner in a monitored setting. Also, since adalimumab and certolizumab pegol are fully humanized monoclonal antibodies, the risk of infusion reactions, hypersensitivity, and development of autoantibodies are less likely than with infliximab. Adalimumab has also been found effective in patients who have previously not responded to infliximab (Armuzzi et al., 2013; Sandborn et al., 2007). Natalizumab, vedolizumab, and ustekinumab should be considered for patients that failed TNF-α therapy and are only available as IV infusions.

Special Population Considerations

Pediatrics

IBD is typically diagnosed early in life, usually during the second or third decade, leading to significant implications of IBD in the pediatric population. Treatment must be aggressive to limit the potential for nutritional deficiencies leading to stunted growth, malnutrition, and anemia. However, many of the medications lead to untoward effects or are not well studied in pediatrics. The use of long-term corticosteroids may lead to growth abnormalities, whereas ciprofloxacin use is contraindicated in children because it can cause arthropathy, resulting in poor bone formation. Infliximab is indicated for inducing or maintaining remission of CD and UC in children older than age 6. Certolizumab pegol has not been studied in children. Adalimumab is indicated for inducing and maintaining remission of CD in children over the age of 6. Adalimumab has been studied in children for UC, but is not indicated in children at this time. Supplemental therapy including proper nutrition, iron therapy, and adequate hydration should also be considered to maintain growth and general health. Treating IBD in children involves aggressively managing the condition as well as the side effects with the limited options.

Pregnancy

The fertility rate in women with IBD is similar to the general population, but spontaneous abortions, stillbirths, and developmental defects are more common in pregnant women with active disease. Therefore, IBD should be treated aggressively in pregnant women to limit dehydration, anemia, and nutritional deficiencies that could adversely affect fetal outcomes. However, treatment options are limited for pregnant women due to the risk of teratogenicity or unwanted effects on the fetus. Methotrexate is absolutely contraindicated in pregnancy and lactation due to its potential for spontaneous abortions and teratogenicity. Data are controversial regarding the use of mercaptopurine and azathioprine during pregnancy. If either of these agents is necessary during pregnancy, an azathioprine dosage of 2 mg/kg/d or less is recommended to limit pancytopenia in the fetus. Azathioprine and mercaptopurine are contraindicated during nursing due to the potential of fetal immunosuppression. The use of cyclosporine should be reserved for severe refractory cases because it can cause growth retardation. The TNF-α inhibitors for IBD are all pregnancy category B. Studies have shown serum levels of TNF-α inhibitors are detectable in the serum of infants for up to 6 months post in utero exposure. It is

recommended to hold therapy after 30 weeks of gestational age, and all pregnant patients exposed to TNF-α inhibitors should be enrolled into their respective registries (Gisbert, 2010; Zelinkova et al., 2011). Selective adhesion molecule inhibitors have not been studied in pregnancy. Ciprofloxacin and metronidazole should also be avoided in pregnancy and lactation because they can cause fetal malformations. Corticosteroids may be used at the lowest doses possible to induce remission for the shortest period of time to limit adrenal suppression of the fetus. Women taking sulfasalazine should be given higher dosages of folate (2 mg/d) because sulfasalazine interferes with folate absorption. Preconception counseling is imperative to discuss the condition, lifestyle changes, nutritional issues, and treatment options with the patient. Special attention should be given to maintaining body weight before conception and preventing exacerbations during pregnancy.

MONITORING PATIENT RESPONSE

Various parameters must be monitored to detect efficacy and toxicity associated with therapy. Efficacy parameters include signs and symptoms of CD and UC, which are well defined in the Working Definition of Crohn's Disease Activity and Criteria for Severity of Ulcerative Colitis. Nutritional parameters such as weight, albumin, vitamin B_{12} levels, iron levels, and transferrin saturation should also be followed. Mental status and quality-of-life issues such as frequency of social interactions, attendance at work, and completion of activities of daily living all may indicate effectiveness of therapy. Although there are no definitive guidelines for the frequency of monitoring, it is important to monitor these endpoints when adjustments are made in drug therapy or when exacerbations occur.

Specific monitoring of drug toxicities is imperative for all pharmacologic agents. CBC and liver function tests should be performed periodically to detect asymptomatic undesired reactions in patients taking sulfasalazine. In addition, renal function (i.e., blood urea nitrogen, serum creatinine) should be monitored routinely with aminosalicylates to identify nephrotoxicity.

Corticosteroid treatment is associated with significant drug toxicities, but most occur with long-term use. In general, short-term corticosteroid treatment does not require intense monitoring. However, patients who have uncontrolled hypertension or who are glucose intolerant must have their blood pressure or fasting blood glucose level monitored periodically while taking corticosteroids. For patients taking corticosteroids on a long-term basis, baseline tests including a lipid panel, electrolytes, and fasting blood glucose studies should be performed every 6 to 12 months. A baseline bone density scan may be judicious and may be repeated yearly.

Azathioprine and 6-mercaptopurine are both associated with significant side effects, so it is important to acquire a baseline CBC with differential and serum creatinine, amylase, and liver function tests. The CBC should be monitored more frequently during the initiation of therapy (every 1 to 2 weeks for the first 3 months) and then less frequently (every 3 to 6 months) for the duration of therapy. Liver function tests should be monitored every 3 months for the first year or until a stable dosage has been achieved, then every 4 to 6 months for the duration of treatment. Creatinine clearance is an important parameter in guiding the dosing regimen of azathioprine or 6-mercaptopurine, so serum creatinine and creatinine clearance should be monitored annually if renal function is stable and more often if fluctuations in dosages or renal function occur. Amylase is not routinely ordered, but it may be checked upon patient complaints due to the risk of pancreatitis.

During the initial phase of methotrexate therapy, CBC and liver function tests should be performed every 2 to 4 weeks. If methotrexate therapy is continued beyond 16 weeks, CBC and liver function tests should be monitored every 4 to 8 weeks for the duration of therapy. Dosage adjustments must be made based on creatinine clearance, so serum creatinine must be monitored at baseline and at every dosage change. If renal function is stable, serum creatinine should be monitored annually at a minimum. Liver biopsies may be obtained once yearly if the patient is taking methotrexate, although formal recommendations have not been made.

IV cyclosporine therapy requires daily monitoring of cyclosporine blood levels (200 to 400 ng/mL), blood urea nitrogen, serum creatinine, and blood pressure. Although cyclosporine is extensively metabolized by the liver, it is eliminated by the kidneys and is highly associated with permanent renal dysfunction; therefore, renal function must be monitored closely. Dosages should be adjusted daily based on renal function and cyclosporine blood levels. Opportunistic infections may occur with high-dose cyclosporine use, so CBC, signs of infection, and temperature should also be monitored daily.

Biologics are associated with many side effects; however, most do not occur commonly. Due to the rare incidence of serious side effects, routine laboratory monitoring is not indicated; however, a heightened awareness of the clinical symptoms of adverse events is warranted. Patients and health care professionals should routinely monitor for symptoms of heart failure, vasculitis, TB, infection, hepatotoxicity, and lupus-like syndrome. Autoantibodies to the TNF-α inhibitors are known to develop and can be monitored via serum levels. Patients who develop autoantibodies may be more likely to develop lupus-like syndrome or have reduced efficacy with the agents (West et al., 2008). Routine administration of biologics and concomitant administration of immunosuppressants limit the development of autoantibodies.

Metronidazole and ciprofloxacin do not require significant drug monitoring, but long-term antibiotic treatment may lead to superinfection, so signs and symptoms of infection should be noted and treated. Patients receiving metronidazole therapy should also be monitored for peripheral paresthesias.

PATIENT EDUCATION

Drug Information

Patients and caregivers need to understand that uncontrolled IBD may affect quality of life, psychological well-being, and general physical health, so adherence to medication therapy is imperative. In addition, due to the increased GI transit time during an exacerbation, patients may not fully absorb oral medications for any of their conditions, which may lead to poor control of their other conditions during an IBD exacerbation.

Patients should swallow the enteric-coated sulfasalazine or mesalamine tablets and capsules whole so that the dosage form can penetrate the affected area. Sulfasalazine can discolor body fluids (e.g., urine and tears), which may stain clothing and contact lenses. When taking metronidazole, patients must abstain from alcohol to avoid severe nausea and vomiting.

Often, patients request chronic corticosteroid therapy because of its beneficial results, but these patients need to be informed of the long-term complications of corticosteroids and should be advised regarding other medications that may be more appropriate for chronic therapy. Patients also need to be aware that immunosuppressants (azathioprine, 6-mercaptopurine, methotrexate) take 10 to 15 weeks to take effect; therefore, adherence to the medication regimen is imperative even though resolution of symptoms will not be apparent until weeks later.

Although the biologics are quite efficacious for IBD, patients must be made aware of the significant risks associated with them. In addition, if patients are prescribed either adalimumab or certolizumab pegol, they must be instructed on the proper self-administration of a subcutaneous injection as well as sterile technique and safe needle disposal.

Patient-Oriented Information Sources

Along with their health care professionals, there are many other resources available for patients who are seeking information on IBD. A local support group may be a good resource for patients having trouble dealing with the illness. Many local hospitals as well as the Crohn's and Colitis Foundation of America organize support groups for patients with IBD. For general medical information regarding IBD, the following Web sites offer helpful patient-specific information:

- AGA: www.gastro.org
- American College of Gastroenterology: www.acg.gi.org
- Crohn's and Colitis Foundation of America: www.ccfa.org
- MedlinePlus: www.nlm.nih.gov/medlineplus/
- National Institute of Diabetes, Digestive, and Kidney Diseases: www.niddk.nih.gov

Preventive Care

Nutritional Status

Nutritional status is a significant issue for patients with active IBD and those with surgical resections. Patients with IBD are at risk for stunted growth, malnutrition, dehydration, weight loss, iron deficiency anemia, macrocytic anemia, osteopenia, and other conditions. Nutrient deficiencies of iron, vitamin B_{12}, zinc, folate, calcium, and vitamin D may result from decreased oral intake, malabsorption, excessive losses, hypermetabolism due to infection, or drug-induced side effects. Concurrent administration of folate with methotrexate and sulfasalazine and administration of calcium and vitamin D with corticosteroids are recommended to limit the potential for nutritional deficiencies. Also, due to folate deficiencies, patients with IBD are at risk of hyperhomocysteinemia, resulting in an elevated potential for thrombosis. Vitamin B_6 and vitamin B_{12} supplementation is recommended to decrease homocysteine levels. Folate supplementation is especially important in women of child-bearing age.

Many special dietary agents have been studied in patients with IBD with varying results. Diets high in short-chain fatty acids are associated with a small decrease in disease severity, potentially due to an anti-inflammatory effect. Fish oils have been associated with a decreased frequency of exacerbations potentially due to their anti-inflammatory properties. An area of new research interest is the role of probiotics such as *Lactobacillus* and *Saccharomyces* in the treatment of IBD. By altering the GI flora, it is theorized that probiotic agents assist with controlling IBD exacerbations.

Enteral and parenteral routes of nutrition have been routinely used to improve the nutritional status of IBD patients. In general, enteral nutrition is preferred due to the complications of infection, thrombosis, and pancreatitis associated with parenteral nutrition. Along with correcting nutritional deficiencies, enteral nutrition has also been studied as a primary treatment measure in combination with aminosalicylates. Parenteral nutrition, however, is advocated in severe exacerbations when bowel rest is in order for proper healing of the IBD. In general, nutritional supplementation plays a large role in the management of IBD. Depending on the severity of weight loss and general health status of the patient, a combination of vitamin and mineral supplementation along with either enteral or parenteral nutrition should be advocated.

Vaccination

Vaccination status in patients with IBD is critical. Since IBD is an autoimmune disease and treatment is focused on immunosuppressant therapy, patients are at higher risk for developing infections. Vaccination records should be reviewed routinely and updated as necessary. Patients on biologic therapy are at risk for hepatitis B reactivation; therefore, screening patients prior to therapy may be prudent. Patients taking an immunosuppressant cannot receive live vaccines; however, they are eligible for inactivated vaccines such as influenza, pneumococcal, meningococcal, tetanus, and hepatitis B (Kornbluth & Sachar,

2010). Prior to the initiation of any biologics, consider bringing all immunizations up to date.

Cancer Screening

Patients with IBD are at a higher risk for colorectal cancer (Eaden et al., 2001). The extent of the risk depends on the extent, course, and duration of the disease in a particular individual (Jesse et al., 2012). Due to the increased risk, patients with IBD for a minimum of 8 years should be screened for colorectal cancer with a colonoscopy and biopsy. Although the data are conflicting as to how often patients should be screened, the American College of Gastroenterology recommends either annually or biannually (Kornbluth & Sachar, 2010).

Complementary and Alternative Therapies

Alternative therapies are used by many patients with IBD: according to one study, 47% of patients with IBD had used alternative therapies for their condition. The most common alternative therapies used were Acidophilus and flaxseed, along with massage therapy, even though data are limited regarding the efficacy of these agents in IBD. Omega-3 fatty acids have also been studied for use in IBD. The National Institutes of Health reported variable results with the use of omega-3 fatty acids for IBD, so widespread use cannot be endorsed at this time (Cabre et al., 2012).

Surgical options are considered in patients who are at risk for a further decline in physical health and quality of life resulting from frequent exacerbations that are unresponsive to conventional therapy. Surgical options include proctocolectomy for UC and a variety of ostomy procedures for patients with CD, depending on the location of disease (**Table 31.6**). Proctocolectomy, the removal of the entire colon and rectum, is a curative intervention for UC. However, surgical procedures for CD are not curative because exacerbations may recur in existing areas of the GI tract, and surgery is used only to maintain remission.

For patients who have undergone surgery, the practitioner must pay close attention to general drug therapy issues. Because of the resection of the GI tract, these patients have issues similar to those of patients with short bowel syndrome. Rectally administered agents such as suppositories and enemas are ineffective in patients with any type of lower GI resection. Depending on the site of resection, sustained-release agents and medications targeted to specific areas of the GI tract also are ineffective in general.

TABLE 31.6	
Surgical Interventions	
Procedure	**Area of Resection**
Sigmoid colostomy	Distal end of large intestine
Descending colostomy	Descending colon and rectum
Transverse colostomy	Small portion of transverse colon
Proctocolectomy/ileostomy	Entire rectum and large intestine

CASE STUDY*

B.F., age 28, presents with diarrhea and abdominal pain. He says he feels weak and feverish. His symptoms have persisted for 5 days. He tells you he has 8 to 10 bowel movements each day, although the volume of stool is only about "half a cupful." Each stool is watery and contains bright red blood. Before this episode, he had noticed a gradual increase in the frequency of his bowel movements, which he attributed to a new vitamin regimen. He has not traveled anywhere in the past 4 months and has taken no antibiotics recently. His medical history is significant for UC; his most recent exacerbation was 2 years ago. He is taking no medications except vitamins.

Examination findings include a tender, slightly distended abdomen. His BP is 122/84 sitting, 110/78 standing; HR 96 bpm; and temperature 100°F. Otherwise, physical findings are unremarkable. Laboratory study results reveal hemoglobin, 12 g/dL; hematocrit, 38%; white blood cell count, 12,000/mm³; platelet count, 242 k; sodium, 132; and potassium, 3.6. All other study results are within normal limits. The most recent colonoscopy findings (4 years ago) revealed granular, edematous, friable mucosa with continuous ulcerations extending throughout the descending colon.

DIAGNOSIS: EXACERBATION OF ULCERATIVE COLITIS

1. List specific goals of treatment for **B.F.**
2. What drug therapy would you prescribe? Why?
3. What are the parameters for monitoring success of the therapy?
4. Discuss specific patient education based on the prescribed therapy.
5. List one or two adverse reactions for the selected agent that would cause you to change therapy.
6. What would be the choice for the second-line therapy?
7. What over-the-counter and/or alternative therapies might be appropriate for **B.F.**?
8. What lifestyle changes would you recommend to **B.F.**?
9. Describe one or two drug–drug or drug–food interactions for the selected agent.

* Answers can be found online.

Bibliography

Starred references are cited in the text.

*Armuzzi, A., Pugliese, D., Nardone, O. M., et al. (2013). Management of difficult-to-treat patients with ulcerative colitis: Focus on adalimumab. *Drug Design, Development and Therapy, 7,* 289–296. Retrieved from http://doi.org/10.2147/DDDT.S33197

Cabre, E., & Gassull, M. A. (2003). Nutritional and metabolic issues in inflammatory bowel disease. *Current Opinions in Clinical Nutrition and Metabolic Care, 6,* 563–576.

*Cabre, E., Manosa, M., & Gassull, M. A. (2012). Omega-3 fatty acids and inflammatory bowel diseases—A systematic review. *British Journal of Nutrition, 107*(Suppl. 2), S240–S252. doi: 10.1017/S0007114512001626.

Colombel, J. F., Lemann, M., Cassagnou, M., et al. (1999). A controlled trial comparing ciprofloxacin with mesalamine for the treatment of active Crohn's disease. *American Journal of Gastroenterology, 94,* 674–678.

*Crockett, S., Porter, C., Martin, C., et al. (2010). Isotretinoin use and the risk of inflammatory bowel disease: A case–control study. *American Journal of Gastroenterology, 105,* 1986–1993. doi: 10.1038/ajg.2010.124.

*Eaden, J. A., Abrams, K. R., & Mayberry, J. F. (2001). The risk of colorectal cancer in ulcerative colitis: A meta-analysis. *Gut, 48,* 526–535.

*Everhart, J. E. (Ed.). (2008). *The burden of digestive diseases in the United States.* U.S. Department of Health and Human Services, Public Health Service, National Institutes of Health, National Institutes of Diabetes and Digestive and Kidney Diseases. Washington, DC: U.S. Government Printing Office; NIH Publication No. 09-6443.

Faegan, B. G., Rutgeerts, P., Sands, B. E., et al. (2013). Vedolizumab as induction and maintenance therapy for ulcerative colitis. *New England Journal of Medicine, 369,* 699–710.

Friedman, S., & Regueiro, M. D. (2002). Pregnancy and nursing in inflammatory bowel disease. *Gastroenterology Clinics of North America, 31,* 265–273.

Friend, D. R. (1998). Review article: Issues in oral administration of locally acting glucocorticosteroids for treatment of inflammatory bowel disease. *Alimentary Pharmacology and Therapeutics, 12,* 591–603.

Gassull, M. A. (2003). Nutrition and inflammatory bowel disease: Its relation to pathophysiology, outcome, and therapy. *Digestive Disorders, 211,* 220–227.

*Gisbert, J. P. (2010). Safety of immunomodulators and biologics for the treatment of inflammatory bowel disease during pregnancy and breast-feeding. *Inflammatory Bowel Diseases, 16,* 881–895. doi: 10.1002/ibd.21154.

Graham, T. O., & Kandil, H. M. (2002). Nutritional factors in inflammatory bowel disease. *Gastroenterology Clinics of North America, 31,* 203–218.

*Halfverson, J., Jess, T., Bodine, L., et al. (2007). Longitudinal concordance for clinical characteristics in a Swedish-Danish twin population with inflammatory bowel disease. *Inflammatory Bowel Disease, 13,* 1536–1544.

Irvine, E. J. (1997). Quality of life issues in patients with inflammatory bowel disease. *American Journal of Gastroenterology, 92,* 18S–24S.

*Jesse, T., Simonsen, J., Jorgensen, K., et al. (2012). Decreasing risk of colorectal cancer in patient with inflammatory bowel disease over 30 years. *Gastroenterology, 143*(2), 375–381.

*Kappelman, M. D., Rifas-Shiman, S. L., Kleinman, K., et al. (2007). The prevalence and geographic distribution of Crohn's disease and ulcerative colitis in the United States. *Clinical Gastroenterology and Hepatology, 5*(12), 1424–1429.

*Khalili, H., Higuchi, L. M., Ananthakrishnan, A. N., et al. (2013). Oral contraceptives, reproductive factors and risk of inflammatory bowel disease. *Gut, 62*(8), 1153–1159. Retrieved from http://doi.org/10.1136/gutjnl-2012-302362

Klotz, U. (2000). The role of aminosalicylates at the beginning of the new millennium in the treatment of chronic inflammatory bowel disease. *European Journal of Clinical Pharmacology, 56,* 353–362.

*Kornbluth, A., & Sachar, D. B. (2010). Ulcerative colitis practice guidelines in adults: American College of Gastroenterology, Practice Parameters Committee. *American Journal of Gastroenterology, 105,* 501–523.

Lee, S. D., & Cohen, R. D. (2002). Endoscopy in inflammatory bowel disease. *Gastroenterology Clinics of North America, 31,* 119–132.

Lesko, S. M., Kaufman, D. W., Rosenberg, L., et al. (1985). Evidence for an increased risk of Crohn's disease in oral contraceptive users. *Gastroenterology, 89,* 1046–1049.

Lichtenstein, G. R., Abreu, M. T., Cohen, R., et al. (2006). American Gastroenterological Association Institute technical review on corticosteroids, immunomodulators, and infliximab in inflammatory bowel disease. *Gastroenterology, 130*, 940–987.

*Lichtenstein, G. R., Diamond, R. H., Wagner, C. L., et al. (2009). Clinical trial: Benefits and risks of immunomodulators and maintenance infliximab for IBD-subgroup analyses across four randomized controlled trials. *Alimentary Pharmacology and Therapeutics, 30*, 210–226.

*Lichtenstein, G. R., Hanauer, S. B., Sandborn, W. J., et al. (2009). Management of Crohn's disease in adults. *American Journal of Gastroenterology, 104*, 465–483.

Liu, Y., van Kruiningen, H. J., West, A. B., et al. (1995). Immunocytochemical evidence of *Listeria, Escherichia coli,* and *Streptococcus* antigens in Crohn's disease. *Gastroenterology, 108*, 1396–1404.

Lunney, P. C., & Leong, R. W. L. (2012), Review article: Ulcerative colitis, smoking and nicotine therapy. *Alimentary Pharmacology & Therapeutics, 36*, 997–1008. doi: 10.1111/apt.12086.

Molodecky, N. A., & Kaplan, G. G. (2010). Environmental risk factors for inflammatory bowel disease. *Gastroenterology & Hepatology, 6*(5), 339–346.

Murray, A., Oliaro, J., & Schlup, M. (1995). *Mycobacterium paratuberculosis* and inflammatory bowel disease: Frequency distribution in serial colonoscopic biopsies using the polymerase chain reaction. *Microbios, 83*, 217–228.

*National Institute of Diabetes and Digestive and Kidney Diseases. (2013). *Digestive disease statistics for the United States.* U.S. Department of Health and Human Services, Public Health Service, National Institutes of Health, National Digestive Disease Information Clearinghouse. NIH Publication No. 10-3873. Retrieved from http://www.niddk.nih.gov/health-information/health-statistics/Pages/digestive-diseases-statistics-for-the-united-states.aspx#12

Orholm, M., Munkholm, P., Langholz, E., et al. (1991). Familiar occurrence of inflammatory bowel disease. *New England Journal of Medicine, 324*, 84–88.

Park, K. T., & Bass, D. (2011). Inflammatory bowel disease-attributable costs and cost-effective strategies in the United States: A review. *Inflammatory Bowel Disease, 17*, 1603–1609.

*Pederson, N., Duricova, D., Elkjaer, M., et al. (2010). Risk of extra-intestinal cancer in inflammatory bowel disease: Meta-analysis of population-based cohort studies. *American Journal of Gastroenterology, 105*, 1480–1487.

Pullan, R. D., Rhodes, J., Ganesh, S., et al. (1994). Transdermal nicotine for active ulcerative colitis. *New England Journal of Medicine, 330*, 811–815.

Rahier, J.-F., Moutschen, M., Van Gompel, A., et al. (2010). Vaccinations in patient with immune-mediated inflammatory diseases. *Rheumatology, 49*, 1815–1827. doi: 10.1093/rheumatology/keq183.

*Reddy, D., Siegel, C. A., Sands, B. E., et al. (2006). Possible association of isotretinoin and inflammatory bowel disease. *American Journal of Gastroenterology, 101*, 1569–1573.

Rubin, D. T., & Hanauer, S. B. (2000). Smoking and inflammatory bowel disease. *European Journal of Gastroenterology and Hepatology, 12*, 855–862.

Safdi, M., DeMicco M., Sninsky, C., et al. (1997). A double-blind comparison of oral vs. rectal mesalamine vs. combination therapy in the treatment of distal ulcerative colitis. *American Journal of Gastroenterology, 92*, 1867–1871.

Sandborn, W. J., Colombel, J. F., Enns, R., et al. (2005). Natalizumab induction and maintenance therapy for Crohn's Disease. *New England Journal of Medicine, 353*, 1912–1925.

Sandborn, W. J., Feagan, B. G., Rutgeerts, P., et al. (2013). Vedolizumab as induction and maintenance therapy for Crohn's Disease. *New England Journal of Medicine, 369*, 711–721.

Sandborn, W. J., Feagan, B. G., Stoinov, S., et al. (2007). Certolizumab pegol for the treatment of Crohn's disease. *New England Journal of Medicine, 357*, 228–238.

Sandborn, W. J., Gasink C., Gao, L., et al. (2012). Ustekinumab induction and maintenance therapy in refractory Crohn's disease. *New England Journal of Medicine, 367*, 1519–1928.

*Sandborn, W. J., Rutgeerts, P., Enns, R., et al. (2007). Adalimumab induction therapy for Crohn's disease previously treated with infliximab: A randomized trial. *Annals of Internal Medicine, 146*, 829–838.

Sandborn, W. J., & Targan, S. R. (2002). Biologic therapy of inflammatory bowel disease. *Gastroenterology, 122*, 1592–1608.

Sands, B. E. (2000). Therapy of inflammatory bowel disease. *Gastroenterology, 118*, S68–S82.

Schreiber, S., Khaliq-Kareenmi, M., Lawrance, I. C., et al. (2007). Maintenance therapy with certolizumab pegol for Crohn's disease. *New England Journal of Medicine, 357*, 239–250.

Themistocles, D., Sultan, S., Falck-Ytter, Y. T., et al. (2013). American Gastroenterological Association Institute technical review on the use of thiopurines, methotrexate, and anti-TNF-α biologic drugs for the induction and maintenance of remission in inflammatory Crohn's disease. *Gastroenterology, 145*, 1464–1478.

Thoreson, R., & Cullen, J. (2007). Pathophysiology of inflammatory bowel disease: An overview. *Surgical Clinics of North America, 87*, 575–585.

Ursing, B., Alm, T., Barany, F., et al. (1982). A comparative study of metronidazole and sulfasalazine for active Crohn's disease: The Cooperative Crohn's Disease Study in Sweden. II: Results. *Gastroenterology, 83*, 550–562.

von Schilde, M. A., Hormannsperger, G., Weiher, M., et al. (2012). Lactocepin secreted by *lactobacillus* exerts anti-inflammatory effects by selectively degrading proinflammatory chemokines. *Cell Host & Microbe, 11*(4), 387–396.

Walker, E. A., Roy-Byrne, P. P., Katon, W. J., et al. (1990). Psychiatric illness and irritable bowel syndrome: A comparison with inflammatory bowel disease. *American Journal of Psychiatry, 147*, 1656–1661.

*West, R. L., Zelinkova, Z., Wolbink, G. J., et al. (2008). Immunogenicity negatively influences the outcome of adalimumab treatment in Crohn's disease. *Alimentary Pharmacology and Therapeutics, 28*(9), 1122–1126.

*Zelinkova, Z., de Haar, C., de Ridder, L., et al. (2011). High intra-uterine exposure to infliximab following maternal anti-TNF treatment during pregnancy. *Alimentary Pharmacology & Therapeutics, 33*, 1053–1058. doi: 10.1111/j.1365-2036.2011.04617.x.

Pharmacotherapy for Genitourinary Tract Disorders

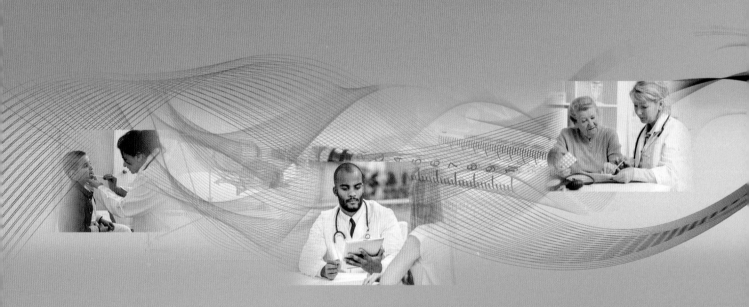

32

Urinary Tract Infection

Virginia P. Arcangelo

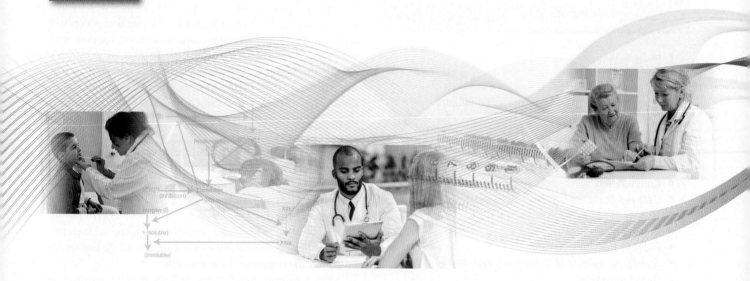

Urinary tract infection (UTI) is a broad term used to describe inflammation of the urethra, bladder, and kidney. Bacteria, yeast, or chemical irritants can cause inflammation in the urinary tract. UTIs are a common problem encountered in health care. It is estimated that each year, there are at least 150 million cases of symptomatic UTIs worldwide (Foxman, 2014). UTIs occur across the life span. As many as 10% of women experience at least one episode of acute uncomplicated urinary infection in a year, and 60% have at least one episode during their lifetime. The peak incidence of infection occurs in young, sexually active women ages 18 to 24. Recurrent episodes are experienced by as many as 5% of women at some time during their life.

The clinical spectrum of UTIs ranges from asymptomatic bacteriuria, to symptomatic and recurrent UTIs, to sepsis associated with UTI requiring hospitalization. Recent evidence helps differentiate asymptomatic bacteriuria from symptomatic UTI. Asymptomatic bacteriuria is transient in older women, often resolves without any treatment, and is not associated with morbidity or mortality. The diagnosis of symptomatic UTI is made when a patient has both clinical features and laboratory evidence of a urinary infection. Absent other causes, patients presenting with any two of the following meet the clinical diagnostic criteria for symptomatic UTI: fever, worsened urinary urgency or frequency, acute dysuria, suprapubic tenderness, or costovertebral angle pain or tenderness. A positive urine culture (≥ 105 CFU/mL) with no more than two uropathogens and pyuria confirms the diagnosis of UTI. Risk factors for recurrent symptomatic UTI include diabetes, functional disability, recent sexual intercourse, prior history of urogynecologic surgery, urinary retention, and urinary incontinence. Testing for UTI is easily performed in the clinic using dipstick tests.

CAUSES

Women contract UTIs in a 30:1 ratio to men because of their short urethra and its proximity to the rectum. Sexual intercourse is a contributing factor. With intercourse, periurethral and urethral bacteria may ascend into the bladder. After age 65, the ratio of UTIs in women to men becomes closer to 1. Risk factors for UTIs in men include homosexuality, intercourse with an infected partner, and an uncircumcised penis.

Normal urine is sterile. Infection occurs when microorganisms, usually bacteria from the digestive tract, cling to the opening of the urethra and multiply. *Escherichia coli* is the causative pathogen in 85% to 90% of community-acquired UTIs. *Staphylococcus saprophyticus* accounts for approximately 5% to 15% of UTIs in young women. The microbial spectrum of complicated UTIs is broader and also includes *Pseudomonas, Enterococcus, Staphylococcus, Serratia, Providencia*, and fungi.

Bacterial growth is decreased by dilute urine and a low urine pH. Glucose in urine is an enhanced medium for the growth of *E. coli*. The urine from pregnant women has a more suitable pH for growth of *E. coli*. Diaphragm and spermicide use (nonoxynol 9), estrogen deficiency, and constipation also are risk factors for UTIs. Inefficient bladder emptying causes UTIs because of stagnating urine. Underlying conditions that predispose to UTI are listed in **Box 32.1**.

In the normal male urethra, the distance between the end of the urethra and the bladder is too long to allow ascending transport of bacteria to the bladder. Therefore, bacteriuria in men should always be considered an abnormal finding, and men cannot have uncomplicated infections.

> **BOX 32.1 Underlying Conditions That Predispose Individuals to Urinary Tract Infections**
>
> - Female sex
> - Pregnancy
> - Diabetes
> - Chronic degenerative neurologic conditions
> - Paralysis
> - Recurrent UTI
> - Ineffective bladder emptying
> - Estrogen deficiency
> - Constipation
> - Delayed postcoital micturition
> - History of recurrent childhood UTI
> - Sickle cell disease
> - Polycystic kidney disease
> - Structural defects of the urinary system
> - Renal transplant

PATHOPHYSIOLOGY

The development of a UTI depends on the virulence of the organism, the inoculum size, and the adequacy of the host's defense mechanisms. In general, the urinary tract is resistant to invading bacteria and rapidly eliminates organisms that reach the bladder. When bacteria enter the bladder, there is increased micturition and diuresis to empty the bladder.

Most pathogens enter the urinary tract and ascend the urethra to the bladder. Most of the microorganisms are from fecal flora, but the vagina is an important source of infecting organisms. Bacteria that cause UTIs originate in the fecal flora, colonize the vagina and periurethral introitus, and ascend to the urethra and bladder. In the bladder, the bacteria multiply and travel up the urethra to the renal pelvis and parenchyma, especially if there is vesicoureteral reflux. With cystitis, there is silent involvement of the kidneys in approximately 50% of cases.

The longer urethra in men increases the distance between the rectum and the urethral meatus, and the drier environment around the urethra and the antibacterial activity of prostatic fluid also decrease the risk of UTIs in men.

DIAGNOSTIC CRITERIA

In women of childbearing age, the most frequent presentation of cystitis is the classic triad of urinary urgency, frequency, and dysuria, with symptoms of abrupt onset. There may also be pressure or fullness in the suprapubic area and back pain. Pyelonephritis presents with flank pain, nausea and vomiting, and temperature greater than 100.4°F (38°C) with or without symptoms of cystitis.

Differentiation must be made between complicated and uncomplicated UTI before progressing with diagnostic evaluation. An uncomplicated UTI is defined as occurring in a premenopausal, sexually active, nonpregnant woman who has not recently had a UTI. A complicated UTI is one that occurs in a man, a postmenopausal or pregnant woman, or a patient with urinary structural defects, neurologic lesions, or a catheter. A UTI also is considered complicated if symptoms have persisted for more than 7 days. In sexually active men with symptoms of cystitis, urethritis must be ruled out. Pyelonephritis presents with recurrent fevers, chills, flank pain, and a positive urine culture.

The diagnosis of UTI is made after a careful history, physical examination, and limited laboratory studies. Because UTI is the most common infection for which adults receive antibiotics, its evaluation and management must be cost-effective. Cultures do not need to be performed if the criteria for an uncomplicated UTI are met, because antimicrobial susceptibility profiles are predictable and culture results do not return until after the symptoms have resolved.

The leukocyte dipstick test is 75% to 95% sensitive in detecting pyuria. Examination of spun or unspun urine that does not show leukocytes should suggest a diagnosis other than UTI. Hematuria occurs in approximately half of all acute UTIs. Pretreatment and posttreatment cultures should be performed for male patients. Pretreatment cultures are ordered in suspected pyelonephritis; posttreatment cultures are performed only if symptoms recur within 2 weeks or if the symptoms do not resolve with treatment initially.

INITIATING DRUG THERAPY

Without treatment, 25% to 42% of uncomplicated acute cystitis cases in women resolve spontaneously. However, the standard therapy for all UTIs is antibiotic treatment.

A urine culture with 10^5/mL organisms or greater is a diagnostic indicator of UTI with or without symptoms. A patient who has symptoms and a culture with 10^2/mL organisms or greater is treated. All symptomatic UTIs should be treated. The purpose of early treatment of cystitis is to reduce the risk of progression to pyelonephritis, although the incidence is small. Treatment does not affect the duration of symptoms, which is 3 to 4 days. In patients with pyelonephritis, early treatment is important to reduce the duration of symptoms, eliminate microorganisms from the renal parenchyma, and reduce the risk of dissemination to the blood.

For some patients with cystitis, a urinary analgesic may be useful to relieve discomfort caused by severe dysuria. A 2-day course is usually sufficient to allow time for symptomatic response to antimicrobial therapy and minimize inflammation. Dysuria is usually diminished within a few hours after the start of antimicrobial therapy.

Although most UTIs resolve spontaneously if not treated, they are treated for symptom relief. The treatment for UTI is antibiotics. The choice of antibiotic and the length of treatment depend on whether the infection is uncomplicated or complicated and on the sex and age of the patient.

A short course of treatment increases compliance and decreases the cost and side effects. For women infected with susceptible *E. coli*, cure rates of 90% to 95% are achieved with 1 to 3 days of therapy. There is no benefit to treatment exceeding 3 days in uncomplicated UTIs in women unless nitrofurantoin is used; the length of treatment for this drug is 5 to 7 days.

Current resistance to ampicillin is near 50% in most regions of the United States. Therefore, it is not recommended for first-line therapy unless the organism is shown to be sensitive to it. Resistance to trimethoprim–sulfamethoxazole (TMP–SMZ) is up to 20% in some areas of the United States, but resistance to nitrofurantoin remains low.

Goals of Therapy

The goals of therapy for UTIs are to destroy the offending organism, relieve symptoms, and prevent complications.

Antibiotics are discussed in detail in Chapter 8. Those used to treat UTIs are listed in **Table 32.1**.

Urinary Analgesics

This class of drugs is used for the symptomatic relief of pain, urgency, burning, frequency, and discomfort associated with trauma to the lower urinary tract mucosa. They are used in infection, trauma, surgery, endoscopic procedures, and catheterization. They should not be used for more than 2 days and are not used for treatment of a UTI per se, but for symptom relief.

TABLE 32.1

Overview of Selected Agents for Urinary Tract Infection

Generic (Trade) Name and Dosage	Selected Adverse Events	Contraindications	Special Considerations
Antibiotics			
trimethoprim–sulfamethoxazole (Bactrim) Children: 5 mg/kg/d in divided doses for 10 d Adults: 1 DS q12h for 10d	Nausea/vomiting, anorexia, megaloblastic anemia, hallucinations, depression, seizures	Megaloblastic anemia Pregnancy (category C) Breast-feeding mother Not recommended for children <2 mo G6PD deficiency	May consider newer macrolide antibiotics, such as clarithromycin and azithromycin
trimethoprim (Trimpex) 100 mg q12h for 3 d	Same as above	Megaloblastic anemia Pregnancy (category C) Breast-feeding mother Sulfa allergy	G6PD-deficient patients can have hemolysis. May cause falsely elevated creatinine Increase fluid intake.
nitrofurantoin (Macrobid, Macrodantin) Macrobid—100 mg q12h for 7 d Macrodantin—100 mg qid for 7 d	Nausea, pulmonary allergic reaction, dizziness, hemolytic anemia Diarrhea, vaginitis, rhinitis, headache	Anuria Oliguria Pregnancy at term Nursing mother Caution if hepatic impairment	Take with food to increase absorption. Avoid use with live vaccines
ciprofloxacin (Cipro) 100–250 mg q12h for 3 d for uncomplicated cystitis and 7 d for complicated cystitis and 500 mg for 10–14 d for uncomplicated pyelonephritis	Nausea, diarrhea, altered taste, dizziness, drowsiness, headache, insomnia, agitation, confusion Serious: pseudomembranous colitis, Stevens-Johnson syndrome	Allergy to fluoroquinolones Avoid in patients <18 y Pregnancy Use with caution in renal disease, central nervous system disease, breast-feeding (safety not established)	Raises serum level of theophylline Avoid taking with aluminum- or magnesium-containing antacids. Food slows absorption. Drug interacts with antacids, theophylline, warfarin, probenecid, digoxin, foscarnet, glucocorticoids.
ofloxacin (Floxin) 200 mg q12h for 3 d for uncomplicated cystitis and 7 d for complicated cystitis and 200–300 mg for 10–14 d for uncomplicated pyelonephritis	Nausea, diarrhea, headache, insomnia, photosensitivity	Pregnancy (category C) Breast-feeding Not recommended in children	Take at least 30 min before or 2 h after meal. Avoid taking with aluminum- or magnesium-containing antacids or sucralfate, iron, and multivitamins with zinc because these can decrease absorption. Increase fluid intake significantly.

(Continued)

TABLE 32.1

Overview of Selected Agents for Urinary Tract Infection (*Continued*)

Generic (Trade) Name and Dosage	Selected Adverse Events	Contraindications	Special Considerations
levofloxacin (Levaquin) 250 mg qd for 3 d for uncomplicated cystitis and 7 d for complicated cystitis and 10–14 d for uncomplicated pyelonephritis	Nausea, diarrhea, photosensitivity	Same as above	Increase fluid intake significantly. Avoid taking with aluminum- or magnesium-containing antacids or sucralfate, iron, and multivitamins with zinc because these can decrease absorption.
norfloxacin (Noroxin) 400 mg q12h for 3 d for uncomplicated cystitis and 7 d for complicated cystitis and 10–14 d for uncomplicated pyelonephritis	Seizures, dizziness, nausea, headache, tendinitis/tendon rupture	Same as above	Same as above
cefixime (Suprax) 400 mg qd for 3 d for uncomplicated cystitis and 7 d for complicated cystitis and 10–14 d for uncomplicated pyelonephritis	Diarrhea GI upset, rash, drug fever, pruritus, headache, dizziness, vaginitis	Known allergy to cephalosporins Use with caution in penicillin-allergic patients. Use with caution in patients with renal impairment, continuous ambulatory peritoneal dialysis, dialysis, GI disease.	Pregnancy category B
Urinary Analgesics methenamine (Urised) 2 tabs qid	Rash, anticholinergic effects, xerostomia, flushing, difficulty in urinating, acute urinary retention with benign prostatic hyperplasia, tachycardia, dizziness, blurry vision, urine or fecal discoloration	Glaucoma Not recommended in patients <6 y Pregnancy (category C) Breast-feeding Bowel obstruction Urinary obstruction Cardiospasm	May cause blue-green discoloration of urine or feces Is not antibacterial
phenazopyridine (Pyridium) 200 mg tid	Headache, rash, GI upset, hemolytic anemia	Renal insufficiency	Discolors urine and clothes (red-orange) Is not antibacterial Take after meals. Reduce dose on improvement.
flavoxate (Urispas) 100–200 mg tid–qid	Nausea and vomiting, anticholinergic side effects, vertigo, headache, drowsiness, urticaria, confusion, tachycardia	GI obstruction Obstructive uropathies Glaucoma	

G6PD, glucose-6-phosphate dehydrogenase.

The azo dye in this class is excreted in the urine and exerts a rapid topical analgesic effect on the mucosa of the urinary tract. The urinary analgesics are used with caution in pregnancy and lactation and are contraindicated in renal insufficiency. For additional information, see **Table 32.1**.

Selecting the Most Appropriate Agent

Antibiotics are selected by identifying the uropathogen, knowing local resistance rates, and considering adverse effect profiles. A 3-day course of TMP–SMZ or trimethoprim alone continues to be recognized as first-line treatment. There are concerns, however, about rare but serious skin reactions to the sulfa component and about growing resistance (about 10% in Canada). This drug should be avoided in patients treated within 6 months because they are more likely to have resistant organisms.

Nitrofurantoin has a long history of good efficacy and continues as a first-line choice, even though a 7-day course is required. Despite heavy use, very little resistance to nitrofurantoin has developed.

Another choice for first-line therapy is fosfomycin. This is a powder dissolved in water. The advantage of this drug is the one-time dosing.

Fluoroquinolones have more recently been introduced to treat UTIs, and they are very effective in a 3-day course. Their cost and the potential for developing resistance, however, suggest that they should remain a second-line choice for treatment. Cephalosporins, ampicillin, and amoxicillin should not be used unless the cultured organism is sensitive to these agents.

Cystitis and pyelonephritis are treated with the same antibiotic, but the treatment course for pyelonephritis is longer. The most desirable antibiotic is one that is low in cost with an infrequent dosing schedule, lack of resistance in local pathogens, long duration in the urinary tract, and the potential to decrease the number of *E. coli* in the vaginal and fecal reservoirs. The antibiotic selected should spare the protective, natural bacterial flora of the vagina and gastrointestinal tract, and there should be a low side effect profile. Nonpregnant women with uncomplicated cystitis may be treated with a 3-day course of antibiotics (except with nitrofurantoin, which is 5 to 7 days). Postmenopausal women should be treated for 7 days (**Figure 32.1**; **Tables 32.2** and **32.3**). Men also require a 7-day treatment because of the increased chance of a complicated infection and prostatic infection.

First-Line Therapy

The first-line choice for cystitis is TMP–SMZ (Bactrim). This drug combination has little impact on normal vaginal flora but decreases the number of *E. coli* in vaginal and fecal reservoirs,

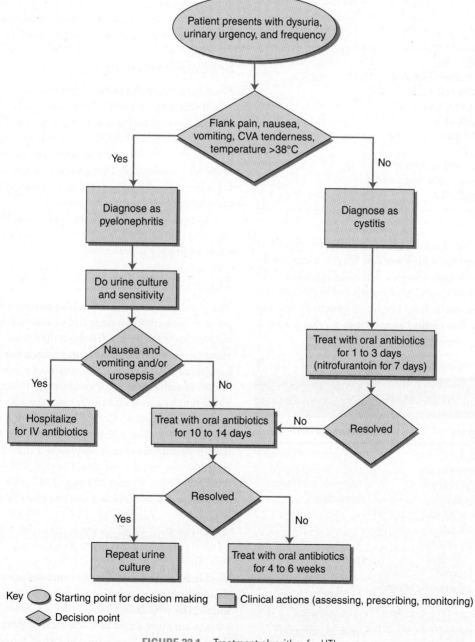

FIGURE 32.1   Treatment algorithm for UTI.

TABLE 32.2

Recommended Order of Treatment for Uncomplicated Cystitis

Order	Agent	Comments
First line	3-day oral therapy of	Drink at least 8 glasses of fluids.
	• TMP–SMZ	Initiate 7-day therapy in postmenopausal women and in men.
	Or 7-day therapy of nitrofurantoin	May use urinary analgesics in combination with antibiotics
		Higher incidence of treatment failure with nitrofurantoin for 3 d, so 7-day use is recommended
Second line	7-day oral therapy of • TMP–SMZ May also use 7-day oral therapy of: • ciprofloxacin • levofloxacin • ofloxacin • norfloxacin	
Third line	Culture and sensitivity/ testing, then treat based on results	

decreasing the chance of reinfection. Trimethoprim appears to be similar in efficacy but with fewer side effects; it can also be used in patients with sulfa allergies. The sulfa ingredient may be more important for complicated cystitis and pyelonephritis.

Nitrofurantoin has a long history of good efficacy and continues as a first-line choice, even though a 7-day course is

TABLE 32.3

Recommended Order of Treatment for Uncomplicated Pyelonephritis

Order	Agents	Comments
First line	Oral for 10–14 d: • ciprofloxacin • levofloxacin • enoxacin • norfloxacin • ofloxacin • sparfloxacin • TMP–SMZ • cefixime • cefpodoxime proxetil	Urine culture and sensitivity testing should be performed before treatment.
Second line	Oral therapy for 2–6 wk	
Third line	Hospitalization for IV therapy	For severe illness or possible urosepsis

required. Despite heavy use, very little resistance to nitrofurantoin has developed.

Fosfomycin (Monaural) is also used in first-line therapy. It is dissolved in water. This is a one-time drug. The disadvantage is that the price is high. There is no generic substitute.

Patients with cystitis can also be given urinary tract analgesics. This group includes methenamine (Urised), phenazopyridine (Pyridium, Uristat), or flavoxate (Urispas).

Uncomplicated pyelonephritis is usually treated in the outpatient setting because of the available oral antibiotics. The patient with pyelonephritis is admitted to the hospital only if he or she cannot take oral fluids or oral antibiotics, has a high fever or marked debility, or has a social situation incompatible with outpatient treatment. First-line therapy for pyelonephritis is an antibiotic, as mentioned previously, for 10 to 14 days. Fluoroquinolones are usually given first if culture results are not available because of their broad spectrum of activity. No follow-up is required if the symptoms resolve.

Second-Line Therapy

Fluoroquinolones are options for empiric therapy of recurrent cystitis. If symptoms of cystitis do not resolve after 3 days of therapy, a 7-day course of antibiotics is recommended. Fluoroquinolones are not recommended as first-line agents for uncomplicated cystitis because of the increased cost and concerns over development of quinolone resistance. They should be reserved for treatment of UTIs in men and postmenopausal women and for patients with complicated UTIs and pyelonephritis.

In pyelonephritis, a culture is obtained after treatment. If the urine is not free of bacteria after initial therapy, 4 to 6 more weeks of therapy is prescribed.

Third-Line Therapy

The recurrence rate for UTIs is approximately 20%. At this point, a urine culture is done and treatment is based on the culture results. If the patient has fewer than two UTIs a year, treatment can be based on the previous culture results. Women who have three or more recurrences annually may be offered the option of self-treatment of recurrences. Postcoital use of antibiotic prophylaxis is effective for women who have recurrences related to intercourse. Continuous antibiotic prophylaxis in a single bedtime dose is also accepted practice for women who have frequent recurrences. Antibiotics that have been shown to reduce the number of recurrences to 0.3 or fewer per year are TMP–SMZ 40 mg/200 mg, TMP 100 mg, norfloxacin 200 mg, and nitrofurantoin macrocrystals 50 to 100 mg.

Special Population Considerations

Geriatric

In elderly patients, UTIs are commonly asymptomatic, but should be strongly considered as a diagnostic possibility for individuals who have changes in mentation. Postmenopausal women are more prone to UTIs because there is uropathogen-dominant vaginal flora with the loss of estrogen. Lactobacilli diminish and pH increases. Elderly patients are at increased risk for UTIs. Vaginal estrogen therapy effectively reduces symptomatic UTI episodes in the elderly population.

Approximately 10% to 20% of the population older than age 65 has bacteriuria related to factors such as fecal incontinence, incomplete bladder emptying, malnutrition, and increased urine pH. Any UTI in a man is considered complicated. *E. coli* and *Enterobacter* species are the usual organisms. In elderly men, *Proteus, Klebsiella, Serratia, Pseudomonas,* and *Enterococcus* species are also responsible for UTIs. UTIs in men are most often seen in conjunction with prostatic hyperplasia with partial obstruction or persistent prostatitis.

Nitrofurantoin is not recommended in the elderly because it requires a creatinine clearance of 40 mL/min. Treatment is for 7 to 10 days in women and 10 to 14 days in men with uncomplicated UTIs.

Pregnancy

Asymptomatic bacteriuria occurs in approximately 7% of pregnant women. Of these, pyelonephritis develops in 30% if the bacteriuria is not treated. Untreated UTIs can contribute to prematurity or stillbirth. Amoxicillin is effective in approximately two thirds of UTIs in pregnant women and is safe for the fetus. Also safe are cephalexin and nitrofurantoin (only during the first and second trimesters). Sulfonamides are safe except in the last trimester. In pregnancy, the urine is cultured 1 week after treatment and every 4 to 6 weeks during the pregnancy.

Physiologic changes in pregnancy increase the risk for pyelonephritis. The ureters become obstructed because of blockage from the enlarged uterus. In addition, increased progesterone relaxes the smooth muscles of the ureter and bladder. Bacteriuria in pregnancy has been associated with a 20% to 30% incidence of pyelonephritis and premature delivery, intrauterine growth retardation, increased risk for death in the perinatal period, and congenital anomalies.

In 5% to 10% of women with UTI, there are no symptoms. Pregnant women should be screened for UTIs, and they must be treated regardless of whether they are symptomatic.

Children

UTIs in children may indicate a genitourinary anomaly. Accurate diagnosis usually requires invasive collection of urine, especially in very young children. It is important to start treatment quickly, especially in young children, because there is an increased risk of renal scarring in children under age 5 from UTIs. UTIs recur in 32% to 40% of children.

UTI should be suspected in febrile infants without an obvious source. Urine specimens collected with a bag are considered insufficient to make a diagnosis. Transurethral and suprapubic catheterization are accepted methods of urine collection in children. All children younger than 3 years diagnosed with a first UTI should have a renal ultrasound scan and a voiding cystourethrogram (VCUG). Boys older than 3 years can either have ultrasonography with VCUG or a renal cortical scan with follow-up VCUG as indicated based on the results. Girls between the ages of 3 and 7 years should have

either ultrasonography with VCUG or a renal scan if febrile or observation without imaging if afebrile. Girls older than 7 years can be observed without imaging.

First-line antimicrobial agents include the β-lactams amoxicillin–clavulanate (25–45 mg/kg/d divided every 12 hours), cephalexin (25–50 mg/kg/d, divided every 6–12 hours), and cefpodoxime (10 mg/kg/d divided every 12 hours) as well as TMP–SMX (8–10 mg/kg/d divided every 12 hours). Two-day to 4-day courses have been shown to be as effective as 7 to 14 days.

MONITORING PATIENT RESPONSE

Prescribers need to evaluate for cystitis that does not resolve or that recurs within a week after treatment requires culture and sensitivity testing and treatment with a fluoroquinolone for 7 days. UTIs recur within a year in approximately half of all women, although there is a very low incidence of pyelonephritis that develops as a result.

If pyelonephritis recurs within 2 weeks after treatment, a urine culture and sensitivity test and renal ultrasound or computed tomography scan should be performed to determine whether there is a urologic abnormality. If the organism is the same as the first, a 4- to 6-week course of antibiotics is recommended.

Patients who have three or more UTIs a year should be given prophylaxis, either continuous or postcoital. Continuous prophylaxis usually consists of TMP–SMZ 40 to 200 mg daily or three times a week. Postcoital therapy is indicated in women who identify intercourse as the cause of infection; the selected therapy is taken after intercourse. The use of estrogen replacement therapy in postmenopausal women decreases the number of recurrent UTIs. In cases of true relapse, the culture is repeated and therapy is prescribed for 2 to 4 weeks.

In pyelonephritis, a culture is repeated 1 to 2 weeks after completion of therapy. If there is a recurrence, therapy is recommended for 6 to 12 months.

PATIENT EDUCATION

Drug Information

Patients can get information about UTIs at http://www.nlm.nih.gov/medlineplus/urinarytractinfections.html, http://kidney.niddk.nih.gov/KUDiseases/topics/uti.aspx, and http://www.healthline.com/health/urinary-tract-infection-adults.

Lifestyle Changes

The most important advice is for sexually active women to urinate shortly after sexual intercourse. In doing so, they wash out the increased number of bacteria in the distal urethra. Another useful suggestion is for patients with recurrent UTIs to practice double or triple voiding and changing position while urinating helps rid the bladder of residual urine.

Other behavioral factors to consider are the direction of toilet paper use after bowel movements, type of menstrual protection

CASE STUDY*

J.S., a 65-year-old woman with diabetes, seeks treatment for dysuria, frequent urination, flank pain, and costovertebral angle tenderness. She has a temperature of 102°F, and under the microscope, her spun urine contains a large number of leukocytes.

DIAGNOSIS: CYSTITIS WITH POSSIBLE PYELONEPHRITIS

1. List specific goals for treatment for **J.S.**
2. What drug therapy would you prescribe? Why?
3. What are the parameters for monitoring success of the therapy?

4. Discuss specific patient education based on the prescribed therapy.
5. List one or two adverse reactions for the selected agent that would cause you to change therapy.
6. What would be the choice for second-line therapy?
7. What over-the-counter and/or alternative medications would be appropriate for **J.S.**?
8. What lifestyle changes would you recommend to **J.S.**?
9. Describe one or two drug–drug or drug–food interactions for the selected agent.

* Answers can be found online.

used, and method of contraception. The use of spermicides changes the vaginal flora, increasing the colonization of *E. coli* and the frequency of UTIs. Women with recurrent UTIs should use a method of birth control that does not involve spermicides.

Other preventive measures include avoiding bubble baths and "feminine hygiene" products. Urinating every 2 hours, taking the time to empty the bladder completely, also helps prevent UTIs. Foods that irritate the bladder should be avoided, including tea, coffee, alcohol, cola, chocolate, and spicy foods.

Patients with frequently recurring cystitis can benefit from early self-treatment if they are well informed and compliant. If treatment is started very shortly after the onset of symptoms, a 3-day course or even a single dose of antimicrobial provides rapid relief of symptoms.

Complementary and Alternative Medicine

Cranberry juice concentrate or cranberry concentrate capsules have been recognized as alternatives to antibiotics or for the prevention of UTIs. Cranberry is believed to have antiadherence properties in the urinary tract and acidifies urine. Small studies have reported that a daily intake of 150 to 750 mL of cranberry juice is effective in preventing recurrent UTIs (Kontiokari et al., 2001). An alternative to juice is one 300- to 400-mg capsule taken two times a day with a glass of water. Additionally, 8 to 16 ounces of preparations with at least 30% cranberry juice can be taken. Vitamin C, 500 mg every 4 hours for the duration of the UTI, has been suggested, with 1,000 to 1,500 mg/d for prevention of UTIs.

Probiotics may decrease UTIs by restoring normal vaginal flora. Lactobacillus is thought to prevent colonization with *E. coli.*

Bibliography

*Starred references are cited in the text.

Beerepoot, M. A., ter Riet, G., Nys, S., et al. (2011). Cranberries vs antibiotics to prevent urinary tract infections: A randomized double-blind noninferiority trial in premenopausal women. *Archives of Internal Medicine,* *171*(14), 1270–1278.

Clark, C., Kennedy, W., & Shortliffe, L. (2010). Urinary tract infections in children: When to worry. *Urologic Clinics of North America, 37*(2), 229–241.

Ebell, M. H. (2013). Most antibiotics similar in efficacy for lower UTI. *American Family Physician, 88*(2), 137–142.

Flores-Mireles, A., Walk, J., Caparon, M., et al. (2015). Urinary tract infections: Epidemiology, mechanisms of infection and treatment options. *Nature Reviews. Microbiology, 13,* 269–284. doi: 10.1038/nrmicro.3432.

*Foxman, B. (2014). Urinary tract infection syndromes: Occurrence, recurrence, bacteriology, risk factors, and disease burden. *Infectious Disease Clinics of North America, 28,* 1–13. Retrieved from http://dx.doi.org/10.1016/j.idc.2013.09.003

Guptal, K., Hooton, T. M., Naber, K. G., et al. (2011). International clinical practice guidelines for the treatment of acute uncomplicated cystitis and pyelonephritis in women: A 2010 update by Infectious Diseases Society of America and the European Society for Microbiology and Infectious Diseases. *Clinical Infectious Diseases, 52*(5), e103–e120.

Hooton, T. M. (2012). Uncomplicated urinary tract infection. *New England Journal of Medicine, 366*(10), 1028–1037.

Kodner, C. M., & Gupton, E. K. (2010). Recurrent urinary tract infections in women: Diagnosis and management. *American Family Physician, 82*(6), 638–643.

*Kontiokari, T., Sundqvist, K., Nuutinen, M., et al. (2001). Randomised trial of cranberry–lingonberry juice and Lactobacillus GG drink for the prevention of urinary tract infections in women. *British Medical Journal, 322*(10), 1571.

Mody, L., & Juthani-Mehta, M. (2014). Urinary tract infections in older women: A clinical review. *JAMA, 311*(8), 844–854.

Wang, A., Nizran, P., Malone, M. A., et al. (2013). Urinary tract infections. *Primary Care; Clinics in Office Practice, 40*(3), 687–706.

33 Prostatic Disorders and Erectile Dysfunction

Virginia P. Arcangelo

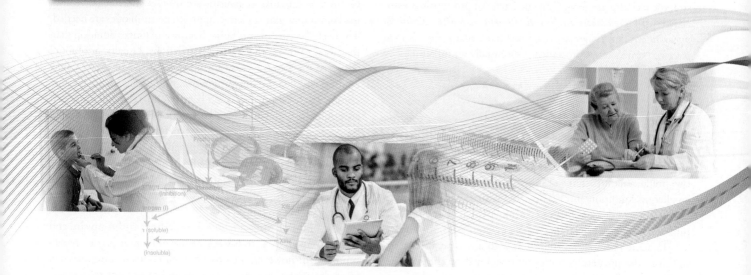

Disorders of the prostate appear as part of the normal aging process and also as abnormalities distinct from normal aging. Often, it is not until age 40 that a man begins to show some form of noncancerous prostatic disorder, whereas prostate cancer usually is found after age 50. At 70, approximately 40% of men report lower urinary tract symptoms (LUTS), increasing to 50% at the age of 75, most often from benign prostatic hypertrophy (BPH).

Prostate cancer is the second most common type of cancer affecting men, with a lifetime prevalence of 15%. Black men have the highest incidence of prostate cancer. Asian and Hispanic men are at lower risk than White men. In addition to race, other risk factors for prostate cancer are age and family history. The disease rarely occurs before age 45, but the incidence rises exponentially thereafter; nearly 70% of cases are diagnosed in men age 65 and older. There are 147.8/100,000 cases of newly diagnosed prostate cancer per year.

Prostate disorders are diagnosed through clinical manifestations and screening procedures used to detect or rule out prostate cancer. Lack of knowledge about prostate cancer and lack of available screening procedures are the major deterrents to accurate and timely diagnosis of prostate cancer.

Treatment of prostatic disorders itself may result in some untoward side effects, which must then also be managed. Often, the man postpones seeking medical intervention and blames aging for many of the manifestations, thus delaying treatment. Some difficulties in seeking treatment can relate to the man's culture; sexuality—specifically, masculinity—can be perceived as synonymous with virility. For this reason, a man may choose not to discuss (even with a health care worker) clinical manifestations.

Prostatic disorders and LUTS occur because of inflammation or infection (prostatitis), BPH, and prostate cancer; prostatitis can involve the bladder neck, thus becoming prostatocystitis. A bacterial infection is often the cause of prostatitis, although some nonbacterial forms of prostatitis do exist. Inflammation can be chronic or acute.

Adenocarcinoma is the most common type of prostate cancer. Metastasis can follow slowly or quickly, and often, the symptoms of metastasis are what lead the man to seek medical intervention.

Presenting manifestations of prostatic disorders are usually specific to the urinary tract and include difficulty in onset of urine flow with or without a low flow of urine, frequency or urgency in voiding, incontinence, distention of the bladder, and hematuria. Management of prostatic disorders is specific to the particular disorder (cancerous vs. noncancerous), with some overlap in treatment.

PROSTATITIS

CAUSES

Prostatitis is one of the most common urological infections afflicting adult men and has recently been divided into four different categories based on the National Institutes of Health (NIH) consensus classification (Weidner & Anderson, 2008). This category system includes category I (acute bacterial prostatitis); category II (chronic bacterial prostatitis); category III chronic nonbacterial prostatitis and pelvic pain syndrome, including inflammatory and noninflammatory types (CP/CPPS); and category IV (asymptomatic inflammatory prostatitis). Acute and chronic bacterial prostatitis affects less than 5% of men with prostatitis. Most patients with prostatitis are found to have either nonbacterial prostatitis or prostatodynia. This disorder can be acute or chronic. With acute bacterial prostatitis, the chief organisms involved are *Escherichia coli* and *Pseudomonas* species, although strains of staphylococci or streptococci also are seen. Chronic bacterial prostatitis is associated with *Pseudomonas*, *E. coli*, *Proteus mirabilis*, *Klebsiella pneumoniae*, and *Enterococcus* species, particularly *Enterococcus faecalis*. Nonbacterial prostatitis is essentially an inflammatory disorder.

PATHOPHYSIOLOGY

Often chronic, nonbacterial prostatitis is nonetheless problematic for the patient. Primary etiologies of this condition include two predominant patterns of inflammation. The first is that of an allergic condition and is associated with eosinophil infiltration. The second is a nonspecific form in which granulomatous inflammation by peculiar, large, pale macrophages is found.

In acute bacterial prostatitis, as with any type of bacterial invasion, the prostate becomes overwhelmed by the bacteria, leading to inflammatory response activation. Usually, acute bacterial prostatitis is seen as an infection ascending up the urinary tract, and younger men, ages 30 to 50, can be affected with this illness.

DIAGNOSTIC CRITERIA

Symptom manifestation revolves around urinary tract signs. There is pain in the lower abdomen, difficulty in bladder emptying with or without a small stream during urination, nocturia, and fever to 104°F (40°C). Along with the febrile state, as with other infections, general arthralgia and malaise can occur.

On examination and interview, the man often admits to painful ejaculation and pain in the rectal or perineal areas. All the symptoms are due to the edema associated with acute inflammation of the prostate. Because of the risk of generalized septicemia, pharmacotherapeutics are urgently warranted.

Culture isolation of prostatic urine is the most accurate method of diagnosis. Prostatic urine is defined as the third and fourth (urine) secretion specimens of four serial urine sample because prostatic fluid is at a significantly higher concentration in these last two of four serial voids. The four urine samples are obtained sequentially, beginning with the initial void, followed by a midstream urine specimen, prostatic massage secretion, and finally the urine voided after the prostatic massage. Standard laboratory culture techniques are applied to establish the causative organism.

Nonbacterial prostatitis is confirmed by negative prostatic urine cultures with a positive elevated white blood cell count and the presence of inflammatory cells in prostatic secretions. This condition and another nonbacterial type of prostatitis known as *prostatodynia* have the same symptoms as does bacterial prostatitis. Treatment of the nonbacterial forms usually consists of symptom management without the use of antibiotics.

INITIATING DRUG THERAPY

Antibiotics are the required pharmacotherapy. (See Chapter 8.) Given that causative organisms are usually gram negative and, less commonly, gram positive, appropriate antibiotics are needed. The overall course of antibiotic therapy is of longer duration than that used to treat other systemic infections. Usually, antibiotics are given for 4 to 6 weeks, but up to 12 weeks of therapy may be necessary due to poor penetration of prostate tissue. Because chronic bacterial prostatitis is a bacterial infection, an appropriate antibiotic with good tissue penetration in the prostate should be selected. Fluoroquinolones have demonstrated the best tissue concentration and are recommended as first-line agents. Although trimethoprim–sulfamethoxazole (TMP-SMZ) may be considered, the tissue penetration may not be as effective, and in many areas of the United States, there is evidence of increasing uropathogenic resistance.

Second-line drugs include doxycycline, azithromycin, and clarithromycin. A 4- to 6-week course of therapy is usually recommended; however, a 6- to 12-week course is often needed to eradicate the causative organism and to prevent recurrence, especially if symptoms persist after completion of the initial therapy. No guidelines exist for treating gram-positive organisms, but ciprofloxacin and levofloxacin have adequate gram-positive coverage as well as excellent gram-negative coverage, and both medications penetrate the prostate tissue well.

Adjunctive therapies that may be beneficial include the use of sitz baths, analgesics, stool softeners, and antipyretics, along with rest. Prostatic massage, voiding in a warm bath (to relax pelvic muscles), and discontinuation of alcohol and caffeinated beverages can also help to relieve symptoms. If possible, withdrawal from antidepressants, anticholinergics, or sedatives may also help bladder function.

Goals of Drug Therapy

The goal of pharmacotherapy for prostatitis is to eradicate the causative organism and restore the prostate to health. Prostatitis often becomes chronic, and therefore, repeated trials with antibiotics or prolonged dosage schedules may be warranted.

Anti-Infectives

Table 33.1 depicts dosage information, adverse events, contraindications, and special considerations for the anti-infective management of bacterial prostatitis.

Trimethoprim–Sulfamethoxazole

This drug is a bacteriostatic combination product and is considered to be more powerful than its two components given separately. Also, when given as the combined form, resistance on the part of the causative organism arises less frequently. This agent ultimately adversely affects the production of proteins and nucleic acids of bacteria at the target (prostate) site. TMP-SMZ further inhibits growth of bacteria because of its antimetabolite property toward PABA (*para*-aminobenzoic acid). Drug–drug interactions can present when the patient is also

TABLE 33.1			
Overview of Selected Antibiotics Used to Treat Acute Bacterial Prostatitis			
Generic (Trade) Name and Dosage	**Selected Adverse Events**	**Contraindications**	**Special Considerations**
trimethoprim–sulfamethoxazole (TMP-SMZ, Septra, Bactrim) 160 mg of TMP with 800 mg SMZ PO q12h	GI distress, rash	Allergy to sulfa and sulfa products	May prolong the INR for patients on oral anticoagulants
fluoroquinolones ciprofloxacin (Cipro) 500 mg bid norfloxacin (Noroxin) 400 mg bid levofloxacin (Levaquin) 250 mg daily	Headache, diarrhea, nausea, drowsiness, altered taste, insomnia, agitation, confusion Serious: pseudomembranous colitis, Stevens-Johnson syndrome	Allergy to macrolides Pregnancy and lactation Use with caution in patients with severe hepatic or renal disease.	May interfere with theophylline metabolism
doxycycline (Vibramycin) 200 mg PO as first dose, thereafter 100–200 mg PO q12h	GI distress, potential acute hepatotoxicity, potential for nephrotoxicity	Hypersensitivity to any of the tetracyclines Pregnancy and lactation	Decreased effectiveness with food and dairy products, so do not take with food unless side effects are significant Can lead to diabetes insipidus because of antagonistic effect with antidiuretic hormone

taking phenytoin (Dilantin), oral hypoglycemics, or warfarin (Coumadin). Close monitoring of the seizure threshold, serum glucose level, or partial thromboplastin time is important in the patient on TMP-SMZ who is also taking these other agents.

Fluoroquinolones

Fluoroquinolones are also effective for bacterial prostatitis. Effective against gram-negative anaerobes and some gram-positive bacteria, these agents decrease the growth and replication of bacteria by inhibiting bacterial deoxyribonucleic acid (DNA) during synthesis. These agents may be the first choice for someone sensitive or allergic to TMP-SMZ.

The absorption of fluoroquinolones is reduced by milk, antacids (aluminum or magnesium based), iron or zinc salts, and sucralfate. For the patient who is also taking any of these medications, the dose should be taken either 2 hours after or 4 hours before the other medication.

Fluoroquinolones also affect the use of theophylline and warfarin. Elevated levels can occur, and thus, a lower dosage of theophylline or warfarin may be necessary.

Doxycycline

A long-acting tetracycline, doxycycline (Vibramycin) acts by inhibiting protein synthesis: binding of peptidyl transfer ribonucleic acid (tRNA) is blocked at ribosomal mRNA.

Many of the metal ions—aluminum, calcium, iron, magnesium, and zinc—can interfere by creating chelates with doxycycline. Thus, if these metals are given (and they often are as components of antacids), at least 2 hours should separate their use from the ingestion of doxycycline.

Azithromycin and Clarithromycin

These are macrolide antibiotics. Macrolides inhibits RNA-dependent protein synthesis by reversibly binding to the 50S ribosomal subunits of susceptible microorganisms. They induce dissociation of tRNA from the ribosome during the elongation phase. Thus, RNA-dependent protein synthesis is suppressed, and bacterial growth is inhibited. Macrolides are mainly bacteriostatic but can be bacteriocidal depending on bacterial sensitivity and antibiotic concentration.

Selecting the Most Appropriate Agent

Oral antibiotics are the treatment agents of choice.

First-Line Therapy

The primary choice for first-line antibiotic therapy is a fluoroquinolone (**Table 33.2**). Therapy lasts for 4 to 6 weeks. See **Figure 33.1** for more information. TMP-SMZ may also be considered if treatment is in an area where there is not a high incidence of resistance.

Second-Line Therapy

Doxycycline, azithromycin, and clarithromycin are second-line agents. If the infection is not resolved with 4 to 6 weeks of drug treatment, therapy can be continued for up to 12 weeks.

Special Population Considerations

In older men who are taking fluoroquinolones, creatinine clearance must be monitored.

TABLE 33.2

Recommended Order of Treatment for Prostatitis

Order	Agents	Comments
First line	Fluoroquinolones or TMP-SMZ	Ineffective against enterococci Treat for 4–6 wk.
Second line	Doxycycline or azithromycin or clarithromycin	

MONITORING PATIENT RESPONSE

As a group, anti-infective agents should begin to elicit results after the first week of therapy. Subjective response from the patient indicating alleviation of symptoms is helpful in monitoring the effectiveness of these medications. Some patients may not notice symptom resolution until after 2 weeks; they should be told this and encouraged to continue taking the medication. Ultimately, 12 weeks of therapy may be required. Follow-up cultures may be obtained at the practitioner's discretion. Further diagnostic criteria may also be recommended for ongoing symptom manifestation.

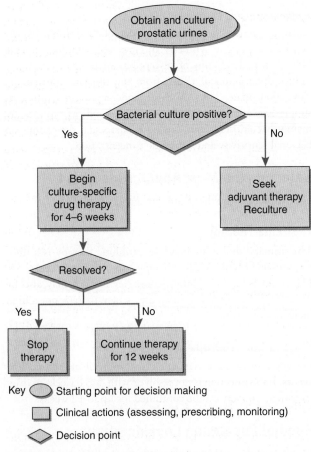

FIGURE 33.1 Treatment algorithm for prostatitis.

PATIENT EDUCATION

The patient should understand potential side effects, interactions, and appropriate use of the medications. Literature can provide patients with a guide for such potential concerns as well as dosing information. With a prepared and knowledgeable patient, these medications are effective against prostatitis. Cost also can be a factor of concern to the patient. The practitioner should be aware of any financial constraints the patient may have, because compliance with medication is important for effective treatment of bacterial prostatitis.

BENIGN PROSTATIC HYPERPLASIA

Benign prostatic hyperplasia (BPH) is the most common prostate problem in men older than age 50; the disease rarely causes symptoms before age 40. As life expectancy rises, so does the occurrence of BPH—an estimated 6.3 million men have BPH. In the United States alone, the disease accounts for 6.4 million doctor visits and more than 400,000 hospitalizations annually. Approximately 90% of men age 80 and older have histologic evidence of BPH, and more than 80% have BPH-related symptoms. Approximately 25% of men older than age 55 and 50% of men older than age 75 experience decreased urinary flow.

CAUSES

The cause of BPH is not well understood. It has been observed that BPH does not develop in men whose testes were removed before puberty. For this reason, some researchers believe that factors related to aging and the testes may spur the development of BPH. Men produce both testosterone and small amounts of estrogen. As men age, the amount of active testosterone in the blood decreases, leaving a higher proportion of estrogen. Studies performed on animals have suggested that BPH may occur because the higher amount of estrogen within the gland increases the activity of substances that promote cell growth. Another theory focuses on dihydrotestosterone (DHT), a substance derived from testosterone in the prostate, which may help control its growth. Some research has indicated that even with a drop in the blood's testosterone level, older men continue to produce and accumulate high levels of DHT in the prostate. This accumulation of DHT may encourage the growth of cells. Researchers have also noted that men who do not produce DHT do not develop BPH.

PATHOPHYSIOLOGY

The dynamic component of BPH and LUTS is based on autonomic input to the smooth muscles in the lower urinary tract, including the bladder, prostate, and urethra. These areas have a large concentration of α_1-adrenergic receptors that, when stimulated by various stressors, cause increasing smooth muscle tone. This increased smooth muscle tone leads to increased urethral resistance and contributes to the bladder outlet obstructive symptoms of BPH. This physiology leads to the basis for a main class of drugs to treat BPH, the use of α_1-adrenergic blockers.

An underlying pathophysiologic process of BPH is the formation of large, nonmalignant lesions at the periurethral region of the prostate gland. Prostatic hyperplasia is an overgrowth of normal cells in the stromal and epithelial tissues of the prostate gland. The hyperplasia originates in the transition zone of the prostate, which surrounds the prostatic urethra between the bladder and the anus. The etiology of the hyperplastic process is unknown, but it has been speculated that it is hormone related because it occurs only in older men. The male aging process involves a decrease in testosterone production with a concomitant increase in estrogen; estrogen may be a sensitizer for the escalating hyperplasia. Bladder control involves reflex activity of the peripheral autonomic nervous system (ANS). The reflex for normal micturition is housed in the brain stem and supported by descending and ascending pathways from the spinal cord. Both the external sphincter and the detrusor muscle are needed for bladder control. Reflex micturition is innervated at the S2 to S4 and T1 to L1 levels in the spinal cord. The cortical center of the brain appears to be important for inhibition or control of the micturition center to modulate contractile, filling, and expulsion activity.

Parasympathetic and sympathetic innervation is crucial to the role of the ANS in voiding. Parasympathetic interplay allows for the detrusor muscle to maintain tone and to contract, whereas sympathetic interplay allows for the bladder to expand and maintain a large filling capacity. The dynamic component of BPH and LUTS is based on autonomic input to the smooth muscles in the lower urinary tract, including the bladder, prostate, and urethra. These areas have a large concentration of α_1-adrenergic receptors that, when stimulated by various stressors, cause increasing smooth muscle tone. This increased smooth muscle tone leads to increased urethral resistance and contributes to the bladder outlet obstructive symptoms of BPH. This physiology leads to the basis for a main class of drugs to treat BPH, the α_1-adrenergic blockers.

BPH disease manifests as urinary tract symptoms. Obstructed urine outflow, the predominant pattern, includes diminished force of the urine stream, an urgent need for nocturnal voiding, residual urine with or without overflow incontinence, and even a feeling of pressure in the abdomen. These manifestations result from either partial or complete compression of the urethra by the hyperplastic prostate. Bladder wall hypertrophy occurs, and herniation into the bladder can occur. Ultimately, if treatment is not initiated, a postrenal cause of acute renal failure can develop because of back pressure on the renal system (i.e., the ureters) and the onset of hydronephrosis.

DIAGNOSTIC CRITERIA

Diagnosis of BPH usually begins with the patient seeking medical intervention because of the annoying symptoms. Along with a complete social history and physical examination, a digital rectal examination (DRE) is performed to palpate the prostate. The degree of prostate enlargement has not been found to correlate with the severity of symptoms; rather, the location of the enlargement is what leads to symptom manifestation.

BPH severity is assessed using validated, self-administered symptom questionnaires such as the American Urological Association Symptom Index (AUASI) (http://www.urology-health.org/_media/_pdf/AUA%20Symptom%20Score.pdf) (**Table 33.3**) or International Prostate Symptom Score (http://www.urospec.com/uro/Forms/ipss.pdf). Mild or nonbothersome symptoms do not require treatment. Bothersome symptoms are managed with lifestyle modifications, medications, and surgery.

In the AUASI, symptoms are scored as mild (0 to 7 points), moderate (8 to 19 points), or severe (20 to 35 points). The American Urological Association (AUA) recommends that this scale be used on initial assessment and then for following the course of illness by periodic ongoing assessment of the patient. Such follow-up management enables the practitioner to initiate more acute or intensive therapy when the score increases. Patients with severe BPH symptoms should not be managed by this scale.

Postvoid catheterization is performed to ascertain the degree of urine retention; any amount of residual urine beyond 100 mL is considered significant. Uroflowmetry provides information about the force of the urine stream. Urodynamics can also be assessed using noninvasive pneumatic technology. Other diagnostic tools include x-ray films, digital ultrasound, computed tomography (CT) scans, magnetic resonance imaging (MRI), and radionuclide scans. Biopsies can be added to the diagnostic workup for further clinical assessment of any hardened prostatic areas found by DRE. Laboratory monitoring of creatinine and blood urea nitrogen should be incorporated to determine whether renal involvement exists and, if so, to what degree. Prostate-specific antigen (PSA) levels can be elevated in patients with BPH.

Many symptoms of BPH stem from obstruction of the urethra and gradual loss of bladder function, which results in incomplete emptying of the bladder. The symptoms of BPH vary, but the most common ones involve changes or problems with urination, including a hesitant, interrupted, or weak stream; urgency, dribbling, or urinary retention; more frequent urination, especially at night; painful urination; and incontinence.

It is extremely important to evaluate men at risk for these symptoms. In 8 out of 10 cases, these symptoms suggest BPH, but they also can signal more serious conditions, such as prostate cancer.

INITIATING DRUG THERAPY

There are three major classes of drugs used to treat BPH. One group is α-adrenergic antagonists or α-blockers (doxazosin, terazosin, tamsulosin, alfuzosin, and silodosin). Tamsulosin,

TABLE 33.3

AUA Symptom Index Scale

Questions to Be Answered	AUA Symptom Score (Circle 1 Number on Each Line)					
	Not at All	Less Than 1 Time in 5	Less Than Half the Time	About Half the Time	More Than Half the Time	Almost Always
1. Over the past month, how often have you had a sensation of not emptying your bladder completely after you finished urinating?	0	1	2	3	4	5
2. Over the past month, how often have you had to urinate again <2 h after you finished urinating?	0	1	2	3	4	5
3. Over the past month, how often have you found that you stopped and started again several times when you urinated?	0	1	2	3	4	5
4. Over the past month, how often have you found it difficult to postpone urination?	0	1	2	3	4	5
5. Over the past month, how often have you had a weak urinary stream?	0	1	2	3	4	5
6. Over the past month, how often have you had to push or strain to begin urination?	0	1	2	3	4	5
7. Over the past month, how many times did you most typically get up to urinate from the time you went to bed at night until the time you got up in the morning?	0 (None)	1 (1 time)	2 (2 times)	3 (3 times)	4 (4 times)	5 (5 times or more)

silodosin, and alfuzosin are selective α_1-adrenoreceptor antagonists, selective for α_{1A}-adrenergic receptor. While causing smooth muscle relaxation in the lower urinary tract, it minimizes blood pressure–related adverse effects. These relax the smooth muscle fibers of the bladder neck and prostate, thereby reducing the dynamic components of prostatic obstruction.

Another group is 5-α-reductase inhibitors (finasteride and dutasteride). Five-α-reductase inhibitors decrease levels of intracellular DHT (the major growth-stimulatory hormone in prostate cells) without reducing testosterone levels. This leads to prostatic size reduction of 20% to 30%. Symptom relief occurs within 2 weeks of initiating α-blockers, compared with several months with finasteride.

The third category is PDE type 5 inhibitor. The only drug in this class approved for this use is tadalafil (Cialis). PDE5 inhibitors have been found to regulate smooth muscle tone in human prostate. These are useful in patients who do not respond to α-blockers, especially in men with concomitant erectile dysfunction (ED).

Management of BPH can include medical, surgical, and a combination of medical and surgical intervention. Choosing the right treatment should be guided by patients' symptoms, comorbidities, and potential side effects of available drugs. Silodosin is a valid option for elderly and for people taking antihypertensive drugs. BPH patients affected by ED can target both conditions with continuous tadalafil therapy.

Pharmacotherapy is prescribed with both medical and surgical approaches to care. The progression of BPH is unique to the individual; the man often will "watch and wait" before proceeding further into active therapy because the process of hyperplasia can be slow. This is acceptable as long as the AUA score is 19 or less.

The Medical Therapy of Prostatic Symptoms (MTOPS) trial tested whether finasteride (Proscar), doxazosin (Cardura), or a combination of the drugs could prevent progression of BPH and the need for surgery or other invasive treatments (Slawin, 2003; Marberger, 2006). Physicians at 17 MTOPS medical centers treated 3,047 men with BPH for an average of 4.5 years. Participants were randomly assigned to receive doxazosin, finasteride, combination therapy, or a placebo. Vital signs, urinary symptoms, urinary flow, adverse effects, and medication use were assessed every 3 months. DRE, serum PSA level, and urinalysis were performed yearly. Prostate size was measured by ultrasound at the beginning and end of the study. Progression of disease was defined by one of the following: a four-point rise in the AUA score, urinary retention, recurrent urinary tract infection, or urinary incontinence.

Finasteride, a 5-α-reductase inhibitor, and doxazosin, an α1-receptor blocker, together reduced the overall risk of BPH progression by 66% compared with a placebo. The combined drugs also provided the greatest symptom relief and improvement in urinary flow rate. Doxazosin alone reduced the overall risk of progression by 39% and finasteride alone by 34% relative to a placebo. The risk of urinary retention was reduced by 81% with combination therapy and 68% with finasteride alone. Doxazosin alone did not reduce the risk of urinary retention. The risk of incontinence was reduced by 65% with combination therapy. Only five men developed urinary tract or blood infections. No patients developed impaired kidney function related to BPH.

Twenty-seven percent of men taking doxazosin, 24% of men taking finasteride, and 18% of men taking combination therapy stopped treatment early, primarily because of adverse effects. The most common adverse effects included sexual dysfunction in men treated with finasteride and dizziness and fatigue in men treated with doxazosin.

Goals of Therapy

The goals of therapy include reduced bladder outlet obstruction, improved quality of life, fewer symptoms, and decreased residual urine volume.

The mainstay of medical management is pharmacotherapy. Pharmacotherapy is used for both controlling hyperplasia and managing annoying side effects, either as primary therapy or as an adjunct to surgical intervention. Management of hyperplasia is based on the premise that there are hormonal changes related to aging and that alpha-adrenergic receptors are present in prostate tissue, specifically smooth muscle. Pharmacotherapeutic interventions consist of hormonal manipulation and blocking effects achieved by alpha-adrenergic blockers. For dosage, adverse events, contraindications, and special considerations of drugs used for BPH, see **Table 33.4**.

5-Alpha-Reductase Inhibitors

Finasteride (Proscar) and dutasteride (Avodart), androgen hormone inhibitors, are used for managing the symptoms of BPH. They aid in the inhibition of androgen transformation from their steroid precursors. On average, most men achieve 20% to 40% reduction in prostate size after at least 6 months of use. In general, these agents are most effective in men with prostate glands more than 30 g (or cm^3). Both drugs lower PSA levels by about 50% after 6 months of use. This is critical to take into account when screening for prostate cancer. If the PSA level does not fall by one half and the patient has been compliant with medication, the patient should be referred to an urologist for a workup.

TABLE 33.4			
Overview of Selected Agents Used to Treat Benign Prostatic Hyperplasia			
Generic (Trade) Name and Dosage	**Selected Adverse Events**	**Contraindications**	**Special Considerations**
Alpha-Adrenergic Blockers			
terazosin (Hytrin) 1–20 mg PO qd	Orthostatic hypotension, somnolence, dizziness	Hypersensitivity to terbutaline Tachyarrhythmias, hypertension, pregnancy, lactation Use with caution in patients with cardiac insufficiency.	Take at bedtime to avoid hypotension.
doxazosin (Cardura) 4–8 mg PO qd	Dizziness, headache, fatigue, malaise	Lactation Use with caution in patients with CHF, renal failure, hepatic impairment.	May have secondary benefit to client with cardiac disease Avoid combination with alcohol, nitrates, or other antihypertensive drugs.
tamsulosin HCl (Flomax) 0.4 mg/d PO qd; increase to 0.8 mg/d PO qd silodosin (Rapaflo) 8 mg PO qd	Orthostasis, headache, problems with ejaculation Orthostatic hypotension, priapism, headache, URI symptoms	Allergy to tamsulosin Prostatic cancer, pregnancy, lactation Hepatic impairment, Severe renal impairment	Ejaculatory problems more common in higher dosage (0.8 mg/d) Interaction with cimetidine decreases clearance of tamsulosin. Contraindicated with clarithromycin
5-α-Reductase Inhibitor			
finasteride (Proscar) 5 mg daily dutasteride (Avodart) 0.5 mg daily dutasteride/tamsulosin (Jalyn) 1 capsule (0.5/0.4) qd	Impotence, decreased libido, smaller ejaculate Orthostatic hypotension, priapism, increased risk for prostate cancer	Not to be handled by pregnant women Caution if sensitivity to sulfonamides	Inform patient that effective outcome of therapy may take up to 6 mo. Avoid handling if pregnant or potentially pregnant.

Mechanism of Action

5-α-reductase inhibitors act by specifically blocking 5-α-reductase, the enzyme that activates testosterone in the prostate. It impairs prostate growth by inhibiting the conversion of testosterone to DHT and causes changes in the epithelial cells of the transition zone. By preventing testosterone activation, 5-α-reductase inhibitors lessen or prevent urinary system symptoms. They also decrease prostatic volume and prevent the progression of the disease in men with a significantly enlarged prostate. There is a slow reduction of 80% to 90% in the serum DHT level. As a result, prostatic volume decreases by about 20% over 3 to 6 months of treatment. Dutasteride blocks both types 1 and 2 5-α-reductase.

Studies have been done to determine the efficacy of finasteride and placebo. The larger Proscar Safety Plus Efficacy Canadian Two-Year Study (PROSPECT) found that treatment with finasteride led to significant improvements in urinary symptoms and flow rates (Nickel et al., 1996). However, in the PROSPECT study, the improvements with finasteride were significantly less than those with any α-blocker or surgery.

5-α-reductase inhibitors decrease PSA levels by 40% to 50%. In a patient taking finasteride who has PSA screening, PSA levels should be doubled and then compared in the usual fashion to age-related norms.

Dosage

The dosage for finasteride is 5 mg/d; that for dutasteride is 0.5 mg/d. These dosages are recommended for use as long-term therapy; studies have shown benefit beyond the usual 2-year period, with beneficial effects in the third year.

Adverse Events

Adverse events include decreased libido, impotence, ejaculatory failure, and gynecomastia. Finasteride can also falsify the PSA level after 6 months of therapy.

Alpha-Adrenergic Blockers

Alpha-adrenergic blockers include terazosin (Hytrin), doxazosin (Cardura), prazosin (Minipress), tamsulosin (Flomax), and silodosin (Rapaflo). It is recommended to use α-blockers in men with smaller prostate glands (less than or equal to 30 to 35 g or cm^3), in younger men, and in patients in whom rapid effect is needed. Side effects of this class include headache, dizziness, asthenia, drowsiness, and retrograde ejaculation. Silodosin is an α$_1$-adrenoreceptor antagonist that is selective for α$_{1A}$-adrenergic receptor. While causing smooth muscle relaxation in the lower urinary tract, it minimizes blood pressure–related adverse effects.

Mechanism of Action

As a pharmacologic classification, α-adrenergic blockers are functional antihypertensives with potential effects on glomerular filtration rate, renal perfusion, and heart rate. They are strongly linked with fluid retention. These agents relax the smooth muscle of the prostate and bladder neck without interfering with bladder contractility, thereby decreasing bladder resistance to urinary outflow. In general, weeks to months may pass before benefits from these medications are noted. However, benefits may last for up to 2 years, in some cases longer.

Adverse Events

Side effects can be a major concern, especially considering the potential for hypotension, specifically orthostatic hypotension, and fluid retention. However, cardiac output can actually improve, thus preventing heart failure. Of the four agents, prazosin has more potential for causing orthostatic hypotension than the others.

Side effects such as dizziness, postural hypotension, fatigue, and asthenia affect 7% to 9% of patients treated with nonselective α-blockers. Side effects can be minimized by bedtime administration and slow titration of the dosage.

Tamsulosin (Flomax) is a highly selective α$_{1A}$-adrenergic antagonist that was developed to avoid the side effects of nonselective agents. Some patients who do not respond to nonselective α-blockers may respond to tamsulosin and, because of the selectivity, may have fewer side effects.

Dutasteride/tamsulosin (Jalyn) is a combination 5-α-reductase inhibitor and α$_1$-adrenergic antagonist for the treatment of symptomatic BPH. The complementary mechanisms affect hormonal and smooth muscle pathways, inhibiting enlargement of the prostate and producing muscular relaxation resulting in a decrease of symptoms. Although monotherapy with dutasteride or tamsulosin is beneficial for many men, the combination drug is slightly better than either component alone at decreasing symptom scores. In carefully diagnosed, selected, and monitored patients who do not respond to monotherapy, Jalyn may produce clinical benefit.

Phosphodiesterase-5 Inhibitors (See Erectile Dysfunction)

The use of tadalafil (Cialis) at a dose of 5 mg daily has been approved for BPH.

Selecting the Most Appropriate Agent

The most appropriate agent is the one that achieves symptom control and produces the fewest adverse effects (**Table 33.5** and **Figure 33.2**).

First-Line Therapy

If symptoms are mild (AUA score less than 7), no medical treatment is recommended. The man should limit his fluid intake after dinner, avoid decongestants, massage the prostate after intercourse, and void frequently.

Second-Line Therapy

Pharmacotherapy is initiated when the AUA score is more than 7. An α-adrenergic blocker is effective first-line pharmacotherapy. The addition of a 5-α-reductase inhibitor is effective in men with moderate to severe symptoms and a documented

TABLE 33.5

Recommended Order of Treatment for Benign Prostatic Hyperplasia

Order	Agents	Comments
First line	If AUA score is 7 or less, watchful waiting	
Second line	α-adrenergic blocker or 5-α-reductase inhibitor or PDE5 inhibitor	α-adrenergic blocker can be prescribed for patients with hypertension; 5-α-reductase inhibitor is recommended if prostate enlargement exceeds 40 g.
Third line	Combination of α-blocker and 5-α-reductase inhibitor or PDE5 inhibitor	

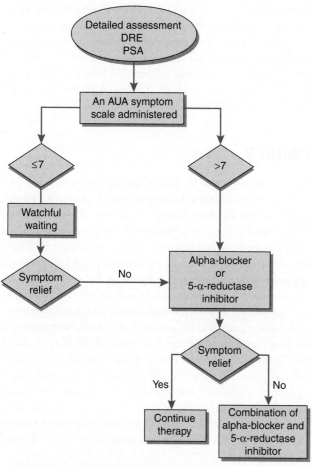

Key ⬭ Starting point for decision making

▭ Clinical actions (assessing, prescribing, monitoring)

⬦ Decision point

FIGURE 33.2 Treatment algorithm for benign prostatic hyperplasia (BPH).

enlarged prostate when an α-adrenergic blocker is not effective. Choosing the right treatment should be guided by patients' symptoms and comorbidities and potential side effects of available drugs. Silodosin is a valid option for elderly and for people taking antihypertensive drugs. BPH patients affected by ED can target both conditions with continuous tadalafil therapy.

Third-Line Therapy

Combination therapy with a 5-α-reductase inhibitor and alpha blocker may show greater improvement.

Fourth-Line Therapy

Referral to urology for possible surgery is recommended if other therapy fails.

The prevailing surgical intervention is prostatic resection or prostatectomy. Transurethral resection of the prostate (TURP) is the most common surgical intervention. Regardless of the surgical technique used (i.e., retrograde, perineal, or suprapubic approach), removal of the prostate is not without potential complications. The primary side effect, which can be permanent, is impotence from nerve damage. Incontinence is rare and usually only temporary; retrograde ejaculation can occur. Prostatectomy using laser technique is also an option, as is balloon dilation or urethral stent implantation. Laser surgery requires only an overnight stay; stent insertion is recommended for the man with cardiac or pulmonary morbidities, although it does not address the underlying problem of BPH itself.

Transurethral microwave thermotherapy is performed on an outpatient basis. Although anesthesia is not required, use of a local or general antianxiety agent may be helpful because the procedure is performed by catheter insertion into the prostate, through the urethra. This procedure uses heat derived from microwave energy (approximately 45°C) to remove or destroy excess cells of the prostate while cool water is circulated to preserve surrounding tissue.

MONITORING PATIENT RESPONSE

As noted previously, the AUA symptom score can be used to monitor men with mild or even moderate BPH. A three- or four-point improvement in the AUASI score is clinically significant. Abatement of symptoms is used to evaluate the success of pharmacotherapy. If side effects become evident with a chosen agent, a different agent can be tried. The patient's blood pressure should be monitored frequently during the first 2 weeks of treatment to observe for an untoward hypotensive response. In addition, the practitioner should not pass off subjective complaints related to sexual health, because it could lead to medication noncompliance.

PATIENT EDUCATION

Drug Information

With terazosin use, an improvement in urine flow may begin within 1 to 2 weeks; thus, the patient must be informed that urine flow improvement will not occur overnight. The man should rise slowly from a sitting or standing position and quickly sit down or recline if abrupt vertigo occurs.

Lifestyle Changes

Patients with BPH can obtain symptomatic relief with regular, relaxed, and frequent voiding; decreasing fluid intake several hours before bedtime; and avoiding diuretics and alcohol. Other medications to avoid include anticholinergics, antihistamines, and antidepressants.

Alternative Therapies for BPH

Many men are using herbal and nutritional therapies to support prostate health although there is no scientific proof that these are effective. Men are encouraged to lose weight if overweight; to eat a low-fat, high-fiber diet; and to drink a minimum of two quarts of water daily. Supplements to maintain prostate health include saw palmetto, pygeum, and zinc (**Table 33.6**). Because these are not found in standard pharmacologic compendiums, dosages for saw palmetto and pygeum should follow the manufacturer's recommendations.

Saw palmetto, a herb derived from the dark berries of a palm tree native to the southern United States, is reported to have been in use since the 1700s. Purportedly, it is useful for the management of prostate inflammation by a threefold mechanism. First, it inhibits testosterone conversion to DHT, resulting in the prevention of prostate enlargement. Second, it stops DHT binding to receptor sites; third, it has a general inhibitory effect on both estrogen and androgen receptors. There is no evidence of deleterious effects on PSA levels with the use of saw palmetto. Saw palmetto is available in capsule, liquid, or softgel form and as a tea; the tea is not believed to be effective for BPH. Saw palmetto often is used in combination with pygeum (http://www.sawpalmetto.com).

Pygeum is the ground and powdered bark of the pygeum tree, an evergreen of Southern Africa. It is prepared as a tea for easing complaints related to the genitourinary system. Widely used in Europe for symptom relief in BPH and thus postponement of surgery or the use of stronger medications, the efficacy of pygeum is being researched at the University of Southern California. Dosage recommendations are 50 to 100 mg twice daily; gastrointestinal irritation is a rare side effect (http://www.mothernature.com).

Zinc also plays a role in BPH, improving general prostate health by preventing or even decreasing prostate enlargement. Research has supported that doses of zinc sulfate lead to the inhibition of 5-α-reductase, the enzyme for conversion of testosterone to DHT. The recommended dosage for zinc sulfate is 150 mg/d for 2 months followed by a maintenance dose of 50 to 100 mg/d.

PROSTATE CANCER

In the decade from 1980 to 1990, the incidence of prostate cancer increased by 50%, although this is actually perceived as a positive development, indicating enhanced screenings rather than a truly increased incidence of disease. This disease is more common in African American men than in White men and, in general, in men from North, Central, and South America, Africa, and the Near East. Ironically, in African American men, prostate cancer develops at a significantly higher rate than in their native African counterparts. Men of Asian heritage have a low incidence of prostate cancer and low death rates from the disease. Once again, Asian American men have a slightly higher incidence of prostate cancer than their native Asian counterparts.

As men age, the overall risk of developing prostate cancer also increases. Incidence reports estimate that 6 or 7 of every 100 men who are currently 60 years old have a 6.29% chance of developing prostate cancer by the age of 70 (Howlader et al., 2014; U.S. Cancer Statistics Working Group, 2015).

CAUSES

The disease seems to be closely aligned with the aging process; the exact cause is not well understood, although a genetic predisposition has been found. Thus, sons of men who have had prostate cancer are at higher risk for developing prostate cancer themselves. No link between prostate cancer and BPH has been uncovered. From an environmental and occupational perspective, association with cadmium in the workplace is correlated with the later onset of prostate cancer.

Essentially, 95% of prostate cancers are adenocarcinomas, with most occurring at the prostate's periphery. How aggressive the neoplasm becomes seems to be more highly correlated with the degree of anaplasia, or lack of differentiation, of the cancer cells as opposed to tumor size. Progression of the cancer begins with local extension, but metastasis to distant sites occurs through blood and lymphatic vessels. Given the anatomic location of the prostate, it is easily understood how progression to the pelvis and rectum, lumbar and thoracic spine and ribs, and femur can ensue.

PATHOPHYSIOLOGY

In many cases, symptoms present only with advanced disease. As with BPH, bladder-associated problems occur first—slow urine stream, inadequate emptying of bladder, painful

TABLE 33.6	
Alternative Therapies for Benign Prostatic Hyperplasia	
Agent	**Dosage**
Saw palmetto	Doses vary based on manufacturer.
Pygeum	50–100 mg PO bid
Zinc	150 mg PO qd for 2 mo, 50–100 mg qd thereafter

urination, frequency, and nocturia. However, with prostate cancer, unlike BPH, there is no remission from these symptoms. Difficulty in defecation, and even obstruction of the large bowel, can also occur depending on how the tumor is spreading, but again this is usually seen with advanced disease.

DIAGNOSTIC CRITERIA

While early detection of prostate cancer is crucial, routine screening is controversial depending on age, and according to the U.S. Preventive Services Task Force (USPSTF), AUA, and needs to be a shared decision for men between 55 and 69 years of age (Eggener et al., 2015). That being said, prostate cancer remains a significant problem specifically for African American men who tend to be diagnosed at a more advanced stage, and their rate of survival is poorer than among Whites (Carter et al., 2010; Lehto et al., 2010). Thus, public education targeting African American men is of paramount importance.

Three screening methods are commonly used. The first is the DRE; the second is the serum level of PSA. When either result is abnormal, an ultrasound study is performed transrectally. The man should be cautioned to avoid ejaculation for 48 hours before obtaining a PSA because false-positive results may be obtained. The diagnostic yield rises dramatically when ultrasound is incorporated with DRE and PSA. It is recommended that all men older than age 45 undergo an annual DRE and all men older than age 50 have a conversation about annual testing of their PSA level in addition to the DRE. Normal PSA values should be less than 2.7 in men younger than age 40 and 4.0 or less in men older than age 40.

However, for confirmation of cancer, and with suspect findings, further diagnostic investigation is warranted. This includes a biopsy to confirm the diagnosis and identify the cancer's histologic type, after which MRI and CT scans are necessary to determine the extent of metastasis.

Treatment options include surgery, chemotherapy, and radiation, either alone or in combination. Regardless of the treatment modality, loss of physiologic function can occur. This loss of function varies from temporary loss of urinary control to permanent incontinence. In addition to loss of urinary control, fecal incontinence can also result. Sexual dysfunction frequently occurs and involves the ability to attain an erection or have emission or ejaculation. Return to normal physiologic function often occurs over time, but some permanent dysfunction can result.

INITIATING DRUG THERAPY

Pharmacologic intervention can also help the patient return to normal physiologic function after other treatments, such as partial or radical prostatectomy, which are options based on the cancer's histologic type and the extent of metastasis. Often, surgery is performed after a period of radiation or chemotherapy. A main postoperative concern is that bladder dysfunction will persist; this manifests as incomplete emptying, incontinence, decreased force of stream, and urinary scarring.

Bilateral orchiectomy has also been used for advanced disease to decrease the risk of complications and spread of prostate cancer, but it is not considered curative in the setting of metastasis or advanced disease. Bilateral orchiectomy is radical surgery used to extend the man's life; it provides relief from symptoms. There is minimal morbidity and mortality associated with the surgery, but it may have a negative impact on the man's self-esteem and sense of identity. Postsurgical pharmacologic management is crucial to promoting the man's self-esteem and correcting, as much as possible, the altered physiologic function.

ERECTILE DYSFUNCTION

ED is the most common sexual problem in men. It is defined as the repeated inability to achieve or maintain an erection that is firm enough for sexual intercourse. ED can be a total inability to achieve erection, an inconsistent ability to do so, or a tendency to sustain only brief erections. Approximately 18 million men in the United States over age 20 are affected by ED. The prevalence ranges from 20% to above 50% with increasing age. The prevalence is also increased threefold in men with diabetes. An organic cause can be found in about 80% of men with ED. The other 20% have psychogenic causes.

ED treatment costs in the United States are estimated at $328 million annually. Even with insurance, a patient may spend from $119 to $30,000 for ED therapy in 1 year.

Lifestyle choices associated with ED include being sedentary, obese, smoking, and abuse of either illicit substances (e.g., cocaine) or alcohol. Lower education levels are also associated with higher prevalence of ED.

CAUSES

An erection requires a precise sequence of events, and ED can occur when any of the events are disrupted. The sequence includes nerve impulses in the brain, the spinal column, and the area around the penis and response in muscles, fibrous tissues, veins, and arteries in and near the corpora cavernosa. As men age, libido decreases, probably because of a decline in testosterone levels. Cardiovascular diseases encompass vascular damage associated with diabetes, hypertension, coronary heart disease, and dyslipidemia. Any history of psychological or psychiatric problems including depression, anxiety, sexual abuse, or stress predisposes to developing ED. Damage to nerves, arteries, smooth muscles, and fibrous tissues (often as a result of disease) is the most common cause of ED. Chronic diseases such as diabetes, kidney disease, chronic alcoholism, multiple sclerosis, atherosclerosis, vascular disease, and neurologic disease account for about 70% of ED cases. Between 35% and 50% of men with diabetes experience ED. Psychological issues can also lead to ED, and it is often a combination of physical and psychological issues. See **Box 33.1** for a list of risk factors for ED.

BOX 33.1 Risk Factors for Erectile Dysfunction

Advancing age
Cardiovascular disease
Cigarette smoking
Diabetes mellitus
History of pelvic irradiation or surgery, including radical prostatectomy
Hormonal disorders (e.g., hypogonadism, hypothyroidism, hyperprolactinemia)
Hypercholesterolemia
Hypertension
Illicit drug use (e.g., cocaine, methamphetamine)
Medications (e.g., antihistamines, benzodiazepines, selective serotonin reuptake inhibitors)
Neurologic conditions (e.g., Alzheimer disease, multiple sclerosis, Parkinson disease, paraplegia, quadriplegia, stroke)
Obesity
Peyronie disease
Psychological conditions (e.g., anxiety, depression, guilt, history of sexual abuse, marital or relationship problems, stress)
Sedentary lifestyle
Venous leakage

Surgery (especially radical prostate surgery for cancer) can injure nerves and arteries near the penis, thus causing ED. Injury to the penis, spinal cord, prostate, bladder, and pelvis can lead to ED by harming nerves, smooth muscles, arteries, and fibrous tissues of the corpora cavernosa.

Many common drugs such as antihypertensives, antihistamines, antidepressants, tranquilizers, appetite suppressants, and cimetidine can have ED as an adverse event. Psychological factors such as stress, anxiety, guilt, depression, low self-esteem, and fear of sexual failure cause 10% to 20% of ED cases. Other possible causes of ED include smoking, which affects blood flow in veins and arteries, and hormonal abnormalities, such as low testosterone levels.

PATHOPHYSIOLOGY

Sexual performance in men has four stages: libido (desire), erection (arousal or engorgement), ejaculation, and detumescence. Problems in any stage can result in male sexual dysfunction. The basic mechanical or primary focus of ED is in stage 2. Erection is a complex neuroendocrine psychophysiological event that can occur even during sleep, indicating that sexual stimulation is not required.

Nitric oxide (NO) is essential for erection. The release of NO in the cells of the corpus cavernosa following parasympathetic stimulation leads to the conversion of guanylate cyclase to cyclic guanosine monophosphate (cGMP). This causes smooth muscle relaxation that permits the influx of blood causing engorgement of the penis. This mechanism also slows the outflow of venous blood from the penis thus enhancing penile engorgement. Other contributors to vasodilation during erection include vasoactive intestinal peptide (VIP) and prostaglandins E1 and E2 (PGE1 and PGE2).

The penis is innervated by both autonomic and somatic nerves. Sympathetic and parasympathetic fibers in the cavernous nerves regulate blood flow into the corpus cavernosum during erection and detumescence. Erection, at the level of the penis, begins with transmission of impulses from parasympathetic nerves and nonadrenergic, noncholinergic nerves. This neural stimulus leads to the release of nitric oxide from the nonadrenergic, noncholinergic nerves and possibly the endothelial cells. Nitric oxide increases intracellular levels of cGMP in the cavernosal smooth muscle, which acts to relax cavernosal tissue, perhaps by activating protein kinase G and stimulating phosphorylation of the proteins that regulate corporal smooth muscle tone. The actions of the parasympathetic nervous system, nitric oxide, and cGMP permit rapid blood flow into the penis and the development of an erection. As pressure within the corporal body increases, small emissary veins traversing the tunica albuginea are occluded, trapping blood in the corpus cavernosum. The erection is maintained until ejaculation, which usually leads to detumescence.

Phosphodiesterases (PDEs) are hydrolytic enzymes that play a critical role in regulating physiologic processes by terminating signal transduction through their hydrolytic action on cyclic nucleotides. They play a key role in the physiology of erection.

Significant changes in penile structure occur with aging. Collagen and elastic fibers in the tunica albuginea are key structures that permit increases in the girth and length of the penis during tumescence, and ultrastructural analysis of penile biopsies has shown that the concentration of elastic fibers decreases with age. This decrease results in a reduction in elasticity, which could contribute to ED in elderly men. Additionally, there is a decrease of up to 35% in the smooth muscle content of the penis in men older than age 60. Decreases in the ratio between corpus cavernosum smooth muscle and connective tissue have been associated with increased likelihood of diffuse venous leak that may contribute to ED. It has also been noted that the concentration of type III collagen decreases and that of type I collagen increases in the aging penis. It has been suggested that this change makes the corpus cavernosum less compliant, reduces filling of vascular spaces, and also contributes to veno-occlusive dysfunction. It has also been hypothesized that changes in the collagen content of the penis may result in chronic ischemia that leads to loss of smooth muscle cells. Any condition, disease, medication, or injury or surgery that affects the ability to initiate erections or to fill the lacunar space or store blood may cause ED.

ED involves multiple organic and psychogenic factors, which often coexist. Psychogenic factors are the most common causes of intermittent ED in younger men, but these are usually secondary to or may coexist with organic factors in older men. Other factors contributing to ED include vasculogenic, neurogenic, endocrinologic, structural (traumatic), and pharmacologic causes and lifestyle factors, such as obesity, a sedentary lifestyle, and alcohol and tobacco use. Many of the conditions that contribute to ED are chronic and systemic, involving multiple avenues of damage. These conditions include cardiovascular disease, hypertension, diabetes mellitus, and depression. Many of the diseases linked to ED involve endothelial dysfunction.

There are many drugs that can affect erectile function. These include

- alcohol
- analgesics
- anticholinergics
- anticonvulsants
- antidepressants
- antihistamines
- antihypertensives
- anti-Parkinson agents
- corticosteroids
- diuretics
- nicotine
- tranquilizers

DIAGNOSTIC CRITERIA

A thorough history is paramount to diagnosing ED. Every male patient should be asked about medical conditions, medications, and sexual function. Initial diagnostic workup should usually be limited to a fasting serum glucose level and lipid panel, thyroid-stimulating hormone test, and morning total testosterone level.

INITIATING DRUG THERAPY

ED can be very traumatic to men. There are now drugs that can assist with achieving and maintaining an erection that is firm enough for sexual intercourse. Testosterone levels should be determined, and a complete cardiac history and evaluation should be done to determine whether there are contraindications to these medications. Approximately one third of men with ED do not respond to therapy with phosphodiesterase-5 (PDE5) inhibitors.

Goals of Drug Therapy

The goals of drug therapy for ED are to enable the patient to achieve sexual satisfaction and to achieve and maintain an erection.

Phosphodiesterase-5 Inhibitors

PDE5 inhibitors promote penile erection by inhibiting the breakdown of one of the messengers involved in the erectile response. PDE5 is the main cGMP-catalyzing enzyme in human trabecular smooth muscle. It is also expressed in vascular smooth muscle, lung, platelets, and a wide variety of other tissues but is not present in cardiac muscle cells. Human corpus cavernosum also contains PDE types 2, 3, and 4 enzymes. PDE5 inhibitors are contingent on the presence of cGMP in the smooth muscle cell. In the presence of sexual stimulation, PDE5 inhibitors reinforce the normal cellular signals that increase cyclic nucleotide concentrations by blocking cyclic nucleotide hydrolysis, thereby facilitating the initiation and maintenance of an erection.

Dosage

The recommended dosage of sildenafil is 50 mg 30 to 60 minutes before intercourse, but doses range from 25 to 100 mg. The maximum is one dose a day. Food can delay absorption, especially if taken close to a fatty meal.

The recommended dose of tadalafil is 10 mg, but doses range from 5 to 20 mg. Tadalafil can be taken without restriction on food or alcohol intake.

The recommended dose of vardenafil is 10 mg, but doses range from 2.5 to 20 mg. It is taken 60 minutes before intercourse. Food can delay absorption.

Avanafil (Stendra) is a new novel second-generation PDE5 inhibitor with a much shorter half-life. The recommended dose is 100 mg, but doses range from 50 to 200 mg. It is taken 15 minutes prior to intercourse. Dosing is not restricted by food intake, but alcohol intake should be limited.

Time Frame for Response

Sildenafil (Viagra) and vardenafil (Levitra) are rapidly absorbed, reaching maximum plasma concentrations within 30 to 120 minutes (median 60 minutes) of oral dosing in the fasted state; a high-fat meal has been found to reduce the rate of absorption. The elimination half-life is approximately 4 hours, and no more than one dose should be taken per 24-hour period.

Tadalafil (Cialis) has an onset of action of 30 minutes and allows intercourse for at least 30 hours. This is significant because it may eliminate the need for planning sexual activity.

Avanafil (Stendra) has an onset of action of 30 to 45 minutes. Absorption occurs quickly following oral administration elimination half-life of 5 hours. As with sildenafil and vardenafil, no more than one dose should be taken in 24 hours.

Contraindications

PDE5 inhibitors can potentiate the vasodilatory properties of nitrates, so their administration in patients who use nitrates in any form is contraindicated. In an emergency situation, nitrates can be used 24 hours after administration of sildenafil and vardenafil and 48 hours after tadalafil.

PDE5 inhibitors are contraindicated in patients with unstable angina, hypotension with a systolic blood pressure below 90 mm Hg, uncontrolled hypertension of more than 170/110 mm Hg, history of recent stroke, life-threatening arrhythmia, myocardial infarction (MI) within 6 months, and severe cardiac failure. They are also contraindicated in patients

TABLE 33.7

Overview of Selected Agents Used to Treat Erectile Dysfunction

Generic (Trade) Name and Dosage	Selected Adverse Events	Contraindications	Special Considerations
tadalafil (Cialis) 5–20 mg/d	Headache, flushing, GI disturbance, nasal congestion, rash, priapism	Nitrates and α-blockers except tamsulosin 0.4 mg once a day	Food and alcohol make no difference in absorption. May remain in system for 36 h.
vardenafil (Levitra, Staxyn) 5–20 mg/d	As above	Nitrates and α-blockers	High-fat meal delays absorption.
sildenafil (Viagra) 25–100 mg/d	As above and color disturbances	Nitrates and within 4 h of an a blocker and at a dose no >25 mg	As above
avanafil (Stendra) 50–200 mg/d	As above	Nitrates and α-blockers	Food makes no difference in absorption. Caution with alcohol.

with severe hepatic impairment or end-stage renal disease requiring dialysis.

Sildenafil has a relative contraindication with the concomitant use of α-blockers and should not be taken within 4 hours of an α-blocker and at a dose no greater than 25 mg. Tadalafil should not be taken with an α-blocker other than tamsulosin, 0.4 mg once a day. Vardenafil is contraindicated with any α-blocker. Avanafil should be administered cautiously with an α-blocker, preferably at the 50 mg dose.

Adverse Events

Most adverse events are vasodilatory, including headache, flushing, and nasal congestion. Dyspepsia has also been reported. With sildenafil, abnormal color vision has been reported.

Interactions

Potent CYP3A4 inhibitors can cause increased levels of PDE5 inhibitors. They may also be affected by amlodipine, beta blockers, cimetidine, diuretics, and erythromycin.

Selecting the Most Appropriate Agent

It is important to include the significant other in counseling about ED. A complete cardiac history must be taken. If there is any question as to the stability of the cardiac status, further testing must be done. Testosterone, serum glucose (or alternatively glycosylated hemoglobin), and serum lipid levels must be determined in all cases of ED. Depending on patient history and physical examination findings, more extensive laboratory tests may be necessary. If testosterone levels are abnormal, testosterone replacement is needed. See **Table 33.7** for selected agents.

The patient with the following factors is considered at low risk for a cardiac event with the use of PDE5 inhibitors: fewer than three risk factors for coronary artery disease; controlled hypertension; mild, stable angina; uncomplicated MI more than 8 weeks previously; mild valvular disease; and New

York Heart Association class 1 heart failure. See **Box 33.2** and **Figure 33.3**.

First-Line Therapy

First-line therapy for ED is aimed at lifestyle changes and modifying pharmacotherapy that may contribute to ED. A PDE5 inhibitor is also prescribed (**Table 33.8**).

Second-Line Therapy

If PDE5 inhibitors are not successful in treating ED, the patient should be referred to an urologist. Alternative therapies include penile intracavernosal injection therapy, a medical intraurethral system for erections, a vacuum erection device, and penile prostheses.

MONITORING PATIENT RESPONSE

The patient should be followed in 6 months to determine the effectiveness of therapy and to re-evaluate his cardiac status. If the patient does not meet the criteria for low risk, the PDE5 inhibitors are discontinued.

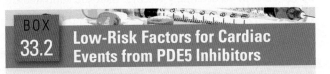

BOX 33.2 **Low-Risk Factors for Cardiac Events from PDE5 Inhibitors**

Fewer than three risk factors for coronary artery disease
Controlled hypertension
Stable angina
Uncomplicated MI more than 8 weeks previously
Mild valvular disease
New York Heart Association class 1 heart failure (see Chapter 22)

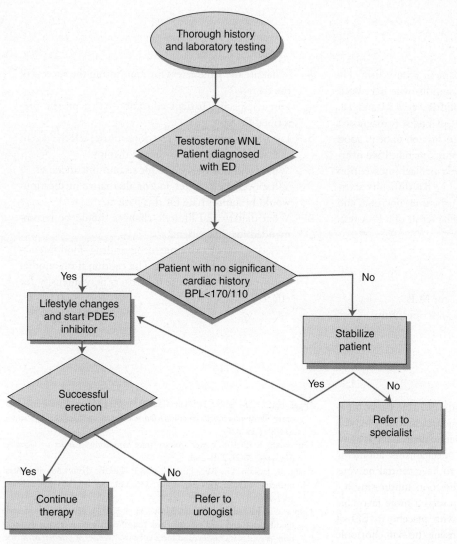

FIGURE 33.3 Treatment algorithm for erectile dysfunction (ED).

TABLE 33.8		
Recommended Order of Treatment for Erectile Dysfunction		
Order	**Agent**	**Comment**
First line	PDE5 inhibitors	Contraindicated if on nitrates, unstable hypertension, unstable cardiac condition
Second line	Referral to urologist	Procedures available include penile intracavernosal injection therapy, medical intraurethral system for erections, vacuum erection device, penile prostheses

PATIENT EDUCATION

Drug Information

With sildenafil and vardenafil, a high-fat meal has been found to reduce the rate of absorption. Food and alcohol have no effect on the absorption of tadalafil.

Sildenafil has a relative contraindication with the concomitant use of α-blockers and should not be taken within 4 hours of an α-blocker and at a dose no greater than 25 mg. Tadalafil should not be taken with an α-blocker other than tamsulosin 0.4 mg once a day. Vardenafil is contraindicated with any α-blocker.

Complementary and Alternative Medicine

Yohimbine, an agent derived from the bark of the African yohimbe tree, has been found to be beneficial in some cases of ED. It is reported to act by both peripheral and central mechanisms,

CASE STUDY*

M.P., age 45, works as an accountant in a busy firm. He is of African American descent. He and his wife have been married for 25 years and have 2 children, ages 21 and 18. His father is alive and well at age 68 but was diagnosed with BPH 5 years ago. **M.P.** considers himself to be in good health and has no allergies; he is approximately 15% overweight. His wife insisted that he seek medical intervention because of urinary symptomatology: he has difficulty starting his stream of urine, burning on urination, nocturia, and lower back and pelvic discomfort. The result of a PSA test, his first in over 2 years, is 3.1.

DIAGNOSIS: BPH

1. List specific goals for treatment for **M.P.**
2. What drug therapy would you prescribe? Why?

3. What are the parameters for monitoring the success of the therapy?
4. Discuss specific patient education based on the prescribed therapy.
5. List one or two adverse reactions for the selected agent that would cause you to change therapy.
6. What would be the choice for second-line therapy?
7. What over-the-counter and/or alternative medications would be appropriate for this patient?
8. What dietary and lifestyle changes should be recommended for this patient?
9. Describe one or two drug–drug or drug–food interactions for the selected agent. Use caution if on another antihypertensive because α-blockers may intensify the effect.

*Answers can be found online.

acting peripherally as a presynaptic stimulant at parasympathetic nonnoradrenergic, noncholinergic transmitter (NANC) nerves and presynaptically as an adrenergic depressant at sympathetic alpha₁-adrenoceptors, both mechanisms augmenting penile blood flow. It also appears to have central nervous system activity, with blockade of the erection-suppressing α_2-adrenoceptors; several studies have reported a more favorable response with yohimbine compared with placebo in ED of psychogenic origin. Ginkgo biloba, ginseng, human chorionic gonadotropin (HCG), and L-arginine are some of the popular supplements advertised for ED. Patient should be asked about use of these therapies, and those patients who choose to continue use should be monitored for adverse effects and potential drug–drug interactions.

Bibliography

*Starred references are cited in the text.

Ahuja, S. (2014). Chronic bacterial prostatitis. Retrieved from http://emedicine.medscape.com/article/458391-overview#a8

Barry, M. (2009). Screening for prostate cancer—The controversy that refuses to die. New England Journal of Medicine, 360, 1351–1354.

Bullock, B. A., & Henze, R. L. (2000). Focus on pathophysiology. Philadelphia, PA: Lippincott Williams & Wilkins.

Carter, V., Tippett, F., Anderson, D., et al. (2010). Increasing prostate cancer screening among African American men. Journal of Health Care for the Poor and Underserved, 21(3), S91–S106. doi: 10.1353/hpu.0.0366.

Deters, L. (2015). Benign prostatic hypertrophy. Retrieved from http://emedicine.medscape.com/article/437359-overview

Djavan, B., Ekersberger, E., Finklestein, J., et al. (2010). Benign prostatic hyperplasia: Current clinical practice. Primary Care: Clinics in Office Practice, 37(3), 583–597.

Eardley, I., Donatucci, C., Corbin, J., et al. (2010). Pharmacotherapy for erectile dysfunction. Journal Sex Medicine, 7, 524–540. doi: 10.1111/j.1743-6109.2009.01627.x.

*Eggener, S., Cifu, A., & Nabhan, C. (2015). JAMA clinical guidelines synopsis: Prostate cancer screening. Journal American Medical Association, 314(8), 825–826.

Gammoch, J. (2010). Lower urinary tract symptoms. Clinics in Geriatric Medicine, 26(2), 249–260.

Grant, P., Jackson, G., Baig, I., et al. (2013). Erectile dysfunction in general medicine. Clinical Medicine, 13(2), 136–140. doi: 10.7861/clinmedicine.13-2-136.

Gupta, B.P., Murad, M., Clifton, M. M., et al. (2011). The effect of lifestyle modification and cardiovascular risk factor reduction on erectile dysfunction: A systematic review and meta-analysis. Archives of Internal Medicine, 171(20), 1797–1803. doi: 10.1001/archinternmed.2011.440.

Heidelbaugh, J. (2010). Management of erectile dysfunction. American Family Physician, 81(3), 305–312.

Howlader, N., Noone, A. M., Krapcho, M., et al. (2014). SEER Cancer Statistics Review, 1975-2011, National Cancer Institute. Bethesda, MD, http://seer.cancer.gov/csr/1975_2011/, based on November 2013 SEER data submission, posted to the SEER web site, April 2014.

Katz, E., Tan, R., Rittenberg, D., et al. (2014). Avanafil for erectile dysfunction in elderly and younger adults: Differential pharmacology and clinical utility. Therapeutics and Clinical Risk Management, 10, 701–711. Retrieved from http://dx.doi.org/10.2147/TCRM.S57610

*Lehto, R., Song, L., Stein, K., & Coleman-Burns, P. (2010). Prostate cancer screening in African American men. Western Journal of Nursing Research, 32(6), 779–793. doi: 10.1177/0193945910361332.

McNicholas, T., & Kirby, R. (2012). Benign prostatic hyperplasia and male lower urinary tract symptoms. American Family Physician, 86(4), 359–360.

*Marberger, M. (2006). The MTOPS study: New findings, new insights, and clinical implications for the management of BPH. European Urology Supplements, 5, 628–633. doi: 10.1016/j.eursup.2006.05.002.

McVary, K. T., Roehrbom, C. G., Avins, A. L., et al. (2010). American Urological Association guideline: Management of benign prostatic hyperplasia (BPH). Retrieved from http://www.auanet.org/common/pdf/education/clinical-guidance/Benign-Prostatic-Hyperplasia.pdf

Mobley, D., Feibus, A., & Baum, N. (2015). Benign prostatic hypertrophy and urinary symptoms: Evaluation and treatment. Postgraduate Medicine, 127(3), 301–307.

*Nickel, J. C., Fradet, Y., Boake, R., et al. (1996). Efficacy and safety of finasteride therapy for benign prostatic hyperplasia: Results of a 2-year randomized controlled trial (the PROSPECT study). *Canadian Medical Journal*, *155*(9), 1251–1259.

Pearson, R., & Williams, P. M. (2014). Common questions about the diagnosis and management of benign prostatic hyperplasia. *American Family Physician*, *90*(11), 769–774B.

Russo, A., LaCroce, G., Capogrosso, P., et al. (2014). Latest pharmacotherapy options for benign prostatic hyperplasia. *Expert Opinion on Pharmacotherapy*, *15*(16), 2319–2328.

*Slawin, K. M. (2003). The medical therapy of prostatic symptoms study: What will we learn? *Reviews in Urology*, *5*(Suppl. 4), S42–S47.

Sharp, V., Takas, E., & Powell, C. (2010). Prostatitis: Diagnosis and treatment. *American Family Physician*, *82*(4), 397–406.

*U.S. Cancer Statistics Working Group. *United States Cancer Statistics: 1999–2012 incidence and mortality web-based report*. Atlanta, GA: Department of Health and Human Services, Centers for Disease Control and Prevention, and National Cancer Institute; 2015.

*Weidner, W., & Anderson, R. (2008). Evaluation of acute and chronic bacterial prostatitis and diagnostic management of chronic prostatitis/chronic pelvic pain syndrome with special reference to infection/inflammation. *International Journal of Antimicrobial Agents*, *31S* (2008), S91–S95.

34 Overactive Bladder

Jennifer A. Reinhold

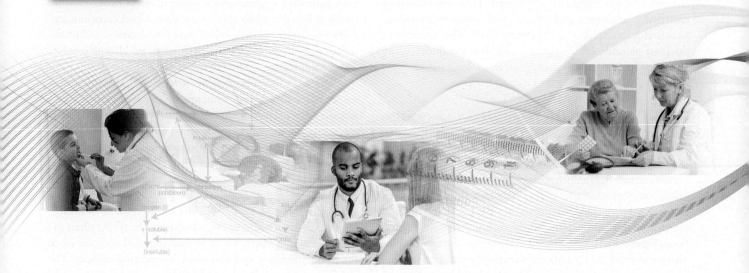

Overactive bladder (OAB) is a highly prevalent yet under-reported condition that transcends the boundaries of race, gender, and socioeconomic class. OAB is loosely defined by the International Continence Society (ICS) as a constellation of symptoms that include primarily urinary urgency usually accompanied by frequency (voiding eight or more times per 24 hours) and nocturia (awakening two or more times at night to void), with or without urge urinary incontinence (UUI). It is a symptom syndrome and not a discrete diagnosis. The most recent data suggest that OAB affects between 16% and 17% of adults in the United States, or about 34 million people. However, given the substantial underreporting and the inherent challenges in identifying sufferers of OAB, the actual prevalence is likely markedly higher. Women and men tend to be affected by OAB proportionately; however, women are more likely than men to present with the symptom of incontinence as part of their clinical picture. The incidence of OAB increases linearly with age and is predicated on a number of factors that are impacted by aging. However, OAB with or without incontinence is not considered a normal part of aging; OAB symptomatology and any instance of urgency are always considered pathologic.

OAB syndrome has extensive ramifications with respect to morbidity, mortality, and economic impact. A preponderance of literature supports the assertion that OAB is associated with increased rates of depression, decreased self-esteem, social isolation, general fragility, and falls and fracture. Upon development of OAB symptoms, patients tend to engage in avoidance behaviors in order to escape the social stigma and embarrassment associated with urinary incontinence (UI) or urinary urgency. Eventually, this translates into substantial lifestyle changes and the potential for social isolation. Total costs attributable to OAB are estimated to be $65.9 billion ($49.1 billion

direct medical, $2.3 billion direct nonmedical, and $14.6 billion indirect) (Ganz et al., 2010). A leading cause of morbidity in the elderly population and the most commonly cited reason for assisted living and long-term care facility admission, OAB needs to be assessed in the primary care setting preemptively.

The terms OAB, detrusor overactivity (DO), and UI are frequently used interchangeably erroneously. UI is a possible symptom as part of the symptomatology construct that constitutes OAB; it does not necessarily need to be present in patients diagnosed with OAB. While urgency is the cardinal symptom of OAB and must be present in order to yield a diagnosis of OAB, only about 25% to 35% of patients experience *incontinence* as well. DO implies an involuntary and inappropriate contraction of the bladder; however, it is considered a surrogate marker of OAB that may or may not correlate with urgency. DO is further delineated into idiopathic (absence of an identifiable cause) or neurogenic (an underlying neurological condition, deficit, or injury is the causative factor). There is considerable overlap between nonpharmacologic and pharmacologic treatments for OAB, UI, and DO; therefore, UI subtypes will be discussed. The accepted nomenclature for UI differentiates between the underlying pathophysiology and the nature of the urine loss. UUI implies a strong and sudden urge to urinate that cannot be deferred and results in involuntary loss of urine. Stress urinary incontinence (SUI) occurs when an internal or external force impacts the bladder or the musculature that supports it. Common examples of such pressures include coughing, sneezing, heavy lifting, or prolapsed pelvic organs. Mixed UI is a combination of both SUI and UUI. The historical term *overflow incontinence*, which suggested some level of obstruction or voiding difficulty, has been replaced with bladder outlet obstruction (BOO) and is no longer part of the classification schema.

CAUSES

The exact cause of the OAB symptom constellation is multifactorial and not completely elucidated. There are numerous underlying anatomic, physiologic, and comorbidity-related factors that precipitate or exacerbate OAB. The majority of cases are considered idiopathic, with the remainder being attributed to myogenic or neurogenic causation.

PATHOPHYSIOLOGY

The bladder and the corresponding micturition cycle are controlled by a complex, coordinated interplay among the central nervous system (CNS), peripheral nervous system, and the anatomic components of the lower urinary tract (LUT). The LUT is composed of the bladder, urethra, bladder outlet, internal and external urethral sphincters, and the musculature of the pelvic floor (**Figure 34.1**). The discord between the continuous production of urine (1 to 2 L/d) and the episodic nature of voiding necessitates the storage of urine. The bladder (detrusor muscle) is a highly compliant, viscoelastic hollow organ that expands to accommodate the storage of urine while maintaining a constant pressure throughout this filling phase. As the bladder fills, it maintains a pressure that is lower than that of the urethra, therefore facilitating the development of a pressure gradient that prevents urine from being expelled. The normal urge to void is under voluntary control, and therefore, only when the bladder reaches a critical volume, or about 75% of total capacity, will an individual feel the desire to void. This urge, which is different from pathologic urgency and is under different neural control, can be deferred until an appropriate time. Upon conscious and deliberate urination, the urethral resistance decreases and phasic contractions in the bladder result in increased bladder pressure and the subsequent voiding of urine.

The LUT is innervated by efferent and afferent neuronal complexes involving sympathetic, parasympathetic, and somatic nerves. The *sympathetic* nervous system primarily stimulates urethral sphincter closure and detrusor relaxation during filling, while the *parasympathetic* system influences contraction of the detrusor and relaxation of the urethral sphincters during the emptying phase. Somatic innervation maintains the tone of the striated pelvic floor muscles and the external urethral sphincter (**Table 34.1**). The bladder is continuously bombarding the CNS with afferent signals during the filling phase via $A\delta$ fibers and C fibers. These normal impulses indicate when the bladder is filling and also when it is nearing capacity. The impulses are transmitted to higher brain centers such as the cortex, pons, and brain stem, which also exert some level of control over micturition. The sensations generated by this neurotransmission will result in variable degrees of the normal urge to urinate. The $A\delta$ fibers generally respond to the mechanical stretch of the bladder during the filling phase. However, during pathologic conditions, it is thought that the unmyelinated C

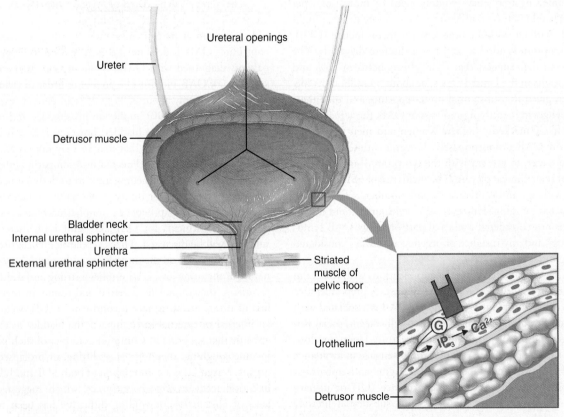

FIGURE 34.1 M_3 receptors are coupled to G proteins, which activate phospholipase, generating inositol triphosphate (IP_3). IP_3 causes the release of stored Ca^{2+}, which stimulates bladder contraction.

TABLE 34.1

Bladder and Urethral Innervation

Nerve	Anatomic Location	Nervous System	Spinal Cord Origin	Physiologic Function
Pudendal	External sphincter	Somatic	S2, S3, S4	Maintains tone in pelvic floor Excitatory innervation to external urethral sphincter
Pelvic	Urethra	Parasympathetic	S2, S3, S4	Relaxes sphincter
Hypogastric	Urethra	Sympathetic	T1–L2	Stimulates sphincter closure
Pelvic	Bladder neck	Parasympathetic	S2, S3, S4	Relaxes sphincter
Hypogastric	Bladder neck	Sympathetic	T1–L2	Stimulates sphincter closure
Pelvic	Bladder	Parasympathetic	S2, S3, S4	Contraction of detrusor during micturition
Hypogastric	Bladder	Sympathetic	T1–L2	Relaxes detrusor during filling phase

sensory fibers may precipitate abnormal OAB sensations. The C sensory fibers are dappled with vanilloid receptors (which can be stimulated by capsaicin), purinergic receptors or P2X$_2$ and P2X$_3$ (which can be stimulated by adenosine triphosphate), and neurokinin receptors (which can be stimulated by neurokinin A and substance P). (see **Figure 34.2**).

Acetylcholine-mediated activation of muscarinic receptors is the predominant physiologic mediator of detrusor

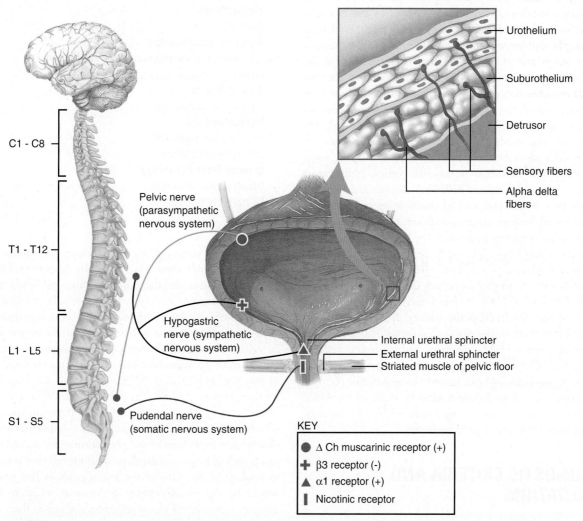

FIGURE 34.2 The bladder is innervated by the sympathetic, parasympathetic, and somatic nervous systems. The pudendal nerve maintains external sphincter and pelvic muscle tone. The pelvic nerve stimulates bladder contraction. The hypogastric nerve stimulates internal sphincter closure and detrusor relaxation.

contraction. Muscarinic receptor subtypes M_1, M_2, and M_3 are found in the urinary bladder; however, it is the M_3 subtype that is primarily responsible for bladder contraction. These receptors, particularly the M_3 subtype, have become drug targets for purposes of treating OAB.

Any aberration of any individual component or combination of components involved in the micturition reflex can result in OAB or UI, as can separate comorbid conditions or physiologic states. Transient and reversible conditions or behaviors may contribute to symptoms consistent with OAB, namely, increases in fluid intake or increases in caffeine or alcohol consumption. Benign prostatic hyperplasia (BPH) or obstruction can manifest in incontinence. Sacral nerve damage can lead to urinary retention. Irrespective of the etiology of OAB, the common themes include increased bladder pressure at low volumes during filling, altered response to stimuli, amplified myogenic activity and contraction, and changes in the smooth muscle anatomy.

Owing to the poor electrical coupling between smooth muscle bundles in the bladder, the highly innervated bladder is able to ignore some of the errant impulses that would otherwise cause unwanted contraction. Patchy denervation and morphologic changes in the electrical coupling may result in bladder hypertrophy and incomplete emptying. Abnormal micturition can be stimulated by damage to the afferent neurons in the dorsal root ganglia as well, which can then confer an abbreviated delay in the micturition reflex. Ischemic conditions such as diabetic neuropathy, peripheral vascular disease, and urethral stricture may also result in compromised blood flow and ultimately neuronal death with subsequent detrusor hyperactivity. Inevitable physiologic changes that occur during the aging process may also contribute to impaired cortical inhibition of bladder contraction. Stroke, Alzheimer disease, and multiple sclerosis have been implicated in contributing to the disease process as well. Nonneurogenic conditions may also yield OAB symptoms; polyuria may be produced by uncontrolled diabetes, and nocturia may be precipitated by sleep apnea (**Box 34.1**).

Once OAB symptoms have emerged, a self-propelling cycle of factors can further exacerbate the condition. Urgency, a central feature of OAB, increases the frequency of micturition and therefore reduces the volume of each micturition provided that fluid intake remains constant. This sometimes leads to incomplete bladder emptying and subsequent residual volume that promotes the urgency and increased frequency of urination. Similarly, DO can result from neurogenic or myogenic causes. The contractions tend to be weak, which results in incomplete bladder emptying, a reduced bladder capacity, and therefore increased urinary frequency.

DIAGNOSTIC CRITERIA AND EVALUATION

OAB is a markedly underreported condition, owing mostly to the embarrassment and stigma with which it is associated. It tends to elude the typical clinical assessments and patient

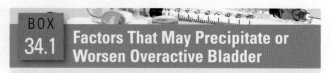

BOX 34.1 Factors That May Precipitate or Worsen Overactive Bladder

Neurologic Conditions
Stroke
Spinal cord injury
Diabetic neuropathy
Alzheimer disease
Multiple sclerosis

Systemic or Metabolic Conditions
Sleep disorders (apnea)
Venous insufficiency/heart failure
Diabetes mellitus

Behavioral Considerations
Excessive fluid or caffeine consumption
Constipation
Impaired mobility

Psychological Conditions
Depression

Medications
Diuretics
Narcotic pain relievers
Calcium channel blockers
Alpha-adrenergic antagonists
Anticholinergics
Alpha-adrenergic agonists

Miscellaneous
Prostate enlargement
Estrogen deficiency

Urinary Tract Pathology
Urinary tract infection
Urinary obstruction

interviews that constitute the primary care visit and is generally diagnosed only when it is reported by the patient. The only diagnostic criteria that have been firmly established are the presence of urgency with or without nocturia and frequency. These criteria are inherently subjective; however, there have been attempts to impose objective measurements and ratings in order to determine whether a symptom is pathologic.

Current recommendations suggest that pointed questioning should be integrated into the patient interview during routine primary care visits in order to capture urinary symptoms that may otherwise be overlooked. If patient complaints or interview-generated information is suggestive of OAB, the practitioner should perform a genitourinary exam and urinalysis as well as a more in-depth medical history that is germane to urinary health. One of the major goals of this interview would be the establishment of potential causative factors acutely or chronically (acute infection, changes in fluid intake, menstrual history, obstetric history, prostate pathology). The urinalysis is intended to assist in ruling out hematuria or an infection.

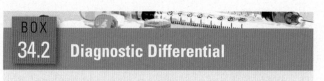

BOX
34.2   **Diagnostic Differential**

Bladder cancer, bladder calculus, interstitial cystitis
Endometriosis
Prostate cancer
Urethral calculus
Bacterial cystitis, prostatitis, urethritis
Urinary retention, polyuria, psychogenic urinary
    frequency

Since abnormalities or pathology in the LUT can precipitate OAB symptoms, it is imperative to evaluate the bladder, urethra, and pelvic floor muscles as well. In patients at risk for urinary retention (diabetics, spinal cord injury patients, patients with BPH), more invasive testing may be required. A residual urine volume of more than 100 mL suggests urinary retention, and these patients may need to be evaluated by cystoscopy to rule out malignancy. OAB is a constellation of symptoms, all of which could be reasonably attributed to other conditions. Therefore, OAB is often diagnosed after the exclusion of other pathology. Primarily, infections, cancers (bladder, prostate), structural abnormalities (urethral, prostate), and urinary retention should be ruled out during the evaluation process.

A neurologic exam, with emphasis on the sacral neuronal pathways, is recommended because OAB may be caused by neurogenic LUT dysfunction. In addition to assessments of gait, abduction/dorsiflexion of toes, and sensory innervation to the LUT, a rectal exam will provide some information relevant to voluntary sphincter control. In males specifically, a measurement of prostate-specific antigen (PSA) and administration of the American Urological Association's subjective symptoms assessment (AUA-7) should occur (**Box 34.2**).

One of the tools with the highest level of clinical evidence is the "bladder diary" or "voiding diary," a patient-generated daily log that includes fluid intake and urinary output with corresponding times. Typically, entries are made by the patient over either a 3- or 7-day period. It yields information regarding urinary habits, estimation of bladder capacity, volume voided with each micturition, diurnal and nocturnal frequency, urgency, and incontinence. A number of clinical trials have used this tool to assess outcomes and have found that bladder diaries are an accurate measure of OAB symptoms, including urgency. Another parameter that is thus far not validated is "warning time," the length of time between an initial perception of the urge to void and the time at which it can no longer be deferred.

The use of urodynamic testing (UDT), the comprehensive evaluation of bladder and urethral performance during micturition, has been met with some controversy. UDT consists of a collection of urodynamic assessments that range from simple direct observations to complex, sophisticated, invasive evaluations. In order to best assess a LUT dysfunction or OAB, the symptoms need to be reproducible in a clinical setting. **Table 34.2** provides a list of the possible components of UDT. UDT is not required for a diagnosis of OAB; however, it may be indicated if there is suspicion of a BOO, neurogenic voiding dysfunction, or an uncertain diagnosis.

TABLE 34.2

Urodynamic Testing

Component	Description	Clinical Utility
Uroflowmetry	Measurement of the volume over urine voided, speed at which voiding occurs, and duration of void	Obstruction is likely if speed is <10 mL/s.
Postvoid residual (PVR)	After voiding, determination of PVR made via ultrasound or through catheterization	<25 mL is considered normal and >100 mL is abnormal.
Multichannel filling cystometry	Evaluation of bladder capacity, bladder compliance, and at what volume the urge to void occurs; accomplished by filling the bladder with normal saline and measuring detrusor pressure	Bladder pressure during filling should be <10 cm H_2O; dysfunction is diagnosed if the pressure rises at an unacceptable rate.
Leak point pressure	Evaluation of the first urine leakage and the abdominal pressure at which it occurs; the patient is instructed to perform Valsalva maneuver (e.g., coughing); patient is observed for urine leakage.	Low readings (<40 cm H_2O) are associated with sphincter weakness.
Pressure flow study	Assesses the interaction among the bladder, bladder outlet, pelvic floor, and urethra during voiding; patient is instructed to void with all catheters in place (catheters include urethral catheterization and possibly vaginal or rectal catheterization).	Useful for diagnosing bladder outlet obstructions
Electromyography	Assessment of the coordination between the perineal muscles and the bladder	Useful in diagnosing neurogenic etiology of OAB

INITIATING DRUG THERAPY

Once a diagnosis of OAB has been established, the subsequent steps include an assessment of the degree of impairment or annoyance resulting from OAB, initiation of empiric or disease-specific therapy if required, treatment of comorbid conditions, and referral to a specialist if warranted. If it is determined that the patient is significantly bothered by OAB and/or has begun to engage in avoidance behaviors that are compromising quality of life, therapy should be initiated. The 2014 American Urological Association

(AUA) recommends utilizing behavioral therapies as the first-line intervention, a series of behaviors that change patient behavior or the environment. The most common behavioral interventions are bladder training, pelvic floor muscle exercises, and weight loss. The nondrug therapies usually are ultimately combined with pharmacologic therapy (**Table 34.3** and **Figure 34.3**).

The *anticholinergic* or antimuscarinic drugs (oxybutynin, tolterodine, trospium, darifenacin, solifenacin, fesoterodine) have the greatest level of evidence with respect to their safety and efficacy in treating OAB and are recommended as first-line

TABLE 34.3

OAB Medication Overview

Medication	Usual Dose	Uroselectivity	Clinical Considerations	Level of Evidence
Anticholinergics/Antimuscarinics				
oxybutynin (Ditropan)	5–15 mg orally three times daily	No	Dry mouth occurs in up to 66% of patients. Indicated for neurogenic and nonneurogenic detrusor overactivity	1A
oxybutynin ER (Ditropan XL)	5–15 mg orally once daily	No	Dry mouth occurs in up to 66% of patients. Indicated for neurogenic and nonneurogenic detrusor overactivity	1A
oxybutynin (Oxytrol transdermal patch)	3.9 mg/patch twice weekly (every 3–4 d)	No	Dry mouth occurs half as frequently as compared to the oral formulation.	1A
tolterodine (Detrol)	2 mg orally twice daily	Yes	Incidence of dry mouth is 20% to 25%.	1A
tolterodine ER (Detrol LA)	4 mg orally once daily	Yes	Dry mouth occurs in <20% of patients.	1A
trospium (Sanctura)	20 mg orally twice daily	Yes	Take before meals or on an empty stomach. No CYP P-450 metabolism	1A
trospium extended release (Trospium XR)	60 mg orally once daily	Yes	Take before meals or on an empty stomach. No CYP P-450 metabolism	1A
solifenacin (VESIcare)	5–10 mg orally once daily	Yes		1A
darifenacin hydrobromide (Enablex)	7.5–15 mg once daily (may titrate up to 15 mg after 2 wk if tolerated)	Yes	Possibly less impact on cognitive function than other antimuscarinics	1A
fesoterodine (Toviaz)	4–8 mg orally daily	No	Less CYP2D6 interaction potential	1A
Beta-3-Adrenoreceptor Agonists				
mirabegron (Myrbetriq)	25–50 mg orally once daily	Yes	Less incidence of anticholinergic and cognitive adverse effects	1B
onabotulinumtoxinA 100U injections (interval undetermined but generally every 6–9 mo) OnabotulinumtoxinA (Botox)		Yes	Efficacy maintained for several months; possible risk of urinary retention and voiding dysfunction	B, C
Serotonin Norepinephrine Reuptake Inhibitors				
duloxetine (Cymbalta)	40–80 mg orally once daily	No	Avoid concomitant administration with other serotonergic drugs.	1A
Alpha-Adrenergic Antagonists				
alfuzosin (Uroxatral)	2.5 mg orally three times daily	No	4D	
doxazosin (Cardura)	1–16 mg orally once daily	No	Dizziness occurs in up to 20% of patients.	4D
prazosin (Minipress)	1–10 mg orally twice daily	No	4D	
tamsulosin (Flomax)	0.4–0.8 mg orally once daily		No	4D
terazosin (Hytrin)	1–10 mg orally at bedtime	No	4D	
silodosin (Rapaflo)	8 mg orally once daily	No	Retrograde ejaculation occurs in up to 28% of patients.	4D

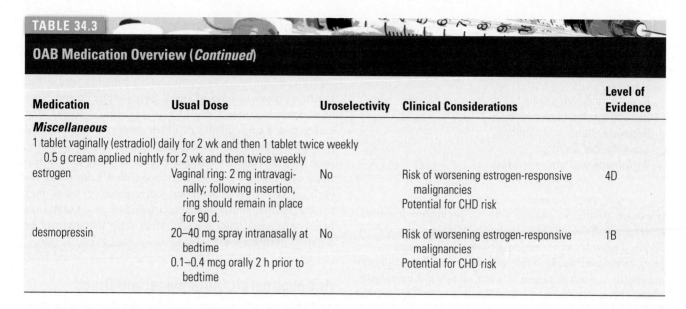

TABLE 34.3

OAB Medication Overview (*Continued*)

Medication	Usual Dose	Uroselectivity	Clinical Considerations	Level of Evidence
Miscellaneous				
1 tablet vaginally (estradiol) daily for 2 wk and then 1 tablet twice weekly				
0.5 g cream applied nightly for 2 wk and then twice weekly				
estrogen	Vaginal ring: 2 mg intravaginally; following insertion, ring should remain in place for 90 d.	No	Risk of worsening estrogen-responsive malignancies Potential for CHD risk	4D
desmopressin	20–40 mg spray intranasally at bedtime	No	Risk of worsening estrogen-responsive malignancies Potential for CHD risk	1B
	0.1–0.4 mcg orally 2 h prior to bedtime			

pharmacologic therapy by the 2014 AUA guidelines. Their clinical use is sometimes limited, however, by their inherent anticholinergic adverse effects, most commonly dry mouth, blurred vision, constipation, cognitive dysfunction, and urinary retention. This is particularly challenging because the population with the highest prevalence of OAB is the elderly, an age cohort that is also more predisposed to cognitive dysfunction, urinary retention, and visual disturbances.

If tolerability issues preclude the use of anticholinergic drugs, tricyclic antidepressants (TCAs; imipramine), desmopressin, topical estrogens for females, and alpha-adrenergic antagonists for males are appropriate alternatives. There is emerging evidence about the role of selective serotonin reuptake inhibitors

(SSRIs) and serotonin norepinephrine reuptake inhibitors (SNRIs) in treating OAB syndrome. Vanilloids and afferent nerve inhibitors such as capsaicin or resiniferatoxin are in the investigation phases to assess their utility in managing OAB.

The combination of pharmacologic and nonpharmacologic treatment tends to yield superior outcomes and clinical success. "Bladder training" encompasses pelvic floor exercises, scheduled voiding, urge suppression skills, and extensive patient education. Over 70% of patients who are considered cognitively competent experience a meaningful reduction in incontinence episodes over a 2- to 3-month period as a result of employing bladder training and pelvic floor exercises (Ouslander, 2004). Benefit may still be derived from prompted

FIGURE 34.3 Treatment algorithm for overactive bladder.

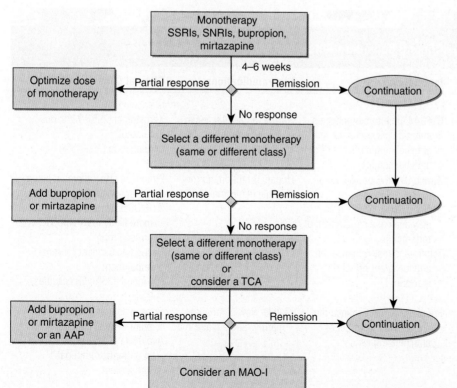

BOX 34.3   Behavioral Modifications

Reduce fluid consumption.
Reduce alcohol consumption.
Reduce caffeine consumption.
Start bladder training.
Perform pelvic floor exercises.

scheduled voiding in patients who are cognitively impaired. In refractory cases of OAB, biofeedback devices that deliver electrical stimulation via vaginal or rectal probes augment the pelvic floor exercises. In severe or refractory patients, surgical interventions, such as neural ablation, slings, and neuromodulating device implantation, may be attempted. This will be further discussed.

Compensatory behaviors such as limiting fluid intake or reducing the frequency of diuretics are not recommended, although patients frequently engage in these behaviors. Self-imposed fluid restriction may precipitate dehydration and subsequent increased fall risks, cognitive impairment, worsened renal function, and changes in drug metabolism. Altering diuretic administration could negatively impact the treatment of other conditions or result in fluid overload. The use of absorbent pads or undergarments may help to mitigate the social stigma aspect of OAB, especially in patients who experience incontinence. Rushing to find a restroom when urgency occurs also predisposes patients to falls and fractures (**Box 34.3**).

Goals of Drug Therapy

The intended outcome of pharmacologic therapy is primarily resolution of symptoms (urgency, frequency, nocturia), cessation of incontinence episodes (if present), and a full return to previous level of social functioning. In the event of a comorbid mood disorder (depression, anxiety) that emerged as a consequence of OAB, goals of therapy would include resolution of this disorder as well. Patients suffering from OAB are at an increased risk for urinary tract infections, and those with associated incontinence are at risk for perineal skin infections. These corresponding issues may resolve spontaneously upon treatment of the OAB and/or incontinence; however, additional drug therapy may be required (**Table 34.4**).

Anticholinergic/Antimuscarinic Drugs

As a class, antimuscarinic drugs are the mainstay of pharmacologic therapy for OAB and UI. Anticholinergic drugs are considered first-line therapy and typically will be used even after clinical failure or intolerance to an initial anticholinergic medication. The class is divided into tertiary and quaternary amines, differing with respect to lipophilicity, molecular size, and charge. High lipophilicity, small molecular size, and low charge confer upon the tertiary amines (oxybutynin, tolterodine, solifenacin, darifenacin, fesoterodine) easy transfer into the CNS via the blood–brain barrier. The quaternary amine trospium tends to not be as well absorbed and has limited ability to cross the blood–brain barrier (**Table 34.5**).

TABLE 34.4

Medication Pharmacokinetics and Clinical Considerations

Drug	Metabolism	Interactions	Contraindications	Clinical Considerations
Antimuscarinics				
oxybutynin	Minor substrate of CYP3A4	CYP3A4 inhibitors or inducers Pramlintide may enhance the anticholinergic effects of anticholinergics.	Narrow-angle glaucoma, urinary retention	Xerostomia (29%–71%; dose related) Constipation (7%–15%)
tolterodine	Major substrate of CYP2D6 and 3A4 Minor substrate of CYP2C9 and 2C19	Strong CYP2D6 or 3A4 inhibitors or inducers Systemic azole antifungals may decrease metabolism of tolterodine. Tolterodine may enhance the anticoagulant effect of warfarin.	Urinary retention, narrow-angle glaucoma	Prolonged QTc interval at supratherapeutic doses CYP2D6 poor metabolizers more likely to exhibit QTc prolongation Dosage adjustment for renal impairment Dry mouth (35%; ER capsules, 23%)
trospium	Not fully elucidated; thought to be metabolized by esterase hydrolysis and conjugation	Pramlintide may enhance the anticholinergic effect of anticholinergics.	Bladder flow obstruction, narrow-angle glaucoma	Dosage adjustment of IR trospium in renal impairment Avoid use of ER trospium in patients with renal impairment.

TABLE 34.4

Medication Pharmacokinetics and Clinical Considerations (*Continued*)

Drug	Metabolism	Interactions	Contraindications	Clinical Considerations
solifenacin	Major CYP3A4 substrate	Major inhibitors or inducers of CYP3A4 Grapefruit juice may increase the serum level effects of solifenacin.	Bladder flow obstruction, narrow-angle glaucoma	Dosage adjustment for severe renal impairment (CrCl < 30 mL/min)
darifenacin	Major substrate of CYP3A4 and minor substrate of 2D6 Moderate inhibitor of 2D6 and minor inhibitor of 3A4	CYP3A4 or 2D6 inhibitors or inducers	Uncontrolled narrow-angle glaucoma; urinary retention, paralytic ileus, GI or GU obstruction Concomitant administration of thioridazine	Xerostomia (19%–35%), constipation (15%–21%)
fesoterodine	Parent compound metabolized to active metabolite (5-HMT) by nonspecific esterases 5-HMT metabolized by CYP2D6 and CYP3A4	CYP3A4 or 2D6 inhibitors or inducers	Bladder flow obstruction, narrow-angle glaucoma	Dose adjustment in patients with severe renal impairment (CrCl < 30 mL/min)

OnabotulinumtoxinA

onabotulinumtoxinA (Botox). No metabolism. Neuromuscular blocking agents and aminoglycoside antibiotics can potentiate the neuromuscular effect of onabotulinumtoxinA.			Hypersensitivity to onabotulinumtoxinA	Black box warning for distant spread (can result in muscle weakness, life-threatening breathing issues)

Serotonin Norepinephrine Reuptake Inhibitors

duloxetine	Major substrate of CYP1A2 and 2D6 Moderate inhibitor of 2D6	CYP1A2 or 2D6 inhibitors or inducers MAO inhibitors or thioridazine	Concomitant use or within 2 wk of MAO inhibitors; uncontrolled narrow-angle glaucoma	Ulcerogenic potential increased with NSAIDs (increased risk of bleeding) Serotonin syndrome or neuroleptic malignant syndrome risk Not recommended when CrCl <30 mL/min

Alpha-Adrenergic Antagonists

alfuzosin	Major substrate of CYP3A4	Strong CYP3A4 inhibitors	Strong CYP3A4 inhibitors (itraconazole, ketoconazole, ritonavir)	Avoid concomitant use with other alpha-1-antagonists. Potential to cause dizziness
doxazosin	Major substrate of CYP3A4	Strong CYP3A4 inhibitors	Strong CYP3A4 inhibitors (itraconazole)	Dizziness may occur in up to 28% of patients.
prazosin	Major substrate of CYP3A4	Strong CYP3A4 inhibitors	Strong CYP3A4 inhibitors (itraconazole)	Dizziness
tamsulosin	Major substrate of CYP3A4	Strong CYP3A4 inhibitors	Strong CYP3A4 inhibitors (itraconazole)	Dizziness
terazosin	Major substrate of CYP3A4	Strong CYP3A4 inhibitors	Strong CYP3A4 inhibitors (itraconazole)	Dizziness
silodosin	Major substrate of CYP3A4	Strong CYP3A4 inhibitors	Strong CYP3A4 inhibitors (itraconazole)	Retrograde ejaculation

Mechanism of Action

The mechanism of action of each of the medications is relatively similar, with the exception of oxybutynin. Generally, anticholinergics mediate a pharmacologic action by antagonizing the parasympathetic muscarinic receptors in the bladder with relative selectivity for the M_3 and M_1 subtypes. Antagonism of the M_3 muscarinic receptors manifests as a reduction in spontaneous myocyte activity, a decrease in

frequency, and a reduction in contraction intensity. They effectively increase bladder capacity, decrease the intensity and frequency of bladder contractions, and delay the initial urge to void. Oxybutynin is both an antimuscarinic and an antispasmodic (secondary to direct muscle relaxation) as well as a local anesthetic.

Oxybutynin boasts a lengthy and robust history of efficacy with respect to OAB and UI. A tertiary amine, oxybutynin is

TABLE 34.5

Molecular Properties of Antimuscarinic Drugs

Drug	Molecular Classification	Corresponding Molecular Characteristics	Clinical Characteristics
Oxybutynin Tolterodine Solifenacin Darifenacin Fesoterodine	Tertiary amine	High lipophilicity Small molecular size Low charge	Extensive transfer into CNS Increased risk of cognitive adverse effects
Trospium	Quaternary amine	Low lipophilicity Large molecular size High charge	Limited transfer into CNS Reduced risk of cognitive adverse effects

highly lipophilic and easily crosses the blood–brain barrier, thereby conferring higher rates of CNS and anticholinergic adverse effects. The potential for cytochrome P-450 (CYP) enzyme interactions is relatively high as well. Secondary to these adverse effects and interaction potential, oxybutynin may not be well tolerated in all patient populations. Oxybutynin undergoes extensive first-pass metabolism to its active metabolite, N-desmethyl oxybutynin, which is purported to produce most of the pharmacologic activity and adverse effects. Up to 80% of patients will report at least one significant muscarinic-mediated adverse effect during therapy, up to 20% of whom will subsequently discontinue therapy. Xerostomia, experienced by up to 70% of patients, is dose related but is also the most common reason cited for discontinuing oxybutynin therapy. Despite these inherent limitations, the use of oxybutynin remains prevalent among all available formulations. The extended-release (ER; Ditropan XL) formulation of oxybutynin has been clinically shown to be equally efficacious but is associated with less adverse effects than the conventional formulation. The transdermal oxybutynin patch (Oxytrol) causes roughly 75% less dry mouth as compared to ER tolterodine and is now available without a prescription. The transdermal system releases drug constantly over 96 hours at which time the patch is replaced.

Tolterodine (Detrol) is a competitive antagonist of muscarinic receptors that causes increased residual urine volume and decreased detrusor pressure. It is associated with clinically meaningful reductions in micturition frequency as well as incontinence episodes. In comparison to oxybutynin, tolterodine use yields less dosage changes, adverse effects, and treatment-related therapy discontinuations. Tolterodine ER (Detrol LA) is 18% more effective in reducing the incidence of incontinence as compared to the regular formulation and is responsible for 23% less xerostomia (Robinson & Cardozo, 2010). ER oxybutynin, however, is significantly more efficacious than ER tolterodine in reducing micturition frequency.

Trospium (Sanctura) is a nonselective muscarinic receptor antagonist that improves urinary frequency, episodes of incontinence, urgency, and volume voided. A quaternary ammonium compound, trospium crosses the blood–brain barrier only to a limited extent, which confers a reduced likelihood of cognitive sequelae. Trospium may possess a therapeutic advantage in patients with comorbidities that require drug therapy, given its negligible hepatic metabolism and low risk of drug interactions.

Solifenacin (VESIcare) is a bladder-selective M_3 receptor antagonist that has been shown to be statistically significantly more efficacious than ER tolterodine with respect to urge incontinence, overall incontinence, and urgency. In another pivotal study, solifenacin was shown to reduce episodes of urgency and increase warning time. It is postulated that solifenacin may provide a greater level of efficacy as compared to other drugs within the class. However, despite its bladder selectivity, solifenacin causes dose-related dry mouth in over 20% of patients and xerostomia-related treatment discontinuation in almost 5%, a frequency that is of clinical importance but is lower than other members of this class (Cipullo, 2014).

Darifenacin (Enablex), a tertiary amine, is a highly selective M_3 receptor antagonist that is effective in reducing frequency of micturition, increasing bladder capacity, reducing frequency and severity of urgency, and reducing the number of episodes of incontinence. A comparative advantage associated with darifenacin is its lack of cognitive impairment, as evidenced in multiple randomized controlled trials.

Fesoterodine (Toviaz), a prodrug, is converted to its active metabolite 5-hydroxymethyl tolterodine (5-HMT), which exerts a pharmacologic effect as a competitive antagonist at the muscarinic receptors. Tolterodine (Detrol) is metabolized to 5-HMT via a CYP2D6-mediated oxidation, and both tolterodine and 5-HMT are responsible for the pharmacologic effect of Detrol. Fesoterodine, however, does not require CYP2D6 activation and therefore may have less potential for pharmacokinetic variability and CYP2D6-specific drug interactions.

The AUA recommends initiating an ER anticholinergic as first-line therapy but does not recommend a specific product.

Time Frame for Response

Expected therapeutic response is variable among members of this class. Generally, a meaningful response would be realized within about 2 weeks. However, evidence suggests that patients taking tolterodine ER experienced reduced micturition, urgency episodes, and incontinence by day 5 of therapy. Trospium may exert a clinical effect as early as day 1 with regard to incontinence, day 3 for urgency, and day 5 for micturition frequency.

Contraindications

Anticholinergic medications are capable of precipitating or worsening urinary retention as well as worsening narrow-angle glaucoma. Both of these conditions, if present in the patient prior to therapy, represent contraindications to the use of antimuscarinics. Antagonism of muscarinic receptors and subsequent down-regulation of acetylcholine activity can result in paralysis of smooth muscle in the bladder or gastrointestinal tract. Additionally, mydriasis can occur with increased intraocular pressure; therefore, anticholinergics should be avoided in patients with narrow-angle glaucoma. Tolterodine, trospium, solifenacin, and fesoterodine require a dosage reduction in the case of severe renal impairment (creatinine clearance [CrCl] less than 30 mL/min). However, the ER formulation of trospium should be avoided in patients with severe renal impairment (**Table 34.6**).

Adverse Events

The expected adverse event profile includes traditional anticholinergic effects such as xerostomia, constipation, and urinary retention. Antimuscarinic drugs exert an action mainly during the storage phase of the micturition cycle when there is an absence of parasympathetic activity in the detrusor. During the emptying phase of micturition, there is a massive release of acetylcholine, which effectively blunts the drug's action. If this did not occur, the presence of the active drug would undoubtedly decrease the ability of the bladder to contract to promote urinary retention. Prescribing these drugs within the confines of acceptable dosing typically does not precipitate urinary retention; however, overdose or pharmacokinetic interactions may do so.

Interactions

Most antimuscarinic drugs are metabolized by one or more CYP P-450 isoenzymes, the most common of which are CYP3A4 and CYP2D6. Heterozygous or CYP2D6 homozygous patients are considered "extensive metabolizers," which implies an innate ability to appropriately metabolize drugs via this isoenzyme. However, patients who are poor metabolizers with respect to CYP2D6 may be at an increased risk for drug-related toxicity secondary to their inability to fully metabolize CYP2D6-metabolized drugs. Trospium is metabolized

TABLE 34.6						
Antimuscarinic Medication Dosing Considerations						
	Oxybutynin	**Tolterodine**	**Trospium**	**Solifenacin**	**Darifenacin**	**Fesoterodine**
Usual dose	IR: 5–15 mg orally three times daily ER: 5–15 mg orally once daily Patch: 3.9 mg/patch twice weekly (every 3–4 d)	IR: 2 mg orally twice daily ER: 4 mg orally once daily	IR: 20 mg orally twice daily ER: 60 mg once daily ≥75: 20 mg orally once daily	5–10 mg orally once daily Dosage adjustment with concomitant CYP3A4 inhibitors: Maximum dose 5 mg/d	7.5–15 mg once daily Dosage adjustment with concomitant potent CYP3A4 inhibitors (e.g., azole antifungals, erythromycin, protease inhibitors): 7.5 mg/d	4–8 mg orally daily
Renal insufficiency		**CrCl 10–30 mL/min: IR: 1 mg twice daily ER: 2 mg daily **Use with caution	CrCl ≤30 mL/min: IR: 20 mg once daily at bedtime ER: Use not recommended	CrCl <30 mL/min: Maximum dose 5 mg/d		Severe renal impairment (CrCl <30 mL/min): 4 mg
Hepatic insufficiency		IR: 1 mg twice daily ER: 2 mg daily		Moderate (Child-Pugh class B): Maximum dose 5 mg/d Severe (Child-Pugh class C): Use not recommended	Moderate impairment (Child-Pugh class B): Daily dosage should not exceed 7.5 mg/d. Severe impairment (Child-Pugh class C): Use not recommended	Severe hepatic impairment (Child-Pugh class C): Use not recommended
CYP interactions	CYP3A4 inhibitors or inducers	Strong CYP2D6 or 3A4 inhibitors or inducers Azole antifungals		Major inhibitors or inducers of CYP3A4	CYP2D6 and 3A4 inhibitors	Strong CYP3A4 inhibitors

exclusively by nonspecific esterases independent of the hepatic CYP P-450 system. Notable drug interactions within the anticholinergic class tend to involve pharmacokinetic interactions at the enzyme level and typically manifest as increases or decreases in drug metabolism. Solifenacin and tolterodine are capable of causing prolonged QTc, particularly in supratherapeutic dosing. Concomitant administration of other QTc-prolonging medications can potentiate a pharmacodynamic interaction that may result in arrhythmia.

Beta-Adrenoreceptor Agonists

Mirabegron (Myrbetriq) is a selective beta-3-adrenoreceptor agonist that increases bladder capacity and decreases the frequency of micturition without impacting micturition pressure or residual volume. Detrusor relaxation is achieved in part by activation of beta-3-adrenoreceptors by norepinephrine, which subsequently results in activation of adenylyl cyclase, and formation of cAMP, which produces smooth muscle relaxation. Bladder relaxation is crucial during the storage phase of micturition as it allows for compliance and low intravesical pressure during filling. Mirabegron, through its interaction with the beta-3-adrenoreceptor, promotes relaxation during filling and therefore increases bladder capacity, which then influences frequency of micturition. This is the first novel compound for the treatment of OAB, which has been able to produce a therapeutic effect without engaging the muscarinic receptors and producing anticholinergic adverse effects, a limiting factor associated with the mainstay of therapy, the antimuscarinic drugs.

Mirabegron, in daily doses of 25 to 200 mg, was evaluated in several 12-week randomized, placebo-controlled phase III studies, which support its efficacy, safety, and tolerability. Treatment with mirabegron resulted in decreased incontinence episodes, decreases in the number of micturitions, decreases in urgency episodes, and increases in mean volume voided per urination. Therapeutic effects were observed as early as week 4 and persisted throughout the duration of the studies. Meaningful and statistically significant improvements in these micturition parameters and in quality of life measures were observed in patients who were treatment naive and in patients who had failed or were intolerant to the antimuscarinics. Several studies that utilized tolterodine ER 4 mg as an active control reported similar efficacy and tolerability among the mirabegron and tolterodine groups, although no direct statistical comparisons occurred. Rates of xerostomia were significantly higher in patients treated with tolterodine, however. Evaluation of the available literature suggests that mirabegron is similar in efficacy to the antimuscarinics but with a lower incidence of adverse effects.

Dosage

Mirabegron is available as a 25- or 50-mg extended-release 24-hour tablet, which is formulated as an oral-controlled absorption system (OCAS). Generally, 25 mg daily is sufficient to control symptoms of urgency, frequent urination, and UI.

An increase to 50 mg daily can be considered dependent upon observed efficacy and tolerability in the individual patient. Maximum daily doses of 25 mg are recommended for patients with severe renal impairment or moderate hepatic impairment. It is not recommended in patients with end-stage renal disease or severe hepatic impairment. Mirabegron is approximately 70% bound to albumin and alpha-1-acid glycoprotein and is extensively metabolized through multiple pathways including dealkylation, glucuronidation, oxidation, and hydrolysis, as well as enzymatically metabolized through CYP3A4 and CYP2D6. Metabolism of mirabegron produces 10 pharmacologically inactive metabolites. The 50-hour elimination half-life allows for once-daily dosing.

Time Frame for Response

A therapeutic effect is usually realized within the first 8 weeks of therapy, at which point a decision regarding the need to a dosage increase can be considered. Meaningful improvements in parameters of micturition were observed in studies as early as week 4, however.

Contraindications

Mirabegron does not have specifically labeled contraindications; however, dose-related QT prolongation has been observed in clinical studies. Prolongation of the QT interval was observed in female patients on the 200-mg dose of mirabegron, a dose that is supratherapeutic and is not available in the market. Doses of 50 to 100 mg daily did not elicit any electrocardiogram abnormalities in any evaluation. However, patients with QT prolongation or at risk of QT prolongation (taking concurrent medications that prolong QT) should avoid mirabegron.

Adverse Events

Long-term safety and tolerability studies suggest that the rate of treatment-emergent adverse effects is similar between mirabegron and placebo and tends to be mild to moderate in intensity. As compared to tolterodine, mirabegron causes less xerostomia, constipation, urinary retention, and blurred vision. It also does not induce neurological adverse effects such as cognitive impairment, which tends to be associated with the antimuscarinics. Meaningful increases in blood pressure were observed during clinical studies, although hypertension is not considered a contraindication. Monitoring blood pressure is recommended, however.

Interactions

There are no clinically meaningful drug interactions related to the hepatic metabolism with the exception of drugs metabolized by CYP2D6, as mirabegron is a moderate inhibitor of this isoenzyme.

Given mirabegron's efficacy in treatment-experienced and treatment-naive patients as well as its low potential for drug interactions, mild adverse effect profile, and absence of cognitive impairment-related sequelae, mirabegron may become a first-line option. Mirabegron can be considered an appropriate intervention in patients at risk of cognitive impairment and those who are elderly. Treatment discontinuation is a frequent and unfortunate reality with regard to the antimuscarinic drugs, the current treatment of choice. There is no evidence thus far related to treatment adherence with mirabegron, though one of its advantages is its low incidence of adverse effects.

OnabotulinumtoxinA (Botox)

Botulinum toxin serotype A, a purified version of *Clostridium botulinum*, is a neurotoxin, which has demonstrated utility in OAB and DO. Two noninterchangeable products are currently approved and marketed for both neurogenic bladder and urge incontinence: Botox (onabotulinumtoxinA) and Dysport (abobotulinumtoxinA). The preponderance of evaluation and evidence focuses on the Botox product. Generally, the use of injectable botulinum toxin is reserved for patients who have failed more than one of the recommended initial drug therapies (anticholinergics or mirabegron) and are considered refractory. The 2014 AUA guidelines have officially incorporated botulinum toxin into its therapeutic recommendations and consider it a third-line option.

Mechanism of Action

Botulinum toxin, when injected into the detrusor muscle, inhibits calcium-dependent release of acetylcholine, adenosine triphosphate, and substance P and reduces the expression of capsaicin receptors on motor neurons. The resulting desensitization of the motor neurons ultimately causes inhibition of the afferent and efferent pathways that influence DO. In addition to the motor effects, botulinum toxin also modulates the sensory aspect of DO by reducing the expression of vanilloid and muscarinic (M_1, M_2, and M_3) receptors in the suburothelium. The resulting flaccid paralysis in the detrusor reduces bladder pressure, increases bladder capacity, reduces incontinence episodes, and reduces perceived urgency. The effect is permanent and persists until the motor endplate units regenerate after 3 to 24 months, necessitating additional treatment.

Randomized controlled studies have demonstrated onabotulinumtoxinA's sustained efficacy over 6 months in reducing incontinence episodes, improving nocturia, improvement in voiding frequency, improvement in urgency episodes, and improvement in quality of life indicators. Clinical success was achieved in upwards of 70% of patients. Voiding dysfunction and urinary tract infections were the most commonly reported adverse effects.

Optimal dosing and dosing interval have yet to be established; however, there appears to be a balance between efficacy and tolerability at doses of 100 U per injection. Higher doses demonstrated similar efficacy much appreciably higher rates of adverse effects, namely, urinary retention. The duration of therapeutic effect is dependent upon the regrowth of the motor end units on the affected neurons and, therefore, is highly variable. Most patients require retreatment after 6 to 9 months.

Contraindications, Adverse Events, and Interactions

Adverse effects tend to be restricted to urinary tract infections and urinary retention secondary to the localized placement of the botulinum toxin. Urinary tract infection has been observed in 18% to 49% of patients and urinary retention in 6% to 17% of patients. A condition of treatment, as recommended by the product labeling and the AUA guidelines, is willingness and ability of the patient to self-catheterize. Education on technique should be provided prior to initiating therapy. Systemic adverse effects do not occur unless there is unintended spread of the botulinum toxin beyond the site of injection. A black box warning includes statements related to the blurred vision, dysarthria, muscle weakness, ptosis, dysphagia, and life-threatening breathing difficulties that could indicate unintentional spread of the toxin from its injection site.

Contraindications include sensitivity to the product or patients with existing urinary retention. Botulinum toxins are not metabolized, and therefore, interactions are limited to other drugs that may potentiate the neuromuscular-blocking effects such as anticholinergics, neuromuscular-blocking drugs, and aminoglycoside antibiotics.

Serotonin Norepinephrine Reuptake Inhibitors

Venlafaxine (Effexor) and duloxetine (Cymbalta), SNRIs, have been evaluated as nontraditional therapies for OAB.

Mechanism of Action

Serotonin facilitates urine storage, augmenting parasympathetic innervation and inhibiting sympathetic innervation to the bladder. During the filling phase, glutamate is released and acts upon Onuf nucleus. Onuf nucleus is a discrete confluence of neurons in the anterior horn of the sacral region of the spinal cord, which is involved in the micturition reflex, continence, and muscular contraction during orgasm. The action of glutamate in Onuf nucleus activates the pudendal nerve and subsequent release of acetylcholine, which elicits contraction of the external urethral sphincter. The dense population of the nucleus with serotonin and norepinephrine receptors implies a facilitator role for these monoamines with regard to the micturition reflex and urine storage. Duloxetine enhances urethral sphincter activity and is associated with dose-dependent decreases in episodes of incontinence and improvements in quality of life. It is believed that duloxetine exerts this effect by increasing the availability of serotonin and norepinephrine in the synaptic clefts of Onuf nucleus. Nausea occurs in about 25% of patients but tends to subside by day 7 of treatment. Numerous studies support the use of SNRIs alone or in combination with pelvic floor muscle exercises.

Contraindications, Adverse Events, and Interactions

Duloxetine may not be used concurrently with MAO inhibitors or within 2 weeks of discontinuing an MAO inhibitor. Duloxetine is metabolized in the liver by CYP3A4 and

CYP2D6 and therefore is subject to pharmacokinetic interactions with strong inhibitors of these isoenzymes. It is not to be coadministered with thioridazine because there is a significant CYP2D6-mediated interaction that may result in increased concentrations and toxicity in both drugs. Concomitant administration of duloxetine with other medications that have serotonergic or noradrenergic actions may increase the risk of serotonin syndrome or neuroleptic malignant syndrome.

Alpha-Adrenergic Antagonists

The alpha-adrenergic antagonists have proven efficacy and tolerability with respect to treating BPH in males. However, some studies suggest that tamsulosin may reduce bladder pressure, increase the flow rate, and provide symptomatic improvement in patients with OAB and a confirmed obstruction. The extent to which OAB symptoms are relieved is appreciably less than the resolution of symptoms of obstruction. Use in women is controversial because alpha-adrenergic antagonists may precipitate stress incontinence in female patients.

Mechanism of Action

Alpha-adrenergic antagonists, or alpha-blockers, competitively inhibit postsynaptic alpha-1-adrenergic receptors in prostate and bladder tissue. The antagonism reduces the sympathetic-mediated urethral stricture that is associated with BPH or BOO symptoms.

Adverse Events

Postural hypotension is one of the most clinically relevant adverse effects that may occur. All of the drugs in this class have the potential to induce this effect; however, doxazosin precipitates postural hypotension in upwards of 30% of patients. It is of special concern since the majority of patients who would likely be taking an alpha-1-antagonist are elderly and are predisposed to postural hypotension and subsequent falls.

Interactions

The alpha-1-antagonists are metabolized by CYP3A4, and concomitant administration with strong CYP3A4 inhibitors should be avoided. Also, secondary to the potential to cause hypotension, more than one alpha-blocker should not be used concurrently.

Estrogens

Despite the dearth of anecdotal evidence supporting the use of estrogens for symptomatic improvement of OAB and incontinence in females, randomized, controlled trials have yielded contradictory results at best. Unopposed systemic estrogen therapy or combination estrogen/progesterone therapy is associated with an increase in SUI and UUI episodes, as was evidenced by several large multinational studies. Topical estrogen therapy in the form of vaginal estradiol tablets (Vagifem) or the estrogen-releasing vaginal ring (Estring) has, however, demonstrated some symptomatic improvement. The vaginal tablet improved urgency, frequency, urge incontinence, and stress incontinence. The vaginal ring improved urge incontinence, stress incontinence, and nocturia. The therapeutic effect is attributed to increasing the maximum urethral pressure, although some clinicians hypothesize that it is due to reversal of urogenital atrophy and not direct bladder or urethral activity.

Mechanism of Action

Topical estradiol exerts a local action that improves tone and elasticity of female urogenital anatomy by increasing secretion of the cervical mucosa, thickening vaginal mucosa, and proliferation of the endometrium. Both the vaginal tablet and the vaginal ring are indicated for urinary urgency and dysuria.

Contraindications

Patients with undiagnosed vaginal bleeding, a history of breast carcinoma or estrogen-dependent tumors, and thromboembolic disorders (deep vein thrombosis, pulmonary embolism, stroke, myocardial infarction) and patients who are pregnant should not use estrogens.

Adverse Events

Administration of topical estrogens for OAB and incontinence symptoms is not without risk. Well-designed, large-scale, randomized, controlled trials have clearly demonstrated the cardiovascular sequelae that can result from utilizing hormone replacement therapy (HRT) for primary prevention of cardiovascular disease. Since the advent of the Women's Health Initiative study, the use of HRT has dramatically declined. However, in selected individuals, HRT is still used for the treatment of menopause-related symptoms, which include urogenital complaints (vaginal atrophy, dysuria, incontinence).

Risks of administration include the potential for thromboembolic complications, aggravation of existing estrogen-responsive malignancies or development of estrogen-responsive cancers, changes in libido, mood dysregulation, irritability, or syncope.

Antidiuretic Drugs

Mechanism of Action

Desmopressin (1-desamino-8-D-arginine vasopressin; DDAVP), a synthetic vasopressin analogue, had been indicated for nocturnal enuresis in adults and children. It possesses profound antidiuretic properties without any appreciable pressor activity; DDAVP can diurese without impacting blood pressure in a clinically significant way. Exploiting the hypothesis that a relative absence of nocturnal vasopressin and subsequently increased nocturnal urine production underlies the predisposition to suffer from enuresis, DDAVP reduces urine volume and osmolality. In addition to the established indication for enuresis in children, DDAVP has been shown to be efficacious in treating adult patients with nocturia of polyuric origin.

Contraindications and Adverse Events

Patients with hyponatremia or a history of hyponatremia or moderate to severe renal impairment (CrCl less than 50 mL/min) should avoid DDAVP. Adverse effects are mild and rare.

However, there is a risk of water retention with or without hyponatremia. Sodium monitoring is recommended in elderly patients prior to treatment and several days into therapy.

Interactions

There are no significant drug interactions associated with DDAVP. Several medications (lithium, TCAs, SSRIs, nonsteroidal anti-inflammatory drugs, carbamazepine) may enhance the toxic effects of DDAVP, but none of the risks are particularly likely.

New and Emerging Therapies

Vanilloid receptors on afferent neurons that innervate the bladder and urethra may be acted upon by capsaicin or resiniferatoxin. Capsaicin-mediated activation of the afferent neurons results in an initial excitation phase immediately followed by a protracted blockade that effectively desensitizes the neurons to normal stimuli. A capsaicin analogue, resiniferatoxin, can also impact the afferent neurons and the Aδ fibers. This transient physiologic "damage" to sensory nerves results in more prolonged retention of urine and improvement in OAB and DO of neurogenic and idiopathic origin.

Botulinum toxin A blocks the release of acetylcholine from the presynaptic neuron, which, in turn, decreases muscle contractility and increases muscle atrophy locally.

Selecting the Most Appropriate Agent

First-Line Therapy

The AUA 2014 guidelines for the management of OAB recommend initiating behavioral therapy in all patients prior to commencing drug therapy. In the absence of contraindications, anticholinergic medications are considered first-line pharmacologic therapy for OAB and symptoms of incontinence. Nonpharmacologic interventions, such as bladder training, typically are recommended prior to initiating drug therapy. Oftentimes, if the behavioral modifications do not suitably resolve the symptoms of OAB, a medication will be added to the nondrug intervention.

Antimuscarinics as a class have an established reputation with regard to efficacy and safety. They effectively reduce bladder pressure, increase bladder capacity and compliance, increase the volume threshold for desire to urinate, and reduce inappropriate bladder contractions. Tolerability issues involving anticholinergic adverse effects (dry mouth, constipation) may limit clinical utility in some patient populations but largely does not significantly impact therapy. There is no unequivocal evidence that recommends the use of one member of this class over another; however, there have been smaller studies that suggest some differential benefits. In terms of efficacy, the larger body of literature supports relative equivalence among antimuscarinics. ER formulations have demonstrated improved efficacy compared to their immediate-release (IR) counterparts. Some recent meta-analyses have insinuated that solifenacin may offer superior clinical efficacy compared to oxybutynin ER and tolterodine ER (Robinson & Cardozo, 2010). When considering

the anticholinergic side effect potential, oxybutynin is undeniably responsible for the most xerostomia and constipation. Trospium and darifenacin promote fewer cognitive sequelae than oxybutynin, tolterodine, or solifenacin. Trospium is not metabolized by the CYP P-450 system and therefore is associated with far fewer drug interactions than the rest of this class, which is metabolized primarily by CYP. New evidence suggests that fesoterodine may be more effective than tolterodine in terms of efficacy and improvement in quality of life. Tolterodine is currently the market leader in the majority of countries. The AUA recommends initiating an ER formulation of any of the anticholinergic drugs. If therapeutic failure occurs or tolerability issues arise, it is recommended that another member of the class be initiated before attempting another drug class.

Mirabegron is now also considered an appropriate first-line pharmacologic intervention, according to the guidelines. Mirabegron is a novel entity, which acts upon beta-3-adrenoreceptors in the detrusor muscle to promote relaxation during the filling phase, thereby reducing urgency, increasing the bladder capacity, and decreasing the number of micturitions. Clinical studies have consistently demonstrated efficacy that is similar to that of the anticholinergics and also improved tolerability comparatively, with a remarkably decreased risk of anticholinergic adverse effects and cognitive impairment. The once-daily dosing, coupled with the efficacy and tolerability advantages, low incidence of drug–drug interactions, and absence of anticholinergic effects, confers upon mirabegron a possible therapeutic advantage.

Second- and Third-Line Therapy

Failure or intolerance to the initial anticholinergic medication generally warrants the trial of a second anticholinergic medication. Since there are some appreciable differences among anticholinergics in terms of side effect profiles and tolerability, a switch to another anticholinergic typically precedes a switch to a different class. The transdermal oxybutynin patch is available without a prescription and may also be considered if oral therapy is not well tolerated but is not recommended as the initial pharmacologic intervention.

Botulinum A toxin is indicated for neurogenic and non-neurogenic DO as well as neurogenic spasm of the urethra due to spinal cord injury or secondary to DO. Injections of 100 U directly into the detrusor muscle promote an effect for 6 to 9 months secondary to the resulting flaccid paralysis of the bladder. Retreatment after dissipation of therapeutic effect is recommended and the interval at which this occurs has not been established. There is a low risk of drug–drug interactions but a relatively significant risk of serious adverse effects such as urinary retention requiring catheterization. Botulinum toxin is recommended after failure of at least two first-line pharmacologic options.

Duloxetine has demonstrated some success in OAB, but to a greater extent with stress incontinence. Incontinence (generally urge incontinence) is part of the OAB symptom constellation and is alleviated by duloxetine treatment. A similar scenario exists for the use of estrogens for OAB. Estrogens are primarily used for SUI and other urogenital symptoms but have demonstrated utility in OAB. Neither the SNRIs nor estrogen is recommended in the guidelines.

Surgical intervention is arguably the last option in terms of management of OAB; it is generally attempted after failure of all reasonable pharmacologic options. This is mostly due to the inherent risks in abdominal or pelvic operation, namely, impacts on renal function, on sexual function, and on any abdominal or pelvic pathology. In addition, surgical intervention is generally most effective in cases of isolated stress incontinence where there is underlying bladder or urethral pathology. In females, surgery usually involves repositioning the urethra so that it is more amenable to pressure changes or providing artificial support or resistance to the urethra by way of a sling. In males, surgery involves implantation of a manually controlled artificial silicone urethral sphincter.

Refractory Overactive Bladder

Depending upon the underlying etiology of OAB, some patients may not be successfully treated with first- or even second-line options. If multiple antimuscarinic drugs fail, as well as appropriate second- and third-line options, more invasive interventions might become necessary. Implantable neurostimulator devices or sacral neuromodulator placement is moderately successful but costly alternatives. Electrical stimulation of the peripheral nervous system has been shown to positively impact urinary urgency and urge incontinence. Both anal and vaginal transcutaneous stimulation play a role in the treatment of OAB. Direct electrical stimulation of the third and sometimes fourth sacral nerves via a surgically implanted modulator delivers continuous stimulation directly to a nerve with which it is in close contact. Augmentation cystoplasty surgery involves the anastomosis of a segment of bowel to the bisected bladder. This procedure increases bladder capacity and decreases bladder pressure. Serious risks include kidney or bladder infections, new recurrent urinary tract infections, or metabolic abnormalities. Surgical augmentation cystoplasty, neobladder construction, and urinary diversion techniques involve more risk and tend to be reserved for severe, refractory cases.

Another therapeutic consideration is the somewhat controversial dual antimuscarinic drug therapy. This has been studied in both adults and children and has been found to be safe and effective. Dual therapy does not appear to contribute to increased incidence of adverse effects; however, in some patients, the addition of a second anticholinergic drug precipitated postvoid residual volume increases but not urinary retention (Bolduc et al., 2009).

In male patients with OAB in the setting of BOO secondary to BPH, the combination of alpha-adrenergic blockers and 5-α-reductase inhibitors (finasteride, dutasteride) may offer some clinical utility. (See Chapter 33 for further discussion of BPH.)

Special Considerations
Pediatric

Isolated incontinence tends to manifest in young children as nocturia or enuresis. This is generally due to underlying deficits in learned neural control, delayed development of the nervous system, or potentially a more complex issue involving multiple systems. OAB symptoms of urgency or frequency in children commonly occur as a result of fecal impaction or underlying structural abnormalities. Children can present with voiding dysfunction, urgency, frequency, or incontinence. Oxybutynin IR and ER formulations are the only pharmacologic options approved by the U.S. Food and Drug Administration for OAB in children, although tolterodine IR and ER and trospium have been evaluated in clinical trials. All of the medications yielded successful outcomes in terms of reductions in diurnal incontinence, urgency episodes, micturition, and increases in bladder capacity. The adverse effects are similar to those experienced by adults and consisted mainly of dry mouth. Cognitive effects are not significant with respect to memory, cognition, speed of processing, or attention. DDAVP nasal spray has been the cornerstone of therapy for children with enuresis and has demonstrated clinical efficacy, safety, and tolerability.

Geriatric

As was previously mentioned, there is an inherent challenge with regard to OAB in the elderly patient. Numerous nonurinary factors such as anatomic, physiologic, age-related, or iatrogenic elements predispose elderly patients to the development of OAB or the worsening of existing OAB. The incidence of OAB is highest in the elderly population, and yet, the preferred pharmacologic modality for treating this syndrome tends to impact cognition to an extent that may limit utility in this population. Despite these clinical considerations, antimuscarinic therapy is still considered first line. If the adverse effects are intolerable or if the antimuscarinic agent aggravates an existing condition, an alternate medication should be given. If pharmacologic options are exhausted or are not feasible, surgical interventions can be considered in surgical candidates or the syndrome can be managed less aggressively. Less aggressive options include scheduled voiding, bladder training, and the use of absorbent pads or undergarments.

Women

True OAB syndrome affects men and women relatively equally; however, the symptom of incontinence tends to present more frequently in women. Furthermore, within postmenopausal symptomatology, vaginal atrophy and other urogenital changes may underlie urgency, frequency, and urge or stress incontinence that frequently accompanies menopause. SUI affects 78% of women with incontinence episodes (Basu & Duckett, 2009). SUI may be predicated on intrinsic urethral sphincter deficiency or urethral hypermobility secondary to the loss of vaginal support structures. Antimuscarinic medications are first line; however, in appropriately selected patients, topical estrogens may offer some therapeutic benefit. Duloxetine has been extensively studied in women with stress incontinence secondary to urethral dysfunction or vaginal atrophy. There is an established correlation between SUI and female sexual dysfunction.

MONITORING PATIENT RESPONSE

Despite the seemingly impressive efficacy of anticholinergic drug therapy, there is roughly a 50% placebo response rate, which complicates the assessment of patient response. As the majority of OAB symptomatology is subjective in nature, patient-generated feedback is the most valuable assessment tool with which to measure success. The domains related to the pathology itself that should be assessed include symptoms, symptom severity, and quality of life. If drug therapy has been initiated, drug-specific parameters such as treatment-emergent side effects or drug interactions need to be assessed as well.

There are numerous validated symptom inventories and quality of life assessment tools that have been employed in clinical trials as well as in practice to monitor patient response to treatment. The ICS highly recommends that symptom assessment and quality of life inventories be used throughout the treatment process in order to assess and guide therapy. The OAB-q assesses both the symptoms and quality of life impact in men and women. The reduced version of this scale includes 8 bladder symptom items and 25 health-related quality of life (HRQOL) items, which include symptom bother, coping skills, concerns and worries, sleep, social interaction, and HRQOL total. In females, the Urogenital Distress Inventory (UDI-6), the Incontinence Severity Index (ISI), and the BFLUTS questionnaire are used to assess the symptom of UI specifically. In males, the ICS$_{male}$ and DAN-PSS will assess the symptom of UI. The UDI-6 assesses 19 LUT symptoms as well as the degree of anxiety or bother that is experienced as a result of the incontinence episodes. This scale may have predictive value with respect to urodynamic studies, especially in stress incontinence, BOO, and DO. The ISI is a simple index that generates a numerical product based on frequency and volume of urine loss. The product is associated with the level of severity of the incontinence. BFLUTS evaluates incontinence symptoms and LUT symptoms as well as the degree of bother associated with each. Both the ICS$_{male}$ and DAN-PSS assess LUT symptoms and the extent to which the patient is bothered. Unfortunately, there is no consensus regarding at which point or how frequently these assessment tools should be administered to yield optimal information about treatment response.

Ongoing assessment of potential treatment-related adverse effects is highly recommended. This can be accomplished by clinician-led patient interviews or patient-generated complaints. The drugs most frequently used to treat OAB have the potential to cause bothersome or sometimes serious adverse effects. Since the patient population most often affected by OAB is usually also affected by polypharmacy,

multiple medical conditions, predisposition to falls, and predisposition to anticholinergic adverse effects, diligent monitoring of iatrogenic effects is paramount. Upwards of 60% of patients discontinue drug therapy for OAB within 12 months, which underscores the importance of anticipating and then mitigating adverse effects and other barriers to successful treatment (Wagg et al., 2012).

PATIENT EDUCATION AND PATIENT-ORIENTED INFORMATION SOURCES

Although OAB tends to affect the elderly more frequently than younger patients and may be partially caused or worsened by seemingly normal processes associated with aging, OAB is *not* considered a normal part of aging. Patients need to be made aware of this and their symptoms need to be validated. One of the challenges in diagnosing OAB is the reluctance of patients to complain of the symptoms or the patient's misconception about the symptoms being a normal part of aging. Once a patient is diagnosed with OAB, it is exceptionally important to emphasize that the symptoms need not be tolerated and that ongoing assessment of symptoms and symptom bother is essential to successful treatment.

Once a treatment modality has been mutually agreed upon by the patient and the care provider, the risks and benefits need to be clearly explained to the patient. More often than not, the treatment will consist of a medication and lifestyle changes or bladder training. The medications used to treat OAB (usually anticholinergics) will likely cause at least some minor anticholinergic adverse effects such as dry mouth or constipation. Severe xerostomia can be treated with adequate hydration as well as saliva substitutes. Constipation can be avoided by maintaining adequate hydration or remedied by using a stool softener (docusate) or a stimulant laxative (senna, bisacodyl). Patients should be warned about potentially severe anticholinergic effects such as urinary retention and advised to seek medical attention if symptoms consistent with urinary retention present. Antimuscarinic drugs may potentially augment anticholinergic effects of other anticholinergic medications. Therefore, in the case of multiple physicians, patients should be advised to make their care providers aware of any and all medications prescribed by all members of the health care team.

Aside from the OAB and medication information that may be provided by the patient's care provider, there are numerous reputable sources for patient-oriented information. The American Urogynecology Society maintains a patient-friendly Web site that explains pelvic floor disorders, incontinence, and OAB. It also provides a list of frequently asked questions, tools for patients, bladder diary support, medications and other treatment options, and a search engine for locating a care provider. The National Association for Continence is another reputable Web site that offers useful information regarding underlying causes of OAB, treatment options, frequently asked questions, and a public bathroom finder. The bathroom finder tool is a Google Maps™–powered application that allows the user to input a city or zip code and will then generate a graphical representation of the location of public restrooms.

Nutrition/Lifestyle Changes

Generally before the initiation of drug therapy, patients will be encouraged to adopt some clinician-guided lifestyle changes to minimize the impact of diet or behavior on OAB. It is *not* recommended that patients attempt to remedy OAB on their own by modifying behavior as was previously discussed. Uninformed and unmonitored changes (such as cessation of diuretic use) may detrimentally impact other aspects of the patient's care or may instigate a nascent problem. All of the nutritional or lifestyle changes should be recommended by the care provider and should be monitored; none of these changes should be initiated by the patient.

Compounds that irritate the bladder may exacerbate or precipitate OAB. Tomatoes, artificial sweeteners, grapes, carbonated beverages, strawberries, apple juice, vinegar, weight loss supplements, and spicy foods all may contribute to OAB pathology. Alcohol and caffeine not only act as bladder irritants but also inhibit antidiuretic hormone (ADH) release, which, in turn, will increase the production of urine and contribute to urgency and frequency. Moderation of the consumption of these foods, beverages, or products will likely reduce some of the added pressures that may be contributing to OAB symptoms.

Maintenance of a healthy body weight will also aid in the mitigation of OAB symptoms as excess weight puts increased pressure on the bladder. Pelvic floor exercises and bladder training are also shown to be effective in treating OAB as monotherapy or in combination with medications.

Complementary and Alternative Medications

Numerous natural compounds and botanicals have been evaluated for purposes of treating OAB; however, there is a paucity of evidence to support their use. OAB or urinary dysfunction that is associated with BPH may be further remedied by adjunctive treatment with saw palmetto extract. Saw palmetto or American dwarf plant (*Serenoa repens*) is thought to inhibit 5-α-reductase as its primary pharmacologic action. 5-α-reductase is responsible for the conversion of testosterone to dihydrotestosterone (DHT). DHT is among the androgens that contribute to prostate growth and, in BPH, contributes to pathologic prostate growth. Inhibition of 5-α-reductase opposes the pathologic enlargement of the prostate and subsequently eases the pressure on the urethra at the bladder neck. This effectively reduces or removes the BOO and improves LUT symptoms in males. Saw palmetto extract would not be an appropriate therapeutic option in patients who do not have an underlying BPH-mediated BOO.

To date, three active comparator trials have evaluated the efficacy and safety of saw palmetto extract as compared to 5-α-reductase inhibitors or alpha-1-receptor antagonists. Saw palmetto and finasteride both improved the score on the International Prostate Symptom Score (IPSS), improved quality of life, and increased peak urinary flow rate. Unlike finasteride, saw palmetto did not impact prostate volume or PSA. The trial comparing saw palmetto to tamsulosin did not find a difference between the two groups in terms of IPSS reduction, maximal flow rate, and irritative or obstructive symptoms (Suzuki et al., 2009).

CASE STUDY*

C.J. is a 55-year-old postmenopausal woman presenting with a 2-year history of incontinence. She reports that she often cannot get to the bathroom in time when she feels the urge to urinate. She also experiences incontinence most frequently when she laughs or sneezes. This has caused significant embarrassment and has decreased her social interactions. She drinks four cups of coffee daily. Current prescription medications include hydrochlorothiazide for hypertension. **C.J.** denies the use of any nonprescription medications or supplements.

DIAGNOSIS: STRESS INCONTINENCE

1. List specific goals for treatment for **C.J.**
2. What drug therapy would you prescribe? Why?

3. What are the parameters for monitoring the success of the therapy?
4. Discuss specific patient education based on the prescribed therapy.
5. List one or two adverse reactions for the selected agent that would cause you to change therapy.
6. What would be the choice for second-line therapy?
7. What OTC and/or alternative medications would be appropriate for this patient?
8. What dietary and lifestyle changes should be recommended for this patient?
9. Describe one or two drug–drug or drug–food interactions for the selected agent.

---

* Answers can be found online.

Bibliography

Starred references are cited in the text.

Banakhar, M. A., Al-Shaiji, T. F., & Hassouna, M. M. (2012). Pathophysiology of overactive bladder. *International Urogynecology Journal, 23*(8), 975–982.

Bartoli, S., Aguzzi, G., & Tarricone, R. (2010). Impact on quality of life of urinary incontinence and overactive bladder: A systematic literature review. *Urology, 75*(3), 491–500.

*Basu, M., & Duckett, J. R. (2009). Update on duloxetine for the management of stress urinary incontinence. *Clinical Interventions in Aging, 4*, 25–30.

*Bolduc, S., et al. (2009). Double anticholinergic therapy for refractory overactive bladder. *Journal of Urology, 182*(4 Suppl.), 2033–2038.

Campbell, J. D., et al. (2009). Treatment success for overactive bladder with urinary urge incontinence refractory to oral antimuscarinics: A review of published evidence. *BMC Urology, 9*, 18.

*Cipullo, L. M., et al. (2014). Pharmacological approach to overactive bladder and urge urinary incontinence in women: An overview. *European Journal of Obstetrics, Gynecology, and Reproductive Biology, 174*, 27–34.

Fry, C. H., Meng, E., & Young, J. S. (2010). The physiological function of lower urinary tract smooth muscle. *Autonomic Neuroscience, 154*(1–2), 3–13.

*Ganz, M. L., et al. (2010). Economic costs of overactive bladder in the United States. *Urology, 75*(3), 526–532, 532.e1–e18.

Gillespie, J. I., et al. (2009). On the origins of the sensory output from the bladder: The concept of afferent noise. *BJU International, 103*(10), 1324–1333.

International Continence Society. (2009). *4th International Consultation on Incontinence*. Plymouth, UK: Health Publications Ltd.

Jayarajan, J., & Radomski, S. B. (2014). Pharmacotherapy of overactive bladder in adults: A review of efficacy, tolerability, and quality of life. *Research and Reports in Urology, 6*, 1–16.

Leone Roberti Maggiore, U., et al. (2014). Mirabegron in the treatment of overactive bladder. *Expert Opinion on Pharmacotherapy, 15*(6), 873–887.

Michel, M. C., & Chapple, C. R. (2009). Basic mechanisms of urgency: Preclinical and clinical evidence. *European Urology, 56*(2), 298–307.

Miller, J., & Hoffman, E. (2006). The causes and consequences of overactive bladder. *Journal of Women's Health, 15*(3), 251–260.

*Ouslander, J. G. (2004). Management of overactive bladder. *New England Journal of Medicine, 350*(8), 786–799.

*Robinson, D., & Cardozo, L. (2010). New drug treatments for urinary incontinence. *Maturitas, 65*(4), 340–347.

*Suzuki, M., et al. (2009). Pharmacological effects of saw palmetto extract in the lower urinary tract. *Acta Pharmacologica Sinica, 30*(3), 227–281.

Tincello, D. G., Rashid, T., & Revicky, V. (2014). Emerging treatments for overactive bladder: Clinical potential of botulinum toxins. *Research and Reports in Urology, 6*, 51–57.

Tsakiris, P., Oelke, M., & Michel, M. C. (2008). Drug-induced urinary incontinence. *Drugs & Aging, 25*(7), 541–549.

*Wagg, A., et al. (2012). Persistence with prescribed antimuscarinic therapy for overactive bladder: A UK experience. *BJU International, 110*(11), 1767–1774.

Ward-Smith, P. (2009). The cost of urinary incontinence. *Urologic Nursing, 29*(3),188–190, 194.

Yamaguchi, O., et al. (2009). Clinical guidelines for overactive bladder. *International Journal of Urology, 161*(2), 126–142.

Yoshimura, N., et al. (2014). Neural mechanisms underlying lower urinary tract dysfunction. *Korean Journal of Urology, 55*(2), 81–90.

35

Sexually Transmitted Infections

Virginia P. Arcangelo

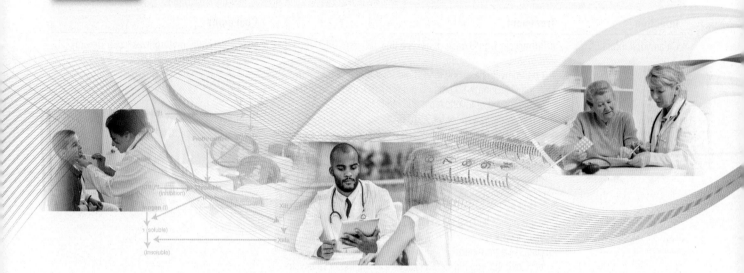

Sexually transmitted infections (STIs) are among the most common illnesses in the world. They have far-reaching health, social, and economic consequences. Our knowledge about the global prevalence and incidence of these infections is limited by the quality and quantity of data available from throughout the world. STIs remain a major public health concern in the United States. The economic burden is impressive: Centers for Disease Control and Prevention's (CDC) new estimates show that there are about 20 million new infections in the United States each year, with a total of more than 110 million among men and women. STIs cost the American health care system nearly $16 billion in direct medical costs alone (CDC, 2013).

It is estimated that half of all new STIs in the country occur among young men and women. Those at the highest risk for contracting STIs are those between 15 and 24 years, and gay and bisexual men. Gay and bisexual men have the highest rate of syphilis infections. While most STIs will not cause harm, some have the potential to cause serious health problems, especially if not diagnosed and treated early.

In 2015, the CDC updated the guidelines for treating STIs (**Table 35.1**). Available from the CDC, these guidelines are one of the most widely used documents published by that organization. The guidelines emphasize the development of management strategies that are adaptable to the managed care environment. Because the guidelines are considered the gold standard for treating STIs, most of the information in this chapter is based on them. The goals of therapy for all STIs are to eradicate the causative organism and prevent complications.

The accurate and timely reporting of STIs is integrally important for assessing morbidity trends, targeting limited resources, and assisting local health authorities in partner notification and treatment. STIs, human immunodeficiency virus (HIV), and acquired immunodeficiency syndrome (AIDS)

cases should be reported in accordance with state and local statutory requirements. Syphilis, gonorrhea, chlamydia, chancroid, HIV infection, and AIDS are reportable diseases in every state. The requirements for reporting other STIs differ by state, and clinicians should be familiar with state and local reporting requirements. Reporting can be provider or laboratory based.

Intrauterine or perinatally transmitted STIs can have severely debilitating effects on pregnant women, their partners, and their fetuses. All pregnant women and their sex partners should be asked about STIs, counseled about the possibility of perinatal infections, and ensured access to treatment, if needed.

All pregnant women in the United States should be tested for HIV infection as early in pregnancy as possible. Testing should be conducted after the woman is notified that she will be tested for HIV as part of the routine panel of prenatal tests, unless she declines the test.

CHLAMYDIAL INFECTION

Chlamydial infection is the most prevalent STI in the United States, with 2 to 3 million new cases reported annually. The detection and treatment of this disease is important because the complications can be serious.

CAUSES

Chlamydial infection is caused by *Chlamydia trachomatis*, which shares properties of both bacteria and viruses. The organism is transmitted sexually or perinatally. Repeated infections are common.

TABLE 35.1

Pharmacotherapy for Sexually Transmitted Infections

Infection	Treatment	Comments
Chlamydial infection	azithromycin 1 g PO once *or* doxycycline 100 mg PO bid for 7 d *Alternative:* erythromycin base 500 mg PO qid for 7 d *or* erythromycin ethylsuccinate 800 mg PO qid for 7 d *or* ofloxacin 300 mg bid for 7 d *or* levofloxacin 500 mg PO for 7 d	Use amoxicillin, erythromycin, *or* azithromycin in pregnancy.
Genital herpes	*Initial episode treatment* for 7–10 d acyclovir 400 mg PO tid *or* acyclovir 200 mg PO 5 times a day *or* valacyclovir 1 g PO bid *Recurrent treatment:* acyclovir 400 mg PO tid for 5 d *or* acyclovir 800 mg bid for 5 d *or* acyclovir 800 mg tid for 2 d *or* famciclovir 125 mg PO bid for 5 d *or* famciclovir 100 mg bid for 1 d valacyclovir 500 mg PO bid for 3 d *or* valacyclovir 1 g once a day for 5 d *Suppressive treatment:* acyclovir 400 mg bid *or* famciclovir 250 mg bid *or* valacyclovir 500 mg or 1,000 mg qd	Treatment can be extended if healing is not complete after 10 d.
Gonorrhea	ceftriaxone 250 mg IM once *PLUS* azithromycin 1 g PO once *or* doxycycline 100 mg PO bid for 7 d *Alternative:* cefixime 400mg once	
Human papillomavirus	*Patient applied:* podofilox 0.5% solution or gel for 3 d and then 4 d of no therapy imiquimod 5% cream three times a week up to 16 wk *Provider applied:* podophyllin resin 10%–25% in compound of tincture of benzoin weekly as needed trichloroacetic acid or bichloracetic acid 80%–90% weekly as needed	Solution applied with cotton swab and gel with finger to visible warts. This is done for 3 d and then 4 d with no therapy and may be repeated four times. Area should be washed with mild soap and water 6–10 h after application. Allow to air-dry. Wash off 1–4 h after application. Apply only to warts and let dry; white "frosting" appears; powder with talc or sodium bicarbonate to remove unreacted acid.
Pelvic inflammatory disease	ceftriaxone 250 mg IM once *or* cefoxitin 2 g IM *and* probenecid 1 g PO once *and* doxycycline 100 mg PO bid for 14 d PLUS doxycycline 100 mg PO bid for 14 d WITH OR WITHOUT metronidazole 500 mg PO bid for 14 d	
Syphilis	*Early primary, secondary, or latent syphilis <1 y* Adult: benzathine penicillin G 2.4 million U, IM single dose Child: 50,000 U/kg, IM, single dose up to 2.4 mil unit *Latent disease >1 y or unknown duration* Adult: benzathine penicillin G 2.4 million U, IM, for 3 doses at 1-wk intervals Child: 500,000 U/kg, IM, for 3 doses at 1-wk intervals *Allergic to penicillin and not pregnant:* doxycycline 100 mg PO bid for 14 d *or* tetracycline 500 mg PO bid for 14 d *Allergic to penicillin and pregnant:* desensitization followed by treatment with penicillin	

From Centers for Disease Control and Prevention. (2006). Sexually transmitted treatment guidelines, 2006. *Morbidity and Mortality Weekly Reports, 59*(RR-12), 1–110.

In infants, perinatal exposure to the mother's cervix causes the infection. The prevalence is greater than 5% regardless of race, ethnicity, or socioeconomic status. In preadolescent children, sexual abuse must be considered as a causative factor for chlamydial infection; infection of the nasopharynx, urogenital tract, and rectum may persist for greater than 1 year. Because criminal investigation is always a possibility, cultures should be confirmed by microscopic fluoroscopy, which can detect conjugated monoclonal antibodies specific for *C. trachomatis*.

Chlamydial infections occur most frequently in women younger than age 25. All adolescents and young women should be screened for chlamydia yearly, as should any woman who has new or multiple sex partners.

PATHOPHYSIOLOGY

Chlamydial organisms are like viruses in that they are obligate intracellular parasites. They resemble bacteria by containing both deoxyribonucleic acid (DNA) and ribonucleic acid, by dividing by binary fission, and by having cell walls that resemble those of gram-negative bacteria. Species of chlamydial organisms include *Chlamydia psittaci* and *C. trachomatis*, the latter of which has a number of serotypes. These species cause numerous diseases, including lymphogranuloma venereum, blinding trachoma, conjunctivitis, nongonococcal urethritis, cervicitis, salpingitis, proctitis, epididymitis, and newborn pneumonia.

DIAGNOSTIC CRITERIA

The infection may be silent: more than half of infected patients have no clinical signs or symptoms. In symptomatic women, the clinical presentation includes vaginal discharge, mucopurulent cervicitis with edema and friability, urethral syndrome or urethritis, pelvic inflammatory disease (PID), ectopic pregnancy, infertility, and endometritis. Men may report a thin, clear discharge and dysuria. Chlamydial organisms are the major causes of nongonococcal urethritis and epididymitis in young men.

In infants aged 1 to 3 months, chlamydial infection presents in the mucous membranes of the eye, oropharynx, urogenital tract, and rectum and as subacute, afebrile pneumonia; in neonates, it presents as an asymptomatic infection of the oropharynx, genital tract, and rectum. However, chlamydial infection most commonly presents as conjunctivitis 5 to 12 days after birth and is the most frequent identifiable infectious cause of ophthalmia neonatorum. Therefore, for all infants with conjunctivitis who are no older than 30 days, a chlamydial etiology should be considered.

Diagnostic tests for chlamydial ophthalmia neonatorum include tissue cultures and nonculture tests. Ocular exudate should also be tested for *Neisseria gonorrhoeae*.

Chlamydial infection is diagnosed by examination, culture, and antigen detection methods, including direct fluorescent monoclonal antibody staining, enzyme-linked immunosorbent assay, DNA probe assay, and polymerase chain reaction.

INITIATING DRUG THERAPY

Treatment for all STIs consists of antimicrobial therapy followed by preventive education.

Goals of Drug Therapy

Patients are treated to eradicate the organism and prevent transmission to sex partners or to a newborn during birth. Because chlamydial infections often are accompanied by gonococcal infections, patients may be treated for both infections.

Antibiotic Therapy

Antibiotic treatments are prescribed to cure infection and usually relieve symptoms (CDC, 2015). Azithromycin (Zithromax) and erythromycin (E-Mycin), macrolide antibiotics; doxycycline (Vibramycin), a tetracycline antibiotic; and ofloxacin (Floxin), a fluoroquinolone, are drugs of choice for chlamydial infections.

If therapeutic compliance is in question, azithromycin should be used for treatment because it is prepared as a single-dose drug. Doxycycline, however, has been used more extensively and is less expensive. An alternative regimen can be erythromycin, but it is less efficacious and has gastrointestinal (GI) side effects. Other alternatives include fluoroquinolones such as ofloxacin and levofloxacin (**Table 35.2**).

In infants, erythromycin base treatment has an efficacy of 80%. A second course of therapy may be required, and follow-up of the infant is recommended.

Mechanism of Action

Azithromycin and erythromycin bind to bacterial ribosomes to block protein synthesis. The drugs are also bactericidal, depending on their concentration. (For more information on antibiotic actions, see Chapter 8.) Doxycycline is thought to act in a similar way, whereas ofloxacin kills bacteria by blocking DNA gyrase and inhibiting DNA synthesis.

Dosages

A single 1-g dose of azithromycin or 100 mg of doxycycline twice a day for 7 days is the usual initial therapy.

Contraindications

Sensitivity to erythromycin or other macrolides is the main contraindication to therapy.

The safety and efficacy of azithromycin in pregnant and lactating women are not known. Doxycycline and ofloxacin are contraindicated in pregnant women.

Adverse Events

In some patients, GI side effects (nausea, vomiting, diarrhea, abdominal discomfort) cause them to discontinue therapy.

TABLE 35.2

Overview of Drugs Used to Treat Chlamydial Infections*

Generic (Trade) Name and Dosage	Selected Adverse Events	Contraindications	Special Considerations
azithromycin (Zithromax) Adult: 1 g PO single dose Pregnancy: 1 g PO in a single dose Child (≥45 kg, <8 y): 1 g PO in a single dose Child (≥8 y): 1 g PO in a single dose (or doxycycline as below)	GI upset, abdominal pain, pseudomembranous colitis, angioedema, cholestatic jaundice	Hypersensitivity to azithromycin, erythromycin, or any macrolide antibiotic Use with caution with impaired hepatic or renal function.	Do not take with aluminum- or magnesium-containing antacids.
doxycycline (Vibramycin) Adult: 100 mg bid for 7 d Child (≥8 y): 100 mg PO bid for 7 d	Superinfection, photosensitivity, GI upset, enterocolitis, rash, blood dyscrasias, hepatotoxicity	Pregnancy, lactation, hypersensitivity to any of the tetracyclines	Monitor blood, renal, and hepatic function in long-term use. Use of drug during tooth development may discolor teeth. Advise patient to avoid excessive sunlight or ultraviolet light. Caution patient that drug absorption is reduced when taken with food or bismuth subsalicylate.
amoxicillin (Augmentin) Pregnancy: 500 mg tid for 7 d	Hypersensitivity reactions, pseudomembranous colitis, GI upset, rash, urticaria, vaginitis	History of Augmentin-associated cholestatic jaundice, hepatic dysfunction, or allergic reactions to any penicillin	Monitor blood, renal, and hepatic function in long-term use.
ofloxacin (Floxin) 300 mg bid for 7 d	Rash, hives, rapid heartbeat, difficulty swallowing or breathing, photosensitivity, angioedema, dizziness, light-headedness	Pregnancy, hypersensitivity to ofloxacin or quinolones Use with caution with hepatic or renal insufficiency.	Do not take with food. Drink fluids liberally.
levofloxacin (Levaquin) 500 mg daily for 7 d	Same as above	Same as above	Same as above
erythromycin base (E-Mycin) Adult: 500 mg qid for 7 d Pregnancy: 500 mg qid for 7 d or 250 mg qid for 14 d Children: 50 mg/kg/d PO divided into 4 doses daily for 10–14 d	GI upset, pseudomembranous colitis, hepatic dysfunction, cardiac dysrhythmias, CNS disturbances, urticaria, skin eruptions, hearing loss, superinfection and local irritation	Known hypersensitivity to erythromycin Prescribe with caution for patients with impaired hepatic function and children who weigh <45 kg.	Effectiveness of treatment is ~80%; a second course of therapy may be required. Use for prophylaxis of ophthalmia neonatorum and infant pneumonia.
erythromycin ethylsuccinate (E.E.S.) Adult: 800 mg qid for 7 d Pregnancy: 800 mg qid for 7 d or 400 mg qid for 14 d	Same as above	Same as above	Same as above

*In adults, pregnant women, children, ophthalmia neonatorum, and infant pneumonia.

Selecting the Most Appropriate Agent

The most appropriate therapy is the one that best matches the needs of the patient in different situations or stages of life. **Figure 35.1** and **Tables 35.1** and **35.2** summarize treatment options.

Special Population Considerations
Pediatric

To prevent chlamydial infection among neonates, prenatal screening is recommended. In general, patients appropriate for screening include pregnant women younger than age 25 with new or multiple sex partners.

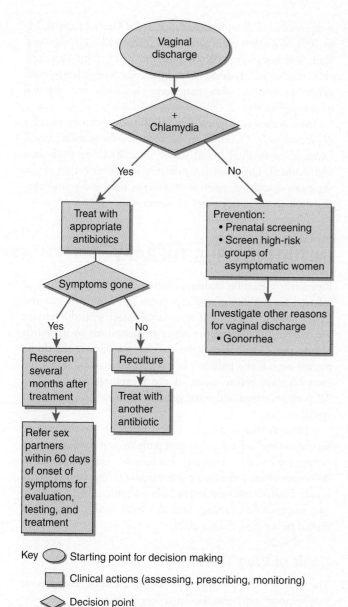

Key ⬭ Starting point for decision making

⬜ Clinical actions (assessing, prescribing, monitoring)

◇ Decision point

FIGURE 35.1 Treatment algorithm for chlamydial infection.

C. trachomatis infection of neonates results from perinatal exposure to the mother's infected cervix. The prevalence of *C. trachomatis* infection among pregnant women does not vary by race/ethnicity or socioeconomic status. Neonatal ocular prophylaxis with silver nitrate solution or antibiotic ointments does not prevent perinatal transmission of *C. trachomatis* from mother to infant. However, ocular prophylaxis with those agents does prevent gonococcal ophthalmia and therefore should be continued.

Initial *C. trachomatis* perinatal infection involves mucous membranes of the eye, oropharynx, urogenital tract, and rectum. *C. trachomatis* infection in neonates is most often recognized by conjunctivitis that develops 5 to 12 days after birth. Chlamydia is the most frequent identifiable infectious cause of ophthalmia neonatorum. *C. trachomatis* also is a common cause of subacute, afebrile pneumonia with onset from

ages 1 to 3 months. Asymptomatic infections also can occur in the oropharynx, genital tract, and rectum of neonates.

A chlamydial etiology should be considered for all infants aged 30 days or less who have conjunctivitis. Sexual abuse should be considered for infants and children who test positive for chlamydial infections.

Pregnancy

The recommended regimen for pregnancy is a single dose of azithromycin 1 g or amoxicillin 500 mg orally three times daily for 7 days.

Alternative regimens are erythromycin base 250 mg orally four times a day for 14 days, erythromycin ethylsuccinate 800 mg orally four times a day for 7 days or 400 mg orally four times a day for 14 days, or azithromycin 1 g orally, single dose. Erythromycin estolate is contraindicated during pregnancy because of drug-related hepatotoxicity. Doxycycline is contraindicated in the second and third trimester. All pregnant women who have chlamydia should be retested 3 to 4 weeks and then 3 months after their treatment, which is contrary to the discussion in monitoring patient responses. If infection persists, it can severely affect the mother and neonate.

MONITORING PATIENT RESPONSE

Because therapy with azithromycin or doxycycline is highly efficacious, patients do not need to be retested after treatment is completed, unless they are pregnant (see section "Pregnancy"). If alternative agents, such as erythromycin, are used for treatment, repeat testing for cure is no longer recommended unless therapeutic adherence is in question, symptoms persist, or reinfection is suspected (CDC, 2015).

Screening for *C. trachomatis* should be performed in high-risk groups when the practitioner performs a pelvic examination. High-risk groups include sexually active adolescents and women ages 15 to 24, particularly those who have new or multiple sex partners; those attending family planning clinics, prenatal clinics, or abortion facilities; or those in juvenile detention centers. Screening for high-risk men should be considered when they seek health care.

PATIENT EDUCATION

The patient's sex partner must be treated. The newest guidelines (CDC, 2015) recommend presumptive treatment for all partners. Patients should abstain from sexual intercourse for 7 days after single-dose therapy or until the 7-day regimen is completed. Abstinence should also continue until the patient's sex partner has been treated, to prevent reinfection. Sex partners should be treated if they have had sexual contact with the patient during the 60 days preceding onset of symptoms in the patient or the diagnosis of chlamydial infection. The most recent sex partner should be treated even if the time of the last sexual contact was greater than 60 days before onset or diagnosis.

GONORRHEA

Approximately 820,000 new infections with *N. gonorrhoeae* occur each year in the United States. They are the major causes of PID, tubal scarring, infertility, ectopic pregnancy, and chronic pelvic pain in the United States. Most men seek treatment before serious complications develop, but not soon enough to prevent transmission to others. In women, symptoms may not develop until complications such as PID occur. Screening of men and women at high risk for STIs is an important component of gonorrhea control (CDC, 2015). Patients infected with *N. gonorrhoeae* frequently are coinfected with *C. trachomatis*; this finding has led to the recommendation that patients treated for gonococcal infection also be treated routinely with a regimen that is effective against uncomplicated genital *C. trachomatis* infection. Because the majority of gonococci in the United States are susceptible to doxycycline and azithromycin, routine cotreatment might also hinder the development of antimicrobial-resistant *N. gonorrhoeae*.

CAUSES

Gonorrhea is caused by *N. gonorrhoeae*, a gram-negative diplococcal bacterium. It is transmitted by sexual contact, and the rate of male-to-female transmission is higher than female-to-male or male-to-male. Women with gonorrhea have a high prevalence of other STIs, including chlamydial infection, trichomoniasis, bacterial vaginosis, and herpes genitalis.

Uncomplicated anogenital gonorrhea in women can involve the endocervix, urethra, Skene glands, Bartholin glands, and anus. The endocervix is the most common site of infection. Pharyngeal infection can also occur and is usually asymptomatic.

PATHOPHYSIOLOGY

Several strains of gonorrhea have been identified. Gonococcal sensitivity and resistance to antibiotics are clinically significant. Certain strains of the organism are resistant to sulfonamides. Penicillinase-producing *N. gonorrhoeae* and chromosomal-resistant *N. gonorrhoeae* are resistant to penicillin, and tetracycline-resistant *N. gonorrhoeae* is resistant to tetracycline.

DIAGNOSTIC CRITERIA

In the United States, an estimated 820,000 new *N. gonorrhoeae* infections occur each year. Most infections among men produce symptoms that cause them to seek curative treatment soon enough to prevent serious sequelae, but this may not be soon enough to prevent transmission to others. Among women, many infections do not produce recognizable symptoms until complications such as PID have occurred. Up to 30% of women with gonorrheal infection have symptoms. Signs and symptoms include purulent or mucopurulent cervical discharge, dysuria, anal bleeding, menorrhagia, and pelvic discomfort. Men may have discharge and regional lymphadenopathy.

Gonorrhea is diagnosed by examination and culture for *N. gonorrhoeae*. Culture can be obtained from endocervical (women) or urethral (men) swabs, or urine (from both men and women). Diagnosis is confirmed by identification of the organism on culture, positive oxidase reaction, and gram-negative diplococcal morphology on Gram stain.

INITIATING DRUG THERAPY

Preventive education is always offered. Sex partners should be referred for evaluation and treatment of *N. gonorrhoeae* and *C. trachomatis* infection if their last contact with the patient was within 60 days before onset of symptoms or diagnosis of infection. The patient's most recent sex partner should be treated even if the patient's last sexual intercourse was more than 60 days before onset of the symptoms or diagnosis. All patients diagnosed with gonorrhea should be tested for syphilis.

Patients treated for gonococcal infection are also treated for chlamydial infection because patients with gonorrhea are commonly coinfected with *C. trachomatis*. The occurrence of fluoroquinolone-resistant *N. gonorrhoeae* in the United States is rare. Patients with treatment failure should undergo culture and susceptibility testing, and the local health department should be notified (CDC, 2015).

Goals of Drug Therapy

The goal of drug therapy is to eradicate disease and prevent complications and spread of infection to others.

Antibiotics

The CDC describes recommended regimens for uncomplicated gonococcal infections of the cervix, urethra, and rectum (**Table 35.3**).

Cefixime

Cefixime (Suprax) covers an antimicrobial spectrum similar to that of ceftriaxone (Rocephin). A dose of 400 mg orally once is an alternative therapy to ceftriaxone. The advantage of cefixime is that it can be administered orally, and clinical trials have shown a 97.1% cure rate for uncomplicated urogenital and anorectal gonococcal infections.

Ceftriaxone

A single injection of 250 mg of ceftriaxone provides sustained, high antibacterial levels in the blood. Extensive clinical experience shows that the drug is safe and effective for treating

TABLE 35.3

Overview of Selected Drugs Used to Treat Uncomplicated Gonococcal Infections in Adults and Children*

Generic (Trade) Name and Dosage	Selected Adverse Events	Contraindications	Special Considerations
ceftriaxone (Rocephin) Adult: 125 mg IM in a single dose	Pseudomembranous colitis, rash, GI upset, hematologic abnormalities	Known allergy to cephalosporins Prescribe with caution to penicillin-sensitive patients.	Use for uncomplicated gonococcal infection of the pharynx.
Child: ophthalmia neonatorum: 25–50 mg/kg IV or IM in a single dose, not to exceed 125 mg Child: 125 mg IM in a single dose or 50 mg/kg (maximum dose 1 g) IM or IV in a single dose daily for 7 d or 50 mg/kg (maximum dose 2 g) IM or IV in a single dose daily for 10–14 d Child (<45 kg with bacteremia or arthritis): 50 mg/kg, max 1 g IM or IV in a single daily dose for 7 d Child (>45 kg with bacteremia or arthritis): 50 mg/kg, max 2 g, IM or IV in a single daily dose for 10–14 d		Prescribe with caution to hyperbilirubinemic infants, especially premature infants.	Prescribe prophylactically in infants whose mothers have gonococcal infection.
cefixime (Suprax) 400 mg po in single dose	Pseudomembranous colitis, GI upset, skin rash, headache, dizziness	Known allergy to cephalosporins Prescribe with caution to penicillin-sensitive patients and patients with renal impairment or GI disease Prescribe with caution in patients on dialysis	
azithromycin (Zithromax) 2 g PO Uncomplicated gonococcal infection of the pharynx: 1 g PO in a single dose	GI upset, abdominal pain, pseudomembranous colitis, angioedema, cholestatic jaundice	Hypersensitivity to azithromycin, erythromycin, or any macrolide antibiotic Prescribe with caution in patients with impaired hepatic or renal function.	Take 1 h before or 2 h after meals for greatest absorption. Avoid taking with aluminum- or magnesium-containing antacids. Comes in powder form
doxycycline (Vibramycin) 100 mg PO bid for 7 d	Superinfection, photosensitivity, GI upset, enterocolitis, rash, blood dyscrasias, hepatotoxicity	Pregnancy, lactation, hypersensitivity to any of the tetracyclines	Monitor blood, renal, and hepatic function in long-term use. Because of photosensitivity, patients should avoid sunlight or UV light. Use of drug during tooth development may discolor teeth. Absorption is reduced when drug is taken with food or bismuth subsalicylate (Pepto-Bismol). Prescribe for uncomplicated gonococcal infection of the pharynx.

*Infections of the cervix, urethra, and rectum; uncomplicated gonococcal infection of the pharynx; ophthalmia neonatorum; and gonococcal infection in children.

uncomplicated gonorrhea at all sites, with a cure rate of 99.1% in clinical trials for uncomplicated urogenital and anorectal infections.

The CDC also recognizes other antimicrobials for use against *N. gonorrhoeae*. If there is a severe cephalosporin allergy, a single dose of azithromycin (Zithromax) 2 g orally is effective for uncomplicated gonococcal infection, but it is expensive and causes GI distress. If there is a Zithromax allergy, doxycycline can be considered; however, some isolates are resistant to this class of antibiotic.

The regimen recommended by the CDC for uncomplicated gonococcal infections of the pharynx is summarized in **Table 35.1** and **Figure 35.2**. These infections are more difficult to treat than urogenital and anorectal infections. Few drugs can reliably cure these infections more than 90% of the time. Treatment for gonorrhea and chlamydial infection is suggested, even though chlamydial coinfection of the pharynx is unusual.

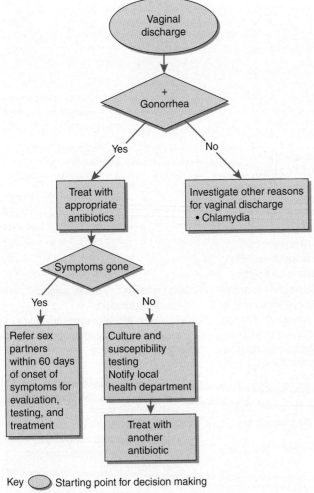

FIGURE 35.2   Treatment algorithm for gonorrheal infection.

Selecting the Most Appropriate Agent

Therapy for uncomplicated gonococcal infections includes a cephalosporin or fluoroquinolone, as follows:

- Single-dose ceftriaxone 250 mg IM

    PLUS:

- Single-dose azithromycin 1 g
- Doxycycline 100 mg orally twice daily for 7 days

The choice is based on the practitioner's assessment of the patient's reliability, allergies, and preferences. If there is a question regarding the patient's reliability, ceftriaxone IM may be the treatment of choice because it is administered in the office.

Special Population Considerations
Pediatric

Gonococcal infection may be transmitted to infants exposed to infected cervical exudate at birth. The infection presents as an acute illness 2 to 5 days after birth. The prevalence in infants depends on the prevalence of infection in pregnant women, whether pregnant women are screened for gonorrhea, and whether newborns receive prophylactic treatment. Manifestations of the infection in newborns include ophthalmia neonatorum, which may result in perforation of the ocular globe and blindness, sepsis with arthritis, and meningitis, rhinitis, vaginitis, urethritis, and inflammation at fetal monitoring sites. Cultures should be taken when typical gram-negative diplococci are identified in conjunctival exudate, and testing for chlamydial organisms should be done in all cases of neonatal conjunctivitis. Presumptive treatment can be given for newborns who are at increased risk for gonococcal ophthalmia or who have conjunctivitis but no gonococci in a Gram-stained smear of conjunctival exudate. Infants with gonococcal ophthalmia should be hospitalized and monitored for signs of disseminated infection. Many physicians prefer to continue therapy until cultures are negative for gonococcal organisms at 48 to 72 hours.

To prevent ophthalmia neonatorum, erythromycin is used as a prophylactic agent, installed in the eyes within 24 hours of delivery; this is required by law in most states, regardless of whether delivery was vaginal or cesarean (**Table 35.4**).

In preadolescent children, sexual abuse is the most frequent cause of gonococcal infection. Vaginitis is the most common manifestation, followed by anorectal and pharyngeal infections, which are commonly asymptomatic. Standard culture procedures should be used to diagnose the infection, and nonculture gonococcal tests should not be used alone.

Follow-up cultures are not needed if ceftriaxone is used. Only parenteral cephalosporins are recommended for use in children. Quinolones are not approved for use in children because of concerns regarding toxicity. A follow-up culture is needed to ensure that treatment was effective if spectinomycin is used. All children with gonococcal infections should be evaluated for syphilis and chlamydial coinfection.

TABLE 35.4

Prophylaxis for Ophthalmia Neonatorum

Topical Agent	Adverse Events	Contraindications	Special Considerations
erythromycin (Ilotycin) 0.5% ophthalmic ointment in a single application	Sensitivity reactions	Hypersensitivity to erythromycin	Instill into both eyes as soon as possible after birth Use single tubes administration

MONITORING PATIENT RESPONSE

Patients who have had uncomplicated gonorrhea and who were treated with any of the recommended regimens do not need to return for test of cure. If symptoms persist after treatment, the patient is evaluated by culture for *N. gonorrhoeae*, and isolated gonococci should be tested for antimicrobial susceptibility. If infection is identified, its source is usually reinfection rather than treatment failure. In patients treated with spectinomycin for pharyngeal infection, culture should be performed 3 to 5 days after treatment because spectinomycin is not highly effective against these infections.

PATIENT EDUCATION

Patient education concentrates on prevention. All patients should be encouraged to adopt meticulous hygiene and practice safe sex, to insist that partners seek treatment, and to schedule and keep follow-up health care appointments.

SYPHILIS

In the 1990s, syphilis reemerged in endemic forms in the United States, with a significant increase in the incidence of primary, secondary, and congenital syphilis. The increase has been attributed to greater use of illicit drugs, most notably crack cocaine, and high-risk sexual behavior related to drug use. Approximately 55,000 new cases of primary and secondary syphilis occur annually in the United States (CDC, 2013). Gay and bisexual men are at greatest risk.

CAUSES

Syphilis is a chronic, infectious disease caused by the spirochete *Treponema pallidum*. Infection may be active, and characterized by symptoms, or inactive (latent). The latent stage has no clinical symptoms. During the latent stage, infections can be detected by serologic testing. Early latent syphilis is defined as latent syphilis acquired within the preceding year. Any other cases of latent syphilis are either late latent syphilis or syphilis of unknown duration (CDC, 2015).

PATHOPHYSIOLOGY

T. pallidum is considered a bacterium because of its cell wall and response to antibiotic therapy. *T. pallidum* is not readily grown in vitro and cannot be seen by light microscopy.

DIAGNOSTIC CRITERIA

Patients who contract syphilis may seek treatment for signs or symptoms of primary infection, which include an ulcer or chancre at the infection site. The chancre erupts approximately 3 weeks after exposure. Signs and symptoms of secondary syphilis are low-grade fever, malaise, sore throat, hoarseness, headache, anorexia, rash, mucocutaneous lesions, alopecia, and adenopathy. Signs and symptoms of tertiary infection include cardiac, neurologic, ophthalmic, auditory, or gummatous lesions. Definitive methods for diagnosing early syphilis include dark-field examination and direct fluorescent antibody study of the chancre's exudate or tissue. The serologic tests used to confirm the syphilis diagnosis are nontreponemal and treponemal. The nontreponemal tests are the Venereal Disease Research Laboratory (VDRL) test and the rapid plasma reagin test. The treponemal tests include the fluorescent treponemal antibody absorption test and the microhemagglutination assay for antibody to *T. pallidum*. The two serologic tests are necessary because false-positive nontreponemal test results occur on occasion secondary to certain medical conditions. Treponemal test antibody titers do not correlate accurately with disease activity and should not be used to assess treatment response.

A single test cannot be used to diagnose all cases of neurosyphilis. The diagnosis is made using a combination of tests, including combinations of reactive serologic test results; abnormalities of cerebrospinal fluid (CSF) cell count or protein; or reactive VDRL-CSF with or without clinical manifestations (CDC, 2015).

INITIATING DRUG THERAPY

Although sexual transmission occurs only when mucocutaneous syphilitic lesions, including the rash, are present, people exposed in any stage should be evaluated clinically and serologically. Treatment should be given to those who were exposed within 90 days preceding the diagnosis of primary, secondary, or early latent syphilis in a sex partner, because the partner might be infected even if he or she is seronegative. Treatment should also be given to those who were exposed more than 90 days before the diagnosis of primary, secondary, or early latent syphilis in a sex partner if serologic test results are unavailable and follow-up tests and treatments are uncertain. Patients who have syphilis of unknown duration and who have high nontreponemal serologic test titers are considered to have early syphilis. Sex partners should be notified and treated. Long-term partners of patients with late syphilis should have a clinical and serologic evaluation and should be treated based on the findings.

For all stages of syphilis, penicillin is the preferred treatment. The stage and clinical manifestations of the disease determine the preparation used as well as the dosage and duration of treatment. However, no adequate trials have been performed to determine the optimal penicillin regimen. The only therapy with documented efficacy for syphilis during pregnancy or neurosyphilis is parenteral penicillin G benzathine. Penicillin G has been used for the past five decades to achieve a local cure and to prevent late sequelae.

Goals of Drug Therapy

The goal of treatment for primary and secondary syphilis is cure. The goal of treatment for latent syphilis is to prevent occurrence or progression of late complications. There is limited evidence supporting specific regimens for penicillin, even though clinical experience has shown the effectiveness of penicillin in achieving these goals.

Antibiotics

Penicillin

Adults with primary or secondary syphilis should be treated with penicillin G benzathine (Bicillin). Other choices for unusual situations include doxycycline, tetracycline (Achromycin), ceftriaxone, and erythromycin (**Table 35.5**).

Mechanism of Action
Penicillins are bactericidal. They disrupt synthesis of the bacterial cell wall and bind to enzyme proteins, interfering with the biosynthesis of mucopeptides and preventing the structural components of the cell wall from leaking out. As such, the bacteria cannot lay protein cross-links in the cell wall. In

TABLE 35.5

Overview of Selected Drugs Used to Treat Syphilis

Generic (Trade) Name and Dosage	Selected Adverse Events	Contraindications	Special Considerations
Nonallergic Adults penicillin G benzathine (Bicillin) *Primary, secondary, and early latent infection:* 2.4 million U IM single dose *Late latent infection, infection of unknown duration, or tertiary infection:* 7.2 million U; total 3 doses of 2.4 million U IM each at 1-wk intervals	Hypersensitivity, urticaria, laryngeal edema, fever, eosinophilia, serum sickness–like reactions, anaphylaxis, hemolytic anemia, leukopenia, thrombocytopenia, neuropathy, nephropathy	Hypersensitivity to any penicillin or procaine	Use with caution with patients with allergies or asthma. Do not inject into or near an artery or nerve.
Nonallergic Children *Primary, secondary, and early latent infection:* 50,000 U/kg IM up to adult dose of 2.4 million U in a single dose *Late latent infection, infection of unknown duration:* 50,000 U/kg IM up to adult dose of 2.4 million U administered as 3 doses at 1-wk intervals (total 150,000 U/kg up to adult dose of 7.2 million U)	Same as above	Same as above	Same as above

TABLE 35.5

Overview of Selected Drugs Used to Treat Syphilis (*Continued*)

Generic (Trade) Name and Dosage	Selected Adverse Events	Contraindications	Special Considerations
Nonpregnant, Penicillin-Allergic Patients			
doxycycline (Vibramycin) 100 mg PO bid for 2 wk *Latent syphilis:* 100 mg PO bid for 4 wk (if infection is <1 y, give for 2 wk)	Superinfection, photosensitivity, GI upset, enterocolitis, rash, blood dyscrasias, hepatotoxicity	Pregnancy, lactation Hypersensitivity to any of the tetracyclines	Monitor blood, renal, and hepatic function in long-term use. Avoid sunlight or UV light. Use of drug during tooth development may cause dental discoloration. Absorption is reduced when taken with food or bismuth subsalicylate.
tetracycline (Achromycin) 500 mg PO qid for 2 wk *Latent syphilis:* 500 mg PO qid for 4 wk (if infection is <1 y, give for 2 wk)	Photosensitivity, GI upset, glossitis, dysphasia, enterocolitis, pancreatitis, anogenital lesions, elevated hepatic enzymes, hepatic toxicity, rash, hypersensitivity, dizziness, tinnitus, visual disturbances	Hypersensitivity to any tetracyclines	Use of drug during tooth development may cause dental discoloration. Use of tetracycline may render oral contraceptives less effective.
ceftriaxone (Rocephin) 1 g PO qd for 8–10 d	Pseudomembranous colitis, rash, GI upset, hepatologic abnormalities	Known allergy to cephalosporins	Prescribe with caution to penicillin-sensitive patients.
erythromycin (Ilosone) 500 mg PO qid for 2 wk	GI upset, abdominal pain, anorexia, hepatic dysfunction, rash, superinfection, pseudomembranous colitis	Hypersensitivity to erythromycin Hepatic disease	Prescribe with caution in patients with hepatic disease or myasthenia gravis, or patients who are breast-feeding.

addition, autolytic enzymes, which promote lysis of bacteria, are activated.

Contraindications

Penicillin is contraindicated in patients with allergies to penicillin, cephalosporin, or imipenem (Primaxin).

Adverse Events

Hypersensitivity, urticaria, laryngeal edema, fever, eosinophilia, anaphylaxis, hemolytic anemia, leukopenia, thrombocytopenia, neuropathy, and nephropathy are some of the adverse effects of the penicillins.

Interactions

Penicillin decreases the effect of oral contraceptives. Hyperkalemia can result from concurrent use of potassium-sparing diuretics, angiotensin-converting enzyme inhibitors, and potassium supplements with parenteral penicillin G.

Doxycycline, Tetracycline, and Others

Nonpregnant patients with latent syphilis who are allergic to penicillin should be treated with doxycycline or tetracycline. Both drugs should be given for 2 weeks if the infection is of less than 1 year's duration; otherwise, they should be given for 4 weeks. Patients who are not pregnant but who are allergic to penicillin and who have primary or secondary syphilis should be treated with doxycycline or tetracycline. For patients who

cannot tolerate these, ceftriaxone is recommended. Although erythromycin is less effective than other regimens, it can be used for nonpregnant, compliant patients. Patients whose compliance is questionable or pregnant patients who are allergic to penicillin should be desensitized and treated with penicillin. For more information, see Chapter 8.

Selecting the Most Appropriate Agent

Penicillin G therapy is the first and usually only choice for patients who have syphilis and who are not allergic to penicillin. For patients who are allergic to penicillin and who are not pregnant, first-line therapy relies on doxycycline or tetracycline. There are no proven alternative drugs for pregnant women who have syphilis and who are allergic to penicillin. These women should be desensitized and then treated with penicillin (**Figure 35.3**).

Special Population Considerations

Pediatric

Children with syphilis should have a CSF examination for asymptomatic neurosyphilis. To assess for congenital or acquired syphilis, birth and maternal records should be reviewed. Children who have primary or secondary syphilis should have an evaluation, consultation with child protection services, and treatment with a pediatric regimen.

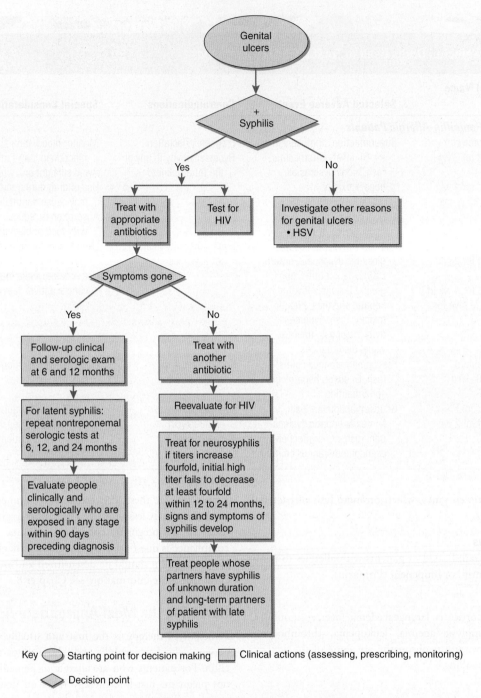

FIGURE 35.3 Treatment algorithm for syphilis.

Women

Pregnant women should be screened and treated for syphilis to protect the fetus and the newborn from exposure to syphilis. Screening is performed at the time pregnancy is confirmed. If the patient is in a high-risk group, testing should also occur at 28 weeks and at delivery. Pregnant patients who are allergic to penicillin should be desensitized and treated with penicillin.

At-Risk Populations

All patients with syphilis should be tested for HIV infection. In areas where the prevalence of HIV is high, patients with

primary syphilis should be retested for HIV after 3 months if the first HIV result was negative.

MONITORING PATIENT RESPONSE

Patients should have a clinical and serologic examination at 6 and 12 months, or more frequently if follow-up results are uncertain. Those who fail to respond to treatment or who were reinfected, those who have signs that persist or recur, or those who have a sustained fourfold increase in nontreponemal test titer values within 6 months after treatment for

TABLE 35.6			
Overview of Drugs Used to Treat Neurosyphilis			
Generic (Trade) Name and Dosage	**Selected Adverse Events**	**Contraindications**	**Special Considerations**
aqueous crystalline penicillin G 18–24 million U/d, give as 3–4 million U IV q4h for 10–14 d	Similar to penicillins	Hypersensitivity to penicillin	This penicillin preparation is the drug of first choice in treating neurosyphilis; second-line therapy is procaine penicillin.
procaine penicillin (Bicillin with probenecid, Benemid) 2.4 million U IM/d, plus probenecid 500 mg PO qid, both for 10–14 d	Similar to other penicillins *Probenecid:* Headache, dizziness, GI upset, hypersensitivity reactions, acute gouty arthritis, nephrotic syndrome, uric acid stones	Hypersensitivity to penicillin or probenecid Children <2 y: blood dyscrasias, uric acid kidney stones	If compliance can be ensured, avoid IV, intravascular, or intra-arterial administration. *Probenecid:* Use caution in prescribing for patients with peptic ulcer.

primary or secondary syphilis should be retreated after evaluation for HIV infection. Treatment with three weekly injections of penicillin G benzathine is recommended if additional follow-up results are uncertain, unless CSF examination identifies neurosyphilis.

Patients with latent syphilis should be evaluated for tertiary disease. All patients with latent syphilis should have quantitative nontreponemal serologic tests repeated at 6, 12, and 24 months.

Patients should be evaluated for neurosyphilis and treated if titer values increase fourfold, an initially high titer fails to decrease at least fourfold within 12 to 24 months, or signs and symptoms related to syphilis develop. Patients with symptoms of neurologic or ophthalmic disease should be evaluated for neurosyphilis and syphilitic eye disease and treated appropriately according to the results (**Table 35.6**).

PATIENT EDUCATION

Teaching patients about preventive strategies is important in deterring the transmission of disease. All patients with a diagnosis of syphilis should be advised to undergo HIV testing as well.

GENITAL HERPES SIMPLEX VIRUS INFECTION

In the United States, genital herpes simplex (HSV) is the most prevalent genital ulcer disease with approximately 50 million persons infected. It is associated with a higher risk of HIV infection. More than 500,000 new cases occur each year. Most infected people remain undiagnosed. They have mild or unrecognized infections that shed the virus in the genital tract intermittently. Although some first episodes of genital herpes may be characterized by severe disease requiring hospitalization, many people are unaware they have the infection or are asymptomatic when transmission occurs. The disease can be controlled, not cured. It recurs periodically. Viral infections, for which

curative therapy is not available, have been stable or increasing in prevalence. With 500,000 new cases each year, herpes simplex virus (HSV) is one of the most common viral STIs.

CAUSES

Genital herpes simplex is caused by HSV, which has two serotypes: HSV-1 (genital) and HSV-2 (anorectal). The infection is transmitted by contact with an infected person by kissing or sexual intercourse, or during vaginal birth. Recurrent outbreaks may be triggered by injury to the infected area, an illness that alters immune status, emotional stress, or menses.

PATHOPHYSIOLOGY

Recurrent genital herpes is usually caused by HSV-1, while anorectal is HSV-2. After the virus enters the body through a susceptible mucosal surface, it resides and remains dormant in the cells of the nervous system until activated later. Exacerbations of varying frequency may or may not occur. In general, recurrent outbreaks are less severe than the initial episode.

DIAGNOSTIC CRITERIA

A diagnostic evaluation for herpes includes a health history and physical examination. In addition to serologic testing for HSV, patients should have a serologic test for syphilis. HIV testing should be considered as well. Specific tests for genital herpes include culture or antigen test for HSV. In addition, a POCkit HSV-2 test can be performed.

The patient seeking treatment may report any one of three genital HSV syndromes. The first is primary infection, which is the first infection with genital HSV characterized by no preexisting antibodies to either HSV-1 or HSV-2. Symptoms include genital pain, vesicles, fever, malaise, regional adenopathy, and, in women, lesions on the cervix. The second syndrome is nonprimary first episode infection, which is the first clinically evident infection in women who have had a previous infection with the heterologous strains. The symptoms include fewer lesions, few constitutional symptoms, and a shorter, milder course. The third syndrome is recurrent infection, which usually has no constitutional symptoms, a shorter duration of viral shedding, and a shorter healing time.

INITIATING DRUG THERAPY

The only effective therapy for genital herpes is drug therapy. Patient education is an important measure for preventing spread of the disease.

Goals of Drug Therapy

Treatment goals for first clinical episodes, recurrent episodes, and daily suppressive therapy aim to control the symptoms of the herpes episodes. The drugs *do not eradicate* the latent virus, and once discontinued, they do not affect the risk, frequency, or severity of recurrences. Treatment trials show acyclovir (Zovirax), valacyclovir (Valtrex), and famciclovir (Famvir) to be beneficial for treating genital herpes. The use of topical acyclovir is discouraged because it is substantially less effective than the systemic drug. The recommended acyclovir dosing regimens have been approved by the U.S. Food and Drug Administration and reflect substantial clinical experience and expert opinion for initial and recurrent episodes (**Table 35.7**).

Antivirals: Acyclovir, Famciclovir, and Valacyclovir

The three first-line systemic agents used to control genital herpes infections are acyclovir, famciclovir, and valacyclovir. These drugs inhibit viral DNA replication and are highly effective.

Acyclovir, which has low bioavailability, works only in the cells infected by HSV. Famciclovir, a prodrug of penciclovir, is well absorbed. It is converted to penciclovir by first-pass metabolism. Valacyclovir, a prodrug of acyclovir, is converted rapidly by first-pass metabolism to acyclovir. It has a 50% bioavailability; it also deactivates viral DNA polymerase.

Because antiviral medications are excreted by the renal system, caution should be used in patients with renal disease. They should also be prescribed cautiously for pregnant patients and are contraindicated in breast-feeding patients. These antivirals interact with probenecid, which increases the effect of the antiviral agent, and with zidovudine (Retrovir), which may cause drowsiness. For a detailed discussion of the roles that acyclovir, famciclovir, and valacyclovir play in controlling HSV-1 and HSV-2, see Chapter 13.

Selecting the Most Appropriate Agent

Therapy progresses from selecting treatment for the first clinical episode of infection to prescribing an antiviral agent for suppressive therapy (**Figure 35.4**).

TABLE 35.7			
Overview of Selected Drugs to Treat Genital Herpes			
Generic (Trade) Name and Dosage	**Selected Adverse Events**	**Contraindications**	**Special Considerations**
acyclovir (Zovirax) *First clinical episode:* 400 mg tid for 7–10 d or 200 g five times a day for 7–10 d *Recurrence:* 400 mg tid for 5 d or 200 mg five times a day for 5 d or 800 mg bid for 5 d Daily *suppressive therapy:* 400 mg bid *Severe disease:* 5–10 mg/kg IV q8h for 5–7 d or until clinical resolution occurs	GI upset (nausea, vomiting), headache, CNS disturbances, rash, malaise, vertigo, arthralgia, fatigue, viral resistance	Hypersensitivity to acyclovir Use with caution with renal impairment, pregnancy, breast-feeding mothers.	Do not exceed maximum dose.
famciclovir (Famvir) *First clinical episode:* 250 mg tid for 7–10 d *Recurrence:* 125 mg bid for 5 d Daily *suppressive therapy:* 250 mg bid	Headache, fatigue, GI upset With chronic use: pruritus, rash, laboratory test abnormalities, paresthesias	Hypersensitivity to famciclovir Pregnancy, lactation Use with caution in patients with renal dysfunction.	Easy to administer for prolonged treatment May be affected by drugs metabolized by aldehyde oxidase
valacyclovir (Valtrex) *First clinical episode:* 1 g PO bid for 7–10 d *Recurrent episodic infection:* 500 mg PO bid for 5 d Daily *suppressive therapy:* 500 mg PO qd (<9 episodes a year) or 1,000 mg PO qd	GI upset, headache, dizziness, abdominal pain	Hypersensitivity to valacyclovir Do not use in children. Use with caution with renal impairment, pregnancy, lactation.	Valacyclovir 500 mg qd is less effective than other valacyclovir regimens in patients with ≥10 episodes yearly. Be alert for renal or CNS toxicity in patients taking other nephrotoxic drugs.

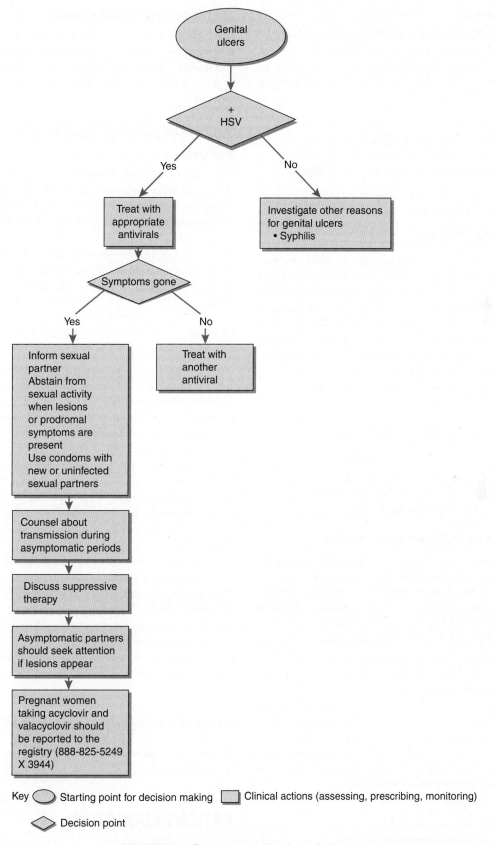

FIGURE 35.4 Treatment algorithm for genital herpes.

First-Line Therapy

Treatment for the first clinical episode of genital herpes includes antiviral therapy and counseling about the natural history of the virus, sexual and perinatal transmission, and methods to reduce transmission. Antiviral therapy for the initial outbreak includes the following:

- Acyclovir 400 mg three times daily for 7 to 10 days
- Acyclovir 200 mg five times a day for 7 to 10 days
- Famciclovir 250 mg three times a day for 7 to 10 days
- Valacyclovir 1.0 g two times a day for 7 to 10 days

The choice is based on the cost of medication, patient preference, or scheduling issues.

Second-Line Therapy (Recurrent Episodes)

Most patients with genital herpes infection have recurrent episodes of genital lesions. Episodic or suppressive antiviral therapy may shorten the duration of lesions or prevent recurrences. Episodic therapy is beneficial for recurrent disease if the treatment is started during the prodromal phase or within 1 day after onset of the lesions. When given episodic treatment, the patient should also be given additional antiviral therapy so the treatment can be initiated at the first sign of prodrome or genital lesions. Recurrent episodes are treated with:

- Acyclovir 400 mg three times a day for 5 days
- Acyclovir 800 mg two times a day for 5 days
- Acyclovir 800 mg three times a day for 2 days
- Famciclovir 125 mg two times a day for 5 days
- Famciclovir 1,000 mg twice a day for 1 day
- Valacyclovir 500 mg two times a day for 3 days
- Valacyclovir 1.0 g once a day for 5 days

Third-Line Therapy (Suppressive Therapy)

Third-line therapy is also known as suppressive therapy for HSV. The frequency of recurrent symptoms, or outbreaks, can be reduced by 75% or more with daily suppressive therapy, although suppressive therapy does not eliminate subclinical viral shedding. This therapy is used for patients with more than six episodes a year. Acyclovir has documented safety and efficacy for use for as long as 6 years, and valacyclovir and famciclovir for 1 year. Discontinuation of therapy should be discussed with the patient after 1 year of continuous suppressive therapy to determine the rate of recurrence and the patient's psychological adjustment. In many patients, the frequency of recurrence decreases over time.

Asymptomatic viral shedding is reduced but not eliminated with suppressive treatment with acyclovir. Therapy is not discontinued in patients who are HIV positive.

Suppressive therapy is as follows:

- Acyclovir 400 mg two times a day
- Famciclovir 250 mg two times a day
- Valacyclovir 500 or 1,000 mg once a day

Valacyclovir 500 mg once a day may be less effective than other regimens for prolonged suppression.

Severe or Complicated Disease

For patients with severe disease or complications requiring hospitalization, intravenous (IV) therapy is indicated. The recommended regimen is acyclovir 5 to 10 mg/kg body weight IV every 8 hours for 5 to 7 days or until clinical resolution is attained.

Special Population Considerations
Pediatric

The risk of HSV infection in the neonate is not completely eliminated with cesarean delivery. Infants exposed to HSV during birth should be followed carefully. Before clinical signs develop, the CDC recommends that the infant have surveillance cultures of mucosal surfaces to detect HSV infection. Infants born to women who acquired genital herpes near term should receive acyclovir therapy. Infants with neonatal herpes should be treated with acyclovir 30 to 60 mg/kg/d for 10 to 21 days.

Women

During pregnancy, the first clinical episode of genital herpes may be treated with oral acyclovir. IV administration of acyclovir is indicated for life-threatening maternal HSV infection. Acyclovir is not recommended for routine administration in pregnant women who have a history of recurrent genital herpes. The safety of systemic acyclovir and valacyclovir in pregnant women is unknown.

Women who acquire genital herpes close to the time of delivery (30% to 50%) are at high risk for transmitting the disease to the neonate. Those who have recurrent herpes at term or those who acquire genital HSV during the first half of pregnancy (3%) are at low risk for transmitting the disease to the neonate.

Sex partners who are symptomatic should have an evaluation and treatment similar to patients who have genital lesions. Most people who have genital HSV infection have no history of genital lesions. Therefore, asymptomatic sex partners of patients with newly diagnosed genital herpes should be interviewed regarding histories of typical and atypical genital lesions and encouraged to perform examinations and seek medical attention immediately if lesions appear.

MONITORING PATIENT RESPONSE

Response to therapy is monitored by symptom relief and resolution of lesions.

PATIENT EDUCATION

Patients should inform their sex partners that they have genital herpes and should abstain from sexual activity when lesions or prodromal symptoms are present. The practitioner can also discuss use of condoms with sex partners. Patients should also be counseled about transmission of HSV during asymptomatic periods. A diagnosis of genital herpes can be devastating to the individuals involved, so counseling should include helping patients cope with their infection and prevention of transmission.

Effective episodic treatment of recurrent herpes requires initiation of therapy within 1 day of lesion onset or during the prodrome that precedes some outbreaks. The patient should be provided with a supply of drug or a prescription for the medication with instructions to initiate treatment immediately when symptoms begin.

The risk of neonatal infection should be discussed with both sexes, and women who are pregnant should advise their health care providers about the infection. Patients should also be advised that episodic antiviral therapy may shorten the duration of lesions during recurrent episodes and that recurrent outbreaks can be ameliorated or prevented with suppressive antiviral therapy. Prevention of neonatal herpes should be emphasized during late pregnancy and counseling provided regarding unprotected genital and oral sexual contact at this time.

Patients who have genital herpes should be educated about the natural history of the disease, with emphasis on the potential for recurrent episodes, asymptomatic viral shedding, and the attendant risks of sexual transmission. All persons with genital HSV infection should be encouraged to inform their current sex partners that they have genital herpes and to inform future partners before initiating a sexual relationship. Persons with genital herpes should be informed that sexual transmission of HSV can occur during asymptomatic periods. Asymptomatic viral shedding is more frequent in genital HSV-2 infection than genital HSV-1 infection and is most frequent in the first 12 months of acquiring HSV-2.

PELVIC INFLAMMATORY DISEASE

It is estimated that PID affects 1 million women each year. Approximately 250,000 of these women are hospitalized and more than 150,000 major surgical procedures are performed. The disease is associated with significant long-term consequences, including tubal factor infertility, ectopic pregnancy, and chronic pelvic pain. Risk factors for PID include previous episodes of PID, presence of *N. gonorrhoeae*, *C. trachomatis*, or bacterial vaginosis in the lower genital tract, multiple sex partners, use of an intrauterine contraceptive device, adolescence, sexual intercourse during the last menstrual period, douching, and cigarette smoking. Oral contraceptives are thought to afford some protection against PID.

CAUSES

The most common etiologic agents for PID are *N. gonorrhoeae* and *C. trachomatis*. Other microorganisms that are part of the vaginal flora can also cause PID, as well as *Mycobacterium hominis* and *Ureaplasma urealyticum*.

PATHOPHYSIOLOGY

PID consists of several inflammatory disorders of the upper female genital tract that include any combination of endometritis, salpingitis, tubo-ovarian abscess, and pelvic peritonitis. It is an ascending infection that spreads from the lower genital tract to the endometrium, to the fallopian tubes, and to the peritoneal cavity.

DIAGNOSTIC CRITERIA

In all settings, no single historical, physical, or laboratory finding is sensitive and specific enough to make the diagnosis of acute PID. Many cases of PID are not recognized because they are asymptomatic or because the patient or health care provider fails to recognize mild or nonspecific symptoms.

The following diagnostic criteria are from the CDC (2015) guidelines. Empiric treatment of PID should be given to sexually active young women and others who are at risk for STIs if all of the following minimum criteria are present with no other causes for the illness: lower abdominal tenderness, adnexal tenderness, and cervical motion tenderness. Additional criteria may be used to enhance the specificity of the minimum criteria, including oral temperature exceeding 101°F (38.3°C), abnormal cervical or vaginal discharge, elevated erythrocyte sedimentation rate, elevated C-reactive protein, and laboratory documentation of cervical infection with *N. gonorrhoeae* or *C. trachomatis*. In selected cases, the following definitive criteria for diagnosing PID are warranted: histopathologic evidence of endometritis on endometrial biopsy; transvaginal sonography or other imaging techniques showing thickening, fluid-filled tubes with or without free pelvic fluid or tubo-ovarian complex; and laparoscopic abnormalities consistent with PID.

INITIATING DRUG THERAPY

Treatment for PID is prescribed when the patient's signs and symptoms meet the diagnostic criteria. Treatment includes empiric, broad-spectrum coverage of likely pathogens, including *N. gonorrhoeae*, *C. trachomatis*, anaerobes, gram-negative facultative bacteria, and streptococci. The CDC (2015) recommends patients be hospitalized when surgical emergencies cannot be excluded and when the patient is pregnant; does not respond clinically to oral antimicrobials; cannot tolerate an outpatient oral regimen; has severe illness, nausea and vomiting, or high fever; has a tubo-ovarian abscess; or is immunodeficient. There are no efficacy data that compare parenteral with oral regimens, and clinical experience should guide the decision to switch from parenteral to oral therapy, which may occur within 24 hours of clinical improvement.

Goals of Drug Therapy

In addition to ameliorating infection or preventing the progression of disease, the goal of drug therapy is to preserve the patient's reproductive health or at least minimize the effects of infection. Treatment should begin as promptly as possible because prevention of long-term sequelae has a direct correlation with immediate antibiotic coverage. Factors to consider in selecting treatment include drug availability and cost, patient acceptance, and antimicrobial susceptibility.

Antimicrobials and Appropriate Treatment Choices

For the most part, antimicrobial regimens for PID are those used for patients with chlamydial and gonorrheal infections. Refer to the sections on chlamydial infection and gonorrhea in this chapter, and also see **Table 35.8** for an overview of drug therapy in PID and **Figure 35.5** for a synopsis of the treatment. For women with PID of mild or moderate severity, parenteral therapy and oral therapy appear to have similar clinical efficacy.

Special Population Considerations

So that the mother and fetus can be closely monitored, pregnant women with suspected PID should be hospitalized and treated with parenteral antibiotics.

MONITORING PATIENT RESPONSE

Patients treated with oral or parenteral therapy should demonstrate substantial clinical improvement within 3 days after therapy has been initiated. Those who do not improve in this period usually require additional diagnostic tests or surgical intervention. The patient should be seen after 1 week of antibiotic therapy to check for residual pelvic abnormalities. Outpatient oral or parenteral therapy also requires a follow-up examination performed within 72 hours, using the criteria for clinical improvement.

TABLE 35.8

Overview of Selected Drugs to Treat Pelvic Inflammatory Disease

Generic (Trade) Name and Dosage	Selected Adverse Events	Contraindications	Special Considerations
cefoxitin (Mefoxin) Mefoxin plus probenecid (Benemid) 2 g IV q6h	*cefoxitin:* Pseudomembranous colitis, thrombophlebitis, rash, pruritus, eosinophilia, fever, dyspnea, hypotension, GI upset	Hypersensitivity to cefoxitin or cephalosporins Pregnancy, lactation, hypersensitivity to any of the tetracyclines	Prescribe with caution to penicillin-sensitive patients and those with GI disease. Monitor blood, renal, and hepatic function in long-term use. Avoid sunlight or UV light. Use of drug during tooth development may cause dental discoloration. Absorption is reduced when taken with food or bismuth subsalicylate.
Mefoxin plus doxycycline (Vibramycin) 100 mg PO for 14 d	*doxycycline:* Superinfection, photosensitivity, GI upset, enterocolitis, rash, blood dyscrasias, hepatotoxicity		
doxycycline (Vibramycin) 100 mg PO bid for 14 d or	Same as above	Same as above	Parenteral therapy may be discontinued 24 h after patient improves clinically.
clindamycin (Cleocin) 450 mg PO qid for 14 d			Clindamycin is used with tubo-ovarian abscess rather than doxycycline.
ofloxacin (Floxin) 400 mg PO bid for 14 d	Rash, hives, rapid heartbeat, difficulty swallowing or breathing, photosensitivity, angioedema, dizziness, light-headedness	Pregnancy Hypersensitivity to ofloxacin or fluoroquinolones	Use with caution with hepatic or renal insufficiency. Do not take with food.
metronidazole (Flagyl) 500 mg PO bid for 14 d	CNS stimulation, phototoxicity, GI upset, insomnia, headache, dizziness, tendinitis or tendon rupture, local reactions	Hypersensitivity to metronidazole Pregnancy, lactation	Take on empty stomach with full glass of water and maintain adequate hydration throughout therapy. Avoid excessive sunlight or UV light. Monitor blood, renal, and hepatic function in long-term use. Use with caution with CNS disorders that increase seizure risk and in renal or hepatic impairment.
ceftriaxone (Rocephin) 250 mg IM once	Pseudomembranous colitis, rash, GI upset, hematologic abnormalities	Known allergy to cephalosporins	Prescribe with caution to penicillin-sensitive patients.

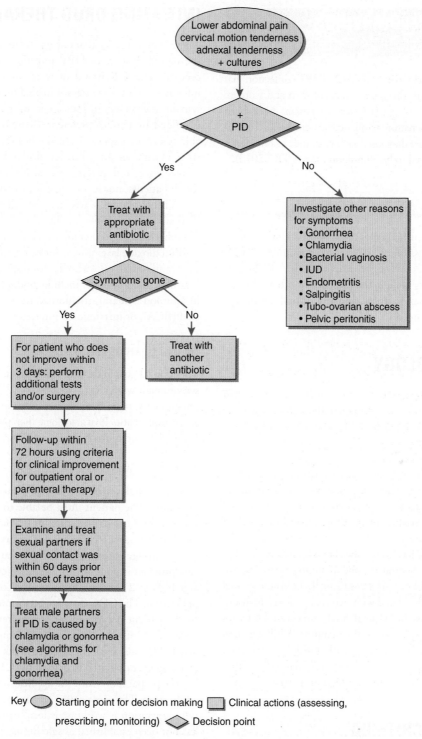

FIGURE 35.5   Treatment algorithm for pelvic inflammatory disease (PID).

PATIENT EDUCATION

If *N. gonorrhoeae* or *C. trachomatis* is present, the practitioner needs to explain to patients with PID that their sex partners should be examined and treated if they have had sexual contact with the patient during the 60 days before the onset of the patient's symptoms. Male partners of women with PID caused by *C. trachomatis* or *N. gonorrhoeae* are often asymptomatic and should be treated empirically with regimens that are effective against both infections.

HUMAN PAPILLOMAVIRUS INFECTION

The detection of human papillomavirus (HPV) infection has increased in frequency in the genital tracts of men and women. Genital warts, known as *condylomata acuminata,* have been detected with widely increasing frequency as well. About 14 million new cases of HPV are diagnosed each year, and the prevalence of this disease is estimated to be 79 million cases (CDC, 2013).

CAUSES

There are over 100 identified types of HPV, which 40 are genital. The sexual transmission of HPV is well documented, with the highest prevalence in young, sexually active adolescents and adults. Risk factors include the presence of other STIs, an increased number of sex partners, and use of oral contraceptives without other protection.

PATHOPHYSIOLOGY

Most HPVs cause no symptoms, are subclinical, or remain unrecognized. Warts that are visible in the genital tract are usually caused by HPV types 6 or 11, which also cause warts (that cannot be seen externally) on the uterine cervix and in the vagina, urethra, and anus. These viruses, which can produce symptoms, have also been associated with conjunctival, nasal, oral, and laryngeal warts. They are rarely associated with invasive squamous cell carcinoma of the external genitalia. Genital warts can be painful, friable, or pruritic, depending on their size and anatomic location.

Cervical dysplasia has been strongly associated with other HPV types in the anogenital region, including types 16, 18, 31, 33, and 35. These are found occasionally in visible genital warts and have been associated with external genital squamous intraepithelial neoplasia and vaginal, anal, and cervical intraepithelial dysplasia and squamous cell carcinoma. Visible genital warts can be infected simultaneously with multiple HPV types. The body's immune system clears most HPV naturally within 2 years (about 90%), though some infections persist.

DIAGNOSTIC CRITERIA

Genital warts are diagnosed definitively by biopsy, which is needed only if the diagnosis is uncertain, if the lesions do not respond to standard therapy, if the disease worsens during therapy, if the patient is immunocompromised, or if the warts are pigmented, indurated, fixed, and ulcerated. The literature does not support HPV nucleic acid tests for use in the routine diagnosis or management of visible genital warts. For women who have exophytic cervical warts, high-grade squamous intraepithelial lesions must be ruled out before initiating treatment for genital warts (CDC, 2006).

INITIATING DRUG THERAPY

There is no evidence that current treatments eradicate or affect the natural history of HPV infection or the development of cervical cancer. Removal of warts may or may not decrease infectivity. Warts that are not treated may resolve on their own, remain unchanged, or increase in number and size. Treatment is guided by patient preference, cost of treatment and available resources, experience of the health care practitioner, wart size and number, anatomic location of wart, wart morphology, convenience, and adverse effects. No single treatment is ideal for all patients, nor is one superior to another.

Visible genital warts may be self-treated by the patient if they are accessible or by the health care practitioner. Nonpharmacologic therapies include surgery or laser therapy. Carbon dioxide laser is used for extensive warts or intraurethral warts and for patients who do not respond to other treatments. Pharmacotherapy may include podophyllin resin (Podofin), imiquimod (Aldara), trichloroacetic acid (TCA), bichloracetic acid (BCA), or intralesional interferon (Intron A).

Goals of Drug Therapy

The primary goal in treating visible genital warts is the removal of symptomatic warts and prevention of HPV transmission. Removal can induce wart-free periods in most patients. Often, genital warts are asymptomatic. Pharmacologic therapy may include podofilox (Condylox), imiquimod, TCA, and BCA (**Table 35.9**).

Podofilox and Podophyllin Resin

Visible genital warts can be self-treated by the patient with podofilox. The patient must be able to identify and reach the warts to be treated. Podofilox in 0.5% solution or gel is safe, inexpensive, easy to use, and efficacious on mucosal surfaces.

A stronger preparation for application only by the health care provider is podophyllin resin, which may be administered at a 10% to 25% concentration in a compound with tincture of benzoin. The CDC does not recommend use of podophyllin by the patient because of rare but potential toxicity involving systemic absorption, bone marrow suppression, or serious GI upset. The preparation is applied weekly as needed. Again, to guard against potential toxicities, the CDC recommends washing the preparation from the application site 1 to 4 hours after application. The most common adverse effect, which indicates the preparation is working, is local irritation. The preparation has not been established as safe for use during pregnancy.

Imiquimod

Like podofilox, imiquimod may be self-administered by the patient. This antimitotic preparation enhances the immune response to HPV. Imiquimod can be topically applied three times weekly for 3 to 4 months. As with podophyllin, the imiquimod site should be washed with mild soap and water 6 to 10 hours after application. Warts should disappear in 8 to 10 weeks. During imiquimod therapy, sexual contact should be avoided to prevent viral transmission. Adverse effects include

TABLE 35.9

Overview of Selected Drugs and Procedures Used to Treat Genital Warts

Generic (Trade) Name and Dosage	Selected Adverse Events	Contraindications	Special Considerations
Patient Applied			
podofilox solution or gel (Condylox) 0.5% bid for 3 d followed by 4 d of no therapy; repeat cycle as needed for a total of 4 cycles.	Mild or moderate pain or local irritation	The safety of podofilox during pregnancy has not been established.	Apply solution with cotton swab or apply gel with finger. Total wart area should not exceed 10 cm², and total volume of podofilox should not exceed 0.5 mL/d.
imiquimod cream (Aldara) 5% cream applied three times a week for up to 16 wk	Mild to moderate local inflammatory reactions	The safety of imiquimod during pregnancy has not been established.	Apply with finger at bedtime. Wash area with mild soap and water 6–10 h after application of cream. May clear area of warts in 8–10 wk or sooner.
Practitioner Applied			
cryotherapy	Pain, necrosis, blistering	Use of cryoprobe in the vagina is not recommended because of risk of vaginal perforation and fistula formation.	Repeat applications every 1–2 wk. Use local anesthetic. Indicated for urethral meatus warts, anal warts, oral warts
podophyllin or resin in compound tincture of benzoin 10%–25% (Podofin)	Local irritation	The safety of podophyllin during pregnancy has not been established. Use with caution vaginally because of potential systemic absorption.	Apply small amount to each wart and allow site to air-dry. Limit to ≤0.5 mL of podophyllin or ≤10 cm² of warts per therapy session. Wash off preparation 4 h after application to reduce local irritation. Repeat application weekly if necessary. With vaginal warts, allow to dry before removing speculum and treat with ≤2 cm² per session. For warts on the urethral meatus, treatment area must be dry before preparation comes in contact with normal mucosa.
trichloroacetic acid or bichloracetic acid 80%–90%	Can spread rapidly and damage adjacent tissue; pain		Apply small amount only to warts and allow site to dry. White "frosting" will develop. Use talc with baking soda to remove unreacted acid if an excess amount is applied. Repeat treatment weekly as needed. Indicated for vaginal warts

a local inflammatory reaction. The safety of use during pregnancy has not been established.

Trichloroacetic Acid (TCA) and Bichloracetic Acid (BCA)

TCA and BCA are applied by the health care provider. These are strong 80% to 90% acids that flow onto the wart site quickly, and the fluid can spread equally quickly. Application requires particular care and skill. The acid is applied only to the warts and left to air-dry. A white "frosting" appears at the site. The practitioner can use talc or sodium bicarbonate powders to neutralize acid that falls on healthy tissue. TCA and BCA can be used effectively on keratinized areas and are safe for use during pregnancy. They are associated with low systemic toxicity.

Intralesional Interferon

Interferon is ineffective when used systemically. However, the use of intralesional interferon appears to be effective, and recurrence rates after therapy are comparable to those with other treatment modalities. Intralesional therapy appears to be effective because of interferon's antiviral or immunostimulating effects.

Selecting the Most Appropriate Agent

Treatment of genital warts should be guided by the preference of the patient, the available resources, and the experience of the health care provider. No definitive evidence suggests that any one of the available treatments is superior to the others, and no single treatment is ideal for all patients or all warts. Most patients have 10 or fewer genital warts. These warts respond to most treatment modalities. Factors that may influence selection of treatment include wart size, wart number, and anatomic site of wart, wart morphology, patient preference, and cost of treatment, convenience,

adverse effects, and provider experience. Many patients require a course of therapy rather than a single treatment. In general, warts located on moist surfaces or in intertriginous areas respond better to topical treatment than do warts on drier surfaces. **Figure 35.6** outlines the most appropriate patient- or practitioner-applied drug therapies in the most appropriate order.

Special Population Considerations

Pediatric

Laryngeal papillomatoses in infants and children are caused by HPV 6 and HPV 11. The prevention value of cesarean section is unknown, and the route of transmission is not completely understood.

Women

Many experts recommend removing warts during pregnancy because they can proliferate and become friable.

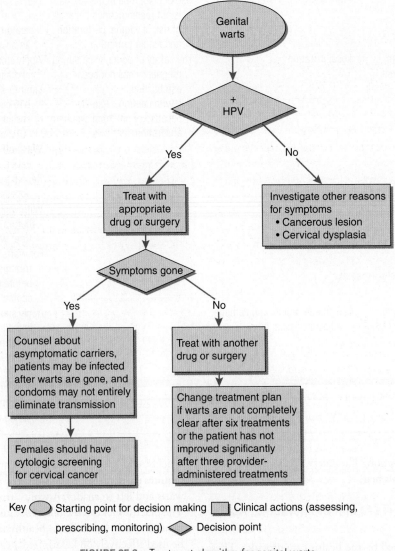

FIGURE 35.6 Treatment algorithm for genital warts.

CASE STUDY*

J.R. is a 36-year-old white, middle-class woman who has been sexually active with one partner for the past 2 years. She and her partner have no history of STIs, but her partner has a history of fever blisters. She reports genital pain, genital vesicles and ulcers, and fever and malaise for the last 3 days. Examination reveals adenopathy and vaginal and cervical lesions.

DIAGNOSIS: GENITAL HERPES

1. List specific goals for treatment for **J.R.**
2. What drug therapy would you prescribe? Why?
3. What are the parameters for monitoring the success of the therapy?
4. Discuss specific education for **J.R.** based on the diagnosis and prescribed therapy.
5. List one or two adverse reactions for the selected agent that would cause you to change therapy.
6. What, if any, would be the choice for second-line therapy?
7. What OTC or alternative medicines would you recommend?
8. What dietary and lifestyle changes should be recommended for this patient?
9. Describe one or two drug–drug or drug–food interactions for the selected agent.

* Answers can be found online.

MONITORING PATIENT RESPONSE

If the warts are not completely clear after six treatments or the patient has not improved significantly after three practitioner-administered treatments, the treatment plan should be changed. Evaluation of the risk/benefit ratio of treatment should occur throughout the course of therapy to avoid over-treatment. Women with genital warts should have cytologic screening for cervical cancer.

Once warts are eradicated, follow-up evaluations are not mandatory. Patients should monitor for recurrences, especially in the first 3 months. Patients who have concerns regarding recurrences can have a follow-up evaluation 3 months after treatment. Earlier follow-up visits may help to verify a wart-free state and monitor or treat complications and can be used for patient education and counseling.

PATIENT EDUCATION

Most sexually active men and women will get HPV at some point in their lives. This means that everyone is at risk for the potential outcomes of HPV and many may benefit from the prevention that the HPV vaccine provides. HPV vaccines are routinely recommended for 11- or 12-year-old boys and girls and protect against some of the most common types of HPV that can lead to disease and cancer, including most cervical cancers. CDC recommends that all teen girls and women through age 26 get vaccinated, as well as all teen boys and men through age 21 (and through age 26 for gay, bisexual, and other men who have sex with men). HPV vaccines are most effective if they are provided before an individual ever has sex.

The practitioner needs to provide precise instruction and guidance for applying topical antimitotic preparations, such as by showing how to apply podofilox solution with a cotton swab and the gel with a finger to visible warts. Patients should also be informed that HPV organisms persist despite resolution of lesions. Sex partners do not need to be examined because reinfection is most likely minimal and treatment to reduce transmission is not realistic in the absence of curative therapy. However, partners should be counseled about having a partner with genital warts and should be informed that the patient may remain infectious even when the warts are gone. The use of condoms may not eliminate the risk of transmission.

Patients should be warned that ablative therapies may cause scarring in the form of persistent hypopigmentation or hyperpigmentation. Depressed or hypertrophic scars rarely occur. Disabling chronic pain syndromes can also occur but are rare.

Bibliography

Starred references are cited in the text.

*CDC Fact Sheet: Incidence, prevalence, and cost of sexually transmitted infections in the United States. Retrieved from http://www.cdc.gov/std/stats/sti-estimates-fact-sheet-feb-2013.pdf

*CDC Fact Sheet. (2013). Reported STDs in the United States: 2013 national data for chlamydia, gonorrhea, and syphilis. Retrieved from http://www.cdc.gov/nchhstp/newsroom/docs/std-trends

*Centers for Disease Control and Prevention. (2015). Sexually transmitted treatment guidelines, 2015. *Morbidity and Mortality Weekly Report, 64*(RR3), 1–137.

Gibson, E. J., Bell, D. L., & Powerful, S. A. (2014). Common sexually transmitted infections in adolescents. *Primary Care; Clinics in Office Practice, 41*(3), 631–650.

LeFevre, M. L. (2014). Behavioral counselling interventions to prevent sexually transmitted infection: U.S. Preventive Services Task Force recommendations. *Annals of Internal Medicine, 161*(12), 894–901.

O'Connor, E. A., Lin, J. S., Burda, B. U., et al. (2014). Behavioral sexual risk-reduction counseling in primary care to prevent sexually transmitted infections: A systematic review for the U.S. Preventive Services Task Force. *Annals of Internal Medicine, 161*(12), 874–883.

Rompalo, A. (2011). Preventing sexually transmitted infections: Back to basics. *Journal of Clinical Investigation, 121*(12), 4580–4583.

UNIT 8

Pharmacotherapy for Musculoskeletal Disorders

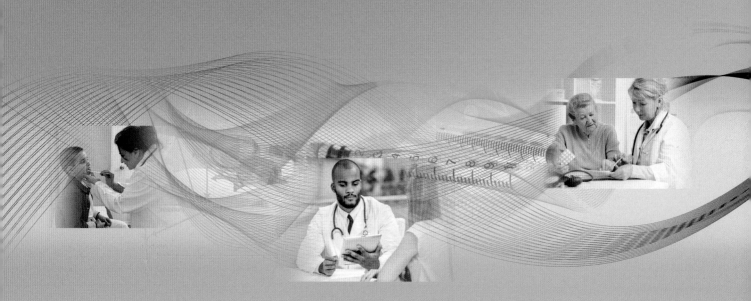

36 Osteoarthritis and Gout

Sarah F. Uroza ■ Lauren K. McCluggage ■ Carol Gullo Mest

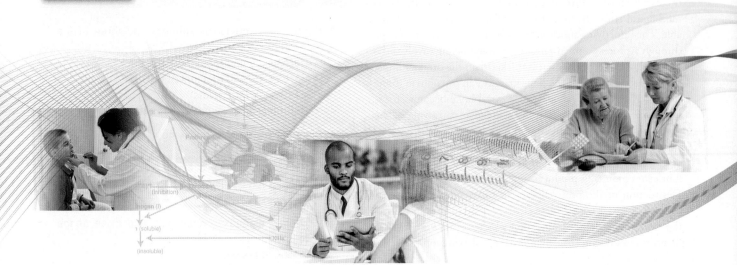

Osteoarthritis (OA), formerly known as *degenerative joint disease*, is the most common joint problem in the United States. Based on U.S. data from 2005, OA affects approximately 14% of adults older than age 25 and one third of adults older than age 65. Although prevalent, OA is often undiagnosed because clinical signs and symptoms are typically attributed to the normal aging process. In population-based studies in which asymptomatic patients were screened, the incidence of radiographic-defined OA was consistently higher than the incidence of symptomatic OA in the hands, knees, and hips.

OA is a progressive disease that can result in chronic pain, restricted range of motion, and muscle weakness, especially if a weight-bearing joint is affected. The joints commonly affected by OA include the knees, hips, cervical and lumbar spine, distal interphalangeal (DIP) joints, and the carpometacarpal joint at the base of the thumb.

CAUSES

There are two forms of OA. *Primary*, or idiopathic, OA arises from physiologic changes that occur with normal aging. *Secondary* OA usually results from traumatic injuries or inherited conditions and may present as hemochromatosis, chondrodystrophy, or inflammatory OA.

There are several modifiable and nonmodifiable risk factors that contribute to the development of OA. Of all the risk factors, obesity is the greatest in the development of OA of the knees and hips, especially in women. This is due to mechanical stress on weight-bearing joints. There may also be a metabolic effect of excess fat on articular cartilage that may account for some of the significance of obesity as a systemic risk factor.

Other modifiable risk factors include prior joint injury and occupations that require excessive mechanical stress or heavy lifting. For patients with a past knee injury, the lifetime risk of knee OA is 57% compared to 45% in patients with no previous injury.

The nonmodifiable risk factors include gender, age, race, and genetics. Women have a higher overall risk for developing OA, but men tend to have disease onset at an earlier age. Increasing age is a risk factor until age 75, at which point the risk equilibrates. OA of the DIP and carpometacarpal joints is more common in White women; OA of the knees occurs more frequently in African American women. Genetics may determine approximately one fourth of knee OA cases and one half of hip and hand OA cases.

PATHOPHYSIOLOGY

OA must be differentiated from other forms of arthritis because the physiologic changes specific to the condition dictate disease management. Although most forms of arthritis, including OA, result in degeneration of articular cartilage, the subsequent formation of new bone is a change specific to OA.

The physiologic changes associated with OA begin with deterioration of the articular cartilage, which reduces joint friction during movement by diffusing mechanical stress to the underlying bone. Normal articular cartilage is smooth and is supported by subchondral bone. The subchondral bone serves as a flexible base to absorb mechanical force.

Articular cartilage consists of chondrocytes, connective tissue cells that are embedded in an extracellular matrix. The matrix is made up of collagen, water, and proteoglycans (macromolecules). The proteoglycans provide elasticity and flexibility to the matrix, which allows the articular cartilage to resist direct pressure. In OA, there is a reduction in proteoglycans in the extracellular matrix, leading to a decrease in resiliency to mechanical stress. In time, the articular cartilage becomes friable. The underlying subchondral bone responds to this change through a process termed *remodeling*. Remodeling involves the production of new bone that is thicker than the original bone. If remodeling occurs at the joint margins, an osteophyte (bone spur) may develop. The adjacent cortical bone becomes fortified with new bone, resulting in an irregular narrowing of the joint space. Sclerosing and cyst formation may ensue.

In addition to cartilaginous changes, concomitant changes in the synovial fluid must be considered. Synovial fluid, the main lubricant of joints, is produced and excreted from the cartilage. Destruction of the proteoglycans in OA renders the mechanism of synovial release ineffective, thereby further impairing the smooth mechanical operation of the joint. **Figure 36.1** demonstrates the mechanism of cartilage destruction.

DIAGNOSTIC CRITERIA

Joints commonly affected by OA include the hip, knee, hand, and cervical and lumbosacral spine. The American College of Rheumatology (ACR) published criteria for the diagnosis of OA of the knee (1986), hip (1991), and hand (1990) (**Box 36.1**). Often, a thorough history and physical examination provide enough data to diagnose OA. The most common symptom is joint pain; the patient in an early stage of OA usually describes the pain as insidious, intermittent, and mild. As the disease progresses, the patient may describe the pain as more constant and more disabling. Most patients report remittance of pain with rest and exacerbation of pain with joint movement.

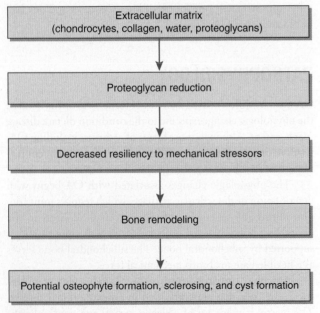

FIGURE 36.1 Destruction of cartilage in osteoarthritis.

BOX 36.1 Diagnostic Criteria for Osteoarthritis

- Hand: Pain, aching, or stiffness and three of the following:
  - Hard tissue enlargement of >2 joints
  - Hard tissue enlargement of >2 DIP joints
  - <3 swollen MCP joints
  - Deformity of >1 selected joint

- Hip: Pain and 2 of the following
  - ESR < 20 mm/h
  - Radiographic femoral or acetabular osteophytes
  - Radiographic joint space narrowing

- Knee
  - Clinical diagnosis: Knee pain and three of the following
    - >50 years old
    - Stiffness < 30 minutes
    - Crepitus
    - Bony tenderness
    - Bony enlargement
    - No palpable warmth
  - Clinical and radiographic diagnosis: Knee pain + osteophytes and one of the following:
    - >50 years old
    - Stiffness < 30 minutes
    - Crepitus
  - Clinical and laboratory diagnosis: Knee pain and five of the following:
    - Age > 50 years old
    - Stiffness < 30 minutes
    - Crepitus
    - Bony tenderness
    - Bony enlargement
    - No palpable warmth
    - ESR < 40 mm/h
    - RF < 1:40
    - Synovial fluid signs of OA (clear, viscous, or WBC count < 2,000/mm³)

MCP, metacarpophalangeal joint; ESR, erythrocyte sedimentation rate.

Although the symptoms of OA are localized, associated pain may be referred. For example, it is common for OA of the hip to be referred to the medial knee. Another symptom associated with OA is crepitus, a painless "crackling" in the joint. Crepitus most commonly affects the knee, but it may be heard in other joints affected by OA as well. As OA progresses to later stages of articular damage, deformity of the joint may be observed. The deformity usually appears as an enlargement of the joint, which may result from either increased bone production or synovitis. Other deformities resulting from OA of the knee include varus (bow-legged knees) and valgus (knock-kneed legs).

OA of the cervical spine may present with pain that radiates to the supraclavicular or upper trapezius areas. Depending on the level of nerve involvement, symptoms may progress to include pain in the distal upper extremities. OA of the lumbar spine may produce symptoms of neurogenic claudication.

On physical examination, decreased range of motion is the most common finding. This finding may be absent in the early stages of the disease but gradually progresses as the condition worsens. In later stages of the disease, joint contractures may occur, resulting in varus and valgus deformities. Patients with severe OA of the hip may present with gait disturbances.

Because OA is a progressive disease, complications such as joint effusion and enlargement may occur. Occasionally, radicular problems may occur secondary to changes in the cervical vertebrae.

Joint enlargement due to the formation of osteophytes may be observed. Osteophyte formation in the DIP joint is called *Heberden nodes*; in the proximal interphalangeal joint, it is referred to as *Bouchard nodes*.

Radiologic findings in OA may be used to confirm the suspected diagnosis. Narrow joint spaces with osteophyte formation are common findings.

INITIATING DRUG THERAPY

Before initiating drug therapy, the practitioner should recommend appropriate physical activity or physical therapy. The goals of physical therapy are to reduce pain, improve motion, and maintain functional ability (**Box 36.2**). In addition, for hip and knee OA, overweight patients should be counseled on the need for weight loss.

The goals of pharmacotherapy for OA are to maintain function, prevent further joint damage, and diminish associated pain. The degree of joint involvement and the severity of the symptoms usually dictate proper interventions for individual patients.

Acetaminophen

First-line pharmacotherapy for OA is geared toward analgesia, specifically with acetaminophen (Tylenol). Due to acetaminophen's cost-effectiveness and safety, it is currently the first-line treatment recommended in guidelines by the ACR, the European League Against Rheumatism (EULAR), and others.

Mechanism of Action

Acetaminophen exerts its action within the central nervous system (CNS). It is thought to inhibit central cyclooxygenase (COX), which results in decreased prostaglandin synthesis. Through this prostaglandin inhibition, acetaminophen exerts analgesic and antipyretic effects but does not have anti-inflammatory effects.

Dosage

The recommended dose is 650 mg every 4 to 6 hours or 1,000 mg every 6 to 8 hours around the clock. The key to acetaminophen dosing for OA is to schedule the dose regardless of the patient's pain. To be most effective, it must be taken regularly.

The recommended dose of up to 4 g/d is safe for patients with normal liver function. Higher doses have been associated with hepatotoxicity. Patients with a history of liver disease or who are chronic alcohol drinkers should not take more than 1,800 to 2,000 mg/d. All patients should be counseled regarding the need to avoid other products that contain acetaminophen.

Time Frame for Response

If taken as scheduled, patients can experience pain relief within 1 week of initiation.

Contraindications

The only absolute contraindication to acetaminophen use is hypersensitivity to acetaminophen. Acetaminophen should be used cautiously in patients with hepatic disease or who drink more than three alcoholic drinks daily.

Adverse Events

Acetaminophen is typically well tolerated with the most common adverse events being dizziness and rash. For patients who take more than the recommended daily dose, acetaminophen can induce hepatic failure as a result of the accumulation of the hepatotoxic metabolite acetylimidoquinone. Also, patients need to be educated about the risk of accidental overdose with combination products that also contain acetaminophen. Renal toxicity has also been observed with chronic overdosages.

BOX 36.2 **Nonpharmacologic Therapies for Osteoarthritis**

- Moist heat to help diminish muscle spasm and relieve stiffness
- Weight loss if the patient is overweight
- Exercises to strengthen the muscles surrounding the involved joint(s) and a fitness program to maintain flexibility of the involved joint through swimming, walking, cycling, and isometric exercises
- Use of assistive devices to help with ambulation and activities of daily living

Interactions

With chronic doses of greater than 1.3 g daily, acetaminophen can increase the international normalized ratio (INR) of a patient on warfarin. If a patient is on chronic acetaminophen and warfarin, the INR should be monitored more frequently upon initiation and discontinuation of acetaminophen. Isoniazid may increase the risk of hepatotoxicity of acetaminophen.

Nonsteroidal Anti-inflammatory Drugs

Second-line therapy for OA includes nonsteroidal anti-inflammatory drugs (NSAIDs), the most commonly used class of drugs in the world. NSAIDs are further classified according to their chemical structure (**Table 36.1**). Although these classes have subtle differences, they all basically act by inhibiting COX. These drugs may be prescribed if patients do not respond well to acetaminophen or if an inflammatory process has begun.

Mechanism of Action

There are two mechanisms by which NSAIDs exert their anti-inflammatory action. One is by inhibiting the conversion of arachidonic acid to prostaglandin, prostacyclin, and thromboxanes—all of which are mediators of pain and inflammation. The other is by interfering with protein kinase activation (especially when taken at higher doses).

COX is the enzyme that converts arachidonic acid to prostaglandin G_2. The COX enzyme is present in two forms, COX-1 and COX-2. Most NSAIDs nonselectively inhibit both COX-1 and COX-2, except for celecoxib, which is more selective for COX-2. COX-1 enzymes are found in the gastrointestinal (GI) tract and kidney and produce protective prostaglandins, which is why most research focuses on preserving the activity of COX-1. COX-2 is produced at nonspecific sites of inflammation as well as in the kidneys. Inhibition of COX-2 produces anti-inflammatory and analgesic effects without affecting the GI tract. COX-2 produces protective prostaglandins in the kidney that are responsible for maintaining

TABLE 36.1

Overview of Selected Nonsteroidal Anti-inflammatory Agents Used to Treat Osteoarthritis and Rheumatoid Arthritis

Generic (Trade) Name	Dosage	Contraindications	Special Considerations	Short, Intermediate, or Long Acting
Acetic Acid NSAIDs				
etodolac (Lodine)	IR: 600–1,000 mg/d PO in 2 or 3 divided doses ER: 400–1,000 mg/d PO	Pregnancy and lactation; use cautiously with allergies, renal, hepatic, CV, and GI conditions.		Intermediate
indomethacin (Indocin)	50–200 mg/d PO in 2–3 divided doses	Same as above, and also GI bleeding with history of proctitis or rectal bleeding	Decreased diuretic effect with loop diuretics; potential decreased antihypertensive effect with beta blockers; increased CNS adverse effects due to lipophilicity	Short
nabumetone (Relafen)	750–2,000 mg/d PO in 1–2 divided doses	Pregnancy and lactation; use cautiously with allergies, hepatic, CV, and GI conditions; significant renal impairment	May be taken in divided dose	Long
sulindac (Clinoril)	300 mg/d PO in 2 divided doses	Pregnancy and lactation; use cautiously in patients with asthma, chronic urticaria, CV dysfunction, hypertension, GI bleeding, peptic ulcer, impaired hepatic or renal function.	May take with meals if GI upset occurs.	Intermediate
tolmetin (Tolectin)	600–2,000 mg/d PO in 3–4 divided doses	Pregnancy, lactation; use cautiously with allergies, renal, hepatic, CV, and GI conditions	May affect results (false positive) of proteinuria tests using acid precipitation tests; patient should have ophthalmic examination periodically during long-term therapy.	Intermediate

TABLE 36.1

Overview of Selected Nonsteroidal Anti-inflammatory Agents Used to Treat Osteoarthritis and Rheumatoid Arthritis (*Continued*)

Generic (Trade) Name	Dosage	Contraindications	Special Considerations	Short, Intermediate, or Long Acting
Enolic Acid NSAIDs				
piroxicam (Feldene)	10–20 mg/d PO	Pregnancy and lactation; use cautiously with allergies, renal, hepatic, CV, and GI conditions	Because therapeutic response progresses over several weeks, evaluate response after 2 wk. NSAID with the longest half-life.	Long
Fenamic Acid NSAID				
meclofenamate (Meclomen)*	200–400 mg/d PO in 3–4 divided doses	Same as above	Patient should have ophthalmic examination periodically during long-term therapy.	Short
Phenylacetic Acid NSAIDs				
diclofenac sodium (Voltaren) diclofenac potassium (Cataflam)	OA: 100–150 mg/d PO in 2–3 divided doses RA: 100–200 mg/d PO in 2–4 divided doses	Significant renal impairment, pregnancy, lactation; use cautiously with impaired hearing; allergies; hepatic, CV, and GI conditions.	NSAID with the shortest half-life	Short
Propionic Acid NSAIDs				
fenoprofen (Nalfon)	800–3,200 mg/d PO in 3–4 divided doses	Same as above	Patient should have ophthalmic examination periodically during long-term therapy.	Short
ibuprofen (Motrin)	1,200–3,200 mg/d PO in 3–4 divided doses	Same as above	Therapeutic response may occur over several weeks.	Short
naproxen (Naprosyn)	500–1,500 mg/d PO in 2 divided doses	Same as above	May take with meals if GI upset occurs.	Intermediate
Salicylic Acid NSAIDs				
diflunisal (Dolobid)	500–1,500 mg/d PO in 2–3 divided doses	Pregnancy and lactation; use cautiously with allergies, renal, hepatic, CV, and GI conditions.		Intermediate
aspirin (Bayer, others)	2.4–3.6 g/d PO in 4–6 divided doses; maximum daily dose is 5.4 g	Allergy to salicylates, other NSAIDs, tartrazine, hemophilia, and other bleeding disorders, pregnancy (possibly teratogenic), and more; do not use in children after illness because of association with Reye syndrome.	Increased risk of bleeding when taken concomitantly with anticoagulants and other NSAIDs. Consult package insert for extensive list of interacting drugs and effects.	Short
COX-2 Selective NSAIDs				
celecoxib (Celebrex)	200–400 mg/d PO in 2 divided doses	Allergy to the drug or to sulfonamides, NSAIDs, or aspirin; significant renal impairment; pregnancy, lactation	Elimination of the drug occurs primarily through hepatic metabolism; therefore, patients with symptoms suggesting liver dysfunction should be carefully monitored.	Intermediate

*Brand name only available in Canada.

adequate blood perfusion via vasodilation of the afferent arteriole. Therefore, inhibition of either COX-1 or COX-2 can result in decreased renal perfusion and impaired kidney function.

Dosage

Dosing of NSAIDs is variable. The drugs are classified into short-, intermediate-, and long-acting categories. NSAIDs require five half-lives to reach peak therapeutic levels and five half-lives to be fully excreted. Categories with a longer half-life require longer periods to reach therapeutic levels.

Some common agents used to treat OA are diclofenac, ibuprofen, and the COX-2 inhibitor celecoxib. Diclofenac is given at 50 mg twice daily, and ibuprofen is usually given at 400 mg four times daily. The typical dose of celecoxib is 100 mg twice daily or 200 mg once daily. Patients should be encouraged to use the prescribed NSAID consistently for 2 to 3 weeks to determine its effectiveness. **Table 36.1** gives information about other agents and dosing considerations.

Time Frame for Response

Patients' responses to NSAIDs are quite variable. Patients who do not respond to one NSAID may respond to another, even one in the same class. This response variability is also seen in the side effect profile of NSAIDs. The practitioner should be familiar with several of the NSAIDs from each class and should try to individualize therapy based on symptom management and side effects.

Contraindications

NSAIDs are contraindicated in patients allergic to aspirin, in patients with alcohol dependence, or in pregnant patients. Further, since celecoxib contains a sulfa moiety, it is contraindicated in patients with a sulfa allergy. Caution should be used when prescribing NSAIDs to patients with renal or hepatic impairment or the elderly. Due to the increase in cardiovascular adverse events, all NSAIDs carry a black box warning emphasizing that they are contraindicated for perioperative pain treatment in patients undergoing coronary artery bypass graft surgery.

Adverse Events

NSAIDs have gained a reputation as innocuous agents because of their over-the-counter (OTC) availability and widespread use. However, this class of drugs is far from benign, and patient education materials should highlight potential adverse events. The side effect profile of NSAIDs is quite extensive.

Visual changes, weight gain, headache, dizziness, nervousness, photosensitivity, weakness, tinnitus, easy bruising or bleeding, and fluid retention are adverse events that have been associated with use of NSAIDs. Again, cautious use and frequent monitoring, particularly of elderly patients, is of paramount importance for safe NSAID use. The most common adverse events of NSAIDs occur in the GI and renal systems.

Adverse GI events may run the gamut from minor GI irritation to ulcers, GI bleeding, perforation, and gastric outlet obstruction. These GI effects are why NSAIDs remain a second-line approach to OA treatment. Concomitant use of misoprostol

(Cytotec) has been shown to decrease the incidence of ulcer disease and GI complications. Misoprostol, a prostaglandin analog, is given at 200 mg four times daily. Its use should be limited to patients at high risk for GI complications (age > 65, comorbid medical conditions, history of peptic ulcer disease or upper GI bleeding, oral glucocorticosteroids, or anticoagulants).

Studies of the treatment of GI effects as a result of NSAIDs have compared the efficacy of proton pump inhibitors and histamine-2 (H_2) receptor antagonists. Yeomans et al. (1998) determined that omeprazole (Prilosec), a proton pump inhibitor, healed existing ulcers and prevented further ulcer development more effectively than did ranitidine (Zantac), an H_2 receptor antagonist. Similarly, Hawkey et al. (1998) found omeprazole and misoprostol equally successful at treating ulcers and other GI symptoms associated with NSAID use. However, omeprazole was better tolerated and was associated with an improved relapse rate.

Another option for patients experiencing GI adverse events with nonselective NSAIDs is celecoxib. In a study conducted by Chan et al. (2010), patients randomized to celecoxib had a lower incidence of upper or lower GI events compared with patients treated with diclofenac plus omeprazole.

Patients with renal disease, congestive heart failure (CHF), cirrhosis, and volume depletion may experience renal aberrations, particularly related to renal blood flow. These adverse events underscore the need for frequent monitoring of patients on long-term NSAID therapy.

Controversy surrounds the issue of increased risk of cardiovascular events, including thrombotic events, myocardial infarction, and stroke due to NSAID use. This increased risk led to the market removal of two COX-2 selective agents, rofecoxib and valdecoxib. All NSAIDs have a black box warning regarding this increased risk and warn that patients with cardiovascular disease risk factors may be at an increased risk. In multiple analyses, naproxen seems to have little to no increased cardiovascular risk, whereas diclofenac consistently demonstrates an increased risk.

Interactions

NSAIDs have the potential to increase bleeding so they need to be used cautiously with other anticoagulants, specifically warfarin. Also, due to the risk of hypertension, NSAIDs may counteract the effect of antihypertensives. If possible, patients with hypertension should not be on NSAIDs. The combination of NSAIDs and angiotensin-converting enzyme inhibitors or angiotensin receptor blockers may result in decreased renal function and should be avoided. For patients who take aspirin daily, ibuprofen must be taken 30 minutes to 2 hours after or 8 hours before the aspirin in order for the aspirin to be cardioprotective. If taken concurrently with lithium, NSAIDs may increase the drug concentrations of lithium and caution is advised.

Nonacetylated Salicylates

Nonacetylated salicylates (**Box 36.3**) are especially beneficial in patients who are sensitive to the GI irritation caused by long-term aspirin use. Diflunisal (Dolobid), the most commonly used nonacetylated salicylate, is an effective COX-1 inhibitor with anti-inflammatory and analgesic properties, but its antipyretic activities are weak. In terms of symptom relief, the

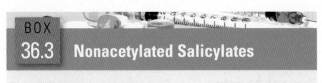

BOX 36.3 | Nonacetylated Salicylates

- Diflunisal
- Sodium salicylate
- Choline salicylate
- Magnesium salicylate
- Choline magnesium trisalicylate
- Salsalate

nonacetylated salicylates are probably as effective as aspirin in treating inflammatory disorders.

Analgesics

When the pain associated with OA progresses and is no longer responsive to acetaminophen or NSAIDs, analgesics are the next option. Analgesics can also be used in patients who cannot tolerate acetaminophen or NSAIDs or in whom they are contraindicated. Analgesics only decrease pain and have no effect on inflammation. These drugs should be prescribed for a limited time because of potential dependence and withdrawal symptoms. Analgesics used for OA other than tramadol and tapentadol, detailed below, include codeine in combination with acetaminophen.

Tramadol

Mechanism of Action
Tramadol exerts multiple effects to induce pain relief. It is a mu opioid receptor agonist similar to other opioids such as morphine. By binding to the mu opioid receptor, ascending pain pathways are inhibited, resulting in decreased pain sensation. In addition, tramadol also inhibits the reuptake of serotonin and norepinephrine. These neurotransmitters are also involved in the ascending pain pathway.

Dosage
Tramadol is available as an immediate-release tablet (Ultram), extended-release tablet (Ultram ER), and in combination with acetaminophen (Ultracet). For the immediate-release tablet, patients can take 50 to 100 mg every 4 to 6 hours as needed for pain with a maximum daily dose of 400 mg. For patients taking the extended-release tablet, the starting dose is 100 mg daily with an increase every 5 days to the maximum of 300 mg/d. All forms of tramadol need to be dose adjusted for renal and hepatic dysfunction.

Time Frame for Response
Patients may feel a decrease in pain as soon as 1 hour after taking an immediate-release tramadol dose with a maximum effect at 2 hours. The extended-release tablet takes about 12 hours for the maximum effect to be seen.

Contraindications
Patients with an opioid dependency should not take tramadol since it has opioid effects. Also, patients with acute intoxication with alcohol, hypnotics, central-acting analgesics, opioids, or psychotropic drugs should not be given tramadol. Tramadol has the ability to lower the seizure threshold. Therefore, tramadol should not be used in patients with a history of seizures and needs to be used cautiously with other medications that may lower the seizure threshold.

Adverse Events
Unlike NSAIDs, tramadol does not produce serious GI adverse events nor does it aggravate existing hypertension, CHF, or renal disease. The most common side effects of tramadol include nausea, dizziness, drowsiness, and sweating. Due to the opioid receptor agonism, tramadol has the potential to exert similar adverse events as other opioids, such as constipation, dependency, euphoria, and respiratory depression.

Interactions
Tramadol is metabolized by CYP2D6, and any medication that inhibits or induces this enzyme will interact with tramadol. Also, because it inhibits serotonin reuptake, tramadol has the potential to induce serotonin syndrome when used in combination with other serotonergic agents, such as selective serotonin reuptake inhibitors, tricyclic antidepressants, monoamine oxidase (MAO) inhibitors, or linezolid.

Tapentadol

Mechanism of Action
Similar to opioids, tapentadol is an agonist for the mu opiate receptor. In addition, tapentadol also inhibits the reuptake of norepinephrine.

Dosage
For patients starting tapentadol (Nucynta), the recommended dose for the first day of therapy is 50 to 100 mg every 4 to 6 hours as needed with the option of giving the second dose as soon as 1 hour after the first dose, if needed. After the first day of therapy, the recommended dose is 50 to 100 mg every 4 to 6 hours as needed with a maximum daily dose of 600 mg. The dosing interval should be increased to every 8 hours or longer in patients with moderate hepatic impairment. Tapentadol is not recommended in patients with severe hepatic or renal impairment (clearance less than 30 mL/min).

Tapentadol is also available in an extended-release formulation. For opioid-naïve patients, the recommended starting dose is 50 mg by mouth twice daily. The dose can be increased by 50 mg per dose every 3 days to a maximum daily dose of 500 mg.

Time Frame for Response
Patients are likely to experience pain relief within 1 to 2 hours of taking the dose. The ER formulation peaks after 3 to 6 hours of ingestion.

Contraindications
Due to the opioid receptor agonism, tapentadol is contraindicated in patients with impaired pulmonary function who are not in a monitored setting. Also, patients with paralytic ileus should avoid use due to the risk of opioid-induced constipation. Last, since tapentadol inhibits norepinephrine reuptake, it cannot be used within 14 days of a MAO inhibitor.

Adverse Events

The adverse event profile of tapentadol is similar to that of other opioids and tramadol. The most common adverse events are dizziness, somnolence, constipation, nausea, and vomiting. There is a risk of respiratory depression and CNS depression.

Interactions

Tapentadol needs to be used cautiously with other CNS depressants due to additive effects. As mentioned above, tapentadol and MAO inhibitors cannot be used within 14 days of each other. Using tapentadol with serotonergic agents increases the risk of serotonin syndrome.

Ethanol may increase the tapentadol concentrations if patients are taking the extended-release product. Therefore, patients taking extended-release tapentadol need to refrain from alcohol and any medication containing ethanol.

Duloxetine

Mechanism of Action

Duloxetine is a serotonin and norepinephrine reuptake inhibitor. By enhancing serotonin and norepinephrine, duloxetine works in the CNS to reduce pain transmission. Duloxetine is a relatively balanced serotonin and norepinephrine reuptake inhibitor.

Dosage

The FDA-approved dosing for chronic musculoskeletal pain is 30 mg by mouth daily for 7 days and then increase to 60 mg by mouth daily, which is the listed maximum dose for this indication. However, the trials that resulted in duloxetine's approval for this indication increased the dose to 120 mg by mouth daily in patients not having an adequate response to the 60 mg dose.

Time Frame for Response

The benefit of duloxetine was seen as early as 4 weeks in the clinical trials. Time points sooner than this were not assessed, so it is not known if its effect starts sooner.

Contraindications

Due to the risk for serotonin syndrome, duloxetine should not be started while a patient is on a monoamine oxidase inhibitor (MAOI) or within 14 days of stopping an MAOI. Also, starting duloxetine while a patient is receiving linezolid and intravenous methylene blue may increase the risk of serotonin syndrome and is contraindicated.

Adverse Effects

Some of the precautions and warnings associated with duloxetine risk include hepatotoxicity, orthostatic hypotension, serotonin syndrome, abnormal bleeding, and activation of mania. These are considered the more rare but serious adverse effects. More common adverse effects seen in the clinical trials include nausea, constipation, somnolence, and hyperhidrosis.

Interactions

Duloxetine is metabolized through CYP1A2 and CYP2D6; therefore, medications that inhibit these enzymes may cause increased duloxetine concentrations. Due to the serotonergic effects of duloxetine, there is a risk for serotonin syndrome if other serotonergic agents are used concomitantly. Heavy alcohol use should be discouraged due to an increased risk of hepatotoxicity.

Topical Agents

Capsaicin

Mechanism of Action

For the relief of arthritic pain, capsaicin exerts its effect through the depletion of substance P. Initially, capsaicin releases substance P from the peripheral sensory neurons. However, with repeated use, substance P becomes depleted, and capsaicin prevents reaccumulation of substance P. Substance P is a chemomediator responsible for pain transmission from the periphery to the CNS. Therefore, by depleting peripheral neurons of substance P, the pain impulse will not be transmitted centrally.

Dosage

Capsaicin is available as an OTC product in a patch, cream, gel, liquid, or lotion. The directions for the patch are to apply it to the affected area three to four times a day for 7 days. The patch can remain on the area for up to 8 hours. The cream, gel, liquid, and lotion forms should be applied at least three times a day for maximal efficacy.

Time Frame for Response

The maximal effect is seen after 2 to 4 weeks of continual use.

Contraindications

There are no absolute contraindications for topical capsaicin. Patients should be advised to not apply capsaicin to broken or irritated skin.

Adverse Events

The most common adverse event is burning and irritation at the application site. The burning typically subsides within days of continual use. Due to the initial release of substance P, patients may experience some pain with initial use and should be advised to expect this.

Topical NSAIDs

Diclofenac is currently the only commercially available topical NSAID. It is available as a 1.5% solution (Pennsaid) for the relief of OA pain of the knee and as a 1% topical gel (Voltaren) for the relief of OA pain in joints amenable to topical therapy.

Mechanism of Action

The mechanism of action for topical diclofenac is the same as for oral NSAIDs. The benefit is that minimal diclofenac is absorbed when applied topically, which then decreases the risk of adverse events. Data has shown that only 6% to 10% of the topical gel and 2% to 3% of the solution is absorbed.

Dosage

The dosage of topical diclofenac is dependent on the formulation and location. For the gel, if used on the lower extremities, 4 g should be applied four times a day; if used on the upper extremities, 2 g should be applied four times a day. The entire total daily dose should not exceed 32 g/d. For the topical solution, 40 drops should be applied to the affected knee(s) four times a day. The solution should be applied in 10-drop increments to limit spillage. It can be first applied to the hand and then rubbed on the knee. Regardless of formulation, it is imperative that the entire affected area be covered to achieve maximal effect.

Contraindications

Topical diclofenac carries the same warnings and contraindications as oral NSAIDs, although the risk is less. Also, topical diclofenac is contraindicated on nonintact or damaged skin.

Adverse Events

The most common adverse events are application site reactions and include pruritus, rash, dry skin, pain, and exfoliation.

Interactions

Topical diclofenac should be used cautiously with medications that interact with oral NSAIDs since some of the topical medication is absorbed.

Corticosteroids

If symptoms of OA are restricted to one or two joints that have not responded to first- or second-line treatment, intra-articular corticosteroids may be helpful. Aseptic technique and a local anesthetic are required. The amount of drug injected depends on the size of the joint. Careful technique that avoids the surrounding soft tissues is imperative to avoid tissue atrophy. The side effect of localized pain may be treated with an NSAID or

another appropriate analgesic. Injection of corticosteroids usually produces symptom relief within a few days, and the relief may last up to several months. Because of the potential for cartilage destruction and osteonecrosis with repeated injections, this therapy should be used judiciously.

SELECTING THE MOST APPROPRIATE AGENT

In 2012, the ACR published guidelines for the treatment of hand, hip and knee OA. In these guidelines, it is specified that patient specific characteristics need to be assessed and care should be individualized. In selecting therapies for OA, the prescriber should consider patient variables such as age, childbearing status, progression of arthritis, and underlying illnesses. These guidelines provide recommendations for initial therapy but do not provide recommendations for subsequent treatment sequences if initial therapy fails.

With the 2012 ACR guidelines, multiple agents were listed as first-line therapies based on the location of the OA (**Table 36.2**). For hand OA, the initial recommended treatments are topical capsaicin, topical NSAIDs, oral NSAIDs, and tramadol. For knee OA, initial recommended treatments include acetaminophen, oral NSAIDs, topical NSAIDs, tramadol, and intra-articular corticosteroid injections. For patients 75 years or older, topical NSAIDs are preferred over oral NSAIDs. Also, if a patient has a history of upper GI ulcer

TABLE 36.2
Guideline Recommendations for the Treatment of OA

	ACR	EULAR	OARSI
Hand	Initial treatment options: • Topical capsaicin • Topical NSAIDs • Oral NSAIDs	1st line: topical NSAIDs, capsaicin 2nd line: APAP 3rd line: NSAIDs IA steroids for painful flares	
Hip	Initial treatment options: • APAP • Oral NSAIDs • Tramadol • IA steroids	1st line: APAP 2nd line: NSAIDs +/– gastroprotection 3rd line: opioid +/– APAP IA steroids for flares unresponsive to analgesia and NSAIDs	1st line: APAP 2nd line: oral NSAIDs 3rd line: weak opioid analgesics Moderate to severe pain unresponsive: IA steroids
Knee	Initial treatment options: • APAP • Oral NSAIDs • Topical NSAIDs • Tramadol • IA steroids	1st line: APAP, topical NSAIDs, capsaicin 2nd line: NSAIDs +/– gastroprotection 3rd line: opioid +/– APAP IA steroids for flares with effusions	Without comorbidities • IA steroids • Topical NSAIDs • Oral NSAIDs • capsaicin • duloxetine • APAP With comorbidities • IA steroids • Topical NSAIDs

ACR, American College of Rheumatology; APAP, acetaminophen; EULAR, European League Against Rheumatism; IA, intra-articular; NSAIDs, nonsteroidal anti-inflammatory drugs; OARSI, Osteoarthritis Research Society International.

within a year, the recommendation is to use a COX-2 selective NSAID in addition to a proton pump inhibitor. For patients who have a history of upper GI ulcers greater than a year prior to initiating therapy, a selective NSAID can be used or a non-selective NSAID with a proton pump inhibitor. The ACR recommendations for hip OA are similar to that of knee except they do not recommend topical NSAIDs as initial therapy.

Also the EULAR has guidelines for the treatment of hip (2005), knee (2003), and hand (2007) OA. These guidelines outline first-line and subsequent treatment recommendations. The Osteoarthritis Research Society International (OARSI) has published guidelines regarding the treatment of hip and knee OA. **Table 36.2** compares the recommendations of these three guidelines. **Figure 36.2** outlines a general treatment algorithm for patients with hip or knee OA.

First-Line Therapy

Historically, acetaminophen 1 gram every 6 to 8 hours has been the first-line treatment for OA due to its effectiveness in reducing the pain of OA within 4 weeks and lasting for up to 2 years. However, there is conflicting data regarding the analgesic effect of acetaminophen compared to NSAIDs for OA pain. Many trials indicate that NSAIDs are superior, especially in patients with more severe disease; however, NSAIDs are associated with more adverse reactions. The EULAR continues to recommend acetaminophen as first-line therapy for hip and knee OA. Due to the relative safety of acetaminophen compared to NSAIDs, a trial of acetaminophen for most patients with OA remains first line.

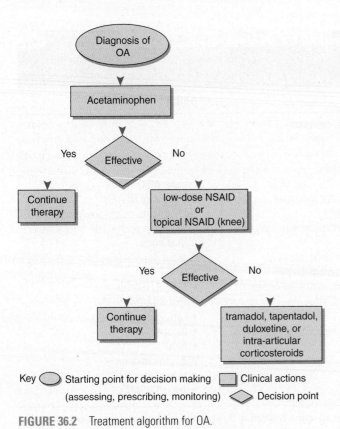

Key ⬭ Starting point for decision making ◻ Clinical actions
 (assessing, prescribing, monitoring) ◇ Decision point

FIGURE 36.2 Treatment algorithm for OA.

Second-Line Therapy

For patients without risk factors for GI disturbance, if acetaminophen therapy fails to provide relief, ibuprofen or a similar nonselective NSAID should be considered for second-line therapy as monotherapy or in combination with acetaminophen. Since there is no evidence that one NSAID is more effective than another, the choice of the specific NSAID should be based on the cost and convenience of therapy. For patients at increased risk for GI disorders, such as peptic ulcer disease, a COX-2 inhibitor may be a better second-line choice. Alternatively, the use of a traditional NSAID coupled with a proton pump inhibitor may be sufficient to provide analgesia along with gastric protection.

Third-Line Therapy

For patients who have failed to obtain pain control with acetaminophen or NSAIDs or those in which these therapies are contraindicated, opioid or nonopioid analgesia can be tried. The addition of codeine to acetaminophen may further reduce pain, but often, patients discontinue this combination due to the side effects associated with codeine (constipation, drowsiness). Tramadol or tapentadol may be tried, realizing that patients may experience similar adverse effects as they do to opioids. Duloxetine is another alternative to analgesics that can be tried as monotherapy or as adjunct to acetaminophen or NSAIDs. Most of the data regarding the use of duloxetine is for knee OA and showed modest improvement in pain scores.

Intra-articular steroids may be useful when an effusion is present and there are clear signs of local inflammation.

Special Populations
Geriatric

For elderly patients, the practitioner usually prescribes an NSAID with a shorter half-life in a smaller dosage than for a younger adult. Patients over age 65 should be considered at risk for GI hemorrhage and treated with either a COX-2 inhibitor or a combination of a nonselective NSAID and a gastric protective agent, such as misoprostol or a proton pump inhibitor.

Women

Many of the NSAIDs are pregnancy category C agents during the first 30 weeks of gestation. After gestational week 30, most NSAIDs are categorized as class D agents, indicating that there is evidence of harm to the fetus and should only be used in life-threatening illnesses.

MONITORING PATIENT RESPONSE

In addition to routine questions about the efficacy of the drug (e.g., pain relief), baseline and ongoing monitoring for specific drug therapy should be done. If a patient is taking acetaminophen, baseline liver function tests should be checked and monitored periodically. Monitoring for NSAID therapy includes a complete blood count (CBC), urinalysis, and serum creatinine. These studies should be repeated at 1 to 3 months and then every 3 to 6 months thereafter for the duration of therapy. In patients at risk for GI hemorrhage, the clinician should consider evaluating the patient for stool occult blood, anemia, and other signs of bleeding.

PATIENT EDUCATION

Drug Information

For patients taking acetaminophen, they need to be educated that it is most effective if taken around the clock regardless of pain. Also, patients need to be cognizant of other products that may contain acetaminophen and ensure they are not exceeding the daily limit. Last, for patients taking scheduled acetaminophen, alcohol intake should be minimized or avoided.

Patients taking NSAIDs need to be aware of their potentially harsh effects on the GI system, ranging from mild GI discomfort to gastric bleeding. The practitioner may emphasize strategies for dealing with some of these adverse events, including taking NSAIDs with food or milk or at meals. Patients should be reminded that a specific NSAID should be used regularly for 2 to 3 weeks before switching to another NSAID. This period is needed to assess whether the medication is effective.

Patients receiving a corticosteroid injection for joint pain need to be informed that a single joint should not be injected more frequently than every 6 months. Patients should be cautioned to limit activity of the injected joint for several days after the injection. Otherwise, the reduced pain perception of the joint may allow the patient to cause further joint damage, enhancing the progression of OA.

Patient-Oriented Information Sources

The National Institute of Arthritis and Musculoskeletal and Skin Diseases (NIAMS) is a government-sponsored group that provides information on OA and its treatment (http://www.niams.nih.gov/hi/topics/arthritis/oahandout.htm). This information is also available in Spanish. The Arthritis Foundation (http://www.arthritis.org/about-arthritis/types/osteoarthritis/) provides information on the web and in print.

Nutrition/Lifestyle Changes

The practitioner should provide the patient with information about the continued use of physical therapy, exercise, and weight loss. All of the guidelines stress the importance of nonpharmacologic recommendations in the treatment of OA.

Complementary and Alternative Medications

Glucosamine, a form of an amino acid, is a naturally occurring substance in the body. It is believed to be involved in the development and repair of cartilage. Exogenous replacement of this substance is thought to help build on existing cartilage. Evidence-based reviews of this agent suggest that moderate improvements in pain relief and function can be achieved when administered at 1,500 mg/d. This effect is thought to be similar in magnitude to that of low-dose NSAIDs or acetaminophen.

Chondroitin, a large protein-like molecule that can impart elasticity to collagen, has shown similar, but slightly less, efficacy compared to glucosamine. The dosage of chondroitin used in most of the studies was 800 to 1,200 mg/d.

The most common adverse effects associated with these products are GI discomfort, including diarrhea, heartburn, nausea, and vomiting. A concern exists that glucosamine may negatively affect blood glucose; however, this has not been proven in trials. Also, because of its uncertainty, glucosamine is not recommended in patients with poorly controlled diabetes. Since they are considered food supplements, there is little U.S. Food and Drug Administration regulation, and the preparations may vary in potency and effectiveness.

Trials that have examined the use of glucosamine and chondroitin for the treatment of OA have failed to consistently show a benefit of the combination versus placebo. In a subgroup analysis of the GAIT trial conducted by Clegg et al. (2006), patients with moderate to severe symptoms, the use of combination glucosamine and chondroitin resulted in decreased pain scales. However, this was a subgroup analysis that has not yet been verified with a subsequent trial. The ACR guidelines conditionally recommend against the use of glucosamine for the treatment of hip and knee OA.

GOUT

Historically, gout has been called the "disease of kings." For years, it was believed that gout was caused by an overindulgence in food and alcohol that only the rich could afford. While dietary factors can play a role, they are not the only risk factor leading to the development of gout.

Gout is the most common form of inflammatory arthritis in the United States. The incidence of gout in America has increased over the last 20 years and is now estimated to affect 8.3 million Americans (4%). This increase is thought to be due to the improved diagnosis but also the increasing number of patients with obesity, hypertension, thiazide diuretic use, and alcohol intake.

Gout is an inflammatory condition that results from monosodium urate crystals precipitating in the synovial fluid between joints due to hyperuricemia. The monosodium urate crystals form due to hyperuricemia either from overproduction or underexcretion of uric acid. The most common joint affected is the metatarsophalangeal joint. Other common affected joints include the midtarsal joints, ankles, knees, fingers, wrists, and elbows.

CAUSES

The overproduction or underexcretion of uric acid in the body leads to hyperuricemia. Hyperuricemia is defined as serum urate concentrations greater than 6.8 mg/dL. At levels greater than 6.8 mg/dL, serum uric acid concentrations exceed the natural saturation point, which leads to the development of monosodium urate crystals. These crystals precipitate in patients' joints causing pain, arthritis, and inflammation.

The underexcretion of uric acid through insufficient renal clearance is the most common cause of hyperuricemia. Patients with diseases that can affect the kidneys (i.e., diabetes, chronic kidney disease [CKD], etc.) or those taking drugs that can alter uric acid excretion such as thiazide diuretics and aspirin can also have insufficient renal clearance of uric acid leading to hyperuricemia.

Genetic and dietary factors play a role in the overproduction of uric acid. Typically, dietary factors alone will not cause a significant enough increase in serum urate levels to cause hyperuricemia. Foods and beverages associated with increasing urate levels can cause an acute elevation in patients who are already experiencing hyperuricemia due to genetic overproduction or renal underexcretion leading to a gout attack. A further discussion of dietary modifications that can be made to decrease gout attacks can be found in the Nutrition/Lifestyle Changes section of this chapter.

There are many other factors that can play a role in the development of gout. Female sex hormones increase the excretion of uric acid in premenopausal women. This may explain why gout is seen more in male patients than in female patients. As female patients go through menopause and sex hormones change, this can decrease their excretion of uric acid leading to postmenopausal women developing gout. Gout is also associated with advancing age in men, obesity, and comorbidities such as hypertension, CHF, and organ transplantation. A full list of risk factors for the development of gout can be found in **Box 36.4.**

BOX 36.4 | **Risk Factors for the Development of Gout**

- Males
- Advancing age
- Menopausal women
- Obesity
- Dietary factors
  - Organ meat
  - Seafood
  - Sweetened Beverages
  - Fructose
  - Ethanol
- Drugs
  - Thiazide diuretics
  - Loop diuretics
  - Cyclosporine
  - Aspirin (<1 g/d)
- Insulin resistance
- Renal insufficiency
- Hypertension
- Congestive heart failure
- Organ transplantation

PATHOPHYSIOLOGY

When hyperuricemia leads to the development of monosodium urate crystals being released into joint spaces, these crystals are phagocytized by macrophages. This phagocytosis causes the activation and release of IL-1β. IL-1β binds to synovial endothelium and causes the release of proinflammatory cytokines. Neutrophils are recruited to the synovium, which causes further release of IL-1β and other proinflammatory cytokines that perpetuates the gouty arthritis inflammatory process.

In some cases, the monosodium urate crystals alone may not be sufficient to trigger the activation and release of IL-1β from macrophages. In these cases, they require additional stimulation from free fatty acids or lipopolysaccharides to release IL-1β. When patients consume alcohol or a large meal, this can increase the free fatty acid concentration in the body and trigger the release of IL-1β.

Chronic gout and acute inflammation from gouty flares can lead to chronic pain, joint damage, and potential disability. As the disease progresses, joints may look deformed due to the development of tophi. Tophi are nodules created by monosodium urate crystals in a matrix of lipids, proteins, and mucopolysaccharides, and they may form in joint spaces. Tophi are most commonly found in the metatarsophalangeal joint, but they can also be found in other common joints affected by gout and throughout the body. Tophi can protrude through the skin and resemble a chalky substance. These urate crystals can also be found in other areas of the body, such as soft tissue, vertebrae, or skin. When they are located outside of the common joints, these crystals can mimic other disease states.

DIAGNOSTIC CRITERIA

Diagnosis of gout usually occurs clinically when a patient is experiencing rapid monoarticular arthritis, typically in the first metatarsophalangeal joint. This arthritis is accompanied by swelling and redness of the joint. The ACR diagnostic criteria that were developed in 1977 are still the most widely used form of diagnosis for patients with gout. Patients experiencing six or more of the clinical, laboratory, or radiologic criteria found in **Box 36.5** are considered to have gout.

Confirmation of a gout diagnosis can be made by aspirating monosodium urate crystals from the synovial fluid of the inflamed joint, but this is a painful and often unnecessary procedure if the patient is already displaying characteristic symptoms. Radiography can also be done using ultrasounds, MRIs, or computed tomography, but often it takes over 10 years of untreated chronic gout before crystals can be seen using one of these methods.

INITIATING DRUG THERAPY

The treatment of gout can be divided into treatment of chronic gout and treatment of acute gout attacks. The goals of drug therapy in chronic gout are to decrease the serum urate level

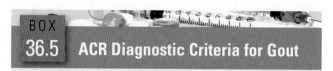

BOX 36.5 — ACR Diagnostic Criteria for Gout

More than one acute arthritis attack
Maximum joint inflammation develops within 1 day
Monoarticular arthritis attack
Joint redness
Pain or swelling of first metatarsophalangeal joint
Unilateral first metatarsophalangeal joint attack
Unilateral tarsal joint attack
Suspected tophus
Hyperuricemia
Radiography of asymmetric swelling within a joint
Radiography of subcortical cysts without erosions
Monosodium urate crystals in joint fluid during attack
Negative culture for organisms within joint fluid during an attack

to less than 6 mg/dL and to decrease the occurrence of acute gout attacks. The goal of less than 5 mg/dL may be preferred in patients with multiple risk factors or with a history of frequent acute gout attacks. Decreasing the serum urate level will help to reach the clinical goal of less pain and inflammation in the joints. For an acute gout attack, the goals are to relieve pain, terminate the attack, and maintain joint function.

The sections that follow are divided based on chronic gout treatment and acute gout attack treatment.

Chronic Gout

Urate-lowering therapies (ULT) are the primary pharmacologic treatment for chronic gout. Often, gout flares can occur when initiating ULT due to the redistribution of uric acid. To prevent these gout flares, patients should take NSAIDs or colchicine for the first 6 months of therapy. After 6 months, the number of gout flares should decrease due to the initiation of ULT. At this time, NSAIDs and colchicine can be discontinued until it is required for gouty flares.

Xanthine Oxidase Inhibitors

According to the 2012 ACR guidelines, the first-line therapy for the management of chronic gout is xanthine oxidase inhibitors (XOIs). There are currently two XOIs on the market, allopurinol and febuxostat. While allopurinol has been the mainstay of therapy for years, it does have an increased risk for hypersensitivity reactions and must be dose adjusted in patients with kidney failure. When febuxostat came to the market in 2010, it gave those patients at risk of developing hypersensitivity reactions or with kidney impairment another option for chronic gout treatment.

Mechanism of Action

XOIs decrease uric acid levels by selectively inhibiting xanthine oxidase. Xanthine oxidase is the enzyme responsible for the conversion of hypoxanthine to xanthine to uric acid.

Hypoxanthine and xanthine are then excreted in the urine with little risk of precipitation. By inhibiting the conversion to uric acid, uric acid levels are decreased, thereby reducing the risk of crystallization and a gout attack.

Dosage

Allopurinol is initially dosed 100 mg once daily and should be gradually titrated by 100 mg/d in 2- to 5-week increments until uric acid is less than 6 mg/dL. The usual dosage is 300 mg daily either once daily or taken in divided doses up to four times daily. The max dose is 800 mg/d. Patients with stage 4 or worse CKD should start at 50 mg/d and titrate up to a therapeutic dosage.

Febuxostat is dosed 40 mg once daily and may be increased to the FDA-approved max dose of 80 mg once daily in patients who do not achieve a serum uric acid level less than 6 mg/dL after 2 weeks. According to the ACR guidelines and international standards, febuxostat can be increased up to 120 mg daily in refractory cases. Febuxostat is metabolized through the liver and can be used in patients with mild to moderate kidney impairment without dose reduction.

Time Frame for Response

Serum urate levels can begin to fall as early as 2 weeks following initiation of chronic gout therapy. Serum uric acid levels should be drawn every 2 to 5 weeks during dose titration until desired level is reached, which may take up to 6 months. Once goal serum uric acid levels are achieved, the patient should have levels drawn every 6 months throughout treatment.

Contraindications

Pegloticase should not be administered with allopurinol or febuxostat. Using both agents could increase the risk of infusion site reactions or anaphylaxis with the pegloticase. Allopurinol should not be used with didanosine as it may increase the serum concentrations of didanosine leading to toxicity. Allopurinol and febuxostat can inhibit the metabolism of azathioprine and mercaptopurine leading to toxic doses and should not be used concurrently.

Adverse Events

Common adverse reactions that can occur with the use of XOIs include rash, arthralgias, and GI complications, which can be reduced by taking the medication with food. Allopurinol and febuxostat have been associated with liver function abnormalities. Liver function tests should be performed at baseline periodically throughout treatment.

Allopurinol, although generally well tolerated, does have a risk of hypersensitivity reactions. Allopurinol hypersensitivity syndrome consists of a rash (Stevens-Johnson syndrome and toxic epidermal necrolysis), fever, impaired liver and kidney function, leukocytosis, and eosinophilia. The risk of allopurinol hypersensitivity syndrome increases in patients with kidney dysfunction or those of certain ethnic populations that are more genetically predisposed to the reaction. Prior to initiating allopurinol, Koreans with stage 3 or worse CKD, Han Chinese, and Thai patients should receive genetic testing for the HLA-B*5801 allele. Patients that report HLA-B*5801 positive should be prescribed alternative therapy to allopurinol. Patients should be counseled to report a rash immediately to their health care provider.

Interactions

The use of ACE inhibitors, thiazide, and loop diuretics along with allopurinol may increase the levels of allopurinol and increase the risk of allopurinol hypersensitivity syndrome. Before initiating allopurinol with patients on antineoplastic agents, interactions should be evaluated. Multiple antineoplastic agents are affected by allopurinol, and the effects can range from noneffective antineoplastic treatment to toxicity. INR levels should be monitored when patients are taking both allopurinol and warfarin as allopurinol may increase bleeding risk due to decreased warfarin metabolism.

As previously mentioned, both allopurinol and febuxostat inhibit the metabolism of mercaptopurine and azathioprine. Concurrent use should be avoided if possible. Febuxostat is contraindicated with these agents. However, allopurinol can be used, but the azathioprine or mercaptopurine dose needs to be reduced to 1/3 to 1/4 of the typical dose and monitored closely for toxicity.

Probenecid

If at least one XOI is contraindicated or not tolerated well, practitioners should use probenecid for the treatment of chronic gout.

Mechanism of Action

Probenecid increases the excretion of serum uric acid by competitively inhibiting the reabsorption of uric acid at the proximal convoluted tubule.

Dosage

The initial dose is 250 mg twice daily for 1 week, and the dose is then increased to 500 mg twice daily if needed. The dose can be increased in 500-mg increments every 4 weeks to a maximum of 2 g/d. Once serum uric acid levels are within normal limits and no gout attacks have occurred for 6 months, the dose can be reduced by 500 mg every 6 months.

Time Frame for Response

As with the XOIs, serum uric acid levels will begin to decrease within 2 weeks but may take up to 6 months to see full effect.

Contraindications

Probenecid should not be given during an acute gout attack as it could exacerbate the symptoms when initiated. It also should not be given to patients who have been diagnosed with blood dyscrasias, uric acid kidney stones, children less than 2 years old, or anyone who has a past medical history of a reaction with probenecid. Patients should also not use ketorolac while taking probenecid, because it may increase the concentration of ketorolac leading to toxic symptoms such as nausea, gastric ulcers, headache, and edema.

Adverse Events

There are many adverse effects associated with probenecid. Serious reactions that can occur include hemolytic anemia and aplastic anemia in patients with G6PD deficiency, hepatic necrosis, and anaphylaxis. Other less serious but common reactions include headache, dizziness, anorexia, nausea vomiting, gingival soreness, urinary frequency, renal colic, nephrotic syndrome, dermatitis, pruritus, flushing fever, and gout exacerbations.

Interactions

Avoid the use of probenecid with antibiotics including penicillin derivatives, cephalosporins, and fluoroquinolones as probenecid may increase the concentrations of the antibiotics increasing the risk of adverse effects and toxicities associated with these drugs. The use of methotrexate with probenecid may result in methotrexate toxicity including leukopenia, thrombocytopenia, anemia, and nephrotoxicity. Using citalopram with probenecid may increase citalopram concentrations, increasing the risk of QT prolongation, and its use with lorazepam can also increase lorazepam concentrations leading to toxicity. The use of probenecid with aspirin and other salicylates may reverse the uricosuric effect of probenecid. As with XOIs, probenecid should not be used with pegloticase due to an increased risk of anaphylaxis and infusion reactions of the pegloticase.

Pegloticase

Pegloticase is used as last-line therapy for patients with chronic gout that has not successfully been treated with either XOIs or probenecid. It must be administered intravenously in a health care facility every 2 weeks and costs more than $5,000 per dose.

Mechanism of Action

Pegloticase is a pegylated recombinant form of uricase. Uricase is an enzyme typically absent in humans but is found in high levels in primates. Uricase converts uric acid to allantoin, which is an inactive, water-soluble metabolite of uric acid allowing uric acid to be easily excreted by the kidneys.

Dosage

The recommended dose for pegloticase is 8 mg IV over at least 2 hours every 2 weeks. Before beginning pegloticase infusions, patients should discontinue the use of any oral antihyperuricemic agents and should not begin taking oral medications for chronic gout throughout the course of therapy.

Gouty flares can occur from initiating a new therapy and can be prevented by using NSAIDs or colchicine. It is recommended to begin this prophylaxis at least 1 week prior to initiating pegloticase and to continue for 6 months.

Patient should also be pretreated with antihistamines and corticosteroids prior to the infusion. This will help patients with any infusion reactions and potential anaphylaxis.

Time Frame for Response

The reduction of uric acid concentrations can be seen as soon as 1 day after the infusion. For patients who are responders to pegloticase, the reduction can be maintained for at least 6 months.

Contraindications

Pegloticase is contraindicated in patients with glucose-6-phosphate dehydrogenase deficiency.

Adverse Events

As with all of the chronic gout medications, pegloticase can cause potential gout flares within the first few months of treatment. Prophylaxis for these gout flares is recommended for the first 6 months of treatment with colchicine or an NSAID.

Injection site reactions such as, bruising, urticaria, erythema, and pruritus are also common. Administering antihistamines and corticosteroids with each infusion can decrease these injection site reactions in most patients.

Some patients also experience GI-related symptoms such as nausea, vomiting, and constipation with pegloticase.

Antipegloticase antibodies form in 92% of patients and anti-PEG antibodies in 42%. These antibodies may result in a loss of response to pegloticase as early as 4 months into treatment.

Pegloticase does hold a black box warning for hypersensitivity and anaphylaxis reactions. Anaphylaxis has been reported during and after administration. Due to these reactions, patients should receive pegloticase infusions in a health care facility while being closely monitored during and for a period of time after administration. Most reactions occur within 2 hours of administration, but some patients have had delayed hypersensitivity reactions. The risk of these infusion reactions increases in patients whose uric acid level is greater than 6 mg/dL. Health care practitioners should monitor serum uric acid levels prior to infusion and discontinuing treatment if patients' concentrations are greater than 6 mg/dL on two consecutive measurements.

Interactions

Patients taking pegloticase should discontinue all other chronic gout medications. Allopurinol, febuxostat, and probenecid may increase the levels of pegloticase and increase the risk of infusion reactions and anaphylaxis.

SELECTING THE MOST APPROPRIATE DRUG

In 2012, the ACR developed guidelines for the management of gout and the treatment of hyperuricemia (Khanna, 2012a). In addition to outlining the treatment options, they defined which patients should be initiated on chronic ULT. The criteria for initiating long-term ULT include patients with a diagnosis of gouty arthritis and one of the four following criteria: tophi or tophus, two or more gouty attacks yearly, CKD stage 2 or worse, or past urolithiasis. For those meeting criteria for chronic ULT, the options include XOIs, probenecid, and pegloticase.

First-Line Therapy

The initiation of either allopurinol or febuxostat should be used as first-line therapy for chronic gout. The ACR did not provide preference of one agent over the other. These agents can effectively lower serum uric acid in patients who are underexcretors

or overproducers. If a patient has an intolerance or adverse effect to one XOI, the other one can be substituted. The XOIs are considered first-line agents due to their efficacy and relative safety.

As previously mentioned, regardless of the agent selected, patients need to be initiated on acute gout prophylaxis when chronic ULT is started. This acute gout prophylaxis could include NSAIDs or colchicine and should be continued for 6 months.

Second-Line Therapy

If at least one XOI is contraindicated or not tolerated well, probenecid is the second-line agent. Probenecid is associated with more drug interactions and cannot be used in patients with a history of urolithiasis.

If a patient is on a XOI at maximal appropriate dose and the goal serum urate concentration is not achieve, probenecid can be added to the XOI and titrated to goal.

Third-Line Therapy

For patients who are on both a XOI and probenecid and are unable to achieve their uric acid goal and continue to have disease activity, pegloticase can be initiated after discontinuation of other ULT.

Acute Gout

Patients with chronic gout will commonly experience gout attacks. Making dietary modifications and discontinuing the usage of medications that can induce gout attacks, weight loss, and controlling other diseases states will help decrease the frequency of attacks, but they will occur in gout patients. When an acute gout attack occurs, patients can rest the joint and apply ice as needed to help with the pain. They can also use short courses of NSAIDs, corticosteroids, or colchicine to reduce the pain.

NSAIDs

NSAIDs can help decrease inflammation and pain during acute gout attacks. Naproxen, indomethacin, and sulindac are the three NSAIDs indicated for the treatment of acute gout. NSAIDs should be initiated at onset of the gout attack and continued for 24 hours after the resolution of symptoms. The usual course of treatment is 3 to 7 days. See the discussion of NSAIDs in the OA section of this chapter for more information about NSAIDs. See **Table 36.3** for appropriate dosing for acute gout attacks.

TABLE 36.3

NSAID Dosing for Acute Gout

Drug	Dose
naproxen	750 mg initially followed by 250 mg every 8 h until attack subsides
indomethacin	50 mg three times daily until pain is tolerable then reduce dose
sulindac	200 mg twice daily

Systemic Corticosteroids

Systemic corticosteroids can be given to patients to help decrease inflammation during an acute gout attack. Most patients will tolerate a short duration of oral corticosteroids; those that do not may benefit from an intramuscular dose. If a patient's gout attack is focused in 1 to 2 large joints, the clinician may choose to provide an intra-articular dose alone or in addition to oral corticosteroids.

Mechanism of Action

Corticosteroids decrease inflammation by suppressing the migration of polymorphonuclear leukocytes. Leukocytes cause a further release of IL-1β and other proinflammatory cytokines that lead to the inflammation associated with gouty arthritis.

Dosage

For oral doses, patients can take prednisone or methylprednisolone. Patient taking prednisone should use 0.5 mg/kg for 5 to 10 days or 0.5 mg/kg for 2 to 5 days and then taper 7 to 10 days. Clinicians can also choose to use a methylprednisolone dose pack. This dose pack contains (21) 4-mg tablets. These are tapered from six tablets on day 1, five tablets on day 2, and so forth until the patient is only taking one tablet on day 6.

For patients unable to take oral corticosteroids, an intramuscular dose of methylprednisolone 0.5 to 2 mg/kg for one dose can be given. This dose can be repeated as clinically indicated.

For patients experiencing pain in 1 to 2 large joints, an intra-articular dose of triamcinolone acetonide can be given. The dose is dependent on the size of the joint being treated. Large joints such as knees can be given 40 mg of triamcinolone, medium joints such as wrist ankles and elbows can be given 30-mg injections, and smaller joints can be given 10-mg injections.

Time Frame for Response

Patients should start to feel pain relief in 1 to 2 days. It may take up to a week for complete resolution.

Contraindications

Oral corticosteroids should be used with caution in patients with suppressed immune systems, diabetes, uncontrolled HTN, cardiovascular disease, and psychiatric disorders. If patients are requiring a corticosteroid and have one of these conditions, they may be a good candidate for an intra-articular dose as these will have less of a systemic effect.

Adverse Events

Adverse effects of corticosteroids are extensive. By limiting the duration of treatment, many of the more chronic adverse effects will be avoided. However, even using corticosteroids for 5 to 10 days may results in acute adverse effects. These acute adverse effects include hyperglycemia, hypertension, fluid retention, CNS stimulation, and dyspepsia. Patients at risk for these conditions need to be monitored closely while on corticosteroids.

Interactions

Interactions associated with corticosteroids are more severe when associated with long-term treatment. With the short-term use of corticosteroids being used to treat gout, there are few interactions.

The interactions that should be monitored are with specific disease states. Diabetic patients should monitor their blood sugar more closely as corticosteroids may cause an increase in blood sugar levels. Patients with hypertension, CHF, and fluid retention should also monitor their blood pressure and symptoms as corticosteroids can cause edema leading to worsening HTN and CHF. Corticosteroids also cause immunosuppression so use caution in patients where immunosuppression needs to be avoided.

Colchicine

Colchicine has been used for the treatment of gout, Mediterranean fever, and multiple cardiovascular diseases for centuries. Although colchicine has had widespread use for many years, it was only approved by the FDA in 2009 under the unapproved drugs initiative. With this approval, there were changes to the dosing regimen and a new focus on safety related to comorbidities and drug–drug interactions.

Mechanism of Action

Colchicine inhibits the activation, degranulation, and migration of neutrophils to the area of a gout attack. This then decreases the inflammation and pain associated with a gout attack.

Dosage

For acute gout attacks, patients should be given their first dose within 24 hours of symptom onset. Colchicine is not recommended if symptoms started more than 36 hours prior. Patients should take 1.2 mg at first sign of gout flare followed by 0.6 mg 1 hour later. They can then take 0.6 mg daily or BID starting 12 hours later and continue until the attack resolves. Patients with severe renal failure (CrCl < 30 mL/min) should have the dose reduced to 0.3 mg daily. These patients should be monitored closely for adverse effects and should not repeat treatment more than once every 2 weeks.

Prophylactic doses of colchicine to prevent gout attack during initiation of chronic gout treatment are 0.6 mg once or twice daily for up to 6 months after achieving target serum urate levels. If a patient is receiving prophylactic dosing and experiences a gout attack, they can begin the acute gout dose. They should wait 12 hours from their last dose of acute gout treatment before resuming the prophylactic dosing.

When patients are also taking P-glycoprotein (P-gp) or CYP3A4 inducers, their dosing needs to be altered to prevent colchicine toxicities. See **Table 36.4** for dosage adjustments with P-gp or CYP3A4 inducers (**Figure 36.3**).

Time Frame for Response

Colchicine begins to provide its pain relief within 18 to 24 hours. It can take up to 48 hours to have its full anti-inflammatory effect.

Contraindications

Patients who have renal or hepatic impairment or those taking P-gp inhibitors or strong CYP3A4 inhibitors should use caution and possible lower doses of colchicine. Patients with both renal and hepatic impairments and also taking a P-gp inhibitor or strong CYP3A4 inhibitor should not take colchicine as it may cause fatal colchicine toxicity.

TABLE 36.4

Prophylactic Colchicine Dosing Dependent on Interactions

Usual Treatment	Strong 3A4 Inhibitor	Moderate 3A4 Inhibitor	P-gp Inhibitor	CrCl < 30 mL/min
0.6 mg twice daily	0.3 mg daily	0.3 mg BID or 0.6 mg daily	0.3 mg daily	0.3 mg daily
0.6 mg daily	0.3 mg every other day	0.3 mg daily	0.3 mg every other day	

Adverse Events

The most common adverse effects of colchicine are GI effects in particular diarrhea. Some patients also experience pharyngolaryngeal pain, fatigue, and headache when being treated for gout flares. Other more uncommon but serious adverse effects of colchicine include blood dyscrasias and neuromuscular toxicity including rhabdomyolysis.

Interactions

Colchicine is a substrate of the efflux transporter P-gp, and it is mainly metabolized by CYP3A4. Because of these pharmacokinetic properties, colchicine has many drug interactions with P-gp and CYP3A4 inhibitors. If P-gp or CYP3A4 inhibitors are coadministered with colchicine, it can cause increased

concentrations of colchicine, which can potentially be fatal. In addition to its anti-inflammatory effects, colchicine inhibits cell mitosis. Inhibition of cell mitosis can lead to organ system dysfunction and failure. Cardiac effects are most commonly seen in patients who have taken increased concentrations of colchicine. Since many drugs are P-gp and CYP3A4 inhibitors, it is important to be aware of the strength of the inhibition. This will help the clinician to judge if the drug should be avoided, if the dose should be adjusted, or if the patient should just be monitored while taking the drugs concomitantly. **Figure 36.3** lists common drug interactions with colchicine and the degree to which the drug inhibits P-gp or CYP3A4. **Table 36.4** lists the dose adjustments for colchicine based on the clinician's assessment of the drug interaction and renal function.

SELECTING THE MOST APPROPRIATE DRUG

The ACR created guidelines for the treatment of acute gout attacks in 2012 (Khanna, 2012b). Prior to determining appropriate therapy, the patient's attack needs to be classified as mild, moderate, or severe. This is determined based on the patient's reported pain score with mild being less than or equal to 4, moderate being 5 to 6, and severe being greater than or equal to 7. Also, the location needs to be considered. The ACR breaks down the extent of the attack into one or few small joints, 1 or 2 large joints (ankle, knee, wrist, elbow, hip or shoulder), or polyarticular

	CYP 3A4 Inhibitors	P-glycoprotein inhibitors
Strong Inhibitors	Clarithromycin	Cyclosporine
	Telithromycin	Ketoconazole
	Nefazodone	Tacrolimus
	Indinavir	Amiodarone
	Saquinavir	Clarithromycin
	Ritonavir	Verapamil
	Atazanavir	Telaprevir
	Ketoconazole	Ranolazine
	Itraconazole	Itraconazole
	Grapefruit juice	Grapefruit juice
	Erythromycin	Saquinavir
	Fluconazole	Lovastatin
	Verapamil	Simvastatin
	Diltiazem	Atorvastatin
	Fluoxetine	Erythromycin
	Cimetidine	
	Atorvastatin	
Weak Inhibitors	Amiodarone	

FIGURE 36.3 Drug interactions with colchicine.

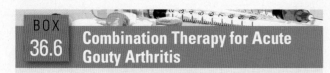

BOX 36.6 Combination Therapy for Acute Gouty Arthritis

Colchicine + NSAID
Oral corticosteroid + colchicine
Intra-articular steroid + (NSAID or colchicine or oral corticosteroid)

(4 or more joints). Based on the location and severity of pain, the appropriate treatments can be determined.

First-Line Therapy

For patients with mild to moderate pain in small joints or 1 to 2 large joints, initial therapy includes NSAIDs, systemic corticosteroids, or colchicine. If the pain started more than 36 hours prior, then colchicine is no longer a preferred agent. For patients with diabetes, heart failure, hypertension, or other conditions predisposing them to adverse effects of corticosteroids, steroids would not be the preferred agent. Patients may want to also supplement pharmacologic treatment with topical ice applied to the affected joint(s) as needed.

For patients with severe pain or polyarticular attacks, combination therapy is recommended as initial therapy. **Box 36.6** lists common combinations recommended for acute gout treatment.

Second-Line Therapy

If monotherapy is not effective, the patient can switch to another first-line therapy or switch to combination therapy (**Box 36.6**). NSAIDs and corticosteroids are not recommended as a combination due to the overlap in toxicities and should be avoided in the treatment of gout.

SPECIAL CONSIDERATIONS

Ethnic/Genomics

As mentioned in the discussion of allopurinol, Korean, Han Chinese, and Thai patients have a higher probability of having an allopurinol hypersensitivity reaction due to the HLA-B*5801 genetic allele. All Han Chinese and Thai patients and Korean patients with stage 3 or worse CKD should be genetically tested for the HLA-B*5801 allele before beginning allopurinol therapy. If the patients test positive, they should be given alternative therapy to allopurinol.

MONITORING PATIENT RESPONSE

Patients should have their serum urate levels monitored during the titration of XOIs or probenecid every 2 to 5 weeks. Once target serum urate level is achieved (less than 6 mg/dL or less than 5 mg/dL), the patients should be monitored every 6 months.

It is very common for patients with gout to also have hypertension and renal insufficiency, so it is important that they also undergo appropriate assessments for their renal and cardiovascular systems. Baseline lab tests should include complete blood cell count, urinalysis, serum creatinine, blood urea nitrogen, and serum uric acid measurements.

Nephrolithiasis occurs in approximately 10% to 25% of patients with primary gout. The solubility of uric acid crystals increases when the urine pH becomes more alkaline. Acidic urine saturated with uric acid crystals may result in spontaneous stone formation. Patients should be warned about this complication and should be treated appropriately if stones occur.

PATIENT EDUCATION

To prevent acute gout attacks, patients can follow some nutritional and lifestyle modifications listed below. During an acute attack, patients should be counseled to elevate, ice, and rest the affected joint(s).

Drug Information

Patient-Oriented Information Sources

The ACR Web site has a section targeted to patients (https://www.rheumatology.org/practice/clinical/patients/diseases_and_conditions/gout.as). There is a page regarding gout that includes basic facts and lists of other resources for patients.

Nutrition/Lifestyle Changes

Dietary modifications can help to decrease the risk and frequency of acute gout attacks. Decreasing purine-rich foods, sweetened beverages, and alcohol will help decrease the serum urate levels. **Box 36.7** has a full list of foods to decrease or avoid the consumption of in patients with gout. Patients should also increase their consumption of water, vegetables,

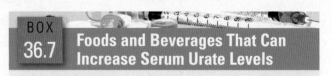

BOX 36.7 Foods and Beverages That Can Increase Serum Urate Levels

Red meat: (specifically organ meat)
    Kidney
    Liver
    Sweetbreads
Seafood:
    Sardines
    Shellfish
High-fructose corn syrup:
    Sodas or sports drinks
    Foods containing high levels
Alcohol
    Especially beer
    Also wine and spirits

CASE STUDY*

G.P., a 66-year-old, right-handed white man, seeks treatment for swelling and decreased range of motion in the right knee. He tells you he retired at age 65 after 40 years of assembly-line work. He reports that his physical activity has decreased and his weight has increased 20 pounds since retiring. His hobbies include woodworking and playing cards and playing with his two grandchildren. He denies tobacco use and alcohol use.

Although he describes several years of joint pain that gradually worsened, his activities were not limited until approximately 6 months ago, when he noted an insidious onset of swelling in the right knee. Over the years, he has sporadically taken acetaminophen, aspirin, and ibuprofen to control the pain. He reports that none of the drugs provided better relief than the others. His medical history is remarkable for hypertension and three episodes of gout.

DIAGNOSIS: OSTEOARTHRITIS

1. List specific goals of treatment for G.P.
2. What drug therapy would you prescribe, and why?
3. What are the parameters for monitoring success of the therapy?
4. Discuss specific patient education based on the prescribed therapy.
5. List one or two adverse reactions for the selected agent that would cause you to change therapy.
6. What would be the choice for second-line therapy?
7. What over-the-counter and/or alternative medications would be appropriate for G.P.?
8. What lifestyle changes should be recommended for G.P.?
9. Describe one or two drug–drug or drug–food interactions for the selected agent.

* Answers can be found online.

and nonfat dairy as they have been shown to lower the risk of gout. Improving overall health status through weight loss and smoking cessation and closely monitoring and treating comorbidities, such as coronary artery disease, obesity, diabetes, hyperlipidemia, and hypertension, can also help decrease the risk of gout and prevent gouty flares.

Complementary and Alternative Medicine

Studies have shown that vitamin C inhibits uric acid synthesis and lowers serum uric acid levels. In a 2011 meta-analysis by Juraschek et al. (2011) of 13 trials, researchers studied the effect of oral vitamin C supplementation on serum uric acid levels. This trial showed that a mean dose of 500 mg/d of vitamin C reduced serum urate levels 0.32 mg/dL. This dose is well over the recommended dietary allowance for vitamin C (90 mg/d men; 75 mg/d women) but is still under the maximum tolerable intake of 2 g/d. Vitamin C along with dietary modifications may be an option for some patients who do not tolerate pharmacologic therapy or wish to have an additional benefit with their pharmacologic therapy.

Bibliography

*Starred references are cited in text.

Altman, R., Alarcon, G., Appelrouth, D., et al. (1991). The American College of Rheumatology criteria for the classification and reporting of osteoarthritis of the hip. Arthritis and Rheumatism, 34, 505–514.

Altman, R., Asch, E., Bloch, D., et al. (1986). The American College of Rheumatology criteria for the classification and reporting of osteoarthritis of the knee. Arthritis and Rheumatism, 29, 1039–1049.

Altman R. D., Barthel H. R. (2011). Topical therapies for osteoarthritis. Drugs, 71(10), 1259–1279.

American College of Rheumatology. (1977). Criteria for the classification of acute arthritis of primary gout. Retrieved from https://www.rheumatology.org/ACR/practice/clinical/classification/gout.asp on May 15, 2015.

Bannuru R. R., Schmid C. H., Kent D. M., et al. (2015). Comparative effectiveness of pharmacologic interventions for knee osteoarthritis: A systematic review and network meta-analysis. Annals of Internal Medicine, 162, 46–54.

*Chan, F. K., Lanas, A., Scheiman, J., et al. (2010). Celecoxib versus omeprazole and diclofenac in patients with osteoarthritis and rheumatoid arthritis (CONDOR): A randomized trial. Lancet, 376, 173–179.

Chappell, A. S., Desaiah, D., Liu-Seifert, H., et al. (2010). A double-blind, randomized, placebo-controlled study of the efficacy and safety of duloxetine for the treatment of chronic pain due to osteoarthritis of the knee. Pain Practice, 11(1), 33–41.

*Clegg, D. O., Reda, D. J., Harris, C. L., et al. (2006). Glucosamine, chondroitin sulphate, and the two in combination for painful knee osteoarthritis. New England Journal of Medicine, 354(8), 795–808.

Cymbalta [package insert]. (2014). Indianapolis, IN: Eli Lilly and Company.

Danelich, I. M., Wright, S. S., Lose, J. M., et al. (2015). Safety of nonsteroidal anti-inflammatory drugs in patients with cardiovascular disease. Pharmacotherapy. doi: 10.1002/phar.1584.

Doherty, M., Hawkey, C., Goulder, M., et al. (2011). A randomised controlled trial of ibuprofen, paracetamol or a combination tablet of ibuprofen/paracetamol in community-derived people with knee pain. Annals of the Rheumatic Diseases, 70, 1534–1541.

Felson, D. T. (2015). Osteoarthritis. In D. Kasper, A. Fauci, S. Hauser, et al., (Eds.), Harrison's principles of internal medicine (19th ed.). Retrieved from http://accesspharmacy.mhmedical.com/content.aspx?bookid=1130&Sectionid=79751047 on May 07, 2015.

Finkelstein, Y., Aks, S. E., Juurlik, D. N., et al. (2010). Colchicine poisoning: The dark side of the ancient drug. Clinical Toxicology, 48(5), 407–414.

Grosser, T., Smyth, E., & FitzGerald, G. A. (2011). Anti-inflammatory, antipyretic, and analgesic agents; pharmacotherapy of gout. In L. L. Brunton, B. A. Chabner, & B. C. Knollmann, (Eds.), Goodman & Gilman's the pharmacological basis of therapeutics (12th ed., Chapter 34). Retrieved May 18, 2015. New York, NY: McGraw-Hill.

Gonzalez, E. B. (2012). An update on the pathology and clinical management of gouty arthritis. Clinical Rheumatology, 31, 13–21.

Hainer, B. L., Matheson, E., & Wilkes, R. T. (2014) Diagnosis, treatment, and prevention of gout. American Family Physician, 90(12), 831–836.

*Hawkey, C. J., Karrasch, J. A., Szczepanski, L., et al. (1998). Omeprazole compared with misoprostol for ulcers associated with nonsteroidal anti-inflammatory drugs. New England Journal of Medicine, 338, 727–734.

Helmick, C. G., Felson, D. T., Lawrence, R. C., et al. (2008). Estimates of the prevalence of arthritis and other rheumatic conditions in the United States: Part 1. *Arthritis and Rheumatism, 58*(1), 15–25.

Hochberg, M. C., Altman, R. D., April, K. T., et al. (2012). American College of Rheumatology 2012 recommendations for the use of nonpharmacologic and pharmacologic therapies in osteoarthritis of the hand, hip and knee. *Arthritis Care and Research, 64*(4), 465–474.

Hochberg, M. C., Martel-Pelletier, J., Monfort, J., et al. (2015). Combined chondroitin sulphate and glucosamine for painful knee osteoarthritis: A multicentre, randomised, double-blind, non-inferiority trial versus celecoxib. *Annals of the Rheumatic Diseases.* doi: 10.1136/annrheumdis-2014-206792.

Jordan, K. M., Arden, N. K., Doherty, M., et al. (2003). EULAR recommendations 2003: An evidence based approach to the management of knee osteoarthritis: Report of a Task Force of the Standing Committee for International Clinical Studies Including Therapeutic Trials (ESCISIT). *Annals of the Rheumatic Diseases, 62,* 1145–1155.

*Juraschek, S. P., Miller, E. R., Gelber, A. C. (2011) Effect of oral vitamin C supplementation on serum uric acid: A meta-analysis of randomized controlled trials. *Arthritis Care and Research, 63*(9), 1295–1306.

*Khanna, D., Fitzgerald, J. D., Khanna, P. P., et al. (2012a). American College of Rheumatology guidelines for management of gout. Part 1: Systematic nonpharmacologic and pharmacologic therapeutic approaches to hyperuricemia. *Arthritis Care and Research, 64*(10), 1431–1446.

*Khanna, D., Khanna, P. P., Fitzgerald, J. D., et al. (2012b). American College of Rheumatology guidelines for management of gout. Part 2: Therapy and anti-inflammatory prophylaxis of acute gouty arthritis. *Arthritis Care and Research, 64*(10), 1447–1461.

Kim, S. C., Newcomb, C., Margolis, D., et al. (2013). Severe cutaneous reactions requiring hospitalization in allopurinol initiators: A population-based cohort study. *Arthritis Care and Research, 65*(4), 578–584.

Loeser, R. F., Goldring, S. R., Scanzelloo, C. R., et al. (2012). Osteoarthritis: A disease of the joint as an organ. *Arthritis and Rheumatism, 64*(6), 1697–1707.

McAlindon, T. E., Bannuru, R. R., Sullivan, M. C., et al. (2014). OARSI guidelines for the non-surgical management of knee osteoarthritis. *Osteoarthritis and Cartilage, 22*(3), 363–388.

Murphy, L., & Helmick, C. G. (2012). The impact of osteoarthritis in the United States: A population-health perspective. *American Journal of Nursing, 112*(3), S13–S17.

Myers, J., Wielage, R. C., Han, B. (2014). The efficacy of duloxetine, non-steroidal anti-inflammatory drugs, and opioid in osteoarthritis: A systematic literature review and meta-analysis. *BMC Musculoskeletal Disorders, 15,* 76.

National Center for Chronic Disease Prevention and Health Promotion. (2010). *Arthritis: Meeting the challenge.* Retrieved from www.cdc.gov/arthritis

Neogi, T. (2011). Gout. *New England Journal of Medicine, 364,* 443–452.

Singh, J. A., Reddy, S. F., & Kundukulam, J. (2011). Risk factors for gout and prevention: A systematic review of the literature. *Current Opinion in Rheumatology, 23*(2), 192–202.

Silverstein, F. E., Faich, G., Goldstein, J. L., et al. (2000). Gastrointestinal toxicity with celecoxib vs nonsteroidal anti-inflammatory drugs for osteoarthritis and rheumatoid arthritis: The CLASS study: A randomized controlled trial. *Journal of the American Medical Association, 284*(10), 1247–1255.

Slobodnick, A., Shah, B., Pillinger, M. H., et al. (2015). Colchicine: Old and new. *The American Journal of Medicine, 128,* 461–470.

Sundy, J. S., Baraf, H. S., Yood, R. A., et al. (2011). Efficacy and tolerability of pegloticase for the treatment of chronic gout in patients refractory to conventional treatment: Two randomized controlled trials. *Journal of the American Medical Association, 306*(7), 711–720.

Towheed, T., Maxwell, L., Judd, M., et al. (2009). Acetaminophen for osteoarthritis (review). *Cochrane Database of Systematic Reviews, 1,* CD004257.

U.S. Food and Drug Administration. (2012). Full Prescribing Information for colchicine. Retrieved from http://www.accessdata.fda.gov/drugsatfda_docs/label/2014/022352s017lbl.pdf on May 15, 2015.

Wallace, S. L., Robinson, H., Masi, A. T., et al. (1977). Preliminary criteria for the classification of the acute arthritis of primary gout. *Arthritis and Rheumatism, 20*(3), 895–900.

*Yeomans, N. D., Tulassay, Z., Laszlo, J., et al. (1998). A comparison of omeprazole with ranitidine for ulcers associated with nonsteroidal anti-inflammatory drugs. *New England Journal of Medicine, 338,* 719–726.

Zhang, W., Doherty, M., Arden, N., et al. (2005). EULAR evidence based recommendations for the management of hip osteoarthritis: Report of a Task Force of the Standing Committee for International Clinical Studies Including Therapeutic Trials (ESCISIT). *Annals of the Rheumatic Diseases, 64,* 669–681.

Zhang, W., Doherty, M., Leeb, B. F., et al. (2007). EULAR evidence based recommendations for the management of hand osteoarthritis: Report of a Task Force of the Standing Committee for International Clinical Studies Including Therapeutic Trials (ESCISIT). *Annals of the Rheumatic Diseases, 66,* 377–388.

Zhang, W., Moskowitz, R. W., Nuki, G., et al. (2008). OARSI recommendations for the management of hip and knee osteoarthritis, Part II: OARSI evidence-based, expert consensus guidelines. *Osteoarthritis and Cartilage, 16,* 137–162.

Zhu, Y., Pandya, B. J., & Choi, H. K. (2011). Prevalence of gout and hyperuricemia in the US general population. *Arthritis and Rheumatism, 61*(10), 3136–3141.

37 Rheumatoid Arthritis

Lauren K. McCluggage ■ Carol Gullo Mest

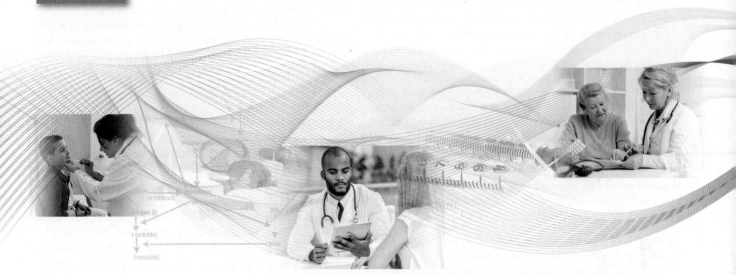

Rheumatoid arthritis (RA) is a chronic autoimmune inflammatory disease characterized by symmetric polyarthritis and joint changes, including erythema, effusion, and tenderness. The course of RA is characterized by remissions and exacerbations. RA can affect several organs, but it usually involves synovial tissue changes in the freely movable joints (diarthroses). RA most commonly affects small joints, including the wrists, second through fifth metatarsophalangeal joints, proximal interphalangeal joints, and metacarpophalangeal joints. RA may also affect large joints, including the elbows, shoulders, neck, hips, knees, and ankles.

In 2008, approximately 0.6% of the adult population in the United States had RA, with the prevalence in women about twice of that in men (Helmick et al., 2008). New onset of RA is seen throughout the life span, including infancy, but most cases occur in the fifth or sixth decade. Recent data have shown that diagnosis is occurring later in life, and the overall prevalence is decreasing. Previous data have shown that patients with RA have a higher rate of disability and mortality compared to patients of similar age without RA. However, with the increased use of disease-modifying antirheumatic drugs (DMARDs), especially early in the disease process, these risks appear to have normalized (Kroot et al., 2000).

CAUSES

The cause of RA continues to be the subject of research. Theories of causation include genetic factors, infectious agents, environmental factors, and an antigen–antibody response. It is unlikely that a single factor is responsible for all cases of RA.

PATHOPHYSIOLOGY

The major physiologic changes associated with RA include synovial membrane proliferation followed by erosion of the subarticular cartilage and subchondral bone. Although the precise etiology of RA is unknown, mounting evidence points to a series of immunologic events. It is unclear whether an infectious, viral, or genetic agent prompts these events.

Specific major histocompatibility complex class II alleles and human leukocyte antigen are seen more frequently in patients with RA. These molecules are responsible for processing and presenting antigenic material to CD4+ T cells. The exact antigen that initiates the following cascade is unknown but could be an exogenous or endogenous protein. T-cell activation stimulates monocytes, macrophages, and synovial fibroblasts to produce proinflammatory cytokines, including tumor necrosis factor (TNF) alpha, interleukin (IL)-1, and IL-6. During this process, matrix metalloproteinases are also released, causing major destruction in the joint cartilage. The activated T cells stimulate B cells, which then produce immunoglobulins, including rheumatoid factor (RF) and anti–citrullinated protein antibody (ACPA). The activation of the macrophages, monocytes, and synovial fibroblasts along with the release of cytokines stimulates angiogenesis in the synovial membrane. TNF-alpha is a key inflammatory mediator because it induces further production of proinflammatory cytokines and stimulates expression of adhesion molecules on endothelial cells. The expression of adhesion molecules promotes recruitment of leukocytes and more inflammatory cells. The result is a self-perpetuating inflammatory cycle.

Early Phase

In the early phase of RA, the synovium becomes more vascularized, and proliferation and hypertrophy begin. This results in the synovial tissue becoming edematous and exhibiting frond-like villi. As leukocytes proliferate, the synovial fluid becomes less viscous.

Progression

As RA progresses to the chronic form, continued hyperplasia and hypertrophy of the synovial lining occur. The thickness of the synovial lining increases up to fivefold from the normal one or two cell layers. The proliferation of the synovium persists, with lymphocytic tissue and plasma cells forming around blood vessels. This proliferative tissue extends into the joint space, joint capsule, ligaments, and tendons.

Severe, Chronic Rheumatoid Arthritis

In severe RA, pannus forms as a result of the release of lysosomal enzymes. Pannus is granulation tissue composed of lymphocytes, plasma cells, fibroblasts, and macrophages. Growing much like a tumor, pannus can invade the cartilage, activate chondrocytes, and release enzymes that can degrade cartilage and bone. This destructive process begins at the synovium and extends to the unprotected area at the junction of the cartilage and subchondral bone. These inflammatory cells can erode surrounding tissue, tendons, and cartilage. When pannus invades the joint margins, decreased range of motion and ankylosis may ensue. Pannus is a specific feature of RA, differentiating it from other forms of arthritis.

DIAGNOSTIC CRITERIA

In 2010, the American College of Rheumatology (ACR) and the European League Against Rheumatism (EULAR) collaborated on defining classification criteria for RA (**Table 37.1**). The goal of the criteria is to identify patients early who have a high probability of persistent RA and in whom early treatment would be beneficial. The emphasis of the classification criteria is on new patients with synovitis not explained by other conditions. Components of these criteria include joint involvement, serologic testing, acute phase reactants, and duration of symptoms.

The serology test can be either RF or ACPA, and the acute phase reactant test can be either erythrocyte sedimentation rate (ESR) or C-reactive protein (CRP). For serology tests, results are divided into three categories: negative, low positive (above normal but less than three times the upper limit of normal [ULN]), or high positive (greater than three times the ULN). The acute phase reactants are either normal or abnormal. None of these tests alone are sufficient to diagnose RA, but each is a component of diagnosis.

Other classic symptoms experienced by patients with RA include morning stiffness in involved joints persisting for at least 1 hour and subsiding with activity, symmetric joint involvement, and painful, swollen joints. Although RA characteristically affects joint structures, it is a systemic disease

with potential extra-articular manifestations. Throughout the disease, the patient also may have generalized symptoms such as weakness, fatigue, mild fever, anorexia, and weight loss. End-organ involvement may occur in patients with high RF titers.

The most common extra-articular manifestation of RA is joint nodules. These occur in 15% to 20% of patients with RA and are most commonly seen in patients with erosive disease. These subcutaneous nodules may develop in any area of the body exposed to pressure. Some of these areas are the olecranon bursa, knuckles, ischial spines, Achilles tendon, extensor surfaces of the forearm, and the bridge of the nose (in patients who wear glasses). These nodules may also form internally on the heart, lungs, and intestinal tract. The nodules are firm and rubbery, occur in clusters, and may be either freely mobile or attached to underlying connective tissue. The treatment of the nodules is confined to the treatment of the underlying disease. These nodules may occur in other connective tissue diseases (e.g., systemic lupus erythematosus), so alone they are not criteria for diagnosing RA.

An ocular manifestation of RA is sicca syndrome; patients have a sensation of grittiness in the eyes, accumulation of dried mucus, and decreased tear production. Scleritis and episcleritis are occasional sequelae of sicca syndrome. Additional extra-articular manifestations of RA include vasculitis, pulmonary fibrosis, and pericarditis.

INITIATING DRUG THERAPY

Physical and occupational therapies are considered mainstays of nonpharmacologic therapy in patients with RA. These therapies help protect the joints and maintain strength, function, and mobility. Reduction of joint stress is an additional goal of therapy. Patients should engage in activity to their fullest possible extent with adequate rest after activity, but they should avoid vigorous exercise and heavy labor during acute exacerbations of the disease. Hydrotherapy and hot and cold packs may be used to relax muscle spasms and facilitate joint movement. Warm showers and paraffin treatments may help relieve morning stiffness.

In 2012, the ACR updated their guidelines for the use of nonbiologic and biologic DMARDs, and in 2013, the EULAR provided updated recommendations for the treatment of RA. Both organizations indicated the importance of starting patients on DMARDs as early in the disease process as possible. Evidence has shown that the earlier in the disease process that DMARDs are started, the greater the chance of reducing disability and disease progression. Ideally, patients should be started on DMARD therapy within 3 months of diagnosis. The use of nonsteroidal anti-inflammatory drugs (NSAIDs) can still be considered for symptom control, but these do not have disease-modifying characteristics.

Goals of Drug Therapy

The goals of drug therapy for RA include reducing pain, stiffness, and swelling; preserving mobility and joint function; and preventing further joint damage. Due to advancements in the treatment of RA, the ACR and EULAR now recommend treating

TABLE 37.1

2010 American College of Rheumatology/European League Against Rheumatism Classification Criteria for Rheumatoid Arthritis

	Score
Target population (Who should be tested?): patients who	
1. Have at least one joint with definite clinical synovitis (swelling)*	
2. With synovitis not better explained by another disease[†]	
Classification criteria for RA (score-based algorithm: add score of categories A–D; a score ≥6/10 is needed for classification of a patient as having definite RA)[‡]	
A. Joint involvement[§]	
1 large joint[ǀ]	0
2–10 large joints	1
1–3 small joints[#]	2
4–10 small joints	3
>10 joints with at least 1 small joint**	5
B. Serology (at least one test is needed for classification)[††]	
Negative RF and negative ACPA	0
Low-positive RF or low-positive ACPA	2
High-positive RF or high-positive ACPA	3
C. Acute phase reactants (at least 1 test results is needed for classification)[‡‡]	
Normal CRP and ESR	0
Abnormal CRP or abnormal ESR	1
D. Duration of symptoms[§§]	
<6 wk	0
≥6 wk	1

*The criteria are aimed at classification of newly presenting patients. In addition, patients with erosive disease typical of RA with a history compatible with prior fulfillment of the 2010 criteria should be classified as having RA. Patients with long-standing disease, including those whose disease is inactive (with or without treatment) and who, based on retrospectively available data, have previously fulfilled the 2010 criteria, should be classified as having RA.

[†]Differential diagnosis varies among patients with different presentations but may include conditions such as systemic lupus erythematosus, psoriatic arthritis, and gout. If it is unclear about the relevant differential diagnoses to consider, an expert rheumatologist should be consulted.

[‡]Although patients with a score <6/10 are not classifiable as having RA, their status can be reassessed and the criteria might be fulfilled cumulatively over time.

[§]Joint involvement refers to any swollen or tender joint on examination, which may be confirmed by imaging evidence of synovitis. Distal interphalangeal joints, first carpometacarpal joints, and first metatarsophalangeal joints are excluded from assessment. Categories of joint distribution are classified according to the location and number of involved joints, with placement into the highest category possible based on the patter of joint involvement.

[ǀ]Large joints refer to shoulders, elbows, hips, knees, and ankles.

[#]Small joints refer to metacarpophalangeal joints, proximal interphalangeal joints, second through fifth metatarsophalangeal joints, thumb interphalangeal joints, and wrists.

**In this category, at least one of the involved joints must be a small joint; the other joints can include any combination of large and additional small joints, as well as other joints not specifically listed elsewhere (e.g., temporomandibular, acromioclavicular, sternoclavicular, etc.).

[††]Negative refers to IU values that are less than or equal to the ULN for the laboratory and assay; low positive refers to IU values that are higher than the ULN but less than or equal to three times the ULN for the laboratory and assay; high positive refers to IU values that are greater than three times the ULN for the laboratory and assay. When RF is only available as positive or negative, a positive result should be score as low positive for RF.

[‡‡]Normal/abnormal is determined by local laboratory standards.

[§§]Duration of symptoms refers to patient self-report of the duration of signs and symptoms of synovitis (e.g., pain, swelling, tenderness) of joints that are clinically involved at the time of assessment, regardless of treatment status.

RF, rheumatoid factor; ACPA, anticitrullinated protein antibody; CRP, C-reactive protein; ESR, erythrocyte sedimentation rate.

Redrawn with permission from Aletaha, D., Neogi, T., Silman, A. J., et al. (2010). 2010 rheumatoid arthritis classification criteria. *Arthritis and Rheumatism, 62*(9), 2569–2581.

to a goal of remission or if remission is not possible then low disease activity. In 2011, the ACR and EULAR developed a definition for remission, which includes a swollen joint count, tender joint count, CRP level and patient global assessment of ≤1 each, or a simplified Disease Activity Score of ≤3.3. Low disease activity can be assessed in a variety of ways via the Patient Activity Scale (0.28 to 3.7), Clinical Disease Activity Index (greater than 2.8 to 10.0), Disease Activity Score in 28 joints (2.6 to 3.2), or the simplified Disease Activity Index (greater than 3.3 to 11).

Nonsteroidal Anti-inflammatory Drugs

NSAIDs are typically used to help relieve pain and improve symptoms during the diagnostic process. These agents are continued through the initiation of a DMARD to maintain reduced symptoms. This approach allows NSAIDs to exert their anti-inflammatory action while the DMARD takes effect. See the discussion of NSAIDs in Chapter 36 Osteoarthritis and Gout (**Table 36.1**).

Corticosteroids

Low-dose corticosteroids (prednisone 10 mg or equivalent) are beneficial in patients who are beginning DMARD therapy. Because the therapeutic effect of DMARDs may not be seen until several weeks to months after initiating therapy, corticosteroids may be used to provide almost immediate symptom relief. Corticosteroids are also indicated in elderly patients with recent onset of RA. Last, higher doses of corticosteroids are beneficial in acute flares to regain control of inflammation and pain.

Corticosteroids have been proven to slow the progression of erosions when initiated early in treatment. Most of the trials have examined this benefit in combination with other DMARD therapy, and monotherapy is only recommended if patients have contraindications to other DMARD therapy. The extended-release prednisone has been examined for use in RA patients. The hypothesis is that if the extended-release prednisone is dosed at night, then the medication would be released at the time when proinflammatory cytokines become activated. The studies showed that this formulation resulted in reduced morning stiffness and a reduction in IL-6.

The difficulty in therapy with corticosteroids lies in the fine dosing line that divides therapeutic effects from long-term side effects. Low doses, such as prednisone 5 to 7.5 mg every morning, may be beneficial. The lowest dose possible should be given by gradually decreasing the dose in 1-mg decrements.

Injectable corticosteroids can be used if symptoms are restricted to one or two joints that have not responded to first-line treatment. They may also be of limited benefit for acute flare-ups of RA.

The most common adverse events of corticosteroid therapy include cataracts, glaucoma, mild glucose intolerance, and cutaneous atrophy. Less common adverse events include myopathy, hypothalamic–pituitary–adrenal axis dysfunction, and osteoporosis. Osteoporosis may be avoided by taking a calcium supplement (1,500 mg/d) along with vitamin D (800 mg/d).

Disease-Modifying Antirheumatic Drugs

As stated previously, the early use of DMARDs is advocated because of the high degree of inflammation that is present early in the disease (**Table 37.2**). Radiographic evidence of joint

TABLE 37.2

Overview of Selected Disease-Modifying Antirheumatic Drugs

Generic (Trade) Name and Dosage	Selected Adverse Events	Contraindications	Special Considerations
Preferred csDMARDs			
methotrexate (Rheumatrex) 7.5 mg/wk in single dose, up to 25 mg/wk	GI effects, leukopenia, oral ulcers, thrombocytopenia, pulmonary toxicity, hepatotoxicity	Pregnancy and 1 mo before conception; caution in alcohol drinkers and liver disease	May take 3–8 wk to achieve clinical benefit; can induce spontaneous abortion and birth defects; monitoring includes CBC, serum creatinine, and liver function tests at 4- to 8-wk intervals
sulfasalazine (Azulfidine) 500–1,000 mg/d in divided doses; may increase up to maximum 3 g/d	GI effects, heartburn, dizziness, headache, rash, neutropenia, thrombocytopenia, orange-yellow color of skin	Contraindicated in intestinal or urinary obstruction. Safety in pregnancy not established in RA treatment, although drug has proved safe in patients with inflammatory bowel disease in pregnancy	May take 1–4 mo to achieve clinical effect; causes reversible sterility in men; recommend that men cease therapy 90 d before starting a family; monitoring includes liver enzyme evaluation; CBC is necessary early in therapy but required less with prolonged use.
hydroxychloroquine (Plaquenil) 400–600 mg/d in divided doses	GI effects, rash, CNS effects, ocular effects	Use caution in pregnancy and with lactation.	Six months may be needed for clinical effect. Can trigger exacerbation of psoriasis; prolonged therapy may cause retinal damage. Monitoring should include periodic CBC and eye examination every 3–6 mo to monitor for retinal damage.
leflunomide (Arava) 100 mg PO daily for 3 d; 20 mg daily thereafter	Diarrhea, hair loss, weight loss, rash, infection	Pregnancy	If 20 mg daily is not tolerated, then 10 mg daily may be used. Long half-life; cholestyramine will enhance elimination if agent is to be discontinued.

TABLE 37.2

Overview of Selected Disease-Modifying Antirheumatic Drugs (*Continued*)

Generic (Trade) Name and Dosage	Selected Adverse Events	Contraindications	Special Considerations
Nonpreferred csDMARDs			
D-Penicillamine (Depen, Cuprimine) 125 mg/d as single dose; may increase at monthly intervals to maximum daily dose of 1.5 g	GI effects, rash, itching, renal effects, autoimmune reactions, cytopenia	Not recommended in pregnancy or lactation—causes damage to fetal connective tissue	From 4 to 6 mo may be needed to establish clinical effect of therapy. Monitoring should include CBC with differential and platelets and urinalysis every 2–6 wk.
azathioprine (Imuran) 50–100 mg in single daily dose; can increase after 6–8 wk; 3.5 mg/kg is maximum daily dose	GI effects, bone marrow suppression, infection, hepatotoxicity, alopecia	Renal disease; avoid during pregnancy and lactation	From 6 to 8 and up to 12 wk may be needed to establish clinical effect. Monitoring should include CBC with differential and platelets weekly for the first month, then biweekly for the second and third months, then monthly.
cyclophosphamide (Cytoxan, Neosar) 1 mg/kg/d increased to 2 mg/kg/d after 6 wk	Alopecia, hemorrhagic cystitis, sterility, GI effects, increased susceptibility to infection, thrombocytopenia	Contraindicated for RA during pregnancy and lactation	In renal impairment, decrease dose. Four months may be needed to establish clinical effect. Monitoring includes CBC with differential, platelets, urinalysis for blood repeatedly, ESR, BUN, serum creatinine.
cyclosporine A (Sandimmune, Neoral) 5 mg/kg/d divided into 2 doses	Hypertension, tremor, nephrotoxicity, hepatotoxicity, increased susceptibility to infection, hyperkalemia	Contraindicated for RA during pregnancy and lactation	Approximately 8 wk may be needed to establish clinical effect. Decrease dose by 50% if hypertension or nephrotoxicity results. Monitoring includes CBC with differential, BUN, serum creatinine, serum bilirubin, liver enzymes repeatedly.
Gold compounds *Injectable*: aurothioglucose (Solganal); gold sodium thiomalate (Myochrysine) 10 mg/wk IM, up to a total dose of 1 g; maintenance dose ~50 mg/mo *Oral*: auranofin (Ridaura) 3 mg bid	GI effects, rash, itching, stomatitis, vasomotor reactions, bone marrow suppression, nephritis, pneumonitis, exfoliative dermatitis, proteinuria	Uncontrolled diabetes; liver and renal disease, systemic lupus erythematosus, blood dyscrasias; lack of long-term studies in pregnant women, so not recommended during pregnancy or lactation	May take 6–8 wk for injectable form and 3–6 mo for oral form of drug to establish effectiveness. Monitoring includes routine CBC with differential, platelet count; urinalysis to measure protein; renal and liver function tests.
tsDMARD			
tofacitinib (Xeljanz) 5 mg PO twice a day	Bone marrow suppression (lymphopenia, neutropenia, anemia), GI perforations, infections	Coadministration with strong CYP3A4 inducers, known malignancy, history of interstitial lung disease	Not to be used in combination with bDMARDs. Dose adjustments for coadministration with CYP3A4 inhibitors and CYP2C19 inhibitors
Biologic DMARDs			
etanercept (Enbrel) 25 mg SQ twice weekly or 50 mg SQ weekly	Upper respiratory tract infections, pain at the injection site, headache	Concurrent infections or hypersensitivity to medication	Use caution in patients predisposed to infection. Concomitant immunosuppressants can increase risk of serious infection.

(Continued)

TABLE 37.2

Overview of Selected Disease-Modifying Antirheumatic Drugs (*Continued*)

Generic (Trade) Name and Dosage	Selected Adverse Events	Contraindications	Special Considerations
infliximab (Remicade) 3 mg/kg IV infusion at baseline, 2 wk, 6 wk, then every 8 wk thereafter	Urticaria, infusion reactions, dyspnea, hypotension	Same as above	Same as above
adalimumab (Humira) 40 mg SQ every other week; 40 mg weekly as monotherapy	Redness, swelling, bruising, or pain at the site of injection, headache, upset stomach, diarrhea, infection, rash	Same as above	Same as above
golimumab (Simponi) 50 mg SQ monthly in combination with methotrexate	Injection site reactions, infection, dizziness, antibody formation	Same as above	Same as above
certolizumab pegol (Cimzia) 400 mg SQ at weeks 0, 2, and 4 then 200 mg every other week	Injection site reactions, headache, nausea, infection	Same as above	Same as above
anakinra (Kineret) 100 mg SQ daily	Redness, swelling, bruising, or pain at the site of injection, headache, upset stomach, diarrhea, infection, rash	Sensitivity to *E. coli*–derived proteins; pre-existing infection	Routine monitoring of WBCs is recommended; concomitant immunosuppressants can increase risk of serious infection.
abatacept (Orencia) 500–1,000 mg (based on weight) IV at weeks 0, 2, and 4, and then every 4 wk; 125 mg SQ weekly	COPD exacerbations, headache, hypertension, infusion reactions, infections, anaphylaxis	Hypersensitivity to abatacept; use caution in patients with history of infections or COPD.	Concomitant immunosuppressants increase risk of infection. Reserved for patients unresponsive to other therapy
tocilizumab (Actemra) 4–8 mg/kg IV every 4 wk; 162 mg SQ every other week—weekly (weight based)	Increased LDL and transaminase, decreased WBC, infusion-related reactions	Untreated latent TB or hepatitis	Indicated for patients who did not respond to TNF-alpha inhibitor

damage usually is present in the first year of the disease, and functional deterioration due to this damage may be irreversible. Therefore, early initiation of DMARD therapy may be the best course of action to take in meeting the long-range goals of treatment. DMARD therapy should be initiated within 3 months after onset of symptoms. There are several DMARDs to select from; the ones described here are the DMARDs currently recommended by the ACR. Due to lack of data or high adverse events profile, cyclophosphamide, D-penicillamine, cyclosporine, azathioprine, gold compounds, and anakinra are not currently recommended for patients with RA. They can be used in patients who have failed the traditional treatments discussed below.

Due to the development of new DMARDs, a modified nomenclature for the DMARDs has been developed. DMARDs are first divided into synthetic and biologic DMARDs. The synthetic DMARDs are then further divided in conventional synthetic DMARDs (csDMARDs) (methotrexate, leflunomide, sulfasalazine, hydroxychloroquine) and targeted synthetic DMARDs (tsDMARD) (tofacitinib).

Biologic DMARDs are also further divided into biologic originator DMARD (boDMARD) and biosimilar DMARD (bsDMARD).

Methotrexate

The most commonly prescribed DMARD is methotrexate (Rheumatrex). The patient best suited for treatment with methotrexate is one who has morning stiffness and synovitis.

Mechanism of Action

Methotrexate, a folic acid antagonist, is thought to affect leukocyte suppression, decreasing the inflammation that results from immunologic by-products. When treatment stops, exacerbation of symptoms may occur as early as 2 weeks after cessation.

Dosage

Methotrexate is available for oral, subcutaneous, intramuscular, or intravenous (IV; reserved for chemotherapy) use. For most patients, a starting dose of 7.5 mg orally once per week is recommended. If a significant decrease in symptoms is not noted, the dose should be increased every few weeks to a maximal dose of 25 to 30 mg weekly. The patient needs to be on the maximal dose for at least 8 weeks before someone can be considered a methotrexate failure. Most patients respond to 12.5 to 15 mg/wk. Injectable methotrexate may be used if there is an inadequate response to oral therapy or if the weekly dose needs to exceed 25 mg.

Time Frame for Response

Approximately 70% to 75% of patients respond favorably to methotrexate therapy, but it may take 3 to 8 weeks before improvement is noted. More than 50% of patients stay on the treatment for more than 5 years. However, if patients have difficulty tolerating side effects, methotrexate should be discontinued or the dosage should be lowered.

Contraindications

Methotrexate is contraindicated in pregnant and breast-feeding patients and those with leukopenia (white blood cell [WBC] count of less than 3,000 cells/mm³), acquired immunodeficiency syndrome, renal impairment (creatinine clearance less than 30 mL/min), or liver disease (liver enzymes greater than two times the ULN). Methotrexate also has many black box warnings, including the risk of hepatotoxicity, renal impairment, pneumonitis, bone marrow suppression, diarrhea, ulcerative stomatitis, dermatologic reactions, and opportunistic infections. The ACR also lists acute serious bacterial infections, latent tuberculosis (TB), active fungal infections, active herpes zoster viral infection, platelets less than 50,000 cells/mm³, treated lymphoproliferative disease within 5 years, and acute or chronic hepatitis B or C as contraindications to methotrexate therapy.

Adverse Events

The most commonly reported adverse events of methotrexate are nausea and abdominal pain. These effects may be minimized by switching to parenteral therapy. Oral ulcers, leukopenia, anemia, and thrombocytopenia are also common. However, these adverse reactions may be minimized by administering 1 mg of folic acid daily. Although methotrexate may inhibit folic acid metabolism, it does not seem to affect the efficacy of the therapy.

The most serious adverse event of therapy is liver toxicity, which occurs more frequently in patients with diabetes, obesity, alcohol use, and existing liver disease. Pneumonitis is another potentially serious side effect of therapy. A baseline chest x-ray may be obtained, and patients should be instructed to report the new onset of a dry cough, dyspnea, or fever. Methotrexate should be immediately discontinued if the patient has pulmonary problems because immutable pulmonary damage may occur.

Baseline laboratory values should be obtained before initiation of therapy and should include a CBC, liver function tests, blood urea nitrogen (BUN), and serum creatinine. During therapy, the CBC should be monitored every 4 weeks, and creatinine, BUN, and liver function tests should be monitored every 3 months. A transient yet marked increase in liver enzymes may be seen, with stabilization occurring with continued treatment or dose reduction. If liver enzymes persist at concentrations of two to three times the ULN, then methotrexate should be discontinued and a liver biopsy obtained.

Methotrexate is classified as pregnancy category X due to the risk of fetal death or severe abnormalities and has implications for both males and females. Therefore, women who wish to conceive should stop taking methotrexate at least one ovulatory cycle before attempting to become pregnant. Men must discontinue methotrexate at least 3 months before trying to conceive. Men and women of childbearing age who are not sterilized should use a reliable form of contraception.

Interactions

Concurrent use with NSAIDs may increase the risk of bone marrow suppression and gastrointestinal (GI) toxicity. The combination should be avoided when taking moderate to high doses of methotrexate. Medications such as penicillins, tetracyclines, probenecid, and sulfonamides that compete with methotrexate for renal tubular secretion will enhance the effects of methotrexate and should be used cautiously. Methotrexate may increase the concentrations of mercaptopurine and theophylline. Concomitant use of cholestyramine decreases the absorption of methotrexate.

Sulfasalazine

Like methotrexate, sulfasalazine (Azulfidine) is an effective DMARD that relieves symptoms relatively quickly. The best candidates for treatment are patients with significant synovitis but no poor prognostic factors.

Mechanism of Action

Sulfasalazine's mechanism of action is not clearly understood but is thought to be due to its conversion to sulfapyridine and 5-acetylsalicylic acid in the gut. The sulfapyridine component is thought to be responsible for the disease-modifying activity. Research has shown the anti-inflammatory features of this conversion, as well as its ability to decrease inflammatory cytokine production.

Dosage

Sulfasalazine is available in oral form in 500-mg tablets. Dosing is started at 1,000 mg/d in two divided doses. The daily divided dose is gradually increased to 2,000 mg over 2 weeks. After 12 weeks of 2,000 mg daily, if the response is still not adequate, then the dose can be increased to 3,000 mg daily. Enteric-coated tablets are recommended for the treatment of RA to reduce the risk of GI-related adverse events.

Time Frame for Response

Patients may start to notice an effect as early as 1 month, but the full effect may take up to 4 months.

Contraindications

Due to its sulfa component, sulfasalazine is contraindicated in patients with a sulfa allergy. Also, once a pregnant woman is at full term, sulfasalazine is classified as a pregnancy category D and should be avoided. Patients with a GI or genitourinary tract obstruction or those with porphyria should not use this medication. Platelet count of less than 50,000 cells/mm^3, liver enzymes greater than two times the ULN, and hepatitis B or C infection resulting in Child-Pugh class B or C hepatic function are contraindications, according to the ACR guidelines.

Adverse Events

The most common adverse events to sulfasalazine are dose dependent and include nausea and diarrhea. Other reported adverse events include dizziness, intestinal or urinary obstruction, oral ulcers, thrombocytopenia, orange-yellow pigmentation of the skin, headache, and depression. Any of these common adverse events may become intolerable and cause discontinuation of the drug. Reversible sterility has been reported in men; therapy should be discontinued 3 months before attempting to father a child.

Agranulocytosis, the gravest adverse event to sulfasalazine, has been reported in fewer than 2% of patients, but it dictates immediate discontinuation. Before initiating sulfasalazine therapy, the practitioner should obtain baseline laboratory test values, including a CBC and liver enzymes. These values should be monitored every 2 weeks for 1 month after initiation of therapy and then monthly for 5 months. If laboratory values remain stable for the first 6 months of therapy, a CBC should be checked every 3 months.

Interactions

The risk of bone marrow suppression will be enhanced if used with other suppressive agents such as azathioprine, methotrexate, or mercaptopurine, and additional monitoring is warranted. Sulfasalazine may increase the effects of oral hypoglycemics and oral anticoagulants; therefore, patients should be monitored closely if on concurrent therapy. Sulfasalazine may decrease the concentration of cyclosporine.

Antimalarials

The antimalarial agents hydroxychloroquine (Plaquenil) and chloroquine are attractive because of their tolerable adverse event profile, with the drugs being discontinued in fewer than 9% of patients. However, because these drugs cannot limit the progression of RA, they are currently used as an adjunct to methotrexate therapy or as single-agent therapy in early, mild RA without bone erosion. Hydroxychloroquine is the preferred agent in this class.

Mechanism of Action

Antimalarials inhibit antigen processing by elevating cellular pH, which changes antigen degeneration. Thus, the presentation of the antigen to T cells is impaired.

Dosage

Hydroxychloroquine and chloroquine are available in oral form and are rapidly and completely absorbed. Dosing is calculated by patient weight, but the typical dosage for hydroxychloroquine is 200 mg twice daily or 400 mg daily.

Time Frame for Response

Therapeutic effects are usually noted within 2 to 6 months of treatment.

Contraindications

Patients with pre-existing retinal field changes should not use antimalarials due to the ocular effects of long-term therapy.

Adverse Events

The most common adverse events associated with antimalarials are nausea, diarrhea, and abdominal discomfort. Less common adverse events include photosensitivity and skin pigmentation changes. A maculopapular, pruritic rash encompassing the entire body may occur and cause extreme discomfort. Although neuromyopathy has been reported rarely, deep tendon reflexes should be monitored regularly for diminished activity.

After absorption, these drugs concentrate in the retina, kidneys, bone marrow, and liver. The concentration of antimalarials in specific organs dictates baseline and ongoing monitoring during therapy. Specifically, patients need a baseline eye examination with a follow-up exam 5 years later and then annually thereafter because of potential retinal accumulation of the drug. A CBC should be performed periodically.

Interactions

Antimalarial agents can decrease the metabolism of beta blockers with some exceptions, including atenolol and nadolol. For patients on beta blockers, consider switching to atenolol prior to initiating antimalarial therapy. Also, cyclosporine and digoxin concentrations may be increased, requiring more frequent monitoring. Antimalarial doses should be separated from magnesium-containing products by 2 to 4 hours due to decreased absorption of the antimalarials.

Leflunomide

Leflunomide (Arava) exerts anti-inflammatory and antiproliferative actions, retarding erosions and joint space narrowing.

Mechanism of Action

Leflunomide is a prodrug that undergoes rapid conversion to its active metabolite. The drug is a competitive inhibitor of dihydrofolate reductase. This inhibition decreases the production of pyrimidines (amino acid building blocks), decreasing T-cell and B-cell proliferation. This action is similar to methotrexate, making this agent a reasonable alternative for patients who cannot tolerate or who have an inadequate response to methotrexate. Since leflunomide inhibits pyrimidine synthesis and methotrexate inhibits purine synthesis, these agents may be used in combination.

Dosage

Since the half-life of the active metabolite is 15 to 18 days, therapy with leflunomide is usually initiated with a 100-mg daily loading dose for 3 days, and then the agent is continued at 20 mg/d if tolerated. If the patient cannot tolerate 20 mg/d, the dose can be lowered to 10 mg/d. The loading dose can be omitted in patients at increased risk for hepatic or hematologic toxicity.

Time Frame for Response

Benefit from leflunomide can be seen as early as 4 weeks but may take up to 3 months.

Contraindications

Like other DMARDs, leflunomide is contraindicated in pregnancy. Since the half-life is so long, a typical washout period for women who wish to conceive is about 2 years. However, agents interrupting the enterohepatic recirculation (e.g., activated charcoal or cholestyramine) can be used to reduce the half-life of the metabolite to about 1 day. The dosing of cholestyramine, as recommended by the manufacturer, is 8 g three times a day for 11 days. To ensure appropriate clearance, plasma concentrations should be less than 0.02 mg/L measured twice at least 14 days apart.

Due to hepatotoxicity, patients with a history of alcoholism or with pre-existing liver disease should not take leflunomide.

Adverse Events

About 5% of patients receiving leflunomide monotherapy have elevated liver enzymes. While this number appears low, there are reports of more than 10 patients dying while on leflunomide therapy; the deaths are thought to be related to the hepatotoxicity of the agent.

More common adverse events include GI symptoms, weight loss, alopecia, and hypertension. Leflunomide also has been associated with bone marrow suppression, including anemia, thrombocytopenia, and agranulocytosis.

A CBC and liver function tests should be taken as a baseline and then monthly for the first 6 months of therapy. If test results remain stable, monitoring can be every 6 to 8 weeks thereafter.

Interactions

Leflunomide is a weak inhibitor of the CYP2C9 enzyme and therefore may increase the levels of agents metabolized through this pathway, including warfarin. Rifampin may increase the concentration of leflunomide's active metabolite. The use of bile acid sequestrants decreases the enterohepatic recycling of leflunomide, decreasing its effectiveness.

Tofacitinib

Tofacitinib is the first tsDMARD available and targets Janus kinase (JAK) activity.

Mechanism of Action

Tofacitinib interferes with JAK1, JAK2, JAK3, and Tyk2 but has higher potency for JAK3. It is a competitive, reversible inhibitor. Tofacitinib prevents the phosphorylation and activation of signal transducers and activators of transcription. This results in decreased signal transduction for cytokines and decreases propagation of the inflammatory response via decrease leukocyte maturation and activation and cytokine production.

Dosage

The typical dose is 5 mg orally twice daily. However, if used in combination with a strong CYP3A4 inhibitor or concomitant moderate CYP3A4 inhibitor with a potent CYP2C19 inhibitor, the recommended dose is 5 mg by mouth daily. Also, for patients with moderate to severe renal or hepatic impairment, the dose is 5 mg by mouth daily.

Contraindications

There are no absolute contraindications to tofacitinib therapy; however, there are many warnings associated with its use. Due to the risk of bone marrow suppression, tofacitinib should not be initiated if a patient has a lymphocyte count less than 500 cells/mm^3 and absolute neutrophil count of less than 1,000 cells/mm^3. A CBC should be monitored at baseline, 4 to 8 weeks after initiation and then every 3 months thereafter. Tofacitinib may cause hepatotoxicity and patients should be monitored for this. Similar to other DMARDs, tofacitinib may increase the risk of infection including TB, fungal infections, and opportunistic infections. Patients should be screened for latent TB prior to initiating therapy.

Adverse Events

Common adverse effects include headache, diarrhea, hypertension, and upper respiratory infections. Tofacitinib may increase lipid parameters such as total cholesterol, LDL, and HDL, and a lipid panel should be checked 4 to 8 weeks after initiating therapy.

Interactions

Tofacitinib is a major substrate of CYP3A4 and a minor substrate of CYP2C19. Tofacitinib is not recommended to be used with strong CYP3A4 inducers such as rifampin. Due to the risk of infection, tofacitinib should not be used with any biologic DMARDs. Live vaccines should not be administered while a patient is receiving tofacitinib.

Biologic Disease-Modifying Antirheumatic Drugs

Biologic agents are developed from living sources, such as humans, animals, or microorganisms. The introduction of various biologics effective against RA has changed the management of RA. These agents target multiple components involved in the pathogenesis of RA, such as TNF-alpha, T-cell activation, IL-1, and IL-6. Prior to initiating bDMARDs, patients should be screened for latent TB due to the increased reactivation of TB and hepatitis B.

Tumor Necrosis Factor Inhibitors

Etanercept (Enbrel), infliximab (Remicade), adalimumab (Humira), golimumab (Simponi), and certolizumab pegol (Cimzia) are TNF-alpha inhibitors used in RA treatment.

Mechanism of Action

These agents act by binding the circulating TNF-alpha and render it inactive. This then reduces the chemotactic effect of TNF-alpha by reducing IL-6 and CRP, resulting in reduced infiltration of inflammatory cells into joints. Also, when these agents bind to surface TNF-alpha, cell lysis occurs.

Dosage

All five of these agents are injectables. Etanercept is self-administered subcutaneously at 25 mg twice weekly or 50 mg weekly as combination therapy or monotherapy. Infliximab is an IV infusion with a recommended dose of 3 mg/kg at 0, 2, and 6 weeks and then every 8 weeks thereafter. Doses of infliximab have ranged from 3 to 10 mg/kg every 4 to 8 weeks. Infliximab is indicated in conjunction with methotrexate because infliximab antibodies develop when administered as monotherapy. Adalimumab is given at 40 mg every other week as a subcutaneous injection. Adalimumab may be administered concomitantly with methotrexate, glucocorticoids, or NSAIDs. It may also be used as monotherapy; however, the dose may need to be increased to 40 mg weekly. Certolizumab pegol is administered as a subcutaneous injection at a dose of 400 mg at 0, 2, and 4 weeks and then 200 mg every other week thereafter. An alternative maintenance dosing regimen is 400 mg every 4 weeks. Golimumab is only indicated for use in combination with methotrexate, and the recommended dose is 50 mg subcutaneously one time a month.

Time Frame for Response

All of the TNF-alpha inhibitors produce a rapid response, within days to weeks.

Contraindications

Patients should be assessed at baseline for infections or risk factors for infections. There have been reports of TB developing in patients taking infliximab; the theory is that the immunomodulation allows latent TB to flare. This usually occurs within the first 2 to 5 months of therapy. Therefore, all patients must be evaluated for latent TB with a tuberculin skin test or interferon gamma release assay prior to beginning therapy. Other serious infections, including fungal and opportunistic infections, have also occurred with these agents, and careful consideration of the patient's history is important when prescribing them. This class of medications is not recommended for patients with untreated hepatitis B or treated hepatitis B with Child-Pugh score of B or higher. In addition, patients with New York Heart Association class III or IV heart failure should not be initiated on TNF inhibitors.

Adverse Events

Adverse events include injection-site reactions (certolizumab pegol, golimumab, etanercept, adalimumab) or infusion reactions (infliximab). Caution must be used when administering these agents to patients predisposed to infection. Sepsis and fatal infections have occurred in patients receiving TNF-alpha inhibitors. If a patient develops an infection while taking a TNF-alpha inhibitor, the agent should be discontinued until the infection resolves. Other serious but more rare adverse events include demyelinating central nervous system diseases, autoimmune disorders such as lupus-like syndrome, and lymphomas. The risk of lymphoma is increased in children and adolescents, and it is not elucidated if the increased risk is due to the medication or the disease. Due to this risk, these agents are not recommended for the treatment of RA in patients with a treated solid malignancy within the last 5 years or treated lymphoproliferative malignancy.

Interactions

TNF-alpha inhibitors should not be used in combination with other biologic DMARDs due to the increased risk of infection. As a result of immunosuppressive effects, patients should not receive live vaccinations while being treated with a TNF-alpha inhibitor. Also, the response to other vaccines may be diminished while on therapy.

Anakinra

Anakinra (Kineret) is a recombinant form of human IL-1 receptor antagonist but differs by the addition of methionine at one of the N-terminals.

Mechanism of Action

The levels of naturally occurring IL-1 receptor antagonists are not adequate to compete with the elevated amount of IL-1 present in the synovium of RA patients. With limited competition, IL-1 can promote inflammation and degrade cartilage. By exogenously providing this antagonist to RA patients, the joint inflammation process is interrupted.

Dosage

Anakinra is given 100 mg subcutaneously daily. In patients with severe renal dysfunction (creatinine clearance below 30 mL/min), it should be administered every other day.

Time Frame for Response

In patients who responded to anakinra, the effect was seen within 12 weeks.

Contraindications

The primary contraindication to anakinra is sensitivity to *Escherichia coli*–derived proteins. Similar to the other immunomodulators, pre-existing infection or risk of infection may be a contraindication since there is an increased risk of infection in patients taking anakinra. Anakinra should not be administered in combination with TNF-alpha inhibitors due to the increased risk of infection.

Adverse Events

The most common adverse event of anakinra is skin irritation, including erythema, inflammation, and pain at the injection site. This occurs in more than half of patients and usually resolves within a few weeks. Although rare, there is a possibility of hypersensitivity reactions, including anaphylaxis and angioedema. Also, patients are at an increased risk for infection.

Patients also may experience a decrease in WBCs. Routine monitoring is recommended at baseline and then monthly for the first 3 months, and then quarterly for the first year.

Interactions

No known pharmacokinetic drug interactions exist. Pharmacodynamically, agents that suppress the immune system should be used with caution, if at all, due to the increased risk of serious infections. Anakinra should not be used in combination with TNF-alpha inhibitors.

Abatacept

Abatacept (Orencia) is indicated for the treatment of moderate to severe RA as monotherapy or in combination with csDMARDs.

Mechanism of Action

Abatacept is a costimulation modulator that binds to CD80 and CD86 on antigen-presenting cells. This binding blocks the CD28 interaction between the antigen-presenting cell and T cells necessary for T-cell activation. Therefore, abatacept decreases the activation of T cells.

Dosage

Abatacept is given as an IV infusion over 30 minutes and is dosed based on weight (less than 60 kg, 500 mg; 60 to 100 kg, 750 mg; greater than 100 kg, 1,000 mg). It is dosed at weeks 0, 2, and 4 and then every 4 weeks thereafter. It is also available as a subcutaneous injection with can be initiated with or without receiving an IV dose. If a patient receives an IV loading dose (based on weight), the subcutaneous dose is 125 mg within 24 hours of the IV dose followed by 125 mg weekly thereafter. If the patient does not receive an IV loading dose, the dose is 125 mg subcutaneously weekly. If a patient had been receiving the IV formulation and wishes to convert to the subcutaneous formulation, the recommendation is to start the 125 mg subcutaneous weekly at the time of their next scheduled IV dose.

Time Frame for Response

The onset of action for abatacept ranges from 1 to 3 months.

Contraindications

The only absolute contraindication associated with abatacept is hypersensitivity to it or any component of the formulation. Abatacept should be used cautiously in patients with a history of infection or chronic obstructive pulmonary disease (COPD). Patients need to be screened for hepatitis and latent TB prior to initiation due to the risk of reactivation.

Adverse Events

Patients with COPD experienced a higher rate of exacerbations, cough, pneumonia, and dyspnea. Common adverse events include headache, hypertension, and infusion-related reactions. Similarly to other immunomodulators, abatacept is associated with a higher risk of infections. Although rare, abatacept can cause anaphylaxis.

Interactions

Patients should not receive a live vaccine while on abatacept or for up to 3 months after discontinuing the drug. Abatacept should not be used in combination with other bDMARDs due to the increased risk of immunosuppression.

Tocilizumab

Tocilizumab (Actemra) is the first IL-6 receptor inhibitor on the market and is indicated for adult patients with moderate to severe RA after not responding to one or more DMARDs.

Mechanism of Action

Tocilizumab is a humanized anti-IL-6 receptor monoclonal antibody. By inhibiting IL-6 activity, B-cell and T-cell activation is decreased as well as acute phase reactant production and osteoclast activation.

Dosage

Tocilizumab is available as an IV infusion or a subcutaneous injection. For the IV infusion, tocilizumab is initiated at a dose of 4 mg/kg every 4 weeks with an option to increase to 8 mg/kg if needed based on clinical response. For the subcutaneous formulation, the dose for a patient weighing less than 100 kg is 162 mg every other week with the option to increase to weekly dosing if needed. For patients weighing more than 100 kg, the recommended starting dose is tocilizumab 162 mg subcutaneously every week. For a patient wishing to transition from IV to subcutaneous, they would initiate the subcutaneous dose at the time of their next scheduled IV dose.

Time Frame for Response

It may take up to 3 months for symptomatic improvement with tocilizumab.

Contraindications

Tocilizumab should not be initiated if patients have an absolute neutrophil count of less than 2,000 cells/mm^3, platelets less than 100,000/mm^3, or ALT or AST greater than 1.5 times the ULN. Similar to the other biologic agents, patients should be screened for TB and hepatitis prior to initiation.

Adverse Events

Overall, tocilizumab is well tolerated. There have been laboratory abnormalities associated with tocilizumab that include increased low-density lipoprotein cholesterol, elevated transaminase, and decreased WBCs. Approximately 8% of patients experienced an infusion-related reaction.

Based on laboratory abnormalities, a CBC and liver function tests need to be monitored at baseline and then every 4 to 8 weeks while on therapy. A lipid panel should be checked at baseline, 4 to 8 weeks into therapy, and then every 6 months while being treated with tocilizumab.

Interactions

Avoid using tocilizumab with leflunomide due to concern for increased hematologic toxicity. Patients should not receive live vaccines while on therapy and for at least 3 months after discontinuing treatment. Also, patients may not be able to respond appropriately to inactivated vaccines administered while on therapy. Due to the risk of infection, tocilizumab should not be used with any TNF-alpha inhibitors, anakinra, abatacept, or other immunosuppressants.

Selecting the Most Appropriate Agent

In 2008, the ACR published recommendations regarding the use of nonbiologic and biologic DMARDs for the treatment of RA, and this guideline was updated in 2012. It is important to note that gold and anakinra were not included due to infrequent use and lack of relevant new data. Decisions regarding appropriate therapy are based on disease duration, poor prognostic factors, and disease activity. Disease duration is divided into early (less than 6 months) or established (greater than 6 months). Poor prognostic factors include functional limitation, extra-articular disease, RF positivity, positive ACPA, or bony erosions on radiography. Last, disease activity is divided into low, moderate, or high based on several questionnaire instruments. Treatment algorithms are displayed in **Figures 37.1** and **37.2**.

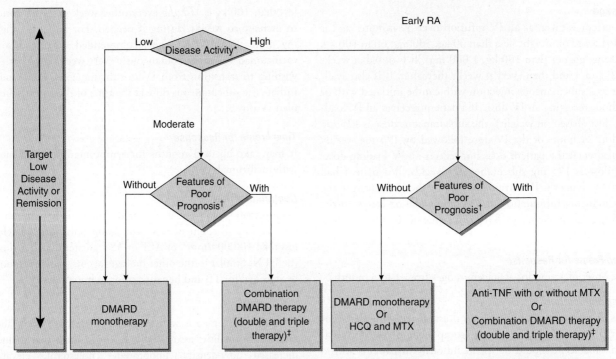

FIGURE 37.1   2012 American College of Rheumatology recommendations update for the treatment of early rheumatoid arthritis (RA) defined as a disease duration less than 6 months. DMARD, disease-modifying antirheumatic drug (includes hydroxychloroquine [HCQ], leflunomide [LEF], methotrexate [MTX], minocycline, and sulfasalazine); anti-TNF, anti–tumor necrosis factor. *Definitions of disease activity are discussed in the full text of the reference and were categorized as low, moderate, or high. †Patients were categorized based on the presence or absence of one or more of the following poor prognostic features: functional limitation (e.g., Health Assessment Questionnaire score or similar valid tools), extra-articular disease (e.g., presence of rheumatoid nodules, RA vasculitis, Felty syndrome), positive rheumatoid factor or anti–cyclic citrullinated peptide antibodies, and bony erosions by radiograph. ‡Combination DMARD therapy with two DMARDs, which is most commonly MTX based, with some exceptions (e.g., MTX + HCQ, MTX + LEF, MTX + sulfasalazine, and sulfasalazine + HCQ) and triple therapy (MTX + HCQ + sulfasalazine). (Reprinted from Singh, J. A., Furst, D. E., Bharat, A., et al. (2012). 2012 Update of the 2008 American College of Rheumatology Recommendations for the use of disease-modifying antirheumatic drugs and biologic agents in the treatment of rheumatoid arthritis. *Arthritis Care & Research*, *64*(5), 625–639, with permission.)

FIGURE 37.2 (*Continued*)   biologics include adalimumab, certolizumab pegol, etanercept, infliximab, and golimumab. Non-TNF biologics include abatacept, rituximab, or tocilizumab (therapies listed alphabetically). *Definitions of disease activity are discussed in the full text of the reference and were categorized as low, moderate, or high. †Features of poor prognosis include the presence of one or more of the following: functional limitation (e.g., Health Assessment Questionnaire score or similar valid tools), extra-articular disease (e.g., presence of rheumatoid nodules, RA vasculitis, Felty syndrome), positive rheumatoid factor or anticyclic citrullinated peptide antibodies, and bony erosions by radiograph. ‡Combination DMARD therapy with two DMARDs, which is most commonly MTX based, with some exceptions (e.g., MTX + HCQ, MTX + LEF, MTX + sulfasalazine, and sulfasalazine + HCQ) and triple therapy (MTX + HCQ + sulfasalazine). §Reassess after 3 months and proceed with escalating therapy if moderate or high disease activity in all instances except after treatment with non-TNF biologic (rectangle D), where reassessment is recommended at 6 months due to a longer anticipated time for peak effect. ¶LEF can be added in patients with low disease activity after 3 to 6 months of minocycline, HCQ, MTX, or sulfasalazine. #If after 3 months of intensified DMARD combination therapy or after second DMARD has failed, the option is to add or switch to an anti-TNF biologic. **Serious adverse events were defined per the U.S. Food and Drug Administration (FDA); all other adverse events were considered nonserious adverse events. ††Reassessment after treatment with a non-TNF biologic is recommended at 6 months due to anticipation that a longer time to peak effect is needed for non-TNF compared to anti-TNF biologics. ‡‡Any adverse event was defined as per the U.S. FDA as any undesirable experience associated with the use of a medical product in a patient. The FDA definition of serious adverse events includes death, life-threatening event, initial or prolonged hospitalization, disability, congenital anomaly, or an adverse event requiring intervention to prevent permanent impairment or damage. (Reprinted from Singh, J. A., Furst, D. E., Bharat, A., et al. (2012). 2012 Update of the 2008 American College of Rheumatology Recommendations for the use of disease-modifying antirheumatic drugs and biologic agents in the treatment of rheumatoid arthritis. *Arthritis Care & Research*, *64*(5), 625–639, with permission.)

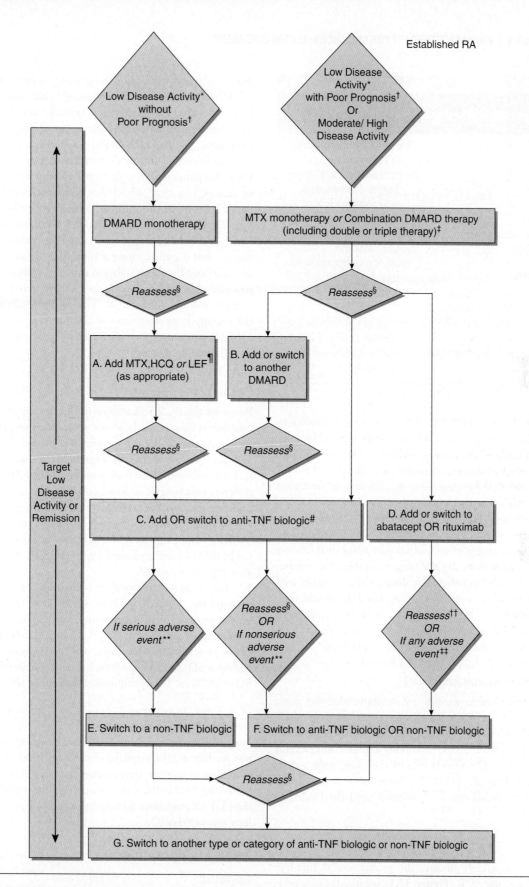

FIGURE 37.2 2012 America College of Rheumatology (ACR) recommendations updated for the treatment of established rheumatoid arthritis (RA), defined as a disease duration ≥6 months or meeting the 1987 ACR classification criteria. Depending on a patient's current medication regimen, the management algorithm may begin at an appropriate rectangle in the figure, rather than only at the top of the figure. Disease-modifying antirheumatic drugs (DMARDs) include hydroxychloroquine (HCQ), leflunomide (LEF), methotrexate (MTX), minocycline, and sulfasalazine (therapies are listed alphabetically; azathioprine and cyclosporine were considered but not included). DMARD monotherapy refers to treatment in most instances with HCQ, LEF, MTX, or sulfasalazine; in few instances, where appropriate, minocycline may also be used. Antitumor necrosis factor (anti-TNF)

TABLE 37.3

EULAR Treatment Recommendations

Phase I	Initial treatment	Methotrexate monotherapy or combination
		If contraindication to methotrexate: leflunomide or sulfasalazine alone or combination
Phase II	Failure of phase I	With poor prognostic factors: bDMARD
		Without poor prognostic factors: change csDMARDs
	Failure of second csDMARD regimen	bDMARD
Phase III	Failure of first bDMARD	Replace bDMARD with alternative bDMARD
	Failure of ≥2 bDMARD	Replace bDMARD with tofacitinib

In 2013, the EULAR published recommendations regarding the management of RA with synthetic and biologic DMARDs (**Table 37.3**). These guidelines break treatment into three phases based on response to therapy. Similar to the ACR guidelines, the EULAR guidelines do differentiate treatment for patients with or without poor prognostic factors.

In selecting a DMARD or combining DMARDs, the clinician needs to consider the toxicities of the medications, including the interactions with other prescribed drugs. Some patients may have difficulty adhering to monitoring requirements for some of the more toxic drugs. Other patients may not be able to adhere to a strict dosing schedule. In addition, the time required to achieve benefit can be protracted with certain DMARDs, which may be unacceptable to the patient. Finally, the cost of the various therapies varies widely.

Symptomatic Treatment

NSAIDs and/or corticosteroids are recommended for acute symptoms associated with RA. These agents are particularly helpful while a patient is undergoing diagnostic assessment. NSAIDs do not have disease-modifying abilities, and steroids often have intolerable adverse effects; therefore, once a definite diagnosis is made, DMARD therapy should be started. NSAIDs and steroids can be continued until the DMARD takes effect.

First-Line Therapy

For patients with early disease, the recommended first-line treatment from the ACR (**Figure 37.1**) is monotherapy csDMARD for patients with low disease activity regardless of poor prognostic factors or patients with moderate disease activity without poor prognostic factors. For patients with moderate disease activity with poor prognostic factors, combination csDMARD therapy is recommended. This combination can be double or triple therapy and typically will be methotrexate based. For patients with high disease activity without poor prognostic factors, csDMARD monotherapy or combination methotrexate with hydroxychloroquine is recommended. Lastly, for patients with high disease activity and poor prognostic factors, treatment with either combination csDMARD or anti-TNF with or without methotrexate is first line.

The EULAR guidelines state that methotrexate should be a part of the initial treatment strategy for patients with active disease, and if patients have a contraindication to methotrexate, leflunomide or sulfasalazine can be substituted. However, patients with mild or low disease activity may be sufficiently treated with an antimalarial. The recommendation for initial therapy is monotherapy or combination therapy of csDMARDs without explicit advice of when to use monotherapy or combination therapy.

Second-Line Therapy

Based on the ACR recommendations, options for those with established disease or those not responding to primary treatment vary depending on previous treatments, disease activity, and poor prognostic factors. **Figure 37.2** outlines the specific recommendations based on previous treatments. For many patients, switching or adding a csDMARD is sufficient for second-line therapy. However, for patients with more advanced, symptomatic disease who have already failed combination csDMARD, advancing to a bDMARD may be beneficial. The initial bDMARD recommended by the ACR are TNF inhibitors, abatacept or rituximab.

For those not responding to first-line treatment appropriately, the EULAR outlines second-line treatment based on the presence of poor prognostic factors. For those patients without poor prognostic factors, changing csDMARD strategy is preferred, and for those with poor prognostic factors, adding a bDMARD is preferred. The recommended first-line bDMARDs are TNF inhibitors, abatacept or tocilizumab.

Third-Line Therapy

For patients who have been treated with a bDMARD and have not yet met treatment goals, recommendations include either switching to another agent within the same class or switching to another bDMARD class. Another option recommended by the EULAR guidelines is initiating tofacitinib after failure of at least one bDMARD.

Special Populations
Geriatric

Caution should be used when starting elderly patients on NSAIDs due to the increased risk of GI hemorrhage. Further, many elderly patients have decreased renal function, and

NSAIDs may contribute to a decline in this function. Several DMARDs and some immunomodulators are renally excreted, and doses should be adjusted in the elderly due to decreased renal function.

Women

Women with RA who plan on having children need to discuss treatment options with their physician and understand the risks of conception. Certain medications, including methotrexate, leflunomide, abatacept, and rituximab, cannot be used during pregnancy because of known teratogenicity. DMARDs with the most data to support their use during pregnancy are antimalarials, sulfasalazine, azathioprine, and cyclosporine. These medications can be used as monotherapy or in combination with corticosteroids or NSAIDs. If corticosteroids are used during pregnancy, the dose should not exceed 15 mg/d because higher doses increase the risk of intrauterine infection and premature delivery. NSAIDs should be avoided after 30 weeks of gestation because of the increased risk of premature closure of the ductus arteriosus in the fetus. TNF-alpha inhibitors are all classified as pregnancy category B, indicating there were no teratogenic effects in animals and limited or no data in humans. There have been case reports of congenital malformations in children exposed to TNF-alpha inhibitors as a fetus. Therefore, TNF-alpha inhibitors need to be used cautiously in pregnant women.

MONITORING PATIENT RESPONSE

Because the drugs used for treating arthritis have many adverse events and because most are used for long-term treatment, monitoring should include baseline studies against which later results can be compared. CBC with differential, urinalysis, creatinine, serum bilirubin, liver enzymes, ESR, BUN, platelet studies, and eye examinations are among the tests performed periodically during therapy.

Patients should follow the treat-to-target approach, which requires more intensive follow-up and monitoring. Patients started on DMARD therapy should be assessed at least every 3 months and as soon as 1 month to have disease activity assessed. If goals are not met at 3 months, therapy should be adapted until the goal or remission or low disease activity is met. Once the goal is met, patients can be reassessed every 3 to 6 months to ensure their goals are sustained.

PATIENT EDUCATION

Patient education depends on the type of agent selected. The patient should know that routine blood work is important to detect adverse events before they become serious and life threatening. Patients taking DMARDs and immunomodulators should report illness immediately, as the risk of serious infections is increased in these patients. Patients need to understand that there is a delay between initiating therapy and experiencing the full clinical effects and that therapy must be continued in order to be effective.

Patient-Oriented Information Sources

Support groups, education of family members, and assistive devices can help with activities of daily living. The ACR has patient information available on their Web site regarding a variety of topics such as medications, research, advocacy, and exercise (www.rheumatology.org/Pratice/clinical/patients/information_for_patients). In addition, the Arthritis Foundation has information directed at patients regarding different aspects of living with arthritis (www.arthritis.org). The National Institutes of Health, in conjunction with the American Society of Health-System Pharmacists and the United States Pharmacopeia, has a drug information Web site with information about thousands of medications (http://www.nlm.nih.gov/medlineplus/druginformation.html).

Nutrition/Lifestyle Changes

Weight loss programs and healthy habits such as adequate rest are key to the success of a treatment program. Patients should consider occupational therapy as needed to help with household chores. The patient should avoid repetitive joint motion and vibrations from electrical appliances or tools to reduce exacerbations. Splinting the affected joint helps relieve pain and prevent deformity. Patients should remove the splint at least once daily and for any exercise activities. Patients should be instructed on strategies to avoid physical and emotional stress, which may precipitate an exacerbation.

Complementary and Alternative Medications

Folk remedies have been used for RA for many years. Although most of these remedies cause no harm, there is little scientific evidence supporting their efficacy. Some of the more commonly used approaches include shark cartilage, chondroitin, herbs, vitamins, acupuncture, magnet therapy, climate therapy, and several diets. Clinicians should be aware of the therapies being considered or used by the patient; joint treatment goals should be established and monitored. Just as in traditional medicine, patients using complementary approaches either alone or as adjunctive therapy require ongoing monitoring for safety and efficacy of the selected approach.

A recent review of the literature suggests that gamma linolenic acid (GLA) may have a moderate effect on reducing pain and joint tenderness. This agent is found in borage seed oil (9% GLA), black currant oil (6% GLA), or evening primrose oil (2% GLA). The dose should be about 540 mg/d of GLA.

CASE STUDY*

J.W., a 46-year-old African American woman, presents to your office with the chief complaint of bilateral stiffness of the shoulders, hands, and wrists in the morning. She reports she is otherwise healthy, takes no medications, and is employed as a systems analyst for a large bank. She recalls having some minor flulike symptoms approximately 3 weeks before her visit. The stiffness makes it difficult for her to work for any extended period. She has also started wearing a wig because she cannot raise her arms in the morning to fix her hair. She has lost 10 pounds over the past 8 months but has not consciously dieted. She finds it increasingly difficult to drive, particularly when making turns and driving in reverse.

Pertinent laboratory results:

ESR 89 mm/hr (0 to 29 mm/hr), ACPA 65 EU/mL (less than 20 EU/mL), SCr 1.0 mg/dL

DIAGNOSIS: RHEUMATOID ARTHRITIS WITH MODERATE DISEASE ACTIVITY

1. List specific goals of treatment for J.W.
2. Which drug therapy would you prescribe, and why?
3. What are the parameters for monitoring success of the therapy?
4. Discuss specific patient education based on the prescribed therapy.
5. List one or two adverse reactions for the selected agent that would cause you to change therapy?
6. What would be the choice for second-line therapy?
7. What over-the-counter and/or alternative medications would be appropriate for J.W.?
8. What lifestyle changes should be recommended for J.W.?
9. Describe one or two drug–drug or drug–food interactions for the selected agent.

* Answers can be found online.

Bibliography

*Starred entries are cited in text.

Aletaha, D., Neogi, T., Silman, A. J., et al. (2010). 2010 rheumatoid arthritis classification criteria. *Arthritis and Rheumatism, 62*(9), 2569–2581.

American College of Rheumatology Ad Hoc Committee on Clinical Guidelines. (1996). Guidelines for monitoring drug therapy in rheumatoid arthritis. *Arthritis and Rheumatism, 39*, 723–731.

Anderson, J. J., Wells, G., Verhoeven, A. C., et al. (2000). Factors predicting response to treatment in rheumatoid arthritis: The importance of disease duration. *Arthritis and Rheumatism, 43*(1), 22–29.

Feist, E., & Burmester, G. R. (2013). Small molecules targeting JAKs—A new approach in the treatment of rheumatoid arthritis. *Rheumatology, 52,* 1352–1357.

Felson, D. T., Smolen, J. S., Wells, G., et al. (2011). American College of Rheumatology/European League Against Rheumatism provisional definition of remission in rheumatoid arthritis for clinical trials. *Arthritis and Rheumatism, 63*(3), 573–586.

*Helmick, C. G., Felson, D. T., Lawrence, R. C., et al. (2008). Estimates of the prevalence of arthritis and other rheumatic conditions in the United States: Part 1. *Arthritis and Rheumatism, 58*(1), 15–25.

Kavanaugh, A., & Wells, A. F. (2014). Benefits and risks of low-dose glucocorticoid treatment in the patient with rheumatoid arthritis. *Rheumatology, 53,* 1742–1751.

*Kroot, E. J., van Leeuwen, M. A., van Rijswijk, M. H., et al. (2000). No increased mortality in patients with rheumatoid arthritis: Up to 10 years of follow up from disease onset. *Annals of the Rheumatic Disease, 59,* 954–958.

McInnes, I. B., & Schett, G. (2011). The pathogenesis of rheumatoid arthritis. *The New England Journal of Medicine, 365,* 2205–2219.

Nell, V. P., Machold, K. P., Eberl, G., et al. (2004). Benefit of very early referral and very early therapy with disease-modifying anti-rheumatic drugs in patients with very early rheumatoid arthritis. *Rheumatology, 43*(7), 906–914.

Ostensen, M. (2009). Management of early aggressive rheumatoid arthritis during pregnancy and lactation. *Expert Opinion on Pharmacotherapy, 10*(9), 1469–1479.

Ruderman, E. M. (2012). Overview of safety of non-biologic and biologic DMARDs. *Rheumatology, 51,* vi37–vi43.

Saag, K. G., Teng, G. G., Patkar, N. M., et al. (2008). American College of Rheumatology 2008 recommendations for the use of nonbiologic and biologic disease-modifying antirheumatic drugs in rheumatoid arthritis. *Arthritis and Rheumatism, 59*(6), 762–784.

Soeken, K. K., Miller, S. A., & Ernst, E. (2003). Herbal medicines for the treatment of rheumatoid arthritis. *Rheumatology, 42*(5), 652–659.

Singh, J. A., Furst, D. E., Bharat, A., et al. (2012). 2012 Update of the 2008 American College of Rheumatology Recommendations for the use of disease-modifying antirheumatic drugs and biologic agents in the treatment of rheumatoid arthritis. *Arthritis Care & Research, 64*(5), 625–639.

Smolen, J. S., Aletaha, D., Bijlsma, J. W., et al. (2010). Treating rheumatoid arthritis to target: Recommendations of an international task force. *Annals of the Rheumatic Diseases, 69*(4), 631–637.

Smolen, J. S., van der Heijide, D., Machold, K. P., et al. (2014). Proposal for a new nomenclature of disease-modifying antirheumatic drugs. *Annals of the Rheumatic Diseases, 73*(1), 3–5.

Upchurch, K. S., & Kay, J. (2012). Evolution of treatment of rheumatoid arthritis. *Rheumatology, 51,* vi28–vi36.

Wahl, K., & Schuna, A. A. (2014). Rheumatoid arthritis. In J. T. Dipiro, et al. (Eds.). *Pharmacotherapy: A pathophysiologic approach* (9th ed.). New York, NY: McGraw Hill.

Pharmacology for Neurological/ Psychological Disorders

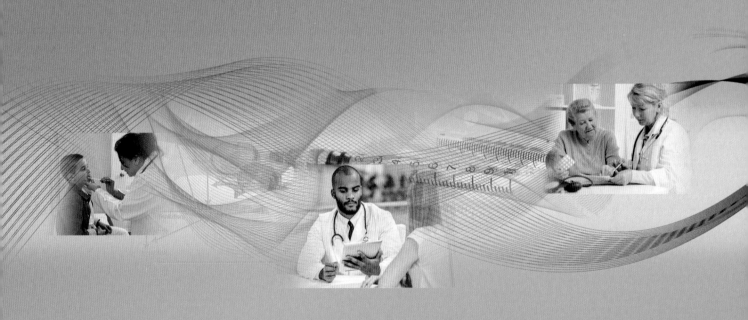

38 Headaches

Kelleen N. Flaherty

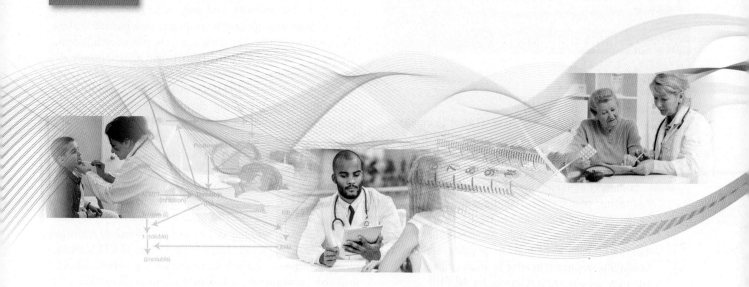

Headache is one of the most common complaints presenting in primary care. The pain of a headache can range from mild to severe, can be acute or chronic, and may last hours to days in duration. Severe headache and migraine are estimated to afflict one in seven individuals in the United States based on multiple population-wide studies and have a significant impact on quality of life and health care resource utilization (Burch et al., 2015). While there are three main categories of headaches according to the most recent International Classification of Headache Disorders (ICHD-3; Headache Classification Subcommittee of the International Headache Society [IHS], 2013), the most commonly encountered headaches seen in primary care are the primary and secondary headaches (**Box 38.1**). A primary headache is one with no identifiable underlying organic disease process; a secondary headache is one for which a specific etiology has been identified. The practitioner must first rule out a secondary headache (or more serious cause of headache pain) and then accurately diagnose the type of primary headache. In some instances, a primary and secondary headache can occur simultaneously. Primary headaches include tension-type headache (TTH), migraine, and cluster headache (CH). This chapter will focus on diagnosing and treating TTH and migraine, the most common forms of primary headache presenting in clinical practice.

Tension headaches have a dull quality, with pain that radiates bilaterally from the forehead to the occiput in a band-like fashion. The pain often radiates down the neck and sometimes even into the trapezius muscle. The pain is mild to moderate and can last from 30 minutes to several days in severe cases. Tension headaches are not typically present upon awakening, but begin later in the day and progress with time. The pain of these headaches is rarely debilitating, but it can affect a person's ability to function, especially if prolonged or chronic. There are no associated symptoms of nausea, vomiting, photophobia, or phonophobia.

Migraine is a neurologic syndrome causing not only throbbing head pain but also often nausea, appetite change, photophobia, and phonophobia. The pain generally ranges from moderate to severe and can be disabling. The Global Burden of Disease Study in 2010 ranked migraine as the third most prevalent and seventh highest specific cause of disability in the world (ICHD-3, 2013). According to epidemiologic studies, migraine occurs in one in seven individuals in the United States and is two to three times more common in females than males. The National Health Interview Survey (2005–2015) estimated a national prevalence of 13.8%, 18.9% in females and 9% in males, with migraine occurring disproportionately higher in at-risk groups such as the unemployed, the uninsured, or those in lower socioeconomic strata (Burch et al., 2015). The age of onset is from 15 to 35, but peak prevalence is from ages 35 to 45. A family history of migraine has shown to be diagnostic in 60% of cases and is considered to be a significant risk factor. Significant comorbidity has also been demonstrated in population studies, including musculoskeletal complaints, cardiovascular disorders, psychiatric disorders, and epilepsy (Merikangas, 2013). Combined direct and indirect costs for migraine are estimated to be $3.2 billion in the United States, plus $700 million for emergency department visits and $375 million for in-patient treatment (Merikangas, 2013). Decreased productivity is a significant contribution to the indirect cost burden of migraine. Approximately 53% of migraine visits are to primary care offices, with another 16.7% presenting in emergency departments—adding to the financial burden (Burch et al., 2015). It is estimated that half of the individuals suffering from migraine do not report it or seek help for it, and many who do will discontinue treatment (Merikangas, 2013).

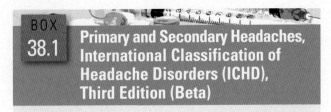

BOX 38.1 Primary and Secondary Headaches, International Classification of Headache Disorders (ICHD), Third Edition (Beta)

Primary Headaches
Migraine
Tension-type headache (TTH)
Trigeminal autonomic cephalalgias (TACs) (includes CH, paroxysmal hemicranias, short-lasting unilateral neuralgiform headache attacks, hemicranias continua)
Other primary headache disorders (primary cough headache, primary exercise headache, primary headache associated with sexual activity, primary thunderclap headache, cold-stimulus headache, external pressure headache, primary stabbing headache, nummular headache, hypnic headache, and new daily-persistent headache [NDPH])

Secondary Headaches
Headache attributed to trauma or injury to the head and/or neck
Headache attributed to cranial or cervical vascular disorder
Headache attributed to nonvascular intracranial disorder
Headache attributed to a substance or its withdrawal
Headache attributed to infection
Headache attributed to disorder of homeostasis
Headache or facial pain attributed to disorder of cranium, neck, eyes, ears, nose, sinuses, teeth, mouth, or other facial or cranial structure
Headache attributed to psychiatric disorder

Painful Cranial Neuropathies, Other Facial Pains, and Other Headaches
Cranial neuralgias and central causes of facial pain
Other headache, cranial neuralgia, central or primary facial pain

Modified from Headache Classification Committee of the International Headache Society (IHS). (2013). The International Classification of Headache Disorders, 3rd ed. (beta version). *Cephalalgia, 33*(9), 629–808.

CHs may be chronic or acute and episodic and are far less common than migraine or tension headaches, occurring in less than 1% of the population. They are approximately three times more common in males than in females, and the acute/episodic variety is approximately six times more common than chronic CH (Fischera et al., 2008). The pain is disabling, burning, or boring and centered around one eye and is described by patients as being more severe than childbirth or passing a kidney stone. Attacks are unilateral, generally lasting from 15 to 180 minutes, and may occur one to eight times per day. Associated ipsilateral symptoms may include lacrimation, nasal congestion, rhinorrhea, miosis, ptosis, eyelid edema, or conjunctival injection. Restlessness and agitation may also accompany an attack; individuals often cannot lie down and instead pace the floor (ICHD-3, 2013). Significant disability and comorbidity (including cognitive impairment, anxiety, depression, agoraphobia, and even suicidal tendencies) may be associated with CH (Torkamani et al., 2015). A patient with symptoms suggestive of CH should be referred to a neurologist or headache specialist. Episodic CH occurs in a series of repeated headaches, with periods lasting anywhere from 1 week to 1 year, interrupted by periods of pain-free remission. Chronic CH, on the other hand, lasts at least for 1 year without remission, or without at least one full month of remission (ICHD-3, 2013). While the pathophysiology of CH is incompletely understood, hypothalamic dysfunction is believed to be involved; consequently, circadian rhythms are disrupted. CHs often occur at specific times during sleep–wake cycles, another indication of hypothalamic involvement (Francis et al., 2010).

CAUSES OF TENSION HEADACHES

Tension headaches are highly prevalent in the population, with a lifetime prevalence of 30% to 78% demonstrated in a variety of population studies. Prevalence is approximately twice as high in females as it is in males (Haque et al., 2012; ICHD-3, 2013). The high prevalence of TTH results in a more significant and costly socioeconomic burden than that of migraine (Bezov et al., 2010; ICHD-3, 2013). Chronic TTH has a global prevalence of 0.5% to 4.8%. While stress has been shown to be the most common precipitant of TTH, other precipitants have been identified (ICHD-3, 2013; Yu & Han, 2015). Sleep dysregulation has been shown to have a bidirectional relationship with TTH, with lack of sleep being a precipitant of TTH and TTH being a precipitant of insomnia (Rains et al., 2015). Other precipitants reported include sunlight, fatigue, anxiety, temperature (cold and warm), activity, traveling, and reading. Unlike migraine, food does not appear to be a trigger (Haque et al., 2012). Cigarette smoking has also been correlated with an increased number of days of headache per week.

Although more common in migraine patients, one cause of recurrent tension headaches is the overuse of over-the-counter (OTC) and prescription analgesic medications, leading to medication overuse headache (MOH; ICHD-3, 2013). The headache recurs as each dose of medication wears off, causing the patient to take another analgesic and thus continue the cycle of pain. Treating more than two headaches with an OTC analgesic for either migraine or TTH per week can lead to development of chronic daily headache. Other modifiable risk factors include obesity, caffeine overuse, alcohol consumption, and temporomandibular issues. Nonmodifiable risk factors include female gender, genetics, socioeconomic status, head or neck injury, age, and life events (Cho & Chu, 2015; Yu & Han, 2015).

PATHOPHYSIOLOGY OF TENSION HEADACHES

While TTH was originally assumed to be psychogenic in nature, evidence now suggests that these headaches have neurobiologic etiologies (ICHD-3, 2013) and may be a consequence of both centrally (chronic) and peripherally (episodic) processed pain. Central pain processing may result in increased tenderness and lower pain thresholds in pericranial and myofascial muscles. There may also be genetic, comorbid (e.g., chronic pain, depression, etc.), vitamin D deficiency, and vascular components to TTH. Other research has implicated nitric oxide (a vasodilator) as a local mediator of TTH. In one study, blocking nitric oxide production led to decreased pericranial muscle hardness and headache pain in patients with chronic TTH (Ashina et al., 1999).

DIAGNOSTIC CRITERIA

The first step in determining the type of headache a patient has is to take a detailed headache history. The history should include the patient's age; the time of day when the attack(s) occur(s); the duration and frequency of attacks; precipitating or relieving factors; the quality, location, and intensity of the pain; use of OTC analgesics; and associated symptoms. The social history and family history are also important. The results of physical and neurologic examinations should be unremarkable in a patient with primary headache, other than revealing possible tenderness of pericranial muscles. Diagnosis is mostly of exclusion: all possible secondary headaches, migraine headache, and CHs are ruled out. Tension headaches may be diagnosed as primary, secondary, or both. The Headache Classification Committee of the International Headache Society characterizes TTH by "frequent episodes of headache, typically bilateral, pressing or tightening in quality and of mild to moderate intensity, lasting minutes to days. The pain does not worsen with routine physical activity and is not associated with nausea, but photophobia or phonophobia may be present (ICHD-3, 2013)."

Diagnostic alarms in the evaluation of a headache patient that require further testing include headache onset after age 50, sudden-onset headache, accelerating headache pattern, headache with fever and stiff neck, and abnormal results on the neurologic examination. With regard to other types of diagnostic testing, the American Headache Society's (AHS) "Choosing Wisely" recommendations counsel against the use of neuroimaging studies in patients with stable headaches

| BOX 38.2 | Diagnostic Criteria for Frequent Episodic Tension Headache, International Classification of Headache Disorders (ICHD), Third Edition (Beta) |

A. At least 10 episodes of headache occurring on 1 to 14 days per month on average for >3 months (≥12 and <180 days per year) and fulfilling criteria B–D
B. Lasting from 30 minutes to 7 days
C. At least two of the following four characteristics:
  1. Bilateral location
  2. Pressing or tightening (nonpulsating) quality
  3. Mild or moderate intensity
  4. Not aggravated by routine physical activity such as walking or climbing stairs
D. Both of the following:
  1. No nausea or vomiting
  2. No more than one of photophobia or phonophobia
E. Not better accounted for by another ICHD-3 diagnosis

Source: Headache Classification Committee of the International Headache Society (IHS). (2013). The International Classification of Headache Disorders, 3rd ed. (beta version). *Cephalalgia*, *33*(9), 629–808.

that meet criteria for migraine and against the use of CT imaging for headache when MRI is available, except in the emergency setting (Loder et al., 2013). The ICHD-3 diagnostic criteria for frequent episodic tension headache can be seen in **Box 38.2**.

INITIATING DRUG THERAPY FOR TENSION HEADACHES

Before initiating drug therapy, it is critical to determine the type and frequency of OTC medication use. Patients with tension headaches and headaches in general frequently self-medicate and may be presenting with MOH. Again, treating more than two headaches per week for more than a few consecutive weeks can lead to development of a chronic daily headache pattern. Caffeine and butalbital products are notorious contributors to MOH. The initial treatment of MOH consists of withholding all OTC analgesics for 1 to 2 weeks.

It is also important to help identify headache triggers and to encourage a healthy lifestyle. Often, simple changes, such as eating and sleeping in a consistent pattern, decreasing alcohol and tobacco use, and using good posture, can decrease headache severity and frequency.

Adjuncts to pharmacotherapy include relaxation therapy, biofeedback, self-hypnosis, cognitive therapy, and manual therapy (massage). Data from a large meta-analysis show positive results with the use of biofeedback, particularly when combined with relaxation (Nestoriuc et al., 2008). Patients may also benefit from acupuncture or cervical physical therapy in the case of chronic tension headaches.

Headache sufferers (TTH and migraine) use a substantial amount of complementary and alternative medicine (CAM) for the self-management of headache. The alternative approaches include acupuncture, chiropractic, massage, yoga, homeopathy, and use of dietary supplements such as herbal compounds and vitamins. In one large literature review, some 30% to 70% of CAM users report the therapy to be effective. Most practitioners use CAM as adjunctive therapy to pharmacotherapy, rather than prior to or after treatment with medications. While there have been some studies on the efficacy of CAM, they are methodologically weak. Further, many patients are using CAM therapies concomitantly with conventional treatment and may not report its use to the health care practitioner. Health care practitioners should be vigilant and inquire about CAM use, to anticipate and avoid any potential adverse reactions (Adams et al., 2012).

Goals of Drug Therapy for Tension Headaches

The primary goals of drug therapy should be to reduce the severity and frequency of headaches, thus improving the patient's quality of life and ability to function. The goals for patients with episodic tension headaches are to select appropriate analgesic agents that will have the fewest side effects. Prophylactic therapy should be considered in addition to abortive analgesic agents for patients with more than two significant headaches per week. In a patient with MOH, it is appropriate to start a prophylactic agent and abruptly stop abortive analgesic medications simultaneously (other than barbiturate drugs, which must be tapered). It is important to educate patients about MOH and to limit the use of analgesics to 2 days per week. Again, regular and frequent treatment with analgesics may cause development of chronic headache. It is important that patients do not overuse analgesics, as this is likely to interfere with the efficacy of preventive treatment (ICHD-3, 2013).

Acetaminophen and Aspirin

Acetaminophen at a dose of 1,000 mg can be very effective in treating mild to moderate tension headaches, although given the hepatotoxic qualities of the drug, a U.S. Food and Drug Administration (FDA) advisory committee in 2009 voted to lower the recommended single dose to 650 mg (making 1,000-mg tablets available by prescription only) and to lower the maximum daily limit from its presently recommended 4,000 to 3,250 mg (Schilling et al., 2010). Consequently, in 2011, McNeill Consumer Healthcare lowered the maximum recommended dose of Tylenol and increased the dosing interval for some of their OTC medications (DIH, 2014). Injectable acetaminophen carries a black box warning as of 2013 for potential liver failure, transplant, and death (DIH, 2014). The advantages of acetaminophen are that it is well tolerated and has few drug–drug interactions and side effects. Acetaminophen should be avoided in patients with heavy alcohol consumption, alcoholic liver disease, or chronic liver disease, as the drug is metabolized through the liver. Consumption of three or more alcoholic drinks a day in conjunction with acetaminophen use can have hepatotoxic effects. Chronic use of acetaminophen or use of acetaminophen at high doses can cause liver damage, particularly in older persons; the leading cause of acute liver failure in the United States is acetaminophen overdose (and the leading drug overdose seen in emergency departments is with acetaminophen). Acetaminophen overdose is often accidental; patients need to be cautioned not to exceed 4,000 mg/d and to take care not to take other acetaminophen-containing medications in the same day (Schilling et al., 2010). Prolonged use of acetaminophen and aspirin or nonsteroidal anti-inflammatory drugs (NSAIDs) should be avoided.

Aspirin can also alleviate mild to moderate tension headaches. It inhibits prostaglandin synthesis via nonspecific and irreversible deactivation of both cyclooxygenase 1 (COX-1) and cyclooxygenase 2 (COX-2), reducing the inflammatory response and platelet aggregation. Contraindications to aspirin use include a history of bleeding disorders, asthma, and hypersensitivity to salicylates or NSAIDs. Patients should avoid combining aspirin with other NSAIDs because decreased serum concentrations of NSAIDs result when these drugs are used together. The most common adverse effects associated with aspirin are gastrointestinal in nature, such as nausea, vomiting, or heartburn. Aspirin has also been recommended as first-line treatment for TTH and migraine, regardless of headache severity (Lampl et al., 2012).

Nonsteroidal Anti-inflammatory Drugs (NSAIDs)

NSAIDs work well for moderate tension headaches. They work by selectively inhibiting COX-2, responsible for prostaglandin synthesis, thereby reducing inflammation. These drugs take effect in 30 to 60 minutes, similar to aspirin and acetaminophen. Commonly used NSAIDs for the management of TTH include ibuprofen, naproxen, ketoprofen, diclofenac, and indomethacin.

Common side effects of NSAIDs are abdominal cramps, nausea, indigestion, and even headache. Occasionally, these drugs cause peptic ulcers and GI hemorrhage. Many NSAIDs contain boxed warnings about cardiovascular effects, GI effects, and/or use in patients with renal impairment. COX-2-specific inhibitors are not indicated specifically for headache, but are indicated for acute pain and have shown efficacy in stabbing headache (Ferrante et al., 2010) and migraine (Wentz et al., 2008). Its specificity for COX-2 tends to decrease GI effects, but COX-2 inhibitors also carry black box warnings, particularly for cardiovascular events.

Any given NSAID should be tried in a patient twice before deciding whether it is successful or not. It is not uncommon for a patient to respond poorly to one NSAID and extremely well to another. Route of administration may also be a consideration to improve NSAID response (Barbanti et al., 2014).

Antiemetic Agents

Although patients with tension headaches rarely suffer from nausea, antiemetic agents can augment the pain-relieving properties of analgesics by decreasing gastric emptying, therefore improving analgesic absorption (Barbanti et al., 2014). Commonly used antiemetics are promethazine and prochlorperazine. These medications can be sedating and have numerous other potential side effects, including rare but serious neurologic and bone marrow effects. Promethazine carries a boxed warning for use in children 2 years old and younger and for its injectable formulation. Prochlorperazine carries a boxed warning for use in older patients with dementia-related psychosis who are being treated with antipsychotics (DIH, 2014). Patients should be educated about these possible effects before starting on these medications and should be encouraged to use them sparingly.

Other Abortive Agents

For patients whose headaches do not respond to the above agents, certain combination agents can be considered. Some patients have a good response to OTC agents containing acetaminophen, aspirin, and caffeine (such as Excedrin Extra Strength). However, these agents have a high rate of analgesic MOH when used regularly and should not be used more than 1 to 2 days per week.

Prescription combinations that can be used include butalbital/acetaminophen/caffeine (Fioricet and others) and butalbital/aspirin/caffeine (Fiorinal and others). Butalbital is a barbiturate, which is sedating and potentially habit forming; these medications should not be used in patients with a history of substance abuse. Fiorinal and Fioricet very commonly cause MOH and should not be used for more than 3 days per month. If a patient is taking many butalbital-containing pills per day, they must be slowly tapered to avoid withdrawal symptoms. Patients taking these medications should be closely monitored.

Combination acetaminophen/narcotic products such as Vicodin and Percocet are not recommended; FDA has recommended their removal from the market or an inclusion of a black box warning if the drugs remain on the market (FDA, 2009). Opioid- or butalbital-containing medications should not be prescribed as first-line treatment for recurrent headache disorders (Loder et al., 2013). **Table 38.1** gives an overview of selected drugs used to abort TTH.

TABLE 38.1

Overview of Selected Drugs to Abort Tension-Type Headaches

Generic (Brand) Name and Dosage	Selected Adverse Events	Contraindications	Special Considerations
acetaminophen (Tylenol) 325–650 mg q4h–6h limit dose to 3,250 mg/d	Severe hepatotoxicity on acute overdose, potential liver damage w/ chronic daily dosing, nephrotoxicity, agranulocytosis, rash (including potentially fatal Stevens-Johnson syndrome)	Chronic alcohol use, alcoholic liver disease, impaired liver or renal function, G6PD deficiency	Avoid using w/ alcohol
aspirin 325–650 mg q4h–6h, not to exceed 4,000 mg/d	GI upset (stomach pain, nausea, heartburn, vomiting); GI bleeding and angioedema (uncommon)	Platelet or bleeding disorders, renal dysfunction, erosive gastritis, peptic ulcer disease, asthma, rhinitis, nasal polyps, severe hepatic or renal failure, or sensitivity to salicylates	Avoid using w/ NSAIDs, alcohol, during pregnancy, and in children <16 y with viral infections; discontinue 1–2 wk prior to surgery
NSAIDs ibuprofen (Advil) 200–400 mg q4h–6h, not to exceed 1,200 mg/d; under clinical supervision not to exceed ≤2,400 mg/d *Note:* Use lower doses in patients w/ renal or hepatic disease	3%–9%: Dizziness, rash, epigastric pain, heartburn, nausea, tinnitus	**WARNING: NSAIDs are associated with an increased risk of adverse cardiovascular thrombotic events, including MI, stroke, and new onset or worsening of pre-existing hypertension. Use is contraindicated for treatment of perioperative pain in the setting of CABG surgery.** Recent GI bleed, third trimester of pregnancy, renal disease	Use w/ caution if history of CHF, HTN, GI bleeding; monitor for anemia w/ long-term use; older persons are at increased risk for AEs even at low doses; withhold for at least 4–6 half-lives prior to dental or surgical procedures; may increase risk of GI irritation, inflammation, ulceration, bleeding, and perforation

(Continued)

TABLE 38.1

Overview of Selected Drugs to Abort Tension-Type Headaches (*Continued*)

Generic (Brand) Name and Dosage	Selected Adverse Events	Contraindications	Special Considerations
naproxen (Aleve) Initial: 500 mg, then 250 mg q6h–8h not to exceed 1,250 mg/d *Note*: Enteric-coated formulations not recommended for tx of acute migraine	3%–9%: Edema, dizziness, drowsiness, headache, pruritus, skin eruption, ecchymosis, fluid retention, abdominal pain, constipation, nausea, heartburn, hemolysis, tinnitus, dyspnea	Same as above, including **BOXED WARNING**	Same as above
ketoprofen 25–50 mg q6h–8h	>10%: Dyspepsia, abnormal LFTs; 3%–9%: Headache, abdominal pain, constipation, diarrhea, flatulence, nausea, renal dysfunction	Same as above, including **BOXED WARNING**	Same as above
Barbiturates butalbital 50 mg, caffeine 40 mg, acetaminophen 325 mg (Fioricet) 1–2 tabs q4h, not to exceed 6 tabs/d *Note*: Do not use butalbital for the management of acute migraine	Drowsiness, light-headedness, dizziness, sedation, shortness of breath, nausea, vomiting, abdominal pain, intoxicated feeling	Hepatic or renal dysfunction, peptic ulcer disease, history of substance abuse, porphyria, pregnancy, concomitant use w/ alcohol or other CNS depressants	Contains acetaminophen; use w/ caution when taking other acetaminophen-containing drugs; do not exceed a total daily dose of 3,250 mg acetaminophen; may be habit forming or subject to abuse; avoid prolonged use or using w/ other sedating medications; not recommended for use in older persons
butalbital 50 mg/caffeine 40 mg/aspirin 325 mg (Fiorinal) 1–2 tabs q4h, not to exceed 6 tabs/d *Note*: Do not use butalbital for management of acute migraine	Same as above	Hemorrhagic diathesis (e.g., hemophilia, hypoprothrombinemia, von Willebrand disease, thrombocytopenias, thrombasthenia and other ill-defined hereditary platelet dysfunctions, severe vitamin K deficiency, and severe liver damage); nasal polyps, angioedema and bronchospastic reactivity to aspirin or other NSAIDs; peptic ulcer or other serious GI lesions; porphyria	Use w/ caution in the debilitated; severe impairment of renal or hepatic function, coagulation disorders, head injuries, elevated intracranial pressure, acute abdominal conditions, hypothyroidism, urethral stricture, Addison's disease, or prostatic hypertrophy; not recommended for use in older persons

Prophylaxis of Tension Headaches

If a patient has more than two tension headaches per week, prophylaxis should be considered. Antidepressant medications are commonly used for headache prophylaxis. In meta-analyses, individuals with chronic headache taking antidepressants are twice as likely to report improvement of symptoms (Dharmshaktu et al., 2012). Abundant evidence exists for the efficacy of amitriptyline, with individuals experiencing relief even at low doses. Its antinociceptive effects are independent from its antidepressant effects (Yu & Han, 2015). There are data supporting the use of venlafaxine and mirtazapine, but data supporting the use of other antidepressants for headache

prophylaxis (including migraine) are lacking. Smaller noncontrolled trials or case studies have shown efficacy with other tricyclic antidepressants (TCAs), such as imipramine, doxepin, and protriptyline. While there have been trials conducted on the efficacy of fluoxetine as headache prophylaxis, neither it nor the other selective serotonin reuptake inhibitors (SSRIs) have been shown to be effective as headache prophylaxis despite having a more favorable side effect profile compared with TCAs. Other antidepressants, such as monoamine oxidase inhibitors (MAOIs) and serotonin antagonists, have been studied, but safety issues and side effect profiles make them an inappropriate choice for headache prophylaxis. Antidepressants for which little support exists for the management of headache should only be considered if the headache being treated is comorbid with depression. Alleviation or palliation of one comorbidity, however, will not necessarily resolve the other (Smitherman et al., 2011). Prophylactic medications should be started at low dosages and increased slowly. It can take 4 to 8 weeks before the full effect of these medications is seen. Finding the appropriate prophylactic agent for a patient is a process of trial and error, as medications work differently in different patients.

Amitriptyline, a TCA, is the medication most commonly used to prevent tension headaches and considered to be a first-line, gold standard drug. It can be used in doses much lower than those used for treating depression, ranging from 10 to 75 mg. Common side effects include sedation, constipation, blurred vision, and dry mouth. Amitriptyline should be used with caution in patients with a history of coronary artery disease, urinary retention, glaucoma, and seizures. Usually, only low doses of amitriptyline are needed, making discontinuation because of side effects uncommon. Higher doses of amitriptyline are typically used in headache patients with concomitant depression (Smitherman et al., 2011). Given its anticholinergic properties, amitriptyline is an inappropriate choice for use in older patients.

Second-line drugs that have been determined to be effective include venlafaxine (Effexor, a serotonin/norepinephrine reuptake inhibitor or SNRI) and mirtazapine (Remeron, a tetracyclic antidepressant) at 150 and 30 mg, respectively (Barbanti et al., 2014; Bendtson & Jensen, 2011).

These drugs may also concurrently treat depression and anxiety. Common side effects of venlafaxine include nausea, somnolence, and insomnia, which often diminish after a few weeks. Patients may also experience sexual dysfunction, increased sweating, or nervousness, which may or may not diminish with time. Venlafaxine can also interact with many medications and should be tapered upon discontinuation, as withdrawal symptoms may occur with abrupt discontinuation. Mirtazapine has been used for its analgesic properties in chronic headache and has the added benefit of sometimes controlling nausea (Smith, 2015). An additional caution when considering the use of any antidepressant is that of suicidal ideation, particularly in adolescents. In 2007, the FDA required black box warnings in all antidepressant-prescribing information "…about increased risks of suicidal thinking and behavior, known as suicidality, in young adults ages 18 to 24 during initial treatment (generally the first 1 to 2 months)" (FDA, 2007).

Recently, data have emerged on the use of local anesthetics injected into pericranial myofascial trigger points. Lidocaine and bupivacaine are the most commonly used, with the most commonly injected muscles being the trapezius, sternocleidomastoid, and temporalis. While there aren't many data on this approach, some studies have shown substantial efficacy in headache prophylaxis. Contraindications include pregnancy, infection, open skull defect, or any condition in which injection landmarks become difficult to identify (e.g., obesity). Adverse events are typically mild (associated with injection in general), and severe adverse events are rare (but have been reported, e.g., pneumothorax; Robbins et al., 2014). **Table 38.2** lists prophylactic agents for TTH.

First-Line Therapy for Tension Headaches

Aspirin and acetaminophen are appropriate first-line agents. They should be used no more than 2 days per week, as with any other analgesic agent, to avoid MOH. Acetaminophen should be used at a maximum single dose of 650 mg and a maximum daily dose of 3,250 mg. If used judiciously, these agents have few adverse effects and are very well tolerated. They work best for mild to moderate headaches. Again, the AHS's "Choosing Wisely" guideline specifically counsels against the use of opioid- or butalbital-containing analgesics as first-line therapy (Loder et al., 2013).

Second-Line Therapy for Tension Headaches

NSAIDs are the next option for treatment of TTH. If one agent fails for two consecutive headaches, another agent in this class should be tried. NSAIDs seem to work well for more stubborn TTHs. If they provide incomplete relief, an antiemetic agent may be added to augment their effect.

Caffeine-containing analgesics available OTC such as Excedrin Extra Strength can also be an effective treatment. These medications should be used infrequently to obviate MOH and may be alternated with NSAIDs for different headaches.

Third-Line Therapy for Tension Headaches

If the above agents fail, then butalbital-containing compounds (Fioricet or Fiorinal) may be used in patients without specific risk factors for these medications. These agents may also be reserved as backup if the abovementioned agents fail to relieve a more severe TTH. Again, butalbital-containing agents should never be used more than 3 days per month, as they easily trigger MOH. As mentioned earlier, any patient requiring treatment for two or more headaches per week or who has particularly severe TTH should be considered for a prophylactic agent.

CAUSES OF MIGRAINE HEADACHE

The ICHD-3 beta characterizes migraine headaches as a "recurrent headache disorder manifesting in attacks lasting 4 to 72 hours. Typical characteristics of the headache are unilateral location, pulsating quality, moderate or severe intensity, aggravation by routine physical activity and association with nausea and/or photophobia and phonophobia (ICHD-3, 2013)." Why some patients experience migraines while others do not is unknown, but it is clear that there is a genetic component to migraines and that migraines tend to cluster in families (Cho & Chu, 2015). There are many possible migraine triggers, and each patient's triggers are unique. Triggers range from certain foods to too much or too little sleep to medications to hormonal factors and others. In some patients, no obvious triggers are found. Estrogen is thought to play a role in the development of migraines, which explains the predominance of migraines in females. About 25% of migraine attacks occur within 4 days

TABLE 38.2

Overview of Selected Drugs Used to Prevent Tension-Type Headaches

Generic (Brand) Name and Dosage	Selected Adverse Events	Contraindications	Special Considerations
amitriptyline (Elavil) Initial: 10–25 mg qhs, usual dose 150 mg qhs; reported dosing ranges 10–400 mg/d (higher doses in patients w/ concomitant depression)	Degree of anticholinergic effects (urinary retention, dry mouth, constipation) are higher in amitriptyline than in other TCAs; drowsiness/sedation (sometimes significant), orthostasis, conduction abnormalities	**WARNING: Antidepressants increase the risk of suicidal thinking and behavior in children, adolescents, and young adults (ages 18–24) with major depressive disorder and other psychiatric disorders.** Not FDA approved for children < age 12	Most widely used; use w/ caution in patients w/ history of CVD (stroke, MI, tachycardia, or conduction abnormalities); use w/ caution in patients w/ BPH, glaucoma, urinary retention, xerostomia, visual problems, constipation, or history of bowel obstruction; use w/ caution in patients with diabetes, seizures, hyperthyroidism (or thyroid supplementation), or hepatic or renal dysfunction; effects may be intensified by use of other CNS drugs or alcohol; use w/ caution in older persons
venlafaxine XR (Effexor XR) 150 mg/d; taper discontinuation to obviate discontinuation syndrome	>10%: Nausea, somnolence, insomnia (often diminish after a few weeks); sexual dysfunction, increased sweating, nervousness (may or may not diminish with time)	**WARNING: Antidepressants increase the risk of suicidal thinking and behavior in children, adolescents, and young adults (18–24 y of age) with major depressive disorder (MDD) and other psychiatric disorders.** Not FDA approved for use in children; monitor for serotonin syndrome, tachycardia, hypertension, and bleeding	Often used because it usually has fewer side effects than amitriptyline; use with caution in older persons
mirtazapine (Remeron) 15–30 mg/d; taper discontinuation to obviate discontinuation syndrome	>10%: Somnolence, increased cholesterol, xerostomia, increased appetite, constipation, weight gain	**WARNING: Antidepressants increase the risk of suicidal thinking and behavior in children, adolescents, and young adults (18–24 y of age) with major depressive disorder (MDD) and other psychiatric disorders.** Not FDA approved for use in children; monitor for serotonin syndrome	Use w/ caution in seizure disorders or in patients predisposed to seizure (e.g., brain damage, alcoholism, concomitant use with drugs that lower seizure threshold), hepatic or renal dysfunction, and in older persons; may actually help with nausea

of menses, when estrogen has fallen to a low level. The best way to pinpoint triggers is to have the patient keep a diary of what he or she ate and did in the 12 hours before getting the headache to see if any patterns emerge. A large literature review covering 15 studies evaluating triggers (in males and females, with either spontaneous reporting of triggers or selection from

a list) identified a large variety of triggers experienced by individuals reporting them anywhere from 8% of the time to 90% of the time. Some triggers are nonmodifiable (e.g., menstruation, gender, age, etc.), while others are modifiable (e.g., sleep deprivation) (Cho & Chu, 2015; Lipton et al., 2014; Pavlovic et al., 2014). **Box 38.3** lists migraine triggers.

BOX 38.3 Factors That May Trigger Migraine Headaches

PSYCHOLOGICAL FACTORS

Anxiety
Depression
Stress (and relaxation after stress, or the "letdown" hypothesis)
Intense emotion
Crisis; postcrisis letdown

MEDICATIONS

Vasodilators (e.g., blood pressure medications, medications for erectile dysfunction)
Hormones (contraceptives, hormone replacement therapy)
Caffeine
Vitamins

DIETARY FACTORS

Alcohol
Aspartame
Caffeine
Chocolate
Monosodium glutamate
Tyramine-containing foods (e.g., red wine)
"Certain foods" (patient-specific reports)

ENVIRONMENTAL/MECHANICAL FACTORS

Head movements
Bright, flashing lights, glare, or sunlight; photophobia
High altitude
Loud noises; phonophobia
Strong odors, perfume
Tobacco smoke (smoking or passive smoking); nicotine
Weather changes (hot or cold)

LIFESTYLE FACTORS

Dieting, skipping meals or fasting; hunger
Obesity
Strenuous exercise/physical effort
Sleep problems: too much or too little sleep, insomnia, bruxism, snoring, daytime sleepiness
Fatigue
Smoking
Excessive alcohol consumption

HORMONAL FACTORS

Ovulation
Menopause
Menses
Pregnancy

Sources: Cho, S. J., & Chu, M. K. (2015). Risk factors of chronic daily headache or chronic migraine. *Current Pain and Headache Reports*, 19(1), 465; Lipton, R. B., Pavlovic, J. M., Haut, S. R., et al. (2014). Methodological issues in studying trigger factors and premonitory features of migraine. *Headache*, 54(10), 1661–1669; Pavlovic, J. M., Buse, D. C., Sollars, C. M., et al. (2014). Trigger factors and premonitory features of migraine attacks: Summary of studies. *Headache*, 54(10), 1670–1679.

PATHOPHYSIOLOGY OF MIGRAINE HEADACHES

The pathophysiology of migraine is incompletely understood. Studies have shown an interaction of a large number of factors that result in the phenomenon, including genetics, afferent pain processing, anatomy and physiology of the trigeminal system, modulatory influence on trigeminal pain transmission, and various pain processing phenomena (Goadsby, 2012). While previously believed to be vasculogenic in nature ("a good story ruined by the facts," as Goadsby says), neurogenic mechanisms are now recognized as the underlying cause of migraine pathophysiology, including atypical pain processing, central sensitization, hyperexcitability in the cortex, and inflammation (Schwedt, 2014). Recurring migraine may serve to sensitize the trigeminal system, lowering pain thresholds, and possibly contributing to chronic migraine. A network of primarily unmyelinated nerve fibers largely arising from the ophthalmic branch of the trigeminal nerve surrounds large cranial blood vessels, blood sinuses, the pia, and the dura in close proximity. The trigeminovascular

system is an initiator and promoter of tissue inflammation and, when activated, releases neuropeptides such as substance P and calcitonin gene–related peptide that cause vasodilation and inflammation. Stimulation of these vessels and sinuses has been shown to be quite painful. Noradrenergic (from the locus caeruleus) and, more significantly, serotonergic neurons (from the dorsal raphe) regulate this activity; the periaqueductal gray region also contributes to pain modulation. Once triggered, impulses travel out through cranial nerve V and ultimately result in dilated meningeal blood vessels and release of neuroinflammatory and nociceptive compounds (Goadsby, 2012; Schwedt, 2014).

Some 80% of migraineurs report premonitory symptoms (e.g., nausea, bloating, fatigue, stiff neck, etc.) prior to the development of aura. Approximately 30% of migraines are accompanied by a prodromal aura, a focal neurologic phenomenon associated variously with visual, sensory, or motor symptoms, but typically affecting the visual field in a spreading fashion, traveling at approximately 3 mm/min from central to peripheral vision. Aura is not typically associated with pain (Charles, 2013; Goadsby, 2012).

<table>
<tr><td>

BOX 38.4

Diagnostic Criteria for Migraine, International Classification of Headache Disorders (ICHD), Third Edition (Beta)

MIGRAINE WITHOUT AURA

A. At least five attacks fulfilling criteria B–D
B. Headache attacks lasting 4 to 72 hours (untreated or unsuccessfully treated)
C. Headache has at least two of the following four characteristics:
  1. Unilateral location
  2. Pulsating quality
  3. Moderate or severe pain intensity
  4. Aggravation by or causing avoidance of routine physical activity (e.g., walking or climbing stairs)
D. During headache, at least one of the following:
  1. Nausea and/or vomiting
  2. Photophobia and phonophobia
E. Not better accounted for by another ICHD-3 diagnosis

MIGRAINE WITH AURA

A. At least two attacks fulfilling criteria B and C
B. One or more of the following fully reversible aura symptoms:
  1. Visual
  2. Sensory
  3. Speech and/or language
  4. Motor
  5. Brain stem
  6. Retinal
C. At least two of the following four characteristics:
  1. At least one aura symptom spreads gradually over ≥5 minutes, and/or two more symptoms occur in succession
  2. Each individual aura symptom lasts 5 to 60 minutes
  3. At least one aura symptom is unilateral
  4. The aura is accompanied, or followed within 60 minutes, by headache
D. Not better accounted for by another ICHD-3 diagnosis, and transient ischemic attack has been excluded

</td></tr>
</table>

Modified from Headache Classification Subcommittee of the International Headache Society. (2013). The International Classification of Headache Disorders, 3rd ed. (beta version). *Cephalalgia, 33*(9), 629–808.

In summary, migraine is a heritable disorder of episodic sensory sensitivity, associated with acute, throbbing pain and enhanced sensitivity to light, motion, sound, and odors. Migraine can be accompanied by nausea and unsteadiness. In different migraineurs, migraines can occur more or less frequently and vary in duration.

DIAGNOSTIC CRITERIA FOR MIGRAINE HEADACHE

The first step in making a precise diagnosis of migraine is to obtain a thorough headache history. Evaluation of the history should include age at onset; time of day when attacks occur; duration of attacks; precipitating or relieving factors; nature, intensity, and location of headache pain; and any associated symptoms. The patient should also be questioned about any aura symptoms, such as visual symptoms (flashing lights, loss of peripheral vision, diplopia, etc.) or other sensory symptoms (vertigo, tinnitus, paresthesias, or hemiparesis). Having patients keep a migraine diary helps identify triggers and premonitory symptoms. Because a family history is evident in many patients, asking if anyone in the family experiences migraines aids in the diagnosis. Note that some patients may fulfill criteria for both migraine with aura and migraine without aura (ICHD-3, 2013). Specific diagnostic criteria for migraine with aura (classic migraine) and without aura (common migraine) are given in **Box 38.4**.

Patients most frequently experience migraines in the early morning, but a migraine attack can come at any time of the day. Migraines are more often unilateral than bilateral, with the pain occurring around the eye or the temple. Migraine pain generally peaks 2 to 12 hours into the attack. Common symptoms accompanying migraine include nausea, anxiety, depression, irritability, fatigue, light and noise sensitivity, diarrhea or constipation, and hunger or anorexia. Patients may describe the pain of migraine as pounding, pulsating, or throbbing. A migraine sufferer often seeks refuge in a dark, quiet place.

INITIATING DRUG THERAPY FOR MIGRAINE HEADACHES

Practitioners must consider many factors when designing a treatment regimen for patients with migraine, such as the severity of the pain, duration of attack, concomitant disease states, current medication use, and any triggers. Migraine treatment needs to be highly individualized. **Table 38.3** gives an overview of selected drugs used for abortive treatment of migraine headaches.

The most effective treatment for migraines involves both nonpharmacologic and pharmacologic approaches. Nonpharmacologic approaches include various psychological techniques that aid in managing the migraine attack. Relaxation, stress management, and biofeedback are some techniques used to reduce migraine severity and frequency. Progressive muscle relaxation and the use of autogenic phrases are examples of relaxation techniques (see section on tension headaches).

TABLE 38.3

Overview of Selected Drugs for Acute/Abortive Migraine Treatment

Generic (Trade) Name and Dosage	Selected Adverse Events	Contraindications	Special Considerations
aspirin 325–900 mg q4h–6h, not to exceed 4,000 mg/d	GI upset (stomach pain, nausea, heartburn, vomiting); GI bleeding and angioedema (uncommon)	Platelet or bleeding disorders, renal dysfunction, erosive gastritis, peptic ulcer disease, asthma, rhinitis, nasal polyps, severe hepatic or renal failure, or sensitivity to salicylates	Avoid using w/ NSAIDs, alcohol, during pregnancy, and in children < 16 y with viral infections; discontinue 1–2 wk prior to surgery
NSAIDs			
See **Table 38.1**.	See **Table 38.1**.	See **Table 38.1**. (including **BOXED WARNING**)	See **Table 38.1**.
OTC caffeine-containing compounds (Excedrin Extra Strength or Excedrin Migraine; acetaminophen 250 mg/aspirin 250 mg/caffeine 65 mg) 1–2 tabs q24h; do not use for longer than 48 h.	Insomnia, agitation	Uncontrolled HTN	Avoid use with other vasoconstrictive agents; use sparingly to obviate MOH
Triptans			
sumatriptan (Imitrex and Alsuma) 25, 50, 100 mg PO at headache onset, may repeat dose up to 100 mg in 2 h 6 mg subcutaneous, may repeat dose in 2 h 5 or 20 mg intranasal spray; may repeat dose in 2 h Oznetra Xsail; 22 mg intranasal; may repeat dose in 2 h	PO: 3%–>10%: Malaise/fatigue, jaw pain/lightness/pressure, paresthesia, pressure/lightness/heaviness, warm/cold sensation SC: >10%: Dizziness, warm/hot sensation, pain at injection site, paresthesia; 3%–10%: chest pain/lightness/heaviness/pressure, burning, feeling of heaviness, flushing, pressure sensation, feeling of tightness, drowsiness, neck, throat, and jaw pain/lightness/pressure, mouth/tongue discomfort, weakness, numbness, throat discomfort IN powder: >2%: Abnormal taste, nasal discomfort, rhinorrhea, and rhinitis IN: >10%: Bad taste, nausea, vomiting; 5%–10%: nasal discomfort/disorder	Pregnancy, uncontrolled HTN, ischemic heart disease, stroke, TIA, PVD, severe hepatic impairment, basilar or hemiplegic migraine; use within 24 h of use of ergot derivatives, or within 2 wk of (or concomitant) use of MAOIs; do not use as prophylactic treatment for migraine; not for IV use OZNETRA's contraindications are: ischemic coronary artery disease (CAD) or coronary artery vasospasm, including Prinzmetal's angina; or Wolff-Parkinson-White syndrome or arrhythmias associated with other cardiac accessory conduction pathway disorders History of stroke, transient ischemic attack (TIA), or hemiplegic or basilar migraine; peripheral vascular disease; ischemic bowel disease; or uncontrolled hypertension Recent (i.e., within 24 hours) use of ergotamine-containing or ergot-type medication, or another 5-HT1 agonist; or concurrent or recent (within 2 weeks) use of a MAO-A inhibitor Known hypersensitivity to sumatriptan (angioedema and anaphylaxis seen) or severe hepatic impairment	Use w/ caution in history of CAD, HTN, seizure disorder (or low seizure threshold), or hepatic impairment; use caution with concomitant use of other serotonergic drugs (SSRIs, SNRIs, other triptans) or proserotonergic drugs (e.g., tryptophan); use at lowest possible doses OZNETRA may cause: Myocardial ischemia/infarction, Prinzmetal's angina, arrhythmias: Sensations of chest/throat/neck/jaw pain, tightness, pressure, or heaviness, cerebral hemorrhage, subarachnoid hemorrhage, and stroke, other vasospasm reactions, MOH, serotonin syndrome, increased BP, anaphylaxis, and seizures (use with caution in epilepsy or lowered seizure threshold)

(Continued)

TABLE 38.3

Overview of Selected Drugs for Acute/Abortive Migraine Treatment (Continued)

Generic (Trade) Name and Dosage	Selected Adverse Events	Contraindications	Special Considerations
zolmitriptan (Zomig) Tablet: 2.5 mg at onset Orally disintegrating tablet: 2.5 mg at onset Nasal spray: 1 spray (5 mg) at onset	PO: 3%–10%: Chest pain, dizziness, somnolence, pain, nausea, xerostomia, dyspepsia, paresthesia, weakness, warm/cold sensation, neck/throat/jaw pain, diaphoresis	Pregnancy, ischemic heart disease or vaso-spastic CAD, uncontrolled HTN, symptomatic Wolff-Parkinson-White syndrome or other arrhythmias associated w/ accessory cardiac conduction pathway disorders; do not use within 24 h of (or concomitant with) use of another $5HT_1$ agonist, or use within 2 wk of (or concomitant with) use of MAOIs; do not use with w/ ergot derivatives or sibutramine; do not use for management of basilar or hemiple-gic migraine; additional contraindications for IN use: stroke, TIA, PVD	High risk factors for heart disease (HTN, high cholesterol, obesity, diabetes, smoking, strong family history of heart disease, post-menopausal women, and males > 40 y old)
naratriptan (Amerge) 2.5 mg q4h to max of 5 mg/d	1%–10%: Dizziness, drowsiness, malaise/fatigue, nausea, vomiting, paresthesia, pain/pressure in throat or neck	Pregnancy, uncontrolled HTN, ischemic heart disease, PVD, severe hepatic or renal impair-ment; do not use within 24 h of (or concomi-tant) use of ergot derivatives or sibutramine (no longer available in the United States); do not use for treatment of basilar or hemiplegic migraine	Use w/ caution in patients w/ risk factors for CAD, smoking, cerebral/subarachnoid hemorrhage, stroke, peripheral vascular ischemia, and history of HTN; not recom-mended for use in older persons; use lowest possible dose
rizatriptan (Maxalt oral tablet and Maxalt-MLT, orally disintegrating tablet) Tablet: 5–10 mg q2h to max of 30 mg/d (patients taking concomi-tant propranolol: max of 15 mg/d) Orally disintegrating tablet: 5–10 mg q2h to max of 30 mg (patients tak-ing concomitant propranolol: max of 15 mg/d) *Note:* Patients w/ cardiac risks should be administered first dose in the physician's office under observation	>10%: Dizziness, drowsiness, fatigue (dose dependent); 1%–10%: Increase in BP, chest pain, palpitations, flushing, mild increases in GH, hot flashes, abdominal pain, xerostomia, nausea, dyspnea	Documented ischemic heart disease or Prinzmetal angina or uncontrolled HTN; do not use within 24 h of (or concomitant) use of another $5HT_1$ agonist, or use within 2 wk of (or concomitant) use of MAOIs, or concomitant use w/ ergot derivatives; do not use for treatment of basilar or hemiplegic migraine	Reconsider migraine diagnosis if patient does not respond to first dose; patients w/ symptoms of angina postdose should be evaluated for CAD or Prinzmetal angina before receiving a second dose; do not administer to patients w/ risk factors for CAD (e.g., HTN, hypercholesterolemia, smoking, obesity, diabetes, strong family history of CAD, menopause, males > 40 y) w/o adequate cardiac workup; use w/ caution in older persons or in patients w/ hepatic or renal impairment (including dialysis); evaluate cardiovascular status periodically; avoid concomitant use of other serotonergic drugs (SSRIs/SNRIs, other triptans) and serotonin precursors (e.g., tryptophan)

Drug/Dosage	Adverse Effects	Contraindications	Comments
almotriptan (Axert) 6.25–12.5 mg q2h to max of 25 mg/d *Note:* Patients taking potent CYP3A4 inhibitors should only take 6.25 mg as a starting dose to a max of 12.5 mg/d	3%–10%: Somnolence, dizziness, nausea	Pregnancy, known or suspected ischemic heart disease, stroke TIA, PVD, uncontrolled HTN; do not use within 24 h of (or concomitant) use of another $5HT_1$ agonist or concomitant use w/ ergot derivatives, MAOIs, or sibutramine; do not use for treatment of basilar or hemiplegic migraine	Do not use for migraine prophylaxis or cluster headache; if patient doesn't respond to first dose, reconsider migraine diagnosis; use w/ caution in patients w/ sulfonamide allergy; do not administer to patients w/ risk factors for CAD (e.g., HTN, hypercholesterolemia, smoking, obesity, diabetes, strong family history of CAD, menopause, males > 40 y) w/o adequate cardiac workup; evaluate cardiovascular status periodically; use w/ caution in patients w/ hepatic or renal impairment, avoid concomitant use of other serotonergic drugs (SSRIs/SNRIs, other triptans)
eletriptan (Relpax) 20–40 mg q2h to max of 80 mg/d	3%–10%: Chest pain/tightness, dizziness, somnolence, headache, nausea, xerostomia, weakness, paresthesia	Pregnancy, ischemic heart disease or signs or symptoms of ischemic heart disease, stroke, TIA, PVD, or uncontrolled HTN; do not use in severe hepatic impairment or with concomitant use within 24 h of an ergot derivative or another $5HT_1$ agonist, or within 72 h of potent CYP3A4 inhibitors or sibutramine; do not use for treatment of basilar or hemiplegic migraine or for migraine prophylaxis	If patient doesn't respond to first dose, reconsider migraine diagnosis; do not administer to patients w/ risk factors for CAD w/o adequate cardiac workup; evaluate cardiovascular status periodically; use w/ caution in patients w/ mild to moderate hepatic impairment; avoid concomitant use of other serotonergic drugs (SSRIs/SNRIs, other triptans) or serotonin precursors (e.g., tryptophan)
frovatriptan (Frova) 2.5 mg q2h to max of 7.5 mg/d	3%–10%: Flushing, dizziness, fatigue, headache, hot or cold sensation, xerostomia, paresthesia, skeletal pain	Ischemic heart disease or signs and symptoms of ischemic heart disease, stroke, TIA, PVD, or uncontrolled HTN; do not use w/ concomitant use within 24 h of an ergot derivative or another $5HT_1$ agonist or w/ sibutramine; do not use for treatment of hemiplegic or basilar migraine	Not intended for migraine prophylaxis or cluster headache; rule out underlying neurologic disease in patients w/ atypical headache or migraine (w/ no prior history of migraine), or inadequate clinical response to first dose; do not administer to patients w/ risk factors for CAD w/o adequate cardiac workup; evaluate cardiovascular status periodically; slow onset, longest half-life of the triptans

Ergot Derivatives

Drug/Dosage	Adverse Effects	Contraindications	Comments
ergotamine tartrate (Ergomar) 2 mg SL at start of migraine, then 1 tab q30min if needed, to 3 tab/d and 5 tab/wk	Serious vasoconstrictive distress (ischemia, cyanosis, absence of pulse, cold extremities, gangrene, precordial distress and pain, ECG changes and muscle pains), transient tachycardia or bradycardia and hypertension, nausea, vomiting, paresthesias, numbness, weakness, vertigo, localized edema, itching, rare fibrosis (retroperitoneal, pleuropulmonary, and heart valve)	**WARNING: Serious and/or life-threatening peripheral ischemia has been associated with the coadministration of ergotamine tartrate with potent CYP3A4 inhibitors, including protease inhibitors and macrolide antibiotics. Because CYP3A4 inhibition elevates the serum levels of ergotamine tartrate, the risk for vasospasm leading to cerebral ischemia and/or ischemia of the extremities is increased. Hence, concomitant use of these medications is contraindicated.**	Pregnancy category X; do not use in patients with PVD, coronary heart disease, or HTN, impaired hepatic or renal function, or sepsis. Withdrawal and MOH may occur with prolonged use

(Continued)

TABLE 38.3

Overview of Selected Drugs for Acute/Abortive Migraine Treatment (*Continued*)

Generic (Trade) Name and Dosage	Selected Adverse Events	Contraindications	Special Considerations
dihydroergotamine (Migranal) IM/SC: 1 mg first sign of headache, repeat hourly to a max dose of 3 mg total, to a max dose of 6 mg/wk IV: 1 mg first sign of headache, repeat hourly to a max dose of 2 mg total, to a max of 6 mg/wk Intranasal: 1 spray (0.5 mg) each nostril, repeat q15min if necessary, to a max of 4 sprays to a max of 6 sprays/d and a max of 8 sprays/wk	3%–10%: Dizziness, somnolence, nausea, taste disturbance, vomiting, application site reaction, pharyngitis Nasal spray >10%: Rhinitis	See **BOXED WARNING** above Pregnancy Category X; do not use in patients with ischemic heart disease (angina pectoris, history of MI, or documented silent ischemia), or in patients w/ clinical symptoms or findings consistent w/ coronary artery vasospasm, including Prinzmetal variant angina; do not use in uncontrolled HTN; do not use with concomitant use of 5HT₁ agonists, or other ergotamine-containing or ergot-type medications or methysergide within 24 h; do not use for treatment of hemiplegic or basilar migraine, in PAD, sepsis, following vascular surgery, or in severely impaired hepatic or renal function	Use only when a clear diagnosis of migraine headache has been established; not for prolonged use; use with caution in older persons
caffeine/ergotamine (Cafergot) PO: 1 mg ergotamine/100 mg caffeine; 1–2 tabs at onset; may repeat after 1h to max of 6 tabs/d Rectal: 2 mg ergotamine/100 mg caffeine; 1 supp PR; may repeat after 1 h to max 2 supp/d	Nausea, vomiting, irritability, palpitations, paresthesias, MOH, dizziness, tingling of the extremities, rare MI	**WARNING Serious and/or life-threatening peripheral ischemia has been associated with coadministration of Cafergot with potent CYP3A4 inhibitors (e.g., protease inhibitors, macrolide antibiotics). Because CYP3A4 inhibition elevates serum levels of Cafergot, the risk of vasospasm leading to cerebral ischemia and/or ischemia of the extremities is increased. Concomitant use of these medications is contraindicated.** Pregnancy category X; do not use in HTN, PVD, and CAD; do not use with impaired hepatic or renal function or in sepsis	Use w/ caution with concomitant use of less potent CYP3A4 inhibitors; avoid excessive or prolonged use; not indicated for migraine prophylaxis; monitor use in mild to moderate hepatic impairment; MOH may be associated w/ prolonged and uninterrupted use

Barbiturates—see Table 38.1

Opioids

| butorphanol nasal spray (1 mg) 1 spray in 1 nostril, may repeat in 1 h; can repeat initial dosing sequence q3–4h PRN Adjust for renal and hepatic impairment: 1 mg at onset, 1 mg 60–90 min later, then at intervals of no <6 h | >10%: Somnolence, dizziness, nausea and/or vomiting, nasal congestion, insomnia | History of substance abuse | Use w/ caution in impaired renal, hepatic, or pulmonary function; use w/ caution in older persons; use sparingly—not recommended as a first-line drug |

Drug/Dose	Side Effects	Contraindications	Comments
acetaminophen w/ codeine (Tylenol w/ codeine) 1–2 tabs q4h to a max of 12 tabs/d Tylenol w/ codeine 3: 30 mg codeine, 300 mg acetaminophen Tylenol w/ codeine 4: 60 mg codeine, 300 mg acetaminophen	Severe hepatotoxicity on acute overdose, potential liver damage w/ chronic daily dosing, nephrotoxicity, agranulocytosis, rash, drowsiness, constipation	Chronic alcohol use, alcoholic liver disease, or impaired liver or renal function; G6PD deficiency; history of substance abuse; do not use for pregnancy for prolonged use or high doses at term	May be used sparingly in pregnancy; do not exceed 3,250 mg acetaminophen/d (including concomitant use with other acetaminophen-containing products); decrease dose in patients w/ renal impairment; use w/ caution in patients w/ respiratory disorders, CNS depression/coma, head trauma, morbid obesity, prostatic hyperplasia, urinary stricture, thyroid dysfunction, or severe renal or liver insufficiency; may cause CNS depression or hypotension; use w/ caution in patients w/ hypovolemia or cardiovascular disease; abrupt discontinuation after prolonged use may result in withdrawal
Steroids			
dexamethasone Single dose of 4 or 4 mg bid × 2 d then 4 mg daily × 3 d w/tapered discontinuation	Nausea, GI upset, insomnia, mood swings, rare and serious steroid psychosis, peptic ulcer disease, CHF	Pregnancy; systemic fungal infections or acute head injury; avoid concomitant use w/ aldesleukin, BCG, dronedarone, everolimus, natalizumab, nilotinib, nisoldipine, pazopanib, ranolazine, romidepsin, tolvaptan, and live vaccines	Use as rescue medication only; use w/ caution in thyroid disease, hepatic and renal impairment, CVD, DM, glaucoma, cataracts, myasthenia gravis, GI diseases, and in patients at risk for osteoporosis or seizures; use w/ caution in older persons at the lowest possible dose for a short duration

Goals of Drug Therapy

The main goal of pharmacologic therapy is to prevent or relieve the migraine attacks with minimal or no side effects. Short-term goals include decreasing the severity, frequency, and number of migraine days of the headache and relieving nausea, if present. Long-term goals established by the U.S. Headache Consortium include reducing attack frequency and severity, reducing disability, improving quality of life, preventing headache, avoiding headache medication escalation, and educating and enabling patients to manage their disease (Silberstein et al., 2012). Efficacy endpoints in the management of migraine (i.e., in clinical trials) are generally recognized as being pain free (no pain) or headache relief (improvement) response at 2 hours postdose, reduction in 24-hour recurrence rate, and favorable adverse event profile.

Nonsteroidal Anti-Inflammatory Drugs

First-line (level A strength of evidence) abortive agents for mild to moderate migraines are NSAIDs and aspirin. These medications, like all migraine medications, work best when taken early in the attack. The most common side effects are gastrointestinal. The same doses as used for tension headaches are appropriate for migraines (American Academy of Neurology (AAN) guidelines have not changed since 2000) (Marmura et al., 2015). Aspirin may be used in initial dosages of up to 900 mg. Aspirin alone is effective in up to 40% of migraine patients (Silberstein, 2002). Since AAN guidelines have not been updated since 2000, a starting dose of 1,000 mg acetaminophen is still reported as an effective intervention for acute migraine, although recommended doses of acetaminophen in general have been reduced. As with tension headaches, a given NSAID should be used on more than one occasion before deciding whether it is efficacious.

Caffeine-Containing Compounds

OTC caffeine-containing compounds (such as Excedrin Extra Strength or Excedrin Migraine) are also effective for milder migraines, but they can easily cause MOH and should be used no more than 3 days per month or for more than 48 hours at a time. These preparations also contain acetaminophen (250 mg per tablet), so caution is required if acetaminophen or many of the other OTC or prescription acetaminophen-containing preparations are being used, especially concomitantly (Schilling et al., 2010).

5-HT$_1$ Receptor Agonists (Triptans)

Triptans are migraine-specific drugs that work as 5-HT$_1$ serotonin receptor agonists. These receptors are located on intracranial blood vessels, presynaptically on CNS sensory neurons, and trigeminal terminals. Triptans cause cerebral vasoconstriction and can treat both the pain and nausea of migraine.

Triptans are indicated for acute treatment of migraine with or without aura, and they are used for moderate to severe migraines or for milder migraines that do not respond to NSAIDs, aspirin, or the above combination drugs. Triptans vary in their time to peak concentration, half-lives, adverse event profiles, formulation, and route of administration, which helps guide the selection of a triptan for a particular patient. Given the highly individualized nature of migraine, different medications may be more effective than others in any given patient. If a triptan fails on two separate occasions, another triptan should be tried. Triptans work best when given early in the course of a migraine, but unlike many other agents, they may be effective even when given late in the course of a migraine.

Triptans should not be used more than 9 days per month and should not be used within 24 hours of any other vasoconstricting drug, such as ergotamine. Use of these medications is considered to be a better choice than use of the ergot derivatives, as potency is similar but adverse events are significantly fewer in number (Khoury & Couch, 2010). Triptans should be avoided in patients with basilar, hemiplegic, or retinal migraines; they must also be avoided in patients with coronary artery disease, cerebrovascular disease, or severe peripheral vascular disease. Concomitant use of ergotamines and dihydroergotamine (DHE) is also contraindicated, and, while serotonin syndrome is rare, the possibility for it exists with concomitant use of triptans and SSRIs or SNRIs. No more than one triptan at a time should be used within 24 hours (Pringsheim & Becker, 2014).

The seven triptan drugs are sumatriptan, zolmitriptan, naratriptan, rizatriptan, almotriptan, eletriptan, and frovatriptan. A combination sumatriptan/naproxen formulation is also available. Sumatriptan and zolmitriptan are available as a nasal spray, and sumatriptan is also available in transdermal, subcutaneous, and nasal powder formulations. These are useful for patients with severe nausea who cannot tolerate an oral medication. Rizatriptan is also available as an orally disintegrating tablet. The injectable form of sumatriptan has the fastest onset of action of any of the triptans, but has a short half-life, often giving limited headache relief. Sumatriptan is also associated with more adverse events than the other triptans. Frovatriptan has the longest half-life of the triptans, at 26 hours, making it useful for patients with long-lasting migraines. Use of the triptans in the early, mild stages of migraine (but not during aura) results in greater relief (up to 70% pain free in clinical trials) than does use of the drugs during moderate or severe migraine (up to 30% pain-free in clinical trials), but the patient needs to be able to recognize onset of migraine and distinguish it from TTH. Use of a triptan for more than 9 days per month may result in MOH, during which time preventive therapy will be ineffective (Pringsheim & Becker, 2014).

Sumatriptan

Sumatriptan (Imitrex) was the first triptan on the market (FDA approved in 1992 and now available as a generic) and still offers the fastest relief of all the triptans presently available. In its subcutaneous form, it offers the highest therapeutic gain of all the triptans in clinical trials. It is safe and well tolerated (available OTC in the United Kingdom) (Antonaci et al., 2010; Johnston & Rapoport, 2010; Tfelt-Hansen, 2007). Sumatriptan is available in tablets (25, 50, and 100 mg), a powder nasal spray (20 mg), a nasal powder (11 mg), a subcutaneous injection (6 mg), and transdermally (6.5 mg). See **Table 38.3**.

Injectable sumatriptan offers the quickest onset of action (10 minutes), whereas the effects of the tablet take longer (30 to 90 minutes). Sumatriptan is the only triptan with a subcutaneous formulation, making it the fastest-onset triptan available, but it also has the shortest half-life of the triptans, limiting the longer-term relief associated with some of the other triptans with longer half-lives. Injectable sumatriptan is associated with more adverse events than oral sumatriptan (Johnston & Rapoport, 2010). If the headache recurs, the patient can take a second dose of medication, but only after a certain time and without exceeding the maximum dose of 200 mg/d. Patients with migraine with aura cannot take sumatriptan until the headache actually begins because the drug has no effect on relieving aura symptoms. Patients with nausea and vomiting tend to find the nasal formulations easier to take. Pain relief may be dose dependent, but with increased doses come increased adverse events (Johnston & Rapoport, 2010). Adverse events vary by mode of delivery, but most occurred in less than 10% of trial subjects. Concomitant use of sumatriptan with MAOIs is contraindicated (Pringsheim & Becker, 2014).

Zolmitriptan

Zolmitriptan (Zomig; FDA approved in 1997 and now available as a generic) is available in tablet, nasal spray, and orally disintegrating formulations and can be used for migraine with or without aura. The recommended initial dose of zolmitriptan is 2.5 mg. The onset of effect is attained within 45 minutes, resulting in a rapid therapeutic response. Its half-life is 3 hours, longer than that of sumatriptan, and it is extremely potent at serotonin receptors. Zolmitriptan has been shown in clinical trials to be similar in efficacy to sumatriptan (5 vs. 100 mg, respectively), and at a dose of 2.5 mg, it is similar in efficacy to sumatriptan 50 mg, almotriptan 12.5 mg, eletriptan 40 mg, and rizatriptan 10 mg. Therapeutic gain is slightly higher in nasal and orally disintegrating formulations. Efficacy may be dose dependent, with a concomitant increase in adverse events. Dosage should be adjusted down to 1.25 mg in patients with moderate to severe hepatic impairment. Contraindications and adverse effects are similar to the other triptans; MAOIs should also not be used with zolmitriptan, nor should CYP1A2 inhibitors such as cimetidine, fluvoxamine, and ciprofloxacin. See **Table 38.3**.

Naratriptan

Naratriptan (Amerge; FDA approved in 1998 and now available as a generic) is marketed as an alternative agent for patients who are taking repeated doses of other migraine therapies, specifically those who have recurrent headache or chest tightness when using oral sumatriptan. Naratriptan is available only in 1- and 2.5-mg tablet formulation (see **Table 38.3**) and reaches peak serum concentrations in 2 to 3 hours. While onset is slow (1 to 2 hours), duration of action is longest of all the triptans; because of its long half-life of 6 hours, headache recurrences are not common. An initial dose of 1 to 2.5 mg should be used; if headache does not resolve, a second dose can be administered within 4 hours, not to exceed a total dose of 5 mg. The safety of treating more than four migraines per month with naratriptan has not been established. Therapeutic gain at 4 hours (as compared with 2 hours) tends to be higher in this triptan. In the original clinical trial, headache relief was experienced by 68% of patients 4 hours postdose and was maintained for 8 to 24 hours. Given its availability only in

low dosages, its side effect profile in clinical trials was comparable to placebo, making this triptan a good option for patients experiencing intolerable side effects with other triptans (Johnston & Rapoport, 2010; Pringsheim & Becker, 2014).

Rizatriptan

Rizatriptan (Maxalt; FDA approved in 1998 and now available as a generic) is available in a tablet (5 and 10 mg) and orally disintegrating tablet (Maxalt-MLT; 5 and 10 mg), offering an alternative way to treat a migraine. Onset of action is rapid, particularly with the orally disintegrating tablet. Rizatriptan 10 mg produces faster relief than do sumatriptan 50 mg and naratriptan 2.5 mg and is similar in efficacy to almotriptan 12.5 mg, eletriptan 40 mg, and zolmitriptan 2.5 mg. Effects of rizatriptan can be observed within 30 minutes and last from 14 to 16 hours. In the original clinical trial, 62% of patients taking the 5-mg dose and 71% of patients taking the 10-mg dose experienced pain relief 2 hours postdose. Complete relief was achieved in 33% of patients taking a 5-mg dose and 42% of patients taking the 10-mg dose. The drug is well tolerated, even at 10 tablets per month. A second dose can be taken within 2 hours of the first dose if the headache is not resolving; 30 mg should not be exceeded per 24 hours. Rizatriptan should not be used concomitantly with MAOIs, and if used concomitantly with propranolol, only a 5-mg dose of rizatriptan should be used, to a maximum dosage of 15 mg per 24 hours (DIH, 2014; Pringsheim & Becker, 2014). See **Table 38.3**.

Almotriptan

Almotriptan (Axert; FDA approved in 2001; no generic available, but a generic has received tentative approval from the FDA) is a rapidly absorbed triptan with a moderately long half-life (3 to 4 hours). Its efficacy is similar to that of the other triptans, but its potential for drug–drug interactions is reduced, given that it is metabolized by three separate metabolic pathways. It is a well-tolerated drug with few adverse events and is a good choice for triptan-naïve patients or as an alternate drug for patients who need to be switched over from other triptans due to intolerable side effects (Johnston & Rapoport, 2010). Use of almotriptan is contraindicated in patients with renal impairment with concomitant use of a potent CYP3A4 inhibitor. Dose of almotriptan should be adjusted down to 6.25 mg in a single dose, to a maximum dose of 12.5 mg in any patient taking a potent CYP3A4 inhibitor (e.g., ketoconazole, itraconazole, clarithromycin, etc.). See **Table 38.3**.

Eletriptan

Eletriptan (Relpax; FDA approved in 2002; no generic available but a generic has received tentative FDA approval) is available in 20- and 40-mg tablets. The recommended initial dose is 40 mg at the onset of migraine. If relief is not obtained in 2 hours, the dose may be repeated, to a maximum of 80 mg/d. Onset of action is rapid, and elimination half-life is moderately long (4 hours)—shorter only than naratriptan and frovatriptan. While essentially comparable in efficacy to the other triptans, eletriptan at a dose of 40 mg is the only triptan shown to have greater efficacy than sumatriptan at 100 mg. Both efficacy and adverse events are dose dependent, although trials have reported adverse events to be transient and mild to moderate in nature. Contraindications and adverse effects are similar to those of the other triptans, but eletriptan should also not be used concomitantly within 72 hours of use of potent CYP3A4 inhibitors (e.g., conivaptan, systemic fusidic acid, itraconazole, systemic ketoconazole, posaconazole, and voriconazole; DIH, 2014; Pringsheim & Becker, 2014). See **Table 38.3**.

Frovatriptan

Frovatriptan (Frova; FDA approved in 2001 and now available as a generic) has a half-life of 26 hours, by far the longest of all the triptans. Hence, its therapeutic gain is better assessed at 4 hours rather than 2; the 40-hour headache response rate for frovatriptan is 66%. Like naratriptan, its onset is somewhat slower (although this is not the case in all patients taking the medication in early migraine), but its effects are more sustained. Frovatriptan is also metabolized both by the kidney and hepatic CYP1A2, reducing the likelihood for drug–drug interactions. It has also been shown to be particularly effective in menstrual-related migraine, not only for acute relief but also as a 2-day "miniprophylaxis." It is available as a 2.5-mg tablet, which is the recommended dose. If a first dose provides some relief but the headache recurs, another dose may be taken no sooner than 2 hours after the preceding dose, to a maximum of 7.5 mg/d. Contraindications and adverse effects are similar to the other triptans (Johnston & Rapoport, 2010). See **Table 38.3**.

Sumatriptan and Naproxen

Sumatriptan and naproxen (Treximet; FDA approved in 2008; no generic available) is an oral tablet combination medication containing 85 mg sumatriptan and 500 mg naproxen used for treating migraine with or without aura. It is more efficacious than monotherapy with sumatriptan or naproxen alone (as is combined use of individual sumatriptan and naproxen tablets). Sustained pain relief at 24 hours was also significantly better than monotherapy with either sumatriptan or naproxen in clinical trials. It follows the sumatriptan dosing recommendations (one tablet at migraine onset; if relief is not obtained, a second dose may be taken at least 2 hours later, with a maximum of two tablets in 24 hours), and its adverse events, contraindications, and warnings are the same as those for each of its individual components (including the boxed warning for the naproxen component; Khoury & Couch, 2010). Use of sumatriptan/naproxen is not recommended in patients with a creatinine clearance of less than 30 mL/min, and its use is contraindicated in hepatic impairment (DIH, 2014). See **Table 38.3**.

Ergot Derivatives

The first migraine-specific drugs to be developed were the ergot derivatives (ergotamine tartrate and DHE, with a variety of trade names). They are generally recognized as safe and effective, but have fallen out of favor because of unpredictable patient responses and greater adverse events as compared with the safer triptans. Ergot derivatives have partial agonist,

antagonist, or both types of activity for serotonergic, dopaminergic, and alpha-adrenergic receptors, resulting in constriction of peripheral and cranial vessels. Ergot derivatives are typically used to treat infrequent, long-standing migraines in patients who have had multiple relapses when using triptans, but care should be taken to prescribe the medication infrequently, at recommended doses, and in careful consideration of contraindications (e.g., they are Pregnancy Category X drugs and are absolutely contraindicated in patients with cardiovascular or cerebrovascular disease and in patients taking concomitant medications metabolized by the CYP3A4 pathway, such as protease inhibitors, azole antifungals, and certain macrolide antibiotics). While generally found to be less efficacious than oral sumatriptan in clinical trials, rectal ergotamine was found to have superior efficacy than rectal sumatriptan (73% vs. 63%, respectively; rectal sumatriptan is not available as an approved medication). Ergotamine/caffeine combinations are also available in oral, sublingual, and rectal formulations, although evidence of efficacy for these preparations is inconsistent or conflicting (Bigal & Tepper, 2003; Wilson, 2007).

Ergotamine tartrate (Ergomar; Ergostat has been discontinued) is available in 2-mg sublingual tablets. Ergotamine is not an optimal choice, given its side effect profile (nausea may be sufficient enough for discontinuation). It is associated with more side effects than DHE, and use of the medication more than 10 times per month may cause MOH. DHE (Migranal) is available intramuscularly (1 mg), intravenously (1 mg), subcutaneously (1 mg), and as a nasal spray (0.5 mg). There are no oral formulations. This drug is mainly used to treat severe, refractory migraines; recurring migraines; MOH; or status migrainosus (debilitating migraine attacks lasting longer than 72 hours) and is usually managed by specialists. Cafergot, a combination of caffeine and ergotamine, is available in oral (1 mg ergotamine, 100 mg caffeine) and suppository (2 mg/100 mg) formulations. Cafergot can also increase the incidence of migraines and should be used infrequently (Monteith & Goadsby, 2011; Tfelt-Hansen, 2007; Wilson, 2007). Use of these agents is contraindicated in severe renal impairment (DIH, 2014). See **Table 38.3**.

Barbiturates

Butalbital-containing compounds such as Fiorinal (butalbital 50 mg/aspirin 325 mg/caffeine 40 mg; tablets and capsules) and Fioricet (butalbital 50 mg/acetaminophen 325 mg/caffeine 40 mg; tablets, capsules, or liquid) are C-III controlled substances and should be used sparingly and only if the migraine-specific agents have repeatedly failed. There are no data to support the efficacy of these medications, and if overused (as infrequently as five times per month), these agents can lead to addiction, MOH, development of chronic daily headache, and withdrawal symptoms. These drugs have been removed from the market in the European Union, Asia, and Latin America due to their associated risks and their lack of efficacy. Fioricet should particularly be used with caution given its acetaminophen content if it is used concomitantly with other acetaminophen-containing drugs (Tepper & Spears, 2009). The "Choosing Wisely" Task Force of the American Headache Society identified overuse of butalbital-containing and opioid medications for the treatment of migraine as a problem (Loder et al., 2013). See **Table 38.3** for side effects and contraindications.

Opioids

Opioids have been used as rescue medications for severe migraines that do not respond to the above medications. They are also used in patients who have infrequent migraines and have contraindications to other agents. They are used sparingly for moderate to severe migraines during pregnancy. However, they are in general not recommended for the treatment of migraine and, if used as rescue medications, should be used only a few times per year. Overuse can lead to MOH, status migrainosus, or development of chronic daily headache. These are C-IV medications, and the potential for dependence or abuse should also be taken into account when considering them for use. Examples of these medications include butorphanol (generic nasal spray, 1 mg/spray), tramadol (generic tablet, 100 mg daily; can be titrated to a maximum of 300 mg daily), and acetaminophen plus codeine (Tylenol plus codeine; acetaminophen 300 mg/codeine 30 or 40 mg) for mild to moderate pain. The acetaminophen content per dose is 300 mg, which needs to be considered when used concomitantly with other acetaminophen-containing drugs so that a maximum daily dose of 3,250 mg is not exceeded (Tepper & Spears, 2009; Wilson, 2007). As with the butalbital-containing drugs, use of opioid medications for migraine was the second most identified problem by the "Choosing Wisely" Task Force. Use of opioids is rare (seen most frequently in emergency departments) and has even been described as contributing to disease progression, increased use of health care resources, and comorbidity (Loder et al., 2013; Minen et al., 2014; Tepper, 2012). Opioids are not a good choice for managing migraine pain. See **Table 38.3** for side effects and contraindications.

Steroids

If a patient has a severe, persistent migraine or status migrainosus that seems refractory to any abortive medications, a brief course of steroids (typically dexamethasone 6 mg for 5 days or IV 4 to 16 mg) may be used as a rescue medication until the patient is headache free for 24 hours. There are few good data supporting the efficacy of steroid use (AHS level of evidence category C: "possibly effective"), but they have been used with good results (Marmura et al., 2015; Tepper & Spears, 2009; Wilson, 2007). See **Table 38.3** for side effects and contraindications.

Antiemetic Agents

The antiemetic agents prochlorperazine, metoclopramide, and droperidol as well as the antipsychotic chlorpromazine are effective adjunctive therapies for patients experiencing an acute migraine with or without nausea and vomiting. Prochlorperazine comes in a suppository form, which is useful for patients unable to tolerate oral medications. Droperidol carries a black box warning for QT prolongation and torsade de pointes. These medications augment the effects of abortive agents and may be taken before or together with these medications.

PROPHYLACTIC DRUG THERAPY FOR MIGRAINES

Prophylactic medications are used to prevent the occurrence of migraine by reducing the frequency and severity of migraine attacks. Epidemiologic studies have shown that some 38% of migraineurs require some form of preventive therapy, yet only 3% to 13% are receiving prophylactic treatment (Silberstein et al., 2012). A therapeutic trial of a given agent should last for 2 to 3 months before the efficacy of the agent is assessed. The main classes of agents used for migraine prophylaxis are anticonvulsants, beta-blockers, triptans, angiotensin-converting enzyme inhibitors (ACEIs), angiotensin II receptor blockers (ARBs), calcium channel blockers, antidepressants (TCAs and SSRIs/SNRIs), and antihistamines, although strength of evidence for efficacy has been determined for individual medications and not for entire medication classes. A 2012 AAN Quality Standards Subcommittee report identified divalproex sodium, sodium valproate, topiramate, metoprolol, propranolol, and timolol as the agents with the most support for efficacy for migraine prophylaxis (Silberstein et al., 2012). More recently, onabotulinumtoxinA (Botox) has shown efficacy in the management of chronic migraine (Pedraza et al., 2015). The choice of prophylactic agent should be based on the patient's comorbidities and the efficacy and side effect profile of the medication. **Table 38.4** gives an overview of selected drugs used to prevent migraines.

The current recommendations for starting prophylactic therapy are recurring migraines that affect the patient's functioning and quality of life despite acute symptomatic treatments, intolerance or failure of multiple acute treatments, overuse of acute medications, MOH, special circumstances such as hemiplegic migraines, and more than two headaches per week (Pringsheim et al., 2010; Silberstein, 2002).

Medications should be started at low doses and titrated slowly until the desired effects occur. Dosages may need to be lowered if side effects occur. A full therapeutic trial takes at least 2 months. It may take months until an effective agent is found.

Anticonvulsants

Valproic acid (Depakene) and divalproex sodium (Depakote) can reduce the frequency, severity, and duration of migraines. Use of these drugs is contraindicated in patients with liver disease. Side effects such as tremor, weight gain, nausea, and hair loss may limit their use as agents for prophylaxis. Numerous drug interactions can result when valproic acid or divalproex

TABLE 38.4

Overview of Selected Drugs Used for Migraine Headache Prophylaxis

Generic (Brand) Name and Dosage	Selected Adverse Events	Contraindications	Special Considerations
Beta-Blockers			
propranolol (Inderal) (long acting) Start 80 mg daily; goal 160–240 mg daily; increase dose gradually and taper discontinuation, discontinue after 6 wk if no satisfactory response. *Note*: Adjust dose in hepatic impairment	Common: Drowsiness or fatigue, cold hands and feet, weakness or dizziness, dry mouth, eyes, and skin	**WARNING: Beta-blocker therapy should not be withdrawn abruptly (particularly in patients with CAD), but gradually tapered to avoid acute tachycardia, hypertension, and/or ischemia.** Pregnancy, uncompensated CHF, cardiogenic shock, severe sinus bradycardia or second- or third-degree heart block or with severe asthma or COPD	Useful if there is history of coexisting HTN or CAD; use w/ caution in patients w/ PVD or w/ concomitant beta-blocker use; use w/ caution in patients w/ DM, myasthenia gravis, psychiatric disease, and renal or hepatic dysfunction
timolol Initial: 10 mg bid to a max of 30 mg/d	Anaphylaxis (serious); >3%: fatigue/tiredness, bradycardia; AEs in CAD population more numerous; asthenia or fatigue, heart rate <40 beats/min, cardiac failure—nonfatal, hypotension, claudication, cold hands and feet, nausea or digestive disorders, dizziness	See **BOXED WARNING** above Bronchial asthma or history of bronchial asthma, or severe COPD; sinus bradycardia, second- and third-degree AV block, overt cardiac failure, or cardiogenic shock	Use w/ caution in impaired hepatic or renal function, marked renal failure, muscle weakness, or cerebrovascular insufficiency; use w/ caution w/ concomitant use of catecholamine-depleting drugs, NSAIDs, calcium antagonists, digoxin and either diltiazem or verapamil, quinidine, and clonidine
Tricyclic Antidepressants amitriptyline—see **Table 38.1**			
Anticonvulsants			
valproic acid (Depakene, Stavzor) Depakene 250 mg soft gel capsule Stavzor delayed release 125, 250, and 500 mg soft gel capsules initial: 250 mg bid to a max of 1,000 mg/d	≥5%: Headache, asthenia, fever, nausea, vomiting, abdominal pain, diarrhea, anorexia, dyspepsia, constipation, somnolence, tremor, dizziness, diplopia, amblyopia/blurred vision, ataxia, nystagmus, emotional lability, abnormal thinking, amnesia, flu syndrome, infection, bronchitis, rhinitis	**WARNING: May cause teratogenic effects such as neural tube defects (e.g., spina bifida). Hepatic failure resulting in fatalities has occurred in patients; children < age 2 are at considerable risk. Cases of life-threatening pancreatitis, occurring at the start of therapy or following years of use, have been reported in adults and children.** Hepatic disease or significant hepatic dysfunction or with urea cycle disorders	Monitor for hypothermia and thrombocytopenia; monitor psychiatric patients for suicidal ideation; use w/ caution w/ concomitant use of carbapenem, topiramate, aspirin, or lamotrigine; drug interactions are also known for felbamate, rifampin, amitriptyline/nortriptyline, carbamazepine, clonazepam, diazepam, ethosuximide, phenobarbital, phenytoin, tolbutamide, warfarin, and zidovudine; use w/ caution in older persons
divalproex (Depakote) Initial: 250 mg bid, up to 1,000 mg/d	>10%: Nausea, somnolence, dizziness, vomiting; >5%–10%: Asthenia, abdominal pain, dyspepsia, rash	See **BOXED WARNING** above	Same as above

TABLE 38.4

Overview of Selected Drugs Used for Migraine Headache Prophylaxis (*Continued*)

Generic (Brand) Name and Dosage	Selected Adverse Events	Contraindications	Special Considerations
topiramate (Topamax) Initial: 25 mg qhs for first wk, increased weekly by increments of 25 mg; recommended therapeutic dose 100 mg/d in 2 divided doses *Note*: Taper gradually.	>5%: Paresthesia, anorexia, weight decrease, fatigue, dizziness, somnolence, nervousness, psychomotor slowing, difficulty w/ memory, difficulty w/ concentration/attention, confusion; renal calculi, rare acute-angle glaucoma; >5% in migraine trials: paresthesia, taste perversion	None	Decreases effectiveness of oral contraceptives; monitor for acute myopia, oligohidrosis and hyperthermia, suicidal behavior and ideation, metabolic acidosis, cognitive/neuropsychiatric dysfunction, and hyperammonemia; use caution w/ concomitant administration of valproic acid, oral contraceptives, metformin, lithium, and other carbonic anhydrase inhibitors
Calcium Channel Blockers verapamil 40–80 mg tid	>1%: Headache, URI, fatigue, nausea, constipation, dizziness, edema	Severe left ventricular dysfunction, hypotension or cardiogenic shock, sick sinus syndrome, second- or third-degree AV block, atrial flutter or atrial fibrillation and an accessory bypass tract (e.g., Wolff-Parkinson-White, Lown-Ganong-Levine syndromes)	Useful if there is coexisting HTN; monitor LFTs periodically, use w/ caution in patients w/ impaired renal or hepatic function and in patients w/ decreased neuromuscular transmission; use caution w/ concomitant administration of erythromycin, ritonavir, alcohol, aspirin, grapefruit juice, beta-blockers, digitalis, other antihypertensive agents, disopyramide, flecainide, quinidine, lithium, carbamazepine, and rifampin, phenobarbital, cyclosporine, theophylline, inhalation anesthetics, neuromuscular-blocking agents, telithromycin, or clonidine

sodium is administered with other anticonvulsants. Increased effects or toxicity of valproic acid are seen with the administration of CNS depressants and aspirin. Valproic acid is contraindicated in pregnancy because it is toxic to the fetus (in 2013, FDA changed the pregnancy category for valproate from "D" to "X").

Topiramate (Topamax) has been shown to be effective in migraine prophylaxis and is particularly effective for patients who have chronic daily headache or who have failed to respond to many other prophylactic treatments. Topiramate was also shown in trials to be at least as or more effective as other migraine prophylactic therapies such as propranolol, valproate, and amitriptyline. A retrospective claims analysis of oral migraine prevention medications revealed that topiramate was the most commonly prescribed migraine prevention medication and the preventive agent for which there was the greatest amount of patient adherence (Hepp et al., 2015). Topiramate has many potential side effects that

limit its use, such as concentration and memory impairment, significant somnolence, mood disturbance, and tremor. It should be used with caution in patients with renal or hepatic impairment.

Beta-blockers

Beta-blockers are often considered first-line agents for prophylactic treatment of migraine, with many studies showing a 50% reduction or more in occurrence of migraine. Propranolol (Inderal), metoprolol (Lopressor), and timolol are evidence class A medications, while atenolol (Tenormin) and nadolol (Corgard) are evidence class B medications. They have all been used for migraine, with similar efficacy. Nebivolol (Bystolic) and pindolol are evidence class C ("possibly effective"), and bisoprolol (Zebeta) is evidence class U (inadequate information) (Loder et al., 2012; Marmura et al., 2015). Only propranolol and timolol have been approved by the FDA for migraine prophylaxis. Beta-blockers are contraindicated in patients with uncompensated congestive heart failure, bradycardia, second- or third-degree atrioventricular block, and asthma. Side effects include fatigue, vivid dreams, depression, impotence, bradycardia, and hypotension. Many pathways of the cytochrome P450 enzyme system metabolize beta-blockers. Beta-blockers have numerous drug interactions, so careful consideration of polypharmacy is necessary prior to prescribing them.

Tricyclic Antidepressants

TCAs can also be used as first-line agents for migraine prophylaxis. The agents most commonly used include imipramine (Tofranil), nortriptyline (Pamelor), and amitriptyline (Elavil), although only amitriptyline is recommended by the 2012 AAN/AHS guidelines (Loder et al., 2012). Patients usually need only low doses for prophylaxis, lower than those generally used to treat depression. Patients should avoid use if they are currently taking an MAOI, have glaucoma, or are pregnant. Anticholinergic side effects commonly occur and include sedation, constipation, blurred vision, hypotension, and slowed conduction in the atrioventricular node. TCAs also have many potential drug interactions; prescribers should consult a reference before administering them.

Calcium Channel Blockers

Verapamil (Calan) is the calcium channel blocker most commonly used in migraine prophylaxis; however, it provides only a slight benefit in reducing the frequency of attacks (AAN category U: not recommended; Loder et al., 2012). It is often considered a second- or third-line agent for use when other agents are ineffective or contraindicated. The mechanism of action is believed to be the inhibition of serotonin release, which may not be achieved until after 8 weeks of therapy. Its use is contraindicated in patients with bradycardia, heart block, ventricular tachycardia, or atrial fibrillation. Side effects include constipation, fluid retention, bradycardia, and hypotension. Numerous drug interactions are associated with calcium channel blockers; prescribers must consult a reference before administering.

Other Prophylactic Agents

MAOIs can also be used for migraine prophylaxis, but because they have multiple serious side effects, their use should be managed by a neurologist. Gabapentin (Neurontin) has recently been established to be effective in the treatment of chronic daily headache at dosages of 1,800 to 2,400 mg/d. ACEIs and angiotensin receptor blockers are also being studied as potential prophylactic agents. SSRIs, such as venlafaxine and fluoxetine, have been used with some success, although are classified by the 2012 AAN/AHS guidelines as ineffective. They are particularly useful in patients also suffering from anxiety or depression.

TABLE 38.5

Recommended Order for Treatment of Migraine Headaches

Order	Agents	Comments
First line	NSAIDs (oral) or aspirin	With moderate to severe migraines, can use antiemetic as needed
Second line	Triptans	*First tier* • sumatriptan 50–100 mg • almotriptan 12.5 mg • rizatriptan 10 mg • eletriptan 40 mg • zolmitriptan 2.5 mg *Slower effect/better tolerability* • naratriptan 2.5 mg • frovatriptan 2.5 mg
Third line	Triptans plus an NSAID	Can use antiemetic as needed
	Infrequent headache: • ergotamine 1–2 mg • dihydroergotamine 2 mg nasal spray	*For headache recurrence:* • ergotamine 2 mg, most effective rectally/usually w/ caffeine • naratriptan 2.5 mg • almotriptan 12.5 mg • eletriptan 40 mg

Data from Goadsby, P. J., & Sprenger, T. (2010). Current practice and future directions in the prevention and acute management of migraine. *Lancet Neurology, 9*(3), 285–298.

Selecting the Most Appropriate Agent

It is important to initiate therapy at the first sign of a migraine. The 2015 updated AAN/AHS guidelines have been revised according to level of evidence criteria. The following section discusses the recommended therapy for migraines (**Table 38.5**).

First-Line Therapy

NSAIDs and aspirin are appropriate first-line therapy for mild to moderate migraine. They are inexpensive and generally well tolerated. Triptans are first-line therapy for moderate to severe migraine with or without an antiemetic. NSAIDs may be tried for more severe migraines, but they are often unsuccessful.

Second-Line Therapy

OTC caffeine-containing compounds are appropriate treatment options for mild to moderate migraines that have not responded to the above agents. They can also be used as rescue medications if NSAIDs and aspirin fail to relieve a given attack. For more severe migraines, an ergot derivative along with an antiemetic can be used as second-line therapy if multiple triptans have failed in past treatment efforts.

Third-Line Therapy

If the above agents are ineffective in treating mild to moderate migraines, triptans should be tried. For severe migraines that have not responded to triptans or ergot derivatives and antiemetics, butalbital-containing compounds or opioids may be considered.

CLUSTER HEADACHES

Patients suspected of having CHs should be promptly referred to a neurologist to exclude potentially serious differential diagnoses. There is clinical evidence for the efficacy of several medications for the acute treatment of CH. Subcutaneous sumatriptan 6 to 12 mg (the only drug FDA approved for CH), intranasal sumatriptan 6 to 12 mg, zolmitriptan nasal spray 5 to 10 mg, and 100% inhaled oxygen 10 to 15 L/min are recommended for the management of acute attacks. Subcutaneous octreotide (Sandostatin), a somatostatin receptor agonist, has also been shown to be efficacious at 100 mcg, as has olanzapine 2.5 to 10 mg and intranasal lidocaine 10% solution (Pomeroy & Marmura, 2013). For individuals with repeated CH, preventive medications should be considered. There are data supporting the use of a variety of medications, including verapamil, lithium, melatonin, topiramate, gabapentin, valproic acid, DHE, leuprolide, intranasal capsaicin, and baclofen. Preventive therapies may take some time and possible upward titration to become effective (Pomeroy & Marmura, 2013).

SPECIAL POPULATION CONSIDERATIONS

Pediatric

The most common headache type seen in children is migraine. Migraines may present differently in children than in adults. Prevalence is higher in boys prior to puberty, but higher in girls thereafter. Epidemiologic studies have shown that prevalence increases with age, hitting a peak in adolescence. Average age of onset is 7 in boys and 11 in girls, and the incidence of migraine with aura peaks before migraine without aura. The pain is throbbing and pulsating but tends to be bifrontal or bitemporal. Children may have severe nausea and vomiting along with the pain. The headache usually persists for 1 to 3 hours but may last for longer than a day. A particular challenge with pediatric patients is distinguishing migraine from a host of other possible disorders (e.g., epilepsy or vascular or metabolic disorders), further complicated by interpreting the complaint from the child or his or her parents. Cheese, chocolate, and citrus fruits are common triggers of migraine in children. Nonpharmacologic approaches to migraine management, such as developing good sleeping habits and routines, are important. Biofeedback and relaxation therapy are the most commonly used behavioral approaches and have shown some efficacy in reducing frequency and severity of headaches. Clinical trial data for the pharmacologic management of pediatric

migraine are limited. Pediatric migraines are usually best managed by simple analgesics such as acetaminophen and ibuprofen, with an antiemetic added if necessary. Patients and their caregivers, however, need to be cautioned not to use the medication too frequently; use of OTC analgesics more than five times per week can lead to MOH or development of chronic daily headache. Triptans are not indicated for use in children, although safety and efficacy of the nasal formulations of sumatriptan and zolmitriptan and oral formulations of rizatriptan and almotriptan have been demonstrated in clinical trials in patients ages 12 to 17. Topiramate is presently the only FDA-approved medication for children over the age of 12, but other agents have some limited efficacy. Amitriptyline is a popular drug of choice for prevention of pediatric migraine; nortriptyline is also used, as well as other antiepileptics besides topiramate such as valproic acid, levetiracetam, zonisamide, and gabapentin. Cyproheptadine has also been used, as have the antihypertensives propranolol and verapamil. Children are obviously treated with lower doses. Prophylactic medications may require tapering up or down, and, while most of these agents are well tolerated, patients should be monitored for adverse effects. Many of the pediatric formulations are available as suspensions (Kacperski, 2015).

Tension headaches do occur in children. Recurrent tension headaches should prompt a search for underlying stressors at home or at school. A vision examination should also be performed. Tension headaches are usually best managed by simple analgesics, taking care not to overuse the medication.

Geriatric

New-onset migraines do not often occur in the older population. Changes in renal and hepatic function often occur with advancing age, so if an older patient is experiencing migraines, adjustment of drug dosages is recommended.

A new headache pattern in an older patient should make the practitioner suspicious of organic disease or a medication side effect. Many of the medications used to treat migraine are contraindicated for use in older populations (naratriptan is not recommended for use in older persons, and rizatriptan should be used with caution) or need to be used at a lower dose. Comorbidities and polypharmacy need to be considered carefully prior to choosing pharmacologic management.

Women

As noted earlier, migraines occur more often in women than in men: likely an estrogen-related phenomenon. Pregnancy is a primary concern if drug therapy is to be initiated, even though migraines can diminish during the second and third trimesters. Practitioners should consider drug therapy for pregnant women using the risk-versus-benefit approach. The agents selected should be those that are safe to use during pregnancy. Triptans and ergot derivatives are *strongly contraindicated* in pregnancy. Acetaminophen is the safest analgesic to use during pregnancy, but it is usually minimally effective. For more severe migraines, ibuprofen may be used in the first and second trimester only. Tylenol with codeine may be used sparingly throughout the pregnancy. Valproic acid is category X and is contraindicated in pregnancy for migraine prophylaxis.

Menstrual migraines are a common problem that may be particularly responsive to triptans. Frovatriptan, in particular, has been used with success as "miniprophylaxis" for menstrual-related migraine (Johnston & Rapoport, 2010). Women may also be particularly vulnerable to migraine during perimenopause and menopause, when estrogen levels dramatically decline. In one cross-sectional analysis, women using hormone replacement therapy were found to be 40% more likely to have migraines than those who were not taking hormone replacement (Misakian, 2003). If a woman wishes to stay on hormone replacement therapy despite migraines, she can be given a reduced dose and can be switched to pure estradiol or synthetic ethinyl estradiol. Using continuous dosing instead of interrupted dosing may also reduce migraine frequency.

MONITORING PATIENT RESPONSE

Careful monitoring of therapy is important. The practitioner should document the frequency, intensity, and duration of migraines before starting any new therapy and should evaluate the patient periodically after implementing any drug or lifestyle change to assess its effectiveness. Prescribers should monitor how frequently patients are taking abortive therapies to ensure they are not using them excessively. Patients should return to the office after a few attempts with a therapy to assess its effectiveness, and practitioners should switch to another agent if the therapy is unsuccessful. Practitioners also need to evaluate prophylactic therapies for patient compliance and effectiveness. They should note in the chart side effects to therapy and treatment failures to avoid repeating ineffective therapies. Patients should also be queried directly about the use of dietary supplements, as they may not volunteer the information (i.e., not considering it to be a "drug").

PATIENT EDUCATION

Drug Information

Practitioners need to educate patients about their headaches and what they should realistically expect from treatment. The prescriber should attempt to identify headache triggers (i.e., diet, medication, or environmental factors) by encouraging patients to keep diaries and to pay close attention to when migraines start and should encourage the patient to avoid or minimize these triggers.

Practitioners also must educate patients about their drug therapy. They should tell patients how frequently they can take an abortive therapy, what the maximum daily dose is, and what side effects to expect from the medication. If the patient will be using a nasal spray or injectable medication, the prescriber should demonstrate proper administration technique. Also, prescribers need to encourage patients to take their prophylactic therapies as scheduled, emphasizing that taking prophylactic therapies on an as-needed basis will not improve the condition. If switching to a new therapy, the prescriber should remind the patient to stop using the old therapy and not to use the two therapies simultaneously (unless this is intended). Patients must be strongly cautioned about drug–drug interactions, the dangers of concomitant use with some medications, and the use of any medications or dietary supplements they may not report. Acetaminophen overdose is common; patients must ensure that they are not taking a combined dose of acetaminophen from two or more medications that exceeds a maximum daily dose of 3,250 mg.

Nutrition

Foods that can trigger headaches include aspartame, caffeine, chocolate, monosodium glutamate, and red wine and other alcohol. The patient should be aware of any foods that trigger his or her headaches (a migraine diary is helpful for this) and should avoid them. Some medications should be taken with food, and taking some (oral) medications on a full stomach may slow absorption of the drug.

Complementary and Alternative Medicine

Some patients use feverfew to prevent migraines. The active ingredients in feverfew are the sesquiterpene lactones, which have an anti-inflammatory effect that blocks the transcription of inflammatory proteins and inhibits the release of serotonin. A minimum of 0.2% is the recommended dosage. Side effects include nausea, flatulence, diarrhea, and indigestion. Withdrawal symptoms when stopping long-term use can include muscle stiffness, anxiety, and rebound migraines. It also has anticoagulant properties, so prothrombin time and INR levels should be checked periodically, and it should be stopped 2 weeks before surgical procedures.

Another dietary supplement used for migraine prophylaxis is butterbur. This contains petasin and isopetasin, which have vasodilatory properties and inhibit leukotriene synthesis, reducing inflammation. A dose of 50 mg twice daily has been shown to reduce migraines (Grossman & Schmidramsl, 2001). There should be at least 7.5 mg petasin in the preparation. Side effects include abdominal pain, distended abdomen, and reduced urinary output.

Magnesium, high-dose riboflavin (vitamin B_2), and coenzyme Q10 have also been shown to reduce migraines (Goadsby & Sprenger, 2010).

CASE STUDY*

J.J., age 24, presents to your practice for the first time. She reports constant headaches. She smokes a pack of cigarettes a day but is in good health otherwise. She states that the headaches usually occur in the morning and last a few hours. The pain, localized to an area near her right temple, has a throbbing quality. The headache often results in nausea and vomiting and sensitivity to bright lights. She has tried to treat the headaches with acetaminophen, ibuprofen, and naproxen unsuccessfully. The headaches are causing her to miss work, and she is afraid she will lose her job.

DIAGNOSIS: MIGRAINE HEADACHES WITHOUT AURA

1. List specific goals of therapy for J.J.
2. What drug therapy would you prescribe? Why?
3. What are the parameters for monitoring success of the therapy?
4. Discuss specific patient education based on the prescribed therapy.
5. List one or two adverse reactions for the selected agent that would cause you to change therapy.
6. What would be the choice for the second-line therapy?
7. What OTC and/or alternative medicines might be appropriate for this patient?
8. What dietary and lifestyle changes might you recommend?
9. Describe one or two drug–drug or drug–food interactions for the selected agent.

* Answers can be found online.

Bibliography

*Starred references are cited in text.

*Adams, J., Barbery, G., & Lui, C. W. (2012). Complementary and alternative medicine use for headache and migraine: A critical review of the literature. *Headache, 53*(3), 459–473.

*Antonaci, F., Dumitrache, C., De Cillis, I., et al. (2010). A review of current European treatment guidelines for migraine. *Journal of Headache and Pain, 11*(1), 13–19.

*Ashina, M., Bendtsen, L., Jensen, R., et al. (1999). Muscle hardness in patients with chronic tension-type headaches: Relation to actual headache state. *Pain, 75*(2–3), 201–205.

*Barbanti, P., Egeo, G., Aurilia, C., et al. (2014). Treatment of tension-type headache: From old myths to modern concepts. *Neurological Sciences, 35*(Suppl. 1), 17–21.

Bendston, L., & Jensen, R. (2011). Treating tension-type headache—An expert opinion. *Expert Opinion on Pharmacotherapy, 12*(7), 1099–1109.

*Bezov, D., Ashina, S., Jensen, R., et al. (2010). Pain perception studies in tension-type headache. *Headache, 51*(2), 262–271.

*Bigal, M. E., & Tepper, S. J. (2003). Ergotamine and dihydroergotamine: A review. *Current Pain and Headache Reports, 7*(1), 55–62.

*Burch, R. C., Loder, S., Loder, E., et al. (2015). The prevalence and burden of migraine and severe headache in the United States: Updated statistics from government health surveillance studies. *Headache, 55*(1), 21–34.

*Charles, A. (2013). The evolution of a migraine attack—A review of recent evidence. *Headache, 53*(2), 413–419.

*Cho, S. J., & Chu, M. K. (2015). Risk factors of chronic daily headache or chronic migraine. *Current Pain and Headache Reports, 19*(1), 465.

*Dharmshaktu, P., Tayal, V., & Kalra, B. S. (2012). Efficacy of antidepressants as analgesics: A review. *Journal of Clinical Pharmacology, 52*(1), 6–17.

*DIH. (2014). *Drug information handbook* (23rd ed.). Hudson, OH: Lexicomp Drug Reference Handbooks.

*Ferrante, E., Rossi, P., Tassorelli, C., et al. (2010). Focus on therapy of primary stabbing headache. *Journal of Headache and Pain, 11*(2), 157–160.

*Fischera, M., Marziniak, M., Gralow, I., et al. (2008). The incidence and prevalence of cluster headache: A meta-analysis of population-based studies. *Cephalalgia, 28*(6), 614–618.

*Food and Drug Administration (FDA). (2007). Antidepressant use in children, adolescents, and adults. Retrieved from http://www.fda.gov/drugs/drugsafety/informationbydrugclass/ucm096273.htm. Updated: December 24, 2014. Accessed: May 27, 2015.

*Food and Drug Administration (FDA). (2009). Summary Minutes of the Joint Meeting of the Drug Safety and Risk Management Advisory Committee, Nonprescription Drugs Advisory Committee, and the Anesthetic and Life Support Drugs Advisory Committee June 29 and 30, 2009. Retrieved from http://www.fda.gov/AdvisoryCommittees/Calendar/ucm143083.htm. Updated July 30, 2013. Accessed May 27, 2015.

*Francis, G. J., Becker, W. J., & Pringsheim, T. M. (2010). Acute and preventive pharmacologic treatment of cluster headache. *Neurology, 75*(5), 463–473.

*Goadsby, P. J. (2012). Pathophysiology of migraine. *Annals of Indian Academy of Neurology, 15*(Suppl. 1), S15–S22.

*Goadsby, P. J., & Sprenger, T. (2010). Current practice and future directions in the prevention and acute management of migraine. *Lancet Neurology, 9*(3), 285–298.

*Grossman, W., & Schmidramsl, H. (2001). An extract of *Petasites hybridus* is effective in the prophylaxis of migraine. *Alternative Medicine Review, 6*(3), 303–310.

*Haque, B., Rahman, K. M., Hoque, A., et al. (2012). Precipitating and relieving factors of migraine versus tension type headache. *BioMedCentral Neurology, 12*, 82.

*Headache Classification Committee of the International Headache Society (IHS). (2013). The International Classification of Headache Disorders, 3rd edition (beta version). *Cephalalgia, 33*(9), 629–808.

*Hepp, Z., Dodick, D. W., Varon, S. F., et al. (2015). Adherence to oral migraine-preventive medications among patients with chronic migraine. *Cephalalgia, 35*(6), 478–488.

*Johnston, M. M., & Rapoport, A. M. (2010). Triptans for the management of migraine. *Drugs, 70*(12), 1505–1518.

*Kacperski, J. (2015). Prophylaxis of migraine in children and adolescents. *Paediatric Drugs, 17*(3), 217–226. doi: 10.1007/s40272-015-0125-5.

*Khoury, C. K., & Couch, J. R. (2010). Sumatriptan–naproxen fixed combination for acute treatment of migraine: A critical appraisal. *Journal of Drug Design, Development and Therapy, 18*(4), 9–17.

*Lampl, C., Voelker, M., & Steiner, T. J. (2012). Aspirin is first-line treatment for migraine and episodic tension-type headache regardless of headache intensity. *Headache, 52*(1), 48–56.

*Lipton, R. B., Pavlovic, J. M., Haut, S. R., et al. (2014). Methodological issues in studying trigger factors and premonitory features of migraine. *Headache, 54*(10), 1661–1669.

*Loder, E., Burch, R., & Rizzoli, P. (2012). The 2012 AHS/AAN guidelines for prevention of episodic migraine: A summary and comparison with other recent clinical practice guidelines. *Headache, 52*(6), 930–945.

*Loder, E., Weizenbaum, E., Frishberg, B., et al., American Headache Society *Choosing Wisely Task Force. (2013). Choosing wisely in headache medicine: The American Headache Society's list of five things physicians and patients should question. *Headache, 53*(10), 1651–1659.

*Marmura, M. J., Silberstein, S. D., & Schwedt, T. J. (2015). The acute treatment of migraine in adults: The American Headache Society evidence assessment of migraine pharmacotherapies. *Headache, 55*(1), 3–20.

*Merikangas, K. R. (2013). Contributions of epidemiology to our understanding of migraine. *Headache, 53*(2), 230–246.

*Minen, M. T., Tanev, K., & Friedman, B. W. (2014). Evaluation and treatment of migraine in the emergency department: A review. *Headache, 54*(7), 1131–1145.

*Misakian, A. L. (2003). Postmenopausal hormone therapy and migraine headache. *Journal of Women's Health, 12*(10), 1027–1036.

*Monteith, T. S., & Goadsby, P. J. (2011). Acute migraine therapy: New drugs and new approaches. *Current Treatment Options in Neurology, 13*(1), 1–14.

Morren, J. A., & Galvez-Jimenez, N. (2010). Where is dihydroergotamine mesylate in the changing landscape of migraine therapy? *Expert Opinion on Pharmacotherapy, 11*(18), 3085–3093.

*Nestoriuc, Y., Rief, W., & Martin, A. (2008). Meta-analysis of biofeedback for tension-type headache: Efficacy, specificity, and treatment moderators. *Journal of Consulting and Clinical Psychology, 76*(3), 379–396.

*Pavlovic, J. M., Buse, D. C., Sollars, C. M., et al. (2014). Trigger factors and premonitory features of migraine attacks: Summary of studies. *Headache, 54*(10), 1670–1679.

*Pedraza, M. I., de la Cruz, C., Ruiz, M., et al. (2015). OnabotulinumtoxinA treatment for chronic migraine: Experience in 52 patients treated with the PREEMPT paradigm. *Springerplus, 4*, 176.

*Pomeroy, J. L., & Marmura, M. J. (2013). Pharmacotherapy options for the management of cluster headache. *Clinical Medicine Insights: Therapeutics, 5*, 53–74.

*Pringsheim, T., & Becker, W. J. (2014). Triptans for symptomatic treatment of migraine headache. *British Medical Journal, 348*, g2285.

*Pringsheim, T., Davenport, W. J., & Becker, W. J. (2010). Prophylaxis of migraine headache. *Canadian Medical Association Journal, 182*(7), E269–E276.

*Rains, J. C., Davis, R. E., & Smitherman, T. A. (2015). Tension-type headache and sleep. *Current Neurology and Neuroscience Reports, 15*(2), 520 [abstract only].

*Robbins, M. S., Kuruvilla, D., Blumenfeld, A., et al. (2014). Trigger point injections for headache disorders: Expert consensus methodology and narrative review. *Headache, 54*(9), 1441–1459.

*Schilling, A., Corey, R., Leonard, M., et al. (2010). Acetaminophen: Old drug, new warnings. *Cleveland Clinic Journal of Medicine, 77*(1), 19–27.

*Schwedt, T. J. (2014). Chronic migraine. *British Medical Journal, 348*, g1416.

*Silberstein, S. D. (2002). *Clinician's manual on migraine* (2nd ed.). Philadelphia, PA: Current Medicine, Inc.

*Silberstein, S. D., Holland, S., Freitag, F., et al., Quality Standards Subcommittee of the American Academy of Neurology and the American Headache Society. (2012). Evidence-based guideline update: Pharmacologic treatment for episodic migraine prevention in adults. *Neurology, 78*(17), 1337–1345.

*Smith, J. H. (2015). Mirtazapine for new daily persistent headache—Associated chronic nausea. *Headache, 55*(1), 176–177.

*Smitherman, T. A., Walters, A. B., Maizels, M., et al. (2011). The use of antidepressants for headache prophylaxis. *CNS Neuroscience and Therapeutics, 17*(5), 462–469.

*Tepper, S. J. (2012). Opioids should not be used in migraine. *Headache, 52*(Suppl. 1), 30–34.

*Tepper, S. J., & Spears, R. C. (2009). Acute treatment of migraine. *Neurologic Clinics, 27*(2), 417–427.

*Tfelt-Hansen, P. (2007). Acute pharmacotherapy of migraine, tension-type headache, and cluster headache. *Journal of Headache and Pain, 8*(2), 127–134.

*Torkamani, M., Ernst, L., Cheung, L. S., et al. (2015). The neuropsychology of cluster headache: Cognition, mood, disability, and quality of life of patients with chronic and episodic cluster headache. *Headache, 55*(2), 287–300.

*Wentz, A. L., Jimenez, T. B., Dixon, R. M., et al., and CXA20008 Study Investigators. (2008). A double-blind, randomized, placebo-controlled, single-dose study of the cyclooxygenase-2 inhibitor, GW406381, as a treatment for acute migraine. *European Journal of Neurology, 15*(4), 420–427.

*Wilson, J. F. (2007). In the clinic. Migraine. *Annals of Internal Medicine, 147*(9), ITC11-1–ITC11-16.

*Yu, S., & Han, X. (2015). Update of chronic tension-type headache. *Current Pain and Headache Reports, 19*(1), 469.

39 Seizure Disorders

Quinn A. Czosnowski ■ Craig B. Whitman ■ Laura Aykroyd

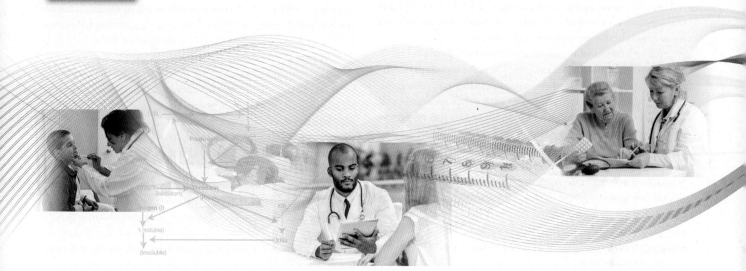

Epilepsy is a common neurologic condition affecting an estimated 2.2 million people in the United States and is the nation's fourth most common neurologic disorder. Every year, approximately 150,000 new cases are diagnosed with the highest rate occurring in children and older adults. Epilepsy is a complex neurologic disorder best defined as recurrent seizure activity. A single seizure does not constitute epilepsy unless a brain abnormality is identified, which may result in future seizure episodes. It is a multifaceted disease with various physical manifestations, prognoses, outcomes, and responses to treatment. Frequent seizures can lead to neuronal damage, which may lead to changes in memory and other cognitive functions. Therefore, it is important for the practitioner to be aware of the various etiologies and to screen patients appropriately with accurate and reliable diagnostic testing. With appropriate diagnosis and treatment, more than 90% of people with epilepsy lead normal, healthy, and productive lives.

CAUSES

Seizures can occur at any age, with etiology varying by age. The most common cause of epilepsy is idiopathic, accounting for about 65% of all cases. Other causes of epilepsy include vascular abnormalities (11%), congenital malformations (8%), and trauma (5%). Seizures from degeneration, infection, and neoplasm are considerably less prevalent. In newborns and infants, perinatal injuries, metabolic defects, congenital malformations, and infection are more likely causes of epilepsy, but still less frequent than the idiopathic diagnoses.

Some cases of epilepsy are hereditary or congenital (present at birth), and some are acquired (e.g., serious head injury, a central nervous system [CNS] infection, stroke, or dementia).

However, not all people with these disorders develop epilepsy. This suggests that there is a certain threshold that plays a role in the development of epilepsy and may be based on individual biochemistry. Why a person may have a seizure at one time rather than another relates to cause. This further suggests that there may be immediate triggers that can provoke an attack in a predisposed person (e.g., sudden seizure activity in people who are playing video games, working with a calculator, or listening to a particular piece of music). These sensory triggers are uncommon and are often referred to as *reflex epilepsy*.

Predisposing factors that may cause epilepsy more often are sleep deprivation, hyperventilation, fever from underlying illness, hormonal changes occurring during menses, and drug or alcohol ingestion. All of these may lower the seizure threshold and provoke seizures in people who are predisposed.

Several acute metabolic, infectious, medication-related, and other disorders (e.g., alcohol or drug withdrawal, viral meningitis, or hypoglycemia from an overdose of insulin) are associated with seizures. However, upon recovery from these disorders, a person is not necessarily predisposed to future seizures. These are known as *secondary* or *acute* seizures rather than epilepsy.

Pathophysiology

To understand the pathophysiologic process of an epileptic seizure, it is necessary to understand normal neuronal conduction. Normal cellular transmission between nerve cells is dependent on a normal distribution of positively or negatively charged ions between the inside and the outside of the cell. In normal human physiology, there is a resting membrane potential (70 μV) that leaves the inside of the cell negatively charged with respect to the outside of the cell. A stimulus is needed to produce a cellular discharge, and once stimulated, an action potential is generated. After the generation of the action potential, there is a brief period during which the nerve cell membrane is hyperpolarized, which makes it more difficult for a second action potential to be generated until the normal resting membrane ionic gradient is restored.

Communication between neurons occurs through highly specialized structures called *synapses*. There are hundreds of synapses on each neuron. In these synapses, neurotransmitters are released from vesicles in the neurons where they are stored and then diffuse across the synaptic region to contact specific receptors. Once stimulated, the receptors can open or close a specific ion channel. There are two types of ion channels—excitatory and inhibitory. The channels consist of a number of different protein substances. The main inhibitory neurotransmitter in the CNS is gamma-aminobutyric acid (GABA). There are several excitatory neurotransmitters as well, including glutamate and aspartate. These chemicals can activate several different receptors that, depending on their action, can excite or inhibit a group of nerve cells.

To produce an actual seizure, a large group of nerve cells (neurons) must fire abnormally and together. It is thought that this firing occurs within certain highly organized areas of the brain that tend to support seizure activity. This is known as an *epileptic focus*. When epileptic discharges (focus) occur, normal inhibitory circuits (GABA-ergic) begin to fire, which tends to limit the size of the focus. The implication is that a seizure may result from impairment of the inhibitory brain nerve cells or conditions in which there is abnormal excitation. The epileptic focus that is produced may lead to a focal seizure only in the involved area of the brain, or the discharge may travel through other pathways to become more generalized and involve the entire brain. Clinical manifestations of a seizure can be classified by type of seizure, but the manifestations depend on the balance between abnormal, excitatory, and inhibitory neuronal firing, the location of the epileptic focus, and the patterns and degree of spread of the epileptic focus.

Classification of Seizures

The International Classification of Epileptic Seizures (ICES) categorizes seizures in two major groups: partial seizures and generalized seizures. The terminology used by the ICES, however, is not always the same as that used by many clinicians. For instance, many practitioners call the ICES "absence" seizure a *petit mal*, and the designation "tonic–clonic" is often referred to as a *grand mal* seizure. A complex partial seizure is often referred to as a *psychomotor* or *temporal lobe* seizure, and a simple partial seizure has been called *focal* or *jacksonian*.

Furthermore, classifying epileptic seizures by seizure type is difficult because seizures often appear within a cluster of other signs and symptoms. To help classify seizure type, physicians may look for precipitating factors, age of onset, severity, chronicity, diurnal or circadian cycling, anatomic location of seizure focus, and physical manifestations to help define the patient's treatment and prognosis.

Partial (Focal, Local) Seizures

Partial seizures begin in a localized area of the brain, although there may be generalization to involve both hemispheres. Simple partial (focal) seizures typically result in no alteration of consciousness, and the first clinical and electroencephalogram (EEG) change indicates an initial activation of nerve cells in a limited part of one cerebral hemisphere.

The patient's symptoms are determined by the anatomic location of the seizure focus. There may be motor, sensory, autonomic, or psychic symptoms. These may evolve into complex partial or secondary generalized tonic–clonic seizures. An EEG recorded during this time may show some low-voltage fast activity, rhythmic spikes, and slow-wave activity.

Complex partial seizures (psychomotor) are associated with impaired consciousness and with some form of automatic behavior (automatisms). This type of seizure can evolve from a simple partial seizure and can generate into a secondarily generalized tonic–clonic seizure. The EEG may show a unilateral or bilateral, low-voltage, fast activity with rhythmic spikes and slow waves. Complex partial seizures may be preceded by an aura.

Generalized (Convulsive or Nonconvulsive) Seizures

Generalized seizures involve both hemispheres of the brain from the onset, and they result in early loss of consciousness. Generalized seizures may involve only loss of consciousness (similar to absence seizures), or they may result in generalized tonic–clonic, clonic, or myoclonic seizures.

Absence seizures (petit mal) usually have a sudden onset, are brief (often lasting less than 10 seconds), and interrupt ongoing activities. The patient exhibits a blank stare and is usually unresponsive when spoken to, although at times the patient may be able to relate what was said to him or her during the initial phase of the seizure. There may be some mild clonic or tonic jerking, but it is not prolonged. There is abrupt onset and discontinuation. There is no postictal confusion, which may be characteristic of other seizure types, and there are no other associated symptoms. The EEG shows a very rhythmic, 3 cycles/s spike-wave discharge during the event. There is often confusion as to the diagnosis of absence seizures versus complex partial seizures. Absence seizures are usually restricted to childhood and are provoked by hyperventilation.

A subtype of absence seizure is the *atypical absence seizure*, in which the alteration of consciousness may not be complete. A child experiencing this type of seizure may continue with some activities. There may be an associated loss of muscle tone of the face and neck muscles, and there may be mild clonic twitching of the eyelids and mouth. The onset and discontinuation of this type of seizure is gradual.

Tonic–clonic seizures (grand mal) are associated with abrupt loss of consciousness. There may be some vague, ill-defined warning signs but no true aura. The patient experiences a sudden, sharp, bilaterally symmetric contraction of muscles and may cry, fall, or do both. The patient's head may be extended and appear cyanotic. There may be associated tongue biting and incontinence. Depressed consciousness that can be prolonged (several hours) characterizes the postictal period, during which the patient exhibits bilaterally symmetric clonic jerking of the extremities, increased salivation and frothing at the mouth, and deep respiration and relaxation of muscles. After the postictal period, the patient usually reports waking with muscle stiffness and headache. The EEG typically shows generalized high-voltage, spike-wave activity.

Clonic seizures consist of rapidly repetitive bilateral jerking of the extremities and facial muscles with loss of consciousness. The postictal phase is usually short.

Atonic seizures (drop attacks or astatic seizures) are characterized by a sudden loss of muscle tone, which may be only fragmentary. This type of seizure may be brief and not associated with loss of consciousness. It can occur in a repetitive, rhythmic, and successive manner and may be seen in patients with more diffuse neurologic insult and psychomotor retardation. Atonic seizures are frequently associated with Lennox–Gastaut syndrome, a pediatric epilepsy associated with multiple seizure types, mental retardation, and abnormal EEG findings.

Myoclonic seizures are sudden, brief, shock-like muscular contractions. They may be generalized or they may be confined to the face and trunk muscles, to one or more of the extremities, or to individual muscle groups. Myoclonic seizures can occur regularly in a repetitive manner, or they can be sporadic. These seizures may accompany other neurologic conditions, such as metabolic or toxic states, as well as epilepsy.

Tonic seizures consist of brief, generalized tonic contractions with associated head extension, possible stiffening of the back, and stiffening of all four extremities. These seizures can be associated with autonomic symptoms, a rapid heart rate, and cessation of breathing followed by cyanosis. This type of seizure is also seen in Lennox-Gastaut syndrome and may be precipitated during slow-wave sleep.

Status Epilepticus

Status epilepticus (SE) is a life-threatening emergency that requires immediate identification and treatment. The standard definition is seizure activity persisting for more than 30 minutes or two or more sequential seizures without recovery between them. Clinical practice and recent guidelines define SE as continuous clinical and/or electrographic seizure activity persisting for more than 5 minutes or recurrent seizure activity without recovery between seizures. Thirty-day mortality of convulsive SE is estimated as 19% to 27% and as high as 65% in nonconvulsive status. Significant morbidity is also associated with SE with the poorest functional outcomes in patients with refractory seizures. Precipitating factors include drug noncompliance and sudden withdrawal from antiepileptic drugs (AEDs), CNS infection, withdrawal from alcohol or sedative drugs, metabolic disturbances, sleep deprivation, stroke, trauma, or encephalitis.

Diagnostic Criteria

The accurate diagnosis of a seizure helps the health care provider decide whether to initiate or withhold drug treatment and which medications to prescribe. A well-conducted history and physical and neurologic examinations may allow a diagnosis of epilepsy to be made without further diagnostic or laboratory testing. The initial assessment should include associated factors (e.g., age, medical history, precipitating events), symptoms during the seizure (e.g., aura, behavior, motor symptoms, loss of consciousness), and symptoms following a seizure (e.g., postictal state). Unfortunately, many of the manifestations of epilepsy are subtle, making diagnosis and classification difficult. In fact, no single test, clinical finding, or symptom is reliable by itself to discriminate between epilepsy and nonepileptic events.

One of the most useful and standard tests for assisting in the diagnosis of epilepsy is the EEG. The EEG is a brain wave tracing showing voltage fluctuations versus time that is recorded from scalp electrodes placed in specific locations on the head (i.e., montages). An EEG is recommended as part of the neurodiagnostic evaluation of children and adults presenting with an apparent unprovoked first seizure.

Neurologic imaging studies also help in the diagnosis of epilepsy. Computed tomography (CT) scanning of the brain is used to detect masses or lesions, bleeding, or stroke-like conditions. Magnetic resonance imaging (MRI), although helpful in diagnosing lesions, bleeding, and stroke-like states, also helps find more subtle brain abnormalities, including medial temporal sclerosis. Current guidelines recommend the use of CT or MRI as part of the initial neurodiagnostic evaluation of adults presenting with an apparent unprovoked first seizure. MRI is the preferred imaging study for use in children. Other less frequently used tests include cerebral arteriography and positron emission tomography (PET). Cerebral arteriography may detect vascular malformation, aneurysms, and significant vascular disease. PET helps particularly in diagnosing partial epilepsy. PET scans measure regional cerebral blood flow and metabolism both during and between seizures. However, PET scanning is expensive, and some insurance carriers do not approve the test for reimbursement.

INITIATING DRUG THERAPY

The selection of the ideal AED depends on several factors, including seizure type and the age and sex of the patient. Treatment with AEDs starts after the diagnosis is confirmed and the patient has experienced two or more seizures. If a patient has one or more risk factors for recurrent seizures (EEG abnormalities, structural lesions, partial seizures, or a family history), then pharmacotherapy can be initiated.

Many epilepsy specialists advocate monotherapy as the first principle of management. If monotherapy fails, replacement by a second AED is recommended. Monotherapy has several advantages, including increased compliance. The most frequent cause of failure to control seizure activity is the patient's lack of adherence to drug therapy. Management of toxicity is easier with monotherapy because adverse events

TABLE 39.1

Recommended Order of Treatment for Epileptic Seizures

	Partial (Both Simple and Complex) Seizures	Generalized Tonic–Clonic Seizures	Absence Seizures	Atypical Absence, Myoclonic, and Atonic Seizures
First-line therapy	carbamazepine, phenytoin, fosphenytoin, valproic acid, lamotrigine, lacosamide, topiramate, oxcarbazepine	carbamazepine, lacosamide phenytoin, valproic acid, fosphenytoin	ethosuximide, valproic acid, lamotrigine	valproic acid
Second-line therapy (alternative therapy)	eslicarbazepine, ezogabine, felbamate, gabapentin, levetiracetam, perampanel, phenobarbital, pregabalin, primidone, tiagabine, vigabatrin	felbamate, gabapentin, lamotrigine, levetiracetam, phenobarbital, primidone, ethotoin, mephobarbital, mephenytoin, vigabatrin	clonazepam, paramethadione, trimethadione, methsuximide, phensuximide	Clonazepam, levetiracetam

often can be correlated with serum drug levels. Some epilepsy specialists report that up to 75% of their patients have had complete seizure control on monotherapy.

Usually, when monotherapy with several drugs has failed, polytherapy may be tried. In contrast to monotherapy, polytherapy may increase the risk of chronic toxicity in the patient.

Whenever two or more drugs are used simultaneously, decisions regarding therapy become more complex, and there is an increased risk of adverse events and drug interactions.

The particular drug selected depends on the seizure type and toxicity. **Table 39.1** and **Figure 39.1** outline the recommended treatment order and algorithm of treatment.

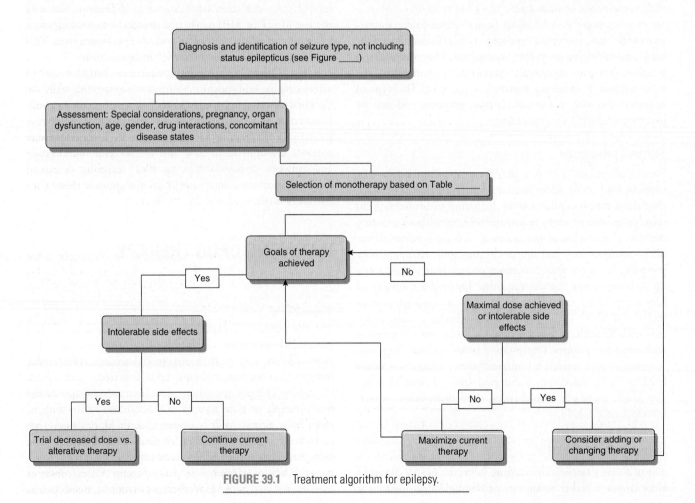

FIGURE 39.1 Treatment algorithm for epilepsy.

Surgical Treatment of Epilepsy

The surgical treatment of epilepsy has become an important therapeutic modality. Candidates for surgery may include patients who have failed multiple medical therapies, with refractory SE or who experience intolerable drug side effects. Various surgical procedures can be performed, including anterior temporal lobectomy, amygdalohippocampectomy, extratemporal focus removal, lesionectomy, corpus callosotomy, and hemispherectomy. Outcomes are generally good with approximately 70% of patients seizure free after a temporal lobectomy.

Goals of Drug Therapy

The drug treatment of patients with epilepsy is designed to reduce the number of seizures. A realistic goal for most patients is to completely control seizures, ideally achieved with monotherapy. In addition to controlling seizures, another goal should be improving the patient's quality of life by allowing a return to normal activities of daily living without restriction (except driving; see Patient Education).

Hydantoins (Phenytoin and Fosphenytoin)
Indications/Uses

One of the oldest and most effective AEDs is phenytoin (Dilantin). Fosphenytoin (Cerebyx), a prodrug, was approved 40 years later and is used for the same indications as its parent compound, phenytoin. Hydantoins are effective in treating a wide range of seizure types, including generalized tonic–clonic as well as simple or partial seizure activity. In either case, they can be used as first-line agents for monotherapy. Phenytoin is one of the most commonly used anticonvulsants for generalized tonic–clonic (grand mal) seizure activity and for simple and complex partial seizures. It can also be used to prevent early posttraumatic seizures occurring within 7 days after a traumatic brain injury.

Mechanism of Action

Phenytoin blocks posttetanic potentiation by stabilizing neuronal membranes. It decreases seizure activity by increasing the efflux or decreasing the influx of sodium ions across cell membranes in the motor cortex during generation of nerve impulses. It also regulates neuronal excitability by inhibiting calcium conduction through altering calcium uptake in presynaptic terminals and preventing cyclic nucleotide accumulation and cerebellar stimulation. Phenytoin is the active moiety of fosphenytoin, after administration fosphenytoin is converted to phenytoin by plasma esterases.

Dosage

Phenytoin is available in multiple dosage forms, including chewable tablets, extended-release capsules, suspension, and intravenous (IV). Regardless of dosage form, a loading dose of phenytoin is typically given to achieve a therapeutic level as quickly as possible. The loading dose is 15 to 20 mg/kg/d in both adults and children. The maximum infusion rate for IV administration of phenytoin is 50 mg/min to avoid cardiovascular collapse or 25 mg/min in patients with preexisting cardiac disease. If given orally, it is divided into three doses given every 2 to 4 hours to increase tolerability with a max of 400 mg per dose secondary to absorption. Following a loading dose, the normal maintenance dose is 4 to 6 mg/kg/d in adults and 5 to 12 mg/kg/d in children based on age. Absorption is also impaired when administered in patients on continuous enteral nutrition; therefore, it is recommended to hold enteral nutrition feeds 1 to 2 hours before and after each phenytoin dose given per feeding tube.

The dose, concentration in solutions, and infusion rates for fosphenytoin are expressed as phenytoin sodium equivalents. Fosphenytoin should always be prescribed in phenytoin sodium equivalents: 75 mg of fosphenytoin sodium = 50 mg of phenytoin sodium (see **Table 39.2**). Fosphenytoin is given as a loading dose of 15 to 20 phenytoin equivalents/kg followed by a maintenance dose of 4 to 6 phenytoin equivalents/kg/d. Advantages include the ability to give it as an intramuscular injection in those without IV access and at a maximum infusion rate of 150 phenytoin equivalents/min.

Phenytoin is unique because it is metabolized in a nonlinear manner, exhibiting Michaelis-Menten enzyme kinetics. The enzymes that metabolize phenytoin are saturable, meaning that as the amount of drug approaches this saturation point, small incremental increases in a dose can result in disproportionately high serum levels. Further, as the concentrations reach closer to the saturation point, the half-life of phenytoin increases. This must be considered when adjusting phenytoin doses.

The therapeutic serum concentration of phenytoin is 10 to 20 mcg/mL in a person with a normal albumin level, while the therapeutic level of free, unbound phenytoin is 1 to 2.5 mcg/mL. In clinical scenarios in which protein binding is impaired, such as hypoalbuminemia, or concurrent medication therapy competes for protein-binding sites, the free fraction and pharmacologically active component are increased. Equations have been developed to help prescribers estimate free fraction in states of hypoalbuminemia, renal failure, and critical illness.

Contraindications

There are no absolute contraindications for phenytoin other than allergy (**Table 39.2**). It carries a black box warning for severe cardiovascular events (hypotension and arrhythmias) with rapid IV administration.

Adverse Events

Phenytoin exhibits adverse effects specific to dosage form and serum concentration in addition to other adverse effects. Common adverse events across dosage forms and concentrations include gingival hyperplasia, hirsutism, coarsening of facial features, rash, ataxia, altered coordination, nystagmus, confusion, peripheral neuropathy, vitamin D deficiency and osteopenia, hepatitis, megaloblastic anemia, thrombocytopenia, and mild sensory polyneuropathy. Serious but less common adverse events include blood dyscrasias (anemia, neutropenia,

TABLE 39.2

Overview of Antiepileptic Drugs

Generic (Trade) Name	Significant Metabolic/ Transporter Interactions	Selected Adverse Events	Contraindications	Special Considerations
phenytoin (Dilantin) Loading dose: 15–20 mg/kg IV. If PO, give in divided doses q2–4h to decrease GI adverse events SE: 20 mg/kg IV loading dose Maintenance dose: 300 mg/d or 5–6 mg/kg/d in three divided doses or qd–bid using an extended-release form of the drug	Strong inducer: CYP2B6, CYP2C19, CYP3A4 Major substrate: CYP2C19, CYP2C9	Nystagmus, ataxia, cognitive impairment, lethargy, gingival hyperplasia, increase in body hair, coarsening of facial features, acne, folate deficiency, skin rash	Heart block; sinus bradycardia Pregnancy Category D	Avoid IM and SQ administration due to pain, erratic absorption, and risk of local tissue damage. An in-line 0.22–5 mcg filter is recommended for IVPB solutions. Therapeutic ranges: Neonates: 8–15 mcg/mL total phenytoin, 1–2 mg/mL free phenytoin Children and adults: Total concentration: 10–20 mcg/mL Free: 1–2.5 mcg/mL
fosphenytoin (Cerebyx) See dosing recommendation above, order in phenytoin equivalents (PE)	See phenytoin	See phenytoin	See phenytoin	See phenytoin
carbamazepine (Tegretol) 6–12 y: 20–30 mg/kg/d in 2–4 divided doses per day; usual dose is 400–800 mg/d, maximum 1 g/d 12 y–adult: usual dose 800–1,200 mg/d in 3–4 divided doses	Strong inducer: CYP1A2, CYP2B6, CYPC19, CYP3A4 Major substrate: CYP3A4 (causes autoinduction starting between days 3 and 5 of therapy and maximal effects within 4 wks)	Hematologic abnormalities, drowsiness, fatigue, ataxia, SIADH, rash (Stevens-Johnson syndrome), GI upset, confusion, nystagmus, and seizures	Hypersensitivity to tricyclic antidepressants, bone marrow suppression, recent use of an MAO inhibitor (≤14 d) Pregnancy Category D	Oral suspension should not be administered simultaneously with other liquid medicinal agents or diluents. To avoid GI upset, take with food or water and divide doses. The appearance of a rash does not automatically rule out using carbamazepine. Therapeutic ranges: 6–12 mcg/mL; 4–8 mg/mL if used in combination with other AEDs; toxic > 15 mcg/mL
oxcarbazepine (Trileptal) Initial dose: 300 mg bid; increased by 600 mg/d at weekly intervals Children 4–16 y: 8–10 mg/kg in 2 divided doses/d, not to exceed 600 mg/d		Dizziness, diplopia, ataxia, headache, weakness, rash, hyponatremia	Pregnancy Category C	Commonly leads to hyponatremia; elderly at higher risk
eslicarbazepine (Aptiom) Initial dose: 400 mg daily; increased to 800 mg/d after 1 wk. Max dose 1,200 mg/d Dose adjustment for CrCl <50 mL/min	Moderate inducer of CYP3A4 Moderate inhibitor of CYP2C19 Substrate of UGT2B4	Dizziness, somnolence, diplopia, fatigue, nausea, ataxia, cognitive dysfunction, vomiting, abnormal vision, abdominal pain, tremor, dyspepsia, abnormal gait, and hyponatremia (decrease > 10 mEq/L)	History or presence of second- or third-degree AV block Oxcarbazepine use Pregnancy Category C	

Drug and Dose	Drug Interactions (CYP)	Side Effects	Contraindications/Precautions	Therapeutic Range/Notes
valproic acid (Depakote, Depakene) Children and adults: 30–60 mg/kg/d in 2–3 divided doses SE: 20–40 mg/kg loading dose Dose adjustment: Reduce dose in hepatic impairment and avoid in severe impairment.	Weak inducer: CYP2A6 Weak inhibitor: CYP2A6 Minor substrate: CYP: 2A6, 2B6, 2C19, 2C9, 2E1	Lethargy, GI upset, weight gain, alopecia, hepatitis	Hepatic dysfunction; hepatic failure resulting in death has occurred, and children <2 y are at considerable risk. Pregnancy Category X for migraine prophylaxis/D for other indications	Therapeutic range: total concentration 50–100 mcg/mL; toxic > 200 mcg/mL Free: 4–15 mcg/mL Seizure control may improve at levels > 100 mcg/mL. Toxicity may occur at levels of 100–150 mcg/mL. Take with food or milk; do not administer with carbonated drinks.
ethosuximide (Zarontin) Children 3–6 y: 15–40 mg/kg/d in 2 divided doses Children > 6 y and adults: 20–40 mg/kg/d in 2 divided doses	Major substrate: CYP3A4	Nausea, GI upset, hiccups, headache	Pregnancy Category C	Seldom-used drug for absence seizures in children Therapeutic range: 40–100 mg/L
phenobarbital Infants: 5–8 mg/kg/d in 1–2 divided doses Children 1–5 y: 6–8 mg/kg/d in 1–2 divided doses Children 5–12 y: 4–6 mg/kg/d in 1–2 divided doses Children >12 y–adults: 1–3 mg/kg/d in 2–3 divided doses or 50–100 mg bid–tid SE: 20 mg/kg loading dose; may give additional 5–10 mg/kg after 10 min	Strong inducer: CYP1A2, CYP2A6, CYP2B6, CYP2C8, CYP2C9, and CYP3A4 and P-glycoprotein Major substrate: CYP2C19	Sedation, ataxia, cognitive impairment, hyperactivity, rash, problems with sleep, megaloblastic anemia (responds to folic acid)	Use caution in patients with hypovolemic shock, congestive heart failure, hepatic impairment, respiratory dysfunction or depression, previous addiction to the sedative/hypnotic group, chronic or acute pain, renal dysfunction, and the elderly. (Because of its long half-life and addiction potential, phenobarbital is not recommended as a sedative in the elderly.) Pregnancy Category D	Avoid rapid IV administration (>50 mg/min). Do not add IV form to acidic solutions. Tolerance, or psychological and physical dependence, may occur with prolonged use. Abrupt withdrawal in patients with epilepsy may precipitate status epilepticus. Therapeutic ranges: Infants and children: 15–30 mcg/mL Adults: 20–40 mg/mL Toxic range: >40 mcg/mL
primidone (Mysoline) Children < 8 y: 10–25 mg/kg/d tid–qid Children > 8 y–adults: Start at 100–125 mg qhs for 3 d; then, increase to 100–125 mg bid for 3 d; then, increase to up to 250 mg tid	Strong inducer: CYP1A2, CYP2A6, CYP2B6, CYP2C8, CYP2C9, and CYP3A4 and P-glycoprotein	Same as phenobarbital	Porphyria Use caution in renal or hepatic impairment or pulmonary insufficiency. Pregnancy Category D	Folic acid as a supplement to avoid folic acid deficiency and megaloblastic anemia: Adults: 5–12 mcg/mL Children <5 y: 7–10 mcg/mL Toxic level: >15 mcg/mL Be consistent with protein intake during primidone therapy. (Low-protein diets increase the duration of action.) Avoid foods high in vitamin C because of displacement of drug from binding sites.
ezogabine (Potiga) 100 mg TID; increase at weekly intervals by no more than 150 mg/d. Max dose 1,200 mg daily—no benefit demonstrated above 900 mg Dose reduction in elderly, CrCl <50 mL/min, or hepatic impairment	Inhibits: OAT3, P-glycoprotein	Loss of visual acuity—black box warning, skin discoloration (bluish, gray-blue, brown), confusion, hallucinations, urinary retention, QT prolongation, drowsiness, impaired coordination, gait disturbances	Pregnancy Category C	If no substantial benefit after adequate titration, then DC and consider other therapies Black box warning—ability to cause retinal abnormalities and loss of visual acuity ~1/3 of patients at 4 y Baseline eye exams and then every 6 mos QT prolongation—credible meds.org

(Continued)

TABLE 39.2

Overview of Antiepileptic Drugs (*Continued*)

Generic (Trade) Name	Significant Metabolic/ Transporter Interactions	Selected Adverse Events	Contraindications	Special Considerations
gabapentin (Neurontin) 900–1,800 mg/d in 3 divided doses Children >12 y: 300 mg on day 1 at bedtime; 300 mg bid on day 2; 300 mg tid on day 3 Dose adjustment: renal failure (CrCl <60 mL/min)		Ataxia, fatigue, dizziness, somnolence, weight gain, GI upset	Pregnancy Category C	Dosage adjustments for patients with renal impairment: CrCl >60 mL/min: 1,200 mg/d CrCl 30–60 mL/min: 600 mg/d CrCl 15–30 mL/min: 300 mg/d CrCl <15 mL/min: 150 mg/d
tiagabine (Gabitril) Children 12–18 y: 4 mg qd for 1 wk; may increase to 8 mg daily in 2 divided doses for 1 wk; then may increase by 4–8 mg weekly to response or up to 32 mg in 2–4 divided doses/d Adults: 4 mg qd for 1 wk; may increase by 4–8 mg/wk to response or up to 56 mg in 2–4 divided doses/d	Major substrate: CYP3A4	Dizziness, somnolence, asthenia, confusion, GI upset, anorexia, fatigue, impaired concentration, speech or language problems, confusion	Pregnancy Category C	Should be taken with food
lamotrigine (Lamictal) Children 2–12 y with concomitant AEDs without valproic acid therapy: 5–15 mg/kg/d; max. 400 mg/d in 2 divided doses Adults: 100–400 mg/d in 1–2 doses/d Dose adjustment: Children 2–12 y with concomitant valproic acid therapy: 1–5 mg/kg/d; max. 200 mg/d in 2 divided doses Adults with concomitant valproic acid therapy: 50–200 mg/d in 2 divided doses	Inhibits OCT2	Dizziness, headache, rash, ataxia, tremor, GI upset, diplopia, Stevens–Johnson syndrome (rare)	Use with caution with lactation, hepatic or cardiac dysfunction, and in children. Pregnancy Category C	Take without regard to meals; drug may cause GI upset. Immediately report development of a rash. Gradually decrease dosage (taper) over 2 wk when discontinuing drug therapy. If doses held for >5 half-lives, consider restarting using initial dosing recommendations
perampanel (Fycompa) Initial dose: 2 mg/d at bedtime; increase by 2 mg every 7 d. Maximum dose 12 mg/d If on enzyme-inducing AEDs: Initial dose 4 mg/d at bedtime Dose reduction in mild to moderate hepatic impairment Avoid if CrCl <30 mL/min	Major substrate: CYP3A4	Perampanel carries a black box warning due to its potential to cause serious life-threatening neuropsychiatric events (aggression, anger, homicidal thoughts, and hostility). Common side effects include dizziness, somnolence, headache, fatigue, gait/balance disturbances, and falls.	Pregnancy Category C	Watch for neuropsychiatric symptoms with initiation and titration.

Drug (dosing)	Metabolism	Adverse effects	Contraindications / Pregnancy Category	Monitoring / Comments
levetiracetam (Keppra) 500 mg twice daily; max 3,000 mg SE: loading dose of 1,000–3,000 mg		Somnolence, asthenia, fatigue, dizziness, ataxia, anorexia, cognitive difficulties	Hypersensitivity to sulfonamides; hypersensitivity to topiramate or any of its components Pregnancy Category C	Limited drug interactions Concentrations only helpful to assess compliance to therapeutic regimen; no therapeutic range Maintain adequate fluid intake.
lacosamide (Vimpat) Initial dose monotherapy: 100 mg twice daily, increased by 100 mg/d at weekly intervals Initial dose adjunctive therapy: 50 mg twice daily; increased by 100 mg/d at weekly intervals Maximum dose of 300 mg/d in patient with CrCl < 30 mL/min or mild/moderate hepatic impairment	Substrate: CYP3A4, CYP2C9, CYP2C19	Common adverse events seen include dizziness, fatigue, somnolence, blurred vision, diplopia, nausea, and tremor. Increases in PR interval, second- and third-degree AV block, syncope, atrial fibrillation, and atrial flutter may occur, especially in patients with a history of cardiovascular disease.	History of/current second- or third-degree AV block Pregnancy Category C	Use caution in patients with cardiac history. Consider ECG monitoring at baseline and when at steady state in patients with significant cardiac history.
topiramate (Topamax) Adults: initial: 50 mg/d; titrate by 50 mg/d at 1-wk intervals to a target dose of 200 mg bid. Dose adjustment: CrCl <70 mL/min: administer 50% of dose and titrate more slowly.		Cognitive difficulties, tremor, dizziness, ataxia, headache, fatigue, GI upset, renal calculi	Hypersensitivity to topiramate or any of its components Pregnancy Category D	Maintain adequate fluid intake.
zonisamide (Zonegran) Initial dose: 100 mg daily, titrated by 100 mg every 2 wk for a maintenance dose of 400–600 mg/d Not recommended in CrCl < 50 mL/min	Major substrate of CYP3A4	Fatigue, dizziness, ataxia, and anorexia Psychiatric symptoms, psychomotor slowing, fatigue, and somnolence more common with doses > 300 mg/d	Sulfonamide allergy	
rufinamide (Banzel) Adults: initial dose 400–800 mg/d divided in two doses. Titrated by 400–800 mg/d every other day until max dose of 3,200 mg/d If on concurrent valproate, start at 400 mg/d. Children: 10 mg/kg/d in two divided doses; titrate by 10 mg/kg/d every other day until 45 mg/kg/d or 3,200 mg reached. Consider supplemental doses following hemodialysis.		Common: QT shortening, somnolence, fatigue, coordination abnormalities, dizziness, gait disturbances, ataxia, nausea, vomiting, status epilepticus, and rash. Less common but clinically important adverse events include multiorgan hypersensitivity reactions, DRESS, SJS, and leukopenia.	Familial short QT syndrome, history or presence of short QT due to risk of sudden cardiac death Hypersensitivity to triazole derivatives Pregnancy Category C	Must be taken with food

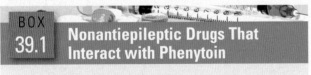

TABLE 39.3

Relationship between Total Serum Concentration of Phenytoin and Adverse Events

Serum Concentration	Adverse Events
>20 mcg/mL	Far lateral nystagmus
>30 mcg/mL	45 degrees lateral gaze nystagmus and ataxia
>40 mcg/mL	Decreased mentation and lethargy
>100 mcg/mL	Lethal

leukopenia, thrombocytopenia), hepatitis, Stevens-Johnson syndrome (SJS), drug reaction with eosinophilia and systemic syndromes (DRESS), and systemic lupus erythematosus (SLE). The IV forms of phenytoin and fosphenytoin carry boxed warnings for cardiovascular events with rapid infusion including hypotension, bradycardia, cardiac arrhythmias, cardiovascular collapse (especially with rapid IV use), venous irritation, thrombophlebitis, and possibly death. The IV formulations of phenytoin are also associated with local tissue necrosis following extravasation. Concentration-specific adverse effects of phenytoin are listed in **Table 39.3**.

Interactions

Phenytoin is a cytochrome P450 CYP2C9 and CYP2C19 enzyme substrate and a CYP1A2, CYP2C9, CYP2D6, and CYP3A3/CYP3A4 enzyme inducer. In addition to enzyme interactions, because of the high protein binding exhibited by phenytoin, it may be displaced by other highly protein-bound drugs, such as valproic acid and salicylic acid. Drug interactions occur frequently with phenytoin and can have a significant impact on therapeutic outcomes. **Box 39.1** contains a list of non-AEDs that interact with phenytoin, and **Table 39.2** lists AEDs that may interact with phenytoin.

BOX 39.1 Nonantiepileptic Drugs That Interact with Phenytoin

NON-AEDs AFFECTING PHENYTOIN LEVELS

Decreases Phenytoin Levels
  Alcohol (long-term use)
  Antacids, folic acid, rifampin, tube feedings
Increases Free Phenytoin Levels
  Aspirin, diazoxide, tolbutamide
Increases Total Phenytoin Levels
  Alcohol (shortly after intake), amiodarone, chloramphenicol, chlordiazepoxide, chlorpheniramine, cimetidine, disulfiram, fluconazole, fluoxetine, imipramine, isoniazid, metronidazole, omeprazole, propoxyphene, sulfonamides, ticlopidine, trazodone

Carbamazepine

Indications/Uses

Carbamazepine is indicated for the treatment of partial and generalized tonic–clonic seizures. It is a first-line drug choice for monotherapy in simple or complex partial seizures with secondary generalization.

Mechanism of Action

Carbamazepine's mechanism of action is not completely understood. It is believed to alter synaptic transmission by limiting the influx of sodium ions across cell membrane channels. Other potential mechanisms of action include depressing activity in the nucleus ventralis of the thalamus or decreasing summation of temporal stimulation.

Dosage

Carbamazepine is available as an immediate-release tablet, extended-release tablet, and oral suspension. The usual starting dosage of carbamazepine is 200 mg twice daily as tablets or 100 mg four times daily as a suspension. Doses should be increased weekly by increments of no more than 200 mg. The usual maintenance dose is 800 to 1,200 mg divided into 2 to 4 doses, depending on the dosage form chosen. The therapeutic plasma concentration is 4 to 12 mg/L. Carbamazepine undergoes autoinduction, which begins 3 to 5 days into therapy and is complete after 21 to 28 days of therapy. This results in a variable drug half-life and time to steady. Patients' serum concentrations will often vary significantly from week 1 of therapy to week 4 of therapy despite remaining on the same dosage of carbamazepine. As a result, frequent monitoring may be required following initiation or changes in dosing. Practitioners should be wary of decreasing a dose for a slightly elevated level during the first month of therapy due to a high likelihood that the serum concentration will decrease as a result of autoinduction. However, if a serum level is low during the first month of therapy, it is highly likely that the patient's level will drop further and a dosage increase is warranted.

Contraindications

Contraindications to carbamazepine include hypersensitivity to carbamazepine or tricyclic antidepressants, bone marrow suppression, recent use of a monoamine oxidase (MAO) inhibitor (≤14 days), and concurrent use of nefazodone, delavirdine, or other nonnucleoside reverse transcriptase inhibitors.

Carbamazepine has black box warnings due to the risk of serious dermatologic reactions in patients with the HLA-B*1502 allele. Asian patients should be screened for the variant HLA-B*1502 allele prior to initiating therapy because this variant is associated with a significantly increased risk of SJS and toxic epidermal necrosis. It also has a black box warning for aplastic anemia and agranulocytosis. Baseline CBC should be checked with periodic monitoring. Those patients demonstrating decreased WBC or platelets should be monitored more closely for the development of significant bone marrow suppression.

Adverse Events

Common adverse events associated with carbamazepine include pruritus, rash, constipation, nausea, vomiting, ataxia, dizziness, somnolence, blurred vision, urinary retention, xerostomia, and hyponatremia. Serious but less common adverse events include blood dyscrasias, syndrome of inappropriate diuretic hormone secretion (SIADH), cardiac conduction abnormalities, SJS, and DRESS (see **Table 39.2**). Carbamazepine is not effective in the treatment of myoclonic seizures and may in fact exacerbate seizures in these patients. Concentration-related adverse effects include dizziness, ataxia, drowsiness, nausea, vomiting, tremors, agitation, nystagmus, urinary retention, arrhythmias, coma, seizures, respiratory depression, and cardiac conduction disturbances.

Interactions

Carbamazepine is a significant inducer of numerous CYP450 enzymes, including CYP1A2, CYP2B6, CYP2C9, CYP2C19, and CYP3A4. Caution should be used when administering other medications metabolized via these pathways. It is also a major substrate of CYP3A4. Since it induces CYP3A4 and is metabolized by CYP3A4, it can induce its own metabolism resulting in decreased serum concentrations over time. This effect is complete after approximately 3 to 4 weeks of therapy. **Table 39.2** and **Box 39.2** list drug interactions among carbamazepine, AEDs, and other drugs.

Oxcarbazepine

Indications/Uses

Oxcarbazepine (Trileptal) is indicated for monotherapy or as adjunctive therapy in treating partial seizures in adults or in children ages 4 to 16 and as adjunctive therapy for partial seizures in children younger than age 2.

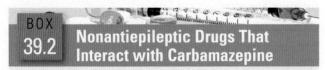

BOX 39.2 Nonantiepileptic Drugs That Interact with Carbamazepine

NON-AEDs AFFECTED BY CARBAMAZEPINE

Decreased Levels due to Carbamazepine
 Benzodiazepines, corticosteroids, cyclosporine, doxycycline, folic acid, haloperidol, oral contraceptives, theophylline, warfarin

NON-AEDs AFFECTING CARBAMAZEPINE LEVELS

Increases Carbamazepine Level
 Cimetidine, danazol, diltiazem, erythromycin, fluoxetine, imipramine, isoniazid, propoxyphene, verapamil, nicotinamide
Decreases Carbamazepine Level
 Alcohol (long-term use), folic acid

Mechanism of Action

Oxcarbazepine's pharmacologic effect is exerted through oxcarbazepine and the 10-monohydroxy metabolite (MHD) of oxcarbazepine. The exact mechanism by which oxcarbazepine and MHD work is unknown. However, studies indicate that the drug blocks sodium channels, resulting in stabilization of hyperexcited neural membranes and inhibition of repetitive neuronal firing. Increased potassium conductance and modulation of high-voltage activated calcium channels may contribute to the anticonvulsant effect.

Dosage

The typical starting dosage is 300 mg twice daily, increasing by 600 mg/d at weekly intervals. The target maintenance dosage is 600 to 2,400 mg/d. There are no therapeutic levels established for this agent.

Contraindications

Oxcarbazepine is contraindicated in patients with a hypersensitivity to the drug or any of its components. Oxcarbazepine should be avoided in patients who have had a hypersensitivity reaction to carbamazepine because there is a cross-reactivity of about 30% and in patients at risk for hyponatremia (2.5% of patients).

Adverse Events

Common adverse events include dizziness, somnolence, diplopia, fatigue, nausea, ataxia, vomiting, abnormal vision, abdominal pain, tremor, dyspepsia, and abnormal gait (see **Table 39.2**). Clinically significant hyponatremia (less than 125 mmol/L) has been reported. Elderly are at an increased risk. Oxcarbazepine has been linked to fatal dermatologic reactions, including SJS, and patients with toxic epidermal necrolysis (TEN) should be monitored for signs and symptoms.

Interactions

Oxcarbazepine is a weak inducer CYP3A4. This leads to potential interactions with numerous AEDs, including valproic acid, lamotrigine, carbamazepine, phenytoin, and phenobarbital. Strong inducers of CYP enzymes (carbamazepine, phenytoin, and phenobarbital) have been shown to decrease plasma levels of the metabolite MHD (29% to 40%). Oxcarbazepine also interacts with non-AEDs metabolized by CYP3A4, including dihydropyridine calcium antagonists and oral contraceptives, leading to decreased plasma concentrations.

Eslicarbazepine

Indications/Uses

Eslicarbazepine is a newer agent approved as an adjunctive therapy for partial-onset seizures in adults 18 years and older.

Mechanism of Action

Eslicarbazepine acetate is primarily converted to the major active metabolite eslicarbazepine along with minor active metabolites of R-licarbazepine and oxcarbazepine. The exact mechanism for eslicarbazepine is unknown but it is thought to block voltage-gated sodium channels resulting in stabilization of hyperexcited neural membranes and inhibition of repetitive neuronal firing.

Dosage

The recommended initial starting dose is 400 mg once daily, which can be increased after 1 week to the recommended maintenance dose of 800 mg once daily. The maximum dose is 1,200 mg once daily. Patients with CrCl < 50 mL/min should receive an initial dose of 200 mg once daily, and titration should occur no more frequently than every 2 weeks by no more than 200 mg with a max dose of 600 mg once daily. There are no published data for use in hemodialysis or severe hepatic impairment.

Contraindications

Contraindications to eslicarbazepine include a history of hypersensitivity to oxcarbazepine or carbamazepine or the presence or history of second- or third-degree AV block.

Adverse Events

Common adverse events include dizziness, somnolence, diplopia, fatigue, nausea, ataxia, cognitive dysfunction, vomiting, abnormal vision, abdominal pain, tremor, dyspepsia, abnormal gait, and hyponatremia (decrease > 10 mmol/L). Severe but less common adverse effects including SJS/TEN, DRESS, severe hyponatremia (less than 125 mmol/L), dose-dependent decreases in serum T3 and T4, and increased liver transaminases and bilirubin have been reported.

Interactions

Eslicarbazepine is a substrate of UGT2B4 as well as a moderate inhibitor of 2C19 and a moderate inducer of CYP3A4. Eslicarbazepine may increase the concentrations of a number of medications that are substrates of CYP2C19; of particular importance is phenytoin. Due to its ability to induce CYP3A4, concomitant use with CYP3A4 substrates should be avoided if possible due to a decrease in their serum concentrations. Eslicarbazepine concentrations may be increased by carbamazepine and decreased by carbamazepine, phenytoin, phenobarbital, and primidone.

Valproic Acid and Derivatives (Divalproex)

Indications/Uses

Valproic acid and its derivatives (divalproex) are approved as monotherapy and adjunctive therapy in complex partial and complex absence seizures and as adjunctive therapy in patients with multiple seizure types, including absence seizures. It is considered first-line therapy for generalized tonic–clonic, simple partial, complex partial, and absence seizures. It has also been used in the treatment of partial myoclonic seizures, atonic seizures, infantile spasms, and SE.

Mechanism of Action

The exact mechanism is not completely understood but is believed to work by affecting GABA. It has been postulated to affect GABA in numerous ways, including increasing GABA availability, enhancing the action of GABA, and mimicking its action at postsynaptic sites.

Dosage

There are three specific forms of valproic acid available in the United States. While the dosage forms and dosing intervals vary, the total daily starting dose is the same (see **Table 39.2**). The recommended initial dose is 15 mg/kg/d increasing at 1-week intervals by 5 to 10 mg/kg/d. The dose is titrated to a desired therapeutic effect or toxicity, whichever occurs first. Doses above 60 mg/kg/d are not recommended. The therapeutic range is 50 to 100 mg/L with some patients requiring levels higher than 100 mg/L to achieve seizure control.

Contraindications

Valproic acid is contraindicated in patients with significant hepatic disease and in those with urea cycle disorders.

It carries several black box warnings including the potential for hepatic failure leading to death in all patients as well as an increased risk of hepatotoxicity in patients with known mitochondrial disorders due to mutations in mitochondrial DNA polymerase gamma (POLG). There is a warning for major congenital malformations, in particular spina bifida. It should not be given to women of childbearing age or during pregnancy unless other medications have failed to control their seizures. The last black box warning is for severe life-threatening pancreatitis that can occur at any time during therapy.

Adverse Events

Common adverse events include fatigue, tremor, GI upset, alopecia, behavioral changes, and weight gain. Severe adverse effects include thrombocytopenia, pancreatitis, hyperammonemia/encephalopathy, and hepatotoxicity, which may occur at various times in therapy. Severe hepatotoxicity has been reported, especially in children age 2 and younger who are also taking other anticonvulsants. Patients taking valproic acid should be monitored for symptoms of hepatotoxicity, including malaise, weakness, facial edema, anorexia, jaundice, and vomiting. Other adverse events include a change in the menstrual cycle, ataxia, drowsiness, impaired judgment, headache, erythema multiforme, prolonged bleeding time, transient increased liver enzymes, tremor, nystagmus, SIADH, and fever. Levels above 100 mg/L are associated with increased adverse effects.

Valproic acid is teratogenic and produces spina bifida in 1% to 2% of pregnancies. It is a Pregnancy Category X drug for migraine prophylaxis and a category D drug for all other indications and should be avoided if possible during pregnancy.

Interactions

Minor interactions may occur with drugs that affect the CYP2C19, CYP2C9, CYP2D6, and CYP3A3/4 enzyme systems. Valproic acid may increase free phenytoin levels through displacement from protein-binding sites. Carbamazepine, lamotrigine, and possibly clonazepam reduce serum concentrations of valproic acid, while aspirin may increase valproic acid levels. Increased effects and possibly toxicity have been associated with the concomitant use of diazepam, CNS depressants, and alcohol.

Concurrent administration with carbapenems (e.g., meropenem) will cause a rapid decline in valproate plasma concentrations, producing an average drop of 66% within 24 hours.

Ethosuximide

Indications/Uses

Ethosuximide (Zarontin) is one of the drugs of choice for absence seizures. It should always be used in combination with another agent. It also is used for managing akinetic epilepsy and myoclonic seizures.

Mechanism of Action

The exact mechanism of ethosuximide is not completely understood, but it suppresses the paroxysmal spike-and-wave pattern in absence seizures and depresses nerve transmission in the motor cortex.

Dosage

The usual adult dosage is 500 mg daily adjusted by 250 mg every 4 to 7 days. The average daily maintenance dose is 20 to 30 mg/kg/d. The initial dose for children ages 3 to 6 is 250 mg daily with the same titration schedule and usual maintenance dose as adults. Doses greater than 1.5 g/d are not recommended. Serum concentrations should be monitored periodically with a therapeutic range of 40 to 100 mg/L (see **Table 39.2**).

Contraindications

Allergy is the only absolute contraindication to taking ethosuximide.

Adverse Events

Common adverse events are GI upset and fatigue. Ethosuximide has been associated with blood dyscrasias, CNS depression, SLE, and cutaneous reactions.

Interactions

Ethosuximide is a major substrate of CYP3A4 and, therefore, serum concentrations are affected by inducers and inhibitors of CYP3A4.

Barbiturates

Barbiturates have a relatively broad spectrum of antiepileptic activity and can be used as alternative monotherapy in generalized tonic–clonic seizures as well as in simple or complex partial seizures with or without secondary generalization. Barbiturates are usually sedating and have long-term cognitive, memory, and behavioral effects, and drug dependence may develop. Therefore, it is usually best to try exhausting other alternatives before initiating barbiturate therapy.

Phenobarbital

Indications/Uses

Phenobarbital is the most commonly used barbiturate-based anticonvulsant. In addition to the indications listed previously, phenobarbital is used for myoclonic epilepsies, SE, and neonatal and febrile seizures in children.

Mechanism of Action

Phenobarbital works by binding to the barbiturate-binding site at the GABA receptor complex, leading to enhanced GABA activity. It interferes with the transmission of impulses from the thalamus to the cerebral cortex, resulting in an imbalance in central inhibitory and facilitatory mechanisms.

Dosage

In SE, phenobarbital is commonly given as a 15 to 20 mg/kg loading dose to more rapidly achieve therapeutic levels. The loading dose should be given no faster than 1 mg/kg/min with a maximum infusion of 30 mg/min for infants and children and 60 mg/min for adults. The recommended adult maintenance dose is 2 to 3 mg/kg/d or 60 to 250 mg/d. The recommended maintenance dose in children is highly variable based on age and ranges from 1 to 5 mg/kg/d. Serum concentrations should be monitored periodically with the usual therapeutic range being 15 to 40 mg/L.

Contraindications

The drug should be administered cautiously to patients with severe liver disease because of increased side effects. It is also contraindicated in patients with porphyria and respiratory disease with dyspnea or obstruction and those with a history of sedative or hypnotic addiction.

Adverse Events

The principal adverse events—drowsiness and fatigue—make phenobarbital difficult to use (see **Table 39.2**). It also may cause ataxia and blurred vision, nausea, vomiting, constipation, and, over a long period, cognitive impairment and behavioral disturbances. Other major adverse events include cardiac arrhythmias, bradycardia, dizziness, light-headedness, CNS excitation or depression, and gangrene with inadvertent intra-arterial injection. To a lesser extent, hypotension, hallucinations, hypothermia, SJS, rash, agranulocytosis, megaloblastic anemia, thrombocytopenia, laryngospasm, respiratory depression, and apnea (especially with rapid IV use) also may occur.

If an overdosage or toxicity occurs, the expected signs and symptoms include unsteady gait, slurred speech, confusion, jaundice, hypothermia, hypotension, respiratory depression, and coma. Patients may require an IV vasopressor to treat hypotension. Repeated doses of activated charcoal significantly reduce the half-life of phenobarbital; the usual dose is 0.1 to

1 g/kg every 4 to 6 hours for 3 to 4 days unless the patient has no bowel movement, causing the charcoal to remain in the GI tract. Urinary alkalinization with IV sodium bicarbonate helps promote elimination. Patients in stage 4 coma due to high serum barbiturate levels may require charcoal hemoperfusion.

Interactions

Phenobarbital is a strong inducer of CYP1A2, CYP2B6, CYP2A6, CYP2C8, CYP2C9, and CYP3A4 and P-glycoprotein. It is also a major substrate of CYP2C19. As a result, it interacts with a number of other AEDs. Other drug interactions include increased toxicity of propoxyphene (Darvon), benzodiazepines, CNS depressants, and methylphenidate (**Box 39.3**).

Primidone
Indications/Uses

Primidone (Mysoline) is structurally related to the barbiturates. It is metabolized to phenobarbital and to phenylethylmalonamide (PEMA). PEMA may enhance the activity of phenobarbital. Primidone is used in the management of grand mal, complex partial, and focal seizures.

Mechanism of Action

Its mechanism of action is similar to phenobarbital and is thought to decrease neuronal excitability and raise the seizure threshold.

Dosage

The adult dose of primidone is 125 mg/d increased by increments of 125 mg every 3 days. The usual dose is 750 to 1,500 mg/d in 3 or 4 divided doses with a maximum recommended dose of 2,000 mg/d. The usual serum level for primidone is 5 to 12 mg/L; however, serum phenobarbital levels are typically used for monitoring purposes (see **Table 39.2**).

Contraindications
See the contraindications for phenobarbital.

Adverse Events
Primidone has an adverse event profile similar to phenobarbital. Dose-related adverse events include fatigue, cognitive impairment, and ataxia. Other adverse events include nausea, vomiting, hematologic abnormalities, and an SLE-like syndrome. A skin rash may develop, and over time, further cognitive impairment and behavioral changes may develop. Patients who have GI upset while taking primidone may take the medication with food.

Interactions
Drug interactions with primidone are similar to those with phenobarbital.

Ezogabine
Indications/Uses

Ezogabine is a newer agent approved as an adjunctive therapy for partial-onset seizures in adults 18 years and older who have responded poorly to other therapies and in whom the benefits may outweigh the risks of decreased visual acuity.

Mechanism of Action

Ezogabine binds to and stabilizes the KCNQ voltage-gated potassium channel in the open position enhancing the M-current and regulating neuronal excitability. It may also have some effect on augmentation of GABA-mediated currents.

Dosage

The initial dose is 100 mg three times daily and should be titrated no more frequently than every week by increments of less than 150 mg/d. The maximum daily dose is 1,200 mg although increased adverse effects and a lack of additional benefit were seen with daily doses exceeding 900 mg/d. If no substantial benefit is seen after reaching target dose, then consider discontinuation and an alternative therapy.

An initial starting dose of 50 mg three times daily should be considered in the elderly, patients with a CrCl < 50 mL/min, and moderate or severe hepatic impairment. In addition, the maximum daily dose varies for the elderly (750 mg), patients with a CrCl < 50 mL/min (600 mg), and patients with moderate hepatic impairment (750 mg) and severe hepatic impairment (600 mg).

Contraindications

Hypersensitivity to pregabalin or any component of the formulation is a contraindication. Ezogabine has a black box warning for its ability to cause retinal abnormalities, which can cause loss of visual acuity.

BOX 39.3 Nonantiepileptic Drugs That Interact with Phenobarbital

NON-AEDs AFFECTED BY PHENOBARBITAL

Decreases Phenobarbital Level
Beta-blockers, chloramphenicol, chlorpromazine, cimetidine, corticosteroids, cyclosporine, desipramine, doxycycline, folic acid, griseofulvin, haloperidol, meperidine, methadone, nortriptyline, oral contraceptives, quinidine, theophylline, warfarin

NON-AEDs AFFECTING PHENOBARBITAL LEVELS

Increases Phenobarbital Levels
Chloramphenicol, propoxyphene, quinine
Decreases Phenobarbital Levels
Chlorpromazine, folic acid, prochlorperazine

INCREASED TOXICITY

Benzodiazepines, CNS depressants, methylphenidate

Adverse Events

Ezogabine use is associated with development of retinal pigment abnormalities in approximately one third of patients after 4 years of therapy. Patients prescribed ezogabine should receive eye exams, which include testing of visual acuity and dilated fundus photography prior to starting therapy and then every 6 months thereafter. Therapy should be discontinued if vision or retinal pigmentary changes are identified unless there are no suitable alternatives. Due to the risk of vision loss, patients who fail to respond to ezogabine after appropriate dosage titration should have therapy discontinued.

Skin discoloration (bluish, gray-blue, or brown) occurs in approximately 10% of patients on prolonged therapy (greater than 2 years). Alternate therapies should be considered if this develops. Neuropsychiatric symptoms (confusion, hallucinations, and psychosis) may occur at any time but typically within the first 8 weeks of therapy and resolve with discontinuation of therapy. Other unique adverse events include urinary retention requiring catheterization, which is typically seen in the first 6 months, and QT prolongation of approximately 8 msec on ECG. More common side effects include dizziness, drowsiness, fatigue, impaired coordination and concentration, gait disturbances, blurred vision, and tremor.

Interactions

Ezogabine inhibits OAT3 and P-glycoprotein and does not have any effects of CYP450 enzymes. Ezogabine may decrease the lamotrigine AUC by approximately 18%. Carbamazepine and phenytoin have been shown to decrease the ezogabine AUC by 31% and approximately 34%, respectively. In addition to enzymatic drug interaction, concomitant treatment with medications that are likely to prolong QT should be avoided. A list of medications with potential to prolong QT intervals can be found at crediblemeds.org. It may also cause a false elevation in serum and urine bilirubin measurements.

Gabapentin

Indications/Uses

Gabapentin (Neurontin) is a safe and well-tolerated anticonvulsant with uncomplicated pharmacokinetics. However, it is uncommonly used in the treatment of epilepsy. It can be used as adjunct therapy in the treatment of complex partial seizures and possibly generalized tonic–clonic seizures. There are insufficient data to support its use as monotherapy.

Mechanism of Action

Gabapentin is structurally related to GABA, but it is not thought to influence synthesis or uptake of GABA. Gabapentin-binding sites have been found throughout the brain in relation to presynaptic voltage-gated calcium channels. It is thought that gabapentin may reduce release excitatory neurotransmitters through its activity at these channels, but the precise mechanism of action in epilepsy is unknown.

Dosage

The mean dosage in adults is approximately 1,800 mg/d, with a maximum of 3,600 mg/d. The therapeutic range is not well defined. It may be given once or twice daily, and its half-life is 5 to 7 hours.

Contraindications

Gabapentin is contraindicated in patients who are hypersensitive to the drug or to any of its components.

Adverse Events

Principal adverse effects are fatigue, dizziness, and blurred vision. In addition, neuropsychiatric events including emotional lability, hostility, and hyperkinesia have been reported in children (see **Table 39.2**). Many of the CNS-like symptoms resolve in a few weeks. The CNS effects are more pronounced with rapid dosage increases or in the setting of renal dysfunction. There have also been reports of modest weight gain. Serious adverse events including DRESS and SJS have been reported with its use.

Interactions

Gabapentin does not have any major drug interactions (antacids decrease its bioavailability), and serum level monitoring is not required.

Pregabalin

Indications/Uses

Pregabalin (Lyrica) is approved as adjunctive therapy for partial-onset seizures in adult patients.

Mechanism of Action

Pregabalin binds to the voltage-gated calcium channels in the brain, inhibiting excitatory neurotransmitter release.

Dosage

Pregabalin is typically started at a dose of 150 mg daily in two or three divided doses and should be titrated based on efficacy and side effects to a maximum dose of 600 mg/d. It requires dosage adjustment in patients with impaired renal function to avoid accumulation and increased adverse effects.

Contraindications

Hypersensitivity to pregabalin or any component of the formulation is a contraindication. Caution should be used in patients with a history of angioedema, heart failure, hypertension, or diabetes due to the risks of weight gain and edema.

Adverse Events

Peripheral edema and weight gain are common adverse effects. Other common adverse events include dizziness, somnolence, ataxia, and blurred vision.

Interactions

Pregabalin may enhance the sedative effects of other CNS depressants and may enhance the fluid-retaining effects of thiazolidinediones.

Lamotrigine

Indications/Uses

Lamotrigine (Lamictal) seems to be efficacious for generalized tonic–clonic, absence (especially atypical), and complex partial seizures. It also may be effective in Lennox-Gastaut syndrome (not approved for use in children younger than age 2).

Mechanism of Action

Although its mechanism of action is not completely clear, lamotrigine stabilizes neuronal membranes by acting on excitatory amino acid release and inhibiting voltage-sensitive sodium channels.

Dosage

The starting dosage for lamotrigine is 25 mg daily, with a slow titration every 2 weeks to a maintenance dose of 300 to 400 mg/d. The titration may even be slower, such as 25 mg every other day, in patients taking valproic acid. This slower titration should help lower the risk for rash.

Contraindications

Lamotrigine is contraindicated in patients with a hypersensitivity to lamotrigine or any of its components.

Adverse Events

Overall, lamotrigine is well tolerated and does not appear to have any long-term cognitive side effects. The principal adverse events include nausea, fatigue, dizziness, diplopia, and ataxia (see **Table 39.2**). In approximately 5% to 10% of patients (most often in children), a rash may develop. If a rash develops, the drug should be discontinued immediately. SJS and TEN have been reported with the majority of cases occurring in the first 8 weeks of therapy. The risk may be increased by coadministration with valproic acid, higher than recommended starting doses, and rapid dose increases. However, isolated cases have been reported with prolonged therapy or without these risk factors. Other adverse events include angioedema, nystagmus, and hematuria.

Interactions

The combined use of lamotrigine and carbamazepine may result in increased serum concentrations of carbamazepine and carbamazepine 10/11 epoxide. Valproic acid inhibits lamotrigine metabolism, whereas carbamazepine and phenytoin induce its metabolism. These enzyme interactions may result in significant changes in the half-life of lamotrigine. When used with valproic acid, the half-life is extended to 48 hours (from 24 hours when used alone), and with carbamazepine or phenytoin, it is reduced to 12 hours. Phenobarbital and primidone tend to decrease lamotrigine levels by approximately 40%. Although acetaminophen (Tylenol) may decrease lamotrigine levels, caution must be used when giving lamotrigine concomitantly with a folate inhibitor because it is an inhibitor of dihydrofolate reductase.

Levetiracetam

Indications/Uses

Levetiracetam (Keppra) has shown efficacy in the adjunctive treatment of adults with partial-onset, myoclonic, or primary generalized tonic–clonic seizures. While it does not have an FDA approval for use as monotherapy, it is approved in Europe for use as monotherapy in the treatment of partial-onset seizures.

Mechanism of Action

The mechanism of action of levetiracetam is not known, but it is theorized to inhibit voltage-dependent N-type calcium channels, facilitate GABA-ergic inhibitory transmission, reduce delayed potassium currents, and bind to synaptic proteins that modulate neurotransmitter release.

Dosage

Levetiracetam is started at a dosage of 500 mg twice daily with immediate-release formulations (1,000 mg daily with extended release) and titrated up to 3,000 mg/d. Dosages of greater than 3,000 mg/d have been used in clinical trials with good tolerability but without evidence of additional benefit. When switching to oral therapy, dose and frequency remain the same.

Contraindications

Levetiracetam is contraindicated in patients with a hypersensitivity to levetiracetam or any of its components.

Adverse Events

The primary adverse events associated with levetiracetam therapy include somnolence, asthenia, headache, and infection. Most of these occur within the first 4 weeks of therapy, with no dose–toxicity relationship seen. Another common adverse event is changes in behavior, including aggression, neurosis, and psychosis, which may require a dose reduction. Serious but rare adverse events include anemia, neutropenia, eosinophilia, and SJS/TEN.

Interactions

Since levetiracetam does not undergo significant metabolism, there are no clinically relevant enzymatic drug interactions with this agent.

Lacosamide

Indications/Uses

Lacosamide is approved for monotherapy and adjunctive therapy of partial-onset seizures.

Mechanism of Action

Lacosamide stabilizes neuronal membranes and enhances the slow inactivation of sodium channels.

Dosage

The initial dose of lacosamide when used as monotherapy is 100 mg twice daily and as adjunctive therapy is 50 mg twice daily. The dose may be increased at weekly intervals by 100 mg/d to a maintenance dose of 200 to 400 mg/d. An initial loading dose of 200 to 400 mg has been used in some patient with SE. When switching to oral therapy, dose and frequency remain the same. In patients with creatinine clearance of less than 30 mL/min or mild to moderate hepatic impairment, the dose should not exceed 300 mg/d. Lacosamide should be avoided in patients with severe liver disease.

Contraindications

There are no contraindications to lacosamide according to the manufacturer.

Adverse Events

Common adverse events seen with lacosamide include dizziness, fatigue, somnolence, blurred vision, diplopia, nausea, and tremor. Less commonly, increases in PR interval, second- and third-degree AV block, syncope, atrial fibrillation, and atrial flutter may occur, especially in patients with a history of cardiovascular disease.

Interactions

Phenytoin, carbamazepine, and phenobarbital may decrease the serum concentration of lacosamide.

Tiagabine

Indications/Uses

Tiagabine (Gabitril) is used as adjunctive therapy in adults and children older than age 12 with partial seizures.

Mechanism of Action

Its mechanism of action is not known; however, in vitro experiments show that it enhances GABA activity.

Dosage

The starting dosage of tiagabine is 4 mg daily and is titrated 4 to 8 mg weekly to response or up to 56 mg daily in 2 to 4 divided doses. The maintenance dose typically ranges from 32 to 56 mg/d.

Contraindications

Avoid using tiagabine in patients with hypersensitivity to any components of the formulation. Caution should be used in patients with hepatic impairment.

Adverse Events

Adverse events of tiagabine include dizziness, headache, somnolence, CNS depression, memory disturbance, ataxia, confusion, tremors, weakness, and myalgia (see **Table 39.2**). Rarely, severe dermatologic reactions such as SJS may occur.

Interactions

Tiagabine is a CYP2D6 and CYP3A3/4 enzyme substrate and is cleared more rapidly when given with other hepatic enzyme–inducing AEDs (i.e., carbamazepine, phenytoin, primidone, and phenobarbital).

Perampanel

Indications/Uses

Perampanel (Fycompa) is used as adjunctive therapy for partial-onset seizures without secondary generalized seizures in patients greater than 12 years of age.

Mechanism of Action

The exact mechanism of perampanel's antiseizure activity is unknown, but it is a noncompetitive antagonist of the AMPA glutamate receptor on postsynaptic neurons.

Dosage

The recommended initial starting dose in patients not on enzyme-inducing AEDs is 2 mg once daily at bedtime, which can be increased in 2-mg increments every 7 days to a maximum recommended dose of 8 to 12 mg daily. Patients on enzyme-inducing AEDs should start on an initial dose of 4 mg with the same titration of 2 mg weekly with a maximum dose of 8 to 12 mg daily. Elderly patients should have their dose titrated no more frequently than every 2 weeks.

Use is not recommended in patients with a CrCl < 30 mL/min or on hemodialysis. Patients with mild to moderate hepatic impairment should be started on no more than 2 mg once daily and titrated no more frequently than every 2 weeks. The maximum dose is 6 mg once daily in Child-Pugh Class A impairment and 4 mg once daily in Class B impairment. Use should be avoided in Class C impairment due to lack of data.

Contraindications

Avoid use in patients with hypersensitivity to perampanel or any component of the formulation. Perampanel carries a black box warning due to its potential to cause serious life-threatening neuropsychiatric events (aggression, anger, homicidal thoughts, and hostility).

Adverse Events

Common side effects include dizziness, somnolence, headache, fatigue, gait/balance disturbances, and falls. Neuropsychiatric events (aggression, anger, homicidal thoughts, and hostility) are more common with initiation of therapy and following dosage titrations. Therapy should be adjusted or discontinued if this develops.

Interactions

Perampanel is a minor substrate of CYP1A2 and 2B6 and a major substrate of CYP3A4. In addition, it is a weak inducer of 3A4. Strong inducers of CYP3A4 should be avoided due to their potential to decrease perampanel concentrations.

The use of other AEDs, which are enzyme inducers (carbamazepine, oxcarbazepine, phenytoin, etc.), may decrease perampanel concentrations and starting doses should be increased as a result. Concomitant use of CNS depressants may increase the risk of sedation.

Topiramate

Indications/Uses

Topiramate (Topamax) is used as monotherapy or adjunctive therapy for partial-onset seizures and primary generalized tonic–clonic seizures. It is also used as adjunctive therapy for seizures associated with Lennox-Gastaut syndrome.

Mechanism of Action

It is thought to decrease seizure frequency by blocking sodium channels in neurons, by enhancing GABA activity, and by blocking glutamate activity.

Dosage

The dosage starts at 25 to 50 mg twice a day and is increased to 200 to 400 mg/d in weekly increases of 25 to 50 mg/d. In patients with a creatinine clearance of below 70 mL/min, the dosage should be lowered by 50%.

Contraindications

Caution must be used in patients with hepatic or renal impairment, during pregnancy, and in breast-feeding mothers.

Adverse Events

Prominent adverse events are fatigue, dizziness, ataxia, somnolence, psychomotor slowing, nervousness, memory difficulties, speech problems, nausea, paresthesias, tremor, nystagmus, and upper respiratory infections (see **Table 39.2**). These may occur more frequently in patients taking more than 600 mg/d of topiramate or when titration occurs too rapidly (3 to 4 weeks to maintenance dose). Other adverse events include chest pain, edema, confusion, depression, difficulty concentrating, hot flashes, dyspepsia, abdominal pain, anorexia, xerostomia, gingivitis, myalgia, back pain, leg pain, rigors, nephrolithiasis, and epistaxis.

Therapy should never be withdrawn abruptly. Proper hydration is essential to decrease the risk of kidney stones.

Interactions

Topiramate is a CYP2C19 enzyme substrate inhibitor; thus, concurrent administration with phenytoin can decrease topiramate concentrations by as much as 48%, administration with carbamazepine reduces them by 40%, and administration with valproic acid reduces them by 14%. Digoxin (Lanoxin) and norethindrone (Aygestin) blood levels are decreased when given with topiramate, and concomitant administration with other CNS depressants increases topiramate's sedative effects. If used with carbonic anhydrase inhibitors, the risk of nephrolithiasis increases.

Zonisamide

Indications/Uses

Zonisamide is a broad-spectrum, sulfonamide-derivative AED approved as adjunctive therapy in partial-onset seizures in adults.

Mechanism of Action

Zonisamide appears to block sodium channels and select calcium channels.

Dosage

The dosage of zonisamide is 100 mg once daily, giving it a distinct compliance advantage over other agents requiring more frequent dosing. The titration to the daily maintenance dose of 400 to 600 mg is slow, at a rate of 100 mg daily every 2 weeks. There are no guidelines for dose adjustment in patients with renal or hepatic impairment, though it is not recommended for use in patients with creatinine clearance of less than 50 mL/min.

Contraindications

Use should be avoided in patients with a history of hypersensitivity to sulfonamide agents or any components of the zonisamide formulation.

Adverse Events

Potentially fatal reactions such as SJS, TEN, and agranulocytosis have been reported. Other important adverse events include fatigue, dizziness, ataxia, and anorexia. In children, there have been reports of high fever secondary to hyperhidrosis; zonisamide is not approved for use in children.

Interactions

Zonisamide is a major substrate of CYP3A4. Concentrations may be decreased when using inducers, such as phenytoin, phenobarbital, and rifampin. Serum levels may be increased when used concomitantly with protease inhibitors, azole antifungals, and macrolide antibiotics.

Felbamate

Indications/Uses

Felbamate can be used as either monotherapy or adjunctive therapy in the treatment of partial seizures. It is also used as adjunctive therapy in the treatment of partial and generalized seizures associated with Lennox-Gastaut syndrome in children. Due to an increased risk of life-threatening adverse effects, the American Academy of Neurology has published a practice advisory directing use.

Mechanism of Action

The mechanism of action is unknown but is believed to have weak inhibitory effects on GABA and benzodiazepine receptor binding.

Dosage

The initial dose of felbamate is 1,200 mg/d in divided doses three or four times a day. The dose may be titrated in 600-mg increments every 2 weeks to 2,400 mg/d based on response and to 3,600 mg/d if clinically indicated. Prior to prescribing felbamate, an "informed consent" form needs to be signed by the patient and physician.

Contraindications

Avoid use in patients with hypersensitivity to felbamate or any component of the formulation or with a known sensitivity to other carbamates. It has black box warnings for an approximately 100-fold increased risk of aplastic anemia in addition to an increased risk of acute hepatic failure. As a result, its use should be avoided in patients with a history of blood dyscrasias or hepatic dysfunction.

Adverse Events

Common adverse effects of felbamate include somnolence, headache, dizziness, ataxia, skin rash, nausea, vomiting, anorexia, and miosis. Rarely, felbamate has been associated with cases of hepatic failure and therefore should not be used in patients with a history of liver disease. An increased risk of developing aplastic anemia is present as well, and routine hematologic monitoring should be performed to detect evidence of bone marrow suppression.

Interactions

Felbamate is a major substrate for CYP3A4 and may be affected by concomitant use of drugs such as phenytoin. In addition, felbamate may increase concentrations of valproic acid and phenobarbital and may decrease the effectiveness of oral contraceptives.

Vigabatrin

Indications/Uses

Vigabatrin (Sabril) is an AED approved for the treatment of infantile spasms and refractory complex partial seizures not controlled with usual treatments. It is only available in the United States through a restricted distribution program called the SHARE program. Only prescribers and pharmacies registered with the program are able to prescribe and distribute the drug.

Mechanism of Action

Vigabatrin irreversibly inhibits GABA transaminase, increasing the levels of GABA in the brain.

Dosage

The adult dose of vigabatrin is 500 mg as an oral tablet twice daily. The dose should be titrated by increments of 500 mg weekly based on the patient's response and adverse effects. The recommended maintenance dose is 1,500 mg twice daily. Upon discontinuation, the drug should be tapered by 1,000 mg weekly. The dose for the treatment of infantile spasms is 50 mg/kg/d divided twice daily titrated by increments of 25 to 50 mg/kg/d every 3 days. The maximum dose for infants is 150 mg/d. Dose adjustments are necessary in renal impairment.

Contraindications

Hypersensitivity to vigabatrin or any component of the formulation contraindicates its use. Vigabatrin has a black box warning for its ability to cause permanent bilateral concentric visual field constriction.

Adverse Events

Common adverse effects of vigabatrin include somnolence, headache, dizziness, irritability, insomnia, weight gain, and diarrhea. Vigabatrin can cause permanent vision loss in patients receiving the drug. Patients who do not show substantial benefit within a short time after initiation (2 to 4 weeks for infantile spasms, less than 3 months for adults) should have the drug discontinued to avoid this adverse effect. Vision loss increases with larger doses and cumulative exposure and can affect more than 30% of patients. Vision should be assessed at baseline, at 4 weeks, and every 3 months thereafter.

Interactions

Vigabatrin may increase the sedative effects of other drugs and alcohol.

Rufinamide

Indications/Uses

Rufinamide (Banzel) is indicated for adjunctive treatment of seizures associated with Lennox-Gastaut syndrome in patients 1 year of age or older

Mechanism of Action

Rufinamide is a triazole derivative whose precise mechanism is unknown. In vitro data suggest it prolongs the inactive state of sodium channels and limits repetitive firing of sodium-dependent action potentials.

Dosage

The starting dose in patients less than 17 years old is 10 mg/kg/d divided into twice-daily doses. The dose should be increased by 10 mg/kg/d every other day until a maximum of 45 mg/kg/d or 3,200 mg, whichever is lower, is reached. Patients on concomitant valproate should start on doses less than 10 mg/kg/d in divided doses.

The starting dose in patients 17 years or older is 400 to 800 mg daily divided into twice daily doses. The dose should be increased by 400 to 800 mg every other day to a maximum dose of 3,200 mg/d. Patients on concomitant valproate should start at 400 mg daily in divided doses.

The extent of absorption is decreased with increasing doses. It should be taken with food as food significantly increases absorption. While no dosage adjustments are provided by the manufacturer, approximately 30% of a dose is removed by a

4-hour run of hemodialysis. A supplemental dose may need to be considered based on clinical response.

Contraindications

Patients with familial short QT syndrome and presence or history of short QT syndrome should not take rufinamide due to a potential for increased risk of sudden cardiac death. It's use is contraindicated in patients with hypersentivity to triazole derivatives or any component of the formulation.

Adverse Events

Common adverse events in clinical trials included QT shortening, somnolence, fatigue, coordination abnormalities, dizziness, gait disturbances, ataxia, nausea, vomiting, SE, and rash. Less common but clinically important adverse events include multiorgan hypersensitivity reactions, DRESS, SJS, and leukopenia.

Interactions

Rufinamide undergoes extensive hydrolysis via carboxylesterases with no appreciable CYP-mediated metabolism. It is a weak inhibitor of CYP2E1 and a weak inducer of CYP3A4. Despite no appreciable CYP-mediated metabolism, carbamazepine, phenytoin, phenobarbital, and primidone may decrease levels of rufinamide. Rufinamide may decrease levels of carbamazepine and estrogen or progestin-based contraceptives. Rufinamide concentrations are significantly increased with concomitant administration of valproic acid. If given together, initiate at lower doses and consider slower dosage titration. Levels of phenytoin and phenobarbital may be increased with coadministration. Food significantly increases the extent of absorption, and patients should be instructed to take it with a meal.

Benzodiazepines

The benzodiazepine antianxiety agents are discussed in depth in Chapter 41.

Clobazam

Indications/Uses

Clobazam (Onfi) is indicated for adjunctive treatment of seizures associated with Lennox-Gastaut syndrome in patients 2 years of age or older.

Mechanism of Action

Clobazam is thought to act as an agonist at the $GABA_A$ receptor to enhance GABA action, thereby depressing nerve transmission in the motor cortex area.

Dosage

Initial clobazam doses are determined by patient weight. Patients weighing 30 kg or less should start on 5 mg daily, while patients weighing more than 30 kg should start on 10 mg/d. Doses greater than 5 mg daily should be given in divided doses twice daily. Dose increases should occur no more frequently than every 7 days and by no more than 100% of the previous dose. Maximum doses per package labeling are 20 mg/d for patients weighing 30 kg or less and 40 mg/d in patients weighing more than 30 kg. Dose decreases should occur slowly and no more frequently than weekly to avoid withdrawal symptoms.

Contraindications

Contraindications include hypersensitivity to clonazepam, any of its components, or other benzodiazepines.

Adverse Events

Constipation, somnolence, sedation, pyrexia, lethargy, and drooling occurred at least 10% more frequently than placebo in clinical trials. Physical and psychological dependence are possible with all benzodiazepines.

Interactions

Clobazam is primarily metabolized by CYP3A4 but also 2C19 and 2B6 to its active metabolite N-desmethyl, which is metabolized by 2C19. Strong 2C19 inducers (e.g., theophylline) may decrease clobazam activity, while strong (e.g., fluconazole) to moderate (e.g., omeprazole) 2C19 inhibitors may increase clobazam activity. Alcohol may increase clobazam concentrations by as much as 50%.

Clobazam is a weak inducer of CYP3A4 and may reduce the effectiveness of some hormonal contraceptives. Nonhormonal forms of contraception should be considered when using clobazam. In addition, clobazam inhibits CYP2D6 in vivo and drugs metabolized by this pathway may require dosage adjustment. Concomitant use of CNS depressants may increase the risk of sedation.

Clonazepam

Indications/Uses

Clonazepam (Klonopin) is effective as an adjunctive drug in some patients with myoclonic, atonic, and generalized tonic–clonic seizures. It also is used for prophylaxis of absence, petit mal, variant (Lennox-Gastaut), akinetic, and myoclonic seizures.

Mechanism of Action

Clonazepam is thought to act at the GABA receptor to enhance GABA action, thereby depressing nerve transmission in the motor cortex area.

Dosage

Clonazepam is given in three divided doses with an initial daily starting dose of up to 1.5 mg in adults and 0.1 to 0.2 mg/kg/d in children. The dose may be increased by 0.5 to 1 mg every 3 day until seizures are controlled or adverse effects are evident (maximum, 20 mg/d). Tolerance to this drug is common.

Contraindications

Contraindications include hypersensitivity to clonazepam, any of its components, or other benzodiazepines, severe liver disease, and acute narrow-angle glaucoma. Caution must be used in patients with chronic respiratory disease or impaired renal function and in patients who are mentally challenged (may have more frequent drug-induced behavioral symptoms).

Adverse Events

Fatigue, sedation, and behavioral changes (e.g., aggressiveness and confusion) are the principal adverse reactions. Tachycardia, chest pain, headache, constipation, nausea, and decreased salivation are other adverse reactions.

Interactions

Medications that induce CYP3A4 enzyme substrates, such as phenytoin and barbiturates, may increase clonazepam clearance. Concomitant use of CNS depressants may increase the risk of sedation.

Lorazepam

Indications/Uses

Lorazepam (Ativan) is used intravenously to treat SE and has an unlabeled use for partial complex seizures.

Mechanism of Action

The drug is believed to depress all levels of the CNS, including the limbic system and reticular formation, probably through the increased action of GABA. Before IV use, the injection must be diluted with an equal volume of compatible diluent. If it is injected intra-arterially, arteriospasm and gangrene may occur. The injectable form contains benzyl alcohol 2%, polyethylene glycol, and propylene glycol, which may be toxic in high doses.

Dosage

In the treatment of SE, lorazepam may be given as a 4-mg slow IV bolus (maximum rate of 2 mg/min). Doses may be repeated every 10 to 15 minutes until seizures stop.

Contraindications

Lorazepam is contraindicated in patients with a hypersensitivity to lorazepam or to any of its components. There is also a risk of cross-sensitivity with other benzodiazepines. It should not be used in comatose patients; patients with preexisting CNS depression, narrow-angle glaucoma, severe, uncontrolled pain, and severe hypertension; and pregnant women. Caution must be used in patients with renal or hepatic impairment, organic brain syndrome, myasthenia gravis, or Parkinson disease.

Adverse Events

Common adverse reactions include tachycardia, chest pain, drowsiness, confusion, ataxia, amnesia, slurred speech, paradoxical excitement, headache, and depression. Light-headedness, rash, decreased libido, xerostomia, bradycardia, cardiovascular collapse, syncope, constipation, nausea, vomiting, decreased salivation, phlebitis, and blurred vision also may occur. Menstrual irregularities, increased salivation, blood dyscrasias, and physical and psychological dependence occur with prolonged use.

Interactions

Lorazepam has a decreased effect with oral contraceptives (combination products), cigarette smoking, and levodopa. Its effects are increased with morphine or other narcotic analgesics. An increased risk of toxicity occurs with the concomitant use of alcohol, CNS depressants, MAO inhibitors, loxapine (Loxitane), and tricyclic antidepressants.

Diazepam

Diazepam is used to treat SE and as an adjunct in convulsive disorders. Its mechanism of action is the same as that of lorazepam.

Dosage

Diazepam may be given intravenously 5 to 10 mg every 5 to 10 minutes 5 or less mg/min to treat SE (maximum dose of 30 mg). It may also be given as a rectal gel out of hospital as a 10-mg, one-time dose and may be repeated once if necessary.

Contraindications

Diazepam should not be used by patients with severe or acute liver disease. Contraindications include hypersensitivity to diazepam or to any of its components. Other contraindications are similar to those for lorazepam. Caution should be used in patients taking other CNS depressants, patients with low albumin levels or hepatic dysfunction, and elderly patients and infants. Because of its long-acting metabolite and the risk for falls in the elderly population, diazepam is not considered a drug of choice.

Adverse Events

Adverse drug effects resemble those of lorazepam.

Interactions

Diazepam is a CYP1A2 and CYP2C9 enzyme substrate. It is also a minor enzyme substrate for CYP3A3/4, and diazepam and desmethyldiazepam are CYP2C19 enzyme substrates. Enzyme inducers may increase the metabolism of diazepam, resulting in decreased efficacy. Increased toxicity, sedation, and respiratory depression may result when diazepam is given with CNS depressants (e.g., alcohol, barbiturates, and opioids). Cimetidine (Tagamet) may decrease the metabolism of diazepam. Valproic acid may displace diazepam from binding sites, which may result in an increase in sedative effects. Selective serotonin reuptake inhibitors (e.g., fluoxetine [Prozac], sertraline [Zoloft], paroxetine [Paxil]) greatly increase diazepam levels by altering its clearance.

Selecting the Most Appropriate Agent

There are several excellent AEDs from which to choose for various seizure types. The goal of monotherapy is to promote patient compliance, minimize side effects and toxicity, and reduce cost. In general, first-line monotherapy drugs are tried before using second-line monotherapy drugs, and first-line drugs may be first combined before trying the various second-line, adjunctive agents. Whether the second-line, adjunctive agents will be effective in monotherapy is still to be determined. The choice of an AED is determined by ease of use (i.e., dosing regimen), pharmacokinetics, interactions, need for monitoring, and toxicity (which could be dose related, idiosyncratic, chronic, or teratogenic). Ultimately, the optimal treatment for a given patient can be established by a process of trial and error and by knowledge of prior AEDs used.

First-Line Therapy

Selecting the appropriate therapy for each patient is difficult, but there is a science to choosing the best treatment:

- Select the appropriate drug and dose for the type and severity of the seizure being treated.
- Consider the patient's characteristics. For example, does the patient have hepatic or renal insufficiency, liver disease, hypoalbuminemia, burns, pregnancy, or malnutrition? What concomitant medications does the patient take? How old is the patient? Does the patient comply with the medication regimen? What adverse events are associated with the medication?
- Determine the patient's socioeconomic status.

If the initial AED fails, the practitioner should taper this drug's dosage while starting another first-line AED, if available. A list of commonly used first-line drugs for different seizure types can be found in **Table 39.1**.

Second-Line Therapy

Before switching to a second-line agent, the practitioner must optimize treatment with the selected first-line drug (unless the patient experiences intolerable adverse effects) and exhaust all possible first-line drug therapy choices. The practitioner at this point may, based on the patient's past medical history, initiate combination therapy with two or more first-line drugs or a first-line drug and a second-line drug. **Table 39.1** contains a list of second-line drugs.

Third-Line Therapy

If all medications fail and the patient experiences intractable seizures, surgery may be a third-line treatment option. Before recommending surgery, the practitioner should make sure drug treatment errors such as inappropriate drug selection, drug interactions, or inappropriate dosage are not contributing.

Special Population Considerations

Status Epilepticus

Guidelines recommend achieving definitive control of SE within 60 minutes of onset. All patients with an epileptic cause will need emergent, abortive therapy, as well as an antiepileptic medication to maintain or achieve seizure control. The goal of treatment is to stop clinical and electrographic seizure as quickly as possible using a combination of benzodiazepines and AEDS (see **Figure 39.2**). Concurrently, acute supportive care measures including airway management, IV access, hemodynamic support, and identification of the underlying cause must be provided.

Benzodiazepines are the first-line treatment option to emergently abort seizure activity. IV administration is preferred; however, if unable to obtain IV access, IM, rectal (PR), or intranasal options can be utilized. First-line therapy, lorazepam 0.1 mg/kg IV up to 4 mg per dose, doses can be repeated as needed based on clinical response. All benzodiazepines can cause respiratory depression; therefore, careful monitoring is required especially with escalating or repeated doses. Midazolam is the preferred IM agent; 0.2 mg/kg up to a maximum of 10 mg can be given to adults. Diazepam PR is often administered in prehospital setting and is often used in pediatric population; adults can receive 0.2 mg/kg up to a maximum of 20 mg. An EEG is necessary to ensure treatment has adequately controlled both convulsive and electrographic seizure activity. If epileptic cause is identified, initial AED therapy should be urgently instituted. Treatment options include phenytoin or fosphenytoin, levetiracetam, valproic acid, midazolam (continuous infusion), or phenobarbital. Refer to **Table 39.2** for additional information regarding loading and maintenance doses in SE.

Refractory SE is defined as either persisting clinical or electrographic seizures after the administration of a benzodiazepine and appropriate antiepileptic medication. Treatment options for refractory patients include midazolam, propofol, pentobarbital, valproic acid, levetiracetam, phenytoin or fosphenytoin, lacosamide, topiramate, and/or phenobarbital. Treatment of refractory SE is a challenge and there is not a defined treatment algorithm for therapy escalation, for treatment duration, or to drive therapeutic selection.

Pharmacogenetics

A patient's response to a given AED is dependent on both environmental and genetic factors. Pharmacogenetic variations exist that may impact therapeutic response, enzyme activity, transporter activity, or even drug-related toxicity. It is an area of increasing focus for many disease states including epilepsy. While pharmacogenetics may have a number of potential impacts on AED therapy, most available data focus on HLA alleles and risk for serious immune-mediated drug reactions. The presence of the HLA-B*1502 allele in patients of Chinese, Thai, Malaysian, and Indian populations has shown a strong association with carbamazepine-induced SJS/TEN. The FDA specifically recommends that HLA testing be completed prior to initiating CBZ in patients of Asian ancestry due to this risk of SJS/TEN. HLA variants and risk of serious immune-mediated reactions have been investigated with other AEDs including oxcarbazepine, lamotrigine, valproic acid, zonisamide, phenytoin, and phenobarbital with variable results. While pharmacogenetic testing is not routine, it is an ever-expanding field and may become a routine part of AED selection. The NIH-funded Web site pharmGKB.org provides useful resources on pharmacogenetics and drug dosing considerations with specific recommendations for carbamazepine and phenytoin.

Pediatric

The most common seizure syndrome in childhood is Lennox-Gastaut syndrome. This usually is associated with mental retardation. Characteristically, multiple seizure types can occur, including atypical absence, atonic (drop attacks), secondarily generalized tonic–clonic, and myoclonic and tonic seizures. EEGs show considerable slow-wave and spike-wave activity. Although patients respond to valproic acid, benzodiazepines, and lamotrigine, there is a poor prognosis for seizure control.

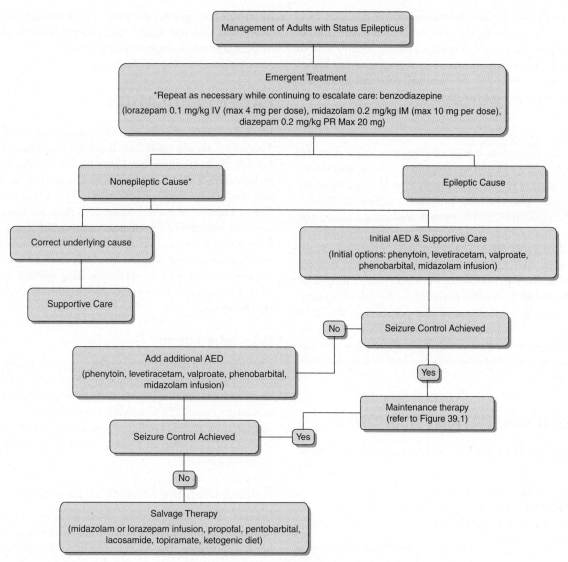

FIGURE 39.2   Treatment algorithm for status epilepticus.

Simple febrile seizures are another important category of seizures that affect children between ages 6 months and 5 years. Febrile seizures occur in 4% of all children and are preceded by high fevers, underlying the importance of controlling high fevers in children. The seizure is generalized and usually lasts under 15 minutes. Approximately 33% of children experience a recurrence, although almost never within the first 24 hours. These patients usually have no preceding neurologic abnormality or family history of epilepsy. Long-term anticonvulsant therapy is not indicated for this seizure type.

Geriatric

Understanding the basic pharmacologic principles involved in the administration of AEDs is the key to the optimal use of these drugs in older patients. Drug clearance and metabolism are significant issues in this population. Many older patients have decreased renal and liver function, which may

have a profound effect on drug metabolism and excretion. Consequently, AED dosages may need to be adjusted.

AEDs are bound to different degrees by plasma proteins, particularly albumin. If a patient has a low albumin level (as elderly adults tend to have), higher free-drug concentrations are present in the blood and may lead to an increased risk of adverse events.

In patients with liver disease, which is common in the geriatric population, the rates of hepatic biotransformation of drugs and of hepatic blood flow are decreased. Therefore, protein binding of AEDs may also be affected by low protein and displacement by bilirubin or other substances. This has the net effect of increasing the serum concentration of free drug. In renal disease, there may be a decrease in the clearance of drugs eliminated entirely by the kidney. Renal failure also may complicate elimination of drugs principally cleared by the liver. Studies have shown that in the patients with uremia who are taking phenytoin, hepatic biotransformation processes continue or accelerate during the renal failure, but renal excretion of metabolites is decreased. Therefore, uremic patients tend to have lower total serum phenytoin concentrations but higher serum concentrations of the oxidized principal metabolite (hydroxyphenyl-phenylhydantoin).

Women

For women taking anticonvulsant therapy, a major point for discussion is the risk during pregnancy. Several anticonvulsants are listed as Pregnancy Category C or D (i.e., phenytoin, fosphenytoin, phenobarbital, primidone, valproic acid, ethosuximide, topiramate, and tiagabine), indicating a greater risk for fetal abnormalities. Pregnancy risk categories for each drug are listed in **Table 39.2**. The practitioner must work closely with women who wish to become, or are, pregnant to assess the risks involved and to choose the most effective drug that's safest for the fetus. In order to minimize the risk of congenital malformations, valproic acid and polytherapy should be avoided during the first trimester of pregnancy. Conversely, topiramate, oxcarbazepine, and lamotrigine may decrease serum concentrations of progestins and lead to oral contraceptive failure.

MONITORING PATIENT RESPONSE

For patients taking an AED, the health care practitioner should monitor

- Frequency and severity of seizures
- Adverse drug events
- Plasma drug levels, if applicable

Therapy is considered to be a failure if the AED dosage achieves and maintains optimal blood concentrations and seizures are still uncontrolled and/or adverse effects become intolerable. Some patients have good clinical responses at serum drug concentrations below the therapeutic range, while others can exhibit toxicity within the therapeutic range. Some require serum concentrations above normal therapeutic values for seizure control, and these patients may tolerate very high levels without signs of toxicity.

Drugs should be added or subtracted as needed. Whenever a new AED is started or a dosage change is made, it takes five elimination half-lives (or the period over which a drug's plasma concentration falls to 50% of the peak level after a single dose) before the new steady-state serum concentration is achieved. It is at this point the full therapeutic impact of the new medication or dosage change can be assessed. Therefore, too much haste in changing an AED or discarding it as ineffective may have significant therapeutic implications.

When AEDs are administered in combination, it is important to note the types of drug interactions that may occur. Even when monotherapy is used, some AEDs alter their own biotransformation when they are administered chronically (e.g., carbamazepine and valproic acid). The existence of these interactions complicates the design of the therapeutic regimen when more than one AED is used, underscoring the desirability of using monotherapy whenever possible.

PATIENT EDUCATION

More than 90% of patients with epilepsy lead normal lives. The patient should avoid sleep deprivation and excessive alcohol use, both of which can lower the seizure threshold and make recurrent seizure activity likely. The patient should avoid jobs that involve working at heights or near heavy machinery, flames, burners, or molten material, so there are some restrictions on careers (e.g., firefighter, commercial driver, or airline pilot). Patients should never swim alone. Most sports are permitted, but those with an increased risk of a sudden loss of consciousness, such as skydiving, hang gliding, mountain climbing, and scuba diving, could be deadly and should probably be avoided.

Drug Information

The American Academy of Neurology's practice guideline center (https://www.aan.com/Guidelines/) provides information about epilepsy and medications for practitioners. Other sources of information on AEDs include the American Epilepsy Society (https://www.aesnet.org/clinical_resources) and the National Institute of Neurological Disorders and Stroke (http://www.ninds.nih.gov/).

Patient-Oriented Information Sources

Patients often have questions about epilepsy prognosis and treatment, first aid, educational needs, pregnancy, and driving and insurance. The American Epilepsy Foundation or the many epilepsy societies around the country can help answer those questions. These organizations provide both professional and lay support assistance, including counseling and psychotherapy, access to social workers, and financial assistance.

Nutrition/Lifestyle Changes

The ketogenic diet has been advocated as a means of treatment for patients with epilepsy. This diet, high in fat and low in carbohydrates, is usually used in children refractory to AEDs. However, there does not appear to be reliable evidence supporting the use of the ketogenic diet in people with epilepsy.

Driving is, of course, one of the most serious restrictions. Laws concerning driving vary from state to state, but in general, driving is not advised for 6 months after the last seizure. Some exceptions are strictly nocturnal seizures or those related to the discontinuation of an anticonvulsant on a physician's advice. Individual state laws regarding the driving restriction need to be reviewed by the practitioner.

First aid for seizure activity consists primarily of protecting the patient's head and body from injury. It usually is not advisable to try to open the patient's mouth or to put objects

CASE STUDY*

Accompanied by her boyfriend, B.C., age 23, visits your office. Her boyfriend states, "She hasn't been herself the last month. She has headaches and is completely confused and tired for no reason." B.C. denies using illicit drugs and any recent traumatic injuries. She thinks her problem started approximately a month ago when she was at a club dancing. Her friends told her that she became confused and began tugging at her clothes. Then she fell down and was unconscious for a few minutes. When she awoke, she felt extremely tired and did not know what was going on. Her boyfriend recalls that she had been hit in the head with a softball during a game the day before they went dancing.

Past medical history discloses insulin use since early childhood (currently 10 units NPH in the morning and 10 units regular insulin before meals), Ranitidine at bedtime, and Ibuprofen (1 or 2 tablets twice a day) for headaches. She is interested in becoming pregnant in the next 12 to 24 months. The patient says she has no allergies and does not drink or use recreational drugs or tobacco.

On physical examination, B.C. is 5 foot 4 inches and 130 lb. Her temperature is 37°C, pulse rate 78, blood pressure 118/76, and glucose level 90. Skin appears normal. Head and neck are normal, chest is clear for anterior and posterior sounds, cardiovascular RRR and (2) r/m/g, and laboratory values are within normal limits. EEG findings include sharp-wave discharges.

At a follow-up visit 2 months later, B.C. and her boyfriend report that things have gotten worse. The boyfriend states that as B.C. was eating dinner one night, she had a seizure. She was completely stiff for a short time, and then her arms and legs began moving. He believes that he was unconscious for a few minutes. B.C. says he could not remember what had happened when she woke up.

DIAGNOSIS: GENERALIZED TONIC–CLONIC SEIZURE

1. Which of the following should be true regarding your initial AED regimen?
    a. Initial combination therapy is warranted due to increased success rates.
    b. Drugs that are taken two to three times daily are preferred due to a lower risk of seizure if a dose is missed.
    c. Levetiracetam is the preferred agent for all seizure types and patients.
    d. The risks of pregnancy must be discussed prior to starting any AED.
2. Which of the following is the most appropriate initial antiepileptic regimen for this patient?
    a. Levetiracetam 500 mg PO daily
    b. Phenytoin 100 mg PO three times daily
    c. Pregabalin 50 mg PO three times daily
    d. Clobazam 5 mg PO twice daily
3. The patient fails to respond and has significant side effects to her initial therapy. Her initial therapy is to be discontinued. Which of the following would be the MOST appropriate replacement?
    a. Valproic acid 500 mg twice daily
    b. Lamotrigine 100 mg twice daily
    c. Lacosamide 100 mg twice daily
    d. Rufinamide 200 mg twice daily
4. After several different AEDs, the patient ends up on carbamazepine and phenytoin. A serum concentration on week 2 of therapy was 6 mcg/mL. The patient presents after 8 weeks of therapy with increased seizures and she is found to have a serum concentration of 2 mcg/mL. Which of the following is a likely cause?
    a. Autoinduction of CYP3A4.
    b. Patient has the HLA-B*1502 subtype.
    c. The oral contraceptive that she recently started.
    d. Coadministration with alcohol.
5. Despite the use of oral contraception, the patient becomes pregnant. Her AED regimen consists of valproic acid and lacosamide. What is the most appropriate treatment intervention?
    a. Discontinue valproic acid and continue lacosamide monotherapy.
    b. Discontinue lacosamide and continue valproic acid monotherapy.
    c. Continue combination therapy.
    d. Discontinue valproic acid and add phenytoin.

* Answers can be found online.

in the patient's mouth. This can result in injury to the patient's mouth and airway as well as to the bystander. However, removing dentures, excessive secretions, and foreign materials from the mouth after a tonic–clonic seizure phase is completed may be helpful. Turning the patient into a semiprone position in the postictal period helps to prevent aspiration.

Complementary/Alternative Medicine

Self-reported use of complementary and alternative medicine (CAM) in patients with epilepsy has been described to be as high as 70%. CAM therapies utilized for epilepsy are wide ranging and include but are not limited to acupuncture, classical music, oxygen, herbal supplements, homeopathic regimens, meditation, aromatherapy, chiropractic manipulation, cranial–sacral therapy, and marijuana. Data showing benefit to these therapies are limited but patient reported satisfaction is often high. One of the most discussed CAM therapies for treatment of refractory seizures are cannabinoids. The cannabinoid, cannabidiol, has received the most interest as it does not bind to the cannabinoid 1 and 2 receptors in the brain and lacks the psychotropic side effects seen with other cannabinoids. Available animal data suggest potential for seizure reduction with the use of cannabidiol; however, clinical data in humans are lacking and are warranted before cannabidiol therapy can be a recommended component of epilepsy treatment.

Bibliography

Birbeck, G. L., French, J. A., Perucca, E., et al. (2012). Evidence based guideline: Antiepileptic drug selection for people with HIV/AIDS. *Neurology*, *78*(2), 139–145.

Bloch, K. M., Sills, G. J., Pirmohamed, M., et al. (2014). Pharmacogenetics of antiepileptic drug-induced hypersensitivity. *Pharmacogenomics*, *15*, 857–868.

Brophy, G. M., Bell, R., Claasseen, J., et al. (2012). Guidelines for the evaluation and management of status epilepticus. *Neurocritical Care*, *17*, 3–23.

De Silva, M., McArdle, B., McGowan, M., et al. (1996). Randomized comparative monotherapy trial of phenobarbitone, phenytoin, carbamazepine or sodium valproate for newly diagnosed childhood epilepsy. *Lancet*, *347*, 709–713.

Devinsky, O., Cilio, M. R., Cross, H., et al. (2014). Cannabidiol: Pharmacology and potential therapeutic roles in epilepsy and other neuropsychiatric disorders. *Epilepsia*, *55*, 791–802.

Fattore, C., & Perucca, E. (2011). Novel medications for epilepsy. *Drugs*, *71*(16), 2151–2178.

French, J. A., Kanner, A. M., Bautista, J., et al. (2004a). Efficacy and tolerability of the new antiepileptic drugs. I: Treatment of new-onset epilepsy: Report of the therapeutics and technology assessment subcommittee and quality standards subcommittee of the American Academy of Neurology and the American Epilepsy Society. *Neurology*, *62*(8), 1252–1260.

French, J. A., Kanner, A. M., Bautista, J., et al. (2004b). Efficacy and tolerability of the new antiepileptic drugs. II: Treatment of refractory epilepsy: Report of the therapeutics and technology assessment subcommittee and quality standards subcommittee of the American Academy of Neurology and the American Epilepsy Society. *Neurology*, *62*(8), 1261–1273.

French, J., Smith, M., Faught, E., et al. (1999). Practice advisory: The use of felbamate in the treatment of patients with intractable epilepsy. *Neurology*, *52*, 1540–1545.

Glauser, T., Ben-Menachem, E., Bourgeois, B., et al. (2013). Updated ILAE evidence review of antiepileptic drug efficacy and effectiveness as initial monotherapy for epileptic seizures and syndromes. *Epilepsia*, *54*, 551–563.

Harden, C. L., Meador, K. J., Pennell, P. B., et al. (2009). Practice parameter update: Management issues for women with epilepsy—Focus on pregnancy. *Neurology*, *73*, 133–141.

Institute of Medicine. Report released March 30, 2012. Epilepsy Across the Spectrum: Promoting Health and Understanding. Retrieved from http://www.iom.edu/Reports/2012/Epilepsy-Across-the-Spectrum/Report-Brief.aspx

Kane, S. P., Bress, A. P., & Tesoro, E. P. (2013). Characterization of unbound phenytoin concentrations in neurointensive care unit patients using a revised winter-tozer equation. *Annals of Pharmacotherapy*, *47*, 628–636.

Krumholz, A., Wiebe, S., Gronseth, G., et al. (2015). Evidence-based guideline: Management of an unprovoked first seizure in adults. Report of the Quality Standards Subcommittee of the American Academy of Neurology and the American Epilepsy Society. *Neurology*, *84*(16), 1705–1713.

LaRoche, S. M., & Helmers, S. L. (2004a). The new antiepileptic drugs: Clinical applications. *Journal of American Medical Association*, *291*(5), 615–620.

LaRoche, S. M., & Helmers, S. L. (2004b). The new antiepileptic drugs: Scientific review. *Journal of American Medical Association*, *291*(5), 605–614.

Lowenstein, D. H., & Allredge, B. K. (1998). Current concepts: Status epilepticus. *New England Journal of Medicine*, *338*(14), 970–976.

Manci, E. E., & Gidal, B. E. (2009). The effect of carbapenem antibiotics on plasma concentrations of valproic acid. *Annals of Pharmacotherapy*, *43*(12), 2082–2087.

Riviello, J. J., Ashwal, S., Hirtz, D., et al. (2006). Practice parameter: Diagnostic assessment of the child with status epilepticus (an evidence based review): Report of the Quality Standards Subcommittee of the American Academy of Neurology and the Practice Committee of the Child Neurology Society. *Neurology*, *67*, 1542–1550.

Schmidt, D., & Schachter, S. C. (2014). Drug treatment of epilepsy in adults. *British Medical Journal*, *348*, G2546.

von Winckelmann, S. L., Spriet, I., & Willems, L. (2008). Therapeutic drug monitoring of phenytoin in critically ill patients. *Pharmacotherapy*, *28*, 1391–1400.

40 Major Depressive Disorder

Jennifer A. Reinhold

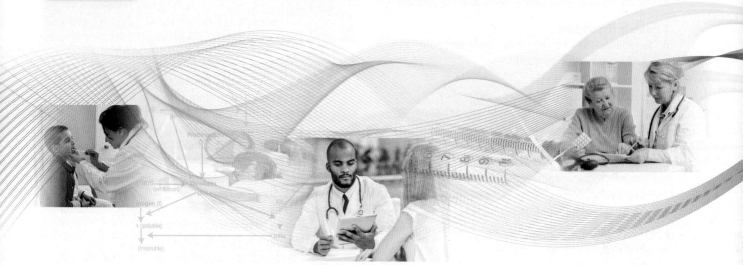

Major depressive disorder (MDD) is a mood disorder characterized by alterations in cognition, behavior, and physical functioning. It is a constellation of symptoms that interfere with normal function and may render an individual unable to perform psychologically, emotionally, and cognitively at previously attainable levels. Among the cardinal symptoms associated with a depressive episode are depressed mood, sadness, hopelessness, sleep disturbance, changes in appetite and weight, loss of interest, guilt, difficulty concentrating, and suicidal ideation. Further delineated by its recurrence and chronicity, depression results in functional impairment in multiple life domains and is a leading predictor of worsened morbidity and mortality. The clinical course is further complicated by the strong correlation of depression to psychiatric and physical comorbidity.

It is estimated that MDD affects 151 million individuals worldwide, with 6.2% lifetime prevalence. In the United States alone, depression is associated with the loss of 225 million missed workdays and indirect annual costs exceeding $83 billion (Donohue & Pincus, 2007). Initial onset of depression may occur at practically any time throughout life; however, the peak onset is considered to be during the fourth decade of life. Earlier onset of presentation is inversely associated with successful treatment outcome; younger patients with depression tend to have a more severe and complicated clinical course with less likelihood of remission and an increased likelihood of recurrence. Today, although 80% to 90% of those affected can be treated effectively, only one third seek treatment.

CAUSES

There has not been a single causative factor for the development of depression elucidated. Rather, the development of depression is thought to be a multifactorial, complicated interplay among numerous physiologic, social, genetic, environmental, and biochemical factors. First-degree relatives of an individual with MDD have a relative risk of developing MDD that is 2.8 times that of the general population. Though not confirmed in large randomized controlled trials, some studies suggest an overall heritability of 37% to 43%. More than 50% of patients who have experienced one episode of major depression will experience a second; over 80% of patients who experience a second episode will experience a third.

PATHOPHYSIOLOGY

Most current research focuses on neurochemical aspects of depression and has spurred several theories relating to the generation and maintenance of specific neurotransmitters in the central nervous system. The basis for these neurochemical theories is the hypothesis that abnormal neurotransmitter release or decreased postsynaptic receptor sensitivity is affected before and during a major depressive episode. At least four theories relate to this hypothesis (**Box 40.1**). Three of the four theories focus on a functional or absolute deficiency in the neurotransmitters serotonin, norepinephrine, or both. A functional deficiency suggests that neurotransmitters are produced but the postsynaptic receptors cannot fully transmit the neural impulse. This is in contrast to an absolute deficiency, in which no neurotransmitters are produced or the postsynaptic receptors cannot transmit the signal at all.

Similar to the theories associated with the monoamine catecholamines norepinephrine and serotonin, new evidence suggests that dopamine may play a significant role in the pathogenesis and symptomatology of MDD. Genetic polymorphisms in the genes associated with dopamine transmission

<table>
<tr><td>

BOX 40.1   Pathophysiologic Hypotheses of Depression

Serotonin Hypothesis
A functional or an absolute deficiency in the neurotransmitter serotonin

Catecholamine Hypothesis
A functional or an absolute deficiency in the neurotransmitters norepinephrine, serotonin, or dopamine

Permissive Hypothesis
Diminished serotonin gives "permission" for a super-imposed norepinephrine deficiency to manifest as depression

Beta-Adrenergic Receptor Hypothesis
Depression results from increased beta-adrenergic receptor sensitivity

</td><td>

BOX 40.2   Diagnostic and Statistical Manual of Mental Disorders 5: Criteria for Diagnosing Major Depressive Episode

A. Five (or more) of the following symptoms have been present during the same 2-week period and represent a change from previous functioning. At least one of the symptoms must be #1 or #2.
1. Depressed mood most of the day. In children or adolescents, the mood can be irritable instead of depressed.
2. Diminished interest or pleasure in all or almost all of usual activities.
3. Significant weight loss or weight gain or decrease or increase in appetite.
4. Insomnia or hypersomnia.
5. Psychomotor agitation or retardation as observed by others.
6. Fatigue or loss of energy.
7. Feelings of worthlessness or excessive or inappropriate guilt.
8. Diminished ability to think or concentrate, indecisiveness.
9. Recurrent thoughts of death, suicidal ideation, suicide attempt, or a specific plan for suicide.

B. The symptoms cause clinically significant distress or impairment in social, occupational, or other important areas of functioning.
C. The symptoms are not due to the direct physiologic effects of a substance or a medical condition.

Reprinted with permission from the *Diagnostic and Statistical Manual of Mental Disorders* (5th ed.), (Copyright ©2013). American Psychiatric Association. All Rights Reserved.

</td></tr>
</table>

may contribute to an increased susceptibility to depression. Deficits in dopamine release or transmission have been linked to dysphoria, one of the most prominent features of MDD. The permissive hypothesis, a more contemporary theory, suggests that reduced serotonin activity sets the stage for a mood disorder, such as depression or mania, depending on the underlying norepinephrine level. A low serotonin level coupled with a low norepinephrine level suggests that depression results from an increased beta-adrenergic receptor sensitivity. This alteration in postsynaptic receptor sensitivity results in an imbalance between the effects of norepinephrine and serotonin and may create a functional deficiency in serotonin. Secondary to the interplay among the catecholamines within the monoaminergic network, any impact on one of the monoamines will likely impact the others. This is applicable to the predisposition and development of MDD as well as the therapeutics of MDD.

DIAGNOSTIC CRITERIA

Mildly depressed patients meet the minimum criteria for diagnosis, whereas moderately depressed patients display a greater degree of dysfunction. Severely depressed patients experience symptoms well in excess of the diagnostic criteria. Their symptoms often greatly interfere with social and occupational functioning. A 2013 update of the American Psychiatric Association's publication, *The Diagnostic and Statistical Manual of Mental Disorders 5* (DSM-5), has established criteria for the diagnosis of depression, which are listed in **Box 40.2**. A patient must exhibit at least five of these signs or symptoms in the same 2-week period along with symptoms of depressed mood or anhedonia, the inability to gain pleasure from normally pleasurable experiences (American Psychiatric Association, 2013).

In addition to the DSM-5 diagnostic criteria, numerous rating scales are employed in clinical practice to assess the severity of depression as well as response to treatment. The 17-item Hamilton Depression Scale (HAM-D) and the Beck Depression Inventory (BDI) are clinician-rated scales that are frequently used for this purpose.

Subtypes of MDD delineate the etiology and severity of the illness or episode. These subtypes include mild, moderate, and severe depression. The descriptors (known as *specifiers*) refer to the severity of dysfunction and delineate comorbid or distinguishing features, such as melancholy, catatonia, and psychosis.

TYPES OF DEPRESSION

The DSM-5 slightly modified the categorization of depressive disorders in its most recent iteration. MDD and dysthymia are now both included under the singular category of persistent depressive disorder. Dysthymia is a chronic but less severe form of depression that is characterized by 2 years of depressive symptoms and functional impairment. It shared the same common core set of features with MDD and potentially did separate clinically from MDD, which led to its absorption into a larger category and its cessation as an independent diagnosis. The diagnostic criteria for MDD did not change; however, two new specifiers (terms or qualifiers that further narrow the MDD presentation and allow for more tailored treatment based on symptomatology) have been added; "with mixed features" refers to MDD with the coexistence of at least three manic symptoms, and "with anxious distress" suggests the presence of an anxious component. The remainder of the depression categories and subtypes remain unchanged. The focus of this chapter will be MDD, as this is the most common presentation; however, the other types are reviewed below.

Postpartum Depression

The onset is usually within 6 weeks after childbirth, and symptoms last from 3 to 14 months. Prevalence of postpartum depression ranges from 5.2% to 74% in developed countries (Norhayati et al., 2015). Women with a history of postpartum depression have a 50% risk of recurrence, and 30% of women with a history of depression not related to childbirth have postpartum depression.

Seasonal Affective Disorder

Seasonal affective disorder (SAD) is a pattern of depressive or manic episodes that occurs with the onset of winter. As the days become shorter and the weather colder, there is an increase in depressive symptoms. SAD causes individuals to eat more, sleep more, experience chronic fatigue, and gain weight. In pronounced cases, significant social withdrawal may occur.

Major Depression with Melancholic Features

Melancholic depression is a severe form of depression characterized by a profoundly depressed mood, nonreactivity, and neurovegetative symptoms. This type of depression is markedly more difficult to treat; however, it tends to be highly responsive to drug therapy.

Major Depression with Psychotic Features

Patients suffering from psychotic depression, in addition to the typical depressive symptoms, will also experience mood-congruent delusions and hallucinations.

INITIATING DRUG THERAPY

The most current guideline for the management of MDD is the American Psychiatric Association's practice guideline for the treatment of patients with MDD, third edition, published in 2010. When prescribing drug therapy, practitioners con-

sider many indicators, among them the severity of symptoms (e.g., mild, moderate, or severe), type of depression (major, acute episode, postpartum, seasonal, dysthymia), duration of therapy, the patient's age, sex, comorbid conditions, and concomitant medications. In addition, if the patient has experienced depressive episodes in the past, the choice of drug may depend on what drug or drug class the patient responded to previously. An abundance of evidence supports the relative efficacy equivalence among antidepressant drug classes. Therefore, selection of the initial drug is generally not based on efficacy but rather on the side effect profile, patient preference, and target symptoms.

Initial staging of depression severity and ongoing assessment of response to treatment is generally accomplished by utilizing patient- or clinician-rated scales. The 17-item clinician-rated HAM-D is traditionally considered the inventory of choice for monitoring response to therapy. Other tools used in assessing the severity or source of depression include a typical health and medication history. Also useful is a physical examination with documentation of the patient's height, weight, and pertinent laboratory test findings, such as a complete blood count with differential, electrolytes, and kidney and liver function. Caution must be exercised in diagnosing MDD since certain medications and illnesses can induce depression. These conditions must be ruled out prior to making the diagnosis (**Box 40.3**).

Nonpharmacologic therapy for depression includes several psychotherapeutic techniques such as cognitive–behavioral therapy and interpersonal therapy. Psychotherapy is traditionally reserved for patients with concurrent psychosocial stressors. Although psychotherapy alone may be effective, patients meeting the criteria for major depression should be evaluated for medication therapy. Moderately depressed patients often need a combination of medication and psychotherapy. Severely depressed patients may be refractory to psychotherapy, and their risk for suicide should be assessed.

Goals of Drug Therapy

Although historically nearly unattainable secondary to poor tolerability of available drugs, the ultimate goal of therapy for depression is *remission* and resolution of residual symptoms. A *response* to therapy, defined as a 50% reduction in the HAM-D score from baseline, was previously accepted as an appropriate therapeutic outcome. However, with the advent of newer and more tolerable drug therapies, the paradigm has shifted such that full remission is considered the only acceptable goal of therapy. Remission represents a complete resolution of depressive symptoms and a full return to previous level of functioning. Patients who have remitted will no longer fulfill the *DSM-5* diagnostic criteria for depression and will score 7 or below on the HAM-D (consistent with normal).

Residual symptoms refer to symptomatology suggestive of depression that persists after a response to treatment. Even upon a successful course of treatment and clinical remission, some patients may continue to experience cognitive depressive

BOX 40.3 Selected Conditions and Medications Associated with Depression

Endocrine disorders
  Addison disease
  Cushing syndrome
  Hypothyroidism

Gastrointestinal disease
  Irritable bowel syndrome
  Inflammatory bowel disease
  Cirrhosis

Infections
  AIDS
  Influenza
  Meningitis

Cardiovascular diseases
  Congestive heart failure
  Myocardial infarction

Neurologic disorders
  Alzheimer disease
  Multiple sclerosis
  Parkinson disease
  Stroke
  Chronic headache

Cancer

Alcoholism

Drug use
  Alcohol
  Antihypertensives
    Reserpine
    Methyldopa
    Diuretics
    Propranolol
    Clonidine
  Oral contraceptives
  Steroids

Rheumatologic
  Systemic lupus erythematosus
  Chronic fatigue syndrome
  Fibromyalgia
  Rheumatoid arthritis

symptoms, such as forgetfulness or apathy, or physical symptoms like fatigue. Patients who do not remit or who continue to have residual symptoms are at a greater risk for relapse or recurrence, have a shorter duration between depressive episodes, and have a worsened overall mortality. Optimal drug therapy not only resolves the acute symptoms of depression but also reduces the risk of relapse (American Psychiatric Association, 2010).

MONITORING PATIENT RESPONSE

Drug therapy for depression consists of three phases: acute, continuation, and maintenance. Usually, the patient needs additional contact with the practitioner or other health care provider (psychologist, social worker) during all phases of drug therapy. Assessments of efficacy, side effects, and adherence to the drug regimen should be made weekly, if possible.

Acute Treatment Phase

The goal of drug therapy in the acute treatment phase is to treat the patient until full remission and a return to the premorbid level of function. The duration of this phase is 6 to 8 weeks and potentially up to 12 weeks with apparent improvements occurring within the first 1 to 2 weeks. Though some clinicians attribute early response to a placebo effect, there is a preponderance of evidence that supports a true therapeutic effect within the first 14 days. In fact, newer research suggests that improvement by week 2 of therapy is a highly sensitive predictor of eventual response and remission.

Patients should have frequent contact with their practitioner throughout therapy, but especially in the first few weeks. Lack of efficacy early on may negatively impact patient adherence and motivation. Early improvements tend to include sleep satisfaction, appetite normalization, and recovery of cognitive function. Eventually, patients will experience an elevation in mood and resolution of anhedonia. Full assessment of the effects of the antidepressant should occur at the 4- to 6-week interval after drug therapy begins. At this point, the practitioner evaluates improvements in the target signs and symptoms, assesses adverse drug effects, and determines whether dosage increases or decreases are necessary. To assist the evaluation, several depression rating scales, such as the HAM-D, the Zung Self-Rating Scale for Depression, and the BDI, may again be used as an objective measure of the change, or lack thereof, in a depressive state.

Continuation Phase

The continuation phase represents the time after a treatment response is seen in the acute phase and usually lasts 9 months to 1 year. The practitioner should continue antidepressant therapy for 4 to 6 months after symptom resolution. Failure to continue medication beyond symptom resolution confers an increased risk of relapse. When therapy is eventually discontinued, the medication is typically tapered over a few weeks to avoid physical or psychological effects that occur with abrupt discontinuation of the medication (discontinuation syndrome). During this time, the patient should be monitored closely for reemergence of symptoms.

Maintenance Phase

For some patients, long-term or even indefinite therapy is indicated. Maintenance therapy should be considered in all patients with three or more prior episodes or any patient with two episodes within the past 5 years, a comorbid substance abuse or anxiety disorder, a family history of recurrent depression, or onset of depression earlier than age 20 or later than age 40. This phase of therapy uses the same effective antidepressant used during the acute and continuation phases for a minimum of 3 and up to 5 years or longer. The risk for recurrence increases with every subsequent episode of depression (Bulloch et al., 2014). Patients who have had two or more episodes of depression are candidates for indefinite antidepressant therapy.

Modification of Drug Therapy

Despite the availability of pharmacologic therapies for depression and the relative equivalence in efficacy among the classes, approximately 50% of patients will not respond to the first trial of a first-line antidepressant (American Psychiatric Association, 2010). Overall response rates to antidepressants in general are 50% to 75%. As evidenced by the pivotal STAR*D trial, subsequent trials of alternate medications after the initial failure yield success rates of 20% with a gradual decrease in rates of response and remission with each trial. Only about one third of patients will remit after the first trial, and almost 30% of patients will not remit even after a series of sequential therapies (Papakostas, 2009; Rush et al., 2003).

Initiation of an appropriate drug at an optimal dose, giving the drug an adequate trial (6 to 12 weeks), and educating the patient about the time frame for response and the importance of adherence are critically essential therapeutic concepts. If the patient is started on an appropriate drug for an adequate period, has been compliant with therapy, and does not respond or remit in a reasonable amount of time, drug therapy may need to be adjusted.

There are four common strategies used to modify drug therapy in the depressed patient: dosage increase/optimization, switching to a different drug within the same class or switching to a drug in a different class, augmenting the current drug, or combining medications. Increasing the dose of a drug is typically recommended if the patient has had a response or a partial response during the first few weeks. If an inadequate response or lack of response occurs within the first few weeks of therapy, a switch to a different drug may be warranted. Within-class and between-class switches are viable options depending upon the patient presentation. Lack of response to one drug within a class does not necessarily confer lack of response to all drugs within a class; therefore, switching within a class may be appropriate. Augmentation of the initial drug preserves any benefit experienced by the patient during the trial and also targets side effects or residual symptoms. The combination of two or more drugs with differing mechanisms of action has also been shown to be efficacious.

Antidepressant Drugs

Several drug classes are available for treating depression: selective serotonin reuptake inhibitors (SSRIs), serotonin norepinephrine reuptake inhibitors (SNRIs), tricyclic antidepressants (TCAs), monoamine oxidase (MAO) inhibitors,

and atypical agents. They all exert a pharmacologic effect by impacting one or more of the primary neurotransmitters theorized to contribute to depression. In theory, each of the antidepressants increases the relative amount of neurotransmitter available in the synapse, either by inhibiting its metabolic degradation or by decreasing the rate at which it is recycled (by the process called *reuptake*) back into the presynaptic neuron (**Figure 40.1**). For example, SSRIs inhibit the reuptake of select isoforms of serotonin, thereby increasing the functional availability of serotonin in the synaptic cleft. SNRIs increase the relative concentrations of both serotonin and norepinephrine, with more serotonergic or noradrenergic activity depending upon the dose. TCAs are thought to work by inhibiting the reuptake of norepinephrine and serotonin from the synaptic cleft, thereby increasing the amount available to stimulate the postsynaptic neuron. Conversely, MAO inhibitors limit the metabolism of monoamines such as dopamine, serotonin, and norepinephrine. This nonselective inhibition also increases the relative amounts of each of these catecholamines available to stimulate the postsynaptic neurons. However, this nonselectivity may contribute to side effects.

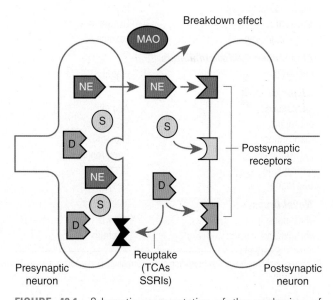

FIGURE 40.1 Schematic representation of the mechanism of action of antidepressant agents. Neurotransmitters (norepinephrine [NE], serotonin [S], dopamine [D]) are released from the presynaptic neuron into the synaptic space. They interact with the postsynaptic receptors and continue the neuronal transmission. After release from the postsynaptic neuron, these agents can be broken down by the enzyme monoamine oxidase (MAO) and the components recycled into the presynaptic neuron, or they can be taken up again through the reuptake mechanism. Antidepressant agents can (1) block the MAO enzymes, MAO inhibitors; (2) inhibit the reuptake of the neurotransmitter; or (3) agonize or antagonize an associated receptor. In effect, each mechanism increases the available concentration of the neurotransmitter.

TABLE 40.1

Classification of Antidepressant Agents and Neurotransmitters Affected

Generic Name	Brand Name	Primary Neurotransmitters Affected		
		NE	5-HT	D
Tricyclic Antidepressants				
amitriptyline	Elavil	++++	++++	0
desipramine	Norpramin	+	+++	0
doxepin	Sinequan	+	+++	0
imipramine	Tofranil	+++	++	0/+
nortriptyline	Pamelor	++	+++	0
protriptyline	Vivactil	+	++++	0
trimipramine	Surmontil	++	++	0
Selective Serotonin Reuptake Inhibitors				
citalopram	Celexa	0	++++	0
fluoxetine	Prozac	0	++++	0
fluvoxamine	Luvox	0	++++	
paroxetine	Paxil	0	++++	0
sertraline	Zoloft	0	++++	0
escitalopram	Lexapro	0	++++	0
Serotonin Norepinephrine Inhibitors				
venlafaxine	Effexor	++++	+++	+
desvenlafaxine	Pristiq	++++	+++	+
duloxetine	Cymbalta	++++	+++	+
levomilnacipran	Fetzima	++++	++++	0
Monoamine Oxidase Inhibitors				
phenelzine	Nardil			
Atypicals				
amoxapine	Asendin	+++	+++	0
bupropion	Wellbutrin	+	0/+	+
maprotiline	Ludiomil	++++	0	0
mirtazapine	Remeron	+	++++	0
nefazodone	Serzone	0/+	+++	0
trazodone	Desyrel	0	++	0
Novel Drugs				
vilazodone	Viibryd	0	++++	0
vortioxetine	Brintellix	0	++++	0

NE, norepinephrine; 5-HT, 5-hydroxytryptamine (serotonin); D, dopamine; ++++, highly potent effect; +, minimally potent effect; 0, no effect.

Table 40.1 presents the antidepressants and the neurotransmitters primarily affected. Because all of these agents appear to have relatively equal efficacy, the practitioner should select the most appropriate initial therapy based on side effect profiles, predicted patient compliance, and cost of therapy. The following discussion and accompanying tables and charts will help the practitioner in selecting the optimal initial agent for treating depression.

Selective Serotonin Reuptake Inhibitors

The development of SSRIs changed the landscape of depression pharmacotherapy. Just as effective as TCAs and older antidepressants, SSRIs boast improved tolerability and reduced lethality in overdose. The leading cause of death in the depressed patient population is suicide, and therefore, utilizing a drug class with minimal risk of successful overdose is paramount. The tolerability profile, relative safety in overdose, and the need for fewer titrations have resulted in SSRIs effectively replacing TCAs as the drug class of choice for treating depression. SSRIs work primarily by binding to the serotonin transporter and inhibiting the reuptake of this neurotransmitter into the presynaptic neurons. Relative efficacy is comparable within the class. **Table 40.2** identifies starting dosages and expected dosage ranges of SSRIs.

Time Frame for Response

The effects of these drugs become apparent within 4 to 6 weeks of treatment. The length of therapy for first episodes of depression is 4 to 6 months after recovery. Continued treatment

TABLE 40.2			
Overview of Antidepressant Agents			
Generic (Trade) Name and Dosage	**Selected Adverse Events**	**Contraindications**	**Special Considerations**
Tricyclic Antidepressants			
amitriptyline (Elavil) Start: 25 mg tid Range: 50–300 mg	Sedation, dry mouth	History of cardiovascular disease	Therapeutic plasma concentration range: 60–200 ng/mL
amoxapine (Asendin) Start: 50 mg tid Range: 100–600 mg	Anticholinergic, sedation	History of epilepsy or cardiac dysfunction	Therapeutic plasma concentration range: 180–600 ng/mL
clomipramine (Anafranil) Start: 25 mg hs Range: 150–200 mg	Sedation, orthostatic hypotension	History of cardiovascular disease	Blood levels not used clinically
desipramine (Norpramin) Start: 25 mg tid Range: 50–300 mg	Sedation, dry mouth	Same as above	Therapeutic plasma concentration range: 125–250 ng/mL
doxepin (Sinequan) Start: 25 mg tid Range: 75–300 mg	Sedation, orthostatic hypotension	Same as above	Therapeutic plasma concentration range: 110–250 ng/mL
imipramine (Tofranil) Start: 25 mg tid Range: 50–300 mg	Sedation, orthostatic hypotension	Risk of falling, history of cardiovascular disease	Therapeutic plasma concentration: 180 ng/mL
maprotiline (Ludiomil) Start: 25 mg tid Range: 50–300 mg	Anticholinergic effects, sedation, seizures	History of epilepsy or cardiac dysfunction	Therapeutic plasma concentration range: 200–400 ng/mL
nortriptyline (Pamelor) Start: 25 mg tid Range: 50–200 mg	Sedation	History of cardiovascular disease	Therapeutic plasma concentration range: 50–150 ng/mL
protriptyline (Vivactil) Start: 5 mg tid Range: 15–60 mg	Sedation, orthostatic hypotension	Same as above	Therapeutic plasma concentration range: 100–200 ng/mL
trimipramine (Surmontil) Start: 25 mg tid Range: 15–90 mg	Sedation, cardiac conduction disturbances	Same as above	
Selective Serotonin Reuptake Inhibitors			
citalopram (Celexa) Start: 20 mg qd Range: 20–40 mg qd	Nausea, dry mouth, increased sweating, somnolence, insomnia	MAO inhibitor therapy	In trials, ~6% of men experienced difficulty with ejaculation, and 3% reported impotence.
fluoxetine (Prozac) Start: 10–20 mg each morning Range: 10–80 mg	Insomnia	Same as above	Take in morning to avoid insomnia.
fluvoxamine (Luvox) Start: 75 mg bid Range: 100–300 mg	Increases in blood pressure	Same as above	Monitor blood pressure.
paroxetine (Paxil) Start: 20 mg qd Range: 10–50 mg	Mild sedation, delayed ejaculation	Same as above	May be useful in patients displaying insomnia as depressive symptom
sertraline (Zoloft) Start: 50 mg qd Range: 50–200 mg	Insomnia	Same as above	Take in morning to avoid insomnia. May be agitating
escitalopram (Lexapro) Start: 10 mg qd Range: 10–20 mg qd	Nausea, diarrhea, increased sweating, somnolence, insomnia, fatigue	Same as above	Extensively metabolized in the liver The dose for hepatic impairment is 10 mg qd.

(Continued)

TABLE 40.2

Overview of Antidepressant Agents (*Continued*)

Generic (Trade) Name and Dosage	Selected Adverse Events	Contraindications	Special Considerations
Serotonin Norepinephrine Reuptake Inhibitors			
venlafaxine (Effexor) Start: 25 mg tid or 37.5 mg bid Range: 75–375 mg	Increases in blood pressure, sexual dysfunction	Do not use within 14 d of MAO inhibitor therapy; caution in narrow-angle glaucoma	Monitor blood pressure closely.
desvenlafaxine (Pristiq) Start: 50 mg Range: 50–100 mg (no additional benefit above 50 mg)	Same as above	Same as above	May cause significant dose-related increases in total cholesterol, LDL, and triglycerides; nausea occurs in up to 30% of patients
duloxetine (Cymbalta) Start: 40–60 mg Range: 60–120 mg (no additional benefit above 60 mg)	Same as above	Same as above	May worsen psychosis in some patients or precipitate a shift to mania or hypomania in patients with bipolar disorder; nausea occurs in up to 30% of patients
levomilnacipran (Fetzima) Start: 20 mg daily (increase by 20–40 mg intervals every 2 d per schedule) Range: 40–120 mg	Orthostatic hypotension (dose related), nausea, erectile dysfunction (dose related)	Same as above	Specific dosing titration over several days
Atypicals			
trazodone (Desyrel) Start: 50 mg tid Range: 50–600 mg	Orthostatic hypotension, priapism	Contraindicated in recovery phase of myocardial infarction	
bupropion (Wellbutrin, Wellbutrin SR, Wellbutrin XL) Start: 100 mg twice daily (IR); 150 mg daily (SR) Range: 300–450 mg	Headache, insomnia, xerostomia	Do not use within 14 d of MAO inhibitors; do not use during an abrupt cessation of sedatives or ethanol.	Lowers seizure threshold at dose >450 mg; avoid concomitant alcohol ingestion
Novel Drugs			
vilazodone (Viibryd) Start: 10 mg daily (increase to 20 mg after 7 d and to 40 mg after more days) Usual dosing: 40 mg daily	Diarrhea, nausea, dizziness	Do not use within 14 d of MAO inhibitors; do not use during an abrupt cessation of sedatives or ethanol	Significantly less risk of sexual dysfunction compared to other antidepressants with similar mechanisms
vortioxetine (Brintellix) Start: 10 mg daily (increase to 20 mg daily as tolerated) Range: 10–20 mg daily (5 mg available for patients intolerant of usual doses)	Sexual dysfunction, nausea	Do not use within 14 d of MAO inhibitors; do not use during an abrupt cessation of sedatives or ethanol.	Metabolized primarily by CYP2D6—specific dosing adjustments recommended when concomitantly prescribed with strong inducers or inhibitors of CYP2D6

beyond the point of recovery drastically reduces the relapse potential over 1 to 3 years. Measures of efficacy include improved scores in the initial rating scales, self-reported improvement in the target symptoms originally described by the patient, and improved affect observed by the practitioner.

Adverse Events

SSRIs are usually administered in the morning because of the potential to induce anxiety and insomnia. Serotonin and serotonin receptors have diverse and variable effects on sleep architecture. SSRI-induced insomnia is thought to be largely related to the suppression of rapid eye movement (REM) sleep, which results in an overall decrease in sleep quality and total sleep time. Insomnia that presents as part of the clinical picture of depression itself or that is treatment emergent may be treated with a sedative–hypnotic drug such as a benzodiazepine or a nonbenzodiazepine GABA-A receptor agonist (zolpidem, etc.). Some patients do, however, experience sedation with an SSRI, and these patients may be advised to take their medication at bedtime.

SSRIs have virtually no potential for inducing orthostatic hypotension or cardiac conduction abnormalities, which makes them ideal for elderly patients or those with a history of arrhythmias. They do have epileptogenic potential, so caution must be used in patients with a history of seizures. Weight gain is another common adverse effect that occurs with various frequencies depending upon the medication. GI upset occurs transiently during the onset of therapy in approximately one third of patients.

Among the most commonly reported SSRI-associated adverse effects is pervasive sexual dysfunction, which may impact any or all of the phases of sexual response and function. This is potentially due to the increased serotoninergic activity at the 5-HT2c receptor. Sexual dysfunction is often a reason cited by patients for prematurely stopping their antidepressants. All SSRIs have the potential to induce sexual dysfunction. The incidence varies from about 24% to 73%, depending on the individual drug. Paroxetine is comparatively associated with the highest rate of sexual side effects, and fluvoxamine may be the least likely in the class to cause sexual dysfunction. The manifestations include reduced libido, arousal difficulties, and delayed or absent orgasm in both men and women. Risk of this side effect must be communicated to the patient prior to starting therapy. Treatment of this dysfunction is available, but lowering the dose without compromising efficacy may be the first strategy. If the symptoms persist, one pharmacologic strategy to consider is the addition of bupropion, which has been successfully used to mitigate the sexual dysfunction and provide an additive and different antidepressant mechanism of action. In addition, sildenafil (Viagra), tadalafil (Cialis), or vardenafil (Levitra) may benefit some male patients who suffer from erectile dysfunction. Patients often become tolerant to the sedation and the gastrointestinal adverse effects, but rarely do patients become tolerant to the sexual dysfunction, and therefore it tends to persist throughout the course of therapy.

The SSRIs are associated with a discontinuation syndrome, particularly upon abrupt discontinuation, but sometimes even after an appropriate taper. The constellation of symptoms include not only a worsening and return of depressive symptoms but also a flu-like presentation, insomnia, irritability, GI effects, and anxiety.

Recently, the question of increased suicidality has been raised with respect to SSRIs and antidepressants in general. SSRIs specifically are associated with an increase in attempted and completed suicide in patients younger than age 25. They have no effect on suicidality in patients ages 25 to 64, and they reduce suicidal behaviors in patients over age 65.

Interactions
The selection of a specific SSRI for an individual patient is determined by the drug interaction profile. SSRIs inhibit various components of the cytochrome P-450 (CYP450) system, thus causing elevations in other medications that are metabolized by this system. Before prescribing an SSRI, the practitioner should conduct a medication history and identify the

potential for altering the pharmacokinetics or pharmacodynamics of medications that the patient will be taking concomitantly. (**Table 40.3** offers a guide to the major drug–drug interactions with common SSRIs.)

Of special note, SSRIs are contraindicated with MAO inhibitors because the combination can lead to a sudden increase in systemic serotonin. The MAO inhibitor–mediated inhibition of the serotonin metabolism (thereby increasing its circulating availability) coupled with the action of the SSRI itself can result in serotonin excess. The manifestation of excessive serotonin, which is potentially life threatening, is termed *serotonin syndrome*. Signs and symptoms include heat stroke, vascular collapse, fever, and tachycardia.

Serotonin Norepinephrine Reuptake Inhibitors
The pharmacologic effect of SNRIs is primarily mediated through the potent inhibition of neuronal uptake of serotonin and norepinephrine and the weak inhibition of dopamine reuptake. SNRIs have no significant activity for muscarinic cholinergic, H_1-histaminergic, or alpha$_2$-adrenergic receptors and do not possess MAO inhibitor activity. Since the inception of SNRIs, there has been clinical debate regarding whether or not this newer class is superior to SSRIs because of its dual inhibition of serotonin and norepinephrine. It is postulated that this confers a broader antidepressant effect. Venlafaxine (Effexor), the first drug developed in this class, has been extensively studied in terms of its comparative efficacy to SSRIs. Numerous studies suggest that there may in fact be a slight but significant advantage in using venlafaxine over SSRIs with respect to remission rates. Literature also supports the use of SNRIs in more severe depression and in treatment-resistant depression (Bauer et al., 2009). There are currently four SNRIs available in the United States: venlafaxine, desvenlafaxine (Pristiq), duloxetine (Cymbalta), and the newly approved levomilnacipran (Fetzima). Desvenlafaxine, the R-isomer of venlafaxine, differs from its parent compound with respect to its simpler dosing regimen, greater bioavailability, and improved ability to inhibit norepinephrine reuptake. Duloxetine has a once-daily dosing schedule, reduced risk of treatment-emergent hypertension, and fewer discontinuation symptoms. An enantiomer of milnacipran, levomilnacipran is a potent and selective inhibitor of serotonin and norepinephrine reuptake, with preferential inhibition of norepinephrine over serotonin. Its efficacy, as evidenced in multiple clinical trials, is similar and possibly slightly less impressive than that of other members of this class. However, it has demonstrated weight neutrality and good tolerability. Please see **Table 40.2**.

Time Frame for Response
Similar to SSRIs, SNRIs require approximately 4 to 6 weeks (and potentially up to 12 weeks) to exert a full pharmacologic effect. Some cognitive and physical symptoms of depression may begin to remit within the first week of therapy, but the full effect is slightly more protracted. As with any of the antidepressants, SNRIs should be taken through the continuation and maintenance phases to reduce the risk of relapse.

TABLE 40.3

Selected Antidepressant Drug Interactions Involving the Cytochrome P-450 System

Agent–Drug Interaction Potential	Isozyme Inhibited	Drugs Affected
Addition of this agent...	*will inhibit this isoenzyme...*	*resulting in increased levels of these drugs:*
fluoxetine—moderate	3A4	Type 1A antiarrhythmics
mirtazapine—low		Clozapine
nefazodone—high		Benzodiazepines (alprazolam, triazolam, clonazepam)
paroxetine—low		Calcium channel blockers
sertraline—low		Cannabinoids
venlafaxine—low		Carbamazepine
		Cyclosporine
		Estrogens
		Fentanyl
		HIV-1 protease inhibitors
		HMG-CoA reductase inhibitors
		Macrolide antibiotics
		Ondansetron
		Tricyclic antidepressants (amitriptyline, clomipramine, imipramine)
		R-warfarin
		Zolpidem
fluoxetine—high	2D6	Narcotic analgesics
mirtazapine—low		Chlorpromazine
paroxetine—high		Fluphenazine
sertraline—low		Haloperidol
venlafaxine—low		Perphenazine
		Risperidone
		Beta-blockers (labetalol, metoprolol, pindolol, propranolol, timolol)
		Benztropine
		Cyclobenzaprine
		Dextromethorphan
		Donepezil
		Glimepiride
		Trazodone
		Tricyclic antidepressants
fluoxetine—low	1A2	Clozapine
fluvoxamine—high		Haloperidol
mirtazapine—low		Thioridazine
nefazodone—low		Olanzapine
paroxetine—low		Chlorpromazine
sertraline—low		Trifluoperazine
venlafaxine—low		Caffeine
		Diazepam
		Metoclopramide
		Ondansetron
		Propranolol
		Tacrine
		Theophylline
		Tricyclic antidepressants (amitriptyline, clomipramine, imipramine)
		Verapamil
		Warfarin
		Zolpidem

Adverse Events

SNRIs have the potential to produce more adverse effects as compared to SSRIs secondary to the noradrenergic activity; there are higher rates of dry mouth, constipation, nausea, and insomnia. Treatment-emergent hypertension has occurred in patients taking venlafaxine, although the majority of cases occur in patients who are predisposed to developing hypertension. Increases in blood pressure of approximately 10 mm Hg have also been reported in patients who are hypertensive prior to starting venlafaxine therapy. Two dose-related side effects occur with venlafaxine: nausea and hypertension. Starting therapy with lower doses and gradually increasing the dose as tolerated minimizes the nausea. The prevalence of sexual dysfunction in patients taking venlafaxine, desvenlafaxine, or duloxetine approximates that of SSRIs.

Abrupt discontinuation of SNRI therapy is not recommended, especially venlafaxine. This can produce a discontinuation syndrome similar to that of SSRIs. Duloxetine has not been shown to elicit these types of symptoms to the extent that the other two members of this class have.

Interactions

SNRIs are metabolized by the CYP450 system, namely, the CYP1A2, CYP3A4, and CYP2D6 isoenzymes. Coadministration of SNRIs with other drugs that are substrates of or that otherwise impact those isoenzymes may result in drug interactions. Concomitant administration of MAO inhibitors with SNRIs is contraindicated because this may result in serotonin syndrome.

Tricyclic Antidepressants

Prior to the emergence of SSRIs, TCAs were the mainstay of therapy for MDD. There are no proven significant differences in terms of efficacy between TCAs and SSRIs; however, the improved tolerability of the SSRIs has served as the impetus for a shift away from the TCAs. TCAs are potent inhibitors of the reuptake of norepinephrine and serotonin, with differences in the extent to which each member of this class impacts each neurotransmitter. Clomipramine (Anafranil) is a potent serotonin reuptake blocker, and its metabolite is a potent norepinephrine reuptake blocker (see **Table 40.2**). Amitriptyline (Elavil), for example, significantly increases the amount of norepinephrine and serotonin available to the postsynaptic neuron. In contrast, nortriptyline (Pamelor) has a relatively low effect on both norepinephrine and serotonin. These drugs, therefore, attempt to restore the balance of neurotransmitters and work in accord with several of the aforementioned theories.

TCAs are also active at acetylcholine and histamine receptors, which contribute to their adverse effect profile. This complex pharmacology, coupled with the anticholinergic side effects, relegates TCAs to second- or third-line therapy for MDD.

Adverse Events

The selection of a TCA for treating depression is based on the adverse effect profile (**Table 40.4**) in addition to response to previous treatments, if applicable. In varying degrees, all TCAs can cause sedation, which is an important consideration, especially if the depression is characterized by insomnia. Administering a TCA at bedtime may help alleviate this symptom.

In addition, the hypotensive effect of each agent varies and should be considered when selecting a particular agent. For example, nortriptyline and desipramine (Norpramin) have less potential for inducing orthostatic hypotension, making them advantageous in elderly patients. Anticholinergic adverse effects are common among this class as is weight gain. Moreover, the epileptogenic potential and life-threatening cardiac conduction abnormalities associated with the TCAs must be considered. TCAs may contribute to atrioventricular block, QT prolongation, and ventricular tachycardia. Preexisting epilepsy and cardiac conduction abnormalities are often considered contraindications to the use of TCAs. TCAs are traditionally lethal in overdose secondary to their proarrhythmic properties.

Therapeutic Ranges

Because the pharmacokinetic properties of the individual agents may vary according to the patient and few TCAs have established therapeutic ranges, routine monitoring of drug levels is not common. However, establishing the drug level at which a patient has improved is reasonable. In this way, the practitioner has documentation of an effective drug concentration for that patient. Later, if needed, changes in drug therapy may be determined based on this baseline information. Otherwise, drug levels should be evaluated only if the practitioner suspects that the patient is not adhering to therapy or if drug toxicity becomes a concern.

Interactions

Drug interactions with TCAs tend to be pharmacodynamic, although some pharmacokinetic interactions do occur. Pharmacokinetically, TCA drug levels may increase in combination with certain SSRIs (see **Table 40.3**) and other CYP450 enzyme inhibitors, such as cimetidine (Tagamet), human immunodeficiency virus protease inhibitors, and some antipsychotic agents. There are additive central nervous system effects with TCAs and anticholinergic drugs, such as diphenhydramine (Benadryl). In addition, TCA–MAO inhibitor interactions may significantly increase the level of circulating catecholamines and lead to a potentially fatal hypertensive crisis.

Atypical Antidepressants

The class of drugs labeled *atypical* represents compounds used to treat depression that elude the traditional classification schema. The mechanisms of action are not consistent within the atypical group but all impact one or more monoamines. These agents are generally considered alternatives to SSRIs, SNRIs, or TCAs; however, the utilization of bupropion has rivaled that of the SSRIs and SNRIs. See **Table 40.2** for starting dosages and dosage ranges.

Bupropion

Bupropion is a structurally distinct compound from the aminoketone class. It is a relatively weak inhibitor of neuronal uptake of norepinephrine and dopamine, and its metabolite also inhibits the reuptake of norepinephrine. It does not inhibit

TABLE 40.4

Major Adverse Event Profile of Antidepressant Agents

Drug	Major Adverse Events					
	Anticholinergic	Cardiac Conduction	Seizures	Orthostatic Hypotension	Sedation	Sexual Dysfunction
Selective Serotonin Reuptake Inhibitors						
citalopram	0	0	+	0	0	++
fluoxetine	0	0	++	0	0	+++
fluvoxamine	0	0	++	0	0	++++
paroxetine	+	0	++	0	+	++++
sertraline	0	0	++	0	0	+++
escitalopram	0	0	++	0	0	++
Serotonin Norepinephrine Inhibitors						
venlafaxine*	+	+	++	0	0	++++
desvenlafaxine*	+	+	+	0	0	++
duloxetine*	+	0	0	0	0	++
levomilnacipran*	+	+	0	++	0	+++
Tricyclic Antidepressants						
amitriptyline	++++	+++	+++	+++	++++	+
desipramine	++	++	++	++	++	+
doxepin	+++	++	+++	++	+++	0
imipramine	+++	+++	+++	++++	+++	+
nortriptyline	++	++	++	+	++	+
protriptyline	++	+++	++	++	+	+
trimipramine	++++	+++	+++	+++	++++	+
Monoamine Oxidase Inhibitors						
phenelzine	++	+	++	++	++	0
tranylcypromine	++	+	++	++	++	0
Atypical Antidepressants						
amoxapine	+++	++	+++	++	+++	0
bupropion	+	+	++++	0	++++	0
maprotiline	+++	++	++++	+++	++++	0
mirtazapine	++	+	+	++++	+	0
nefazodone	0	+	++	+++	++	0
trazodone	0	+	++	++++	++	0
Novel Drugs						
vilazodone*	+	0	0	0	+	+
vortioxetine*	+++	0	0	0	0	++++

*High rate of nausea and diarrhea.

+ + + + + = highly potent effect; + = minimal effect; 0 = no effect.

the reuptake of MAO, and unlike all of the other available drugs, it does not impact the serotonergic system. Bupropion is among the preferred pharmacologic agents, possibly second only to SSRIs and SNRIs. Owing to its virtual absence of sexual adverse effects, bupropion is frequently used in patients who cannot tolerate the sexual adverse effects of SSRIs and SNRIs or may be used adjunctively with these drugs to diminish sexual dysfunction. Rates of somnolence, fatigue, and weight gain are markedly reduced compared to SSRIs, TCAs, and SNRIs (Papakostas, 2009). Bupropion has been implicated in lowering the seizure threshold, especially when combined with alcohol. This tends to occur when dosing exceeds 450 mg daily or more than 150 mg per dose, although the reported risk is less than 1%.

Trazodone

Trazodone (Desyrel) is a weak serotonin receptor antagonist that also blocks serotonin reuptake to a lesser degree. Trazodone is highly sedating at therapeutic doses secondary to its antihistamine properties. Patients whose target symptoms or residual symptoms include insomnia may benefit from the use of trazodone as adjunctive therapy. Trazodone monotherapy is not recommended secondary to modest efficacy. Antidepressant effects will be realized within a few weeks; however, the intended sedative effects occur several hours after the first dose. Also an anxiolytic drug, trazodone has a place in therapy for anxiety disorders as well as depression with comorbid anxiety. Important adverse effects include orthostatic hypotension, nausea, blurred vision, and priapism.

Nefazodone

Nefazodone (Serzone), structurally related to trazodone, acts similarly to trazodone but also inhibits the reuptake of norepinephrine and produces fewer side effects. Because it lacks significant anticholinergic and antihistamine effects, reports of blurred vision, urinary retention, and weight gain are relatively infrequent. Nefazodone interferes with the CYP3A4 system, and caution should be used in patients taking drugs metabolized by this enzyme system. In addition, nefazodone increases the levels of agents such as alprazolam (Xanax) and triazolam (Halcion); practitioners should avoid prescribing these agents concomitantly (see **Table 40.3**). Prior to initiating nefazodone, the washout period after discontinuing an SSRI should generally be 4 to 5 days for paroxetine (Paxil) and sertraline (Zoloft) and several weeks for fluoxetine (Prozac). Nefazodone carries a black box warning for hepatotoxicity, which led to the removal of the brand name product (Serzone) from the market. Generic nefazodone remains available but has fallen out of favor in practice secondary to its risk of liver damage because safer and more efficacious antidepressants are available.

Mirtazapine

Mirtazapine (Remeron) is a selective alpha$_2$-adrenergic receptor antagonist affecting both the norepinephrine and serotonergic systems. The role of mirtazapine in treating depression is similar to that of the TCAs. It has significant histamine-1 receptor blocking activity, thus causing sedation. In addition, because of its appetite stimulation, it may be a good choice for low-weight elderly or ill patients. This agent may be useful in combination therapy because there have been no reports of drug interactions. However, there have been rare cases of reversible agranulocytosis.

Novel Drugs
Vilazodone

Vilazodone is a novel compound and a potent selective serotonin reuptake inhibitor and partial 5-HT1A receptor agonist. Approved in the United States for the treatment of depression at doses of 10 to 40 mg once daily, vilazodone's antidepressant effects are attributed to its modulation of serotonergic activity at pre- and postsynaptic serotonin transporters. Vilazodone is classified as a selective serotonin reuptake inhibitor (SSRI)/5-HT1A receptor partial agonist and not a pure SSRI.

Traditional antidepressants (SSRIs, SNRIs, TCAs) increase the amount of available serotonin by inhibiting its reuptake or otherwise modulating its transmission. In doing so, they also stimulate the 5-HT1A autoreceptors, which acutely decreases the amount of available serotonin, as stimulation of an autoreceptor would facilitate the reuptake of serotonin back into the presynaptic neuron. Only after several weeks do the autoreceptors become desensitized and begin to function normally again,

thereby normalizing serotonergic transmission. Traditional antidepressants' effects at the 5-HT1A autoreceptor may underlie the delay in therapeutic effect (of several weeks). Vilazodone, in contrast, is a *partial* agonist at the 5-HT1A autoreceptor and does not seem to induce this effect, resulting in an onset of effect that is significantly earlier than traditional antidepressants.

Time Frame for Response In multiple randomized, double-blinded, placebo-controlled studies, vilazodone-treated patients experienced a response as early as week 1. This may represent a therapeutic advantage over traditional antidepressants, which generally produce a therapeutic effect after 4 to 6 weeks of treatment. To date, all clinical trials involving vilazodone have been placebo controlled and have not included an active comparator, thereby limiting a comparison to existing therapy with respect to efficacy.

Adverse Events Vilazodone has demonstrated good tolerability and safety in all of the published clinical trials. The most commonly reported adverse effects have consistently been nausea and diarrhea, both occurring in approximately 25% of patients enrolled in trials. These gastrointestinal disturbances emerged early in treatment and tended to dissipate within a few days. Vilazodone does not appear to produce treatment-related effects on sexual function, and, based on score reductions over the course of the pivotal studies, it may have resulted in a slight improvement of sexual functioning. The partial agonism at the 5-HT1A receptor is thought to be the pharmacologic reason for the low risk of sexual dysfunction. Sexual dysfunction is frequently part of the clinical picture in depressed patients, independently of treatment-emergent sexual dysfunction. The majority of pharmacotherapeutic treatment options have the potential to induce some level of sexual dysfunction in patients in whom it exists already and in patients who did not previously experience sexual dysfunction. As previously discussed, the rates of sexual dysfunction associated with the SSRIs are greater than 70%. This is an important consideration when selecting drug therapy, as worsening of existing sexual dysfunction or development of new-onset sexual dysfunction can directly influence medication compliance and therapeutic outcomes.

Another important consideration in the selection of drug therapy for MDD is impact on weight. Many existing drug therapies cause weight gain, sometimes significant, which may influence treatment adherence. Thus far, vilazodone is considered weight neutral, resulting in approximately a 1.7-kg (3.74-lb) increase in weight after 1 year of treatment.

Interactions Vilazodone is a major substrate of CYP3A4, and it weakly inhibits CYP2C8 and weakly induces CYP2C19. The clinically relevant drug–drug interactions are limited to strong CYP3A4 inhibitors, which have the ability to increase serum concentrations of vilazodone. In particular, ketoconazole, a prototypical strong CYP3A4 inhibitor, increases the Cmax and AUC of vilazodone by 50%, necessitating a dose reduction to 20 mg of vilazodone daily. A 20-mg maximum daily dose of vilazodone is recommended when vilazodone is administered concurrently with a strong CYP3A4 inhibitor. Because of extensive hepatic metabolism and lack of renal elimination, mild to moderate renal impairment does not impact vilazodone concentrations. Vilazodone has not been studied in patients with severe renal dysfunction. Mild to moderate hepatic impairment does not result in a clinically meaningful impact on vilazodone concentrations.

Vortioxetine

Vortioxetine is a multimodal antidepressant, which acts as an inhibitor of serotonin reuptake by antagonizing the 5-HT3, 5-HT7, and 5-HT1D receptors, agonizing the 5-HT1A receptor, partially agonizing the 5-HT1B receptor, and inhibiting the 5-HT transporter. Vortioxetine's activity at multiple receptors results in modulation of the serotonergic, noradrenergic, dopaminergic, and histaminic systems, which results in antidepressant effects. Similar to vilazodone, vortioxetine's action at the 5-HT1A receptor is thought to cause an earlier onset of action as compared to traditional antidepressants. Results from several randomized controlled trials are inconsistent with regard to efficacy and tolerability. Response to 2.5 to 20 mg daily was demonstrated in most of the studies, but not all. Remission rates tended to not differ from placebo.

Time Frame for Response Onset of therapeutic effect, as evidenced by available clinical studies, is variable. Some evidence suggests that an onset of effect occurs as early as week 1 of treatment. Other studies failed to see a difference until week 4 or 6; and some studies did not observe a difference at all through study end. To date, there are no published trials that directly compare vortioxetine to another antidepressant.

Adverse Events The most commonly reported adverse effects include dizziness, diarrhea, vomiting, and xerostomia. Sexual dysfunction in men and women occurs at a rate of 34% to 50%.

Interactions Vortioxetine is a major substrate of CYP3A4 and does not inhibit or induce any of the CYP isoenzymes. Bupropion and buspirone, however, should not be used concurrently with vortioxetine due to their ability to enhance the serotonergic effects of vortioxetine.

Monoamine Oxidase Inhibitors

MAO inhibitors were the first effective medications that were developed for the treatment of depression. They work by nonspecifically and irreversibly inhibiting type A and type B MAO, leading to a decreased degradation of norepinephrine, serotonin, and dopamine in the synapse. However, the adverse effect profile and potential for life-threatening hypertensive crises have limited their use and relegated them a last-line treatment in clinical practice. Only skilled practitioners with extensive clinical expertise should prescribe MAO inhibitors. See **Table 40.2** for starting dosages and dosage ranges.

Adverse Events

Adverse reactions to MAO inhibitors are more common than in any other class of antidepressant. Orthostatic hypotension occurring with high-dose therapy is probably the most

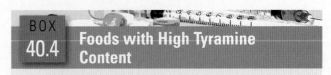

BOX 40.4 **Foods with High Tyramine Content**

- Aged cheese (cheddar, blue, Gouda, Swiss)
- Yeast products
- Aged meats, processed meats, nonfresh meat
- Beef liver or chicken liver
- Sauerkraut
- Licorice
- Tap beer

common adverse effect. Attempts to prevent this reaction by applying support stockings, prescribing stimulants such as methylphenidate, or adding the mineralocorticoid have met with reasonable success. However, caution must be used and the patient must be monitored carefully, especially when receiving the corticoid or the stimulant drug concomitantly. Hypertensive crisis can occur when MAO inhibitors are taken with medications that stimulate excessive release of the neurotransmitters dopamine, epinephrine, and norepinephrine. In addition, patients taking MAO inhibitors must be on a strict diet that eliminates tyramine-containing foods. **Box 40.4** identifies certain foods that have an extremely high tyramine content and, if ingested by patients taking MAO inhibitors, may cause a hypertensive crisis.

Concomitant use of TCAs and MAO inhibitors can lead to a hyperpyretic crisis resulting in seizures and death. Similarly, using SSRIs or SNRIs and MAO inhibitors together can lead to a serotonergic syndrome. Carefully monitored, these agents can be used together safely, but they should be prescribed and monitored only by experienced clinicians.

Selecting the Most Appropriate Drug

Selection of an initial pharmacotherapeutic treatment option involves numerous factors, the most important of which include the patient's target symptoms, comorbid medical or psychiatric conditions, concomitant medications, previous response to an antidepressant, and potential adverse effect and drug interaction profile. A patient's past experience with antidepressants should impact the decision regarding the choice of initial drug because past response tends to predict future response. Another consideration is the patient's perception about the efficacy and side effects she, he, or a family member has experienced. A negative perception of a drug may suggest potential for lack of adherence to drug therapy or an erosion of confidence in the therapy.

Scores of meta-analyses have evaluated the relative efficacy among antidepressants and assert that SSRIs consistently demonstrate relative efficacy as compared to SNRIs, TCAs, bupropion, trazodone, mirtazapine, and nefazodone. Patient-specific considerations will dictate the choice of drug as opposed to efficacy.

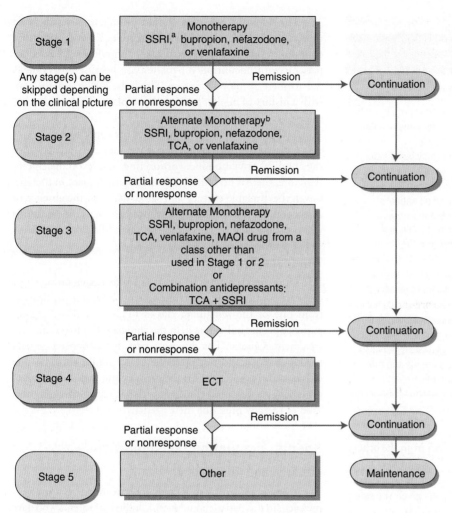

FIGURE 40.2 Amalgam of the Texas Medication Algorithm Project Recommendations (2008) and Recommendations from the American Psychiatric Association (2010). Texas Medication Algorithm Project (TMAP): Major depressive disorder. (Adapted from Suehs, B. T., Argo T. R., Bendele, S. D., et al. (2008). *Texas medication algorithm project procedural manual: Major depressive disorder algorithms.* Austin, TX: Texas Department of State Health Services. [The TMAP algorithms are in the public domain, and this figure may be reproduced without permission, but with the appropriate citation.] American Psychiatric Association (APA). (2011). *Practice guideline for the treatment of patients with major depressive disorder* (3rd ed., p. 152). Arlington, VA: American Psychiatric Association (APA).)

Abbreviations: EC = electroconvulsive therapy, MAOI = monoamine oxidase inhibitor, SSRI = selective serotonin reuptake inhibitor, TCA = tricyclic antidepressant.
a SSRIs preferred.
b Consider TCA or venlafaxine if not tried.

First-Line Therapy

Multiple large-scale trials have demonstrated that efficacy within drug classes and among drug classes is relatively equal, save for a few exceptions. Safety, tolerability, and lethality in overdose are the considerations that tend to drive drug selection, not efficacy. SSRIs and SNRIs are considered first-line therapy for depression and are generally used initially in patients without contraindications. In the absence of specific target symptoms, any of the available SSRIs or SNRIs are acceptable first choices. Recent studies purport the superiority of escitalopram over other members of its class, although this claim has not been substantiated with large randomized, controlled trials. If insomnia is problematic in the patient, paroxetine (Paxil) may be the best choice within the SSRI class. If the patient is taking drugs metabolized by CYP3A4, then avoiding fluoxetine (Prozac) is recommended. If the spectrum of depression-related symptoms includes sexual dysfunction, SSRIs and SNRIs should be avoided. If weight gain needs to be avoided, then bupropion is arguably a more appropriate option versus SSRIs (particularly paroxetine, which has the greatest potential to induce weight gain) or mirtazapine. See **Figure 40.2** and **Table 40.5** for an overview of treating a patient with depression.

Second-Line Therapy

When a patient fails an adequate trial of a first-line antidepressant and therapy needs to be modified, options include dose optimization, augmentation, and switching. If some clinical benefit, but not a true response or remission, is derived from the initial medication and it is well tolerated, an *increase in dose* is appropriate.

If the dose is optimized and some benefit (a response, but not remission) is realized, then *augmentation* with another nonantidepressant may be appropriate. Lithium, thyroid hormone, and stimulant medications have been used traditionally to augment the response to the initial antidepressant. Not common in practice any longer, this recommendation remains in the treatment guidelines.

If a patient fails an SSRI or an SNRI (does not realize any benefit or cannot tolerate the drug), then *switching* to another

TABLE 40.5

Recommended Order of Treatment in Antidepressant Therapy

Order	Agents	Comments
First line	SSRIs	Fluoxetine and sertraline may be good for patients with somnolence. Paroxetine may be good for patients with insomnia. Selection of agent should be based on patient's past experiences with medications and drug interactions. Cost may be a consideration.
Second line	TCA (desipramine or nortriptyline) or atypical antidepressant	These agents have the better side effect profile of the class and should be considered as agents of choice for the TCA class.
Third line	Atypical antidepressant or TCA	Depending on past response to other agents and side effect profile

member of the same class could serve as the second choice, as each member of the class is chemically distinct from the others. Switching to a medication in a different class can also be an option. Atypical antidepressants (bupropion, mirtazapine, etc.) are generally chosen prior to attempting TCAs given the safety and tolerability concerns associated with the TCAs.

Combination therapy implies adding a second drug with a different mechanism of action to the initial therapy. Drugs that are commonly used adjunctively to the initial medication include trazodone, bupropion (though this is often used as initial therapy), mirtazapine, buspirone, and the atypical antipsychotics (AAPs). Generally, the second drug is tailored to address residual symptoms that did not improve on initial therapy; residual symptoms like insomnia or anxious symptoms. There is clinical controversy surrounding the use of AAPs to treat depressed patients that do not have a psychotic component. Even though aripiprazole (Abilify) now carries an FDA indication for the adjunctive treatment of depression, many practitioners are reluctant to use them, given their extensive adverse effect profile. Quetiapine and risperidone are sometimes used off-label as an adjunctive medication. The AAPs have activity at serotonergic, noradrenergic, dopaminergic, and histaminergic receptors; all of which contribute to their therapeutic effects as well as their adverse effects. AAPs as a class are associated with serious and often irreversible metabolic sequelae including significant weight gain, insulin resistance, new-onset diabetes, and dyslipidemia. QT prolongation has also been observed. Given the serious nature of these adverse effects, and the extent to which they occur, the use of AAPs as an augmentation strategy is frequently met with resistance, particularly by psychiatrists.

The definitive selection should include an assessment of the patient's underlying cardiac, neurologic, and comorbid conditions. For example, venlafaxine should be avoided in patients with uncontrolled hypertension because of its potential to increase blood pressure. Similarly, for an elderly man with a history of benign prostatic hyperplasia, TCAs and atypical agents with significant anticholinergic activity should be avoided because this action aggravates the condition.

Current treatment guidelines have not been updated since the approval or vilazodone, vortioxetine, and levomilnacipran; therefore, there is no official guidance on their place in therapy. Given the available efficacy and safety data and the absence of direct comparison to existing therapy, these newer medications will probably be integrated into the second-line tier.

Third-Line Therapy

If the first- and second-line agents fail and augmentation strategies are unsuccessful, the clinician can attempt a medication from one of the remaining classes (TCAs, MAOIs). Again, patient-specific indicators help the clinician decide on the next treatment regimen. For the most part, inexperienced general practitioners should not prescribe MAO inhibitors. The side effects and the potential for dangerous drug and food interactions suggest that only clinicians well versed in managing this kind of therapy prescribe these agents.

Special Population Considerations

Children and Adolescents

The risk for underdiagnosis and undertreatment is extremely prevalent in this patient population. Children of parents who have been diagnosed with serious depression are at risk for developing anxiety and MDD in childhood. Early childhood depression may manifest as acting out, changes in eating or sleeping patterns, or social withdrawal. These patients can seldom communicate a feeling of sadness because of the early language development level. From ages 5 to 8, low self-esteem, underachievement at school, and aggressive or antisocial behaviors (including stealing and lying) may indicate depression. Depressed adolescents experience symptoms similar to depressed adults such as sleep disturbances, irritability, difficulty concentrating, and loss of energy.

Currently, fluoxetine (Prozac) is the only SSRI approved by the US Food and Drug Administration (FDA) for the treatment of depression in children age 8 and up. Escitalopram (Lexapro) is labeled for use in children age 12 and older. Caution has been recommended in using other agents, such as paroxetine (Paxil) or venlafaxine (Effexor), with depressed children and adolescents. Compared to adults, adolescents are more likely to become agitated or to develop a mania while they are taking an SSRI. The FDA has issued a black box warning due to increased risk of suicide in children and adolescents taking SSRIs.

Geriatrics

Late-onset depression commonly occurs in elderly patients, with nursing home residents nearly three times more likely to be depressed than the general population. These patients may also have an underlying neurologic or vascular disorder. Determining the root of the depression is essential to resolution. Elderly patients tend to endorse more vegetative symptoms and cognitive disturbances than they do subjective dysphoria, which differs from the presentation of a younger patient. Recognition and appropriate treatment of depression in this population are essential as the occurrence of depression worsens morbidity and mortality and worsens outcomes of somatic diseases.

Effort should be made to minimize pharmacologic burden on elderly patients and to proactively address possible drug interactions and adverse effects when selecting pharmacotherapy. Geriatric patients often have significant changes in physiologic function, including reduced renal and hepatic function, decreased muscle mass, decreased serum albumin, and dietary alterations. These changes may affect the absorption, distribution, metabolism, and excretion of a variety of drugs, particularly antidepressants. Elderly patients are also more sensitive to anticholinergic effects and orthostatic hypotension; adverse effects that are associated with several of the antidepressant drug classes. Most practitioners agree that antidepressant therapy should be prescribed at one third to one half the usual starting adult dosage.

Women

As noted earlier, younger women are more likely to experience depression than older women or men in general. Women of childbearing age are at the greatest risk; however, some women are especially sensitive to hormonal fluctuations and therefore may experience new-onset depression associated with menopause. The decision to initiate antidepressant medication in a pregnant woman is a difficult one, and the risk of fetal exposure to the drug must be balanced against the risk of continued depression.

Pregnancy-related and postpartum depression is especially prevalent in women with a history of depression and a previous episode of postpartum depression, although the independent prevalence is 10% to 15%. The risk is increased with concomitant marital problems, lack of social support, and medical issues with newborn children. The decision about which drug to use depends on the factors previously discussed as well as on the issue of breast-feeding and the risk of transmission of drugs through breast milk. The potential for antidepressant-associated fetal harm varies by drug and varies by trimester.

Ethnic

There are genetic variations in the metabolism of drugs in patients with varying ethnicity. The CYP2D6 enzyme system, responsible for the metabolism of many psychotherapeutic agents, is influenced by age, gender, and ethnicity. Up to 10% of Whites and nearly 19% of African Americans are considered "poor metabolizers" of drugs via CYP2D6. Similarly, 33% of African Americans and 37% of Asians are poor metabolizers of drugs metabolized by CYP2C19. The result of this poor metabolism can include quicker responses to drugs, greater than expected action of the agent, or even more pronounced side effects. As more data accrue on the effects of genetics on depression and CYP450 metabolism, the effects of race and ethnicity on treating depression and selecting antidepressants will play a more prominent role.

BOX 40.5 Warning Signs of Suicidal Ideation

- Pacing, agitated behavior, frequent mood changes, and chronic episodes of sleeplessness
- Actions or threats of assault, physical harm, or violence
- Delusions or hallucinations
- Threats or talk of death (e.g., "I don't care anymore," or "You won't have to worry about me much longer")
- Putting affairs in order, such as giving possessions away or writing a new will
- Unusually risky behavior (e.g., unsafe driving, abuse of alcohol or other drugs)

Emergencies

Suicide is the most feared consequence of inadequately treated (or unrecognized) depression. Up to two thirds of depressed patients have suicidal ideation, and 10% to 15% actually commit suicide (**Box 40.5**). The practitioner should be ever-vigilant for suicidal ideation and the potential for suicide. This is another reason for frequent contact between the practitioner and the patient. If the patient discloses thoughts of suicide, the practitioner and patient need to develop a plan for psychiatric referral or hospitalization. Contracting with the patient, such as by developing a written agreement to continue treatment without doing self-harm, may also be an effective means for minimizing the risk of suicide. All plans and actions should be documented in the patient's medical record.

PATIENT EDUCATION

Patients and caregivers should be instructed on the full range of issues surrounding depression and antidepressant therapy. Patients should be assured that depression is a biologic illness that occurs in a variety of people, and they should not feel ashamed of the disease. Moreover, the caregivers or significant others should also be counseled on the role they play in aiding in the patient's recovery. The more informed patients and significant others are of the illness, the more likely they will adhere to recommendations.

Expectations for a quick recovery can be detrimental to the healing process. Patients and caregivers should be informed that the antidepressant medication takes several (4 to 6) weeks to begin working and the patient might be required to continue taking the medication.

Teaching patients to recognize early signs and symptoms of behavior that may indicate a recurrence is crucial. Patients and family members should be instructed to contact the clinician if symptoms resume. A support group may also be a good resource for family and patients as a strategy for managing the illness.

Antidepressants and Suicide

Depression is the leading cause of suicide, and up to 80% of depressed patients experience suicidal impulses. Since 1990, whether antidepressant drugs are linked to suicide has been an acrimonious debate. Some argue that depressed adolescents who are suicidal and treated with antidepressants may regain initiative and energy before improvement in cognition and mood, thereby becoming mobilized to attempt suicide. Others argue that the medication prescribed to treat depression is responsible for causing adolescents to attempt suicide. In 2003, British drug regulators warned that SSRIs, with the exception of fluoxetine, were unsuitable in minors experiencing depression. As a result, the FDA began public hearings in February 2004 to discuss this controversy. Currently, fluoxetine (Prozac) is the only FDA-approved antidepressant in patients as young as age 8. However, other antidepressants, such as sertraline (Zoloft), venlafaxine (Effexor), and paroxetine (Paxil), have been widely prescribed for adolescent depression. Current data suggest that the increase in suicidality impacts patients younger than age 25 to a greater extent than patients older than age 25. Therefore, a practitioner needs to be diligent in assessing the patient's risk of suicide.

Patient Information

The National Foundation for Depressive Illness, Inc. (NAFDI) (http://www.depression.org), was established in 1983 to educate the public and health care professionals about depression. This Web site contains useful information on the signs and symptoms of depression and provides public awareness on depression through a national "800" number.

The National Institute of Mental Health's Web site (http://www.nimh.nih.gov/publicat/depressionmenus.cfm), also available in Spanish, is an excellent resource for depression. It describes the different types of depression along with the causes and treatments. This Web site also offers valuable information on how family and friends may contribute and assist in therapy.

The National Mental Health Association (NMHA) (http://www.nmha.org) is a nonprofit organization that provides beneficial information to the public and practitioners on mental illness. This Web site contains news releases along with an online bookstore. A calendar notes coming events relating to mental health. This Web site provides access to comprehensive mental health care and increases public awareness of mental health issues.

The Depression and Bipolar Support Alliance (DBSA) (http://www.dbsalliance.org) is a nonprofit organization that provides a wide range of information and support on depression and bipolar disorders. Their mission, as stated on the Web site, is to improve the lives of those affected by depression and bipolar disorder. The DBSA is a patient-directed national organization focusing on the most prevalent mental illnesses, with a network of approximately 1,000 support groups. This Web site is updated regularly to provide up-to-date, scientifically based information. The DBSA is guided by a scientific advisory board comprising researchers and clinicians in the field of mood disorders.

Complementary and Alternative Medications

The use of herbal products in the United States has dramatically increased in the past few decades, resulting in consumer sales of $250 million in 2007. Subsequent research with respect to drug–drug interactions and safety concerns made available to consumers caused a significant decrease in sales over the next decade. Depression is the most common diagnosis associated with complementary and alternative medication use. Despite the decline in popularity of St. John's wort, herbal sales continue to steadily rise. The FDA does not classify herbal products as drugs, and as such, they are not regulated under the same scrutiny as other medications.

St. John's wort (*Hypericum perforatum*) has been used for centuries for a variety of illnesses, but it is currently used almost exclusively as a herbal antidepressant. Most clinical trials have studied 300 to 1,800 mg/d of standardized extract (usually standardized to 0.3% hypericin content) divided in three daily doses. The clinical effect is usually seen within 2 to 3 weeks of initiating therapy. The mechanism of action is unknown, although it is theorized that it inhibits MAO and the synaptosomal uptake of serotonin, dopamine, and noradrenaline.

St. John's wort appears to be well tolerated, with the most frequent side effects reported as nausea, fatigue, restlessness, rash, and photosensitivity. There have been reported cases of increase in heart rate, but no significant effect was seen on the PR interval. Efficacy has not been well established, with some evidence to support its use and a wealth of studies in which it did not separate from placebo.

St. John's wort may activate hepatic CYP450, so it has the potential to interact with medication that is metabolized by the CYP450 system. Therefore, it has been reported that St. John's wort decreases serum levels of theophylline, cyclosporine, warfarin, oral contraceptives, and indinavir. St. John's wort should not be taken in combination with any other antidepressant because of the risk of serotonin syndrome, especially in the elderly. Symptoms include changes in mental status, tremor, gastrointestinal disturbances, myalgia, restlessness, and headache.

S-adenosylmethionine (SAMe) is a naturally occurring methyl donor in the synthesis of dopamine and serotonin. Though not regulated by the FDA and not recommended in any of the treatment guidelines, there is some data that supports the use of this compound in MDD. Omega-3 fatty acids have also been evaluated as an adjunctive therapy for MDD. Cardiovascular benefits of omega-3 fatty acids have been established and, given their relative safety and tolerability, could be added to conventional therapy. However, their efficacy in MDD has not been affirmed. Folate, however, has been associated with a positive response to antidepressant therapy. When used adjunctively to antidepressants, folate is recommended in patients who have not fully responded to their initial drug therapy. This is considered a low-risk intervention, given its general health benefits and lack of safety concerns.

CASE STUDY*

L.B. is a 55-year-old white female who presents to her family physician's office for a yearly routine physical. Her husband passed away 5 months ago after a 2-year battle with lung cancer. She has three children, two of whom are still in college. Her daughter accompanies her to the doctor's office and says she is concerned about her mother's recent behavior. She explains that her mother has been "sleeping all the time" and has lost 25 lb in the past 2 months without being on a diet. When the doctor examines L.B., she explains that she has become increasingly fatigued and complains of a lack of energy. She no longer has any desire to participate in her lifelong hobbies of painting and photography because of frequent feelings of sadness. L.B.'s medical history is significant for hypothyroidism, hypercholesterolemia, and recently diagnosed hypertension. Her medications are levothyroxine 0.075 mg daily, simvastatin 20 mg daily, hydrochlorothiazide 25 mg daily, lisinopril 10 mg daily, multivitamins 1 tab daily, and aspirin 81 mg daily. In the office today, L.B.'s blood pressure is 138/88 mm Hg.

DIAGNOSIS: MAJOR DEPRESSION

1. List specific goals for treatment for L.B.
2. What drug therapy would you prescribe? Why?
3. What are the parameters for monitoring success of the therapy?
4. Discuss specific patient education based on the prescribed therapy.
5. List one or two adverse reactions for the selected agent that would cause you to change therapy.
6. What would be the choice for second-line therapy?
7. What over-the-counter and/or alternative medications would be appropriate for L.B.?
8. What lifestyle changes would you recommend to L.B.?
9. Describe one or two drug–drug or drug–food interaction for the selected agent.

* Answers can be found online.

Bibliography

Starred references are cited in the text.

*American Psychiatric Association (APA). (2010 Oct). *Practice guideline for the treatment of patients with major depressive disorder* (3rd ed.). Arlington, VA: American Psychiatric Publishing (APA).

*American Psychiatric Association. (2013). *Diagnostic and statistical manual of mental disorders* (5th ed.). Arlington, VA: American Psychiatric Publishing.

American Psychiatric Association (APA). (2011). *Practice guideline for the treatment of patients with major depressive disorder* (3rd ed., p. 152). Arlington, VA: American Psychiatric Association (APA).

*Bauer, M., Tharmanathan, P., Volz, H., et al. (2009). The effect of venlafaxine compared with other antidepressants and placebo in the treatment of major depression: A meta-analysis. *European Archives of Psychiatry and Clinical Neuroscience, 259*(3), 172–185.

Ben-Sheetrit, J., Aizenberg, D., Csoka, A. B., et al. (2015). Post-SSRI sexual dysfunction: Clinical characterization and preliminary assessment of contributory factors and dose-response relationship. *Journal of Clinical Psychopharmacology, 35*(3), 273–278.

*Bulloch, A., Williams, J., Lavorato, D., et al. (2014). Recurrence of major depressive episodes is strongly dependent on the number of previous episodes. *Depression and Anxiety, 31*(1), 72–76.

Butterweck, V. (2003). Mechanism of action of St. John's Wort in depression. *CNS Drugs, 17*(8), 539–562.

*Donohue, J. M., & Pincus, H. A. (2007). Reducing the societal burden of depression: a review of economic costs, quality of care and effects of treatment. *PharmacoEconomics, 25*, 7.

Fava, G. A., Gatti, A., Belaise, C., et al. (2015). Withdrawal symptoms after selective serotonin reuptake inhibitor discontinuation: A systematic review. *Psychotherapy and Psychosomatics, 84*(2), 72–81.

Hamilton, M. (1967). Development of a rating scale for primary depressive illness. *British Journal of Social and Clinical Psychology, 6*, 278–296.

Harris, P. A. (2004). The impact of age, gender, race and ethnicity on the diagnosis and treatment of depression. *Journal of Managed Care Pharmacy, 10*(2, Suppl.), S2–S7.

Koenig, A., & Thase, M. (2009). First-line pharmacotherapies for depression—What is the best choice? *Polskie Archiwum Medycyny Wewnętrznej, 119*(7–8), 478–486.

Matthews, J. D., & Fava, M. (2000). Risk of suicidality in depression with serotonergic antidepressants. *Annals of Clinical Psychiatry, 12*(1), 43–50.

*Norhayati, M. N., Nik Hazlina, N. H., Asrenee, A. R., et al. (2015). Magnitude and risk factors for postpartum symptoms: A literature review. *Journal of Affective Disorders, 175C*, 34–52.

*Papakostas, G. (2009). Managing partial response or nonresponse: Switching, augmentation, and combination strategies for major depressive disorder. *Journal of Clinical Psychiatry, 70*(Suppl. 6), 16–25.

Rickels, K., Athanasiou, M., Robinson, D. S., et al. (2009). Evidence for efficacy and tolerability of vilazodone in the treatment of major depressive disorder: A randomized, double-blind, placebo-controlled trial. *The Journal of Clinical Psychiatry, 70*(3), 326–333.

Robinson, D. S., Kajdasz, D. K., Gallipoli, S., et al. (2011). A 1-year, open-label study assessing the safety and tolerability of vilazodone in patients with major depressive disorder. *Journal of Clinical Psychopharmacology, 31*(5), 643–646.

*Rush, A. J., Trivedi, M., Fava, M. (2003). Depression, IV: STAR*D treatment trial for depression. *The American Journal of Psychiatry, 160*(2), 237.

Tadić, A., Helmreich, I., Mergl, R., et al. (2010). Early improvement is a predictor of treatment outcome in patients with mild major, minor or subsyndromal depression. *Journal of Affective Disorders, 120*(1–3), 86–93.

Trivedi, M. (2009). Tools and strategies for ongoing assessment of depression: A measurement-based approach to remission. *Journal of Clinical Psychiatry, 70*(Suppl. 6), 26–31.

Trivedi, M., Rush, A., Wisniewski, S., et al. (2006). Evaluation of outcomes with citalopram for depression using measurement-based care in STAR*D: Implications for clinical practice. *American Journal of Psychiatry, 163*(1), 28–40.

von Wolff, A., Hölzel, L. P., Westphal, A., et al. . (2013). Selective serotonin reuptake inhibitors and tricyclic antidepressants in the acute treatment of chronic depression and dysthymia: A systematic review and meta-analysis. *Journal of Affective Disorders, 144*(1–2), 7–15.

Willner, P., Scheel-Krüger, J., & Belzung, C. (2013). The neurobiology of depression and antidepressant action. *Neuroscience and Biobehavioral Reviews, 37*(10 Pt 1), 2331–2371.

Zajecka, J. (2003). Treating depression to remission. *Journal of Clinical Psychiatry, 64*(Suppl. 15), 7–12.

41 Anxiety Disorders

Laura A. Mandos ■ Jennifer A. Reinhold

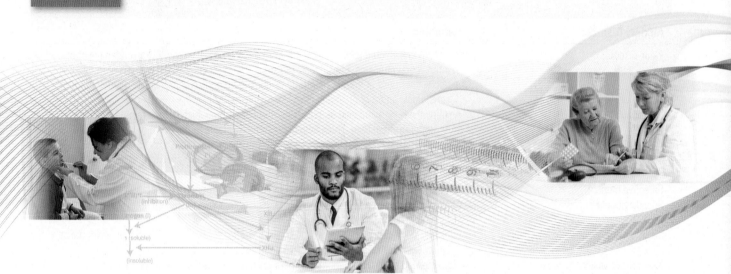

Though related and with some inherent overlap, the anxiety disorders are a compendium of similar but clinically distinct disorders that share clinical features of excessive fear, worry, anxiety, and associated behavioral manifestations. Patients with anxiety disorders generally endorse psychic and somatic symptoms at varying degrees, which may include tension, apprehension, fear, restlessness, and worry along with physical symptoms such as increased heart rate, pupillary dilation, trembling, and increased perspiration.

One of the complications in identifying the presence of an anxiety disorder is that the core symptoms are mainly normal experiences in the human condition; but what delineates "normal" feelings of anxiety, worry, or fear is the extent to which they occur (severity and frequency) and the extent to which they impact functionality.

With 10 different types, the anxiety disorders represent the largest group of psychiatric disorders (**Table 41.1**). The focus of this chapter will be primarily generalized anxiety disorder (GAD), with an additional review of panic disorder (PD) and social anxiety disorder (SAD, also known as social phobia). There were several meaningful changes in the classification of anxiety disorders in the newest iteration of the Diagnostic and Statistical Manual (DSM), with the publication of the DSM-5 in 2013. Obsessive–compulsive disorder is no longer considered part of the anxiety disorder spectrum and will not be covered in this chapter. The agoraphobia specifier has been removed from PD and now is considered an independent diagnosis under the anxiety disorder umbrella.

More than 30 million Americans have a lifetime history of anxiety, and anxiety disorders cost an estimated $42 billion per year in the United States, counting direct and indirect costs. Epidemiologic studies report that 2% to 6% of adults and twice as many women as men have GAD. Approximately 1% of all patients have PD with resulting significant impairment, and 4% to 5% have agoraphobia. Approximately 12% of patients seen in anxiety disorder clinics present with GAD. Between 35% and 50% of individuals with major depression meet criteria for GAD. Coexisting anxious distress (formerly referred to as comorbid GAD in depressed patients), now considered a specifier for major depressive disorder, in depressed patients may worsen the outcome by increasing the suicide rate, worsening overall symptoms, conferring a poorer response to treatment, increasing the number of unexplained symptoms, and increasing functional disability.

The neurobiological and conceptual models that form the basis for anxiety disorders are grounded in the belief that pathologic anxiety is a result of abnormal fear processing, intolerance of uncertainty, anxiety about worry itself, or emotional hyperarousal. Humans have naturally evolved to be able to apply past experiences and responses to new experiences. For a simple example, if an individual had a traumatic experience with a small animal at some point in his or her life and escaped that fearful situation by running away, that individual may repeat that behavior when faced with a small animal in the future. While evolutionarily helpful in some respects, this response may be maladaptive in that the responses may not only be exaggerated and inappropriate but also may extend beyond a specific experience, hence generalization.

Anxiety disorders most commonly begin in early adulthood. They tend to be chronic, with interspersed periods of remissions and relapses of varying degrees, and they frequently

TABLE 41.1

Summary of Anxiety Disorders

Anxiety Disorder	Definition
Panic disorder	Recurrent unexpected panic attacks (discrete periods, in which there is a sudden onset of intense apprehension, fearfulness, or terror, often associated with feelings of impending doom, shortness of breath, palpitations, chest pain or discomfort, choking or smothering sensations, and fear of "going crazy" or losing control).
Agoraphobia	Anxiety about, or avoidance of, places or situations from which escape might be difficult (or embarrassing) or in which help may not be available in the event of having a panic attack or panic-like symptoms.
Separation anxiety	Recurrent, excessive distress when anticipating or experiencing separation from home or from an attachment focus (person, object, etc.) or worry about losing attachment figures.
Selective mutism	Failure to speak in specific social situations in which there is an expectation to do so.
Specific phobia	Clinically significant anxiety provoked by exposure to a specific feared object or situation, often leading to avoidance.
Social anxiety disorder (social phobia)	Clinically significant anxiety provoked by exposure to certain types of social or performance situations, often leading to avoidance behavior.
Generalized anxiety disorder	Characterized by at least 6 months of persistent and excessive anxiety and worry.
Anxiety disorder due to a general medical condition	Characterized by prominent symptoms of anxiety that are judged to be a direct physiological consequence of a general medical condition.
Substance/medication-induced anxiety disorder	Characterized by prominent symptoms of anxiety that are judged to be a direct physiological consequence of a drug abuse, a medication, or toxin exposure.
Anxiety disorder not otherwise specified	Used for coding disorders with prominent anxiety or phobic avoidance that do not meet the criteria for any of the specific anxiety disorders defined in this list (or anxiety symptoms about which there is inadequate or contradictory information).

Adapted from American Psychiatric Association. (2013). *Diagnostic and statistical manual of mental health disorders: DSM-5* (5th ed.). Washington, DC: American Psychiatric Publishing.

continue into old age. Late onset of an anxiety disorder is rare, although the prevalence of GAD increases with increasing age. In the elderly, anxiety disorders as a whole are the most common psychiatric disorders. It is unknown whether they are a continuation of an illness with an onset from a younger age or whether they appear for the first time in old age.

GAD is a highly prevalent, chronic, debilitating, relapsing, and often underdiagnosed anxiety disorder. Characterized by excessive and pathological worry that is difficult to control, a diagnosis of GAD also incorporates physical, psychological, and cognitive symptoms as well as a potentially profound functional impairment. The core symptom of excessive worry must be present for a minimum of 6 months and must occur in conjunction with at least three of six physiological arousal symptoms: restlessness, fatigue, muscle tension, irritability, concentration deficit, and sleep disturbance. As the most commonly occurring anxiety disorder with a lifetime prevalence of 4% to 7%, GAD is characterized by a waxing and waning episodic clinical course with periods of remission and relapse. Many patients with GAD report feeling as though they have "felt anxious" for their entire lives. The median onset, however, is 30 years; though age of onset is spread over a broad age range, this represents the latest age of onset of all the anxiety disorders (APA, 2013).

The pathologic worry is typically based on dangers with an overestimated likelihood of realistically occurring (e.g.,

a loved one being kidnapped), which then rapidly devolves into generalized worry that involves multiple life domains. For some patients, this worry leads to avoidant behavior where activities or places with perceived danger are avoided. Left untreated, the patient's sphere of comfort may continue to constrict until daily activities become limited and normal function is impaired.

CAUSES

Physiologic Factors

The majority of patients with GAD initially seek attention from a primary health care provider with vague somatic complaints, such as pain, headaches, or gastrointestinal (GI) disturbances. Patients also may casually endorse a nonspecific complaint of insomnia, irritability, sexual dysfunction, or trouble concentrating or remembering.

Although the etiology of anxiety disorders is largely unknown, a wide range of medical illnesses, such as cardiovascular disease, respiratory disease, hyperthyroidism, hypothyroidism, hyperadrenocorticism, pheochromocytoma, Cushing disease, hypoglycemia, vitamin B_{12} deficiency, and neurologic conditions, may cause symptoms of anxiety. In addition, amphetamines, cannabis, caffeine, cocaine, bronchodilators, corticosteroids, sympathomimetics, and thyroid hormone may cause substance-induced anxiety.

Genetic Factors

A family history is seen frequently in people with anxiety disorders. Twin studies suggest that heredity accounts for 30% of the cases of various anxiety disorders; environmental factors seem to be responsible for the remaining cases. More than 50% of people with PD have relatives with the disorder. A twin study reported that anxiety disorder with panic attacks occurs five times more frequently in monozygotic twins than in heterozygotic twins.

PATHOPHYSIOLOGY

Anxiety is a phenomenon that all people experience. One type of anxiety, fear, is a normal fight-or-flight response to an observable threat. In contrast, pathologic anxiety is a fight-or-flight response to an internal or external threat that is real or imagined and causes the person to experience an unpleasant emotional state. During this response, the person's autonomic nervous system, which consists of the sympathetic and parasympathetic nervous systems, prepares the person to deal with a threat (**Box 41.1**).

BOX 41.1 Physiologic Reactions to the Fight-or-Flight Response

The fight-or-flight response causes the following:

1. Epinephrine, norepinephrine, and cortisol are released into the blood.
2. The liver releases stored sugar into the blood to meet energy needs.
3. Digestion slows, allowing blood to be shifted to the brain and the muscles.
4. Breathing becomes rapid to allow for greater oxygen supply to the muscles.
5. The heart rate and blood pressure increase.
6. Perspiration increases to cool the body.
7. Muscles tense in preparation for action.
8. The pupils dilate.
9. All senses become more acute.
10. Blood flow to the extremities becomes constricted to protect the body from bleeding from injury.

This response is appropriate for extremely threatening situations, but the response would cause considerable damage to the body if people responded to all stressful situations in this manner.

Neurobiologic Factors

The modulation of normal and pathologic anxiety states is associated with multiple regions of the brain and dysregulation in several neurotransmitter systems (norepinephrine [NE], serotonin [5-HT], gamma-aminobutyric acid [GABA], corticotrophin-releasing factor [CRF], and cholecystokinin). Furthermore, treatment with medications that modulate these systems have produced short-term and sustained anxiolytic responses, further substantiating the implication of noradrenergic, serotonergic, and GABA system involvement.

Norepinephrine, serotonin, and GABA are the major neurotransmitters studied in relation to the pharmacologic treatment of anxiety. People with anxiety disorders, especially PD, are found to have malfunctioning noradrenergic systems with a low threshold for arousal. This, coupled with an unpredictable increase in activity, causes the anxiety symptoms.

GABA and its associated receptors function as central nervous system (CNS) inhibitors. Although psychopharmacologic interventions support this role, the exact pharmacology of GABA receptors is still being examined.

DIAGNOSTIC CRITERIA

Anxiety disorders most commonly begin in early adulthood, tend to be chronic with waxing and waning periods of remission and relapse, and frequently continue into old age. In children, anxiety may develop, particularly in relation to school, and late onset of an anxiety disorder is rare but can occur. In the elderly, anxiety disorders are the most common psychiatric disorders seen.

Prior to diagnosis of an anxiety disorder, a medical evaluation should be conducted to rule out medical disease, neurologic problems, current medications that may be anxiogenic, vitamin B_{12} deficiency, and drug or alcohol misuse. The history should focus on anxiety disorders in family members, environmental factors, family dynamics, cognitive functioning, work or school situations, or exposure to chemical substances.

If the anxiety is not reasonably related to a physical or exogenous chemical (drug, alcohol, etc.) consideration, the practitioner should apply the American Psychiatric Association's (APA) *Diagnostic and Statistical Manual of Mental Disorders, 5th Edition* (DSM-5, 2013) diagnostic criteria. See **Boxes 41.2, 41.3,** and **41.4** for the diagnostic criteria for GAD, PD, and SAD, respectively.

Comorbidity with major depression is common in patients with anxiety. These patients may self-medicate with alcohol or other substances to relieve their symptoms.

INITIATING DRUG THERAPY

A multitude of special challenges exists with respect to the diagnosis and successful treatment of GAD. As previously discussed, many patients present with physical complaints

BOX 41.2 APA DSM-5 Criteria for Diagnosing Generalized Anxiety Disorder

A. Excessive anxiety and worry (apprehensive expectation), occurring more days than not for at least 6 months, about a number of events or activities (such as work or school performance).

B. The person finds it difficult to control the worry.

C. The anxiety and worry are associated with three (or more) of the following six symptoms (with at least some symptoms present for more days than not for the past 6 months).

Note: Only one item is required in children.

1. Restlessness or feeling keyed up or on edge
2. Being easily fatigued
3. Difficulty concentrating or mind going blank
4. Irritability
5. Muscle tension
6. Sleep disturbance (difficulty falling or staying asleep, or restless, unsatisfying sleep)

D. The anxiety, worry, or physical symptoms cause clinically significant distress or impairment in social, occupational, or other important areas of functioning.

E. The disturbance is not attributable to the physiological effects of a substance (e.g., a drug of abuse, a medication) or another medical condition (e.g., hyperthyroidism).

F. The disturbance is not better explained by another mental disorder (e.g., anxiety or worry about having panic attacks in PD, negative evaluation in SAD social phobia, contamination or other obsessions in obsessive–compulsive disorder, separation from attachment figures in separation anxiety disorder, reminders of traumatic events in posttraumatic stress disorder, gaining weight in anorexia nervosa, physical complaints in somatic symptom disorder, perceived appearance flaws in body dysmorphic disorder, having a serious illness in illness anxiety disorder, or the content of delusional beliefs in schizophrenia or delusional disorder).

BOX 41.3 APA DSM-5 Criteria for Diagnosing Panic Disorder

A. Recurrent unexpected panic attacks. A panic attack is an abrupt surge of intense fear or intense discomfort that reaches a peak within minutes and during which time four (or more) of the following symptoms occur:

Note: The abrupt surge can occur from a calm state or an anxious state.

1. Palpitations, pounding heart, or accelerated heart rate
2. Sweating
3. Trembling or shaking
4. Sensations of shortness of breath or smothering
5. Feelings of choking
6. Chest pain or discomfort
7. Nausea or abdominal distress
8. Feeling dizzy, unsteady, lightheaded, or faint
9. Chills or heat sensations
10. Paresthesias (numbness or tingling sensations)
11. Derealization (feelings of unreality) or depersonalization (being detached from oneself)
12. Fear of losing control or "going crazy"
13. Fear of dying

Note: Culture-specific symptoms (e.g., tinnitus, neck soreness, headache, uncontrollable screaming or crying) may be seen. Such symptoms should not count as one of the four required symptoms.

B. At least one of the attacks has been followed by 1 month (or more) of one or both of the following:

1. Persistent concern or worry about additional panic attacks or their consequences (e.g., losing control, having a heart attack, "going crazy")
2. A significant maladaptive change in behavior related to the attacks (e.g., behaviors designed to avoid having panic attacks, such as avoidance of exercise or unfamiliar situations)

C. The disturbance is not attributable to the physiological effects of a substance (e.g., a drug of abuse, a medication) or another medical condition (e.g., hyperthyroidism, cardiopulmonary disorders).

D. The disturbance is not better explained by another mental disorder (e.g., the panic attacks do not occur only in response to feared social situations, as in SAD; in response to circumscribed phobic objects or situations, as in specific phobia; in response to obsessions, as in obsessive–compulsive disorder; in response to reminders of traumatic events, as in posttraumatic stress disorder; or in response to separation from attachment figures, as in separation anxiety disorder).

and no recognition whatsoever of an emotional or psychiatric component. Patients may lack an understanding of mental illness, may deny symptoms or its existence when given the diagnosis of a mental illness, or be so ashamed of the stigma associated with mental illness that they are prevented from

APA DSM-5 Criteria for Diagnosing Social Anxiety Disorder

A. Marked fear or anxiety about one or more social situations in which the individual is exposed to possible scrutiny by others. Examples include social interactions (e.g., having a conversation, meeting unfamiliar people), being observed (e.g., eating or drinking), and performing in front of others (e.g., giving a speech).

B. The individual fears that he or she will act in a way or show anxiety symptoms that will be negatively evaluated (e.g., will be humiliating or embarrassing; will lead to rejection or offend others).

C. The social situation(s) almost always provoke fear or anxiety.
   Note: In children, the fear or anxiety may be expressed by crying, tantrums, freezing, clinging, shrinking, or failure to speak in social situations.

D. The social situation(s) are actively avoided or endured with intense fear or anxiety.

E. The fear or anxiety is out of proportion to the actual threat posed by the social situation and the sociocultural context.

F. The fear, anxiety, or avoidance is persistent, typically lasting 6 or more months.

G. The fear, anxiety, or avoidance cause clinically significant distress or impairment in social, occupational, or other important areas of functioning.

H. The fear, anxiety, or avoidance is not attributable to the physiological effects of a substance (e.g., a drug of abuse, a medication) or another medical condition.

I. The fear, anxiety, or avoidance is not better explained by the symptoms of another mental disorder such as panic disorder, body dysmorphic disorder, or autism spectrum disorder.

J. If another medical condition (e.g., Parkinson disease, obesity, disfigurement from burns or injury) is present, the fear, anxiety, or avoidance is clearly unrelated or is excessive.

Specify if: **Performance only**: If the fear is restricted to speaking or performing in public.

being open to discussing treatment options. Careful, tactful interventions on the part of the clinician will set the stage for a healthy patient–provider relationship, which will increase the likelihood of successful outcomes. This may be achieved by creating an environment in which the patient is comfortable discussing personal and potentially uncomfortable topics. Empathetic listening, open-mindedness, and acknowledgment that psychiatric disease is a legitimate medical disorder and not a personality flaw are critical. Also, aside from misconceptions about mental illness itself, many patients are reluctant to accept drug therapy as a treatment option. Although there is certainly a place in the treatment spectrum for psychotherapy, drug therapy often is a necessary component in achieving true remission of symptoms.

Successful treatment of anxiety disorders also implies a longer-term commitment from the patient and the clinician, as GAD and the other anxiety disorders are chronic illnesses. Thorough explanation at the beginning of therapy is crucial. The patient education from the outset should include not only explanations of the illness itself but also what the patient should expect during treatment in terms of duration of therapy, when to follow-up, expected length of time before pharmacotherapy will be optimized, and how to respond to potential adverse drug effects (ADEs). Nonpharmacologic therapy includes psychoeducation, supportive counseling, behavioral therapy, cognitive therapy, stress management techniques, meditation, and exercise. Today, in many cases, these therapies can be helpful and useful in conjunction with drug therapy.

Behavioral therapists treat anxiety as a learned behavior, arguing that anxiety is an internal conditioned response to a perceived threat or stimulus in the environment. They propose that people with anxiety learn to avoid the stimulus in order to reduce anxiety; therefore, behavior modification is the vehicle for changing behavior. Systematic desensitization is used to control external stimuli and internal sensations as well as anticipation of fear of a panic attack.

Cognitive therapists treat anxiety as a faulty thought pattern that evokes the physiologic symptoms of anxiety, feelings of loss of control, and fear of dying. Cognitive–behavioral therapy (CBT) and drug therapy complement each other and tend to produce a greater therapeutic response. CBT is considered the most effective psychotherapy for GAD, according to the literature. CBT for GAD involves self-monitoring of worry, cognitive restructuring, relaxation training, and rehearsal of coping skills. However, CBT requires special training and may not be readily available to all patients.

Goals of Drug Therapy

The long-term goal of therapy for GAD is remission: a complete resolution of anxious symptoms and a return to premorbid functionality and quality of life. In GAD specifically, *response* to treatment is realized by 50% to 60% of patients, yet *remission* is achieved by approximately one third to one half of patients who respond. Failure to remit fully confers a greater risk of relapse, a reality experienced by 45% of patients with generalized anxiety. Acutely, the goal is to reduce the severity and duration of the anxious symptoms and improve overall functioning. Once target symptoms are improved or resolved, the focus shifts to chronic or maintenance therapy; the goal of which is to completely resolve symptoms and return the patient to a premorbid level of social and occupational functionality (remission). Coupled with the goal of remission is also relapse prevention.

The ideal anxiolytic medication should promote calmness without resulting in daytime sedation and drowsiness and without producing physical or psychological dependence. Pharmacologic options used in the treatment of anxiety disorders can be classified into the following categories: antidepressants, benzodiazepines (BZDs), azapirones, novel antianxiety agents, and atypical antipsychotics (AAPs).

For most anxiety disorders, a single drug, generally an antidepressant, is initiated at a low dose and is titrated upward according to clinical response and tolerability. Four to eight weeks is the generally accepted time at which a preliminary assessment of response can be gauged. Patients who endorse some level of appreciable symptom resolution and are tolerant of the medication are considered to have achieved a durable remission. This is considered predictive of an eventual sustained remission, which persists for several months beyond this acute treatment phase.

Absence of response at the initial 4- to 8-week follow-up visit or intolerance of adverse effects may prompt either a re-evaluation of diagnosis or an adjustment in medication therapy. Reasonable interventions include increasing the dose of medication (if the initial drug was tolerated but the clinical effect was not of the magnitude desired), switching to a different drug within the same pharmacologic class (if there was some level of improvement but questionable tolerability), switching to a drug outside of the pharmacologic class (if there was lack of response and/or poor tolerability), or augmenting the initial drug (if the dose of the initial drug was already optimized but the full therapeutic effect has not been achieved).

Upon resolution of the presenting anxious symptoms, it is recommended that treatment be continued beyond initial symptom resolution for 12 months, particularly in GAD, in order to minimize the risk of relapse. In some anxiety disorders, treatment may continue indefinitely depending on the level of severity. The follow-up intervals also may differ based upon individual patient presentation.

Antidepressants

Antidepressants are generally considered first-line pharmacotherapeutic options for the chronic management of patients with anxiety disorders (see **Table 41.2**).

Selective Serotonin Reuptake Inhibitors

Considered one of the two first-line pharmacotherapeutic options for the management of GAD in the United States, the selective serotonin reuptake inhibitors (SSRIs) are thought to improve anxious symptoms by inhibiting the reuptake of serotonin in the synaptic cleft. While the 2- to 4-week delay until onset of therapeutic effect may be discouraging and may impact patient compliance, significant reductions in "anxious mood" have been documented as early as week 1 in **paroxetine** (Paxil) trials. Remission rates in paroxetine responders at 32 weeks are as high as 73% with only 11% relapsing, a statistic that demonstrates much improvement over the spontaneous remission rate of 20% to 25%. In patients with moderate to severe GAD, **sertraline (Zoloft)** 50 to 100 mg/d has demonstrated superiority to placebo. Clinical response criteria were met by 55% of patients in the sertraline group as compared to 32% in the placebo group by week 12. **Escitalopram** (Lexapro) has been evaluated for the long-term treatment of GAD and prevention of relapse. A randomized, double-blind, placebo-controlled study reported significantly superior results for escitalopram at every time point starting at week 1.

TABLE 41.2

Antidepressants Used in Treating Anxiety Disorders

Generic (Trade) Name	Initial Dose (mg)	Usual Dose (mg)
Tricyclic Antidepressants		
imipramine (Tofranil)	10–50	150–300
Selective Serotonin Reuptake Inhibitors		
citalopram (Celexa)	20	20–40
escitalopram (Lexapro)	10	10–20
fluvoxamine CR (Luvox CR)	100	100–300
paroxetine (Paxil)	10–20	10–60
(Paxil CR)	12.5	12.5–75
sertraline (Zoloft)	25–50	75–200
Serotonin–Norepinephrine Reuptake Inhibitors		
venlafaxine (Effexor, Effexor XR)	37.5–75	75–225
duloxetine (Cymbalta)		
Monoamine Oxidase Inhibitors		
phenelzine (Nardil)	15	45–90

Adverse Events

Class adverse effects include weight gain, insomnia, GI sequelae, and agitation. Sexual dysfunction, often a presenting symptom in anxious patients, may be exacerbated or caused by SSRIs in up to 40% or 50% of patients. Clinical experience shows that this adverse effect is likely underreported. Another unfortunate pharmacologic phenomenon of the SSRI class is its ability to cause agitation and jitteriness in the acute phase of treatment.

Paroxetine (Paxil) may cause more weight gain and sexual inhibition than the other drugs. Approximately 15% of patients discontinue treatment because of side effects. Caution should be used when SSRIs are given in combination with TCAs because SSRIs can inhibit one or more liver microsomal enzyme systems and increase plasma concentrations of the TCA. This can translate into conduction abnormalities due to toxic levels of TCA. The combination of SSRIs and MAO inhibitors has resulted in serious reactions such as hyperthermia, rigidity, and autonomic dysregulation that can be fatal. SSRIs are generally well tolerated, and toxicity in overdose is rare as compared to the TCAs, which partially explains why the SSRIs and serotonin–norepinephrine reuptake inhibitors (SNRIs) have largely supplanted the TCAs as first-line options. See Chapter 40 for more information.

Serotonin–Norepinephrine Reuptake Inhibitors

Members of this class inhibit the reuptake of serotonin and norepinephrine, though the selectivity and balance with respect to the extent of inhibition are variable among the SNRIs. **Venlafaxine** XR 75 mg to 225 mg (Effexor XR) daily consistently demonstrated superior efficacy compared to placebo in improving anxious symptom. The additional benefit of venlafaxine's efficacy in treating anxious symptoms in patients with comorbid depression as well as in pure GAD has made it a commonly prescribed first-line drug. The comorbidity of nonspecific somatic pain complaints is common in patients with GAD, which negatively impacts quality of life, worsens outcomes, hampers achievement of remission, and increases the risk of relapse. Response rates for treatment with venlafaxine approach 70%, and remission rates are as high as 43% acutely and as high as 61% long term.

Duloxetine's (Cymbalta) inhibition of serotonin and norepinephrine is more balanced as opposed to venlafaxine, which is more serotonergic at lower dose and more noradrenergic at higher doses. Its dual impact on anxious symptoms and somatic pain has resulted in 53% to 61% of treated patients achieving symptomatic remission and an approximate 47% achieving functional remission.

Adverse Effects

Adverse effects are similar in scope and magnitude to those of the SSRI class; however, the risk of clinically meaningful increases in blood pressure has also been documented, particularly with venlafaxine.

Tricyclic Antidepressants

TCAs are effective in GAD and PD. **Imipramine** (Tofranil) is the only TCA with an indication for the treatment of GAD and has proven effective in controlling panic attacks in patients with PD and GAD. TCAs are typically most useful in attenuating the psychological symptoms of GAD as opposed to the somatic symptoms. TCAs have largely been supplanted by SSRIs and SNRIs as first-line therapy for the treatment of anxiety disorders.

Mechanism of Action

TCA inhibition of 5-HT and norepinephrine reuptake are thought to produce anxiolytic and antidepressant effects. Imipramine does not have any direct effects on anticipatory anxiety or phobic avoidance behavior. The response is gradual, over a period of weeks.

Adverse Events

TCAs cause anticholinergic adverse effects such as dryness of the mouth and other mucosal surfaces, blurred vision, tachycardia, constipation, and urinary hesitancy. Other adverse effects are postural hypotension, carbohydrate craving, weight gain, and sexual dysfunction. They lower the seizure threshold and are a relative contraindication in patients with seizure disorders. These drugs are contraindicated in patients with narrow-angle glaucoma, urinary hesitancy, BPH, and heart conduction abnormalities. TCAs enhance the CNS effects of alcohol. Plasma measurements of TCAs should be done in selected situations as needed. The profound risk of toxicity in overdose coupled with these undesired effects has resulted in TCAs being replaced by newer, more tolerable, possibly more effective drugs that are less toxic in overdose. See Chapter 40 for more information.

Benzodiazepines

BZDs are important and widely prescribed sedative–hypnotics. Their pharmacologic properties include reduction of anxiety, sedation, muscle relaxation, anticonvulsant, and amnestic effects. Among the prominent BZDs are **alprazolam** (Xanax), **clonazepam** (Klonopin), **diazepam** (Valium), **lorazepam** (Ativan), and **oxazepam** (Serax). They are best utilized in patients with acute anxiety to a time-limited stressor.

Mechanism of Action

BZDs exert a therapeutic effect by binding to GABA-A receptors in the brain. They cause the GABA-A receptors to increase the opening of chloride channels along the cell membrane, leading to an inhibitory effect on cell firing. Other neurotransmitters, such as serotonin and norepinephrine, may play a role in the therapeutic effect of BZDs. The exact mechanism of BZDs' antianxiety effect is not yet fully understood. Most of the drugs in this class possess anxiolytic, sedative–hypnotic, and anticonvulsant properties.

BZDs can be used for treating GAD and PD. Approximately 75% of patients with GAD respond moderately or better to BZDs. Benzodiazepines are indicated for the short-term management of the acute phase of anxiety (first 2 to 4 weeks) as well as any subsequent exacerbations of anxiety during stable treatment with an antidepressant. Their rapid onset and tolerability allow them to ease anxious symptoms when immediate anxiolytic effects are necessary. Although more marked improvement is realized in the first 2 weeks of treatment with BZDs, antidepressants consistently achieve the efficacy of BZDs or even surpass it after 6 to 12 weeks of treatment, particularly in alleviating psychic symptoms. Though still a common practice, the utilization of BZDs long term or as monotherapy is not recommended and is inconsistent with evidence-based guidelines. BZDs are most adept at alleviating somatic symptoms but have no effect to a somewhat detrimental effect on the psychic symptoms of GAD. At this time, there is no evidence that one BZD is superior to another for this disorder. The high-potency BZDs, **alprazolam**, **clonazepam**, and **lorazepam**, have been effective in controlling panic attacks and anticipatory anxiety in panic attacks. The clinical indications for a specific BZD are not absolute, and considerable overlap in their use exists. Not only are they effective in pathologic anxiety but also their calming effect is useful in nonpathologic anxiety states (temporary episodes of anxiety due to fear). BZDs have a wider therapeutic window than most other CNS depressants and are associated with fewer side effects.

The various BZDs differ little in their pharmacologic properties, but they differ significantly in their potency, their ability to cross the blood–brain barrier, and their half-lives. High-potency BZDs, such as **alprazolam**, **clonazepam**, and **lorazepam**, have a great affinity for the BZD receptor. The onset and intensity of action of an oral dose of a BZD is determined by the rate of absorption from the GI tract. BZDs are highly bound to plasma proteins (70% to 90%) and are highly lipid soluble. The duration of action is related to their lipid solubility as well as hepatic biotransformation to active metabolites. **Oxazepam** and **lorazepam** are metabolized to inactive compounds and therefore have shorter half-lives and durations of activity than other BZDs. This one-step inactivation to an inactive compound makes them the preferred drugs for the treatment of anxiety in elderly patients and patients with liver disease.

Accumulation of BZDs with a long half-life (long-acting BZDs) occurs from one dose to another. Long-acting BZDs take a longer time to reach steady-state levels, are removed more slowly, and cause more pronounced side effects (e.g., sedation). However, use of these preparations reduces the likelihood and intensity of withdrawal symptoms when discontinued. Ultra-short–acting BZDs do not accumulate. High lipid solubility results in faster absorption, greater distribution in tissues, and faster entrance and exit from brain sites. Diazepam is a BZD with high lipid solubility used for anxiety. (See **Table 41.3** for more information.)

TABLE 41.3

Overview of Selected Drugs Used to Treat Generalized Anxiety Disorder

Generic Name	Trade Name	Usual Adult Dosage Range (mg/d)	Oral Peak (h)	Half-Life (h) Parent + Active Metabolite	Metabolite Activity	Contraindications
alprazolam	Xanax	0.75–4	1–2	6–20	Inactive	Hypersensitivity to alprazolam or any component of the formulation (cross-sensitivity with other benzodiazepines may also exist), narrow-angle glaucoma, concurrent use of ketoconazole or itraconazole
chlordiazepoxide	Librium	15–40	0.5–4	30–100	Active	Hypersensitivity to chlordiazepoxide or any component of the formulation (cross-sensitivity with other benzodiazepines may also exist)
clonazepam	Klonopin	0.5–3	1–2	18–50	Inactive	Hypersensitivity to clonazepam or any component of the formulation (cross-sensitivity with other benzodiazepines may also exist), narrow-angle glaucoma
clorazepate	Tranxene	7.5–30	1–2	30–100	Active	Hypersensitivity to clorazepate or any component of the formulation (cross-sensitivity with other benzodiazepines may also exist), narrow-angle glaucoma
diazepam	Valium	6–40	0.5–1	30–100	Active	Hypersensitivity to diazepam or any component of the formulation (cross-sensitivity with other benzodiazepines may also exist), myasthenia gravis, severe respiratory insufficiency syndrome, severe hepatic insufficiency syndrome, sleep apnea syndrome, narrow-angle glaucoma

TABLE 41.3

Overview of Selected Drugs Used to Treat Generalized Anxiety Disorder (*Continued*)

Generic Name	Trade Name	Usual Adult Dosage Range (mg/d)	Oral Peak (h)	Half-Life (h) Parent + Active Metabolite	Metabolite Activity	Contraindications
lorazepam	Ativan	1–6	2–4	10–20	Inactive	Hypersensitivity to lorazepam or any component of the formulation (cross-sensitivity with other benzodiazepines may also exist), severe respiratory insufficiency syndrome (except during mechanical ventilation), sleep apnea syndrome (parenteral), narrow-angle glaucoma
oxazepam	Serax	15–120	2–4	8–12	Inactive	Hypersensitivity to oxazepam or any component of the formulation (cross-sensitivity with other benzodiazepines may also exist), narrow-angle glaucoma
buspirone	BuSpar	15–60	—	2–3	Active	Hypersensitivity to buspirone or any component of the formulation
hydroxyzine HCl hydroxyzine pamoate	Atarax Vistaril	75–150	2–4	3	Inactive	Hypersensitivity to hydroxyzine or any component of the formulation

Table is adapted from the following references: Arana, G. W., & Jerrold, R. (2000). *Handbook of psychiatric drug therapy* (4th ed., p. 176). Philadelphia, PA: Lippincott Williams & Wilkins; and Schatzberg, A. F., Cole, J. O., & DeBattista, C. (2010). *Manual of clinical psychopharmacology* (7th ed., pp. 382–384). Washington, DC: American Psychiatric Publishing.

On discontinuation of BZD therapy, relapse may occur. Longer-acting drugs, such as clonazepam, can minimize dose-rebound anxiety. Similarly, rapid-onset agents, such as diazepam or alprazolam, can provide acute anxiolysis, whereas short-acting agents such as lorazepam can minimize accumulation and oversedation. In the elderly, use of long-acting BZDs is discouraged because the active metabolites have a tendency to accumulate.

Tolerance and Dependence Issues

Tolerance to the sedative (but not anxiolytic) effects of BZDs develops at moderate doses. BZDs can cause dependence if used continuously for more than several weeks. If the patient's anxiety is episodic, episodic use of BZDs may control symptoms. If anxiety is prolonged, BZDs may control anxiety, but this therapeutic benefit must be weighed against their capacity to cause dependence. Abuse potential does not appear to be a problem in people who do not abuse alcohol or other substances. See "Monitoring Patient Response" for information on tapering technique and withdrawal issues.

Adverse Events

The major adverse events of BZDs are drowsiness and psychomotor impairment. Mild, transitory cognitive and memory impairments are seen occasionally. This is more significant in elderly people and those with high sensitivity to these drugs. Reactions of rage, excitement, and hostility, although rare, have been reported in children, the elderly, and brain-injured

patients. Other reported side effects include increased depression, confusion, headache, GI disturbances, menstrual irregularities, and changes in libido. Urticaria may occur in people with drug hypersensitivity, and drug interactions may occur with a variety of medications (**Table 41.4**).

Treatment of Benzodiazepine Overdose

Flumazenil (Mazicon) is a competitive BZD receptor antagonist that reverses the sedative effects of BZDs. Antagonism of BZD-induced respiratory depression is less predictable. Flumazenil is the only BZD receptor antagonist available for clinical use. It blocks many of the actions of BZDs but does not antagonize the CNS effects of other sedative–hypnotics such as ethanol, opioids, or general anesthetics. It is used for BZD overdose and after the use of drugs in anesthetic and diagnostic procedures. When given intravenously, it acts rapidly and has a short half-life (0.7 to 1.3 hours). Because all BZDs have a longer duration of action than flumazenil, sedation commonly recurs and repeated doses of flumazenil may be needed. Adverse effects of flumazenil include confusion, agitation, dizziness, and nausea.

Azapirones

Buspirone is a partial agonist at the 5-HT1A receptors and a full agonist at the presynaptic serotonergic autoreceptors. Though buspirone's effectiveness in treating GAD has been demonstrated inconsistently in several studies, its delayed onset of action, tolerability, and relative lack of efficacy with respect

TABLE 41.4

Benzodiazepine Drug Interactions

Drug	Interaction	Description	Management
Alcohol/CNS depressants	↑ BZD levels	Increased CNS effects (sedation, psycho-motor impairment)	Avoid combination
Antacids	↓ BZD levels	Antacids alter the rate but not the extent of GI absorption	Stagger administration times to avoid possible interaction
Azole antifungals (itra-conazole, ketocon-azole, voriconazole)	↑ BZD levels	Azole antifungals decrease the metabo-lism of BZDs, leading into increased CNS depression and sedation	Alprazolam is contraindicated with itraconazole and ketoconazole
Carbamazepine	↓ BZD levels	May increase hepatic metabolism and result in decreased pharmacologic effects	Consider increasing the benzodiazepine dose
Carisoprodol	↑ BZD levels	Increased depressant effects	Strong association between illicit use of carisoprodol, alprazolam, and oxycodone. Be vigilant for legitimacy of the prescriptions
Clozapine	↑ BZD levels	Increased risk of respiratory suppression, delirium, and ataxia	Do not start simultaneously. It may be better to add clozapine to an estab-lished BZD routine
Contraceptives, oral	The clearance rate of benzo-diazepines that undergo glucuronidation may be increased (lorazepam and oxazepam) May see decreased clear-ance and increased free concentrations of chlordiazepoxide, diazepam, and alprazolam, e.g., benzodiazepines that undergo oxidative metabolism		Monitor clinical effects
CYP3A4 inhibitors (cimetidine, diltia-zem, disulfiram, iso-niazid, omeprazole, macrolide antibiotics, metoprolol, proprano-lol, valproic acid)	↑ BZD levels	The elimination of benzodiazepines that undergo oxidative hepatic metabolism (alprazolam, chlordiazepoxide, clonaz-epam, diazepam) may be decreased by the following drugs due to inhibition of hepatic metabolism	May need dosage reduction
Digoxin		Digoxin serum concentrations may be increased	Monitor digoxin levels
Hydantoins (e.g., phenytoin)	↓ BZD levels	Serum concentrations of benzodiazepines may be decreased due to induction of hepatic metabolism by hydantoins. Pharmacologic effects of hydantoins may be increased by benzodiazepines	Monitor clinical effects carefully—consider monitoring serum levels of phenytoin
Probenecid	↑ BZD levels	Probenecid may interfere with benzodi-azepine conjugation in the liver, resulting in prolonged effect	Consider decreasing BZD dose

TABLE 41.4

Benzodiazepine Drug Interactions (*Continued*)

Drug	Interaction	Description	Management
Protease inhibitors (e.g., ritonavir, nelfinavir)	↑ BZD levels	May decrease the oxidative metabolism of benzodiazepines leading to severe sedation and respiratory depression	Decrease BZD dose
Ranitidine	↓ Diazepam	Ranitidine may reduce the GI absorption of diazepam	Stagger doses
Rifampin	↓ BZD levels	The oxidative metabolism may be increased due to enzyme induction. Pharmacologic effects of BZDs may be decreased	Monitor clinically
Sodium oxybate	↑ BZD levels	Concurrent use may result in an increase in sleep duration and CNS depression	Avoid combination
Theophylline	↓ BZD levels	Theophylline may antagonize the sedative effects of benzodiazepines	

to most comorbid conditions (with the exception of MDD) has resulted in buspirone being used primarily as adjunctive therapy. It has comparable but slightly weaker efficacy compared to diazepam, clorazepate, lorazepam, and alprazolam but has a clearly slower onset of action. Buspirone's utility is mainly associated with its propensity to relieve the cognitive aspects, but it lacks long-term efficacy, particularly in managing the behavioral and somatic manifestations. It is rapidly absorbed from the intestinal tract but undergoes extensive first-pass metabolism. People with liver dysfunction have a decreased clearance of buspirone. Buspirone has no hypnotic, anticonvulsant, or muscle relaxant properties. Patients taking buspirone do not acquire a cross-tolerance for alcohol or BZDs. It is generally well tolerated, with only a few patients experiencing adverse effects. When adverse effects do occur, they include nausea, dizziness, and headache (see **Table 41.3**). Doses over 70 mg have caused jitteriness and dysphoria.

In contrast to BZDs, buspirone's therapeutic effect may take 2 to 3 weeks. Because of its delayed effects, this drug is not useful in patients who need immediate relief from anxiety, and patient education is needed to enhance compliance with the medication regimen.

Novel Drugs

Recently, a number of novel entities and also existing medications not initially labeled for use in GAD have been evaluated. **Pregabalin** (Lyrica) has shown some promise in clinical trials, but does not have an indication for the treatment of any anxiety disorder. Two similarly designed randomized, placebo and active comparator-controlled double-blinded studies evaluated the efficacy of pregabalin versus lorazepam for the treatment of GAD. The pregabalin groups and the lorazepam group all experienced improvements by week 4 as compared to placebo, with no observed statistically significant differences among the active groups. Pregabalin at its highest study dose (600 mg) produced statistically superior reductions in the psychic and

somatic symptoms compared to placebo, whereas the lorazepam group only reached statistical significance versus placebo with respect to the somatic symptoms. The relative efficacy and early onset of effect of pregabalin versus commonly used BZDs have been established, and this may represent a new therapeutic intervention for GAD as both a monotherapy (after failure of an initial monotherapy) or as an augmentation strategy.

Monoamine Oxidase Inhibitors

MAO inhibitors are effective in controlling panic attacks in most patients with PD. Their effectiveness in GAD has not been explored because of the necessary dietary restrictions and dangerous drug interactions that make their use cumbersome.

Mechanism of Action

MAO inhibitors inhibit the breakdown of 5-HT and norepinephrine in the synaptic cleft. The most commonly used MAO inhibitor is **phenelzine** (Nardil), which is given in a dose range of 45 to 90 mg/d.

Adverse Events

MAO inhibitors have anticholinergic side effects such as blurred vision, dry mouth and other mucosal surfaces, constipation, urinary hesitancy, and tachycardia. Weight gain, insomnia, and sexual dysfunction frequently occur. Hypotension that is aggravated by postural changes may develop, but it usually diminishes in a few weeks. Palliative measures such as increased fluid intake, salt tablets, and low-dose fludrocortisone (Florinef) can be used to manage hypotension. The greatest danger with MAO inhibitors is hypertensive crisis, which can be caused by food or drug interaction and can result in cerebral hemorrhage and death. MAO inhibitors prevent the breakdown of monoamines, so the patient taking an MAO inhibitor must avoid sympathomimetic substances and foods that contain tyramine, such as cheese, liver, yogurt, yeast, soy sauce, red wine, and beer. For further information, see Chapter 40.

Other Antianxiety Medications

Hydroxyzines are sometimes used to relieve anxiety and tension associated with an anxiety state or as an adjunct in organic disease states with anxiety.

The use of hydroxyzine for long-term treatment of anxiety (more than 4 months) has not been assessed. **Hydroxyzine hydrochloride** (Atarax) and **hydroxyzine pamoate** (Vistaril) are drugs more commonly used for sedating patients before and after surgery and for managing pruritus, chronic urticaria, and atopic contact dermatitis. See **Table 41.3** for doses and adverse events.

Atypical Antipsychotics

The AAPs have been evaluated mostly for purposes of adjunctive therapy when patients do not respond to, are intolerant of, or do not fully remit with conventional therapies. None of the AAPs have labeled indications for any anxiety disorder, though some do as adjunctive treatments for major depressive disorder. Of the eight available AAPs, there are studies evaluating the benefit of five of them in GAD (**aripiprazole**, **quetiapine**, **risperidone**, **ziprasidone**, and **olanzapine**). Thus far, AAPs have mostly been studied in short-term trials as adjunctive therapies in treatment-resistant GAD; however, some monotherapy studies exist. The unfavorable side effect profiles limit their use as first-line long-term drug of choice.

Selecting the Most Appropriate Agent

General Anxiety Disorder

First-Line Therapy

SSRIs and SNRIs are considered drugs of choice for GAD. No evidence exists to support the superiority of any of these drugs individually; however, there are significant differences in adverse effects and drug interactions. Patients may have to try several SSRIs or SNRIs prior to realizing a therapeutic benefit balanced with appropriate tolerability.

Antidepressants all require several weeks to become effective, so BZDs may be given along with an antidepressant until it begins to work. Once this occurs, the patient is slowly tapered off the BZD. BZDs also have a role chronically for purposes of treating exacerbations of anxiety when quick relief is desired. BZDs are considered first-line therapy only for acute anxiety related to a time-limited stressor. The BZDs used most frequently are alprazolam, clonazepam, and diazepam. There is no evidence that one BZD is superior to another in this disorder. When choosing the specific BZD for treatment, the practitioner must consider the drug's onset of action and its half-life and the patient's metabolism (**Figure 41.1** and **Table 41.5**).

Second-Line Therapy

After confirmed failure or intolerance to multiple members of the SSRI and SNRI classes at appropriate doses for an appropriate period of time, imipramine or buspirone may be considered.

Buspirone may be more appropriate if sedation or psychomotor impairment would be dangerous. Buspirone differs from the SSRIs in its efficacy spectrum and side effect profile and has fewer adverse effects compared to BZDs and minimal abuse potential. However, the therapeutic effect of the drug may take 1 to 4 weeks. Buspirone may be the most appropriate drug for patients with a history of substance abuse, personality disorder, or sleep apnea.

Third-Line Therapy

Third-line therapy consists of a TCA alone or buspirone.

Fourth-Line Therapy

After the SSRIs, SNRIs, buspirone, and imipramine are exhausted; combination or adjunctive therapy may be considered. Practitioners may even consider combination or adjunctive therapy prior to attempting buspirone or imipramine (third line). Generally, buspirone, pregabalin (not approved for this indication in the United States), or an AAP (not approved for this indication in the United States) could be added to standard therapy in the event that a therapeutic effect is not realized with monotherapy. An SSRI or SNRI plus an AAP, an SSRI or SNRI plus an antihistamine (hydroxyzine), a combination of an SSRI and imipramine, or a combination of an SSRI and a BZD are all reasonable strategies.

Panic Disorder

First-Line Therapy

Nonpharmacologic therapy is especially critical in the treatment of PD. Patients need to be educated on the avoidance of substances that can precipitate panic attacks; these include caffeine, drugs of abuse, and nonprescription stimulants. CBT is associated with short-term improvement in symptoms.

PD is episodic, and patients with PD frequently do well with SSRIs or venlafaxine. Alprazolam (Xanax) is the only BZD that is approved by the U.S. Food and Drug Administration (FDA) for PD, but clonazepam or lorazepam can also be used. These drugs are used along with an SSRI if rapid relief from anxiety is needed and there is no history of substance abuse. The practitioner needs to monitor symptoms, assess for side effects, and gradually increase the dosages of SSRIs, venlafaxine, alprazolam, lorazepam, or clonazepam if needed (**Figure 41.2**).

Second-Line Therapy

Patients who do not respond to SSRIs may be changed to another SSRI or venlafaxine and monitored for effectiveness in decreasing panic attacks and controlling the severity of anxiety or panic symptoms while causing tolerable adverse events.

Third-Line Therapy

Patients who do not respond to venlafaxine or several SSRIs may be switched to yet another SSRI, imipramine, or an MAO inhibitor. MAO inhibitors can be very effective in controlling panic attacks. Before the patient begins therapy, however, the practitioner must assess his or her willingness to avoid the many tyramine-containing sympathomimetic drugs and foods, which can interact with MAO inhibitors to precipitate serious, life-threatening reactions. Washout periods are critical before beginning an MAO inhibitor due to the risk of serotonin syndrome. In addition, the patient should be referred to a psychiatrist for

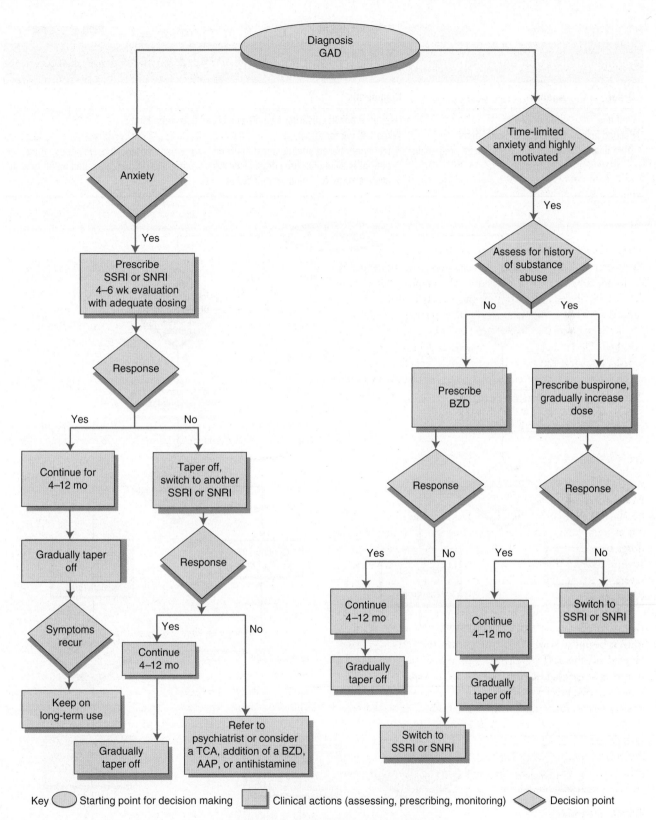

FIGURE 41.1 Treatment algorithm for GAD.

TABLE 41.5

Recommended Order of Long-Term Treatment for Generalized Anxiety Disorder

Order	Agents	Comments
First line	SSRI or SNRI	Useful for anxiety disorder as well as a coexisting comorbidity.
Second line	Buspirone or imipramine	Takes 1–2 wk for effect.
Third line	Adjunctive therapy with pregabalin, buspirone	Select agent based on drug onset, half-life, and patient metabolism. Do not use if the patient is alcohol or drug dependent. May be first-line drug in motivated patients with acute anxiety to a time-limited stress.

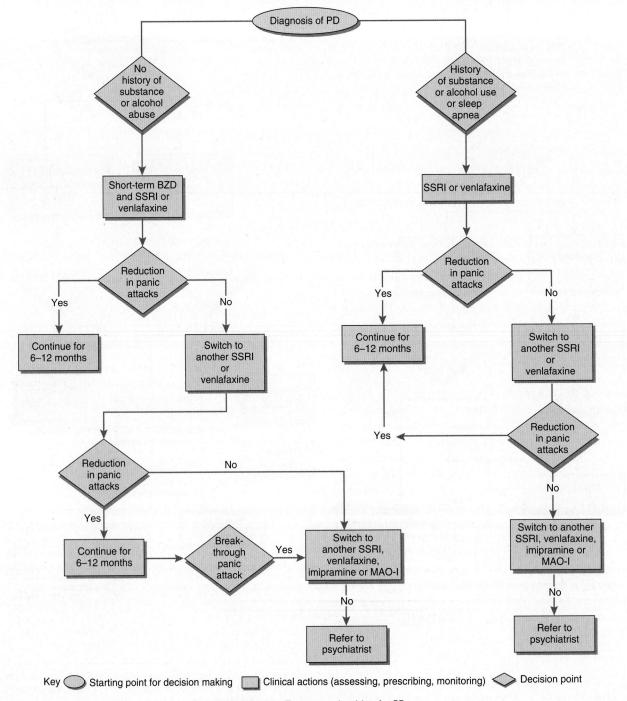

FIGURE 41.2   Treatment algorithm for PD.

intensive therapy, particularly if combination therapy is required. When a TCA is given for PD, approximately 33% of patients feel overstimulated when treatment begins. To reduce this problem, the patient may need to start with a lower dose and gradually increase the dose until a therapeutic dose response occurs. BZDs can be used on a short-term basis to lessen these initial symptoms. Because PD is episodic, it is considered a chronic condition that requires long-term management with TCAs. However, approximately 33% of patients on TCAs discontinue their treatment because they cannot tolerate the side effects of the drugs.

Social Anxiety Disorder (SAD, or Social Phobia)

Social anxiety disorder or social phobia is characterized by an intense, irrational fear of scrutiny or negative evaluation of others in social situations. In generalized SAD, fear and avoidance extend to various social situations, but in the specific form of socialized and anxiety disorder, fear and avoidance are confined to only one or two social situations, such as performing in public. Symptoms most commonly experienced include blushing, shaking, sweating, and heart palpitations.

First-Line Therapy

Generally, the SSRIs and venlafaxine are considered first-line therapies for SAD. Cognitive behavioral therapy is also a potential initial therapy along with a medication or as monotherapy.

Second-Line Therapy

After failure of cognitive behavioral therapy and an adequate trial of either an SSRI or venlafaxine, the MAO-I phenelzine can be attempted in selected patients (see **Figure 41.3**). Given the adverse effect profile, toxicity in overdose, and drug and food interaction potential, phenelzine should be reserved for refractory cases. **Table 41.6** summarizes drug therapy for GAD, PD, and SAD.

Special Population Considerations

Patients who have previously been treated for an anxiety disorder may have had drug treatment or psychotherapy that they found unsatisfactory. The practitioner should review with them what the treatments were, what adverse reactions they had, and the number of previous health care providers who treated them. Check with them for any history of drug withdrawal symptoms. If they report that a drug or treatment was unacceptable, plan a different but effective treatment. Assess for adverse effects to the new program. Also assess for drug-seeking behavior to rule out BZD dependence. Sometimes, patients "shop around" for new health care providers when their previous provider has advised withdrawing from BZDs.

Patients with a history of prescription medication abuse and substance or alcohol abuse can become drug dependent. Buspirone, a nonaddicting drug, is a choice for their treatment regimen.

Pediatric

Four BZDs—clorazepate, chlordiazepoxide, diazepam, and alprazolam—have been approved by the FDA for use in children. Doses vary according to the child's age and weight. Similar

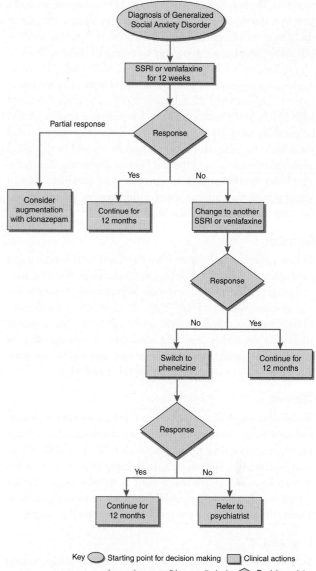

FIGURE 41.3 Treatment algorithm for social anxiety disorder.

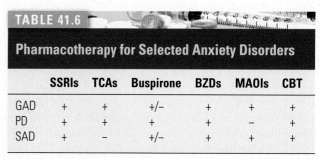

TABLE 41.6

Pharmacotherapy for Selected Anxiety Disorders

	SSRIs	TCAs	Buspirone	BZDs	MAOIs	CBT
GAD	+	+	+/−	+	+	+
PD	+	+	+	+	−	+
SAD	+	−	+/−	+	+	+

GAD, generalized anxiety disorder; PD, panic disorder; SAD, social anxiety disorder; SSRIs, selective serotonin reuptake inhibitors; TCAs, tricyclic antidepressants; BZDs, benzodiazepines; MAOIs, monoamine oxidase inhibitors; CBT, cognitive–behavioral therapy.

to adults, the first-line treatment for GAD in children are SSRI antidepressants. SNRI and TCA have also shown efficacy in the treatment of pediatric anxiety disorders but, due to their side effect profiles, are less easily tolerated. A meta-analysis of 16 randomized trials found a number of SSRI and SNRI antidepressants superior to placebo in the treatment of pediatric anxiety (Uthman and Abdulmalik, 2010). The risks associated with SSRIs/SNRI antidepressants for pediatric anxiety should be carefully weighed against their potential benefits whenever their use is considered. Risks and benefits should be discussed with both the parent and the child before beginning treatment. The FDA recommends close monitoring of the child's clinical status during the early weeks of antidepressant treatment and limiting the duration of their use.

Geriatric

Elderly patients may have decreased liver and renal function and metabolize and excrete drugs more slowly. They also may have neurologic disorders, cardiac disease, hypertension, hypotension, and glaucoma and may be taking drugs for these conditions. Elderly patients may be started on low doses of shorter-acting BZDs, TCAs, SSRIs, and buspirone, and the dosage may be gradually increased. Elderly patients may also experience paradoxical reactions to drugs (see **Tables 41.3 and 41.4**).

Women

Women are more likely than men to seek treatment for anxiety and depression. Women who are taking oral contraceptive drugs may have adverse drug interactions with BZDs (see **Table 41.4**). The practitioner needs to be alert for signs of anxiety disorders in men because they are not as likely as women to report these symptoms. Rather, men are likely to report physical signs of anxiety and not identify the problem as emotional in origin.

Pregnancy

Treatment considerations (to use or not to use antidepressants) during pregnancy *may* pose both maternal and fetal risks: risk of untreated depression or anxiety in the mother and the risk of teratogenicity, malformations, and low birth weight in the fetus, respectively. All antidepressants cross the placenta; however, this does not consistently equate with a risk of teratogenicity. Though somewhat contradictory and arguably not completely clear, some studies have found a modestly increased risk of fetal cardiovascular malformations in fetuses exposed to SSRIs in utero. Other studies have failed to demonstrate this increased risk and suggest that the risk of the aforementioned issues is consistent with that of the general, unexposed population. Thus far, SSRIs have not been associated with maternal complications with the exception of postpartum hemorrhage. The newest evidence, resulting from a large-scale meta-analysis, reveals that fluoxetine may cause fetal heart wall defects and craniosynostosis and paroxetine may cause fetal heart defects, anencephaly, and abdominal wall defects (Reefhuis et al., 2015). The SNRIs, trazodone, bupropion, and the TCAs are also not generally associated with teratogenicity. The observed cases of fetal defects seem to be dependent on the trimester; therefore, the potential risks associated with antidepressant use

during pregnancy vary over the course of the pregnancy. All of the antidepressants discussed in this chapter are pregnancy category C, with the exception of bupropion, which is category B, and paroxetine, which is category D.

The risks of not treating depression in pregnant patients include premature delivery, low birth weight, miscarriage, preeclampsia, and gestational hypertension. Unfortunately, pregnant patients sometimes self-discontinue their antidepressants due to a fear of harming their baby. This can lead to withdrawal in some cases and also rebound or worsened anxious symptoms. Fetal organs begin developing early in pregnancy, and therefore, a conversation as early as possible is recommended. The patient and practitioner need to design a plan that is acceptable for all parties and will minimize risks to the fetus as well as the patient.

Ethnic

Understanding a patient's cultural orientation or ethnic background is necessary for making a correct diagnosis and establishing an appropriate treatment plan. What we view as a problem such as anxiety or depression is not always perceived the same way by patients from other cultures. Complaints of anxiety or depression may not be reported by some patients because this is considered to be a mental disorder that is to be kept secret from people outside the family.

Research findings indicate that people from various racial or ethnic groups may metabolize some drugs differently because of their genetic makeup. An example of a drug that is metabolized differently is the antitubercular drug isoniazid (Laniazid). Researchers are beginning to examine other drug classifications for variations. Practitioners need to keep current with research that examines genetic differences in the metabolism of drugs (see Chapters 2 and 3).

Monitoring Patient Response

Patients need to be monitored for self-reports of decreased anxiety symptoms. The practitioner should monitor patients closely for compliance with the medication regimen as well as side effects.

Most side effects from SSRIs are transient. Dose-related sexual effects, such as decreased libido or delayed ejaculation in men and anorgasmia in women, are common and typically do not resolve without intervention. Management of treatment-related sexual dysfunction includes reducing the SSRI dosage reduction and adding or switching to an antidepressant not associated with sexual dysfunction, such as bupropion (Wellbutrin, Wellbutrin SR), nefazodone, or mirtazapine (Remeron). Another strategy includes the use of sildenafil (Viagra) or buspirone.

A non–life-threatening discontinuation syndrome of flu-like symptoms may occur after abrupt cessation of an SSRI. This syndrome can be minimized by gradually tapering the dose.

An overdose of TCAs can lead to anticholinergic delirium, ventricular arrhythmias, significant hypotension, seizures, and death. A TCA overdose is a medical emergency and requires close clinical and cardiac monitoring.

Many patients do not like buspirone because it takes 1 to 4 weeks to take effect. Frequently, patients stop taking this medication because they think it is not helping their symptoms. Patient education and monitoring for compliance must be ongoing.

There have been no well-documented fatal overdoses of BZDs, but deaths have resulted from the ingestion of multiple drugs and overdoses of BZDs and other drugs. Prolonged use of BZDs can lead to dependence and withdrawal on discontinuation. Although the duration of therapy is not standardized, most clinicians prescribe the medication for 4 to 6 months and then try decreasing the dosage; however, the relapse rate of anxiety is approximately 60% to 80% within the first year that the patient is off the medication.

There are three components of a withdrawal syndrome: relapse is the return of the original symptoms of anxiety, rebound is a return of symptoms at greater severity than originally experienced, and withdrawal is the appearance of new symptoms.

When a BZD is discontinued, the severity of the withdrawal syndrome depends on how rapidly the drug is tapered, the half-life of the drug, and the duration of therapy. The withdrawal syndrome increases in severity with increased dosage and duration of use: for instance, more patients experience withdrawal symptoms after taking a BZD for 8 months than those taking it for less than 3 months. Withdrawal is relatively infrequent with short-term use, but it can occur with therapy as brief as 3 weeks. Abrupt discontinuation is frequently associated with withdrawal, usually of greater severity. Therefore, the rate of discontinuation should be slowed to moderate the symptoms. Drugs with shorter half-lives are also more associated with withdrawal phenomena than those with longer half-lives. The tapering period should be at least 4 weeks, and the rate of tapering should be approximately a 10% dosage decrease every 3 to 4 days. **Box 41.5** lists BZD withdrawal symptoms.

Patients on long-term (more than 4 months) BZD therapy need periodic blood counts and liver and thyroid function testing. BZDs can cause elevations in lactate dehydrogenase, alkaline phosphatase, alanine aminotransferase, and aspartate aminotransferase levels. Use of BZDs may cause leukopenia, blood dyscrasias, anemia, thrombocytopenia, eosinophilia, and decreased uptake of I^{125} and I^{131} sodium iodide. (See **Table 41.3**; see also Chapter 40 for a discussion of monitoring concerns related to antidepressant medications.)

PATIENT EDUCATION

Drug Information

The patient should know the name of the drug prescribed, dose, frequency of administration, expected outcome of therapy, drug interactions, adverse events, and the amount of time it will take for the drug to take effect. The patient should also know how to report adverse events to the primary caregiver. The patient should be taught to take the drug as ordered and not to increase the dose or stop the drug without first contacting the primary care provider.

The patient should know that the therapeutic effect of the drug needs to be monitored and that the dosage may need to be increased or another drug may be more helpful. If laboratory tests are needed, the patient should know the name of the laboratory test, what the test is, and the frequency of monitoring. The patient also needs to tell all health care providers what medications he or she is taking.

The National Institutes of Health's Web site (www.nih.gov/medlineplus/anxiety.html) provides useful patient information, as does the Anxiety Disorder Association of America's Web site (www.adaa.org).

Lifestyle Information

The patient should know that the physical symptoms of anxiety (e.g., increased heart rate, palpitations, pupillary dilatation, trembling, increased perspiration, muscle tension, and sleep disturbances) are not life threatening. The practitioner should instruct the patient about how combination treatment consisting of medications, psychotherapy, and relaxation therapy can control anxiety. Instruction on performing relaxation exercises is helpful. The practitioner should describe the various psychotherapeutic modalities so that the patient may select the one thought to be most appropriate. If the patient does not seek psychotherapy, the primary caregiver may need to provide emotional support. The patient who does not respond well to drug and relaxation therapy must be referred to a psychiatric specialist.

Providing written instructions is important because the patient may have trouble concentrating on or fully comprehending verbal instructions. After providing all instructions and materials, the practitioner should review the patient's comprehension of the instructions and willingness to comply with the medication regimen. This review should be part of each patient visit.

BOX 41.5 Symptoms of Benzodiazepine Withdrawal

Frequent
Anxiety
Insomnia
Irritability
Muscle problems

Common
Nausea
Depression
Ataxia
Hyperreflexia
Blurred vision
Fatigue

Rare
Psychosis
Seizures
Delirium
Confusion

Adapted with permission from Schweizer, E., & Rickels, K. (1998). Benzodiazepine dependence and withdrawal: A review of the syndrome and its clinical management. *Acta Psychiatrica Scandinavica, Supplementum, 393*, 95–101. Copyright © John Wiley and Sons.

CASE STUDY*

L.P., age 23, is a white woman who graduated from college last year. She began working as an accountant 1 month after graduating. Approximately 2 months ago, she moved into a two-bedroom apartment with another woman who works at the same accounting firm. She states that her roommate recommended that she see a doctor to find out if she has anemia or "some sort of fatigue syndrome." She states that she has felt "restless" and "on edge" for most of the past 9 months. She becomes easily fatigued and irritable and has difficulty concentrating and falling asleep. She states that sometimes her mind "just goes blank," and she is worried that her work performance is no longer excellent. She reports that all her life she had good grades in school and was very successful in everything she attempted. Although she has been "a worrier from the day I was born," now she worries more than she ever has and feels nervous "all the time." **L.P.** reports that she has a good relationship with her boyfriend, but they do not get to see each other very often because he is attending graduate school 100 miles away. She reports having a satisfying sexual relationship with him. She denies having any problems with relationships with her parents, roommate, or peers. She denies having any financial worries unless she is fired from her job for poor work performance. She reports that she has always been healthy and has taken good care of herself. The only medication she takes is birth control pills, which she has taken for the past 4 years without any adverse effects.

DIAGNOSIS: GENERALIZED ANXIETY DISORDER

1. List specific treatment goals for **L.P.**
2. What drug therapy would you prescribe? Why?
3. What are the parameters for monitoring the success of the therapy?
4. Describe specific patient monitoring based on the prescribed therapy.
5. List one or two adverse reactions for the selected agent that would cause you to change therapy.
6. What would be the choice for second-line therapy?
7. What dietary and lifestyle changes should be recommended for this patient?
8. Describe one or two drug–drug or drug–food interactions for the selected agent.

* Answers can be found online.

Bibliography

**Starred references are cited in the text.*

*American Psychiatric Association. (2013). *Diagnostic and statistical manual of mental health disorders: DSM-5* (5th ed.). Washington, DC: American Psychiatric Publishing.

Baldwin, D. S., Anderson, I. M., Nutt, D. J., et al. (2014). Evidence-based pharmacological treatment of anxiety disorders, post-traumatic stress disorder and obsessive-compulsive disorder: A revision of the 2005 guidelines from the British Association for Psychopharmacology. *Journal of Psychopharmacology, 28*(5), 403–439.

Bandelow, B., Zohar, J., Hollander, E., et al.; WFSBP Task Force on Treatment Guidelines for Anxiety, Obsessive-Compulsive and Post-Traumatic Stress Disorders. (2008). World Federation of Societies of Biological Psychiatry (WFSBP) guidelines for the pharmacological treatment of anxiety, obsessive-compulsive and post-traumatic stress disorders—First revision. *World Journal of Biological Psychiatry, 9*(4), 248–312.

Bandelow, B., Sher, L., Bunevicius, R., et al.; WFSBP Task Force on Mental Disorders in Primary Care; WFSBP Task Force on Anxiety Disorders, OCD and PTSD. (2012). Guidelines for the pharmacological treatment of anxiety disorders, obsessive-compulsive disorder and posttraumatic stress disorder in primary care. *International Journal of Psychiatry in Clinical Practice, 16*(2), 77–84.

Bandelow, B., Boerner, J. R., Kasper, S., et al. (2013). The diagnosis and treatment of generalized anxiety disorder. *Deutsches Ärzteblatt International, 110*(17), 300–309.

Carleton, R. N. (2012). The intolerance of uncertainty construct in the context of anxiety disorders: Theoretical and practical perspectives. *Expert Review of Neurotherapeutics, 12*(8), 937–947.

Combs, H., & Markman, J. (2014). Anxiety disorders in primary care. *The Medical Clinics of North America, 98*(5), 1007–1023.

Dunsmoor, J. E., & Paz, R. (2015). Fear generalization and anxiety: Behavioral and neural mechanisms. *Biological Psychiatry.* pii: S0006-3223(15)00318-2. doi: 10.1016/j.biopsych.2015.04.010 [Epub ahead of print].

Duval, E. R., Javanbakht, A., & Liberzon, I. (2015). Neural circuits in anxiety and stress disorders: A focused review. *Therapeutics and Clinical Risk Management, 11*, 115–126.

Fava, G. A., Gatti, A., Belaise, C., et al. (2015). Withdrawal symptoms after selective serotonin reuptake inhibitor discontinuation: A systematic review. *Psychotherapy and Psychosomatics, 84*(2), 72–81.

Gadot, Y., & Koren, G. (2015). The use of antidepressants in pregnancy: Focus on maternal risks. *Journal of Obstetrics and Gynaecology Canada, 37*(1), 56–63.

Katzman, M. A. (2009). Current considerations in the treatment of generalized anxiety disorder. *CNS Drugs, 23*(2), 103–120.

Khan, A., Joyce, M., Atkinson, S., et al. (2011). A randomized, double-blind study of once-daily extended release quetiapine fumarate (quetiapine XR) monotherapy in patients with generalized anxiety disorder. *Journal of Clinical Psychopharmacology, 31*(4), 418–428.

Martin, E. I., Ressler, K. J., Binder, E., et al. (2009). The neurobiology of anxiety disorders: Brain imaging, genetics, and psychoneuroendocrinology. *The Psychiatric Clinics of North America, 32*(3), 549–575.

Nardi, A. E., Freire, R. C., Mochcovitch, M. D., et al. (2012). A randomized, naturalistic, parallel-group study for the long-term treatment of panic disorder with clonazepam or paroxetine. *Journal of Clinical Psychopharmacology, 32*(1), 120–126.

*Reefhuis, J., Devine, O., Friedman, J. M., et al.; National Birth Defects Prevention Study. (2015). Specific SSRIs and birth defects: bayesian analysis to interpret new data in the context of previous reports. *British Medical Journal, 351*, h3190.

Reinhold, J. A., Mandos, L. A., Rickels, K., et al. (2011). Pharmacological treatment of generalized anxiety disorder. *Expert Opinion on Pharmacotherapy, 12*(16), 2457–2467.

Rickels, K., Etemad, B., Khalid-Khan, S., et al. (2010). Time to relapse after 6 and 12 months' treatment of generalized anxiety disorder with venlafaxine extended release. *Archives of General Psychiatry, 67*(12), 1274–1281.

Rickels, K., Shiovitz, T. M., Ramey, T. S., et al. (2012). Adjunctive therapy with pregabalin in generalized anxiety disorder patients with partial response to SSRI or SNRI treatment. *International Clinical Psychopharmacology, 27*(3), 142–150.

Rickels, K., Etemad, B., Rynn, M. A., et al. (2013). Remission of generalized anxiety disorder after 6 months of open label treatment with venlafaxine XR. *Psychotherapy and Psychosomatics, 82*, 363–371.

Robinson, G. (2015). Controversies about the use of antidepressants in pregnancy. *Journal of Nervous and Mental Disease, 203*(3), 159–163.

Schweizer, E., & Rickels, K. (1998). Benzodiazepine dependence and withdrawal: A review of the syndrome and its clinical management. *Acta Psychiatrica Scandinavica Supplementum, 393*, 95–101.

Stein, D. J., Bandelow, B., Merideth, C., et al. (2011). Efficacy and tolerability of extended release quetiapine fumarate (quetiapine XR) monotherapy in patients with generalised anxiety disorder: An analysis of pooled data from three 8-week placebo-controlled studies. *Human Psychopharmacology, 26*(8), 614–628.

*Uthman, O. A., & Abdulmalik, J. (2010). Comparative efficacy and acceptability of pharmacotherapeutic agents for anxiety disorders in children and adolescents: A mixed treatment comparison meta-analysis. *Current Medical Research and Opinion, 26*(1), 53–59.

42

Insomnia and Sleep Disorders

Veronica F. Wilbur

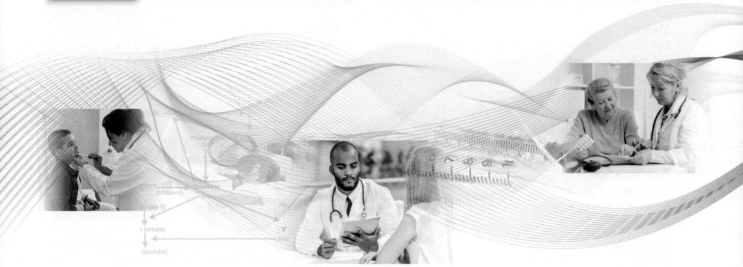

Sleep, a naturally recurring state of restfulness for the body, is a necessary element of our daily life and occurs in a daily rhythmic pattern. Sleep disorders can affect the quality of sleep and therefore how individuals function on a daily basis. Poor sleep can often be a symptom of other underlying physical or psychiatric problems. Sleep disorders include insomnia, snoring and sleep apnea, narcolepsy, and chronic sleep deprivation. Pharmacologic therapy is not appropriate for snoring and sleep apnea but has a role in the management of the other diagnoses. The key to an appropriate treatment plan is to recognize the type of sleep disorder.

INSOMNIA

Although most people occasionally have problems falling or staying asleep, insomnia can be defined as persistent trouble sleeping. Some experts argue, however, that problems sleeping at any time may be referred to as *insomnia*; they define the condition as loss of sleep for a short period. The loss of sleep may be due to physiologic causes such as restless leg syndrome, gastroesophageal reflux, or fibromyalgia, or sleep loss may simply be due to ignoring sleep cues. Sleep that is not refreshing also can be classified as insomnia. According to the Sleep in America Poll (The National Sleep Foundation, 2014), over 45% of respondents between ages of 18 and 64+ reported problems with sleep, but only 17% discussed their complaints with a health care professional. The 2014 Sleep Poll compared sleep complaints among African Americans, Whites, Asians, and Hispanics, finding variations in bedtime routines, meeting sleep needs, sleep partners, and general health related to sleep. Results also show that African Americans and Hispanics are more likely to have poor sleep. Complaints are more prevalent in women and increase with age,

especially in those over age 65; up to 67% of elderly people have frequent sleep problems, but only 17% are diagnosed and treated (The National Sleep Foundation, 2014).

Insomnia can have social and economic consequences, as measured through direct and indirect costs. The America Insomnia Survey (2012) estimated that the cost of sleep deprivation and sleep disorders equals 63.2 to 100 billion annually. This cost is seen in lost productivity, medical expenses, sick leave, and property and environmental damages (Rosekind et al., 2010). Up to 40% of people medicate themselves, commonly treating their insomnia with a host of over-the-counter (OTC) drugs and other remedies before seeking the help of a health care provider. In the United States, more than $1 billion is spent yearly on sleep medications. According to a more recent Sleep in America Poll, little has changed regarding these demographics since the early 1990s.

CAUSES

Insomnia can be of physiologic or psychological origin, and it is important to rule out the physiologic causes before labeling insomnia as psychological (**Box 42.1**). Changes in a patient's biological clock can contribute to insomnia (e.g., hyperarousal states, time zone, and schedule changes), as can the sleep environment. Estimates are that up to half of all cases of insomnia are psychological in origin. Previously, the *International Classification of Sleep Disorders,* second edition (2001) classified insomnia as primary or secondary; however, experts found it difficult to differentiate each category due to overlapping of symptoms and associated features. Therefore, the *International Classification of Sleep Disorders (ICSD),* third edition (2014), changed the categories to *chronic insomnia disorder, short-term*

721

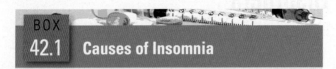

BOX 42.1   Causes of Insomnia

Medical
Cardiac problems (e.g., ischemia and congestive heart failure)
Endocrine problems (e.g., hypothyroidism, hyperthyroidism, degenerative disease)
Neurologic problems (e.g., stroke, degenerative conditions, dementia, peripheral nerve damage, myoclonic jerks, restless leg syndrome (Willis-Ekbom disease), hypnic jerk, and central sleep apnea)
Pulmonary problems (e.g., COPD, obstructive sleep apnea)
Renal problems (e.g., urinary frequency)
Pain

Psychiatric
Anxiety
Excess stress
Major depression
Maladaptive sleep habits
Sleep performance anxiety

Drug and alcohol abuse
Sedatives and stimulants

Primary sleep disorders
Excessive arousal and wakefulness
Poor sleep hygiene: related to lifestyle
Sleep state misperception: achievement of adequate sleep but not perceived by patient

BOX 42.2   Stages of Sleep

Stage I
Light NREM: dreamlike state and lasts a few minutes

Stage II
Relatively light NREM: fragmented thoughts and lasts 15–20 min

Stages III–IV
Deep NREM: lowering of blood pressure, cerebral glucose metabolism, heart rate, and respiratory rate, starts 35–40 min after falling asleep, and lasts 40–70 min

REM sleep
Starts after 90 min of sleep and lengthens toward the end of the night
This cycle alternates throughout the night at intervals of 90–100 min, four to six times per night.

Characteristics of chronic insomnia include somatized tension and acquired habits that prevent either the initiation or maintenance of sleep. Life stresses such as shift work, a family tragedy, or physical pain can exacerbate chronic insomnia. More recent neurobiologic research about insomnia points to a dysregulation of the neurotransmitters in the brain that regulate wakefulness, NREM, and REM sleep contributing to chronic insomnia. Insomnia can start with an initially stressful event, but the hyperarousal state of chronic insomniacs extends well beyond the heightened levels of stress.

Short-Term Insomnia Disorder

The prevalence among adults is 15% to 20% of the general population, more often in women than men and those who are older. Short-term insomnia has been previously classified as acute or adjustment insomnia. Diagnosis is similar to chronic insomnia, but with fewer question categories, see **Box 42.3**. The essential feature here is short-term difficulty initiating or maintaining sleep with general sleep dissatisfaction. Short-term insomnia can be in isolation or as a comorbid with mental disorders, medical conditions, or substance abuse (ICSD, 2014). Short-term insomnia is often related to environmental factors, such as sleeping in an unfamiliar place or excessive heat, noise, light, or movement of the bed partner. Additionally, short-term insomnia can be related to stress either positive or negative. Many features of short-term insomnia are shared with chronic insomnia with the primary difference of duration. Circadian rhythm disorders, jet lag, and rotating shift work should be considered in the differential.

Other Insomnia Disorders

The use of *other insomnia disorders* is reserved for those who have difficulty with initiating and maintaining sleep but do not meet the full criteria for either chronic or short-term

insomnia disorder, and *other insomnia disorder*. In general, insomnia is a serious problem that can adversely impact comorbid conditions. Whether insomnia is labeled as short term or chronic, Rosekind (2015) argued that insomnia is significant for any length of time and needs thoughtful evaluation and possible treatment. Finally, ICSD third edition standardizes the diagnostic criteria for all types of insomnia and does not differentiate between pediatric, adult, and geriatric populations.

Chronic Insomnia

The prevalence of chronic insomnia in the general public is between 10% and 35% and affects more women than men (ICSD, 2014). Previously classified as primary, secondary, or comorbid insomnia, chronic insomnia is a more accurate nomenclature due to difficulties with overlapping symptoms and features. To make the diagnosis of chronic insomnia, specific criteria assist the provider and help to define the features of the disorder (see **Box 42.2**). While all criteria are important for diagnosis, the most essential feature per the ISCD (2014) is frequent and persistent difficulty with initiating sleep and general sleep dissatisfaction.

- What kind of work does the patient do? Is there shift work involved, and which shift?
- What time does the patient go to bed?
- What kind of bed partner does the patient have (restless, still, wakeful sleeper), if any?
- Does the patient regularly take any prescription or over-the-counter drugs?
- How many times during the night does the patient awaken?
- What does the patient do if he or she cannot go to sleep?
- Does the patient take daytime naps?

insomnia. Other sleep disorders, such as restless leg syndrome (Willis-Ekbom disease) and obstructive sleep apnea, should be considered for patients within this category.

PATHOPHYSIOLOGY

To understand how insomnia develops, it is first necessary to understand the physiologic process of sleep. The brain seeks to balance alertness and sleepiness on a continuum between sleep debt, biological alerting, and environmental stimulation. Sleepiness is a function of the brain fighting to get enough sleep to cover the debt. This system of sleep debt versus sleep arousal is intricately linked to circadian rhythms and exposure to light. Additionally, various internally regulated biologic systems govern the circadian pattern of the sleep–wake cycle. The interaction of these biologic systems includes changes in body temperature, cardiac and renal functions, and hormone secretion throughout the day. The term *circadian* means "approximately 1 day" and refers to the fact that endogenous rhythms last approximately 24 hours.

Normal sleep is divided into two phases: rapid eye movement (REM) sleep and non-REM (NREM) sleep. During the REM stage, which accounts for approximately 20% of the sleep cycle, the brain is active and most dreaming occurs. NREM, which constitutes approximately 80% of the sleep cycle, is a phase of deep rest in which pulse, respiration, and brain activity all slow. NREM sleep can be divided into four phases. Stages I and II are called light NREM sleep. Stage I is the lightest sleep, and fleeting dreams often occur during the transition between the awake state and stage I. Stage II, which accounts for 50% of NREM sleep, lasts approximately 15 to 20 minutes and is characterized by fragmented thoughts with distinctive EEG changes. Hypnotics commonly increase stage II. Stages III and IV are called delta or deep NREM sleep. This stage begins after approximately 30 to 45 minutes and lasts 40 to 70 minutes. During stages III and IV, blood pressure, cerebral glucose metabolism, and heart and respiratory rates are at the lowest in the circadian cycle. The total sleep pattern begins with light NREM, by deep NREM, and then by REM. This cycle lasts approximately 90 to 100 minutes and occurs four to six times per night. **Box 42.2** summarizes the sleep stages.

Required amounts of sleep and of NREM sleep vary with age. Newborns sleep approximately 17 to 18 hours each day but have only two phases of sleep: NREM and REM. These two phases cycle every 60 minutes instead of every 90 minutes like adults. Children require 10 hours of sleep. In the early adult years, the total amount of sleep decreases to around 8 hours, which is normal for older adults as well as younger adults, with some variation among individuals. The total amount of REM sleep stays more constant at 15% to 20% throughout an adult's lifetime. Deep NREM sleep constitutes approximately 20% to 30% of total sleep in young children.

Insomnia is seen more often in people over age 65. The stages and architecture of sleep change, resulting in lighter stage II and decreases in stage III and IV sleep. This results in a decrease in deep NREM sleep. The circadian clock also becomes advanced, causing early morning awakening in the elderly.

Light cues are important in the process of sleep. The absence of light cues tends to promote longer sleep–wake cycles. Two peaks in the daily need for sleep have been identified: the first at bedtime and the second in midafternoon. A study by Regestein et al. (1993) suggested that insomniacs have higher daytime alertness compared with normal subjects, which leads to higher hyperarousal states. Desseilles et al. (2008) studied normal sleepers and found that sleep deprivation reduces metabolism in the prefrontal and parietal areas of the brain and produces a primary hyperarousal state. They concluded that insomniacs become more aware of small defects in the quality of sleep and daytime fatigue.

DIAGNOSTIC CRITERIA

Typical complaints of insomnia are malaise, fatigue, and too little sleep. These problems can lead to mild or moderate impairment in concentration and psychomotor abilities. The diagnosis is based on the patient's history, although a complete workup includes evaluating all potential medical and psychological causes. The practitioner must determine the onset and duration of symptoms, along with the patient's regular sleeping schedule and general quality of sleep. The practitioner should interview other family members and significant others regarding any psychiatric or substance abuse problems. If the patient does not sleep alone, the practitioner also should elicit information from the bed partner. Questions about sleep also should be included in the review of systems; **Box 42.4** lists suggested questions.

A complete physical examination is important to rule out medical causes of insomnia. Insomnia can be drug related (e.g., stimulating medications or alcohol). Finally, the practitioner should investigate psychiatric causes of insomnia.

The use of sleep questionnaires or diaries and screening tools for depression and anxiety can add to the evaluation of insomnia. Sleep patterns may be measured by using a special wristwatch that measures wrist movements, a process called

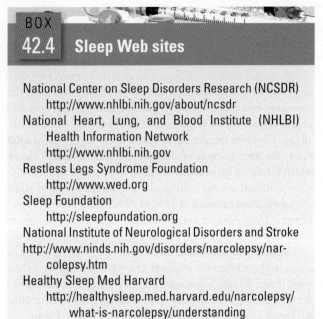

BOX 42.4 Sleep Web sites

National Center on Sleep Disorders Research (NCSDR)
    http://www.nhlbi.nih.gov/about/ncsdr
National Heart, Lung, and Blood Institute (NHLBI)
    Health Information Network
    http://www.nhlbi.nih.gov
Restless Legs Syndrome Foundation
    http://www.wed.org
Sleep Foundation
    http://sleepfoundation.org
National Institute of Neurological Disorders and Stroke
http://www.ninds.nih.gov/disorders/narcolepsy/nar-
    colepsy.htm
Healthy Sleep Med Harvard
    http://healthysleep.med.harvard.edu/narcolepsy/
        what-is-narcolepsy/understanding

actigraphy. In humans, movement of the wrist throughout the night is much less frequent than during the day, which enables the practitioner to estimate the patient's sleep and wake times. This tool, however, is not very accurate in assessing total sleep time of insomniacs. Polysomnography (all-night monitoring of EEG, respiration, muscle activity, and other physiologic parameters) may reveal shallow sleep that is fragmented by multiple arousals. If the patient is depressed, the polysomnogram manifests changes in the REM latency stage. Polysomnograms are indicated when the primary suspected cause of insomnia is sleep apnea. The American Sleep Disorders Association, however, does not recommend the routine use of polysomnography because a patient may not sleep normally at a sleep disorder center.

INITIATING DRUG THERAPY

In combination with behavioral management, the practitioner can consider using certain pharmacologic agents, but only with caution. According to the most recent clinical guidelines for evaluation and management of sleep (Schutte-Rodin et al., 2008), hypnotics should be used at the lowest dose for the shortest time. There is a potential for the drugs that treat insomnia to be habit forming; therefore, it should be used only for brief periods.

A wide range of therapies may be necessary to treat insomnia, because multiple causes of insomnia are the rule rather than the exception. Nonpharmacologic therapy includes evaluating for the key causes and treating with the appropriate intervention first: counseling, behavioral management, and lifestyle alterations for psychiatric problems. Patients with insomnia often have major depression, anxiety, obsessive disorders, or dysthymic disorders, and psychotherapy needs to focus on the specific psychiatric disorder.

Adjunctive to drug therapy, reviewing proper sleep hygiene can enhance the patient's sleep pattern. A thorough examination of sleep hygiene issues can help identify important lifestyle changes that may enhance sleep, and its importance should not be underestimated. The practitioner should implement only one or two behavioral changes at a time. Follow-up and a strong patient–provider relationship are key. Additional measures, such as exposure to bright light, may help those with circadian rhythm disturbances. Light therapy can retrain the light pacemaker and may be effective for night-shift workers, travelers, and those with delayed or advanced sleep phase disorders.

Goals of Drug Therapy

There are two goals of pharmacotherapy. The first goal is to improve sleep quality and quantity, and the second goal is to improve the insomnia-related daytime impairment. The selection of drugs is based on matching the onset and duration to the sleep defect. If given in adequate doses, all hypnotics promote sleep, and the key is to determine the *minimal* dose that will provide efficacy with few or no side effects. Factors in selecting a pharmacologic agent should be directed by (1) symptom pattern, (2) treatment goals, (3) past treatment responses, (4) patient preference, (5) cost, (6) medication interactions, and (7) side effects. An additional goal of pharmacologic treatment is to achieve a favorable balance between therapeutic effects and potential side effects (Schutte-Rodin et al., 2008).

Hypnotics are the primary drugs used for insomnia, including benzodiazepines and benzodiazepine receptor agonists. Other drugs utilized to treat insomnia are orexin receptor agonists, melatonin receptor agonist, and first-generation antihistamines. Some sedating antidepressants are useful if the patient has comorbid depression. The practitioner should carefully consider selection of a hypnotic and prescribe use for as short a time as possible. Short-term use is defined as no more than 2 to 3 weeks combined with behavioral interventions; however, specific patients require occasional chronic hypnotic therapy. They may need to use a hypnotic agent two or three times a week over longer periods than 2 to 3 weeks. Further, it is important to wean patients off of hypnotics when not needed due to rebound effects. Careless use of sedative–hypnotics can be dangerous in patients with sleep apnea or a history of substance abuse.

Benzodiazepines

Benzodiazepines are synthetically produced sedative–hypnotics. This group of structurally related chemicals selectively acts on polysynaptic neuronal pathways throughout the CNS. Benzodiazepines appear to enhance the effects of gamma-aminobutyric acid (GABA) in the ascending reticular activating system, which increases inhibition and blocks thalamic, hypothalamic, and limbic arousal.

When choosing a benzodiazepine, the practitioner should select an agent with an onset of action that matches the patient's complaint yet has a short duration of effect, lacks rebound insomnia, and causes few or no cognitive problems (e.g., hangover, lack of motor coordination, or memory disturbance) (see **Table 42.1**). The prescriber also should consider

TABLE 42.1

Overview of Selected Drugs Used to Treat Insomnia

Generic (Trade) Name and Dosage	Selected Adverse Events	Contraindications	Special Considerations
Benzodiazepines			
alprazolam (Xanax) tablets 0.25, 0.5, 1, 2 mg Start: 0.25–0.5 mg PO tid; maximum 4 mg/d in divided doses Range: 0.25–2 mg tid–qd	*CNS:* transient mild drowsiness, sedation, depression, lethargy, apathy, fatigue, light-headedness, disorientation, headache, mild paradoxical excitatory reaction in first 2 wk *GI:* constipation, diarrhea, dry mouth, nausea	Hypersensitivity to benzodiazepines, acute narrow-angle glaucoma, pregnancy, lactation	Use cautiously with impaired liver or kidney function Drug dependence and withdrawal result when abruptly discontinued, especially when used for longer than 4 mo Use cautiously with elderly patients and gradually increase as tolerated
estazolam (ProSom) tablets 1, 2 mg Start: 0.5–1 mg qhs Range: 0.5–2 mg qhs	*CNS:* transient mild drowsiness, sedation lethargy, apathy, fatigue, light-headedness, asthenia, mild paradoxical excitatory reaction in first 2 wk *GI:* constipation, diarrhea, dyspepsia *CV:* bradycardia, tachycardia *GU:* incontinence, urinary retention, changes in libido	Same as above	In addition to above, drug–drug interactions: increased CNS depression with ethanol, omeprazole; increased effects of estazolam with cimetidine, increased sedative effects of estazolam with theophylline Drug dependence, withdrawal syndrome
flurazepam (Dalmane) 15–30 mg PO qhs Start: 15 mg PO qhs Range: 15–30 mg PO qhs	*CNS:* transient mild drowsiness, sedation lethargy, apathy, fatigue, light-headedness, asthenia *GI:* constipation, diarrhea, dyspepsia *CV:* bradycardia, tachycardia *GU:* incontinence, urinary retention, changes in libido	Same as above	Same as above Has a long half-life
lorazepam (Ativan) 2–4 mg PO qhs	*CNS:* transient mild drowsiness, sedation, depression, lethargy, apathy, fatigue, light-headedness, disorientation, headache, mild paradoxical excitatory reaction in first 2 wk *GI:* constipation, diarrhea, dry mouth, nausea	Same as above	Use cautiously with patients with impaired liver or kidney function Debilitation, drug dependence, and withdrawal result when abruptly discontinued, especially when used for more than 4 mo Use cautiously with elderly patients and gradually increase as tolerated
quazepam (Doral) 7.5–15 mg PO qhs	*CNS:* transient mild drowsiness, sedation, depression, lethargy, apathy, fatigue, light-headedness, disorientation, restlessness, confusion *GI:* constipation, diarrhea *CV:* bradycardia, tachycardia *GU:* incontinence, urinary retention, changes in libido	Same as above	Drug–drug interactions: increased CNS depression with ethanol, quazepam; increased effects of cimetidine, disulfiram, oral contraceptives; increased sedative effects with theophylline
temazepam (Restoril) Start: 15 mg PO qhs Range: 15–30 mg PO qhs	Same as above	Same as above	Drug–drug interactions: increased CNS depression; increased sedative effects with theophylline
triazolam (Halcion) Start: 0.125 mg PO qhs Range: 0.125–0.5 mg PO qhs Elderly: 0.125–0.25 mg PO qhs	Same as above	Hypersensitivity to benzodiazepines, acute narrow angle glaucoma, pregnancy, lactation	Same as above

(Continued)

TABLE 42.1

Overview of Selected Drugs Used to Treat Insomnia (*Continued*)

Generic (Trade) Name and Dosage	Selected Adverse Events	Contraindications	Special Considerations
Benzodiazepine Receptor Agonist			
eszopiclone (Lunesta) Start: 1–2 mg PO qhs Range: 1–3 mg Elderly: start at 1 mg	*CNS:* morning drowsiness, headache, dizziness *GI:* nausea	Hypersensitivity to eszopiclone	Caution in patients taking strong inhibitors or inducers of CYP3A4
zolpidem (Ambien, Ambien CR) Ambien Start: 10 mg PO qhs Range: 5–10 mg PO qhs Ambien CR *Female:* 6.25 mg PO qhs; max 12.5 mg *Male:* 6.25–12.5 mg PO qhs	*CNS:* morning drowsiness, hangover, headache, dizziness, suppression of REM sleep *GI:* nausea Same as above Same as above	Hypersensitivity to zolpidem Use with sodium oxybate (Xyrem)	Use cautiously in patients with acute intermittent porphyria, impaired hepatic or renal function, in addiction-prone patients, and in pregnancy and lactation Useful for patients with problems falling asleep and middle night awakening
zolpidem tartrate (Intermezzo) Starting: 3.75 mg SL Elderly: 1.75 mg SL			Pregnancy category C Used for middle night awakening but must have more than 4 h to sleep Caution with elderly and hepatic impairment
zaleplon (Sonata) Start: 10 mg PO qhs Range: 5–20 mg PO qhs	*General:* back pain, chest pain *CV:* migraine *GI:* constipation, dry mouth *MS:* arthritis *CNS:* depression, hypertonia, nervousness *Derm:* rash, pruritus	Pregnancy, lactation	Pregnancy category C Patient must use just before bedtime because of quick onset
Orexin Receptor Antagonist			
Suvorexant (Belsomra) Start: 10 mg PO within 30 min of bed Maximum: 20 mg	Most common side effects were somnolence, headache, dizziness	Obese women have increased side effects Care with patients with respiratory compromise	Risk of impaired alertness and motor coordination Must have 7 h to sleep Re-evaluate for persistent insomnia after 7–10 d treatment Caution with depression

the patient's metabolic requirements. Benzodiazepines can be categorized as short acting, intermediate acting, and long acting as defined by the pharmacokinetic characteristics. The most commonly used short-acting agent was triazolam, but now, it is not commonly used due to high incidence of rebound insomnia even after using only a short time, as well as neuropsychiatric adverse effects. Temazepam and lorazepam are examples of intermediate-acting agents, with flurazepam in the long-acting category. When a drug has a longer half-life, there is greater potential for untoward effects such as excessive residual sedation or dizziness. Agents with short-term effects and rapid onset are best for patients who have difficulty falling asleep. Agents with intermediate onsets and usually longer half-lives are useful for patients with sleep maintenance issues. These include temazepam (Restoril) and estazolam (ProSom). Two agents with a rapid onset of action, flurazepam and quazepam, assist with falling asleep and also have a longer duration of action, which can assist in maintaining sleep.

Adverse Events

Benzodiazepines have various actions, depending on their half-lives and affinity for the receptor. Drugs of this class can produce drowsiness and impaired motor function, which may be persistent due to metabolites and subsequent hepatic and renal accumulation. Other side effects can include short-term memory loss, confusion, and shakiness. Prolonged use of benzodiazepines can lead to physical dependency; abrupt discontinuance can trigger withdrawal symptoms. Drugs in this category are all classified as controlled substances due to having a potential for addiction in addition to the physical dependency. The newer agents in the class have fewer side effects, but caution should still be exercised when prescribing, and for optimal therapy, the drug selected should address the patient's specific sleep problem.

Interactions

Patients taking benzodiazepines must be cautious with the concomitant use of alcohol. Use of low-dose contraceptives may slightly decrease clearance of lorazepam and temazepam; the patient may need to alter the dosage or switch to oxazepam. Use of erythromycin (E-mycin) can decrease triazolam clearance by 50%; thus, prescribers must consider reducing the dosage of triazolam in patients taking both drugs concomitantly.

Benzodiazepine Receptor Agonists

This class of hypnotic was developed to improve the safety profile of the barbiturate-type and longer-acting benzodiazepine compounds. Benzodiazepine receptor agonists (BRZA) pharmacologically are similar to benzodiazepines but instead mimic the action of GABA, an inhibitory transmitter, which induces sleepiness. The difference between BZD and BRZA is which GABA-A receptor subunits are affected. BZDs act on the subunit of alpha-1, alpha-2, and alpha-3, while BZRAs are selective for alpha-1, which induces sleepiness but not anxiolysis or muscle relaxation. Initially, benzodiazepine receptor agonists (BZRA) were thought to have one of the safest profiles with little or no long-term side effects; however, with more experience,

this proved not to be so. There is some evidence that long-term use of these drugs can alter sleep architecture (Mazza et al., 2014) as well as worsen Alzheimer dementia (Billioti de Gage et al., 2014). Complex sleep-related behaviors, defined as completing activities in an altered state of consciousness, also have been reported with the BZRAs. These activities include sleep walking or eating and driving a car. Some other side effects of this class include decreased motor coordination, confusion, and anterograde amnesia, which were all thought to be less than BZDs.

Eszopiclone

Eszopiclone (Lunesta) is a benzodiazepine receptor agonist indicated for the treatment of insomnia.

Mechanism of Action

While the exact mechanism of action is unknown, eszopiclone is thought to work by interacting with GABA receptors located near benzodiazepine receptors and thus shares some of the same pharmacologic properties. It is classified as a Schedule IV controlled substance.

Dosage

For nonelderly adults, eszopiclone should be started at 2 mg immediately before retiring for bed. The dose may be started or increased to 3 mg to aid in sleep maintenance. For elderly patients, the doses should be started at 1 mg to help patients fall asleep and 2 mg if sleep maintenance is the issue. Limited use of the 3-mg dose is recommended due to impairment of driving ability, coordination, and memory for over 11 hours, even if patients do not realize it (PL-Detail Document, 2014)

Time Frame for Response

The onset of action is rapid, with a peak plasma concentration occurring within 1 hour of dosing. This peak concentration can be delayed if eszopiclone is taken with or shortly after a high-fat meal.

Contraindications

There are no known contraindications to eszopiclone. However, patients should be cautioned against the concomitant use of alcohol due to the sedative effects and the potential for enhancing anterograde amnesia.

Adverse Events

Headache, dry mouth, dizziness, respiratory system infections, and unpleasant taste have occurred in patients taking 2- to 3-mg doses of eszopiclone.

Interactions

Eszopiclone is metabolized by the cytochrome P (CYP) 3A4 enzyme system. Therefore, agents that inhibit (e.g., ketoconazole) or induce (e.g., rifampin) this system will affect eszopiclone metabolism.

Zolpidem

Zolpidem tartrate (Ambien), extended-release zolpidem tartrate (Ambien CR), sublingual zolpidem tartrate (Intermezzo), and zolpidem tartrate oral solution (Zolpimist) are also benzodiazepine receptor agonist products.

Mechanism of Action

Zolpidem is also thought to modulate the GABA-A receptors, and further postulation is that it modulates the chloride channel macromolecular complex responsible for sedative, anticonvulsant, anxiolytic, and myorelaxant drug properties, therefore, causing sedation and relaxation. Zolpidem has a strong hypnotic component and improves the overall quality of sleep while producing less daytime impairment than other hypnotics. The onset of action of zolpidem is rapid; however, regular-release zolpidem peaks quickly while extended-release zolpidem has a biphasic release assisting with sleep onset and sleep maintenance. Zolpidem has no anxiolytic effects, which makes it less desirable for patients with concomitant anxiety. These drugs are also controlled substances (class IV) due to the potential for abuse.

Dosage

Starting doses of zolpidem are lower for females than males. Zolpidem is started at 5 mg for females and 10 mg for males, while extended-release zolpidem starts at 6.25 mg for females and 12.5 mg for males. Dosing can be increased but with the understanding this increases the potential for side effects. Dosing should be altered for patients with hepatic impairment but is not necessary for those who are renally impaired.

Time Frame for Response

Onset of action for zolpidem is 10 to 15 minutes of administration and last for 2 to 3 hours. Extended-release zolpidem has the same onset, but 60% is initially released with the remaining over the next 6 to 8 hours. The sublingual and oral solution products are taken immediately prior to bedtime as their onset of action is rapid.

Contraindications

Contraindications to zolpidem include anaphylactic reactions and angioedema. In addition, the FDA (1/10/2013) put forth a safety communication bulletin that patients should be cautioned about complex behaviors that include sleep-driving activities and other activities.

Adverse Events

The most common adverse events for both drugs are drowsiness, headache, and dizziness. The incidence of complex sleep behaviors can affect up to 15% of those taking zolpidem.

Interactions

Care should be exercised when prescribing zolpidem with other central nervous system drugs that have depressive effects. Other drugs that inhibit the CYP3A4 isoenzymes may increase the exposure to zolpidem.

Zaleplon

Another benzodiazepine receptor agonist is zaleplon (Sonata), which is chemically unrelated to benzodiazepines, barbiturates, and other drugs with hypnotic properties.

Mechanism of Action

Zaleplon is known to interact with the GABA-BZ omega 1 receptor, which causes sedation; however, there are no myorelaxant, anxiolytic, or anticonvulsant properties. This interaction is also hypothesized to be responsible for the pharmacologic properties of benzodiazepines. Zaleplon works well for patients who have difficulty falling asleep. It may not be the agent of choice for patients who have difficulty maintaining sleep because of its short elimination half-life. However, provided that at least 4 hours of sleep remains, this drug can be dosed a second time when patients have a nighttime awakening.

Dosage

The dose of zaleplon should be individualized and can range from 5 to 20 mg. The risk of adverse effects is dose dependent.

Time Frame for Response

The onset of action is rapid, within 1 hour after oral administration, but the medication has a short half-life of 1 hour. Zaleplon can be taken as little as 5 hours before the scheduled wake-up time, with no lingering effects of daytime sedation.

Contraindications

Hypersensitivity and severe hepatic impairment are contraindications to use of zaleplon. Dose adjustment is not necessary for renal impairment.

Adverse Events

Headache is the most commonly reported adverse event followed by dizziness, nausea, and abdominal pain. Postmarketing reports include anaphylaxis and nightmares. Other adverse effects include depression, amnesia, and sleep-related activities.

Interactions

Zaleplon is contraindicated in concomitant use with sodium oxybate (Xyrem) and any type of fentanyl or valerian. Close monitoring is required with use of drugs that are metabolized by the CYP3A4 isoenzyme of the cytochrome P450 system.

Orexin Receptor Antagonists

Orexin receptor antagonists are a new class in the treatment of insomnia. The only agent in the class is suvorexant (Belsomra).

Mechanism of Action

The hypothalamic neuropeptide orexin system was discovered in 1998 and the influence on sleep–wake cycle (De Lecea et al., 1998; Sakurai et al., 1998). Orexin neuropeptides (orexin-A and orexin-B) are found in the hypothalamus and other areas of the brain and perform a role in arousal, appetite, metabolism, reward, stress, and autonomic function (Dubey et al., 2015). Early study of the orexin system discovered that blockage resulted in severe sleepiness, which established the role of orexin in wakefulness. Suvorexant is a selective dual orexin receptor agonist (DORA) with a binding mechanism to both orexin receptors, thus inhibiting the arousal system. Through this inhibitory action, sleep induction and maintenance are facilitated. Suvorexant has been studied for over 1 year showing favorable outcomes and lack of physical dependence and withdrawal syndrome on continuation (Michelson et al., 2014).

Dosage

The starting dose for suvorexant is 10 mg and can be increased to a maximum of 20 mg. For patients taking other drugs that inhibit the CYP3A4 isoenzyme, suvorexant should start at

5 mg and go no higher than 10 mg. Administration should occur within 30 minutes of bedtime, and patients need to have at least 7 hours of planned sleep due to potential complex sleep behaviors. Dose adjustment for hepatic and renal impairment is not required.

Time Frame for Response

Onset of action occurs within 30 minutes of administration with peak concentrations in 2 hours. Suvorexant can last up to 6 hours.

Contraindications

Suvorexant is contraindicated with narcolepsy, alcohol use, and hypersensitivity to the class. Caution should be used with obese female patient, depression, concomitant use of other CNS depressants, and impaired respiratory function.

Adverse Events

The most common adverse reactions to suvorexant include headache, somnolence, and dizziness.

Interactions

Drugs that are CYP3A inhibitors such as ketoconazole and clarithromycin are not recommended for concomitant use. Additionally, drugs that are CPY3A inducers, carbamazepine and phenytoin, may reduce the efficacy of suvorexant.

Melatonin Receptor Agonists

Ramelteon (Rozerem) was introduced as an option to treat insomnia in 2005. There are a few drugs in this class; however, it is the only one approved by the FDA for use in the United States. To illustrate the efficacy of ramelteon, a study of 110 healthy subjects randomized to placebo versus ramelteon (Rozerem) was done; results of the study showed a significant decrease in sleep latency in the ramelteon group (Zee et al., 2010).

Mechanism of Action

Endogenous melatonin is secreted from the pineal gland and regulates the circadian sleep cycle, which is found in the suprachiasmatic nucleus (SCN) of the hypothalamus. Secretion of melatonin signals the timing of darkness via specific receptors (MT_1 and MT_2) and decreases neural firing to the SCN. Ramelteon is a synthetic derivative that has high selectivity and affinity for the MT_1 and MT_2 receptors, which block the receptors and shorten the latency to sleep onset. It does not affect other sleep neurotransmitters such as GABA, dopamine, or serotonin.

Dosage

The dose for ramelteon is 8 mg and should be administered within 30 minutes of going to bed. Avoid administration with a high-fat meal.

Time Frame for Response

Onset of action for ramelteon is within 45 minutes and half-life is 1 to 2.6 hours. There are no accumulating effects with repeated use of ramelteon due to the short half-life.

Administration with a high-fat meal can increase the area under the curve (total exposure).

Contraindications

Ramelteon is contraindicated for patients with hypersensitivity to the class, severe sleep apnea, severe hepatic impairment, and angioedema. Caution should be exercised with mild to moderate hepatic impairment, depression, and severe chronic obstructive pulmonary disease.

Adverse Events

The most common adverse reactions include somnolence, dizziness, fatigue, nausea, and exacerbated insomnia.

Interactions

Ramelteon interacts with rifampin, ketoconazole, fluconazole, donepezil, doxepin, and alcohol.

Antihistamines

Antihistamines are one of the most commonly used classes of OTC sleep-inducing agents. These drugs often come in combination with analgesics such as acetaminophen and ibuprofen. One of the most commonly used agents is diphenhydramine (Benadryl). The main mechanism of diphenhydramine is to competitively inhibit histamine at the H_1 receptor with substantial sedative and anticholinergic effects. No scientific evidence exists in the literature supporting the use of diphenhydramine to relieve insomnia or prolong sleep.

Some side effects of diphenhydramine include excessive daytime drowsiness, impaired psychomotor function, and increasing tolerance to the drug. A better approach may be to use one of the sedating antidepressants before using a trial of diphenhydramine. If a patient taking diphenhydramine is stopped while driving under the influence (DUI) of antihistamines, in many states, he or she can be charged with DUI.

Another first-generation antihistamine agent used for insomnia is doxylamine succinate (Unisom). The mechanism of action is to competitively inhibit histamine at the H_1 receptor with substantial sedative and anticholinergic effects. As an OTC sedative, doxylamine succinate is stronger in the effects of sedation and anticholinergic pharmacodynamics than diphenhydramine. The only formulation of the brand Unisom that contains doxylamine succinate is Unisom SleepTabs, and all other delivery methods, gel caps, minis, liquid, and combination with analgesic, contain diphenhydramine. Precautions also include excessive drowsiness can affect coordination, therefore impairing psychomotor coordination.

Antidepressants

Sedating antidepressants also may be used in the treatment of insomnia, but only for patients with comorbid depression. The most commonly used antidepressants in this category are mirtazapine (Remeron), trazodone, and doxepin (Silenor). If the patient has comorbid panic or anxiety, some newer agents may assist with sleep. This includes trazodone, which also has some sedating as well as antianxiety effects (see Chapter 40).

Selecting the Most Appropriate Agent

As previously discussed, the goal of therapy is to improve sleep quality and quantity along with improvement of insomnia-related daytime impairments. Additionally, selection of the appropriate agent is directed by symptom pattern, treatment goals, past treatment responses, patient preference, and cost, availability of other treatments, comorbid conditions, contraindications, concurrent medication interactions, and side effects. For treatment of short-term insomnia, the suggested duration of hypnotic use is 10 to 14 days, but some patients may need a longer course. Practitioners should schedule follow-up visits to monitor the effectiveness of therapy. The time between follow-up visits can vary, but in general, they should fall between every 1 and 2 weeks. Starting the medication at the lowest possible dosage is always a good practice and should minimize side effects. The practitioner should ask the patient about the effects the drug is having on sleep and daytime functioning. Changes may exist with dreaming, learning, memory, and adaptation to stress. Having the patient complete and bring in a sleep log for review can help pinpoint initial management needs and can continue to assist with evaluation for signs of improvement (**Table 42.2** and **Figure 42.1**). Pharmacologic therapy should be associated with patient education and cognitive therapy (Schutte-Rodin et al., 2008).

First-Line Therapy

As stated previously, the key to pharmacologic therapy is identifying the sleep defect. The practitioner should match the patient's need for an agent to both the classification of insomnia and the aspect of sleep that is altered. The recommended first-line therapy for short-term insomnia is from the benzodiazepine, benzodiazepine receptor agonist classes, or ramelteon. Examples of these medications include zolpidem, eszopiclone, zaleplon, and temazepam.

Doxylamine succinate is the only agent designated as pregnancy category A to treat any sleep defect in pregnant women. The practitioner must assess the potential side effects and benefits for both the fetus and mother before instituting therapy.

Second-Line Therapy

If therapy is unsuccessful, as evidenced by a lack of improvement in the achievement of treatment goals, alternate short-acting BZRAs or ramelteon (Schutte-Rodin et al., 2008). If the patient has a comorbid condition such as depression, consider sedating antidepressants such as trazodone, amitriptyline, doxepin, and mirtazapine. These agents may be helpful especially with patients who have anxiety. Again, the prescriber must consider the kind of sleep defect being treated and select a drug with the appropriate onset and half-life.

Third-Line Therapy

Various combinations of therapy can be considered for third line based on lack of goal achievement. The practitioner should reassess the insomnia situation for patients who fail to respond to both first- and second-line therapies. Insomnia that has become chronic benefits most from continual evaluation and behavioral therapy. Consider other sedating agents in the antiepilepsy class such as gabapentin and atypical antipsychotics including quetiapine and olanzapine. For discussion of these agents, see Chapters 39 and 40.

Suvorexant is the newest class of hypnotic agents with a new mechanism of action but possesses pharmacodynamics similar to other known agents already on the market. Even though approved by the FDA, the preclinical trials exposed less than 2,000 patients to the drug leading to limited population exposure. The cost of suvorexant should be a consideration with prescribing.

Special Population Considerations
Pediatric

Use of barbiturates in the pediatric population is usually limited to those who have seizure disorders. In general, benzodiazepines are not indicated for children younger than age 15. Controlled studies of pharmacologic treatment in this population are lacking, and use of many drugs is off label. Caution is necessary when very young patients use antihistamines because of potential delirium or paradoxical excitation. Melatonin may

TABLE 42.2		
Recommended Order of Treatment for Insomnia		
Order	**Agents**	**Comments**
First line	Benzodiazepine (e.g., alprazolam, lorazepam, temazepam), benzodiazepine receptor agonists (BZRAs) (zolpidem, zaleplon, escitalopram), or ramelteon	Agent selected should match the sleep deficit
	First-generation antihistamine—doxylamine succinate	For pregnant women—Category A
Second line	Alternating short-acting BZRAs (zaleplon, eszopiclone) with ramelteon	Consider short-acting agents, especially with patients who have renal or hepatic problems.
	Sedating antidepressants (trazodone, amitriptyline, doxepin, mirtazapine)	Consider antidepressant with comorbid depression
Third line	Sedating antiepilepsy agents (gabapentin) or atypical antipsychotics (quetiapine, olanzapine)	
	Orexin receptor antagonist (suvorexant)	

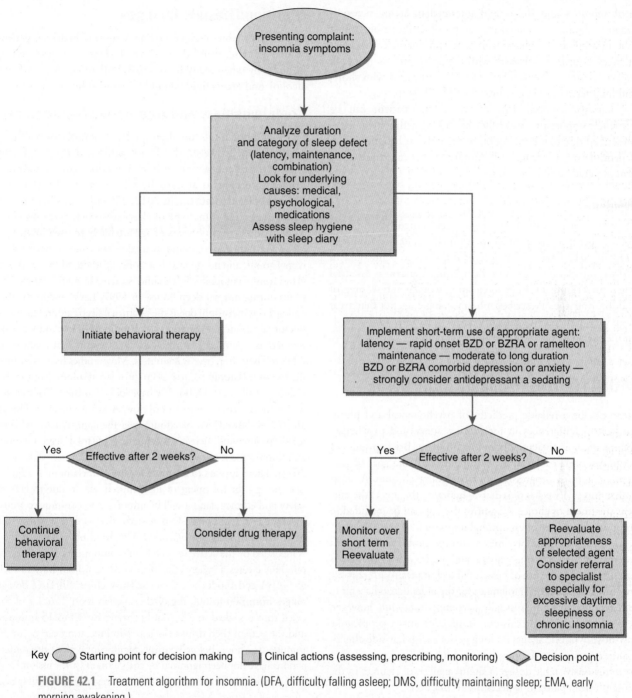

FIGURE 42.1 Treatment algorithm for insomnia. (DFA, difficulty falling asleep; DMS, difficulty maintaining sleep; EMA, early morning awakening.)

be considered as treatment for a limited time (Buscemi et al., 2004; Shamseer & Vohra, 2009).

Geriatric

Older adults may report early morning awakening or general sleep disturbances. Central nervous system (CNS) changes are also thought to affect the sleep of the elderly. Frequent nighttime awakenings may result from secondary changes in circadian rhythms and loss of effective circadian regulation of sleep. Such changes can affect the quality of life. Many elderly

patients exhibit daytime sleepiness, which shows that age does not diminish the need for sleep but reduces the ability to sleep.

It is important to evaluate the geriatric patient for underlying comorbidities that contribute to insomnia. Treating the underlying illnesses is important and may assist with re-establishing good sleeping patterns. Extreme caution is essential when prescribing hypnotic medications to elderly patients because these drugs can increase the potential for delirium and subsequent falls. According to the most recent Beers Criteria (American Geriatric Society, 2015), first-generation antihistamines and short- and intermediate-acting benzodiazepines should be avoided if at all possible. Prescribing must take in account the pharmacokinetic and pharmacodynamics changes in drug metabolism with the aging process (McCall, 2004). There is also an increase in falls associated with short- and long-term benzodiazepines (McCall, 2004, p. 12).

Consistent monitoring of the elderly patient can be extremely important, especially when a long-acting hypnotic is prescribed due to accumulation in the renal or hepatic system depending on the drug used. Antihistamines can cause delirium or paradoxical excitation.

Women

Pharmacokinetic differences have been noted when select BZRA agents are prescribed for women. Guidance from the FDA in 2013 lowered the dose of zolpidem to 5 mg, and in 2014 eszopiclone to no more than 2 mg. Caution is essential when prescribing all drugs to lactating women and women of childbearing age. Prescribed pharmacologic agents that treat sleep vary in pregnancy category risk designations. Only doxylamine succinate has a category A designation.

MONITORING PATIENT RESPONSE

Sleep can be a reliable predictor of psychological and physical health. Differences in monitoring are related to whether the insomnia is an acute or chronic problem. Brief episodes of acute insomnia can warrant treatment, with the goal of preventing it from progressing and becoming chronic. A short course (up to 4 weeks) of sedative–hypnotic therapy is the current treatment of choice. Cognitive therapy can be included to improve the chance of an optimal response.

When insomnia becomes a chronic problem, consistent interaction between the patient and health care provider is important, as is the use of behavioral techniques. With chronic insomnia, issues of drug tolerance for the older benzodiazepines and rebound insomnia usually become paramount; however, few studies have borne this out. In practice, many people take low-dose hypnotic agents for long periods with few side effects. Caution is warranted, however, if a patient requires escalation of a previously stable dosage. Careful analysis of changes in the patient's sleep patterns is necessary in this event.

Patient Education

Patient education plays a key role in the treatment of insomnia. A key side effect of most hypnotic agents is excessive drowsiness or hangover from the medication. The clinician must alert the patient to this possibility and monitor the side effects of each agent prescribed (see **Tables 42.1** and **42.2**).

Patient-Oriented Information Sources

Major sleep centers across the country have Web sites that are useful resources for patients and health care providers. These sites can provide information about diagnosis of sleep disorders and current research and therapies (**Box 42.4**).

Nutrition/Lifestyle Changes

Good sleep habits include setting a routine bedtime, getting regular exercise, using the bed for sleeping only, and getting in bed only when ready for sleep. Stimulants such as caffeine, alcohol, and excess fluids should be avoided before bedtime.

Complementary and Alternative Medications

Herbs and botanicals are often used as a "natural" way of promoting sleep. However, this is not without danger, especially if these treatments are taken in conjunction with prescription drugs. According to analysis by Clarke et al. (2015) of the National Health Statistics in 2012, 32% of adults between 18 and 44 years use some type of alternative therapy/drugs while 31% of adults over 65 years of age are likely to use CAM.

One of the most commonly used nonvitamin agents for sleep is melatonin, an endogenous hormone, synthesized by the pineal gland from tryptophan. It is mainly secreted at night and its level peaks during normal sleep hours. In 1997, Lavie discovered that endogenous melatonin opens the nocturnal sleep gate and increases nocturnal melatonin secretion. Melatonin does not induce sleep but acts as a gatekeeper in the cascade of events that enables the CNS to favor sleep over wakefulness. Most studies have examined the use of melatonin to treat sleep disorders resulting from jet lag (Choy & Salbu, 2011), but few have looked at the use of melatonin in short-term insomnia until now. A further meta-analysis of 19 studies showed that melatonin over the counter reduced time for sleep onset and increased sleep efficiency, total sleep duration, and improvement in overall quality of sleep (Ferracioli-Oda et al., 2013). There appears to be a role for use of melatonin as adjunctive therapy for treatment of insomnia; however, due to lack of safety and efficacy data, it will be important to continue to study. Valerian is a traditional sleep remedy that is derived from the perennial herb *Valeriana officinalis*. The direct physiologic activity is mediated by the active sesquiterpene components of the volatile oil. This creates a synergistic effect with neurotransmitters such as GABA and produces a direct sedative effect. Effective dosage ranges from 300 to 600 mg of the valerian root; 2 to 3 g of the dried root is soaked in a cup of hot water for 10 to 15 minutes, and the patient then drinks the tea. Administration can occur 30 minutes to 2 hours before bedtime. Significant herb or drug interactions have not been reported by the German Commission E.

As with melatonin, few studies exist regarding the safety and efficacy of valerian. Meta-analysis of those studies that exist found more *subjective* improvement of sleep rather than objective measures (Fernandez-San-Martin et al., 2010). Overall, the clinical guidelines do not support use of herbal or nutritional substance due to the lack of efficacy and safety data (Schutte-Rodin et al., 2008).

RESTLESS LEG SYNDROME/WILLIS-EKBOM DISEASE AND PERIODIC LIMB MOVEMENT DISORDER

In 2011, restless leg syndrome (RLS/WED) was renamed Willis-Ekbom Disease to better reflect the neurologic process and underlying pathophysiology. Periodic limb movement disorder (PLMD) is another neurologic disorder that represents repetitive movements and may or may not be associated with RLS/WED. RLS/WED is characterized by an intense need to move the legs, but can also affect the arms and trunk, and may be accompanied by paresthesias and dysesthesias that worsen usually in the evening. Sometimes, the sensations can occur in other large muscle groups, but most often, the legs are involved. Moving around relieves the feeling, but only for a short time, as the sensation soon returns. These sensations interfere with sleep. PLMD is characterized by episodes of highly repetitive and stereotyped limb movements only during sleep.

Both disorders can interfere with sleep and contribute to sleep deprivation and decreased alertness and daytime function. Indications are that in the United States, more than 10 million adults and 1.5 million children and adolescents are affected by RLS/WED (Allen et al., 2005; Berger & Kurth, 2007). PMLD is more common in adults over 60 years of age and is rare in children. Additionally, while 80% to 90% of RLS/WED patients have PMLD, only 30% of PLMD have restless leg (Natarajan, 2010).

CAUSES

Generally, RLS/WED is an idiopathic disorder classified as a central neurologic disorder. Secondary causes of RLS/WED can be associated with end-stage renal disease, iron deficiency, and, sometimes, pregnancy (Natarajan, 2010). RLS/WED can also be hereditary or drug induced. A definitive link has been shown between iron deficits and RLS/WED (Allen et al., 2013a).

PATHOPHYSIOLOGY

RLS/WED and PLMD are chronic sensory–motor disorders that are not fully understood. However, recent advances show strong evidence linking RLS/WED to low iron/transferrin, dopaminergic abnormalities, and excessive glutamate. Primary RLS/WED has a strong hereditary component, with 40% to 60% of patients having a familial association. Genome studies have linked evidence of this familial trait to six distinct different genes for RLS/WED. Onset of RLS/WED before age 45 is consistent with a familial link. Secondary RLS/WED can be associated with neuropathies from changes in axonal and small fiber neural pathways. Patients with rheumatoid arthritis and diabetes also have shown a greater prevalence of RLS/WED, again presumably from changes due to neuropathy. Parkinson disease is frequently associated with RLS/WED, pointing to a commonality in reduced dopaminergic functioning (Peeraully & Tan, 2012). A strong link has been established to the dopaminergic system by the positive response to the dopaminergic agonist classification of drugs (Earley et al., 2011).

The pathophysiology of PMLD is also uncertain, but the projection is there are changes in the descending inhibitory

pathways with neuronal hyperexcitability. Dopamine transmission is also decreased, which supports use of dopaminergic therapy (Earley et al., 2011).

DIAGNOSTIC CRITERIA

RLS/WED is diagnosed primarily through the patient history. Clinical criteria have been established by the International Restless Legs Syndrome Study Group (**Box 42.5**).

PLMD is associated more with stereotypical repetitive movements of limbs (legs alone or legs more than arms) that occur only during sleep. PLMD is generally diagnosed only through a sleep test.

The physical examination for RLS/WED and PLMD should include a full neurologic examination with emphasis on the spinal cord and peripheral nerve function. A vascular examination is also necessary to rule out vascular disorders. Secondary causes of RLS/WED should be evaluated by a serum ferritin level and serum chemistry to rule out uremia and diabetes. Polysomnography is not routinely indicated for RLS/WED but can be helpful to establish the diagnosis. **Box 42.6** lists other possible diagnoses.

> **BOX 42.5 Diagnostic Criteria for Restless Leg Syndrome**
>
> 1. A compelling urge to move limbs associated with paresthesias/dysesthesias
> 2. Motor restlessness as evidenced by:
>   - Floor pacing
>   - Tossing and turning in bed
>   - Rubbing legs
> 3. Symptoms worse or exclusively present at rest with variable and temporary relief by activity
> 4. Symptoms worse in the evening and at night

> **BOX 42.6 Differential Diagnoses for RLS/WED and PLMD**
>
> 1. Nocturnal leg cramps
>   - Painful, palpable involuntary muscle contractions
>   - Focal with sudden onset
>   - Unilateral
> 2. Akathisia
>   - Excessive movement without accompanying sensory complaints
> 3. Peripheral neuropathy
>   - Usually tingling, numbness, or pain sensations
>   - Not associated with motor restlessness
>   - Not helped by movement
>   - Evening or nighttime worsening

INITIATING DRUG THERAPY

Pharmacotherapy should be tailored for each patient. Patients with relatively mild symptoms may not need medications. Nonpharmacologic therapy should be instituted, including mental alerting activities and cessation of alcohol, nicotine, and caffeine. Any medications that may precipitate or worsen RLS/WED symptoms, such as antidepressants and dopamine antagonists, should be avoided. Correction of underlying serum iron deficits may be helpful. Short-term studies have shown that drug therapy has significant benefits, but little is known about long-term treatment. A 3-year study of 70 patients by Clavadetscher et al. (2004) found that a good long-term response with drug therapy can be achieved in 80% of patients. This study helped to establish the benefit of pharmacologic therapy in RLS/WED.

Goals of Drug Therapy

The goal of drug therapy is to calm the restless legs or periodic limb movements. Some patients can be refractory to pharmacologic treatment but still achieve partial relief of their symptoms. Pharmacologic agents for RLS/WED include dopaminergic agents, dopamine agonists, opioids, benzodiazepines, anticonvulsants, and iron (see **Table 42.3**). Other than dopamine agonists, many of these drugs are being used in an "off-label" manner.

Dopaminergic Agents

These drugs are dopamine precursor combinations such as ropinirole (Requip) and pramipexole (Mirapex). These drugs are the only agents of this class approved for RLS/WED. These agents are useful for intermittent RLS/WED because they have a quicker onset than dopamine agonists. This is useful for relief of sleep-onset insomnia and RLS/WED that occurs during long car or airplane journeys. Dosage of these agents is lower than used for Parkinson disease. See Chapter 45 for full discussion of these agents

Adverse Events

The carbidopa–levodopa agents may actually worsen RLS/WED symptoms in up to 80% of patients. The therapeutic effect may be reduced if taken with high-protein food. Insomnia, sleepiness, and gastrointestinal problems are other adverse events.

Dopamine Agonists

The initial dopamine agonists used for RLS/WED were bromocriptine and pergolide, which were prone to side effects. Pergolide is no longer available in the United States and has been replaced by the newer dopamine agonists. These agents include pramipexole and ropinirole, which are not ergot based; while they have fewer side effects, they can cause initial nausea and light-headedness, nasal stuffiness, edema, and rarely, daytime

TABLE 42.3

Overview of Selected Drugs Used to Treat Willis-Ekbom Disease/Restless Leg Syndrome

Generic (Trade) Name and Dosage	Selected Adverse Events	Contraindications	Special Considerations
Dopaminergic Agents			

ropinirole (Requip)
   Start: 0.25 mg q pm × 2 d, then
      0.5 mg × 5 d; increase by 0.5 mg
      weekly until at maximum.
   Range: 3–4 mg
	Common side effects include nausea, somnolence, abdominal pain, dizziness, orthostatic hypotension	Hypersensitivity to class, caution with alcohol use, concomitant CNS depressant, renal and liver impairment	Use cautiously with elderly
			Extended-release form not approved to WED/RLS
			Augmentation is common with this class

pramipexole (Mirapex)
   Start: 0.125 mg/d
   Range: 0.125–0.5 mg
   Max: 0.5 mg
	Same as above	Same as above	Start with lower dose for CrCl 20–60 and increase only every 14 d

rotigotine transdermal (Neupro)
   Start: 1 mg/24 h patch q 24 h
   Range: 1–3 mg/24 h
   Max: 3 mg/24 h
	Same as above	Same as above	Same as above

Anticonvulsants: Alpha-2-Delta Ligands			
gabapentin enacarbil (Horizant)	Common side effects include somnolence, dizziness, headache, and nausea	Same as above	Monitor for baseline creatinine, depression and suicidal ideation, give with food around 5 PM, do not cut/crush/chew Only approved anticonvulsant drug for WED/RLS

sleepiness. Increasing the dose slowly will help to mitigate these side effects. See Chapter 45 for full discussion of these agents.

Opioids

Research is limited with the use of opioids in RLS/WED or PMLD. Opioids are reserved for the most severe cases of RLS/WED or PLMD that are refractory to treatment with other pharmacologic agents. Opioids have been used off label without solid support of efficacy. Trenkwalder et al. (2013) led a randomized placebo-controlled trial of refractory RLS/WED patients in the United Kingdom who were treated with combination prolonged-release oxycodone–naloxone (Targiniq). The results show improvement of the quality of life indicators, which included reduction of sensory, restlessness, pain, and sleep. In 2013, the FDA approved the drug as extended release but only for the indication of severe pain and to help prevent prescription narcotic abuse (FDA News Release, 2013). Practitioners need to be judicious in the selection of patients in whom to prescribe potent narcotics. Revised guidelines for the treatment of RLS/WED support the use of careful opioid usage with careful monitoring (Silber et al., 2013). See Chapter 7 for pain management.

Benzodiazepines

Benzodiazepines (see **Table 42.1**) are used concomitantly with a dopamine agonist when use of a sole agent has failed. Clinical experience is particularly crucial with clonazepam and temazepam. These drugs may be helpful for patients who cannot tolerate the other medications. Caution is necessary when using these agents in the elderly, and they can cause daytime sleepiness and cognitive impairment.

Anticonvulsants

Anticonvulsants are considered when dopamine agonists have failed and in patients who describe the RLS/WED discomfort as pain. Gabapentin is helpful in patients with RLS/WED and peripheral neuropathy but is considered "off label." As with the dopamine agonists, lower dosages of gabapentin (100 to 600 mg one to three times daily) can be successful. The side effect of hypersomnia often limits the dosage. Other side effects can include nausea, sedation, and dizziness. Gabapentin enacarbil is a prodrug of gabapentin and is the only anticonvulsant drug approved for RLS/WED. The starting and continuing dose is 600 mg daily. Adverse effects of the drug are the same as gabapentin (see **Table 42.2**). See Chapter 39 for further discussion of other anticonvulsants.

Selecting the Most Appropriate Agent

For treatment purposes, RLS/WED can be classified as *intermittent* (not often enough to require drug therapy), *daily* (troublesome enough to require drug therapy), and *refractory* (not adequately treated by a dopamine agonist). The ideal agent will minimize or abate the symptoms of RLS/WED. No one pharmacologic agent appears to be efficacious in all patients, and

BOX 42.7	Considerations in Pharmacologic Agent Selection in RLS/WED
Age of patient	Benzodiazepines can cause cognitive impairment in elderly.
Severity of symptoms	Mild symptoms: no medication or levodopa or dopamine agonist
	Severe symptoms: strong opioid
Frequency/regularity of symptoms	Patients with infrequent symptoms may benefit from prn medication.
Presence of pregnancy	No safety and efficacy clinical trials on treatment of RLS/WED with medications in pregnancy
Renal failure	Need to decrease dosage if drugs are renally excreted

often, a combination of medications is needed. The severity of RLS/WED can vary, and pharmacologic treatment needs to be individualized. See **Box 42.7** for considerations when selecting a pharmacologic agent (**Figure 42.2**).

First-Line Therapy

Dopaminergic antagonists such as low-dose carbidopa–levodopa should be reserved for patients with intermittent RLS/WED. The first choice of therapy for daily RLS/WED is one of the dopamine agonists. Comparative analysis of all dopamine agonists (ropinirole, pramipexole, and rotigotine) showed clinically significant improvement in RLS/WED symptomatology (AHRQ, 2012). Nausea, dizziness, dyskinesia, and somnolence are potential side effects of both the dopaminergic antagonists and agonists. One problem with the dopaminergic antagonists is augmentation (worsening of RLS/WED symptoms), which can occur as early as 10 weeks of therapy. Another new first-line therapy (2015) is gabapentin enacarbil (Horizant), which is a prodrug of gabapentin. It is the only drug in the anticonvulsant category that is specifically approved for RLS/WED.

Second-Line Therapy

Pharmacologic agents approved for neuropathic pain such as gabapentin (Neurontin) or pregabalin (Lyrica) can be used alone or in conjunction with other agents, but they are also off label. It is especially helpful for patients who describe RLS/WED symptoms as painful. Other anticonvulsant agents such as carbamazepine (Tegretol) can be considered, but the older agents carry an increased risk of adverse effects such as dizziness, drowsiness, and lack of coordination. Patients also may experience nausea with these older agents. An opioid or opioid receptor agonist, tramadol (Ultram), may be added or used alone at low doses. If either the anticonvulsant or opioid fails, a repeat trial of dopamine agonists should be attempted (Silber et al., 2013).

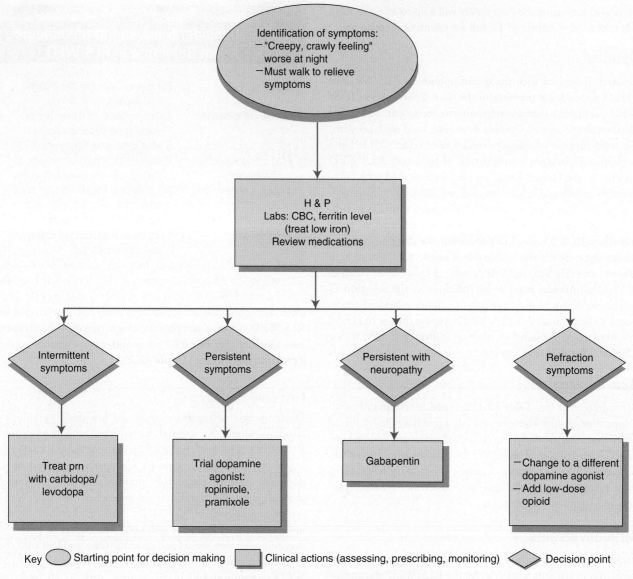

FIGURE 42.2   Algorithm for treatment for RLS/WED.

Third-Line Therapy

Patients who continue to have symptoms may be refractory to treatment. Therapeutic doses may not have been obtained, or the patients could not tolerate the side effects of the medications. Substitution of different medications in the dopamine agonist class or adding higher-potency opioids should be considered. Consultation with a sleep specialist should be considered.

Monitoring Patient Response

Most patients will have remittance of symptoms with the first therapeutic dose of medication. This supports the theory that dopaminergic abnormality is a cause of this disorder. Another indicator of improvement is a decrease in excessive daytime sleepiness from lack of REM sleep. Patients need to be monitored for side effects of the pharmacologic agents.

The long-term efficacy of these pharmacologic agents is uncertain, and monitoring for relapse of symptoms is important. It is also important to monitor for dependence when benzodiazepines or opioids are used.

PATIENT EDUCATION

Many patients who have RLS/WED use OTC sleep medications, and poor sleep hygiene may contribute to the lack of sleep in RLS/WED sufferers. Implementing cognitive sleep hygiene techniques may provide a modest improvement in short-term sleep symptoms (Edinger, 2003). Patients should inform all of their health care providers about their RLS/WED diagnosis, and health care providers should be aware that the patient's inability to keep his or her limbs still is not due to lack of cooperation. Improper restraint of patients with this syndrome has resulted in mortality and morbidity.

Drug Information

A higher dosage of ropinirole (Requip) is needed compared to pramipexole (Mirapex) to achieve the same therapeutic effect. This may contribute to side effects and tolerability of the drug.

Patient-Oriented Information Sources

The Willis-Ekbom Disease Foundation supports research and provides information for patients and health care providers. Extensive international research is also being conducted on this serious sleep problem (see **Box 42.4**).

NARCOLEPSY

Narcolepsy is a sleep disorder caused by poor sleep–wake cycles that can greatly impact the daily activities of those affected. Individuals with narcolepsy sleep the same amount as the average person but cannot control the timing of their sleep. The other features of narcolepsy can include excessive daytime sleepiness, cataplexy (attacks of muscle weakness), sleep paralysis, and hypnagogic hallucinations. Narcolepsy is the second leading cause of excessive daytime sleepiness and has an overall incidence in the world of 0.2 to 1.6 per thousand individuals (Leschziner, 2014). Narcolepsy can have a dramatic impact on virtually all areas of life. Unfortunately, the diagnosis of narcolepsy is often mislabeled as other chronic sleep disorders especially if cataplexy is absent.

CAUSES

Narcolepsy currently lacks distinct etiology and usually starts in the second or third decade of life; however, it has been identified in children as young as age 3. Excessive daytime sleepiness or cataplexy may be the first symptoms, but most often, cataplexy is delayed 2 to 3 years or may be totally absent. Cataplexy attacks are often precipitated by highly specific situations or triggers of strong emotions. Hypnagogic hallucinations can be present but are rarely the first manifestation of narcolepsy.

PATHOPHYSIOLOGY

The pathophysiology of narcolepsy is not well understood but is evolving. Current research has focused on the loss of hypocretinergic neurons in the lateral hypothalamus. These neurons stimulate various histaminergic neurons in the basal forebrain, which increase the arousal state and involve activation of the cerebral cortex. This loss creates an instable

neuronal network that is responsible for maintaining wakefulness and preventing REM sleep (Leschziner, 2014). There is also increasing knowledge about the role of genetics in narcolepsy. Demonstration of a strong genetic component is found through the human leukocyte antigen (HLA), especially when there is a first-degree relative who has narcolepsy and cataplexy.

DIAGNOSTIC CRITERIA

Patient presentations include complaints of excessive daytime sleepiness (EDS), cataplexy, and sleep-related hallucinations along with sleep paralysis. These criteria are commonly known as the narcoleptic triad. *The International Classification of Sleep Disorders,* third edition (2014), now classifies narcolepsy as type 1 or type 2 with subtypes. Diagnosis is based on the presence of excessive daytime sleepiness (EDS), levels of hypocretin in the cerebral spinal fluid, and multilatency sleep test (MLST) (**Box 42.5**).

INITIATING DRUG THERAPY

There is no cure for narcolepsy, and pharmacologic therapy must be initiated to control the attacks (**Table 42.4**). Evaluation for cataplexy, sleep-related hallucinations, and sleep paralysis is important to identify the best agent for treatment. Most often, antidepressants are used to block the REM paralysis of cataplexy. The mainstay of pharmacologic therapy until now has been amphetamines and amphetamine-like drugs such as methylphenidate (Ritalin). Newer drugs on the market now focus on treating the symptoms and the neurobiologic deficit. Pharmacologic agents used in treatment of narcolepsy can be classified into psychostimulants (wake-promoting agents), amphetamines, sodium oxybate, and antidepressants.

Goals of Drug Therapy

Pharmacologic therapy should be titrated to promote the optimal dose of stimulation. The health care provider needs to work with the patient to identify personal treatment goals such as staying awake in a classroom or social situation or while driving. The main goal is to achieve as normal a life as possible, staying awake in situations of normal daily living.

Psychostimulants (Wake-Promoting Agents)

Modafinil and armodafinil (the R-enantiomer of modafinil) are psychostimulants with unique properties to promote wakefulness. The potential for abuse of these agents is much lower than with other stimulants, although it still needs to be monitored. The mechanism of action of modafinil and armodafinil is not well understood, but it appears to attenuate the central alpha-1 adrenergic system. The primary sites of action are the

TABLE 42.4

Overview of Selected Drugs Used to Treat Narcolepsy

Generic (Trade) Name and Dosage	Selected Adverse Events	Contraindications	Special Considerations
Psychostimulants			
armodafinil (Nuvigil) Start: 150–250 mg qam	*Serious:* arrhythmias, syncope, visual changes, abuse/dependency *Common:* headache, nausea/vomiting, rhinitis, diarrhea	Hypersensitivity to modafinil and armodafinil	Reduce dose in patients with severe hepatic dysfunction. Consider low doses in elderly
modafinil (Provigil) Start: 200 mg qam; maximum 400 mg daily	Same as above	Sensitivity to class, caution with coronary artery disease, mitral valve prolapse, impaired liver failure	Start at 100 mg daily in elderly
sodium oxybate (Xyrem) Start: dose 1–2.25 g at hs. Dose 2–2.25 g 2.5–4 h later Increase dose by interval 1.5 g nightly. Range: 6–9 g nightly	*Serious:* CNS and respiratory depression, abuse/dependency, depression, suicidal ideation, psychosis, paranoia, hallucinations, apnea *Common:* nausea, dizziness, vomiting, somnolence enuresis	Sensitivity to class; caution with CNS depressant use; alcohol intake; hepatic, renal, pulmonary, cardiac impairment; psychiatric disorders; drug abuse history	Black box warning for appropriate use—only distributed through Xyrem Success Program and centralized pharmacy Abuse potential due to relation to gamma-hydroxybutyrate (GHB)

subregions of the hippocampus, the centrolateral nucleus of the thalamus, and the central nucleus of the amygdala. Modafinil can produce euphoria and psychoactive effects similar to other CNS stimulants. Absorption of the drug occurs rapidly, with peak plasma concentration in 2 to 4 hours and a half-life of 15 hours. Distribution of the drug is throughout the tissues, and it is moderately bound to plasma proteins. The drug is metabolized in the liver and excreted in the urine (see **Table 42.4**).

Amphetamines

Various amphetamine drugs are used to promote wakefulness in narcolepsy. The most commonly used agent is methylphenidate (Ritalin), which is approved for use in narcolepsy. The mechanism of action is generally unknown but thought to stimulate central nervous system activity and block the reuptake while increasing the release of norepinephrine with dopamine. This agent is metabolized in the liver but not through the CYP450 system. The average half-life of methylphenidate is 3.5 hours and administration can be adjusted to daily activities.

Sodium Oxybate

Sodium oxybate (Xyrem) is approved to treat two common symptoms of narcolepsy, excessive daytime sleepiness (EDS) and cataplexy. The active ingredient of sodium oxybate is gamma-hydroxybutyrate (GHB) that has potential to depress the central nervous system. The drug is only distributed through the manufacturer in a restricted risk evaluation and mitigation strategy (REMS) distribution program due to potential for abuse. While the primary care provider may not be the prescriber of this medication, it is important to have knowledge about the drug.

Antidepressants

Venlafaxine (Effexor) and duloxetine (Cymbalta) act on the serotonergic and noradrenergic systems and may be useful when cataplexy is present (see Chapter 40).

Selecting the Most Appropriate Agent

For treatment purposes, narcolepsy can be classified as *type 1N* or *type 2* (**Box 42.8**). The ideal agent will minimize the triad of symptoms associated with the disease. As with insomnia and RLS/WED, no one pharmacologic agent appears to help all patients, and often, a combination of medications is needed. Individualizing therapy is also important with narcolepsy. The primary care provider most likely will not prescribe these drugs initially but will continue to be part of the health care team and need knowledge about the disease and treatment.

SPECIAL POPULATIONS

Pediatrics

Narcolepsy is rare and difficult to diagnose in children. There are limited drug choices, but drugs that are used in ADHD may be useful (see Chapter 43). Modafinil has not been studied in children. The alternative drug of choice would be methylphenidate.

Geriatrics

Care must be taken when prescribing modafinil to the elderly population. The oral clearance of modafinil is reduced in the elderly by 20% to 50%. Renal failure does not influence the pharmacokinetics of the drug but does increase the inactive metabolite accumulation. Liver impairment can reduce the modafinil clearance and double serum concentrations.

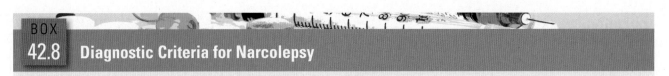

BOX 42.8 Diagnostic Criteria for Narcolepsy

Type 1 N	Type 2
Required:	**Required:**
Hypersomnolence daily × 3 mo	Hypersomnolence daily × 3 mo
Low CSF hypocretin levels (≤110 pg/mL) **OR** cataplexy	Hypocretin not measured **OR** ≥110 pg/mL
Short sleep latency (≤8 min)	Absence of cataplexy
Two or more sleep-onset rapid eye movement (REM) episodes on the multiple sleep latency test (MSLT)	Short sleep latency (≤8 min)
	Two or more sleep-onset REM episodes on the multiple sleep latency test (MSLT)
Subtype	**Subtype**
Type 1 due to a medical condition	Type 2 due to a medical condition
Narcolepsy without cataplexy but low hypocretin.	

MONITORING PATIENT RESPONSE

Narcolepsy is a lifelong disease process, and patients must use the medications for their entire lives. Patient response is monitored by improvement in the disease's severity. Achieving the goals identified by the patient can help to improve compliance.

PATIENT EDUCATION

Patients and their families need to be aware of all available options to treat narcolepsy. Psychological distress is a consequence, not the cause, of the disease. Discussion of potential side effects of the drugs is important for compliance.

Offering counseling and support groups when necessary is important.

Drug Information

Patients who are switched from amphetamine stimulants to modafinil may not experience the same euphoric effects, and this may make the switch undesirable to the patient. Amphetamines tend to produce a feeling of improved well-being and arousal, while modafinil increases arousal without a change in affect.

Patient-Oriented Sources

Health care providers and patients can find information about narcolepsy from a variety of sources. Online support groups exist (see **Box 42.4**).

CASE STUDY*

S.H., age 47, reports difficulty falling asleep and staying asleep. These problems have been ongoing for many years, but she has never mentioned them to her health care provider. She has generally "lived with it" and self-treated the problem with OTC Tylenol PM. Currently, she is also experiencing perimenopausal symptoms of night sweats and mood swings. Current medical problems include hypertension controlled with medications. Past medical history includes childhood illnesses of measles, chickenpox, and mumps. Family history is positive for diabetes on the maternal side and hypertension on the paternal side. Her only medication is an angiotensin-converting enzyme inhibitor and diuretic combination for hypertension control. She generally does not like taking medication and does not take any other OTC products.

DIAGNOSIS: INSOMNIA

1. List specific goals of therapy for **S.H.**
2. What drug therapy would you prescribe? Why?
3. What are the parameters for monitoring the success of the therapy?
4. Discuss specific patient education based on the prescribed therapy
5. List one or two adverse reactions for the selected agent that would cause you to change therapy.
6. What would be the choice for second-line therapy?
7. What OTC and/or alternative medicines might be appropriate for this patient?
8. What dietary and lifestyle changes might you recommend?
9. Describe one or two drug–drug or drug–food interactions for the selected agent.

* Answers can be found online.

Bibliography

Starred references are cited in the text.

AHRQ. (2012). Comparative effectiveness review: Number 86 treatment for restless legs syndrome. *Executive Summary*, Publication No. 12(13)-EHC146-1.

*Allen, R. P., Auerbach, S., Bahrain, H., et al. (2013a). The prevalence of impact of restless legs syndrome on patients with iron deficiency anemia. *American Journal of Hematology*, 88(4), 261–264.

Allen, R. P., Barker, P., Horska, A., et al. (2013b). Thalamic glutamate/glutamine in restless legs syndrome: Increase and related to disturbed sleep. *Neurology*, 80(22), 2028–2034. doi: 10.1212.WNL.0b013e31294b3f6.

Allen, R. P., Chen, C., Garcia-Borreguero, D., et al. (2014). Comparison of pregabalin with pramipexole for restless legs syndrome. *New England Journal of Medicine*, 370, 621–631.

*Allen, R. P., Walters, A. S., Montplasir, J., et al. (2005). Restless legs syndrome prevalence and impact: REST general population study. *Archives of Internal Medicine*, 165(11), 1286–1292.

Allison, M. (2012). Evaluation of insomnia in the adult client. *Journal for Nurse Practitioners*, 8(4), 330–331. doi: 10.1016/j.nurpra.2012.02.009.

Alshaikh, M. K., Tricco, A. C., Tashkandi, M., et al. (2012). Sodium oxybate for narcolepsy with cataplexy: Systematic review and meta-analysis. *Journal of Clinical Sleep Medicine*, 8(4), 451–458. doi: 10.5664/jcsm.2048.

American Academy of Sleep Medicine. (2001). *The International Classification of Sleep Disorders revised: Diagnostic and coding manual*. Chicago, IL: American Academy of Sleep Medicine.

*American Geriatric Society. (2015). American Geriatric Society 2015: Updated beers criteria for potentially inappropriate medication use in older adults. *Journal of American Geriatrics Society*, 63(11), 2227–2246. doi: 10.1111/jgs.13702.

American Psychiatric Association. (2013). *Diagnostic and Statistical Manual of Mental Disorders* (5th ed., pp. 410–413). Arlington, VA: American Psychiatric Association.

Amos, L., Grekowicz, M., Kuhn, E., et al. (2014). Treatment of pediatric restless leg syndrome. *Clinical Pediatrics*, 53(4), 331–336. doi: 10.1177/0009922813507997.

Aurora, R. N., Kristo, D. A., Bista, S. R., et al. (2012). The treatment of restless legs syndrome and periodic limb movement disorder in adults—An update for 2012: Practice parameters with evidence-based systematic review and meta-analyses. *Sleep*, 35(8), 1039–1062.

Avidan, A. (2005). Epidemiology, assessment, and treatment of insomnia in elderly. *Medscape Neurology*, 7(2). Retrieved from http://www.medscape.org/viewarticle/516282 on August 28, 2015.

Baglioni, C., Spiegelhalder, K., Lombardo, C., et al. (2011). Sleep and emotions: A focus of insomnia. *Sleep Medicine Reviews*, 14(4), 227–238. doi: 10.1016/j.smrv.2009.10.007.

Baldwin, D., Atchison, K., Bateson, A., et al. (2013). Benzodiazepines: Risks and benefits. A reconsideration. *Journal of Psychopharmacology*, 27(11), 967–971. doi: 10.1177/0269881113503509.

Bateson, A. (2004). The benzodiazepine site of the GABA_A receptor: An old target with new potential? *Sleep Medicine*, 5(Suppl. 1), S9–S15.

Bent, S., Paudal, A., & Moore, D. (2006). Valerian for sleep: A systematic review and meta-analysis. *American Journal of Medicine*, 119(12), 1005–1012.

*Berger, K., & Kurth, T. (2007). RLS epidemiology-frequencies, risk factors and methods in population studies. *Movement Disorders*, 22(Suppl. 118), S420–S423.

*Billioti de Gage, S., Ducruet, T., Kurth, T., et al. (2014). Benzodiazepine use and risk of Alzheimer's disease: Case-control study. *BMJ*, 349, g520s.

Bluestein, D., Rutledge, C., & Healey, A. (2010). Psychosocial correlates of insomnia severity in primary care. *Journal of the American Board of Family Medicine*, 23, 204. doi: 10.3122/jabfm.2010.02.090179.

Bonnet, M., & Arand, D. (2009). Hyperarousal and insomnia: State of the science. *Sleep Medicine Reviews*, 14(1), 9–15. doi: 10.1016/j.smrv.2009.05.002.

Bozorg, A. (2015). Narcolepsy treatment and management. *EMedicine Drugs & Disease*. Retrieved from http://emedicine.medscape.com/article/1188433 overview on August 24, 2015.

Bozorg, A. (2014). Restless legs syndrome. *EMedicine Drugs & Disease*. Retrieved from http://emedicine.medscape.com/article/1188327-overview on July 8, 2015.

Bozorg, J., & Benbadis, S. (2014). Restless legs syndrome clinical presentation. *Medscape: Drugs & Diseases*. Retrieved from http://emedicine.medscape.com/article/1188327-clinica on July 11, 2015.

Brostrom, A., Stromberg, A., Dahlstrom, U., et al. (2004). Sleep difficulties, daytime sleepiness, and health-related quality of life in patients with chronic heart failure. *Journal of Cardiovascular Nursing*, 19(4), 234–242.

Brezinski, A., Vangel, M. G., Wurtman, R. J., et al. (2005). Effects of exogenous melatonin on sleep: A meta-analysis. *Sleep Medicine Reviews*, 9(1), 41–50.

Burbank, F., Buchfuhrer, M., & Kopjar, B. (2013a). Improving sleep for patients with restless legs syndrome. Part II: Meta-analysis of vibration therapy and drugs approved by the FDA for treatment of restless legs syndrome. *Journal of Parkinsonism and Restless Legs Syndrome*, 3, 11–22. doi: 10.2147/JPRLS.S40356.

Burbank, F., Buchfuhrer, M., & Kopjar, B. (2013b). Sleep improvement for restless legs syndrome patients. Part I: Pooled analysis of two prospective, double-blind, sham-controlled, multi-center, randomized clinical studies of the effects of vibrating pads on RLS symptoms. *Journal of Parkinsonism and Restless Legs Syndrome*, 3, 1–10. doi: 10.2147/JPRLS.S40354.

*Buscemi, N., Vandermeer, B., Randya, R., et al. (2004). Melatonin for treatment of sleep disorders. *Evidence Report/Technology Assessment, No. 108*. Bethesda, MD: AHRQ Publication No. 05-E002-2.

Buyssee, D. (2004). Insomnia, depression, and aging: Assessing sleep and mood interactions in older adults. *Geriatrics*, 59(2), 47–51.

Buysse, D., Cheng, Y., Germain, A., et al. (2011a). Night-to-night sleep variability in older adults with and without chronic insomnia. *Sleep Medicine*, 11(1), 56. doi: 10.1016/j.sleep.2009.02.010.

Buysse, D., Germain, A., Hall, M., et al. (2011b). A neurobiological model of insomnia. *Drug Discovery Today. Disease Models*, 8(4), 129–137. doi: 10.1016/j.ddmopd.2011.07.002.

Carlucci, M., Smith, M., & Simmons, J. (2015). The diagnosis and management of narcolepsy. *Consultant*, 614–616; 622–623.

Chawla, J. (2014). Insomnia. *EMedicine Drugs & Disease*. Retrieved from http://emedicine.medscape.com/article/1187829-overview on June 30, 2015.

*Choy, M., & Salbu, R. (2011). Jet lag: Current and potential therapies. *P & T*, 36(4), 221–231.

*Clarke, T. C., Black, L. I., Stussman, B. J., et al. (2015). Trends in the use of complementary health approaches among adults: United States, 2002–2012. National health statistics reports; no 79. Hyattsville, MD: National Center for Health Statistics.

*Clavadetscher, S., Gugger, M., & Bassetti, C. (2004). Restless legs syndrome: Clinical experience with long-term treatment. *Sleep Medicine*, 5, 495–500.

*Desseilles, M., Dang-Vu, T., Schabus, M., et al. (2008). Neuroimaging insights into the pathophysiology of sleep disorders. *Sleep*, 31(6), 777–794.

De la Herran-Arita, A. K., & Garcia-Garcia, F. (2013). Current and emerging options for the drug treatment of narcolepsy. *Drugs*, 73, 1771–1781. doi: 10.1007/s40265-013-0127-y.

*De Lecea, L., Kilduff, T. S., Peyron, C., et al. (1998). The hypocretins: Hypothalamus-specific peptides with neuroexcitatory activity. *Proceedings of the National Academy of Sciences of the U S A*, 95(1), 322–327.

Doghramji, K. (2005). Longitudinal course of insomnia: Progression of symptoms over time. *Medscape Internal Medicine*, 7(2), 1–6. Retrieved from http://www.medscaped.org/viewarticle/515654_3 on July 3, 2015.

*Dubey, A. K., Handu, S. S., & Mediratta, P. K. (2015). Suvorexant: The first orexin receptor antagonist to treat insomnia. *Journal of Pharmacology and Pharmacotherapeutics*, 6(2), 118–121. Retrieved from http://doi.org/10.4103/0976-500X.155496.

Dyken, M., Afifi, A., & Lin-Dyken, D. (2012). Sleep-related problems in neurologic diseases. *Chest*, 141(2), 528–544. doi: 10.1378/chest.11-0773.

*Earley, D., Kuwabara, H., Wong, D., et al. (2011). The dopamine transporter is decreased in the striatum of subjects with restless legs syndrome. *Sleep*, 34(3), 341–347.

Ebrahim, I. O., Howard, R. S., Kopelman, M. D., et al. (2002). The hypocretin/orexin system. *Journal of the Royal Society of Medicine*, *95*(5), 227–230.

*Edinger, J. (2003). Cognitive and behavioral anomalies among insomnia patients with mixed restless legs and periodic limb movement disorder. *Behavioral Sleep Medicine*, *1*(1), 37–53.

*FDA News Release. (2013). *FDA approves new extended-release oxycodone with abuse-deterrent properties*. Silver Spring, MD: Author.

FDA News Release. (2014). FDA approves new type of sleep drug, Belsomra.

Fernandez-Mendoza, J., Calhoun, S., Bixler, E., et al. (2011). Sleep misperception and chronic insomnia in the general population: The role of objective sleep duration and psychological profiles. *Psychosomatic Medicine*, *73*(1), 88–97. doi: 10.1097/PSY.0b013e3181fe365a.

Fernandez-San-Martin, M. I., Masa-Font, R., Palacious-Soler, L., et al. (2010). Effectiveness of valerian on insomnia: A meta-analysis randomized placebo-controlled trials. *Sleep Medicine*, *11*(6), 505–511.

*Ferracioli-Oda, E., Qawasmi, A., & Bloch, M. H. (2013). Meta-analysis: Melatonin for the treatment of primary sleep disorders. *PLoS One*, *8*(5), E63773. doi: 10.137/journal.pone.0063773.

Freeman, A. A., & Rye, D. B. (2013). The molecular basis of restless legs syndrome. *Current Opinion in Neurobiology*, *23*, 895–900.

Garcia-Borreguero, D., Paul Stillman, P., Benes, H., et al. (2011). Algorithms for the diagnosis and treatment of restless legs syndrome in primary care. *BMC Neurology*, *11*, 28. Retrieved from http://www.biomedcentral.com/1471-2377/11/28 on June 8, 2015.

Gentili, A. (2014). Geriatric sleep disorder. *EMedicine Drugs & Disease*. Retrieved from http://emedicine.medscape.com/article/292498-overview on June 21, 2015.

Gulyani, S., Salas, R., & Gamaldo, C. (2012). Sleep medicine pharmacotherapeutics overview today, tomorrow, and the future (Part 1: Insomnia and circadian rhythm disorders). *Chest*, *142*(6), 1659–1668. doi: 10.1378/chest.12-0465.

Halloran, L. (2013). Can't sleep? Insomnia treatment. *Journal for Nurse Practitioners*, *9*(1), 68–69. doi: 10.1016/j.nurpra.2012.11.007.

Hara, C., Stewart, R., Lima-Costa, M. F., et al. (2011). Insomnia subtypes and their relationship to excessive daytime sleepiness in Brazilian community-dwelling older adults. *Sleep*, *34*(8), 1111–1117.

Hening, W., Walthers, A., Allen, R., et al. (2004). Impact, diagnosis and treatment of restless legs syndrome (RLS/WED) in a primary care population: The REST (RLS/WED Epidemiology, Symptoms, and Treatment) primary care study. *Sleep Medicine*, *5*, 237–240.

Hirshkowitz, M., Dautovich, N., Hillygus, S., et al. (2014). 2014 Sleep Health Index. Retrieved from http://sleepfoundation.org/sleep-health-index on June 19, 2015.

*International Classification of Sleep Disorders (ICSD) (3rd ed.). (2014). Darien, IL: American Academy of Sleep Medicine.

Jeffrey, S. (2014, May 30). FDA okays first device for restless legs syndrome. Retrieved from http://www.medscape.com/viewarticle/825971 on July 2, 2015.

John Hopkins Medicine. (2015). Center for restless leg syndrome. Retrieved from http://www.hopkinsmedicine.org/neurology_neurosurgery/centers_clinics/restless-legs-syndrome/ on July 11, 2015.

Joo, E. Y., Seo, D. W., Tae, W. S., et al. (2008). Effect of modafinil on cerebral blood flow in narcolepsy patients. *Sleep*, *31*(6), 868–873.

Kelso, C. (2014). Primary insomnia. *EMedicine Drugs & Disease*. Retrieved from http://emedicine.medscape.com/article/291573-overview on June 30, 2015.

Klingelhoefer, L., Cova, A., Gupta, B., et al. (2014). A review of current treatment strategies for restless legs syndrome (Willis–Ekbom disease). *Clinical Medicine*, *14*(5), 520–524. Retrieved from www.clinmed.rcpjournal.org/content/14/5/520.full.pdf on July 8, 2015.

Kume, A. (2014). Gabapentin enacarbil for the treatment of moderate to severe primary restless legs syndrome (Willis-Ekbom disease): 600 or 1,200 dose? *Neuropsychiatric Disease and Treatment*, *10*, 249–262. doi: 10.2147/NDT.S30160.

Kryger, M., Monjan, A., Bliwise, D., et al. (2004). Sleep, health and aging: Bridging the gap between science and clinical practice. *Geriatrics*, *59*(1), 24–30.

Late-life insomnia: Psychiatric and medical comorbidity common. (2004). *Geriatric Psychopharmacology Update*, *8*(7), 1–7.

*Lavie, P. (1997). Melatonin: Role in gating nocturnal rise in sleep propensity. *Journal of Biological Rhythms*, *12*, 657–668.

*Leschziner, G. (2014). Narcolepsy: A clinical review. *Practical Neurology*, *14*, 323–331. doi: 10.1136/practneurol-2014-000837.

Maheswaran, M., & Kushida, C. (2006). Restless legs syndrome in children. *Medscape General Medicine*, *8*(2), 79–79. Retrieved from http://www.ncbi.nlm.nih.gov/pmc/articles/PMC1785221/?report=printable on June 30, 2015.

*Mazza, M., Losurdo, A., Testani, E., et al. (2014). Polysomnographic fidings in a cohort of chronic insomnia patients with benzodiazepines abuse. *European Psychiatry*, *29*(Suppl. 1), 1.

*McCall, W. V. (2004). Sleep in the elderly: Burden, diagnosis, and treatment. *Primary Care Companion to the Journal of Clinical Psychiatry*, *6*(1), 9–20.

Meoli, A., Rosen, C., Kristo, D., et al. (2005). Oral nonprescription for treatment for insomnia: An evaluation of products with limited evidence. *Journal of Clinical Sleep Medicine*, *1*(2), 173–187.

*Michelson, D., Snyder, E., Paradis, E., et al. (2014). Safety and efficacy of suvorexant during 1-year treatment of insomnia with subsequent abrupt treatment discontinuation: A phase 3 randomised, double-blind, placebo-controlled trial. *Lancet Neurology*, *13*(5), 461–471. doi: 10.1016/S1474-4422(14)70053-3.

Morin, C., Belleville, G., Bélanger, L., et al. (2011a). The insomnia severity index: Psychometric indicators to detect insomnia cases and evaluate treatment response. *Sleep*, *34*(5), 601–608.

Morin, C., Vallières, A., Guay, B., et al. (2011b). Cognitive-behavior therapy, singly and combined with medication, for persistent insomnia: Acute and maintenance therapeutic effects. *Journal of the American Medical Association*, *301*(19), 2005–2015. doi: 10.1001/jama.2009.682.

Morin, C., & Benca, R. (2012). Chronic insomnia. *Lancet*, *379*, 1129–1141. doi: 10.1016/S0140-6736(11)60750-2.

Morrish, E., King, M., Smith, I., et al. (2004). Factors associated with a delay in the diagnosis of narcolepsy. *Sleep Medicine*, *5*, 37–41.

Narcolepsy. (2015). Medications for treating daytime sleepiness in narcolepsy. Retrieved from http://healthysleep.med.harvard.edu/narcolepsy on August 23, 2015.

*Natarajan, R. (2010). Review of periodic limb movement and restless leg syndrome. *Journal of Postgraduate Medicine*, *56*, 157–162. doi: 10.4103/0022-3859.65284.

Ohayon, M., O'Hara, R., & Vitiello, M. (2011). Epidemiology of restless legs syndrome: A synthesis of the literature. *Sleep Medicine Reviews*, *16*(4), 283–295. doi: 10.1016/j.smrv.2011.05.002.

National Institutes of Health State-of-the-Science. (2005). Conference on manifestation and management of chronic insomnia in adults. *NIH Consensus and State-of-the-Science Statements*, *22*(2), 1–30.

National Sleep Foundation. (2015). *Melatonin: The basic facts*. Available online at http://sleepfoundation.org/sleep-topics/melatonin-and-sleep

Nissen, C., Kloepfer, C., Feige, B., et al. (2011). Sleep-related memory consolidation in primary insomnia. *Journal of Sleep Research*, *20*, 129–136. doi: 10.1111/j.1365-2869.2010.00872.x.

*Peerauily, T., & Tan, E.-K. (2012). Linking restless legs syndrome with Parkinson disease: Clinical, imaging, and genetic evidence. *Translational Neurodegeneration*, *1*(6). Retrieved from http://www.translationalneurodegeneration.com/content/1/1/6 on August 24, 2015.

Perusse, A., Turcotte, I., St-Jean, G., et al. (2013). Types of primary insomnia: Is hyperarousal also present during napping? *Journal of Clinical Sleep Medicine*, *9*(12), 1273–1280. doi: 10.5664/jcsm.3268.

Pearson, N. J., Johnson, L. L., & Nahin, R. L. (2006). Insomnia, trouble sleeping, and complementary and alternative medicine: Analysis of the 2002 national health interview survey data. *Archives of Internal Medicine*, *166*(16), 1775–1782.

*PL-Detail Document. (2014). Comparison of insomnia treatments. *Pharmacist's Letter/Prescriber's Letter*.

Quan, S., & Zee, P. (2004). A sleep review of systems: Evaluating the effects of medical disorders on sleep in the older patient. *Geriatrics*, *59*(3), 37–42.

*Regestein, Q., Dambrosia, J., Hallett, M., et al. (2003). Daytime alertness in patients with primary insomnia. *American Journal of Psychiatry*, *150*(10), 1529–1534.

Restless Legs Syndrome Foundation. (2008). Diagnosis and treatment in primary care. Retrieved from http://www.rls.org

Restless legs syndrome fact sheet. (2010, September 1). Retrieved from http://www.ninds.nih.gov/disorders/restless_legs/detail_restless_legs.htm on July 5, 2015.

Richards, K., Shue, V., Beck, C., et al. (2010). Restless legs syndrome risk factors, behaviors, and diagnoses in persons with early to moderate dementia and sleep disturbance. *Behavioral Sleep Medicine, 8*(1), 48–61. doi: 10.1080/15402000903425769.

*Rosekind, M. (2015, January 14). Awakening a nation: A call to action. *National Transportation Safety Board.* doi: 10.1016/j.sleh.2014.12.005.

Rosekind, M., & Gregory, K. (2010). Insomnia risks and costs: Health, safety, and quality of life. *American Journal of Managed Care, 16*(8), 617–626.

*Rosekind, M., Gregory, K., Mallis, M., et al. (2010). The cost of poor sleep: Workplace productivity loss and associated costs. *Journal of Occupational and Environmental Medicine, 52*(1), 91–98.

Ruoff, C., & Black, J. (2014, January). The psychiatric dimensions of narcolepsy. *Psychiatric Times.* Retrieved from http://www.psychiatrictimes.com/sleep-disorders/psychiatric-dimensions-narcolepsy/page/0/1 on August 26, 2015.

*Sakurai, T., Amemiya, A., Matsuzaki, I., et al. (1998). Orexins and orexin receptors: A family of hypothalamic neuropeptides and G protein-coupled receptors that regulate feeding behavior. *Cell, 92*(4), 573–585. doi: 10.1016/S0092-8674(00)80949-6.

Salas, R., & Kwan, A. (2012). The real burden of restless legs syndrome: Clinical and economic outcomes. *American Journal of Managed Care, 18*, S207–S212. Retrieved from http://www.ajmc.com/journals/supplement/2012/a409_12oct_rls/a409_12oct_salas_s207/ on June 18, 2015.

Sethi, K., & Mehta, S. (2012). A clinical primer on restless legs syndrome: What we know, and what we don't know. *American Journal of Managed Care, 18*(5 Suppl.), S83–S88.

Schutte-Rodin, S., Broch, L., Buysse, D., et al. (2008). Clinical guideline for the evaluation and management of chronic insomnia in adults. *Journal of Clinical Sleep Medicine, 4*(5), 487–504. Retrieved from http://www.ncbi.nlm.nih.gov/pmc/articles/PMC2576317/ on June 15, 2015.

Schwartz, J., Feldman, N., Fry, J., et al. (2003). Efficacy of modafinil for improving daytime wakefulness in patients treated previously with psychostimulants. *Sleep Medicine, 4*, 43–49.

Shahid, A., Chung, S., Phillipson, R., et al. (2012). An approach to long-term sedative-hypnotic use [Dove Press, open access]. *Journal of Nature and Science of Sleep, 4*, 53–61.

Shamseer, L., & Vohra, S. (2009). Complementary, holistic, and integrative medicine: Melatonin. *Pediatrics in Review, 30*(6), 223–228. doi: 10.1542/pir.30-6-223.

Silber, M., Becker, P., Earley, C., et al. (2013). Willis-Ekbom disease foundation revised consensus statement on the management of restless legs syndrome. *Mayo Clinic Proceedings, 88*(9), 977–986. doi: 10.1016/j.mayocp.2013.06.016.

Stevens, M. S. (2013). Normal sleep, sleep physiology, and sleep deprivation. Retrieved from http://emedicine.medscape.com/article/1188226-overview#a3 on July 15, 2015.

Terzano, M., Rossi, M., Palomba, V., et al. (2003). New drugs for insomnia: Comparative tolerability of zopiclone, zolpidem and zaleplon. *Drug Safety, 26*(4), 261–282.

*The National Sleep Foundation. (2014). *2014 Sleep Health Index.* Arlington, VA: Author.

Toro, B. (2014). New treatment options for the management of restless leg syndrome. *Journal of Neuroscience Nursing, 46*(4), 227–232. doi: 10.1097/JNN.0000000000000068.

Tsujinom, N., & Sakurai, T. (2009). Orexin/hypocretin: A neuropeptide at the interface of sleep, energy homeostasis, and reward system. *Pharmacological Reviews, 61*(2), 162–176. doi: 10.1124/pr.109.001321.

Treatment for restless legs syndrome: Research focus for clinicians. (2013). Minnesota Evidence-based Practice Center under Contract No. 290-2007-10064-I, Review No. 86. Retrieved from www.effectivehealthcare.ahrq.gov/restless-legs.cfm on July 7, 2015.

*Trenkwalder, C., Benes, H., Grote, L., et al. (2013). Prolonged release oxycodone-naloxone for treatment of severe restless legs syndrome after failure of previous treatment: A double-blind, randomised, placebo-controlled trial with an open-label extension. *Lancet Neurology, 12*(12), 1133.

Trenkwalder, C., Garcia-Borreguero, D., Montagna, P., et al. (2004). Therapy with ropinirole: Efficacy and tolerability in RLS/WED 1 Study Group. *Journal of Neurology, Neurosurgery, and Psychiatry, 75*(1), 92–97.

Trevena, L. (2004). Practice corner: Sleepless in Sydney—Is valerian an effective alternative to benzodiazepines in the treatment of insomnia? *ACP Journal Club, 141*(1), 14.

Vitiello, M., Larsen, L., & Moe, K. (2004). Age-related sleep change: Gender and estrogen effects on the subjective-objective sleep quality relationships of healthy, noncomplaining older men and women. *Journal of Psychosomatic Research, 56*, 503–510.

Walters, A., Gabelia, D., & Frauscher, B. (2013). Restless legs syndrome (Willis–Ekbom disease) and growing pains: Are they the same thing? A side-by-side comparison of the diagnostic criteria for both and recommendations for future research. *Sleep Medicine, 14*, 1247–1252. doi: 10.1016/j.sleep.2013.07.013.

What are the risks when elderly patients combine herbal and prescription medications? (2004). *Geriatric Psychopharmacology Update, 8*(1), 1–6.

Wickwire, E., & Collop, N. (2010). Insomnia and sleep-related breathing disorders. *Chest, 137*(6), 1449–1463. doi: 10.1378/chest.09-1485.

Wilson, S., Nutt, D., Alford, C., et al. (2010). British Association for Psychopharmacology consensus statement on evidence-based treatment of insomnia, parasomnias and circadian rhythm disorders. *Journal of Psychopharmacology, 24*(11), 1577–1600. doi: 10.1177/0269881110379307.

Wong, E., & Nguyen, T. (2014). Zolpidem use in the elderly and recent safety data. *Journal for Nurse Practitioners, 10*(2), 140–141. doi: 10.1016/j.nurpra.2013.09.012.

Won, C., Mahmoudi, M., Qin, L., et al. (2014). The impact of gender on timeliness of narcolepsy diagnosis. *Journal of Clinical Sleep Medicine, 10*(1), 89–95. doi: 10.5664/jcsm.3370.

*Zee, P. C., Wang-Weigan, S., Wright, K. P., et al. (2011). Effects of ramelteon on insomnia symptoms induced by rapid, eastward travel. *Sleep Medicine, 11*, 525–533.

Zhdanova, I. V., Wurtman, R. J., Regan, M., et al. (2001). Melatonin treatment for age-related insomnia. *Journal of Clinical Endocrinology and Metabolism, 86*(10), 4727–4730.

43 Attention Deficit Hyperactivity Disorder

Jennifer A. Reinhold

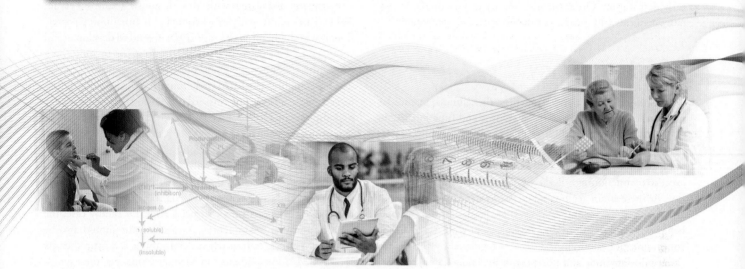

Attention deficit hyperactivity disorder (ADHD) is defined as a cluster of characteristics or behaviors that are related to several heterogeneous biopsychosocial behaviors and neurodevelopmental processes, which ultimately negatively influence one's social, occupational, or academic function (Feifel & MacDonald, 2008; Goodman et al., 2012). In children, the clinical presentation typically includes a combination of the inattentive and the hyperactivity–impulsivity components. This population tends to endorse symptoms of difficulty concentrating, failure to follow through, forgetfulness, and distractibility, the hallmarks of the inattentive symptom's domain. Many patients also endorse symptoms related to the inability to remain seated, fidgetiness, excessive running or climbing in inappropriate situations, trouble awaiting turn, and propensity to interrupt, the hallmarks of hyperactivity and impulsivity. The majority of children present with the combined subtype, that is, a combination of the inattentive and the hyperactive–impulsive subtypes.

But it is this inherent heterogeneity, particularly evident in adults, that complicates the diagnosis and contributes to the lack of uniformly recognized criteria in this population. In adults, however, clinical presentation and functional impacts vary greatly from their child and adolescent counterparts (Montano & Young, 2012). In addition to the heterogeneity with which ADHD presents, the core symptoms are arguably "normal" depending upon the age of the patient, environmental and social demands, and also the extent to which they occur. It is when the symptoms occur more frequently than is considered normal and to an extent that causes functional impairment and is inconsistent with developmental level that it is considered ADHD. For example, poor concentration in an academic setting could be considered normal in a child

who is under the age of 5, particularly when the poor attention occurs sporadically. If an intervention from a parent or a teacher resolves this issue, then this would not be considered ADHD. If, however, a child of a similar age consistently does not pay attention and does so in the context of parental or teacher intervention and disciplinary action, then this may be considered maladaptive and inconsistent with developmental level.

In 2011, it was estimated that approximately 11% of children 4 to 17 years of age (6.4 million) in the United States are diagnosed with ADHD, with a CDC-estimated prevalence of 5.6% to 15.9% of children. In 2013, the worldwide prevalence of ADHD in children was estimated at 5.6%, a contrast to our domestic statistics (American Psychiatric Association, 2013). Clinically meaningful symptoms persist into adulthood in 60% to 80% of patients, which suggests that ADHD is not exclusively a condition of childhood that resolves spontaneously but rather is a chronic illness.

CAUSES

A multitude of potential underlying causes of ADHD have been suggested, but none has yet to be fully validated. Secondary to the vast and diverse clinical manifestations, it is likely that the causes are multifactorial. Evidence suggests that the disorder may have a genetic component as parents and siblings of children with ADHD have a two to eight times greater chance of being diagnosed with ADHD. There have been advances in genetic studies of ADHD (Smith et al., 2009). ADHD has been associated with the dopamine transporter gene (DAT1, SLC6A3) and the dopamine 4 (D4) receptor gene (DRD4)

743

(Franke et al., 2012). Possible nongenetic causes are neurobiological, such as perinatal stress, low birth weight, traumatic brain injury, maternal smoking during pregnancy, and severe early deprivation. Other theories involve dietary intake of certain chemicals and sugars, but the evidence is inconsistent.

PATHOPHYSIOLOGY

The pathophysiology that underlies the clinical manifestations of ADHD involves reduced volume and functionality in the prefrontal cortex (PFC), caudate, and cerebellum. These brain regions are collectively primarily responsible for regulating attention, behavior, emotion, distraction inhibition, and executive functioning. Reduced volume or impaired function in these brain regions manifests as deficits in cognition, attention, motor planning, processing speed, and the complex behavioral complications that are consistent with ADHD. The communication among these areas is regulated by the neurochemicals dopamine and norepinephrine and a complex interaction among their multiple receptor subtypes. Dopamine governs reward, motivation, attention, and emotion, and when the available concentrations of dopamine are appropriate, there is sustained focus and on-task behavior and cognition. Norepinephrine, at appropriate levels, improves executive functioning and increases inhibition of thoughts and behavior. Functionally, norepinephrine enhances relevant signals, while dopamine suppresses irrelevant signals. Therefore, a relative balance between the two is critical for optimal function.

Both a hypoactive and a hyperactive norepinephrine and dopamine theory have been proposed, but an integration of the two may be the most realistic theory. The concentrations of available dopamine and norepinephrine relative to one another and the functionality of their receptors influence the expression of ADHD symptoms. The PFC functions optimally under conditions of moderate catecholamine release, as overstimulation results in impaired cognition as does understimulation. Acquired damage to the aforementioned brain regions produces behavioral disinhibition, distractibility, impulsivity, organizational deficits, and loss of working memory.

The symptom clusters that tend to emerge in a patient with ADHD include behavioral, cognitive, social–emotional, and deficits in executive function. The behavioral symptoms may include hyperactivity, impulsivity, disinhibition, novelty seeking, risk behaviors, and reward dependence. The cognitive features may include organizational issues, poor planning and execution skills, slower or impaired information processing, and deficits in time management. The social–emotional component may include emotional impulsivity, dysphoria, anger, anxiety, emotional lability, trouble reading social cues, and issues with making or keeping friends. Executive functioning refers to a wide range of central control processes that evolve during the process of aging and maturation. Executive function includes self-regulation, sequencing behaviors, planning and organization, working memory, and internalized speech.

Adult patients previously diagnosed and those with undiagnosed ADHD may develop and depend on compensatory mechanisms in order to overcome some of the functional impairments associated with this diagnosis (Santosh et al., 2011). Particularly, patients who are highly functioning professionals with higher than average IQs will tend to develop useful coping mechanisms to overcome symptoms or to hide them from others. Some patients become compulsive list-makers or develop a highly structured daily routine in order to minimize forgetting details, completing tasks, or losing belongings. They may unknowingly rely on coworkers or family members to an inappropriate extent for purposes of reminders or assistance in completing tasks or fulfilling responsibilities. Though compensatory mechanisms are generally therapeutic for the patient, they may cloud the clinical picture particularly in cases where the patient does not self-suspect ADHD but rather a family member or the practitioner suspects ADHD. In any case, the use of appropriate compensatory mechanisms should also be taken into consideration when determining if a drug therapy is indicated. Some patients can adequately manage their symptoms without clinically significant functional impact by relying on compensatory mechanisms and are able to avoid drug therapy.

As patients mature and roles and responsibilities evolve, the functional impairments and symptom presentation evolve in response, thereby presenting a barrier to fulfilling diagnostic criteria (Montano & Young, 2012). Adults are exposed to a variety of social and professional situations, which may provide an opportunity for previously unnoticed symptoms to manifest (Taylor et al., 2011). Inattentive symptoms may manifest as difficulty completing tasks, poor time management, difficulty sustaining attention in work-related activities, distractibility and forgetfulness, and poor concentration. Occupational performance and professional interpersonal relationships may suffer and may ultimately result in frequent job changes, unemployment, failure to live up to one's occupational potential, and lower salaries. Perhaps, the most significant evolution of symptoms occurs in the hyperactivity–impulsivity domain. It is often assumed that these symptoms fade or resolve entirely in adults. However, in adults, these symptoms manifest as interrupting conversations, frequent job changes, irritability, quick to anger, relationship discord, dangerous driving habits, and a low frustration tolerance. Maturation results in a shift in this symptom cluster, and it evolves from behavioral to cognitive; patients will feel restless as opposed to running around and leaving their seat (Santosh et al., 2011). An overwhelming majority of adult patients, somewhere on the order of 90%, will endorse symptoms of inattention.

DIAGNOSTIC CRITERIA

The most contemporary multidimensional approach to a relatively objective diagnosis in children and adolescents is the DSM-5 (*Diagnostic and Statistical Manual of Mental Health Disorders*, Fifth Edition) criteria, which assess symptomatology in all three domains (American Psychiatric Association, 2013). All iterations of the DSM criteria have failed to be validated in the adult population, and therefore, up until the release of the DSM-5 in May of 2013, there was very little consideration for the assessment of adult patients, though the DSM-IV had been used for this purpose. The DSM-5 has adapted the previous set of diagnostic criteria such that they are more accurately applied to adults and adult symptom presentation. The verbiage related to the criteria and the descriptors thereof have been changed to reflect more adult-specific situations, though the use of these criteria in adults has been widely criticized. Even considering the newest iteration of the criteria, practitioners are still in a position of having to make a retrospective evaluation of the presence of ADHD in childhood in order to establish a diagnosis in adulthood. This was cited as one of the most problematic components of the criteria as many patients either could not recall the childhood symptoms or could not produce documentation that would substantiate a childhood diagnosis. As ADHD is considered a developmental disorder, the presence of current symptoms as well as a history of previous symptoms (in childhood) needs to be established. Patients with ADHD, by nature of the illness, have impaired short- and long-term memory capabilities, and therefore, recall bias may impact the accuracy of assessments (Taylor et al., 2011). The practitioner is also faced with the challenge of determining if this was an established childhood diagnosis, a missed diagnosis in childhood, or a late-onset adult ADHD.

There are a host of validated rating scales for assessing the adult patient with suspected ADHD, although each has inherent limitations. The Adult Self-Report Scale (ASRS) is an 18-item screening tool that is based on the DSM-IV criteria (**Box 43.1**). Patients rate the items based on the frequency and degree to which they occur. The Conners' Self-Report Scale is a multidimensional assessment scale that both the patient and an observer complete. The long version of this scale is a 66-item toll that assesses symptoms consistent with inattention and memory deficits, impulsivity and emotional lability, hyperactivity and restlessness, and problems with self-conceptualization. Having multiple perspectives is ideal in that the observer may contribute critical data that the patient may either be unaware of or not willing to disclose. One of the most significant limitations of self-report scales is that they are generally not sufficient independently for establishing a diagnosis in the absence of more objective data or documentation (Modesto-Lowe et al., 2012).

Another challenge in the evaluation of patients is the degree of *symptom overlap* between ADHD and several other psychiatric diagnoses, namely, mood and anxiety disorders. Patients tend to associate poor concentration with ADHD alone and typically would not consider that an untreated or undiagnosed anxiety disorder can produce similar levels of concentration impairment. It is recommended that practitioners include an assessment for mood and anxiety disorders in their initial evaluations of these patients in order to rule out the presence of an additional psychiatric disorder.

In addition to symptom overlap with other psychiatric illnesses, ADHD is frequently *comorbid* with other psychiatric conditions. A determination of whether ADHD is present alone or whether it is present in addition to another psychiatric diagnosis is critical, as mood or anxiety disorders may be the sole diagnosis, which is producing ADHD-like symptoms. Patients with ADHD tend to have high rates of comorbidity with anxiety, depression, and substance abuse disorders with prevalence rates that are more than double those observed in patients without ADHD. In 2005 study, a staggering 87% of adult patients had at least one psychiatric comorbidity and 56% had two.

Substance use disorders (SUDs) are more common in patients with ADHD and the clinical course of ADHD tends to be more challenging in this patient population.

INITIATING DRUG THERAPY

Current guidelines and practice advocate for a multimodal treatment plan, which accounts for variations in response. The Multimodal Treatment Study (MTA) reported that children receiving intensive behavioral management combined with medication fared better than those receiving intensive behavioral management alone. The core symptom clusters of ADHD (inattention, hyperactivity, and impulsivity) respond to medication, with or without the behavioral intervention. Behavioral symptoms seem to respond to environmental modification, while skills in sports, academics, and social situations may not respond to medication or behavior modification. Relationship problems usually can be treated through psychotherapy.

Nonpharmacologic aspects of a multimodal treatment plan consist of behavior modification, parent training, family therapy, social skills training, academic skills training, individual psychotherapy, cognitive behavior modification, and therapeutic recreation. These are discussed further in the Nutrition/Lifestyle section later in this chapter.

The American Association of Pediatrics (AAP) has an established guideline for the treatment of ADHD, most recently published in 2011 (Wolraich et al., 2011). There is no domestic guideline that governs the treatment of ADHD in adults at this time; however, the National Institute for Health and Clinical Excellence (NICE) guideline from the British Psychological Society and the Royal College of Psychiatrists (2009) does include adult guidance (NCCMH, 2009). The NICE guideline for adults parallels the AAP guideline for children, and clinical practice for adult patients in the United States generally aligns with the pediatric/adolescent guidelines and the European guidelines. The AAP guidelines (children 4 to 18 years old) recommend initiating behavioral therapy in children 4 to 5 years old and only initiating methylphenidate if the symptoms are severe. In children older than 5 years (and up to 18 years), the initiation of a stimulant medication +/- behavioral interventions is considered first-line therapy. Preference is not given to one stimulant over another except in

A. A persistent pattern of inattention and/or hyperactivity–impulsivity that interferes with functioning or development, as characterized by (1) and/or (2):

1. **Inattention**: Six (6) or more of the following symptoms have persisted for at least 6 months to a degree that is inconsistent with developmental level and that negatively impacts directly on social and academic/occupational activities.

   Note: The symptoms are not solely a manifestation of oppositional behavior, defiance, hostility, or failure to understand tasks or instructions. For older adolescents and adults (age 17 and older), at least five symptoms are required.

   a. Often fails to give close attention to details or makes careless mistakes in schoolwork, work, or during other activities (e.g., overlooks or misses details, work is inaccurate)

   b. Often has difficulty sustaining attention in tasks or play activities (e.g., has difficulty remaining focused during lectures, conversations, or lengthy reading)

   c. Often does not seem to listen when spoken to directly (e.g., mind seems elsewhere, even in the absence of any obvious distraction)

   d. Often does not follow through on instructions and fails to finish schoolwork, chores, or duties in the workplace (e.g., starts tasks but quickly loses focus and is easily sidetracked)

   e. Often has difficulty organizing tasks and activities (e.g., difficulty managing sequential tasks; difficulty keeping materials and belongings in order; messy, disorganized work; has poor time management; fails to meet deadlines)

   f. Often avoids or is reluctant to engage in tasks that require sustained mental effort (e.g., schoolwork or homework; for older adolescents and adults, preparing reports, completing forms, reviewing lengthy papers)

   g. Often loses things necessary for tasks or activities (e.g., school materials, pencils, books, tools, wallets, keys, paperwork, eyeglasses, mobile telephones)

   h. Is often easily distracted by extraneous stimuli (e.g., for older adolescents and adults, may include unrelated thoughts)

   i. Is often forgetful in daily activities (e.g., doing chores, running errands; for older adolescents and adults, returning calls, paying bills, keeping appointments)

2. **Hyperactivity and impulsivity**: Six (or more) of the following symptoms have persisted for at least 6 months to a degree that is inconsistent with developmental level and that negatively impacts directly on social and academic/occupational activities.

   Note: The symptoms are not solely a manifestation of oppositional behavior, defiance, hostility, or failure to understand tasks or instructions. For older adolescents and adults (age 17 and older), at least five symptoms are required.

   a. Often fidgets with or taps hands or squirms in seat

   b. Often leaves seat in situations when remaining seated is expected (e.g., leaves his or her place in the classroom, in the office or other workplace, or in other situations that require remaining in place)

   c. Often runs about or climbs in situations where it is inappropriate (e.g., in adolescents or adults, may be limited to feeling restless)

   d. Often unable to play or engage in leisure activities quietly

   e. Is often "on the go" acting as if "driven by a motor" (e.g., is unable to be or uncomfortable being still for extended time, as in restaurants, meetings; may be experienced by others as being restless or difficult to keep up with)

   f. Often talks excessively

   g. Often blurts out answers before questions have been completed (e.g., completes people's sentences; cannot wait for turn in conversation)

   h. Often has difficulty awaiting turn (e.g., while waiting in line)

   i. Often interrupts or intrudes on others (e.g., butts into conversations, games, or activities; may start using other people's things without asking or receiving permission; for adolescents and adults, may intrude into or take over what others are doing)

B. Several inattentive or hyperactive–impulsive symptoms were present prior to age 12 years.

C. Several inattentive or hyperactive–impulsive symptoms are present in two or more settings (e.g., at home, school, or work; with friends or relatives; in other activities).

D. There is clear evidence that the symptoms interfere with, or reduce the quality of, social, academic, or occupational functioning.

E. The symptoms do not occur exclusively during the course of schizophrenia or another psychotic disorder and are not better explained by another mental disorder (e.g., mood disorder, anxiety disorder, dissociative disorder, personality disorder, substance intoxication or withdrawal).

TABLE 43.1

Recommended Order of Treatment for ADHD (All Ages)

Order	Agents	Comments
First line	Stimulants	Methylphenidate or amphetamine works quickly with first dose, is available in extended release, and is easy to titrate. If treatment with one member of the class is unsuccessful, attempt subsequent drugs from this class before initiating second-line therapy.
Second line	Nonstimulants	Atomoxetine should be the next drug utilized in patients who have failed stimulants; this is also appropriate for patients who have contraindications to stimulants.
		Guanfacine or clonidine has less impressive efficacy but can be added on to existing stimulant or atomoxetine therapy if monotherapy is insufficient. (This could also occur in third-line treatment.)
Third line	Bupropion	Takes a few weeks to have a therapeutic effect. May worsen anxiety and lower seizure threshold.

the case of children <6 years of age, in which methylphenidate is recommended (due to increased availability of evidence in this age group). Second-line therapy includes the nonstimulant medications with preference given to atomoxetine, then guanfacine, and then clonidine.

The NICE guidelines include recommendations for pediatric patients, adolescents, and adults. Only in cases of moderate impairment should drug therapy be initiated in children or adolescent patients per the NICE guidelines. Preference is not given to methylphenidate, amphetamine salts (referred to as dexamphetamine in Europe), or atomoxetine. In adults, however, drug therapy is considered first-line and methylphenidate is recommended as initial therapy over the other available stimulants. Amphetamine salts and atomoxetine are considered second-line therapies in situations where patients do not respond to or are intolerant of methylphenidate. Therapy (drug and/or nondrug) should continue for as long as it remains clinically effective.

In practice, but not necessarily suggested by any guideline, practitioners tend to initiate intermediate- to long-acting stimulant medications in children, adolescents, and adults. Medication products that have an extended duration of action tend to have a positive influence on tolerability, provide convenience, and improve compliance. It is also reasonable to start therapy with a short-acting medication product to establish an effective dose and then transition to a longer-acting version of the same drug, if available. There is no guideline that governs initiation of immediate-release versus longer-acting drug products, only guidelines that recommend starting doses and titration schedules. The prescriber determines which product to initiate based upon experience, patient preference, and other patient-specific factors.

Goals of Drug Therapy

Upon initiation of drug therapy with or without nondrug therapy, the expectation is that the core symptoms of ADHD will abate and the patient will no longer experience functional deficits in social, occupational, or academic domains. This result tends to emerge relatively quickly, particularly after the initiation of medication therapy. It is not uncommon to realize

this therapeutic success after the first attempt at drug therapy, and it is also not uncommon to utilize several pharmacotherapeutic modalities before the patient is adequately controlled (**Table 43.1**). There is a careful balance between resolving the core symptoms of ADHD and minimizing the risk of transient or serious adverse effects.

Stimulant Medications

Psychostimulants remain the drug class of choice in treating adults and children with ADHD (Modesto-Lowe et al., 2012). Most product formulations available are derived from one of two parent molecules: methylphenidate or amphetamine. See **Tables 43.2** and **43.3**.

Clinical trials have demonstrated a 68% to 97% patient response rate for a stimulant in *either* the amphetamine or methylphenidate subclass and a 12% to 71% response rate for *both* subclasses (Hodgkins et al., 2012).

Mechanism of Action

Pharmacologically, the stimulants inhibit the reuptake of dopamine and norepinephrine, thereby increasing concentrations in the presynaptic cleft. Amphetamines also directly stimulate the release of dopamine and norepinephrine. There are about 13 products currently available in the US market, some of which are immediate-release formulations and some of which are extended-release variations.

TABLE 43.2

Neurotransmitters Affected by Pharmacotherapy

	NE	DA	Comments
Methylphenidate	↑	↑	Blocks reuptake
Amphetamine	↑↑	↑	Blocks reuptake
			Causes release of NE
Atomoxetine	↑		Blocks reuptake of NE
Clonidine			Stimulates alpha2-adrenoceptors
Guanfacine			Stimulates alpha2-adrenoceptors
Bupropion	↑	↑	Weak blocker of NE, DA reuptake

TABLE 43.3

Overview of Agents Used to Treat ADHD

Generic (Trade) Name and Dosage	Selected Adverse Events	Contraindications	Special Considerations
atomoxetine (Strattera) Start: Children and adolescents <70 kg: 0.5 mg/kg/d for 4 d, then 1 mg/kg/d for 4 d, then 1.2 mg/kg/d	Increased heart rate and blood pressure, abdominal pain, decreased appetite, nausea, sedation Urinary retention in adults	Patients on MAO inhibitors, narrow-angle glaucoma	Atomoxetine does not appear to promote the development of new tics and therefore may be a good choice for patients unable to take stimulant medications due to preexisting tics
bupropion (Wellbutrin) Children: Start: Children and adolescents <70 kg: 0.5 mg/kg/d for 4 d, then 1 mg/kg/d for 4 d, then 1.2 mg/kg/d Range: 3–6 mg/kg/d or 150–300 mg/d Adults: 100 mg bid, then 100 mg tid; max. 4.5 mg/d	Insomnia, anorexia, dizziness, anxiety, confusion, xerostomia, constipation, nausea, agitation, fever, headache, vomiting, seizures	Seizure disorders, bulimia, anorexia nervosa Within 14 d of MAO inhibitors	Monitor weight
clonidine (Catapres) Children: Start: <45 kg: 0.05 mg hs, then titrate in 0.05 mg increments bid >45 kg: 0.1 mg hs, then titrate in 0.1 mg increments bid to qid Range: 27–40.5 kg: 0.05–0.2 mg; 40.5–45 kg: 0.05–0.3 mg; >45 kg: 0.05–0.4 mg Adults: 0.1 mg bid; max 2–4 mg/d	Dizziness, drowsiness, anxiety, confusion, xerostomia, constipation, impotence, nausea, hypotension	Hypersensitivity to clonidine	Monitor blood pressure (standing and supine), respiratory rate and depth, and heart rate
Long acting: dexmethylphenidate (Focalin XR 5-, 10-, 15-, 20-, 30-, 40-mg cap) 10 mg/d; max 40 mg/d dextroamphetamine (Dexedrine Spansule 5-, 10-, 15-mg cap) 5 mg/d, titrate 5 mg/d weekly; max 40 mg/d dextroamphetamine/amphetamine (Adderall XR 5-, 10-, 15-, 20-, 25-, 30-mg cap) 10 mg/d; max 30 mg/d lisdexamfetamine (Vyvanse 20-, 30-, 40-, 50-, 60-, 70-mg cap) 30 mg qd; max 70 mg/d methylphenidate; max 60 mg/d: Concerta (18-, 27-, 36-, 54-mg cap) 10 mg/d; titrate 18 mg/d weekly Daytrana (10, 15, 20, 30 mg/9 h patch) Metadate CD (10-, 20-, 30-, 40-, 50-, 60-mg cap) 20 mg qam Ritalin LA (10-, 20-, 30-, 40-mg cap) 20 mg qam	Nervousness, insomnia, arrhythmias, dry mouth, anorexia	Cardiovascular disease, hypertension, arteriosclerosis, hyperthyroidism, glaucoma, alcohol or drug abuse	Monitor growth and CNS activity High abuse potential Not recommended for children <3 y Avoid late evening dosing
Short acting: dexmethylphenidate (Focalin 2.5, 5, 10 mg) 2.5 mg bid; max 20 mg/d dextroamphetamine (Dexedrine 5-, 10-, 15-mg cap) 5 mg/d, titrate 5 mg/d weekly; max 40 mg/d dextroamphetamine/amphetamine (Adderall 5-, 7.5-, 10-, 12.5-, 15-, 20-, 30-mg tab) 5 mg qd to bid; max 40 mg/d methylphenidate; >6 y: 5 mg bid (before breakfast and lunch), titrate 5–10 mg/d weekly; max 60 mg/d methylphenidate (5-, 10-mg tab) Methylin (5-, 10-, 20-mg tab) Ritalin (5-, 10-, 30-mg tab)	Tachycardia, nervousness, insomnia, anorexia, dizziness, drowsiness	Marked anxiety, tension, or agitation Glaucoma History of tics or Tourette syndrome in patient or family	Monitor blood pressure, weight, height, heart rate, tics, sleep habits May potentiate effects of anticoagulants and anticonvulsants Abuse potential Not recommended for children <6 y

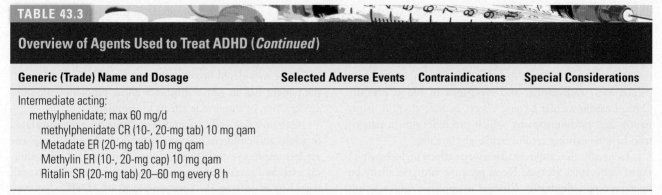

Generic (Trade) Name and Dosage	Selected Adverse Events	Contraindications	Special Considerations

Intermediate acting:
   methylphenidate; max 60 mg/d
     methylphenidate CR (10-, 20-mg tab) 10 mg qam
     Metadate ER (20-mg tab) 10 mg qam
     Methylin ER (10-, 20-mg cap) 10 mg qam
     Ritalin SR (20-mg tab) 20–60 mg every 8 h			

bid, twice daily; cap, capsule; CBC, comprehensive metabolic panel; CR, controlled release; ER, extended release; hs, at bedtime; max, maximum; qam, every morning; qd, every day; qid, four times a day; tab, tablet; tid, three times a day; y, year.

Stimulant medications mitigate the traditional ADHD symptoms and have demonstrated utility in improving interpersonal relationships, self-esteem, cognition, as well as symptoms of comorbid anxiety disorders (Minzenberg, 2012). Prescribing stimulant medications to adults has been a clinical controversy in primary care as well as in psychiatry. This class is arguably the most efficacious in resolving symptoms of ADHD and comorbid psychopathology; however, the risk of adverse effects and abuse potential may impact the rates at which these drugs are prescribed in the adult population.

Though none of the medications within the stimulant class have demonstrated superiority over another member of the class, there are some within-class pharmacokinetic differences that may impact product selection. The immediate-release products generally have a faster onset of action (which can be palpable by the patient) and a more abrupt cessation of effect (which can also be observed by the patient). This may be advantageous for patients who only have a discrete period of time during which they require medication action (during the school day, etc.). It can also be problematic for patients who cannot tolerate the abrupt start and stop of drug action.

The intermediate- and long-acting products have a less pronounced (and therefore less abrupt) onset and offset of therapeutic effect. Extended-release products are formulated to release defined amounts of drug over a 24-hour period. Ritalin LA releases 50% of the dose in two bursts, whereas Concerta releases 22% immediately and 78% later, and Metadate CD releases 30% immediately and 70% later. In addition to their more innocuous presentation, the extended-release products also afford patients a convenience factor, only having to dose once or twice daily (as compared to multiple daily doses with some immediate-acting products). Lisdexamfetamine (Vyvanse), in particular, has a 10- to 12-hour duration of action, which necessitates once-daily dosing. In addition to the convenience factor, this drug product is formulated as a prodrug that requires enzymatic degradation in the GI tract to become active. As a result, Vyvanse is far more difficult to misuse.

The risk of abuse or misuse of stimulants is a legitimate concern, which may ultimately impact treatment. SUDs occur comorbidly with ADHD at an odds ratio of 1.5 to 7.9 (Simon et al., 2015). Utilization of extended-release products minimizes, but does not completely negate, the risk of abuse.

Dosage

It is generally recommended that drug therapy, particularly in adults, should consist of an extended-release product in order to maximize compliance and minimize the risk of abuse. In children, many practitioners may decide to begin with a short-acting product in order to gauge response and tolerability and then switch to a longer-acting product. Initiation of drug therapy, irrespective of the nature of the release of the product, begins at the lowest dose (or the labeled starting dose) and is gradually titrated upward until the benefit is maximized and the patient is without adverse effects.

Time Frame for Response

Most patients taking a therapeutic dose of any stimulant medication will experience an effect on the day of the first dose and certainly within the first few days. If there is no appreciable improvement, then the dose should be increased, provided that it was well tolerated. As the recommended or maximum dose of the selected drug is approached and there is still an absence of effect, then either (1) the medication should be changed or (2) the diagnosis of ADHD should be re-evaluated.

Contraindications

The stimulants are contraindicated in children with certain comorbid disorders. Practitioners should not prescribe methylphenidate to patients with marked anxiety, tension, or agitation; glaucoma; or a history of tics or Tourette syndrome. Stimulants are contraindicated in patients who have existing cardiovascular disease, moderate to severe hypertension, hyperthyroidism, or history of substance abuse. In practice, the presence of a history of substance abuse may be overlooked if the risk of recurrence is determined to be low and the benefit of treatment is determined to be reasonable.

Adverse Events

The most common adverse events related to stimulant therapy tend to be cardiovascular, gastrointestinal, or neurologic in nature. Common, transient adverse effects include sleep disturbance, appetite suppression and associated weight loss, agitation, and nervousness. These are typically minimized by taking the drugs with food and using an extended-release formulation. Serious concerns exist related to the potential cardiotoxicity associated with the stimulants. Patients may experience palpitations, tachycardia, and elevations in blood pressure. Critical cardiovascular adverse effects include rhythm disturbances and cardiomyopathy, which precludes use in patients who have an existing cardiovascular abnormality.

Generally, the cardiovascular adverse effects include palpitations, tachycardia, elevated blood pressure, and potentially but uncommonly arrhythmias. Changes in appetite, nausea, vomiting, and other gastrointestinal (GI) disturbances may occur, particularly at the onset of therapy or upon a dosage increase. The neurologic adverse events range from headache and insomnia to seizure activity, particularly in patients predisposed to seizures.

In general, adverse events are manageable, results are quick and predictable with the first dose, and the medications are easy to titrate. The adverse events of the stimulants, such as headaches, dizziness, appetite suppression, tics, dyskinesias, sleep disturbances, abuse potential, and in particular growth retardation (below height or weight on normal growth charts), may be of concern, though the evidence related to growth suppression is sparse and contradictory. Determining the long-term effect of stimulants on children and adults is challenging. To minimize these effects, it is reasonable for the patient to take drug-free periods, usually over the summer. These periods also allow for reassessment of ADHD. Because children frequently seem to show symptoms in structured settings such as school, weekend "drug holidays" are also reasonable, permitting dosage adjustments and disease assessment. Rebound hyperactivity may be more prominent. No studies have been done to compare the effectiveness of weekend holidays versus summer holidays.

Other data indicate that there is less likelihood of substance abuse later in life when ADHD children take stimulant medication (NSDUH, 2013).

Nonstimulant Medications

Owing to their less impressive efficacy rates as compared to the stimulants, the nonstimulant medications tend to be prescribed less frequently among all age groups. Generally, practitioners do not initiate drug therapy with a nonstimulant unless the patient has a contraindication to stimulants (cardiac abnormalities, previous or current substance abuse) or is intolerant to or has failed the stimulant class. Currently, the nonstimulant therapeutic class includes atomoxetine (Strattera), immediate- and extended-release guanfacine (Tenex and Intuniv, respectively), clonidine and extended-release clonidine (Catapres and Kapvay, respectively), bupropion (Wellbutrin), and the tricyclic antidepressants.

Atomoxetine

Atomoxetine (Strattera) is the first nonstimulant approved by the U.S. Food and Drug Administration (FDA) for treating ADHD. It is not a controlled substance, and existing data suggest no real potential for abuse or diversion. While stimulants have greater treatment effect than atomoxetine, there are fewer adverse effects on appetite and sleep when compared to stimulants. However, there is more nausea and sedation, and it may be considered first-line therapy for ADHD treatment if the patient has an active substance abuse problem, comorbid anxiety, tics, or severe side effects to stimulants.

Atomoxetine's efficacy and safety have been demonstrated in adults and children; however, its associated rates of response are less impressive than those of the stimulants. In most clinical trials and meta-analyses, it has separated from placebo with regard to improving the core symptoms of ADHD; however, the clinical relevance of the improvements is debatable. It remains an appropriate option in patients who have contraindications to stimulants or who have a comorbid anxiety disorder, as anecdotal evidence suggests some level of anxiolytic activity.

Mechanism of Action

Atomoxetine selectively inhibits the reuptake of norepinephrine by inhibiting the presynaptic norepinephrine transporter. This translates into improved function in the PFC.

Dosage

The medication is available in 10-, 18-, 25-, 40-, 60-, 80-, and 100-mg capsules. For adolescents and adults over 70 kg, the starting dose is 40 mg; the dose is increased to an 80-mg target dose after a minimum of 3 days. The maximum recommended dose is 1.8 mg/kg/d for children and 100 mg for adolescents and adults; dosages should be adjusted only after 2 to 4 weeks of treatment at the lower dose. Since this agent undergoes significant metabolism via the CYP2D6 system, in slow metabolizers or patients taking agents with strong CYP2D6 effects (e.g., paroxetine, fluoxetine), the starting dose should be maintained for up to 4 weeks before dose adjustments are made. Patients with significant hepatic impairment should be started on a dose 50% of the usual starting dose.

Time Frame for Response

Atomoxetine is rapidly absorbed from the GI tract, leading to 63% bioavailability in extensive metabolizers and 94% bioavailability in poor metabolizers. The onset of action is quick, and dose adjustments are made in the first week. Despite the short half-life in extensive metabolizers, the duration of activity remains consistent throughout the day.

Contraindications

Atomoxetine should not be taken with MAO inhibitors because it increases synaptic norepinephrine concentrations. Further, due to the risk of angle closure, this agent should not be administered to patients with narrow-angle glaucoma.

Adverse Events

The increase in norepinephrine leads to an increase in blood pressure and heart rate; therefore, atomoxetine should be used cautiously in hypertensive patients or those with underlying cardiovascular disorders. Atomoxetine, like stimulants, should not be administered to patients with uncontrolled hypertension, structural cardiac abnormalities, cardiomyopathy, and abnormalities of the heart rhythm. In adults, there was a 3% rate of urinary retention or hesitation. Other common adverse effects include abdominal pain, vomiting, decreases in appetite, headache, irritability, and dermatitis. Atomoxetine does not appear to promote the development of new tics and therefore may be a good choice for patients who cannot take stimulant medications due to preexisting tics. Boxed warnings regarding rare hepatotoxicity and suicidal ideation in children and adolescents were issued by the FDA in 2005.

Interactions

Atomoxetine is a substrate of the CYP2D6 isoenzyme, and levels of this drug can be increased when CYP2D6 inhibitors are administered.

α-Agonists: Guanfacine and Clonidine

The α-agonists, a decades-old drug class, are traditionally used for the treatment of hypertension. For many years, they have been used off-label, particularly in children, for the adjunctive management of ADHD. Their purpose is largely limited to the treatment of behavioral manifestations, aggression, insomnia, and tics, and not for the core inattentive symptoms of ADHD. Both guanfacine and clonidine now are available in extended-release dosage forms, which are approved for the treatment of ADHD (Intuniv and Kapvay, respectively). Drugs in this therapeutic class are considered inferior to the stimulants with regard to efficacy and tolerability.

Mechanism of Action

Both guanfacine and clonidine act as postsynaptic α2-agonists, which are proposed to regulate subcortical activity in the PFC, the area of the brain responsible for emotions, attention, and behaviors. In some patients, this translates into reduced hyperactivity, impulsivity, and distractibility. Guanfacine demonstrates greater selectivity for the postsynaptic α2a receptor, which may confer improved efficacy and tolerability as compared to clonidine. Guanfacine also has a longer half-life, which is associated with less sedation and dizziness as compared to clonidine.

Dosage

Clonidine is dosed at 0.1 mg at bedtime with a 0.1 mg increase every 7 days until a therapeutic effect is realized (maximum of 0.4 mg daily; ideally dosed twice daily). Guanfacine is dosed at 1 mg daily with a weekly increase of 1 mg until clinical response is achieved (7 mg maximum daily dose). Dose adjustment for guanfacine may be necessary when administered concomitantly with strong CYP3A4 inhibitors or inducers.

Time Frame for Response

Generally, any therapeutic effects would be realized after approximately 4 weeks of treatment, but possibly after several months.

Contraindications

There are no absolute contraindications aside from hypersensitivity to the drug or any other component in the product.

Adverse Events

The adverse effects are generally mild and include fatigue, drowsiness, bradycardia, constipation, dizziness, hypotension, and headache. A gradual upward titration may minimize the emergence of these effects. It is also recommended that a downward taper be employed when discontinuing these medications as abrupt discontinuation may potentiate a hypertensive crisis. For the aforementioned reasons, it is important to educate the patient and/or caregiver about the importance of adherence.

Interactions

Given the central nervous system depressant action of clonidine and guanfacine, other concomitant CNS depressants should be avoided.

Bupropion

Bupropion has been evaluated in a small number of studies involving children, adolescents, and adults in which its efficacy compared to placebo or to an active stimulant comparator has been established. This is not an approved indication for bupropion in any age group. Bupropion may be a therapeutic alternative in adults who have contraindications or are intolerant to stimulant medications or in patients who have a comorbid depressive illness.

Mechanism of Action

Bupropion is an aminoketone antidepressant, which is commonly used for the treatment of depressive disorders as well as smoking cessation. It inhibits the reuptake of norepinephrine and dopamine (like the stimulants) but does so less intensely via a mechanism that is not fully understood. Bupropion is not associated with dependence, abuse, or misuse, which provides a therapeutic advantage in patients who have substance abuse issues.

Dosage

An appropriate dose for the treatment of ADHD has not been established, as the treatment of ADHD is an off-label use. In practice, the antidepressant dose (150 to 450 mg daily) is generally used, though rarely do patients titrate upward to the maximum dose. Bupropion is available as an immediate-release tablet, sustained-release tablet (SR), and extended-release tablet (XL). The XL tablets are dosed once daily and the SR and immediate-release tablets are both dosed twice daily.

Time Frame for Response

The onset of response is not well documented, but it is considered to be more rapid than the α2-agonists (weeks to months) but less rapid than stimulants (same day or a few days).

Contraindications

Bupropion may lower the seizure threshold in predisposed individuals. Therefore, patients with a known seizure disorder or patients taking a medication that has additive effects on the seizure threshold (benzodiazepines, alcohol) should avoid bupropion. This would also include patients who are abruptly discontinuing alcohol or other drugs. Bupropion's labeling includes a boxed warning regarding the risk of suicidal thinking or behavior that is associated with the antidepressant drugs.

Adverse Effects

Common adverse effects include dry mouth, nausea, insomnia, dizziness, anxiety, dyspepsia, sinusitis, and tremor. Bupropion may increase the risk of seizures, particularly with higher doses and shorter-acting formulations. Consideration should be given to patients who have a comorbid anxiety disorder, as bupropion has the potential to worsen anxiety.

Interactions

Bupropion is a major substrate and strong inhibitor of CYP2D6, and therefore, concurrent use of strong CYP2D6 substrates, inhibitors, or inducers is discouraged. Secondary to its impacts on metabolism, bupropion should not be used concomitantly with vortioxetine or the tricyclic antidepressants.

SELECTING THE MOST APPROPRIATE DRUG

Because of the number of therapeutic options available, this section suggests only a general outline to follow. Nonpharmacologic therapy differs for children and adults and may not always be included in the treatment plan (see **Table 43.1**). **Figure 43.1** outlines the therapeutic plan for a child, adolescent, and adult.

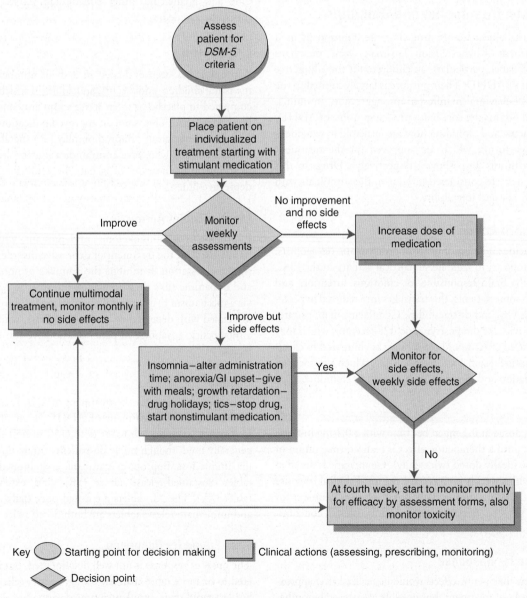

FIGURE 43.1 Treatment algorithm for attention deficit hyperactivity disorder.

Medication therapy is indicated in all patients who fulfill the diagnostic criteria and do not have contraindications to the selected medications.

First-Line Therapy

Stimulant medications are considered first-line therapy in children, adolescents, and adults without contraindications. There is no preference given to methylphenidate-type versus amphetamine-type stimulants, though methylphenidate appears to be favored in young children. There is no established difference in efficacy or tolerability among the members of this class. Product selection tends to be driven by duration of action and individual patient response (efficacy and tolerability). The longer-acting products confer improved convenience, owing to their less complex dosing regimens and possible improved compliance. Lisdexamfetamine (Vyvanse) boasts the longest duration of action and the least abuse potential secondary to its prodrug status, which requires enzymatic activation in the GI tract.

Failure of, or intolerance to, one stimulant does not necessarily mean that the entire therapeutic class is exhausted. In the event that a patient does not realize improvement or is unable to tolerate the initial drug, a different stimulant should be initiated (either from within the subclass of amphetamine-type or methylphenidate-type or from the other subclass).

Second-Line Therapy

Upon clinical failure or intolerance of the stimulants as a therapeutic class, atomoxetine is generally considered second-line therapy. Some practitioners may elect to initiate an α2-agonist at this time; however, guidelines generally recommend atomoxetine first.

Third-Line Therapy

Bupropion or the α2-agonists may be attempted after failure of, or intolerance to, the stimulants and atomoxetine. At this point, these drugs may also be considered as adjunctive therapy to a partially successfully stimulant or atomoxetine. In the past, the tricyclic antidepressants were also considered third- or fourth-line therapy but they are generally no longer used for this purpose.

After failure of several drugs (even if only the stimulants have been attempted), the diagnosis of ADHD should be re-evaluated. The response rates for stimulants exceed 90%, and therefore, a lack of efficacy is suspicious and may suggest an alternate diagnosis.

MONITORING PATIENT RESPONSE

To determine the efficacy of the drugs used to treat ADHD, practitioners must use the rating scales mentioned previously; no laboratory values or diagnostic tests can determine the patient's improvement. Usually, follow-up visits are scheduled monthly after initiation of a medication and until the patients

have achieved a response. When the medication regimen is stable and tolerated, the follow-up visits tend to occur at longer intervals but at least every 6 to 12 months.

Treatment is indicated for as long as the patient is showing core symptoms of ADHD. Practitioners can best determine the need to continue treatment by considering the patient's response during the "drug holidays." If symptoms are no longer present, treatment may not be needed. Continued assessment of the patient even when he or she is not using medication is essential. Medication should be given at the lowest effective dosage.

Studies show that stimulants' general side effects of insomnia, decreased appetite, dizziness, stomachache, and headache are usually mild and do not necessitate discontinuation of the drug. Sleep difficulties may actually be related to the ADHD, which causes symptoms that prevent the child from sleeping. Because sleep disturbances cannot be generalized, it is reasonable to assess the patient and determine whether altered bedtimes or altered medication times are appropriate interventions.

In reviewing the complication of tics and dyskinesias, one study determined that transient tics develop in approximately 9% of children. The development of tics does not depend on prior personal or family history. Even though this study showed that tics or dyskinesias are not a contraindication, most health care professionals use stimulants cautiously in patients with prior histories.

Most of the other adverse events were discussed earlier. If any adverse event occurs that is disturbing to the patient, reasonable alternatives are to lower the dose or discontinue the medication. If the patient is using a stimulant and the outcome is poor, substituting another stimulant is reasonable before trying another medication class.

PATIENT EDUCATION

Medications prescribed for ADHD must be taken exactly as prescribed to get the full benefit. If any adverse events occur that are disturbing, the patient should contact the health care provider immediately. Parents and adult patients should be aware of adverse events to watch for, as previously discussed. Patients need to be evaluated on a regular basis to determine their treatment needs.

Drug Information

The FDA's Web site (www.fda.gov) is a good source of initial prescribing information. Sources such as Facts and Comparisons can also provide information about the use of these agents.

Patient-Oriented Information Sources

The National Institute of Mental Health (NIMH) has an excellent Web site related to ADHD (http://www.nimh.nih.gov/health/topics/attention-deficit-hyperactivity-disorder-adhd/index.shtml). This site provides access to booklets describing strategies for dealing with ADHD directed at parents of young children as well as adolescents. There are also links to local providers, clinical research trials, and other resources. CHADD (Children and Adults with Attention Deficit Disorder) at www.chadd.org is a great source of information and support for parents and patients with ADHD.

Nutrition/Lifestyle Changes

Dietary additives and supplements, such as dyes and preservatives, have long been implicated as a cause of ADHD symptoms. Literature is equivocal regarding whether or not removal of these from the diet in certain children is helpful. At this time, there is no recommendation to limit or exclude dyes from the diet.

Parent training involves teaching parents to recognize situations in which their child could learn or improve social skills. Parents must actively participate in the child's social life, using punishment effectively by clear instruction, positively reinforcing good behavior, ignoring some behaviors, and using negative reinforcement, such as time out, to decrease the child's stimulation. This method has been shown useful for the short term and is an alternative for parents who do not want to proceed directly to medication therapy.

As mentioned previously, the parents also may have ADHD. Family therapy can help teach all members how to negotiate and solve problems together as a unit. Because family therapy may be expensive, parent support groups can promote effective problem-solving techniques and unity.

Social skills training is based on the patient's deficits. Studies show that group training is more effective than individual training because self-observation usually is impossible for this patient population—both children and adults. Academic skills training helps to refine a child's ability to organize, take notes, improve study habits, and prioritize activities. This methodology has not been tested, but in clinical practice, it has been found useful if academic deficiencies are present. Adult patients may also benefit from reappraising their own social, academic, and occupational skill sets. Developing and adhering to a schedule, making commitments to observe deadlines, and accepting consequences when tasks or responsibilities are not successfully completed or maintained will assist in reinforcing good behaviors and minimizing bad behaviors. Adult patients may delay diagnosis by developing compensatory mechanisms and/or relying on others, actively avoiding compensatory mechanisms and not utilizing friends, family, or coworkers as a pathologic support system may also provide a therapeutic benefit.

Psychotherapy is not useful as treatment of ADHD but can help patients with moralization, self-esteem, and compliance problems. It may also be useful for patients with comorbid illnesses such as anxiety and depression. Psychotherapy may be needed only as difficulties arise.

Cognitive behavior modification teaches stepwise problem solving and self-monitoring by using the reinforcement techniques of rewarding for good behavior and removing rewards for unwanted behavior. Although initially believed to be a good strategy, cognitive behavior modification was later found not to improve outcomes when added to medication therapy.

CASE STUDY*

S.B., age 8, is always interrupting his teacher, jumping out of his seat in class, fidgeting relentlessly, and butting into other children's games. At home, he runs around recklessly and is uncontrollable. His mother comes to you and wonders why he will not listen. She is concerned because his grades at school are worsening and he has had disciplinary issues with his teachers. After medical evaluation, you find nothing wrong with **S.B.** physically, and he is taking no other medications. Through questioning, you determine that he has trouble concentrating on his homework, often forgets he has homework, does not complete assignments when he remembers them, loses pieces of games frequently, and hates to sit and read. His mother is unsure of the time frame over which these behaviors developed, but she thinks it has been since her second child was born 4 years ago. While in your office, **S.B.** did not seem to be hyperactive or inattentive, but you notice he is easily distracted by people passing in the hallway because the door is slightly ajar.

DIAGNOSIS: ADHD

1. List specific goals of treatment for **S.B.**
2. What would be the first-line drug therapy for **S.B.**? Why?
3. What monitoring parameters would you institute? **S.B.** parents and teachers should be aware of changes in sleep, appetite, and mood (monitoring for adverse effects) as well as improvements in organization, memory, and follow-through (monitoring for efficacy).
4. Discuss specific patient education you would provide to **S.B.** parents based on the prescribed therapy.
5. Describe one or two drug–drug or drug–food interactions that you would be wary of when prescribing this agent.
6. List one or two adverse reactions to the agent you selected that would cause you to change therapy.
7. If the adverse reactions you described above occurred, what would be your second-line therapy for **S.B.**? Why?
8. What over-the-counter and/or alternative medications would be appropriate for **S.B.**?
9. What dietary and lifestyle changes would you recommend to **S.B.** parents?

* Answers can be found online.

All these techniques offer different benefits, so individual assessment and reassessment are important to determine which techniques (if any) are making a difference for the patient. Some parents may want to try one or more of these methods before trying medication, and practitioners should permit the parents to try whatever methods they feel will be best for their child.

As with children, nonpharmacologic treatment also is beneficial for adults. "Coaching" involves daily encouragement to progress toward set goals. Educational programs help adults to identify their problem, understand it, and not blame themselves for it. Cognitive remediation also is used to teach attention enhancement, memory, problem solving, family relationships, time management, organization skills, and anger control. Medication should not be used as a substitute for treating behaviors with behavior modification. Each patient's therapeutic plan should be assessed and reassessed for success and usefulness.

Complementary and Alternative Medications

There are several herbal medications that may have an impact on a person with ADHD. Ginkgo biloba, a plant-derived medication, has shown some efficacy in improving memory and improving concentration when added to stimulant therapy in children and adolescents (Shakibaei et al., 2015). Supplementation with polyunsaturated acids has also been evaluated as a possible natural adjunctive therapy, but its efficacy has yet to be established.

Bibliography

Starred references are cited in the text.

Adamo, N., Seth, S., & Coghill, D. (2015). Pharmacological treatment of attention-deficit/hyperactivity disorder: Assessing outcomes. *Expert Review of Clinical Pharmacology, 8*(4), 383–397.

*American Psychiatric Association. (2013). *Diagnostic and statistical manual of mental health disorders: DSM-5* (5th ed.). Washington, DC: American Psychiatric Publishing.

Bloch, M. H., & Mulqueen, J. (2014). Nutritional supplements for the treatment of ADHD. *Child and Adolescent Psychiatric Clinics of North America, 23*(4), 883–897.

Brikell, I., Kuja-Halkola, R., & Larsson, H. (2015). Heritability of attention-deficit hyperactivity disorder in adults. *American Journal of Medical Genetics Part B: Neuropsychiatric Genetics.* doi: 10.1002/ajmg.b.32335 [Epub ahead of print].

Chen, L. Y., Crum, R. M., Strain, E. C., et al. (2015). Patterns of concurrent substance use among adolescent nonmedical ADHD stimulant users. *Addictive Behaviors, 49*, 1–6.

Childress, A. C., & Sallee, F. R. (2012). Revisiting clonidine: An innovative add-on option for attention-deficit/hyperactivity disorder. *Drugs of Today (Barcelona, Spain), 48*(3), 207–217.

Culpepper, L., & Mattingly, G. (2010). Challenges in identifying and managing attention-deficit/hyperactivity disorder in adults in the primary care setting: A review of the literature. *The Primary Care Companion—Journal of Clinical Psychiatry, 12*(6).

Estévez, N., Dey, M., Eich-Höchli, D., et al. (2015). Adult attention-deficit/hyperactivity disorder and its association with substance use and substance use disorders in young men. *Epidemiology and Psychiatric Sciences, 20*, 1–12.

*Feifel, D., & MacDonald, K. (2008). Attention-deficit/hyperactivity disorder in adults: Recognition and diagnosis of this often-overlooked condition. *Postgraduate Medicine, 120*(3), 39–47.

*Franke, B., Faraone, S. V., Asherson, P., et al.; International Multicentre persistent ADHD CollaboraTion. (2012). The genetics of attention deficit/hyperactivity disorder in adults, a review. *Molecular Psychiatry, 17*(10), 960–987.

*Goodman, D. W., Surman, C. B., Scherer, P. B., et al. (2012). Assessment of physician practices in adult attention-deficit/hyperactivity disorder. *The Primary Care Companion for CNS Disorders, 14*(4).

*Hodgkins, P., Shaw, M., Coghill, D., et al. (2012). Amfetamine and methylphenidate medications for attention-deficit/hyperactivity disorder: Complementary treatment options. *European Child and Adolescent Psychiatry, 21*(9), 477–492.

Hurt, E. A., & Arnold, L. E. (2014). An integrated dietary/nutritional approach to ADHD. *Child and Adolescent Psychiatric Clinics of North America, 23*(4), 955–964.

Jarrett, M. A. (2015). Attention-deficit/hyperactivity disorder (ADHD) symptoms, anxiety symptoms, and executive functioning in emerging adults. *Psychological Assessment* [Epub ahead of print].

*Minzenberg, M. J. (2012). Pharmacotherapy for attention-deficit/hyperactivity disorder: From cells to circuits. *Neurotherapeutics, 9*(3), 610–621.

*Modesto-Lowe, V., Meyer, A., & Soovajian, V. (2012). A clinician's guide to adult attention-deficit hyperactivity disorder. *Connecticut Medicine, 76*(9), 517–523.

*Montano, C. B., & Young, J. (2012). Discontinuity in the transition from pediatric to adult health care for patients with attention-deficit/hyperactivity disorder. *Postgraduate Medicine, 124*(5), 23–32.

*NCCMH. (2009). *Attention deficit hyperactivity disorder: Diagnosis and management of ADHD in children, young people and adults.* Leicester and London: The British Psychological Society and the Royal College of Psychiatrists [Full guideline].

*NSDUH. (2013). *Substance abuse and mental health services administration, results from the 2012 National Survey on Drug Use and Health: Summary of National Findings, NSDUH Series H-46, HHS Publication No. (SMA) 13-4795.* Rockville, MD: Substance Abuse and Mental Health Services Administration.

Richardson, M., Moore, D. A., Gwernan-Jones, R., et al. (2015). Non-pharmacological interventions for attention-deficit/hyperactivity disorder (ADHD) delivered in school settings: Systematic reviews of quantitative and qualitative research. *Health Technology Assessment, 19*(45), 1–470.

*Santosh, P. J., Sattar, S., & Canagaratnam, M. (2011). Efficacy and tolerability of pharmacotherapies for attention-deficit hyperactivity disorder in adults. *CNS Drugs, 25*(9), 737–763.

*Shakibaei, F., Radmanesh, M., Salari, E., et al. (2015). Ginkgo biloba in the treatment of attention-deficit/hyperactivity disorder in children and adolescents. A randomized, placebo-controlled, trial. *Complementary Therapies in Clinical Practice, 21*(2), 61–67.

*Simon, N., Rolland, B., & Karila, L. (2015). Methylphenidate in adults with attention deficit hyperactivity disorder and substance use disorders. *Current Pharmaceutical Design, 21*(23), 3359–3366.

*Smith, A. K., Mick, E., & Faraone, S. V. (2009). Advances in genetic studies of attention-deficit/hyperactivity disorder. *Current Psychiatry Reports, 11*(2), 143–148.

*Taylor, A., Deb, S., & Unwin, G. (2011). Scales for the identification of adults with attention deficit hyperactivity disorder (ADHD): A systematic review. *Research in Developmental Disabilities, 32*(3), 924–938.

*Wolraich, M., Brown, L., Brown, R. T., et al.; Subcommittee on Attention-Deficit/Hyperactivity Disorder; Steering Committee on Quality Improvement and Management. (2011). ADHD: Clinical practice guideline for the diagnosis, evaluation, and treatment of attention-deficit/hyperactivity disorder in children and adolescents. *Pediatrics, 128*(5), 1007–1022.

44

Alzheimer Disease

Emily R. Hajjar

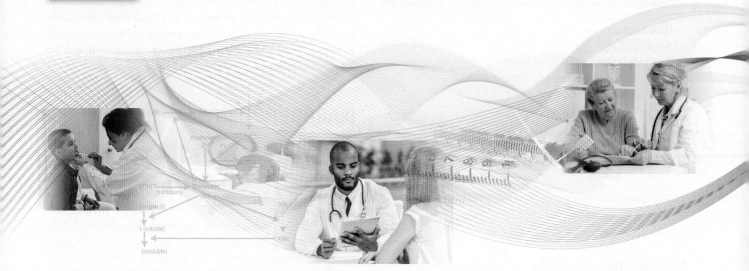

Alzheimer disease (AD), also known as neurocognitive disorder due to Alzheimer disease, is the most common cause of dementia accounting for approximately 60% to 80% of all dementias. AD is characterized by a slow, progressive decline in cognition. Patients initially complain of short-term (recent) memory loss, forgetfulness, and a decreased ability to learn and retain new information.

Estimates suggest that approximately 5.5 million people in the United States and 35 million people worldwide have AD (Quefurth & LaFerla, 2010). The number is expected to grow to 13.2 to 16 million in the United States by 2050 as the population continues to age (Quefurth & LaFerla, 2010). A majority of individuals with AD are residing in the community, which represents a huge emotional and financial burden on the patient, friends, and family members, as well as on society as a whole. The cost of care is estimated at approximately $260 billion each year in the United States. This number does not include the cost of unpaid care given by family members or loved ones.

Early-onset AD occurs in patients younger than 65 years of age and is less common, whereas late-onset AD is more common and occurs in patients age 65 or older. Familial AD is also a less common form of AD and affects patients with genetic mutations of amyloid precursor protein (APP), presenilin-1, and presenilin-2. Familial AD may be of early or late onset (Lendon et al., 1997). Genetic causes (e.g., apolipoprotein E4 allele, presenilin-1, and presenilin-2 gene mutations) have also been linked to late-onset AD. Symptoms of AD can be divided between cognitive symptoms and noncognitive symptoms, and treatment is based on the particular domain of the symptoms. Cognitive symptoms, such as loss of short-term memory, usually present first in mild AD, whereas the noncognitive behavioral symptoms are seen in more moderate-to-severe AD. Currently, AD is incurable although pharmacologic agents

have been used to modestly slow the progression of the disease. The average life span for patients with AD is reduced by as much as 70% with a mean duration of approximately 10 years from the time of diagnosis (Kua et al., 2014). In the United States, AD is the sixth leading cause of death. Women are at a slightly higher risk for developing AD than men. Prevalence increases with age, with AD affecting approximately 40% to 50% of those older than age 85. Patients with AD commonly die from causes such as cardiovascular disease, pneumonia, cancer, and diabetes (Kua et al., 2014).

CAUSES

Apolipoprotein E (ApoE), a protein involved in cholesterol transport, is linked to the development of AD. The E4 allele (homozygote E4/E4) is thought to increase the risk of AD, whereas the E2 allele may be protective. Advanced age and family history are the most significant risk factors for AD, and other risk factors are listed in **Box 44.1.**

PATHOPHYSIOLOGY

Pathologic changes in AD include formation of neurofibrillary tangles and plaques, cortical atrophy, and neuronal (cholinergic, glutamatergic) destruction and loss. In AD patients, acetylcholine levels are decreased, and an excessive stimulation of glutamate causes neuronal toxicity. These changes affect several areas of the brain, including the hippocampus, the amygdala, the cerebral cortex, and, ultimately, the motor cortex. As a result of these changes, short- and long-term memory, learning, language, behavior, and, eventually, motor skills are impaired.

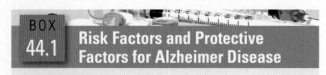

Neurofibrillary Tangles

Neurofibrillary tangles and neuritic or β-amyloid plaques are the hallmark pathologic lesions in AD. Tau protein, the principal component of neurofibrillary tangles, becomes hyperphosphorylated in AD. The abnormal phosphorylation of tau protein leads to the formation of paired helical filaments and finally neurofibrillary tangles. As a result, microtubule assembly is inhibited and critical organelles may collapse, causing abnormal intracellular transport and neuronal cell death.

Plaques

Plaques are brain lesions that contain a core of β-amyloid protein (BAP) and a shell of damaged neurites. APP is the parent protein of BAP. Proteases normally cleave APP through the BAP region, which prevents intact BAP from entering the extracellular fluid. When abnormal proteolysis occurs, leaving BAP intact, increased extracellular BAP becomes involved in plaque formation and neuronal degeneration. Plaques are also composed of neurofibrillary tangles, ApoE, and glial cells, which may be involved in the pathologic process of AD and are areas of interest to researchers. Neurofibrillary tangles and plaque density correlate with increased severity of AD.

Neuronal Destruction

The neuronal cell damage and death seen in AD result in impaired neurotransmitter function. The cholinergic and glutamatergic systems are significantly involved. Destruction of cholinergic neurons leads to decreased levels of acetylcholine, a neurotransmitter that aids in learning and memory. The symptomatic presentation of AD (memory loss and cognitive impairment) appears to be associated with acetylcholine deficiency. The cholinergic system has been the subject of a vast amount of research and pharmacologic development (e.g., acetylcholinesterase inhibitors). Overstimulation or erratic stimulation of the glutamatergic system in the synapse causes

neuronal toxicity leading to neuronal death. This disruption is thought to impair learning and memory.

The autoimmune system or inflammatory mediators may be linked to late-onset AD. Glial cells, complement cascade components, and cytokines are present in plaque areas. These cells and inflammatory mediators may contribute to neuronal cell damage and loss. Their role in AD is under investigation, as is the use of intravenous immunoglobulins for the treatment of AD.

DIAGNOSTIC CRITERIA

The clinical diagnosis of AD can be made using the *Diagnostic and Statistical Manual of Mental Disorders* (5th ed.), known as the *DSM-5*. The diagnosis can be *confirmed* only by autopsy. Diagnostic criteria include concern for loss of memory by the patient, caregiver, or provider; insidious onset; performance below normal on standardized cognition assessments; deficits in one or more cognitive domains; and the absence of other diseases that may account for the symptoms of AD.

Patients and their caregivers should be closely involved in the diagnostic process. A complete history and physical examination that includes a neurologic and mental status evaluation is essential. The Mini Mental State Examination (MMSE) or the Montreal Cognitive Assessment (MOCA) may be used to screen for cognitive impairment. The clock drawing task (CDT) is another initial evaluation tool that is quick and can be performed by any health care professional (**Figure 44.1**).

INITIATING DRUG THERAPY

A careful assessment of baseline diagnostic findings is essential before initiating drug therapy. The patient, family, and caregiver should be informed of the severity of cognitive and functional impairment. Baseline scores on cognitive testing and functional status can help guide decisions related to drug therapy. Reversible causes of dementia must also be considered and eliminated because several medications and medical conditions may cause or aggravate dementia (**Box 44.2**).

Before starting drug therapy for the cognitive symptoms of AD, the patient or family should demonstrate a clear understanding of the efficacy and expected outcomes of treatment, as well as the potential adverse events, costs, and incurability of the disease. The choice not to initiate drug therapy is also a reasonable option as many patients only experience modest benefits from drug therapy and incur side effects and expenses from the medications.

Pharmacologic management of the noncognitive symptoms is tailored to the individual symptom. These medications are usually initiated when the patient progresses to the moderate-to-severe stages of AD. The use of both noncognitive and cognitive therapies may be necessary as the disease progresses.

Nonpharmacologic psychotherapies, such as behavior-oriented, emotion-oriented, cognition-oriented, and stimulation-oriented approaches, can be useful for some patients with AD. Other nonpharmacologic interventions include using calendars,

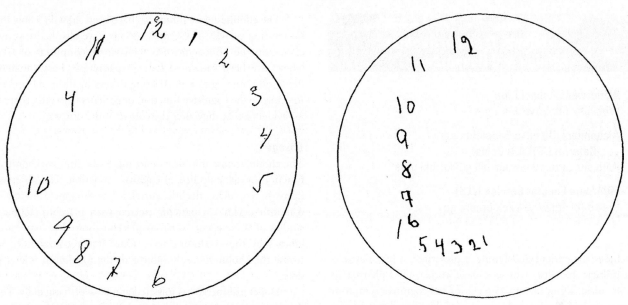

FIGURE 44.1   Clock drawing task completed by various elderly subjects. (Reproduced from Agrell, B., & Dehlin, O. (1998). The clock-drawing test. *Age and Ageing, 27*, 399–403; by permission of Oxford University Press.)

BOX 44.2 Potentially Reversible Causes of Dementia

Medications
Anticholinergics (e.g., benztropine, diphenhydramine)
Antipsychotics (e.g., olanzapine, thioridazine)
Benzodiazepines (e.g., diazepam, lorazepam)
Histamine (H_2) blockers (e.g., cimetidine)

Metabolic Disorders
Dehydration
Hyperthyroidism and hypothyroidism
Hyponatremia
Hypercalcemia

Intracranial Infection or Disease
Meningitis
Neurosyphilis
Normal pressure hydrocephalus
Subdural hematoma
Tumor
Toxoplasmosis

Miscellaneous
Toxins (e.g., lead, mercury, alcohol)
Vitamin B_{12} deficiency
Depression
Psychoses

Data from Wiser, T. H. (1994). Alzheimer's disease. *US Pharmacist, 63* and AGS 2012 Beers Criteria.

clocks, and written notes or instructions. The caregiver should attempt to maintain a predictable routine with the patient. Drastic changes in the environment, as well as confrontation and arguments, should be avoided. Recognition of precipitants of agitation, psychosis, and anxiety can assist the caregiver and health care provider to best develop a patient-specific treatment plan.

The patient's ability to drive should be evaluated, and as AD progresses, the patient should be advised to stop driving because dementia may increase the risk of accidents. The patient's use of a stove should be evaluated because, if left on and unattended, it can be harmful. Families should be taught how to prevent falls and wandering. They should also be informed about the possibility of physical violence and caregiver stress associated with more severe disease. Capable patients may want to discuss with their families advance directives, living wills, desires for nursing home placement, and powers of attorney.

Patient and family education are the most important nonpharmacologic interventions for AD. Depending on the stage of impairment, the patient requires some or full assistance with activities of daily living (ADL), such as dressing, toileting, and, particularly, driving. Support for patients and families is vitally important at any stage of AD (**Box 44.3**), and anyone involved with a patient with AD should be educated on the availability of support groups to deal with the wide variety of issues associated with AD. Other resources for the caregiver include the use of respite care centers and day care centers.

Goals of Drug Therapy

The optimal goal of drug therapy is to maintain and maximize the patient's functional ability, quality of life, and independence for as long as possible while minimizing adverse events and cost (APA, 2014). A multidisciplinary approach to therapy, which

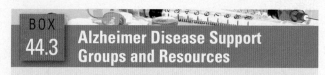

includes the patient and family, a prescriber, a psychiatric or neurologic specialist, a nurse, a social worker, and a pharmacist, is the ideal. Drug therapy choices for the cognitive symptoms primarily include the cholinesterase inhibitors and memantine.

Selected Agents for Cognitive Symptoms

Cholinesterase Inhibitors

Cholinesterase inhibitors, also known as the *acetylcholinesterase inhibitors*, play a key role in the pharmacologic treatment of AD. This drug class includes donepezil (Aricept), rivastigmine (Exelon), and galantamine (Razadyne, Razadyne ER). These agents are used to slow the progression of the cognitive, functional, and behavioral domains of AD.

If no effect is seen within 3 to 6 months of treatment or the patient is experiencing an adverse effect, another agent from this class may be tried. These medications are not curative and it is unknown how long treatment with these agents should be continued. However, once a patient progresses to severe AD, these agents are no longer solely recommended or may be discontinued due to lack of benefit. Additional pharmacologic therapy may be necessary once the disease progresses into the moderate-to-severe stages. Thoughtful discussions with caregivers or families may guide the decision to discontinue therapy.

Cholinesterase inhibitors inhibit one or both types of the cholinesterase enzymes, butyrylcholinesterase or acetylcholinesterase. Butyrylcholinesterase is primarily found in the periphery, and inhibition of this enzyme leads to many of the adverse effects of the cholinesterase agents. Acetylcholinesterase is found more centrally and thus is the primary focus of inhibition for the use in AD.

Rivastigmine is a cholinesterase inhibitor with its potential advantage of being pseudoirreversible. It inhibits the enzyme for about 10 hours, making this an intermediate-acting agent. It is notable that rivastigmine is the only cholinesterase inhibitor that is approved to treat both mild-to-moderate AD as well as mild-to-moderate dementia associated with Parkinson disease. Galantamine is a cholinesterase inhibitor on the market and is indicated to treat mild-to-moderate AD. Besides inhibiting the cholinesterase enzyme, it also allosterically modulates the nicotinic receptor.

The cholinesterase inhibitors have been shown to slow the progression of AD. These medications have also had positive effects on the noncognitive or behavioral symptoms of AD. They have been shown to reduce apathy, psychosis, anxiety, depression, and agitation. Although these medications appear to improve the cognitive function of patients with AD, there is no evidence that they alter the course of the disease.

Dosage

The cholinesterase inhibitors may modestly improve cognitive function or delay decline in cognitive function. The observed delay in cognitive decline correlates with approximately a 6-month decline in patients treated with placebos. Clinical studies of these agents versus a placebo show that maximum efficacy by the maximum dose. Thus, it is recommended to titrate the cholinesterase inhibitor to the maximum tolerated dose.

Donepezil therapy is initiated at a dose of 5 mg daily. The dosage may be increased after 4 to 6 weeks to a maximum dose of 10 mg/d if tolerated. Donepezil 10 mg/d is slightly more effective than the 5-mg dose; therefore, increasing to 10 mg/d is appropriate for patients who do not respond within 6 weeks of treatment with the 5-mg dose. A 23-mg dose may be tried in moderate-to-severe patients that have been stable on 10 mg daily for at least 3 months. Donepezil is available as a tablet as well as an orally disintegrating tablet for patients who have trouble swallowing. Rivastigmine doses should be started at 1.5 mg twice a day and should increase to 3 mg twice a day after 2 weeks of treatment for the capsule and oral solution formulations. Further dose increases should be based on clinical response and can be attempted on a biweekly basis. The maximum dose is 6 mg twice a day for the capsule and oral solution formulations. If the patch formulation of rivastigmine is started, the dose should be 4.6 mg/24 hours and can be titrated to 9.5 mg/24 hours after 4 weeks and then to 13.3 mg/24 hours after another 4-week period, if tolerated. Galantamine is available as an immediate-release tablet and oral solution as well as in extended-release capsules. The immediate-release forms of galantamine are started at a dose of 4 mg twice a day and titrated up every 4 weeks as tolerated to a maximum dose of 24 mg/d (12 mg twice daily). The extended-release formulation of galantamine is started at 8 mg daily and can be titrated up to a dose of 24 mg/d in 4-week intervals.

Time Frame for Response

Cholinesterase inhibitors may slow the progression of AD, but the effects may not be immediately noticeable. Patients and families may report improvement—or lack of continued decline—within 3 to 6 weeks of beginning treatment. Response may also be seen in repeated cognitive assessment measures done in 3- to 6-month intervals.

Contraindications

Contraindications to using a CI include hypersensitivities to any of the compounds. Precautions to using the CIs include anorexia, neuroleptic malignant syndrome, bradycardia, peptic ulcer disease, conduction abnormalities, asthma or chronic obstructive pulmonary disease, and seizure disorder. Patients weighing less than 55 kg may also experience more profound GI side effects such as nausea and vomiting.

Adverse Events

The major adverse effects of the cholinesterase inhibitors are cholinergic, most commonly nausea, vomiting, and diarrhea (5% to 47%). Oral formulations of rivastigmine have been associated with the highest incidence of these gastrointestinal (GI) disturbances (19% to 47%); the patch is associated with much lower rates (6% to 20%). These effects are dose dependent and can be minimized by slowly titrating to higher doses (**Table 44.1**).

Bradycardia can occur with the use of the cholinesterase inhibitors, and they should be used with caution in patients with sick sinus syndrome. Hyperacidity can also occur with cholinesterase inhibitors, and they should be used with caution in patients with a history of peptic ulcer disease and who currently take nonsteroidal anti-inflammatory drugs (NSAIDs). Cholinesterase inhibitors should also be used cautiously in patients with a history of or current seizure disorder. Although

these effects are not common, they are of concern and should be closely monitored in patients who are at risk. Donepezil is also associated with insomnia or nightmares. If these conditions occur, the dosing of donepezil before bed should be changed to a morning administration. Despite the GI effects associated with a rapid increase in dose, these agents appear to be well tolerated.

Interactions

Drug interactions with cholinesterase inhibitors include synergy with other cholinergic agents (e.g., succinylcholine). Concomitant use of any anticholinergic agents (e.g., diphenhydramine) may negate the effects of the CI and should be avoided for optimal medication benefit. Donepezil and galantamine are metabolized by the P450 enzyme system. Donepezil and galantamine are substrates for 2D6 and 3A4. A potential advantage of rivastigmine is that it is metabolized by hydrolysis and thus is not susceptible to the drug interactions associated with the P450 enzyme system. Inhibitors of these isoenzymes would cause an increased drug concentration of the cholinesterase inhibitor and thus more susceptible to cholinergic adverse effects.

TABLE 44.1
Overview of Cholinesterase Inhibitors and Memantine

Generic (Trade) Name and Dosage	Selected Adverse Events	Contraindications	Special Considerations
donepezil (Aricept) Start: 5 mg every day Range: 5–23 mg/d Start 5 mg every day × 4 wk, then 10 mg daily. If stable for 3 mo, may increase to 23 mg/d	*GI:* nausea, vomiting *CV:* bradycardia, syncope	Hypersensitivity to agent or piperidine derivatives	If nightmares occur, dose in the morning
rivastigmine (Exelon) Oral: Start 1.5 mg bid for 2 wk, then increase by 1.5 mg bid; max. 6 mg bid Range: 3–6 mg bid Patch: Start one patch (4.6 mg/24 h) daily × 4 wk, then increase to one patch (9.5 mg/24 h) daily × 4 wk, then increase to one patch (13.3 mg/24 h)	Nausea, vomiting, anorexia, dyspepsia, fatigue, headache, malaise	Hypersensitivity to agent or carbamate derivatives	Initial response seen within 12 wk of therapy Patches are removed and replaced every 24 h
galantamine (Razadyne, Razadyne ER) IR: Start 4 mg PO bid × 4 wk Range: 4–12 mg PO bid ER: Start 8 mg daily × 4 wk Range: 8–24 mg	Nausea, vomiting, diarrhea, anorexia, abdominal pain, dyspepsia, dizziness, sleep disturbances	Hypersensitivity to agent Severe hepatic, renal impairment	Moderate hepatic, renal impairment should not exceed a dose of 16 mg/d
memantine (Namenda, Namenda XR) IR: Start 5 mg PO daily, increase by 5 mg daily every week to a target of 20 mg PO daily XR: Start 7 mg PO daily; increase dose 7 mg each week to a maximum dose of 28 mg PO daily	Dizziness, confusion, headache, anxiety, hypertension, diarrhea	Hypersensitivity to agent	XR capsules may be opened up and sprinkled on applesauce

ER, extended release; INR, international normalized ratio; IR, immediate release; XR, extended release.

Memantine (Namenda)

Memantine is an *N*-methyl-D-aspartate (NMDA) receptor antagonist. This drug was approved for the treatment of moderate-to-severe AD. It has a novel mechanism of action, which focuses on the glutamatergic system as compared to the cholinesterase inhibitors' effect on the cholinergic system. Memantine blocks the activation of the NMDA receptor during an abundance of glutamate. Thus, this blocks overstimulation of the NMDA receptor, and neuronal degeneration is inhibited. It does not interfere with the pathologic activation of the NMDA receptor during learning and memory formation.

Clinical trials have shown that memantine used alone in patients with moderate-to-severe AD has produced reduced clinical deterioration over 28 weeks. When memantine was added to donepezil therapy, it resulted in significantly better cognition and ADL compared to a placebo over 24 weeks. The immediate-release form of memantine should be started at 5 mg once daily and titrated every week, if tolerated, to a maximum dose of 10 mg twice daily. The extended-release product is started at a dose of 7 mg daily and increased by 7 mg each week to a maximum dose of 28 mg daily. Food has no effect on the onset or absorption of memantine. In general, memantine was well tolerated compared to a placebo. Memantine is minimally metabolized by the P450 enzyme system and thus not susceptible to P450 enzyme interactions. It is largely excreted renally via tubular secretion and, thus, there is the potential for decreased renal clearance with other drugs that undergo tubular secretion (e.g., amantadine, ranitidine).

Overall, clinical trials have been positive regarding the use of memantine for moderate-to-severe AD. With a different mechanism of action and indication for moderate-to-severe AD, memantine has a unique role for treatment of AD. In the past, once a cholinesterase inhibitor failed, no other viable option for therapy was available. Now, the addition of memantine to a cholinesterase inhibitor may be an option.

Selected Agents for Noncognitive Symptoms

Antipsychotic Agents

The noncognitive symptoms of AD include agitation, psychosis, anxiety, depression, and sleep disorders. Approximately one half of patients with dementia experience agitation. Many patients with AD also experience psychotic symptoms, such as delusions, hallucinations, and paranoia. Agitation and psychosis, which may be particularly frightening for families and caregivers, should be treated if the patient is causing harm to self or others.

The choice of an antipsychotic agent is based on cost and adverse events. Choosing an agent with a low degree of anticholinergic activity seems warranted in patients with AD. Atypical antipsychotics are associated with less extrapyramidal symptoms than the typical agents; thus, these agents are preferred.

Although atypical antipsychotics are preferred, none of the agents are approved to treat the noncognitive symptoms of dementia, and they all contain a black box warning alerting patients and caregivers to the fact that they are associated with an increased risk of death in patients with dementia-related psychosis. Risperidone (Risperdal) and olanzapine (Zyprexa) have also been associated with an increased risk of stroke in patients using these agents for behavioral disturbances associated with dementia. It is important for the practitioner to weigh the risks versus benefits of using these agents. Regardless of the agent chosen, the lowest effective dose should be used. The practitioner should reassess the need for these medications periodically (every 3 to 6 months).

Benzodiazepines

Benzodiazepines have been prescribed to treat behavioral problems related to dementia. Because they do not appear to be as effective as the antipsychotics for treating behavioral problems, benzodiazepines are often reserved for treating symptoms of anxiety or for episodic agitation. These agents can be used as needed in situations that precipitate acute anxiety.

If a benzodiazepine is prescribed, lorazepam (Ativan) or alprazolam (Xanax) are appropriate choices. They are inexpensive and have a short half-life, and hepatic metabolism is not significantly altered in the elderly. All benzodiazepines should be started at the lowest dose. The advantage of lorazepam is that it is available parenterally.

Adverse effects of benzodiazepines include falls, sedation, delirium, and loss of inhibition. Routine use is not recommended because of limited efficacy, adverse effects, and potential for worsening AD symptoms. The use of benzodiazepines for anxiety associated with dementia should be re-evaluated periodically.

Data on using various other agents (trazodone [Desyrel], valproate [Depakene], carbamazepine [Tegretol], buspirone [BuSpar], SSRIs, and beta-blockers) for treating anxiety associated with AD are limited. These agents may have a role in treating agitation in patients who do not tolerate or respond to antipsychotic agents or benzodiazepines.

Antidepressants

Because there is a high incidence of depression associated with dementia, pharmacologic treatment is often necessary. Patients may not meet explicit criteria for a depressive syndrome, but it is recommended that these patients still be offered treatment. Treatment may improve cognition, mood, apathy, function, behavior, appetite, sleep, and overall quality of life. Because there is no evidence that one class of antidepressants is superior to another in treating depression, the prescriber may base the choice of an agent on the individual patient, cost, side effect profile, and potential drug interactions.

In many clinical practices, SSRIs, such as sertraline or citalopram, have become a first-line therapy for clinically significant depression in the elderly with AD (APA, 2014). Patients who experience anxiety or insomnia with this agent can be given a trial of paroxetine, which is more sedating. Citalopram, in addition to its antidepressant effects, has proved beneficial in improving certain emotional symptoms of AD (panic, bluntness, depressed mood, confusion, irritability, anxiety, and restlessness) in patients with and without depression. SSRIs in general have fewer side effects (particularly anticholinergic) than TCAs or MAO inhibitors and are better tolerated.

Selecting the Most Appropriate Agent for Cognitive Symptoms

First-Line Therapy

Once the decision has been made to initiate drug therapy, cholinesterase inhibitors may be tried. Donepezil is often considered the first choice because fewer adverse events are associated with its use and the once-daily dosing schedule is easier to follow. However, any CI dosed once per day may be tried as a first-line option. These medications may be expensive and only modestly benefit cognitive function. Patients with severe AD may be offered memantine in conjunction with a cholinesterase inhibitor (**Table 44.2**). The combination therapy is expensive and could only provide moderate benefit.

Second-Line Therapy

Second-line therapy is a trial of a different cholinesterase inhibitor. In conjunction, some providers may add vitamin E. Vitamin E has a benign side effect profile and minimal cost and may be added to acetylcholinesterase inhibitor regimens in patients with mild-to-moderate AD.

MONITORING PATIENT RESPONSE

Primary care appointments involving both patients with AD and families every 3 to 6 months may be used to monitor cognitive and behavioral symptoms and to assess the patient's response to pharmacotherapy. If clinical improvement does not occur with a cholinesterase inhibitor after 3 to 6 months of treatment, the practitioner may consider switching to another cholinesterase inhibitor. The MMSE or MOCA are useful objective measures of cognitive response to therapy, but input from family and

caregivers must also be recognized. Discontinuing the medication may be considered at any time during therapy if there is a perceived lack of efficacy. If a marked decline in cognitive function is noted within the first 3 to 6 weeks after discontinuing drug therapy, the practitioner may consider restarting the acetylcholinesterase inhibitor. When patients progress to severe impairment, addition of memantine may be an option.

Ability to perform ADLs, such as bathing, dressing, toileting, and feeding, and instrumental ADLs, such as transferring, housekeeping, shopping, and paying bills, should be assessed to help determine the functional status of the patient and response to treatment. Assessment of the noncognitive symptoms of AD could be a sign of disease progression.

In patients receiving antipsychotic medications, response is usually seen within the first day of therapy. If patients continue to have delusions, hallucinations, or agitation, doses can be gradually increased at 4- to 7-day interval. In contrast, response to antidepressant medications is seen within 4 to 6 weeks. Evidence of suicidal ideation should be taken seriously and immediately addressed by the practitioner.

Treatment with any of these agents may be continued until the risk of pharmacotherapy outweighs the benefit to the patient or family. Clear communication with the patient, family, and caregivers cannot be overemphasized because evaluation of pharmacotherapeutic efficacy and decisions to stop or continue treatment depend on this input.

PATIENT EDUCATION

Regardless of the agents chosen for AD treatment, patients, families, and caregivers must have realistic goals of drug therapy. Their goals should include increasing length of time of self-sufficiency, delaying the need for nursing home placement, and reducing the burden on the caregiver. It is important that the family and patients understand the available agents are expected to slow the disease progression. They need to understand that no currently available agents are curative and only modest improvements can be expected.

Donepezil may be taken with or without food, and patients taking donepezil should be instructed that if insomnia or nightmares occur, the drug may be given in the morning. Rivastigmine should be taken with food to have a slow dose titration to minimize the GI side effects. Galantamine can be taken without regard to food and should be slowly titrated to minimize adverse effects. Memantine appears to be well tolerated. Because vitamin E may predispose certain patients (e.g., those with vitamin K deficiency) to bleeding, patients and families should be informed to report unusual bruising, blood in urine or stool, bleeding gums, and the like immediately to their health care provider.

Patient-Oriented Information Sources

The various support resources available for patients and families of patients with AD are shown in **Box 44.3**.

TABLE 44.2

Recommended Order of Treatment of the Cognitive Symptoms Associated with Alzheimer Disease

Order	Agents	Comments
First line	Cholinesterase inhibitors (CIs)	Once daily CIs will be most likely first-line agents for mild-to-moderate AD
	Memantine	Memantine is reserved for patients with moderate-to-severe AD; may be used in conjunction with a CI
Second line	CIs	A trial of second CI may be warranted
	Vitamin E	Use of vitamin E may be added to the CI or used as monotherapy in patients who cannot afford CIs

CASE STUDY*

M.W. is a 70-year-old white woman with a medical history of hypertension, osteoarthritis, atrial fibrillation, and total hysterectomy who lives by herself in a two-story row home. She visits the primary care clinic with her daughter, who is concerned because **M.W.** has "bounced" a few checks and can no longer pay her bills without assistance. **M.W.** admits that she has been forgetful and appears anxious as she describes an incident in which she went shopping and could not remember where she parked her car. Her daughter states that her mother's memory has progressively worsened over the past year. **M.W.'s** medications include fosinopril 20 mg PO daily, metoprolol succinate ER 50 mg PO daily, warfarin 5 mg PO daily, vitamin D 1,000 IU PO daily, and acetaminophen 325 mg 2 tablets (650 mg) PO tid. A careful evaluation and workup was ordered.

DIAGNOSIS: MILD AD WITH AN MMSE SCORE OF 22

1. List specific goals of treatment for **M.W.**
2. What drug therapy would you prescribe for **M.W.**? Why?
3. What are the parameters for monitoring success of therapy?
4. Discuss specific patient education based on the prescribed therapy.
5. List one or two adverse reactions for the selected agent that would cause you to change therapy.
6. What would be the choice for second-line therapy?
7. Would there be any over-the-counter and/or alternative agents appropriate for **M.W.**?
8. What lifestyle changes would you recommend to **M.W.**?
9. Describe one or two drug–drug or drug–food interactions for the selected agent.

* Answers can be found online.

Complementary and Alternative Medications

Vitamin E

Vitamin E, an antioxidant, may be useful in AD treatment. Due to its antioxidant effects, vitamin E can stabilize free radicals and the damage they produce. Patients with moderate AD started on vitamin E may expect approximately a 7-month delay in reaching a poor functional outcome or end point (i.e., death, institutionalization, loss of the ability to perform basic ADLs, or severe dementia; Sano et al., 1997). This difference is seen within 2 years of initiating treatment. Indefinite treatment with vitamin E is a reasonable approach.

Vitamin E may be effective because of its antioxidant effects. A starting dose of 1,000 international units given orally twice a day appears to be appropriate because this was the regimen used in the trial supporting its efficacy (Sano et al., 1997). Vitamin E, because of its benign side effect profile, minimal cost, and lack of significant drug interactions, has become a good choice for treating AD.

Minimal adverse effects are associated with vitamin E. Because vitamin E may worsen coagulation problems (causing bleeding) in patients with vitamin K deficiency or taking warfarin (Coumadin), it is suggested that these patients receive lower doses (200 to 800 international units/day). An increase in syncope and falls was also noted for vitamin E (and selegiline) in the study by Sano and colleagues (1997). Patients should be monitored for an increase in such events if they are receiving either of these agents.

Herbal Agents

Ginkgo biloba extract, thought to have antioxidant properties, has been studied in patients with mild-to-severe AD or multi-infarct dementia. Modest improvement of cognition was recorded in the results of the Alzheimer's Disease Assessment Scale. Caregivers also recognized improvement in function (Le Bars et al., 1997).

Treatment was well tolerated, with some GI side effects reported. Additional well-designed studies should be conducted before routine use is recommended. Because this product is not regulated by the FDA as a medication, its safety remains unknown, and *Ginkgo biloba* products may vary in extract concentrations and contents. Patients who choose to take this product should be cautioned that it may interact with warfarin or aspirin, increasing their risk of bleeding.

Bibliography

*Starred references are cited in the text.

Agrell, B., & Dehlin, O. (1998). The clock-drawing test. *Age and Ageing, 27,* 399–403.

American Psychiatric Association. (2007). American Psychiatric Association practice guideline for the treatment of patients with Alzheimer's disease and other dementias, 2nd ed. *American Journal of Psychiatry, 164*(Suppl. 12), 5–56.

American Psychiatric Association. (2013). *Diagnostic and statistical manual of mental disorders* (5th ed.). Washington, DC: American Psychiatric Association.

*American Psychiatric Association. (2014). American Psychiatric Association practice guideline for the treatment of patients with Alzheimer's disease and other dementias. *American Journal of Psychiatry.* Retrieved from http://psychiatryonline.org/pb/assets/raw/sitewide/practice_guidelines/guidelines/alzheimerwatch.pdf

Birks, J. (2006). Cholinesterase inhibitors for Alzheimer's disease. *Cochrane Database of Systematic Reviews,* (1), CD00593.

De-Paula, V. J., Radanovic, M., Diniz, B. S., et al. (2012). Alzheimer's disease. *Subcellular Biochemistry, 65,* 329–352.

*Kua, E. H., Ho, E., Tan, H. H., et al. (2014). The natural history of dementia. *Psychogeriatrics, 14,* 196–201.

Kurz, A., & Grimmer, T. (2014). Efficacy of memantine hydrochloride one-daily in Alzheimer's disease. *Expert Opinion on Pharmacotherapy, 15,* 1955–1960.

*Le Bars, P. L., Katz, M. M., Berman, N., et al. (1997). A placebo-controlled, double-blind, randomized trial of an extract of ginkgo biloba for dementia. *Journal of the American Medical Association, 278*, 1327–1332.

*Lendon, C. L., Ashall, F., & Goate, A. M. (1997). Exploring the etiology of Alzheimer's disease using molecular genetics. *Journal of the American Medical Association, 277*, 825–831.

McShane, R., Areosa Sastre, A., & Minakaran, N. (2006). Memantine for dementia. *Cochrane Database of Systematic Reviews, (2)*, CD003154.

Nyth, A. L., & Gottfries, C. G. (1990). The clinical efficacy of citalopram in treatment of emotional disturbances in dementia disorders: A Nordic multicenter study. *British Journal of Psychiatry, 157*, 894–901.

*Quefurth, H. W., & LaFerla, F. M. (2010). Alzheimer's disease. *New England Journal of Medicine, 362*, 329–344.

*Sano, M., Ernesto, C., Thomas, R. G., et al. (1997). A controlled trial of selegiline, alpha-tocopherol, or both as treatment for Alzheimer's disease. *New England Journal of Medicine, 336*, 1216–1222.

Shah, S., & Reichman, W. E. (2006). Treatment of Alzheimer's disease across the spectrum of clinical activity. *Clinical Interventions in Aging, 1*, 131–142.

Talbot, C., Lendon, C., Craddock, N., et al. (1994). Protection against Alzheimer's disease with ApoE2. *Lancet, 343*, 1432–1433.

Wiser, T. H. (1994). Alzheimer's cognitive disturbances: A case study. *U. S. Pharmacist, 19*, 52–78.

45 Parkinson Disease

Karleen Melody ■ Anisha B. Grover

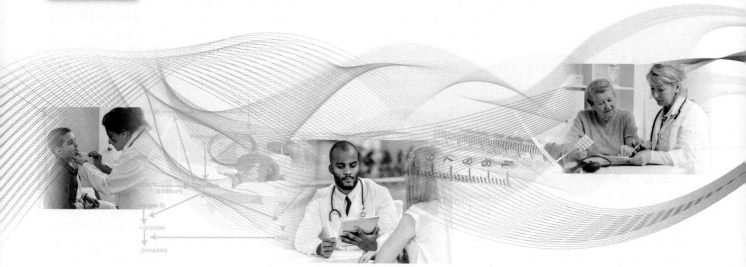

Parkinson disease (PD) is a neurodegenerative disorder characterized by a set of hallmark motor and nonmotor symptoms and was originally described in the "Essay on the Shaking Palsy," written by James Parkinson in 1817 (Parkinson, 1817). The mean age of onset is 65 years, with the typical age of diagnosis ranging between 55 and 65 years. The incidence is reportedly higher in males, with a male-to-female ratio of 1.5:1. The estimated prevalence among the total population is 0.3%, and the prevalence increases with age, affecting 1% of patients over the age of 60 years. Up to 1 million people live with PD in the United States (Connolly & Lang, 2014).

CAUSES

The underlying etiologies of PD are not well understood but likely include factors related to aging, genetic expression, and the environment.

As a preliminary step, drug-induced parkinsonism (DIP) must be considered and ruled out prior to the initiation of treatment for PD. The prevalence and incidence are difficult to determine, as it can be challenging to differentiate DIP from PD. Existing research has demonstrated that DIP may be the second most common etiology of parkinsonism (Shin & Chung, 2012). DIP is associated with agents that deplete or antagonize dopamine, such as first-generation "typical" antipsychotics or neuroleptic drugs. This drug class includes chlorpromazine, promazine, haloperidol, perphenazine, fluphenazine, and pimozide. Up to 80% of patients taking a drug from this class present with more than one kind of extrapyramidal side effect (EPS). Second-generation or "atypical" antipsychotic drugs, such as risperidone, olanzapine, and aripiprazole, were thought to carry a decreased risk than first-generation

antipsychotic drugs; however, studies have shown otherwise. Of the available second-generation antipsychotics, only clozapine and quetiapine are associated with lower rates of DIP among elderly patients. Other offending agents include metoclopramide, valproic acid, methyldopa, and prochlorperazine. Amiodarone and lithium may cause tremor, which can appear similar to Parkinson-like symptoms (Shin & Chung, 2012). Management of these cases involves discontinuation of the responsible medication, as the associated parkinsonism is typically reversible. Up to 10% of patients with DIP may experience persistent symptoms, even after discontinuation of the offending drug, but this is usually explained as an unmasking of symptoms rather than a direct cause of the drug therapy. The reversibility can occur within hours or days but can take up to 2 years. These agents can also worsen symptoms in existing idiopathic PD and should be avoided when possible in diagnosed patients (Shin & Chung, 2012).

The natural aging process is likely associated with some of the neuron degeneration seen in PD. Other contributors include oxidative stress, which may be associated with increased monoamine oxidase-B (MAO-B) metabolism or decreased glutathione clearance of free radicals, mitochondrial dysfunction, inflammation, and signal-mediated apoptosis.

Approximately 15% of patients with PD have a first-degree relative with the disease. The inheritance of Mendelian genes has been linked to 10% or less of PD cases but may be associated with both familial and sporadic PD. At this point, approximately 18 loci and 8 validated genes have been identified. More recently, two causative genes may have been identified (Lesage & Brice, 2012).

Although PD is typically considered sporadic or familial, there is a broad body of epidemiologic research related to PD, which associates environmental factors, such as chronic pesticide exposure, with an increased risk for developing PD. A compound called 1-methyl-4-phenyl-1,2,3,5-tetrahydropyridine (MPTP) is converted in humans to 1-methyl-4-phenylpyridium ion (MPP+), which is a neurotoxic agent. MPTP is structurally similar to many synthetic pesticides (Wirdefeldt et al., 2011).

Interestingly, some studies have shown an inverse association of caffeine intake with the development of PD (Liu et al., 2012). Experimental studies have shown that caffeine may protect dopaminergic neurons. The protective nature of caffeine has been identified more clearly in men, but evidence in women is conflicting. Recently, a large prospective study showed that higher caffeine intake was clearly associated with lower PD risk among women receiving hormone therapy (Ascherio et al., 2003). The same was not seen in women who had never used hormones. Some studies have also found cigarette smoking to be a protective factor; however, this factor does not have as clear of an association and needs to be evaluated separately. There are a limited number of studies that have evaluated the joint effect of caffeine and smoking status. Individuals who drink coffee are more likely to smoke cigarettes, and they often smoke more than noncoffee drinkers; however, cigarette smoking actually increases the metabolism and clearance rates of caffeine in humans, resulting in a higher plasma caffeine concentration in nonsmokers versus smokers who consume identical amounts (Liu et al., 2012). When considering the relationships between these variables, it is important to control for confounders, in order to evaluate true associations and relationships.

PATHOPHYSIOLOGY

PD is associated with several cardinal pathologic findings within the substantia nigra pars compacta (SNpc), including the depigmentation, or degeneration, of dopaminergic neurons, autophagy dysfunction, and the formation of Lewy bodies in the residual neurons.

The extrapyramidal motor system regulates the movement of muscles. Dopamine is a neurotransmitter associated with movement control and is produced and stored in cells within the midbrain structure called the SNpc. At the point of diagnosis, patients have typically already lost at least half of the dopaminergic neurons in the SNpc. This leads to the depletion of dopamine in the corpus striatum, resulting in a breakdown of communication to the motor regulators within the brain. Additional neuronal dysfunction typically manifests in the basal ganglia, neurocortex, and spinal cord.

Autophagy describes an intracellular process in which cytoplasmic proteins and organelles are gathered in vacuoles that are transported into lysosomes, where they can be degraded and recycled. This process facilitates the elimination of damaged proteins and organelles. Dysfunction in this process may also be linked with the neurodegeneration of dopaminergic neurons, contributing to the pathogenesis of PD (Muñoz et al., 2012).

Lewy bodies, named for Frederick Lewy, are round, eosinophilic aggregates located within neuronal nuclei. These structures are made primarily of alpha-synuclein and ubiquitin and consist of a dense core, surrounded by fibrillary elements. Lewy bodies are found in a small percentage of normal older adult brains and are also found in patients with Down syndrome, Alzheimer disease, dementia, and other neurodegenerative conditions. In PD, Lewy bodies can be found within the SNpc, cerebral cortex, basal ganglia, cardiac plexus, and gastrointestinal (GI) system. The distribution and anatomical location of these protein inclusions vary among individuals with PD and are closely linked to the presentation and extent of clinical features (Halliday et al., 2012). The early stages of PD involve Lewy body formation in the medulla oblongata, locus coeruleus, raphe nuclei, and even in the olfactory bulb. This is directly associated with depression, anxiety, difficulty sleeping, and sensory impairment that may manifest initially. PD progression is marked by Lewy body presence in the SNpc, correlating with hallmark motor symptoms. In advanced cases, Lewy bodies form in the cortex, resulting in cognitive changes. Lewy body accumulation in the lateral collateral pathway within the sacral spinal dorsal horn may contribute to urinary urgency and frequency and constipation associated with PD (VanderHorst et al., 2015). Nonmotor symptoms may also result from the loss of a wide range of neurotransmitters, including dopamine, norepinephrine, serotonin, and acetylcholine, which can decrease as various regions of the brain degenerate.

DIAGNOSTIC CRITERIA

The clinical history of the patient, including risk factors, medical history, medication history, and review of systems, will provide the most useful information for the diagnostic process, despite technological advances in imaging and nuclear techniques (Pedrosa & Timmermann, 2013). In evaluating the patient, it is important to first exclude DIP. Patients and caregivers provide valuable information when establishing a diagnosis, including the onset of tremor, stiffness or rigidity in arms or legs, speed of movement, and description of changes in facial expressions, posture, and gait. Hallmark or cardinal motor symptoms include a slowing of movement termed bradykinesia, resting or postural tremor, cogwheel rigidity, and difficulty maintaining balance, also known as postural instability. A neurological exam includes the assessment of facial expressiveness, posture, tone, balance, tremor, and speed of extremity movements (Lyons & Pahwa, 2011). Patients should also be evaluated for any associated nonmotor symptoms or conditions, including depression, anxiety, psychosis, fatigue, sleep disturbances, urinary complaints, increased salivation, orthostatic hypotension, cognitive changes, and GI problems, such as constipation.

Functional magnetic resonance imaging (MRI) or nuclear imaging techniques may be useful in ruling out other conditions, such as essential tremor, vascular parkinsonism, multiple systems atrophy, and progressive supranuclear palsy. These tools can also help form an earlier and more precise diagnosis, preventing a delay in therapy and helping to continually improve the individualization of disease management strategies for patients with PD. Dopamine transporter (DAT) imaging, sometimes used in combination with contrast agents, can be used to assess the degree of DAT loss in patients with PD, which correlates with disease staging, severity, and duration (Eggers et al., 2012). Although patients diagnosed with PD can look similar at baseline, the clinical subtypes can be differentiated by the variances in dopaminergic degeneration. DAT imaging can be used to diagnose presynaptic parkinsonism because even in early PD, DAT uptake in the striatum is significantly decreased. Utilizing DAT imaging can help to differentiate PD from DIP, which involves drug-induced changes in postsynaptic dopaminergic receptors (Shin & Chung, 2012). It can also guide the formation of patient-specific treatment strategies. Additional studies have explored whole-brain functional connectivity.

The Movement Disorder Society–sponsored revision of the Unified Parkinson's Disease Rating Scale (MDS-UPDRS) is a tool that is not designed for diagnostic purposes, but it can be used to monitor the degree of disability and impairment (Goetz et al., 2008). This tool can be used at the time of diagnosis to establish a baseline score, so that patient progress can be measured over time. This 65-item tool has demonstrated validity and reliability and is accompanied by a detailed set of instructions to standardize the use of the tool internationally. It contains four parts, including (1) nonmotor experiences of daily living, (2) motor experiences of daily living, (3) motor examination, and (4) motor complications. The patient or caregiver completes a total of 20 questions from parts I and II. Both rater and patient involvement are required for the remaining portions. The total rater time requirement to administer the tool is 30 minutes.

INITIATING DRUG THERAPY

Traditionally, treatment of patients with newly diagnosed PD would be deferred until the patient developed functional disability interfering with activities of daily living (Clarke et al., 2011). This is largely driven by the lack of available disease-modifying or neuroprotective agents; however, in recent years, there is emerging evidence that points to several advantages of initiating pharmacotherapy early on in PD. Early intervention may delay or diminish both motor and nonmotor symptoms, as well as delay the initiation of levodopa (**Figure 45.1**). Although not conclusively proven, some trials suggest that early treatment may slow the progression of PD because the rate of disease progression is much faster in the early stages than the later stages (Murman, 2012). By the time motor symptoms present, dopamine has been depleted by 60% to 80%, further strengthening the recommendation to initiate treatment earlier rather than waiting for functional disability (Lyons & Pahwa, 2011).

Patients with untreated or inadequately treated PD will experience significant symptomatic deterioration contributing to a reduced quality of life. Even though motor symptoms are more identifiable in PD, nonmotor symptoms have been shown to have a more negative impact on quality of life because they represent the majority of PD symptoms and tend

to emerge early in PD often before motor symptoms appear. A patient presenting with significant nonmotor symptoms may warrant early treatment intervention to improve quality of life (Murman, 2012).

There are several factors that need to be considered in determining when to initiate treatment as well as which treatment option to use. These factors include age, cognitive function, psychiatric issues, comorbidities, lifestyle, symptom severity, and employment, with the latter two factors being the strongest predictors of need for dopaminergic therapy. The patient's symptom severity and levels of impairment and disability should be assessed upon diagnosis and throughout treatment using a validated scale such as the MDS-UPDRS, to objectively evaluate the motor features of PD (Lyons & Pahwa, 2011).

Goals of Drug Therapy

The ultimate goal of drug therapy for PD is to maintain quality of life by alleviating motor and nonmotor symptoms. Other desired outcomes include maintaining patient independence, preserving the ability to perform activities of daily living, and minimizing adverse drug events and treatment complications (Murman, 2012). As with any disease state, it is important to provide cost-effective therapy; involve and educate the patient, family, and caregivers when creating a patient-centered treatment plan; and connect the patient with reliable and accurate resources.

Selected Agents for Motor Symptoms (Table 45.1)

Mild-Potency Drugs

Anticholinergics

Indications/Use The use of anticholinergics in PD is controversial. There is some evidence that they are useful in some patients with PD, particularly for symptoms of drooling and tremor (Abramowicz et al., 2013). However, other randomized controlled studies conclude that the benefits on tremor are inconclusive (Connolly & Lang, 2014). They are indicated for PD symptoms as well as drug-induced EPS.

Mechanism of Action Anticholinergics antagonize acetylcholine receptors to decrease the release of acetylcholine, which regulates muscle movement. The resulting decrease in activity of acetylcholine muscarinic receptors can also decrease salivation, providing an explanation for its potential role for the management of drooling.

Dosage Two anticholinergics used in PD include trihexyphenidyl and benztropine. Trihexyphenidyl, available in an oral tablet and an elixir, is initiated at 1 mg and is titrated in 2 mg increments every 3 to 5 days. A typical maintenance dose is 6 to 10 mg daily in 3 to 4 divided doses to a maximum dose of 15 mg/d. Benztropine, available in an oral tablet, injection, and solution formulation, should be started at 1 mg daily,

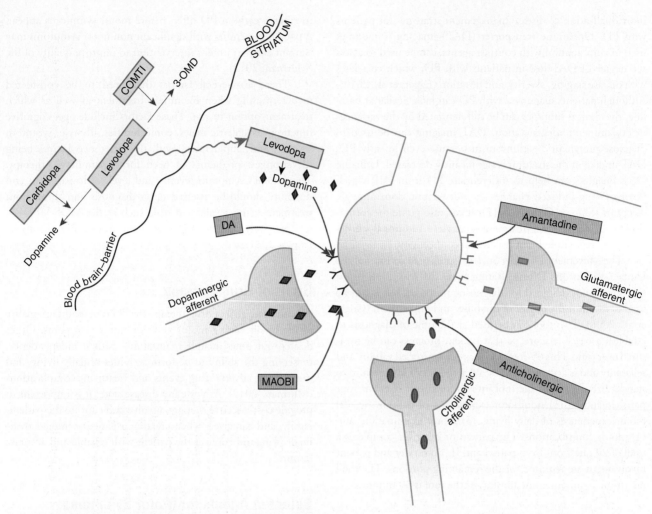

FIGURE 45.1   Sites of action of drugs used in the management of PD. PD is characterized by a deficiency in dopamine, and many drugs work to increase the activity of this neurotransmitter. In the periphery, catechol-*O*-methyltransferase inhibitors (COMTIs) block the degradation of levodopa to 3-O-methyldopa (3-OMD) and carbidopa prevents the conversion of levodopa into dopamine, increasing the amount of levodopa that can cross the blood–brain barrier. Once levodopa has entered the striatum, it undergoes central conversion to dopamine. Other drugs that act primarily in the striatum include dopamine agonists (DAs), which bind to and activate dopamine receptors, and monoamine oxidase type B inhibitors (MAOBIs), which inhibit the breakdown of dopamine. In addition to dopamine, other neurotransmitters serve as drug targets in PD. Anticholinergic drugs bind to and block acetylcholine receptors. Amantadine binds to and blocks *N*-methyl-d-aspartate (NMDA) glutamate receptors and increases the release of dopamine in other ways.

which can be divided into 2 to 4 divided doses. Benztropine can be gradually increased every 5 to 6 days by increments of 0.5 mg to a maximum of 6 mg daily. Abrupt discontinuation of either agent can exacerbate adverse effects, so it is recommended to taper the dose.

Time Frame for Response Anticholinergics have an onset of approximately 1 hour.

Contraindications Both agents are contraindicated in narrow-angle glaucoma. Benztropine is also contraindicated in children less than 3 years of age.

Adverse Drug Events Anticholinergics commonly cause impaired memory, confusion, hallucinations, nausea, blurred vision, dry mouth, urinary retention, and constipation, which often limit their use in PD.

Interactions Potassium chloride should be avoided with anticholinergics because concurrent use increases the risk of ulcers. The risk of GI adverse effects may also be increased in patients on anticholinergics when glucagon is administered. Due to additive side effects, other anticholinergics such as ipratropium, tiotropium, and umeclidinium should be avoided in patients on benztropine or trihexyphenidyl.

Amantadine
Indications/Uses Amantadine is indicated for the treatment of mild PD and most frequently used in a patient experiencing dyskinesia. Evidence supporting the use of amantadine in PD is conflicting. Expert opinion supports its use as monotherapy and adjunctive therapy; however, a 2009 Cochrane review concludes that there is insufficient evidence for its use (Connolly & Lang, 2014).

TABLE 45.1

Overview of Drugs Used in the Management of PD

Generic (Trade) Name and Initial Dosage	Dose Adjustments	Selected Adverse Events	Contraindications	Special considerations
trihexyphenidyl (Artane) 1 mg once daily; titrate by 2 mg every 3–5 d; max. 15 mg/d	None	Impaired memory, confusion, hallucinations, nausea, blurred vision, dry mouth, urinary retention, constipation	Narrow-angle glaucoma	Avoid with potassium chloride, glucagon, and other anticholinergics
benztropine (Cogentin) 1 mg once daily; titrated by 0.5 mg. Max. 6 mg/d	None	Same as trihexyphenidyl	Narrow-angle glaucoma; use in <3 y of age	Same as trihexyphenidyl
amantadine (Symmetrel) 100 mg twice daily; max. 400 mg/d	Serious concomitant illness or high doses of other PD drugs: start 100 mg once daily. CrCl 30–50 mL/min: 200 mg × 1 and 100 mg daily thereafter. CrCl 15–29 mL/min: 200 mg × 1 and 100 mg every other day thereafter. CrCl <15 mL/min or HD: 200 mg every 7 d	Hallucinations, confusion, ankle edema, livedo reticularis, blurred vision, dry mouth, constipation, insomnia	None	Caution with use with memantine or drugs that prolong the QT interval
selegiline (Eldepryl) 5 mg twice daily	None	Headache, nausea, dizziness, hallucinations, dyskinesia, insomnia	Meperidine, methadone, propoxyphene, tramadol, St. John's wort, cyclobenzaprine, dextromethorphan, other MAO-B inhibitors, carbamazepine, SSRIs, SNRIs, clomipramine, imipramine	Caution with use with other serotonergic agents, alcohol, and tyramine-containing foods
rasagiline (Azilect) 1 mg once daily; max. 1 mg/d	If used with levodopa, initial dose should be decreased to 0.5 once daily.	Headache, nausea, dizziness, hallucinations, dyskinesia, orthostatic hypotension, dyspepsia, depression, flulike symptoms, and arthralgia	Meperidine, methadone, propoxyphene, tramadol, St. John's wort, cyclobenzaprine, dextromethorphan, and other MAO-B inhibitors	Same as selegiline
pramipexole IR (Mirapex) 0.125 mg three times daily, titrated every 5–7 d	CrCl 30–50 mL/min: start 0.125 twice daily. CrCl 15–29 mL/min: start 0.125 once daily	Fatigue, nausea, constipation, orthostatic hypotension, hallucinations, lower extremity edema, ICD, sleep attacks	None	
pramipexole ER (Mirapex ER) 0.375 mg once daily; titrated by 0.75 mg every 5–7 d; max. 4.5 mg	CrCl 30–50 mL/min: start 0.375 mg every other day	Same as pramipexole IR	None	Dose should be tapered before discontinuing
ropinirole IR (Requip) 0.25 mg three times daily; titrated weekly; max 24 mg/d	HD: 0.25 mg three times daily; max. 18 mg/d	Same as pramipexole IR	None	Avoid use with CYP1A2 inhibitors and inducers

(Continued)

TABLE 45.1

Overview of Drugs Used in the Management of PD (*Continued*)

Generic (Trade) Name and Initial Dosage	Dose Adjustments	Selected Adverse Events	Contraindications	Special considerations
ropinirole ER (Requip XL) 2 mg once daily; titrated weekly by 2 mg; max 24 mg/d	HD: 2 mg once daily; max. 18 mg/d	Same as pramipexole IR	None	Dose should be tapered before discontinuing. Avoid use with CYP1A2 inhibitors and inducers
rotigotine (Neupro) 2 mg/24 h; titrated by 2 mg/24 h weekly; max. 6 mg/24 h	None	Same as pramipexole IR	None	Dose should be tapered before discontinuing
apomorphine (Apokyn) 2- or 4-mg test dose; titrated by 1 mg every few days; max 6 mg/dose	Renal impairment: start 1-mg test dose	Same as pramipexole IR	None	4-mg test dose administered 2 h after 2-mg test dose if tolerates but does not respond
carbidopa/levodopa IR (Sinemet) or ODT (Parcopa) Preferred: 25/100 mg three times daily; alternative: 10/100 mg three to four times daily; titrated by 1 tablet daily or every other day; max 8 tablets/d or 200 mg/d carbidopa or 2,000 mg/d levodopa	None	Nausea, vomiting, constipation, dizziness, headache, peripheral edema, insomnia, orthostatic hypotension, dyskinesias	Narrow-angle glaucoma	Protein consumption and constipation may reduce the absorption of levodopa, so patients should avoid meals high in protein, take levodopa 1 h before or 2 h after meals, and maintain appropriate bowel regimen
carbidopa/levodopa CR (Sinemet CR) 50/200 mg twice daily; titrated by 1 tablet every 3 d. Max. 8 tablets/d	Levodopa doses >700 mg should be divided into at least 3 daily doses	Same as carbidopa/levodopa IR	Narrow-angle glaucoma	Same as carbidopa/levodopa IR
carbidopa/levodopa ER (Rytary) 23.75/95 mg three times daily for 3 d, then 36.25/145 mg three times daily starting day 4; titrated as tolerated to max. 612.5/2,450 mg/d	None	Same as carbidopa/levodopa IR	Narrow-angle glaucoma	Same as carbidopa/levodopa IR
entacapone (Comtan) 200 mg with each dose of levodopa; max 8 doses/d	None	Dyskinesia, hypotension, nausea, diarrhea, dark-colored urine, somnolence, sleep disorders, hallucinations, headache, confusion	None	Only used adjunct to carbidopa/levodopa therapy. May be necessary to reduce dose of levodopa when adding COMTI
tolcapone (Tasmar) 100 mg three times daily	None	Same as entacapone Black box warning for hepatotoxicity	None	Same as entacapone Bioavailability is decreased by 10%–20% when taken with food

CrCl, creatinine clearance; IR, immediate release; ER, extended release; CR, controlled release; d, day; max., maximum; COMTI, catechol-*O*-methyltransferase inhibitor.

Mechanism of Action The precise mechanism of amantadine in PD is unknown, although it is hypothesized that its inhibition on N-methyl-d-aspartate (NMDA) receptors potentiates dopaminergic responses to reduce PD symptoms.

Dosage Amantadine is available as an oral capsule and tablet and is typically started at a dose of 100 mg twice daily. It can be titrated to a maximum of 400 mg daily in divided doses with careful monitoring. In the presence of a serious concomitant illness, or for patients who are receiving high doses of other PD drugs, an initial dose of 100 mg daily is recommended, which can be titrated to 100 mg twice daily after 1 to 2 weeks. The dose of amantadine needs to be adjusted in patients with renal dysfunction. For patients with a creatinine clearance (CrCl) of 30 to 50 mL/min, a loading dose of 200 mg should be started, followed by 100 mg/d as a maintenance dose. For patients with a CrCl between 15 and 29 mL/min, a 200-mg loading dose should be given, followed by 100 mg every other day. Patients with a CrCl less than 15 mL/min or on hemodialysis (HD) should be given 200 mg every 7 days.

Time Frame for Response The onset of amantadine is within 48 hours of administration.

Contraindications There are no absolute contraindications for amantadine.

Adverse Drug Events Adverse effects of amantadine include hallucinations, confusion, ankle edema, livedo reticularis, a blotchy, purple-colored skin condition with a net-like pattern, in addition to anticholinergic effects like blurred vision, dry mouth, and constipation. Amantadine may also affect sleep–wake cycles, causing insomnia or reduction in daytime sleepiness.

Interactions Caution should be used when amantadine is used concurrently with memantine because of an increased risk of QT prolongation and psychosis. Other drugs that prolong the QT interval should also be used with caution in combination with amantadine.

MAO-B Inhibitors

Indications/Uses MAO-B inhibitors are used for mild PD. When used as monotherapy in early PD, MAO-B inhibitors provide a modest improvement in motor symptoms, which may be seen as early as 1 week after initiation. In more advanced PD, MAO-B inhibitors are used as adjunctive therapy. MAO-B inhibitors also delay the need for levodopa by a few months, but they do not prevent or delay clinical progression of PD (Goetz & Pal, 2014). The MAO-B inhibitors available for the treatment of PD are selegiline and rasagiline.

Mechanism of Action MAO-B plays a major role in the metabolism of dopamine. By inhibiting this metabolism, concentrations of dopamine are increased, allowing more dopamine to reach the brain and ultimately reducing motor symptoms of PD. Selegiline also inhibits the uptake of catecholamines and the release of catecholamine by amphetamine metabolites.

Dosage Selegiline is available in multiple formulations, including an oral capsule, oral tablet, a patch, and an orally disintegrating tablet (ODT), whereas rasagiline is only available as an oral tablet. Of note, the patch is only indicated for depression and the ODT has insufficient efficacy for symptom improvement in PD, so these dosage forms will not be discussed further. Selegiline therapy is initiated at a dose of 5 mg twice daily with breakfast and lunch. The recommended dose of rasagiline as monotherapy or adjunctive therapy (except with levodopa) is 1 mg once daily, which is the maximum daily dose. If rasagiline is used adjunctively with levodopa, the initial dose is 0.5 mg once daily, which could be increased to 1 mg once daily based on response and tolerability.

Time Frame for Response MAO-B inhibitors have an onset of approximately 1, with moderate improvement in motor symptoms seen within 1 week after initiation.

Contraindications MOA-B inhibitors are contraindicated with meperidine, methadone, propoxyphene, tramadol, St. John's wort, cyclobenzaprine, dextromethorphan, and other MAO-B inhibitors. Additional contraindications with selegiline only include concomitant therapy with carbamazepine, selective serotonin reuptake inhibitors (SSRIs), serotonin–norepinephrine reuptake inhibitors (SNRIs), clomipramine, and imipramine.

Adverse Drug Events Adverse effects seen with MOA-B inhibitors include headache, nausea, dizziness, hallucinations, or dyskinesia. Selegiline can also cause insomnia because it is metabolized to amphetamines, which is not true of rasagiline. Rasagiline may additionally cause orthostatic hypotension, dyspepsia, depression, flulike symptoms, and arthralgia.

MAO-B inhibitors have additional adverse event concerns that warrant caution with their use. The risk of developing melanoma is increased in patients with PD, although no clear association with dopaminergic drugs has been established. New or worsening mental status or behavioral changes, including impulse control disorders (ICDs), have also been noted with MAO-B inhibitor use. Somnolence, which may impair physical or mental abilities, has been reported with MAO-B inhibitor use particularly in elderly patients, patients with current sleep disorders, and patients taking concomitant sedating medications. MAO-B inhibitors may also potentiate the dopaminergic side effects of levodopa and may cause or worsen dyskinesia. Rasagiline labeling also contains a warning that it can exacerbate or precipitate hypertension. Proper screenings for the concerns listed above should be conducted regularly.

Interactions The impact of cytochrome P450 (CYP) isoforms on the metabolism of MAO-B inhibitors is important to consider. Selegiline is metabolized primarily by CYP2B6 and to a lesser extent by CYP3A4. Selegiline does not inhibit enzymes in the CYP450 system; however, CYP3A4 inducers, such as phenytoin and carbamazepine, could reduce selegiline concentrations. Rasagiline is metabolized by CYP1A2; therefore, CYP1A2 inhibitors, such as ciprofloxacin and cimetidine, will reduce rasagiline concentrations. Rasagiline does not inhibit or induce enzymes in the P450 system. Caution should be used when MAO-B inhibitors are used concomitantly with alpha/beta agonists, stimulants, and buprenorphine. Additionally, potentially fatal serotonin syndrome has occurred when serotonergic agents are used concomitantly with MAO-B inhibitors. Alcohol- and tyramine-containing foods should also be avoided due to their increased risk of serotonin syndrome.

Moderate-Potency Drugs

Dopamine Agonists

Indications/Uses Compared to levodopa, dopamine agonists (DAs) are less effective but cause dyskinesia or motor fluctuations less frequently (Abramowicz et al., 2013). They are classified as either ergot or nonergot derivatives. The nonergot-derived agents have superior safety profiles and are therefore the preferred choice, so they will be the focus of this section. Pramipexole, ropinirole, and rotigotine are the DAs available to treat moderate symptoms of PD. Apomorphine is an injectable DA that is only approved to treat acute intermittent hypomobility in patients with advanced PD. DAs used as monotherapy can improve UPDRS scores by 4 to 5 points (Lyons & Pahwa, 2011). When used adjunctively to levodopa, a DA has improved efficacy compared to monotherapy and can reduce "wearing-off" phenomena but has an increased risk of dyskinesia (Connolly & Lang, 2014).

Mechanism of Action The exact mechanism of action of DAs is unknown; however, it is believed that stimulation of dopamine D2-type receptors result in improved dopaminergic transmission in the motor area of the basal ganglia.

Dosage Pramipexole and ropinirole are available in immediate-release (IR) and extended-release (ER) oral tablet formulations. Pramipexole IR tablet is initiated at 0.125 mg three times daily and titrated every 5 to 7 days. The typical maintenance dose is 0.5 to 1.5 mg three times daily. The ER formulation of pramipexole is started at 0.375 mg daily and titrated by 0.75 mg daily every 5 to 7 days to a maximum dose of 4.5 mg once daily. Patients with renal impairment will require a dose reduction. Pramipexole IR should be initiated at 0.125 mg twice daily and 0.125 mg once daily for patients with a CrCl of 30 to 50 mL/min and CrCl of 15 to 29 mL/min, respectively. Pramipexole IR should not be used in patients with a CrCl less than 15 mL/min or in those requiring HD. For patients with a CrCl of 30 to 50 mL/min, pramipexole ER should be initiated at 0.375 mg every other day, which can be titrated to 0.375 mg daily after at least 1 week of therapy. Pramipexole ER can further be titrated by 0.375 mg every 7 days to a maximum dose of 2.25 mg daily. Patients with a CrCl less than 30 mL/min or on HD should not take pramipexole ER. To discontinue pramipexole, it is recommended to decrease the dose by 0.75 mg/d until the daily dose is 0.75 mg once daily and then to reduce the dose by 0.375 mg once daily.

The starting dose of ropinirole IR tablet is 0.25 mg three times daily. For the first month of therapy, the daily dosage should increase by 0.75 mg (divided into 3 doses) on a weekly basis. After week 4, the daily dosage may be increased by 1.5 mg/d on a weekly basis up to a dose of 9 mg/d and then by

3 mg/d on a weekly basis up to a total dose of 24 mg/d. When discontinuing ropinirole, it must be tapered over 7 days by reducing the administration to twice daily for 4 days and then once daily for the remaining 3 days. The starting dose of the ER tablet is 2 mg once daily for 1 to 2 weeks, which is then titrated by 2 mg/d on a weekly basis to a maximum of 24 mg daily. Neither formulation has been studied in patients with a CrCl less than 30 mL/min, and use of these agents should be avoided in this population. For patients requiring HD, the initial dose of ropinirole IR should be 0.25 mg three times daily and ropinirole ER should be 2 mg once daily. The maximum daily dose in patients requiring HD for both formulations is 18 mg daily.

Rotigotine is available as a transdermal patch and should be initiated at 2 mg/24 hours. The dose may be increased by 2 mg/24 hours on a weekly basis to a maximum dose of 6 mg/24 hours. If discontinuation of rotigotine is warranted, the dose should be reduced by 2 mg/24 hours every other day.

Since apomorphine is used for acute hypomobility, this medication is administered three times daily as needed. When initiating apomorphine, a test dose of 2 mg subcutaneously is administered under medical supervision. If the patient tolerates the dose, but does not respond, a second test dose of 4 mg should be administered 2 hours later. If the 4-mg dose is tolerated and the patient responds, a maintenance dose of 3 mg should be administered thereafter. If the patient tolerates and responds to either the 2- or 4-mg test dose, the maintenance dose can be titrated in 1-mg increments every few days to a maximum of 6 mg. For patients with mild to moderate renal impairment, the initial test dose and starting dose should be reduced to 1 mg as needed.

Time Frame for Response Pramipexole and ropinirole have an onset of action within 1 hour of administration. Rogigotine has a slower onset action of 4 to 18 hours with a full treatment benefit seen within 1 week. Apomorphine has a rapid onset of action of 10 to 20 minutes.

Contrainidcations There are no contraindications for pramipexole, ropinorole, or rotigotine. Apomorphine is contraindicated with concomitant use of 5-HT3 antagonists.

Adverse Drug Events Adverse effects are similar among all DAs and include fatigue, nausea, constipation, orthostatic hypotension, hallucinations, and lower extremity edema. Severe side effects may include ICD, or sleep attacks. ICD may improve upon reduction or discontinuation of the DA, but switching to a different agent is not recommended as all DAs have a similar risk of ICD. Since sleep attacks can occur at any time, including while driving, eating, and talking, patients should be counseled about driving safety. Because of these significant adverse drug events, DAs are typically avoided in the elderly.

Interactions Pramipexole and rotigotine do not have any major drug interactions, but caution should be used with antipsychotics as the efficacy of both agents can be diminished. Ropinirole is a major substrate of CYP1A2, so its use should be avoided with any CYP1A2 inducers, such as carbamazepine and rifampin, or inhibitors, such as ciprofloxacin and cimetidine.

High-Potency Drugs

Levodopa

Indications/Uses Nearly all patients with PD will require treatment with levodopa, as it is the most effective treatment for symptomatic relief of PD. Levodopa also has the fastest onset of action compared to other PD medications. After several years of levodopa treatment, patients can begin to experience a "wearing-off" phenomenon, which involves the return of motor and nonmotor symptoms prior to the next dose of levodopa. As PD progresses, patients may find a shortening in the length of time with a good response to the medication, also known as "on time," and a lengthening of time with a poor response, also known as "off time." As PD progresses, patients have a diminished capacity to produce dopamine and store converted levodopa for release when needed, resulting in a reappearance of symptoms. Although "wearing off" can occur with many different drugs, it is most commonly associated with levodopa. At high doses and with continued use, patients' inability to store excess dopamine can manifest in the form of motor fluctuations and dyskinesia, so it is typically reserved for severe motor symptoms of PD.

Mechanism of Action Dopamine itself is not used to treat PD because it cannot cross the blood–brain barrier. Levodopa, a dopamine precursor, can cross the blood–brain barrier, where it is then converted via decarboxylation to dopamine. The converted dopamine is then stored in the presynaptic neurons until stimulated for release, when it will bind to dopamine receptors. Levodopa is administered in combination with carbidopa, which limits the peripheral breakdown of levodopa. This allows roughly a fourfold increase in circulating levodopa to cross the blood–brain barrier and reduces the undesirable adverse effects of nausea and vomiting caused by dopamine in the periphery.

Dosage Carbidopa/levodopa is available in many formulations including an IR tablet, an ODT, a controlled-release (CR) tablet, a suspension, and an ER tablet and capsule. The CR formulation has a more variable absorption profile, resulting in a slower and less predictable onset of action than the IR formulation. The half-life of levodopa is only 60 to 90 minutes, so the daily dosage is divided into 3 to 6 doses.

The preferred initial dosing of the IR or ODT formulations is carbidopa 25 mg/levodopa 100 mg three times daily, although carbidopa 10 mg/levodopa 100 mg three to four times daily may also be initiated. This can be titrated upward by 1 tablet daily or every other day as necessary to a maximum of 8 tablets of any strength or 200 mg of carbidopa and 2,000 mg of levodopa.

Patients initiating the CR formulation should start at a dose of carbidopa 50 mg/levodopa 200 mg twice daily at intervals not less than 6 hours apart. If doses of levodopa are greater than 700 mg daily, it should be divided into three or more daily doses. Intervals between doses should be 4 to 8 hours while awake, with the smaller doses given toward the end of the day, if the divided doses are not equal. This can be titrated upward by 1 tablet every 3 days to a maximum of 8 tablets daily.

For levodopa-naïve patients, ER capsule dosage should be initiated at carbidopa 23.75 mg/levodopa 95 mg three times daily for 3 days and then increased to carbidopa 36.25 mg/levodopa 145 mg three times daily on the 4th day. Since ER tablets are not interchangeable with other carbidopa/levodopa products, patients switching from other formulations to the ER formulation are dosed based on their previous total daily dose (TDD) of levodopa. If the TDD was between 400 and 549 mg, initiate 3 capsules of carbidopa 23.75 mg/levodopa 95 mg three times daily; if the TDD was between 550 and 749 mg, initiate 4 capsules of carbidopa 23.75 mg/levodopa 95 mg three times daily; if the TDD was between 750 and 949 mg, initiate 3 capsules of carbidopa 36.25 mg/levodopa 145 mg three times daily; if the TDD was between 950 and 1,249 mg, initiate 4 capsules of carbidopa 36.25 mg/levodopa 145 mg three times daily; if the TDD is ≥1,250 mg, initiate 4 capsules of carbidopa 48.75 mg/levodopa 195 mg three times daily. Titration of the ER formulations as tolerated can continue to a maximum daily dose of carbidopa 612.5 mg/levodopa 2,450 mg.

Time Frame to Response The onset of levodopa is approximately 1 hour.

Contraindications Carbidopa/levodopa is contraindicated in patients with narrow-angle glaucoma.

Adverse Drug Events The most common side effects of carbidopa/levodopa include nausea, vomiting, constipation, dizziness, headache, peripheral edema, insomnia, and orthostatic hypotension. Carbidopa/levodopa can also cause motor fluctuations and dyskinesia, which are more commonly seen when initiated in younger patients.

Interactions Carbidopa/levodopa does not have any major drug interactions, but caution should be used with antipsychotics as the efficacy of both agents can be diminished. Additionally, levodopa may enhance the effect of MAO-B inhibitors. In some cases, protein consumption may reduce the absorption of levodopa from the intestine, so patients should avoid meals high in protein. Patients may also try taking levodopa 1 hour before or 2 hours after meals. It is important for patients to increase fluid and fiber intake, as constipation may reduce levodopa absorption, as well.

Catechol-O-Methyltransferase Inhibitors

Indications/Uses Catechol-O-methyltransferase inhibitors (COMTIs) are used in combination with levodopa to decrease PD-associated disability by improving "wearing-off" phenomena; however, they can increase the risk of dyskinesia.

Mechanism of Action COMT breaks down levodopa in the periphery. By inhibiting this action, levodopa plasma levels are increased and the half-life is prolonged.

Dosage Two oral COMTIs, entacapone and tolcapone, are available for adjunctive therapy to carbidopa/levodopa in the treatment of patients with PD who experience "wearing-off" symptoms. Tolcapone was withdrawn from the market in Canada; however, it is still available in the United States for patients who have tried and failed entacapone. The initial dose of entacapone is 200 mg, administered with each dose of levodopa, to a maximum of 8 doses daily. Tolcapone should be initiated at 100 mg three times daily and does not have to be taken at the same times as levodopa. If no benefit is seen after 3 weeks, tolcapone should be discontinued. COMTIs can exacerbate the adverse effects of levodopa, so it may be necessary to reduce the dose of levodopa when adding a COMTI to the patient's regimen.

Time Frame to Response The onset of COMTIs is approximately 1 hour.

Contraindications There are no contraindications to COMTIs.

Adverse Drug Events Common adverse effects of COMTIs include dyskinesia, hypotension, nausea, diarrhea, dark-colored urine, and central nervous system (CNS) disturbances such as somnolence, sleep disorders, hallucinations, headache, and confusion. These adverse effects are more prevalent with tolcapone. Additionally, tolcapone has a black box warning for hepatotoxicity and requires written consent for its use as well as liver function tests every 2 to 4 weeks for the first 6 months of therapy and periodically thereafter.

Interactions Because COMTIs commonly cause CNS disturbances, they should be used with caution with other CNS depressants. The bioavailability of tolcapone is decreased by 10% to 20% when taken with food. Therefore, it should be administered at least 1 hour before or 2 hours after meals.

Selecting the Most Appropriate Drug

There are no pharmacologic agents that provide disease-modifying or neuroprotective effects; therefore, therapy selection is based on symptoms causing the greatest disability, age, comorbidities, and side effect profile (Goetz & Pal, 2014). Patients requiring therapy for mild motor symptoms should be started first on a MAO-B inhibitor before trying a DA or levodopa due to the increased risk of major adverse drug events with the latter agents. Patients who are experiencing moderate to severe impairment will usually be initiated on a DA or levodopa. Although levodopa is more efficacious than a DA and is associated with less hallucinations, somnolence, and ICDs, DAs have a decreased risk of dyskinesia. DAs are typically chosen over levodopa in younger patients, because the onset of PD at a younger age is a risk factor for developing dyskinesia (Connolly & Lang, 2014). Careful consideration must be given to the patient's age, level of disability, treatment goals, and potential for late complications of dyskinesia and hallucinations before starting levodopa (Goetz & Pal, 2014).

The stepwise treatment approach of PD is dependent on the symptom that is causing the greatest disability. An algorithm that outlines treatment options deemed first-, second-, and third-line therapies for treating PD is shown in **Figure 45.2**. If symptoms are uncontrolled on an adequate trial of therapy and if there were other treatment options listed in the previous step,

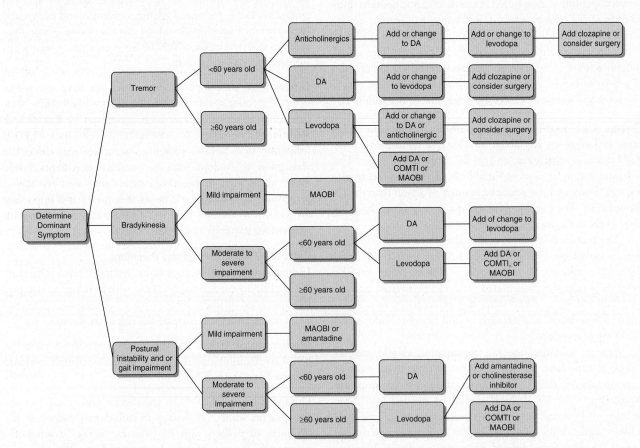

FIGURE 45.2 Treatment algorithm for PD. (MAOBI, monoamine oxidase type B inhibitors; COMTI, catechol-*O*-methyltransferase inhibitors; DA, dopamine agonists.)

all of those alternative agents should be tried before moving to the next step in the algorithm. For a patient with a suboptimal benefit, defined as an improvement in symptoms yet still experiencing bothersome or disabling symptoms, the current medication dose should be increased until maximized before moving to the next step in the algorithm. If the patient is not experiencing any improvement with the medication, the agent should be discontinued and an agent listed in the next step should be initiated (Connolly & Lang, 2014).

Considerations with Mild- and Moderate-Potency Agents

Because of the cognitive side effects associated with anticholinergics and the conflicting evidence related to efficacy, the use of these agents is generally avoided. In younger patients presenting with tremor and fatigue, amantadine should be chosen over MAO-B inhibitors. However, MAO-B inhibitors are favored over amantadine in elderly patients and those with renal dysfunction. Selegiline may be preferred over rasagiline if cost or a positive urine test for amphetamine is a concern (Goetz & Pal, 2014).

Considerations with Moderate-Potency Agents

Cost and convenience typically direct the selection of a therapeutic option because there is no strong evidence of any agent being more effective than another in this class. Since most adverse drug effects are class effects, switching to another agent within the same class is unlikely to alleviate the problem. If adherence is an issue, selecting an ER formulation is recommended. The transdermal DA can reduce the risk of food or drug interactions within the GI system (Goetz & Pal, 2014).

Considerations with High-Potency Agents

The IR formulation is most effective particularly in early PD, since the other formulations have a more variable absorption rate, resulting in a less predictable improvement in symptoms. Patients having difficulty with nighttime mobility may benefit from the CR formulation because the peak concentration is lower, causing less insomnia (Goetz & Pal, 2014).

Other Considerations

Mild- and even moderate-potency agents may not be the most appropriate choice for employed patients, regardless of symptom severity, since they can take several weeks to see the full effect, whereas levodopa has a rapid onset of action (Goetz & Pal, 2014).

For patients who experience the "wearing-off" phenomena, a few recommended management strategies include increasing the dose of the dopaminergic agent, adding on another dopaminergic medication, increasing the number of daily administrations, or adding a MAO-B or COMTI. Studies have compared the effectiveness of adding a MAO-B or COMTI, which has concluded that both therapeutic options similarly reduce "wearing-off" time (Connolly & Lang, 2014).

Special Considerations

Geriatric

A DA used as monotherapy can cause confusion and psychosis in the elderly and should be avoided, especially in patients with dementia. Geriatric patients, specifically those with cognitive dysfunction, are at the greatest risk for developing psychiatric adverse drug events and may benefit more from levodopa than a DA. Adverse effects of anticholinergics contribute to poor tolerability of this class of medications and it is therefore not recommended in the elderly (Connolly & Lang, 2014).

Genomics

As mentioned previously, there is a genetic link in the development of PD. Researchers have identified more than 24 genetic risk factors contributing to PD, including five "PARK" genes (Nalls et al., 2014). Because of this discovery, it is hypothesized that pharmacogenomics is going to play a huge role in emerging therapies for PD. One particular area of clinical development is using viral vectors to silence overexpressing genes that contribute to PD (Tarazi et al., 2014).

Treatment of Selected Nonmotor Symptoms

Psychological symptoms

Psychological symptoms include depression, psychosis, and dementia, which occur in about 25%, 55%, and 80% of patients, respectively (Connolly & Lang, 2014). Evidence in the literature for treating depression in PD is conflicting. Pramipexole and venlafaxine have been shown to be efficacious, while tricyclic antidepressants and dopaminergic drugs have been labeled as likely efficacious. There is unsatisfactory evidence to support the use of other agents including SSRIs, MAO-B inhibitors, omega-3 fatty acids, atomoxetine, and nefazodone. Clozapine and quetiapine have the most evidence to support their use in psychosis. Quetiapine is typically preferred, due to the agranulocytosis and frequent blood monitoring requirements associated with clozapine. Olanzapine, risperidone, and aripiprazole should not be used in PD because they do not reduce the incidence of hallucinations and actually increase the risk of motor deterioration. Donepezil, rivastigmine, and ziprasidone were also shown to be effective in reducing hallucinations. Patients with PD often develop cognitive impairment due to cholinergic dysfunction. Unfortunately, there are no published articles involving cholinesterase inhibitors in the treatment of PD-related cognitive impairment. Expert opinion concludes that although cholinesterase inhibitors provide variable and unpredictable benefit in patients with PD-related cognitive impairment, some patients experience marked improvement, and therefore, a trial is warranted (Connolly & Lang, 2014).

Sleep Problems

Insomnia, involving difficulty with initiation, duration, and/or maintenance of sleep, is the most common sleep disorder that affects patients with PD. Only the short-term treatment of insomnia in PD has been assessed with agents including carbidopa/levodopa, eszopiclone, melatonin, and modafinil. Of these agents, melatonin and the CR formulation of carbidopa/levodopa have been deemed possibly useful. Similarly, only short-term studies have evaluated the treatment of fatigue in PD with modafinil and methylphenidate, which have inconclusive efficacy (Connolly & Lang, 2014).

Autonomic or Other Problems

A patient with PD should be regularly evaluated for orthostatic hypotension, as it can be a significant issue in PD. Hypotension is not only a nonmotor symptom, but it is also an adverse effect of some PD drugs. This can complicate the treatment of hypertension in a patient with PD, so it is essential to monitor supine blood pressure in these patients. Fludrocortisone, midodrine, and indomethacin have been shown to be mildly effective at treating hypotension in patients with PD. Drooling can be an embarrassing nonmotor symptom that may affect patients with PD. Sublingual atropine drops and botulinum toxin injections can aid in reducing drooling symptoms. Constipation is a significant problem in patients with PD. Not only can it be very uncomfortable for the patient, but over time, it can also lead to more serious complications, such as bowel obstruction, if left untreated (Connolly & Lang, 2014). To alleviate symptoms of constipation, stimulant laxatives and stool softeners can be utilized.

MONITORING PATIENT RESPONSE

The monitoring of patient response is multifactorial, considering the broad range of associated symptoms. The previously mentioned scales, such as MDS-UPDRS, can be used to assess disability and impairment, including motor and nonmotor symptoms, complications, and impact on daily living (Goetz et al., 2008). Monitoring plans should engage patients and caregivers, and symptom journals might help provide therapy-guiding information. It is important to establish appropriate therapy expectations early on, so that patients and caregivers understand the progressive nature of PD and which symptoms may be more likely to respond to drug therapy. Patient responses to varying medication doses, presence of dyskinesia, "on" and "off" time, dizziness, nausea, visual hallucinations, "wearing-off" effects, falls, sleep disturbances, abnormal behaviors, and mood or memory changes should be recorded and discussed. Practitioners should ensure that the patient and caregivers understand the prescribed medication regimen and administration instructions and treatment adherence should be gauged. Practitioners should evaluate and remedy adherence barriers, such as cost, adverse effects, regimen convenience, or understanding of regimen. Additionally, all health care professionals should monitor for drugs that can exacerbate parkinsonism or cognitive ability.

PATIENT EDUCATION

For a patient with PD, navigating a complex daily routine of medications and symptom management can be challenging. Patient needs and priorities will continue to change throughout disease progression, and it is important that patients have access to accurate, reliable information that is conveyed in understandable terms.

Drug Information

In 2011, the Movement Disorder Society released evidence-based medicine review updates for motor and nonmotor symptoms of PD (Fox et al., 2011; Seppi et al., 2011). A recent review of pharmacological treatment of PD written by Connolly et al. was published in the Journal of the American Medical Association in 2014 (Connolly & Lang, 2014). This publication contains several figures, tables, and algorithms that clarify the complex approaches to the medication management of PD. The American Academy of Neurology lists current guidelines and tools for both health care professionals and patients (AAN, 2015).

Patient-Oriented Information Sources

Organizations that provide patient-oriented information sources include the American Academy of Neurology, Parkinson's Disease Foundation, and Michael J. Fox Foundation for Parkinson's Research. The National Parkinson Foundation offers several publications, including manuals and checklists. This Web site also offers a smartphone application and allows patients to search for local chapters by indicating their state or zip code. The American Parkinson Disease Association also offers many patient-oriented publications, including books, educational supplements, and brochures. The U.S. Department of Transportation has a posting on their Web site entitled "Driving when you have Parkinson's Disease."

Nutrition/Lifestyle Changes

Nutrition and lifestyle considerations will vary based on patient-specific factors and should complement drug therapy. In more advanced stages of PD, patients may have speech or swallowing difficulties. Dysarthria is a motor speech disorder comprised of an assortment of speech characteristics. Speech therapy may show benefit with some symptoms of dysarthria, specifically with reduced vocal volume, imprecise articulation, and monotony of both pitch and loudness. Other elements of dysarthria, including hoarseness, may not improve. Speech therapy can also focus on drooling and swallowing issues, which can include slowed chewing, choking on liquids, and inability to eat food of various consistencies. The Lee Silverman Voice Treatment (LSVT) can have positive effects on voice quality, respiration, articulation, and even swallowing (Nijkrake et al., 2007). For patients with swallowing issues, a speech therapist can provide individualized dietary recommendations and recommend appropriate management strategies.

Patients may also have to manage bowel irregularities, which may develop with disease progression or as a result of medication side effects. For constipation, patients can make dietary adjustments to help alleviate this symptom. Increased fluid intake and consumption of high-fiber foods, such as fruits, vegetables, whole grains, beans, and prunes, can be helpful in maintaining bowel regularity. If dietary measures are insufficient in managing constipation, patients can use pharmacological agents, as mentioned previously.

Additional medication side effects that may require management include nausea and loss of appetite. These side effects may diminish over time, but patients can take some medications with a small snack to alleviate discomfort, initially. Other nutrition-related medication considerations involve treatment with levodopa. As mentioned previously, high-protein meals can decrease the effectiveness of levodopa. Patients should not aim to eliminate dietary protein but can instead limit protein portions to 3 to 4 ounces per meal, which is approximately the size of a bar of soap or a deck of cards. Additionally, patients should separate the administration of levodopa from meals, as described previously, and could shift protein consumption to the evening. Iron supplements may also decrease levodopa absorption, so patients should separate these by at least 2 hours. Long-term effects of altered diets should be carefully considered, along with the possible inconveniences.

Patients taking MAO-B inhibitors such as rasagiline or selegiline should avoid or limit tyramine-rich foods, as this can increase the risk of serotonin syndrome. These include aged cheeses, soybean products, red wine, tap beer, and cured, fermented, or air-dried meats or fish. Patients should work with nutritionists or dieticians when making significant dietary adjustments.

It is important for patients with PD to maintain bone density, as these individuals may be at a higher risk for developing osteoporosis and may also have an increased fall risk due to motor symptoms, which can result in fractures. Adults over 50 years of age should incorporate calcium-rich products, such as low-fat milk or yogurt or hard cheeses. Patients should also consume vitamin D in the form of fortified dairy or juice products, egg yolks, breakfast cereal, or fatty fish, such as salmon, trout, mackerel, tuna, and eel. A 3-ounce salmon fillet contains approximately 450 IU of vitamin D. Sun exposure can increase vitamin D, although this should be balanced with the risk for skin cancer. Weight-bearing exercise can also contribute to the maintenance of bone health.

In addition to fortifying bones, high-intensity resistance exercises can improve muscle force production and mobility. A variety of exercise regimens have been studied, including progressive resistance exercise, which has a proposed impact on the mechanisms impacting bradykinesia and muscle weakness (David et al., 2012). Physical therapy is also beneficial in improving mobility and strengthening muscles for patients with PD. Benefits of physiotherapy have been described in six core areas including (1) gait; (2) transfers, such as rising from a chair or rolling over in bed; (3) balance; (4) body posture; (5) reaching and grasping; and (6) physical inactivity (Nijkrake et al., 2007).

There appears to be insufficient evidence to support or refute the use of acupuncture, biofeedback, manual therapy including chiropractic and osteopathic manipulation, or Alexander technique, which involves the development of awareness of posture in order to make improvements; however, this may result from a general lack of conducted studies (Nijkrake et al., 2007; Sucherowsky et al., 2006). These therapies are unlikely to induce harm, and patients may find them helpful in the establishment of a holistic PD management plan. Examples of other complementary therapies include tai chi to improve balance, qigong to help patients focus on breathing patterns, meditation and massage to help with relaxation, and acupuncture to help with sleep disturbances. Approximately 40% of patients with PD in the United States reportedly use at least one of these complementary therapies (Nijkrake et al., 2007). The extent of benefit may vary among patients, but patients should be encouraged to work with their health care team to individualize and optimize their PD management strategies.

Complementary and Alternative Medications

Several nonstandard pharmacologic and nonpharmacologic therapies have been explored in patients with PD. The seeds of the *Mucuna pruriens* plant contain levodopa. Although several small trials demonstrated effectiveness, the American Academy of Neurology concluded that there is currently insufficient evidence to support or refute the use of *M. pruriens* (AAN, 2015; Sucherowsky et al., 2006). Variability in standardization and preparation of this product may also lead to unreliable effects. A more recent study in primates suggested that this natural substance might act according to a different mechanism than levodopa (Lieu et al., 2012). *Vicia faba*, also known as fava beans, has also been shown to contain a minimal amount of levodopa and have been suggested for short-term benefit in PD, but evidence is lacking for the benefit of this product in PD (Sucherowsky et al., 2006).

In the early stages of PD, creatine has been explored as an option to strengthen muscles and slow the progression of PD; however, its benefit has not been demonstrated with this product. Neuroprotective effects of vitamin E at doses of 2,000 IU and coenzyme Q10 at doses ranging from 300 to 2,400 mg/d have been studied, but effectiveness has not been demonstrated for either supplement.

For patients experiencing orthostatic hypotension, increasing salt and fluid consumption, along with elevating the head of the bed, and wearing compression stockings can be beneficial. Rapid consumption of two 8-ounce glasses of cold water can also result in a prompt response.

A successful PD treatment approach, management strategy, and monitoring plan should ideally incorporate a complete team of interprofessional experts. This team may include, but is not limited to, primary care and specialist physicians, pharmacists, nurse practitioners, nurses, physician assistants, psychologists, occupational therapists, physical therapists, speech language pathologists, nutritionists, dieticians, social workers, and chaplains.

CASE STUDY*

M.P. is a 66-year-old man with past medical history of hypertension and hyperlipidemia presenting to the clinic describing problems with balance and gait that have worsened in the past few months. A gait assessment reveals reduced arm swing while walking and a single halt hesitation when turning. During straight walking, he continues smoothly without freezing. The MDS-UPDRS reveals slight impairment related to postural instability and mild impairment related to both gait and freezing. Based on his history and physical exam, he is diagnosed with PD. Following his diagnosis, he mentions that he is considering retirement.

DIAGNOSIS: PARKINSON DISEASE

1. Which of the following is *not* an appropriate goal of therapy for **M.P.**?
   a. Maintain patient independence by alleviating motor symptoms.
   b. Preserve patient ability to perform activities of daily living.
   c. Reverse disease progression.
   d. Maintain patient quality of life by alleviating non-motor symptoms.

2. What is the *most* appropriate initial therapy for **M.P.**?
   a. Amantadine 100 mg twice daily
   b. Carbidopa/levodopa IR 25 mg/100 mg three times daily
   c. Pramipexole IR 0.125 mg three times daily
   d. Benztropine 0.5 mg twice daily

3. In addition to the pharmacologic recommendation mentioned above, which of the below recommendations is *most* appropriate for **M.P.**?
   a. Referral to a speech therapist
   b. High-intensity resistance exercises
   c. Qigong
   d. Initiation of coenzyme Q10 300 mg daily

* Answers can be found online.

Bibliography

Starred references are cited in the text.

*Abramowicz, M., Zucchotti, G., Pflomm, J. M., et al. (2013). Drugs for Parkinson's disease. *Treatment Guidelines from the Medical Letter, 11*(135), 101–106.

*American Academy of Neurology. (2015). *Practice guidelines: Movement disorders.* Retrieved from https://www.aan.com on April 24, 2015.

American Parkinson's Disease Association. (2015). *Download publications.* Retrieved from http://www.apdaparkinson.org/resources-support/download-publications on April 24, 2015.

*Ascherio, A., Chen, H., Schwarzschild, M. A., et al. (2003). Caffeine, postmenopausal estrogen, and risk of Parkinson's disease. *Neurology, 60*(5), 790–795.

Berardelli, A., Wenning, G. K., Antonini, A., et al. (2013). EFNS/MDS-ES/ENS [corrected] recommendations for the diagnosis of Parkinson's disease. *European Journal of Neurology, 20*(1), 16–34.

Chaudhuri, K. R., Rojo, J. M., Schapira, A. H., et al. (2013). A proposal for a comprehensive grading of Parkinson's disease severity combining motor and non-motor assessments: Meeting an unmet need. *PLoS One, 8*(2), e57221.

Chen, Y., Yang, W., Long, J., et al. (2015). Discriminative analysis of Parkinson's disease based on whole-brain functional connectivity. *PLoS One, 10*(4), e0124153.

*Clarke, C. E., Patel, S., Ives, N., et al. (2011). Should treatment for Parkinson's disease start immediately on diagnosis or delayed until functional disability develops? *Movement Disorders, 26*(7), 1187–1193.

*Connolly, B. S., & Lang, A. E. (2014). Pharmacological treatment of Parkinson disease: A review. *Journal of the American Medical Association, 311*(16), 1670–1683.

*David, F. J., Rafferty, M. R., Robichaud, J. A., et al. (2012). Progressive resistance exercise and Parkinson's disease: A review of potential mechanisms. *Parkinson's Disease, 2012,* 124527.

Dibble, L. E., Foreman, K. B., Addison, O., et al. (2015). Exercise and medication effects on persons with Parkinson disease across the domains of disability: A randomized clinical trial. *Journal of Neurologic Physical Therapy, 39,* 85–92.

*Eggers, C., Pedrosa, D. J., Kahraman, D., et al. (2012). Parkinson subtypes progress differently in clinical course and imaging pattern. *PLoS One, 7*(10), e46813.

Ferreira, J. J., Katzenschlager, R., Bloem, B. R., et al. (2013). Summary of the recommendations of the EFNS/MDS-ES review on therapeutic management of Parkinson's disease. *European Journal of Neurology, 20,* 5–15.

*Fox, S. H., Katzenschlager, R., Lim, S. Y., et al. (2011). The movement disorder society evidence-based medicine review update: Treatments for the motor symptoms of Parkinson's disease. *Movement Disorders, 26*(S3), S2–S41.

*Goetz, C. G., & Pal, G. (2014). Initial management of Parkinson's disease. *British Medical Journal, 349,* g6258.

*Goetz, C. G., Tilley, B. C., Shaftman, S. R., et al. (2008). Movement Disorder Society-sponsored revision of the Unified Parkinson's disease rating scale (MDS-UPDRS): Scale presentation and clinimetric testing results. *Movement Disorders, 23*(15), 2129–2170.

*Halliday, G., McCann, H., & Shepherd, C. (2012). Evaluation of the Braak hypothesis: How far can it explain the pathogenesis of Parkinson's disease? *Expert Review of Neurotherapeutics, 12*(6), 673–686.

Hickey, P., & Stacy, M. (2011). Available and emerging treatments for Parkinson's disease: A review. *Drug Design, Development and Therapy, 5,* 241–254.

Lacy, C., Armstrong, L. L., Goldman, M. P., et al. (2015–2016). *Drug information handbook* (24th ed.). Hudson, OH: Lexicomp, Inc.

*Lesage, S., & Brice, A. (2012). Role of Mendelian genes in "sporadic" Parkinson's disease. *Parkinsonism & Related Disorders, 18*(Suppl. 1), S66–S70.

*Lieu, C. A., Venkiteswaran, K., Gilmour, T. P., et al. (2012). The antiparkinsonian and antidyskinetic mechanisms of *Mucuna pruriens* in the MPTP-treated nonhuman primate. *Evidence-Based Complementary and Alternative Medicine, 2012,* 840247.

*Liu, R., Guo, X., Park, Y., et al. (2012). Caffeine intake, smoking, and risk of Parkinson disease in men and women. *American Journal of Epidemiology, 175*(11), 1200–1207.

*Lyons, K. E., & Pahwa, R. (2011). Diagnosis and initiation of treatment in Parkinson's disease. *International Journal of Neuroscience, 121*(Suppl. 2), 27–36.

Michael J. Fox Foundation. (2015). *Parkinson's books and resources.* Retrieved from https://www.michaeljfox.org/understanding-parkinsons/resources.html on April 24, 2015.

Movement Disorder Society-sponsored revision of the Unified Parkinson's Disease Rating Scale (MDS-UPDRS). (2008). Retrieved from http://www.movementdisorders.org/MDS-Files1/PDFs/Rating-Scales/MDS-UPDRSfinal_Update.pdf on April 24, 2015.

*Muñoz, P., Huenchuguala, S., Paris, I., et al. (2012). Dopamine oxidation and autophagy. *Parkinson's Disease, 2012,* 920953.

*Murman, D. L. (2012). Early treatment of Parkinson's disease: Opportunities for managed care. *American Journal of Managed Care, 18,* S183–S188.

*Nalls, M. A., Pankratz, N., Lill, C. M., et al. (2014). Large-scale meta-analysis of genome-wide association data identifies six new risk loci for Parkinson's disease. *Nature Genetics, 46*(9), 989–993.

National Parkinson Foundation. (2015). *Education for patients.* Retrieved from http://www.parkinson.org/Improving-Care/Education/Education--For-Patients on April 24, 2015.

*Nijkrake, M. J., Keus, S. H. J., Kalf, J. G., et al. (2007). Allied health care interventions and complementary therapies in Parkinson's disease. *Parkinsonism & Related Disorders, 13*(Suppl. 3), S488–S494.

*Parkinson, J. (1817). *An essay on the shaking palsy.* London, UK: Sherwood, Neely, and Jones.

Parkinson's Disease Foundation. (2015a). *Living with Parkinson's.* Retrieved from http://www.pdf.org/living_pd on April 24, 2015.

Parkinson's Disease Foundation. (2015b). *Understanding Parkinson's.* Retrieved from http://www.pdf.org/understanding_pd on April 24, 2015.

*Pedrosa, D. J., & Timmermann, L. (2013). Review: Management of Parkinson's disease. *Neuropsychiatric Disease and Treatment, 9,* 321–340.

Pezzoli, G., & Cereda, E. (2013). Exposure to pesticides or solvents and risk of Parkinson disease. *Neurology, 80*(22), 2035–2041.

Schröder, S., Martus, P., Odin, P., et al. (2012). Impact of community pharmaceutical care on patient health and quality of drug treatment in Parkinson's disease. *International Journal of Clinical Pharmacy, 34*(5), 746–756.

*Seppi, K., Weintraub, D., Coelho, M., et al. (2011). The movement disorder society evidence-based medicine review update: Treatments for the non-motor symptoms of Parkinson's disease. *Movement Disorders, 26*(S3), S42–S80.

*Shin, H. W., & Chung, J. S. (2012). Drug-induced parkinsonism. *Journal of Clinical Neurology, 8*(1), 15–21.

*Sucherowsky, O., Gronseth, G., Perlmutter, J., et al. (2006). Practice parameter: Neuroprotective strategies and alternative therapies for Parkinson disease (an evidence–based review): Report of the Quality Standards Subcommittee of the American Academy of neurology. *Neurology, 66,* 976–982.

*Tarazi, F. I., Sahli, Z. T., Wolny, M., et al. (2014). Emerging therapies for Parkinson's disease: From bench to bedside. *Pharmacology & Therapeutics, 144*(2), 123–133.

U.S. Department of Health and Human Services, National Institute of Neurologic Disorders and Stroke. (2015). *NINDS Parkinson's disease information page.* Retrieved from http://www.ninds.nih.gov/disorders/parkinsons_disease/parkinsons_disease.htm on April 24, 2015.

U.S. Department of Transportation. (2015). *Driving when you have Parkinson's disease.* Retrieved from http://www.nhtsa.gov/people/injury/olddrive/Parkinsons%20Web on April 24, 2015.

*VanderHorst, V. G., Samardzic, T., Saper, C. B., et al. (2015). α-Synuclein pathology accumulates in sacral spinal visceral sensory pathways. *Annals of Neurology, 78*(1), 142–149. doi: 10.1002/ana.24430.

*Wirdefeldt, K., Adami, H. O., Cole, P., et al. (2011). Epidemiology and etiology of Parkinson's disease: A review of the evidence. *European Journal of Epidemiology, 26*(Suppl. 1), S1–S58.

UNIT 10

Pharmacotherapy for Endocrine Disorders

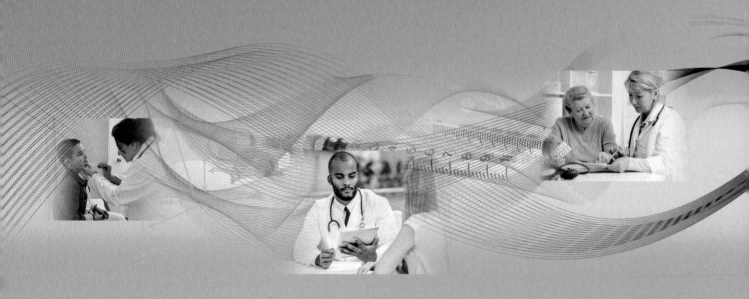

Pharmacotherapy for
Enteric Disorders

10

46 Diabetes Mellitus

Lorraine Nowakowski-Grier ■ Veronica F. Wilbur

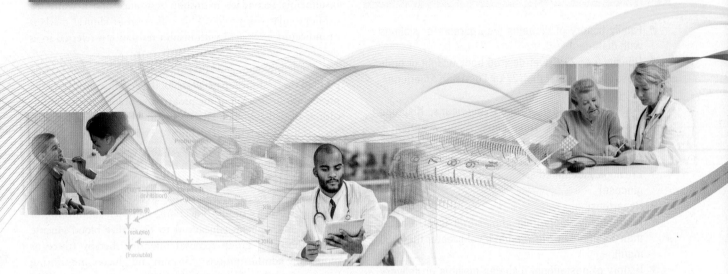

Diabetes mellitus is the term used to represent a clinically and genetically heterogeneous group of disorders characterized by abnormally high blood glucose levels (hyperglycemia) as a result of either insulin deficiency or cellular resistance to the action of insulin. Four major classifications of diabetes have been defined: type 1 diabetes mellitus (formerly known as *insulin-dependent diabetes mellitus*), type 2 diabetes mellitus (formerly known as *non–insulin-dependent diabetes mellitus*), gestational diabetes mellitus, and diabetes secondary to other conditions (e.g., hormonal abnormalities and pancreatic diseases).

According to the Centers for Disease Control and Prevention (CDC, 2014), there are more than 29.1 people with diabetes in the United States. Of this number, 90% to 95% have type 2 diabetes. Additionally, there is another 86 million who have a condition called *prediabetes* (CDC, 2014). The National Institute of Diabetes and Digestive and Kidney Diseases and the American Diabetes Association (ADA) found that diabetes was the seventh leading cause of death in the United States in 2006. Overall, the risk of death among people with diabetes is approximately twice that of people without diabetes. The annual medical costs for diabetes in the United States in 2013 were $245 billion in direct and indirect costs. This is a 41% increase in the overall dollar amount spent on all aspects of diabetes care.

CAUSES

Type 1 diabetes is thought to be an autoimmune disease in which pancreatic beta cells are destroyed. The beta cells are responsible for secreting insulin, a major hormone that promotes cellular uptake and use of glucose and maintains

metabolic functions throughout the body. If the beta cells are destroyed, the pancreas produces no insulin, causing glucose levels in the blood to skyrocket. Onset can occur at any time, but most patients are younger than age 30.

Although type 1 diabetes is one of the most common chronic diseases in children, its etiology remains unclear. Suggested etiologies include genetic predisposition to the destruction of beta cells, infection, autoimmunity, and environmental factors. Viral agents are highly suspected in the pathogenesis of type 1 diabetes because mumps, rubella, varicella, measles, influenza, coxsackievirus, cytomegalovirus, and viral pneumonia have been reported to precede its onset. Furthermore, the incidence increases in the United States during the fall and winter, when viral infections are prevalent. Autoimmunity is evident because 80% of patients with type 1 diabetes test positive for specific human leukocyte antigen. It is likely that a combination of these factors contributes to the destruction of beta cells and the subsequent absence of insulin.

In type 2 diabetes, adipose and muscle cells become less sensitive to the actions of insulin or the pancreas produces less insulin than the body needs. In either situation, glucose levels in the blood escalate. Most patients with type 2 diabetes are older than age 30. **Box 46.1** lists risk factors for type 2 diabetes; the major risk factors are obesity and family history. Both beta cell defects and insulin resistance are found in patients with type 2 diabetes.

In gestational diabetes, pregnancy causes the woman to become intolerant to glucose. The causes are not fully clear, but they appear to be related to the anti-insulin effects created by progesterone, cortisol, and human placental lactogen. Usually, once the woman has delivered her infant, blood glucose levels

BOX
46.1 **Major Risk Factors for Type 2
Diabetes Mellitus**

- Family history of diabetes (i.e., parents or siblings with diabetes)
- Obesity (i.e., 20% over desired body weight or body mass index greater than 27 kg. For Asian Americans, it is greater than 23 kg)
- Race/ethnicity (e.g., African Americans, Hispanic Americans, Native Americans, Asian Americans, Pacific Islanders have increased risk)
- Age older than 45 years
- Previously identified as having IFG (impaired fasting glucose)
- Hypertension
- High-density lipoprotein cholesterol level greater than 35 mg/dL or triglyceride level greater than 250 mg/dL
- History of gestational diabetes mellitus or delivery of babies weighing greater than 9 lb
- Sedentary lifestyle

return to normal; however, women who have had gestational diabetes have a 20% to 50% chance of developing diabetes in the next 5 to 10 years.

PATHOPHYSIOLOGY

In type 1 diabetes, the pancreatic beta cells are destroyed, causing a subsequent absence of insulin. In genetically susceptible people, an autoimmune attack occurs in which monocytes/macrophages and activated cytotoxic T cells infiltrate the islets. Multiple antibodies against beta cell antigens develop in the blood, and insulin reserve steadily decreases until the amount is insufficient to maintain a normal blood glucose level.

The pathogenesis of type 2 diabetes involves insulin resistance, impaired insulin secretion, elevated glucose production by the liver, or all these components. With insulin resistance, circulating insulin concentrations increase as compensation. Researchers have hypothesized that in type 2 diabetes, the ability of insulin to inhibit hepatic glucose production and to stimulate its uptake and use by adipose and muscle cells is diminished. In lean patients with type 2 diabetes, the primary defect appears to occur in the beta cells. In overweight patients, who represent most patients with type 2 diabetes, the most likely primary defect is impairment of the target cells. Although abnormal hepatic glucose metabolism plays an important role in maintaining the diabetic state, it is probably not the earliest development and most likely follows impaired insulin sensitivity in the muscle.

Insulin affects many body systems, and chronic hyperinsulinemia contributes to the pathogenesis and worsening

of hypertension, dyslipidemia, and coronary heart disease. Hypertension, high plasma triglyceride levels, and low high-density lipoprotein (HDL) plasma levels correlate with hyperinsulinemia secondary to insulin resistance and a worsened cardiovascular risk profile. This collection of clinical markers or indicators associated with insulin resistance is referred to as *metabolic syndrome.*

Epidemiologic and interventional studies consistently point to the relationship between good glycemic control and the prevention or slowing of the progression of long-term complications of diabetes. The Diabetes Control and Complications Trial (DCCT) presented definitive evidence to support the hypothesis that diabetic complications are related to the degree of hyperglycemia. In this landmark study, patients with type 1 diabetes were randomized to two groups and followed for an average of 6.5 years. One group received conventional therapy (one or two daily insulin injections, daily self-monitoring of glucose, and diabetes education) to normalize blood glucose levels; the other group received intensive therapy (three or more daily administrations of insulin and glucose monitoring four times daily). The incidence of microvascular complications was 60% lower in the group that received intensive therapy than in the patients who received conventional therapy. Hence, intensive therapy delayed the onset of complications and slowed their progression. The UK Prospective Diabetes Study (UKPDS) Group answered the question as to whether the DCCT results could be extrapolated to include type 2 diabetes. In the UKPDS, patients with type 2 diabetes were randomized to intensive or conventional therapy and followed over a 10-year period. As in the DCCT, there was a significant (25%) risk reduction in microvascular end points with tight control.

DIAGNOSTIC CRITERIA

Patients with marked hyperglycemia present with the classic symptoms of polyuria (excessive urination), polydipsia (increased thirst), weight loss, polyphagia (increased hunger and caloric intake), and blurred vision. In type 1 diabetes, the onset of these symptoms usually is sudden and often preceded by ketoacidosis. In contrast, the course of development for type 2 diabetes is gradual, insidious, and frequently undiagnosed for years. The onset and sometimes the presence of symptoms often go unnoticed. Therefore, screening for diabetes as part of a routine medical examination is appropriate if a patient has one or more risk factors (see **Box 46.1**). The more risk factors that the individual has, the greater the chances are for him or her to develop or have diabetes. Because early detection and prompt treatment may reduce the impact of diabetes and its complications, screening is recommended for those at risk.

The new consensus for diagnosis includes use of hemoglobin A_{1C} (HbA_{1C}). Fasting plasma glucose (FPG) can also be used; less often, the oral glucose tolerance test (OGTT) is employed. Diagnosis can also be made on presentation with classic overt signs and symptoms of diabetes. FPG and now the HbA$_{1C}$ are generally the easiest and least expensive diagnostic tests. Fasting is defined as no intake of food or beverage other than water for at least 8 hours before testing. The OGTT is still the preferred test for pregnant women, and it can be performed in either a one-step or two-step method. The key with pregnant women is careful risk assessment in the early stages of pregnancy regarding their risk of diabetes.

Normal glucose is defined as an FPG level of less than 100 mg/dL and a 2-hour post load glucose (PG) value in the OGTT of less than 140 mg/dL. A normal HbA$_{1C}$ is less than 5.7 and can be obtained regardless of the last oral intake. Those who test higher than or equal to 6.5% should have repeat testing to confirm the diagnosis. An FPG level of 126 mg/dL or more or a 2-hour PG value in the OGTT of 200 mg/dL or more warrants repeat testing on a different day to confirm the diagnosis. Patients with an FPG of at least 100 mg/dL but less than 126 mg/dL have impaired fasting glucose (IFG). Patients with a 2-hour PG value of at least 140 mg/dL but less than 200 mg/dL in the OGTT are considered as having impaired glucose tolerance (IGT). Patients with IFG or IGT are now referred to as having *prediabetes*, indicating the relatively high risk of developing diabetes. Diagnostic criteria are presented in **Table 46.1**.

Plasma glucose levels can be obtained from patients regardless of the time the patients last ate. Such levels are referred to as random plasma glucose levels. Any random plasma glucose level of 200 mg/dL or more is considered positive for diabetes and warrants additional testing, preferably by the FPG test on another day.

Many medications have adverse effect on glucose metabolism. While medications are not usually a true etiologic factor for diabetes, they can unmask less obvious glucose intolerance that had not yet been detected. Diuretics are one type of medication that is commonly blamed for "causing" diabetes.

When used for hypertension therapy in people with diabetes, they may cause worsening of glucose control, probably facilitated by a loss of potassium. Often times, maintaining proper potassium replacement will eliminate some of the diuretic-induced glucose intolerance.

INITIATING DRUG THERAPY

Effective treatment programs for diabetes mellitus require comprehensive training in self-management, ongoing support from the clinical care team, and, for many, intensive pharmacologic regimens. These programs must be individualized according to each patient's needs and should include the following features:

- Self-monitoring of blood glucose (SMBG)
- Medical nutrition therapy
- Regular exercise
- Drug therapy individualized for each patient
- Oral glucose-lowering agents for some patients with type 2 diabetes
- Instruction in the prevention and treatment of acute and chronic complications, including hypoglycemia
- Continuing patient education and support
- Periodic assessment of treatment goals

Treatment of abnormal glucose levels consists of diet and exercise. The cornerstone of therapy for all patients with diabetes is diet, but the goals of therapy differ between types 1 and 2 diabetes. In general, patients with type 1 diabetes are usually thin and present at or below ideal body weight. Therefore, the goals of diet are directed toward regulation of caloric intake and proper spacing of meals and snacks. In the presence of exogenously administered insulin, these patients require proper timing of meals and routine activities to prevent episodes of hypoglycemia. Patients taking insulin should carry a source of simple sugar at all times in the event of hypoglycemia.

Because most patients with type 2 diabetes are overweight, the goal of treatment is directed toward weight reduction. Weight loss leads to improved glucose tolerance by enhancing the sensitivity of peripheral glucose receptors. Patients with type 2 diabetes can control the condition through diet and exercise alone. Physical activity and exercise are important in both prevention and the treatment of type 2 diabetes. Regular physical activity can prevent or delay the onset of type 2 diabetes and its complications. The Diabetes Prevention Program (DPP) was a landmark randomized clinical trial of 3,234 overweight individuals with prediabetes in the United States (2002). The DPP found lifestyle intervention to be more effective than metformin in preventing type 2 diabetes. The trial reported that intensive lifestyle intervention decreased the incidence of type 2 diabetes by 58%, compared with 31% in the group taking metformin.

If these interventions fail to achieve desirable glycemic control, practitioners should initiate drug therapy.

TABLE 46.1

Criteria for the Diagnosis of Diabetes Mellitus

Normoglycemia	Impaired Glucose Metabolism (Prediabetes)	Diabetes Mellitus
HbA$_{1C}$ 4%–5.6%	5.7%–6.4%	HbA$_{1C}$ ≥ 6.5%
FPG <100 mg/dL	FPG 100–125 mg/dL (IFG)	FPG ≥ 126 mg/dL
OGTT PG < 140 mg/dL	OGTT 140–199 mg/dL (IGT)	≥200 mg/dL
Random plasma glucose ≥200 mg/dL and symptoms of diabetes mellitus		>200 mg/dL

FPG, fasting plasma glucose; HbA$_{1C}$, hemoglobin A$_{1C}$; IFG, impaired fasting glucose; IGT, impaired glucose tolerance; PG, plasma glucose.

Goals of Drug Therapy

The major goals of drug therapy in diabetes mellitus have been established by the ADA and the American Association of Clinical Endocrinology (AACE), and while they are similar, there is some variance as follows:

GLYCEMIC CONTROL

American Diabetes Association

HBA$_{1C}$ <7.0%. Individualized based on duration of disease, age/life expectancy, comorbid conditions, known CVD or advanced microvascular complications, hypoglycemia unawareness, individual patient considerations.

More (6.5%) or less (8.0%) stringent glycemic goals may be appropriate based on the above criteria.

American Association of Clinical Endocrinologist (AACE)

- **HBA$_{1C}$** ≤6.5% Individualized based on age, comorbidities, duration of disease
- Closer to normal for healthy
- Less stringent for "less healthy"

Both ADA and ACCE

- Preprandial plasma glucose level 80 to 130 mg/dL
- Postprandial plasma glucose level less than 180 mg/dL

BLOOD PRESSURE

- <140/90 mm Hg (125/75 for patients with proteinuria)

LIPIDS

- Low-density lipoprotein (LDL) level less than 100 mg/dL—no overt CVD
  LDL level less than 70 mg/dL—overt CVD
- Triglyceride level less than 150 mg/dL
- HDL level greater than 40 mg/dL (men)
  HDL level greater than 50 (women)

MICROALBUMIN (RANDOM COLLECTION)

- <30 µg/mL creatinine

In type 1 diabetes, insulin is the mainstay of drug therapy. When diet and exercise alone do not achieve glycemic control of type 2 diabetes, drug therapy is indicated. In type 2 diabetes, oral agents with glucose-lowering effects are used. The ADA suggests that pharmacologic therapy be selected with consideration to the following factors:

- Degree of hyperglycemia and the presence or absence of symptoms
- Presence of comorbidity
- Patient motivation
- Patient preference

Sulfonylureas

Sulfonylureas are a major group of oral hypoglycemic agents used to treat type 2 diabetes (see **Table 46.2**). They correct derangements of carbohydrate, lipid, and protein metabolism.

Mechanism of Action

Sulfonylureas bind to specific receptors on beta cells, causing adenosine triphosphate (ATP)-dependent potassium channels to close. The calcium channels subsequently open, leading to increased cytoplasmic calcium, which stimulates the release of insulin. Theorists have hypothesized that these drugs also have extrapancreatic effects involving the liver, muscle, and adipose cells, but because these agents are ineffective in patients with type 1 diabetes, it appears that their predominant hypoglycemic action is on the beta cells. When used alone, these agents have the most significant effect on blood sugar, especially in patients who are lean and insulinopenic.

Dosage

Sulfonylureas are divided into first- and second-generation agents. All of this class should be started at the lowest dose and titrated as needed to reach target blood glucose levels. Second-generation drugs are more potent and more widely used than first-generation agents. Comparison of these drugs by potency and other pharmacologic properties is presented in **Table 46.3**.

Approximately one third of patients with type 2 diabetes fail to respond adequately to sulfonylureas, most often because of markedly impaired beta cell function, not adhering to diet, or stressful events such as infection. After 10 years of therapy, only 50% of initial responders have adequate glycemic control. For optimal response, careful patient selection should include the following criteria: duration of disease less than 5 years, no history of prior insulin therapy or good glycemic control on less than 40 units/day of insulin, close to normal body weight, and FPG less than 180 mg/dL.

Adverse Events

The most important complication of the use of sulfonylureas is hypoglycemia. In the elderly population, this risk is greatest secondary to comorbidity, polypharmacy, or poor social situations (e.g., isolation, financial constraints). In younger patients, hypoglycemia may be associated with alcohol abuse or overexertion. Sulfonylureas are classified in pregnancy category C. However, prospective studies with glyburide (pregnancy category B) in rats and rabbits revealed no harm to the fetus, and retrospective human data suggest that glyburide may be suitable option for pregnant women unable or unwilling to use insulin. Many drugs are excreted in human milk; sulfonylureas should not be administered to nursing women. Safety and efficacy of sulfonylureas have not been established for children.

TABLE 46.2

Overview of Oral Antidiabetic Agents

Generic (Trade) Name and Dosage	Selected Adverse Events	Contraindications	Special Considerations
Sulfonylureas			
FIRST GENERATION			
tolbutamide (Orinase) 0.25–3 g in 1 or 2 divided doses	Hypoglycemia, increased risk of cardiovascular disease	Ketoacidosis, sulfa allergy	Onset occurs within 1 h, lasts 6–12 h. Give with morning meal. Effectiveness may decrease over time. Increased hypoglycemia may occur in elderly or debilitated patients. Signs and symptoms of hypoglycemia may be masked in patients taking beta-blockers.
chlorpropamide (Diabinese) 100–750 mg qd. Elderly start at 100 mg/d and others at 250 mg/d	Hypoglycemia	Same as above	Onset is 1 h, lasts 72 h. Same as above.
tolazamide (Tolinase) Initially 100–250 mg qd; increase weekly by 100–250 mg/d until desired blood glucose Maximum dose 1,000 mg/d	Hypoglycemia, increased risk of cardiovascular mortality	Same as above	Onset occurs within 4–6 h, lasts 10–14 h. Same as above.
SECOND GENERATION			
glyburide (DiaBeta, Micronase) Initially 2.5–5 mg qd; increase by 2.5 mg/wk until desired blood glucose Elderly patients start at 1.25 mg/d Maximum dose 20 mg/d	Hypoglycemia	Same as above	Onset occurs within 1.5 h, lasts 18–24 h. Same as above.
glyburide, micronized (Glynase) Initially 1.5–3 mg qd; 0.75 mg in elderly Maximum dose 12 mg/d	Same as above	Same as above	Onset occurs within 1.5 h, lasts 18–24 h. Same as above.
glipizide (Glucotrol) Initially 5 mg qd (2.5 mg in elderly); increase weekly to a maximum of 40 mg/d to desired blood glucose	Same as above	Same as above	Patients should take medication 30 min before a meal. Onset occurs within 1 h, lasts for 10–24 h. Same as above.
glimepiride (Amaryl) Initially 1–2 mg with breakfast; increase by 2 mg/wk until desired blood glucose Maximum dose 8 mg/d	Same as above	Same as above	Onset occurs within 2–4 h, lasts 24 h. Same as above.
BIGUANIDE			
metformin (Glucophage) Initially 500 mg bid; increase by 500 mg/wk until desired blood glucose	GI distress: diarrhea, nausea, bloating, flatulence Rare lactic acidosis	Renal dysfunction, CHF, metabolic acidosis, ketoacidosis, impaired hepatic function, excess alcohol consumption, pregnancy	Patients should take with meals to minimize GI side effects. Medication must be temporarily held when the patient is undergoing IV iodinated contrast study.

(Continued)

TABLE 8.2

Overview of Oral Antidiabetic Agents (*Continued*)

Generic (Trade) Name and Dosage	Selected Adverse Events	Contraindications	Special Considerations
Maximum dose 2,550 mg/d in divided doses			Modest synergistic effect may occur when given with sulfonylurea. Medication should be held for patients undergoing surgery.
Thiazolidinediones			
rosiglitazone (Avandia) Initially 4 mg/d in single dose; if response is inadequate after 12 wk, increase to 8 mg/d in single dose	Anemia, edema, headache, reversible increase in ALT	Children, ketoacidosis	Monitor ALT at baseline, every 2 mo for the first 12 mo and periodically thereafter. Discontinue medication if ALT is greater than three times the upper limit of normal or if jaundice occurs. Medications may increase plasma volume; caution is necessary for patients with New York Heart Association class III and IV heart failure. Monitor for increased risk of myocardial infarction. Resumption of premenopausal ovulation may occur in anovulatory women. Unintended pregnancy may result. Use restricted for patients unable to take pioglitazone or to manage their blood sugar.
pioglitazone (Actos) 15–30 mg/d Maximum 45 mg/d as monotherapy and 30 mg/d as combined therapy	Same as above	Same as above	Same as above. Increased risk of CHF but without myocardial infarction.
α-Glucosidase Inhibitors			
acarbose (Precose) Initially 25 mg tid with the first bite of a meal; increase by 25 mg at 4- to 8-wk intervals to a maximum of 300 mg in three divided doses (150 mg if weight <60 kg)	Flatulence, diarrhea, abdominal pain/distention	Renal dysfunction, ketoacidosis, inflammatory bowel disease, colonic ulceration; predisposition to intestinal obstruction; disorders of digestion	Patient should take with first bite of each meal.
miglitol (Glyset): Same as above	Same as above	Same as above	Same as above.
Meglitinide Analogs			
repaglinide (Prandin) Initially 0.5 mg with two to four meals daily if the patient has never received other treatment for diabetes; if previous treatment, 1–2 mg with two to four meals daily Double dose weekly to a maximum of 16 mg/d	Hyperglycemia, upper respiratory tract infection, headache, diarrhea, constipation, arthralgia, back or chest pain	Type 1 diabetes, ketoacidosis	As monotherapy or in conjunction with metformin, medication is to be taken within 30 min of a meal. Patient should skip a dose if he or she skips a meal and add a dose if he or she adds a meal.
nateglinide (Starlix) Initially 120 mg before each meal to a maximum dose of 360 mg/d	Same as above	Same as above	Same as above.

Drug (Dose)	Side Effects	Contraindications	Monitoring
DIPEPTIDYL PEPTIDASE-4 INHIBITORS			
sitagliptin (Januvia) 100 mg oral daily or 50 mg oral daily	Common to both acute upper respiratory infection, urinary tract infection, headache	Type 1 diabetes	Same as above
	Must adjust dosage to mild renal insufficiency		
	Increases tendency toward hypoglycemia when combined with sulfonylureas		
	Potential for acute pancreatitis, hypersensitivity to medication		
saxagliptin (Onglyza) 2.5 or 5 mg daily	Same as above	History of pancreatitis	
alogliptin (Nesina) 6.25 ng, 12.5 mg, or 25 mg daily	Same as above		
linagliptin (Tradjenta) 2.5 or 5 mg daily	Same as above		
vildagliptin (Galvus) 50 or 100 mg daily			
Sodium–Glucose Cotransporter 2 Inhibitors			
canagliflozin (Invokana) 100 or 300 mg daily	Hyperkalemia mycotic infections, urinary tract infections, and renal insufficiency, hypotension	Type 1 diabetes or DKA, severe kidney disease (eGFR 30 mL/min/1.73), or on hemodialysis	Monitor potassium and LDL cholesterol monitoring. Check blood pressure and symptoms of mycotic infections.
dapagliflozin (Farxiga) 5 or 10 mg daily			
empagliflozin (Jardiance) 10 or 25 mg daily			
ipragliflozin (Suglat) 25, 50, or 100 mg daily			

TABLE 46.3

Comparison of Oral Sulfonylureas

Drug	Equivalent Therapeutic Dose (mg)	Duration of Action (h)	Doses per Day	Adverse Events (%)	Hypoglycemic Reactions (%)
First Generation					
tolbutamide	1,000	6–12	2–3	3	<1
tolazamide	250	12–24	1–2	2	<1
acetohexamide	500	12–18	2	4	<1
chlorpropamide	250	24–72	1	8	<4–6
Second Generation					
Long-acting glipizide	10	12–24	1–2	5	<2–4
Long-acting glipizide	5–10	24	1	5	<1
Long-acting glyburide	5	16–24	1–2	7	<4–6

Contraindications

Long-acting agents (e.g., chlorpropamide [Diabinese]) place elderly patients with other underlying disorders at risk for prolonged and sometimes fatal hypoglycemic episodes. Drugs with active metabolites also may increase the risk of hypoglycemia in patients with impaired renal function. Hence, patient education must include recognition of symptoms as well as prevention and treatment plans for hypoglycemia. Sulfonylureas can cause weight gain of about 2 to 3 kg. They cannot be used in patients with sulfa allergies. Baseline renal and hepatic function levels should be documented prior to starting sulfonylurea therapy.

Interactions

Patients taking sulfonylureas may enhance sensitivity to sunlight, so patients should be advised to use appropriate sun protection. Certain drugs may increase the effectiveness of sulfonylureas resulting in hypoglycemia; a select list of commonly prescribed includes ciprofloxacin (especially with glyburide), clofibrate, gemfibrozil, H_2 antagonists, probenaid, sulfonamides, and tricyclic antidepressants. Drugs that may decrease the effectiveness of the sulfonylureas, resulting in hyperglycemia, include the following: beta-blockers, calcium channel blockers, cholestyramine, corticosteroids, diazoxide, estrogens, hydantoins, isoniazid, nicotinic acid, oral contraceptives, phenothiazines, rifampin, sympathomimetics, thiazide diuretics, thyroid medications, and urinary alkalinizers.

Biguanides

Biguanides are not considered hypoglycemic agents, because their major pharmacologic action does not increase insulin secretion. They can be used in conjunction with diet as first-line monotherapy or in combination with other classes of diabetic drugs, including insulin, to treat type 2 diabetes (see **Table 46.2**). Their mechanisms of action and side effect profiles differ from those of sulfonylureas, offering notable advantages.

Biguanides do not cause hypoglycemia (when used as monotherapy) and do not promote hyperinsulinemia or weight gain.

Mechanism of Action

This class inhibits hepatic glucose production and moderately improves peripheral sensitivity to insulin. Gluconeogenesis and glycogenolysis are inhibited in the liver. Glycemic control is achieved without stimulating insulin secretion, so hypoglycemia does not develop. Metformin can also decrease intestinal absorption of glucose and improve insulin sensitivity in skeletal muscle. The oral bioavailability is 50% to 60%, and food decreases the bioavailability with a slight delay in the absorption of metformin. Metformin does not bind to liver or plasma proteins and is primarily excreted by the kidneys. Other advantages of biguanides over sulfonylureas include their tendency to induce weight loss and promote favorable effects on lipid profiles. In addition, in certain patients, biguanides can be combined effectively with sulfonylureas, thiazolidinediones (TZDs), or insulin because their mechanisms of action differ. Biguanides are the agents of choice in patients who exhibit secondary failure to sulfonylureas. In view of their many beneficial effects, biguanides appear to be a more rational choice than sulfonylureas for first-line therapy in patients with newly diagnosed type 2 diabetes. Metformin is available in over 100 combinations with other oral agents from sulfonylureas, TZDs, dipeptidyl peptidase-4 inhibitors (DPP4-i), and sodium–glucose cotransporter 2 (SGLT-2) inhibitors, refer to the discussion about cited drugs further in this chapter for review of individual agents.

Dosage

The dose of metformin is started low and increased weekly as needed to the maximum. Patients usually take the medication before meals in the morning and evening. The dose is carefully titrated in elderly patients. With metformin, the starting dose is 500 or 850 mg daily or twice daily, with increases every 1 to 2 weeks to a maximum of 2,550 mg/d. Peak action is within 2 to 2.5 hours, and the effects last for 10 to 16 hours. Steady-state levels of the drug are achieved in 24 to 48 hours. Metformin also comes in an extended-release formula. It is started at 500 mg daily with the evening meal and increased to a maximum of 2,000 to 2,550 mg daily.

Contraindications

Metformin is contraindicated in males with a serum creatinine levels of greater than 1.5 mg/dL and in females with levels greater than 1.4 mg/dL, heart failure, and pregnancy. This class also is contraindicated in children, alcoholics, binge drinkers, those over age 80, and those with dehydration. The presence of hepatic dysfunction can predispose patients receiving metformin to lactic acidosis. Metformin is classified in pregnancy category B. It is not known whether metformin is excreted in human milk. Nursing women should discontinue nursing to avoid hypoglycemia in breast-feeding infants. Patients must stop taking metformin when undergoing radiologic studies with iodinated contrast the day of and restart the metformin in 2 days when renal function has returned. Patients should also stop taking metformin, when experiencing metabolic acidosis and before surgery until they resume normal oral intake. Metformin may restore ovulation in women, who were anovulatory due to insulin resistance.

Adverse Events

The most common side effect of metformin therapy is gastrointestinal (GI) upset, which includes diarrhea, nausea, vomiting, abdominal bloating, flatulence, anorexia, and a metallic taste in the mouth. Such problems occur in approximately 30% of patients during the initiation of therapy and usually resolve with continued treatment. To minimize these adverse effects, treatment is started with a low dose and increased slowly at no less than weekly intervals. Instruct patients to take metformin with meals to reduce GI side effects.

Because GI upset is rare late in therapy, any sudden onset of severe vomiting or diarrhea at that time should alert providers to the possibility of lactic acidosis, a rare but potentially fatal complication of metformin therapy. In such cases, patients should discontinue metformin immediately until they can be evaluated and stabilized. From the data collected in Europe over 20 years, the reported worldwide incidence of metformin-induced lactic acidosis is 0.03 cases/1,000 patient-years. The risk of lactic acidosis increases with advancing age and worsening renal function. Therefore, metformin is contraindicated in patients with renal disease or dysfunction and acute or chronic metabolic acidosis. Renal dysfunction may be secondary to a variety of comorbid conditions such as cardiopulmonary insufficiency, liver disease, alcoholism, and infection. These conditions predispose patients to impaired perfusion of tissues and decreased elimination of lactate and are therefore contraindications to the use of metformin. In addition, patients should temporarily discontinue metformin during any situation in which an acute decline in renal function may occur (e.g., aggressive diuresis, dehydration from gastroenteritis, surgery).

The concomitant use of metformin with cimetidine increases the risk of hypoglycemia. The concomitant use of metformin with glucocorticoids or alcohol increases the risk of lactic acidosis.

Metformin use over the age of 80 is not contraindicated, but due to the deterioration of renal function of the elderly, glomerular filtration rate (GFR) testing should be done at the beginning of therapy and periodically thereafter.

Interactions

While metformin itself does not cause hypoglycemia, combination therapy with sulfonylureas, meglitinides, or insulin can be associated with hypoglycemia.

Thiazolidinediones

This class of antidiabetic agents (**Table 46.2**) reduces insulin resistance at sites of insulin action.

Mechanism of Action

TZDs bind to the nuclear steroid hormone receptor peroxisome proliferator–activated receptor gamma and increase insulin sensitivity in the skeletal muscle and fat. Clinically, they decrease peripheral insulin resistance and at higher doses may decrease hepatic glucose production. Like biguanides, they improve the action of insulin without directly stimulating insulin secretion from the pancreatic beta cells. There is an improvement of endothelial function, preservation of beta cell function, and a decrease in albumin excretion.

Dosage

Therapy is usually started at the lowest dose, with gradual increases to reach plasma glucose goals. TZDs should be taken with the main meal of the day. The dose varies according to the agent used.

TZDs are classified in pregnancy category C and are not indicated for use during pregnancy, for breast-feeding women, or children. In addition, increased risk fracture in women and macular edema has also been observed with TZD therapy.

There may be small increases in HDL-C, and LDL-C may occur with rosiglitazone.

A concern specific to pioglitazone is the possible increased risk of bladder cancer. Interim results reported an increased risk of bladder cancer with increasing cumulative dose and duration of therapy. Based on these and other data, pioglitazone was withdrawn from use in France 2011, and no new prescriptions are authorized for patient in Germany. The studies done here in the United States have not been able to reproduce this statistical significance; therefore, it is considered safe to use in the United States.

In 2011, access to rosiglitazone was restricted by the FDA due to meta-analysis from the RECORD trial findings, which suggested that rosiglitazone may increase the relative risk of myocardial infarction. Later in 2014, the FDA re-evaluated the data determining that an increased risk of myocardial infarction could not be attributed specifically to the use of rosiglitazone; therefore, restricted distribution was removed.

Currently, rosiglitazone is available alone and in combination with metformin in the United States.

Adverse Events

Pioglitazone may cause reduced concentrations of combined oral contraceptives; therefore, patients using oral contraceptives should consider alternative contraception methods.

In premenopausal anovulatory women with insulin resistance, ovulation may resume when drugs of this class are used. Thus, the patient may be at risk of unintended pregnancy, and contraception should be considered. Because of increased plasma volume from this class of drugs, TZDs are not recommended for patients with New York Heart Association class III or class IV heart failure. Another contraindication is active liver disease. TZDs can stimulate weight gain from plasma volume expansion and generation and redistribution of fats into the subcutaneous compartments.

Adverse Effects

Serum transaminase levels (AST, ALT) should be monitored prior to initiating therapy and periodically thereafter per the clinical judgment of the health care provider. Liver function studies should also be obtained in the presence of hepatic dysfunction symptoms such as abdominal pain, fatigue nausea, vomiting, or dark urine. TZD therapy should be discontinued in the presence of jaundice. Edema, shortness of breath, rapid weight gain, and other signs and symptoms of heart failure should be included in assessing TZD therapy. Hypoglycemia may develop in patients taking this class of drug with insulin or sulfonylureas because TZDs are potent sensitizers of insulin. If this occurs, the drug should be discontinued or the dose of insulin or sulfonylurea should be reduced. TZDs require several weeks to achieve the maximum benefit from a dosage level. Patients experiencing edema/swelling, shortness of breath, or muscle aches should contact their health care provider.

Interactions

As a class, TZDs are effected by other drugs that are strong CYP2C8 inhibitors, such as gemfibrozil, and other drugs that induce CYP2C8, such as rifampin. Others to be used with caution include digoxin, fexofenadine, midazolam, nifedipine, and warfarin. α-Glucosidase inhibitors

Alpha-glucosidase Inhibitors

Mechanism of Action

The enzyme α-glucosidase, found on the brush border of the intestine, is necessary for the absorption of starch and disaccharides. This class of drugs (**Table 46.2**) acts by slowing the absorption of carbohydrates from the intestines, minimizing the postprandial rise in blood sugar. The result of this delay is decreased levels of postprandial glucose and HbA_{1C}. The α-glucosidase inhibitors are most useful in patients with postprandial hyperglycemia and patients with very high HbA_{1C} levels and poor dietary adherence. They are useful in patients from

ethnic groups with high-carbohydrate diets, such as Asians and Hispanics. Due to the limited ability of these drugs to lower HBA_{1C} and their side effect profile, they are not commonly used as monotherapy but as adjuncts to existing therapy.

Dosage

Agents from this class Acarbose (Precose) and Miglitol (Glyset), can be prescribed alone or with a sulfonylurea. Patients should take each dose with the first bite of each meal. Dosages are increased gradually (at 4- to 8-week intervals) to avoid GI side effects. The starting dose is 25 mg three times a day at the start of each meal. This regimen lasts for 4 to 8 weeks; then, the dose may be increased to 50 mg three times a day. After 3 months at 50 mg, the dose can be increased to 100 mg three times a day. Peak concentration occurs in 2 to 3 hours. Patients using alpha-glucosidase inhibitors should be encouraged to maintain physical movement, especially after a meal to limit the buildup of GI tract gas. The medication should be taken with the first bite of food.

Contraindications

Patients with inflammatory bowel disease, colonic ulceration, obstructive bowel disorders, or chronic intestinal disorders of digestion or absorption should not use these agents. Acarbose is contraindicated in patients with cirrhosis of the liver and not recommended in patients with serum creatinine levels of greater than 2.0 mg/dL or a creatinine clearance of less than 25 mL/min. Alpha-glucosidase inhibitors are classified in pregnancy category B. This drug should be used during if pregnancy only if clearly needed. These drugs should not be administered to nursing women. Elevation of serum transaminases (AST or ALT) has been observed in clinical trials in patients taking acarbose at a dose of 200 to 300 mg daily. Liver function should be periodically monitored. A 2-hour postprandial glucose measurement is useful to assess the therapeutic response during the dosage titration period. Additional monitoring should include serum aminotransferases every 3 months during the first year of therapy and periodically thereafter to monitor for liver toxicity.

Adverse Events

The most common side effects involve the GI tract. Increased fermentation secondary to the delay in carbohydrate absorption increases intestinal gas, causing flatulence, diarrhea, and abdominal distention.

Interactions

Intestinal adsorbents such as charcoal antagonize this class of drugs. The α-glucosidase inhibitors may decrease the levels of propranolol and ranitidine.

Meglitinide Analogs

Mechanism of Action

Meglitinide analogs are rapid-acting insulin secretagogues that stimulate the release of insulin from the pancreas in response to a meal (see **Table 46.2**). Binding at characterized sites closes the ATP-dependent potassium channels in the membranes of the beta cells. This causes a depolarization of the beta cells and an opening of calcium channels. The resulting increased influx of calcium causes insulin secretion.

Meglitinide analogs are effective in patients who become hypoglycemic while taking sulfonylureas and have acceptable FPG readings but high postprandial blood glucose levels. They also are effective for patients with irregular meal schedules because patients take them at meals. Repaglinide (Prandin) and nateglinide (Starlix) are the two drugs available in this class. They lower postprandial blood glucose concentrations without any significant effects on FPG level.

Dosage

Meglitinide analogs can be used as monotherapy or in combination with other oral agents. The starting dose of repaglinide is 0.5 mg before meals if the HbA_{1C} level is less than 8.0. If the HbA_{1C} concentration is greater than 8.0, the starting dose is 1 to 2 mg, taken 15 minutes (but no longer than 30 minutes before each meal). Patients must add a dose if they add another meal or skip a dose if they skip a meal. The dose may be doubled to 4 mg before meals to a maximum of 16 mg a day. Nateglinide is similarly administered with a starting dose of 60 to 120 mg before meals.

The peak level is achieved in 1 hour. In 96 hours, the body excretes 90% of the medication. Meglitinide analogs are contraindicated in patients with diabetic ketoacidosis. Take right before eating. Due to potential for hypoglycemia, those taking this medication should be advised to monitor blood glucose levels.

Contraindications

Type 1 diabetes, DKA, severe infection, surgery, trauma, or other severe stressors. Repaglinide and nateglinide are classified in pregnancy category C and are not indicated for use during pregnancy, for breast-feeding women, or for children. Elderly, debilitated, or malnourished patients and those with adrenal, pituitary, or hepatic insufficiency are susceptible to the hypoglycemic effects.

Adverse Events

Adverse events include hypoglycemia, GI disturbances, upper respiratory infections, headache, diarrhea, constipation, arthralgias, and back or chest pain.

Interactions

Concomitant use with beta-blockers or alcohol increases the risk of hypoglycemia. Ketoconazole, miconazole, erythromycin, and other cytochrome P-450 (CYP450) 3A4 inhibitors may potentiate the drug, as may nonsteroidal anti-inflammatory drugs, aspirin, sulfonamides, and warfarin. Drugs such as rifampin, barbiturates, thiazides, phenothiazines, phenytoin, sympathomimetics, calcium channel blockers, and isoniazid may antagonize it.

Dipeptidyl Peptidase-4 Inhibitors
Mechanism of Actions

Physiologically in response to a glucose load, two incretin hormones, glucose-dependent insulinotropic polypeptide and glucagon-like peptide 1 (GLP-1), are released from the distal bowel. These hormones account for up to 50% of the response to postprandial glucose. However, dipeptidyl peptidase-4 (DPP-4), which is a surface enzyme, inactivates GLP-1, therefore decreasing the levels of circulating GLP-1 and glucoregulatory functions. The class of agents called DPP-4 inhibitors acts to block the effect against GLP-1 and ultimately increase the amount of native active circulating incretins (see **Table 46.2**).

Currently, there are five DPP-4 inhibitors (DPP-4i), sitagliptin (Januvia) and saxagliptin (Onglyza), linagliptin (Tradjenta), vildagliptin (Galvus), and alogliptin (Nesina), on the market. These medications are indicated for daily administration and coadministration with other oral antidiabetic agents and insulin.

Dosage

DPP-4i drugs are administered once daily. Sitagliptin has one starting dose of 100 mg daily. Dosage should be decreased to 50 mg daily for patients with moderate renal insufficiency, defined by creatinine clearance greater than 30 mL/min but less than 50 mL/min. Sitagliptin has also been precombined with metformin. The sitagliptin dose is 50 mg with either 500 or 1,000 mg of metformin. It is also approved in combination therapy with sulfonylureas, TZDs, and insulin.

Saxagliptin has two doses, 2.5 or 5 mg, also prescribed daily. The starting dose of 2.5 mg is used for patients with mild renal insufficiency. Saxagliptin is a strong CYP3A4/5 inhibitor, which interacts with other drugs that use that pathway. Like sitagliptin, it is approved for combination therapy with sulfonylureas and TZDs but not insulin.

Contraindications

The contraindications for both medications are similar and include hypersensitivity to the agent and type 1 diabetes; caution should be used in patients with renal impairment. Only sitagliptin is contraindicated in the patient with a history of pancreatitis. All the DPP-4i inhibitors are classified in pregnancy category B. This drug category is not approved for children.

Adverse Events

The most common adverse effects are the same for sitagliptin and saxagliptin and include upper respiratory infection, urinary tract infection, and headaches when compared to placebos. Both drugs have potential for hypoglycemia when given in combination therapy with sulfonylureas. Additional postmarketing reports for sitagliptin include hypersensitivity reactions, such as anaphylaxis, angioedema, rash, urticaria, cutaneous vasculitis, and exfoliative skin conditions including Stevens-Johnson syndrome; hepatic enzyme elevations; and potentially fatal pancreatitis.

Interactions

Sitagliptin has no pharmacokinetic drug–drug interactions, but it pharmacodynamically potentiates the action of sulfonylureas and insulin. As a potent CYP3A4/5 inhibitor, saxagliptin interacts with drugs such as ketoconazole, erythromycin, and diltiazem. When DPP-4i drugs are used on combination with sulfonylureas, doses of the sulfonylureas may be reduced to avoid hypoglycemia.

Incretins

This class is also called glucagon-like peptide 1 receptor (GLP-1R) and used as adjunctive therapy to diet and exercise in type 2 diabetes.

Mechanism of Action

The mechanism of action is to stimulate glucose-dependent secretion of insulin from pancreatic beta cells while suppressing the inappropriate release of glucagon from alpha cells. It slows gastric emptying, therefore increasing satiety. Fasting and postprandial glucose are reduced with the use of incretins. As euglycemia is approached, insulin secretion subsides, therefore avoiding hypoglycemia by the response of glucagon. Incretins are not a substitute for insulin, but augment the natural physiologic responses to elevated blood sugar levels. There are presently five GLP-1R agonists available: exenatide (Byetta, Bydureon), liraglutide (Victoza), albiglutide (Tanzeum), and dulaglutide (Trulicity).

Dosage

Exenatide (Byetta) is only available as an injectable and can be used as monotherapy or in conjunction with other oral agents, metformin, sulfonylureas, TZDs, and insulin. The starting dose is 5 mcg, administered within the 60 minutes before morning and evening meals or prior to the largest meals of the day and spaced more than 6 hours apart. Based on response, in 1 month, the dose can be increased to 10 mcg twice a day. If a dose is missed, the treatment should be restarted at the next scheduled dose time.

Liraglutide may be administered once daily at any time. The initial dose of 0.6 mg/d is not effective for glycemic control, but should be administered for 1 week to reduce GI symptoms; once initial dose is tolerated, it should be increased to 1.2 mg daily; if glycemic goals are still not met after 2 to 4 weeks, the dose may be increased to the maximum 1.8 mg/d.

The extended release of exenatide (Bydureon) is dosed once weekly, and timing of the injection may be performed without regard to meals.

Albiglutide (Tanzeum) is a long-acting GLP-1R agonists; it can be given once a week. Its fusion with albumin extends its half-life. The initial dose is 30 mg once weekly. It can be increased to 50 mg with or without food. There is no adjustment of renal impairment. There are less GI effects with this GLP-1R.

Dulaglutide (Trulicity) may be administered once weekly. What makes this unique is it has a hidden needle and requires

not reconstitution. When used with a hypoglycemic agent, GLP-1R agonists may cause hypoglycemia; therefore, patients should be cautioned to monitor blood glucose levels carefully.

Contraindications

Contraindications to GLP-1R agonists include type 1 diabetes, ketoacidosis, and allergy. GLP-1R agonists should be avoided in patients with severe GI disorders, including gastroparesis. GLP-1R is classified in pregnancy category C, and nursing women should either discontinue the drug or discontinue nursing. Both exenatide and liraglutide may delay and reduce the peak concentration of digoxin, lisinopril, lovastatin, and acetaminophen. Exenatide is associated with acute pancreatitis, including fatal and nonfatal, and hemorrhagic or necrotizing pancreatitis based on postmarketing data.

Liraglutide causes thyroid C-cell tumors in both male and female mice and rats; it is unknown whether liraglutide causes thyroid C-cell tumors in humans.

Patients with a personal or family history of medullary thyroid carcinoma or multiple endocrine neoplasia syndrome type 2 should not take liraglutide. Alternative therapy should be considered.

Adverse Events

The most common adverse reactions to exenatide are GI related, including nausea, vomiting, diarrhea, and dyspepsia. Hypoglycemia is also a concern when exenatide is prescribed in combination with a sulfonylurea. Caution should be exercised with any dose increase to monitor for signs and symptoms of pancreatitis, especially severe abdominal pain with or without vomiting. Exenatide should be stopped immediately with any of these signs.

Interactions

Due to the decrease in gastric emptying, exenatide should not be administered close to drugs that have a narrow therapeutic window. Caution should be exercised when patients are taking warfarin, and the international normalized ratio should be monitored closely with drug initiation and dose changes. Exenatide can possibly decrease in the ethinyl estradiol component of oral contraceptives; therefore, exenatide and oral contraceptives should not be administered within 1 hour of each other.

After initiation of therapy or dose increases with GLP-1R agonists, patients should be monitored for signs and symptoms of pancreatitis.

Dopamine Receptor Agonists

Dopamine receptor agonists are used as monotherapy in type 2 diabetes or secondary diabetes with substantial capacity for insulin production. The mechanism by which dopamine receptor agonists improve glycemic control is unknown. Following morning administration of bromocriptine mesylate (Cycloset), postprandial glucose levels are improved without increasing plasma insulin concentrations.

Dosage

The dose of bromocriptine mesylate is 0.8 mg taken 2 hours after waking with the first meal of the day. The dose may be increased by 0.8 mg each week until the maximal tolerated daily dose of 1.6 to 4.8 mg is achieved. Bromocriptine mesylate should be taken 2 hours after waking with the first meal of the day. Patients should notify their health care provider regarding symptoms of orthostatic hypotension such as dizziness, nausea, or diaphoresis.

Contraindications

Bromocriptine mesylate is classified in pregnancy category B. It also inhibits lactation and should not be administered to nursing women. Additionally, there may be an increased risk of hypotension and syncope with bromocriptine upon increase in dose. Exacerbation of psychotic disorders or reduction in the effectiveness of drug that treat psychosis may occur when bromocriptine is coadministered.

Concomitant use of bromocriptine mesylate with other dopamine receptor agonists indicated for the treatment of Parkinson disease, restless leg syndrome, acromegaly, and other disorders is not recommended. Bromocriptine mesylate is highly bound to serum proteins and may increase unbound fraction of other highly protein-bound drugs (e.g., salicylates, sulfonamides, chloramphenicol, and probenecid), resulting in altered effectiveness.

Adverse Events

The most common side effects include somnolence, nausea, fatigue, dizziness, vomiting, and headache. Monitoring blood glucose monitoring should include some premeal and postmeal readings to assess the effectiveness of the medication. Patients should also be assessed for signs and symptoms of orthostatic hypotension.

Interactions

Bromocriptine mesylate is highly bound to serum proteins; therefore, it may increase the unbound fraction of other concomitantly used highly protein-bound therapies (e.g., salicylates, sulfonamides, chloramphenicol, and probenecid), which may alter their effectiveness and risk for side effects.

Amylin Analog

A recombinant form of amylin is pramlintide (Symlin). This is an injectable agent that is a synthetic of the pancreatic neurohormone amylin, which is cosecreted with insulin from beta cells in response to food. Pramlintide has three actions as an amylinomimetic agent. First, it helps to delay gastric emptying into the small intestine, which delays the rise in postprandial glucose release. This effect lasts for approximately 3 hours and does not alter nutrient absorption. Second, pramlintide alters the release of additional inappropriate glucagon by pancreatic alpha cells, which is abnormal in diabetes. Finally, there is an increase in satiety, which decreases the total calorie intake and promotes weight loss. Pramlintide can be used to treat type 1 or type 2 diabetes. It is also approved for use with insulin.

Dosage

The initiation and dosage of pramlintide differs for type 1 and type 2 diabetes; however, the management of changes in dosage, side effects, and monitoring blood sugar levels is the same for both. The starting dose for those with type 1 diabetes is 15 mcg just prior to any major meal. If tolerated, pramlintide is titrated by 15 mcg increments to a total dose of 30 to 60 mcg. Patients with type 2 diabetes also administer pramlintide just prior to any major meal at 60 mcg per injection. The dose is increased to 120 mcg in 3 to 7 days if there is no nausea. Both patients with type 1 and type 2 diabetes must reduce their current insulin regimen by 50%. The titration of pramlintide is based on blood glucose levels and the presence or absence of nausea. Close monitoring of blood glucose levels is very important to detect hypoglycemia. If significant nausea occurs, the dosage should be decreased until the drug is tolerated. If nausea persists even at the lowest dose, pramlintide should be discontinued.

Contraindications

Few physiologic contraindications exist for those whom pramlintide is appropriate; however, it is critical to select appropriate patients. Those with poor adherence to diabetic care regimens, those with HbA_{1C} greater than 9%, those taking drugs that increase gastric motility gastroparesis, and pediatric patients should not take pramlintide. Additional precaution exists for anyone with known hypersensitivity to the product. Studies have shown no effects on the drug in those with renal or liver disease and are approved as safe. Pramlintide is categorized in pregnancy category C. The major concern is the risk of hypoglycemia. This effect is not actually due to the pramlintide, but rather secondary to making the insulin more effective.

Adverse Events

Nausea is the most common side effect. Gradual titration to the recommended dose reduces this reaction. Other side effects include nausea, vomiting, headache, and anorexia.

Interactions

Pramlintide must not be mixed together with regular, NPH, or 70/30 insulin in the same syringe and must be administered as separate injections. It also has the potential to delay the absorption of concomitantly administered oral medications such as analgesics, antibiotics, and oral contraceptives. Patients who are taking drugs that alter gastric motility such as anticholinergics should not take pramlintide or alpha-glucosidase inhibitors. Interaction can also occur with oral antidiabetic products, ACE inhibitors, and fibrates, fluoxetine, and sulfonamide antibiotics.

Sodium-Glucose Co-transporter 2 (SGLT2) Inhibitors

This category of medication functions to induce glycosuria through the kidneys independent of insulin secretion by inhibiting the SGLT-2 system. Normally, 90% of filtered glucose is reabsorbed through SGLT-2 transport system in the proximal tubule of the kidney. A normal glucose load in the tubules is approximately 120 mg/min, and due to reabsorption there is almost no glucose excretion in the urine. To promote blood sugar control, SGLT-2 inhibitors will cause an approximately 60% excretion of glucose in the urine. The SGLT-2 inhibitors include empagliflozin (Jardiance), canagliflozin (Invokana), and dapagliflozin (Farxiga).

Mechanism of Action

All drugs in this class block the action of SGLT—resulting in increased excretion of glucose in the urine. The reduced ability to reabsorb tubular glucose results in lower plasma glucose and potentially excess calorie in fat accumulation. Using canagliflozin (Invokana), one study showed a weight loss of ≥5% from baseline occurred for the 100-mg dose and the 300-mg dose (Cefalu et al., 2015). Glucose control is enhanced by allowing increased insulin sensitivity and uptake of glucose in the muscle cells, decreased gluconeogenesis, and improved first-phase insulin release from the beta cells.

Dosage

Empagliflozin is started at 10 mg po in the morning and can be titrated up to 25 mg. The medication should be discontinued for persistent estimated glomerular filtration rate (eGFR) less than 45. The initial dose of canagliflozin is 100 mg before the first meal for the day. The dose can be increased to 300 mg daily in patients with normal kidney function, defined as eGFR greater than 60 mL/min/1.73 m. The dose should remain at 100 mg daily for patients with impaired kidney function (eGFR between 45 mL/min/1.73 m and 60 mL/min/1.73 m). The initial dose for dapagliflozin is 5 mg with or without food. The dose can be increased to 10 mg. Do not initiate or discontinue dapagliflozin if eGFR less than 60 mL/min/1.73 m.

Contraindications

SGLT-2 inhibitors should not be used to treat type 1 diabetes or diabetes ketoacidosis (DKA). Patients with severe kidney disease (eGFR, 30 mL/min/1.73) or on hemodialysis should not use SGLT-2 inhibitors.

Adverse Events

This class of drug can cause hyperkalemia, mycotic infections, urinary tract infections, and renal insufficiency. SGLT-2 inhibitors are classified in pregnancy category C and should not be administered to nursing women or children. Risk of hypotension may be increased in patients with low volume status, which can be found in patients taking diuretics, angiotensin-converting enzyme inhibitors, or angiotensin receptor blockers. These patients should be carefully monitored and have fluid status corrected before starting an SGLT-2. The increased glucose excretion is associated with increased urinary frequency. The high urinary glucose concentration also predisposes patients to genital mycotic infections and urinary tract infections. SGLT-2 inhibitors may cause hyperkalemia, especially in patients with decreased kidney function; therefore, careful monitoring of potassium is indicated. Increases in LDL cholesterol have also been observed. Routine HBA_{1C} monitoring should be accompanied by potassium and LDL cholesterol monitoring. Check blood pressure and symptoms of mycotic infections.

Interactions

Some of the commonly prescribed drugs that need to be monitored with this class include sulfonylureas, amlodipine, carvedilol, and cortisone. See **Table 46.2** for further information.

Combination Oral Medication for Type 2 Diabetes

There are many fixed-dose combination products of two or three different drug classes available to treat type 2 diabetes. Many patients find it easier to take a single medication as opposed to two separate medications, therefore improving overall drug adherence. Fixed-dose combinations are generally tried after a patient has failed to reach reduction of their hyperglycemic goals based on one drug alone. The drawback of using these combination medications is the cost. In some cases, the combinations cost more than each drug separately. In addition, starting combination therapy in drug-naive patients can create problems determining the specific cause of drug-induced side effects or allergic reactions.

Insulin

Insulin is the only drug therapy of choice for all patients with type 1 diabetes and for those patients with type 2 diabetes who cannot control their condition with diet and exercise alone or in whom oral therapy fails. Other clinical situations in which insulin therapy is appropriate include newly diagnosed cases of type 2 diabetes presenting with severe, symptomatic hyperglycemia, pregnancy, and surgery.

Just like the insulin normally produced by the pancreas, insulin as drug therapy regulates glucose metabolism in the muscle and other tissues (except the brain). It causes the rapid transport of glucose and amino acids intracellularly, promotes anabolism, and inhibits protein catabolism. In the liver, it promotes the uptake and storage of glucose in the form of glycogen, inhibits gluconeogenesis, and promotes the conversion of excess glucose into fat.

The major characteristics of insulin preparations are onset of action and duration of action (**Table 46.4**). Semisynthetic insulin, which is produced by recombinant deoxyribonucleic acid technology, has the identical amino acid composition as human

TABLE 46.4

Insulins

Preparation	Brand	Onset (h)	Peak (h)	Duration (h)
Very Rapid Acting				
Insulin analog	Humalog	<0.5	0.5–3	3–5
	NovoLog	<0.5	1–3	3–5
	Glulisine	<0.5	1	2–4
Short Acting				
Insulin injection				
	Humulin R	0.5	2–4	6–8
Regular (R)	Novolin R	Same	Same	Same
Intermediate Acting				
NPH	Humulin N	1–4	4–12	14–26
	Novolin N			
Long Acting				
Insulin extended zinc suspension (U)	Humulin U	4–6	8–20	24–36
Insulin glargine	Lantus	1–2	None	24
	Toujeo	3–4	None	>24
Insulin detemir	Levemir	1	None	24
Combination				
Fixed combination	70/30 (NPH/regular ratio)	30–60 min	Dual	10–16 h
	50/50 (NPH/regular ratio)	5–15 min	Dual	10–16 h
	75/25 (NPL/lispro ratio)	5–15 min	Dual	10–16 h
	70/30 (NPA/aspart ratio)	5–15 min	Dual	10–16 h

endogenous insulin and is therefore referred to as *human insulin*. Human insulin preparations lower the risk of local reactions. An insulin analog, lispro insulin, is a two amino acid modification of regular human insulin. Aggregates do not form when lispro insulin is injected subcutaneously, allowing for a more rapid onset and shorter duration than regular insulin and minimizing the postprandial rise in blood sugar and the risk of late hypoglycemia. Another human insulin analog is insulin glargine.

Insulins are categorized as basal (NPH, glargine, and detemir) or bolus (regular, lispro, and aspart). Initial insulin doses should be individualized in patients previously untreated with insulin. The preferred method of insulin therapy administration is through a basal insulin plus a bolus insulin 15 minutes before the start of each meal.

Insulin harvested from animal sources is no longer manufactured. Human insulin is less antigenic than beef insulin and slightly less antigenic than pork insulin. Insulin analogs and U-500 insulin all require a prescription.

The concentrations of insulin currently available in the United States are U-100 and U-500, indicating 100 units/mL and 500 units/mL. U-500 insulin is available for patients with extreme insulin resistance. A goal of insulin therapy is to mimic, as nearly as possible, the physiologic profile of insulin secretion (basal/bolus). The evolution of insulin management has moved from a single daily injection therapy to multiple injections with multiple insulin products. This pattern allows the opportunity to adjust the prandial insulin (rapid-acting or

regular) doses based on the results of the blood glucose checks and food quantity consumed while targeting specific glucose levels. Most programs are very similar in terms of the prandial insulin (see **Figure 46.1**).

There are various ways to providing the basal insulin. One common regimen for programs using insulin injections is providing a basal insulin that is long acting and peakless such as glargine or detemir, then adding short-acting insulin for meals. Another method of administration is to utilize an insulin pump with only short-acting insulin. The pump provides continuous insulin subcutaneously as an infusion in very small doses. Basal insulin and boluses are administered through the pump to cover for ingestion of carbohydrates and blood sugars out of range from normal. The goal is to normalize the blood sugars with insulin administration as much as possible

In the past, multiple doses of an intermediate insulin, neutral protamine hagedorn (NPH), have provided basal insulin before the availability of peakless basal insulins. While NPH can still work well as a basal insulin for some people, the ease of the new peak less basal insulins has led to best practice and predominance of usage.

Premixed insulins that contain both basal and prandial (biphasic) insulins are commercially available as 70/30, 50/50, or 75/25. This insulin regimen may be appropriate for patients who have difficulty mixing their own insulins or for those in whom these ratios are effective. However, for intensive insulin regimens, these insulins are usually not recommended.

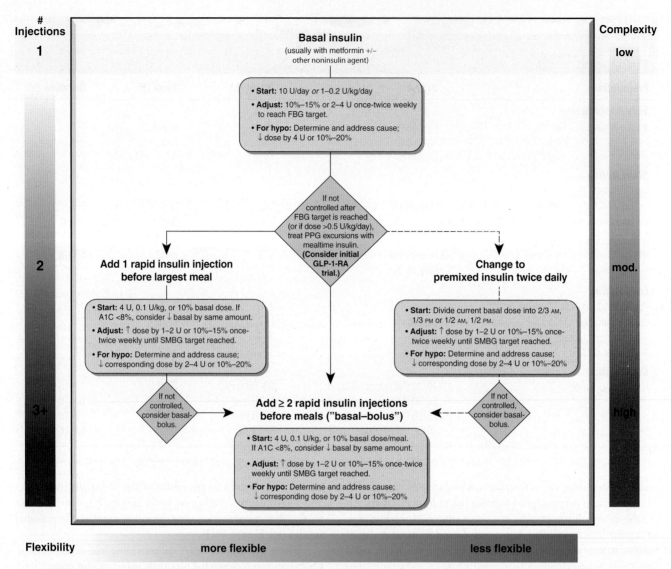

FIGURE 46.1 Algorithm for pharmacotherapy for insulin management. (Reprinted with permission from American Diabetes Association. (2015). Approaches to glycemic treatment. Diabetes care. *Diabetes Care, 38*(Suppl. 1), S41–S48. doi: 10.2337/dc15-S010. Copyright © 2015, American Diabetes Association.)

Dosage

When staring insulin therapy, take the total daily amount of insulin that can be determined based on this general calculation: 0.55 × Total Weight in Kilograms. For example, total daily insulin dose = 0.55 × 70 kg = 38.5 units of insulin/day. For type 2 diabetes, there are two ways to start insulin. First, insulin may be supplemental or as an additional agent added to one or more oral agents. Typically, single daily injections are used, commonly starting between 10 and 20 units depending on the size of the person and the degree of hyperglycemia.

Secondly, type 2 diabetes can also be treated with insulin as the sole pharmacologic agent requiring at least two or more injections per day. In two injection regimens, insulin is administered in the morning before breakfast and before the evening meal or at bedtime. This regimen may include only intermediate-acting insulin; doses of regular or rapid acting

can be added. Insulins mixed with long-acting or intermediate-acting insulin, or premixed formulations (i.e., mixtures such as Humalog Mix 75/25 or NovoLog Mix 70/30), are dosed twice a day. One injection before breakfast and one injection before dinner. Rapid-acting or regular insulin doses are adjusted based on glucose levels in the targeted range of about 100 to 150 mg/dL. Algorithmic adjustments can be up or down by amount such as 1 or more units for every 50 to 100 mg/dL glucose increment:

- 2 units if FBG greater than 120 mg/dL
- 4 units if FBG greater than 140 mg/dL
- 6 units if FBG greater than 180 mg/dL

Insulin doses should be individualized and closely monitored. In lieu of empiric estimations, however, the following guidelines can be used for total daily dosage:

- Children and adults: 0.5 to 0.6 units/kg/d
- Adults during illness or adolescents: 0.5 to 0.75 units/kg/d
- Adolescents during a growth spurt: 1.25 to 1.5 units/kg/d
- Pregnancy: 0.7 units/kg/d

If two doses are given a day, it is recommended that two thirds of the total daily dose be given in the morning with a 2:1 ratio of intermediate- to short-acting insulin and one third of the total daily dose be given before dinner with a 1:1 ratio of short-acting insulin and intermediate-acting insulin.

Doses should be adjusted based on the patient's clinical response, as evidenced by blood glucose levels. Adjustments are made in 1 to 2 unit increments. Insulin must be decreased with hypoglycemia and increased with hyperglycemia. **Table 46.5** provides some suggestions on when dosages need adjusting. For information on time frame for response, see **Table 46.4**. Insulin glargine and detemir is given at bedtime and cannot be mixed with other insulins. The advantage of using the basal insulins includes:

- Provides a smooth basal effect than patterns using multiple injections for intermediate insulin
- Provides moderate flexibility in timing of meals
- Very effective in mimicking normal physiologic acting patterns
- Very effective in controlling the fasting glucose without increasing nocturnal hypoglycemia
- Less weight gain than NPH-based regimens

The 1,500 rule can be used to determine the change needed in the insulin dose. The insulin sensitivity factor (ISF) is determined by dividing a constant (1,500) by the total daily dose (TDD) of insulin. This determines the change in blood glucose from 1 unit of insulin. The formula is as follows:

ISF = 1,500/TDD. For example, if the patient takes 50 units of insulin in 24 hours, the ISF is 1,500/50 = 30.

Therefore, each unit of insulin lowers the blood glucose level of 30 mg/dL. If the SMBG at noon is 170, an addition of 2 units in the morning should lower the blood glucose level to 110 mg/dL.

Adverse Events

Hypoglycemia, hypokalemia, lipodystrophy, and local or systemic allergic reaction can occur with insulin. The dawn phenomenon, so-called for worsening hyperglycemia that occurs in the early morning hours, is caused by growth hormone surges that occur during sleep. The Somogyi effect, which also may be mistaken for inadequate control, is a rebound of hyperglycemia that occurs after an early morning episode of insulin-induced hypoglycemia. The hypoglycemia goes unnoticed because it happens while the patient is sleeping, at approximately 3:00 AM. Signs and symptoms include night sweats, nightmares, sleep disturbances, and early morning headaches. Monitoring of blood glucose when hypoglycemia is thought to be occurring helps make the diagnosis.

Interactions

There are many drugs that can interact with insulin either causing hypoglycemia or hyperglycemia. The following are the most common drug interactions associated with the use of insulin:

Salicylates, beta-blockers, monoamine oxidase inhibitors, alcohol, and sulfa drugs potentiate insulin. Corticosteroids, isoniazid, niacin, estrogens, thyroid hormones, thiazides, phenothiazines, and sympathomimetics antagonize it.

TABLE 46.5

Adjusting Insulin Dosages Based on Clinical Response

Problem	Time Experienced	Possible Solutions
Hyperglycemia	Fasting	If the patient is receiving a single dose of an intermediate-acting insulin, split into two doses: ⅔ of total dose before breakfast, ⅓ of total dose before supper.
		If the patient is receiving split-dose insulin, increase presupper dose or move to later in the evening.
	Midmorning	Add Regular to morning dose to achieve a ratio of 2:1 (intermediate to Regular).
	Midafternoon	Increase morning NPH or Lente dose.
		Add Regular at lunch.
	Bedtime	Add or increase Regular with presupper dose.
	Early morning (2:00–3:00 AM)	Give the presupper dose later in the evening.
		Give Regular at bedtime.
Hypoglycemia	Fasting	Decrease evening insulin dose.
	Midmorning	Decrease or omit prebreakfast dose of Regular.
	Midafternoon	Decrease morning NPH or Lente.
	Bedtime	Add a bedtime snack.
		Decrease presupper dose of Regular.
	Early morning (2:00–3:00 AM)	Consider Somogyi effect—decrease evening NPH.

Continuous Glucose Monitoring

Glucose monitoring has come a long way from dipstick measurements of urine glucose, to glucose meters and strips, to the present era in continuous glucose monitoring or "CGM." CGM uses a disposable sensor that measures interstitial glucose every few minutes, 24 hours a day. The patient inserts the sensor subcutaneously just underneath the skin, replacing it every 3 to 7 days. The sensor transmits glucose readings to a separate receiver or insulin pump. These glucose readings can provide both the patient and clinician a "video" perspective on the overall glucose patterns throughout the day and night. The blood sugars can then be correlated with factors such as food intake or activity and can assist with achieving glycemic control. Indications for CGM include frequent hypoglycemia, hypoglycemia unawareness, and elevated HBA_{1C} despite multiple adjustments in treat plan.

Special Considerations

Pediatric/Adolescent

Until the mid-1990s, type 1 diabetes was the prevalent type of diabetes in children and adolescents. Type 2 diabetes for children is on the rise worldwide, and the mean age is approximately 13.5 years (Rosenbloom et al., 2009). The greatest risk factors are childhood obesity and inactivity. Diabetes is often discovered with glycosuria on a random urinalysis. A red flag for type 2 diabetes in adolescents is acanthosis nigricans, dark pigmentation in skin creases and flexural area. This is a sign of insulin resistance and is present in 60% to 90% of adolescents with type 2 diabetes. It is often easier to see on a physical exam of non-Caucasians, due to having more skin pigmentation. Hypertension is present in 20% to 30% of adolescents with type 2 diabetes. In type 1 diabetes, children present with inappropriate polyuria, dehydration, poor weight gain, and ketonuria.

Treatment for type 1 diabetes in children is insulin therapy. Doses are:

- 0.7 mg/kg before puberty
- 1.0 mg/kg midpuberty
- 1.2 mg/kg after puberty

These children should be treated by a specialist.

Treatment for type 2 diabetes is weight loss, medical nutritional therapy, exercise, and, in many cases, medication. The only drugs approved for adolescents are insulin and metformin.

Geriatric

Diabetes in the elderly is often complicated by coexisting conditions. Complications develop at an accelerated rate probably because poor glycemic control has been long standing. Also, the elderly usually have a decrease in renal function. Exercise programs for the elderly have to be started carefully with comorbid conditions in mind.

Pregnancy

There are two types of diabetes during pregnancy. One is pregestational diabetes, present before the pregnancy. This is treated by a specialist during pregnancy and is considered very high risk. The most common is gestational diabetes, which is glucose intolerance detected during pregnancy and associated with probable resolution after pregnancy. Experts now believe that high-risk women found to have diabetes at pregnancy should be diagnosed with overt diabetes, not just gestational diabetes.

During pregnancy, human placental lactogen plays a pivotal role in triggering glucose intolerance. It has an anti-insulin and lipolytic effect. Peripheral insulin sensitivity decreases to 50% of the first trimester while during the third trimester, while basal hepatic glucose output increases by 30%.

Screening is recommended between weeks 24 and 48. There are two choices for screening. Women can have a two-step test, with a 50-g one-hour glucose load, followed by a 3-hour glucose tolerance test if necessary. A second alternative is a one-step test, with a 75-g two-hour test.

In the gestational diabetic, multiple daily SMBG is required, and it can often be controlled by diet and medical nutritional therapy. If this does not control glucose levels, insulin is required.

Potential neonatal complications include shoulder dystocia, hypoglycemia, polycythemia, and respiratory distress.

Selecting the Most Appropriate Agent

Insulin is necessary in all cases of type 1 diabetes. In patients with type 2 diabetes, various oral agents as monotherapy or in combination therapy can be prescribed, because the oral agents act in different ways. **Table 46.6** lists the potential decrease in HbA_{1C} with each agent. **Table 46.7** shows first- and second-line agents for patients with type 1 diabetes. **Table 46.8** shows first-, second-, and third-line therapy for patients with type 2 diabetes (**Figure 46.2**). The ultimate goal of controlling glycemia is to avoid hyperosmotic symptoms of hyperglycemia, instability of blood sugar over time, and prevent or delay complications from diabetes.

TABLE 46.6

Capacity to Decrease HbA_{1C} by Agent/Class of Drugs

Agent	Decrease in HbA_{1C}
insulin	>2%
sulfonylurea	1%–2%
biguanide	1.5%–2%
TZD	0.5%–1.8%
α-glucosidase inhibitor	0.5%–1%
meglitinide	0.6%–1.8%
sitagliptin	1%
sitagliptin with biguanide	1.8%
saxagliptin	0.1%–0.3%
GLP-1 agonists	0.4%–0.9%
SGLT-2 inhibitors	0.5%–0.9%

TABLE 46.7

Recommended Order of Treatment for Type 1 Diabetes Mellitus

Order	Agents	Comments
First line	Four-injection regimen, a long-acting insulin such as insulin glargine once a day and a rapid-acting or short-acting insulin administered at mealtimes or a combination of intermediate and short acting; dose is 0.5–0.6 units/kg/d	Several schedules are used to administer insulin (see **Table 46.5**). The most commonly used regimen is four injections a day. This regimen best duplicates normal physiologic insulin. The second regimen would be two injections a day, one in the morning and one in the evening. This promotes glycemic control both during the day and while sleeping. The insulin dose required is divided into ⅔ of the dose in the morning and ⅓ of the dose in the evening. The morning dose is divided into ⅔ intermediate insulin and ⅓ short- or rapid-acting insulin. The evening dose is ½ intermediate insulin and ½ short- or rapid-acting insulin.
Second line	Insulin dose is gradually increased	Adjustments are made at 1 to 2 units at a time over 3 d. Adjustments are based on SMBG records.

TABLE 46.8

Recommended Order of Treatment for Type 2 Diabetes Mellitus

Order	Agents	Comments
Entry HBA₁c <7.5		
First line	Monotherapy with an oral agent: biguanides, GLP-1, DPP4-i, and AG-i	The rule for initiating therapy with any of these agents is to start slowly and increase the dose every 1–2 wk as needed. The patient can be switched to another drug or class after 1 mo if the therapy is not effective in achieving glycemic control. Biguanides are the drugs of choice in the patient with metabolic syndrome X and when the blood glucose levels are <250 mg/dL. The α-glucosidase inhibitors are most effective in patients with postprandial hyperglycemia but only mild fasting glucose elevations.
Second line	SGLT-2, TZD, and SU/GLN	Sulfonylureas are the best choice if the patient is thin, older than age 40, has had diabetes for <5 y, and has a blood glucose >250 mg/dL. Glyburide is most effective in patients with fasting hypoglycemia, and glipizide is most effective in patients with postprandial hyperglycemia. Start with a single timed dose of 10 units of insulin with dose adjusted weekly (2 units if FPG >120 mg/dL; 4 units if FPG >140 mg/dL; 6 units if FPG >180 mg/dL).
Entry HBA₁c >7.5		
First line Second line	Metformin or another first-line agent, combinations of sulfonylureas and biguanides, TZDs, or α-glucosidase inhibitors are effective. Also, metformin can be combined with a meglitinide or TZD for effective control	Again, the dose is started at the lowest level and increased every 1–2 wk as needed.
Entry HBA₁c >9.0%		
First line	Consider starting insulin therapy and slowing wean back Triple oral therapy and consider additional basal insulin and short-acting boluses	Oral medications at the same dose.

FIGURE 46.2 Algorithm for type 2 oral therapy management.

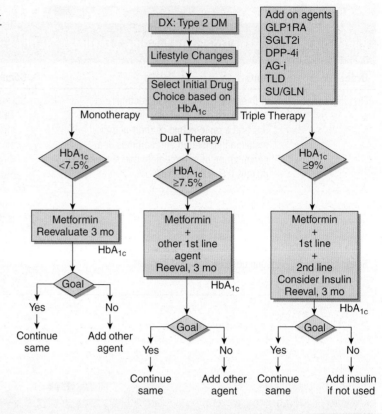

First-Line Therapy

In type 1 diabetes, insulin is the only first-line therapy due to absolute insulin deficiency. There are several schedules that can be used for administering acting insulin (see **Table 46.9**). The most common regimen is a program that provides basal insulin coverage, using a peakless basal insulin and a rapid-acting insulin before breakfast, lunch, and dinner (see **Figure 46.1**). The dosage is 0.5 to 0.6 units/kg/d. This promotes glycemic control during the day and while the patient sleeps. Approximately 25% to 50% of daily

total as basal insulin is given once a day. Premeal (prandial) insulin (rapid acting or regular insulin) is distributed as 40% before breakfast, 30% before lunch, and 30% before dinner. A second regime is a combination of intermediate- and short-acting insulin. This consist of two injections a day, one in the morning and one in the evening (see **Table 46.9**). The morning dose is divided into two-thirds intermediate-acting insulin and one-third short- or rapid-acting insulin. The evening dose is one-half intermediate-acting insulin and one-half short- or rapid-acting insulin.

TABLE 46.9		
Various Insulin Regimens		
No. of Daily Injections	**How Administered**	**Comments**
2	Two thirds of insulin 15–30 min before breakfast and ⅓ 15–30 min before the evening meal In AM, ⅔ intermediate, ⅓ short or rapid acting In PM, ½ intermediate, ½ rapid or short acting	This regimen is the most commonly prescribed. It is the most desirable to patients. There may be too little coverage at noon and too much insulin during the night. There is less dawn phenomenon and Somogyi effect.
3	40% intermediate and 15% short or rapid acting 15–30 min before breakfast 15% short or rapid acting before dinner 30% intermediate acting at bedtime	There is too little coverage at noon.
4	20%–25% of daily dose with rapid or short acting before each meal 25%–40% intermediate or long acting at bedtime	Use of insulin glargine or detemir provides most predictable basal control.

First-line therapy for type 2 diabetes with HBA$_{1C}$ ≥6.5% is monotherapy with metformin if not contraindicated and tolerated. The goal is to achieve or maintain a targeted HBA$_{1C}$ of less than 7.0%. If the HBA$_{1C}$ in patients with markedly elevated blood sugars consider starting insulin therapy. Other agents used for first-line therapy and have few adverse events include GLP-1RA, DPP4-i, and α-glucosidase inhibitors. Meglitinides, SGLT-2i inhibitors, sulfonylureas, and TZDs are used with caution. The rule for initiating therapy with any of these agents is to start slowly and increase the dose every 1 to 2 weeks as needed. If intensification of treatment is required to meet goals (i.e., HbA$_{1C}$ <7.0%), the addition of another drug from a different class is recommended.

Biguanides and TZDs are the drugs of choice in patients with metabolic syndrome. The α-glucosidase inhibitors are most effective in patients with postprandial hyperglycemia but only mild fasting glucose elevations.

Second-Line Therapy

With failure to achieve optimal blood glucose levels in type 1 diabetes, practitioners must gradually increase the insulin dose, making adjustments 1 to 2 units at a time over 3 days. They must base their adjustments on SMBG records. **Figure 46.1** and **Table 46.9** list how to determine adjustments.

Failure to achieve optimal blood glucose levels in type 2 diabetes with an HBA$_{1C}$ greater than 7.5 necessitates the addition of another oral agent. Combinations of sulfonylureas and biguanides, TZDs, or α-glucosidase inhibitors may be added. SGLT-2 inhibitors, DPP-4 inhibitors, and GLP1 agonist may also be considered as therapy.

Third-Line Therapy

In patients with type 2 diabetes, and an HBA$_{1C}$ greater than 9.0 with no symptoms, a third agent can be added. If the goal of decreasing the HBA1C is not achieved in 3 months, proceed to insulin therapy. An intermediate or basal insulin at bedtime added to the daytime oral regimen can be very effective in treating those with type 2 diabetes. Patients with type 1 diabetes may be appropriate candidates for an insulin pump.

Combination Therapy

Many combination products of two different drug classes are available to treat type 2 diabetes. The following are some of the most common combinations:

- **A sulfonylurea and a biguanide** combination produces mealtime stimulation of endogenous insulin with the sulfonylurea and gluconeogenesis with the biguanide. This is recommended for an HbA$_{1C}$ level above 8%.
- **A sulfonylurea and a TZD** combination improves insulin resistance and may enable a decrease in the sulfonylurea dose.
- **A biguanide and a TZD** combination provides a synergistic effect on glycemic reduction. Liver and renal function must be monitored with this regimen.

- **A DPP-4i and a biguanide** combination improves insulin resistance and helps to lower postprandial blood sugars, which are best used with an elevated postprandial blood glucose level.
- **Meglitinide and a TZD or biguanide** combination promotes a stimulation of insulin release and a decrease in peripheral insulin resistance and fasting hyperglycemia.

The provider must weigh the risks and benefits of using combinations medications. In some cases, the combination products cost more.

MONITORING PATIENT RESPONSE

Prolonged hyperglycemia of diabetes gives rise to long-term complications that involve lesions of the small (microvascular) and large (macrovascular) blood vessels. Microvascular complications include retinopathy, nephropathy, and neuropathy.

Control is measured using the patient's levels of blood glucose and HbA$_{1C}$. Patients use SMBG to keep a daily record of blood glucose. HbA$_{1C}$ measures blood glucose over 3 months. **Table 46.10** lists the desired levels and levels that require changes in drug regimen.

PATIENT EDUCATION

Drug Information

Education is a hallmark of diabetes therapy. SMBG is essential for monitoring therapeutic response. Practitioners must educate patients about the signs and symptoms of hypoglycemia and instruct them to carry a source of glucose with them at all times. Possible sources are hard candy (not sugarless) or 4 oz. of orange juice. All patients with diabetes should have medical identification in the form of a Medic Alert bracelet or necklace.

In patients taking insulin, meals are to be eaten on a regular basis. If a rapid-acting insulin is used, it is taken immediately before eating. The α-glucosidase inhibitors are only taken if a meal is eaten.

Here are some patient-oriented sources for information and Apps that can be downloaded to a smartphone:

- www.diabetes.org is the site from the ADA with information for managing the diabetic's life.

TABLE 46.10		
Measures of Control of Fasting Blood Glucose		
Measure of Glucose	**Goal**	**Levels When Adjustment to Regimen Is Indicated**
Fasting glucose	80–130 mg/dL	<80 or >140 mg/dL
Bedtime glucose	110–150 mg/dL	<110 or >160 mg/dL
HbA$_{1C}$	<7	≥7

- www.niddk.nih.gov/health/diabetes.htm is a site from National Institutes of Health that serves as an information clearinghouse.
- www.diabetes.com provides information for the diabetic individual.

1. CDC national Web site for diabetes

Diabetes Apps

- Glucose Buddy
- Diabetes In Check
- Calorie King Food Search
- My Fitness Pal

Nutritional and Lifestyle Changes

Diabetes management includes medical nutrition therapy, exercise, and, in most cases, drug therapy. Foods high in processed sugar and fat are to be avoided, as is alcohol. Regular daily exercise helps to control blood sugar levels.

Patients with diabetes must follow "sick day guidelines" for the treatment of their condition when dealing with other illnesses. In general, practitioners should instruct people with diabetes not to stop their medication when they are ill. Infection, stress, and other variables increase plasma glucose levels, even though oral intake may be reduced. Practitioners should instruct patients to increase their fluid intake to approximately 8 oz of water or sugar-free beverage every hour,

especially if they have a fever. Patients should monitor blood glucose levels at home more frequently, as often as every 4 hours. Urine also requires testing for ketones. If the blood glucose concentration is greater than 300 mg/dL on two consecutive readings, fever is persistently high, and symptoms of severe dehydration and ketonuria develop, the patient requires formal evaluation. Sick day plans should be developed with patients before illness occurs.

Complementary and Alternative Medicine

Many people with diabetes combine alternative and traditional medicine. Some of the most common forms of alternative dietary supplements is cinnamon. The use of cinnamon is a popular dietary supplement by many people with diabetes to help lower blood glucose levels. Cinnamon is thought to enhance insulin sensitivity and reduce postprandial glucose levels. In a recent study conducted at the U.S. Department of Agriculture, cinnamon reduced serum glucose levels and improved lipid profiles in patients with type 2 diabetes. Patients were randomized into six groups that received 1, 2, or 3 g of cinnamon or a placebo. All groups receiving cinnamon had a decrease of 18% to 30% in fasting serum glucose values and a reduction of 23% to 30% in triglycerides and 7% to 27% reduction in LDL levels. Total cholesterol level declined from 12% to 26%. Doses used have ranged from 1 to 6 g. Overall cinnamon used as a food is safe.

CASE STUDY*

R.S. is a 55-year-old moderately obese Hispanic woman (body mass index is 29). She was referred to you when her gynecologist noted glucose on a routine urinalysis. She subsequently has an FPG of 190 and 200 mg/dL on two separate occasions. She is thirstier than usual and has more frequent urination. She also complains of decreased energy over the last several months and numbness and tingling in her left lower extremity.

- Family history: sister, mother, and maternal grandmother have diabetes
- Social history: nonsmoker, drinks alcohol socially (1 drink about three times a month), and does not exercise
- **Review of systems**: 20 lb weight gain over the past 2 years, has some blurred vision, has had two urinary tract infections in the past year, and has frequent vaginal yeast infections
  - Gestational diabetes in last two pregnancies
- **Physical exam**: unremarkable except blood pressure of 150/90
  - Height: 5.2 inches
  - Weight: 200 lb

- Laboratory results: FPG 200 mg/dL, HbA$_{1C}$ 10%, LDL 160 mg/dL, HDL 35 mg/dL, and triglycerides 266 mg/dL

DIAGNOSIS: TYPE 2 DIABETES MELLITUS

1. List specific goals for the treatment for **R.S.**
2. What dietary and lifestyle changes would you recommend for **R.S.**?
3. What drug therapy would you prescribe? Why?
4. What is the goal for the FPG? Postprandial glucose? HbA$_{1C}$?
5. Discuss specific education for **R.S.** based on the prescribed therapy.
6. List one or two adverse reactions for the therapy selected that would cause you to change the therapy.
7. If the HbA$_{1C}$ after 3 months on the prescribed therapy is 8.8%, what would be the next line of therapy?
8. What over-the-counter or herbal medicines might be appropriate for **R.S.**?
9. Describe one or two drug–drug or drug–food interactions for the selected agent.

* Answers can be found online.

Bibliography

Starred references are cited in the text.

Abdul-Ghani, M., Norton, L., & DeFronzo, R. (2011). Role of sodium-glucose cotransporter 2 (SGLT2) inhibitors in the treatment of type 2 diabetes. *Endocrine Reviews, 32,* 515–531. doi: 10.1210/er.2010-0029.

Adler, A. I., Stratton, I. M., Neil, H. A., et al. (2000). Association of systolic blood pressure with macrovascular and microvascular complications of type 2 diabetes (UKPDS 36): Prospective observational study. *British Medical Journal, 321,* 412–419.

ALLHAT Collaborative Research Group. (2000). Major cardiovascular events in hypertensive patients randomized to doxazosin vs. chlorthalidone: The Antihypertensive and Lipid-Lowering Treatment to Prevent Heart Attack Trial (ALLHAT). *Journal of the American Medical Association, 283,* 1967–1975.

ALLHAT Study Group. (2002). Major outcomes in high-risk hypertensive patients randomized to angiotensin-converting enzyme inhibitor or calcium channel blocker vs. diuretic: The Antihypertensive and Lipid-Lowering Treatment to Prevent Heart Attack Trial (ALLHAT). *Journal of the American Medical Association, 288,* 2981–2997.

American Diabetes Association. (2015a). Standards of medical care in diabetes—2015. *Diabetes Care, 38*(Suppl. 1), S1–S94. doi: 10.2337/dc15-S003.

American Diabetes Association. (2015b). Classification and diagnosis of diabetes mellitus. *Diabetes Care, 38*(Suppl. 1), S8–S16. doi: 10.2337/dc15-S005.

Bacha, F., Lee, S., Gungor, N., et al. (2010). From pre-diabetes to type 2 diabetes in obese youth. *Diabetes Care, 33*(10), 2225–2231. doi: 10.2337/dc10-0004.

Bailey, C., & Kodack, M. (2011). Patient adherence to medication requirements for therapy of type 2 diabetes. *International Journal of Clinical Practice, 65*(3), 314–322. doi: 10.1111/j.1742-1241.2010.02544.x.

Barteis, D. (2004). Adherence to oral therapy for type 2 diabetes: Opportunities for enhancing glycemic control. *Journal of the American Academy of Nurse Practitioners, 16*(1), 8–16.

Beaser, S. R. (2010). *Joslin's diabetes deskbook: A guide for primary care providers.* Boston, MA: Lippincott Williams & Wilkins.

*Cefalu, W., Stenlöf, K., Leiter, L., et al. (2015). Effects of canagliflozin on body weight and relationship to HbA$_{1C}$ and blood pressure changes in patients with type 2 diabetes. *Diabetologia, 58,* 1183–1187. doi: 10.1007/s00125-015-3547-2.

*Centers for Disease Control and Prevention. (2014). *National diabetes statistics report: Estimates of diabetes and its burden in the United States.* Atlanta, GA: U.S. Department of Health and Human Services. Retrieved from http://www.cdc.gov/diabetes/pubs/statsreport14/national-diabetes-report-web.pdf

Chiasson, J. L., Josse, R. G., Gomis, R., et al. (2002). Acarbose for prevention of type 2 diabetes mellitus: The STOP-NIDDM randomized trial. *Lancet, 359,* 2072–2077.

Chyan, Y., & Chuang, L. (2007). Dipeptidyl peptidase IV inhibitors: An evolving treatment for type 2 diabetes mellitus from the incretin concept. *Recent Patents on Endocrine, Metabolic & Immune Drug Discovery, 1*(1), 15–24.

Copeland, K., Silverstein, J., Moore, K., et al. (2013). Management of newly diagnosed type 2 diabetes mellitus (T2DM) in children and adolescents. *Pediatrics, 131,* 364–382. doi: 10.1542/peds.2012-3494.

DCCT Research Group. (1995). Effect of intensive therapy on the development and progression of diabetic nephropathy in the Diabetes Control and Complications Trial (DCCT). *Kidney International, 47,* 1703–1720.

DCCT/EDIC Research Group. (2000). Retinopathy and nephropathy in patients with type 1 diabetes four years after a trial of intensive therapy. *New England Journal of Medicine, 342,* 381–389.

Diabetes Control and Complications Trial Research Group. (1993). The effect of intensive treatment of diabetes on the development and progression of long-term complications in insulin-dependent diabetes mellitus. *New England Journal of Medicine, 329,* 977–986.

Diabetes Prevention Program Research Group. (2002). Reduction in the incidence of type 2 diabetes with lifestyle intervention or metformin. *New England Journal of Medicine, 346,* 393–403.

Eknoyan, G., Hostetter, T., Bakris, G. L., et al. (2003). Proteinuria and other markers of chronic kidney disease: A position statement of the National Kidney Foundation (NKF) and the National Institute of Diabetes and Digestive and Kidney Diseases (NIDDK). *American Journal of Kidney Disease, 42,* 617–622.

FDA. (2011). *FDA drug safety communication: Avandia (rosiglitazone) labels now contain updated information about cardiovascular risks and use in certain patients.* Retrieved from http://www.fda.gov/Drugs/DrugSafety/ucm241411.htm

FDA. (2013). *FDA drug safety communication: FDA requires removal of some prescribing and dispensing restrictions for rosiglitazone-containing diabetes medicines.* http://www.fda.gov/Drugs/DrugSafety/ucm376389.htm

Flint, A., & Arslanian, S. (2011). Treatment of type 2 diabetes in youth. *Diabetes Care, 34*(Suppl. 2), S177–S183. doi: 10.2337/dc11-s125.

Garber, J. A., Abrahamson, M., Barzilay, J., et al. (2015). AACE/ACE Comprehensive diabetes management algorithm. *Endocrine Practice, 21*(4), 438–447. doi: 10.4158/EP15693.CS.

García-Pérez, L. -E., Álvarez, M., Dilla, T., et al. (2013). Adherence to therapies in patients with type 2 diabetes. *Diabetes Therapy, 4*(2), 175–194. Retrieved from http://doi.org/10.1007/s13300-013-0034-y

Heart Outcomes Prevention Evaluation (HOPE) Study Investigators. (2000). Effects of ramipril on cardiovascular and microvascular outcomes in people with diabetes mellitus: Results of the HOPE study and MICRO-HOPE study. *Lancet, 355,* 253–259.

Heart Protection Study Collaborative Group. (2003). MRC/BHF Heart Protection Study of cholesterol-lowering with simvastatin in 5963 people with diabetes: A randomized placebo-controlled trial. *Lancet, 361,* 2005–2016.

Homko, C., Zamora, L., Kerper, M., et al. (2012). A single HBA1C ≥ 6.5% accurately identifies type 2 diabetes/impaired glucose tolerance in African Americans. *Journal of Primary Care and Community Health, 3*(4), 235–238. doi: 10.1177/2150131011435526.

James, P., Oparil, S., Carter, B., et al. (2014). 2014 evidence-based guideline for the management of high blood pressure in adults. Report from the panel members appointed to the eighth joint national committee (JNC 8). *Journal of the American Medical Association, 311*(5), 507–520. doi: 10.1001/jama.2013.284427.

Janumet. (2010). *Janumet: Full prescribing information.* Whitehouse Station, NJ: Mercke, Sharp, & Dohme.

Januvia. (2010). *Januvia: Full prescribing information.* Whitehouse Station, NJ: Mercke, Sharpe & Dohme.

Jones, M., & Patel, M. (2006). Insulin detemir: A long acting insulin product. *American Journal of Health-System Pharmacy, 63*(24), 2466–2472.

Mensing, C. (2014). *The art & science of diabetes self-management education desk reference* (3rd ed.). Chicago, IL: American Association of Diabetes Educators.

Nathan, D., Buse, J., Davidson, M., et al. (2009). Medical management of hyperglycemia in type 2 diabetes mellitus: A consensus algorithm for the initiation and adjustment of therapy. *Diabetes Care, 32,* 193–203.

Ninomiya, T., Perkovic, V., deGalan, B., et al. (2009). Albuminuria and kidney function independently predict cardiovascular and renal outcome sin diabetes. *Journal American Society of Nephrology, 20,* 1813–1821. doi: 10.1681./ASN.2008121270.

Nolan, C., Damm, P., & Prentki, M. (2011). Type 2 diabetes across generations: From pathophysiology to prevention and management. *Lancet, 378,* 169–81. doi: 10.1016/S0140-6736(11)60614-4.

*Rosenbloom, A., Silverstein, J., Amemiya, S., et al. (2009). Type 2 diabetes in the children and adolescents. *Pediatric Diabetes, 10*(Suppl. 12), 17–32.

Schwarts, E., Koska, J., Mullin, M., et al. (2010). Exenatide suppresses postprandial elevations in lipids and lipoproteins in individuals with impaired glucose tolerance and recent onset type 2 diabetes mellitus. *Atherosclerosis, 212*(1), 217–222. doi: 10.1016/j.atherosclerosis.2010.05.028.

Sosenkjo, J., Skyler, J. Herold, K., et al. (2011). The metabolic progression to type 1 diabetes as indicated by serial oral glucose tolerance testing in the diabetes prevention trial—type 1. *Diabetes, 61,* 1331–1337. doi: 10.2337/db11-1660.

Sullivan, M., & Mechcatie, E. (2010). Limits on rosiglitazone may effectively end use. *Clinical Endocrinology News, 5*(10), 1.

Taylor, S., & Harris, K. (2013). The clinical efficacy and safety of sodium glucose cotransporter-2 inhibitors in adults with type 2 diabetes mellitus. *Pharmacotherapy, 33*(9), 1–16. doi: 10.1002/phar.1303.

The Diabetes Prevention Program (DPP) Research Group. (2002). The Diabetes Prevention Program (DPP): Description of lifestyle intervention. *Diabetes Care, 25*(12), 2165–2171.

Tuomilehto, J., Lindstrom, J., Eriksson, J. G., et al. (2001). Prevention of type 2 diabetes mellitus by changes in lifestyle among subjects with impaired glucose tolerance. *New England Journal of Medicine, 344,* 1343–1350.

UK Prospective Diabetes Study Group. (1998a). Effect of intensive blood-glucose control with metformin on complications in overweight patients with type 2 diabetes (UKPDS 34). *Lancet, 352,* 854–865.

UK Prospective Diabetes Study Group. (1998b). Intensive blood-glucose control with sulfonylureas or insulin compared with conventional treatment and risk of complications in patients with type 2 diabetes (UKPDS 33). *Lancet, 352,* 837–853.

Whittemore, R., Melkus, G., Wagner, J., et al (2009). Translating the diabetes prevention program to primary care: A pilot study. *Nursing Research, 58*(1), 2–12. Retrieved from http://doi.org/10.1097/NNR.0b013e31818fcef3

Zopopini, G., Targher, G., Chonchol, M., et al. (2012). Predictors of estimated GFR decline in patient with type 2 diabetes and preserved kidney function. *Clinical Journal of the American Society of Nephrology, 7,* 401–408. doi: 10.2215/CJN.07650711.

47 Thyroid Disorders

Louis R. Petrone

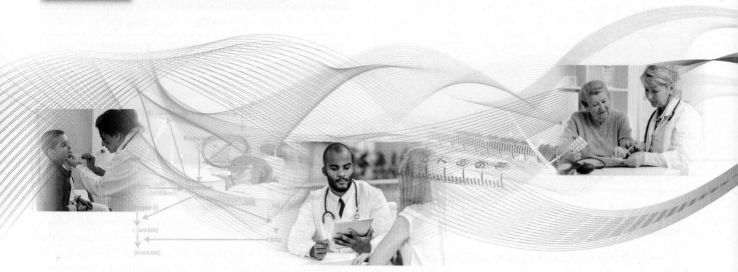

Diseases of the thyroid gland are common clinical conditions, accounting for many office visits each year. Population-based studies have found that hypothyroidism exists to some degree in 4.6% to 9.5% of individuals, with higher rates occurring in the elderly (Canaris et al., 2000; Hollowell et al., 2002; Rodondi et al., 2010); prevalence also varies according to the availability of iodine in individual communities. These studies and others found a 1.2% to 2.2% rate of hyperthyroidism. Both hypothyroidism and hyperthyroidism have been associated with adverse cardiovascular outcomes (Hak et al., 2000; Iervasi et al., 2007; Rodondi et al., 2010). If these conditions are not treated properly, their morbidity can be high. Thyroid nodules are common, occurring clinically in approximately 5% of patients but found using ultrasound studies in 22% of patients and in autopsy studies in 50% of patients. Although most thyroid nodules are nonmalignant and most thyroid cancers are not very aggressive, approximately 298,000 new cases are diagnosed worldwide annually (Ferley et al., 2012), and 1,900 deaths per year are attributed to thyroid malignancy in the United States (American Cancer Society, 2014). Therefore, clinicians should understand the therapeutic options for these conditions.

To diagnose and treat thyroid disease, a basic understanding of thyroid anatomy and physiology is necessary (**Figures 47.1** and **47.2**). The gland is divided into two lobes that are separated by an isthmus. Histologically, the thyroid is composed of follicles that are made of cells that are cuboidal at rest but column shaped when activated by thyroid-stimulating hormone (TSH). These follicular cells encircle a mass of colloid that contains thyroglobulin, a glycoprotein that the follicular cells secrete. Iodine, which is consumed in the diet, is reduced to iodide in the gastrointestinal (GI)

tract and readily absorbed. Iodide is then carried to the thyroid, where it is taken up by the follicular cells. In these cells, iodide is oxidized and incorporated into tyrosine residues of thyroglobulin to form monoiodothyronine (MIT). Two MITs are paired to make diiodothyronine (DIT), and combinations of MIT with DIT produce triiodothyronine (T_3) and thyroxine (T_4).

The pituitary gland secretes TSH, which controls the rate of release of T_3 and T_4. The hypothalamus secretes thyrotropin-releasing hormone (TRH), which modulates the release of TSH. All of these hormones work in a negative feedback system, in which low levels of thyroid hormones in the blood cause increased secretion of TRH, TSH, and, subsequently, T_3 and T_4.

Once T_3 and T_4 are secreted into the bloodstream, proteins known as *thyroid-binding globulins* (TBGs), which are synthesized by the liver, bind most of these hormones. Only a small amount of T_3 and T_4 is in the "free" or unbound state; the hormones in this state are the clinically significant ones. Free T_3 and free T_4 act at the cellular level to regulate metabolism by binding to nuclear receptors and affecting gene expression and protein synthesis. Any condition that can affect TBGs also can affect the level of free T_3 and free T_4. The thyroid produces only approximately 20% of circulating T_3, whereas monodeiodination of T_4 in the periphery produces the remainder.

Clinically, measurement of serum TSH and free T_4 are used most commonly to assess thyroid function. Given the availability of the free T_4 assay, total T_4 is used less frequently because actual thyroid function depends on the level of free T_4 rather than total T_4. **Table 47.1** depicts relative levels of TSH and free T_4 in disorders of thyroid function.

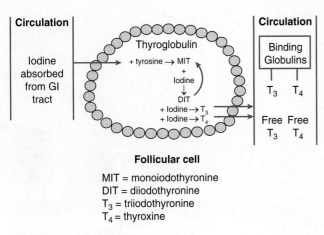

MIT = monoiodothyronine
DIT = diiodothyronine
T₃ = triiodothyronine
T₄ = thyroxine

FIGURE 47.1   Thyroid hormone synthesis.

TABLE 47.1

Thyroid Function Testing in Common Thyroid Disorders

	TSH	Free T$_4$
Primary hypothyroidism	Increased	Decreased
Secondary or tertiary hypothyroidism	Decreased	Decreased
Mild thyroid failure	Increased	Normal
Hyperthyroidism	Decreased	Increased (or normal in T$_3$ thyrotoxicosis)
Subclinical hyperthyroidism	Decreased	Normal

HYPOTHYROIDISM

Hypothyroidism is a relatively common clinical entity, occurring in up to 5.9% of women and 0.2% of men. Patients may complain of symptoms of fatigue, constipation, weight gain, or change in menstrual periods, among others. Physical examination may reveal thyromegaly, bradycardia, or peripheral edema (**Box 47.1**). Total cholesterol and low-density lipoprotein (LDL) levels may be elevated in 90% to 95% of patients.

CAUSES

Hypothyroidism has several causes (**Box 47.2**). In the United States and other developed countries, hypothyroidism nearly always results from a problem with the production or release (or both) of thyroid hormones. Worldwide, iodine deficiency is most commonly the cause. Hashimoto (or autoimmune) thyroiditis is the most common precipitant

of hypothyroidism in the United States. It results from the infiltration of the thyroid gland by lymphocytes, which results in progressive fibrosis and decreased function of the gland. Patients may present with goiter and be euthyroid or hypothyroid initially; antithyroid antibodies are often positive in high titers.

Posttherapeutic (after treatment for hyperthyroidism) hypothyroidism is another common cause, whereas other entities such as subacute thyroiditis or postpartum thyroiditis can produce brief periods of hypothyroidism. Subacute and postpartum thyroiditis are discussed at the end of this chapter.

Many drugs may interfere with thyroid function and induce hypothyroidism (**Box 47.3**). These include amiodarone (Cordarone) and lithium (Eskalith). If patients discontinue these drugs, thyroid function should return to normal; however, many patients taking these drugs have serious coexisting conditions and cannot stop using them. Therefore, clinicians should monitor these patients regularly for hypothyroidism and treat them with thyroid replacement if appropriate.

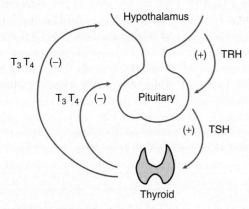

TRH = thyroid-releasing hormone
TSH = thyroid-stimulating hormone
T₃ = triiodothyronine
T₄ = thyroxine
(+) = positive effect
(−) = negative effect

FIGURE 47.2   Hypothalamic–pituitary–thyroid axis.

BOX 47.1   Symptoms and Signs of Hypothyroidism

Fatigue	Bradycardia
Constipation	Delayed deep tendon reflexes
Menorrhagia	Hyperlipidemia
Weight gain	Goiter
Hair loss	Hypothermia
Cold intolerance	Periorbital swelling
Hoarseness	Jaundice
Depression	Ataxia
Dry skin	Edema
Infertility	Myalgias
Difficulty with memory and concentration	

BOX 47.2 Causes of Hypothyroidism

PRIMARY HYPOTHYROIDISM

Thyroid dysgenesis
Destruction of thyroid tissue
Chronic autoimmune thyroiditis—atrophic and goitrous forms
Radiation—[131]I therapy for thyrotoxicosis, Graves disease; external radiotherapy to the head and neck for nonthyroid malignant disease
Subtotal and total thyroidectomy
Infiltrative diseases of the thyroid (amyloidosis, scleroderma)
Defective thyroid hormone biosynthesis
Congenital defects in thyroid hormone biosynthesis
Iodine deficiency

Drugs with antithyroid actions—lithium, iodine, and iodine-containing drugs and radiographic contrast agents

CENTRAL HYPOTHYROIDISM

Pituitary disease
Hypothalamic disease

TRANSIENT HYPOTHYROIDISM

Silent (painless) thyroiditis including postpartum thyroiditis
Subacute thyroiditis
After withdrawal of thyroid hormone therapy in euthyroid patients/inadequate thyroid hormone replacement

Reprinted with permission from Braverman, L. E., & Cooper, D. S. (2013). Introduction to hypothyroidism. *Werner & Ingbar's the thyroid; A fundamental and clinical text* (10th ed.). Philadelphia, PA: Lippincott Williams & Wilkins.

PATHOPHYSIOLOGY

Hypothyroidism results from a relative deficit of thyroid hormones, usually free T_4. The deficit may result from failure of the thyroid gland itself (primary hypothyroidism) or, less commonly, from failure of the pituitary gland or hypothalamus (secondary or tertiary hypothyroidism, respectively). Presenting symptoms of thyroid hormone deficiency are similar in all types of hypothyroidism.

BOX 47.3 Drugs that May Alter the Levothyroxine Dose Required by a Patient by Affecting T_4 Metabolism or Transport

Drugs That Alter T_4 Metabolism	Drugs That Alter T_4 Transport	
	Increased TBG	Decreased TBG
Phenobarbital	Estrogen	Androgens
Phenytoin	Tamoxifen	Anabolic steroids
Carbamazepine	Raloxifene	Glucocorticoids
Rifampin	Clofibrate	
Sertraline	Opioids	
Imatinib	Mitotane	
Amiodarone	Fluorouracil	
	Capecitabine	

Reprinted with permission from: Jonklaas, J. (2013). Treatment of hypothyroidism. *Werner & Ingbar's the thyroid; A fundamental and clinical text* (10th ed.). Philadelphia, PA: Lippincott Williams & Wilkins.

DIAGNOSTIC CRITERIA

Primary hypothyroidism is confirmed, in the appropriate clinical setting, by the finding of an elevated TSH and a low free T_4 level. Secondary hypothyroidism, as a result of pituitary dysfunction, results in low free T_4 and low TSH levels. Tertiary hypothyroidism results from decreased production of TRH by the hypothalamus. Secondary hypothyroidism can be distinguished from tertiary hypothyroidism by imaging of the pituitary and hypothalamus. There is a TRH stimulation test in which exogenous TRH is administered and serum TSH response is measured, but this test is of limited value. Secondary hypothyroidism and tertiary hypothyroidism are not very common.

INITIATING DRUG THERAPY

The only course of treatment for hypothyroidism is replacement with thyroid hormone. **Figure 47.3** shows an algorithm for the evaluation and treatment of hypothyroidism.

Goals of Drug Therapy

The goal of therapy is to return the patient to the euthyroid state with a TSH in the range of 0.5 to 4.0 mIU/mL. However, there is some debate regarding the optimal range of TSH; some organizations favor a top normal level of 2.5. Also, there is a

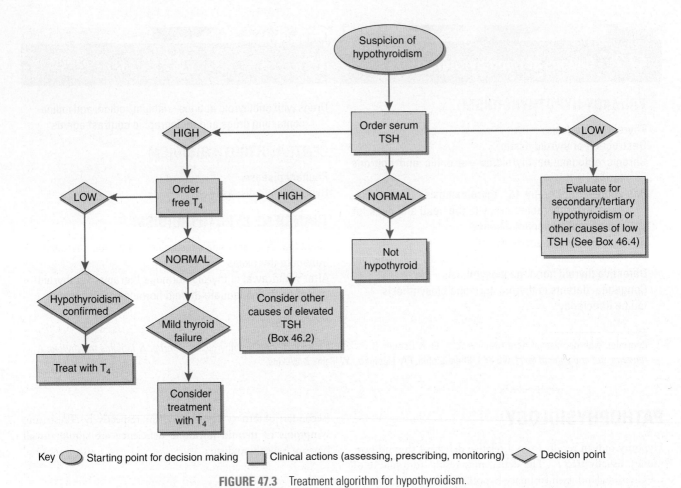

FIGURE 47.3 Treatment algorithm for hypothyroidism.

natural rise of TSH levels in the elderly, which must be considered when treating and monitoring this group of patients (Cappola et al., 2015). Clinicians should exercise caution not to overtreat hypothyroidism by suppressing the TSH to lower than normal levels because such overtreatment will put the patient at risk for hyperthyroidism and its attendant morbidities. Treatment of most cases of hypothyroidism usually is lifelong; exceptions include those cases that occur transiently in patients with postpartum or subacute thyroiditis (discussed later in this chapter).

Thyroid Hormone

Once they have made a diagnosis of hypothyroidism, practitioners should initiate treatment with thyroid hormone replacement in the form of levothyroxine (T_4). **Table 47.2** lists the various preparations available. Natural thyroid extract is derived from porcine thyroid glands and is a combination of T_3 and T_4. This preparation is not used much because of variability in the amount of T_3. T_3 replacement alone is available (liothyronine [Cytomel]) but also is not prescribed frequently because of its association with an increased risk of iatrogenic hyperthyroidism. It is sometimes given for short-term use before radioactive iodine scanning and as augmentation therapy in treatment-resistant depression. A combination product of

T_3 and T_4 (liotrix [Thyrolar]) exists but offers no advantage over T_4 alone. Furthermore, this product increases serum T_3 above physiologic levels within several hours, leading to palpitations.

Several branded preparations of T_4 are available, any one of which may be used. Historically, authorities have recommended against the use of generic T_4. A study of the bioavailability of generic preparations compared with brand name T_4, however, found no significant difference between generic and nongeneric T_4 and concluded that generic drugs may be used safely; however, experts consider it beneficial for the patient to receive the same brand or generic preparation to limit variability in bioavailability, especially in children and pregnant women. Furthermore, in 2007, the U.S. Food and Drug Administration (FDA) required that all manufacturers of levothyroxine products provide evidence of potency between 95% and 105%, a narrower window than the previous 90% to 110%, to limit the variability among the various products (U.S. Food and Drug Administration, 2015).

Levothyroxine is readily absorbed from the GI tract. Serum T_4 levels peak at 2 to 4 hours, although the rise in serum T_3 levels is slower because of the time needed for conversion from T_4. Synthetic T_4 has a half-life of 1 week and requires approximately 6 to 8 weeks of therapy to reach steady state; therefore, patients may not notice improvement in symptoms for 1 week or more.

TABLE 47.2

Overview of Drugs Used for Treatment of Hypothyroidism

Generic (Trade) Name and Dosage	Selected Adverse Events	Contraindications	Special Considerations
levothyroxine (Synthroid, others) Start: 12.5–100 mcg/d Maintenance: 75–150 mcg/d	Only with excessive dosing: arrhythmias, palpitations, nervousness, tremor, weight loss	Untreated thyrotoxicosis, hypersensitivity to thyroid hormones, uncorrected adrenal cortical insufficiency	Goal TSH 0.5–4.0 milliunits/L
liothyronine (Cytomel) Start: 25 mcg/d Maintenance: 25–75 mcg/d	Only with excessive dosing	Same as above	Goal TSH 0.5–4.0 milliunits/L
liotrix (Thyrolar) (liothyronine and levothyroxine) Start: levothyroxine 50 mcg/d + liothyronine 12.5 mcg/d Maintenance: levothyroxine 100 mcg/d + liothyronine 25 mcg/d	Only with excessive dosing	Same as above	Goal TSH 0.5–4.0 milliunits/L
thyroid, desiccated (Armour) (liothyronine and levothyroxine) Start: 60 mcg/d Maintenance: 60–120 mcg/d	Only with excessive dosing	Same as above	Goal TSH 0.5–4.0 milliunits/L; not used much because of variability of T_3 content

Dosage

When initiating therapy, clinicians must consider the patient's age, the duration of hypothyroidism, and any concomitant conditions. For adolescents and young adults, treatment can begin with the full replacement dose (100 to 125 mcg/d, or 1.6 mcg/kg/d, or approximately 0.75 mcg/lb/d). Children require approximately 4 to 10 mcg/kg/d depending on age. In older adults or patients at risk for cardiac disease, thyroid hormone replacement should begin at 25 or even 12.5 mcg/d. Prescribers should increase the dosage incrementally (by 25 mcg/d every 4 to 6 weeks) until reaching the full replacement dose. Clinicians must monitor serum TSH levels and adjust the dose of T_4 accordingly. Many different dosage strengths (25 to 300 mcg) are available to allow titration to appropriate levels.

Interactions

Some drugs interfere with the absorption of thyroid hormone from the GI tract. (See **Box 47.3.**) These include cholestyramine (Questran), sucralfate (Carafate), aluminum-containing antacids, and calcium carbonate. Patients should not take T_4 several hours before or after ingesting these agents.

The concentration of total T_4 and T_3 depends on the concentration of serum TBGs. Any drug or condition that interferes with TBG levels can affect the interpretation of thyroid function tests. Furthermore, in patients who are taking T_4, the changing concentration of TBGs may necessitate adjustment of the dose. The most common causes of an increased serum TBG concentration are increased estrogen production (e.g., as in pregnancy) and the administration of estrogen, in the form of either an oral contraceptive or as estrogen replacement therapy. Patients receiving these therapies will likely need higher doses of T_4 to maintain the euthyroid state because the estrogen

increases the level of TBGs, and more thyroid hormone is in the bound, inactive state rather than in the free, active state. Androgens and niacin can decrease TBG concentrations and have opposite effects on thyroid function tests; patients taking these drugs will likely need lower doses of T_4.

Several drugs decrease the affinity of T_4 and T_3 to TBGs, causing displacement of hormones and resulting in a transient increase in free T_4 and free T_3 levels. Salicylates and high doses of furosemide (Lasix) can exert this effect.

Another concern is for the patient taking oral anticoagulants. When hypothyroid patients become euthyroid, metabolism of vitamin K–dependent clotting factors increases. Therefore, the patient's prothrombin time may increase, as does the risk of bleeding. The opposite occurs in patients treated for hyperthyroidism. Thus, clinicians need to monitor carefully coagulation studies in patients taking warfarin (Coumadin) who are being treated for thyroid disease.

Drugs like phenytoin (Dilantin) and carbamazepine (Tegretol) alter the metabolism of thyroid hormones. Patients who use these agents require more frequent monitoring of thyroid function.

Patients on some chemotherapeutic agents (e.g., sunitinib and imatinib) may develop or experience worsening of hypothyroidism. Clinicians should monitor these patients carefully and may need to start or adjust the dose of T4.

Special Population Considerations
Pediatric

In children, developmental defects like thyroid aplasia or hypoplasia or inborn errors in thyroid hormonogenesis may result in thyroid deficiency. Routine screening of newborns allows early identification and treatment of this potentially devastating condition. Children with congenital hypothyroidism require referral to a pediatric endocrinologist for treatment. Older children also may become hypothyroid as a result of lymphocytic (Hashimoto) thyroiditis or secondary to irradiation or surgery on the thyroid. Treatment is similar to that for adults, but children may require doses of up to 4.0 to 10.0 mcg/kg/d of T_4 due to rapid metabolism (Buck, 2008).

Geriatric

Clinicians need to maintain a high level of suspicion for thyroid disease in older adults because the presentation of illness may differ from that in younger patients. This difference is partly because of alterations in the rate of hormone secretion and clearance as well as increased nodularity and fibrosis of the thyroid gland. Furthermore, concomitant illnesses and medications can modify thyroid function in older adults. Symptoms of hypothyroidism may be subtle or nonexistent. Ataxia, paresthesias, and carpal tunnel syndrome may be the presenting symptoms of hypothyroidism in older adults. Psychiatric manifestations of thyroid disease (e.g., depression or change in sensorium) also are more common in this age group. Older adults also are more susceptible to complications of therapy. Treatment should be initiated at a lower dose for elderly patients.

Pregnancy

Hypothyroidism in pregnancy deserves special mention. Because of the increased amount of thyroglobulin during pregnancy, more T_4 is bound in the circulation. Total T_4 and T_3 increase early in the first trimester, even in women without hypothyroidism. The free T_4 consequently declines to such a degree that symptoms of hypothyroidism may develop in many pregnant women with previously controlled hypothyroidism treated with T_4, necessitating a dose increase by approximately 50 mcg until after delivery. Clinicians should evaluate thyroid function in pregnant women during every trimester by means of a TSH level. The serum total T_3 level returns to normal approximately 1 week after delivery, whereas the total T_4 level declines by 3 to 4 weeks if the patient is not using an oral contraceptive.

MONITORING PATIENT RESPONSE

Patients require clinical and laboratory evaluation with a serum TSH 6 to 8 weeks after initiating therapy or adjusting the dose of T_4. Because it takes this long for the TSH level to decline in response to T_4 replacement, a TSH test should not be ordered before this time. Clinicians should perform an interval history and physical examination, focusing on symptoms and signs of hyperthyroidism, which suggest overdosage, and residual symptoms of hypothyroidism to assess for underdosage.

Practitioners should check TSH levels 6 months after normalization to ensure stable metabolism of T_4, then annually unless new symptoms or medical conditions develop or new drugs are prescribed that may interact with T4 in the interim. Therapy is usually lifelong (although spontaneous recovery

may occur in up to 20% of patients with hypothyroidism related to Hashimoto thyroiditis), so clinicians must encourage patients to comply with their medication regimens. The finding of a very high TSH but a normal free T_4 level suggests intermittent compliance with T_4 therapy.

PATIENT EDUCATION

Patients with primary hypothyroidism most likely will require lifelong replacement with thyroid hormone. Patients should not expect to see a difference in their symptoms until 2 to 4 weeks after beginning therapy. Follow-up laboratory testing is necessary relatively frequently until a therapeutic dosage that results in a stable TSH is reached; at that point, testing should be done annually.

Drug Information

Patients are advised against taking excessive thyroid hormone replacement because of the increased risk of drug-induced hyperthyroidism, which would put patients at risk for osteoporosis and arrhythmias. Thyroid replacement should be taken on an empty stomach 30 minutes to 1 hour before ingestion of the first food of the day.

Patients on thyroid hormone replacement therapy should limit the use of adrenergic agents (e.g., nonprescription decongestants). Patients should not take thyroid hormone at the same time as iron or calcium supplements, antacids, bile acid sequestrants, or simethicone; these preparations require administration at least 2 hours before or after administration of thyroid hormone. Finally, clinicians should reassure patients that although hypothyroidism is a chronic condition, treatment is usually safe and effective.

HYPERTHYROIDISM

Hyperthyroidism results from the presence of an excess amount of thyroid hormone(s), which may result in thyrotoxicosis, a term that refers to the effect of inappropriately high thyroid hormone levels on tissues. Overt hyperthyroidism occurs in up to 2.2% of the population (Bahn et al., 2011; Hollowell et al., 2002), with a female-to-male ratio of 5:1 (Kahaly et al., 2011).

CAUSES

Graves disease, an autoimmune disease that occurs most commonly in patients ages 20 to 50 with a female-to-male ratio of 4 to 8:1, is the most common cause of overt hyperthyroidism (**Box 47.4**). It develops as a result of stimulation of the thyroid gland by TSH receptor autoantibodies on the follicular cell surface. The autoantibodies act like TSH in stimulating thyroid gland function. The gland is not susceptible to the usual negative feedback mechanism of the thyroid hormones; thus, levels of thyroid hormone escalate.

BOX 47.4   Drugs and Conditions that May Alter the Levothyroxine Dose Required by a Patient by Affecting Levothyroxine Absorption

Drugs, Supplements, and Inert Ingredients	Food and Beverages	Medical and Physiologic Conditions
Calcium carbonate	Meals	Gastritis
Phosphate binders	Timing with regard to meals	Celiac disease
Inert ingredients (contained in different LT$_4$ products)	Fiber	Lactose intolerance
Antacids	Soy products	Aging
Ferrous sulfate	Espresso coffee	Severe obesity
Cholestyramine		
Colesevelam		
Sucralfate		
Raloxifene		
Proton pump inhibitors		
Orlistat		

Reprinted with permission from Jonklaas, J. (2013). *Treatment of hypothyroidism. Werner & Ingbar's the thyroid; A fundamental and clinical text* (10th ed.). Philadelphia, PA: Lippincott Williams & Wilkins.

Toxic nodular goiter (Plummer disease) is another frequent cause of hyperthyroidism, especially in older adults. In this condition, one or more thyroid nodules begin to "hyperfunction" and are not dependent on the feedback mechanisms of the pituitary–thyroid axis. As a result of the increased systemic T$_4$ produced by the nodule, TSH is suppressed, and the remainder of the gland begins to atrophy. Eye findings (i.e., exophthalmos and lid lag sometimes found with Graves disease) are absent in this condition.

A less common cause of hyperthyroidism is thyrotoxicosis factitia, in which patients intentionally take T$_4$ in doses high enough to suppress their TSH. This finding is more common among those in the medical profession with access to prescription medications. These patients may want to use T$_4$ to help with weight loss or to treat fatigue or depression.

Several forms of thyroiditis may result in hyperthyroidism with a characteristically low radioactive iodine uptake. These are discussed in a later section.

Amiodarone and other drugs that contain iodine, including radiographic contrast agents, may induce hyperthyroidism in patients with autonomously functioning nodules. Clinicians must monitor such patients closely to evaluate ongoing need for these agents.

DIAGNOSTIC CRITERIA

The patient with hyperthyroidism classically exhibits symptoms of enhanced metabolic activity (i.e., palpitations, sweating, heat intolerance, weight loss). Examination may reveal elevated blood pressure, tachycardia, a bruit over the thyroid gland, or exophthalmos in patients with Graves disease

(**Box 47.5**). The diagnosis is confirmed by finding a low, or suppressed, TSH level with an elevated free T$_4$ level. A nuclear ^{123}I thyroid scan can confirm Graves disease, which causes a diffuse increase in uptake of radioactive iodine. Hyperthyroidism caused by a hyperfunctioning nodule appears as a localized area of increased radioiodine uptake (a "hot" nodule), with the remainder of the gland exhibiting generalized decreased uptake of the isotope.

INITIATING DRUG THERAPY

There are three main options to treat hyperthyroidism: (1) antithyroid drugs, (2) radioactive iodine ablation with ^{131}I, and (3) surgery (**Table 47.3** and **Figure 47.4**). In general, radioactive iodine is the treatment of choice for patients older than age 40; it often is used in younger patients as well. Because of the high rate of permanent hypothyroidism after treatment and the eventual need for lifelong thyroid replacement, as well as concerns about subsequent cancers after exposure to radioiodine at a young age, many clinicians initially attempt to treat younger patients with antithyroid medications. Data on this issue have been conflicting, but many providers are now using radioactive iodine as first-line therapy in young patients (Bahn et al., 2011). Radioactive iodine is contraindicated in pregnancy; however, it may be used in women of childbearing age and in children. Women should postpone pregnancy until 6 months after radioiodine therapy. Lactating women should not receive radioiodine because it passes into breast milk.

Practitioners should follow patients treated with ^{131}I every 4 to 6 weeks for 3 months after radioiodine treatment, then less frequently. Because most patients with Graves

BOX 47.5 Causes of Hyperthyroidism/Thyrotoxicosis

THYROTOXICOSIS ASSOCIATED WITH A NORMAL OR ELEVATED RADIOIODINE UPTAKE OVER THE NECK

Graves disease
Toxic adenoma or toxic multinodular goiter
Trophoblastic disease
TSH-producing pituitary adenomas
Resistance to thyroid hormone (T3 [triiodothyronine] receptor mutation)[b]

THYROTOXICOSIS ASSOCIATED WITH A NEAR-ABSENT RADIOIODINE UPTAKE OVER THE NECK

Painless (silent) thyroiditis
Amiodarone-induced thyroiditis
Subacute (granulomatous, de Quervain) thyroiditis
Iatrogenic thyrotoxicosis
Factitious ingestion of thyroid hormone
Struma ovarii
Acute thyroiditis
Extensive metastases from follicular thyroid cancer

Reprinted with permission from Bahn, R. S., et al. (2011). Hyperthyroidism and other causes of thyrotoxicosis: Management Guidelines of the American Thyroid Association and American Association of Clinical Endocrinologists. *Thyroid 21.* Mary Ann Liebert, Inc. doi: 10.1089/thy.2010.0417. Retrieved on April 26, 2015. Copyright 2011, with permission from the American Association of Clinical Endocrinologists.

disease become hypothyroid after treatment, clinicians must screen for symptoms and measure TSH and free T_4 levels intermittently. Conversely, when radioactive iodine is used to treat toxic nodules, the rate of posttherapeutic hypothyroidism is lower, likely related to the degree of suppression of the remainder of the gland by the nodule. If the free T_4 becomes low and the TSH elevated, patients should start T_4 supplementation with the goal of reaching the replacement dosage and maintaining euthyroidism. TSH levels should be done yearly or more frequently if the patient's clinical condition changes.

Surgery is reserved for patients with large goiters that compress vital structures or for those in whom there is a concern about a malignancy in the gland. It also may be used in pregnant women who are unable or unwilling to take antithyroid drugs. Before surgery, patients are often treated with antithyroid drugs until they are euthyroid, with inorganic iodide (discussed later) added 10 days after surgery.

Potential complications of surgery include hypoparathyroidism and injury to the recurrent laryngeal nerve, although in experienced hands, these complications are rare. Hypothyroidism develops after thyroidectomy in up to 70% of cases depending on the extent of surgery, so postsurgical patients need regular follow-up and supplementation with T_4 as necessary.

Goals of Drug Therapy

The goals of therapy are to restore patients to the euthyroid state and eliminate the risks associated with chronic hyperthyroidism. Pharmacologic therapy for hyperthyroidism is usually not lifelong. Patients usually stop taking antithyroid drugs after 1 to 2 years. If permanent hypothyroidism develops as a result of radioactive iodine treatment or surgery, however, then treatment of hypothyroidism (discussed previously) is lifelong.

Antithyroid Drugs

Antithyroid drugs commonly used in the United States are methimazole (Tapazole) and propylthiouracil (PTU [Propyl-Thyracil]; **Table 47.4**).

Mechanism of Action

These drugs act by inhibiting iodine organification. They also block the conversion of T_4 to T_3 in the periphery, although this mechanism has minimal clinical relevance. The drugs are rapidly absorbed and concentrated in the thyroid follicular

TABLE 47.3 Recommended Order of Treatment for Hyperthyroidism

Order	Agents	Comments
First line	Radioactive iodine	Usually recommended in patients older than age 40 but may be used for younger patients
		High incidence of hypothyroidism when used to treat Graves disease; less when used for toxic nodules
Second line	Antithyroid drugs	Often used in younger patients to induce remission of Graves disease; also used to prepare some patients for treatment with radioiodine or surgery
Third line	Surgery	Usually reserved for patients with large goiters or suspected malignancy

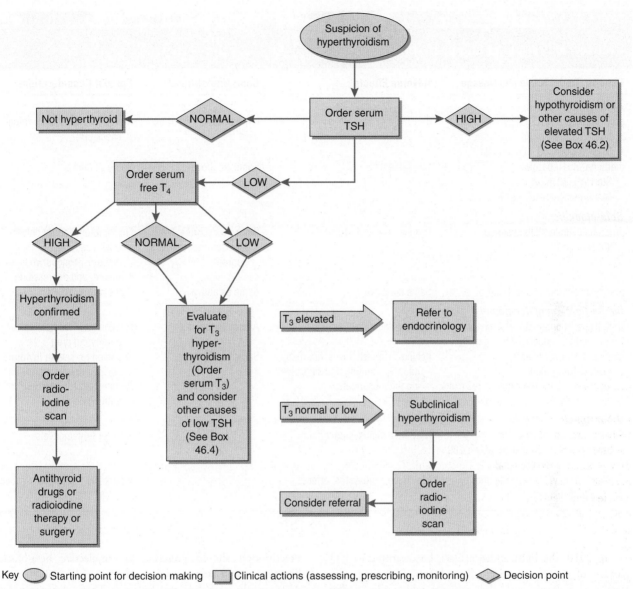

FIGURE 47.4 Treatment algorithm for hyperthyroidism.

cells. PTU has a short duration of action and thus requires multiple doses per day. Methimazole has a longer duration and may be dosed once a day, making it the drug of choice in most instances.

Dosage

The starting dose for PTU is 200 to 400 mg/d, whereas the initial dose of methimazole is 10 to 30 mg/d. Treatment usually continues for 12 to 24 months. Success rates for antithyroid drugs range from 10% to 75%, with remission rates inversely related to the duration of hyperthyroidism and the size of the goiter.

Antithyroid drugs also are used to prepare patients with severe hyperthyroidism for ablative therapy with either radioactive iodine or surgery, especially in those at risk for cardiac complications. The drugs usually are given for several weeks then stopped several days before definitive therapy, although

some patients may need to continue the drugs for several months after ^{131}I therapy to control persistent hyperthyroidism.

Adverse Events

Side effects are fairly minimal (**Table 47.5**), with the most common being rash, arthralgias, itching, and hepatic abnormalities. Patients who have difficulty with one medication may be given a trial of another, although cross-sensitivity among the antithyroid drugs may occur. Rarely (0.3% of patients), a potentially fatal agranulocytosis may result, which occurs somewhat more often with PTU than with methimazole. Clinicians should consider routine monitoring of the complete blood count (CBC) during the first 3 months of therapy. They should warn patients who are taking these drugs to report symptoms of sore throat and fever immediately; they should obtain a CBC and stop the drug if the patient's white blood cell count is low.

TABLE 47.4

Overview of Drugs Used to Treat Hyperthyroidism

Generic (Trade) Name and Dosage	Adverse Effects	Contraindications	Special Considerations
Antithyroid Drugs			
propylthiouracil (PTU [Propyl-Thyracil]) Start: 100–600 mg/d Maintenance: 50–100 mg q8h	See Table 47.5.	Hypersensitivity to drug	Monitor for fever, sore throat; check CBC
methimazole (Tapazole) Start: 15–30 mg/d Maintenance: 5–15 mg/d	See Table 47.5.	Same as above	Same as above
Beta-blockers			
propranolol (Inderal) long acting: 80–160 mg/d	Fatigue, sexual dysfunction	Sinus bradycardia, heart block greater than first degree	For symptom control only Use with caution in asthma, diabetes, congestive heart failure, and depression
atenolol (Tenormin) 50–200 mg/d	Same as above	Same as above	Same as above
Iodine-Containing Compounds			
SSKI (Lugol solution) 0.1–0.3 mL tid sodium iodide (Iodopen) 0.5–1 g q12h	Rash, sialadenitis, vasculitis	Allergy to iodine	Administer after starting antithyroid drug
Iodinated contrast agents: ipodate (Oragrafin) iopanoate acid (Telepaque) 0.5–2 g/d	Itching, skin rash, hives, diarrhea, nausea, vomiting; bruising/bleeding with iopanoate	Same as above	Reserved for severe thyrotoxicosis or thyroid storm Administer after starting antithyroid drug
Other Agents			
lithium (Eskalith, others) Starting and maintenance: 900–1,200 mg/d in divided doses	May have multisystem effects		Monitor lithium levels
Glucocorticoids dosage depends on agent selected	May have multisystem effects		Adjunctive therapy for thyroid storm

In 2010, the FDA added a black box warning to PTU because of reports of severe liver injury, including some deaths, in pediatric and adult patients taking this medication. The FDA also recommends that PTU be reserved for patients who cannot tolerate other therapies for hyperthyroidism (http://www.fda.gov/Drugs/DrugSafety/PostmarketDrugSafetyInformationforPatientsandProviders/ucm209023.htm).

Interactions

Because antithyroid drugs decrease iodine uptake and organification, they can interfere with subsequent radioactive iodine therapy. Higher doses of ^{131}I may be needed to increase success rates in these patients.

Adjunctive Agents Used to Manage Hyperthyroidism

Beta-Blockers

Beta-blockers are used to treat the symptoms of hyperthyroidism. They do not affect thyroid hormone synthesis; rather, they act by decreasing the symptoms of adrenergic stimulation caused by the increased concentration of thyroid hormones.

Practitioners should prescribe a nonselective beta-blocker like long-acting propranolol starting at a dose of 80 mg/d. Alternatively, atenolol may be used. These drugs can help prevent hyperthyroid-induced atrial fibrillation or control the ventricular rate in patients with established atrial fibrillation. Clinicians should consider anticoagulation to reduce the risk of stroke in patients with atrial fibrillation; treatment of these patients should be in consultation with a cardiologist. Prescribers should taper beta-blockers gradually and discontinue them as soon as the patient is euthyroid and asymptomatic. Patients in whom beta-blockers are not tolerated or are contraindicated (e.g., those with asthma) may be treated with calcium channel blockers like diltiazem.

Iodine-Containing Compounds

Other agents used adjunctively in the treatment of hyperthyroidism are iodine-containing compounds like potassium iodide (in the form of saturated solution of potassium iodide [SSKI] 35 mg/drop or Lugol solution 7 mg/drop) and the iodinated contrast agents ipodate (Oragrafin) and iopanoate acid (Telepaque). These drugs are reserved for the treatment of severe thyrotoxicosis or thyroid storm. Such patients are

TABLE 47.5

Side Effects of Antithyroid Drugs

Minor
Common (1%–5%)
Urticaria or other rash
Arthralgia
Fever
Transient granulocytopenia

Uncommon (<1%)
Gastrointestinal upset
Abnormalities of taste and smell
Arthritis

Major
Rare (0.2%–0.5%)
Agranulocytosis

Very rare (<0.1%)
Aplastic anemia
Thrombocytopenia
Toxic hepatitis (PTU)
Cholestatic hepatitis (methimazole)
Vasculitis, systemic lupus-like syndrome
Hypoprothrombinemia (PTU)
Hypoglycemia (due to anti-insulin antibodies) (methimazole)

Reprinted with permission from Cooper, D. S. (2013). *Treatment of thyrotoxicosis. Werner & Ingbar's the thyroid; A fundamental and clinical text* (10th ed.). Philadelphia, PA: Lippincott Williams & Wilkins.

usually treated in an intensive care unit under the care of an endocrinologist, intensivist, or both. Pharmacologic doses of iodine inhibit the release of thyroid hormones from the gland in the short term; however, because new hormone synthesis proceeds during treatment with iodine, iodine must be used in combination with antithyroid drugs, which are given 1 hour before the iodine compound.

Lithium

Lithium, which is chemically similar to iodine, is used rarely to block the release of thyroid hormone from the gland in those patients who are intolerant of antithyroid drugs. The dose is 900 to 1,200 mg/d, divided, and clinicians should monitor lithium levels.

Glucocorticoids

Glucocorticoids are occasionally used in thyroid storm. They reduce peripheral conversion of T_4 to T_3.

Treatment of Ophthalmopathy of Graves Disease

None of the aforementioned therapies for hyperthyroidism affects the ophthalmopathy of Graves disease. Anti-inflammatory drugs, immunosuppressive drugs (e.g., prednisone and dexamethasone), and surgery are offered to patients as treatment for the ophthalmopathy. Sunglasses and artificial tears are used adjunctively for comfort.

Special Population Considerations

Geriatric

The term *apathetic hyperthyroidism* has been used to describe the atypical presentation of hyperthyroidism in some older patients. Rather than the usual symptoms of increased metabolic rate, these patients may present with weakness, dyspnea, anorexia, depression, or constipation. Physical examination may be unrevealing. Occasionally, new-onset atrial fibrillation or congestive heart failure is the initial presentation of hyperthyroidism in the older person.

Pregnancy

Radioactive iodine is contraindicated during pregnancy because it crosses the placenta and adversely affects fetal thyroid development. Because of an increased risk of birth defects related to methimazole use during the first trimester of pregnancy, PTU is the drug of choice for hyperthyroidism during and just before this time. Since it enters the breast milk less than methimazole, PTU may be a safer alternative for a lactating woman. During pregnancy, practitioners should prescribe the lowest dosages possible of antithyroid drugs that still maintain euthyroidism. The dosage usually decreases as pregnancy progresses and the severity of Graves disease lessens, then increases again after delivery. Clinicians should treat pregnant patients who have hyperthyroidism in consultation with an endocrinologist.

MONITORING PATIENT RESPONSE

Patients usually become euthyroid within 6 to 12 weeks of beginning antithyroid drugs; however, permanent hypothyroidism may develop many years after a course of therapy, so long-term follow-up is necessary. Patients taking antithyroid drugs should be evaluated every 1 to 3 months after starting treatment depending on the degree of hyperthyroidism and comorbid conditions. Once euthyroidism is achieved, practitioners can decrease the dose of antithyroid drugs and reevaluate the patient in 3 to 4 months. Clinicians should order free T_4 levels to monitor the patient because the TSH level remains suppressed for several months after the patient becomes euthyroid. They should continue to reduce and eventually discontinue the antithyroid drugs, after which they should see patients every 4 to 6 weeks for 3 to 4 months and less frequently thereafter.

PATIENT EDUCATION

Patients with hyperthyroidism may have very troublesome symptoms that resemble those of anxiety disorders, such as panic attacks. Clinicians should advise them that these symptoms (which can be severe) will resolve with treatment of their thyroid disease.

Practitioners should review all treatment options with patients. They should tell patients that antithyroid drugs will put their disease into remission, but that the relapse rate is high. They should discuss the high likelihood of permanent hypothyroidism after radioactive iodine therapy. Patients will likely gain weight after therapy for hyperthyroidism, even if they do not become hypothyroid. Clinicians should emphasize the chronic nature of the condition and the importance of long-term follow-up regardless of the chosen treatment.

Drug Information

There can be increased effects of digoxin, metoprolol, and propranolol when the patient becomes euthyroid. The effects of anticoagulants can be altered. Drugs should be taken at equal intervals.

Complementary and Alternative Medicine

Bugleweed has been shown to treat a mildly overactive thyroid. It decreases thyroid hormone activity and increases the absorption and storage of thyroid hormone, causing a decreased metabolism. This is not used in patients with hypothyroidism.

Lemon balm is used in hyperthyroidism for its sedative effects.

Special Populations

Women of childbearing age with Graves disease may want to consider definitive treatment (radioiodine or surgery) before conception. It is recommended to prescribe PTU during the first trimester of pregnancy. Clinicians must monitor thyroid function closely because of variations in the course of the disease in pregnancy.

THYROID NODULES

Thyroid nodules are encountered relatively often in clinical practice. The gland may have one or multiple nodules. Most are the result of adenomas, cysts, large collections of colloid, or focal areas of thyroiditis. Five percent of solitary nodules result from thyroid cancer, with higher rates in the very young and older age groups. Fine-needle aspiration biopsy (FNAB) is the initial diagnostic procedure to rule out carcinoma in a solitary nodule.

INITIATING DRUG THERAPY

Treatment of thyroid cancer is beyond the scope of this work; however, clinicians should be aware that high doses of T_4 are used in patients who have been treated for thyroid cancer in an effort to suppress the growth of any remaining cancer cells. Once a thyroid nodule is proved benign histologically, some clinicians previously attempted to reduce the size of the

nodule medically (**Figure 47.5**). T_4 was given in higher than replacement doses (2.2 mcg/kg/d) in an attempt to turn off the secretion of TSH by the pituitary, with the presumption that growth of the nodule depends on TSH. With less circulating TSH, the nodule in theory will not increase in size and may decrease. The literature yields conflicting results in this regard, with some studies showing a significant effect on nodule size but most showing no effect. Therefore, this therapy is no longer utilized.

Radioactive iodine and surgery are appropriate for patients with large single nodules or multiple nodules.

MONITORING PATIENT RESPONSE

Patients with thyroid nodules should be monitored at least annually. If there are ongoing concerns about malignancy, practitioners should perform a repeat FNAB. Patients with hyperthyroidism as a result of toxic nodules respond to antithyroid drugs either in conjunction with or in lieu of ablative therapy.

PATIENT EDUCATION

Patients with thyroid nodules often are unaware of a problem. Therefore, practitioners need to emphasize the potential (although small) for malignancy and the need for further evaluation with FNAB.

If the nodule is found to be benign, clinicians must discuss treatment options. Patients need to follow up at least annually with a physical examination and an ultrasound to evaluate whether the existing nodule has enlarged or if new nodules have developed.

SUBCLINICAL THYROID DISEASE

The entity of subclinical hypothyroidism presents a therapeutic challenge. This condition is defined as an elevated TSH level with a normal free T_4 concentration, usually in a patient with no symptoms. Many authorities believe that subclinical hypothyroidism requires the same treatment as overt hypothyroidism because both entities have been associated with adverse cardiovascular outcomes (Franklyn, 2013).

Proponents of therapy for mild thyroid failure cite studies showing higher levels of LDL cholesterol and lower levels of high-density lipoprotein cholesterol in these patients, as well as increased systolic time intervals and decreased cognitive function. After treatment with T_4, some of these problems show improvement. Patients who have coexisting cardiovascular disease or dysrhythmias probably should not be treated for subclinical hypothyroidism because the risks of therapy outweigh the potential benefits. If treatment is attempted, it should be with T_4 at doses to lower the TSH level to the normal range. The incidence of subclinical hypothyroidism is higher in older

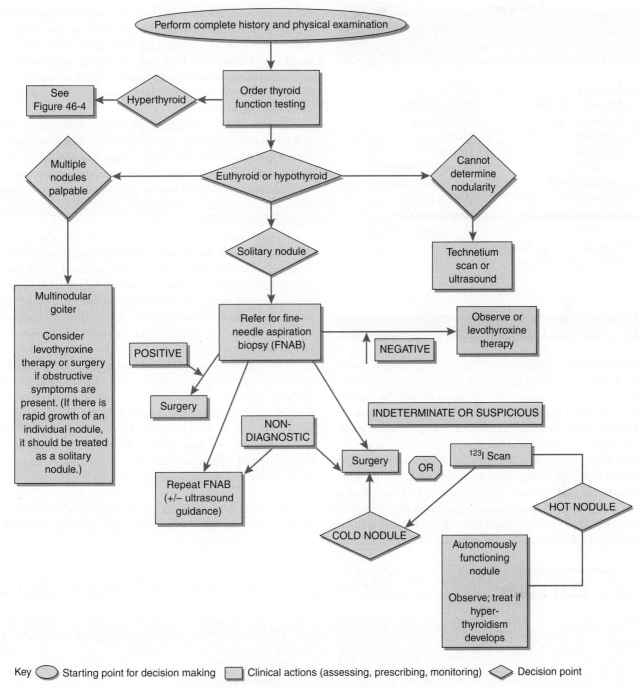

FIGURE 47.5 Evaluation and management of thyroid nodules.

adults, occurring in up to 20% of people older than age 60; however, since TSH levels have been found to rise naturally in geriatric populations, this may be an overestimate of the prevalence.

A subclinical hyperthyroid entity has been defined by normal free T_4 and T_3 concentrations with a low TSH level in asymptomatic patients. This condition results from over-replacement of T_4, Graves disease, autonomously functioning nodules, surreptitious intake of T_4, nonthyroid illness, or certain medications that decrease TSH. (See **Box 47.6**.) Risks of

subclinical hyperthyroidism include increased bone turnover, which may predispose to osteoporosis and an increased risk of atrial fibrillation and other adverse cardiovascular outcomes. The risk of progression to overt hyperthyroidism is higher in patients with undetectable TSH levels, compared with low but detectable levels. Antithyroid therapy similar to that of overt hyperthyroidism should be considered in consultation with an endocrinologist. Treatment recommendations are based on age of the patient, coexistent conditions, and level of TSH suppression (Palmeiro et al., 2013).

BOX 47.6 Symptoms and Signs of Hyperthyroidism

Dyspnea	Goiter
Heat intolerance	Brisk reflexes
Palpitations	Tachycardia
Infertility	Tremor
Insomnia	Lid lag
Irritability	Exophthalmos (with
Nervousness	Graves disease)
Sweatiness	Weight loss
Frequent bowel	Amenorrhea or
movements	oligomenorrhea
Pretibial myxedema (with	
Graves disease)	

THYROIDITIS

After delivering a child, up to 10% of women without previous thyroid disease have postpartum (also known as *painless* or *silent*) thyroiditis, a variant of Hashimoto thyroiditis. Patients present within 1 year after delivery with nonspecific symptoms of fatigue, palpitations, and depression. Tachycardia and goiter may be present on examination.

Patients often go through a hyperthyroid phase that resolves in a few months. Some then have transient hypothyroidism that can last from 2 to 6 months. This condition is usually self-limited, so treatment is indicated only to relieve the symptoms of hyperthyroidism. Beta-blockers are the treatment of choice. Antithyroid drugs are not helpful because the hyperthyroidism that develops is a result of the gland's spilling of preformed thyroid hormone. Some patients require replacement doses of T_4 during the hypothyroid phase of their condition. Women with high titers of antithyroid peroxidase antibodies during or after the pregnancy are at increased risk for development of permanent hypothyroidism; these women should be followed closely.

Women with postpartum thyroiditis may experience symptoms similar to postpartum depression; therefore, practitioners should reassure these women that their symptoms will resolve once the condition subsides. Clinicians should encourage those women at higher risk for permanent hypothyroidism (those with a high titer of antithyroid peroxidase antibodies) to return for periodic follow-up.

Patients sometimes develop subacute (de Quervain) thyroiditis several weeks after an upper respiratory tract infection. They present with a painful, enlarged gland and symptoms and signs of hyperthyroidism, which is the result of leakage of thyroid hormones from the inflamed gland. If a radioiodine scan is performed, it shows diffusely *decreased* uptake of tracer (as opposed to the increased uptake seen in Graves disease).

This condition is self-limited and requires symptomatic treatment only. As in postpartum thyroiditis, beta-blockers are used to reduce tachycardia, tremor, and nervousness. Aspirin or other nonsteroidal anti-inflammatory drugs can reduce the pain in the gland. Rarely, steroids are needed to reduce swelling and pain. These patients may experience a brief period of hypothyroidism but do not usually become permanently hypothyroid, so that vigilant follow-up is not required.

Clinicians should reassure patients with subacute thyroiditis that their condition will resolve spontaneously, but may take weeks.

CASE STUDY*

M.E. is a 29-year-old woman with a 7-month history of heavy, irregular menses, a 5-lb weight gain, constipation, and decreased energy. Her past history is unremarkable. She takes no prescription medications but uses iron and calcium supplements. She has a family history of thyroid disease. On examination, her weight is 152 lbs, her heart rate is 64 bpm, and her blood pressure is 138/86. Her thyroid gland is mildly enlarged, without nodularity. She has trace edema in her lower extremities, and her reflexes are slow. Laboratory studies are as follows: TSH is 15.3 mIU/mL (elevated), free T_4 is 0.3 mIU/mL (decreased), total cholesterol is 276 mg/mL.

DIAGNOSIS: PRIMARY HYPOTHYROIDISM

1. List specific goals of treatment for **M.E.**
2. What drug therapy would you prescribe? Why?
3. What are the parameters for monitoring the success of the therapy?
4. Discuss specific patient education based on the prescribed therapy.
5. List one or two adverse reactions for the selected agent that would cause you to change therapy.
6. What would be the choice for second-line therapy?
7. What over-the-counter and/or alternative medications would be appropriate for **M.E.**?
8. What lifestyle changes would you recommend to **M.E.**?
9. Describe one or two drug–drug or drug–food interactions for the selected agent.

* Answers can be found online.

Bibliography

Starred references are cited in the text.

*American Cancer Society. (2014). *Cancer Facts & Figures 2014*. Atlanta, GA: American Cancer Society. Retrieved from Cancer.org on March 15, 2015.

*Bahn, R. S., Burch, H. B., Cooper, D. S., et al.; The American Thyroid Association and American Association of Clinical Endocrinologists Taskforce on Hyperthyroidism and Other Causes of Thyrotoxicosis. (2011). Hyperthyroidism and other causes of thyrotoxicosis: Management guidelines of the American Thyroid Association and American Association of Clinical Endocrinologists. *Thyroid, 21,* 593–646. Mary Ann Liebert, Inc. doi: 10.1089/thy.2010.0417.

Brander, A., Viikinkoski, P., Nickels, J., et al. (1991). Thyroid gland: US screening in a random adult population. *Radiology, 181,* 683–687.

Braverman, L. E., & Cooper, D. S. (2013). *Introduction to hypothyroidism. Werner & Ingbar's the thyroid; A fundamental and clinical text* (10th ed.) Philadelphia, PA: Lippincott Williams & Wilkins.

*Buck, M. (2008). Levothyroxine use in infants and children with congenital or acquired hypothyroidism. In K. Hofer & M. McCarthy (Eds.), *Medscape—Pediatric Pharmacology, 14*(10). Retrieved from http://www.medscape.com/viewarticle/585291_9

*Canaris, G. J., Manowitz, N. R., Mayor, G., et al. (2000). The Colorado thyroid disease prevalence study. *Archives of Internal Medicine, 160,* 526–534.

*Cappola, A. R., Arnold, A. M., Wulczyn, K., et al. (2015). Thyroid function in the euthyroid range and adverse outcomes in older adults. *Journal of Clinical Endocrinology and Metabolism, 100,* 1088–1096.

Cooper, D. S. (2003). Hyperthyroidism. *Lancet, 362,* 459–468.

*Cooper, D. S. (2013). *Treatment of thyrotoxicosis. Werner & Ingbar's the thyroid; A fundamental and clinical text* (10th ed.) Philadelphia, PA: Lippincott Williams & Wilkins.

*Ferlay, J., Soerjomataram, I., Ervik, M., et al. (2013). GLOBOCAN 2012 v1.0, Cancer Incidence and Mortality Worldwide: IARC CancerBase No. 11 [Internet]. Lyon, France: International Agency for Research on Cancer. Retrieved from http://globocan.iarc.fr on March 30, 2016.

*Franklyn, J. (2013). The thyroid—Too much and too little across the ages: The consequences of Subclinical thyroid dysfunction. *Clinical Endocrinology, 78*(1), 1–8. Retrieved from http://www.medscape.com/viewarticle/776505_3

*Hak, A. E., Pols, H. A., Visser, T. J., et al. (2000). Subclinical hypothyroidism is an independent risk factor for atherosclerosis and myocardial infarction in elderly women: The Rotterdam study. *Annals of Internal Medicine, 130,* 270–278.

*Hollowell, J. G., Staehling, N. W., Flanders, W. D., et al. (2002). Serum TSH, T_4, and thyroid antibodies in the United States Population (1988 to 1994): National Health and Nutrition Examination Survey (NHANES III). *Journal of Clinical Endocrinology and Metabolism, 87,* 489–499.

*Iervasi, G., Molinaro, S., Landi, P., et al. (2007). Association between increased mortality and mild thyroid dysfunction in cardiac patients. *Archives of Internal Medicine, 167,* 1526–1532.

Jonklaas, J. (2013). *Treatment of hypothyroidism. Werner & Ingbar's the thyroid; A fundamental and clinical text* (10th ed.). Philadelphia, PA: Lippincott Williams & Wilkins.

Jonklaas, J., Bianco, A. C., Bauer, A. J., et al. (2014). Guidelines for the treatment of hypothyroidism; Prepared by the American Thyroid Association Task Force on thyroid hormone replacement. *Thyroid, 24,* 1670–1751.

Kahaly, G. J. (2000). Cardiovascular and atherogenic aspects of subclinical hypothyroidism. *Thyroid, 10,* 665–679.

Kahaly, G. J., Grebe, S. K., Lupo, M. A., et al. (2011). Graves' disease: Diagnostic and therapeutic challenges (multimedia activity). *American Journal of Medicine, 124*(6), S2–S3. doi: 10.1016/j.amjmed.2011.03.001.

Lee, S. (2014). Hyperthyroidism. *eMedicine Medscape*. Retrieved from http://emedicine.medscape.com/article/121865-overview

LeFevre, M. L. (2015). Screening for thyroid dysfunction: U.S. Preventive Services Task Force Recommendation Statement. *Annals of Internal Medicine, 162,* 641–650.

Mandel, S. J., Brent, G. A., & Larsen, P. R. (1993). Levothyroxine therapy in patients with thyroid disease. *Annals of Internal Medicine, 119,* 492–502.

Mitrou, P., Raptis, S., & Dimitriadis, G. (2011). Thyroid disease in older people. *Maturitas, 70*(2011), 5–9. doi: http://dx.doi.org/10.1016/j.maturitas.2011.05.016.

Mokshagundam, S., & Barzel, U. S. (1993). Thyroid disease in the elderly. *Journal of the American Geriatrics Society, 41,* 1361–1368.

Mulder, J. E. (1998). Thyroid disorders in women. *Medical Clinics of North America, 82,* 103–125.

*Palmeiro, C., Davila, M. I., Bhat, M., et al. (2013). Subclinical hyperthyroidism and cardiovascular risk: Recommendations for treatment. *Cardiology in Review, 21,* 300–308.

Parle, J. V., Maisonneuve, P., Sheppard, M. C., et al. (2001). Prediction of all-cause and cardiovascular mortality in elderly people from one low serum thyrotropin result: A 10-year cohort study. *Lancet, 358,* 861–865.

Pearce, E. N., Farwell, A. P., & Braverman, L. E. (2003). Current concepts: Thyroiditis. *New England Journal of Medicine, 348,* 2646–2655.

*Rodondi, N., den Elzen, W. P., Bauer, D. C. et al. (2010). Subclinical hypothyroidism and the risk of coronary heart disease and mortality. *Journal of the American Medical Association, 304,* 1365–1377. doi: 10.1001/jama.2010.1361.

Sawin, C. T., Geller, A., Wolf, P. A., et al. (1994). Low serum thyrotropin concentrations as a risk factor for atrial fibrillation in older persons. *New England Journal of Medicine, 331,* 1249–1252.

Subclinical hypothyroidism: An update for primary care physicians. (2009). Retrieved from http://www.mayomedicallaboratories.com/articles/communique/2009/03.html

Surks, M. I., Ortiz, E. O., Daniels, G. H., et al. (2004). Subclinical thyroid disease: Scientific review and guidelines for diagnosis and management. *Journal of the American Medical Association, 291,* 228–238.

U.S. Food and Drug Administration. (2015). *Postmarket drug safety information for patients and providers: Levothyroxine sodium product information*. Retrieved from http://www.fda.gov/Drugs/DrugSafety/PostmarketDrugSafetyInformationforPatientsandProviders/ucm161257.htm

Uzzan, B., Campos, J., Cucherat, M., et al. (1996). Effects on bone mass of long term treatment with thyroid hormones: A meta-analysis. *Journal of Clinical Endocrinology and Metabolism, 81,* 4278–4289.

UNIT 11

Pharmacotherapy for Immune Disorders

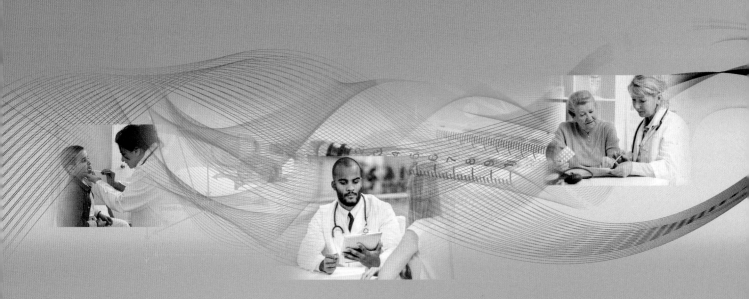

48 Allergies and Allergic Reactions

Lauren M. Czosnowski ■ Andrew M. Peterson

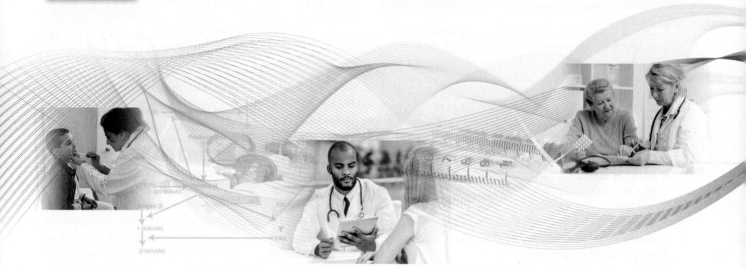

The term *allergy* is derived from the Greek words *allos* (differing from the normal or usual) and *ergon* (work or energy). To describe it in simple, nonclinical terms, allergy is an abnormal release of energy in the body. In clinical or physiologic terms, allergy is an exaggerated immune response resulting from an antibody–antigen reaction.

Antibodies are soluble protein molecules made by B lymphocytes in response to foreign substances. Antibodies, also referred to as *immunoglobulins*, are tailored specifically and uniquely to bind to each foreign substance and remove it from the circulation. Invasion or contact with a foreign substance results in the production and secretion of antibodies. Therefore, the foreign substance is an *anti*body *gen*erator—hence the term *antigen*. Antigens also are referred to as *allergens*; the terms are interchangeable.

All people come in contact with the same antigens, yet not all people display allergic symptoms. Allergy symptoms appear when the immune response is exaggerated or inappropriate, causing inflammation and tissue damage. This exaggerated response to an antigen is referred to as *hypersensitivity*. Hypersensitivity is a characteristic of an individual. It is manifested on the second or a subsequent contact with a particular antigen.

Allergens can be food based, chemical, or environmental. Typical food allergens include milk or egg protein, peanut, shellfish, and wheat or soy. Parabens and lanolin, commonly found in makeup and sunscreens; thimerosal, a preservative found in contact lens solutions; and fragrance enhancers found in perfumes are common chemical allergens. Drugs, such as the local anesthetics lidocaine and benzocaine, are also chemical allergens. Environmental allergens include mold, pollen, and dust.

In contrast to allergy, *anergy* is the term used to describe the unexpected failure of the immune system to respond to the challenge of a foreign substance (antigen or allergen). Several skin test antigens may be applied to the skin (an anergy panel) to determine the status of the immune system. The antigens selected are those to which a majority of the population would exhibit a reaction. Examples of these include *Candida* species and histoplasmin. If the characteristic wheals do not appear in the prescribed period, it can be interpreted that the patient has not had prior exposure to the antigen or potentially has a compromised immune system.

CLASSIFICATION OF ALLERGIC REACTIONS

The medical literature describes four types of hypersensitivity reactions (Coombs and Gell classification) that are listed and described in **Box 48.1** (Nairn & Helbert, 2007). There are four types of reactions under this classification system. Type I reactions involve the interaction between an antigen and a specific immunoglobulin (Ig) E antibody. These antibodies are bound to member receptors on mast cells and basophils. When an antigen binds to these antibodies, the cell releases histamine, leukotrienes, and prostaglandins. These vasoactive substances produce vasodilation and increase capillary permeability, both of which allow for eosinophils and other inflammatory cells to infiltrate tissues, furthering the allergic response. The first contact results in the formation of the antibody. Subsequent contact with the same antigen results in the antibody–antigen reaction, resulting in this type I hypersensitivity reaction. The antibody–antigen reaction triggers the immune response that

BOX 48.1 Coombs and Gell Classification of Hypersensitivity

- Type I (immediate hypersensitivity)—Immunoglobulin (Ig) E attached to mast cells binds with an antigen, inducing degranulation and release of histamine and other mediators of inflammation. (Asthma and allergic rhinitis are examples of type I hypersensitivity.)
- Type II—IgG attached to a T lymphocyte killer cell is directed against antigens on target cell. This leads to direct cytotoxic action or complement-mediated lysis.
- Type III—Immune complexes of antibody and antigen are deposited in the tissue. Complement is activated, and polymorphonuclear leukocytes are attracted to the site of the complex. Local tissue damage occurs. (Autoimmune disease is an example of type III hypersensitivity.)
- Type IV (delayed hypersensitivity)—Antigen-sensitized T cells release inflammatory substances after a second contact with the same antigen. (Contact dermatitis, such as poison ivy, and the tuberculin skin test [PPD] are examples of delayed hypersensitivity.)

results in allergic symptoms (**Figure 48.1**). Allergies can affect the airways, eyes, skin, or the entire body. Type I reactions are typically anaphylactic in nature and can be life-threatening.

Type II reactions, also known as *cytotoxic reactions*, occur when an antibody reacts with an antigenic component of a cell. This antibody–antigen reaction in turn activates killer T cells or macrophages to aid in the destruction of the antigenic cell. Complement activation is also involved in this process, furthering the cytotoxic process leading to tissue destruction. Transfusion reactions are typically type II allergic reactions.

Type III reactions result from immune complexes that activate the complement system. Activating this system promotes the migration and release of cells such as polymorphonuclear cells that can release proteolytic enzymes and factors

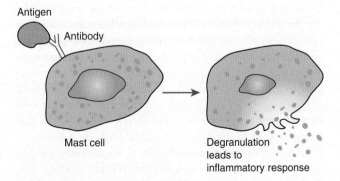

FIGURE 48.1 Antibody–antigen reaction.

that promote tissue permeability. Systemic lupus erythematosus is a form of a type III allergic reaction.

Type IV reactions are also called delayed hypersensitivity reactions. These cell-mediated reactions are the result of sensitized T lymphocytes coming into contact with a specific antigen. The delay typically takes 2 to 3 days or up to a week. Allergic dermatitis is an example of a type IV reaction.

Immunologic Versus Nonimmunologic Reactions

Some cutaneous reactions, such as contact dermatitis, may appear to be allergic reactions, but they do not involve the immune system. Irritant contact dermatitis is the most common cutaneous reaction and is often caused by skin irritants such as powders or chemicals found in gloves.

Contact dermatitis differs from allergic dermatitis in that there is direct tissue insult from the skin irritant that causes the release of inflammatory mediators from skin cells. A common example of irritant contact dermatitis is a reaction to repeated hand-washing with soap or other cleaners. In some instances, the cracked, dry skin occurring with contact dermatitis no longer can prevent allergens from entering the systemic circulation. With latex allergies, for example, the powder already present in the glove can give rise to a contact dermatitis, thus allowing for the latex antigens to enter the circulation. This in turn increases the likelihood of an allergic reaction, resulting in allergic contact dermatitis. Because of this phenomenon, it is often difficult to distinguish allergic from nonallergic contact dermatitis. See Chapter 11 for more details on dermatitis.

General Treatment Overview of Allergic Reactions

The first step in treating an allergic reaction is to remove the allergen, if possible. This may involve removing the person from the environment causing the allergy, stopping the offending drug, or washing off the offending chemical. Most allergic reactions clear up within a few days of removing the cause. Symptomatic cutaneous reactions, such as pruritic rash, urticaria, or morbilliform eruptions as well as reactions involving multiple organs, should be treated.

Cutaneous Reactions

Cutaneous reactions such as urticaria, pruritus, and hives are often secondary to the release of histamine, making antihistamine therapy the mainstay of treatment. There are two types of antihistamines used in the general treatment of allergic reactions: first generation and second generation. The first-generation antihistamines include diphenhydramine, hydroxyzine, and chlorpheniramine, among others. These agents are typically very effective, but they may also be very sedating. The second-generation agents, such as loratadine and fexofenadine, are nonsedating antihistamines (NSAs) that work fairly well at controlling mild to moderate symptoms of cutaneous reactions. However, if the symptoms persist for more than a few

CHAPTER 48 | ALLERGIES AND ALLERGIC REACTIONS **829**

days, or are not well controlled, a first-generation antihistamine may be substituted, or added, to the NSA. Close communication with the patient regarding resolution of the symptoms is necessary, along with balancing quality-of-life issues related to side effects, such as sedation, dry mouth, and urinary retention. If the reaction is moderate to severe or if there is no relief from antihistamine therapy, systemic glucocorticoids may be used. Short courses of treatment with oral prednisone or methylprednisolone are usually used. See Chapter 11 for more information on the use of oral steroids for treating cutaneous reactions.

Anaphylaxis and Anaphylactoid Reactions

Anaphylaxis is a type I hypersensitivity reaction involving IgE-mediated release of histamine, leukotrienes, and other mediators from already sensitized mast cells and basophils. The release of these mediators initiates a systemic chain of events that includes symptoms such as angioedema, flushing, pruritus, urticaria, nausea, vomiting, and wheezing. The onset of the reaction is quick, generally within 1 to 30 minutes. The histamine release causes a smooth muscle contraction and vasodilation. The wheezing resulting from smooth muscle contraction in the lungs decreases oxygenation, whereas vasodilation results in a release of fluids into the tissues, thus causing a lower effective plasma volume, leading to shock. Prolonged vasodilation, coupled with decreased oxygenation, can lead to arrhythmias, convulsions, and death.

Anaphylactoid reactions are similar in appearance to anaphylaxis but may occur after the *first* injection of certain drugs and contrast media. They are non-IgE mediated, and the agent causes a direct release of histamine and other inflammatory toxins. They have a dose-related, idiosyncratic mechanism rather than an immunologically mediated one. A classic example of an anaphylactoid reaction is the "red man syndrome" associated with vancomycin. Patients may experience itching, redness, and hives with rapid infusion of vancomycin due to histamine release; slowing the infusion rate usually improves the reaction.

Treatment

Immediate treatment with epinephrine is imperative. Epinephrine effectively increases the blood pressure and is an antagonist to the effects of histamine on smooth muscle and other tissues.

At the onset of anaphylactic symptoms, such as generalized pruritus, urticaria, angioedema, or wheezing, 0.01 mL/kg aqueous epinephrine 1:1,000 (1 mg/mL) subcutaneously or intramuscularly (usual dose, 0.2 to 0.5 mL in adults; 0.3 mL maximum for children) should be given. This dose may be repeated every 5 to 15 minutes as necessary to control symptoms. Intramuscular injection into the lateral thigh muscle results in a shorter time to peak concentrations of epinephrine in the blood, compared to subcutaneous injection or intramuscular injection into the deltoid muscle. An injectable antihistamine such as diphenhydramine (usual dose for adults, 25 to 50 mg; children, 1 mg/kg) may also be given in addition

to epinephrine to treat symptoms related to anaphylaxis such as itching and hives. These agents alone do not treat airway obstruction, hypotension, or shock.

If the reaction does involve the cardiovascular system, then intravenous fluids should be rapidly infused to maintain volume. Hypovolemia is usually the major cause of the hypotension due to fluid moving out of the intravascular space. Colloid plasma expanders such as dextran are rarely necessary. Normal saline is an appropriate choice for most patients, and 1 to 2 L should be given as an initial bolus. Fluids may be continued as necessary to maintain hemodynamic stability. If fluid replacement is ineffective at restoring blood pressure, then dopamine or norepinephrine may be *cautiously* introduced. Alternatively, if the patient is experiencing bradycardia, atropine may be used to increase heart rate. Patients with severe reactions should be observed in the hospital for 24 hours after recovery in case of relapse.

Systemic corticosteroids may help prevent late-phase reactions in some cases of anaphylaxis, although they will not have an effect for 4 to 6 hours. Typically, methylprednisolone 1 to 2 mg/kg/d divided every 6 to 8 hours for adults and 1 to 2 mg/kg/d divided every 8 to 12 hours for children is needed to prevent the onset of late-phase reactions. For milder attacks, oral prednisone dosed at 0.5 mg/kg/d may be administered, although there are not strong data to support in administering glucocorticoids.

Prophylaxis

The primary means of preventing an allergic reaction is avoidance. However, when this is not feasible or practical, immunotherapy is an effective means of preventing reactions, particularly anaphylactic reactions from insect bites. This form of "desensitization" is only effective when a specific allergen can be identified. Some ragweed and pollen allergies respond well to immunotherapy, though it may take several months before immunity is conferred.

Desensitization may be rapidly achieved in patients requiring drug therapy to which they have an established allergy. For example, patients with anaphylactic reactions to penicillin may be desensitized by administering increasing concentrations of penicillin every 15 minutes. To ensure patient safety, desensitization is best done under constant supervision and in consultation with an experienced allergist. There are numerous protocols for penicillin desensitization and an increasing number for patients who are allergic to sulfa drugs.

ALLERGIC RHINITIS (HAY FEVER OR POLLEN ALLERGY)

Allergic rhinitis is an *airway allergy*. (Asthma, also an airway allergy, is discussed in Chapter 25.) Many people have hay fever. The National Institute of Allergy and Infectious Diseases states that pollen allergy may affect approximately 7% of adults and 9% of children in the United States. (NIAID July 2015).

CAUSES

Common inhaled allergens that cause allergic rhinitis in sensitized people include pollen (grass, trees, weeds), dust mites, mold spores, enzymes (in detergents), and insect body parts. The two most common types of allergic rhinitis are seasonal and perennial (**Table 48.1**). The incidence of seasonal rhinitis is approximately 10 times greater than that of perennial rhinitis.

In seasonal allergic rhinitis, symptoms correspond with seasonal peaks in tree, grass, and weed pollens. During the spring, tree pollens such as alder, birch, and oak cause problems for many people. In the summer, grass pollens, such as timothy grass, can cause allergies. Weeds, such as mugwort and ragweed, pollinate in late summer and autumn. Pollens usually are windborne, and patients with seasonal allergic rhinitis often are said to have "hay fever." The most common cause of seasonal allergic rhinitis is ragweed pollen.

Patients with perennial allergic rhinitis have symptoms throughout the year, instead of only during certain months. They usually require chronic treatment. The most common causes of perennial rhinitis are animal dander and dust mites. In many cases, causative agents are difficult for patients to avoid because many such agents are indoor allergens. Perennial rhinitis may worsen when patients are exposed to nonnatural irritants such as paint, cleaners, or tobacco smoke.

Genetic predisposition plays a major role in the development of allergic rhinitis. The genetically determined tendency to produce increased quantities of IgE expresses itself after prolonged exposure to an allergen. Consequently, allergic rhinitis is uncommon before age 3. Those in later childhood or young adulthood are at greatest risk for development of new symptoms. In general, neither sex exhibits more of a predilection for allergic rhinitis; however, some sources indicate that the perennial form is more common in women.

Patients with a family history of asthma or eczema are more likely to have an allergic basis for rhinitis. The incidence of allergic rhinitis increases by approximately 20% to 30% when one parent has a history and is even higher when both parents have allergic disorders. Studies of pediatric

populations have uncovered certain factors that may increase the expression of allergy: maternal smoking, especially during pregnancy, female gender, and exposure to air pollution (Corren et al., 2014).

PATHOPHYSIOLOGY

Initial exposure to the antigen/allergen stimulates the B lymphocytes (plasma cells) to produce an antigen-specific antibody (IgE) that binds to mast cell membranes (tissue-fixed antibody). The person is now sensitized to that specific antigen and susceptible to allergic reactions when re-exposed to it. On subsequent exposure, the antigen binds to the tissue-fixed IgE antibody and triggers breakdown of the mast cells (degranulation) and release of mediators (histamine, prostaglandins, leukotrienes, kinins, thromboxanes, and serotonin). Histamine, which is stored primarily in mast cells and basophils, is believed to be the mediator most responsible for the clinical signs and symptoms of allergic rhinitis.

Common symptoms in patients with allergic rhinitis are ocular pruritus (itching of the eyes) and conjunctival inflammation (inflammation of the membrane lining the eyelids). Other symptoms of allergic rhinitis are irritability, lethargy, fatigue, and loss of appetite. Once released into the nasal mucosa, the mediators cause vasodilation, increased capillary permeability, increased mucus production, and stimulation of nerve endings. The resulting symptoms are rhinorrhea (profuse, watery nasal discharge), nasal congestion (obstruction by mucus), and nasal pruritus. The most severe symptoms include violent episodes of sneezing (often a dozen or more times in a row) and total obstruction of nasal airflow resulting from copious amounts of mucus (**Figure 48.2**).

The specific IgE antibody made in response to the allergen also may attach to eosinophils. Antigen-provoked degranulation of eosinophils also causes allergic symptoms. The symptoms associated with eosinophils are related to a late-phase allergic response, occurring hours to days after the initial reaction.

DIAGNOSTIC CRITERIA

The diagnosis of allergic rhinitis begins with a thorough history determining the presence of classic signs and symptoms and the time, place, and circumstances under which they occur. A family history is also important because it may establish the familial predisposition to allergy.

Physical examination of the patient with suspected allergic rhinitis begins with assessment of facial appearance, which often includes teary eyes and a red, swollen nose with scaling and crusting from frequent blowing and rubbing with facial tissues. There also may be dark circles under the eyes (allergic shiners), pinched nostrils, and a gaping mouth (from mouth breathing). The nasal mucous membranes are typically pale,

TABLE 48.1

Seasonal Versus Perennial Allergies

Causes of Seasonal Allergies	Causes of Perennial Allergies
Tree pollen (spring)	Mold (indoor)
Grass pollen (spring through fall)	Dust (dust mites)
Weeds (late summer)	Animal dander (skin flakes)
Leaf mold (early spring and late summer)	Animal fur
	Foods (nuts, shellfish, milk, eggs)

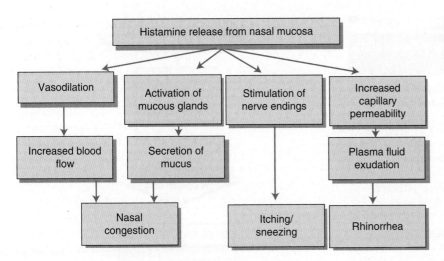

FIGURE 48.2 Results of histamine release in the nasal mucosa.

swollen, and coated with a clear, watery secretion. Some erythema and bleeding may be noted. Swelling, streaks of erythema, and mucus may be present in the posterior pharynx. Other positive physical findings include swelling around and watery discharge from the eyes.

Nasal Smears

Practitioners may use the Wright stain for nasal secretions to detect eosinophils. Although eosinophilia suggests an allergic etiology for rhinitis symptoms (in infectious rhinitis, neutrophils predominate), it is not diagnostic. Conversely, an absence of eosinophilia does not rule out allergy. Eosinophilia may be absent in patients who have superimposed infections or have not had a recent exposure to allergens.

Skin Testing

Skin testing with extracts of suspected allergens usually provides the most effective means of identifying specific sensitivities in patients with allergic rhinitis. In this test, a superficial scratch or prick is made in the skin and a diluted extract of antigen is applied. If the patient has allergen-specific IgE antibodies bound to tissue mast cells, a classic wheal-and-flare reaction appears over the next 15 to 30 minutes. To avoid false-negative results, patients should discontinue the use of antihistamines before they undergo skin testing. Clinicians should individualize this time frame based on the pharmacokinetics of the specific antihistamine that the patient is taking. In most cases, it is adequate to stop taking antihistamines 48 to 72 hours before testing. If patients do not stop taking antihistamines before skin testing, practitioners may mistakenly exclude a diagnosis of allergic rhinitis and subject patients to unnecessary further evaluations.

If the results of the scratch test are negative or unclear, practitioners may administer a more dilute extract of antigen intradermally. Clinicians should not use the intradermal test in patients with a positive response to scratch testing because of the risk of significant allergic reaction, including anaphylaxis.

Radioallergosorbent Testing

Radioallergosorbent testing (RAST) permits in vitro detection of serum IgE antibodies to allergens. Because only 1% of IgE molecules circulate in the blood (the remainder are bound to tissue), RAST results may not reflect the biologic situation. Although RAST is more specific, skin testing is less costly, more sensitive, and simpler to perform. Despite these shortcomings, RAST is helpful when the results of skin testing are unclear. The test is likewise useful when patients are unable to undergo skin testing because of dermatologic conditions or a history of anaphylactic reaction to the suspected allergen. RAST is also indicated for evaluating children younger than age 2 as well as for patients unable to discontinue using antihistamines, as required before skin testing.

Differential Diagnosis

Symptoms similar to those of allergic rhinitis may result from *mechanical nasal obstruction* (foreign body or anatomic factors); as a *side effect of medications* (oral contraceptives, hormone replacement therapy, tricyclic antidepressants, propranolol [Inderal], reserpine [Serpasil], methyldopa [Aldomet], and aspirin-containing compounds); or from *medical conditions associated with increased vasodilation* (e.g., hypothyroidism, cystic fibrosis, tumors, alcoholism, or pregnancy). **Table 48.2** compares the symptoms of seasonal rhinitis with common cold symptoms to illustrate the similarities and differences between these conditions.

Although seasonal rhinitis usually is relatively easy to diagnose, identification of perennial rhinitis may be more elusive. Other nonallergic conditions could cause similar symptoms. *Vasomotor rhinitis* (congestion of the nasal mucosa without infection or allergy) could be difficult to differentiate from perennial rhinitis. In vasomotor rhinitis, however, irritants (e.g., fumes, cold air, high humidity, alcoholic beverages, or emotional stress) rather than allergens usually trigger symptoms. Moreover, vasomotor rhinitis is associated with an absence of nasal, palatal, or conjunctival pruritus. In *nonallergic rhinitis with eosinophilia*, testing likewise fails to indicate a specific allergen.

TABLE 48.2

Symptoms of Seasonal Allergies Versus Respiratory Infections

Symptoms	Seasonal Allergy (Hay Fever)	Upper Respiratory Infection
Head congestion/ runny nose	Yes	Yes
Sneezing	Yes	Sometimes
Itchy, watery eyes	Yes	No
Cough	Usually dry	Dry or productive
Predictable seasonal patterns	Yes	Uncommon
Fever	No	Yes
Short duration (3–7 d)	No	Yes
Long duration (weeks)	Yes	No
Productive cough	Uncommon (except in asthma)	Yes

INITIATING DRUG THERAPY

Allergic rhinitis may be treated through avoidance of the allergen, pharmacologic agents, and immunotherapy. The basic approach to pharmacologic management of allergic rhinitis is the use of antihistamines, nasal decongestants, and intranasal corticosteroids (**Figure 48.3**).

The ideal treatment for allergic rhinitis is avoidance of the offending allergen. Complete avoidance often is not feasible, but most patients usually can reduce exposure. Basic strategies include the use of air conditioners in homes and automobiles to lessen exposure to pollen by keeping windows closed and use of dehumidifiers to discourage the growth of molds and mites. If possible, humidity should be maintained at 30% to 40% throughout the year. Patients can lessen exposure to mites by encasing mattresses in plastic, washing all bedding in very hot water each week, and removing carpeting and upholstered furniture. They can use high-efficiency particulate air (HEPA) cleaners to help filter out dust molds and pollen. Ideally, pets should be removed from the home; however, many patients and their families find doing so unacceptable. At a minimum, families should keep pets out of the allergic person's bedroom, as well as away from heating and cooling systems.

Immunotherapy, also known as *desensitization, hyposensitization,* or *allergy shots,* has been used for decades for the treatment of allergic rhinitis and asthma. It consists of repeated subcutaneous injections of gradually increasing concentrations of the allergens considered to be specifically responsible for the patient's allergy symptoms. However, patients must have documented IgE antibodies to these allergens. The injections are purified extracts of the "trigger" substances, such as ragweed, grass, dust mite, and animal dander. Clinical benefits are related to the administration of high doses of allergens weekly or every other week. The duration of treatment is typically 3 to 5 years, but if there is no improvement after 1 year,

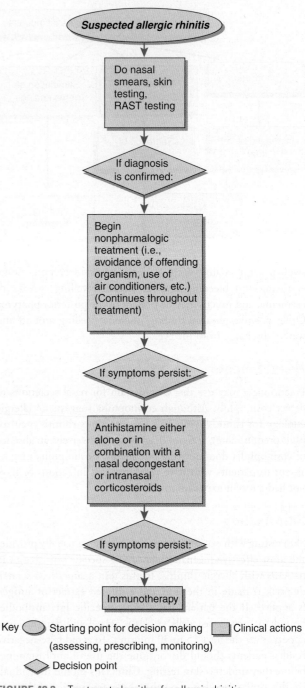

FIGURE 48.3 Treatment algorithm for allergic rhinitis.

consider discontinuing immunotherapy. Treatment is discontinued based on minimal symptoms over two consecutive seasons of exposure. The benefit is derived from a reduction in the percentage of histamine released after immunotherapy compared with before treatment. The result is milder or no symptoms of allergy. Immunotherapy is not the first-line treatment. It is usually initiated when avoidance of the triggers and drug therapy fail to control the symptoms of hay fever and other allergies.

Goals of Drug Therapy

The goal of drug therapy for patients with allergies is to alleviate the symptoms with a little to no adverse effects from medications. This is accomplished primarily through decreasing the release or inhibiting the effect of histamine release and other mediators of inflammation from mast cells. Mast cells are distributed throughout the body; however, the greatest concentration of histamine occurs in the skin, respiratory system, and gastrointestinal (GI) mucosa. Relief of symptoms with minimal drug side effects should lead to an improved quality of life.

Histamine released in the GI tract does not cause allergic symptoms. It may result in hyperacidity by stimulating histamine type 2 (H_2) receptors and lead to peptic ulcer disease or gastroesophageal reflux disease. Treatment of these conditions is with H_2 blockers. It is the histamine released in the skin and respiratory tract (H_1 receptors) that causes classic allergic symptoms. The medications used to treat these symptoms are antihistamines (H_1 blockers), nasal decongestants, intranasal corticosteroids, and intranasal cromolyn. Suggestions for their selection are outlined in the following sections. The decision to treat with medications will depend on the severity of symptoms and patient tolerance of symptoms, as well as the balance of symptoms versus medication side effects. If drug treatment is chosen by the patient, it will be required as long as exposure to the triggers continues or until the patient becomes desensitized to the trigger, either naturally ("outgrowing the allergy") or through immunotherapy (described earlier).

Antihistamines

Antihistamines are classified according to their sedative effects or as first generation (older) and second generation (newer) depending on when they were marketed. The older antihistamines cross the blood–brain barrier, causing the greatest degree of sedation as well as other central nervous system (CNS) effects. These agents can be subclassified on the basis of chemical structure. The main groupings include the ethanolamines, alkylamines, phenothiazines, piperazines, and piperidines.

Mechanism of Action

Antihistamines are drugs that exert their effect in the body primarily by blocking the actions of histamine at receptor sites. They are classified as pharmacologic antagonists of histamine. They do not prevent histamine release, but act by competitive inhibition. Most antihistamines can be classified as either H_1-receptor blockers, which block the smooth muscle response, or H_2-receptor blockers, which block the histaminic stimulation of gastric acid. In general, H_2-receptor blockers are not used for patients with allergies. If the concentration of antihistamine drug at the receptor site exceeds the concentration of histamine, then the effects of histamine are blocked. Antihistamines usually ameliorate itching, sneezing, ocular symptoms, and nasal discharge but do not always reduce nasal congestion.

First-Generation Antihistamines

The first-generation antihistamines, such as diphenhydramine, chlorpheniramine, and brompheniramine, are the older antihistamines. As noted earlier, these tend to be more sedating than newer, second-generation agents such as loratadine or cetirizine.

Dosage

The dosage varies depending on the age and weight of the patient. The frequency of dosing is typically every 4 to 6 hours as needed, but can be upward of every 12 hours depending on the half-life of the drug and the formulation. For example, diphenhydramine (Benadryl) is given every 4 to 6 hours, but brompheniramine is dosed every 12 to 24 hours. These are often over-the-counter (OTC) agents and are supplied as tablets, capsules, elixirs, or suspensions. Further, these formulations come in a variety of flavors, and some are even free of dye.

Time Frame for Response

The onset of action of these agents typically ranges from 15 to 30 minutes and lasts nearly as long as the dosing interval. Those agents with a longer half-life will take longer to get to steady state, but the initial effect is often seen fairly rapidly.

Some regular users of antihistamines find that tolerance, or drug failure, develops after several weeks or months. One reason for this decreased effectiveness is that some antihistamines are capable of hepatic enzyme induction, resulting in increased metabolism in the liver. Essentially, the antihistamine drug hastens its own destruction and removal from circulation. The various antihistamine classes differ in their capacity to induce hepatic enzymes. Some practitioners have found that if tolerance develops, patients may benefit by switching to another antihistamine in a different chemical category. The effectiveness of this technique has not been evaluated by controlled studies.

Contraindications

First-generation antihistamine therapy is contraindicated in lactating mothers. Additionally, the anticholinergic side effects of the first-generation antihistamines put patients with narrow-angle glaucoma at risk for an increase in intraocular pressure. Similarly, men with benign prostatic hyperplasia (BPH) should avoid these agents due to the drug's ability to decrease urine flow. The sedating effects of these agents should also be considered when patients are required to perform hazardous tasks or drive. Because of the sedating and anticholinergic properties, first-generation antihistamines are on the Beers list, a list of drugs that should be avoided or used with extreme caution in elderly patients (AGS, 2012). Antihistamines are recommended for the treatment of itching and rhinitis in pregnant women; diphenhydramine is pregnancy category B.

Adverse Events

Knowledge of the chemical category to which an antihistamine belongs can help determine the relative degree of sedation and anticholinergic effects associated with the particular agent. In general, the ethanolamine derivatives, such as diphenhydramine, and the phenothiazine derivatives, such as promethazine (Phenergan), cause the greatest degree of sedation and anticholinergic effects. The most problematic anticholinergic effects are dry mouth, blurred vision, urinary hesitancy, constipation, confusion, and mental cloudiness.

The sedative effects of the older antihistamines vary among patients and may not cause problems for some. Tolerance to the sedative effect develops, and many patients find that sedation either disappears or becomes less bothersome after several days of continued use. Nonetheless, sedation may affect the patient's acceptance of the older antihistamine drugs.

Less Sedating Antihistamines

More recently, antihistamines have been developed that do not cross the blood–brain barrier to the extent exhibited by the older agents. These newer antihistamines, commonly referred to as *NSAs*, are considered to act peripherally and do not produce sedation or cause clinically important changes in mental status. In general, the anticholinergic effects of these agents are also minimal. Cetirizine, a metabolite of the antipruritic hydroxyzine (Atarax), is not always accepted as an NSA because it is reported to have a higher incidence of sedation than the other newer antihistamines. It is generally classified as a peripherally acting antihistamine and is often still listed in the same category. Nonetheless, it is an effective antihistamine approved by the U.S. Food and Drug Administration (FDA) for seasonal and perennial rhinitis. The NSAs are listed and compared in **Table 48.3**.

TABLE 48.3

Overview of Selected Antihistamines and Decongestants

Generic (Trade) Name and Dosage	Selected Adverse Events	Contraindications	Special Considerations
Nonsedating Antihistamines			
cetirizine (Zyrtec) 5–10 mg PO daily Children 2–6 y: 2.5 mg daily 6–11 y: 5–10 mg daily	Somnolence, dry mouth, pharyngitis, dizziness	Known hypersensitivity to cetirizine or hydroxyzine	Renal or hepatic impairment: Adults—5 mg qd; Children—not recommended Pregnancy category B
levocetirizine (Xyzal) 2.5–5 mg PO daily Children 2–5 y: 1.25 mg daily 6–11 y: 2.5 mg PO daily	Same as cetirizine	Known hypersensitivity to levocetirizine or cetirizine, end-stage renal disease, renal impairment in children	Use with caution in patients with renal impairment. Pregnancy category B
fexofenadine (Allegra) 60 mg PO bid 180 mg tablet PO daily Children 2–11 y: 30 mg bid	Viral infection (cold, influenza), nausea, dysmenorrhea, drowsiness, dyspepsia, fatigue	Known hypersensitivity to any of its ingredients	Erythromycin and ketoconazole may increase plasma levels of fexofenadine. Pregnancy category C
loratadine (Claritin) 10 mg PO qd Children 2–5 y: 5 mg daily	Headache, somnolence, fatigue, dry mouth	Known hypersensitivity to any of its ingredients	Give same dose every other day in renal or hepatic impairment. Pregnancy category B
desloratadine (Clarinex) 5 mg PO daily Children 2–5 y: 1.25 mg daily 6–11 y: 2.5 mg daily	Same as loratadine	Known hypersensitivity to any ingredients or loratadine	Give same dose every other day in renal or hepatic impairment. Pregnancy category C
Intranasal Antihistamines			
olopatadine (Patanase) two sprays per nostril twice daily Children 6–11 y: One spray per nostril twice daily	Headache, somnolence, cough, epistaxis, throat irritation, bitter taste, dry mouth	None	Amount of drug per actuation (spray): 127 mcg
azelastine (Astelin or Astepro nasal spray) 1–2 sprays in each nostril bid; 100 doses per bottle	Bitter taste, headache, somnolence, nasal burning, pharyngitis, dry mouth, paroxysmal sneezing, nausea, rhinitis, fatigue, dizziness	Known hypersensitivity	Amount of drug per spray: 137 mcg (Astelin), 205.5 mcg (Astepro) Astepro may be dosed two sprays once daily rather than BID. Not recommended in children 6–12 y

TABLE 48.3

Overview of Selected Antihistamines and Decongestants

Generic (Trade) Name and Dosage	Selected Adverse Events	Contraindications	Special Considerations
Oral Nasal Decongestants			
pseudoephedrine 60 mg q6h (240 mg); extended release, 120 mg q12h; controlled release 240 mg q24h Children 6–12 y: 30 mg q6h (120 mg) Children 2–6 y: 15 mg q6h (60 mg)	Headache, insomnia, dry mouth, somnolence, nervousness, dizziness, fatigue, dyspepsia, nausea, pharyngitis, anorexia, thirst	Hypersensitivity to drug or its components, use within 14 days of an MAO inhibitor	Extended release should not be recommended for children <12 y. Pregnancy category C
phenylephrine 10–20 mg q4h Children 6–12 y: 10 mg q4h	Same as pseudoephedrine	Same as pseudoephedrine	Pregnancy category C
Intranasal Cromolyn			
cromolyn (Nasalcrom nasal solution) Patients ≥2 y: one spray in each nostril three to six times a day until symptom relief, then every 8–12 h	Common: burning, stinging, or irritation inside nose, increase in sneezing Rare: cough, headache, unpleasant taste, bloody nose	Hypersensitivity to cromolyn or the formula; acute asthma attacks	Comes in 13-mL bottle and 26-mL bottle—13-mL bottle = 100 sprays, 26-mL bottle = 200 sprays Not recommended in children <2 y

Dosage

Loratadine (Claritin) is dosed as 10 mg once daily for adults and children ages 6 and older. For children ages 2 to 5, the dose is 5 mg once daily. Cetirizine (Zyrtec) is given 5 to 10 mg once daily for children older than age 6 and adults. The lower dosage can be used for younger children or for patients with less severe symptoms. Children ages 2 to 5 should be started on 2.5 mg once daily. Levocetirizine and desloratadine are generally half the dose of cetirizine and loratadine. Fexofenadine (Allegra) doses are for adults and children age 12 and older. The starting dose is 60 mg twice daily or 180 mg once daily for the extended-release formulation. Children ages 6 to 11 should start at 30 mg twice a day.

Time Frame for Response

This class of agents has a rapid onset of action, with a time to maximum effect ranging from 1 to 2.5 hours. The half-life of these drugs is 8 to 28 hours, leading to a 1- to 3-day delay in reaching a steady state. Food can delay the time to peak of cetirizine and loratadine, but not fexofenadine.

Contraindications

The lower propensity for anticholinergic effects allows for wider use of NSAs in the elderly, patients with glaucoma, and men with BPH because they do not share the same contraindications. NSAs are contraindicated in patients with previous hypersensitivity to these drugs and are not recommended in lactating mothers. Using antihistamines is generally considered safe during pregnancy, although the NSAs are generally considered second line.

Adverse Events

Overall, this class of drugs is well tolerated in patients. Common adverse events include headache, dry mouth, dyspepsia, nausea, and fatigue. See **Table 48.3** for specific agents. It is important to note that cetirizine and levocetirizine are known to be more sedating than the other drugs in this class. More serious but rare side effects include dizziness, myalgia, somnolence, and dysmenorrhea.

Interactions

While loratadine and desloratadine do not have any significant drug interactions, fexofenadine does have some interactions that should be clinically considered. Fexofenadine concentrations may be increased by azole antifungals and erythromycin. Antacids and grapefruit juice administered with fexofenadine may decrease the absorption of fexofenadine. There is also a remote possibility that fexofenadine may prolong the QT interval on an electrocardiogram when administered with other drugs that concurrently prolong the QT interval. Cetirizine or levocetirizine administered with sedating drugs may increase sedation.

Intranasal Antihistamines

Azelastine (Astelin) and olopatadine (Patanase) intranasal antihistamines are also available to treat allergic rhinitis. In placebo-controlled trials, they significantly improved the symptoms of rhinorrhea, sneezing, and nasal pruritus. The adverse events that occurred more frequently than in the patients treated with placebos were bitter taste (19.7% vs. 0.6% for placebo) and somnolence (11.5% vs. 5.4%) (Astelin Package Insert, 2014). These agents still have some systemic absorption, so it is important to remember that they may cause side effects and interact with allergy skin tests. Intranasal prescribing information is noted in **Table 48.3**.

Nasal Decongestants

Mechanism of Action

Nasal decongestants are sympathomimetic amines chemically related to norepinephrine, a major neurotransmitter of the sympathetic nervous system. These drugs are vasoconstrictors. They offer relief from nasal congestion by constricting the blood vessels of the nasal mucosa that have been dilated by histamine and are available in either oral or topical nasal formulations. The results are a shrinking of swollen nasal passages and more air movement to make breathing easier. However, just as norepinephrine is a CNS stimulant, so are the synthetic oral and topical (nasal) decongestants, which is an important clinical consideration.

Dosage

Dosing for common nasal decongestant products is noted in **Table 48.3**. Many decongestants are available in combination with antihistamines. Fixed combination products containing antihistamines and sympathomimetic amines are convenient, but the effective dose of oral decongestants varies among patients. If use of a fixed combination causes side effects or does not relieve symptoms, then clinicians should titrate with single agents to achieve the required dosage.

Because these agents are available OTC, counsel patients to read all labels carefully in order to select a product with only the components that they need to treat symptoms. Many of these combination products may also contain pain relievers or caffeine in addition to antihistamines and decongestants. If patients are also taking separate doses of pain relievers, they could be in danger of overdose.

Starting in September 2006, the sale of OTC pseudoephedrine has been restricted to "behind-the-counter" status, which means that customers may not directly access any products containing this drug. This could be behind the pharmacy counter or in a locked cabinet. This change was the result of the "Combat Methamphetamine Epidemic Act of 2005," which sought to deter citizens from synthesizing illicit methamphetamine from pseudoephedrine-containing products. Purchasers are not required to have a prescription, but must present photo identification. The seller must keep a record of the purchaser's name and information, along with the quantity purchased. The quantity limits may vary per state, but most states have a maximum of 3.6 g that may be purchased in a 24-hour period; many states set a limit of 9 g in a 30-day period (FDA, 2014). Some states have also imposed a minimum age for purchasing pseudoephedrine (e.g., 18 years and older).

Time Frame for Response

The onset of action for these agents, in immediate-release form, is typically 15 to 30 minutes with a peak response within 30 to 60 minutes. The half-life of pseudoephedrine is 9 to 16 hours, but the effect of the decongestant activity wears off within 4 to 6 hours after administration.

Contraindications

Caution should be used when recommending OTC oral decongestants. Patients with high blood pressure, heart disease, hyperthyroidism, narrow-angle glaucoma, seizure disorders, and BPH may see exacerbation of their disease. In addition, use of oral decongestants is contraindicated in patients taking monoamine oxidase (MAO) inhibitors within 14 days of the administration of pseudoephedrine. Pseudoephedrine and phenylephrine cause the release of norepinephrine into the synapse, and MAO inhibitors inhibit the enzymatic degradation of norepinephrine. As such, the concomitant use of these agents increases the sympathetic activity of the nervous system and can lead to hypertensive crisis. Nasal decongestants are not recommended during pregnancy, and pseudoephedrine should be avoided during the first trimester of pregnancy.

Adverse Events

Oral decongestants constrict blood vessels throughout the body and also act as CNS stimulants, thus increasing blood pressure and heart rate and causing palpitations. Stimulation of the CNS can lead to insomnia, irritability, restlessness, and headache. Many patients find that they can use oral decongestants only during the daytime because the stimulatory effects of these drugs can cause nervousness, agitation, and insomnia.

Topical (Intranasal) Decongestants

Intranasal application (sprays or drops) of sympathomimetic amines provides a prompt and dramatic decrease of nasal congestion. A rebound phenomenon (rhinitis medicamentosa), however, often follows topical application of these drugs. In this scenario, the nasal mucous membrane becomes even more congested and edematous as the drug's vasoconstrictor effect wears off. This secondary congestion is believed to result from ischemia caused by the drug's intensive local vasoconstriction and local irritation of the agent itself. If the use of a topical decongestant is limited to 3 or 4 days, rebound congestion is minimal. With chronic use or overuse of these drugs, rebound nasal stuffiness may become quite pronounced. This phenomenon may begin a vicious cycle, leading to more frequent use of the drug that causes the problem. Should this occur, patients should discontinue topical decongestant therapy. They may use an oral decongestant, isotonic saline drops or spray, or both instead (**Table 48.4**). Side effects from topically administered agents include local irritation and rebound congestion.

TABLE 48.4

Topical Nasal Decongestants

Generic	Trade	Concentration (%)	Patient Age			
			>6 mo	2–6 y	6–12 y	>12 y
phenylephrine	Neo-Synephrine	0.125	Yes	Yes	Yes	Yes
	Neo-Synephrine	0.25	No	No	Yes	Yes
	Neo-Synephrine	0.5	No	No	No	Yes
naphazoline	Privine	0.05	No	No	No	Yes
oxymetazoline	Afrin	0.05	No	Yes	Yes	Yes
tetrahydrozoline	Tyzine Pediatric	0.05	No	Yes	Yes	Yes
	Tyzine	0.1	No	No	Yes	Yes
xylometazoline	Triaminic Nasal and Sinus Congestion	0.05	No	Yes	Yes	Yes

Intranasal Corticosteroids

Nasal-inhaled corticosteroids are the most effective forms of therapy for allergic rhinitis. They help to relieve congestion and rhinorrhea by limiting the late-phase response and reducing inflammation. Corticosteroids have a wide range of inhibitory activities against multiple cell types (e.g., mast cells, eosinophils, neutrophils, macrophages, and lymphocytes) and mediators of inflammation (e.g., histamine, eicosanoids, leukotrienes, and cytokines).

Mechanism of Action

Corticosteroids exert their anti-inflammatory effect by disabling the cells that present antigen to antibody. Interfering with the antigen–antibody reaction reduces the stimulus for mast cell degranulation. With reduced mast cell degranulation, secretion of cytokines is diminished. The result is a weaker inflammatory reaction with milder or no symptoms of runny nose, nasal congestion, itching, and sneezing.

Dosage

The dosage of the individual intranasal steroids is listed in **Table 48.5**. In general, mometasone furoate, fluticasone propionate, and budesonide have been rated as most potent in vitro. However, these differences have not been shown to translate into meaningful clinical differences in patients. Intranasal corticosteroids must be primed before initial use. Clinicians should counsel patients to squeeze the pump a few times until a fine spray appears. If patients do not use the pump for more than 1 week, they should reprime it.

Time Frame for Response

The therapeutic effects of intranasal corticosteroids are not immediate, but will begin working within 3 to 12 hours. Clinicians must counsel patients that they may not experience maximal effects for 1 to 2 weeks if they are using intranasal steroids continuously. Although continuous use is more

efficacious, as-needed dosing has also been shown to be useful in patients with seasonal allergic rhinitis. Intranasal corticosteroids should be initiated 2 to 4 weeks before the start of allergy season in patients with recurrent seasonal allergic rhinitis for maximal benefit.

If nasal blockage is severe, patients should use a topical nasal decongestant for the first 2 to 3 days to reduce the swelling and increase the delivery of corticosteroid to the nasal mucosa. Use of nasal corticosteroids should not continue beyond 3 weeks in the absence of significant symptomatic improvement, according to the manufacturers' professional product information.

Contraindications

All intranasal corticosteroids are designated as pregnancy category C. This means that either animal reproduction studies have shown adverse effects on the fetus and there are no controlled studies in women or there are no studies in women or animals. The drug should be given only if potential benefit justifies potential risk.

Adverse Events

These agents are supplied as aqueous solutions in manually activated metered-dose nasal spray pumps, with separate patient instructions for use with every package. Some of these formulations have a flowery odor that some patients may find annoying. Local side effects such as irritation, bleeding, and septal perforation may occur but are rare; ensure that patients are using these products correctly in order to minimize these side effects.

Overall, intranasal steroids do not achieve significant systemic concentrations, although the effects of long-term systemic absorption could be concerning. Probably, the most concerning adverse effects of intranasal steroids are the possibility of decreasing the rate of growth and suppressing the hypothalamic–pituitary–adrenal axis. Transient effects on growth in children have been noted, but the studies looking at this

TABLE 48.5

Intranasal Corticosteroid Prescribing Information

Drug	Brand Name (Manufacturer)	Amount of Drug per Spray/Doses per Bottle	How Supplied	Suggested Dose Adult	Suggested Dose Pediatric (6–12 y)
beclomethasone	Beconase AQ (GlaxoSmithKline)	42 mcg/200	25-g amber glass bottle with spray pump	One or two sprays in each nostril bid spray pump	Same as adult
budesonide	Rhinocort Aqua (Astra)	32 mcg/120	8.6-g bottle with spray pump	One to four sprays in each nostril daily	Same as adult
ciclesonide	Omnaris (Sepracor)	50 mcg/120	12.5-g bottle with spray pump	Two sprays in each nostril daily	Same as adult
flunisolide	N/A	25 µg/200	25-mL bottle with spray pump	Two sprays in each nostril bid	Same as adult
fluticasone	Flonase (GlaxoSmithKline)	50 mcg/120	16-g bottle with spray pump, available OTC	Two sprays in each nostril daily	One spray in each nostril daily
	Veramyst (GlaxoSmithKline)	27.5 mcg/120	10-g bottle with spray pump	Two sprays in each nostril daily	One spray in each nostril daily
mometasone	Nasonex (Schering)	50 mcg/120	17-g bottle with spray pump	Two sprays in each nostril daily	One spray in each nostril daily
triamcinolone	Nasacort AQ (Aventis)	55 mcg/100	10-g aerosol canister	One spray up to four sprays in each nostril daily	One spray up to two sprays in each nostril qd

end point have varied widely. At normal recommended doses, fluticasone, mometasone, and budesonide have not shown growth suppression. The only study to show growth suppression used higher than recommended doses for long periods, so this should not be a serious concern in clinical practice.

All aqueous preparations contain preservatives. Benzalkonium chloride, which may cause ciliary dysfunction, is the preservative in the beclomethasone, flunisolide, fluticasone, mometasone, and triamcinolone products, whereas budesonide contains potassium sorbate as the preservative.

Interactions

Interactions with other drugs are generally not a concern due to low systemic absorption of intranasal corticosteroids.

Intranasal Cromolyn

Cromolyn is classified as a mast cell stabilizer. It prevents antigen-induced degranulation, thereby inhibiting the release of histamine and other cytokines that mediate inflammatory cell function. Cromolyn is of no value in treating acute allergic rhinitis. It is helpful only in preventing the nasal symptoms of allergic rhinitis. Treatment is more effective if it begins 2 to 4 weeks before exposure and continues throughout the exposure period. Intranasal cromolyn is available to patients as Nasalcrom 4% Nasal Solution. It does not require a prescription. Patient use information is noted in **Table 48.3**.

Selecting the Most Appropriate Agent

Nasal symptoms of allergic rhinitis include watery rhinorrhea (runny nose), paroxysmal sneezing (sudden fits of sneezing), nasal congestion (stuffy nose, sinus headache, or both), and postnasal drip that may cause coughing. Allergic rhinitis also may involve the conjunctiva (allergic conjunctivitis). The resulting symptoms are ocular pruritus (itching eyes), lacrimation (watery eyes), conjunctival hyperemia (bloodshot eyes), and chemosis (swollen eyelids). Drug treatment must be tailored to address the most bothersome symptoms. See **Box 48.2** and **Figure 48.3** for a stepwise approach to treating allergic rhinitis. **Table 48.6** lists the recommended treatment order for allergies.

First-Line Therapy

Intranasal corticosteroids are the most potent agents available for the relief of *established* seasonal or perennial rhinitis. They provide efficacy with substantially reduced side effects compared with oral corticosteroids. Selection of the best agent mostly depends on the patient's insurance formulary.

However, due to the long time frame for response and that they may not be as effective for systemic symptoms, these agents are often given in combination with antihistamines. First-generation antihistamines were considered first-line agents for the prevention and treatment of allergic symptoms. However, the sedative side effects of the traditional antihistamines limit

> ## BOX 48.2
> ### A Stepwise Approach Is Used to Manage the Symptoms of Allergic Rhinitis
>
> 1. Identify the offending allergens by history with confirmation of the allergy by skin test.
> 2. Teach the patient to avoid the offending allergens.
> 3. For mild symptoms, prophylactic treatment with cromolyn nasal spray (Nasalcrom) or treatment with an antihistamine/decongestant combination may be necessary.
> 4. For prominent symptoms, begin with topical corticosteroid nasal spray.
> 5. For treatment failures despite avoidance and pharmacotherapy, progress to immunotherapy.

their usefulness in patients who must remain awake and alert. Fortunately, NSAs, also known as *newer* or *second-generation antihistamines*, cause minimal sedation because they do not cross the blood–brain barrier into the CNS.

The various first- and second-generation antihistamines are equally effective in treating symptoms of allergic rhinitis. Product selection is based on dosing frequency (i.e., duration of action), potential for adverse effects, and cost. Second-generation antihistamines may be given only once or twice a day, and they are relatively nonsedating. First-generation antihistamines are given three to four times a day. Some products

TABLE 48.6

Recommended Order of Treatment for Allergies

Order	Agents	Comments
First line	Intranasal corticosteroids	Intranasal corticosteroids are the most potent agents available for relief of established seasonal or perennial rhinitis
Second line	Antihistamines/ nasal decongestants	Either first- or second-generation agent can be used
		Product selection is based on dosing frequency, potential for adverse effects, and cost
		Second-generation antihistamines may be given only once or twice a day, and they are relatively nonsedating. First-generation antihistamines are given three to four times a day. Pseudoephedrine and phenylephrine are the most popular oral nasal decongestants
Third line	Intranasal cromolyn	Must be used prophylactically

are available in long-acting dosage forms that may be given only twice a day. While more sedating, first-generation antihistamines are also significantly less expensive than the second-generation drugs. These agents have the best results when patients take them before exposure to a known allergen. During seasonal attack, patients may need to take antihistamines around-the-clock for maximal effectiveness.

Second-Line Therapy

Because antihistamines do not reduce nasal congestion, they are often used in combination with nasal decongestants. Pseudoephedrine and phenylephrine are the most popular oral nasal decongestants. Nasal decongestants are α-adrenergic receptor agonists. As such, they stimulate α-adrenergic receptors, causing vasoconstriction in the nasal mucosa, decreasing congestion, and opening nasal passages. Side effects include CNS and cardiovascular stimulation. Elevation in blood pressure may also occur. Many prescription and nonprescription drugs contain a combined antihistamine and nasal decongestant. Some examples are given in **Table 48.3**.

Topical (intranasal) decongestants avoid systemic adverse effects. Prolonged use leads to rebound nasal congestion, however, so they are impractical for seasonal or perennial allergies. Their use should be limited to short periods (a few days).

Third-Line Therapy

Cromolyn, in the form of a metered-dose nasal spray, could be considered a first-line treatment for allergic rhinitis, but it is a prophylactic measure only. It is classified as a mast cell stabilizer in that it prevents or attenuates the allergen activation of nasal mast cells. To be efficacious, cromolyn must be administered continuously (usually four times a day) during seasonal allergen exposure or immediately before an anticipated exposure such as animal dander.

Intranasal cromolyn is an alternative to antihistamines and nasal decongestants for allergic rhinitis. It generally is considered less effective than intranasal corticosteroids, but it is virtually free of side effects.

Special Population Considerations
Pediatric

If one parent has allergies, the child has a 50% chance of having allergies. Allergies may also be more common in children who were formula fed, of low birth weight, or exposed to tobacco smoke early in life. In childhood, more boys have allergic rhinitis than do girls, but this difference begins to disappear after adolescence. No sex differences are found in adults.

To determine the dose of allergy medication for a child, practitioners should use weight if possible. Otherwise, they may base according to age. The official product literature usually provides child dosage recommendations by age and weight. Parents should also be counseled to look at package labeling carefully and use dose recommendations for their child's weight if the directions specify. Also, parents should use appropriate teaspoon or tablespoon measurements rather than kitchen utensils. Counsel patients to ask the pharmacist at their local pharmacy if they are not sure if they have an accurate measuring tool.

In determining the dose of medication for a child, practitioners must recognize that infants and small children are not merely "scaled-down" adults. Organs such as the GI tract, liver, and kidneys are not developed enough in children for them to handle medications. Estimating a child's dose based on the adult dose is not always safe. Most pharmaceutical manufacturers do not provide such comprehensive pediatric dosing guidelines. Usually, an age range for children's doses is stated in the official package insert or on the commercial package. If not, prescribers should contact the manufacturer or consult with a specialist who is experienced with the treatment.

As noted earlier, a major consideration in prescribing intranasal steroids in children is the impact on growth. The FDA has approved the use of mometasone and fluticasone furoate for children older than age 2, fluticasone propionate for children older than age 4, and ciclesonide, budesonide, and flunisolide for children age 6 and older. The other agents are approved for use in children older than age 6.

Geriatric

Although few factors provoke rhinitis in older adults, treatments need to be more tailored because of slower metabolism and the potential for side effects, especially in the CNS. Also, this population is more likely to be taking multiple medications and therefore runs a greater risk of drug interactions than most other patients.

Women

In women, allergic rhinitis symptoms may worsen during pregnancy. The antihistamines diphenhydramine, loratadine, and cetirizine are pregnancy category B agents, whereas desloratadine and fexofenadine are category C agents. All intranasal steroids are category C agents.

MONITORING PATIENT RESPONSE

Assessing the efficacy of treatment requires monitoring the patient's adherence to the drug therapy plan, quality of life, and degree of satisfaction with the care provided. **Box 48.3** could be a useful office tool for this purpose.

PATIENT EDUCATION

Patient education is extremely important in the prevention and management of allergy symptoms. Teaching each patient about the causes of allergic reactions, how triggers evoke symptoms, the various medications available and their use, when to self-treat and when to seek medical help, and how to assess whether treatment is working is highly desirable and appropriate during an office visit. But comprehensive teaching may not be practical because of time constraints. It may be more efficient to

determine what the patient *does not* understand and fill in the gaps at that time. For example, at the end of the visit, practitioners could ask the patient three very basic questions about treatment:

- What is the name of the medication you are taking for allergy symptoms?
- What beneficial effects do you expect, and what side effects may occur?
- How do you take the medication (i.e., dose, time of day, with meals, and what to avoid taking with it)?

If the patient can articulate the correct answers to these questions, little more needs to be discussed about treatment. Practitioners could provide verbally or in writing those things that the patient does not know or understand. Also, they should encourage patients to accept written materials that pharmacists provide when they fill prescriptions and to question any ambiguous or contradictory information.

Drug Information

A variety of sources provide information regarding the treatment of allergic rhinitis. The American Association of Allergies, Asthma, and Immunology provides practice parameters for the treatment of allergic rhinitis (www.aaaai.org). Further, the FDA provides drug information specific to the product, particularly in relation to children or pregnant women.

Patient-Oriented Information Sources

The American Association of Allergies, Asthma, and Immunology provides patient-directed information (http://www.aaaai.org/patients/resources/fastfacts/rhinitis.stm). Similarly, the FDA has information regarding medications in an easy-to-use format for patients.

Complementary and Alternative Medications

There is some suggestion that acupuncture and biofeedback may be effective means of treating allergic rhinitis. However, controlled studies evaluating the effectiveness of these treatment modalities are lacking. Further, although few studies have examined the effectiveness of specific homeopathic therapies, *nux vomica* has been used to help in the treatment of nasal congestion and discharge.

ALLERGIC CONJUNCTIVITIS

The signs and symptoms of allergic conjunctivitis result from the same allergens that cause allergic rhinitis. Mast cells are abundant in the eyelid and conjunctiva, but are infrequently found in the eye. This limits allergic ocular inflammation to the lining of the eyelid and the ocular surface (the conjunctiva).

Histamine and arachidonic acid derivatives are the mediators that probably cause most ocular signs and symptoms. Mast cell activation, however, also leads to recruitment of

MONITORING SIGNS, SYMPTOMS, AND FUNCTIONAL STATUS

- Has your allergy been better or worse since your last visit?
- In the past 2 weeks, how many days have you had: (*Ask the patient to tell you how symptoms developed, what they were like, and how long they lasted.*)

  A runny, stuffy, or itchy nose?

  Any wheezing or coughing?

  Any hives or swelling?

  Eczema or other skin rashes?

  Reactions to foods?

  Reactions to insects?

- Since your last visit, how many days has your allergy caused you to:

  Miss work or school?

  Reduce your activities?

  (For caregivers) change your activity because of your child's allergies?

- Since your last visit, have you had any unscheduled or emergency department visits or hospital stays?
- Since your last visit, have you had any times when your allergy symptoms were a lot worse than usual?

  If yes, what do you think caused the symptoms to get worse?

  If yes, what did you do to control the symptoms?

- Have there been any changes in your home, school, or work environment (e.g., new smokers or pets)? Any new hobbies or recreational activities?

- Has there been difficulty sleeping at night due to symptoms of allergy?

MONITORING PHARMACOTHERAPY

- What medications are you taking?
- How often do you take each medication? How much do you take each time?
- Have you had any unusual reactions to your medications?
- Have you missed or stopped taking any regular doses of your medications for any reason?
- Have you had trouble filling your prescriptions (e.g., for financial reasons, not on formulary)?
- Have you tried any other medications?
- Has your allergy medicine caused you any problems (e.g., sleepiness, bad taste, sore throat)?
- Have you had any nighttime awakenings?

MONITORING PATIENT–PROVIDER COMMUNICATION AND PATIENT SATISFACTION

- What questions do you have about your allergy management?
- What problems have you had in following your allergy management plan, such as taking your medications or reducing your exposure to allergens?
- Has anything prevented you from getting the treatment you need for your allergies?
- Have the costs of your allergy treatment interfered with your ability to get appropriate care?
- How can we improve your allergy care?

This information is provided by the Asthma and Allergy Foundation of America (AAFA) as part of its educational outreach to patients and their caregivers. The information was adapted from the 2007 National Asthma Education and Prevention Program's Guidelines for the Diagnosis and Treatment of Asthma published by the National Heart, Lung, and Blood Institute.

eosinophils, which can be found in the conjunctiva 3 to 5 hours after mast cell degranulation.

Many patients experience ocular symptoms only when allergens directly contact the eyes. For example, patients with sensitivity to cat dander may not have reactions in a room with cats but experience symptoms if they bring their hands to their face. Patients who have symptoms even without direct contact need to be particularly rigorous in their efforts to eliminate or avoid allergens in their homes, workplaces, or schools. Eye rubbing not only introduces allergens into the eye but also may degranulate mast cells mechanically.

Practitioners should encourage patients to apply cool compresses to their eyelids rather than rubbing their eyes to alleviate symptoms. Artificial tears also may reduce symptoms

and wash away allergens and inflammatory mediators from the conjunctiva. Often, however, these approaches are inadequate. In such cases, patients require pharmacologic intervention. The types of eye drop medications used to treat allergic conjunctivitis are corticosteroids, antihistamines, vasoconstrictor/antihistamine combinations, mast cell stabilizers, and nonsteroidal anti-inflammatory drugs (NSAIDs).

First-generation oral antihistamines, which can help reduce ocular itching, may cause more problems by decreasing tear production due to anticholinergic effects. NSAIDs provide temporary relief of ocular itching due to seasonal allergic conjunctivitis. They work by inhibiting biosynthesis of prostaglandin, a mediator of pain and inflammation. See Chapter 17 for more information on treating Allergic Conjunctivitis.

CASE STUDY*

G.B. an 18-year-old African American female college student, lives on campus with three other students. Her home is approximately 100 miles away. She has been at college since the beginning of the fall semester, approximately 2 weeks. She presents today with a chief complaint of fits of sneezing (sometimes 10 in a row); a runny, itchy, stuffy nose; and red, tearing eyes. Her temperature is 99°F; blood pressure is 118/78. She denies cough and headache. Her chest is clear. Her past medical history is unremarkable, except for "hay fever" when she was younger, which she "outgrew" during high school. These symptoms are the same. She is having difficulty studying because of the sneezing and itching nose, and she is embarrassed to be in class with these symptoms. She was nervous about meeting the challenges of college and making new friends. Her local physician prescribed lorazepam (Ativan) 1.0 mg as needed for stress, anxiety, or both. So far, she has taken two doses of a prescription for 30 tablets.

DIAGNOSIS: ALLERGIC RHINITIS/CONJUNCTIVITIS

1. List specific goals for treatment for G.B.
2. What drug therapy would you prescribe? Why?
3. What are the parameters for monitoring success of the therapy?
4. Discuss specific patient education based on the prescribed therapy.
5. List one or two adverse reactions for the selected agent that would cause you to change therapy.
6. What would be the choice for second-line therapy?
7. What over-the-counter and/or alternative medications would be appropriate for G.B.?
8. What lifestyle changes would you recommend to G.B?
9. Describe one or two drug–drug or drug–food interaction for the selected agent.

* Answers can be found online.

Bibliography

*Starred references are cited in the text.

*Astelin Package Insert. (2014). MEDA Pharmaceuticals, Somerset, NJ. October 2014.

Choo K. J., Simons F. E., & Sheikh A. (2012). Glucocorticoids for the treatment of anaphylaxis. *Cochrane Database of Systematic Reviews, 4,* CD007596.

*Corren J., Baroody F. M., & Pawankar R. (2014). Allergic and nonallergic rhinitis. In *Middleton's allergy: Principles and practice* (8th ed.). St. Louis, MO: Elsevier.

Dipiro, J. (2008). Allergic and pseudoallergic drug reactions. In J. T. Dipiro (Ed.), *Pharmacotherapy: A pathophysiologic approach* (7th ed.). New York, NY: McGraw-Hill Medical.

Gendo, K., & Larson, E. B. (2004). Evidence-based diagnostic strategies for evaluating suspected allergic rhinitis. *Annals of Internal Medicine, 140,* 278–289.

Lichtenstein, L., & Fauci, A. (1996). *Current therapy in allergy, immunology, and rheumatology* (5th ed.). St. Louis, MO: Mosby-Year Book.

Lieberman, P., Kemp, S. F., Oppenheimer, J., et al. (2010). The diagnosis and management of anaphylaxis: An updated practice parameter. *Journal of Allergy and Clinical Immunology, 115,* S483–S523.

Middleton, E., Reed, C., Ellis, E., et al. (Eds.). (1998). *Allergy: Principles and practice* (5th ed., Vols. I and II). St. Louis, MO: Mosby-Year Book.

*Nairn, R., & Helbert, M. (2007). Hypersensitivity reactions. In R. Nairn & M. Helbert(Eds.), *Immunology for medical students.* St. Louis, MO: Elsevier.

National Institute of Allergy and Infectious Disease. (1997). *Disease state management sourcebook.* New York, NY: Faulkner and Gray.

*National Institute of Allergy and Infectious Disease. (2015). Pollen allergy fact sheet. Retrieved from http://www.niaid.nih.gov/topics/allergicDiseases/Documents/PollenAllergyFactSheet.pdf on July 2015.

Patterson, R., Grammar, L., & Greenberg, P. (1997). *Allergic diseases: Diagnosis and management* (5th ed.). Philadelphia, PA: Lippincott-Raven.

*The American Geriatrics Society (AGS) 2012 Beers Criteria Update Expert Panel. (2012). American Geriatrics Society updated Beers Criteria for potentially inappropriate medication use in older adults. *Journal of American Geriatrics Society, 60,* 616–631.

*U.S. Food and Drug Administration. (2014). *Legal requirements for the sale and purchase of drug products containing pseudoephedrine, ephedrine, and phenylpropanolamine.* Retrieved from http://www.fda.gov/Drugs/DrugSafety/InformationbyDrugClass/ucm072423.htm on August 2015

Wallace, D. V., Dykewicz, M. S., Bernstein, D. I., et al. (2008). The diagnosis and management of rhinitis: An updated practice parameter. *Journal of Allergy and Clinical Immunology, 122,* S1–S84.

Wheatley, L. M., & Togias, A. (2015) Allergic rhinitis. *New England Journal of Medicine, 372*(5), 456–463.

Wingard, L., Brody, T., Larner, J., et al. (1991). *Human pharmacology: Molecular to clinical.* St. Louis, MO: Mosby-Year Book.

Yanez, A., & Rodrigo, G. J. (2002). Intranasal corticosteroids versus topical H_1 receptor antagonists for the treatment of allergic rhinitis: A systematic review with meta-analysis. *Annals of Allergy, Asthma & Immunology, 89,* 479–484.

49 Human Immunodeficiency Virus

Linda M. Spooner

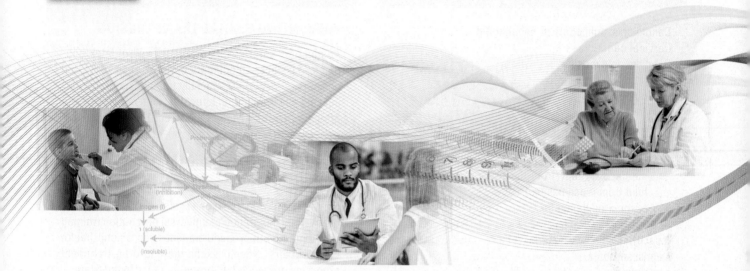

The first known case of human immunodeficiency virus (HIV) infection was documented in 1959 in a man from Kinshasa, Congo. How he became infected with the virus is unknown. Furthermore, how the disease grew to epidemic proportions also is unclear. In the United States, HIV infection was first recognized in 1981 after it was discovered that young homosexual men were contracting unusual cases of pneumonia and rare cancers that typically were not seen in immunocompetent patients.

HIV is the virus that causes acquired immunodeficiency syndrome (AIDS). A diagnosis of AIDS is based on the presence of an AIDS-defining condition (**Box 49.1**) or a CD4+ T-cell count of less than 200/mm³ (Centers for Disease Control and Prevention [CDC], 1992). Although rates of progression from HIV infection to AIDS vary greatly among individuals, the median is approximately 10 years in patients not receiving antiretroviral medications.

The two types of HIV that have been identified are HIV-1 and HIV-2. HIV-1 accounts for the majority of cases worldwide, including in the United States, whereas HIV-2 is primarily found in West Africa. HIV-2 is less efficiently transmitted and results in a slower disease progression than HIV-1. Unfortunately, since there are no randomized clinical trials that have assessed the efficacy of antiretroviral medications for treatment of HIV-2 infection, the ideal initial treatment regimen is unknown. It appears reasonable to base a regimen on a protease inhibitor (PI) boosted with ritonavir or an integrase inhibitor for patients with HIV-2 infection (Panel on Antiretroviral Guidelines, 2016).

Over the past three decades, HIV infection has reached epidemic proportions. The World Health Organization (WHO) estimates that approximately 35 million people worldwide are infected with HIV, with more than two thirds of cases occurring in sub-Saharan Africa (WHO, 2015). Of these, 3.2 million children younger than age 15 are infected. In 2013, 2.1 million people were newly infected with HIV, and there were 1.5 million deaths attributed to HIV throughout the world. Explanations for these overwhelming numbers include limited access to health care and antiretroviral medications as well as lack of education about prevention and transmission of HIV.

According to the most recent estimates, 1.1 million individuals were living with HIV in the United States at the end of 2010 (CDC, 2012). The number of new infections occurring annually has remained stable at approximately 50,000 per year.

The management of patients infected with HIV is challenging for several reasons. First, selection of antiretroviral therapy (ART) regimens can be complex, requiring the practitioner to individualize treatment selection based upon genotypic resistance testing results, comorbidities, concomitant medications, and patient preferences. Second, adverse effects of the medications may affect a patient's ability to tolerate and comply with therapy. Third, nonadherence to ART results in treatment failure as well as the development of resistance due to suboptimal serum concentrations of antiretroviral drugs. The health care practitioner should collaborate with the individual patient to select a regimen that the patient can take successfully and still manage potential adverse effects and drug interactions.

CAUSES

HIV is transmitted through four types of contact: sexual intercourse, blood-borne contact, perinatal transmission, and breast-feeding. *Prevention is the key to avoiding transmission* (**Box 49.2**). The most common route of transmission worldwide is through sexual contact with an infected person's genital fluids. The virus is also transmitted via intravenous (IV)

BOX
49.1   **AIDS-Defining Conditions**

Candidiasis, pulmonary or esophageal
Cervical cancer
Coccidioidomycosis
Cryptococcosis
Cryptosporidiosis
Cytomegalovirus
Herpes simplex virus
Histoplasmosis (microscopy [histology or cytology],
    culture, or detection of antigen in a specimen
    obtained directly from the tissues affected or a
    fluid from those tissues)
HIV-associated dementia
HIV-associated wasting
Isosporiasis
Kaposi sarcoma
Lymphoma
Mycobacterium avium infection
Pneumocystis jiroveci pneumonia
Other pneumonias, recurrent (more than one episode
    in a 1-year period)
Progressive multifocal leukoencephalopathy
Salmonella septicemia
Toxoplasmosis
Tuberculosis

Adapted from Centers for Disease Control and Prevention. (1992). 1993 revised classification system for HIV infection and expanded surveillance case definition for AIDS among adolescents and adults. *Morbidity and Mortality Weekly Report, 41*(RR-17), 1–19.

BOX
49.2   **Preventing HIV Transmission**

PREVENTING SEXUAL TRANSMISSION

Abstinence, safer sexual practices, use of latex condoms, risk factor modification, notification of sexual partners, education (especially to adolescents), treating sexually transmitted infections, and consistent and effective use of ART may be used to prevent sexual transmission of HIV.

PREVENTING BLOOD EXPOSURE TRANSMISSION

Since 1985, all donated blood is tested for the presence of HIV. Implementation of universal precaution training programs has decreased transmission among health care workers. Needle exchange and drug treatment programs are available throughout the United States.

PREVENTING PERINATAL TRANSMISSION

Lowering antepartum viral load in the mother with combination ART, combined with pre- and postexposure prophylaxis of the infant with ART, aggressive family planning services (e.g., HIV testing, counseling), and recommending against breast-feeding for infected women.

transfer of infected blood through transfusions, IV drug use and needle sharing, or occupational exposure. An infected mother may transmit the virus to her baby prior to or during birth as well as during breast-feeding. It is important to note that HIV is *not* transmitted through casual contact (e.g., contact with tears, saliva, toilet facilities).

Effective treatment with ART reduces the risk of transmission to sexual partners, as lower concentrations of HIV ribonucleic acid (RNA) in plasma are associated with decreased levels of HIV in genital secretions. Therefore, consistent use of ART leading to sustained reductions in HIV viral loads should be combined with safer sexual and drug use practices to prevent HIV transmission.

PATHOPHYSIOLOGY

HIV is a retrovirus; each viral particle contains two single-stranded molecules of RNA rather than deoxyribonucleic acid (DNA). Following infection of host cells, the viral enzyme

reverse transcriptase allows synthesis of a DNA molecule that is then inserted into the DNA of the host cell, allowing the virus to replicate. In the case of HIV, the host cells are $CD4^+$ T lymphocytes, a white blood cell involved in cell-mediated immunity. As the virus replicates, it destroys the $CD4^+$ T lymphocytes, thereby leading to immune deficiency.

HIV incorporates itself into the host cell through a number of steps. A viral envelope surrounding the HIV RNA contains proteins on its outer surface that react specifically with the $CD4^+$ receptor on the T lymphocyte ($CD4^+$ T cell). Additionally, the viral membrane uses coreceptors (CCR5 or CXCR4) to attach to the $CD4^+$ T cell. Once this is completed, the viral envelope fuses to the host cell and allows the HIV RNA to enter the host cell. Next, reverse transcriptase catalyzes the formation of a single-stranded DNA intermediate from the viral RNA. This step is followed by duplication of the single-stranded DNA to form a double-stranded DNA. Catalyzed by the enzyme integrase, viral DNA is integrated into the host cell's nucleus. After the DNA is transcribed and translated back to RNA, the virus then makes long chains of polyproteins that are split by the enzyme protease to form new copies of HIV RNA. To protect the viral RNA, a protective core protein called a *capsid* surrounds the genetic material. This process is rapidly repeated, producing an estimated 10 billion new particles each day. The average half-life of a viral particle is 6 hours. The largest concentration of viral particles can be found in lymph node tissue and genital secretions.

DIAGNOSTIC CRITERIA

The signs and symptoms of HIV disease vary among patients. The acute retroviral syndrome occurs 2 to 3 weeks following exposure to the virus. During this time, the number of CD4+ T lymphocytes (CD4+ count) declines dramatically, and the number of HIV RNA particles in the plasma (viral load) increases greatly. Clinically, the patient may experience fever, swollen lymph nodes, sore throat, skin rash, muscle soreness, headache, nausea, vomiting, and diarrhea. The specific symptoms and their duration vary among patients, and their presence alone does not constitute a diagnosis. Diagnosis of HIV is based on the presence of HIV RNA or p24 antigen in the plasma or serum, often with a negative or indeterminate HIV antibody test (Panel on Antiretroviral Guidelines, 2016).

The currently used method for diagnosing HIV-1 infection is a combination immunoassay, which detects circulating antibodies to the virus and p24 antigen. This assay is highly sensitive and specific for established infection (99% to 100% sensitivity and specificity), but false-positive results may occur in patients who recently received hepatitis B or rabies vaccines, have acute infections, or have autoantibody formation. False-negative results may occur in newly infected patients whose antibody titer has not risen to detectable levels. Antibodies develop within 6 months after infection in 95% of patients, and the median time for antibody development is 2 months. If the initial test is reactive, further testing is performed to determine HIV RNA concentrations.

Laboratory Parameters

Once the diagnosis of HIV has been confirmed using the above tests, initiation of therapy should be guided by the patient's clinical status as well as two main laboratory parameters, including the CD4+ T-cell count, the plasma HIV RNA (viral load), and viral resistance testing. Determination of these results allows the clinician to understand the patient's risk of opportunistic infections and risk for disease progression and to monitor response to the selected drug therapy.

CD4+ T-Cell Count

The CD4+ T-cell count indicates the extent to which HIV has damaged the immune system. Normally, the CD4+ T-cell count ranges between 500 and 1,600/mm^3. As the viral infection progresses, the CD4+ count declines, correlating with increasing immunosuppression. Its value is especially important *before* initiating ART. CD4+ T-cell counts of less than 200/mm^3 are associated with an increased risk of AIDS malignancies, such as Kaposi sarcoma, and opportunistic infections, such as *Pneumocystis jiroveci* pneumonia, toxoplasmosis, and cytomegalovirus infection.

Plasma HIV RNA (Viral Load)

Quantification of HIV replication is determined by measuring the viral load in number of copies per milliliter of plasma. The primary assay used is the HIV-1 reverse transcriptase polymerase chain reaction assay, which has a lower limit of detection of 20 to 75 copies/mL. Clinical trials demonstrate that viral loads that are undetectable (e.g., <20 to 75 copies/mL) are associated with longer duration of suppression of viral replication as compared with detectable levels. The viral load is a useful tool to monitor a patient's virologic status, disease progression, and ART regimen.

HIV Drug Resistance Testing

Because of the significant association between the presence of drug-resistant HIV and failure of antiretroviral treatment regimens, HIV resistance assays have become useful mechanisms for guiding the selection of appropriate therapy. When used in combination with medication histories and patient counseling, these assays have assisted in the attainment of more efficient and sustained viral suppression. Drug resistance testing is recommended for all patients in the initial laboratory testing they receive as they enter into care.

The two methods used to assess resistance include genotypic and phenotypic assays. Genotypic assays detect genetic mutations that may confer viral resistance. Interpretation of these genotypes requires an understanding of the mutations and their correlation with resistance to specific classes of antiretroviral medications. Results are typically available within 1 to 2 weeks. Phenotypic assays calculate the concentrations of antiretroviral drugs required to inhibit HIV replication by 50%. This value is known as the *median inhibitory concentration* and is abbreviated as the IC_{50}. The ratio of the IC_{50} of the patient's and reference virus is noted as the fold increase in IC_{50} for a variety of antiretroviral medications. Results of phenotypic assays are available within 2 to 3 weeks due to automation techniques, but they are more expensive to perform than genotypic assays and more complicated to interpret. Both assays may be unsuccessful in patients with low viral loads (<500 to 1,000) due to inadequate presence of the virus.

Several limitations exist with HIV drug resistance testing. First, there is no standardized method for quality assurance for the available genotypic and phenotypic assays. Second, they are expensive to perform. Lastly, if drug-resistant virus comprises less than 10% to 20% of a patient's total virus population, the assays will not detect the resistant virus. Overall, these assays provide a method for making decisions on initiating ART, changing ART in patients experiencing virologic failure or suboptimal response, and selecting ART in pregnant women.

INITIATING DRUG THERAPY

When considering treatment of patients with HIV infection, it is important to note that all patients, regardless of CD4+ count, should be offered treatment with ART (Panel on Antiretroviral Guidelines, 2016). Additionally, regardless of CD4+ count, effective ART reduces the risk of sexual transmission of HIV infection.

Initiation of ART should be provided for any individual with AIDS-defining illnesses, pregnancy, HIV-associated nephropathy, early HIV infection, hepatitis B or C coinfection, and rapidly declining CD4⁺ counts.

Before therapy is started for any patient, a thorough history and physical examination should be performed, in addition to a complete blood count, basic chemistry profile, liver function tests, fasting lipid profile and glucose, urinalysis, CD4⁺ T-cell count, viral load, genotypic resistance testing, and additional evaluation of various serologies (e.g., hepatitis B and C).

Goals of Therapy

Because currently available antiretroviral regimens cannot achieve eradication of HIV, goals of therapy primarily focus on sustained suppression of viral replication to undetectable levels. There are five main goals of ART (Panel on Antiretroviral Guidelines, 2016). These include maximal and sustained suppression of viral load, restoration and preservation of immune system function, enhancement of quality and duration of

life, reduction in morbidity and mortality from HIV-related complications, and prevention of HIV transmission. Patients' responses to ART are variable, although successful regimens initiated in treatment-naive patients can decrease viral loads to undetectable levels within 12 to 24 weeks. Virologic success is improved with high-potency ART, excellent treatment adherence, low baseline viral load, higher baseline CD4⁺ count, and rapid reduction of viral load in response to treatment.

To maximize the benefits of ART, it is important to select drug regimens carefully based on drug resistance testing, pretreatment viral load (e.g., greater than or less than 100,000 copies/mL), adverse effects, convenience, patient preference, drug interaction profile, pregnancy or pregnancy potential, comorbidities, and cost. There are several recommended regimens that may be used as initial therapy for HIV infection, as they have potent efficacy in suppressing viral replication. These include nonnucleoside reverse transcriptase inhibitor–based regimens, protease inhibitor–based regimens, and integrase inhibitor–based regimens. **Table 49.1** lists the characteristics of all of the currently available antiretroviral medications.

TABLE 49.1

Overview of Drugs Used to Treat HIV Infection

Generic (Trade) Name and Adult Dosage in Treatment-Naive Patients	Selected Adverse Effects	Contraindications	Special Considerations
Nucleoside Reverse Transcriptase Inhibitors			
abacavir (Ziagen) 300 mg PO bid or 600 mg PO daily	Hypersensitivity reaction (fever, rash, malaise, fatigue, nausea, vomiting, respiratory symptoms), possible increased risk of myocardial infarction	Hypersensitivity to any component Moderate-to-severe hepatic impairment Rechallenge following the hypersensitivity reaction	Take without regard to meals. Hypersensitivity reaction can be fatal (black box warning) Discontinue immediately. Do not rechallenge Requires HLA-B*5701 screening prior to use Available in combination with lamivudine (Epzicom), zidovudine + lamivudine (Trizivir), and lamivudine + dolutegravir (Triumeq)
didanosine (Videx) ≥60 kg: 400 mg PO daily; with tenofovir, 250 mg PO daily <60 kg: 250 mg PO daily; with tenofovir, 200 mg PO daily	Pancreatitis, peripheral neuropathy, optic neuritis, lactic acidosis with hepatic steatosis, noncirrhotic portal hypertension	Concomitant use of allopurinol or ribavirin	Take 30 min before or 2 h after a meal Dose adjustment is required for renal insufficiency
emtricitabine (Emtriva) 200 mg PO daily	Skin hyperpigmentation, severe acute exacerbation of hepatitis B in coinfected patients who discontinue treatment	Hypersensitivity to any component	Take without regard to meals. Dose adjustment is required for renal insufficiency Available in combination with tenofovir (Truvada), tenofovir + efavirenz (Atripla), tenofovir + rilpivirine (Complera), and tenofovir + elvitegravir/cobicistat (Stribild) and tenofovir alafenamide + elvitegravir/cobicistat (Genvoya)

TABLE 49.1

Overview of Drugs Used to Treat HIV Infection (*Continued*)

Generic (Trade) Name and Adult Dosage in Treatment-Naive Patients	Selected Adverse Effects	Contraindications	Special Considerations
lamivudine (Epivir) 150 mg PO bid or 300 mg PO daily	Severe acute exacerbation of hepatitis B in coinfected patients who discontinue treatment	Hypersensitivity to any component	Take without regard to meals Dose adjustment is required for renal insufficiency Available in combination with zidovudine (Combivir), abacavir (Epzicom), zidovudine + abacavir (Trizivir), and abacavir + dolutegravir (Triumeq)
stavudine (Zerit) ≥60 kg: 40 mg PO bid <60 kg: 30 mg PO bid	Peripheral neuropathy, pancreatitis, lactic acidosis with hepatic steatosis, lipoatrophy, hyperlipidemia	Hypersensitivity to any component	Take without regard to meals Do not use with zidovudine Dose adjustment is required for renal insufficiency
tenofovir disoproxil fumarate (Viread) 300 mg PO daily	Nausea, vomiting, diarrhea, headache, asthenia, renal insufficiency, decreased BMD, severe acute exacerbation of hepatitis B in coinfected patients who discontinue treatment	Hypersensitivity to any component	Take without regard to meals Dose adjustment is required for renal insufficiency Available in combination with emtricitabine (Truvada), emtricitabine + efavirenz (Atripla), emtricitabine + rilpivirine (Complera), and emtricitabine + elvitegravir/cobicistat (Stribild)
zidovudine (Retrovir) 200 mg PO tid or 300 mg PO bid	Nausea, headache, malaise, bone marrow suppression, lactic acidosis with hepatic steatosis, nail pigmentation	Hypersensitivity to any component	Take without regard to meals Dose adjustment is required for renal insufficiency Available in combination with lamivudine (Combivir) and lamivudine + abacavir (Trizivir)
Nonnucleoside Reverse Transcriptase Inhibitors			
efavirenz (Sustiva) 600 mg PO hs	Neuropsychiatric symptoms (hallucinations, abnormal dreams, suicidality, dizziness, impaired concentration, euphoria, confusion), rash, elevated liver function tests, hyperlipidemia, false-positive cannabinoid and benzodiazepine screening tests, teratogenic	Hypersensitivity to any component Avoid pregnancy Numerous drug interactions; see **Table 49.2** for contraindicated combinations	Take on empty stomach at bedtime Available in combination with emtricitabine + tenofovir (Atripla)
etravirine (Intelence) 200 mg PO bid	Rash (including Stevens–Johnson syndrome), hypersensitivity reactions, nausea	None	Take following a meal
nevirapine (Viramune, Viramune XR) 200 mg PO daily for 14 d, followed by 200 mg PO bid or XR tablet 400 mg PO daily	Rash (including Stevens–Johnson syndrome), fatal hepatic necrosis (significantly higher risk in treatment-naive women with CD4+ count > 250 and men CD4+ count > 400)	Moderate–severe hepatic impairment	Take without regard to meals. Lead-in period can be extended in patients who develop a rash without constitutional symptoms but should not exceed 28 d
rilpivirine (Edurant) 25 mg PO daily	Rash, depression, headache, insomnia, hepatotoxicity	Coadministration of anticonvulsants (phenytoin, phenobarbital, carbamazepine, oxcarbazepine), rifampin Numerous drug interactions; see **Table 49.2** for contraindicated combinations	Take with a meal Available in combination with tenofovir + emtricitabine (Complera) and tenofovir alafenamide + emtricitabine (Odefsey)

(*Continued*)

TABLE 49.1

Overview of Drugs Used to Treat HIV Infection (*Continued*)

Generic (Trade) Name and Adult Dosage in Treatment-Naive Patients	Selected Adverse Effects	Contraindications	Special Considerations
Protease Inhibitors	Class adverse effects: lipo-dystrophy, GI intolerance, hepatotoxicity, hyperlipidemia, hyperglycemia	Numerous drug interactions; see **Table 49.2** for contraindicated combinations	
atazanavir (Reyataz) 300 mg PO daily plus ritonavir 100 mg PO daily OR 300 mg PO daily plus cobicistat 150 mg PO daily	Prolonged PR interval with 1st-degree AV block, indirect hyperbilirubinemia, nephrolithiasis, cholelithiasis, rash	Hypersensitivity to any component	Take with food Use caution when dosing with acid-reducing agents Available coformulated with cobicistat (Evotaz) Dose adjustment is required in hepatic insufficiency
darunavir (Prezista) 800 mg PO daily plus ritonavir 100 mg PO daily OR 600 mg PO bid plus ritonavir 100 mg PO bid OR 800 mg PO daily plus cobicistat 150 mg PO daily	Rash (Stevens–Johnson syndrome and erythema multiforme reported), headache		Take with food. Available coformulated with cobicistat (Prezcobix)
fosamprenavir (Lexiva) 1,400 mg PO bid **or** 1,400 mg PO daily plus ritonavir 100–200 mg PO daily **or** 700 mg PO bid plus ritonavir 100 mg PO bid	Rash, headache, nephrolithiasis	Same as above	Take with a meal if boosted with ritonavir. Dose adjustment is required for hepatic insufficiency
indinavir (Crixivan) 800 mg PO q8h or 800 mg PO bid plus ritonavir 100–200 mg PO bid	Nephrolithiasis, hyperbilirubinemia, headache, dizziness, metallic taste, rash	Same as above	Should be taken 1 h before or 2 h after meals when unboosted. Take without regard to meals when boosted with ritonavir Drink 1.5 L fluid daily to avoid renal stones Dose adjustment is required for hepatic insufficiency
lopinavir/ritonavir (Kaletra) 400/100 mg PO bid or 800/200 mg PO daily	Prolonged PR interval or QT interval, asthenia	Same as above	Take with food Alternative dosing is required in patients taking concomitant efavirenz or nevirapine
nelfinavir (Viracept) 1,250 mg PO bid or 750 mg PO tid	Diarrhea	Same as above	Take with food
ritonavir (Norvir) Use only as a booster with other PIs; 100–400 mg PO daily in 1–2 divided doses	Circumoral and peripheral paresthesias, taste perversion, asthenia	Same as above	Take with food
saquinavir (Invirase) 1,000 mg PO bid plus ritonavir 100 mg PO bid	Prolonged PR interval, prolonged QT interval, headache	Same as above, plus severe hepatic impairment	Take with large meal Avoid use in patients with pretreatment QT interval > 450 msec
tipranavir (Aptivus) 500 mg PO bid plus ritonavir 100 mg PO bid	Hepatotoxicity (including hepatic decompensation and fatal hepatitis) rash, fatal and non-fatal intracranial hemorrhage	Same as above, plus moderate-to-severe hepatic impairment	Take without regard to meals Must be boosted with ritonavir

TABLE 49.1

Overview of Drugs Used to Treat HIV Infection (*Continued*)

Generic (Trade) Name and Adult Dosage in Treatment-Naive Patients	Selected Adverse Effects	Contraindications	Special Considerations
Fusion Inhibitors			
enfuvirtide (Fuzeon) 90 mg subcutaneously bid	Local injection site reactions (almost 100% of patients), increased rate of bacterial pneumonias, hypersensitivity reaction (<1%)	Hypersensitivity to any component	Store reconstituted solution in refrigerator and use within 24 h
Integrase Inhibitors			
dolutegravir (Tivicay) 50 mg PO once daily or 50 mg PO bid	Hypersensitivity reactions, insomnia, headache	Hypersensitivity to any component Concomitant use with dofetilide	Take without regard to meals Twice-daily dosing used when coadministered with efavirenz, fosamprenavir/ritonavir, tipranavir/ritonavir, rifampin. Also used for treatment-experienced patients with resistance mutations Available coformulated with abacavir + lamivudine (Triumeq)
elvitegravir (Vitekta) 150 mg PO daily plus cobicistat 150 mg PO daily	Nausea, diarrhea, renal impairment	None listed	Take with a meal Not recommended for patients with baseline creatinine clearance <70 mL/min Available coformulated with tenofovir + emtricitabine + cobicistat (Stribild) and tenofovir alafenamide + emtricitabine + cobicistat (Genvoya) Numerous drug interactions
raltegravir (Isentress) 400 mg PO bid	Nausea, diarrhea, headache, creatine kinase elevation, muscle weakness, fever	Hypersensitivity to any component	Take without regard to meals When dosed with rifampin, administer raltegravir 800 mg PO bid Use caution with concomitant agents that cause myopathy
CCR5 Antagonists			
maraviroc (Selzentry) 150 mg PO bid with strong CYP450 3A inhibitors (including PIs other than tipranavir/ritonavir); 300 mg PO bid with nonstrong CYP450 3A inhibitors or inducers; 600 mg PO bid with CYP450 3A inducers (efavirenz, etravirine)	Hepatotoxicity, cough, dizziness, rash, orthostatic hypotension	Severe renal impairment or end-stage renal disease with concomitant use of potent CYP450 3A inhibitors or inducers Numerous drug interactions; see **Table 49.2** for contraindicated combinations	Take without regard to meals

Reverse Transcriptase Inhibitors

There are two subclasses of reverse transcriptase inhibitors (RTIs): the nucleoside reverse transcriptase inhibitors (NRTIs) and the nonnucleoside reverse transcriptase inhibitors (NNRTIs).

Nucleoside Reverse Transcriptase Inhibitors

There are six NRTIs marketed in the United States. These include abacavir (Ziagen), didanosine (Videx), emtricitabine (Emtriva), lamivudine (Epivir), stavudine (Zerit), and zidovudine (Retrovir). There is one nucleotide RTI, tenofovir, available as tenofovir

disoproxil fumarate and tenofovir alafenamide, which is similar in mechanism of action but is slightly different in structure than the nucleoside analogs. In addition, several combination products are available for dosing convenience; these are listed in **Table 49.1**.

Mechanism of Action

The NRTIs must be phosphorylated in the target cells before becoming active. This intracellular phosphorylation results in an active triphosphorylated form that interferes with the transcription of viral RNA to DNA. This interference can occur through two mechanisms: chain termination and competitive inhibition.

The *chain termination* process results in the reverse transcriptase enzyme adding the NRTI to the growing chain of HIV viral DNA instead of the needed DNA nucleoside. The NRTI acts as a nucleoside analog in the DNA production, and its addition is relatively simple. Once this is accomplished, no more DNA nucleosides can be added to the chain, thus terminating its growth and halting the production of viral DNA.

Competitive inhibition occurs when the active (phosphorylated) NRTI competes with the cell's own nucleoside building block. By competing for the cell's building block, these agents also halt the production of viral DNA.

Dosing

With the exception of abacavir, all NRTIs require elimination by the kidneys and therefore must be dose adjusted for patients with renal insufficiency. This is an important concept because it helps to minimize the incidence of adverse effects.

The first NRTI that received U.S. Food and Drug Administration (FDA) approval in the United States was zidovudine. It has been studied extensively as a component of ART and has proven to be effective in delaying progression of the disease, reducing the incidence of opportunistic infections, and prolonging survival. Significant adverse effects of zidovudine include bone marrow suppression, which can lead to clinically significant anemia and neutropenia, gastrointestinal (GI) toxicity, fatigue, and lactic acidosis with hepatic steatosis. Thus, it is not recommended as a component of initial treatment of nonpregnant adults.

Lamivudine is one of the better-tolerated NRTIs and was the second NRTI to receive FDA approval. Other NRTIs have been available for many years, including didanosine and stavudine. The bioavailability of didanosine is decreased in the presence of gastric acidity. Therefore, it is formulated as an enteric-coated capsule or as a solution that is reconstituted with liquid antacid to allow for improved absorption. Dosing of didanosine and stavudine should be based on weight (see **Table 49.1**). Both of these NRTIs have similar toxicities, including pancreatitis, peripheral neuropathy, and GI disturbances. Didanosine also has been associated with noncirrhotic portal hypertension. Neither of these agents is recommended as part of initial treatment for treatment-naive patients.

Contraindications

Abacavir is an effective component of ART. Patients who initiate treatment with this agent must be cautioned about the hypersensitivity reaction that occurs in 2.5% to 8% of patients. Symptoms of the hypersensitivity reaction include fever, rash, GI disturbances, lethargy, and malaise. These can occur at any time after initiating therapy (median, 9 days), although the majority of reactions occur within the first 6 weeks of therapy. Symptoms resolve after discontinuation of the drug but may recur and result in death if abacavir is restarted. The risk of this reaction is correlated with the presence of the HLA-B*5701 allele. As a result, pretreatment screening for this allele should be performed before initiating therapy. Abacavir should not be used in those individuals who test positive for the HLA-B*5701 allele on the screening test, and they should be considered allergic to abacavir. Patients who test negative for the allele should still be counseled about the signs and symptoms of the hypersensitivity reaction. Additionally, there is controversy over an association between abacavir and cardiovascular disease, as some analyses have demonstrated increased risk of myocardial infarction, while others have not. At this time, it is recommended to use caution when considering initiation of abacavir in patients with risk factors for cardiovascular disease.

Tenofovir and emtricitabine are the two newest NRTIs available for use as a part of an ART regimen. Both are well tolerated, are dosed once daily, and can be taken without regard to meals. Tenofovir may cause renal insufficiency, with a higher risk in patients with advanced HIV infection, long treatment duration, low body weight, and preexisting renal impairment. Baseline and periodic assessment of serum creatinine and phosphorous, along with urinary glucose and protein, should be performed. Tenofovir and emtricitabine, which are also available in a coformulated tablet (Truvada), are recommended as one of the dual NRTI combinations for treatment-naive patients, as they are very potent in suppressing viral replication and are superior to zidovudine plus lamivudine in virologic efficacy and adverse effect profile. Also, since both tenofovir and emtricitabine exhibit activity against hepatitis B virus, they are the agents of choice for the management of patients who are coinfected with HIV and hepatitis B.

Dual NRTIs are used as part of ART in combination with a boosted PI, an NNRTI, or an integrase inhibitor. Recommended dual NRTIs include tenofovir/emtricitabine (coformulated as Truvada) and abacavir/lamivudine (coformulated as Epzicom). Triple NRTI regimens are less effective than PI- or NNRTI-based regimens; therefore, they should not be used in routine clinical practice.

Adverse Effects

A class adverse effect observed with all NRTIs includes lactic acidosis with hepatic steatosis. Although this adverse effect is rare, especially with newer NRTIs, it results in a high risk of death. This may be due to mitochondrial dysfunction that occurs on administration of NRTIs. The clinical presentation of lactic acidosis varies greatly among patients but often includes nonspecific GI symptoms (nausea, vomiting, abdominal pain) as well as generalized weakness, myalgias, and paresthesias that can progress to tachycardia, tachypnea, mental status changes, and multiorgan failure. Hepatic steatosis may manifest as an enlarged fatty liver on computed tomography scan as well as increased liver transaminases.

Risk factors for development of this syndrome include female gender, pregnancy, obesity, regimen components (stavudine, didanosine, zidovudine), and prolonged use of NRTIs. If this syndrome develops, the NRTIs should be discontinued immediately, and supportive care should be initiated. Because other clinical interventions such as administration of thiamine, riboflavin, and levocarnitine have not been adequately assessed in clinical trials, their efficacy cannot be determined at this time. Patients taking NRTIs should be cautioned about the signs and symptoms of lactic acidosis, and if these are observed, the patient should notify the practitioner immediately. It is optimal to use NRTIs with less risk of mitochondrial toxicity, such as tenofovir, emtricitabine, lamivudine, or abacavir, instead.

Additionally, all NRTIs can decrease bone mineral density (BMD). The risk is greater with regimens containing tenofovir. BMD assessment can be considered for individuals with a history of fractures or other risk factors for osteoporosis or BMD loss. Calcium and vitamin D supplementation can also be considered.

Nonnucleoside Reverse Transcriptase Inhibitors

Mechanism of Action and Clinical Use

By binding to reverse transcriptase, NNRTIs also interfere with the conversion of RNA to DNA. The five available NNRTIs are delavirdine (Rescriptor), efavirenz (Sustiva), etravirine (Intelence), nevirapine (Viramune), and rilpivirine (Edurant). This class of agents demonstrates a low genetic barrier for resistance development. Delavirdine is the least potent NNRTI and therefore is not recommended as part of initial ART. Nevirapine has a higher incidence of rash and hepatotoxicity than efavirenz; thus, it is no longer recommended for initial treatment. It can be continued in patients who are stabilized on the drug already. Etravirine has primarily been studied in treatment-experienced patients with prior virologic failure, and its use is reserved for this purpose. Trials have shown that efavirenz-based regimens have similar virologic efficacy as compared with PI- and integrase inhibitor–based regimens, although some studies show that other regimens are superior to efavirenz because of fewer discontinuations due to central nervous system side effects and possible association with suicidality. Thus, the DHHS Panel considers efavirenz as an alternative agent in NNRTI-based regimens. Rilpivirine is also an alternative NNRTI, since it was shown to be noninferior to efavirenz overall. However, its use should be restricted to individuals with a pretreatment viral load of less than 100,000 copies/mL and CD4+ count above 200 cells/mm³. This is because comparative clinical trials with rilpivirine and efavirenz showed a higher rate of virologic failure with rilpivirine in patients with very high viral loads or low CD4+ counts, due to the development of resistance mutations. Both efavirenz and rilpivirine are available in coformulations with tenofovir and emtricitabine in order to reduce pill burden.

Adverse Effects

The most frequently reported adverse effects of NNRTIs include GI disturbances, rash, and elevations in hepatic transaminases. Efavirenz commonly causes central nervous system adverse effects, including dizziness, impaired concentration, abnormal dreams, and hallucinations. These events occur within the first few days of initiating therapy but resolve over 2 to 4 weeks with continued treatment. Dosing at bedtime is helpful in minimizing these adverse effects. Congenital defects have been observed in offspring of both animals and humans exposed to efavirenz during pregnancy; therefore, this agent must be avoided in pregnant women in their first trimester of pregnancy or those of childbearing potential who are not using consistent and effective contraception.

Nevirapine has been associated with severe, life-threatening hepatotoxicity, including hepatic necrosis and hepatic failure, primarily occurring within the first few weeks of initiation. This may also occur along with a hypersensitivity reaction that includes rash and fever. A black box warning in the nevirapine labeling notes that women with CD4+ counts greater than 250 cells/mm³ and men with CD4+ counts greater than 400 cells/mm³ have a considerably higher risk of hepatotoxicity. Therefore, all patients who initiate therapy with nevirapine should initiate dosing once daily for 14 days followed by twice daily, and they should receive close monitoring of liver function tests and clinical symptoms throughout the treatment course. If hepatotoxicity occurs, nevirapine should be discontinued permanently.

Etravirine demonstrates activity against some HIV viruses that express mutations conferring resistance to the other four NNRTIs and is reserved for treatment-experienced patients. Its adverse effects include nausea, rash, and hypersensitivity reactions associated with organ dysfunction.

Rilpivirine is the newest NNRTI on the market; it causes fewer central nervous system adverse effects than efavirenz. Its side effects include depression, headache, insomnia, and rash.

Drug Interactions

All of the NNRTIs are metabolized by the cytochrome P-450 (CYP450) 3A4 isoenzyme system in the liver. Each NNRTI also has variable effects on inhibiting or inducing this enzyme system. Therefore, caution should be used when administering NNRTIs with drugs dependent on CYP450 3A4 for metabolism, including PIs, phenytoin, phenobarbital, and clarithromycin. Concomitant use of rifampin with etravirine or rilpivirine is contraindicated because of increased metabolism of etravirine that results in reduced serum concentrations and reduced efficacy. Rifampin may be used with caution with nevirapine. Rifampin must be used with an increased dose of efavirenz (800 mg daily). Concomitant use of St. John's wort is contraindicated with all NNRTIs due to risk of virologic failure secondary to the resulting suboptimal NNRTI concentrations. Use of rilpivirine with proton pump inhibitors is contraindicated due to reduced absorption and subsequent decreased concentrations of rilpivirine. Additional contraindicated concomitant medications can be found in **Table 49.2**.

Protease Inhibitors

Mechanism of Action

Introduced in the mid-1990s, PIs have demonstrated potent virologic efficacy, durable effects, and high barriers to resistance. They act near the final stage of HIV viral replication through inhibiting the protease-mediated cleavage of the polyproteins.

TABLE 49.2

Nonantiretroviral Medications That Are Contraindicated for Concomitant Use with NNRTIs, PIs, or INSTIs

Class/Drug	Contraindicated Medications and/or Classes	Comments
All NNRTIs	St. John's wort	Results in virologic failure
	rifapentine	Results in tuberculosis treatment failure
	simeprevir, dasabuvir, ombitasvir, paritaprevir	Results in concomitant medication toxicity
efavirenz	cisapride, pimozide, midazolam, triazolam	Results in concomitant medication toxicity
etravirine	rifampin, carbamazepine, phenytoin, phenobarbital	Results in decreased etravirine concentrations
rilpivirine	proton pump inhibitors, rifampin	Results in virologic failure
	rifampin, carbamazepine, oxcarbazepine, phenytoin, phenobarbital	Results in decreased rilpivirine concentrations
All PIs	simvastatin, lovastatin	Results in increased risk of rhabdomyolysis
	amiodarone, dronedarone, ranolazine, cisapride, pimozide, midazolam, triazolam, lurasidone, ergot alkaloids, alfuzosin, salmeterol, fluticasone, salmeterol, simeprevir, dasabuvir, ombitasvir, paritaprevir, sildenafil (when used for pulmonary arterial hypertension)	Results in concomitant medication toxicity
	rifampin	Results in virologic failure
	rifapentine	Results in tuberculosis treatment failure
	St. John's wort	Results in virologic failure
atazanavir	Proton pump inhibitors	When used with unboosted atazanavir, results in decreased atazanavir concentrations
darunavir	carbamazepine, oxcarbazepine, phenytoin, phenobarbital	Results in concomitant medication toxicity
		Results in decreased concentrations of phenytoin and phenobarbital
dolutegravir	dofetilide	Results in concomitant medication toxicity
	carbamazepine, oxcarbazepine, phenytoin, phenobarbital	Results in virologic failure
elvitegravir/ cobicistat	cisapride, pimozide, ranolazine, midazolam, triazolam, lurasidone, ergot alkaloids, alfuzosin, salmeterol, fluticasone, salmeterol, simeprevir, ledipasvir, dasabuvir, ombitasvir, paritaprevir sildenafil (when used for pulmonary arterial hypertension)	Results in concomitant medication toxicity

These polyproteins are responsible for creating new HIV RNA copies. Inhibiting this final stage by the use of PIs decreases the production of HIV RNA copies.

Nine PIs are available: atazanavir (Reyataz), darunavir (Prezista), fosamprenavir (Lexiva), indinavir (Crixivan), lopinavir/ritonavir (Kaletra), nelfinavir (Viracept), ritonavir (Norvir), saquinavir (Invirase), and tipranavir (Aptivus). These agents vary greatly in terms of their potency, adverse effects, and pharmacokinetic characteristics.

Dosing

PI-based regimens provide excellent efficacy in virologic suppression. Either ritonavir or cobicistat, potent CYP450 3A4 isoenzyme inhibitors, can be used to increase the concentrations of other PIs, allowing greater exposure of the virus to the PI. These "boosted" regimens demonstrate more potent virologic activity while reducing pill burden and adverse effects. However, it is important to note that there are numerous drug–drug interactions that result from the presence of these pharmacokinetic enhancing agents in a regimen. Despite this, boosting regimens with low-dose ritonavir or cobicistat is now the standard of care in PI-based ART regimens.

The pharmacokinetic characteristics of the PIs vary greatly across the class. Food affects the bioavailability of many of the PIs (see **Table 49.1**). For example, administration of atazanavir with food increases its bioavailability substantially and therefore should be administered with a meal. In contrast, concentrations of indinavir decrease by 77% with food, resulting in the requirement that this drug be taken on an empty stomach or with a small, low-fat snack (e.g., pretzels) when used without ritonavir booster doses.

Adverse Effects

The adverse effects of all PIs include GI disturbances, such as nausea, vomiting, and diarrhea, occurring upon treatment initiation. All PIs can cause increases in levels of hepatic transaminases. Clinical hepatitis and hepatic decompensation are more common in patients receiving regimens containing tipranavir/ritonavir. Risk factors for hepatotoxicity with PIs include hepatitis B or C coinfection, alcohol abuse, underlying liver disease, and concomitant use of hepatotoxic agents. This should be monitored carefully.

A class effect of the PIs includes fat maldistribution, also known as *lipodystrophy*. This results in accumulation of fat in the abdomen, breasts, and dorsocervical fat pad ("buffalo hump"). This occurs in a large percentage of patients receiving ART, depending upon the regimen used and the duration of treatment. Fat maldistribution may be accompanied by metabolic abnormalities such as hyperlipidemia and hyperglycemia. Management of lipodystrophy includes use of diet and exercise as well as administration of tesamorelin, a growth hormone–releasing factor. Improvements have been demonstrated in clinical trials of patients changed from lopinavir/ritonavir to atazanavir.

All of the PIs, with the exception of unboosted atazanavir, have been associated with hyperlipidemia, including increased levels of triglycerides, total serum cholesterol, and low-density lipoproteins. Lopinavir/ritonavir and fosamprenavir/ritonavir cause a substantial increase in triglycerides when compared to atazanavir/ritonavir or darunavir/ritonavir. These lipid abnormalities may be associated with accelerated coronary artery disease in HIV patients. Management includes dietary modifications, exercise, smoking cessation, and changing to agents with a lower likelihood of lipid abnormalities, as well as the addition of lipid-lowering treatments, such as 3-hydroxy-3-methylglutaryl-coenzyme A (HMG-CoA) reductase inhibitors (statins). However, it is important to note that most statins cause drug interactions with the PIs, and some are contraindicated (**Table 49.2**). Therefore, pravastatin is the preferred agent because it does not have as many interaction concerns.

Another class effect of PIs includes hyperglycemia, which may lead to new-onset diabetes mellitus as a result of insulin resistance in approximately 3% to 5% of patients. Patients should be cautioned about warning signs of hyperglycemia, including polydipsia, polyphagia, and polyuria. Management of hyperglycemia includes lifestyle modifications (diet and exercise), consideration of NNRTI or integrase inhibitor use as an alternative, and pharmacologic management according to the American Diabetes Association.

Clinical Use

Based upon virologic efficacy and durability data, dosing convenience and low pill burden, and good tolerability, the guidelines published by the Panel on Antiretroviral Guidelines (2016) list darunavir/ritonavir as the recommended component of an initial PI-based regimen (**Table 49.3**). Clinical trials comparing darunavir/ritonavir to lopinavir/ritonavir demonstrated superior virologic efficacy with darunavir/ritonavir after 96 weeks of treatment. Darunavir contains a sulfa moiety and therefore can cause a rash. The rash is typically mild to moderate in severity and self-limited. However, the agent should be discontinued if the rash is severe or in the presence of fever or elevated liver function tests. Atazanavir/ritonavir has fewer adverse effects on lipids when compared to other PI-based regimens, but it has a higher rate of discontinuation due to adverse effects when compared to darunavir/ritonavir or raltegravir; thus, it is considered to be an alternative agent for initial therapy. The primary adverse effect of atazanavir is hyperbilirubinemia with or without jaundice or icteric sclerae. It may also cause nephrolithiasis, nephrotoxicity, and cholelithiasis. Since it requires an acidic GI environment for dissolution, acid-reducing agents such as antacids, histamine$_2$

receptor antagonists, and proton pump inhibitors may inhibit the absorption of atazanavir, requiring staggered dosing and limitations on the use of these agents.

Drug Interactions

All PIs are metabolized by the CYP450 3A4 isoenzyme system in the liver. Each of the PIs has a different effect on inducing or inhibiting the efficiency of this isoenzyme system. Therefore, caution must be used when combining PIs with any medications that are metabolized by CYP450 3A4 or that induce or inhibit this system. Concurrent use of PIs with ergot alkaloids, simvastatin, lovastatin, rifampin, and St. John's wort is contraindicated. A summary of these contraindicated medications is provided in **Table 49.2**.

Fusion Inhibitors

Enfuvirtide (Fuzeon) is the only available agent in this class of antiretroviral drugs. It inhibits fusion of the virus to the cell membrane of the CD4$^+$ T cell, thereby preventing HIV from entering the cell. Because its mechanism of action is distinct from the intracellular agents previously discussed, it may be useful for highly treatment-experienced patients with the virus that is resistant to other currently available antiretroviral agents.

Enfuvirtide must be injected subcutaneously twice daily. Adverse effects include local injection site reactions, such as erythema, induration, and pain, which occur in almost all patients. Less than 1% of patients experience hypersensitivity reactions, including rash and fever. Enfuvirtide significantly increases tipranavir/ritonavir concentrations, resulting in an increased risk of adverse effects.

Integrase Inhibitors

Three integrase strand transfer inhibitors (INSTIs) are available for treatment of HIV infection. These include dolutegravir (Tivicay), elvitegravir (Vitekta), and raltegravir (Isentress). They prevent the integration of viral DNA into the host cell's genome. Each of these agents is recommended for use with a dual NRTI backbone as initial therapy in treatment-naive individuals, per the Panel's guidelines (2016), as they have similar virologic efficacy as other recommended regimens and are well tolerated.

Raltegravir was the first INSTI approved, and it is dosed twice daily. It is metabolized via UGT1A1-mediated glucuronidation and therefore exhibits minimal drug–drug interaction risk. This agent can cause elevations in creatine kinase with possible rhabdomyolysis and should be used with caution in patients receiving concomitant medications that have similar adverse effects. Rare cases of hypersensitivity reactions have been documented in postmarketing surveillance.

Elvitegravir is marketed as a single agent or coformulated with the booster agent cobicistat and tenofovir, emtricitabine (Stribild or Genvoya), which permits the product to be dosed once daily but results in numerous drug interactions. The most common adverse effects of elvitegravir include nausea, headache, and diarrhea. Additionally, because cobicistat inhibits the active renal tubular secretion of creatinine, increases in serum creatinine and decreases in creatinine clearance occur without reducing renal function. This combination product is not recommended for use in individuals with baseline creatinine clearance of less than 70 mL/min, and it should be discontinued if creatinine clearance decreases to less than 50 during treatment.

Dolutegravir is the newest INSTI available for use and is considered a second-generation INSTI, in that it may have a higher genetic barrier to resistance. The dosing is once daily for treatment-naive patients and twice daily in treatment-experienced patients. It is available as a single agent or coformulated with abacavir and lamivudine (Triumeq). It is well tolerated, causing insomnia or headache in rare cases. Because its absorption is affected by agents containing polyvalent cations (e.g., calcium supplements, antacids, iron supplements), its dosing should be 2 hours before or 6 hours after administration of these products.

CCR5 Antagonists

Maraviroc (Selzentry) is the only available agent in this class of antiretrovirals. It blocks the CCR5 receptor on the membrane of CD4+ T cells, preventing entry of the HIV virus. Prior to use, a coreceptor tropism assay (e.g., Trofile) must be performed to determine if the patient's virus utilizes the CCR5 receptor, since not all HIV strains do. Maraviroc has a black box warning in its package insert describing hepatotoxicity that may be preceded by a systemic allergic reaction. This agent may also cause cough, orthostatic hypotension, rash, and fever. It also has a multitude of drug–drug interactions associated with its use, requiring dose adjustment. At this time, the Panel (2016) does not recommend maraviroc-based regimens as initial therapy for treatment-naive patients.

Selecting the Most Appropriate Regimen

Although guidelines exist for the combinations of agents to be used in ART, each patient must have a highly individualized regimen. Although current regimens are effective at keeping the viral load at undetectable levels, eradication of the virus is not yet attainable. This is due to the early development of latently infected CD4+ T cells with a long half-life that, even with prolonged therapy, persist.

Previously Untreated Patients

One of the most important therapeutic interventions in the care of the patient with HIV infection is the initial treatment regimen (**Tables 49.1** and **49.3**). It is essential to select the most potent and appropriate therapy possible, keeping in mind adverse effects and adherence issues. Discontinuing recommended therapy due to nonadherence increases the risk of drug resistance and failure with alternate regimens.

"Recommended regimens" have been selected by the DHHS Panel based on optimal efficacy and durability demonstrated in clinical trials as well as tolerability and convenience of use. "Alternative regimens" demonstrate efficacy and tolerability but have disadvantages or less evidence supporting their use. The list of alternative regimens is brief because the list of recommended regimens has been expanded, permitting most treatment-naive patients to receive a recommended agent.

Recommended initial therapy is comprised of two NRTIs (also known as the dual nucleoside "backbone") plus a third drug, either a boosted PI or INSTI (**Table 49.3**). Recommended dual NRTI backbones include either tenofovir/emtricitabine or abacavir/lamivudine. Since they are each available as coformulated tablets with once-daily dosing, selection depends upon consideration of clinical data, adverse effects, and comorbidities. Since tenofovir can cause nephrotoxicity and decreased BMD, use of abacavir/lamivudine can be considered in patients at increased risk of these adverse effects. Prior to initiation of abacavir, testing for the HLAB*5701 allele to determine risk of hypersensitivity should be performed. If a patient is coinfected with HIV and hepatitis B, tenofovir/emtricitabine is the preferred backbone due to its activity against hepatitis B virus.

Selection of the third drug in the regimen, either a boosted PI or INSTI, depends upon clinical data, adverse effects, dosing convenience, genetic barrier to resistance, comorbid conditions, and drug interaction potential. PI-based regimens contain a PI with a booster dose of ritonavir or cobicistat in combination with two NRTIs. These combinations have proven to be effective in numerous clinical trials. The recommended PI-based regimen is darunavir/ritonavir plus tenofovir/emtricitabine (**Table 49.2**). Darunavir contains a sulfa group and may cause rash. It also has a higher pill burden than some of the coformulated INSTI products discussed below.

The INSTI-based regimens of raltegravir, elvitegravir, or dolutegravir plus a dual NRTI backbone are also recommended as initial regimens in treatment-naive patients. Their advantages include comparable virologic efficacy to other regimens with fewer adverse effects and lipid abnormalities. They also have fewer drug interactions than PI-based regimens.

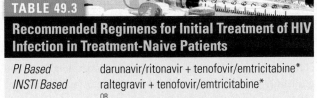

TABLE 49.3

Recommended Regimens for Initial Treatment of HIV Infection in Treatment-Naive Patients

PI Based	darunavir/ritonavir + tenofovir/emtricitabine*
INSTI Based	raltegravir + tenofovir/emtricitabine*
	OR
	elvitegravir†/cobicistat/tenofovir disoproxil fumarate/emtricitabine
	OR
	elvitegravir#/cobicistat/tenofovir alafenamide/emtricitabine
	OR
	dolutegravir + abacavir‡/lamivudine*
	OR
	dolutegravir + tenofovir/emtricitabine*

*May substitute lamivudine for emtricitabine or vice versa.
†Do not initiate if creatinine clearance <70 mL/min.
‡Do not use abacavir in patients who are HLA-B*5701 positive.
#Do not initiate if creatinine clearance <30 mL/min.
Panel on Antiretroviral Guidelines for Adults and Adolescents. (2015). Guidelines for use of antiretroviral agents in HIV-1–infected adults and adolescents. Department of Health and Human Services [Online]. Retrieved from http://www.aidsinfo.nih.gov/ContentFiles/AdultandAdolescentGL.pdf

Raltegravir requires twice-daily dosing and may be less convenient than all of the other recommended options. Elvitegravir is coformulated in a once-daily tablet, but can cause elevations in serum creatinine and more drug interactions than raltegravir. Dolutegravir was shown to be superior to darunavir/ritonavir and efavirenz in virologic efficacy, primarily due to fewer discontinuations for side effects. It appears to have a higher genetic barrier to resistance than other INSTIs, but has more drug interactions than raltegravir.

Treatment-Experienced Patients

When antiretroviral treatment failure occurs, it is necessary to assess why this occurred to determine the appropriate therapy change. Antiretroviral treatment failure is a term that encompasses all potential reasons for suboptimal response to therapy that must be assessed, including patient factors (e.g., incomplete medication adherence, psychiatric illness, presence of resistant virus, interruption of access to ART) and drug-related factors (e.g., drug toxicities, suboptimal pharmacokinetic issues, drug interactions, medication errors) (Panel on Antiretroviral Guidelines, 2016). Treatment regimen failure often results in virologic failure, incomplete virologic response, or virologic rebound. *Virologic failure* is defined as the failure to achieve or maintain HIV RNA plasma levels less than 200 copies/mL. An *incomplete virologic response* results when two consecutive viral loads are above 200 copies/mL after 24 weeks on ART. *Virologic rebound* occurs when the viral load increases to 200 copies/mL or higher after virologic suppression has been achieved. It is also important to note that virologic blips can occur, where an isolated occurrence of detectable virus happens, but is followed by return to undetectable concentrations.

After the practitioner considers the causes and types of treatment failure, the drug regimen should be changed accordingly. The patient's previous treatment experience and current drug resistance pattern must be considered because there may be cross-resistance between agents within the same therapeutic class. In addition, if an adverse effect or unacceptable toxicity caused a cessation of therapy, the practitioner should avoid alternative agents likely to cause that adverse effect. Furthermore, agents with complicated dosing schedules and strict food and timing requirements should be avoided if that is what caused the first treatment failure. Selecting agents that are free of side effects and strict food or timing requirements may not be easy, but each patient must be given the regimen to which he or she will most likely adhere.

When changing therapy, one or more of the agents in the regimen may need to be replaced. This will vary depending on the individual patient's situation. Expert advice from an HIV clinician is crucial to selecting the most appropriate option.

Special Population Considerations

Pediatric

Guidelines exist for treating HIV infection in the pediatric patient (Panel on Antiretroviral Therapy and Medical Management of HIV-Infected Children, 2016). Although the principles remain the same in all HIV-infected individuals, unique considerations in subsets of the pediatric population need brief discussion. These include diagnosis of disease, differences in CD4+ T-cell counts and viral loads, changes in pharmacokinetic parameters, and adherence issues.

Diagnostic testing for suspected HIV-infected infants can be performed as early as at birth and by age 4 months in almost all infants. Testing in high-risk infants should occur by 48 hours of life because in nearly 30% to 40% of infected infants, the diagnosis can be made within this time frame. If the initial test is negative, repeat testing should be performed at age 1 to 2 months and age 4 to 6 months. HIV DNA polymerase chain reaction or RNA assays are the preferred virologic methods for diagnosing HIV in infants. Antibody testing is not accurate due to the transfer of maternal HIV antibodies to the infant.

The CD4+ T-cell counts in children younger than age 5 are typically higher than adult counts. Therefore, monitoring absolute CD4+ counts may not be as reliable as measuring the percentage change in CD4+ counts as disease progresses. Pediatric patients with a positive virologic test should have CD4+ T-cell counts and viral loads monitored every 3 to 4 months if not on ART, or more frequently in those initiating or changing ART. CD4+ counts can be monitored every 6 to 12 months in children who have demonstrated treatment adherence, sustained virologic suppression, stable clinical status, and high CD4+ counts for at least 2 to 3 years. Similarly, because of immunologic differences, particularly in those patients acquiring the disease perinatally, viral loads may be difficult to interpret during the first year of life. Using CD4+ T-cell count and viral load together can more accurately predict prognosis and survival.

Pharmacokinetic variables, particularly volume of distribution and clearance, change as a person ages. These changes should be considered when designing drug therapy regimens for children. Similarly, the issue of medication adherence in this population is crucial. Some of the solution formulations for these agents may be unpalatable, depending on the child's preferences. Also, absorption of drugs can be affected by food, and timing of drug administration around food schedules can be extremely difficult. Mixing medications in bottles with formula may increase palatability but may create compatibility issues. Additionally, children depend upon their caregivers to administer ART; therefore, the complexity and convenience of the regimen must be considered. It is preferable for an HIV expert to manage these patients in order to select optimal treatment and monitor short- and long-term adverse effects and quality of life.

Women/Pregnancy

Thresholds for the initiation of ART in HIV-infected women are the same as those for HIV-infected men. Selection of antiretrovirals in women of childbearing potential should reflect regimen efficacy as well as its potential for teratogenicity if the woman becomes pregnant. For example, efavirenz should be avoided in women considering pregnancy or who are not using reliable contraception. It is also important to note that the efficacy of many oral contraceptives is reduced by ART.

When considering the use of ART in pregnant women with HIV infection, practitioners must consider two main issues: ART of HIV in the mother and prophylaxis to reduce the risk of perinatal HIV infection (Panel on Treatment of HIV-Infected Pregnant Women and Prevention of Perinatal Transmission, 2015). The benefits and risks of using ART must be assessed prior to initiating therapy in a pregnant patient as well as special considerations for dosing, adverse effects, and other medication counseling points.

The acquisition of disease through exposure in utero is a major source of HIV infection in infants. Therefore, early identification of HIV-infected women is crucial before or during pregnancy. Preconception HIV prevention counseling and testing for all pregnant women have been advocated by national organizations, including the American College of Obstetricians and Gynecologists and the CDC.

One of the more remarkable aspects of zidovudine therapy was the discovery that this agent reduced the maternal–fetal transmission of HIV. The pivotal study by Connor and colleagues showed a maternal–fetal transmission rate of 8.3% with zidovudine versus 25.5% with placebo in expectant mothers between 14 and 34 weeks of gestation (Connor et al., 1994). Therefore, antiretroviral chemoprophylaxis with IV zidovudine during labor is recommended for all pregnant women with viral loads greater than 1,000 copies/mL or unknown viral loads at the time of delivery. This is not required for women adherent to ART whose viral loads have remained consistently below 1,000 copies/mL during late pregnancy and delivery. Postnatally, the infant should receive oral chemoprophylaxis in an effort to reduce perinatal transmission. Additionally, breastfeeding is not recommended for any HIV-positive woman in the United States, regardless of ART regimen.

Health Care Workers/Occupational Exposure

The primary means of transmission of HIV in the health care worker population is through an accidental needlestick. However, transmission can occur through exposure of HIV-infected blood or other infected body fluids to a health care worker's nonintact skin or mucous membranes. The risk of HIV transmission after a percutaneous exposure to infected blood is approximately 0.3%; the risk decreases to approximately 0.09% for a mucous membrane exposure.

In theory, initiation of antiretroviral postexposure prophylaxis (PEP) within hours after exposure may prevent or inhibit systemic infection by limiting the replication of virus in the lymphocytes and lymph nodes. As such, the U.S. Public Health Service has published recommendations regarding the initiation and continuation of PEP in health care personnel (Kuhar et al., 2013). The primary role of PEP is to prevent HIV infection after an accidental occupational exposure.

Current guidelines recommend a preferred PEP regimen of tenofovir/emtricitabine plus raltegravir, due to its potency, tolerability, dosing convenience, and minimal drug interactions. Alternative regimens are listed in **Table 49.4**; these can be considered if there are contraindications, cost concerns, or intolerability with the preferred regimen. PEP should be initiated as

TABLE 49.4

Recommended HIV PEP for Occupational Exposure

Column A	Column B
atazanavir 300 mg PO daily + ritonavir 100 mg PO daily	tenofovir/emtricitabine tablet PO daily
darunavir 800 mg PO daily + ritonavir 100 mg PO daily	tenofovir 300 mg PO daily + lamivudine 300 mg PO daily
etravirine 200 mg PO bid	zidovudine/lamivudine tablet PO bid
lopinavir/ritonavir 2 tablets PO bid	zidovudine 300 mg PO bid + emtricitabine 200 mg PO daily
raltegravir 400 mg PO bid	
rilpivirine 25 mg PO daily	

Preferred regimen: tenofovir/emtricitabine tablet PO daily PLUS raltegravir 400 mg PO bid
Alternative regimen: Choose one drug or drug pair from Column A and one drug or drug pair from Column B. May also use elvitegravir/cobicistat/tenofovir/emtricitabine (Stribild) po daily
Adapted from Kuhar, D. T., Henderson, D. K., Struble, K. A., et al. (2013). Updated U.S. public health service guidelines for the management of occupational exposures to HIV and recommendations for postexposure prophylaxis. *Infection Control and Hospital Epidemiology, 34,* 875–892. Courtesy of JSTOR. Retrieved from http://nccc.ucsf.edu/wp-content/uploads/2014/03/Updated_USPHS_Guidelines_Mgmt_Occupational_Exposures_HIV_Recommendations_PEP.pdf

soon as possible after exposure, while awaiting results of source identification, resistance profile, or both. Therapy should be continued for 28 days and should only be discontinued early if the source patient is proven to be HIV negative, if the exposed health care worker is shown to be HIV positive, if the adverse effects of PEP are intolerable and there is no other alternative available, or if the exposed health care worker decides to discontinue treatment based on risks and benefits. HIV antibody testing should be performed at baseline, 6 weeks, 12 weeks, and 6 months after exposure. If a fourth-generation combination HIV antigen/antibody test is used, the final test can be completed at 4 weeks. Extended follow-up (e.g., at 12 months) is recommended for health care workers who become infected with hepatitis C virus following exposure to a coinfected patient.

Nonoccupational Postexposure Prophylaxis (nPEP)

Use of ART within 72 hours of exposure to HIV outside of the workplace, such as through sexual assault, unprotected sexual intercourse, sharing needles during injection drug use, etc., is a method that has never been studied in clinical trials, but is employed to prevent HIV infection. Each case should be considered individually, to assess if the source is HIV negative (nPEP not recommended), unknown (consider nPEP), or HIV positive (nPEP recommended). As with occupational PEP, the preferred regimen is tenofovir/emtricitabine plus raltegravir for 28 days.

Preexposure Prophylaxis

Use of daily preexposure prophylaxis (PrEP) with tenofovir/emtricitabine in sexually active adults at risk of becoming infected with HIV has helped to decrease transmission. The largest clinical trial assessing the efficacy of this approach, known as the iPrEX study, demonstrated a 44% relative risk reduction in HIV infection incidence in HIV-negative men who have sex with men (Grant et al., 2010). Studies in heterosexual populations also show that this strategy is effective in reducing incidence of HIV infection. The decision to use PrEP must be considered carefully. Since the effectiveness of the regimen is linked with adherence, it is crucial to emphasize the importance of taking the regimen every day, not just on days when sexual intercourse would occur. Per recommendations from the U.S. Public Health Service, individuals must test negative for HIV infection within 1 week of PrEP initiation and every 3 months during treatment, to prevent the development of resistance in the presence of HIV infection (U.S. Public Health Service, 2014). Additionally, patients should receive safer sexual practices counseling at each visit, to further reduce the risk of transmission. No more than a 90-day supply of PrEP should be prescribed, and patients should be seen every 3 months for lab work and adherence assessments.

MONITORING PATIENT RESPONSE

The CD4+ T-cell counts are important not only because they indicate the risk of development of opportunistic infections before treatment but also because they help the health care provider initiate or discontinue opportunistic infection prophylaxis during ART. Once ART is started, a CD4+ count should be checked at baseline and after 3 months to assess reconstitution of the immune system. It is important to check CD4+ counts every 3 to 6 months in order to assess response to ART during the first 2 years of treatment and to determine the necessity of opportunistic infection prophylaxis. CD4+ counts may be obtained once yearly in those individuals who are receiving suppressive ART and have CD4+ counts well above the threshold for risk of opportunistic infections, consistently ranging between 300 and 500 cells/mL or higher. More frequent monitoring would be required in patients with changes in clinical status, those who are unable to achieve virologic suppression on ART, or in those initiating treatment with interferon, steroids, or cancer chemotherapeutic agents.

Viral load indicates both initial and sustained responses to treatment with ART, and decreases in viral load correlate with decreased risk of progression to AIDS and death. Viral load should be measured at baseline for all patients, to permit appropriate ART selection. Once therapy has been initiated or changed, viral load should be assessed immediately before treatment and again 2 to 8 weeks later. The viral load should be repeated every 4 to 8 weeks until it becomes undetectable. Subsequent testing should reveal an undetectable viral load by 8 to 12 weeks in those patients adherent to ART. At that point, viral load testing should be repeated every 3 to 4 months to determine continuing effectiveness of the regimen. This duration can be extended to 6 months in those patients who are stable and have fully suppressed viral loads for at least 2 years. If a patient exhibits a suboptimal response, it is important to review medication adherence, drug interactions, and resistance mutations to permit consideration of regimen changes.

Genotypic resistance testing is recommended for all patients at baseline, regardless of when treatment is initiated, in order to optimize regimen selection by determining which drugs still retain activity. It is also useful for patients with suboptimal viral load reduction and virologic failure. Resistance testing is not recommended for patients with viral loads of fewer than 500 copies/mL because the assays cannot consistently determine resistance patterns with such low-level viremia. Recommendations for genotypic resistance testing in pregnant patients include baseline testing prior to therapy as well as testing those with detectable viral loads while taking ART.

PATIENT EDUCATION

To minimize the likelihood of treatment regimen failure and development of drug resistance, the health care professional must be aware of who is at high risk for adherence issues as well as the most common reasons for poor adherence. Risk factors for poor adherence to antiretroviral regimens include active substance abuse, active mental illness, lack of disease and medication education, low levels of literacy, and stigma. Several treatment factors affect adherence, such as pill burden, frequency of dosing, food requirements, adverse effects, and treatment fatigue.

Strategies the practitioner can use to minimize the risk of failure due to nonadherence include encouraging the patient to develop a strong relationship with the health care team, taking an active role in his or her therapy, and involving the patient's family, friends, and peers in the therapy. In addition, counseling on HIV and the goals of achieving viral suppression (e.g., reduction in HIV-related morbidity and mortality, prevention of sexual transmission) may encourage an otherwise indifferent patient to adhere to a regimen.

Another strategy the practitioner should use to promote drug adherence is preparing the patient for adverse events. The patient needs to know which adverse events are likely to occur, how to minimize the risk of experiencing adverse events, and which adverse events demand discontinuation of therapy. The patient also needs to understand the importance of following the dosing schedule in addition to the food requirements for each agent (Panel, 2015). **Table 49.1** provides information on dosing, diet, and fluid requirements of each agent.

Developing a plan for scheduling medications and carefully explaining to the patient how the medication should be taken is imperative. This plan should focus on daily pill taking as well as future events in a patient's life that threaten to interrupt the established schedule (e.g., holidays or vacations). This plan must consider lifestyle factors such as work schedule and privacy issues (e.g., taking medication at work or storage of medication at work). Regardless of how much or little assistance the patient needs in developing strategies for ensuring adherence, success is often determined by the patient's

CASE STUDY*

A.P. is a 36-year-old woman who was diagnosed with HIV infection 2 weeks ago at a community outreach clinic. She has been feeling well for the past 2 years, and she maintains a healthy, active lifestyle by exercising three to four times a week and eating a balanced diet. Her medications include a multiple vitamin and occasional antacids for heartburn, and she does not consistently use birth control methods. She has never received ART. She comes to your office for an initial physical exam and blood work in preparation for treatment initiation. The physical examination is unremarkable, and the laboratory results are as follows:

Electrolytes, serum creatinine, liver function tests: within normal limits

Complete blood count with differential: within normal limits

CD4$^+$ T-cell count: 400 cells/mm^3

Viral load: 110,000 copies/mL

Genotype: No resistance mutations detected

DIAGNOSIS: ASYMPTOMATIC HIV INFECTION

1. List specific goals for treatment for this patient.
2. What drug therapy would you prescribe? Why?
3. What are the parameters for monitoring success of the therapy?
4. Discuss specific patient education based on the prescribed therapy.
5. List one or two adverse reactions for the selected agents that would cause you to change therapy.
6. What would be the choice for the second-line therapy?
7. What over-the-counter and/or alternative medications would be appropriate for **A.P.**?
8. What dietary and lifestyle changes should be recommended for this patient?
9. Describe one or two drug–drug or drug–food interactions for the selected agents.

* Answers can be found online.

outlook. If the patient perceives that therapy will lead to an improved quality of life or increased length of life, chances for adherence are greater (Reynolds, 1998). Therefore, before attacking the logistics of a medication schedule, the health care provider must convince the patient of the benefits of continuing therapy.

Once the daily plan is developed, it should evolve into a long-term plan that allows the patient to adhere to therapy and allows the health care provider to monitor adherence. Aids for adherence include pill boxes that separate doses per day, alarms to remind patients of their doses, or something as simple as a calendar that lists dosing schedules. Whatever method is used, the patient must remain adherent and be checked for adherence. The simplest way to check for adherence is to ask the patient. However, a patient may not confess to missed doses or may not be aware of missed doses. Pill counting is another option, but patients may remove missed doses to appear adherent. Testing the viral load may reveal adherence information, but if levels increase because of resistance, not nonadherence, the results will be misleading. Adherence counseling and effective engagement and retention in care are all closely linked to improving treatment success.

Bibliography

Starred references are cited in the text.

Anonymous. (2014). Drugs for HIV infection. *Treatment Guidelines from the Medical Letter, 12*(138), 7–16.

*Centers for Disease Control and Prevention. (1992). 1993 revised classification system for HIV infection and expanded surveillance case definition for AIDS among adolescents and adults. *Morbidity and Mortality Weekly Report, 41*(RR-17), 1–19.

*Centers for Disease Control and Prevention. (2012). Estimated HIV incidence in the United States, 2007-2010. *HIV Surveillance Supplemental Report, 17.*[Online]. Retrieved from http://www.cdc.gov/hiv/pdf/statistics_hssr_vol_17_no_4.pdf

*Connor, E. M., Sperling, R. S., Gelber, R., et al. (1994). Reduction of maternal-infant transmission of human immunodeficiency virus type 1 with zidovudine treatment. Pediatric AIDS Clinical Trials Group Protocol 076 Study Group. *New England Journal of Medicine, 331*, 1173–1180.

*Grant R. M., Lama J. R., Anderson P. L., et al. (2010). Preexposure chemoprophylaxis for HIV prevention in men who have sex with men. *New England Journal of Medicine, 363*, 2587–2599.

*Kuhar, D. T., Henderson, D. K., Struble, K. A., et al. (2013). Updated U.S. public health service guidelines for the management of occupational exposures to HIV and recommendations for postexposure prophylaxis. *Infection Control and Hospital Epidemiology, 34*, 875–892.

Lacy, C. F., Armstrong, L. L., Goldman, M. P., et al. (2014). *Drug information handbook* (23rd ed.). Hudson, OH: Lexi-Comp.

Marrazzo, J. M., del Rio C., Holtgrave, D. R., et al. (2014). Antiretroviral treatment of adult HIV infection: 2014 recommendations of the international AIDS Society USA Panel. *Journal of the American Medical Association, 312*, 410–425.

Olin, J. L., Spooner, L. M., Klibanov, O. M. (2012). Elvitegravir/cobicistat/emtricitabine/tenofovir disoproxil fumarate single tablet for HIV-1 infection treatment. *Annals of Pharmacotherapy, 46*, 1671–1677.

*Panel on Antiretroviral Guidelines for Adults and Adolescents. (2016). *Guidelines for use of antiretroviral agents in HIV-1-infected adults and adolescents. Department of Health and Human Services* [Online]. Retrieved from http://www.aidsinfo.nih.gov/ContentFiles/AdultandAdolescentGL.pdf

*Panel on Antiretroviral Therapy and Medical Management of HIV-Infected Children. (2016). *Guidelines for the use of antiretroviral agents in pediatric*

HIV infection. HHS Panel on Antiretroviral Therapy and Medical Management of HIV-Infected Children—A Working Group of the Office of AIDS Research Advisory Council (OARAC). Retrieved from http://aidsinfo.nih.gov/contentfiles/lvguidelines/pediatricguidelines.pdf

*Panel on Treatment of HIV-Infected Pregnant Women and Prevention of Perinatal Transmission. (2015). Recommendations for use of antiretroviral drugs in pregnant HIV-1-infected women for maternal health and interventions to reduce perinatal HIV transmission in the United States. [Online]. Retrieved from http://www.aidsinfo.nih.gov/ContentFiles/lvguidelines/PerinatalGL.pdf

*Reynolds, N. R. (1998). Initiatives to get HIV-infected patients to adhere to their treatment regimens. *Drug Benefit, 10*(11), 23–25, 29–30, 32.

*U.S. Public Health Service. (2014). *Preexposure prophylaxis for the prevention of HIV infection in the United States–2014: A Clinical Practice Guideline.* [Online]. Retrieved from http://www.cdc.gov/hiv/pdf/prep-guidelines2014.pdf

*World Health Organization (WHO). (2015). *HIV/AIDS: Data and statistics* [Online]. Retrieved from http://www.who.int/hiv/data/en

UNIT 12
Pharmacotherapy for Hematologic Disorders

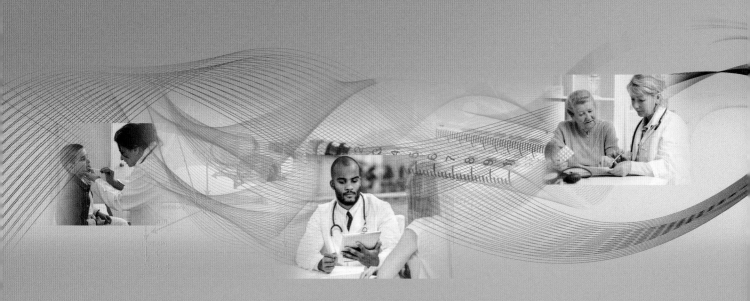

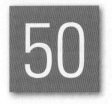

50 Pharmacotherapy for Venous Thromboembolism Prevention and Treatment, Stroke Prevention in Atrial Fibrillation, and Thromboembolism Prevention with Mechanical Heart Valves

Sarah A. Spinler

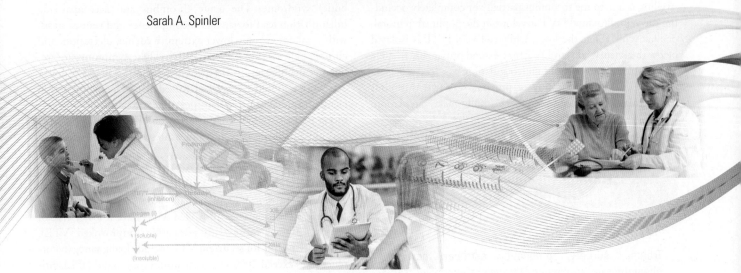

Thromboembolic disease and patients with risk factors for thromboemboli are frequently encountered in the ambulatory population, and an understanding of the pathogenesis of these conditions and underlying patient risk factors, along with the clotting cascade, is essential for determining appropriate treatment. The indications for anticoagulation continue to expand, and treatment for some conditions has now shifted to the outpatient setting. Several disorders warrant anticoagulant therapy, including venous thromboembolism (VTE) prevention and treatment, stroke prevention in atrial fibrillation (SPAF), ischemic stroke, prosthetic cardiac valves, coronary and peripheral vascular disease, and hypercoagulable conditions. Recognizing when prophylaxis for clotting events is appropriate is also important, including during orthopedic surgery and during hospitalization in patients with multiple risk factors for VTE. Anticoagulation practices are an important component of quality metrics and patient safety practices for hospitalized patients. Anticoagulation management strategies for the prevention and treatment of VTE and SPAF and the prevention of systemic thromboembolism in patients with prosthetic heart valves are discussed in this chapter.

DISORDERS REQUIRING ANTICOAGULATION AND THEIR CAUSES

Venous Thromboembolism

VTE is a thromboembolic event occurring in the venous system, and it is manifested as either deep vein thrombosis (DVT)

or pulmonary embolism (PE). VTE contributes significantly to patient morbidity and mortality and is considered a major global disease burden (Raskob et al., 2014). Venous thrombus formation occurs in the setting of venous stasis (sluggish blood flow), vascular endothelial wall injury, and hypercoagulability (propensity for increased blood clotting); these three features are classically referred to as *Virchow triad* (Merli, 2008).

The components of Virchow triad can assist with categorizing the most common causes and risk factors for VTE. Venous stasis, which results in pooling of blood in the lower extremity veins, is precipitated by prolonged immobility occurring during hospitalization, surgery, spinal cord injury, or paralyzing stroke; in conditions that increase venous pressure, including varicose veins or venous insufficiency from the post-thrombotic syndrome; or, less frequently, in obesity or pregnancy. Vascular intimal injury is often related to recent surgery, especially abdominal and orthopedic surgery, recent trauma or fracture to the pelvis or lower extremities, childbirth, and previous venous thrombosis. Imbalances between the body's regulatory mechanisms of procoagulant and anticoagulant proteins can result in hypercoagulable conditions. Hypercoagulability may be present secondary to inherited abnormalities of coagulation (thrombophilia), malignancy, oral contraceptive use, and estrogen therapy (Merli, 2008). In addition, central venous catheters and age older than 40 years also increase the risk of venous thromboembolic disease (Ortel, 2010). The incidence of VTE is approximately 0.75 to 2.69 per 1,000 individuals in the general population and is increased to between 2 and 7 per

1,000 among those ages ≥70 years and to 1 in 200 in patients with active cancer (Easaw et al., 2015; Raskob et al., 2014). Risk factors for VTE should be identified and corrected, if possible (Heit, 2006). Inherited thrombophilia is the most common risk factor in patients presenting with VTE under the age of 50 years (Kreidy, 2014). See **Box 50.1** for more information on predisposing risk factors for VTE.

In DVT, the characteristic symptom of lower extremity swelling is due to the thrombus partially or completely occluding the vein. Proximal DVT develops in the popliteal, femoral, or iliac veins above the knee, while calf vein DVT is isolated below the knee. Calf vein DVT may extend proximally in 40% to 50% of patients without anticoagulation.

The major complication of proximal DVT is thrombus dislodgment and extension into the pulmonary circulation.

BOX 50.1 Risk Factors for Deep Vein Thrombosis and Pulmonary Embolism

REVERSIBLE

Trauma,[§] surgery,[*] pregnancy, estrogen therapy,[±] chemotherapy, prolonged or transient immobility, fractures, central venous catheters, obesity, long-haul air travel[¯]

ACQUIRED

Increasing age >40 years, malignancy,[†] previous venous thromboembolism, hematologic disease, heart failure, stroke, inflammatory bowel disease, nephrotic syndrome, spinal cord injury, varicose veins, superficial vein thrombosis, antiphospholipid antibodies, lupus anticoagulant[¯]

INHERITED DISORDERS

Activated protein C resistance, antithrombin III deficiency, protein C deficiency, protein S deficiency, anticardiolipin antibodies,[‡] factor V Leiden, prothrombin gene mutation

---

[*]Especially orthopedic, gynecologic, neurosurgical, or urologic procedures.
[§]Especially major or lower extremity injury
[±]Oral contraceptives or hormone replacement therapy
[†]Especially of the lung, breast, or viscera
[‡]May also be acquired
[¯]Considered weak factor
Data from Geerts, W. H., Bergqvist, D., Pineo, G. F., et al. (2008). Prevention of venous thromboembolism: American College of Chest Physicians Evidence-Based Clinical Practice Guidelines (8th ed.). *Chest, 133*(6 Suppl.), 381S–453S; and Osinbowale, O., Ali, L., & Chi, Y. W. (2010). Venous thromboembolism: A clinical review. *Postgraduate Medicine, 122*(2), 54–65.

PE is a life-threatening emergency, with an associated mortality rate of 25%. Lower extremity DVTs are the source of 90% of PEs (Piazza & Goldhaber, 2006). Distal DVT isolated to the calf veins has a lower risk of long-term complications. In hospitalized patients, proximal DVT accounts for 80% of cases, with distal DVT comprising 20% (Righini & Bounameaux, 2008).

Nearly 50% of patients experiencing DVT develop chronic venous insufficiency or postphlebitic (postthrombotic) syndrome. The acute thrombus and accompanying inflammation lead to valvular incompetence and venous stasis, with resultant chronic lower extremity edema, ulceration, and chronic pain (Vazquez et al., 2009). These symptoms are frequently debilitating to the patient's quality of life. The lower extremities should be assessed for edema, skin pigmentation changes, spider veins, varicosities, and scarring from previous ulcers to assist with recognizing chronic venous insufficiency and implementing preventive measures if possible (Kelechi & Bonham, 2008).

Patients with a proximal DVT have a higher risk of recurrence than those with a distal DVT, and patients with PE have a higher recurrent VTE risk than those with isolated DVT. Patients presenting with provoked VTE have a lower risk of recurrence than those with idiopathic (unprovoked VTE). Other risk factors for recurrent VTE include malignancy (recurrence rates exceed 20% at 1 year), antiphospholipid (aPL) antibody syndrome, male sex, persistent positive D-dimer (checked 3 weeks to 2 months following cessation of anticoagulation), and residual thrombosis. Several paper score sheets and web-based risk prediction models are available to estimate a patient's risk of recurrent VTE (http://cemsiis.meduniwien.ac.at/en/kb/science-research/software/clinical-software/recurrent-vte/, http://www.mdcalc.com/dash-prediction-score-for-recurrent-vte/, Barnes et al., 2015).

Atrial Fibrillation

Atrial fibrillation is a cardiac arrhythmia characterized by loss of coordination of electrical and mechanical activity in the atria. Thrombi can form in the left atrial appendage due to impaired ventricular filling and incomplete emptying of the atria. Atrial fibrillation may initially present with the embolic complication of stroke, when atrial thrombi dislodge and travel through the bloodstream to the brain. Other major complications of AF include heart failure, dementia, and death (January et al., 2014). Patients with AF caused by conditions other than valvular problems (e.g., nonvalvular AF [NVAF]) have a fivefold risk of ischemic stroke compared with those in sinus rhythm (January et al., 2014). NVAF is defined as AF in the absence of a mechanical or bioprosthetic heart valve, mitral stenoses, or a history of mitral valve repair surgery (January et al., 2014).

Atrial fibrillation is the most common cardiac rhythm disturbance seen in clinical practice. Hospitalization for this arrhythmia is increasing, accounted for by the aging of the population and an increased incidence of chronic heart disease (Mozaffarian et al., 2015). The incidence increases with advancing age and is highest in those older than age 65 or in younger patients with comorbidities of hypertension or underlying heart disease. Other underlying cardiovascular conditions that can cause AF include hypertension with left ventricular hypertrophy, coronary artery disease, heart failure (HF), and rheumatic valvular disease, especially mitral valve disease. Additional cardiac causes include atrial enlargement, atrial septal defect, and coronary artery bypass graft surgery. Noncardiac etiologies include thyrotoxicosis, hypothermia, fever, stroke, chronic pulmonary disease, electrolyte disorders, PE, alcohol intoxication, obesity, and genetic predisposition (Mozaffarian et al., 2015).

The three key components to managing AF include preventing transient ischemic attack (TIA) and stroke with anticoagulant drugs, restoring and maintaining sinus rhythm in selected patients, and controlling the ventricular heart rate. The patient's risk of stroke determines the need for anticoagulation. Patients with a history of stroke or TIA have the highest risk of a recurrent event. Other independent risk factors for stroke in AF are increasing age, hypertension (HTN), HF with impaired systolic function, and diabetes mellitus. Patients older than age 75 comprise over half of AF-associated strokes; thus, the elderly represent a population in which stroke prophylaxis is essential (Fuster et al., 2006). Anticoagulation therapy is the cornerstone for SPAF.

Prosthetic Valvular Heart Disease

Prosthetic heart valves confer a high risk of systemic embolism, and antithrombotic therapy, antiplatelet therapy, anticoagulation, or a combination of antiplatelet and anticoagulation, is warranted in most patients. Valvular heart disease is most commonly caused by degenerative valve disease due to increasing life spans and rheumatic heart disease. Indications for prosthetic heart valve replacement include mitral stenosis, mitral regurgitation, aortic stenosis, and aortic regurgitation, as progressive deterioration of the native valve can lead to syncope, dyspnea, angina, and HF. There are two main types of prosthetic heart valves: mechanical, made from synthetic materials, or bioprosthetic, of porcine or bovine origin. Mechanical prosthetic valves are more thrombogenic than bioprosthetic valves and require lifelong anticoagulation, but they are more durable. Factors contributing to thrombus formation with mechanical valve replacement include disruption of the vessel wall during surgery, leading to altered blood flow and activation of hemostasis, or exposure of circulating blood to the artificial surfaces of the valve prosthesis (Sun et al., 2010).

Prosthetic valves in the mitral position are more thrombogenic than those in the aortic position. In the mitral position, shear stress is low, blood flow is stagnant, and stasis occurs. In the aortic position, blood flow is rapid and shear stress is high, which causes red blood cell hemolysis and activation of platelets and coagulation factors (Sun et al., 2010).

The risk of thromboembolism in native valvular heart disease is influenced by the position of the valve, for example, mitral versus aortic, heart chamber dimension, ventricular performance, and concomitant risk factors such as prior thromboembolism and AF. In native valvular disease, individuals with rheumatic mitral valve disease have the greatest incidence of systemic embolism. Thromboembolism in aortic valve disease has been noted but is uncommon. Without the coexistence of mitral valve disease or AF, anticoagulation is not indicated in these patients (Salem et al., 2008).

Anticoagulant therapy for thromboprophylaxis is recommended in all patients having prosthetic valve replacement. The rate of embolism reported with mechanical valves (St. Jude bileaflet valve) when antithrombotic prophylaxis was not administered ranged from 12%/year with aortic valves to 22%/year with mitral valves (Salem et al., 2008). Bioprosthetic tissue valves present a much lower risk of thromboembolism, averaging 1%/year; the risk of thromboembolic events is highest in the first 3 months following surgery, after which anticoagulant therapy is usually discontinued (Sun et al., 2010).

PATHOPHYSIOLOGY OF COAGULATION AND CLOTTING DISORDERS

Disrupting the body's normal system of checks and balances for hemostasis will lead to either excessive bleeding or inappropriate clotting. The three major components of the coagulation system—endothelial cells, platelets, and coagulation proteins—preserve hemostasis by promoting clot formation in response to vascular injury. The intact vessel wall of the vascular endothelium maintains blood fluidity by inhibiting blood coagulation and platelet aggregation while promoting fibrinolysis. When the vessel wall is injured, substances in the endothelial cell lining stimulate the formation of a hemostatic plug by promoting platelet adhesion and aggregation and by activating blood coagulation, resulting in a fibrin clot (Colman et al., 2006).

Role of Clotting Cascade

In response to tissue injury, a series of complex enzymatic reactions (the clotting cascade, **Figure 50.1**) is initiated that leads to the formation of a stable fibrin clot. Circulating inactive coagulation factors are sequentially converted into activated coagulation factor complexes. The final step in the cascade is the formation of thrombin (factor IIa), which leads to the conversion of fibrinogen to fibrin and the formation of a fibrin clot (Colman et al., 2006).

Platelets also participate in repairing tissue injury by adhering to the site of injured blood vessels, attracting other platelets to the site, and forming large platelet aggregates that help stabilize the platelet–fibrin clot. When platelets are activated, receptors for clotting factors are exposed. This also provides a stable environment for the initiation of the clotting cascade (Colman et al., 2006).

The coagulation system is traditionally divided into the intrinsic and extrinsic pathways. Activity through the extrinsic pathway is initiated by components from the blood and vasculature, with factor VII as the major initiating factor. Activation

COAGULATION PATHWAY

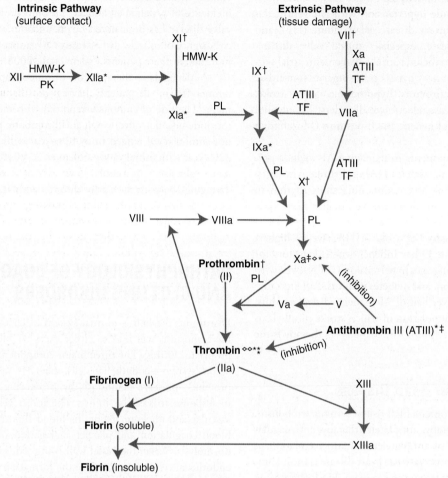

* Major site of activity for unfractionated heparin
† Site of activity for warfarin
‡ Major site of activity for low molecular weight heparin, apixaban rivaroxaban and edoxaban
⁞ Minor site of activity for low molecular weight heparin
◇◇ Major site of activity for dabigatran

HMW-K: high molecular weight kininogen; PK: prekallekrein; PL: phospholipids from activated platelets

FIGURE 50.1   The coagulation system.

occurs when procoagulant components migrate to sites of vascular damage or when blood is exposed to substances released as a result of vascular wall damage. In contrast, activity through the intrinsic coagulation pathway is initiated by activation of factor XII when blood comes in contact with a foreign surface (such as a prosthetic device) or damaged endothelial blood vessels. Once factor X is activated in either the extrinsic or intrinsic pathways, the two pathways merge to form a final common pathway for clot formation by converting prothrombin to thrombin (Colman et al., 2006). (See **Figure 50.1**.)

Several inhibitory processes limit the clotting process. One of the main regulatory proteins of the clotting cascade is antithrombin III, which inhibits the activated clotting factors Xa, VIIa, IXa, XIa, XIIa, and IIa (thrombin). Three other regulatory proteins, proteins C, S, and Z must be present in sufficient

amounts because they prevent excessive clot formation by inactivating factors Va and VIIIa (activated protein C with its cofactor protein S), and preventing the degradation of factor Xa (protein Z). Deficiency in any of these proteins creates a predisposition to pathologic thrombosis (Colman et al., 2006).

Thrombotic Process

Thrombi can form in any part of the cardiovascular system—the veins and arteries (including those of the brain) as well as the heart. Thrombi can cause local complications by obstructing vessels or by breaking off and traveling to a distant site (embolization). Arterial thrombi often form in the setting of preexisting atherosclerosis or other vascular diseases, especially at the sites of ruptured atherosclerotic plaques. In the heart, thrombi can develop on damaged cardiac valves, in a dilated or dyskinetic heart chamber, or on prosthetic valves. Although most intra-cardiac thrombi cause no symptoms, serious consequences can arise if the thrombi migrate to the systemic circulation, espe-cially the brain. In the venous system, thrombi usually occur in the lower extremities as DVT or in the pulmonary circulation as PE. Venous thrombi form in areas of sluggish blood flow (venous stasis) and contain primarily red cells held together with fibrin, with only small amounts of platelets. In contrast, arte-rial thrombi form in areas of high blood flow and are composed primarily of platelets bound with fibrin strands (Colman et al., 2006). The type of thrombus will dictate whether treatment is most appropriate with anticoagulant drugs or antiplatelet drugs.

Hypercoagulable States

Patients with thrombophilia, or hypercoagulable conditions, have an increased tendency to develop thrombosis, most often venous thrombosis. Hypercoagulability may be inherited or acquired. The two most common genetic risk factors for VTE are factor V Leiden mutation and the prothrombin gene muta-tion 20210. The aPL antibody syndrome is the most common nongenetically acquired thrombophilia. Genetic risk factors increase the likelihood of an initial VTE but don't impact the risk of a recurrent event (Goldhaber, 2010).

A mutation in coagulation factor V, one of the key pro-teins in the coagulation cascade, occurs with factor V Leiden. Normally, activated protein C and S will inactivate factor V; in individuals with factor V Leiden, activated factor V is not degraded as efficiently, resulting in increased coagulability (Varga, 2008). Factor V Leiden occurs in 2% to 10% of whites in the United States and increases the risk of VTE two- to five-fold (Coppola et al., 2009).

Another genetic mutation that causes an increased risk of thrombosis is prothrombin gene mutation 20210 or 20210A. Some patients will have increased prothrombin activity, which is thought to contribute to thrombosis. The incidence in the population and the risk of VTE is similar to factor V Leiden. Both the factor V Leiden and prothrombin gene mutation are uncommon in Blacks and Asians (Merli, 2008).

Antithrombin III, activated protein C, and activated pro-tein S are natural anticoagulants, so deficiencies in these clot-ting factors, although very rare, will also induce a prothrombotic state, corresponding to a 5- to 10-fold increase in VTE risk.

Homocysteine is an amino acid formed when the essen-tial amino acid methionine is metabolized. Genetic defects (polymorphism) in the enzymes that regulate homocysteine metabolism can lead to elevated levels (hyperhomocystein-emia), but the exact association between this defect and resul-tant VTE is still uncertain. Hyperhomocysteinemia has been linked to an increased risk of stroke (Goldstein et al., 2011). Hyperhomocysteinemia is likely due to genetic and acquired causes (e.g., dietary deficiencies of folate, vitamin B_6, or vita-min B_{12}) (Coppola et al., 2009).

The presence of a genetic risk factor superimposed with an acquired risk factor significantly increases the risk of VTE

(Coppola et al., 2009). Clues that a patient with VTE has an underlying inherited hypercoagulable condition include thrombosis in patients younger than age 50, a positive family history of VTE, idiopathic or unprovoked thrombosis, recur-rent thrombosis, and thrombosis in unusual locations, such as the adrenal glands, renal veins, or upper extremities (Merli, 2008).

A wide spectrum of acquired hypercoagulable states exist, including aPL antibody syndrome, malignancy, hematologic disorders, and nephrotic syndrome. For the purposes of this chapter, only aPL antibody syndrome will be discussed. aPLs are autoantibodies that bind to membrane phospholipid pro-teins, which are thought to cause the proteins to be antigenic and initiate thrombosis. Several aPLs have been identified, but the two most common are lupus anticoagulant and anticardio-lipin antibodies. Lupus anticoagulant is often found in patients with systemic lupus erythematosus, but can occur in other dis-eases, including syphilis. Lupus anticoagulant is a strong pre-dictor of thrombotic risk for arterial and venous thrombosis. The hallmark characteristics of aPL antibody syndrome are recurrent arterial or venous thrombosis, unexplained fetal loss, and thrombocytopenia with the presence of circulating aPLs. Ischemic stroke is a well-established criterion for the diagnosis of aPL antibody syndrome (Dafer & Biler, 2008).

A workup for thrombophilia is usually deferred until after the acute thrombosis phase because diagnosis does not impact treatment (Goldhaber, 2010). Widespread screening for inher-ited disorders is not recommended unless it is expected to change clinical management. A hematologist referral is required to determine what, if any, laboratory testing is required and whether wider testing of family members is warranted. The presence of certain anticoagulant drugs, in particular warfarin, will dictate the best timing for laboratory testing because war-farin treatment will affect protein C, Z, and S (Merli, 2008).

Although inherited thrombophilia increases the risk of VTE, prophylaxis with long-term anticoagulation is not nec-essary because the risk of bleeding, including fatal bleeding, outweighs the benefits of prophylaxis. However, in the setting of a potential triggering risk factor (e.g., surgery), anticoagu-lation prophylaxis is beneficial during the period of exposure (Coppola et al., 2009).

DIAGNOSTIC CRITERIA

Venous Thromboembolism

Erythema, pain, swelling, venous distention, and warmth in the affected leg are common presenting symptoms of DVT. Other conditions, such as muscle strain, cellulitis, and postphlebi-tic syndrome, may mimic symptoms of DVT. Approximately 50% of patients with DVT have no symptoms. Diagnosing VTE based on clinical factors is often unreliable because only 20% of patients who present with suspected VTE actually have a thrombosis. Therefore, objective confirmatory tests are required (Merli, 2008).

First, the laboratory blood test D-dimer may be measured. D-dimer is the major degradation product released into the circulation when cross-linked fibrin undergoes fibrinolysis. Levels of D-dimer are elevated (>500 μg/L) in most patients with ongoing thrombosis. Current assays for D-dimer are over 95% sensitive but not specific. Therefore, a negative D-dimer (<500 μg/L) test helps to rule out DVT or PE. Clinical prediction models that divide patients into low-, moderate-, or high-risk categories for DVT/PE have been validated. For a first-time DVT, the Wells Score may be calculated to determine the pretest probability of DVT or PE (see http://www.qxmd.com/calculate-online/hematology/wells-dvt-deep-vein-thrombosis and http://www.mdcalc.com/wells-criteria-for-pulmonary-embolism-pe/). Using clinical judgment along with D-dimer assays may decrease the need for unnecessary testing and patient exposure to radiation and contrast dye (Merli, 2008).

The methods used for detecting DVT are contrast-enhanced venography, compression ultrasonography (CUS), and magnetic resonance imaging (MRI). Contrast-enhanced venography is the gold standard for confirming DVT because it is nearly 100% sensitive and specific and can visualize the distal and proximal venous system. However, it is no longer used in the initial diagnosis of DVT due to high cost, invasiveness, and risk of contrast dye–induced allergic reactions and renal impairment. CUS measures the rate and direction of blood flow and can visualize clot formation in the proximal leg veins. CUS is the diagnostic method of choice because it is noninvasive, can be conducted at the bedside, and is relatively easy to perform. In CUS, DVT is diagnosed if the common femoral or popliteal veins cannot be compressed. For CUS, the sensitivity is 95% and specificity is 96% with a first episode of symptomatic proximal DVT. Disadvantages of CUS include decreased accuracy for detecting calf vein thrombi (73% sensitivity), operator variability, and limitations caused by obesity, casts, and immobilization devices. Although MRI is useful for examining pelvic veins, it has limited usefulness for diagnosing DVT because it is expensive and requires the presence of an experienced radiologist (Merli, 2008).

PE is the most serious complication of DVT. The PE mortality rate is related to the size of the thrombus. A massive PE obstructs 50% of the pulmonary vasculature. The term *submassive* is used when less than 50% of the pulmonary circulation is affected. Death occurs from acute right-sided HF in untreated patients. The diagnosis of PE is difficult when based on symptoms because presenting symptoms are not specific. For patients presenting with PE, shortness of breath with or without leg pain may be the first symptom. Other physical findings include sudden onset of dyspnea, pleuritic chest pain, cough, tachycardia, and tachypnea; these symptoms also occur in HF, interstitial lung disease, and pneumonia, so thorough examination and further testing is important. Suspicion of PE is based on symptoms along with such risk factors as immobility, recent trauma or surgery, underlying malignancy, and oral contraceptive use. Baseline tests for evaluating PE include a chest x-ray, an electrocardiogram (ECG) to differentiate between PE and MI, and arterial blood gas evaluations (to assess the severity of hypoxemia). Chest x-ray is often normal, so it is most useful in excluding the diagnosis of other conditions with similar symptoms of PE, including pneumothorax (Merli, 2008).

For PE, ventilation/perfusion (V/Q) lung scanning is used to measure the distribution of blood and air flow in the lungs. The results are reported as high, intermediate, or low probability or normal. A normal scan excludes clinically important PE and is sufficient evidence to withhold anticoagulant therapy. An abnormal scan, even though it might suggest PE, can result from other disease states. V/Q lung scanning previously was the major test for diagnosing PE. However, the combination of clinical suspicion and V/Q scan results is nondiagnostic in 72% of patients. Thus, additional confirmatory testing is required. Pulmonary angiography is the gold standard for confirming PE, but it is invasive and expensive, uses contrast dye, and is not always readily available. It is reserved for patients when noninvasive tests are inconclusive (Merli, 2008). A V/Q scan is reserved for patients with acute kidney injury, chronic kidney disease, or dye allergy who have a relative or absolute contraindication to contrast.

Computed tomography pulmonary angiography (CTPA) has replaced the pulmonary angiogram as the preferred test for diagnosing PE, and it has largely replaced V/Q lung scanning due to higher sensitivity. With CTPA, the sensitivity is 92%, and its specificity is 94%. Disadvantages to CTPA include radiation exposure and the need for injected contrast agent and subsequent risk of renal impairment; V/Q lung scanning is preferred in this setting. CTPA and V/Q lung scanning can reliably exclude the diagnosis of PE (Weitz, 2009).

Imaging of the chest and vascular structures is possible with MRI. In magnetic resonance angiography (MRA), the contrast agent gadolinium is used, which has a lower risk of renal toxicity than the contrast agents used in computed tomography (CT) scans. Disadvantages to MRA include cost and patient physical limitations (e.g., implanted metallic devices and cardiac pacemakers, claustrophobia, obesity) (Merli, 2008).

Atrial Fibrillation

Symptoms associated with AF include palpitations, chest discomfort, shortness of breath, weakness, hypotension, dizziness, and syncope. Clinical signs of AF include acute HF, pulmonary edema, dyspnea, and possibly hemodynamic instability (Fuster et al., 2006). On physical examination, findings of an irregular pulse, irregular jugular venous pulsations, or variations in the intensity of the first heart sound (S_1) can guide the practitioner in suspecting AF (Bentz, 2006). The ECG is used to confirm the diagnosis; an irregularly irregular rhythm is the hallmark of AF. Other ECG characteristics include the absence of P waves and ventricular response rates of 100 to 180 beats/minute. A thorough history and physical examination is needed to rule out underlying causes of AF. Other baseline assessments include evaluation of electrolytes, thyroid function tests, complete blood count (CBC), and chest x-ray. The diagnostic workup also includes a transthoracic echocardiogram, which can detect left ventricular dysfunction, left ventricular hypertrophy, valvular heart disease, and atrial enlargement. In some cases, a stress test is ordered to rule out the presence of ischemic heart disease. Transesophageal echocardiography (TEE) is frequently used to identify left atrial thrombi in preparation for electrical cardioversion, which attempts to restore normal sinus rhythm (Fuster et al., 2006).

Nurses and physician assistants can assist with the initial management of AF by remembering the mnemonic *SALTE*—stabilize (monitor heart rate, blood pressure, respiratory status, and medication), assess (fluid and electrolyte status, medication management, risk factor identification and modification), label/treat (arrhythmia management, reducing anxiety, anticoagulation management), and educate (disease process, anticoagulation teaching, prescribed medications) (McCabe, 2005). Patients with stroke or TIA or risk factors for stroke should be taught the acronym FAST, a mnemonic that stands for facial drooping, arm weakness, speech difficulty, and time to call 911 (http://www.strokeassociation.org/STROKEORG/WarningSigns/Stroke-Warning-Signs-and-Symptoms_UCM_308528_SubHomePage.jsp).

Atrial fibrillation may be classified as "valvular" or "nonvalvular" AF (NVAF). NVAF is defined by the American College of Cardiology (ACC)/American Heart Association (AHA)/Heart Rhythm Society of America (HRSA) AF practice guidelines as "AF in the absence of rheumatic mitral stenosis, a mechanical or bioprosthetic heart valve, or mitral valve repair" (January et al., 2014). Antithrombotic therapy selection for the prevention of stroke is based upon a discussion with the patient about the risk of stroke and the benefits/risks of antithrombotic therapy. Patients with valvular heart disease and AF are at high risk of stroke. For patients with NVAF, an annual risk of stroke is estimated using the CHAS$_2$DS$_2$-Vasc Score (http://www.mdcalc.com/cha2ds2-vasc-score-for-atrial-fibrillation-stroke-risk/ or via a mobile phone app AnticoagEvaluator available from the ACC at http://www.acc.org/tools-and-practice-support/mobile-resources). Risk factors included in this estimate are age, female gender, HF, HTN, prior history of stroke or TIA, diabetes mellitus, and presence of concomitant vascular disease, such as myocardial infarction (MI), peripheral arterial disease, or aortic plaque.

Ischemic Stroke

Ischemic stroke is characterized by a sudden or progressive onset of focal neurologic signs due to an inadequate blood supply to the brain. The resulting neurologic deficits depend on the location of cerebral infarction. Most often, the deficits are confined to one side of the body, right or left. The most common presenting stroke symptom is tingling, numbness, and weakness or paralysis on one side of the body. Incoordination, aphasia, dysarthria, and visual disturbances also can occur. Other manifestations include changes in mental status or loss of consciousness. The time of onset of symptoms is a key piece of historical information to determine from the patient or family members because it will dictate treatment. Neurologic signs or symptoms may progress in approximately 25% of patients

in the first 24 to 48 hours. Approximately 50% of patients are left with a permanent disability (Adams et al., 2007).

The physical examination may show signs of trauma or seizures (e.g., contusions, tongue lacerations) or carotid disease (bruits). A comprehensive neurological exam is necessary to determine the extent of neurological deficit, identify the possible location of the thrombus, and help determine the most appropriate intervention (Adams et al., 2007).

All patients presenting with suspected ischemic stroke require several diagnostic tests, including blood glucose, electrolytes, CBC with platelets, ECG, cardiac enzymes, prothrombin time (PT), international normalized ratio (INR), activated partial thromboplastin time (aPTT), and oxygen saturation (Adams et al., 2007).

Brain imaging studies, including noncontrast CT scan and MRI, are used to detect the presence, extent, and progression of a cerebral infarction and if there is intracranial bleeding. Several tests can help detect the source of a presumed thromboembolic ischemic stroke. Noninvasive carotid ultrasound will show occlusion or stenosis. An ECG differentiates between AF and MI. Transthoracic and transesophageal echocardiograms visualize cardiac function and the presence of an atrial thrombus. Carotid cerebral angiography can be performed to examine the arteries and veins of the brain and neck. This provides the most accurate visualization to detect abnormalities such as stenosis or occlusion that may have caused the ischemic event (Adams et al., 2007).

Native and Prosthetic Valvular Heart Disease

Signs and symptoms of valvular heart disease vary depending on the valve that is affected. In aortic stenosis, the cardinal symptoms are dyspnea, angina, syncope, and HF. Aortic regurgitation is often asymptomatic. Dyspnea is the hallmark symptom of mitral stenosis, although this usually is present with exertion and has a gradual onset over approximately 20 years. Mitral regurgitation also progresses slowly and may be asymptomatic for many years. The initial symptoms may be fatigue, dyspnea on exertion, and palpitations that, in severe cases, may lead to pulmonary edema. Each valvular disorder is associated with a characteristic murmur, but the intensity of the murmur does not always correlate with the severity of the valvular disorder (Maganti et al., 2010).

Findings on physical examination also vary with the severity of the valve calcification, severity of stenosis, and left ventricular dysfunction. The chest x-ray will show cardiomegaly, which can occur with aortic stenosis. An ECG is used to determine the possible cardiac effects of valve incompetence or stenosis such as left ventricular hypertrophy in mitral and aortic regurgitation. Confirmation of the diagnosis of valvular disease is best accomplished by an echocardiogram, which will also give an estimate of disease severity. Cardiac catheterization and angiography are used when noninvasive tests are inconclusive. When physical symptoms of valvular disease lead to limitations in daily activities or if cardiac decompensation occurs despite medical treatment, surgical intervention either with surgical repair, surgical valve replacement or minimally invasive transcatheter aortic valve replacement are recommended (Maganti et al., 2010).

GOALS OF DRUG THERAPY

Preventing the development of a stroke is the primary goal of antithrombotic therapy in patients with AF and prosthetic heart valves and in those with a history of cardioembolic stroke. Anticoagulation treatment in patients with existing DVT/PE is initiated to prevent extension of the thrombus; thromboembolic complications, including postthrombotic syndrome; and development of a new thrombus. Anticoagulation prophylaxis after orthopedic surgery is initiated with aspirin or anticoagulation to decrease the risk of DVT or PE. The goals of antiplatelet therapy are to prevent and treat ischemic strokes from noncardioembolic sources. Other indications for antiplatelet therapy for primary or secondary prevention of CVD events will not be discussed in this chapter.

ANTICOAGULANTS: INDICATIONS

A valid indication for anticoagulation is essential before starting anticoagulant therapy. Unfractionated heparin (UFH) and low molecular weight heparins (LMWHs) are used for treatment and secondary prevention of VTE and treatment of acute coronary syndromes. In addition, UFH is used in hospitalized patients undergoing procedures such as cardiothoracic surgery, electrophysiology arrhythmia catheter ablation, cardioversion for atrial fibrillation, and percutaneous coronary intervention as well as in patients undergoing hemodialysis. Warfarin is used in the prevention of valve thrombosis in patients with mechanical heart valves as well as for SPAF, prevention of VTE in patients undergoing orthopedic surgery, and treatment and secondary prevention of VTE. FDA-approved indications for direct-acting oral anticoagulants (DOACs) are described in **Table 50.1**.

CONTRAINDICTIONS TO ANTICOAGULATION

Absolute contraindications to anticoagulation are as follows: recent hemorrhagic stroke, active major bleeding, recent trauma or traumatic surgery, use in the immediate postoperative period

after CNS or ocular surgery, or the presence of spinal catheters and aneurysms or CNS tumors with a high bleeding risk (Bristol-Myers Squibb, 2010). Warfarin is contraindicated in pregnancy, and there are no data with DOACs in pregnancy. Therefore, UFH or LMWH, which does not cross the placenta, is preferred. Active or a recent (within 100 days) history of heparin-induced thrombocytopenia (HIT) is a contraindication to UFH and LMWHs. Neuraxial anesthesia with spinal or epidural catheter placement or removal poses a risk of spinal hematoma in the anticoagulated patient. Therefore, the American Society of Regional Anesthesia and Pain Medicine released guidelines regarding timing for neuraxial needle placement and removal relative to UFH, LMWH, and DOAC dose were published (Horlocker et al., 2010).

ANTICOAGULANTS: CONSIDERATIONS BEFORE STARTING THERAPY

In addition to a valid indication, several patient factors also warrant consideration to determine if the risk of hemorrhage outweighs the benefit of therapy.

Baseline laboratory values including PT, INR, aPTT, urinalysis, CBC (with platelet count), and a liver profile are recommended before initiating anticoagulation. In women of childbearing age, laboratory testing for β-human chorionic gonadotropin is strongly encouraged to rule out pregnancy. Obtaining the patient's telephone number and an alternative contact, such as a responsible family member or neighbor (obtain consent to contact others per HIPAA guidelines), is also advised. In addition, rule out any active major bleeding from the central nervous system (CNS) or gastrointestinal (GI) tract. A digital rectal examination or guaiac test to detect blood in the stool is recommended. A detailed medical, surgical, and medication history, including over-the-counter (OTC) medications and dietary supplements, is needed to assess the patient's risk of bleeding events or inadequate anticoagulation. It is also important to document the indication for anticoagulation, which determines the duration of therapy, and, if warfarin is selected, to define the corresponding target INR, which defines the intensity of anticoagulation. When all these

TABLE 50.1				
FDA-Approved Indications for DOACs				
Drug	**Dabigatran**	**Rivaroxaban**	**Apixaban**	**Edoxaban**
Stroke and systemic thromboembolism prevention in NVAF	X	X	X	X
Prophylaxis of DVT following hip and knee orthopedic surgery	X	X	X	
Treatment of DVT and PE	X*	X	X	X*
To reduce risk of recurrence of DVT and PE in patients previously treated	X	X	X	

*In patients who have been treated with a parenteral anticoagulant for 5–10 d.
NVAF, nonvalvular atrial fibrillation; DVT, deep vein thrombosis; PE, pulmonary embolism.

issues are addressed, anticoagulation is initiated (Witt, 2010). For patients receiving an LMWH or DOAC, body weight (kg), serum creatinine, and estimation of renal function creatinine clearance (CrCl) should be calculated. For patient receiving UFH, body weight (kg) should also be obtained. Although not currently recommended as a routine practice, a bleeding risk estimate for patients with AF may be obtained from calculating the HAS-BLED score and is discussed later in this chapter (http://www.mdcalc.com/has-bled-score-for-major-bleeding-risk/ or via a mobile phone app AnticoagEvaluator available from the ACC at http://www.acc.org/tools-and-practice-support/mobile-resources). The HAS-BLED score has only been validated in patients taking vitamin K antagonists (VKAs) and not in patients receiving parenteral anticoagulants or DOACs.

ANTICOAGULANTS: MECHANISM OF ACTION AND TIME FRAME FOR RESPONSE, DOSING SELECTION, DRUG–DRUG INTERACTIONS, AND MONITORING

Anticoagulants include the injectable agents unfractionated heparin (UFH) and low-molecular-weight heparins (LMWHs) (e.g., enoxaparin), oral vitamin K antagonist (VKA) warfarin, and the direct-acting oral anticoagulants (DOACs) dabigatran etexilate (a direct thrombin inhibitors), and oral factor Xa inhibitors (rivaroxaban, apixaban, and edoxaban). (See **Figure 50.1.**)

Parenteral Anticoagulants: Unfractionated Heparin and Low Molecular Weight Heparin

UFH and LMWH are used for the treatment of acute venous or arterial thrombosis and prophylaxis of VTE.

Unfractionated Heparin

UFH inhibits reactions that lead to clotting, but it does not alter the concentration of the normal clotting factors of the blood. When UFH binds to antithrombin III, the shape of the structure changes, which increases the inactivation rate of the intrinsic clotting cascade pathway, including activated clotting factors XII, XI, X, and IX and thrombin (factor II). Once active thrombosis has developed, UFH inhibits further coagulation by inactivating thrombin and preventing the conversion of fibrinogen to fibrin. UFH is a very large molecule (i.e., it has an average molecular weight of 15,000 Da with chains of 18 to 50 saccharide units), but only a small portion of the entire structure is necessary for binding with antithrombin III. Because the structure is so large, UFH can bind to both factor Xa and thrombin. Heparin derivatives with smaller structures cannot bind to thrombin, but can bind to and inhibit factor Xa (Hirsh et al., 2008). One disadvantage of heparin's large size is that it cannot inactivate clot-bound thrombin or activated factor X that is bound to platelets. Clot-bound thrombin can continue to generate more thrombin, activate platelets, and

convert fibrinogen into fibrin, promoting clotting. In contrast to UFH, direct thrombin inhibitors do not activate platelets (Spyropoulos, 2008).

Heparin is not absorbed from the GI tract, so it must be administered parenterally. UFH has an immediate onset of action and is administered by intravenous (IV) infusion when rapid anticoagulation is needed, as in acute DVT, PE, or unstable angina. UFH may also be administered subcutaneously with peak levels occurring 2 to 4 hours after administration, depending on the dose. Subcutaneous dosing must be at a sufficient amount to overcome the lower bioavailability, approximately 30%, associated with this route of administration. The duration of action and half-life are dose dependent. The average half-life is 30 to 180 minutes, which may be significantly prolonged at high doses. UFH is metabolized by liver heparinase and the reticuloendothelial system and possibly secondarily in the kidneys. It is then excreted in urine as unchanged drug.

Limitations of UFH include variability in its size, anticoagulant activity, and pharmacokinetic profile. UFH can range in size from 5,000 to 30,000 Da. Agents with higher molecular weights are cleared from the circulation more rapidly than agents with lower molecular weights. UFH is highly bound to plasma proteins and cellular components, including endothelial cells and macrophages, which reduces its therapeutic effect and increases the incidence of immunologic reactions (e.g., HIT). Furthermore, some patients exhibit heparin resistance. This is characterized by no measurable change in anticoagulant effect despite receiving large doses (35,000 units) of heparin daily. UFH also has a nonlinear dose response, so that small changes in dosage can result in large changes in anticoagulant effect (Hirsh et al., 2008).

Before initiating UFH therapy, define the target aPTT, establish the frequency of aPTT monitoring, and determine the duration of therapy. UFH treatment dosing is based on weight. Initial dosing for treatment of VTE is 80 units/kg as an IV bolus and then 18 units/kg/hour as a continuous IV infusion. UFH's effect is monitored by aPTT. Dosage changes should be made based on aPTT levels monitored every 6 hours until the patient is stable and then every 12 to 24 hours. Each individual hospital defines a regent-specific aPTT therapeutic range depending upon an antifactor Xa concentration—aPTT curve. Hospitals construct a dosing algorithm for dose adjustment depending on the resultant aPTT or utilize heparin anti-Xa activity measures directly. One popular method is the weight-based nomogram (Hirsh et al., 2008) shown in **Table 50.2.** Anticoagulation may be subtherapeutic or supratherapeutic despite the use of validated dosing protocols. UFH in a fixed low dose of 5,000 units subcutaneously every 8 to 12 hours is used for VTE prophylaxis. This regimen may be used in postoperative patients and medical patients with decreased mobility (Hirsh et al., 2008).

Low Molecular Weight Heparins

LMWHs are fragments of UFH, prepared by the depolymerization of porcine heparin. Like UFH, LMWHs produce their major anticoagulant effect via thrombin and factor Xa.

TABLE 50.2

Weight-Based Heparin Dosing Nomogram

Activated Partial Thromboplastin Time	Rate Change
Initial dose	80 U/kg bolus, then 18 U/kg/h
<35 s	80 U/kg bolus, then increase infusion by 4 U/kg/h
35–45 s	40 U/kg/h bolus, then increase infusion by 2 U/kg/h
46–70 s	No change (Therapeutic range determined by anti-Xa calibration curve 0.3–0.7 IU/mL)
71–90 s	Decrease infusion rate by 2 U/kg/h
>90 s	Hold infusion for 1 h; then decrease infusion rate by 3 U/kg/h

LMWHs are used for prophylaxis of VTE in patients after orthopedic and abdominal surgery, in medical patients with decreased mobility or increased risk of VTE, and for treatment of DVT/PE. As with UFH, most patients need subsequent treatment with warfarin, depending on the indication for anticoagulation. Other uses that will not be discussed in this chapter include the treatment of acute coronary syndromes. Three LMWHs are available in the United States: dalteparin (Fragmin), enoxaparin (Lovenox), and tinzaparin (Innohep), but the most commonly used in enoxaparin.

LMWHs preferentially inhibit the activation of factor X but have minimal effects on thrombin (factor II) because of their small size. The average molecular weight of LMWHs ranges from 4,000 to 6,500 Da with 13 to 22 saccharide units. (UFH has a mean molecular weight of 12,000 to 15,000 Da with 18 to 50 saccharide units.) Only the LMWHs with saccharide chains having 18 or more units can bind to and inhibit thrombin. UFH has a ratio of anti-Xa to anti-IIa activity of 1:1, and the anti-Xa to anti-IIa activity of LMWHs ranges from 2:1 to 4:1 (Hirsh et al., 2008).

LMWHs given by the subcutaneous route have a bioavailability of greater than 90% of the given dose. In contrast to UFH, LMWHs have minimal binding to cells or plasma proteins, which results in the persistence of free drug in the circulation and a longer half-life of activity. The half-lives of LMWHs range from 108 to 252 minutes. Dosing is fixed in prophylaxis, but is based on weight for treatment. The peak effect occurs at approximately 4 hours following a subcutaneous dose.

As previously noted, the major antithrombotic and bleeding effects of LMWHs arise through their ability to inactivate factor Xa. UFH is monitored using aPTT, which primarily reflects antiactivated factor II (IIa) activity, but LMWHs have minimal effects on the aPTT. Theoretically, LMWHs may be monitored by anti-Xa activity, with a target range for treatment regimens of a chromogenic anti-Xa peak of 0.5 to 1.2 units/mL measured 3 to 4 hours after a subcutaneous dose. Studies have demonstrated that the anti-Xa effect of LMWHs is linearly

related to the dose administered. Therefore, plasma levels are predictable, and anti-Xa activity monitoring is not routinely performed. Monitoring may be considered in selected patients, such as those with renal dysfunction because LMWHs are cleared primarily by the renal route, morbidly obese patients (>150 kg) because weight-adjusted dosing has not been evaluated in patients with severe obesity, and pregnant patients because their weight changes, volume shifts occur, and clearance changes as pregnancy progresses. In addition to the recommendation for monitoring anti-Xa levels in patients with renal dysfunction, a dosing reduction is recommended for enoxaparin. UFH is recommended over LMWH for patients with CrCl < 30 mL/min in the 2012 American College of Chest Physicians Guidelines (Hirsh et al., 2008).

Advantages of LMWHs over UFH include greater bioavailability with subcutaneous administration; longer duration of anticoagulant effect, allowing for once-daily or twice-daily dosing; high degree of correlation between anti-Xa and body weight, allowing for fixed dosing; less intensive nursing care; and less intensive laboratory monitoring and more predictable anticoagulant response, permitting use in the outpatient setting (Hull & Pineo, 2004).

Each LMWH has a unique dosing regimen because of its unique chemical properties and the relative proportions of anti-Xa to anti-IIa activity. Because of differences in the manufacturing process, molecular weight, half-life, ratio of anti-Xa to anti-IIa activity, and dose, the FDA does not consider these agents therapeutically interchangeable (Hirsh et al., 2008). Enoxaparin at 30 mg every 12 hours or 40 mg daily is currently approved for prophylaxis in medical inpatients and patients after hip, knee, and abdominal surgery. Dalteparin at 2,500 units every 12 hours or 5,000 units daily is approved for prophylaxis in patients after hip and abdominal surgery. For VTE treatment, current FDA-approved dosing for enoxaparin is 1 mg/kg subcutaneous every 12 hours or 1.5 mg/kg daily subcutaneous for inpatients with acute DVT with and without PE when administered in conjunction with warfarin and for outpatients with acute DVT without PE when administered in conjunction with warfarin. Dosing adjustment is required for enoxaparin in patients with CrCl <30 mL/min. Dalteparin is dosed at 100 international units/kg subcutaneous every 12 hours or 200 international units/kg every 24 hours for patients with acute DVT with or without PE. Tinzaparin 175 international units/kg subcutaneous daily is FDA approved for inpatient treatment of acute DVT with and without PE when administered in conjunction with warfarin. When LMWHs are used in the outpatient setting, patient education regarding subcutaneous injection is necessary. Establish that the patient or their caregiver can reliably and accurately administer the subcutaneous injection, or consider arranging for home health care visits (www.lovenox.com/docs/pdf/At-Home-With-Lovenox_p.pdf). The use of UFH and LMWH for acute coronary syndromes will not be discussed in this chapter.

Patients are carefully assessed for bleeding including hematuria and GI bleeding/blood in stools or hemoptysis. Monitoring UFH and LMWHs for HIT is the section on Other Adverse Effects below.

TABLE 50.3

Relationship between the Prothrombin Time Ratio and the International Normalized Ratio for Thromboplastins with Varying International Sensitivity Index Values

Hospital	ISI	Control PT (s)	PT (s)	PT ratio	INR
A	1.3	14.8	33.9	2.3	2.9
B	2.3	11.4	18.2	1.6	2.9

The INR takes into account the differences in thromboplastin sensitivity, thus giving a more accurate reflection of the level of anticoagulation.

PT, prothrombin time; PT ratio, observed PT divided by control PT; ISI, International Sensitivity Index; INR, international normalized ratio (INR = PT ratio^{ISI}).

Vitamin K Antagonist (Warfarin)

Warfarin inhibits activation of the clotting factors in the liver that depend on vitamin K for synthesis—factors II, VII, IX, and X and the coagulation inhibitor proteins C, Z and S. Warfarin interferes with the conversion of vitamin K from its inactive form to active vitamin K. Vitamin K is depleted, and the rate of clotting factor formation is decreased, which ultimately prevents clot formation and extension. Warfarin does not affect the function of existing clotting factors and has no effect on an existing thrombus (Ansell et al., 2008).

A significant limitation to warfarin is its long onset of effect. The half-lives of clotting factors range from 6 hours (factor VII) to 60 hours (factor II) (Tran & Ginsberg, 2006). The average half-life of warfarin is 36 to 42 hours. The onset of anticoagulant effect depends on both the half-life of warfarin and the time required to deplete the vitamin K–dependent clotting factors. The anticoagulant effect of warfarin is monitored with the INR, which is derived from the PT **(Table 50.3** and **Box 50.2)**. The INR will show an initial prolongation 1 to 3 days after warfarin is first administered, which is due to the rapid depletion of factor VII. However, the full antithrombotic effect of warfarin won't be seen for 8 to 14 days, when factor II (prothrombin) is depleted. In cases of acute DVT or PE, UFH or LMWHs is often given with warfarin when rapid anticoagulation is needed or in hypercoagulable patients (protein C or S deficiency). Warfarin causes a quick fall in protein C (half-life of 8 to 10 hours), which can induce a temporary hypercoagulable state, putting patients at risk for thrombosis. The injectable anticoagulant is continued until the INR is stable for at least 2 days, which allows for additional reductions in the levels of factors X and II (Ansell et al., 2008). During therapy in hospitalized patients, daily CBCs and platelet counts are usually obtained and daily INRs with warfarin to determine the dose.

Currently, warfarin (Coumadin) is the most widely used oral anticoagulant in the United States. However, it has

BOX 50.2   International Normalized Ratio: Sensitive Test for Clotting Time

The international normalized ratio (INR is the universally accepted laboratory test for monitoring anticoagulation therapy with the vitamin K antagonists. The INR has replaced the previously used prothrombin time (PT) ratio.

PT is the time in seconds for a blood sample to clot after the addition of laboratory reagents, including specific plasma proteins (tissue thromboplastins) that aid in coagulation. PT measures the reduction in three of the four vitamin K–dependent clotting factors (II, VII, and X) of the extrinsic coagulation cascade. The PT ratio is simply the patient's individual PT divided by a laboratory's control PT. A change in the tissue thromboplastin source from human brain to rabbit brain 40 years ago resulted in a reduced sensitivity in the PT test, leading to lower PT values, and accordingly higher PT ratio goals, with subsequent increased bleeding risk. The International Sensitivity Index (ISI) was developed by the World Health Organization (WHO) as a reference standard to correct this problem.

Mathematically, the INR is the PT ratio raised to the power of the ISI, or INR = PT ratio^{ISI}. The ISI for

commercially available tissue thromboplastins varies between individual lots and manufacturers. The WHO reference standard was assigned an ISI of 1.0, although most commercial laboratories use tissue thromboplastins with ISIs ranging from 1.0 to 2.88. The ISI for a particular reagent is identified in the package insert. The INR can be determined using a calculator, if needed.

Most laboratories commonly report PT and INR. However, only the INR should be used for dosing changes. Relying on the INR minimizes variability in reported results if different laboratories, with different thromboplastin preparations, are used **(Table 50.1)**. The INR represents the best method for standardizing results from different thromboplastin reagents. The American College of Chest Physicians has standardized the desired target INR goal for anticoagulation therapy for each clinical indication. Current guidelines recommend an INR range of 2 to 3 for most indications of anticoagulation. INRs of 2.5 to 3.5 are reserved for patients with prosthetic heart valves or hypercoagulable conditions.

Data from Ansell, J., Hirsh, J., Hylek, E., et al. (2008). Pharmacology and management of the VKAs. American College of Chest Physicians Evidence-Based Clinical Practice Guidelines (8th ed.). *Chest, 133*(6 Suppl.), 160S–198S.

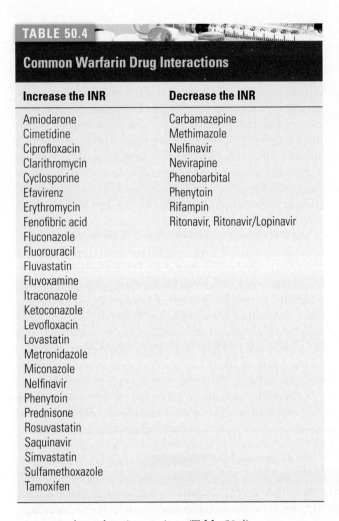

TABLE 50.4

Common Warfarin Drug Interactions

Increase the INR	Decrease the INR
Amiodarone	Carbamazepine
Cimetidine	Methimazole
Ciprofloxacin	Nelfinavir
Clarithromycin	Nevirapine
Cyclosporine	Phenobarbital
Efavirenz	Phenytoin
Erythromycin	Rifampin
Fenofibric acid	Ritonavir, Ritonavir/Lopinavir
Fluconazole	
Fluorouracil	
Fluvastatin	
Fluvoxamine	
Itraconazole	
Ketoconazole	
Levofloxacin	
Lovastatin	
Metronidazole	
Miconazole	
Nelfinavir	
Phenytoin	
Prednisone	
Rosuvastatin	
Saquinavir	
Simvastatin	
Sulfamethoxazole	
Tamoxifen	

numerous drug–drug interactions (**Table 50.4**), a very narrow therapeutic index, and requires routine laboratory monitoring of the INR at least every 4 to 6 weeks. Warfarin is metabolized by the liver isoenzymes CYP2C9, CYP3A4, and CYP1A2. Medications that inhibitor or are a substrate for these isoenzymes may decrease warfarin metabolism and increase the INR. Medications that induce these isoenzymes increase the clearance of warfarin and decrease the INR.

Several herbal preparations can potentially interfere with the anticoagulant effect of warfarin. Although stringently performed clinical trials are lacking, bilberry, feverfew, garlic, and ginger have limited data that show an increased anticoagulant effect when used with warfarin (Nutescu et al., 2006). Fish oil has been noted to increase the INR (Jacobs, 2008). Garlic has platelet inhibitory effects that can increase bleeding risk, and there are anecdotal reports of increases in the PT/INR in patients receiving warfarin. Herbal products that can decrease the effect of warfarin include ginseng and green tea, due to its vitamin K content (Holbrook et al., 2005). Literature and regulatory actions on herbal supplements can be accessed through the U.S. Department of Agriculture Food and Nutrition Information Center Web site at http://fnic.nal.usda. gov. Supplements containing multiple ingredients are a concern because there may be variations in the amount and purity of the substances comprising the product (Wittkowsky, 2008).

Because of its long half-life, warfarin is administered once daily. Warfarin is completely absorbed after oral administration and is metabolized to inactive metabolites by the liver. Warfarin has a narrow therapeutic window; therefore, the dose needed to exert clinical efficacy is similar to the dose that causes adverse effects (Ansell et al., 2008). Individual patients vary widely in their ability to absorb and eliminate warfarin (pharmacokinetic variations) and in their rate of clinical response and dosage requirements (pharmacodynamic variations). Patient variability in the dose response to warfarin is not related to weight or sex but is influenced by age, comorbid disease states, concomitant medications, and one's genetically predetermined rate of metabolism (Ansell et al., 2008; Garcia et al., 2008).

Gene variants have been identified affecting CYP2C9 (warfarin metabolism) as well as vitamin K epoxide reductase complex 1 (VKORC1) (an enzyme involved in the conversion of vitamin K from active to inactive forms affecting the body's sensitivity to warfarin). The prescribing information contains recommended initial doses of warfarin for warfarin-naive patients based upon selected genotypes combinations of CYP2C9 and VCORC1. However, since many other factors affect warfarin clearance and thus INR, and there are no strong scientific data supporting improved outcomes from knowing this pharmacogenetic information prior to starting warfarin, pharmacogenetic testing for these genetic variants prior to starting warfarin is currently not recommended by any professional organization (Kimmel, 2015).

An increased warfarin response can occur in patients with hepatic dysfunction, in which there is impaired synthesis of clotting factors and decreased warfarin metabolism. Likewise, lower warfarin doses may be needed in patients with low serum albumin or those with significant congestive HF (Jacobs, 2008). Other pharmacodynamic factors that may potentiate warfarin response include hypermetabolic states, such as hyperthyroidism, and febrile states when there is an increased catabolic rate of vitamin K–dependent clotting factors. The elderly also seem to be more sensitive to warfarin, possibly because of altered pharmacodynamic parameters, but the etiology is unknown (Jacobs, 2008).

If the patient receives a prescription for warfarin, the prescriber needs to choose among nine different dosage strengths and colors (e.g., a 1-mg tablet is pink, whereas a 5-mg tablet is peach). For safety's sake and to avoid confusing the patient, prescribe only one warfarin tablet strength (e.g., 2.5- or 5-mg tablets, but not both). Patients also need to be taught to remember the tablet color, shape, and tablet strength with each new prescription and refill.

The goal INR for various indications is described in **Box 50.3**. It is difficult to predict an individual's warfarin requirement needed to reach the INR range that is considered therapeutic for the disease state. The initial dose of warfarin is typically 5 to 10 mg/d orally administered for 1 to 3 days. Certain patient populations, such as the elderly, patients with congestive heart failure, those with underlying malignancy, those with severely impaired renal or hepatic function, or those taking interacting drugs that increase warfarin's effect, are at high risk for bleeding and should receive a lower initial dose. Larger starting doses, such as 7.5 to 10 mg, may be used in

<table>
<tr><td>

BOX 50.3   Target INRs for Thrombosis Prevention

INR GOAL 2.0 TO 2.5

Patients with a disease-specific anticoagulation goal of 2.0 to 3.0 (see below) who also are taking concomitant aspirin and a P2Y12 inhibitor

INR GOAL 2 TO 3

Prophylaxis of venous thrombosis
Treatment of deep vein thrombosis
Treatment of pulmonary embolism
Stroke prevention in atrial fibrillation
Tissue (bioprosthetic) heart valves with other risk factors for stroke
Mechanical prosthetic heart valves (bileaflet valves; St. Jude Medical, Medtronic Hall) in the aortic position
Hypercoagulable conditions (antiphospholipid antibodies with lupus anticoagulant)—certain patients with thromboembolism

INR GOAL 2.5 TO 3.5

Mechanical prosthetic heart valves (caged ball, tilting disk) in the mitral position or in the aortic position for patients with additional stroke risk factors (e.g. AF)
Hypercoagulable conditions (antiphospholipid antibodies with lupus anticoagulant)—if a history of thromboembolic events with INR of 2 to 3

</td><td>

BOX 50.4   Questions to Ask When INR Results Are Unexpected

- Have any warfarin doses been missed in the past 3 to 5 days?
- Have extra warfarin tablets been ingested?
- Is the patient taking a warfarin regimen other than prescribed?
- Is the patient experiencing bleeding problems?
- Is the patient experiencing thromboembolic complications?
- Have any new medications (prescription, over the counter, herbal) been started, deleted, or changed from the patient's medication regimen?
- Has the patient's underlying condition changed, as in acute congestive heart failure exacerbation or worsening renal or hepatic impairment?
- Has the patient had a recent acute febrile or GI illness?
- Has thyroid status changed or has a malignancy been diagnosed?

</td></tr>
</table>

younger patients without comorbid conditions if rapid effect is urgently needed, but this is unnecessary for most patients. During the initial titration phase, daily dosage increases or decreases are commonly made in 2- to 2.5-mg increments based on INR values. Administering warfarin at the same time daily is recommended to reduce variability in effects (Ansell et al., 2008). Warfarin is overlapped with an injectable anticoagulant in patients with acute VTE and in patients at higher risk of stroke or recently cardioverted patients with AF (Jacobs, 2008).

Target INRs for various anticoagulation indications are described in **Box 50.3**. The relationship between the warfarin dosage and the INR is not linear. Therefore, minor changes in dose can result in greater than expected changes in the INR. The maintenance warfarin dose varies widely among individuals, and there are no widely accepted patient characteristics that reliably predict the necessary maintenance dose. Warfarin-dosing algorithms for initiation and maintenance therapy can also assist with determining warfarin doses (Witt, 2010). Questions to ask to help determine the cause of an out-of-range INR in a patient previously stabilized on warfarin are described in **Box 50.4**.

For maintenance therapy changes, calculating the total weekly warfarin dose and then increasing or decreasing the weekly regimen by only 10% to 20%, spread over the course of the week, can cause measurable changes in the INR. Some clinicians advocate administering the same dosage daily, whereas others agree that giving varying doses on alternate days is rational. Patients with low educational levels and cognitive impairments or those receiving several other medications may benefit from a simple dosing schedule. If an alternating-day regimen is chosen, defining the actual dosage for each day of the week is recommended (e.g., 5 mg administered on Tuesdays, Thursdays, Saturdays, and Sundays and 7.5 mg on Mondays, Wednesday, and Fridays, rather than 5 mg alternating with 7.5 mg every other day). This helps to reduce patient confusion and avoid fluctuations in the INR. Sensitive patients with reduced requirements should receive warfarin daily rather than alternating between drug and drug-free days, for example, 1.5 mg given every day, rather than 2 mg alternating with 1 mg every other day (Ansell et al., 2008). Once a patient has reached a therapeutic INR with a consistent warfarin dose, INR monitoring should continue at least every 4 weeks (Witt, 2010). Patients using vitamin K supplementation will require frequent INR value checks to avoid the INR dropping below the therapeutic range. Patients also need to be cautioned to not abruptly discontinue the vitamin K supplement due to the risk of excessive anticoagulation (Ansell et al., 2008).

Several dosing nomograms are available that assist in rapidly achieving therapeutic INR values when warfarin is started, and computer software programs are also used (Jacobson, 2008; Witt, 2010 also see www.cfp.ca/content/suppl/2013/08/13/59.8.856.../Warfarin_Tips.pdf). It is important to note that these nomograms were developed in patients who were not taking interacting medications. The addition or subtraction of an interacting medication requires more frequent INR monitoring. If possible, patients taking warfarin should be managed by specialized anticoagulation clinics as the clinic reported patient time spent in the therapeutic INR range is higher than "usual" care and bleeding events lower (Garcia and Hylek, 2008).

Direct-Acting Oral Anticoagulants

Dabigatran etexilate (Pradaxa), rivaroxaban (Xarelto), apixaban (Eliquis), and edoxaban (Savaysa) are DOACs. FDA-approved indications of DOACs are described in **Table 50.1**. Dabigatran etexilate is a prodrug that is metabolized by blood esterases to dabigatran, which binds to and inhibits thrombin that prevents the conversion of fibrinogen to fibrin. Thrombin is also the most potent stimulator of platelet aggregation. (See **Figure 50.1**.) Blocking thrombin is an effective method of inhibiting coagulation since thrombin is needed for fibrin formation and to activate factors V, VII, VIII, IX, and XIII. Dabigatran directly inhibits free and clot-bound thrombin. The direct-acting agents, rivaroxaban, apixaban, and edoxaban, bind directly to factor Xa and do not require antithrombin like LMWHs do. Intravenous direct thrombin inhibitors are available (e.g., bivalirudin, and argatroban) and are administered via infusion in the hospital and used primarily for percutaneous coronary intervention (bivalirudin) or treatment of HIT (argatroban and bivalirudin).

One of the most important advantages of the DOACs over warfarin is that the DOACs have a faster onset of action. The time to anticoagulant effect of a DOAC depends on the time to maximum plasma concentration, which typically occurs within 2 to 4 hours of first dose administration. Therefore, bridging between an injectable anticoagulant and a DOAC is not necessary. Other advantages compared to warfarin include fixed dosing, no dietary interactions, and few indications for coagulation intensity monitoring. The DOACs have fewer drug–drug interactions compared to warfarin (**Table 50.5**).

In contrast to warfarin, these agents have fixed dosing and a predictable anticoagulant response; therefore, dosing adjustments are not necessary.

Disadvantages of DOACs compared to warfarin include lack of a specific antidote for reversal of apixaban, edoxaban and rivaroxaban, a higher acquisition cost, and potentially a faster offset of action so that adherence is key to a sustained effect.

Determining a patient's past history of medication compliance is also recommended because dabigatran and apixaban require twice-daily dosing, and anticoagulant efficacy will be decreased if a patient misses one dose. Dabigatran cannot be crushed or put in weekly pillboxes to help with compliance because it is packaged in moisture-proof containers. Rivaroxaban must be taken with a meal to improve bioavailability. The dosing of rivaroxaban and apixaban for the treatment of NVAF and VTE differs (**Tables 50.6 and 50.7**). Apixaban has the least dependency on renal clearance, and edoxaban has the fewest labeled drug–drug interactions (**Table 50.5**). Edoxaban has a black box warning for stroke prevention in NVAF to avoid use in patients with CrCl >95 mL/min due to reduced efficacy for ischemic stroke. Reduced efficacy was not proportional to CrCl and was not apparent in the primary endpoint of stroke or systemic thromboembolism.

In a patient transitioning from warfarin to a DOAC, warfarin should be discontinued and the DOAC should be started when the INR is at the lower end of the warfarin therapeutic range. In a patient transitioning from UFH to a DOAC, discontinue UFH at the time that the DOAC is administered. In a patient transitioning from LMWH to a DOAC, discontinue the LMWH and administer the DOAC at the time of the next scheduled LMWH dose. When switching between DOACs, give the first dose of the new DOAC at the time the previous DOAC scheduled dose was due.

TABLE 50.5

DOAC Drug Interactions

Type of Interaction and Outcome	Dabigatran	Rivaroxaban	Apixaban	Edoxaban
Pharmacokinetic (increase of at least 50% in AUC plasma concentrations)	Amiodarone Dronedarone Ketoconazole Quinidine Ticagrelor Verapamil	Clarithromycin Itraconazole Ketoconazole Posaconazole Voriconazole Ritonavir	Itraconazole Ketoconazole Posaconazole Voriconazole Ritonavir	No dose reduction for P-gp inhibitors
Pharmacokinetic (decrease of at least 50% in AUC plasma concentrations)	Carbamazepine Rifampin St. John's wort	Carbamazepine Rifampin St. John's wort Phenobarbital Phenytoin	Carbamazepine Rifampin St. John's wort Phenytoin	Rifampin
Pharmacodynamic (increased risk of bleeding)	Aspirin NSAIDs Other antiplatelets (e.g., cilostazol, vorapaxar, dipyridamole) Other anticoagulants Thrombolytics			

TABLE 50.6

Dosing and Renal Adjustment for DOACs for Stroke and Systemic Thromboembolism Prevention in Nonvalvular AF

	Dabigatran	Rivaroxaban*	Apixaban	Edoxaban
SPAF	150 mg bid	20 mg once daily	5 mg bid	60 mg once daily if CrCl 51–95 mL/min
Renal adjustment	75 mg bid if CrCl 15–30 mL/min No dosing recommendation if CrCl <15 mL/min	15 mg daily if CrCl 15–50 mL/min Avoid use if CrCl < 15 mL/min	2.5 mg bid if 2 of the following 3 are present: SCr ≥1.5 mg/dL, age ≥80 years or weight ≤60 kg*	Do not use if CrCl > 95 mL/min 30 mg once daily if CrCl 15–50 mL/min

NOTE: the 2014 AHA/ACC/HRS AF Guidelines note that warfarin is preferred for patients with CrCl <15 mL/min and NOACs are not recommended.
*For NVAF patients with end-stage renal disease, the recommended dose is 5 mg twice daily; reduce dose to 2.5 mg twice daily if one of the following patient characteristics (age ≥ 80 years or body weight ≤60 kg) is present; patients with ESRD with or without dialysis were not studied in clinical efficacy and safety studies; therefore, the dosing recommendations for patients with NVAF are based on pharmacokinetic and pharmacodynamic data in subjects maintained on dialysis.
SPAF, Stroke Prevention in Atrial Fibrillation; CrCl, creatinine clearance; *, taken with a meal.
1. Pradaxa (dabigatran etexilate mesylate) [prescribing information]. Ridgefield, CT: Boehringer Ingelheim Pharmaceuticals Inc.; 01/2015. 2. Xarelto (rivaroxaban) [prescribing information]. Titusville, NJ: Janssen Pharmaceuticals, Inc.; 01/2015. 3. Eliquis (apixaban) [prescribing information]. Princeton, NJ: Bristol-Myers Squibb Company; 6/2015. 4. Savaysa (edoxaban) [prescribing information]. Parsippany, NJ: Daiichi Sankyo, Inc; 01/2015.

ANTICOAGULANTS: PATIENT EDUCATION

Patient education is essential because patients must comply with laboratory follow-up and accurately follow dosing instructions. An assessment of any contraindications to therapy, including active bleeding and pregnancy, is necessary before starting therapy. The risk of bleeding may exceed the benefits of taking warfarin in patients with a previous history of medication nonadherence, falls, significant alcohol consumption, memory impairment, and lack of adequate support from family members or caregivers. Patients and caregivers must agree with the decision to initiate therapy (Witt, 2010). Common elements of anticoagulation patient education are described in **Box 50.5**.

Education concerning food restrictions for patients taking warfarin is essential. Vitamin K_1, the antidote to warfarin,

is naturally found in several plant foods. In contrast, vitamin K_2 is primarily synthesized by normal intestinal flora. The estimated necessary dietary intake of vitamin K_1 is 80 μg/d for men older than age 25 and 65 μg/d for women older than age 25. In the United States, typical American dietary vitamin K_1 intake is 300 to 500 μg (Suttie, 1992). Excessive amounts of dietary vitamin K_1 may antagonize warfarin's clinical effect and decrease the INR. Khan and coworkers (2004) found that for every 100-μg increase in vitamin K_1 intake in the 4 days before an INR measurement, the INR fell by 0.2. In another study, it was found that higher warfarin doses at 5.7 ± 1.7 mg/d were needed by those consuming 250 μg or more of vitamin K daily compared to that of 3.5 ± 1.0 mg/d by those consuming less than 250 μg of vitamin K daily (Khan et al., 2004).

TABLE 50.7

Dosing and Renal Adjustment for DOACs for VTE Treatment and Secondary Prevention of VTE

	Dabigatran	Rivaroxaban	Apixaban	Edoxaban
VTE Treatment				
VTE	150 mg bid (after parenteral therapy)	15 mg bid for 21 days, then 20 mg daily for months	10 mg bid for 7 days, then 5 mg bid	Following parenteral therapy, 50 mg once daily when weight is > 60 kg; 30 mg once daily if ≤ 60 kg
Renal Adjustment	No dosage recommendation if CrCl ≤ 30 mL/min	Avoid use if CrCl <30 mL/min	No adjustment required	30 mg once daily if CrCl ≤15–50 mL/min
VTE Secondary Prevention				
Long-term Secondary Prevention	150 mg bid	20 mg daily	2.5 mg bid	Not approved for this indication
Renal Adjustment	No dosage recommendations for CrCl ≤ 30 mL/min	Avoid use if CrCl < 30 mL/min	No adjustment required	Not approved for this indication

VTE, venous thromboembolism; CrCl, creatinine clearance.
1. Pradaxa (dabigatran etexilate mesylate) [prescribing information]. Ridgefield, CT: Boehringer Ingelheim Pharmaceuticals Inc.; 01/2015. 2. Xarelto (rivaroxaban) [prescribing information]. Titusville, NJ: Janssen Pharmaceuticals, Inc.; 01/2015. 3. Eliquis (apixaban) [prescribing information]. Princeton, NJ: Bristol-Myers Squibb Company; 6/2015. 4. Savaysa (edoxaban) [prescribing information]. Parsippany, NJ: Daiichi Sankyo, Inc; 01/2015.

BOX 50.5   Elements of Anticoagulation Patient Education

Indicate the reason for initiating anticoagulation therapy and how it relates to clot formation.

Review the name of anticoagulant drug(s) (generic and trade) and discuss how they work to reduce the risk of clotting complications.

Discuss the potential duration of therapy.

Describe the common signs/symptoms of bleeding and what to do if they occur.

Describe the common signs/symptoms of clotting complications and what to do if they occur.

Outline precautionary measures to minimize the risk of trauma or bleeding.

Discuss potential drug interactions (prescription and in addition for warfarin over the counter, herbal) and what to do when normal medication regimens change.

Clarify whether or not the patient may take concomitant low-dose aspirin and other NSAIDs.

Discuss the need to avoid or limit alcohol consumption.

Explain the need for birth control measures for women of childbearing age.

Review the importance of notifying all health-care providers (e.g., physicians, dentist) of the use of anticoagulation therapy.

Review the importance of notifying the anticoagulation provider when dental, surgical, or invasive procedures and hospitalization are scheduled.

Explain when to take anticoagulant mediations and what to do if a dose is missed.

Discuss the importance of carrying identification (ID card, medical alert bracelet/necklace).

Document in the patient's medical record that the patient education session occurred.

For warfarin:

Explain the meaning and significance of the INR.

Explain the need for frequent INR testing and target INR values appropriate for the patient's treatment.

Identify the laboratory location where the patient will go for the INR test and the date and time of the next test.

Identify the prescriber who will interpret the INR and the method of communicating those changes to the patient.

Discuss the narrow therapeutic index of warfarin and emphasize the importance of regular monitoring as a way to minimize the risk of bleeding/thrombosis.

Discuss the influence of dietary vitamin K use on the effects of VKA.

For rivaroxaban, apixaban, and edoxaban:

Explain the importance of periodic serum creatinine laboratory tests to monitor renal function.

Identify the prescriber or their designee as the individual to contact regarding questions, bleeding, and refills.

Review the date, time, and location of the patient's next follow-up appointment.

For rivaroxaban

Explain that the dose should be taken with a large meal.

For dabigatran:

Explain that the capsule cannot be crushed and cannot be removed from the original packaging.

Adapted from: Garcia, D. A., Witt, D. M., Hylek, E., et al. (2008). Delivery of optimized anticoagulant therapy: Consensus statement from the anticoagulation forum. *Annals of Pharmacotherapy, 42,* 979–988.

Dark green leafy vegetables (spinach and turnip, collard, and mustard greens), broccoli, Brussels sprouts, and cabbage are the primary sources of vitamin K and contain high amounts, greater than 100 mg/100-g serving. Herbal and green teas may also contain large quantities of vitamin K_1 (1,400 mg/100 g), and high levels of vitamin K_1 (50 mg/100 g) are found in soybean and soy products and olive oils, whereas peanut and corn oils contain minimal amounts. Vitamin K is also found in certain plant oils and prepared foods containing these oils, such as baked goods, margarine, and salad dressings. Food preparation with oils rich in vitamin K may also contribute to total vitamin K intake and affect warfarin action. The *Coumadin Cookbook* (available from amazon.com) is a great resource for patients taking warfarin because it provides tips for monitoring and maintaining a consistent vitamin K intake and provides many recipes with a low vitamin K content. Patients should be encouraged to eat a healthy diet, maintain consistency in their choice of foods, and avoid large fluctuations in

dietary vitamin K_1 intake. Instructing patients to maintain a consistent intake of vitamin K–containing foods, rather than trying to eliminate all sources of dietary vitamin K_1, is essential. Patients must also be educated on portion sizes and their vitamin K content so that they are not only consistent with the frequency of intake of vitamin K foods but also consistent with the number of servings of vitamin K they consume. Fad diets, such as the "cabbage soup" diet, are discouraged, and if diets such as the Atkins diet or low-carbohydrate diets are to be started, the patient must notify the practitioner so that INRs can be monitored more often. These diets, when strictly followed, frequently lead to a change in the intake amount of vitamin K foods. **Table 50.8** lists examples of vitamin K food content and serving sizes.

Hidden sources of excess vitamin K include enteral supplements, which can cause resistance to warfarin. Checking the amount of vitamin K in any nutritional supplement is advised because several of these preparations are now marketed directly

TABLE 50.8

Vitamin K Content of Common Foods

Description	Weight (g)	Common Measure	Vitamin K per Measure (mcg)
Asparagus, frozen, cooked, boiled, drained, without salt	180	1 cup	144
Beans, snap, green, canned, regular pack, drained solids	135	1 cup	53
Beet greens, cooked, boiled, drained, without salt	144	1 cup	697
Broccoli, cooked, boiled, drained, without salt	156	1 cup	220
Broccoli, raw	88	1 cup	89
Broccoli, cooked, boiled, drained, without salt	37	1 spear	52
Broccoli, frozen, chopped, cooked, boiled, drained, without salt	184	1 cup	162
Brussels sprouts, frozen, cooked, boiled, drained, without salt	155	1 cup	300
Brussels sprouts, cooked, boiled, drained, without salt	156	1 cup	219
Cabbage, raw	70	1 cup	53
Cabbage, cooked, boiled, drained, without salt	150	1 cup	163
Cabbage, Chinese (pak choi), cooked, boiled, drained, without salt	170	1 cup	58
Celery, cooked, boiled, drained, without salt	150	1 cup	57
Collards, frozen, chopped, cooked, boiled, drained, without salt	170	1 cup	1,059
Collards, cooked, boiled, drained, without salt	190	1 cup	836
Cowpeas (blackeyes), immature seeds, frozen, cooked, boiled, drained, without salt	170	1 cup	63
Cucumber, with peel, raw	301	1 large	49
Dandelion greens, cooked, boiled, drained, without salt	105	1 cup	579
Endive, raw	50	1 cup	116
Kale, frozen, cooked, boiled, drained, without salt	130	1 cup	1,147
Kale, cooked, boiled, drained, without salt	130	1 cup	1,062
Lettuce, iceberg (includes crisphead types), raw	539	1 head	130
Lettuce, green leaf, raw	56	1 cup	71
Lettuce, cos or romaine, raw	56	1 cup	57
Lettuce, butterhead (includes boston and bibb types), raw	163	1 head	167
Mustard greens, cooked, boiled, drained, without salt	140	1 cup	419
Onions, spring or scallions (includes tops and bulb), raw	100	1 cup	207
Okra, cooked, boiled, drained, without salt	160	1 cup	64
Okra, frozen, cooked, boiled, drained, without salt	184	1 cup	88
Parsley, fresh	10	10 sprigs	164
Peas, green (includes baby and lesuer types), canned, drained solids, unprepared	170	1 cup	63
Peas, edible-podded, frozen, cooked, boiled, drained, without salt	160	1 cup	48
Plums, dried (prunes), stewed, without added sugar	248	1 cup	65
Rhubarb, frozen, cooked, with sugar	240	1 cup	51
Spinach, frozen, chopped or leaf, cooked, boiled, drained, without salt	190	1 cup	1,027
Spinach, canned, regular pack, drained solids	214	1 cup	988
Spinach, cooked, boiled, drained, without salt	180	1 cup	888
Spinach souffle	136	1 cup	172
Spinach, raw	30	1 cup	145
Turnip greens, frozen, cooked, boiled, drained, without salt	164	1 cup	851
Turnip greens, cooked, boiled, drained, without salt	144	1 cup	529
Pie crust, cookie type, prepared from recipe, graham cracker, baked	239	1 pie shell	59
Noodles, egg, spinach, cooked, enriched	160	1 cup	162
Fast foods, coleslaw	99	3/4 cup	70
Bread crumbs, dry, grated, seasoned	120	1 cup	55

Adapted with permission from INRTracker: http://inrtracker.com/articles/diet/vitamin-k-foods

to patients through the lay press. In addition, many OTC vitamin preparations contain vitamin K, and patients should be counseled to read the label or bring in all medication bottles to the practitioner. For example, one Viactiv calcium chew contains 40 mcg of vitamin K; this translates to 80 mcg of vitamin K daily if the recommended dose of two chews is ingested. Questioning patients regarding any changes in dietary habits may provide clues when the INR varies.

MANAGING ANTICOAGULATION-RELATED BLEEDING

Bleeding is the most worrisome adverse event associated with antithrombotic therapy. In patients with AF, the annual risk of major bleeding is approximately 2% to 3% with DOACs and 3% to 4% with warfarin with fatal bleeding occurring in up to 0.5% (Kovacs et al., 2015; Werth et al., 2015). In patients with VTE, the annual risk of major bleeding for warfarin and DOACs is approximately 1% to 2% (Werth et al., 2015). The highest risk of bleeding with warfarin, especially intracranial hemorrhage, occurs when the INR exceeds a 4 to 5 range. The frequency of major bleeding in patients with a target INR of 2 to 3 is half of that seen in patients with a target INR above 3. One of the greatest advantages of DOACs over warfarin for SPAF is that they reduce the risk of intracranial hemorrhage by more than 50% (Werth et al., 2015).

In addition to the intensity of anticoagulation, the other major factors that determine bleeding risk include individual patient characteristics such as elderly age, chronic kidney disease, liver disease, a prior history of stroke (for patients with AF), a labile INR (for patient taking warfarin), anemia, malignancy, uncontrolled HTN (for patients with AF), ethanol use, concomitant antiplatelets (such as aspirin, other NSAIDs, P2Y12 inhibitors such as clopidogrel, prasugrel, and ticagrelor) and concomitant use of selective serotonin reuptake inhibitors (such as sertraline, fluoxetine, and citalopram), ethanol intake, as well as a longer duration of therapy (Schulman et al., 2008). The greatest risk of bleeding occurs within the first months of therapy (Ansell et al., 2008). Coadministration of aspirin plus an anticoagulant increases a patient's bleed risk by about 50%, and therefore, indications for concomitant antiplatelet therapy should be scrutinized carefully (Goodman et al., 2014; Held et al., 2015; Lauffenburger et al., 2015).

Minor bleeding is defined as that which is self-terminating and does not require hospitalization or an office visit or treatment by a health-care provider. Clinically relevant nonmajor bleeding is defined as overt bleeding that does not meet the criteria for major bleeding but does require either hospitalization and prompt physician-guided medical or surgical care or change in antithrombotic therapy. Major bleeding involves bleeding into a major organ, intracranial or epidural bleeding, and pericardial, intraocular, retroperitoneal, intra-articular, or intramuscular with compartment syndrome bleeding. Bleeding that is overt with a 2 g/dL drop in hemoglobin, or requires transfusion of at least 2 units, or requires surgical correction or administration of intravenous vasoactive agents, is also described as major bleeding (Kovacs et al., 2015).

Common locations of antithrombotic bleeding include the oral or nasal mucosa, urine, stool, or soft tissues. Bleeding complications in order of frequency are epistaxis, purpura, hematuria, GI bleeding, and hemoptysis (Jacobs, 2008). Women are more likely to experience minor bleeding than men (Schulman et al., 2008). Minor bleeding is usually managed by temporarily discontinuing warfarin therapy for 1 to 2 days and then restarting warfarin at a reduced dosage or reducing the target INR range.

Patients with a history of falling are commonly thought to have an increased risk of intracranial hemorrhage. One researcher evaluated the risk of elderly patients falling and subsequent development of a subdural hematoma, compared to the benefits of warfarin for stroke prevention in AF. Their conclusion was the risk of stroke if the patient did not receive warfarin (5% per year) was much larger than the risk of developing a subdural hematoma (0.0004 per patient-year). An elderly patient with AF would need to fall 300 times a year for the risk of subdural hematoma to outweigh the benefits of warfarin therapy (Man-Son-Hing et al., 1999).

Management of Warfarin-Associated Bleeding

When the INR is elevated, management depends on the patient's potential risk of bleeding, whether the patient is actively bleeding, and the INR level. Treatment options include simply omitting one or more warfarin doses with more frequent INR testing or administering vitamin K. In the inpatient setting, administering prothrombin concentrates can also be considered. Management of major bleeding focuses on reversing the anticoagulation effects of warfarin, which include administration of either intravenous or oral vitamin K with or without clotting factor replacement. The 2012 ACCP Guidelines for VKA reversal according to INR and presence or absence of bleeding are described in **Box 50.6**. Currently, administration of four factor prothrombin complex concentrates is recommended over fresh frozen plasma for warfarin reversal because of a more rapid and complete effect with similar incidence of thromboembolic events (Goldstein et al., 2015). Any bleeding event should be adequately investigated because an underlying comorbidity, such as malignancy, may be the cause.

Management of DOAC-Associated Bleeding

Currently, there are no available antidotes for apixaban-, edoxaban- or rivaroxaban-associated bleeding. Idarucizumab, a humanized monoclonal antibody fragment against dabigatran was recently approved in October 2015, and andexanet alpha, a recombinant inactive factor Xa derivative against factor Xa inhibitors including apixaban, edoxaban, rivaroxaban, and LMWHs (Gomez-Outes et al., 2014; Pollack et al., 2015) is anticipated to be available in late 2016.

For minor bleeding, the bleeding site should be manually compressed. Rarely should a dose be held given the short half-life and risk of thromboembolic event. The situations should be evaluated to determine whether or not the DOAC should be continued, dose adjusted, or changed to a different DOAC or warfarin.

For major bleeding, the DOAC should be discontinued and manual or mechanical compression of the bleeding site should be performed. If the last administered dose was within 3 hours, administer activated charcoal. For dabigatran, administer

2012 ACCP Guidelines for Reversing the Anticoagulant Effects of VKAs

The reason for bleeding should be evaluated. Consider discontinuing or holding 1–2 doses of VKA. Stop concomitant medications that predispose to bleeding as appropriate (e.g., aspirin). Consider restarting with a lower maintenance dose and monitor the INR more frequently.

INRs 4.5 TO 10 AND NO EVIDENCE OF BLEEDING. NO ADMINISTRATION OF VITAMIN K

For patients with INRs above 4.5 but less than or equal to 10 who are not experiencing significant bleeding, omitting the next one to two doses, monitoring the INR more frequently, and resuming therapy at a lower dose is one approach.

INRs > 10

Patients with INRs above 10 who are not experiencing significant bleeding should have their warfarin held

and receive oral vitamin K (2.5 to 5 mg). The INR will fall substantially in 24 to 48 hours. Frequent INR checks are necessary, and additional doses of oral vitamin K can be given if the INR is still elevated. Once the INR falls within the target range, warfarin can be resumed at a lower dose.

SIGNIFICANT BLEEDING

Patients experiencing significant bleeding, regardless of how high the INR is elevated, or patients with life-threatening bleeding need immediate reversal of the INR and should have their warfarin temporarily discontinued; administration of four-factor prothrombin complex concentrate should be administered (e.g., KCentra; see dosing information based on INR at Kcentra.com), as well as intravenous vitamin K 5–10 mg should be administered via slow intravenous (IV) infusion over 1 hour. Depending on the INR, repeat doses of vitamin K can be given every 12 hours.

Recommendations from Holbrook, A., Schulman, S., Witt, D. M., et al. (2012). Evidence-based management of anticoagulant therapy: Antithrombotic therapy and prevention of thrombosis. American College of Chest Physicians Evidence-Based Clinical Practice Guidelines (9th ed.) *Chest, 141*(2 Suppl.), e152S–e184S.

idarucizumab 5 g by rapid IV bolus or infusion. In patients with chronic kidney disease or acute kidney injury, the DOAC half-life may be prolonged and the patient should be monitored for a longer period of time. In the absence of a direct-acting antidote and clinical trials, experts have advocated discontinuation and administration of four-factor prothrombin complex concentrate to treat major bleeding associated with apixaban, rivaroxaban, and edoxaban (Nutescu et al., 2013). Administration of recombinant factor VIIa is reserved for serious bleeding with either warfarin apixaban, edoxaban, or rivaroxaban when other hemostatic products fail (Nutescu et al., 2013).

Management of Unfractionated Heparin-Associated Bleeding

Excessive anticoagulation with UFH can be reversed with IV protamine sulfate, which is high in arginine and is cationic binding tightly to heparin, which is highly anionic, thus reversing the anticoagulant effect (Hirsh et al., 2008). Unfortunately, protamine has other undesirable effects in some patients, including immediate and delayed allergic response.

Management of LMWH-Associated Bleeding

There is no proven method for reversing excessive anticoagulation occurring with LMWHs, although consensus guidelines provide dosing recommendations for using protamine and

it has been found useful in some, but not all, coagulopathic patients (Van Veen et al., 2011).

OTHER ANTICOAGULANT ADVERSE EFFECTS

Heparin-Induced Thrombocytopenia

Platelet counts should be closely monitored during UFH and LMWH therapy because a drop in platelet count below 150 × 10^9/L or greater than 50% of baseline necessitates an evaluation for HIT, antibody-mediated prothrombotic reaction. This immune-mediated thrombocytopenia, HIT, has been reported in less than 1% of patients. The incidence of thrombocytopenia is much lower with LMWH than with UFH. Clinical effects of HIT can result in DVT, PE, MI, limb ischemia, gangrene requiring limb amputation, cerebral thrombosis, and death. Suspected HIT should be evaluated using the "4Ts" score: thrombocytopenia, Timing, Thrombosis, and oTher where scores above three require that all sources of heparin or LMWH such as heparin flushes and heparin-coated catheters, infusions, and injections are required for platelet counts to normalize. In patients in which HIT is strongly suspected or confirmed, an alternative anticoagulant such as an intravenously administered direct thrombin inhibitor (argatroban and bivalirudin) should be administered. The diagnosis is confirmed using an ELISA antibody test (sensitive but not specific for HIT) and/or the heparin antibody serotonin release assay. The patient should be carefully monitored for the development of thrombosis, and argatroban is administered until platelet counts are above 150×10^9/L (Warkentin, 2010).

ANTIPLATELET AGENTS

Clinical Uses

Antiplatelet agents that have been used in the prevention and treatment of ischemic stroke are aspirin, aspirin/dipyridamole (Aggrenox), and the P2Y12 inhibitor clopidogrel (Plavix). Aspirin has been studied in primary and secondary prevention of VTE. Aspirin has been studied as a sole therapy for stroke prevention in patients with bioprosthetic heart valves and as add-on therapy to warfarin for stroke prevention in patients with mechanical heart valves. Aspirin has been shown to be inferior to warfarin and apixaban for SPAF. Two other P2Y12 inhibitors, prasugrel (Effient) and ticagrelor (Brilinta), as well as clopidogrel are used to prevent CV death, MI, or stroke following acute coronary syndrome and to prevent stent thrombosis following percutaneous coronary intervention. The use of P2Y12 inhibitors for secondary coronary heart disease indications will not be discussed in this chapter.

Mechanism of Action, Dosing, and Adverse Effects of Antiplatelets

Aspirin

Aspirin prevents prostaglandin synthesis in platelets and other tissues by irreversibly modifying and inhibiting the enzyme COX, which catalyzes the conversion of arachidonic acid to thromboxane A_2, a prostaglandin derivative, which is a potent vasoconstrictor and promoter of platelet aggregation. The onset of antiplatelet effects is within 5 min of oral administration. After discontinuing aspirin, platelets are impaired for their normal life span of 7 to 10 days because of the irreversible inhibition of COX. Every 24 hours, 10% of platelets are replaced; 5 to 6 days after aspirin ingestion, approximately 50% of platelets function normally (Patrono et al., 2008).

The optimal aspirin dosage for thrombotic disorders is still controversial because doses ranging from 30 to 1,500 mg/d are effective (Adams et al., 2008; Albers et al., 2008). Inhibition of platelet aggregation can be shown at doses as low as 20 mg/d given over several days. Randomized trials have found lower aspirin doses ranging between 50 and 100 mg/d effective as an antithrombotic agent (Patrono et al., 2008). There is no benefit to higher doses over low-dose aspirin for CVD prevention. Because higher doses may be associated with increased risk for GI bleeding, a lower dose, such as 81 mg orally daily, is preferred (Antiplatelet Trialists' Collaboration, 2009).

Aspirin's contraindications are active GI bleeding (unless a recent coronary stent has been placed) or aspirin allergy or hypersensitivity. The most common adverse effects of aspirin are GI upset, such as nausea, dyspepsia, heartburn, epigastric discomfort, anorexia, and bleeding. These effects are dose related and are more likely to occur at doses greater than 325 mg/d. Although lower aspirin doses cause fewer GI symptoms, they still can cause significant GI bleeding. Aspirin may also potentiate peptic ulcer disease. Caution should be exercised when using aspirin with other drugs that affect platelet function (e.g., NSAIDs, P2Y12 inhibitors, and SSRI antidepressants) or anticoagulants because the bleeding potential will be increased.

Aspirin/Dipyridamole

A combination product containing 25-mg aspirin and 200-mg extended-release dipyridamole (Aggrenox) administered twice daily is available for preventing recurrent stroke in patients who have experienced a TIA or previous ischemic stroke. Dipyridamole inhibits platelet adhesion, but its full mechanism of action is unknown. A European trial conducted in 6,000 patients (ESPS2) was the basis for FDA approval of this agent. Efficacy was also confirmed in a second trial (ESPRIT). The most common adverse effects include GI complaints, diarrhea, and headache. Elevations in hepatic enzymes have also been reported. Contraindications for aspirin with dipyridamole include hypersensitivity or allergy to aspirin or NSAIDs and active peptic ulcer disease.

Clopidogrel

Clopidogrel inhibits adenosine diphosphate (ADP), a promoter of platelet receptor binding (Patrono et al., 2008). A clopidogrel dose of 75 mg/d irreversibly inhibits ADP-mediated platelet aggregation. Dose-dependent inhibition of platelet aggregation is seen 2 hours after a single oral dose with a peak effect about 6 hours after the dose, and platelet aggregation and bleeding time return to baseline approximately 7 days after discontinuing clopidogrel.

Clopidogrel is a prodrug and must be activated (biotransformed) to inhibit platelet aggregation. Clopidogrel is extensively metabolized by the liver primarily by CYP2C19, and moderate or stroke CYP2C19 inhibitors, such as omeprazole, decrease the antiplatelet effect of clopidogrel. Patients vary in their ability to biotransform clopidogrel because the activity of CYP2C19 is controlled genetically. An early communication from the FDA in January 2009 acknowledged that clopidogrel was less effective in some patients and that genetic differences in drug metabolism likely accounted for the reduced effectiveness. Another mechanism for reduced clopidogrel activity is via inhibition of CYP2C19 by interacting drugs. PPIs are frequently given with clopidogrel plus aspirin to protect against GI bleeding. Omeprazole is a strong inhibitor of CYP2C19 and reduces the conversion of clopidogrel to the active form. An FDA public health advisory in November 2009 recommended against using clopidogrel with both omeprazole and esomeprazole. Several retrospective reviews of pharmacy claims databases reported that patients receiving a PPI, most commonly omeprazole, with clopidogrel had reduced effectiveness of the antiplatelet drug, shown by an increase in cardiovascular events, including MI, hospitalization for acute coronary syndrome, and all-cause mortality (Abraham et al., 2010). Only one randomized trial has prospectively examined cardiovascular event rates in patients receiving clopidogrel 75 mg/d with omeprazole 20 mg/d (Bhatt et al., 2010). The study was terminated early due to the manufacturer going into bankruptcy, but an interim analysis showed no significant difference in the incidence of cardiovascular death, MI, or stroke in patients receiving clopidogrel with omeprazole compared to a placebo. The combination did protect against GI bleeding; the number of GI events was similar between a placebo and the antiplatelet/PPI combination. Limitations to the trial include that it was not powered to detect differences in cardiovascular events, and it was terminated early after a median duration of 133 days, which may not have been long enough to show a difference in outcomes. There is ongoing controversy regarding the clinical impact of this drug interaction. Current joint consensus from leading cardiology and gastroenterology groups is that PPIs are appropriate in patients with multiple risk factors for GI bleeding (e.g., history of ulcer disease or prior GI bleeding, dual antiplatelet therapy, concomitant anticoagulant therapy, advanced age) who require antiplatelet therapy (Abraham et al., 2010).

Bruising and bleeding are the primary risks of clopidogrel therapy, and the risk is increased in the setting of dual antiplatelet therapy with aspirin. In the CAPRIE trial, there was no major difference between clopidogrel and aspirin

monotherapy in terms of safety, although there was a slightly higher rate of serious hemorrhage in the patients receiving aspirin. Clopidogrel is considered to have a safety profile similar to that of 325 mg/d dose of aspirin (Patrono et al., 2008). Contraindications to clopidogrel are active major bleeding, including from peptic ulcer or intracranial hemorrhage. Diarrhea is relatively common, occurring in approximately 5%. Rash and thrombotic thrombocytopenic purpura are rare adverse effects of clopidogrel.

SELECTING THE MOST APPROPRIATE AGENT

Treatment of Deep Vein Thrombosis or Pulmonary Embolism

Treatment options for VTE are shown in **Table 50.9**. All patients with a diagnostically confirmed DVT of the proximal leg veins or diagnostically confirmed PE should receive a bolus of IV UFH followed by a continuous IV infusion of UFH, subcutaneous LMWHs, and oral rivaroxaban or oral apixaban as initial therapy. Injectable UFH/LMWH is followed by warfarin, apixaban, dabigatran, edoxaban, or rivaroxaban for at least 3 months. A decision on duration of therapy for treating DVT or PE depends on whether or not the VTE event was considered to be caused by a reversible risk factor ("provoked") or

TABLE 50.9		
Treatment options for VTE		
Agent	**Initial Dosing or Lead In**	**Maintenance Dosing**
Preferred for Renal Insufficiency (<30 mL/min)		
UFH[1]	Weight-based bolus followed by weight-based continuous infusion Fixed subcutaneous: 333 U/kg followed by 250 U/kg bid	
Ideal for Normal Renal Clearance		
LMWH[1]	**Dalteparin:** 200 IU/kg every 24 h or 100 IU/kg bid **Enoxaparin:** 1 mg/kg bid or 1.5 mg/kg every 24 h **Nadroparin:** 86 IU/kg bid or 171 IU/kg every 24 h **Tinzaparin:** 175 IU/kg every 24 h	
Warfarin	Bridge with LMWH or UFH ≥5 d 0.5–10 mg/d	• 0.5–6 mg/d, individualized to INR 2.0–3.0
Apixaban	10 mg bid for 7 d **Coadministration with strong dual CYP3A4 and P-gp inhibitors:** For patients receiving apixaban >2.5 mg bid, reduce the dose by 50% when apixaban is coadministered with drugs that are strong dual inhibitors of cytochrome P450 3A4 (CYP3A4) and P-glycoprotein (P-gp) (e.g., ketoconazole, itraconazole, ritonavir, clarithromycin)	• 5 mg bid • 2.5 mg bid for secondary prevention
Dabigatran	5–10 d parenteral anticoagulant	• 150 mg bid (CrCL >30 mL/min)
Edoxaban	5–10 d parenteral anticoagulant	• 60 mg/d • 30 mg/d (CrCL 15–50 mL/min, ≤60 kg, or with some P-gp inhibitors)
Rivaroxaban	15 mg bid for 21 d with food	• 20 mg/d with food (CrCL >30 mL/min)

[1]Bridged to a DOAC or warfarin.

when no reversible risk factor can be identified ("unprovoked"). For patients with a provoked DVT, the recurrence rate is less than 5% at year 1 and less than 15% at 5 years. A 3-month course of warfarin is sufficient in patients with reversible risk factors, if the provoking risk factor has resolved. Patients with idiopathic VTE are more likely to experience recurrent DVT than provoked events (10% recurrence rate at 1 year and 30% recurrence rate at 5 years); extended warfarin therapy is recommended (Kearon et al., 2008). Provoked VTEs are treated for 3 months and unprovoked VTEs for a minimum of 3 months and often longer than 12 months depending on patient tolerability, continued presence of the clot on ultrasound or CT, or continued elevation of D-dimer measured 3 months off anticoagulation (and then anticoagulation may resume) (Wells et al., 2014). If warfarin is selected, it should be overlapped with UFH or LMWHs for approximately 4 to 5 days while warfarin reaches a therapeutic level (Kearon et al., 2008).

In clinical trials, DOACs have similar efficacy and reduced bleeding compared to warfarin for treatment of VTE (van der Hulle et al., 2014). One area that requires further study is the use of DOACs for treating VTE associated with malignancy, and at this time, LMWH remains the preferred agent (Streiff, 2010; Vedovati et al., 2015).

Nondrug Therapy

An inferior vena cava (IVC) filter or umbrella filter (Greenfield filter) is inserted percutaneously into the IVC and traps thrombi in the leg veins to prevent migration to the lungs (Anderson & Bussey, 2006). IVC filter placement is recommended in patients with proximal DVT or PE in which anticoagulants are contraindicated due to the risk of bleeding. However, the routine use of IVC filters in addition to anticoagulation is not recommended for patients with DVT or PE. If the patient's bleeding risk resolves, a conventional course of anticoagulation should be initiated (Kearon et al., 2008). Vena cava filters have not been shown to decrease mortality. Complications of IVC filters include thrombosis, migration of the filter (rarely to the heart), and obstruction of the vena cava.

Prophylaxis of Deep Vein Thrombosis and Pulmonary

Patients undergoing total hip replacement (THR), total knee replacement (TKR), or hip fracture surgery should receive anticoagulation prophylaxis to reduce the high risk of DVT or PE. Several studies have found the prevalence of total DVT at 7 to 14 days after THR, TKR, and hip fracture surgery to be approximately 50% to 60%. The incidence of PE is less certain, but in studies in which a V/Q scan was performed, about 7% to 11% of THR and TKR patients had a high probability scan within 7 to 14 days after surgery. It has also been found that total DVT rate is greater in TKR than THR. Overall, the data suggest that asymptomatic VTE is common after orthopedic surgery and, in the absence of prophylaxis, will affect at least half of these patients (Geerts et al., 2008). Numerous pharmacologic and nonpharmacologic agents have been used in the postoperative setting to decrease the risk of DVT or

PE. According to the ACCP 2012 guidelines, effective drugs for prophylaxis of VTE following orthopedic surgery include LMWHs (example enoxaparin 40 mg subcutaneous daily), fondaparinux, warfarin, apixaban (2.5 mg twice daily), rivaroxaban (10 mg daily), and aspirin (Falck-Ytter et al., 2012) Recently, dabigatran at an initial dose of 110 mg on day 1 followed by 220 mg daily was FDA-approved for VTE prophylaxis following orthopedic surgery.

For the hospitalized medical patient, LMWH, fondaparinux, or UFH is considered efficacious (Kahn et al., 2012).

VTE prophylaxis is a Joint Commission Core Measure for hospitalized medical and surgical patients at risk (VTE-1), and the incidence of hospital-acquired potentially preventable VTE events is also reported for hospitals (http://www.jointcommission.org/venous_thromboembolism/). The proportion of patients undergoing surgery receiving VTE prophylaxis within 24 hours before to 24 hours after surgery is also a reported quality measure (SCIP-VTE-2) (https://manual.jointcommission.org/pub/Manual/MIF0061/SCIPVTE2).

Nondrug Therapy

Nondrug therapies help prevent or treat the complications of DVT, including venous stasis ulcers and the postthrombotic syndrome. Mechanical measures, including IPC devices and graduated compression stockings, offer the advantage of carrying no risk of bleeding compared to anticoagulants. IPC sleeves applied to the lower extremities periodically inflate and deflate, to squeeze the calf and prevent venous stasis and pooling of blood in the leg veins. Nonambulatory patients can have IPC devices applied to reduce the risk of VTE. Use of IPC alone is recommended in patients with a high risk of bleeding following general orthopedic or general surgery, until the bleeding risk resolves (Geerts et al., 2008).

Secondary Prevention of Noncardioembolic Ischemic Stroke and Transient Ischemic Attack

Pharmacotherapy for secondary prevention of stroke/TIA is described in the 2014 AHA/ASA guidelines (Kernan et al., 2014). Antiplatelet therapy reduces the relative risk of death, MI, or recurrent stroke by 22% (Kernan et al., 2014). These guidelines recommend treatment with either aspirin (50 to 325 mg/d) or aspirin plus dipyridamole (25 mg/200 mg twice daily) as first-line class I indications. Second-line class II agents are either clopidogrel monotherapy (75 mg daily) (class IIa) or clopidogrel plus aspirin (class IIb) combination therapy. If clopidogrel is combined with aspirin for stroke, it should be started within 24 hours poststroke and only continued for 90 days (CHANCE trial). If used later, the combination is associated with an increased risk of hemorrhagic stroke (Kernan et al., 2014).

Although not directly compared in a head-to-head trial, the efficacy of clopidogrel alone (CAPRIE trial) seems comparable to aspirin/dipyridamole (PRoFESS trial) and by inference aspirin (comparable to clopidogrel in CAPRIE).

Because of cost, low-dose aspirin, 81 mg, is often preferred. Side effects may also influence drug selection with aspirin/dipyridamole associated with headache as well as GI intolerance. Aspirin plus clopidogrel may be preferred in patients with acute coronary syndrome or coronary artery stents (Kernan et al., 2014).

Stroke Prevention in Nonvalvular Atrial Fibrillation

Antithrombotic therapy for stroke prevention in NVAF is outlined in the 2014 AHA/ACC/HRS guidelines (January et al., 2014).

The risk of thromboembolic stroke in patients with NVAF should be estimated using the CHA_2DS_2-Vasc score. Patients with a CHA_2DS_2-Vasc Score of 0 have an annual stroke risk of less than 1% and do not require antithrombotic therapy for SPAF. There is controversy with respect to drug selection for patients with a CHA_2DS_2-Vasc Score of 1 who have an annual risk of 1 to 2%, and no therapy, aspirin (81 mg to 325 mg/d) or oral anticoagulation is recommended. Patients with a CHA_2DS_2-Vasc Score of 2 or greater have an annual risk of stroke of 2% to 15%, and anticoagulation is recommended (January et al., 2014). Either warfarin or a DOAC may be selected with warfarin preferred in patients with creatinine clearance less than 30 mL/min.

DOACs have been found to have superior or similar efficacy to warfarin for the prevention of stroke or systemic thromboembolism with similar or lower major bleeding and an approximate 50% reduction in intracranial hemorrhage (Chan et al., 2014; Ruff et al., 2014). Drug selection is often made by patient preference based upon cost (insurance copay) or convenience (dosing frequency, lack of INR monitoring).

Prophylaxis Against Systemic Embolism in Patients with Prosthetic Heart Valves

Antithrombotic therapy for patients with prosthetic heart valves is described in the 2014 AHA/ACC guideline for the management of patients with valvular heart disease (Nishimura et al., 2014). Long-term anticoagulation with warfarin alone or in combination with aspirin is required in patients with mechanical heart valves because the valve itself is thrombogenic and because of the high risk of thromboembolism (Sun et al., 2010). The rate of major thrombotic events in patients who have mechanical heart valves and who are not receiving anticoagulation is 8%; anticoagulation therapy decreases this risk by 75% (Carnetiger et al., 1995). Refer to the professional guidelines for information on anticoagulation in patients with native valvular disease (rheumatic mitral valve disease, mitral stenosis) and other conditions.

Both the position and type of the mechanical valve influence the risk of embolism. The prevalence of thromboembolism is higher with a valve in the mitral position than in the aortic position. Caged ball valves like the Starr–Edwards valves, which are rarely seen today, have the highest risk of thromboembolism, followed by tilting-disk valves (Bjork–Shiley valves)

and then bileaflet valves (St. Jude Medical valves, which are most commonly used today, or Medtronic Hall valves). Patients with double mechanical valves (i.e., aortic and mitral valve replacement) have a higher risk of thromboembolism compared with those with only one prosthetic valve. The risk of thromboembolism is highest in the 3 months following valve replacement surgery, until the valve becomes covered with endothelial tissue. Immediately after surgery, LMWH or UFH is used short term until the INR with warfarin is therapeutic (Sun et al., 2010). Individual patient risk factors that increase the risk of embolic events include AF, previous thromboembolic event, impaired left ventricular systolic function, and concomitant hypercoagulable conditions.

Patients with mechanical valves in the (1) mitral position or (2) patients with aortic valves with additional risk factors such as AF, previous thromboembolism, left ventricular ejection fraction less than 40%, as well as those with older caged ball valves require lifelong therapy with warfarin maintained at a target INR of 2.5 to 3.5 (target INR 3.0). A lower INR of 2 to 3 (target 2.5) is recommended for patients with mechanical bileaflet or Medtronic Hall valves in the aortic position because studies show there is not an increased risk of thromboembolism and the bleeding risk is lower than with a higher target INR (Nishimura et al., 2014).

With warfarin therapy, the risk of thromboembolism is still 1% to 2% per year. Therefore, adding 100 mg/d of aspirin to warfarin therapy is recommended and has been shown to reduce mortality and thromboembolic events without increasing the risk of major bleeding (Nishimura et al., 2014).

For bioprosthetic (e.g., porcine heart valves), warfarin with an INR of 2 to 3 (target 2.5) for the first 3 months for aortic valves and an INR of 2.5 to 3.5 (target 3.0) for the first 3 months following surgery is recommended. Only 3 months of anticoagulation is warranted because after that time frame, the risk of bleeding outweighs the risk of thrombosis. Aspirin monotherapy 75 to 100 mg/d is then recommended lifelong after the first 3 months regardless of the valve position (Nishimura et al., 2014). Following transaortic valve replacement (TAVR), 6 months of aspirin 81 mg/d plus clopidogrel 75 mg/d is recommended (Nishimura et al., 2014).

Patients with mechanical heart valves can experience thromboembolic events even if antithrombotic therapy is administered appropriately; the risk is 0.5% to 1.7%/patient-year. Options in these cases from expert consensus are to increase the target INR for patients on warfarin, to add aspirin to patients not already receiving warfarin, or to add warfarin if the patient is receiving aspirin (Sun et al., 2010).

Dabigatran has been shown to be less effective than warfarin for patients with mechanical heart valves, and therefore, at this time, DOACs are not recommended for use in patients with mechanical heart valves (Eikelboom et al., 2013; Nishimura et al., 2014). Few patients with AF and bioprosthetic heart valves have been included in clinical trials at this time. Product prescribing information for dabigatran, apixaban, and rivaroxaban recommends against their use, while no recommendation is made for edoxaban.

CASE STUDY*

D.G. is a 74-year-old woman who arrives at the emergency room complaining of shortness of breath, palpitations (for 2 days), and lower extremity edema. Her medical history includes diabetes mellitus, hypertension, heart failure with reduced ejection fraction, and osteoarthritis. She had a left heart catheterization and coronary angiography last year and has no significant coronary artery disease. She has a biventricular pacemaker/implantable defibrillator for heart failure symptom treatment and sudden cardiac death prevention. The patient's current medications are losartan 100 mg/d, metoprolol succinate 50 mg/d, metformin 500 mg twice daily, spironolactone 25 mg/d, furosemide 40 mg/d, and naproxen 500 mg twice daily.

Vital signs are as follows: blood pressure of 140/80 mm Hg, respiratory rate of 30 bpm, and heart rate of 120 bpm. ECG shows atrial fibrillation with a rapid ventricular response. Echocardiography reveals a moderately dilated left atrium, left ventricular systolic ejection fraction of 35% (unchanged), chronic kidney disease (baseline serum creatinine 1.01 mg/dL), and moderate mitral regurgitation.

Pertinent laboratory values include the following: hemoglobin 12 g/dL, hematocrit 36%, platelets 300,000/microliter, and serum creatinine 1.20 mg/dL (estimated creatinine clearance 39 mL/min). Her weight is 60 kg (increased from 55 kg), and height is 5 ft 3 inches. She does not smoke and does not drink alcohol. Dietary habits include one can of Ensure daily, with other meals provided by a social service agency (Meals on Wheels). Social concerns include the fact she lives alone, but a son visits every 1 to 2 weeks and transports her to physician appointments. She is living on a limited budget. With regard to her medication adherence, her son states that she occasionally forgets to take her afternoon medications, but overall, she is considered to be reasonably adherent with her drug regimens.

DIAGNOSIS: ATRIAL FIBRILLATION, ACUTE ONSET

1. List specific goals of treatment for **D.G.**
2. What drug therapy would you prescribe for stroke prevention in atrial fibrillation? Why?
3. What are the parameters for monitoring success of the anticoagulant therapy?
4. Discuss specific patient education based on the prescribed therapy.
5. List one or two adverse reactions for the selected agent that would cause you to change therapy.
6. What would be the choice for the second-line therapy?
7. What OTC or alternative medications would be appropriate for **D.G.**?
8. What lifestyle changes would you recommend to **D.G.**?
9. Describe one or two drug–drug or drug–food interactions for the selected agent.

* Answers can be found online.

Bibliography

Starred references are cited in the text.

*Abraham, N. S., Hlatky, M. A., Antman, E. M., et al. (2010). ACCF/ACG/AHA 2010 expert consensus document on the concomitant use of proton pump inhibitors and thienopyridines. *Journal of the American College of Cardiology, 56*, 2051–2066.

*Adams, H. P., del Zoppo, G., Albers, M. J., et al. (2007). Guidelines for the early management of adults with ischemic stroke: A guideline from the American Heart Association/American Stroke Association Stroke Council, Clinical Cardiology Council, Cardiovascular Radiology and Intervention Council, and the Atherosclerotic Peripheral Vascular Disease and Quality of Care Outcomes in Research Interdisciplinary Working Groups: The American Academy of Neurology affirms the value of this guideline as an educational tool for neurologists. *Stroke, 38*, 1655–1711.

*Adams, R. J., Albers, G., Alberts, M. J., et al. (2008). Update to the AHA/ASA recommendations for prevention of stroke in patients with ischemic stroke or transient ischemic attack. *Stroke, 39*, 1647–1652.

*Albers, G. W., Amarenco, P., Easton, J. D., et al. (2008). Antithrombotic and thrombolytic therapy for ischemic stroke: American College of Chest Physicians Evidence-Based Clinical Practice Guidelines (8th ed.). *Chest, 133*(6 Suppl.), 630S–669S.

*Anderson, R. C., & Bussey, H. I. (2006). Retrievable and permanent inferior vena cava filters: Selected considerations. *Pharmacotherapy, 26*(11), 1595–1600.

*Ansell, J., Hirsh, J., Hylek, E., et al. (2008). Pharmacology and management of the vitamin K antagonists. American College of Chest Physicians Evidence-Based Clinical Practice Guidelines (8th ed.). *Chest, 133*(6 Suppl.), 160S–198S.

*Antiplatelet Trialists' Collaboration. (2009). Aspirin in the primary and secondary prevention of vascular disease: collaborative meta-analysis of individual participant data from randomized trials. *Lancet, 373*(9678), 1849–1860.

Barnes, G. D., Kanthi, Y., Froehlich, J. B. (2015). Venous thromboembolism: Predicting recurrence and the need for extended anticoagulation. *Vascular Medicine, 20*(2), 143–152.

*Bentz, B. A. (2006). Gaining control over atrial fibrillation. *RN, 69*(12), 35–38.

*Bhatt, D. L., Cryer, B. L., & Contant, C. F. (2010). Clopidogrel with or without omeprazole in coronary artery disease. *New England Journal of Medicine, 363*, 1909–1917.

Boehringer Ingelheim. (2009). *Product information for Aggrenox*. Ridgefield, CT: Author.

Boehringer Ingelheim. (2010). *Product information for Pradaxa*. Ridgefield, CT: Author.

*Bristol-Myers Squibb. (2010). *Product information for Coumadin*. Princeton, NJ.

*Carnetiger, S. C., Rosendaal, F. R., Wintzen, A. R., et al. (1995). Optimal anticoagulant therapy in patients with mechanical heart valves. *New England Journal of Medicine*, *333*, 11–17.

Chan, N. C., Paikin, J. S., Hirsh, J., et al. (2014). New oral anticoagulants for stroke prevention in atrial fibrillation: Impact of study design, double counting and unexpected findings on interpretation of study results and conclusions. *Thrombosis and Haemostasis*, *111*(5), 798–807.

*Colman, R. W., Clowes, A. W., George, J. N., et al. (2006). Overview of hemostasis. In R. W. Colman (Ed.). *Hemostasis and thrombosis: Basic principles and clinical practice* (5th ed., pp. 13–17). Philadelphia, PA: J. B. Lippincott.

*Coppola, A., Tufano, A., Cerbone, A. M., et al. (2009). Inherited thrombophilia: Implications for prevention and treatment of venous thromboembolism. *Seminars in Thrombosis and Hemostasis*, *35*, 683–694.

*Dafer, R. M., & Biler, J. (2008). Antiphospholipid syndrome: Role of antiphospholipid antibodies in neurology. *Hematology/Oncology Clinics of North America*, *22*, 95–105.

Easaw, J. C., Shea-Budgell, M. A., Wu, C. M. J., et al. (2015). Canadian consensus recommendations on the management of venous thromboembolism in patients with cancer. Part 1: Prophylaxis. *Current Oncology*, *22*, 133–143.

Eikelboom, J. W., Connolly, S. J., Brueckmann, M., et al. (2013). Dabigatran versus warfarin in patients with mechanical heart valves. *New England Journal of Medicine*, *369*, 1206–1214.

Eisai. (2009). *Product information for Fragmin*. Woodcliff Lake, NJ: Author.

Eli Lilly. (2010). *Product information for Effient*. Indianapolis, IN: Author.

Falck-Ytter, Y., Francis, C. W., Johanson, N. A., et al. (2012) Prevention of VTE in orthopedic surgery patients: Antithrombotic therapy and prevention of thrombosis (9th ed.: American College of Chest Physicians Evidence-Based Clinical Practice Guidelines). *Chest*, *141*(Suppl. 2), e278S–e325S.

*Fuster, V., Ryden, L. E., Cannon, D. S., et al. (2006). American College of Cardiology/American Heart Association/European Society of Cardiology 2006 Guidelines for the management of patients with atrial fibrillation. *Circulation*, *114*, e-257–e-354.

*Garcia, D. A., & Hylek, E. (2008). Reducing the risk of stroke for patients who have atrial fibrillation. *Clinical Cardiology*, *26*, 267–275.

*Garcia, D. A., Witt, D. M., Hylek, E., et al. (2008). Delivery of optimized anticoagulant therapy: Consensus statement from the anticoagulation forum. *Annals of Pharmacotherapy*, *42*(9), 79–88.

*Geerts, W. H., Bergqvist, D., Pineo, G. F., et al. (2008). Prevention of venous thromboembolism: American College of Chest Physicians Evidence-Based Clinical Practice Guidelines (8th ed). *Chest*, *133*(6 Suppl.), 381S–453S.

GlaxoSmithKline. (2010). *Product information for Arixtra*. Research Triangle Park, NC: Author.

*Goldhaber, S. Z. (2010). Risk factors for venous thromboembolism. *Journal of the American College of Cardiology*, *56*(1), 1–7.

*Goldstein, L. B., Adams, R., Bushnell, C. D., et al. (2011). Guidelines for the primary prevention of ischemic stroke: A guideline for healthcare professionals from the American Heart Association/American Stroke Association. *Stroke*, *42*, 517–584.

Goldstein, J. N., Refaai, M. A., Milling, T. J., Jr., et al. (2015) Four-factor prothrombin complex concentrate versus plasma for rapid vitamin K antagonist reversal in patients needing urgent surgical or invasive interventions: A phase 3b, open-label, non-inferiority, randomised trial. *Lancet*, *385*(9982), 2077–2087.

Gomez-Outes, A., Suarez-Gea, M. L., Lecumberri, R., et al. (2014). Specific antidotes in development for reversal of novel anticoagulants. *Recent Patents on Cardiovascular Drug Discovery*, *9*, 2–10.

Goodman, S. G., Wojdyla, D. M., Piccini, J. P., et al. (2014). Factors associated with major bleeding events: Insights from the ROCKET AF trial (rivaroxaban once-daily oral direct factor Xa inhibition compared with vitamin K antagonism for prevention of stroke and embolism trial in atrial fibrillation). *Journal of the American College of Cardiology*, *63*(9), 891–900.

Guyatt, G. H., Akl, E. A., Crowther, M., et al. (2012). Executive summary: Antithrombotic therapy and prevention of thrombosis (9th ed.: American College of Chest Physicians Evidence-Based Clinical Practice Guidelines). *Chest*, *141*(2 Suppl.), 7S–47S.

*Heit, J. A. (2006). Epidemiology of venous thromboembolism. In R. W. Colman (Ed.). *Hemostasis and thrombosis: Basic principles and clinical practice* (5th ed., pp. 1227–1233). Philadelphia, PA: J. B. Lippincott.

Held, C., Hylek, E. M., Alexander, J. H., et al. (2015). Clinical outcomes and management associated with major bleeding in patients with atrial fibrillation treated with apixaban or warfarin: Insights from the ARISTOTLE trial. *European Heart Journal*, *36*(20), 1264–1272.

*Hirsh, J., Bauer, K. A., Donati, M. B., et al. (2008). Parenteral anticoagulants. American College of Chest Physicians Evidence-Based Clinical Practical Guidelines (8th ed.). *Chest*, *133*(6 Suppl.), 141S–159S.

*Holbrook, A. M., Pereira, J. A., Labiris, R., et al. (2005). Systematic overview of warfarin and its drug and food interactions. *Archives of Internal Medicine*, *165*, 1095–1106.

Holbrook, A., Schulman, S., Witt, D. M., et al. (2012). Evidence-based management of anticoagulant therapy: Antithrombotic therapy and prevention of thrombosis. American College of Chest Physicians Evidence-Based Clinical Practice Guidelines (9th ed.). *Chest*, *141*(2 Suppl.), e152S–e184S.

Horlocker, T. T., Wedel, D. J., Rowlingson, J. C., et al. (2010). Regional anesthesia in the patient receiving antithrombotic or thrombolytic therapy: American Society of Regional Anesthesia And Pain Medicine Evidence-Based Guidelines (3rd ed.). *Regional Anesthesia and Pain Medicine*, *35*, 64–101.

*Hull, R. D., & Pineo, G. F. (2004). Heparin and low molecular-weight heparin therapy for venous thromboembolism: Will unfractionated heparin survive? *Seminars in Thrombosis and Hemostasis*, *30*(Suppl. 1), 11–23.

*Jacobs, L. G. (2008). Warfarin pharmacology, clinical management, and evaluation of hemorrhagic risk for the elderly. *Cardiology Clinics*, *26*, 157–167.

*Jacobson, A. K. (2008). Warfarin monitoring: Point-of-care INR testing limitations and interpretation of the prothrombin time. *Journal of Thrombosis and Thrombolysis*, *25*, 10–11.

*January, C. T., Wann, L. S., Alpert, J. S., et al. (2014). 2014 AHA/ACC/HRS guideline for the management of patients with atrial fibrillation: A report of the American College of Cardiology/American Heart Association task force on practice guidelines and the heart rhythm society. *Journal of the American College of Cardiology*, *64*, e1–e76.

Kahn, S. R., Lim, W., Dunn, A. S., et al. (2012). Prevention of VTE in nonsurgical patients: Antithrombotic therapy and prevention of thrombosis (9th ed.: American College of Chest Physicians Evidence-Based Clinical Practice Guidelines). *Chest*, *141*(Suppl. 2), e195S–e226S.

*Kearon, C., Kahn, S. R., Agnelli, G., et al. (2008). Antithrombotic therapy for venous thromboembolic disease: American College of Chest Physicians Evidence-Based Clinical Practical Guidelines (8th ed.). *Chest*, *133*(6 Suppl.), 454S–545S.

*Kelechi, T., & Bonham, P. A. (2008). Lower extremity venous disorders: Implications for nursing practice. *Journal of Cardiovascular Nursing*, *23*(2), 132–143.

Kernan, W. N., Pvbiagele, B., Black, H. R., et al. (2014). Guidelines for the prevention of stroke in patients with stroke and transient ischemic attack: A guideline for healthcare professionals from the American Heart Association/American Stroke Association. *Stroke*, *45*(7), 2160–2236.

*Khan, T., Wynne, H., Wood, P., et al. (2004). Dietary vitamin K influences intra-individual variability in anticoagulant response to warfarin. *British Journal of Haematology, 124*(3), 348–354.

Kimmel, S. E. (2015). Warfarin pharmacogenomics: Current best evidence. *Journal of Thrombosis and Haemostasis, 13*(Suppl. 1), S266–S271.

Kovacs, R. J., Flaker, G. C., Saxsonhouse, S. J., et al. (2015). Practical management of anticoagulation in patients with atrial fibrillation. *Journal of the American College of Cardiology, 65*(13), 1340–1360.

Kreidy, R. (2014). Influence of acquired and genetic risk factors on the prevention, management, and treatment of thromboembolic disease. *International Journal of Vascular Medicine, 2014,* 859726. doi: 10.1155/2014/859726.

Lauffenburger, J. C., Rhoney, D. H., Farley, J. F., et al. (2015). Predictors of gastrointestinal bleeding among patients with atrial fibrillation after initiating dabigatran therapy. *Pharmacotherapy, 35*(6), 560–568.

Leo Pharma. (2010). *Product information for Innohep.* Parsippany, NJ: Author.

*Maganti, K., Rigolin, V. H., Enriquez Sarano, M., et al. (2010). Valvular heart disease: Diagnosis and management. *Mayo Clinic Proceedings, 85,* 483–500.

*Man-Son-Hing, M., Nichol, G., Lau, A., et al. (1999). Choosing antithrombotic therapy for elderly patients with atrial fibrillation who are at risk for falls. *Archives of Internal Medicine, 159,* 677–685.

Marsh, J. D., & Keyrouz, S. G. (2010). Stroke prevention and treatment. *Journal of the American College of Cardiology, 56*(9), 683–691.

*McCabe, P. J. (2005). Spheres of clinical nurse specialist practice influence evidence-based care for patients with atrial fibrillation. *Clinical Nurse Specialist, 19*(6), 308–317.

*Merli, G. J. (2008). Pathophysiology of venous thrombosis and the diagnosis of deep venous thrombosis-pulmonary embolism in the elderly. *Cardiology Clinics, 26,* 203–219.

Mozaffarian, D., Benjamin, E. J., Go, A. S., et al. (2015). Heart disease and stroke statistics-2015 update. *Circulation, 131,* e29–e322.

Nishimura, R. A., Otto, C. M., Bonow, R. O., et al. (2014). 2014 AHA/ACC guideline for the management of patients with valvular heart disease: A report of the American College of Cardiology/American Heart Association Task Force on Practice Guidelines. *Journal of Thoracic Cardiovascular and Surgery, 148*(1), e1–e132.

Nutescu, E. A., Dager, W. E., Lewin, J. J., III, et al. (2013). Management of bleeding and reversal strategies for oral anticoagulants: Clinical practice considerations. *American Journal of Health-System Pharmacy, 70,* 1914–1929.

*Nutescu, E. A., Shapiro, N. L., Ibrahim, S., et al. (2006). Warfarin and its interactions with foods, herbs and other dietary supplements. *Expert Opinion on Drug Safety, 5*(3), 433–451.

*Ortel, T. L. (2010). Acquired thrombotic risk factors in the critical care setting. *Critical Care Medicine, 28*(Suppl.), S43–S50.

*Osinbowale, O., Ali, L., & Chi, Y. W. (2010). Venous thromboembolism: A clinical review. *Postgraduate Medicine, 122*(2), 54–65.

*Patrono, C., Baigent, C., Hirsh, J., et al. (2008). Antiplatelet drugs: American College of Chest Physicians Evidence-Based Clinical Practice Guidelines (8th ed.). *Chest, 133*(6 Suppl.), 199S–233S.

*Piazza, G., & Goldhaber, S. Z. (2006). Acute pulmonary embolism. Part 1: Epidemiology and diagnosis. *Circulation, 114,* e28–e32.

Pollack, C. V., Reilly, P. A., Eikelboom, J., et al. (2015). Idarucizumab for dabigatran reversal. *New England Journal of Medicine, 373*(6), 511–520.

Raskob, G. E., Angchaisuksiri, P., Blanco, A. N., et al. (2014). Thrombosis: A major contributor to global disease burden. *Thrombosis Research, 134,* 931–938.

*Righini, M., & Bounameaux, H. (2008). Clinical relevance of distal deep vein thrombosis. *Current Opinion in Pulmonary Medicine, 14,* 408–413.

Rincon, F., & Sacco, R. L. (2008). Secondary stroke prevention. *Journal of Cardiovascular Nursing, 23,* 34–41.

Roche. (2001). *Product information for Ticlid.* Nutley, NJ: Author.

Ruff, C. T., Giugliano, R. P., Braunwald, E., et al. (2014). Comparison of the efficacy and safety of new oral anticoagulants with warfarin in patients with atrial fibrillation: A meta-analysis of randomised trials. *Lancet, 383*(9921), 955–982.

*Salem, D. V., O'Gara, P. T., Madias, C., et al. (2008). Valvular and structural heart disease: American College of Chest Physicians Evidence-Based Clinical Practice Guidelines (8th ed.). *Chest, 133*(6 Suppl.), 593S–626S.

*Sanofi Aventis. (2010). *Product information for Lovenox.* Bridgewater, NJ: Author.

Sawyer, N. A. (2010). Lower extremity edema: To maintain a balance, treat the underlying disease. *Advance for Physician Assistants, 6*(8), 16–20.

*Schulman, S., Beyth, R. J., Kearon, C., et al. (2008). Hemorrhagic complications of anticoagulant and thrombolytic treatment. American College of Chest Physicians Evidence-Based Clinical Practice Guidelines (8th ed.). *Chest, 133*(6 Suppl.), 257S–298S.

Simmons, B. B., Yeo, A., & Fung, K. (2010). Current guidelines on antiplatelet agents for secondary prevention of noncardiogenic stroke. *Postgraduate Medicine, 122*(2), 49–53.

Slusher, K. B. (2010). Factor V Leiden: A case study and review. *Dimensions of Critical Care Nursing, 29*(1), 6–10.

Somarouthu, B., Abbara, S., & Kalva, S. (2010). Diagnosing deep vein thrombosis. *Postgraduate Medicine, 122*(2), 66–73.

*Spyropoulos, A. C. (2008). Brave new world: The current and future use of novel anticoagulants. *Thrombosis Research, 123,* S29–S35.

*Streiff, M. B. (2010). The National Comprehensive Cancer Network (NCCN) guidelines on the management of venous thromboembolism in cancer patients. *Thrombosis Research, 125*(Suppl. 2) S128–S133.

*Sun, J. C., Davidson, M. J., Lamy, A., et al. (2010). Antithrombotic management of patients with prosthetic heart valves: Current evidence and future trends. *Lancet, 374,* 565–576.

*Suttie, J. W. (1992). Vitamin K and human nutrition. *Journal of the American Dietetic Association, 92,* 585–590.

*Tran, H. A., & Ginsberg, J. S. (2006). Anticoagulant therapy for major arterial and venous thromboembolism. In R. W. Colman, (Ed.). *Hemostasis and thrombosis: Basic principles and clinical practice* (5th ed., pp. 1676–1680). Philadelphia, PA: J. B. Lippincott.

Turka, J. (2005). Understanding the INR. *Nursing, 35*(8), 18–19.

Van Veen, J. J., Hampton, R. M., Laidlaw, S., et al. (2011). Protamine reversal of low molecular weight heparin: Clinically effective? *Blood Coagul Fibrinolysis, 22*(7), 565–570.

van der Hulle, T., Kooiman, J., den Exter, P. L., et al. (2014). Effectiveness and safety of novel oral anticoagulants as compared with vitamin K antagonists in the treatment of acute symptomatic venous thromboembolism: A systematic review and meta-analysis. *Journal of Thrombosis and Haemostasis, 12,* 320–328.

*Varga, E. A. (2008). Genetics in the context of thrombophilia. *Journal of Thrombosis and Thrombolysis, 25,* 2–5.

*Vazquez, S. R., Freeman, A., Van Woerkom, et al. (2009). Contemporary issues in the postthrombotic syndrome. *Annals of Pharmacotherapy, 23,* 1824–1835.

Vedovati, M. C., Germini, F., Agnelli, G., et al. (2015). Direct oral anticoagulants in patients with VTE and cancer: A systematic review and meta-analysis. *Chest, 147*(2), 475–483.

Wann, L. S., Alpert, J. S., Curtis, A. B., et al. (2011a). 2011 ACC/AHA/HRS focused update on the management of patients with atrial fibrillation (updating the 2006 guidelines). *Circulation, 123,* 104–123.

*Warkentin, T. E. (2010). Agents for the treatment of heparin-induced thrombocytopenia. *Hematology and Oncology Clinics of North America, 24,* 755–775.

*Weitz, J. I. (2009). Unanswered questions in venous thromboembolism. *Thrombosis Research, 123*(4 Suppl.), S2–S10.

Welch, E. (2006). The assessment and management of venous thromboembolism. *Nursing Standard, 20*(28), 24–30.

Wells, P. S., Forgie, M. A., Rodger, M. A. (2014). Treatment of venous thromboembolism. *Journal of American Medical Association, 311*(7), 717–728.

Werth, S., Breslin, T., NiAinle, F., et al. (2015). Bleeding risk, management and outcome in patients receiving non-VKA oral anticoagulants (NOACs). *American Journal of Cardiovascular Drugs, 15*(4), 235–242.

Weyland, P. (2009). Warfarin management: Tap into new ways to slow the clot. *The Nurse Practitioner, 34*(3), 22–28.

*Witt, D. (2010). Optimizing use of current anticoagulants. *Hematology Oncology Clinics of North America, 24*, 717–726.

*Wittkowsky, A. K. (2008). Dietary supplements, herbs and oral anticoagulants: The nature of the evidence. *Journal of Thrombosis and Thrombolysis, 25*, 72–77.

51 Anemias

Kelly Barranger

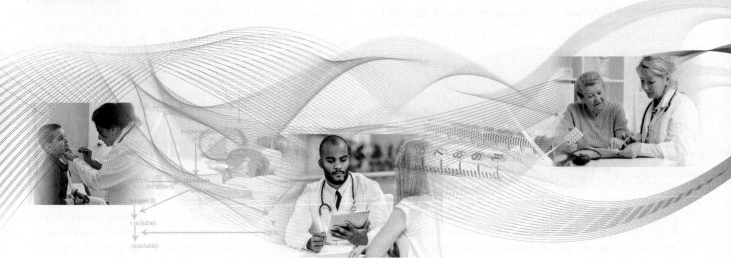

Anemia is a condition in which there is a decrease in the number of red blood cells (RBCs) or hemoglobin in the blood. Anemia can also be defined as a reduced ability to carry oxygen to meet physiologic needs, which varies by age, sex, altitude, and pregnancy status. There is not one set of "normal ranges" for hemoglobin, hematocrit, and RBCs. In general, anemia can be defined as values that are more than two standard deviations below the mean. The World Health Organization (WHO) criteria for anemia in men and women are less than 13.0 and less than 12.0 g/dL, respectively (**Table 51.1**). These values are also supported in the second National Health and Nutrition Examination Survey (Centers for Disease Control and Prevention, 2012).

CAUSES

Anemia may develop through blood loss, nutritional deficiency, or malabsorption syndromes, or concurrently with inflammation or malignancy, or be inherited as in sickle cell disease (SCD), thalassemia, or hemoglobinopathy. Anemia may also occur from the treatment of diseases such as cancer, human immunodeficiency virus (HIV)/acquired immunodeficiency syndrome, or hepatitis C.

PATHOPHYSIOLOGY

RBCs, also known as *erythrocytes*, are formed in the marrow of the ribs, sternum, clavicle, vertebrae, pelvis, and proximal epiphyses of the humerus and femur. RBCs play a vital role in the support of metabolism by transporting oxygen to and removing carbon dioxide from tissue. To maintain proper tissue oxygenation and sustain a normal acid–base balance, an adequate number of RBCs must be available and they must be in specific shape and size. The average adult blood cell concentration for mean corpuscular volume (MCV) is 80 to 96 fL. These values may vary slightly from laboratory to laboratory.

RBCs develop from a pluripotent cell, which differentiates into an erythroid precursor. The cells shed their nuclei and obtain hemoglobin. The production of RBCs is initiated by the hormone erythropoietin (EPO), which is produced by the kidneys in response to a decrease in tissue oxygen concentration. Decreased tissue oxygen then signals the kidneys to increase production and release EPO. This EPO stimulates the stem cell to differentiate into proerythroblasts. EPO also increases the rate of mitosis and increases the release of reticulocytes from the marrow and induces hemoglobin formation. When hemoglobin synthesis is accelerated, the critical hemoglobin concentration necessary for maturity is reached more rapidly, causing an earlier release of reticulocytes. The appearance of reticulocytes in peripheral circulation indicates that RBC production is being stimulated. The maturation process takes about 1 week. Several days are then required for the reticulocyte to become an erythrocyte (**Figure 51.1**). The normal RBC survival time is 120 days; the survival time can be decreased to 18 to 20 days before occurrence of an anemia if the bone marrow functions at maximal capacity. When hemolytic destruction of RBCs exceeds marrow production, anemia will develop, causing the hemoglobin value to decrease.

DIAGNOSTIC CRITERIA

Anemia is a reduction in the number of circulating RBCs (the hemoglobin concentration) or the volume of packed RBCs (hematocrit) in the blood. Anemias are classified according

TABLE 51.1	
Hemoglobin Thresholds	
Age or Gender Group	**Hemoglobin Thresholds (g/dL)**
Children (0.5–4.99 y)	11.0
Children (5.00–11.99 y)	11.5
Children (12.0–14.99 y)	12.0
Nonpregnant women (15.00 y)	12.0
Pregnant women	11.0
Men (15.00 y)	13.0

to their pathophysiologic basis and occur due to decreased production or increased destruction of RBCs. They are also classified according to cell size using the MCV (**Figure 51.2**). Microcytic anemias are those anemias due to RBCs with a lower than normal size. These include iron deficiency anemia, thalassemia, and anemia of chronic disease, infection, inflammation, or malignancy. In contrast, macrocytic anemia may be megaloblastic such as folate or vitamin B$_{12}$ deficiency or nonmegaloblastic causes such as myelodysplasia, liver disease, or reticulocytosis (**Box 51.1**).

The signs and symptoms of anemia depend on the rate of development, age, and cardiovascular status of the patient.

Rapid onset of anemia is most likely to present with cardiorespiratory symptoms (tachycardia, light-headedness, breathlessness). Anemia of a chronic nature may present with vague symptoms including fatigue, weakness, headache, vertigo, faintness, sensitivity to cold, pallor, and loss of skin tone.

Normal ranges may not be appropriate for all populations. Patients living at high altitude have values higher than those living at sea level. Smokers or those who have a significant exposure to secondary smoke have higher than normal levels. African Americans of both sexes have lower values than compared to the Caucasian population.

EVALUATION

Anemia is never normal. A history, physical examination, and simple laboratory testing are useful in evaluating patients with anemia. The first thing to consider in evaluating anemia is the stability of the patient. Secondly, consider whether it is recent or lifelong. Recent anemia is almost always acquired, whereas lifelong anemia is likely inherited (hemoglobinopathies, thalassemia hereditary spherocytosis). Next, obtain a thorough history including recent and past infections, malignancy, renal disease, and a history of autoimmune disease. The review of systems should include weight loss or weight gain, fever, chills or night sweats, change in bowel habits, and black tarry stools.

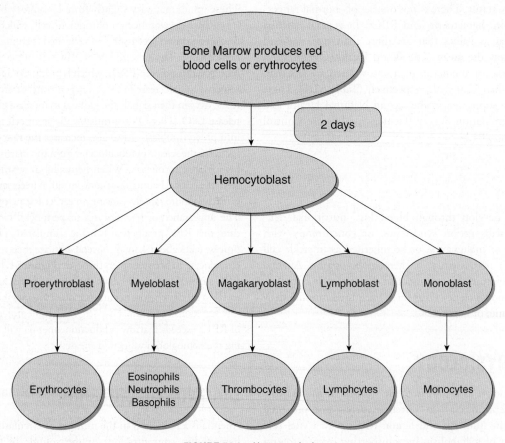

FIGURE 51.1 Hematopoiesis.

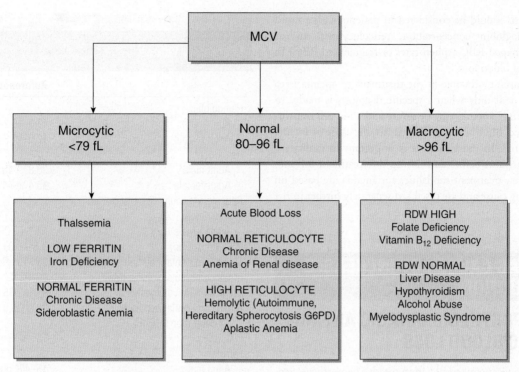

FIGURE 51.2 Anemias classified by mean corpuscular volume (MCV).

The goal of the physical examination is to assess the patient's condition and to find signs of organ or multisystem involvement. During the physical examination, note the presence or absence of tachycardia, dyspnea, fever, or postural hypotension. Also, note the presence or absence of

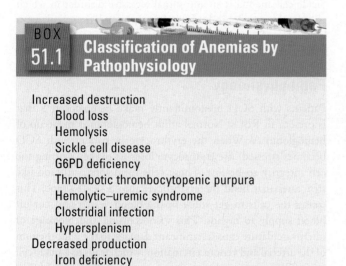

BOX 51.1 Classification of Anemias by Pathophysiology

Increased destruction
 Blood loss
 Hemolysis
 Sickle cell disease
 G6PD deficiency
 Thrombotic thrombocytopenic purpura
 Hemolytic–uremic syndrome
 Clostridial infection
 Hypersplenism
Decreased production
 Iron deficiency
 Thalassemia
 Anemia of chronic disease
 Aplastic anemia
 Myeloproliferative leukemia

G6PD, glucose-6-phosphate dehydrogenase.

lymphadenopathy, hepatosplenomegaly, and bone tenderness, especially over the sternum (chronic myeloid leukemia) or lytic lesion (multiple myeloma or metastatic cancer). Assess the skin for signs of petechiae due to thrombocytopenia, ecchymosis, or coagulation abnormalities. During the physical examination, a stool examination for occult blood should be performed.

Laboratory evaluation should be performed and include a complete blood count (CBC), including differential and reticulocytes.

A low WBC count (leukopenia) may be associated with hypersplenism, cobalamin deficiencies, or bone marrow suppression or replacement, whereas high WBC count may be associated with a primary hematologic malignancy, inflammation, or infection.

The WBC differential, in conjunction with the total WBC count, may show absolute number of various cell types:

- Absolute neutrophil count may be elevated due to infection and may be decreased after having chemotherapy.
- Absolute monocyte count may be elevated in myelodysplasia.
- Absolute eosinophil count may be elevated in certain infection.
- Absolute lymphocyte count may be decreased in HIV infection or following treatment with glucocorticoids.

Pancytopenia is the combination of anemia, thrombocytopenia, and neutropenia. Mild pancytopenia is seen in patients with splenomegaly and splenic trapping. The presence of severe pancytopenia is associated with disorders such as aplastic anemia, folate or cobalamin deficiency, hematologic malignancy, and marrow ablation from chemotherapy or radiation.

Hemolysis should be considered in patients with a rapid fall in hemoglobin concentration, reticulocytosis, and/or abnormally shaped RBC (spherocytes or fragmented RBC) in the absence of blood loss.

An important principle in the treatment of anemia is to initiate treatment only when a specific diagnosis is made. In the acute setting, anemia may be severe and a red cell transfusion is required, but this is rare. Frequently, the cause of anemia is multifactorial. In most cases, it is important to evaluate a patient's iron status before and during the treatment for anemia. Moreover, treatment modalities for anemia are based on the underlying cause and are discussed separately further in the chapter.

ANEMIAS CAUSED BY INCREASED DESTRUCTION

ACUTE POSTHEMORRHAGIC ANEMIA/ CHRONIC BLOOD LOSS

Posthemorrhagic anemia results from massive hemorrhage associated with spontaneous or traumatic rupture or incision of a large blood vessel. It can also be from an erosion of an artery by a lesion (peptic ulcer, neoplasm) or failure to maintain normal hemostasis. The sudden loss of one third of blood volume may be fatal, whereas a two-thirds loss of blood volume slowly over 24 hours is without immediate risk. During and immediately after hemorrhage, the RBC count, hemoglobin value, and hematocrit may be high due to vasoconstriction. Fluid from tissue enters the circulation within a few hours resulting in hemodilution causing a drop in the RBC count and hemoglobin value. This result is proportional to the severity of bleeding. Signs of vascular instability (hypotension and decreased organ perfusion) appear with acute losses of 10% to 15% of the total blood volume. When more than 30% of blood volume is lost suddenly, hypotension and tachycardia occur. When more than 40% of blood volume is lost, signs of hypovolemic shock (confusion, dyspnea, diaphoresis, hypotension, and tachycardia) appear.

Diagnostic Criteria

Initial evaluation of anemia includes a careful history and physical examination. Laboratory evaluation includes CBC, reticulocyte index, iron studies, examination of the peripheral blood smear, and a stool sample for occult blood (**Table 51.2**). Further studies are indicated based on the results of the preliminary evaluation.

Initiating Therapy

Immediate therapy consists of hemostasis, restoration of blood volume, and treatment of shock. In many cases, the blood lost needs to be replaced promptly. Blood transfusion is the only means of rapidly restoring blood volume.

TABLE 51.2	
Laboratory Values	
	Reference Range*
Hemoglobin	
Adult male	13.3–16.2 g/dL
Adult female	12.0–15.8 g/dL
Hematocrit	
Adult male	38.8%–46.4%
Adult female	35.4%–44.4%
Reticulocyte count	
Adult male	0.8%–2.3% RBCs
Adult female	0.8%–2.0% RBCs
WBC (leukocyte)	3.54–9.06 L
Mean corpuscular hemoglobin (MCH)	26.7–31.9 pg
Mean corpuscular volume (MCV)	79–93 fL
Mean platelet volume (MPV)	9.0–12.95 fL
Mean corpuscular hemoglobin concentration (MCHC)	32.3–35.9 g/dL
Platelet	165–415 mn
Ferritin	
Adult male	15–400 ng/mL
Adult female	10–200 ng/mL
Vitamin B$_{12}$	200–600 pg/mL
Folate	3–16 ng/mL

*These values may vary from laboratory to laboratory.

SICKLE CELL ANEMIA

Sickle cell anemia is an autosomal recessive disorder in which abnormal hemoglobin leads to chronic hemolytic anemia with numerous clinical consequences. It most commonly affects African Americans and, to a lesser extent, Hispanics.

Pathophysiology

Patients with SCD predominantly make hemoglobin S that is present in RBCs. Normal adult hemoglobin is made up of hemoglobin A. When the erythrocyte in patient with SCD becomes stressed, the erythrocyte loses its oxygen causing the cell integrity to be lost. These cells form long, stiff rod-like structures that bend the erythrocyte into a sickle shape. This causes the cells to get stuck in the blood vessels and cut off blood supply to organs. This vasoocclusion and blockage of microvasculature causes significant damage to the endothelium of the arterial and venous circulation, which leads to a sickle cell crisis. Crisis occurs when patients are physically stressed (exercise), exposed to high altitude or cold temperatures, or have a high fever or infection. The underlying cause includes hypoxia, dehydration, and acidosis. Sickle cell crises last about a week but may not resolve for several weeks to months. Pain typically occurs in the back, ribs, and limbs. Patients with sickle cell anemia are susceptible to infection, particularly *Streptococcus pneumoniae* and *Haemophilus influenzae*, and are prone to gallstones and renal failure. Other complications include chronic leg ulcer, priapism, aseptic necrosis of the humoral and femoral heads, and chronic osteomyelitis. Long-term effects include stroke, heart failure, and death. Patients should be screened for renal disease, pulmonary hypertension, hypertension, retinopathy, risk of stroke, and pulmonary disease and should receive reproductive and contraception counseling.

Therapeutic transfusion therapy is reserved for individuals with acute stroke, acute chest syndrome, acute multiorgan failure, and acute symptomatic anemia. A lifelong cure for SCD is available through an HLA-matched sibling donor hematopoietic stem cell transplant. However, this treatment is limited to individuals who are younger than age 16 due to toxicities and adverse outcomes including stroke, acute chest syndrome, osteonecrosis, and osteomyelitis and a mortality rate of 10% (Bernaudin et al., 1997).

Diagnostic Criteria

Examination of a peripheral blood smears for sickling and checking a reticulocyte count can provide supportive data for the diagnosis of SCD. Hemoglobin electrophoresis or a sickle cell preparation can also be useful in the diagnosis of SCD. Laboratory findings also show reduced hemoglobin and an RBC count between 2 and 3 million/μL.

For those at risk, techniques such as chorionic biopsy have been used during early gestation (6 to 8 weeks of pregnancy) to identify SCD. Genetic counseling and education must also be offered. Risk of the procedure to mother and fetus, risks of false-positive and false-negative results, and the acceptability of therapeutic abortion should also be discussed.

Initiating Drug Therapy

The management of SCD focuses on primary prevention and treatment of the complication as well as a potential cure. Children with SCD should be immunized against *S. pneumoniae*, *H. influenzae* type B, hepatitis B virus, and influenza. All individuals should be immunized as recommended by the Advisory Committee on Immunization Practices (ACIP). The immunization schedule can be found online and is updated up to four times a year (National Heart, Lung, and Blood Institute, 2014). Infants are at increased risk for pneumococcal disease and should receive 13-valent conjugate pneumococcal vaccine (PCV13) shortly after birth and 23-valent pneumococcal polysaccharide (PPSV23) vaccine at 2 years of age. A second dose should be given at 5 years of age. Other immunizations include hepatitis B and meningococcal vaccine.

Patients are maintained on folic acid supplementation, 1 mg/d, because of accelerated erythropoiesis.

Hydroxyurea

In selected patients, hydroxyurea is used for prophylaxis treatment to reduce the number of crises (acute chest syndrome or greater than three crises per year) in adult and children. The effects of hydroxyurea on RBCs include increasing hemoglobin F levels, increasing water content of RBCs, increasing deformability of sickled cells, and altering the adhesion of RBCs to endothelium. Evidence suggests that hydroxyurea reduces the number of chest syndromes and transfusions and may reverse organ dysfunction (Wong et al., 2014).

The starting dose of hydroxyurea for adults is 15 mg/kg/d (round up to the nearest 500 mg). For patient with chronic kidney disease (CKD), the dose is adjusted to 5 to 10 mg/kg/d. Starting dosage for infants and children is 20 mg/kg/d. While adjusting the dose of hydroxyurea, a CBC with differential and reticulocyte count should be done every 4 weeks. The goal of therapy is for an absolute neutrophil count ≥2,000/μL and a platelet count ≥80,000/μL. In younger patients, an absolute neutrophil count down to 1,250/μL may be safely tolerated. If neutropenia or thrombocytopenia occurs, hydroxyurea should be held and a CBC with differential should be performed weekly. Once blood counts have recovered, reinstitute hydroxyurea at a dose 5 mg/kg/d lower than the dose given before onset of cytopenias. The dose of hydroxyurea should be increased by 5 mg/kg/d every 8 weeks until mild myelosuppression (absolute neutrophil count 2,000 to 4,000/μL) is achieved, up to a maximum of 35 mg/kg/d. Laboratory studies including a CBC with differential, reticulocyte count, and platelet count should be performed every 2 to 3 months. The effectiveness of hydroxyurea depends on adherence, and patients should be counseled not to miss a dose and not to double up on doses. Keep in mind that it may take 3 to 6 months of treatment with hydroxyurea to see a clinical response. Patients should be maintained on a maximum tolerated dose for 6 months before considering discontinuation or treatment failure. During hospitalizations, patients should be continued on hydroxyurea (National Heart, Lung, and Blood Institute, 2014).

Hydroxyurea should not be used in patients likely to become pregnant or those unwilling or unable to follow instructions regarding treatment. Patients should be monitored for myelotoxicity. Serious adverse reactions include myelosuppression and the risk of cancer. Side effects include cutaneous hyperpigmentation, alopecia, xerosis, nail pigmentation, and leg ulcers.

Pain Management

Management of acute painful episodes consists of exclusion of causes (infection), hydration by oral or intravenous (IV) fluid resuscitation, and aggressive pain relief, including analgesics and opiates. Acetaminophen has analgesic and antipyretic effects. The 24-hour maximum daily dose of acetaminophen in four divided dose should not exceed 4 g for healthy individuals and 3 g in individuals with liver disease or who are pregnant. High dosages of acetaminophen can damage the liver and could be fatal (Ballas, 2005).

Nonsteroidal anti-inflammatory agents (NSAIDs) have anti-inflammatory effects in addition to pain and antipyretic proprieties. NSAIDs have potentially serious adverse effects, including gastritis and gastrointestinal (GI) bleeding, which may result in anemia. NSAIDs are contraindicated in patients with history of GI bleed and renal disease (Ballas, 2005). The management of acute painful crisis includes aggressive narcotic analgesia, such as morphine or hydromorphone (see Chapter 7). Adverse effects of opioid analgesics include severe sedation and respiratory depression. Side effects include itching, nausea, and vomiting. Opioid analgesics should be used carefully in patients with asthma, impaired ventilation, liver failure, renal failure, and increased intracranial pressure.

Meperidine should be used with caution in the treatment of acute SCD because multiple doses are associated with the accumulation of its major metabolite, normeperidine, and central toxicity, including twitching, multifocal clonus, and seizures. Coadministration with antipsychotics may cause neuromuscular disorders, including dystonia, tardive dyskinesia, akathisia, and neuroleptic malignant syndrome. Meperidine in combination with monoamine oxidase inhibitors may cause severe adverse reactions, including excitation, hyperpyrexia, convulsions, and death.

Patients with chronic sickle cell pain are managed with long-acting opioids and short-acting opioids for breakthrough pain according to the National Heart, Lung, and Blood Institute's guidelines.

ANEMIAS CAUSED BY DIMINISHED PRODUCTION OF RED BLOOD CELLS

IRON DEFICIENCY ANEMIA

Iron deficiency anemia is the most common nutritional deficiency worldwide. The diagnosis of iron deficiency anemia is made by low hemoglobin and iron stores, whereas iron deficiency is made by low iron stores without anemia. According to the WHO, iron deficiency is most prevalent in young children and women of childbearing age. The goal of treatment is to identify the underlying causes and administer the appropriate therapy.

Causes

The cause of iron deficiency is related to insufficient iron intake, inadequate absorption from the GI tract, and increased iron demands and is exacerbated by chronic intestinal blood loss due to parasitic and malarial infections.

A vegetarian diet and a diet low in consumption of animal protein contribute to inadequate intake of iron. Inadequate absorption from the GI tract is usually related to malabsorption syndromes (celiac disease, Whipple disease, bacterial overgrowth), postgastrectomy, gastric bypass and the presence of certain foods (dietary fiber, coffee, tea, eggs, or milk) or drugs (quinolones, tetracycline, H2 blockers, proton pump inhibitors, calcium supplements), or unrelenting diarrhea. Iron demands are increased in menstrual blood loss, pregnancy, and lactation. Iron requirements are highest during infancy and pregnancy. Iron deficiency in pregnancy has been implicated as a cause of perinatal complications such as low birth weight and premature delivery in affected mothers. In children, long-term

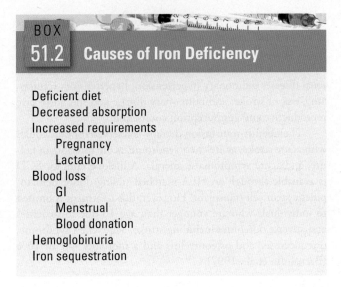

BOX 51.2   Causes of Iron Deficiency

Deficient diet
Decreased absorption
Increased requirements
    Pregnancy
    Lactation
Blood loss
    GI
    Menstrual
    Blood donation
Hemoglobinuria
Iron sequestration

findings include increased susceptibility to infection, poor growth, developmental and behavioral delays, and low mental and motor test scores. Pregnant women should routinely receive iron supplementation and continue into postpartum.

The consequence of chronic alcoholism, food faddism, prolonged illness with anorexia, or poor nutrition also contributes to iron deficiency (**Box 51.2**). Interventions such as foods fortified with iron and iron supplementation are in place to prevent and correct iron deficiency.

Pathophysiology

The predominant use of iron is for the creation of heme groups that are incorporated into hemoglobin and myoglobin. Additionally, iron is involved in the production of cytochromes and other enzymes. Immediately bioavailable, iron is bound in the bloodstream to a specific carrier protein, transferrin. Excess of immediate iron needs is stored in the liver, spleen, and bone marrow as ferritin. Patients with iron deficiency anemia may be asymptomatic or have vague symptoms. Other manifestations include koilonychia (spoon nail), angular stomatitis, glossitis, and pica (eating dirt, paint, clay, ice, or cornstarch).

Diagnostic Criteria

Laboratory findings are critical for the diagnosis. The classic criteria for iron deficiency anemia include low serum iron and ferritin concentrations and a high total iron-binding capacity (TIBC). In mild iron deficiency, the hemoglobin, hematocrit, and RBC indices remain normal. In the later stages, the hemoglobin and hematocrit levels fall below normal values (**Table 51.2**).

A low concentration of ferritin (less than 0 to 120 ng/L) is the earliest and most sensitive indication of iron deficiency. However, patients with renal or liver disease, malignancies, or infectious or inflammatory processes may have elevated ferritin levels that may not correlate with iron stores in the bone marrow. Transferrin saturation (serum iron divided by TIBC) is also used to assess iron deficiency anemia. Low values (less than 15%) indicate iron deficiency anemia, although low serum transferrin saturation values may also be present in inflammatory disorders. In this case, TIBC helps to differentiate the diagnosis. A TIBC over 400 mcg/dL suggests iron deficiency anemia, whereas values below 200 mcg/dL usually represent inflammatory disease. Free erythrocyte protoporphyrin (FEP) can also be used to distinguish between iron deficiency anemia and thalassemia minor. Iron binds with protoporphyrin to form heme. The serum concentration of protoporphyrin not bound to iron is elevated when iron levels are low. Thus, FEP is elevated in patients with iron deficiency anemia, inflammatory disorders, and lead poisoning. Rarely, a bone marrow examination is performed to assess iron stores.

Initiating Drug Therapy

The successful treatment of iron deficiency anemia depends on identifying the underlying cause. The treatment of iron deficiency anemia consists of dietary supplementation and iron preparations (**Table 51.3**). Oral iron is inexpensive and effective in the treatment of anemia. Iron is best absorbed from red meat, fish, and poultry. Plant-based foods are good sources of iron, although they are less easily absorbed. Whole-grain or iron-fortified cereals, breads, and pastas are among the best. Beverages such as tea or milk will reduce the absorption of iron and should be consumed in moderation between meals. Medications such as antacids, proton pump inhibitors, and histamine-2 (H_2) antagonists reduce absorption and should be avoided if possible. Vitamin C (500 mg daily), as well as orange juice, increases the absorption of iron due to increased stomach acidity. They should be given together and are recommended with meals. Transfusion should be considered for patients with iron deficiency anemia complaining of fatigue or dyspnea on exertion.

Indications for the use of IV iron include chronic bleeding, intestinal malabsorption, intolerance to oral iron, nonadherence, or hemoglobin of less than 6 g/dL with signs of poor perfusion.

Goals of Drug Therapy

The goal of therapy is based on how the anemia affects the patient's quality of life, activities of daily living, and general well-being. Treatment with oral iron may take 6 to 8 weeks for the hemoglobin to improve and as long as 6 months to replete iron stores. Minimization of the impact chronic

iron deficiency anemia has on adequate iron replacement has typically occurred when the serum ferritin level reaches 500 ng/L and when the hemoglobin and hematocrit have returned to normal levels.

Iron Replacement Therapy

Dosage

Treatment of iron deficiency anemia in adults should start with 100 to 200 mg of elementary iron (Adamson, 2012). For children, treatment is 3 to 6 mg/kg. Supplemental iron should be administered in divided doses without food. The addition of vitamin C may improve absorption.

Non–enteric-coated ferrous salts containing ferrous sulfate are the least expensive and provide adequate elemental iron. Typically, a dose of 325 mg ferrous sulfate three times daily provides sufficient iron replacement (195-mg elemental iron or about 2.7 mg/kg for a 70-kg adult). Slow-release or sustained-release iron preparations do not dissolve until reaching the small intestines, significantly reducing iron absorption.

Iron dextran is administered intravenously in one large dose of 200 to 500 mg. Safer alternatives include sodium ferric gluconate and iron sucrose. Sodium ferric gluconate is administered intravenously in eight weekly 125-mg doses for a total of 1,000 mg, and iron sucrose is administered intravenously five times over 2 weeks in 200-mg doses. Side effects of intravenous iron supplementation include nausea, vomiting, pruritus, headache, and flushing. Myalgia, arthralgia, and back and chest pain usually resolve in 48 hours.

Blood transfusion should be reserved for those patients who are hemodynamically unstable or show signs of end-organ ischemia from acute GI bleeding.

Time Frame for Response

Therapeutic doses of iron should increase hemoglobin value by 0.7 to 1 g/wk. Reticulocytosis occurs within 7 to 10 days after initiation of iron therapy. Iron therapy should be continued for at least 3 to 6 months. Common causes of treatment failure include noncompliance with therapy, malabsorption, and blood loss equal to the rate of production. Malabsorption can be ruled out by the iron test, which is rarely use, in which plasma iron levels are measured 1 to 2 hours afterward. Refractory responses to treatment may be due to patient with *Helicobacter pylori* infection or celiac disease. By eradicating *H. pylori* or following a gluten-free diet may eliminate the need for iron supplementation.

Adverse Events

Adverse reactions to iron are primarily GI difficulties, consisting of discolored feces, anorexia, constipation or diarrhea, nausea, and vomiting. To minimize the GI side effects, iron supplements should be taken with food. However, the impact of this on bioavailability of agents may be as high as a 66% decrease in iron absorption. Changing to a different iron salt or to a controlled-release preparation may reduce side effects.

TABLE 51.3	
Elemental Iron Content of Various Iron Salts	
Iron Salt	**% Iron**
Ferrous fumarate	33
Ferrous gluconate	11.6
Ferrous sulfate	20
Ferrous sulfate, anhydrous	30

A major adverse reaction of iron dextran is the risk of anaphylaxis, which can be fatal. Delayed reactions include myalgias, headache, and arthralgias.

Interactions

There is a host of drug–drug interactions with iron preparations. Many antibiotics, such as tetracyclines and fluoroquinolones, have a decrease in absorption due to the formation of a chelation product with the ferrous ions. The absorption of iron may be decreased when it is given with products containing aluminum, calcium, or magnesium. This effect may be as much as 30% to 40% reduction in absorption. The theory is that the reduced stomach acidity secondary to the antacid-like properties of products reduces the iron absorption. Similarly, patients taking proton pump inhibitors or H_2 antagonists may also have decreased iron absorption due to the lowered stomach acid. If the patient is taking both medications, space them at least 1 to 2 hours apart. In contrast, acidifying agents such as ascorbic acid (vitamin C) may enhance the absorption of iron-containing salts.

ANEMIA OF CHRONIC RENAL FAILURE

Anemia is a common complication of chronic renal failure and is primarily due to reduced EPO production by the kidney. Anemia occurs when the glomerular filtration rate (GFR) declines below 60 mL/min. Stages of CKD are defined according to the estimated GFR (**Table 51.4**) based on National Kidney Foundation guidelines (Kidney Dialysis Outcomes Quality Initiative [KDOQI, 2007]). Risk factors that increase the risk of CKD include hypertension, diabetes mellitus, autoimmune disease, older age, African ancestry, a family history of renal disease, a previous episode of acute renal failure, and the presence of proteinuria, abnormal urinary sediment, or structural abnormalities of the urinary tract. Measurement of albuminuria is a good test for early detection of renal disease; a 24-hour urine collection is the "gold standard." A first-morning urine sample is often more practical and correlates well, but not perfectly. Persistence in the urine of greater than 17 mg of albumin per gram of creatinine

TABLE 51.4	
Classification of Chronic Kidney Disease	
Stage	**GFR, mL/min/1.73 m²**
0	>90*
1	>90†
2	60–89
3	30–59
4	15–29
5	<15

*With risk factors for CKD.
†With demonstrated kidney damage (e.g., persistent proteinuria, abnormal urine sediments, abnormal blood and urine chemistry, and abnormal imaging studies).

in adult males and 25 mg of albumin per gram of creatinine in adult females usually signifies chronic renal damage.

Progressive renal impairment is associated with worsening systemic inflammation as seen with elevated levels of C-reactive protein, which contributes to the acceleration of vascular disease and comorbidities associated with advanced renal disease. As renal impairment advances, metabolic and endocrine functions are impaired and result in anemia, malnutrition, and abnormal metabolism of carbohydrates, fats, and proteins. Plasma levels of hormones, including parathyroid hormone (PTH), insulin, glucagon, sex hormones, and prolactin, change with renal failure as a result of urinary retention, decreased degradation, and abnormal regulation. Calciphylaxis is a devastating condition seen in patients with advanced kidney disease. It is heralded by livedo reticularis and advances to patches of ischemic necrosis, especially on the legs, thighs, abdomen, and breasts.

Pathophysiology

CKD is characterized by the progressive loss of functioning nephrons. With a reduction in nephron mass, renal vasodilation occurs and leads to hyperperfusion of the remaining glomeruli. Nephrons exposed to prolonged hyperperfusion begin to leak protein, become sclerotic, and eventually are destroyed. Substances that are filtered that are neither secreted nor resorbed by the tubule, such as urea, begin to rise early in the course of renal impairment.

Serum concentration of phosphorus, which is under the influence of PTH, is kept within the normal range until more than 80% of real function is lost. This is because increased PTH reduces the amount of phosphorus resorbed by the tubule. Failure of the kidney to fulfill its excretory, endocrine, and metabolic function results in inadequate quantities of EPO and 1,25-dihydroxy-vitamin D_3. Other hormones, such as PTH, insulin, and prolactin, are present in excess. The primary cause of anemia in patients with CKD is insufficient EPO production by the diseased kidneys. The mechanisms impairing renal EPO production are not well understood.

Initiating Drug Therapy

Patients should be placed on a multivitamin to replace the vitamins lacking in restrictive diets. Adequate bone marrow iron stores should be available before EPO treatment is initiated. Iron supplementation is usually essential to ensure an adequate response to EPO because the demand for iron by the marrow frequently exceeds the amount of iron immediately available for erythropoiesis (measured by percentage of transferring saturation) as well as the amount of iron stores (measured by serum ferritin). Current practice is to target a hemoglobin concentration of 10 to 12 g/dL.

The treatment of anemia caused by chronic renal failure begins with treating reversible causes of deteriorating renal function. Disorders of mineral metabolism (calcium, phosphorus, and bone) are common in CKD. Oral phosphorus-binding agents, calcium carbonate, and calcium acetate are used to treat hyperphosphatemia. Phosphorus-binding agents that do not contain calcium are sevelamer and lanthanum. Vitamin D or vitamin D analogs (calcitriol, paricalcitol) are given to treat secondary hyperparathyroidism.

Many of the immunologically mediated renal diseases (e.g., membranous nephropathy, Wegener disease, Goodpasture syndrome, lupus nephritis) respond to treatment with corticosteroids, cytotoxic agents, or plasmapheresis. This will not be discussed here. These patients should be under the care of a rheumatologist and/or a nephrologist.

When renal disease is associated with a metabolic disorder such as diabetes (Chapter 46) or gout (not discussed here), the treatment is directed at metabolic control to slow the course of renal deterioration.

When a drug (methicillin, indomethacin, NSAID, metformin, meperidine, and oral hypoglycemics) or other toxic substance is identified as the cause of renal failure, the offending agent should be withheld or avoided. Many antibiotics, antihypertensives, and antiarrhythmics require a reduced dosage or a change in the dose interval in patients with kidney disease.

Kidney Disease: Improving Global Outcomes (KDIGO) 2012 recommendations for erythropoiesis-stimulating agents (ESA) therapy in nondialysis and dialysis patient follow the recommendation from the FDA (Kliger et al., 2013). That is, a hemoglobin target range of 10 to 12 g/dL should be replaced by using the lowest possible dose of ESA to prevent transfusion. The concern is that increased blood transfusions will expose eligible kidney transplant recipients to allosensitizing effects of blood transfusions. Furthermore, ESA dose should be reduced or interrupted if the hemoglobin exceeds 11 g/dL. The ESA dosing strategy should be individualized for each patient considering the risks and benefits. KDIGO guidelines add an additional goal to avoid hemoglobin levels of less than 9 g/dL. The Normal Hematocrit Study reported worse outcomes in patients with hemoglobin 13 to 15 g/dL compared to 9 to 11 g/dL. While the FDA removed quality-of-life benefits in the use of ESA, the KDIGO recommendation is that it is still reasonable to start ESA in some patients with a hemoglobin level above 10 g/dL. The disagreement falls in interpreting quality of life.

For the naive pediatric patient with anemia, not on iron or ESA, the KDIGO recommendation is for oral iron when the transferrin is less than 20% and ferritin is less than 100 ng/mL. For pediatric patients on dialysis, oral or IV iron is recommended.

Goals of Drug Therapy

The goals of therapy are to (1) treat the underlying renal disease; (2) slow the progression of renal deterioration by modifying the known or suspected factors that are thought to aggravate the primary process and avoid factors that may aggravate existing renal failure; and (3) treat the specific complications of renal disease and prevent long-term complications of uremia. Correction of anemia decreases morbidity and reduces hospitalization and mortality among patients with CKD. Benefits of correcting anemia include improvements in quality of life, exercise capacity, cognitive function, and sexual function.

Epoetin and Darbepoetin

The KDOQI anemia guidelines 2007 recommend individualizing the risks and benefits of ESA therapy. The goal is to avoid transfusion and for a hemoglobin target of 11.0 to 12.0 g/dL and should not be above 13.0 g/dL.

Recombinant EPO (epoetin, Epogen, Procrit) is indicated for the treatment of anemia due to chronic renal failure, zidovudine administration (in HIV-infected patients), and chemotherapy administration. Other indications include a reduction in blood transfusions in anemic patients undergoing elective, noncardiac, nonvascular surgery. Similarly, darbepoetin is indicated for patients with chronic renal failure and patients receiving chemotherapy. Recombinant EPO is indicated in chronic renal failure to elevate the hemoglobin when the hemoglobin is less than 10.0 g/dL and to decrease the need for transfusion. Epogen should be avoided for a hemoglobin greater than 12.0 g/dL.

Mechanism of Action

Epoetin and darbepoetin are recombinant hormones that stimulate the production of RBCs from the erythroid tissues in the bone marrow. Epoetin also stimulates the division and differentiation of erythroid progenitors in bone marrow. Darbepoetin is a longer-acting erythropoietic agent than epoetin (serum half-life of 25 vs. 8.5 hours).

Dosage

The starting dose of epoetin is 50 to 100 units/kg given subcutaneously three times a week for a hemoglobin less than 10 g/dL for anemia due to CKD (Epogen, 2005). For patient on dialysis, this should be administered intravenously. Dosing should be individualized and the lowest dose used to reduce the need for transfusion. The dose should be reduced or interrupted for a hemoglobin greater than 10 g/dL or if the hemoglobin rises greater than 1 g/dL in a 2-week period. In the latter case, the dose should be reduced by 25% or more.

The recommended starting dose for darbepoetin is 0.45 mcg/kg body weight, administered as a single IV or subcutaneous injection once weekly (Aranesp, 2013). Dosing is the same whether it is given subcutaneously or intravenously. Treat to a target hemoglobin concentration of 10 to 11 g/dL. After initiating therapy, the hemoglobin level should be monitored weekly for at least 4 weeks until the hemoglobin value has stabilized.

All patients receiving erythropoietic stimulation should receive iron supplementation unless iron stores are already in excess. Iron supplementation should be initiated no later than the beginning of treatment and continue throughout the course of therapy. Oral therapy with ferrous sulfate 325 mg once to three times daily is adequate. Monitor the patient's hematocrit, ferritin, transferrin, vitamin B_{12} and folate levels, blood pressure, clotting times, platelet counts, blood urea nitrogen level, and serum creatinine concentration.

Time Frame for Response

Two to 6 weeks may be required to evaluate the effectiveness of epoetin. If the response is not satisfactory in terms of reduced transfusion requirements or increased hematocrit after 8 weeks of therapy, the dose may be increased up to 300 units/kg three times a week. If patients do not respond, it is unlikely that they will respond to higher doses. Maintenance doses are individualized for each patient.

With once-weekly dosing, steady-state serum levels are achieved within 4 weeks with darbepoetin. Dose adjustment should not be increased more frequently than once a month. If the hemoglobin is increasing and approaching 11 g/dL, the dose should be reduced by 25%. If the hemoglobin continues to increase, the dose is withheld temporarily until the hemoglobin begins to stabilize.

Contraindications

Epoetin and darbepoetin are contraindicated in patients with uncontrolled hypertension or hypersensitivity to mammalian cell–derived products or human albumin. In 2011, the Food and Drug Administration (FDA) revised the labeling of ESA warning that the risks may outweigh the benefits in patient who have current malignancy and had previous stoke. The KDIGO 2012 guidelines agree about using caution when using ESA. ESA is not intended for patients with chronic renal failure who require correction of severe anemia or in patients with iron folate deficiencies or GI bleeding.

Adverse Events

Epoetin and darbepoetin are generally well tolerated. Adverse reactions may include hypertension, headache, seizure, arthralgia, nausea, edema, fatigue, diarrhea, vomiting, chest pain, asthenia, and dizziness. Other adverse reactions include infection, hypertension, hypotension, and myalgia. Serious adverse reactions include vascular access thrombosis, heart failure, sepsis, and cardiac arrhythmia. There are no significant drug interactions.

ANEMIA OF CHRONIC DISEASE

Anemia of chronic disease is a hypoproliferative anemia and is associated with infection, organ failure, trauma, inflammation, and neoplasia (**Box 51.3**).

Pathophysiology

Anemia of chronic disease typically occurs despite adequate reticuloendothelial iron stores and is characterized by reduced concentrations of serum iron, transferrin, and TIBC; normal or raised ferritin levels; and high erythrocyte sedimentation rate. RBCs are often normochromic and normocytic. In patients with rheumatoid arthritis and Crohn disease, RBCs are similar to the effects of iron deficiency, with hypochromic and microcytic indices.

Diagnostic Criteria

In anemia of chronic disease, the hematocrit rarely falls below 60% of baseline. The MCV is usually normal or slightly reduced. Serum iron values may be unmeasurable, and transferrin saturation may be extremely low. Serum ferritin

---

BOX 51.3 | **Causes of Anemia of Chronic Disease**

Common Causes

Chronic infections
    Tuberculosis
    Subacute bacterial endocarditis
    Osteomyelitis
Chronic inflammation
    Rheumatoid arthritis and inflammatory osteoarthritis
    Systemic lupus erythematosus
    Collagen vascular diseases
    Gout
Malignancies

Less Common Causes

Alcoholic liver disease
Heart failure
Thrombophlebitis
Chronic obstructive lung disease
Ischemic heart disease

---

values should be normal or increased. A serum ferritin value lower than 300 ng/L suggests coexistent iron deficiency.

Initiating Drug Therapy

Treatment is directed at the underlying cause and at eliminating exacerbating factors such as nutritional deficiencies and marrow-suppressive drugs. Other causes of anemia should be treated before initiating therapy.

Doses of recombinant epoetin are higher than those in renal anemia. Epoetin is administered subcutaneously, and doses may vary from 150 to 1,500 units/kg/wk.

Goals of Drug Therapy

A good response is likely if, after 2 weeks of therapy, the hemoglobin increases more than 0.5 g/dL. If no response has been observed at 900 units/kg/wk, further escalation is unlikely to be effective. Iron supplements are required to ensure an adequate epoetin response.

THALASSEMIA

The thalassemias are hereditary disorders of hemoglobin synthesis, which are considered among the hypoproliferative anemias. The α-thalassemia syndromes are seen primarily in persons from India and China and are less commonly seen in African Americans. The β-thalassemia syndrome affects primarily persons of Mediterranean origin (Italian, Greek). Every year, more than 200,000 babies are born with thalassemia major. They have a life expectancy of less than 30 years and are dependent on blood transfusions. Repeated transfusions result in cirrhosis of the liver, cardiomyopathy, endocrinopathies, and death due to hemosiderosis (Savulescu, 2004).

Pathophysiology

Normal adult hemoglobin is primarily hemoglobin A. Hemoglobin A consists of equal quantities of α- and β-globin chains. Thalassemia is present when a hemoglobinopathy is associated with a decreased production of either the α- or β-globins or a structurally abnormal globin chain. In α-thalassemia, the production of α-globin chains is controlled by four genes. Mutation of all four genes is incompatible with life (hydrops fetalis). Mutation of only one of the four is considered a silent carrier. Mutations of two of the four genes result in both microcytosis and mild anemia. Mutations of three of the four genes allow excess β-chains to form tetramers (hemoglobin H) and result in severe anemia in addition to microcytosis. Physical examination will reveal pallor and splenomegaly. β-Thalassemia is commonly classified by the severity of anemia; many genotypes exist for each phenotype. In β-thalassemia, β-globin chain is controlled by two genes. Mutations of one of two genes results in β-thalassemia trait (β-thalassemia minor). Thalassemia intermedia is associated with dysfunction of both β-globin genes. Clinical severity is intermediate (hemoglobin level of 7 to 10 g/dL), and patients are usually not dependent on transfusions. Thalassemia major (Cooley anemia) results from mutations of both genes and reveals a majority of hemoglobin F, which results in severe anemia, and RBC transfusions are required to sustain life. Clinical problems include growth failure, bony deformities (abnormal facial structure, pathologic fractures), hepatosplenomegaly, jaundice, leg ulcers, and cholelithiasis. As a result of transfusion dependency, iron overload results because of the body's inability to excrete iron from the transfused RBCs. This results in hemochromatosis, heart failure, cirrhosis, and endocrinopathies typically after more than 100 units.

Diagnostic Criteria

α-Thalassemia Trait

Patients with mild anemia have a hematocrit between 28% and 40%. The MCV is low despite modest anemia, and the RBC bound is normal or increased. Peripheral blood smear shows microcytic, hypochromia, target cell and acanthocytes (cell with irregularly spaced bulbous projections). The reticulocyte and iron parameters are normal.

Hemoglobin H

Patients have marked hemolytic anemia with a hematocrit between 22% and 32%. The MCV is low. The peripheral blood smear reveals hypochromia, microcytosis, target cells, and poikilocytosis. The reticulocyte count is elevated. A peripheral blood smear demonstrates the presence of hemoglobin.

β-Thalassemia Minor

Patients have modest anemia with a hematocrit between 28% and 40%. The MCV ranges from 50 to 75 fL, and the RBC count is normal or increased. The peripheral blood smear reveals hypochromia, microcytosis, and target cells, and basophilic stippling may be present. The reticulocyte count is normal or slightly elevated.

β-Thalassemia Major

Patients have severe anemia, and the hematocrit may fall to less than 10%. The peripheral blood smear is bizarre, revealing severe poikilocytosis, hypochromia, microcytosis, target cells, basophilic stippling, and nucleated RBCs.

Initiating Drug Therapy

Patients with mild thalassemia (α-thalassemia trait or β-thalassemia minor) require no treatment. Patients should be identified so that they will not be subjected to repeated evaluation and treatment for iron deficiency. Patients with hemoglobin H should take folate supplements and avoid iron and oxidative drugs such as sulfonamides. Patients with severe thalassemia are maintained on a regular transfusion schedule and receive folate supplementation. Iron chelation therapy with deferoxamine mesylate may be used when transfusions result in tissue iron overload. Deferoxamine is administered by continuous subcutaneous infusion for 10 to 24 hours/day. Adverse reactions include local irritation at the injection site, pruritus, hypotension, tachycardia, abdominal discomfort, diarrhea, nausea, and vomiting. Ocular and auditory disturbances may occur, and patients should have baseline and annual vision and hearing examinations.

VITAMIN B₁₂ DEFICIENCY

Vitamin B_{12} (cyanocobalamin) deficiency, or pernicious anemia, is a disorder of impaired DNA synthesis. Vitamin B_{12} deficiency is considered a macrocytic anemia and may arise because of genetic or acquired abnormalities. Special populations, such as older adults, alcoholics, patients with malnutrition, strict vegans, and patient who had weight loss surgery, namely, Roux-en-Y anastomosis, are at high risk for developing vitamin B_{12} deficiency. Vitamin B_{12} is essential in maintaining the integrity of the neurologic system.

Pathophysiology

Vitamin B_{12} deficiency has several causes, including lack of intrinsic factor, inadequate intake, decreased absorption, and inadequate utilization. Other causes include fish tapeworm infestation, *H. pylori* infection, malignancy, pancreatitis, gluten enteropathy, sprue, and small bowel bacterial overgrowth (**Box 51.4**). More recently, the increased incidence of obesity and the option of gastric bypass surgery raise greater concerns about vitamin B_{12} deficiency. Vitamin B_{12} is water soluble and obtained by ingestion of fish, meat (beef, pork, organ meat), and dairy products. Its absorption occurs in the terminal ileum and requires intrinsic factor (found in gastric mucosa) for transport across the intestinal mucosa. Ileal absorptive sites may be congenitally absent or destroyed by inflammation or surgical resection. Other causes of decreased absorption include

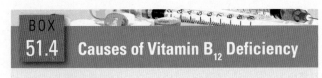

BOX
51.4   **Causes of Vitamin B₁₂ Deficiency**

Dietary deficiency
Decreased production of intrinsic factor
    Pernicious anemia
    Gastrectomy
Helicobacter pylori infection
Fish tapeworm
Pancreatic insufficiency
Surgical resection of ileum
Crohn disease

chronic pancreatitis, malabsorption syndromes, and drugs (oral calcium-chelating drugs, aminosalicylic acid, and biguanides).

Vitamin B₁₂ deficiency can present with gastric mucosal atrophy, neuropsychiatric abnormalities (paranoia, delirium, confusion, irritability, dementia), and yellow-blue color blindness. GI manifestations include anorexia, intermittent constipation and diarrhea, and poorly localized abdominal pain. An early symptom may be glossitis or weight loss. In the early stages, neurologic symptoms include peripheral loss of position and vibratory sensation in the extremities, weakness, and loss of reflexes. Later stages include spasticity, Babinski responses, and ataxia. Early diagnosis is important because neurologic defects, if left untreated, are irreversible.

Diagnostic Criteria

Serum vitamin B₁₂ assay is the most commonly used method for establishing B₁₂ deficiency. There is variability between laboratories as to what is a low normal vitamin B₁₂ level. This ranges from 150 to 200 pg/mL. Serum concentrations of homocysteine as well as serum and urinary concentrations of methylmalonic acid can aid in the detection of vitamin B₁₂ deficiency. These levels are elevated in vitamin B₁₂ deficiency due to a decreased metabolism rate. In patients with an intrinsic factor deficiency, the Schilling test can confirm the diagnosis.

Initiating Drug Therapy

Pernicious anemia, malabsorption syndromes, weight loss surgery, or surgical removal of the stomach causes absence of intrinsic factor. Therefore, dietary vitamin B₁₂ cannot be absorbed. In this case, therapy consists of parenteral administration of vitamin B₁₂. In the case of inadequate intake, dietary allowance and supplementation can be recommended.

Goals of Drug Therapy

Clinical improvement is evidenced by increased alertness, appetite, and cooperation. Reticulocytosis occurs within 2 to 3 days and peaks within 5 to 8 days. The hematocrit begins to rise within 2 weeks and reaches normal values within 2 months.

The MCV will increase initially due to increased reticulocytes and then will gradually decrease to normal.

Vitamin B₁₂ (Cyanocobalamin)

Pernicious anemia is typically treated with parenteral (i.e., intramuscular or deep subcutaneous) cyanocobalamin in a dose of 1,000 mcg (1,000 mcg, 1 mg) every day for 1 week followed by 1 mg every week for 4 weeks. Then, if the underlying disorder persists (e.g., pernicious anemia, surgical removal of the terminal ileum), 1 mg is administered every month for the remainder of the patient's life.

Oral vitamin B₁₂ therapy is not usually recommended for pernicious anemia because of insufficient absorption due to lack of intrinsic factor.

For dietary insufficiency, the recommended daily doses of vitamin B₁₂ are 0.4 mcg for patients ages 0 to 6 months; 0.5 mcg, ages 7 to 12 months; 0.9 mcg, ages 1 to 3; 1.2 mcg, ages 4 to 8; 1.8 mcg, ages 9 to 13; 2.4 mcg, ages 14 and older; 2.6 mcg in pregnant patients; and 2.8 mcg in breast-feeding women.

FOLATE DEFICIENCY

Pathophysiology

Folic acid is necessary for the production of nucleic proteins, amino acids, purines, and thymine. Humans are unable to synthesize total daily folate requirements and depend on a dietary source. Major sources of folate include fresh vegetables and fruits, yeast, mushrooms, and animal organs such as liver and kidney. The minimum daily requirement is 50 to 100 mcg. Folic acid deficiency results in the development of large functionally immature erythrocytes (megaloblasts). Major causes of folic acid deficiency include inadequate intake, inadequate absorption, inadequate utilization, increased requirement (pregnancy, lactation, infancy, malignancy, increased metabolism), and increased excretion (renal dialysis; **Box 51.5**). Folic acid deficiency is associated with poor eating habits as seen in the elderly, alcoholics, food faddists, and those who are

BOX
51.5   **Causes of Folate Deficiency**

Dietary deficiency
Decreased absorption due to
    Phenytoin
    Sulfasalazine
Trimethoprim–sulfamethoxazole
Increased requirements
    Chronic hemolytic anemia
    Pregnancy
    Exfoliative skin disease

chronically ill. It is also seen in patients with malabsorption syndromes, Crohn disease, and celiac disease. Several drugs reported to cause folic acid deficiency include co-trimoxazole, primidone, phenytoin, and phenobarbital.

Symptoms associated with folate deficiency are similar to those in patients with vitamin B_{12} deficiency. Symptoms include weakness, fatigue, difficulty concentrating, irritability headache, shortness of breath, and palpitations. However, the major difference is the absence of neurologic manifestations.

Diagnostic Criteria

Laboratory assessment of folate status includes a serum folic acid level. Serum folic acid levels less than 4 ng/mL suggest deficiency. A low RBC folate level identifies tissue deficiency; however, the values depend on the laboratory method used. Serum homocysteine measurement provides the best evidence of tissue deficiency. Both methylmalonic acid and homocysteine must be measured because B_{12} uses the same pathway. A normal methylmalonic acid level with an elevated homocysteine level confirms the diagnosis of folate deficiency.

Initiating Drug Therapy

A serum folate level less than 4 ng/mL indicates deficiency. Folic acid 1 mg daily is started to replenish the vitamin deficiency. A serum folate level can be followed to evaluate adequate folate stores.

Goals of Drug Therapy

The evaluation of symptomatic improvement is the same as those with vitamin B_{12} deficiency.

Folate Replacement

Folic acid is present in most fruits and vegetables (citrus fruits and green leafy vegetables). The recommended dietary allowances for adult men are 0.15 to 0.2 mg and for women, 0.15 to 0.18 mg. Total body stores are approximately 5 mg and supply requirements for up to 2 to 3 months. Folate deficiency is treated by oral replacement therapy. The usual dose of folate is 1 mg daily. Higher doses up to 5 mg daily may be required for folate deficiency due to malabsorption. The duration of therapy depends on the cause of deficiency. Patients with hemolytic anemia or those with malabsorption or chronic malnutrition should receive oral folic acid indefinitely. Side effects include erythema, skin rash, nausea, abdominal distention, altered sleep patterns, irritability, mental depression, confusion, and impaired judgment.

APLASTIC ANEMIA

Aplastic anemia is a condition of bone marrow failure that can be hereditary or arise from injury to or abnormal expression of the stem cell. Aplastic anemia is defined as pancytopenia

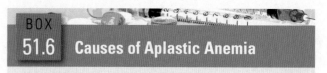

BOX 51.6 Causes of Aplastic Anemia

Congenital
Idiopathic/autoimmune
Systemic lupus erythematosus
Chemotherapy
Radiation therapy
Toxins
    Benzene, toluene, insecticides
Heavy metals
    Gold, arsenic, bismuth, mercury
Drugs
Pregnancy

with a hypocellular bone marrow in the absence of an abnormal infiltrate and with no increase in reticulin (Marsh et al., 2009). There are several causes of aplastic anemia (**Box 51.6**). One cause is direct stem cell injury from radiation, chemotherapy (alkylating agents), antimetabolites, antimitotics, toxins (benzenes), or pharmacologic agents (**Box 51.7**).

BOX 51.7 Drugs Associated with Aplastic Anemia

Antiprotozoals (quinacrine and chloroquine, mepacrine)
NSAIDs (phenylbutazone, indomethacin, ibuprofen, sulindac, aspirin)
Anticonvulsants (hydantoins, carbamazepine, phenacemide, felbamate)
Sulfonamides
    Antithyroid drugs (methimazole, methylthiouracil, propylthiouracil)
    Antidiabetic drugs (tolbutamide, chlorpropamide)
    Carbonic anhydrase inhibitors (acetazolamide, methazolamide)
Antihistamines (cimetidine, chlorpheniramine)
D-penicillamine
Estrogens
Sedatives and tranquilizers (chlorpromazine, prochlorperazine, piperacetazine, chlordiazepoxide, meprobamate, methyprylon)
Allopurinol
Methyldopa
Quinidine
Lithium
Guanidine
Potassium perchlorate
Thiocyanate
Carbimazole

Pathophysiology

Erythrocytes, granulocytes, and platelets, which are normally produced in the bone narrow, decrease to dangerously low levels. The bone marrow becomes hypoplastic with replacement of normal marrow hematopoietic cells by fat cells, and pancytopenia develops. This results in bleeding and increased risk of infection. Patients most commonly present with fatigue, dyspnea, weakness, and skin or mucosal hemorrhage or visual disturbance due to retinal hemorrhage. Physical examination may reveal signs of pallor, purpura, and petechiae.

Diagnostic Criteria

A CBC typically shows pancytopenia. In most cases, the hemoglobin level and neutrophil, reticulocyte, and platelet counts are depressed with a preserved lymphocyte count. The bone marrow aspirate and bone marrow biopsy appear hypocellular with scant amounts of normal hematopoietic progenitors. Magnetic resonance imaging of the vertebrae shows uniform replacement of marrow with fat.

Initiating Drug Therapy

Mild cases of aplastic anemia may be treated with supportive care. Foremost, RBC transfusions and platelets are given for bleeding, and antibiotics are given for infections (Marsh et al., 2009). Antifungals are given prophylactically for a low neutrophil count. Treatment for severe acquired aplastic anemia includes hematopoietic stem cell transplantation and immunosuppression therapy. When the cause of aplastic anemia is related to drugs or chemicals, these should be discontinued. Patients presenting with aplastic anemia should be referred to a hematologist/oncologist.

SPECIAL POPULATION CONSIDERATIONS

Pediatric

The American Academy of Pediatrics recommends hemoglobin screening and risk evaluation for iron deficiency anemia in all children at 1 year of age. The Centers for Disease Control and Prevention recommends screening for low-income or newly immigrated families to begin at 9 to 12 months of age and low-birth-weight infants before 6 months of age if they are not fed iron-fortified formula. Iron deficiency anemia significantly impairs mental and psychomotor development in infants and children. Iron deficiency can be reversed with treatment; however, the reversibility of the mental and psychomotor effects is unclear. Furthermore, iron deficiency increases a child's susceptibility to lead toxicity as lead replaces iron in the absorptive pathway when iron is unavailable.

Young children are at greatest risk for iron deficiency anemia due to rapid growth, increased iron requirements, and lack of iron in the diet. Poverty, abuse, and living in a home with poor household conditions also place children at risk for iron deficiency anemia. Iron deficiency anemia is seen most commonly in children ages 6 months to 3 years. Those at highest risk are low-birth-weight infants after age 2 months, breast-fed term infants who receive no iron-fortified food or supplemental iron after age 4 months, and formula-fed term infants who are not consuming iron-fortified formula. During the first months of life, the newborn rapidly uses iron stores due to an accelerated growth rate and increased blood volume. Maternally derived iron stores are generally sufficient for the first 4 to 6 months; however, sustained growth demands an increased iron supply. By the end of the second year of life, the growth rate decreases and accompanying iron needs level off. During adolescence, growth accelerates and iron needs increase. Adolescent girls are at increased risk and need additional iron to compensate for menstrual loss. Patients with iron deficiency who are responding poorly to the usual dietary supplementation regimens should be screened for lead poisoning. Heavy metal poisoning, as with lead and bismuth, is often overlooked.

Geriatric

Anemia should not be accepted as an inevitable consequence of aging. Mild anemia, less than 10 g/dL as defined by the WHO criteria, is associated with significant negative outcomes including decreased physical performance, increased number of falls, increased frailty, decreased cognition, increased dementia, increased hospitalization, and increased mortality.

Anemia in the elderly is a risk factor of adverse outcomes including hospitalization, morbidity, and mortality. The prevalence of anemia increases after 50 years of age and exceeds 20% of those 85 years and older (Goodnough & Schrier, 2014). There is no specific recommended hemoglobin threshold, but it is prudent to maintain hemoglobin level of 9 to 10 g/dL unless otherwise indicated. The most common causes of anemia in elderly patients are chronic disease (CKD, infections, malignancies, and inflammatory disorders), iron deficiency, and nutritional and metabolic disorders. Anemia resulting from blood loss due to surgery, injury, and GI and genitourinary bleeding is more common in hospitalized patients.

Women

Pregnant women and women who are 4- to 6-week postpartum are at risk for asymptomatic iron deficiency anemia. As such, the American Academy of Family Physician, U.S. Preventative Services Task Force, and the Centers for Disease Control and Prevention recommend routine screening. Pregnant women who are iron deficient are at increased risk for a preterm delivery and delivering a low-birth-weight baby. Two to three times more iron is required in pregnancy and in childhood. In pregnant women who had a previous pregnancy with a fetus or infant with a neural tube defect, the recommended dose of folate is 5 mg daily. Also, women who may become pregnant and have seizure disorders should take folate supplementation.

MONITORING PATIENT RESPONSE

In almost all cases of anemia, evaluation should proceed in an orderly manner and therapy withheld until a specific diagnosis can be made. Patients with significant cardiopulmonary disease, who may be compromised by a decreased oxygen capacity, require immediate correction of anemia. This may require inpatient evaluation and consideration of transfusion therapy when they are experiencing dyspnea, angina, or marked fatigue related to anemia. Once treatment has been initiated, patient response should be evaluated on at least a monthly basis. Correction of anemia decreases morbidity and reduces hospitalization and mortality among patients with CKD. Benefits of correcting anemia include improvements in the patient's quality of life, exercise capacity, cognitive function, and sexual function.

PATIENT EDUCATION

Patients need to be told to what extent the anemia accounts for symptoms, what the possible causes are, and what the appropriate workup will be. Patient education and the importance of adherence to therapy are integral to successful management. Because some cases of anemia require the need for medication, the patient needs to be informed about possible side effects and when to report dangerous side effects.

Nutrition

All patients are encouraged to limit the use of alcohol, to avoid tobacco, to exercise, and to consume a diet of meat, poultry, fish, and fresh fruits and vegetables. To prevent deficiency, all patients are encouraged to eat fortified foods (fortified cereals, dairy products) or take supplements as prescribed by their physician. Patients with specific problems, such as pica, may need additional counseling.

Complementary and Alternative Medications

Herbal medicine to supply iron, iodine, and calcium include yellow dock root, Irish moss, and horsetail in equal parts made into a tea. Other herbal medicines for the treatment of iron deficiency include burdock, devil's bit, meadow sweet, mullein leaves, restharrow, salep, silver weed, stinging nettle, strawberry leaves, and toad flax. Patients should be educated that herbs are not regulated by the U.S. FDA and may interact with prescription medications. Patients must also understand that they should report any adverse reactions and stop the herbal medication immediately.

CASE STUDY*

M.W. is a 69-year-old African American man and was referred to clinic for evaluation of increasing shortness of breath.

Past medical history
    Chronic renal insufficiency
    Hypertension
    Congestive heart failure
    Diabetes mellitus type 2, poor control
    Deep vein thrombosis
    Alcohol abuse
    Chronic obstructive pulmonary disease with respiratory failure
Family history
    Noncontributory
Physical examination
    Height 69 inches, weight 205 lb
    Blood pressure: 138/88
    Pulse 86 beats/min, regular
    Lungs clear, neck supple negative for jugular venous distention
    Lower extremities +1 edema
Laboratory findings
    Scr = 2.8 K$^+$ = 5.1
    BUN = 56 Na$^+$ = 147

WBC = 5.0 Hb = 8.2
Hct = 24.6
Serum ferritin 189 mg/dL
Social history
    Tobacco: 52 pack-years
    Alcohol: distant past

DIAGNOSIS: ANEMIA OF CKD

1. List specific goals of treatment for **M.W.**
2. What drug therapy would you prescribed? Why?
3. What are the parameters for monitoring success of therapy?
4. Discuss specific patient education based on the prescribed therapy.
5. List one or two adverse reactions for the selected agent that would cause you to change therapy.
6. What would be the choice for second-line therapy?
7. What over-the-counter and/or alternative medications would be appropriate for **M.W.**?
8. What dietary and lifestyle changes would you recommended for **M.W.**?
9. Describe one or two drug–drug or drug–food interactions for the selected agent.

* Answers can be found online.

Bibliography

Starred references are cited in the text.

Abramson, J., Jurkovitz, C., Vaccarino, V., et al. (2003). Chronic kidney disease, anemia, and incident stroke in a middle-aged, community-based population: The ARIC study. *Kidney International, 64*, 610–615.

*Adamson, J. (2012). Iron deficiency and other hypoproliferative anemias. In D. Longo, A. Fauci, D. Kasper, et al., (Eds.), *Harrison's principles of internal medicine* (pp. 448–457). New York, NY: McGraw-Hill.

Aigner, E., Feldman, A., & Datz, C. (2014). Obesity as an emerging risk factor for iron deficiency. *Nutrients, 6*, 3587–3600.

Alleyne, M., Horne, M., & Miller, J. (2008). Individualized treatment for iron-deficiency anemia in adults. *The American Journal of Medicine, 121*, 943–948.

Amgen. (2005). *Epogen package insert*. Thousand Oaks, CA: Amgen.

Amgen. (2013). *ARANESP (darbepoetin alfa) package insert*. Thousand Oaks, CA: Amgen.

Andrews, N. (2008). Forging a field: The golden age of iron biology. *Blood, 112*, 219–230.

Angerio, A., & Lee, N. (2003). Sickle cell crisis and endothelin antagonists. *Critical Care Nursing Quarterly, 26*, 225–229.

Bacigalupo, A. (2008). Treatment strategies for patients with severe aplastic anemia. *Bone Marrow Transplantation, 42*, S42–S44.

*Ballas, S. (2005). Pain management of sickle cell disease. *Hematology/Oncology Clinics of North America, 19*, 785–802.

Benoist, B., McLean, E., Egli, I., et al. (2008). *Worldwide prevalence of anaemia 1993–2005*. WHO global database on anaemia. Geneva, Switzerland: World Health Organization.

*Bernaudin, F., Souillet, G., Vannier J., et al. (1997). Report of the French experience concerning 26 children transplanted for severe sickle cell disease. *Bone Marrow Transplantation, 19*, S112–S115.

Borgna-Pignatti, C. (2009). Modern treatment of thalassaemia intermedia. *British Journal of Haematology, 138*, 291–304.

Brawley, O., Cornelius, L., Edwards, L., et al. (2008). National Institutes of Health Consensus Development Conference statement: Hydroxyurea treatment for sickle cell disease. *Annals of Internal Medicine, 148*, 932–938.

Butler, C., Vidal-Alaball, J., Cannings-John, R., et al. (2006). Oral vitamin B_{12} versus intramuscular vitamin B_{12} for vitamin B_{12} deficiency: A systematic review of randomized controlled trails. *Family Practice, 23*, 279–285.

Camaschella, C. (2015). Iron-deficiency anemia. *New England Journal of Medicine, 372*, 1832–1843.

Cao, A., & Galanello, R. (2002). Effect of consanguinity on screening for thalassemia. *New England Journal of Medicine, 347*, 1200–1202.

*Centers for Disease Control and Prevention. (2012). *National health and nutrition examination survey*. Retrieved from http://www.cdc.gov/nchs/nhanes/nhanesii.htm

Cravens, D., Nasheisky, J., Oh, R. (2007). Clinical inquiries. How do we evaluate a marginally low B12 level? *Journal of Family Practice, 56*, 62–63.

*Goodnough, L., & Schrier, S. (2014). Evaluation and management of anemia in the elderly. *American Journal of Hematology, 89*, 88–96.

Guidi, G., & Santonastaso, C. (2010). Advancements in anemias related to chronic conditions. *Clinical Chemistry & Laboratory Medicine, 48*, 1217–1226.

Gurusamy, K., Nagendran, M., Broadhurst, J., et al. (2014). Iron therapy in anaemic adults without chronic kidney disease. *Cochrane Database System Review. 12*, 1–132.

Inker, L., Astor, B., Fox, C., et al. (2014). KDOQI US commentary on the 2012 KDIGO clinical practice guideline for the evaluation and management of CKD. *American Journal of Kidney Disease, 63*, 713–735.

Killip, S., Bennett, J., & Chambers, M. (2007). Iron deficiency anemia. *American Family Physician, 75*, 671–678.

*Kliger, A., Foley, R., Goldfarb, D. S., et al. (2013). KDOQI US commentary on the 2012 KDIGO clinical practice guideline for anemia in CKD. *American Journal of Kidney Disease, 62*(5), 849–859.

Lanzkron, S., Strouse, J., Wilson, R., et al. (2008). Systematic review: Hydroxyurea for the treatment of adults with sickle cell disease. *Annals of Internal Medicine, 12*, 939–950.

Liu, K., & Kaffes, A. (2011). Iron deficiency anaemia: A review of diagnosis, investigation and management. *European Journal of Gastroenterology & Hepatology, 24*, 109–116

*Marsh, J., Ball, S., Cavenagh, J., et al. (2009). Guidelines for the diagnosis and management of aplastic anaemia. *British Journal of Haematology, 147*, 43–70.

Miller, H., Hu, J., Valentine, J., et al. (2010). Efficacy and tolerability of intravenous ferric gluconate in the treatment of iron deficiency anemia in patients without kidney disease. *Archives of Internal Medicine, 167*, 1327–1328.

*National Kidney Foundation. (2007). *KDOQI clinical practice guideline and clinical practice recommendations for anemia in chronic kidney disease: 2007 update of hemoglobin target*. Retrieved from http://www2.kidney.org/professionals/KDOQI/guidelines_anemiaUP/guide1.htm

Poskitt, E. (2003). Early history of iron deficiency. *British Journal of Haematology, 122*, 504–562.

Robinson, A., & Mladenovic, J. (2001). Lack of clinical utility of folate levels in the evaluation of macrocytosis or anemia. *American Journal of Medicine, 110*, 88–90.

*Savulescu, J. (2004). Thalassaemia major: The murky story of deferiprone. *British Medical Journal, 328*, 358–359.

Short, M., & Domagalski, J. (2013). Iron deficiency anemia: Evaluation and management. *American Family Physician, 87*, 98–104.

Tefferi, A. (2003). Anemia in adults: A contemporary approach to diagnosis. *Mayo Clinic Proceedings, 78*, 1274–1280.

*U.S. Department of Health and Human Services. National Heart, Lung, and Blood Institute. (2014). *Evidence-based management of sickle cell disease*. Retrieved from http://www.nhlbi.nih.gov/health-pro/guidelines/sickle-cell-disease-guidelines

U.S. Renal Data System. (2001). *USRDS 2001 annual data report*. Bethesda, MD: National Institute of Diabetes and Digestive and Kidney Diseases, National Institutes of Health.

Vajpayee, N., Graham, S., & Bem, S. (2011). Basic examination of blood and bone marrow. In R. A. McPherson & M. R. Pincus (Eds.), *Henry's clinical diagnosis and management by laboratory methods* (22nd ed.). Philadelphia, PA: Elsevier/Saunders.

*Wong, T., Brandow, A., Lim, W., et al. (2014). Update on the use of hydroxyurea therapy in sickle cell disease. *Blood, 24*, 3850–3857.

Yawn, B., Buchana, G., Afenyi-Annan, A., et al. (2014). Management of sickle cell disease. Summary of the 2014 evidence-based report by expert panel members. *Journal of American Medical Association, 312*, 1033–1048.

Yen, P. (2000). Nutritional anemia. *Geriatric Nursing, 21*, 111–112.

Young, N. (2002). Acquired aplastic anemia. *Annals of Internal Medicine, 136*, 534–546.

Pharmacotherapy in Health Promotion

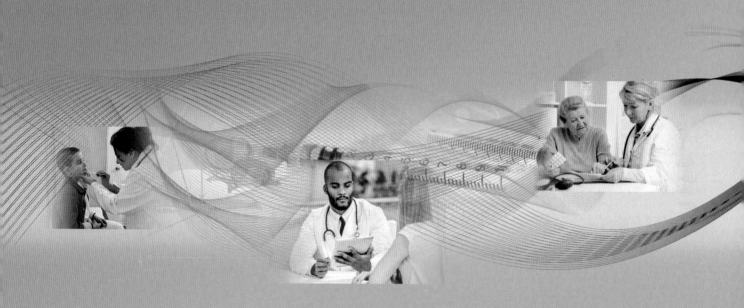

52 Immunizations

Jean M. Scholtz

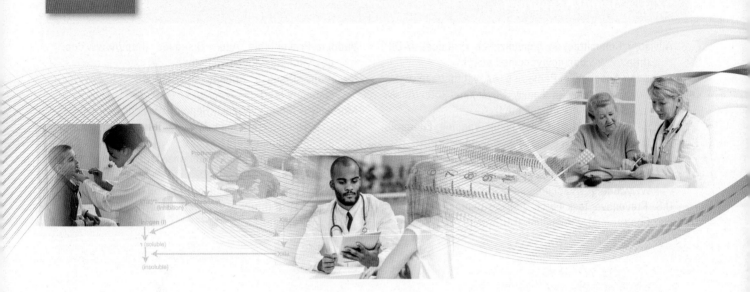

The use of immunizations is described as one of the 10 greatest public health achievements. Immunization rates in the United States are at their highest, with more than 90% of children 3 years of age receiving all required vaccines (Hill et al., 2015). As a result, cases of diphtheria, polio, rubella, mumps, measles, and *Haemophilus influenzae* type B (Hib) are at record low levels. Immunization prophylaxis is important for all age groups—infants through older adults. Unfortunately, immunization rates in adolescents and adults are not as high as those in preschool age children. Immunization rates in persons 18 to 64 years of age against influenza and pneumococcus range from 33% to 69%, with pneumonia and influenza the 8th leading cause of death in the United States (Xu et al., 2014). There are even lower immunization rates in the socioeconomically disadvantaged and various ethnicities. In addition, there are individuals who continue to be antivaccinators due to the fear of autism. Practitioners need to develop a system that facilitates review of immunization status at all health care visits so that no opportunity is missed to educate and update immunizations for those who are not adequately vaccinated and thus inadequately protected against preventable diseases.

Immunization prophylaxis offers an opportunity to prevent disease, improve clinical outcomes for those at high risk, and realize significant savings to the person in terms of cost, time, and resources. Healthy People 2020 continues to promote the movement throughout the United States to increase immunization rates and reduce preventable infectious diseases. They continue to have a significant impact on preventing communicable diseases, reducing preventable complications, and improving clinical outcomes. However, because these diseases persist in other countries, immunization prophylaxis needs to be continued. Recommendations for immunization prophylaxis come from multiple sources, and useful resources are listed in **Box 52.1**. The CDC is responsible for providing vaccine management, technical assistance, information, epidemiology, and assessment. In February of each year, the immunization schedule is reviewed and revised as indicated.

CHARACTERISTICS OF IMMUNIZATIONS

Many infectious diseases can be prevented by immunoprophylaxis, which is accomplished either through active or passive immunization. Active immunization involves giving a person either live or attenuated (live but killed; inactivated) vaccine to stimulate the development of immune system defenses against future natural exposure.

Active immunization involves administration of all or part of a microorganism or a modified product of that microorganism (e.g., toxoid, a purified antigen, or an antigen produced by genetic engineering) to evoke an immune response that mimics the response of the body to natural infection but that usually presents little or no risk to the recipient. Protection may be afforded for a limited time or for a lifetime. If protection is for a limited time, the vaccine must be readministered at specified intervals.

Passive immunization is used for those people who have already been exposed or who have the potential to be exposed to certain infectious agents. Passive immunization involves the administration of a preformed antibody when the recipient has a congenitally acquired defect or immunodeficiency, when exposure is likely to result in high-risk complications, or when time does not permit adequate protection by active immunization (e.g., immunizations against rabies or hepatitis B). In addition, passive immunity can be used therapeutically during active disease states to help suppress the effects of a toxin or the inflammatory response.

BOX 52.1 Useful Resources

Advisory Committee on Immunization Practices (ACIP) (http://www.cdc.gov/vaccines/acip/)

American Academy of Pediatrics (AAP) (http://aap.org)

American Academy of Family Physicians (http://www.aafp.org/online/en/home.html)

Children's Hospital of Philadelphia Vaccine Education Center (http://www.vaccine.chop.edu)

Epidemiology and prevention of Vaccine-Preventable Diseases—The Pink Book 13th Edition (2015) (http://www.cdc.gov/vaccines/pubs/pinkbook/index.html)

U.S. Preventive Task Force and the Centers for Disease Control and Prevention (CDC) (http://www.cdc.gov/vaccines/)

Vaccine-Preventable Adult Diseases (http://www.cdc.gov/vaccines/adults/vpd.html)

Infectious Disease Society of America (http://www.idsociety.org/)

Morbidity & Mortality Weekly Report (www.cdc.gov/mmwr)

National Network for Immunization Information (www.immunizationinfo.org)

Directory of Immunization Coalitions (http://www.izcoalitions.org/)

The Yellow Book: CDC Health Information for International Travel 2016 (http://wwwnc.cdc.gov/travel/page/yellowbook-home)

BOX 52.2 Vaccines Licensed in the United States

Adenovirus type 4 and type 7

Anthrax

BCG

Diphtheria and tetanus toxoid adsorbed

Diphtheria and tetanus toxoids and acellular pertussis vaccine adsorbed

Diphtheria and tetanus toxoids and acellular pertussis vaccine adsorbed and inactivated polio

Diphtheria and tetanus toxoids and acellular pertussis adsorbed, inactivated polio, and *H. influenzae* B conjugate

H. influenzae B conjugate

H. influenzae B conjugate and hepatitis B

Hepatitis A

Hepatitis B

Hepatitis A and hepatitis B

Human papillomavirus quadrivalent (types 6, 11, 16, 18)

Human papillomavirus 9-valent

Human papillomavirus bivalent (types 16, 18)

Influenza A (H1N1)

Influenza (H5N1)

Influenza virus (trivalent, types A and B)

Influenza vaccine (quadrivalent, types A and B, intranasal, live)

Influenza vaccine (quadrivalent, types A and B, injectable)

Japanese encephalitis

Measles and mumps (live)

Measles, mumps, and rubella (live)

Measles, mumps, rubella, and varicella (live)

Meningococcal (groups A, C, Y, and W-135) oligosaccharide diphtheria CRM197 conjugate

Meningococcal polysaccharide (serogroups A, C, Y, and W-135) diphtheria toxoid conjugate

Meningococcal polysaccharide groups A, C, Y, and W-135 combined

Meningococcal (groups C and Y) and *Haemophilus* b tetanus toxoid conjugate and W-135

Meningococcal (groups A, C, Y, and W-135) polysaccharide diphtheria toxoid conjugate

Meningococcal group B

Plague

Pneumococcal polyvalent

Pneumococcal 7-valent conjugate

Pneumococcal 13-valent conjugate

Poliovirus, inactivated

Rabies

Rotavirus (live, oral)

Rotavirus pentavalent (live)

Smallpox (live)

Tetanus and diphtheria toxoids adsorbed for adults

Tetanus toxoid adsorbed

Tetanus toxoid, reduced diphtheria toxoid, and acellular pertussis, adsorbed

Typhoid (live, oral)

Typhoid Vi polysaccharide

Varicella virus (live)

Yellow fever

Zoster (live)

VACCINES

Vaccines are the pharmacologic substances used to provide or boost immunity to disease. The major constituents of vaccines include active immunizing antigens (toxoid, live virus, or killed bacteria), suspending fluid, preservatives, stabilizers, antibiotics, and adjuvants. The differences depend on the manufacturer, and the person prescribing or administering the vaccine should check the package insert for the active and inert ingredients for each product. Potential allergic reactions may result from one or more of the preservatives, stabilizers, adjuvants, or antibiotics in the vaccine, and the recipient's sensitivity to one or more of the additives should be anticipated as a hypersensitivity. Current vaccines licensed in the United States are identified in **Box 52.2**.

The recommended immunization schedule for persons aged 0 through 18 years in the United States is listed in **Figure 52.1**. The schedules have columns added at 4 to 6 years and 11 to 12 years of age to highlight school entry and adolescent age group vaccine recommendations. Footnotes are listed for each vaccine and contain the recommendations for routine vaccination, catch-up, and vaccination to individuals with high-risk conditions or special circumstances. **Figure 52.2** presents the recommended immunizations for persons aged 4 months through 18 years who are behind in immunizations.

Recommendations for hepatitis B; rotavirus (RV1/RV5); diphtheria, tetanus, and pertussis (DTaP); tetanus, diphtheria, and pertussis (Tdap); *H. influenzae* type B (Hib); pneumococcus; poliomyelitis; influenza; measles, mumps, and rubella (MMR); varicella; hepatitis A; human papillomavirus; and meningococcus are included from birth to age 18.

Combination vaccines are available that assist in reducing the number of injections a child must receive at any one time. In addition, recommended acceptable ranges for administration provide some flexibility regarding the number of injections administered at any one time as recommendations for catch-up vaccinations. A consideration for flexible scheduling should include parental or guardian compliance with appointments as well as office follow-up methods used for those patients who do not keep scheduled appointments for immunizations.

Special Circumstances

Preterm infants and children who are immunocompromised, infected with human immunodeficiency virus (HIV), lack a spleen, or have a personal or family history of seizures require special consideration when immunization prophylaxis is reviewed and administered.

These recommendations must be read with the footnotes that follow. For those who fall behind or start late, provide catch-up vaccination at the earliest opportunity as indicated by the green bars in Figure 52.1. To determine minimum intervals between doses, see the catch-up schedule (Figure 52.2). School entry and adolescent vaccine age groups are shaded.

Vaccine	Birth	1 mo	2 mos	4 mos	6 mos	9 mos	12 mos	15 mos	18 mos	19–23 mos	2–3 yrs	4–6 yrs	7–10 yrs	11–12 yrs	13–15 yrs	16–18 yrs
Hepatitis B[1] (HepB)	1st dose	←—2nd dose—→			←——————— 3rd dose ———————→											
Rotavirus[2] (RV) RV1 (2-dose series), RV5 (3-dose series)			1st dose	2nd dose	See footnote 2											
Diphtheria, tetanus & acellular pertussis[1] (DTaP: <7 yrs)			1st dose	2nd dose	3rd dose		←——— 4th dose ———→					5th dose				
Haemophilus influenzae type b[4] (Hib)			1st dose	2nd dose	See footnote 4		3rd or 4th dose See footnote 4									
Pneumococcal conjugate[5] (PCV13)			1st dose	2nd dose	3rd dose		←——— 4th dose ———→									
Inactivated poliovirus[6] (IPV: <18 yrs)			1st dose	2nd dose	←——————— 3th dose ———————→							4th dose				
Influenza[7] [IIV; LAIV]					Annual vaccination (IIV only) 1 or 2 doses							Annual vaccination (LAIV or IIV) 1 or 2 doses		Annual vaccination (LAIV or IIV) 1 dose only		
Measles, mumps, rubella[8] (MMR)					See footnote 8		←— 1st dose —→					2nd dose				
Varicella[9] (VAR)							←— 1st dose —→					2nd dose				
Hepatitis A[10] (HepA)							←——— 2nd dose series See footnote 10 ———→									
Meningococcal[11] Hib-MenCY ≥6 weeks MenACWY-D ≥9 mos; MenACWY-CRM ≥2 mos					See footnote 11									1st dose		Booster
Tetanus, diphtheria & acellular pertussis[12] (Tdap: ≥7 yrs)														(Tdap)		
Human papillomavirus[13] (2vHPV: females only; 4vHPV, 9vHPV males and females)														(3-dose Serials)		
Meningococcal B[11]															See footnote 11	
Pneumococcal polysaccharide[5] (PPSV23)												See footnote 5				

Range of recommended ages for all children	Range of recommended ages for catch-up immunization	Range of recommended ages for certain high-risk groups	Range of recommended ages for non-high-risk groups that may receive vaccine, subject to individual clinical decision making	No recommendation

This schedule indicates recommendations in effect as of January 1, 2016. Any dose not administered at the recommended age should be administered at a subsequent visit, when indicated and feasible. The use of a combination vaccine generally is preferred over separate injections of its equivalent component vaccines. Vaccination providers should consult the relevant Advisory Committee on Immunization Practices (ACIP) statement for detailed recommendations, available online at http://www.cdc.gov/vaccines/hcp/acip-recs/index.html. Clinically significant adverse events that follow vaccination should be reported to the Vaccine Adverse Event Reporting System (VAERS) online (http://www.vaers.hhs.gov) or by telephone (800-822-7967). Suspected cases of vaccine-preventable diseases should be reported to the state or local health department. Additional information, including precautions and contraindications for vaccination, is available from CDC online (http://www.cdc.gov/vaccines/recs/vac.admin/contraindications.html) or by telephone (800-CDC-INFO [800-232-4636]).

This schedule is approved by the Advisory Committee on Immunization Practices (http:www.cdc.gov/vaccines/acip), the American Academy of Pediatrics (http://www.aap.org), the American Academy of Family Physicians (http://www.aafp.org) and the American College of Obstetricians and Gynecologists (http://www.acog.org).

NOTE: The above recommendations must be read along with the footnotes of this schedule.

FIGURE 52.1   Recommended immunization schedule for persons aged 0 through 18 years—United States, 2016 (Centers for Disease Control and Prevention, 2014).

The figure below provides catch-up schedules and minimum intervals between doses for children whose vaccinations have been delayed. A vaccine series does not need to be restarted, regardless of the time that has elapsed between doses. Use the section appropriate for the child's age. Always use this table in conjunction with Figure 52.1 and the footnotes that follow.

Vaccine	Minimum Age for Dose 1	Minimum Interval Between Doses			
		Dose 1 to Dose 2	Dose 2 to Dose 3	Dose 3 to Dose 4	Dose 4 to Dose 5
Children age 4 months through 6 years					
Hepatitis B[1]	Birth	4 weeks	8 weeks *and at least 16 weeks after first dose.* Minimum age for the final dose is 24 weeks.		
Rotavirus[2]	6 weeks	4 weeks	4 weeks[2]		6 months[2]
Diphtheria, tetanus, and acellular pertussis[3]	6 weeks	4 weeks	4 weeks	6 months	6 months[3]
Haemophilus influenzae type b[4]	6 weeks	4 weeks if first dose was administered before the 1st birthday. 8 weeks (as final dose) if first dose was administered at age 12 through 14 months. No further doses needed if first dose was administered at age 15 months or older.	4 weeks[4] if current age is younger than 12 months **and** first dose was administered at younger than age 7 months, **and** at least 1 previous dose was PRP-T (ActHib, Pentacel) or unknown. 8 weeks *and age 12 through 59 months (as final dose)[4]* • if current age is younger than 12 months **and** first dose was administered at age 7 through 11 months (wait until at least 12 months old); OR • if current age is 12 through 59 months **and** first dose was administered before the 1st birthday, and second dose administered at younger than 15 months; OR • if both doses were PRP-OMP (PedvaxHIB; Comvax) **and** were administered before the 1st birthday. (wait until at least 12 months old). No further doses needed if previous dose was administered at age 15 months or older.	8 weeks (as final dose) This dose only necessary for children age 12 through 59 months who received 3 doses before the 1st birthday.	
Pneumococcal[4]	6 weeks	4 weeks if first dose administered before the 1st birthday. 8 weeks (as final dose for healthy children) if first dose was administered at the 1st birthday or after. No further doses needed for healthy children if first dose administered at age 24 months or older.	4 weeks if current age is younger than 12 months and previous dose given at <7months old. 8 weeks (as final dose for healthy children) if previous dose given between 7-11 months (wait until at least 12 months old); OR if current age is 12 months or older and at least 1 dose was given before age 12 months. No further doses needed for healthy children if previous dose administered at age 24 months or older.	8 weeks (as final dose) This dose only necessary for children aged 12 through 59 months who received 3 doses before age 12 months or for children at high risk who received 3 doses at any age.	
Inactivated poliovirus[6]	6 weeks	4 weeks[6]	4 weeks[6]	6 months[6] (minimum age 4 years for final dose).	
Measles, mumps, rubella[8]	12 months	4 weeks			
Varicella[9]	12 months	3 months			
Hepatitis A[10]	12 months	6 months			
Meningococcal[11] (Hib-MenCY ≥ 6 weeks; MenACWY-D ≥ 9 mos; MenACWY-CRM ≥ 2 mos)	6 weeks	8 weeks[11]	See footnote 11	See footnote 11	
Children and adolescents age 7 through 18 years					
Meningococcal[11] (Hib-MenCY ≥ 6 weeks; MenACWY-D ≥ 9 mos; MenACWY-CRM ≥ 2 mos)	Not Applicable (N/A)	8 weeks[11]			
Tetanus, diphtheria, tetanus, diphtheria, and acellular pertussis[12]	7 years[12]	4 weeks	4 weeks if first dose of DTaP/DT was administered before the 1st birthday. 6 months (as final dose) if first dose of DTaP/DT or Tdap/Td was administered at or after the 1st birthday.	6 months if first dose of DTaP/DT was administered before the 1st birthday.	
Human papillomavirus[12]	9 years	Routine dosing intervals are recommended[12]			
Hepatitis A[10]	N/A	6 months			
Hepatitis B[1]	N/A	4 weeks	8 weeks and at least 16 weeks after first dose.		
Inactivated poliovirus[6]	N/A	4 weeks	4 weeks[6]	6 months[6]	
Measles, mumps, rubella[8]	N/A	4 weeks			
Varicella[9]	N/A	3 months if younger than age 13 years. 4 weeks if age 13 years or older.			

NOTE: The above recommendations must be read along with the footnotes of this schedule.

FIGURE 52.2 Catch-up immunization schedule for persons aged 4 months through 18 years who start late or who are more than 1 month behind—United States, 2016.

Preterm Infants

Preterm (<37 weeks' gestation) and low-birth-weight (<2,500 g) infants are at high risk for vaccine-preventable deaths due to an immature immune system and possible decreased maternal antibody levels. Preterm infants born to mothers who are hepatitis B surface antigen (HBsAg) negative should receive their first hepatitis B immunization at 1 month of age or at hospital discharge.

Preterm infants born to mothers who test positive for HBsAg should receive hepatitis B immune globulin within 12 hours of birth and concurrent hepatitis B vaccine (in the appropriate dose per package insert) at a different site. If the maternal HBsAg status is unknown, the vaccine should be given at 1, 2, and 6 months of age. In addition, all preterm infants should receive the influenza vaccine annually in the fall beginning at age 6 months.

Immunosuppressed Children

Children who are immunosuppressed or immunodeficient are at risk for actually contracting the disease or experiencing serious adverse effects from live bacteria or live virus vaccines. Live vaccines are therefore contraindicated. In general, experience with vaccine administration to an immunosuppressed or immunodeficient child is limited. Efficacy is suboptimal because their ability to develop immunogenicity to a specific agent is altered owing to a depressed immune system. Theoretical considerations are the only guide because experiential data are lacking or adverse consequences have not been reported.

Children with a deficiency in antibody-synthesizing capacity cannot respond to vaccines. These children should receive regular doses of immune globulin, usually intravenous immune globulin, that provides passive protection against many infectious diseases. Specific immune globulins (e.g., varicella-zoster immune globulin) are available for postexposure prophylaxis for some infections. An exception appears to be the judicious use of live virus varicella vaccine in children with acute lymphocytic leukemia in remission in whom the risk of natural varicella outweighs the risk from the attenuated vaccine virus. This vaccine may be obtained from the manufacturer on a compassionate use protocol for patients' aged 12 months to 17 years who have acute lymphocytic leukemia in remission for at least 1 year.

Children with Transplants

Transplant recipients (e.g., bone marrow transplant recipients) should also be viewed in a special light. Some experts elect to reimmunize all children without serologic evaluation, and others, because of the limited amount of data, recommend that immunization protocols be developed for these children in conjunction with experts in the fields of infectious disease and immunology. Information about the use of live virus vaccines in organ transplant recipients is also limited. Only inactivated poliovirus vaccine should be given to transplant recipients and their household contacts.

Children Taking Corticosteroids

Children receiving corticosteroids also need careful consideration and thorough review of their medical history, including a review of the underlying disease, the specific dose and schedule of corticosteroids prescribed, and the current immunization status, which includes an evaluation of risk factors relative to infectious disease. In general, children who have a disease (which suppresses the immune response) and who are receiving either systemic or locally administered corticosteroids (which also suppress the immune response) should not be given live virus vaccines except in special circumstances. The guidelines for administering a live virus vaccine to patients receiving corticosteroid therapy are based on the dosage in relation to the child's weight in kilograms and the duration of corticosteroid therapy. The following treatments do not contraindicate administration:

1. Topical therapy or local injections of corticosteroids
2. Physiologic maintenance doses of corticosteroids
3. Low or moderate dosage of systemic corticosteroids (less than 2 mg/kg/d of prednisone [Deltasone] or its equivalent or less than 20 mg/d or on alternate days if the child weighs greater than 10 kg)

Special consideration should be given if high-dose corticosteroids are prescribed. Administration of high-dose corticosteroids ($\geq$2 mg/kg/d of prednisone or its equivalent or $\geq$20 mg/d if the child weighs >10 kg) given daily or on alternate days for 14 days or less preempts the administration of live virus vaccines until the treatment is discontinued. Some experts recommend delaying immunization until 2 weeks after discontinuation of therapy (Centers for Disease Control and Prevention, 2011).

Patients who receive high doses of systemic corticosteroids—daily or on alternate days for 14 days or more—should not receive live virus vaccines until steroid therapy has been discontinued for at least 1 month. In addition, if clinical or laboratory evidence of systemic immunosuppression results from prolonged application, live virus vaccines should not be administered until corticosteroid therapy has been discontinued for at least 1 month.

Children with Seizures

Infants and children with a personal or family history of seizures are at increased risk for having a convulsion after receiving either pertussis (as DTaP) or measles (as MMR) vaccine. Seizures are usually brief, self-limited, and generalized and occur in conjunction with fever (Pickering et al., 2009). However, in the case of DTaP vaccine administered during infancy, administration may coincide with or hasten the inevitable recognition of a seizure-related disorder, such as infantile spasms or epilepsy. This causes confusion about the role of the pertussis vaccine, and in this instance, pertussis immunization should be deferred until a progressive neurologic disorder is excluded or the cause of the seizure diagnosed.

Measles immunization, however, is usually given at an age when the cause and nature of the seizure activity have been

Recommended Adult Immunization Schedule—United States - 2015

Note: These recommendations must be read with the footnotes that follow containing number of doses, intervals between doses, and other important information.

Recommended immunization schedule for adults aged 19 years or older, by vaccine and age group[1]

VACCINE ▼ AGE GROUP ►	19–21 years	22–26 years	27–49 years	50–59 years	60–64 years	≥65 years
Influenza*,[2]	1 dose annually					
Tetanus, diphtheria, pertussis (Td/Tdap)*,[3]	Substitute Tdap for Td once, then Td booster every 10 years					
Varicella*,[4]	2 doses					
Human papillomavirus (HPV) female*,[5]	3 doses	3 doses				
Human papillomavirus (HPV) male*,[5]	3 doses	3 doses				
Zoster[6]					1 dose	1 dose
Measles, mumps, rubella (MMR)*,[7]	1 or 2 doses depending on indication					
Pneumococcal 13-valent conjugate (PCV13)*,[8]						1 dose
Pneumococcal polysaccharide (PPSV23)[6]			1 or 2 doses depending on indication			1 dose
Hepatitis A*,[9]			2 or 3 doses depending on vaccine			
Hepatitis B*,[10]			3 doses			
Meningococcal 4-valent conjugate (Men ACWY) or polysaccharide (MPSV4)*,[11]			1 or more doses depending on indication			
Meningococcal B (Men B)[11]			2 or 3 doses depending on vaccine			
Haemophilus influenzae type b (Hib)*,[12]			1 or 3 doses depending on indication			

*Covered by the Vaccine Injury Compensation Program

Recommended for all persons who meet the age requirement, lack documentation of vaccination, or lack evidence of past infection; zoster vaccine is recommended regardless of past episode of zoster

Recommended for persons with a risk factor (medical, occupational, lifestyle, or other indication)

No recommendation

Report all clinically significant postvaccination reactions to the Vaccine Adverse Event Reporting System (VAERS). Reporting forms and instructions on filling a VARES report are available at www.vaers.hhs.gov or by telephone, 800-822-7967.

Information on how to file a Vaccine Injury Compensation Program claims is available at www.hrsa.gov/vaccinecompensation or by telephone, 800-338-2382. To file a claim for vaccine injury, contact the U.S. Court of Federal Claims, 717 Madison Place, N.W. Washington, D.C. 20005; telephone, 202-357-5400.

Additional information about the vaccines in this schedule, extent of available data, and contraindications for vaccination is also available at www.cdc.gov/vaccines or form the CDC-INFO Contact Center at 800-CDC-INFO (800-232-4636) in English and Spanish, 8:00 a.m. - 8.00 p.m. Eastern Time, Monday–Friday, excluding holidays.

Use of trade names and commercial sources is for identification only and does not imply endorsement by the U.S. Department of Health Services.

The recommendations in this schedule were approved by the Centers for disease Control and Prevention's (CDC) Advisory Committee on immunization Practices (ACIP), the American Academy of Family Physicians (AAFP), the America College of Physicians (ACP), American College of Obstetricians and Gynecologists (ACOG) and American College of Nurse-Midwives (ACNM).

FIGURE 52.3 Recommended adult immunization schedule—United States, 2016.

established. Therefore, measles immunization should not be deferred in children with a history of one or more seizures.

Adolescents

Adolescents continue to be adversely affected by vaccine-preventable disease, including varicella, hepatitis B, measles, meningococcus, HPV, and rubella. Recommendations for adolescents at ages 11 and 12 aim to improve the vaccine coverage and to establish routine visits to health care providers. These strategies reflect the recommendations (see **Box 52.1**) of the Advisory Committee on Immunization Practices (ACIP), American Academy of Pediatrics (AAP), American Academy of Family Physicians, and American Medical Association. In addition to providing an opportunity for administering needed vaccines, such as hepatitis B, varicella, second dose of MMR, tetanus and diphtheria booster, and HPV, this visit provides an opportunity to render other recommended preventive services, including health behavior guidance; screening for biomedical, behavioral, and emotional conditions; and delivery of other health services. For more information, see **Figure 52.1** and **Box 52.1**.

IMMUNIZATION RECOMMENDATIONS FOR ADULTS

Immunization prophylaxis is as important for adults as it is for children. However, the practice of assessing the vaccination status of adults at their routine health visits remains an issue.

As a result, many adults continue to be affected adversely by vaccine-preventable diseases such as varicella, pertussis, measles, and rubella. The guidelines are updated yearly in February, and all schedules are published in *Morbidity and Mortality Weekly Report* (http://www.cdc.gov/mmwr/index.html) and may be found at http://www.cdc.gov/vaccines/schedules/index.html. The ACIP recommendations are available at http://www.cdc.gov/vaccines/hcp/acip-recs/. Each patient's immunization records should be reviewed at each patient visit and determined if any vaccines are required. For more information, see **Figure 52.3** and **Box 52.1**.

DISEASE-SPECIFIC VACCINE RECOMMENDATIONS

Pneumococcal Vaccine 23-Valent (PPSV23)

Pneumococcal infection causes an estimated 5,000 deaths annually in the United States, accounting for more deaths than any other vaccine-preventable bacterial disease. *Streptococcus pneumoniae* colonizes the upper respiratory tract and can cause disseminated invasive infections, including bacteremia and meningitis, pneumonia and other lower respiratory tract infections, and upper respiratory tract infections, including otitis media and sinusitis. The pneumococcal vaccine protects against invasive bacteremic disease, although existing data suggest that it is less effective in protecting against other types of pneumococcal infections.

BOX 52.3 Recommendations for the Use of Pneumococcal Vaccine

Groups for Which Vaccination Is Recommended

People aged 65 y and older

People aged 2–64 y with chronic cardiovascular disease including congestive heart failure and cardiomyopathies, chronic pulmonary disease including chronic obstructive lung disease, emphysema, and asthma, sickle cell disease, diabetes mellitus, and people who smoke

People aged 2–64 y with alcoholism, chronic liver disease including cirrhosis, cochlear implants, or cerebrospinal fluid leaks

People aged 2–64 y with functional or anatomic asplenia

People aged 2–64 y living in nursing homes or other long-term care facilities

Immunocompromised People

Immunocompromised people aged 2 y and older, including those with HIV infection, leukemia, lymphoma, Hodgkin disease, multiple myeloma, generalized malignancy, chronic renal failure, or nephrotic syndrome; those receiving immunosuppressive chemotherapy (including corticosteroids); and those who have received an organ or bone marrow transplant

---

The ACIP recommends giving one dose of pneumococcal vaccine to elderly patients (65 years or older), with an additional dose given earlier to identified high-risk populations (**Box 52.3**). Two available vaccines include a 13-valent pneumococcal conjugate and a 23-valent purified capsular polysaccharide antigens of *S. pneumoniae*. If an elderly patient's vaccination status is unknown, he or she should receive one dose of the vaccine. There are no data to support revaccination beyond two doses.

Response to Vaccine

Antibodies develop within 2 to 3 weeks in healthy young adults; immune responses are not consistent among all 23 serotypes in the vaccine. Antibody concentrations and responses to individual antigens tend to be lower in the following populations:

- People aged 65 years or older
- People with alcoholic cirrhosis, chronic obstructive pulmonary disease, type 1 diabetes mellitus, Hodgkin's disease, or asthma
- People who smoke
- People with chronic renal failure requiring dialysis, renal transplantation, or nephrotic syndrome
- People with acquired immunodeficiency syndrome or HIV infection

Special Circumstances

Antibody response is diminished or absent in people who are immunocompromised or who have leukemia, lymphoma, or multiple myeloma. The antibody levels to most pneumococcal vaccine antigens remain elevated for at least 5 years in healthy adults.

A more rapid decline (within 3 to 5 years) occurs in certain children who have undergone splenectomy after trauma and in those who have sickle cell disease. Antibody concentrations also decline after 5 to 10 years in elderly people, those who have undergone splenectomy, patients with renal disease requiring dialysis, and people who have received transplants. A lower antibody response or rapid decline in antibody levels is also noted in patients with Hodgkin's disease and multiple myeloma. At least 2 weeks should elapse between immunization and the initiation of chemotherapy or immunosuppressive therapy.

Revaccination is recommended once for patients who are aged 2 or older, who are at highest risk for serious pneumococcal infection, and who are likely to have a rapid decline in antibody levels provided that 5 years has elapsed since receiving the first dose of vaccine.

Pneumococcal Conjugate Vaccine

In February 2010, the U.S. Food and Drug Administration licensed a 13-valent pneumococcal conjugate vaccine, PCV13 (Prevnar-13). This vaccine is recommended for universal use in children aged 23 months and younger. The number of doses for the primary series varies with the age of the child at the first dose.

Children ages 24 to 59 months who are at high risk for invasive pneumococcal infection and who have not been previously immunized should also receive 23-valent vaccine to expand the serotype coverage. In June 2012, the ACIP recommended routine use of the PCV13 for adults with immunocompromising conditions. It should be administered in addition to the PPSV23 to all eligible adults.

Influenza Vaccine

Influenza and pneumonia are the eighth leading causes of death in the United States and fifth in older adults. Fatalities from influenza begin to rise in midlife and are highest in persons with chronic disease. Measures available to reduce the incidence of influenza include immunoprophylaxis with inactivated (killed virus) vaccine and chemoprophylaxis. Before the influenza season gets under way, vaccination of people at risk and those likely to transmit influenza to at-risk populations is the most effective measure. The vaccine is associated with a decrease in influenza-related respiratory illness in all age groups, decreased hospitalization and death in people at high risk, decreased incidence of otitis media in children, and decreased work and school absenteeism. Influenza vaccine is recommended in anyone aged 6 months and older.

Two types of influenza vaccine are available—inactivated virus and live attenuated vaccine (in the form of nasal spray). The live virus is recommended for those aged 2 to 49 years and is contraindicated in patients who are immunocompromised and require a protected environment, health care workers, and household members who are in close contact with the immunocompromised individual. If a live virus is given, the patient should not have contact with those who are immunocompromised for 7 days. The antigenic composition of the influenza vaccine changes each year; thus, this vaccine must be administered every year. It provides protection against influenza A and B and is available as either a trivalent inactivated influenza vaccine (IIV3) or a quadrivalent live (LAIV4) or inactivated vaccine (IIV4). The IIV3 vaccine is available in a high-dose formulation for patients 65 years and older, and there is an intradermal IIV4 formulation approved for patients 18 to 64 years. Children aged 6 months through 8 years require 2 doses of influenza vaccine (administered ≥4 weeks apart) during their first season of vaccination to optimize response. Recombinant (RIV3) and cell-cultured (ccIIV3) influenza vaccines should be utilized in patients with severe allergic and anaphylactic reactions to various influenza vaccine components (Centers for Disease Control and Prevention, 2015a, 2015b, 2015d).

Groups at Risk

People at increased risk for influenza-related complications include:

1. Those aged 50 and older
2. Children ages 6 to 23 months
3. Adults and children with pulmonary disease, including asthma
4. Adults and children who have required regular medical follow-up or hospitalization during the preceding year because of chronic metabolic diseases (including diabetes mellitus), renal dysfunction, hemoglobinopathies, or immunosuppression (including immunosuppression caused by medications or HIV infection)
5. Children and teenagers on long-term aspirin therapy who might be at risk for development of Reye syndrome after influenza
6. Women in the second or third trimester of pregnancy during the influenza season
7. Persons who live with or care for persons at high risk, including health care workers and household contacts (including children from birth to age 23 months)

Transmission of Influenza

Just as immunizing people in groups at high risk for flu and its complications is important, so too is immunizing those who are most likely to transmit the disease. Groups that can transmit influenza to people at high risk include health care workers (in hospital and outpatient settings and in emergency response service), employees of nursing homes and chronic care facilities who have contact with patients or residents, employees of assisted living and other residences for people in high-risk groups, providers of home care to people at high risk (e.g., visiting nurses, volunteers), household contacts of high-risk individuals, and providers of essential community services.

Additional populations for consideration include people with HIV infection, breast-feeding mothers, people traveling to foreign countries, students or other people in institutional settings, and the general populace who want to reduce the likelihood of contracting influenza.

The current 2- to 3-month time frame over which patients are traditionally immunized is too short to fully implement immunization recommendations and inconsistent with the duration of influenza activity. Health care providers and patients should re-evaluate their approach to influenza vaccination and recognize the need to extend the immunization time period into January and beyond. To increase influenza immunization rates, the CDC and other professional societies recommend an expanded immunization season, with vaccination offered at every opportunity between October and May.

Antibody development after vaccination can take as long as 2 weeks in healthy adults and as long as 6 weeks in children—or 2 weeks after the second dose. Most persons recommended for influenza vaccination should receive a single dose each year. The exception is children ages 6 months to 9 years who are receiving an influenza vaccine for the first time. They should receive 2 doses administered at least 1 month apart. No influenza vaccine is currently approved for children age 6 months and younger; these vulnerable infants should be protected indirectly through the vaccination of close contacts.

Chemoprophylaxis with antiviral agents, amantadine (Symmetrel), rimantadine (Flumadine), zanamivir (Relenza), and oseltamivir (Tamiflu) can also be helpful. When administered within 48 hours of the onset of illness, they can reduce the severity and shorten the duration of illness in otherwise healthy people. Oseltamivir can be used in the prevention of influenza in adults and children aged 13 and older.

Meningococcal Vaccine

Approximately 3,000 cases of meningococcal diseases occur in the United States each year, with a fatality rate of 10% despite antibiotic therapy early in the illness. During 1991 to 1998, the highest rate occurred among infants younger than age 12 months. The three serogroups of meningococcal disease that are most commonly seen in the United States are serogroups B, C, and Y. Three kinds of meningococcal vaccines are now available in the United States. Meningococcal polysaccharide (MPSV4) and meningococcal conjugate (MCV4) provide coverage against types A, C, Y, and W. MPSV4 is the only vaccine licensed for patients older than 55 years of age, and MCV4 is the preferred vaccine for patients 55 years of age or younger. The recently released serogroup B meningococcal (MenB) vaccines provide short-term protection against most strains of serogroup B meningococcal disease. The Advisory Committee on Immunization Practices recommends routine vaccination of all adolescents aged 11 to 18 years with the quadrivalent meningococcal conjugate vaccine (MCV4). A single dose should be administered at age 11 or 12 years

with a booster dose at age 16 years for persons who receive the first dose before age 16 years. The MenB vaccine series should be administered to persons aged 16 to 23 years (preferred age 16 to 18 years) with routine vaccination of certain persons at increased risk for meningococcal disease with MenACWY and serogroup B meningococcal (MenB) vaccine. Meningococcal vaccine (MCV4) is recommended for high-risk patients (e.g., sickle cell disease, anatomic or functional asplenia, complement deficient) beginning at 2 months of age.

Pertussis Vaccine

Pertussis continues to be poorly controlled in the United States despite high compliance with childhood pertussis vaccination. In 2009, 16,858 pertussis cases and 12 infant deaths were reported. In October 2010, the ACIP expanded the use of tetanus toxoid and reduced diphtheria toxoid and acellular pertussis (Tdap) for adolescents and adults to improve immunity against pertussis. Adolescents aged 11 through 18 years who have completed the recommended childhood diphtheria and tetanus toxoids and pertussis/diphtheria and tetanus toxoids and acellular pertussis (DTaP) vaccination series and any adults greater than 19 years should receive a single dose of Tdap. Pregnant women should receive one dose of Tdap during each pregnancy at 27 to 36 weeks' gestation.

Human Papillomavirus Vaccine

Three human papillomavirus (HPV) vaccines, bivalent (2vHPV), quadrivalent (4vHPV), and 9-valent (9vHPV), are currently available. All three vaccines target HPV types 6 and 11, which are most commonly associated with clinical diseases and cause over 95% of genital warts. Types 16 and 18, believed to be responsible for approximately 66% of cases of cervical cancer, are contained in the quadrivalent and 9-valent vaccines. The 9-valent product provides additional protection against HPV 31, 33, 45, 52, and 58, which account for 14% for females and 4% males of HPV-associated cancers. The ACIP guidelines (Petrosky et al., 2015) recommend 9vHPV, 4vHPV, or 2vHPV for routine vaccination of females 9 through 26 years of age who have not been vaccinated previously or who have not completed the three-dose series. The 9vHPV or 4vHPV is recommended for routine vaccination of males 9 through 21 years of age, who have not been vaccinated previously or who have not completed the three-dose series, and through age 26 years in men who have sex with men and immunocompromised men (including those with HIV infection) through age 26 years if not vaccinated previously. It can be given to immunocompromised women, but the immune response may be reduced. Pregnant women should not receive the HPV vaccine, even if the series has been started before pregnancy. It can be administered to lactating women.

Ideally, the vaccine should be administered before potential exposure to HPV through sexual contact. The vaccine is a series of three doses. The second dose is administered 1 to 2 months after the first dose, and the third dose is administered 6 months after the first dose.

Rotavirus Vaccine

Rotavirus is the most common cause of severe gastroenteritis in children younger than age 5.

Before rotavirus vaccines were available in the United States, more than 200,000 children younger than age 5 received care in hospital emergency departments for rotavirus disease each year, and 55,000 to 70,000 young children were hospitalized. Two years after the introduction of the vaccine in 2006, a significant reduction in rotavirus hospitalization rates ($P < 0.001$) was observed among all age groups (87% reduction in 6 to less than 12 months old, 96% reduction in 12 to less than 24 months old, and a 92% reduction in 24 to less than 36 months old). Multiple studies have continued to show that the U.S. rotavirus season has become less pronounced and shorter since the utilization of the vaccine (Payne et al., 2011).

Rotavirus is very contagious. People who get a rotavirus infection shed large amounts of the virus in their feces. The disease spreads when infants or young children get rotavirus in their mouth. This happens through contact with the hands of other people or objects (such as toys) that have been contaminated with small amounts of rotavirus.

The first dose of the rotavirus vaccine can be given as early as age 6 weeks and needs to be given before an infant is age 15 weeks. Children should receive all doses of rotavirus vaccine before they are age 8 months.

Haemophilus influenzae Type b Vaccine

Haemophilus influenzae type b (Hib) vaccine prevents meningitis and pneumonia caused by Hib. It is given to all infants at 2, 4, and 6 months for a total of two- to three-dose primary series (depending on brand) and a booster dose at age 12 to 15 months. More than 95% of infants will develop protective antibody levels after a primary series with clinical efficacy estimated at 95% to 100%. Invasive Hib disease in a completely vaccinated infant is very uncommon. Unimmunized older children, adolescents, and adults with certain specified medical conditions (anatomic or functional splenectomy, HIV infection, sickle cell disease, immunoglobulin or complement deficiency, chemotherapy recipients, hematopoietic stem cell transplant) should receive additional doses of Hib vaccine, as they have an increased risk for invasive Hib disease.

Hepatitis A Vaccine

Hepatitis A is a serious liver disease caused by hepatitis A virus (HAV) and transmitted by hand-to-mouth contact through eating and drinking. Proper sanitation and good personal hygiene can help prevent its spread. It is typically self-limiting, but may lead to jaundice and, if severe, death (about 3 to 6 deaths per 1,000 cases) (Hamborsky et al., 2015). In 2006, the hepatitis A vaccine became available for the long-term protection of HAV infections. A two-dose series should be routinely administered to children beginning at 12 months of age. This vaccine should also be given to individuals traveling to countries with an intermediate to high prevalence of hepatitis A, men who have sex with men, drug abusers, chronic liver disease, or those treated with clotting factors.

Hepatitis B Vaccine

Hepatitis B is a serious disease caused by hepatitis B virus (HBV) that attacks the liver. The virus is very resilient and is viable outside the body for up to 7 days. It can cause lifelong infection, cirrhosis (scarring) of the liver, liver cancer, liver failure, and death. It is spread through person-to-person contact through blood, semen, or other body fluids. All children should get their first dose of hepatitis B vaccine at birth and complete the vaccine series by 6 to 18 months of age. Children and adolescents younger than 19 years of age who have not yet gotten the vaccine and adults with risk factors (e.g., men who have sex with men, IV drug users, health care and public safety personnel, persons with chronic liver disease, HIV, or undergoing renal dialysis, those residing in correctional facilities, and travelers to endemic regions) should also be vaccinated. A series of 3 or 4 shots should be given over a 6-month period. The hepatitis B vaccine provides greater than 90% protection to infants, children, and adults if they are immunized prior to being exposed to HBV.

Inactivated Poliovirus

Polio is an infectious disease caused by *Enterovirus*. A polio outbreak in the United States in 1952 resulted in over 21,000 cases of paralysis. The incidence fell rapidly following introduction of effective vaccines. The inactivated polio vaccine (IPV) is the only polio vaccine available in the United States. Children should receive a total of 4 doses of IPV beginning at 2 , 4, 6 to 18 months, and a booster dose at 4 to 6 years. The last case of wild-virus polio reported in the United States was in 1979, and global polio eradication may be achieved within the next decade.

Measles, Mumps, and Rubella Vaccine

The measles, mumps, and rubella (MMR) vaccine provides protection against three diseases and has been administered since 1967. Two doses of MMR provide complete protection. Children should be given the first dose of MMR vaccine at 12 to 15 months of age. The second dose can be given 4 weeks later, but is usually given before the start of kindergarten at 4 to 6 years of age. Measles and mumps are contagious diseases transmitted by contact with an infected person through coughing and sneezing, and both spread very easily. The measles consists of an erythematous, maculopapular, pruritic, splotchy rash, which lasts about 5 days and is preceded with a several-day prodrome of malaise, fever, coryza, and conjunctivitis. It may result in encephalitis (permanent brain damage) or death in 1 to 2 of every 1,000 cases (Marshall, 2012). The mumps consists of fever, headache, malaise, myalgias, and bilateral swelling of the parotid glands (parotitis). Testicular swelling and tenderness (orchitis) and aseptic meningitis may occur in 30% and 10% of patients, respectively. Patients with rubella (also called German measles or 3-day measles) exhibit a transient, erythematous, and sometimes pruritic rash, with about 60% of postpubertal women developing arthritis. If a woman in her first trimester of pregnancy contracts rubella, fetal damage is almost 100%. If contracted in second or third trimester, babies are born with congenital rubella syndrome (CRS) at birth. CRS will result in deafness, cataracts, cardiac defects, and CNS abnormalities.

By 2001, administration of the MMR vaccine eradicated measles from the United States, decreased the incidence of mumps by 99%, and provided lifelong protection against rubella. However, due to parents' concern of the MMR vaccine causing autism, mumps and measles cases have increased over the last several years. In 2010, there were 2,600 cases of the mumps, which decreased to 229 in 2012. In 2014, there were over 600 cases of measles reported, which has decreased to 189 cases in the United States from January to September 2015 (Hamborsky et al., 2015; Perry et al., 2015).

Varicella Vaccine

Chickenpox is a highly contagious disease caused by the varicella-zoster virus. In an unvaccinated child, it appears as an itchy, uncomfortable rash with blisters and vesicles. Before the chickenpox vaccine was widely used, nearly 11,000 people were hospitalized each year and about 50 children and 50 adults died every year from chickenpox. A live varicella vaccine was licensed for use in the United States in 1995, and since then, the number of hospitalizations and deaths due to chickenpox has decreased by more than 90% (Hamborsky et al., 2015). Two doses of the chickenpox vaccine are recommended, with the first dose given at age 12 through 15 months old and the second at age 4 through 6 years.

Zoster Vaccine

Herpes zoster, or shingles, occurs when latent varicella-zoster virus (VZV) reactivates and causes recurrent disease. Patients contracting zoster experience a painful, vesicular eruption unilaterally along a sensory nerve. The patient may experience pain and paresthesias a few days prior to the rash. Shingles is typically associated with aging and immunosuppression. A complication that may result after the lesions have resolved is postherpetic neuralgia (PHN) or pain in the area of the occurrence. About 30% of American will develop herpes zoster each year, and the risk of the disease increases with increasing age with more than half the cases occurring in people 60 years or older. In May 2006, the FDA approved herpes zoster vaccine for use in persons 60 years of age and older. It is a live vaccine with 64% efficacy in people aged 60 through 69 years versus about 18% efficacy in people aged 80 years and older. ACIP recommends a one-time dose of the zoster vaccine in patients at least 60 years of age (Hamborsky et al., 2015).

ADVERSE EVENTS ASSOCIATED WITH VACCINES

Risks of vaccination vary from inconvenient to severe and life-threatening. Common vaccine side effects (e.g., fever and local irritation to DTaP vaccine) are usually mild to moderate in severity and without permanent consequences. However, serious side effects and adverse reactions are possible, although the occurrence of an adverse event does not prove causation

by the vaccine (i.e., the adverse event may be caused by factors other than the vaccine).

Reporting of adverse events is important because it may provide clues to unanticipated adverse reactions. It is important to interview the patient or guardian regarding any side effects after past immunizations. Any unexpected, reported, and observed event that required medical attention soon after the administration should be described in detail in the patient's medical record and reported using the Vaccine Adverse Events Reporting System (VAERS) (accessible online, https://vaers.hhs.gov/esub/index).

The VAERS is a result of the National Childhood Injury Act of 1986, which made provisions for health care providers to report occurrences of certain adverse events and to maintain permanent immunization records. Pertinent information to be reported includes a detailed description of the event (signs and symptoms reported and observed) and the time from administration of vaccine to presentation of signs and symptoms.

Pertinent patient history information should be noted regarding any existing physician-diagnosed allergies, medical conditions, and birth defects as well as any illness at the time of vaccine administration. In addition, information about the vaccine must be included. Documentation should identify the type of vaccine; the manufacturer, lot number, site, and route of administration; and any previous doses received.

Staff members from the VAERS contact the provider (reporter) to follow up about the patient's condition at 60 days and at 1 year after the initial reporting of adverse events. **Figure 52.4** contains the VAERS form.

CONTRAINDICATIONS TO VACCINATIONS

The primary contraindications to vaccine administration are acute febrile illness, allergy to a vaccine component, or history of hypersensitivity/anaphylactic reaction to vaccine constituents. **Table 52.1** includes a detailed listing of contraindications by vaccine. The four main types of hypersensitivity reactions include:

1. Allergic reactions to egg-related antigens (e.g., yellow fever, influenza)
2. Mercury sensitivity in some recipients of vaccines or immune globulin
3. Antibiotic-induced allergic reactions (e.g., inactivated poliovirus vaccine—trace streptomycin, neomycin, and polymyxin B; MMR, including single or combined with varicella—trace neomycin; varicella and herpes zoster vaccines-neomycin)
4. Hypersensitivity to other vaccine components, including the infectious agent (e.g., shingles vaccine-gelatin)

Acute febrile illness suggesting a moderate to severe illness is sufficient reason to defer vaccination until the person recovers. Guidelines in this instance are based on the provider's assessment of the illness and the vaccines scheduled for administration. The rationale for withholding vaccination in moderate to severe illness, with or without fever, is that evolving

WEBSITE: www.vaers.hhs.gov   E-MAIL: info@vaers.org   FAX: 1-877-721-0366

| VAERS | **VACCINE ADVERSE EVENT REPORTING SYSTEM**
24 Hour Toll-Free Information 1-800-822-7967
P.O. Box 1100, Rockville, MD 20849-1100
PATIENT IDENTITY KEPT CONFIDENTIAL | *For CDC/FDA Use Only*
VAERS Number _____
Date Received _____ |

Patient Name:	Vaccine administered by (Name):	Form completed by (Name):
Last First M.I.	Responsible Physician _____	Relation ☐ Vaccine Provider ☐ Patient/Parent
Address	Facility Name/Address	to Patient ☐ Manufacturer ☐ Other
		Address *(if different from patient or provider)*
City State Zip	City State Zip	City State Zip
Telephone no. (___) _____	Telephone no. (___) _____	Telephone no. (___) _____

1. State	2. County where administered	3. Date of birth ___/___/___ mm dd yy	4. Patient age	5. Sex ☐ M ☐ F	6. Date form completed ___/___/___ mm dd yy

7. Describe adverse events(s) (symptoms, signs, time course) and treatment, if any	8. Check all appropriate: ☐ Patient died (date ___/___/___) mm dd yy ☐ Life threatening illness ☐ Required emergency room/doctor visit ☐ Required hospitalization (_____days) ☐ Resulted in prolongation of hospitalization ☐ Resulted in permanent disability ☐ None of the above

9. Patient recovered ☐ YES ☐ NO ☐ UNKNOWN	10. Date of vaccination ___/___/___ mm dd yy Time _____ AM/PM	11. Adverse event onset ___/___/___ mm dd yy Time _____ AM/PM
12. Relevant diagnostic tests/laboratory data		

13. Enter all vaccines given on date listed in no. 10

	Vaccine (type)	Manufacturer	Lot number	Route/Site	No. Previous Doses
a.					
b.					
c.					
d.					

14. Any other vaccinations within 4 weeks prior to the date listed in no. 10

	Vaccine (type)	Manufacturer	Lot number	Route/Site	No. Previous doses	Date given
a.						
b.						

15. Vaccinated at: ☐ Private doctor's office/hospital ☐ Military clinic/hospital ☐ Public health clinic/hospital ☐ Other/unknown	16. Vaccine purchased with: ☐ Private funds ☐ Military funds ☐ Public funds ☐ Other/unknown	17. Other medications

18. Illness at time of vaccination (specify)	19. Pre-existing physician-diagnosed allergies, birth defects, medical conditions (specify)

20. Have you reported this adverse event previously? ☐ No ☐ To health department ☐ To doctor ☐ To manufacturer	*Only for children 5 and under*
	22. Birth weight _____ lb. _____ oz.	23. No. of brothers and sisters

21. Adverse event following prior vaccination (check all applicable, specify)	*Only for reports submitted by manufacturer/immunization project*

	Adverse Event	Onset Age	Type Vaccine	Dose no. in series
☐ In patient				
☐ In brother or sister				

24. Mfr./imm. proj. report no.	25. Date received by mfr./imm.proj.
26. 15 day report? ☐ Yes ☐ No	27. Report type ☐ Initial ☐ Follow-Up

Health care providers and manufacturers are required by law (42 USC 300aa-25) to report reactions to vaccines listed in the Table of Reportable Events Following Immunization. Reports for reactions to other vaccines are voluntary except when required as a condition of immunization grant awards.

Form VAERS-1(FDA)

FIGURE 52.4 Vaccine adverse event reporting system form.

TABLE 52.1

Guide to Contraindications and Precautions to Commonly Used Vaccines in Adults (Centers for Disease Control and Prevention, 2014)

Vaccine	Contraindications	Precautions
Influenza, inactivated (IIV)	Severe allergic reaction (e.g., anaphylaxis) after previous dose of any influenza vaccine or to a vaccine component, including egg protein	Moderate or severe acute illness with or without fever History of Guillain-Barré syndrome within 6 wks of previous influenza vaccination
Influenza, recombinant (RIV)	Severe allergic reaction (e.g., anaphylaxis) after previous dose of RIV or to a vaccine component. RIV does not contain any egg protein Severe allergic reaction (e.g., anaphylaxis) after a previous dose or to a vaccine component	Moderate or severe acute illness with or without fever History of Guillain-Barré syndrome within 6 wks of previous influenza vaccination
Influenza, live attenuated (LAIV)	Severe allergic reaction (e.g., anaphylaxis) after a previous dose or to any component of the vaccine Pregnant women Immunosuppressed adults Adults who have taken influenza antiviral medications within the previous 48 h	Moderate or severe acute illness with or without fever History of Guillain-Barré syndrome within 6 wks of previous influenza vaccination Asthma in patients ≥ 5 y Other chronic medical conditions, e.g., other chronic lung diseases, chronic cardiovascular disease (excluding isolated hypertension), diabetes, chronic renal or hepatic disease, hematologic disease, neurologic disease, and metabolic disorders
Tetanus, diphtheria, pertussis (Tdap); tetanus, diphtheria (Td)	Severe allergic reaction (e.g., anaphylaxis) after a previous dose or to a vaccine component For pertussis-containing vaccines: encephalopathy (e.g., coma, decreased level of consciousness, or prolonged seizures) not attributable to another identifiable cause occurring within 7 d of administration of a previous dose of Tdap or diphtheria and tetanus toxoids and acellular pertussis (DTaP) vaccine	Moderate or severe acute illness with or without fever History of Guillain-Barré syndrome within 6 wks after a previous dose of vaccine containing tetanus toxoid component History of Arthus-type hypersensitivity reactions after a previous dose of tetanus or diphtheria toxoid–containing vaccine; defer at least 10 y since the last tetanus toxoid–containing vaccine For pertussis-containing vaccines: progressive or unstable neurologic disorder, uncontrolled seizures, or progressive encephalopathy until condition has stabilized
Varicella	Severe allergic reaction (e.g., anaphylaxis) after a previous dose or to a vaccine component Known severe immunodeficiency Pregnancy	Recent (within 3–11 mo) receipt of antibody-containing blood product (specific interval dependent on product) Moderate or severe acute illness with or without fever Receipt of specific antivirals (i.e., acyclovir, famciclovir, or valacyclovir) 24 h before vaccination; avoid these for 14 d after vaccination
Human papillomavirus (HPV)	Severe allergic reaction (e.g., anaphylaxis) after a previous dose or to a vaccine component	Moderate or severe acute illness with or without fever Pregnancy
Zoster	Severe allergic reaction (e.g., anaphylaxis) after a previous dose or to a vaccine component Known severe immunodeficiency Pregnancy	Receipt of specific antivirals (i.e., acyclovir, famciclovir, or valacyclovir) 24 h before vaccination; avoid these for 14 d after vaccination Moderate or severe acute illness with or without fever
Measles, mumps, rubella (MMR)	Severe allergic reaction (e.g., anaphylaxis) after a previous dose or to a vaccine component Known severe immunodeficiency Pregnancy	Recent (within 3–11 mo) receipt of antibody-containing blood product (specific interval dependent on product) Moderate or severe acute illness with or without fever
Pneumococcal conjugate (PCV13)	Severe allergic reaction (e.g., anaphylaxis) after a previous dose or to a vaccine component, including to any vaccine containing diphtheria toxoid	Moderate or severe acute illness with or without fever
Pneumococcal polysaccharide (PPSV23)	Severe allergic reaction (e.g., anaphylaxis) after a previous dose or to a vaccine component	Moderate or severe acute illness with or without fever
Meningococcal, conjugate (MenACWY); meningococcal, polysaccharide (MPSV4); serogroup B meningococcal (MenB)	Severe allergic reaction (e.g., anaphylaxis) after a previous dose or to a vaccine component	Moderate or severe acute illness with or without fever

(Continued)

TABLE 52.1

Guide to Contraindications and Precautions to Commonly Used Vaccines in Adults (Centers for Disease Control and Prevention, 2014) (*Continued*)

Vaccine	Contraindications	Precautions
Hepatitis A	Severe allergic reaction (e.g., anaphylaxis) after a previous dose or to a vaccine component	Moderate or severe acute illness with or without fever
Hepatitis B	Severe allergic reaction (e.g., anaphylaxis) after a previous dose or to a vaccine component	Moderate or severe acute illness with or without fever
Haemophilus influenzae type b (Hib)	Severe allergic reaction (e.g., anaphylaxis) after a previous dose or to a vaccine component	Moderate or severe acute illness with or without fever

signs and symptoms associated with the illness may be difficult to distinguish from the reaction to the vaccine. Minor illness (minor respiratory, gastrointestinal, or other illness) and low-grade fevers are not contraindications to immunization. The benefit of the immunization at the recommended age, regardless of the presence of mild illness, outweighs the risk of vaccine failure (Pickering et al., 2009).

One needs to use special attention to contraindications when administering live vaccines. Contraindications for all live vaccines include pregnancy and known severe immunodeficiency (e.g., from hematologic and solid tumors, receipt of chemotherapy, congenital immunodeficiency, or long-term immunosuppressive therapy, or patients with human immunodeficiency virus [HIV]

infection who are severely immunocompromised) (see the preceding discussions on immunocompromised children).

PATIENT AND PROVIDER EDUCATION AND ISSUES

Patient and health care provider/practitioner education, updates on immunization protocols, and established office systems with designated areas of responsibility are significant factors in improving immunization rates. Office routines and systems should incorporate pediatric immunization standards (**Box 52.4**) and facilitate the use of all possible opportunities

BOX 52.4   Standards for Pediatric Immunization Practices

Standard 1. Immunization services are readily available.

Standard 2. No barriers or unnecessary prerequisites to the receipt of vaccines exist.

Standard 3. Immunization services are available free or for a minimal fee.

Standard 4. Providers use all clinical encounters to screen and, when indicated, immunize children.

Standard 5. Providers educate parents and guardians about immunization in general terms.

Standard 6. Providers question parents or guardians about contraindications and, before immunizing a child, inform them in specific terms about the risks and benefits of the immunizations their child is to receive.

Standard 7. Providers follow only true contraindications.

Standard 8. Providers administer simultaneously all vaccine doses for which a child is eligible at the time of each visit.

Standard 9. Providers use accurate and complete recording procedures.

Standard 10. Providers co-schedule immunization appointments in conjunction with appointments for other child health services.

Standard 11. Providers report adverse events after immunization promptly, accurately, and completely.

Standard 12. Providers operate a tracking system.

Standard 13. Providers adhere to appropriate procedures for vaccine management.

Standard 14. Providers conduct semiannual audits to assess immunization coverage levels and to review immunization records in the patient populations they serve.

Standard 15. Providers maintain up-to-date, easily retrievable medical protocols at all locations where vaccines are administered.

Standard 16. Providers operate with patient-oriented and community-based approaches.

Standard 17. Vaccines are administered by properly trained individuals.

Standard 18. Providers receive ongoing education and training on current immunization recommendations.

From Centers for Disease Control and Prevention. (1993). Standard for pediatric immunization practices: Recommended by National Vaccine Advisory Committee (ACIP). *Morbidity and Mortality Weekly Report, 42*(RR-5), 1–13.

to review and update the immunization status of each patient (National Vaccine Advisory Committee, 2003). Tickler systems, chart reminders, and flow sheets that identify needed immunizations clearly and visibly are useful adjuncts to patient care.

A team approach to staff involvement also helps to enhance vaccination rates. Support staff should be aware of immunization needs when scheduling return or preventive visits as well as visits for illness or minor health problems. Visual reminders on the patient's chart or visit encounter form can be used to alert the practitioner to review specific vaccine needs or requests. **Box 52.5** presents recommendations related to the immunization schedule, and **Box 52.6** offers answers to frequently asked questions about immunization.

Vaccines should be stored in the office in sufficient amounts to meet the needs of the patients. Staff should have specific assignments to monitor stock levels, lot numbers, and expiration dates. Vaccines should be stored according to the manufacturer's recommendations with a backup system to address times when power outages may have affected vaccines, particularly during nonbusiness hours. Methods can range from plugging in a digital clock in the same outlet to use of alarm systems on the freezer or refrigerator. An inexpensive method of detecting a power outage uses a cup of ice with a penny or other coins placed on top of the ice. The length of a power outage may be judged by how far the coin sinks in the previously completely frozen ice. If power outages occur, the pharmaceutical manufacturer should be contacted for information about vaccine use, revised expiration dates, or unusable vaccine. Staff members should not automatically assume that vaccine should be discarded.

A central log book, maintained by date and time and including lot numbers and expiration dates of the vaccines, is recommended. Used with patient schedule information and chart documentation, the log book helps identify patients should a pharmaceutical company notify the office of a vaccine recall or a need to reimmunize patients receiving a specific lot of vaccine. Immunization screening processes are necessary for all populations to determine if an individual can receive the required vaccines. The screening questions, asked prior to vaccination, should be as follows:

Do you have diarrhea or a substantial fever, or are you vomiting today?
Do you have any drugs or food allergies?
Have you ever had a reaction to any vaccine? If yes, describe it.
Are you being treated by a doctor for a disease?
Do you have cancer or any disease that affects the immune system?

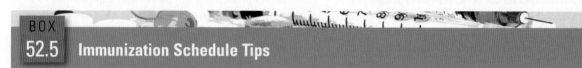

BOX 52.5 Immunization Schedule Tips

Restarting Vaccine Series
With the exception of oral typhoid vaccine, it never is necessary to restart a vaccine series because the interval has been prolonged—although every effort should be made to adhere to the recommended schedule.

Vaccines Given Too Soon
These will not be accepted at school entry and revaccination will be recommended.

Lack of Written Vaccination Record
An attempt should be made to verify vaccination status. If no record can be verified, the child should be considered unimmunized and should be revaccinated as appropriate for age.

Hepatitis B
In the case of an *interrupted* or *incomplete* series, resume the series; do not repeat or restart. Dose should be appropriate in accord with the manufacturer's instructions. The *third dose* should be given at least 2 mo after the second dose and at least 4 mo after the first dose but not before 6 mo of age.

PPD/MMR
PPD can be done before or at the same time as the measles vaccine is administered. Give PPD 4 to 6 wk after measles vaccine, if measles is given first, because measles can reduce the reactivity of PPD. This reduction in reactivity is due to mild suppression of cell-mediated immunity, which can lead to false-negative test results.

DtaP
The fourth dose can be given if a child is ≥12 mo of age and 6 mo has elapsed since DTaP dose 3 (especially if the child is unlikely to return at 15 to 18 mo of age). The fifth dose should be given at 4 to 6 y. Children should not receive more than six doses of diphtheria or tetanus-containing toxoid before their seventh birthday. No pertussis-containing vaccines are licensed for use in people ≥7 y of age.

HIB
No HIB vaccine should be given to infants younger than 6 wk of age and is not recommended after age 5 y. Minimum age for last HIB is 12 mo, if at least 2 mo has passed since the previous dose. DTaP/HIB combination products should not be used for primary series (2, 4, 6 mo of age).

Varicella
Dosage for people 12 mo and older: Single 0.5-mL dose subcutaneously suffices for protection 12 mo to 12 y. People 13 y of age and older should receive two 0.5-mL doses at least 4 wk apart.

BOX 52.6 Questions and Answers About Immunization

Q. How long should the vaccination needle be?
A. Subcutaneous injections for children and adults: ⅝ to ¾ in., 23- to 25-gauge needle.

Intramuscular injections for infants and children: minimum needle length of ⅞ in. for anterolateral thigh and minimum of ⅝ in. for deltoid injection; for adults: 1 to 1½ in. needle (Marshall, 2012).

Q. What are the immunization recommendations for children of parents or household residents who were never vaccinated for polio?
A. If the unvaccinated or inadequately vaccinated person resides in the household, an all-IVP schedule is recommended for the child. Parents and household contacts may receive IVP too.

Q. Which HIB vaccines are the best?
A. Different manufacturers' products are considered interchangeable for the primary series and the booster. However, no HIB vaccine is recommended for infants younger than 6 wk of age. If it is given, it may make the child incapable of responding to subsequent doses.

Q. What are some special concerns related to pregnancy?
A. There are no contraindications to immunization of a household member if another household member is pregnant. However, if a woman in the household wants to become pregnant and also wants to be vaccinated, she should wait to become pregnant at least 1 mo after receiving mumps, measles, varicella and 3 mo after receiving rubella.

Q. What happens if someone has an extra vaccination?
A. Extra doses of live vaccine do not appear to have adverse consequences, and they may boost immunity. Extra doses of inactivated vaccines can induce very high antibody titers. If these people are revaccinated, large local inflammatory reactions may ensue.

Q. Is it harmful to receive vaccines simultaneously?
A. No evidence exists that simultaneous administration of vaccines reduces vaccine effectiveness or increases adverse events.

Q. What are the implications of an error, such as previous administration of a vaccine at the wrong site, in a wrong dose, by a wrong route?

A. Unfortunately, they do not count. Only full doses in acceptable sites should be counted. Revaccinate according to age. The exception to the rule is live vaccines (MMR, varicella), which are recommended to be administered subcutaneously—intramuscular administration of these vaccines is not likely to decrease immunogenicity. *Note:* Reducing or dividing doses of any vaccine including those to preterm or low-birth-weight infants is not indicated.

Q. What is the recommended way to administer multiple injections to infants?
A. The recommended approach is to place the vaccine most likely to cause a local adverse reaction (e.g., DTaP) in one leg and the two less reactive in different sites in the other leg.

Q. How effective is the varicella vaccine?
A. Effectiveness is 70% to 90% protection against infection with 95% protection against severe disease. Protection persists at least 7 to 10 y. The risk of transmission appears low but somewhat higher if the vaccine develops a varicella-like rash after vaccination. Recommend that vaccines avoid contact with immunocompromised people when the rash is present.

Q. Why is the MMR vaccine given twice?
A. The second dose is given because 2% to 5% of people do not develop immunity after the first dose, and 95% of the people who did not respond to the first dose respond to the second.

Note: Birth before 1957 is generally considered evidence of rubella immunity; laboratory evidence of immunity is recommended. Combined MMR vaccine is the drug of choice if vaccination is needed.

Q. What is the standard dosing schedule for hepatitis B vaccine?
A. There is no standard dose. That is why it is so important to read the package insert for hepatitis B vaccine carefully. The formulations vary, and the appropriate microgram dose must be selected.

Have you received blood or antibodies (immune globulins) in the past 3 to 11 months?
Are you pregnant or planning to become pregnant in the next month or so?
Does the infant or child have any neurologic problem (e.g., seizures) that is not resolved or stabilized?

A focus on adolescent and adult populations as well as infants and children is critical. Current recommendations include routine screening at ages 11, 12, and 50. An interim process for high-risk people in combination with aforementioned recommended screenings provides the best mechanism for implementing a comprehensive immunization program.

It is extremely important to keep updated and be familiar with Web sites and organizations that provide vaccine information to be aware of changes that occur.

CASE STUDY*

B.E. is a 58-year-old female with no food or drug allergies. She presents to your clinic on November 10 for a follow-up visit for type 2 diabetes mellitus diagnosed 2 months ago. Her history is significant for the following:

- Type 2 diabetes mellitus controlled with diet and exercise.
- Her daughter is pregnant and **B.E.** plans to care for the infant.
- Vaccination history: oral polio vaccine 1964, Td 2010, physician confirmed chicken pox, mumps, and measles as a child.

1. You assess that **B.E.** requires several vaccines. Which of the following screening questions should you ask to determine if she can be immunized today?
   a. Have you had a fever or diarrhea in the last 24 hours?
   b. Do you have cancer or are you being treated for any immune problem?
   c. Are you a smoker?
   d. A and B
   e. All of the above

2. You determine that **B.E.** can be immunized today. Which of the following vaccines should **B.E.** receive today?
   a. PPSV-23, inactivated influenza, Tdap
   b. Inactivated influenza, Tdap, MMR
   c. Inactivated influenza, Tdap
   d. PPSV-23, Tdap
   e. Live influenza nasal spray, Tdap

3. **B.E.** asks you if she will need any vaccines in the future. How should you respond?
   a. You will need to get a yearly influenza vaccine.
   b. In 2 years, you will qualify for the zoster vaccine to provide protection against shingles.
   c. When you turn 65 years of age, you will require PPSV-23 and PCV-13.
   d. A and B
   e. All of the above

* Answers can be found online.

Bibliography

Starred references are cited in the text.

American Academy of Pediatrics, Committee on Infectious Diseases. (1999). Poliomyelitis prevention: Revised recommendations for use of inactivated and live oral poliovirus vaccines. *Pediatrics, 103*, 171–172.

*Advisory Committee on Immunization Practices recommended immunization schedule for persons aged 0–18 years—United States, 2015. *Morbidity and Mortality Weekly Report, 65*(4), 86–87. Retrieved from http://www.cdc.gov/mmwr/volumes/65/wr/mm6504a4.htm on February 28, 2016.

*Advisory Committee on Immunization Practices recommended immunization schedule for adults aged 19 years or older—United States, 2015. *Morbidity and Mortality Weekly Report, 65*(4), 88–90. Retrieved from http://www.cdc.gov/mmwr/volumes/65/wr/mm6504a5.htm on February 28, 2016.

Centers for Disease Control and Prevention. (1993). Standards for pediatric immunization practices. *Morbidity and Mortality Weekly Report, 42*(RR-5), 1–13.

Centers for Disease Control and Prevention. (2010a). Updated recommendations for prevention of invasive pneumococcal disease among adults using the 23-valent pneumococcal polysaccharide vaccine. *Morbidity and Mortality Weekly Report, 59*(34), 1102–1106.

Centers for Disease Control and Prevention. (2010b). Prevention of pneumococcal disease among infants and children—Use of 13-valent pneumococcal conjugate vaccine and 23-valent pneumococcal polysaccharide vaccine. *Morbidity and Mortality Weekly Report, 59*(RR11), 1–18.

Centers for Disease Control and Prevention. (2011b). Updated recommendations for use of tetanus toxoid, reduced diphtheria toxoid and acellular pertussis (Tdap) vaccine from the Advisory Committee on Immunization Practices, 2010. *Morbidity and Mortality Weekly Report, 60*(1), 13–15.

Centers for Disease Control and Prevention. (2012). Use of 13-valent pneumococcal conjugate vaccine and 23-valent pneumococcal polysaccharide vaccine for adults with immunocompromising conditions. *Morbidity and Mortality Weekly Report, 6*(40), 816–819.

Centers for Disease Control and Prevention. (2013). Prevention and control of meningococcal disease. *Morbidity and Mortality Weekly Report, 62*(RR02), 1–22.

Centers for Disease Control and Prevention. (2014b). Barriers and strategies to improving influenza vaccination among healthcare personnel. Retrieved from http://www.cdc.gov/flu/toolkit/long-term-care/strategies.htm on October 1, 2015.

Centers for Disease Control and Prevention. (2014c). Use of MenACWY-CRM vaccine in children aged 2 through 23 months at increased risk for meningococcal disease. *Morbidity and Mortality Weekly Report, 63*(24), 527–530.

*Centers for Disease Control and Prevention. (2015a). Retrieved from http://www.cdc.gov/vaccines/schedules/hcp/child-adolescent.html on July 15, 2015.

*Centers for Disease Control and Prevention. (2015b). Retrieved from http://www.cdc.gov/vaccines/schedules/hcp/adult.html on July 15, 2015.

Centers for Disease Control and Prevention. (2015c). ACIP vaccine recommendations. Retrieved from http://www.cdc.gov/vaccines/hcp/acip-recs/index.html on July 15, 2015.

*Centers for Disease Control and Prevention. (2015d). Prevention and control of influenza with vaccines: Recommendations of the Advisory Committee on Immunization Practices, United States, 2015–16 Influenza Season. *Morbidity and Mortality Weekly Report, 64*(30), 818–825.

Centers for Disease Control and Prevention. (2015e). Use of serogroup B meningococcal vaccines in persons aged > 10 years at increased risk for serogroup B meningococcal disease. *Morbidity and Mortality Weekly Report, 64*(22), 608–612.

DiazGranados, C. A., Dunning, A. J., Kimmel, M., et al. (2014). Efficacy of high-dose versus standard-dose influenza vaccine in older adults. *New England Journal of Medicine, 371*, 635–645.

*Hamborsky, J., Kroger, A., & Wolfe, C. (Eds.). (2015). *Epidemiology and prevention of vaccine-preventable diseases (The Pink Book)* (13th ed). Washington, DC: Public Health Foundation. Retrieved from http://www.cdc.gov/vaccines/pubs/pinkbook/index.html on July 15, 2015.

*Hill, H. A., Elam-Evans, L. D., Yankey, D., et al. (2015). National, state, and selected local area vaccination coverage among children aged 19–35 months—United States, 2014. *Morbidity and Mortality Weekly Report, 64*(33), 889–896.

Humiston, S., & Atkinson, W. (1998). Immunization schedule changes and clarifications. *Pediatric Annals, 27*(6), 338–348.

Kobayashi, M., Bennett, N. M., Gierke, R., et al. (2015). Intervals between PCV13 and PPSV23 vaccines: Recommendations of the Advisory Committee on Immunization Practices (ACIP). *Morbidity and Mortality Weekly Report, 64*(34), 944–947.

Malone, K. M., & Hinman, A. R. (2003). Vaccination mandates: The public health imperative and individual rights. *In Law in Public Health Practice* (pp. 262–284). New York, NY: Oxford University Press. Retrieved from http://www.cdc.gov/vaccines/imz-managers/guides-pubs/downloads/vacc_mandates_chptr13.pdf on October 15, 2015.

Marshall, G. (2012). *The vaccine handbook: A practical guide for clinicians* (4th ed.). West Islip, NY: Professional Communications, Inc.

National Vaccine Advisory Committee. (2014). Recommendations from the national vaccine advisory committee standards for adult immunization practice. *Public Health Reports, 129*, 115–123.

*National Vaccine Advisory Committee. (2003). Standards for child and adolescent immunization practices. *Pediatrics, 112*, 958–963.

Opel, D. J., & Omer, S. B. (2015). Measles, mandates, and making vaccination the default option. *JAMA Pediatrics, 169*(4), 303–304.

*Payne, D. C., Staat, M. A., Edwards, K. M., et al. (2011). Direct and indirect effects of rotavirus vaccination upon childhood hospitalizations in 3 US counties, 2006–2009. *Clinical Infectious Diseases, 53*(3), 245–253.

Payne, D. C., Wikswo, M., & Parashar, U. M. (2011). Chapter 13: Rotavirus. In *Manual for the surveillance of vaccine-preventable diseases. VPD Surveillance Manual* (5th ed.). Atlanta, GA: Centers for Disease Control and Prevention.

*Perry, R. T., Murray, J. S., Gacic-Dobo, M., et al. (2015). Progress toward regional measles elimination—Worldwide, 2000–2014. *Morbidity and Mortality Weekly Report, 64*(44), 1246–1251.

*Petrosky, E., Bocchini, J. A., Hariri, S., et al. (2015). Use of 9-valent human papillomavirus (HPV) vaccine: Updated HPV vaccination recommendations of the Advisory Committee on Immunization Practices. *Morbidity and Mortality Weekly Report, 64*(11), 300–304.

*Pickering, L., Baker, C., Kimberlin, D., et al. (Eds.). (2009). *The 2009 red book: Report of the Committee on Infectious Diseases* (26th ed.). Elk Grove Village, IL: American Academy of Pediatrics.

Poland, G., & Johnson, D. (2008). Increasing influenza vaccination rates: The need to vaccinate throughout the entire influenza season. *American Journal of Medicine, 121*(7 Suppl. 2), S3–S10.

Ranee, S., Calhoun, K., Knighton C.L., et al. (2015). Vaccination coverage among children in kindergarten—United States, 2014–15 school year. *Morbidity and Mortality Weekly Report, 64*(33), 897–904.

Trimble, C., & Frazer, I. (2009). Development of therapeutic HPV vaccines. *The Lancet Oncology, 10*(10), 975–980.

*Xu, J. Q., Kochanek, K. D., Murphy, S. L., et al. (2014). *Mortality in the United States, 2012. NCHS data brief,* no. 168. Hyattsville, MD: National Center for Health Statistics.

53 | Smoking Cessation

Tyan F. Thomas

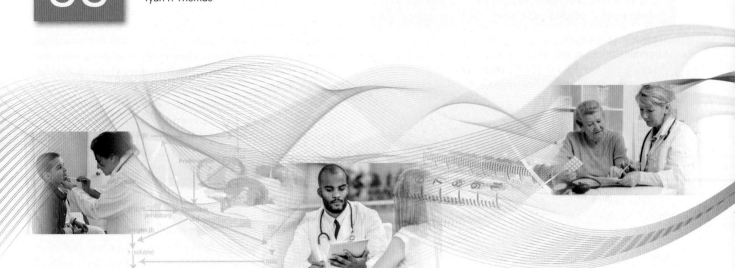

A traditional cigarette is one of many tobacco products. Tobacco products may be categorized as traditional cigarettes or smokeless tobacco. Nicotine is the addictive compound in tobacco products, and it is important to note that nicotine may also be delivered by tobacco-free products, such as electronic cigarettes (e-cigarettes). e-Cigarettes do not contain tobacco but deliver nicotine by vaporizing nicotine-containing liquids. Because the majority of adult tobacco and nicotine users smoke traditional cigarettes, this chapter will focus on cessation of cigarette smoking (CDC, 2014b). **Table 53.1** provides a list of forms of tobacco available in the United States (CDC, 2014a).

Cigarette smoking is a chronic condition. Like sufferers of other chronic conditions, many cigarette smokers cycle through periods of remission (i.e., periods of abstinence from cigarette use) and relapse (i.e., periods of active cigarette use). Similar to other chronic conditions, cigarette smoking contributes to morbidity and mortality and is the leading cause of preventable morbidity and mortality in the United States (U.S. Department of Health and Human Services [USDHHS], 2014).

The U.S. Department of Health and Human Services (USDHHS) estimates that in the United States, cigarette smoking and secondhand exposure to cigarette smoke results in at least 480,000 premature deaths annually. Lung cancer, coronary heart disease (CHD), and chronic obstructive pulmonary disease (COPD) are the three leading causes of smoking-related deaths (USDHHS, 2014). Smoking accounts for a little over 80% of all lung cancer deaths and is attributable to deaths caused by 11 non–lung-related cancers, including oral–pharyngeal and stomach cancers (Siegel et al., 2015). Life expectancy is estimated to be 10 years shorter for smokers compared to lifelong nonsmokers (Jha et al., 2013).

In addition to the variety of cancers, smoking is a major risk factor for cardiovascular diseases, such as CHD and aortic aneurysm, cerebrovascular disease, and peripheral arterial disease. It is estimated that each year, as many as 24% of all deaths related to CHD in American adults 35 years of age and older may be attributable to cigarette smoking (USDHHS, 2014) and that smoking doubles the risk of ischemic stroke (Meschia et al., 2014). Furthermore, smoking increases the risk of acute respiratory infections. It is also a major risk factor for the development of COPD and is estimated to account for nearly 80% of COPD-related deaths (USDHHS, 2014).

In the United States, the total economic burden of smoking is estimated to be at least $289 billion annually, with costs for medical expenditures for care of smoking-related illnesses estimated to be at least $132 billion and costs related to lost earnings and loss of productivity estimated to be at least $151 billion (USDHHS, 2014).

Adverse health effects associated with smoking seem to lessen with smoking cessation. Jha and colleagues found that adult smokers who quit at younger ages gained years of life compared to adults who continued smoking: adults who quit when aged 25 to 34 years gained 10 years of life, compared to 9 years of life gained when quitting from ages 35 to 44 years, and 6 years gained when quitting from ages 45 to 55 years. In fact, adults who quit smoking between 25 and 34 years of age had survival curves similar to adults who never smoked (Jha, 2013).

The CDC estimates that in 2013, approximately 17.8% (42.1 million) of adults in the United States smoked cigarettes, which is down from 20.9% (45.1 million) in 2005 (Jamal et al., 2014). According to the CDC, more men than women in the United States smoke (20.9% of adult males compared to

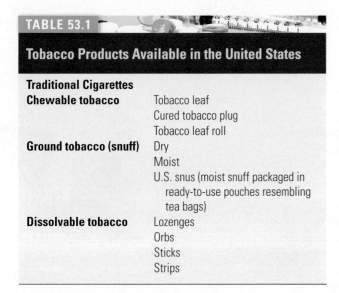

TABLE 53.1

Tobacco Products Available in the United States

Traditional Cigarettes	
Chewable tobacco	Tobacco leaf
	Cured tobacco plug
	Tobacco leaf roll
Ground tobacco (snuff)	Dry
	Moist
	U.S. snus (moist snuff packaged in ready-to-use pouches resembling tea bags)
Dissolvable tobacco	Lozenges
	Orbs
	Sticks
	Strips

15.3% of adult females) (Jamal et al., 2014). Among racial and ethnic populations in the United States, Asians have the lowest rates of cigarette use (9.6%), while American Indians/Alaska natives had the highest rates (26.1%) (Jamal et al., 2014). Smoking rates vary by age group as well, with the lowest rates among those older than age 65 years (8.8%) and higher rates among adults aged 25 to 44 years (20.1%) (Jamal et al., 2014). In 2014, an estimated 24.6% (3.7 million) of U.S. high school students reported on the National Youth Tobacco Survey using tobacco or nicotine products (including e-cigarettes, hookah, traditional cigarettes, and other tobacco products) during the preceding 30 days prior to taking the survey (Arrazola et al., 2015). Use of e-cigarettes was most common, with hookah and traditional cigarettes rounding out the top three most commonly used nicotine-containing products by high school students (Arrazola et al., 2015). While use of traditional cigarettes and other tobacco products has decreased in high schoolers, this decrease is offset by the increased use of e-cigarettes and hookah (Arrazola et al., 2015).

Although nearly 70% of adult smokers report that they would like to quit, only 52.4% will make a quit attempt during any given year, and only 6% are likely to be successful; however, many who attempt to quit smoking do not use recommended cessation methods and most relapse within the first week of quitting (Fiore et al., 2008; Malarcher et al., 2011). Fortunately, most smokers make multiple attempts, and nearly half of users will eventually abstain (American Psychiatric Association [APA], 2013). The U.S. Department of Health and Human Services/Public Health Service guidelines (DHHS/PHS) recommend that all health care professionals, including physicians, pharmacists, nurses, and others, ask about and document their patients' smoking status (Fiore et al., 2008). The 2008 DHHS/PHS guidelines urge clinicians to treat tobacco use disorder as a chronic disease similar in many respects to other diseases such as hypertension, diabetes mellitus, and hyperlipidemia and to provide patients with appropriate advice and pharmacotherapy (Fiore et al., 2008).

PATHOPHYSIOLOGY

Nicotine is the addictive substance in cigarette smoke. It is absorbed and distributed to most tissues of the body, where it binds with nicotinic receptors and produces its physiologic effects on the heart, brain, and other organ systems. Nicotine is a ganglionic cholinergic receptor agonist whose pharmacologic effects are highly dose dependent. These effects include central and peripheral nervous system stimulation and depression, respiratory stimulation, skeletal muscle relaxation, epinephrine release by the adrenal medulla, peripheral vasoconstriction, and increased blood pressure, heart rate, cardiac output, and oxygen consumption (Doering et al., 2014). In addition, nicotine increases dopamine levels in the central nervous system, thus stimulating the reward system and reinforcement of its use (O'Brien, 2011). Activation of nicotine receptors in the brain produces relaxation, decreases stress and anxiety, and improves concentration and reaction times (Benowitz, 2010). Cessation of smoking leads to depressed mood, irritability, difficulty concentrating, and anxiety. Smokers use nicotine to experience the rewarding effects and to avoid the unpleasant effects of nicotine withdrawal.

A common endocrine and metabolic effect of nicotine is weight loss. Smokers tend to weigh 2.4 to 4.5 kg less than nonsmokers (Audrain-McGovern & Benowitz, 2011; Molarius et al., 1997). Additional endocrine effects include increased risk of osteoporosis and earlier menopause (Benowitz, 2008). Finally, smoking alters the liver's metabolic effects by inducing hepatic (cytochrome P-450) enzymes. These effects on hepatic enzymes result in the increased metabolism of certain medications, such as theophylline and acetaminophen, and substances such as caffeine.

DIAGNOSTIC CRITERIA

Chronic nicotine ingestion may lead to physical and physiologic dependence and tolerance to some of its pharmacologic effects. Tobacco use disorder has been defined as a form of substance abuse that can lead to clinically important impairment or distress (American Psychiatric Association [APA], 2013). The key features required for the diagnosis of tobacco use disorder are continued use despite wanting to quit, prior attempts at quitting, persistent use despite the presence of physical illness, tolerance, and presence of withdrawal symptoms (APA, 2013). **Box 53.1** highlights the APA criteria for tobacco use disorder and tobacco withdrawal. Another clinical assessment tool for tobacco/nicotine dependence is the Fagerstrom Test for Nicotine Dependence, which assesses a patient's level of nicotine dependence, in part, by determining the time to first cigarette (TTFC) of the day (Heatherton et al., 1991). Nicotine has a relatively short half-life, and nicotine-dependent tobacco users may experience significant discomfort on waking unless they quickly have their first cigarette (Mallin, 2002). The number of cigarettes

<table>
</table>

BOX 53.1 APA Criteria for Tobacco Use Disorder and Tobacco Withdrawal

TOBACCO USE DISORDER

Tobacco use disorder is defined as a problematic pattern of use of tobacco that leads to clinically important impairment or distress, as demonstrated by the presence of two or more of the following, occurring within a 12-month period:

1. Tobacco is taken in larger amounts over a longer period of time than was intended.
2. There exists a persistent desire to cut down or control tobacco use, or unsuccessful efforts are made to cut down or control tobacco use.
3. A significant amount of time is spent in activities necessary to obtain or use tobacco.
4. Craving, or a strong desire or urge to use tobacco, exists.
5. Recurrent tobacco use results in a failure to fulfill important obligations or responsibilities at work, school, or home.
6. Tobacco use continues despite its contribution to persistent or recurrent social or interpersonal problems (e.g., tobacco use causes or contributes to arguments with others).
7. Tobacco use results in the individual giving up important social, occupational, or recreational activities.
8. Tobacco use recurs in situations that are physically hazardous (e.g., smoking in bed).
9. Persistent tobacco use despite knowledge of having chronic tobacco-related physical or psychosocial problems
10. Tolerance to tobacco exists, with tolerance being defined as either one of the following: (1) the need for a markedly increased amount of tobacco to

produce the intended effect or (2) a markedly diminished effect with the continued use of the same amount of tobacco
11. Withdrawal occurs (see below for characteristics of withdrawal). Withdrawal is manifested by either one of the following: (1) the presence of characteristic tobacco-related withdrawal symptoms; (2) tobacco, or other nicotine-containing products, is taken to relieve or avoid withdrawal symptoms.

WITHDRAWAL

Withdrawal symptoms may be initiated and characterized by the following:

1. Daily use of tobacco for at least several weeks
2. Abrupt cessation of nicotine use, or reduction in the amount of nicotine used, followed within 24 hours by four or more of the following:
   a. Irritability, frustration, or anger
   b. Anxiety
   c. Difficulty concentrating
   d. Increased appetite
   e. Restlessness
   f. Depressed mood
   g. Insomnia
3. The signs and symptoms outlined in item 2 cause clinically significant distress or impairment in social, occupational, or other important areas of functioning.
4. The signs or symptoms are not due to a different medical condition and are not better accounted for by another mental disorder, including intoxication or withdrawal from another substance.

smoked per day and the TTFC both have been shown to correlate with the degree of nicotine dependence. Therefore, the use of the Fagerstrom test may be used (**Box 53.2**) in addition to the APA criteria for diagnosis of tobacco use disorder among smokers.

DEVELOPMENT AND COURSE OF TOBACCO USE DISORDER AND NICOTINE DEPENDENCE

Many teenagers experiment with use of tobacco and nicotine products, and by age 18, 20% use these products at least monthly; many of these individuals will become daily users

(APA, 2013). Commencement of tobacco use after the age of 21 is rare (APA, 2013). Individuals may have some of the APA-defined criteria of tobacco use disorder soon after beginning tobacco use, and many individuals will have a pattern of use that meet the APA's definition of tobacco use disorder by late adolescence (APA, 2013).

Patients who are addicted to nicotine may experience withdrawal symptoms. Onset of these symptoms usually occurs within 24 hours and may last for days, weeks, or longer (Henningfield et al., 2009). Nicotine withdrawal is associated with a well-described syndrome characterized by irritability, awakening from sleep, anxiety, impaired concentration, impaired reaction time, restlessness, drowsiness, confusion, increased appetite, and weight gain (Henningfield et al., 2009; Shiffman et al., 2004). In health care settings, a patient

Write the number of the answer that is most applicable on the line to the left of the question.

_____1. How soon after you awake do you smoke your first cigarette?
3 points: Within 5 minutes
2 points: 6 to 30 minutes
1 point: 31 to 60 minutes
0 points: After 60 minutes

_____2. Do you find it difficult to refrain from smoking in places where it is forbidden such as the library, theater, or doctor's office?
1 point: Yes
0 points: No

_____3. Which cigarette would you hate most to give up?
1 point: The first one in the morning
0 points: Any other cigarette

_____4. How many cigarettes a day do you smoke?
0 points: 10 or less
1 points: 11 to 20
2 point: 21 to 30
3 points: 31 or more

_____5. Do you smoke more frequently during the first hours after waking than during the rest of the day?
1 point: Yes
0 points: No

_____6. Do you smoke when you are so ill that you are in bed most of the day?
1 point: Yes
0 points: No

Scoring Instructions: Add you up your responses to all the items. Total scores should range from 0 to 10, where a score of 6 to 7 suggests a high level of physical dependence to nicotine and a score of 8 to 10 suggests a very high level of physical dependence to nicotine.

TOTAL SCORE: _____

Heatherton, T. F., Kozlowski, L. T., Frecker, R. C., et al. (1991). The Fagerstrom Test for Nicotine Dependence: A revision of the Fagerstrom Tolerance Questionnaire. *British Journal of Addictions, 86,* 1119–1127.

should be asked about his/her tobacco use and responses about use documented every visit. The DHHS/PHS expert panel recommends that tobacco use status be adopted as a new vital sign to be assessed along with blood pressure, temperature, pulse, and respiration rates (Fiore et al., 2008).

INITIATING DRUG AND NONDRUG THERAPY

The DHHS/PHS guidelines recommend that all clinicians aggressively motivate and assist their smoking patients to quit (Fiore et al., 2008). The expert panel's analysis of various studies and trials has found that a wide variety of clinicians can effectively implement these strategies and such interventions as brief as 3 minutes can increase the cessation rate significantly (Fiore et al., 2008). Such interventions should be made by clinicians in patients unwilling to attempt to quit at the time of inquiry because such interventions increase motivation and the likelihood of future attempts (Fiore et al., 2008). The panel reminds clinicians that effective treatment of tobacco dependence now exists and that every patient should receive at least minimal intervention (i.e., as little as 3 minutes of time dedicated to counseling the patient about the benefits of smoking cessation) every time he or she visits a clinician. The first step in this process, identification and assessment of tobacco use status, separates patients into three treatment categories:

1. Patients who use tobacco and are willing to quit should be offered assistance to increase chances of successful cessation and arrange follow-up contact soon after quit date, preferably within the first week after quit date (**Box 53.3**).

Ask every patient about tobacco use and record information in patient's medical record at every visit.

↓

Strongly **advise** every tobacco user to quit, using a personalized approach.

↓

Assess the patient's willingness to make an attempt to quit.

↓

Assist the patient who is willing to make an attempt to quit by offering medication and providing or referring for smoking cessation counseling.

↓

Arrange for follow-up contact within the first week after the quit date. For patients unwilling to make a quit attempt, address willingness to quit at next visit.

Source: U.S. Department of Health and Human Services, Public Health Service, Agency for Health Care Policy and Research. (2008). *Treating tobacco use and dependence: 2008 update.* Rockville, MD: Author.

BOX 53.4 Tobacco Users Unwilling to Quit: The "Five Rs"

Relevance

Encourage patient to discuss why quitting is personally relevant to him or her. Motivational information has the highest impact when it is relevant to a patient's disease status or risk, family or social situation (e.g., having children in the home), health concerns, and other patient factors (e.g., prior quitting experience, personal barriers to cessation).

Risks

The clinician should ask the patient to identify potential negative consequences of tobacco use. The clinician may suggest and highlight the negative consequence that seems most relevant to the patient. The clinician also should emphasize that smoking low-tar/low-nicotine cigarettes or use of other forms of tobacco (e.g., smokeless tobacco, cigars, and pipes) will not eliminate these risks.

Rewards

The clinician should ask the patient to identify potential benefits of stopping tobacco use. The clinicians may suggest and highlight the benefits that seem most relevant to the patient. Examples of rewards include improved health, greater ability to taste food, improved sense of smell, saving money, less smoke-related odors in home, car, clothing, feeling better physically, and improved appearance (less wrinkling/aging of skin and whiter teeth).

Roadblocks

The clinician should ask the patient to identify barriers or impediments to quitting and provide treatment (e.g., problem-solving counseling, medication) that could address barriers. Typical barriers may include withdrawal symptoms, fear of weight gain, lack of support, depression, and being around other tobacco users.

Repetition

The motivational intervention should be repeated every time an unmotivated patient is encountered in a clinical setting. Tobacco users who have failed previous quit attempts should be encouraged by telling them that most people make repeated quit attempts before they are successful.

Source: U.S. Department of Health and Human Services, Public Health Service, Agency for Health Care Policy and Research. (2008). *Treating tobacco use and dependence: 2008 update.* Rockville, MD: Author.

---

2. Patients who use tobacco but are willing to quit at the time of inquiry should go through the five Rs of motivational interventions: Relevance, Risks, Reward, Roadblocks, and Repetition (**Box 53.4**) with the goal to increase motivation to stop smoking.

3. Patients who have quit using tobacco recently should be provided relapse prevention treatment. Clinicians should reinforce the patient's decision to quit, review the benefits of quitting, and assist the patient in resolving any residual problems arising from quitting (Fiore et al., 2008).

Once the diagnosis of tobacco use disorder is made, the next step is to assess the patient's readiness to change (Mallin, 2002). The five-step transtheoretical stages of change (SOC) model are useful for assessing the patient's readiness to quit. The SOC model identifies smoking behavioral change as a process involving movement through a series of five motivational stages (Mallin, 2002):

- Stage 1—Precontemplation: the patient has no intention to quit.
- Stage 2—Contemplation: a smoker is interested in quitting but has no definite plans.
- Stage 3—Preparation: the smoker in this stage is planning to quit within the next month and has made a failed attempt to quit during the previous year.

- Stage 4—Action: the smoker makes a serious effort to quit by modifying his or her behavior and environment. During this stage, the patient has abstained anywhere from 1 day to 6 months. After 6 months of abstinence, the patient enters the final stage.
- Stage 5—Maintenance.

The first step in any cessation program should be to target a quit date with the patient. This date should be identified; otherwise, the patient may never actually make the attempt to stop smoking. In addition, picking a definite date provides the patient with an obtainable goal and avoids overwhelming the patient with the thought of having to change an entire lifestyle.

Nonpharmacologic approaches to smoking cessation consist of various individual and group behavioral interventions, including self-management, group counseling and support, nicotine fading, and aversion techniques (APA, 1996). Behavioral therapy is based on the theory that learning processes operate in the development, maintenance, and cessation of smoking (APA, 1996). The core feature of behavioral therapies is to educate the patient about the benefits of smoking cessation. When used alone, these interventions have low success rates because they do not satiate cravings or prevent withdrawal symptoms. However, patients who are highly motivated or who smoke only a few cigarettes a day may benefit the most from these approaches. The DHHS/PHS recommends combining behavioral therapy and pharmacologic therapy, as the combination yields higher quit rates than behavioral or pharmacologic therapy alone (Fiore et al., 2008).

Self-Management

Self-management techniques are commonly used to make patients more aware of their smoking habits and cues. By becoming more familiar with the environment and events that precede smoking a cigarette, patients may be able to interrupt these patterns by avoiding certain situations. If a relapse occurs, the patient should determine what may have triggered the failed attempt and eliminate those factors. Some nondrug methods to enhance smoking cessation and prevent relapse include getting rid of ashtrays, drinking water and breathing deeply between sips, avoiding places with smoke-filled air, making a dental appointment to get teeth cleaned, exercising, calling on friends or family for support and encouragement, eating a balanced diet, chewing gum or a toothpick, and avoiding the routine that causes craving a cigarette, such as drinking coffee every morning with a cigarette (Mallin, 2002). An analysis of self-help programs showed these programs to be relatively ineffective compared to individual, group, or proactive telephone counseling.

Individual and Group Counseling and Support

The DHHS/PHS expert panel emphasized the strong dose–response relationship between the intensity of tobacco dependence counseling and its effectiveness, meaning that the more intensive interventions are, the more effective they are. Person-to-person contact (via individual, group, or proactive telephone counseling) delivered across four or more sessions seems especially effective in increasing abstinence rates. Two types of counseling and behavioral therapies are recommended by the expert panel to be included in smoking cessation interventions:

a. Provision of practical counseling (problem solving/skills training)
b. Provision of social support as part of treatment (intratreatment social support)

Group counseling programs help to educate the patient on the risks and benefits of smoking cessation. In addition, the patient is presented with strategies to cope with and avoid situations that may lead to relapse. These programs are intended to keep the patient motivated to quit smoking.

Nicotine Fading

Nicotine fading consists of a slow decrease in the intake of nicotine. This can be accomplished by decreasing the number of puffs taken or the number of cigarettes smoked per day or by switching to a brand of cigarettes that contains less nicotine. However, the success rate of this technique is limited because the patient can compensate by inhaling more deeply or for longer periods.

Cutdown to Quit Method with Nicotine Replacement Therapies

Some investigations have shown that the cutdown to quit method may improve sustained abstinence from tobacco (Canadian Agency for Drugs and Technology in Health [CADTH], 2014). This method requires the smoker to reduce the number of cigarettes smoked per day and to supplement cigarettes smoked with a nicotine replacement product, such as nicotine gum. Moreover, this method appears to be less effective than planned, abrupt smoking cessation, but may be an option for smokers who are unwilling to abruptly cease smoking, smokers who failed a previous quit attempt, or smokers who desire gradual cessation from smoking (CADTH, 2014). This method is not endorsed at this time by any U.S. smoking cessation treatment guideline, and no nicotine replacement product currently has the U.S. Food and Drug Administration (FDA) approval for this use.

Aversion Therapy

Finally, aversion techniques have been used to make smoking less desirable to the patient. The first method, satiation, requires the patient to smoke double or triple the usual amount in a short time. In the second method, rapid smoking, the patient must inhale rapidly every 6 to 8 seconds until the cigarette is finished or the patient is nauseated. The use of these methods is limited because of possible health problems and compliance issues. Aversive smoking procedures (e.g., rapid smoking, puffing) have been shown to be more effective than providing no counseling, but this method is not recommended by the DHHS/PHS expert panel.

Other Emerging Approaches to Counseling

Recently, individually tailored materials have been researched. Tailored materials are designed to address variables specific to the smoker, such as letters mailed to patients, or web-based materials such as interactive Web sites. Some components of tailored therapy have been shown to be effective. Computerized interventions via the use of e-health and Internet interventions have the potential to reach a larger portion of the smoking population and are inexpensive to deliver. These computer programs collect information from the smoker and use this information to provide tailored feedback and/or recommendations. However, the most effective features of computerized interventions have yet to be identified, and some Web sites may be confusing and may not tailor information to an individual patient's needs. Stepped care interventions employ the use of low-intensity intervention with progression to more intensive interventions in treatment failures. While each of these interventions is promising, none has been adequately studied to be recommended as standard interventions at this time (Fiore et al., 2008).

A health care professional who merely advises his or her patient to quit smoking is providing at least minimal assistance in the efforts.

Goals of Drug Therapy

All patients attempting to quit should be encouraged to use effective pharmacotherapies for smoking cessation. Long-term smoking cessation pharmacotherapy should be considered as a strategy to reduce the likelihood of relapse (Fiore et al., 2008). As with other chronic diseases, smoking cessation requires repeated intervention and multiple quit attempts (Fiore et al., 2008). The most effective treatment of tobacco dependence requires the use of multiple modalities (Fiore et al., 2008). According to the DHHS/PHS guidelines, clinicians should encourage all patients initiating a quit attempt to use one or a combination of efficacious medications, although medication use requires special consideration in some patient groups (i.e., those with medical contraindications, those who use smokeless tobacco products, pregnant/breast-feeding women, and adolescent smokers; Fiore et al., 2008). Long-term abstinence is the ultimate goal of treatment of tobacco use disorders. Initial goals include moving smokers from precontemplating to contemplating quitting or taking action to quit and actually attempting to quit.

Drug therapy known as *nicotine replacement therapy* (NRT), the most commonly used pharmacotherapy for smoking cessation, aims to control nicotine levels in the bloodstream so that withdrawal does not occur while the patient is adjusting to life without cigarette smoking. The goal of therapy is to maintain the cessation of smoking for a period that allows the patient to develop preventive strategies to avoid relapse.

The primary mechanism of action by which NRT enhances smoking cessation is to obtain plasma levels of nicotine that can relieve or prevent withdrawal symptoms (Benowitz, 2008). The pharmacokinetic effects underlie the concept of nicotine replacement as an aid to smoking cessation, providing that steady-state levels of nicotine can prevent a smoker from experiencing intense withdrawal while not providing the reinforcing peaks achieved from smoking (Le Houezec, 2003). **Figure 53.1** shows the pharmacokinetic profiles of currently available NRT products. Smokers can, therefore, achieve abstinence by dealing with the various behavioral aspects of smoking. Once abstinence is achieved, the smoker can taper of the nicotine by gradual reduction (Le Houezec, 2003).

One benefit of NRT includes not exposing the smoker to the carcinogens and other toxins in cigarette smoke. NRT is approved by the FDA as an aid to smoking cessation for the relief of nicotine withdrawal symptoms when used as part of a comprehensive behavioral program. The guideline panel identifies seven first-line medications (bupropion SR, nicotine gum, nicotine inhaler, nicotine nasal spray, nicotine patch, nicotine lozenge, and varenicline) (**Table 53.2**). Two second-line medications (clonidine and nortriptyline) are also identified for smoking cessation but are not approved by the FDA. The DHHS/PHS expert panel found in research studies that

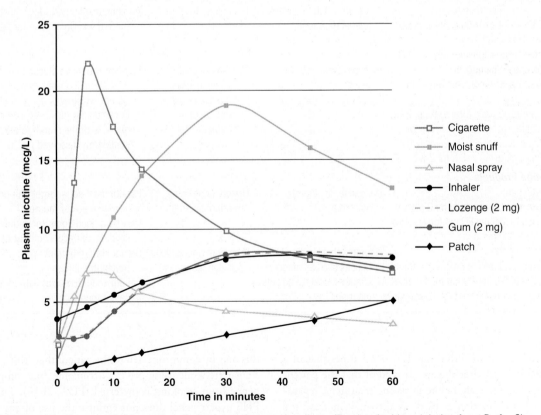

FIGURE 53.1 Pharmacokinetic profiles of nicotine replacement products. (Reprinted with permission from *Rx for Change: Clinician-Assisted Tobacco Cessation* program. Copyright © 1999–2016 The Regents of the University of California. All rights reserved.)

TABLE 53.2

Overview of Selected Agents Used in Smoking Cessation

Generic (Trade) Name and Dosage	Selected Adverse Events	Contraindications	Special Considerations
Nicotine Products			
Nicotine patch (Habitrol and various generic products) ≥10 cigarettes/d: 21 mg for 4 wk, then 14 mg for 2 wk, then 7 mg for 2 wk <10 cigarettes/d: 14 mg for 6 wk, then 7 mg for 2 wk	Cutaneous irritation, GI disturbances, dizziness, headaches	None noted	Patch worn for 16–24 h/d
Nicotine patch (Nicoderm CQ) ≥10 cigarettes/d: 21 mg for 6 wk, then 14 mg for 2 wk, then 7 mg for 2 wk <10 cigarettes/d: 14 mg for 6 wk, then 7 mg for 2 wk	Same as above	Same as above	Same as above
Nicotine polacrilex gum (Nicorette) Start: 2 mg q1–2h for 6 wk 2 mg q2–4h for 2 wk 2 mg q4–8h for 2 wk Range: 1–24 pieces per day	Sore throat, hiccups, undesirable taste	Dentures, temporomandibular joint disease, dizziness	Gum should be chewed until patient feels a tingling sensation, then "parked" between cheek and gum. Repeat chewing every 15–30 min. When given as monotherapy, patient should chew at least 9 pieces each day during the first 6 wks
Nicotine nasal spray (Nicotrol NS) Start: 1–2 sprays in each nasal hourly (one spray = 0.5 mg) Range: 1–40 sprays per day	Nasal irritation, sore throat, dizziness, headache	Hypersensitivity to preservatives Rhinitis, sinusitis	No more than 5 sprays per hour When given as monotherapy, patient should use at least 8 doses each day
Nicotine inhaler (Nicotrol inhaler) Start: 6 cartridges per day; self-titrated to avoid withdrawal Range: 6–16 cartridges per day	Throat irritation, dizziness, headache, cough	Hypersensitivity to menthol	A minimum of 6 cartridges must be used for 3–6 wk. Do not use for >6 mo
Nicotine lozenge (Commit) First cigarette within 30 min of waking: 4 mg First cigarette >30 min after waking: 2 mg One lozenge every 1–2 h for first 6 wk, then one every 2–4 h for 2 wk, and one lozenge every 4–8 h for 2 wk	Hiccups, dyspepsia, dry mouth, and irritation/soreness of the mouth	Those who continue to smoke, chew tobacco, or use other nicotine products	Lozenge should be placed in mouth and allowed to dissolve for about 20–30 min. Do not swallow or chew the lozenge. Occasionally, move the lozenge from one side of the mouth to other until completely dissolved
Nonnicotine Products			
Bupropion (Zyban) Start: 150 mg PO once daily for 3 d, then increase to 150 mg PO bid for 7–12 wk Range: 150–300 mg/d	Headache, dry mouth, insomnia	History of seizures, eating disorders	Patient must set a target quit date the second week of therapy May be a good agent for initial therapy in smokers with concomitant depression
Varenicline (Chantix) Start: 0.5 mg PO once daily for 3 d, then increase to 0.5 mg PO bid for 4 d, then increase to 1 mg PO bid for 12–24 wk	Neuropsychiatric disturbances such as mood changes, anxiety, suicidal ideation	History of anaphylaxis or skin reactions	Do not start in patients with preexisting psychiatric illness Patient should set quit date for eighth day of therapy

the abstinence rate with NRT was 1.5 to 2.3 times that of a placebo at 6 months after therapy. It is ideal that the patient stops smoking completely before initiating treatment, regardless of which formulation is used, as this may increase the patient's risk of nicotine-associated adverse effect and relapse. However, the FDA has found that overlapping use of NRT with an occasional cigarette poses no significant health risks;

this may be communicated to the patient that "slip" with use of a cigarette while using NRT is acceptable, but complete abstinence from smoking is preferred (FDA, 2015). The DHHS/PHS expert panel does not endorse the use of any one NRT over another because of similar effectiveness demonstrated with all products. Patient preference will help guide the clinician's treatment decisions.

Nicotine Replacement Patches

Nicotine Transdermal Patches

Currently, there are two nicotine transdermal systems on the market, and both products are available without a prescription (**Table 53.2**): Nicoderm CQ and Habitrol are available as brand name products and as various generic nicotine transdermal patch products.

Nicoderm CQ varies slightly from other available products in its weaning regimen. The recommended dosing regimen for Nicoderm CQ patches for patients who smoke more than 10 cigarettes daily is 21 mg for 6 weeks, 14 mg for 2 weeks, and 7 mg for 2 weeks. The recommended dosing regimens for Habitrol, for other generic patch products, and for patients who smoke more than 10 cigarettes daily are 21 mg for 4 weeks, 14 mg for 2 weeks, and 7 mg for 2 weeks. For all available products, it is recommended that patients who smoke 10 cigarettes or less per day start at a 14-mg patch for 6 weeks and then decrease to a 7-mg patch for 2 weeks.

All available transdermal products may be worn for 16 to 24 hours and should be applied at the same time each day. Patients who experience nightmares or other sleep disturbances when wearing the patch for 24 hours may be counseled to wear it for 16 hours and to remove the patch prior to falling asleep. Persistence of sleep disturbances despite removing patch before sleeping may signal the presence of nicotine withdrawal. A new patch should then be applied on waking, and only one patch should be applied at a time.

The most common side effects of the transdermal patches include a mild skin reaction with pruritus, burning, and erythema. The skin reactions are usually mild and self-limiting, resolving within 24 hours of removing the patch. Rotating application sites, changing brands, and applying nonprescription strength hydrocortisone cream may reduce the incidence and severity of these events. Transdermal patches should not be used on patients with systemic eczema, atopic dermatitis, or psoriasis because these patients are more likely to develop skin reactions.

The initial patch should be applied immediately on awakening on the patient's targeted quit date. The application site should be clean and dry before applying the patch. The patient should press the patch onto a hairless portion of the upper outer arms or upper chest and hold it for approximately 10 seconds. To decrease irritation that may occur with the patches, the patient should rotate application sites with each new patch. It is common to experience mild tingling, itching, or burning sensations for the first minute after application. If these symptoms persist for more than 4 days, however, the prescriber should be notified and an alternative method should be used.

If the patch gets wet or if it falls off, a new patch should be applied to a different site and then removed at the original time the first patch would have been removed. Proper disposal of the patch is important. After the patch is removed, it should be placed in the wrapper from the newly applied patch and discarded responsibly—out of the reach of children and pets.

It is important to advise patients not to use the patch if they use other nicotine-containing products or continue to smoke or chew tobacco unless informed by their physician. However, the patient may be reassured that health risks appear to be minimal if a tobacco product is used while wearing the patch (FDA, 2015). Instruct patients not to smoke even if they are not wearing the patch because the nicotine in the skin will be entering the bloodstream for several hours after the patch is removed.

Nicotine Gum

Nicotine polacrilex gum (Nicorette) was the first NRT to be approved and is available without a prescription. The patient should chew the gum slowly until he or she senses a peppery, citrus, or minty taste or tingling. Then, the gum should be "parked" between the cheek and the gingiva to increase absorption. This cycle should be repeated with the same piece of gum approximately every minute for 15 to 30 minutes. The gum is more effective if used on a fixed schedule as opposed to an "as-needed" basis (APA, 1996). This may be explained in part by the fact that one piece of gum stays in the bloodstream for 2 to 3 hours. Therefore, a fixed schedule will help to ensure consistent nicotine levels in the blood, and the patient should be advised to chew one piece of gum every 1 to 2 hours (Hukkanen et al., 2005). Chewing at least nine pieces a day during the first 6 weeks of attempting to quit has been shown to increase the patient's chance of success. Most patients should use a 2-mg dose, but a 4-mg dose is also available and may be used as the initial dose in the following:

- Patients with a history of severe withdrawal symptoms
- Patients who smoke their first cigarette within 30 minutes of awakening
- Patients for whom the 2-mg gum failed
- Patients who request it

The initial duration of therapy is 6 weeks regardless of what strength is used. After the first 6 weeks, the patient should be slowly weaned off the gum to avoid withdrawal symptoms. The manufacturer of Nicorette gum recommends that the patient chew a piece of gum every 1 to 2 hours during the first 6 weeks of therapy, then decrease to one piece of gum every 2 to 4 hours during weeks 7 and 8, and then one piece of gum every 4 to 8 hours during weeks 8 to 12. The maximum dose is 24 pieces per day (see **Table 53.2**).

The patient should be advised not to smoke while using the gum; however, the patient may be reassured that a "slip" of smoking a cigarette while using nicotine gum is unlikely to cause harm (FDA, 2015). In addition, food and fluid should not be taken for at least 15 minutes before and after chewing the gum because certain foods (e.g., coffee, tea, carbonated beverages) cause the saliva to become more acidic, consequently decreasing the absorption of the gum. Patients should dispose of the gum and wrapper properly to avoid ingestion by small children and pets.

Common adverse effects of nicotine gum use include jaw muscle aches and fatigue, oral sores, hiccups, belching, throat irritation, and nausea. Some of these events (i.e., hiccups, throat irritation, nausea) result from rapid chewing, leading to excessive nicotine release and absorption. Patient education on the proper use of the gum decreases the incidence of these events.

Nicotine Nasal Spray

The nicotine nasal spray is a prescription product and is marketed under the brand name Nicotrol NS. Compared to other NRT products, nicotine nasal spray has the fastest rate of absorption and thus is the most similar to the onset of the effect that occurs with cigarette smoking (Hukkanen et al., 2005). This formulation may have a role for patients who fail to quit smoking by using the gum or patch or who are highly dependent smokers who require nicotine replacement at a quicker rate than the gum and patch can provide.

Each spray contains 0.5 mg of nicotine, and the minimum dose is 1 mg–delivered as one 0.5-mg spray in each nostril. The recommended initial dosage of the nasal spray is 1 mg (i.e., one spray in each nostril) or 2 mg (two sprays in each nostril) per hour. The dosage may be increased as needed to prevent withdrawal symptoms. The maximum dose is 5 doses (i.e., 5 mg) per hour or 40 sprays per day. A minimum of 8 doses should be used each day to increase the chance of success. After the initial 6 to 8 weeks of treatment, the dosage should be slowly tapered over the next 4 to 6 weeks. No one titration schedule has proven superior; some health care providers may recommend that the patient taper by inhaling half of the dose while maintaining the same dosing frequency used during the initial 8 weeks of therapy or extending the dosing interval (i.e., skipping doses) while maintaining the same dose. Using the nasal spray for longer than 6 months is not recommended because there is no greater efficacy, and the safety of use beyond 6 months has not been well studied.

Before administering the first dose, the patient must prime the pump. This is accomplished by pumping the medication into a tissue six to eight times until a fine spray appears. If the spray is not used for 24 hours or more, the pump must be primed again. Once the pump is ready for use, the patient must follow the manufacturer's directions. For a summary, see **Box 53.5**. The difference between the nicotine nasal spray and other nasal sprays is that the patient must remember not to sniff or inhale while administering Nicotrol NS. If the spray comes in contact with the mouth, eyes, or skin, the patient should rinse the area immediately with cold water to prevent toxicity. The patient must be aware that it takes approximately 1 week to adjust to the side effects.

Common side effects of the nicotine nasal spray include nose and throat irritation, rhinitis, sneezing, coughing, and watery eyes. Other side effects were transient changes in sense of taste or smell, nasal congestion, and transient epistaxis. These events can occur in more than 75% of patients.

Nicotine Inhaler

In 1998, the nicotine inhaler became available as a prescription drug for smoking cessation. The inhaler is thought to improve smoking cessation through two mechanisms: when it is used, it mimics the hand-to-mouth ritual that occurs when smoking a cigarette and it produces a sensation of inhaled smoke on the back of the throat. However, because of the limited evidence, the inhaler is often reserved for patients who have failed initial treatment with other products (see **Table 53.2**).

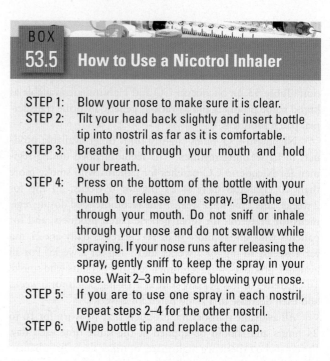

BOX 53.5 How to Use a Nicotrol Inhaler

STEP 1: Blow your nose to make sure it is clear.
STEP 2: Tilt your head back slightly and insert bottle tip into nostril as far as it is comfortable.
STEP 3: Breathe in through your mouth and hold your breath.
STEP 4: Press on the bottom of the bottle with your thumb to release one spray. Breathe out through your mouth. Do not sniff or inhale through your nose and do not swallow while spraying. If your nose runs after releasing the spray, gently sniff to keep the spray in your nose. Wait 2–3 min before blowing your nose.
STEP 5: If you are to use one spray in each nostril, repeat steps 2–4 for the other nostril.
STEP 6: Wipe bottle tip and replace the cap.

The inhaler consists of a mouthpiece and a cartridge. These two separate pieces are pressed together to break the seal on the cartridge. Once the seal is broken, the nicotine-filled air is inhaled into the mouth as a cigarette would be inhaled. The best results have been found when the patient takes shallow, frequent puffs over 20 minutes.

The recommended dose is 6 to 16 cartridges per day. A minimum of six cartridges must be used during the first 3 to 6 weeks of therapy, and therapy should be continued for at least 3 months. After 3 months, the dose should be tapered over the next 6 to 12 weeks. No standard tapering schedule exists; patient and health care provider may devise a patient-specific tapering schedule. Use of the Nicotrol inhaler should not exceed 6 months. Like the nasal spray, the inhaler must be used regularly for 1 week before the patient adjusts to the side effects. Finally, because the cartridges contain high concentrations of nicotine, they should be stored and disposed of in a place that cannot be accessed by children and pets.

The nicotine inhaler is associated with dyspepsia, throat or mouth irritation, oral burning, rhinitis, and cough after inhalation. Patients should adjust to side effects after the first week of continued inhaler use.

Nicotine Lozenge

The newest formulation of NRT is the nicotine lozenge (formerly Commit, now Nicorette), which was approved by the FDA in October 2002 and is available without a prescription. The nicotine lozenge is available in 2-mg and 4-mg strengths. One study found that treatment with the nicotine lozenge results in significantly greater 28-day abstinence at 6 weeks for the 2-mg (46.0% vs. 29.7%; $p < 0.001$) and the 4-mg lozenges compared with a placebo (48.7% vs. 20.8%; $p < 0.001$; Shiffman et al., 2002). Similar treatments were maintained for a full year. Use of more lozenges also resulted in reducing cravings and withdrawal (Shiffman et al., 2002).

The nicotine lozenge helps control cravings by delivering craving-fighting medicine quickly. The lozenge uses a unique method for smokers to determine their degree of physical dependence on nicotine. This indicator is called TTFC. With TTFC, those who smoke their first cigarette within 30 minutes of waking are directed to use the 4-mg strength, whereas those who smoke their first cigarette after 30 minutes of waking are directed to use the 2-mg strength (Shiffman et al., 2002). It is hypothesized that the TTFC is a better method than number of cigarettes smoked per day as a way of identifying patients who are highly nicotine dependent. This is because some patients may not smoke often each day but are physiologically dependent on nicotine since they develop withdrawal symptoms during prolonged periods without smoking (i.e., upon awakening after no cigarette use while sleeping; Shiffman et al., 2002). Utilizing TTFC may allow clinicians to identify more patients with physiologic nicotine dependence and recommend higher, more effective doses of NRT. It is recommended that during the first 6 weeks, an individual should take one lozenge every 1 to 2 hours, for at least 9 days. This dosage is then reduced to one lozenge every 2 to 4 hours in weeks 7 to 9 and every 4 to 8 hours in weeks 10 to 12. The recommended length of treatment of therapy for the nicotine lozenge is 12 weeks. Because it delivers 25% more nicotine per dose, the lozenge may be an alternative for patients who report the presence of withdrawal symptoms with the gum (Shiffman et al., 2002).

The patient should be advised not to eat or drink for 15 minutes before using the nicotine lozenge. The lozenge should be placed in the mouth and sucked on for 20 to 30 minutes to allow the lozenge to slowly dissolve. The lozenge should not be swallowed or chewed. The patient will feel a warm or tingly sensation. Occasionally, the lozenge should be moved from one side of the mouth to the other until it is completely dissolved. Only one lozenge should be used at a time, and patients should not use more than 5 lozenges in 6 hours or more than 20 per day.

The most common side effects of the nicotine lozenge are hiccups, dyspepsia, dry mouth, nausea, and irritation/soreness in the mouth and throat (Shiffman et al., 2002). These effects mainly occurred in patients who chewed or swallowed the lozenge. Patient education on how to properly administer the lozenge can help decrease these incidences. Finally, because the lozenge looks similar to hard candy, it should be stored and disposed properly to avoid access to children.

Nonnicotine Therapies

Bupropion

Bupropion is the first nonnicotine product approved for smoking cessation. The drug has been commonly used as an antidepressant under the brand name Wellbutrin SR. It is available by prescription as an aid to smoking cessation under the brand name Zyban. The exact mechanism of action is unknown; however, it is believed to be related to dopaminergic or noradrenergic properties. In a randomized double-blind, placebo-controlled trial (Dale et al., 2001), 27% of patients who received the active drug were abstinent at 6 months compared with 16% of patients taking a placebo ($p < 0.001$).

The initial dose of bupropion SR is 150 mg/d for 3 days to decrease the incidence of insomnia. After 3 days, the dose can be increased to 150 mg twice a day for 7 to 12 weeks. Dosages higher than 300 mg/d are not recommended because of the increased risk of seizures. Unlike NRT, bupropion SR therapy should be initiated while the patient is still smoking because the drug takes approximately 1 week to reach steady-state plasma concentrations. The patient should set a target quit date during week 2 of therapy. If the patient has not made significant improvements by week 7 of treatment, the attempt is unlikely to be successful and the medication should be discontinued. Additionally, a patient who successfully quits after 7 to 12 weeks of treatment should be considered for continuation of bupropion SR therapy. Tapering the dose is not required when stopping the medication.

The most common side effects of bupropion SR are dry mouth and insomnia. Insomnia may be reduced by avoiding bedtime administration, but the patient must be counseled to allow 8 hours between the 2 daily doses. Other adverse events that can occur include nervousness or difficulty concentrating, rash, and constipation. Seizures have also occurred but are very rare (Dale et al., 2001).

It is important that patients taking bupropion SR participate in behavioral therapy programs that include counseling both during and after therapy. Patients need to be informed not to use Wellbutrin, Wellbutrin SR, or Wellbutrin XL while taking Zyban because these medications all contain bupropion. In addition, monoamine oxidase inhibitors should not be used during or within 14 days of bupropion SR treatment. The interaction between these agents increases bupropion toxicity (i.e., seizures, psychotic changes). Zyban SR should not be chewed or crushed because it will damage the sustained release formulation, which may increase the risk of overdose and adverse events.

Varenicline

Varenicline is the newest approved agent on the market to aid in smoking cessation. It is available in the United States with a prescription under the brand name Chantix. It aids in smoking cessation by binding to a subunit of the nicotinic acetylcholine receptor. When attached to this subunit, varenicline blocks nicotine's binding to the same subunit and blocks nicotine's effects in the brain (i.e., reward, stimulant, depressant affects). Varenicline is also a partial agonist of the nicotine acetylcholine receptor, so it alleviates withdrawal symptoms produced with smoking cessation. In short, varenicline provides patients attempting to quit some of the rewarding effects felt with smoking while blocking the reinforcement effects of continued nicotine use. In one randomized controlled trial, varenicline given for 12 weeks improved successful quit rates during weeks 9 to 12 when compared to a placebo (43.9% vs. 17.6%, $p < 0.001$) and when compared to bupropion (43.9% vs. 29.8%; $p < 0.001$; Jorenby et al., 2006). However, as is the case with many smoking cessation interventions, quit rates during weeks 9 to 52 were lower in all treatment groups but still highest in the varenicline treatment group: 23% varenicline versus 10.3% placebo ($p < 0.001$) and 23% varenicline versus 14.6% bupropion ($p < 0.004$).

To reduce the risk of nausea, varenicline should be titrated over a 1-week period to its effective dose of 1 mg twice daily. The starting dose is 0.5 mg once daily for days 1 to 3, which is then increased to 0.5 mg twice daily for days 4 to 7, and finally increased to the target dose of 1 mg twice daily on day 8. Patients who develop intolerable nausea when taking 1 mg twice daily may have the dose reduced to 1 mg once daily, but a dose titration to 1 mg twice daily should be attempted at a later time. For people with severe renal impairment (creatinine clearance less than 30 mL/min), the starting dose is 0.5 mg once daily, which may be titrated to a target dose of 0.5 mg twice daily. Varenicline should be started 1 week before the patient's set quit date. As with other smoking cessation treatments, varenicline should be given along with behavioral counseling.

The most commonly reported adverse events are nausea, constipation, and abnormal dreams. Other side effects are headaches, difficulty concentrating, somnolence, and visual disturbances. There have been several reports of accidents and near-miss accidents while driving or operating heavy machinery in people taking varenicline, which may have been a result of somnolence and visual disturbances. Patients should be counseled not to drive or operate heavy machinery until they know how varenicline will affect them.

Varenicline use has been reported to cause neuropsychiatric symptoms (e.g., mood changes, psychosis, hallucinations, suicidal ideation, suicide attempts, and completed suicides). Because of this effect, varenicline should not be prescribed to patients with preexisting psychiatric conditions, and patients who experience any changes in mood or behavior or develop suicidal ideation should immediately stop varenicline and contact their health care provider immediately. Recommendations regarding varenicline use in patients with stable depression or previously treated depression may change as more data become available. Anthenelli and colleagues found that varenicline did not exacerbate depression in patients on stable depression treatment (stable treatment = no dose changes to antidepressant for at least 2 months) or patients whose depression was effectively treated within the 2-year period preceding study enrollment (Anthenelli et al., 2013). For now, the recommendation remains that varenicline use should be avoided in patients with a history of psychiatric disorders.

Clonidine and Nortriptyline

Two other nonnicotine products are also available to aid in smoking cessation but are not approved by the FDA for smoking cessation. These two products are clonidine and nortriptyline, which are both available only with a prescription. Clonidine therapy has been examined for use in treatment of nicotine addiction because of its availability to reduce withdrawal symptoms in people addicted to narcotics or alcohol. Clonidine treatment increased the chance of a successful quit attempt when compared to a placebo (odds ratio 2.1, CI: 1.2 to 3.7; Fiore et al., 2008). Clonidine therapy is usually started 3 to 7 days before the quit date. Oral clonidine can be given 0.10 mg orally twice daily initially, and the dosage can then be adjusted as tolerated to 0.1 to 0.75 mg/d administered in divided doses (Fiore et al., 2008). Alternatively, the clonidine transdermal patch can be used at a dosage of 0.1 to 0.2 mg/d. Duration of therapy is for 3 to 10 weeks, during the time acute nicotine withdrawal symptoms would be present. The dose should be tapered over several days in all patients to reduce withdrawal effects from clonidine, but tapering is especially important in patients with hypertension to avoid rebound hypertension and patients with diabetes who may experience relative hypoglycemia (Gourlay et al., 2008). Those with rebound hypertension should not use clonidine. Common side effects include dry mouth, drowsiness, dizziness, and sedation.

Nortriptyline is another second-line nonnicotine agent that has been effective and well tolerated for the treatment of addiction to smoking (Da Costa et al., 2002). Nortriptyline dosage may be started at 25 mg/d and titrated to a target dose range of 75 to 100 mg/d and duration for 12 to 24 weeks (Fiore et al., 2008). It may double the chances of smoking cessation compared to a placebo (odds ratio 1.8, CI: 1.2 to 1.7; Fiore et al., 2008). Nortriptyline is contraindicated in those with risk of arrhythmias. Common side effects include sedation and dry mouth (Da Costa et al., 2002).

The DHHS/PHS guidelines recommend the use of these two products as second-line therapy because they are not FDA approved for the treatment of nicotine dependence and withdrawal and because of concerns with the side effect profiles of these agents.

Uses of Electronic Cigarettes to Aid in Smoking Cessation

A recent systematic review was conducted to analyze published data on the use of e-cigarettes to aid in smoking cessation efforts. The authors concluded that e-cigarette use, when compared to placebo, may improve chances for maintaining smoking cessation at 6 months. However, the recommendation was deemed weak because of the relatively small numbers of patients included in the analysis. There were no observed differences in success rates when e-cigarette use was compared to nicotine transdermal therapy, but this finding may have been the result of small numbers of participants included in the trials (McRobbie et al., 2014).

Because e-cigarettes are not regulated by the FDA, ingredients in various products may be unknown. According to a National Institute of Drug Abuse publication, some e-cigarettes that underwent testing were found to contain formaldehyde, a known carcinogen, and to contain heavy metal nanoparticles from the vaporizing apparatus (National Institute of Drug Abuse, 2014). Use of e-cigarettes should not be recommended to aid in smoking cessation efforts because of unconfirmed effectiveness and potential safety concerns.

FDA-regulated NRT may be considered for the patient who finds appealing the hand-to-mouth ritual associated with the use of e-cigarettes.

Combination Drug Therapy

Although most of the drugs discussed above have only been approved as single pharmacologic agents, combined treatment may be appropriate for smokers who are unable to quit with monotherapy. Three combinations of nicotine replacement have shown to be safe and effective in smoking cessation and are recommended by the DHHS/PHS expert panel: long-term (greater than 14 weeks) nicotine patch + other NRT (gum or spray), nicotine patch + nicotine inhaler, and nicotine patch + bupropion SR (Fiore et al., 2008).

An analysis of three studies showed that compared to treatment with nicotine patch monotherapy, combination therapy with long-term nicotine patch and nicotine gum or nicotine spray doubled smoking cessation rates at 6 months (odds ratio 1.9, CI: 1.3 to 2.7; Fiore et al., 2008). Kornitzer and colleagues studied smoking cessation rates in people given nicotine patch + nicotine gum versus nicotine patch + a placebo (Kornitzer et al., 1995). The group receiving the patch + gum was more likely to have continuously abstained from smoking at 3 and 6 months compared to the group receiving the patch alone (34.2% vs. 22.7% at 3 months, $p = 0.027$; 27.5% vs. 15.3% at 6 months, $p = 0.010$). Incidence of side effects was similar in combination and monotherapy groups. A review of four studies found that combination therapy with nicotine patch and nicotine gum reduced withdrawal symptoms in heavy smokers (Okuyemi et al., 2000). Blondal and colleagues' study results showed the combination of nicotine patch + nicotine spray increased continued smoking cessation at 3 and 6 months when compared to the nicotine patch alone (37% vs. 25%, $p = 0.045$ at 3 months; 31% vs. 16% at 6 months, $p = 0.005$; Blondal et al., 1999).

An analysis of two studies showed that compared to placebo, combination therapy with nicotine patch and nicotine inhaler doubled the chances for smoking cessation at 6 months (odds ratios 2.2, CI: 1.3 to 3.6; cessation rate 25.8%; Fiore et al., 2008). However, this combination does not seem to provide additional benefits over nicotine patch monotherapy. Tonnesen and Mikkelsen found continued abstinence rates were actually lower at 3 and 6 months in the nicotine patch + nicotine inhaler group compared to nicotine patch alone. However, the authors did not report p-values, so we are unable to determine if these differences were statistically significant (14.8% vs. 19.2% at 3 months, 8.7% vs. 14.4% at 6 months; Tonnesen & Mikkelsen, 2000). Adverse events were similar in combination and monotherapy treatment arms. Combination of NRT treatments should be considered for smokers with significant cravings or withdrawal symptoms despite adequate doses of single agents and should be continued for 3 to 6 months (Okuyemi et al., 2000).

Unlike the other combinations previously described, use of combination therapy with the nicotine patch and bupropion is FDA approved. An analysis of three studies showed that compared to nicotine patch alone, the combination therapy with nicotine patch and bupropion increased the chances for continued smoking cessation at 6 months by 30% (odds ratio 1.3, CI: 1.0 to 2.8; Fiore et al., 2008). Jorenby and colleagues found that abstinence rates at 6 and 12 months were higher in the bupropion + nicotine patch group compared to patch monotherapy (38.8% vs. 21.3%, $p < 0.001$ at 6 months; 35.5% vs. 16.4%, $p < 0.001$ at 12 months; Jorenby et al., 1999). Abstinence rates in the combination group were higher compared to bupropion monotherapy, but these differences were not statistically significant. If this combination is initiated, patients should be started on bupropion 150 mg/d for 3 days, then 150 mg twice daily for 1 to 2 weeks prior to quit date. Transdermal nicotine patch therapy should be added starting on the quit date and treatment continued for 3 to 6 months (Okuyemi et al., 2000).

Koegelenberg and colleagues recently published study results showing the combination of varenicline and nicotine transdermal patch to have higher abstinence rates at 12 weeks, compared to varenicline monotherapy (Koegelenberg et al., 2014). This placebo-controlled study included 446 participants and was conducted in South Africa. The continuous abstinence rates at 12 weeks were 55.4% versus 40.9% (OR 1.85; 95% CI: 1.19 to 2.89; $p = 0.007$) in the combination and varenicline monotherapy groups, respectively. Continuous cessation rates were also higher in the combination group at 6 months: 49% versus 32.6% (OR 1.98; 95% CI: 1.25 to 3.14; $p = 0.004$). There were more reports of nausea, sleep disturbances, depression, and skin reactions in the combination group; however, skin reactions were the only adverse effect that was statistically higher than the monotherapy group (14.9% vs. 7.8%; $p = 0.03$). While these results are promising, more studies are needed, and more information about the adverse effect profile with this combination are needed before this combination should be routinely prescribed.

There are also ongoing investigations of bupropion and varenicline combination therapy for smoking cessation. Ebbert and colleagues observed statistically significant differences in long-term smoking cessation (defined as no smoking from 2 weeks after quit date) at 12 and 26 weeks for patients taking the combination of the two medications compared to those participants taking varenicline monotherapy (Ebbert et al., 2014). More patients in the combination group had maintained smoking cessation at 52 weeks, but the difference was not statistically significant. The potential benefit of higher quit rates was offset by increased reports of anxiety and depressive symptoms with combination therapy. At this time, combination therapy with bupropion and varenicline should not be recommended.

Selecting the Most Appropriate Agent

Which therapeutic agent is most effective depends on the patient and the patient's smoking history, among other factors. For a review of the recommended order of treatment and the

TABLE 53.3

Recommended Order of Treatment for Smoking Cessation

Order	Agents	Comments
First line	All nicotine replacement therapies, bupropion, varenicline	There is evidence showing all of these therapies increase abstinence when compared to a placebo. The patch leads to fewer compliance problems, less patient education time, and greater ease of use. Also, the patch provides continuous nicotine replacement without multiple daily dosing, unlike other forms of nicotine replacement (i.e., gum, lozenge, inhaler, nasal spray). It is recommended that the patch be used routinely in clinical practice unless contraindicated or if the patient has failed the patch
Second line	Combination therapy	Combination therapy using the patch plus the gum or the patch plus the nasal spray should be considered if patients fail or suffer withdrawal symptoms with the use of the patch alone. In this case, the patch provides continuous nicotine replacement, and the gum or spray provides relief of "breakthrough" withdrawal symptoms. The patch plus bupropion may also be considered when a single nicotine replacement agent fails. However, data are limited with regard to the efficacy of adding nicotine replacement therapy to bupropion after the patient has failed bupropion monotherapy
Third line	Clonidine, nortriptyline	Because of the side effect profile of these agents, they should be reserved for patients who fail first- and second-line therapies

clinical guidelines for prescribing pharmacotherapy according to the DHHS/PHS guidelines for smoking cessation, see **Tables 53.3** and **53.4** and **Figure 53.2**.

Special Population Considerations

Pregnant Women

Female patients should be monitored for pregnancy because NRT can harm the fetus, and little is known about effects on the fetus with use of bupropion and varenicline Furthermore, no medication intervention has been shown to increase long-term smoking cessation rates in pregnant women (Fiore et al., 2008). The American College of Obstetrics and Gynecology recommends intensive behavioral therapy over medication therapy (ACOG, 2010). If the clinician is considering use of medication therapy for a pregnant smoker, the ACOG recommends that the clinician provides in-depth education about side effect profiles of medications and frequently monitor the patient for adverse effects (ACOG). The nicotine gum and lozenge are classified as pregnancy category C (risk cannot be excluded: animal studies have shown an adverse effect on the fetus, but there are no adequate, well-controlled studies in pregnant women), and the patches, nasal spray, and inhaler are classified as category D (positive evidence of risk: studies in humans or postmarketing have demonstrated a risk to the fetus). Bupropion and varenicline also are classified as category C.

Breast-Feeding Women

No NRT product has been evaluated in breast-feeding women, so it is unknown if these products are excreted in milk. Use of NRT should be considered only if the benefit to the mother outweighs possible harm to the breast-fed infant.

Varenicline has not been evaluated in nursing women, so it is unknown if the product is excreted in breast milk; however, it has been shown to be excreted in milk of lactating animals. For these reasons, the manufacturer recommends to avoid varenicline use in breast-feeding women, unless the benefit to the mother outweighs possible harm to the breast-fed infant. The effects of bupropion on the breast-fed infant are unknown. This agent should be used only if necessary and benefit outweighs risk.

Nicotine replacement therapy should be used with caution in those patients with cardiovascular disease because it can cause tachydysrhythmia and worsen angina. However, the risks are small compared with the cardiovascular effects of smoking. Nicotine concentrations are higher and delivered more rapidly from cigarettes compared with NRT products.

MONITORING PATIENT RESPONSE

Smoking status must be monitored in all patients. As mentioned, patients starting NRT must stop smoking completely before initiating treatment to avoid nicotine toxicity. Common signs of nicotine toxicity include nausea, vomiting, diarrhea, hypersalivation, abdominal pain, perspiration, dizziness, headache, hearing and visual disturbances, confusion, and weakness. On the other hand, patients beginning treatment with Zyban SR or varenicline must set a quit date after the medication has been taken for at least 1 week (1 week for varenicline and 1 to 2 weeks for bupropion SR).

A follow-up telephone call from the practitioner should occur within 1 week after the patient's scheduled quit date. If the patient is aware of the future call, compliance may be improved. In addition, the follow-up call may help

TABLE 53.4

Clinical Guidelines for Prescribing Pharmacotherapy for Smoking Cessation

Who should receive pharmacotherapy for smoking cessation?	All smokers trying to quit, except in the presence of special circumstances. Special consideration should be given before using pharmacotherapy with selected populations: those with medical contraindications, those smoking fewer than 10 cigarettes/d, pregnant/breast-feeding women, those who use smokeless tobacco, and adolescent smokers
What first-line pharmacotherapies are recommended?	All seven of the FDA-approved pharmacotherapies for smoking cessation are recommended, including bupropion SR, nicotine gum, nicotine inhaler, nicotine lozenge, nicotine nasal spray, nicotine patch, and varenicline. The clinician should consider the first-line medication regimens that have been shown to be more effective than the nicotine patch alone—varenicline 2 mg/d or the combination of nicotine patch and as-needed use of nicotine gum or nicotine nasal spray
What factors should a clinician consider when choosing among the seven first-line pharmacotherapies?	Because of the lack of sufficient data to rank order these seven medications, choice of a specific first-line pharmacotherapy must be guided by factors such as clinician familiarity with the medications, contraindications for selected patients, patient preference, previous patient experience with a specific pharmacotherapy (positive or negative), and patient characteristics (e.g., history of depression, concerns about weight gain)
Are pharmacotherapeutic treatments appropriate for lighter smokers (e.g., 10–15 cigarettes/d)?	If pharmacotherapy is used with lighter smokers, clinicians should consider reducing the dose of first-line NRT pharmacotherapies. No adjustments are necessary when using bupropion SR
What second-line pharmacotherapies are recommended?	Clonidine and nortriptyline
When should second-line agents be used for treating tobacco dependence?	Consider prescribing second-line agents for patients unable to use first-line medications because of contraindications or for patients for whom first-line medications are not helpful. Monitor patients for the known side effects of second-line agents
Which pharmacotherapies should be considered with patients particularly concerned about weight gain?	Bupropion SR and nicotine replacement therapies, in particular nicotine gum and nicotine lozenge, have been shown to delay, but not prevent, weight gain
Are there pharmacotherapies that should be especially considered in patients with a history of depression?	Bupropion SR and nortriptyline appear to be effective with this population. NRT also provides some help, but varenicline should be used with caution in this population
Should nicotine replacement therapies be avoided in patients with a history of cardiovascular disease?	No. The nicotine patch in particular is safe and has been shown not to cause adverse cardiovascular effects
May tobacco dependence pharmacotherapies be used long term (e.g., 6 mo or more)?	Yes. This approach may be helpful with smokers who report persistent withdrawal symptoms during the course of pharmacotherapy, who have relapsed in the past after stopping therapy, or who desire long-term therapy. A minority of individuals who successfully quit smoking use ad libitum NRT (gum, nasal spray, inhaler) long term. The use of these medications long term does not present a known health risk. Additionally, the FDA has approved the use of bupropion SR, varenicline, and some NRTs for 6-month use
May pharmacotherapies ever be combined?	Yes. There is evidence that combining the nicotine patch with either nicotine gum or nicotine nasal spray, nicotine patch with nicotine inhaler, and nicotine patch with bupropion increases long-term abstinence rates over a placebo. The use of nicotine patch with either nicotine gum or nicotine nasal spray increases long-term abstinence over the use of a single nicotine replacement product

U.S. Department of Health and Human Services, Public Health Service, Agency for Health Care Policy and Research. (2008). *Treating tobacco use and dependence: 2008 update*. Rockville, MD: Author.

detect ineffective use or adverse events early in the course of treatment. Additional follow-up contacts should occur as needed. If the patient has been successful at the time of the call, the clinician should offer congratulations and additional support. However, if the patient has relapsed, it is important to reassure the patient that it is not indicative of ultimate failure. Many smokers attempt to quit several times before achieving their goal. The reasons for failure should be identified and eliminated for the next attempt, and the patient should be encouraged to try again. Intensification of behavioral counseling may also be warranted. Therapy may be prolonged beyond 3 months if the patient develops cravings or feels he or she may relapse upon discontinuation of therapy. At least one study found that duration of therapy for 6 months or longer was associated with higher quit rates (Stead et al., 2012).

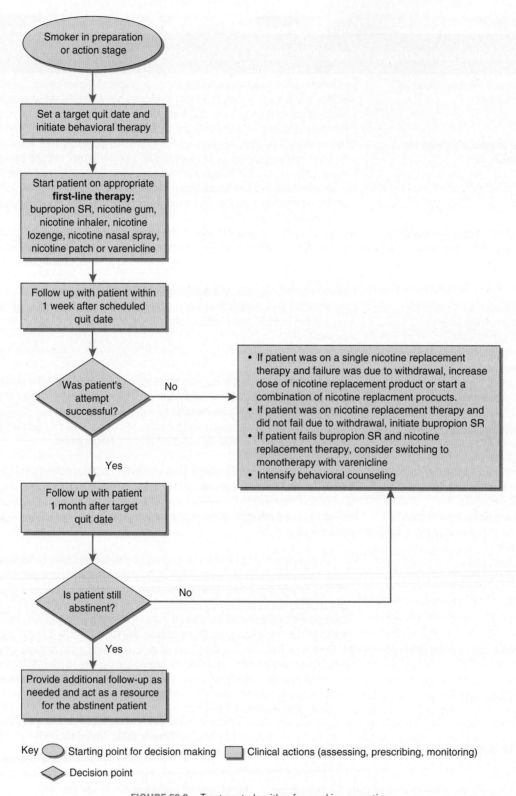

FIGURE 53.2   Treatment algorithm for smoking cessation.

Duration of therapy must be monitored to evaluate if tolerance or physical dependence occurs to NRT. Dependence is most common with the nicotine nasal spray because of its rapid delivery of nicotine. Proper dosage titration and weaning schedule should be monitored as well to prevent withdrawal symptoms from occurring.

PATIENT EDUCATION

The occurrence of adverse events with any medication has a definite correlation with patient compliance. Therefore, it is important that both the practitioner and patient be aware of the common side effects that may occur when using smoking

CASE STUDY*

A.P., a 55-year-old white man, has been smoking 1 pack of cigarettes per day for the last 38 years. He has a very stressful job as executive of a large marketing company. **A.P.** and his coworkers frequently go to "happy hour" at the local bar after a long day at work. When he is at home, **A.P.** has a sedentary lifestyle that consists of lounging by the pool or watching television. He tried to quit smoking "cold turkey" 2 years ago and remained abstinent for approximately 6 months, but has never tried any pharmacologic smoking cessation aids. During his previous attempt to quit, he became very anxious, irritable, and depressed and had trouble sleeping and concentrating at work. He has a medical history of hypertension for the last 10 years and a bout of successfully treated depression 5 years ago after the death of his mother. His family has been encouraging him to stop smoking for years. He is currently at the doctor's office for his blood pressure checkup and inquires about smoking cessation options; he doesn't have a definitive timeline for a quit date.

Smoking habits: He smokes 1 pack per day and describes craving his first cigarette of the day about 10 to 15 minutes after awakening. He has observed that smoking with his morning coffee, smoking when drinking at the bar with his friends, and smoking after meals to be triggers that led to his relapse with his prior smoking cessation efforts. He would like to try something to help with acute cravings.

1. What symptoms experienced by this patient during his previous attempt to quit smoking are consistent with physical dependence to nicotine?
2. What motivational level (stage of change) is this patient in?
3. When **A.P.** reaches the action stage, what pharmacologic options are available for him?
4. Which smoking cessation aid would you recommend starting in this patient? Why?
5. How would your recommendation for smoking cessation aids change if patient reported smoking his first cigarette more than 30 minutes upon awakening?
6. What adverse events could you see with the product that you chose in the previous question?
7. What are some nondrug methods that may enhance smoking cessation in this patient?

* Answers can be found online.

cessation products. In addition, the patient needs to be informed that tolerance to the adverse effects associated with NRT usually occurs.

Weight gain is a common outcome of smoking cessation, and many patients are hesitant to quit for this reason. Many former smokers gain 4 to 5 kg, but as many as 13% gain 11 kg or more (Pisinger & Jorgensen, 2007). The mechanism for this is thought to be a slowing of metabolism. As mentioned earlier, the average smoker weighs 2.4 to 3.0 kg less than the average nonsmoker (Audrain-McGovern & Benowitz, 2011; Molarius et al., 1997). Therefore, with the cessation of smoking, the average former smoker should weigh approximately the same as the average nonsmoker. Patients must be informed that weight gain is possible but not significant. In addition, the health risk of increased weight is small compared with continued smoking. The increase in weight can be addressed after the patient has achieved complete abstinence. If weight gain is a major deterrent to treatment, nicotine replacement therapies, particularly nicotine gum and nicotine lozenge, and bupropion may be used since these agents may delay the weight gain.

Furthermore, patient counseling on the proper use of nicotine products including dose and administration can improve efficacy and safety of the medications. Although the important role of pharmacotherapy is addressed, it should be recognized that a sustained reduction in smoking prevalence will require social desirability of limiting access to cigarettes and increasing availability and use of effective cessation interventions (Stead et al., 2012). Finally, as the effort to promote smoking cessation interventions is sustained, increase in quit rates will be expected as well as an ultimate decrease in smoking-related morbidity and mortality among both children and adults.

Bibliography

Starred references are cited in the text.

*American College of Obstetrics and Gynecologists. (2010, reaffirmed 2013). Smoking cessation during pregnancy. Committee Opinion No. 471. *Obstetrics and Gynecology, 116*, 1241–1244.

*American Psychiatric Association. (1996). Practice guideline for the treatment of patients with nicotine dependence. *American Journal of Psychiatry, 153*(Suppl. 10), 1–31.

*American Psychiatric Association. (2013). Substance-related and addictive disorders. In *Diagnostic and statistical manual of mental disorders* (5th ed.). doi: http://dx.doi.org/10.1176/appi.books.9780890425596.dsm16.

*Anthenelli, R. M., Morris, C., Ramey, T. S., et al. (2013) Effects of varenicline on smoking cessation in adults with stably treated current or past major depression. *Annals of Internal Medicine, 159*, 390–400.

*Arrazola, R. A., Singh, T. S., Corey, C. G., et al. (2015). Tobacco use among middle and high school students–United States, 2011–2014. *Morbidity and Mortality Weekly Report, 64*(14), 381–385.

*Audrain-McGovern, J., & Benowitz, N. L. (2011). Cigarette smoking, nicotine, and body weight. *Clinical Pharmacology and Therapeutics, 9*(1), 164–168. doi: 10.1038/clpt.2011.105.

*Benowitz, N. L. (2008). Tobacco. In L. Goldman (Ed.), *Cecil textbook of medicine* (23rd ed.). Philadelphia, PA: Elsevier.

*Benowitz, N. L. (2010). Nicotine addiction. *New England Journal of Medicine, 362*(24), 2295–2303.

*Blondal, T., Gudmundsson, L. J., Olafsdottir, I., et al. (1999). Nicotine nasal spray with nicotine patch for smoking cessation: Randomized trial with six year follow up. *British Medical Journal, 318*, 285–289.

*Canadian Agency for Drugs and Technology in Health. 2014. *Nicotine replacement therapy for smoking cessation or reduction: A review of the clinical evidence.* Retrieved from https://www.cadth.ca/media/pdf/htis/feb-2014/RC0514% 20%20Smoking%20Cessation%20Update.pdf on June 18, 2015.

*Centers for Disease Control and Prevention (CDC). (2014a). *Type of smokeless tobacco.* Retrieved from http://www.cdc.gov/tobacco/data_statistics/ fact_sheets/smokeless/use_us/types/index.htm on June 20, 2015.

*Centers for Disease Control and Prevention. (2014b). *Smokeless tobacco use in the United States.* Retrieved from http://www.cdc.gov/tobacco/data_ statistics/fact_sheets/smokeless/use_us/index.htm June 20, 2015.

*Da Costa, C. L., Younes, R. N., & Lourenco, M. T. (2002). Stopping smoking: A prospective, randomized, double-blind study comparing nortriptyline to placebo. *Chest, 122,* 403–408.

*Dale, L. C., Glover, E. D., Sachs, D. P., et al. (2001). Bupropion for smoking cessation. *Chest, 119,* 1357–1364.

*Doering, P. L., Doering, L. R., Li, R. M., et al. (2014). Chapter 49. Substance-related disorders II: Alcohol, nicotine, and caffeine. In J. T. DiPiro, R. L. Talbert, G. C. Yee, et al., (Eds.), *Pharmacotherapy: A pathophysiologic approach* (9th ed.). Retrieved from http://accesspharmacy.mhmedical.com.db.usciences. edu/content.aspx?bookid=689&Sectionid=45310500 on June 20, 2015.

*Ebbert, J. O., Hatsukam, D. K., Croghan, I. T., et al. (2014) Combination varenicline and bupropion SR for tobacco-dependence treatment in cigarette smokers. *Journal of the American Medical Association, 311*(2), 155–163.

*Fiore, M. C., Jaen, C. R., Baker T. B., et al. (2008). *Treating tobacco use and dependence: 2008 update.* Clinical Practice Guideline. Rockville, MD: U.S. Department of Health and Human Services, Public Health Service.

*Food and Drug Administration (FDA). (2015). Nicotine replacement therapy labels may change. Retrieved from http://www.fda.gov/ForConsumers/ ConsumerUpdates/ucm345087.htmon June 22, 2015.

Glover, E. D., Glover, P. N., Franzon, M., et al. (2002). A comparison of a nicotine sublingual tablet and placebo for smoking cessation. *Nicotine and Tobacco Research, 4,* 441–450.

Gold, P. B., Rubey, R. N., & Harvey, R. T. (2002). Naturalistic, self-assignment comparative trial of bupropion SR, a nicotine patch, or both for smoking cessation treatment in primary care. *American Journal on Addictions, 11*(4), 315–331.

*Gourlay, S. G., Stead L. F., & Benowitz, N. (2008). Clonidine for smoking cessation (review). *Cochrane Database of Systematic Reviews, 4,* 1–15.

*Heatherton, T. F., Kozlowski, L. T., Frecker, R. C., et al. (1991). The Fagerstrom Test for nicotine dependence: A revision of the Fagerstrom Tolerance Questionnaire. *British Journal on Addiction, 86*(9), 1119–1127.

*Henningfield, J. E., Shiffman, S., Ferguson, S. G., et al. (2009). Tobacco dependence and withdrawal: Science base, challenges and opportunities for pharmacotherapy. *Pharmacology and Therapeutics, 123*(1), 1–16.

*Hukkanen, J., Jacob III, P., & Benowitz, N. L. (2005). Metabolism and disposition kinetics of nicotine. *Pharmacological Reviews, 57,* 79–115.

Hurt, R. D., Sachs, D. P. L., Glover, E. D., et al. (1997). A comparison of sustained-release bupropion and placebo for smoking cessation. *New England Journal of Medicine, 337,* 1195–1202.

*Jamal, A., Agaku, I. T., O'Conner, E., et al. (2014). Current cigarette smoking among adults—United States, 2005–2013. *Morbidity and Mortality Weekly Report, 63*(47), 1108–1112.

*Jha, P., Ramasundarahettige, C., Landsman, V., et al. (2013). 21st century hazards of smoking and benefits of smoking cessation in the United States. *New England Journal of Medicine, 368*(4), 341–350.

*Jorenby, D. E., Hays, J. T., Rigotti, N. A., et al. (2006). Efficacy of varenicline, an α4β2 nicotinic acetylcholine receptor partial agonist, vs placebo or sustained-release bupropion for smoking cessation. *Journal of the American Medical Association, 296*(1), 56–63.

*Jorenby, D. E., Leischow, S. J., Nides, M. A., et al. (1999). A controlled trial of sustained release bupropion, a nicotine patch, or both for smoking cessation. *New England Journal of Medicine, 340,* 685–691.

*Koegelenberg, C. F. N., Noor, F., Bateman, E. D., et al. (2014) Efficacy of varenicline combined with nicotine replacement therapy vs varenicline alone for smoking cessation: A randomized clinical trial. *Journal of the American Medical Association, 302*(2), 155–161.

*Kornitzer, M., Boutsen, M., Thijs, J., et al. (1995). Combined use of nicotine patch and gum in smoking cessation: A placebo controlled clinical. *Preventive Medicine, 24,* 41–47.

*Le Houezec, J. (2003). Nicotine pharmacokinetics in nicotine addiction and nicotine replacement: A review. *International Journal of Tuberculosis and Lung Disease, 7*(9), 809–810.

*Malarcher, A., Dube S., Shaw L., et al. (2011). Quitting smoking among adults–United States, 2001–2010. *Morbidity and Mortality Weekly Report, 60*(44), 1513–1519.

*Mallin, R. (2002). Smoking cessation integration of behavioral and drug therapies. *American Family Physician, 65*(16), 1107–1114.

*Meschia, J. F., Bushnell, C., Boden-Abala, B., et al. (2014). Guidelines for the primary prevention of stroke: A statement for health care professionals from the American Heart Association and the American Stroke Association. *Stroke, 45*(12), 3754–3832.

*McRobbie, H., Bullen, C., Hartmann-Boyce, J., et al. (2014). Electronic cigarettes for smoking cessation and reduction. *Cochrane Database of Systematic Reviews, 2014*(1), 1–57.

McRobbie, H., & Hayek, P. (2001). Nicotine replacement therapy in patients with cardiovascular disease: Guidelines for health professionals. *Addiction, 96,* 1547–1551.

*Molarius, A., Seidell, J. C., Kuulasmaa, K., et al. (1997). Smoking and relative body weight: An international perspective from the WHO MONICA project. *Journal of Epidemiology and Community Health, 51,* 252–260.

*National Institute of Drug Abuse. (2014). *Drug facts: Electronic cigarettes.* Retrieved from http://www.drugabuse.gov/publications/drugfacts/electronic-cigarettes-e-cigarettes on June 19, 2015.

*O'Brien, C. P. (2011). Drug addiction. In L. L. Brunton, B. A. Chabner, & B. C. Knollmann (Eds.), *Goodman & Gilman's the pharmacological basis of therapeutics* (12th ed.). Retrieved from http://accesspharmacy.mhmedical. com.db.usciences.edu/content.aspx?bookid=374&Sectionid=41266230 on June 25, 2015.

*Okuyemi, K. S., Ahluwalia, J. S., & Harris, K. J. (2000). Pharmacotherapy of smoking cessation. *Archives of Family Medicine, 9,* 270–281.

Patterson, F., Jepson, C., Kaufmann, V., et al. (2003). Predictors if attendance in a randomized clinical trial of nicotine replacement therapy with behavioral counseling. *Drug and Alcohol Dependence, 72,* 123–131.

*Pisinger, C., & Jorgensen, T. (2007). Weight concerns and smoking in a general population: The Inter99 study. *Preventive Medicine, 44,* 283–289.

*Shiffman, S., Dresler, C. M., Hajek, P., et al. (2002). Efficacy of a nicotine lozenge for smoking cessation. *Archives of Internal Medicine, 162*(22), 2632–2633.

*Shiffman, S., Dresler, C. M., Rohay, J. M., et al. (2004). Successful treatment with a nicotine lozenge of smokers with prior failure in pharmacological therapy. *Addiction, 99*(1), 83–92.

Shiffman, S., West, R. J., & Gilbert, D. G. (2004). Recommendation for the assessment of tobacco craving and withdrawal in smoking cessation trials. *Nicotine and Tobacco Research, 6*(4), 599–614.

*Siegel, R., Jacobs, E. J., Newton, C. C., et al. (2015). Deaths due to cigarette smoking for 12 smoking-related cancers in the United States. *Journal of the American Medical Association: Internal Medicine, 175*(9), 1574–1576. doi: 10.1001/jamainternmed.2015.2398.

*Stead, L. F., Perera, R., Bullen, C., et al. (2012). Nicotine replacement therapy for smoking cessation: Review. *The Cochrane Library, 11,* 1–231.

Steinberg, M. B., Foulds, J., Richardson, D. L., et al. (2006). Pharmacotherapy and smoking cessation at a tobacco dependence clinic. *Preventive Medicine, 42,* 114–119.

*Tonnesen, P., & Mikkelsen, K. L. (2000). Smoking cessation with four nicotine replacement regimes in a lung clinic. *European Respiratory Journal, 16,* 717–722.

*U.S. Department of Health and Human Services. (2014). *The health consequences of smoking—50 years of progress. A report of the surgeon general.* Atlanta, GA: U.S. Department of Health and Human Services, Centers for Disease Control and Prevention, National Center for Chronic Disease Prevention and Health Promotion, Office on Smoking and Health. Accessed June 1, 2015.

54

Weight Loss

Amy M. Egras

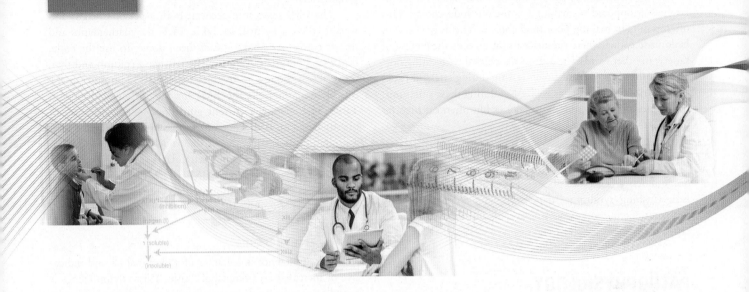

Obesity has reached epidemic proportions, affecting more than 600 million adults worldwide. According to the most recent survey from the National Health and Nutrition Examination Survey (NHANES) for 2009 to 2010, 33.1% of U.S. adults are overweight (body mass index [BMI] from 25 to 29.9 kg/m²) and 35.7% are obese, with a BMI exceeding 30 kg/m².

Since the 1960s, the prevalence of obesity among adults in the United States has more than doubled (13% to 36%) and has more than tripled in children and adolescents (5% to 17%). Looking more closely at the youth, for children and adolescents aged 2 to 19, 31.8% are considered to be overweight or obese, with 16.9% considered to be obese.

CAUSES

The rise in obesity is attributed to physiological and psychological causes as well as social and environmental factors. Overall, obesity is determined by overall body energy stores and the energy balance. When the calories consumed exceed the calories burned, the result is an increase in body fat storage and ultimately obesity. Researchers link obesity to the development of chronic debilitating disease states such as cardiovascular disease, type 2 diabetes mellitus, cancer, sleep apnea, and cognitive dysfunction. Because of these links, the World Health Organization (WHO) and health officials have declared obesity a global epidemic. Additionally, obesity is resulting in a large economic burden. Medical spending for someone who is obese is 42% higher than someone who is normal weight. Overall, the medical burden of obesity is costing the United States as much as $147 billion per year (in 2008 dollars).

Genetic Factors

While genetics is not the primary cause of obesity, it is clear that genetics may predispose people to be obese. In fact, it has been observed that obesity tends to run in families. However, family members share not only the genes but the diet and lifestyle habits that may contribute to obesity. The combination of an imbalance of energy, secondary to psychological/social/environmental factors, plus genetics has created an "obesogenic" environment that results in obesity.

Environmental Factors

Although genetics may play a role in the development of obesity, the environmental influence on both energy intake and energy expenditure is apparent. In regard to energy intake, Americans now live in a world where there is an excess amount of readily available food that is processed (e.g., high in fat and refined sugars) and low in cost. In addition to this, an increase in portion sizes has also contributed to the increase in obesity. Americans are eating more calories than they were 30 to 40 years ago.

On top of the increased consumption of calories is the decrease in energy expenditure. Advancements in technology have moved the American population away from work that demands physical labor to a sedentary lifestyle. This is seen in both the work force and during leisure time.

Psychological Factors

Psychological factors may also influence eating habits. Eating behaviors associated with obesity may include heightened food responsiveness and enjoyment of eating, eating in the absence of hunger, eating disinhibition, and impulsive eating. Other psychosocial issues include heuristic eating, hedonistic eating, and stressful eating.

In heuristic eating, people choose foods based on familiar cues as opposed to making a conscious food choice. This often results in making poor food choices. This is opposed to hedonistic eating where the drive to eat exceeds the feeling of satiety; in other words, the pleasure associated with eating outweighs other factors. And finally, eating during stressful times can contribute to obesity as well. Also, during these situations, people not only consume more calories but often eat high fat or sweets.

Other Causes

Some illnesses can cause obesity. These include hypothyroidism, Cushing syndrome, depression, and some neurologic problems. Certain drugs, such as steroids and some antidepressants, may cause excessive weight gain.

PATHOPHYSIOLOGY

Obesity is more than just a disorder of body weight regulation. If this were the case, it would be easy for people to lose weight. However, losing weight is difficult. This is due to some biological adaptive responses to weight loss. Some of these changes are due to dysfunctional hormonal systems.

Signals from the gut, adipose tissue, liver, and pancreas to the hypothalamus and brain stem control appetite. In particular, peptide YY (PYY) and cholecystokinin (CCK) in the gastrointestinal (GI) tract, and gastric inhibitory polypeptide (GIP) and glucagon-like peptide-1 (GLP-1), which are secreted in response to glucose, signal satiety. In addition to these hormones, ghrelin is an appetite stimulant. And, finally, leptin is an appetite suppressant. Leptin works by inhibiting neuropeptide Y/Agouti-related peptide neurons and activating proopiomelanocortin (POMC)/cocaine- and amphetamine-related transcripts in the arcuate nucleus. This cascade of events leads to decreased food intake and increased energy expenditure. A disruption of this hormonal system, along with reward and emotional factors, is believed to play a role in the pathophysiology of obesity.

Diagnostic Criteria

The main variable in obesity is excess body fat. The best way to measure body fat measurement is densitometry, which determines the density of a body submersed in water. However, the cost and technical requirements limit its usefulness in the clinical setting. The more commonly used measurement of obesity in the clinical setting is the BMI.

Body Mass Index

The BMI is the measurement of choice for clinicians and researchers studying obesity. Besides its simplicity, which eases use in clinical practice, associations have been demonstrated

between BMI and adiposity, disease risk, and mortality. In general, when BMI exceeds 25 kg/m^2, morbidity and mortality rise proportionally.

The BMI takes into account both a person's height and weight (BMI = kg/m^2). In **Table 54.1**, the mathematics and metric conversions have already been done. To use the table, find the appropriate height in the left-hand column and then move across the row to the given weight. The number at the top of the column is the BMI for that height and weight. **Table 54.2** gives the current guidelines for classification of obesity based on BMI. Similar to the weight-for-height tables, a limitation of BMI is that it does not distinguish excess fat from muscle. Therefore, some muscular people may be mistakenly classified as obese using BMI alone. In addition, it does not take body fat distribution into account, which is an independent predictor of health risk.

Waist Circumference

Waist circumference is a marker of abdominal fat and indicative of increased cardiometabolic risk. Waist circumference is found by measuring the circumference around the waist at the level of the iliac crest (just above the hip bone). A waist circumference exceeding 40 inches (102 cm) in men and 35 inches (88 cm) in women signifies increased health risk in those who have a BMI of 25 to 34.9 kg/m^2. It is not necessary to measure waist circumference in patients with a BMI $\geq$ 35 kg/m^2 since it is likely to be elevated and adds no additional information regarding cardiometabolic risk.

INITIATING DRUG THERAPY

Weight loss for those who are overweight and obese can provide many benefits such as prevention of disease and improvements in emotions and function. In fact, even modest weight loss, 5% to 10%, has been shown to significantly improve many health conditions. According to the 2013 American Heart Association (AHA)/American College of Cardiology (ACC)/ the Obesity Society (TOS) Guidelines for the Management of Overweight and Obesity in Adults, those with a BMI of $\geq$30 kg/m^2 or BMI of 25 to 29.9 kg/m^2 with additional cardiovascular disease (CVD) risk factors (e.g., diabetes, prediabetes, hypertension, dyslipidemia, elevated waist circumference) should try to lose weight.

Weight loss requires creating an energy deficit by reducing calorie intake, increased physical activity, and behavioral therapy. All patients recommended to lose weight should be offered a comprehensive lifestyle intervention that involves trained professionals (e.g., registered dietician). A comprehensive lifestyle intervention results in greater weight loss initially and, over the long term, helps minimize weight regain. The lifestyle intervention should include the following:

• Reduced calorie diet: decrease calorie intake by $\geq$500 kcal/d; this is typically prescribed as 1,200 to 1,500 kcal/d for women or 1,500 to 1,800 kcal/d for men.

TABLE 54.1

Body Mass Index Conversion Chart*

Body Mass Index (kg/m²)

19	20	21	22	23	24	25	26	27	28	29	30	35	40
Height (inches) Body Weight (lbs)													
58	91	96	100	105	110	115	119	124	129	134	138	143	167	191
59	94	99	104	109	114	119	124	128	133	138	143	148	173	198
60	97	102	107	112	118	123	128	133	138	143	148	153	179	204
61	100	106	111	116	122	127	132	137	143	148	153	158	185	211
62	104	109	115	120	126	131	136	142	147	153	158	164	191	218
63	107	113	118	124	130	135	141	146	152	158	163	169	197	225
64	110	116	122	128	134	140	145	151	157	163	169	174	204	232
65	114	120	126	132	138	144	150	156	162	168	174	180	210	240
66	118	124	130	136	142	148	155	161	167	173	179	186	216	247
67	121	127	134	140	146	153	159	166	172	178	185	191	223	255
68	125	131	138	144	151	158	164	171	177	184	190	197	230	262
69	128	135	142	149	155	162	169	176	182	189	196	203	236	270
70	132	137	146	153	160	167	174	181	188	195	202	207	243	278
71	136	143	150	157	165	172	179	186	193	200	208	215	250	286
72	140	147	154	162	169	177	184	191	199	206	213	221	258	294
73	144	151	159	166	174	182	189	197	204	212	219	227	265	302
74	148	155	163	171	179	186	194	202	210	218	225	233	272	311
75	152	160	168	176	184	192	200	208	216	224	232	240	279	319
76	156	164	172	180	189	197	205	213	221	230	238	246	287	328

*Each entry gives the body weight in pounds for a person of a given height and body mass index. Pounds have been rounded off. To use the table, find the appropriate height in the left-hand column. Move across the row to a given weight. The number at the top of the column is the body mass index for the height and weight.
From *Understanding adult obesity*. National Institute of Diabetes and Digestive and Kidney Diseases, U.S. Department of Health and Human Services, http://win.niddk.nih.gov/publications/understanding.htm

- Increased physical activity: increased aerobic physical activity for ≥ 150 min/wk (approximately ≥30 min/d, most days of the week).
- Behavior therapy: behavior change program that may include self-monitoring of food intake, physical activity, and weight.

Adjunctive therapy with pharmacotherapy is recommended for patients with a BMI > 30 kg/m² or BMI ≥ 27 kg/m² with comorbidity (e.g., type 2 diabetes, hypertension, dyslipidemia, CVD, nonalcoholic fatty liver disease, osteoarthritis,

TABLE 54.2

Classification of Obesity by Body Mass Index (BMI)

	BMI (kg/m²)
Underweight	<18.5
Normal	18.5–24.9
Overweight	25.0–29.9
Obesity, class	
I	30.0–34.9
II	35.0–39.9
III (extreme)	≥40

major depression, sleep apnea) who are unable to successfully lose weight or sustain weight loss (**Table 54.3**). Furthermore, for those patients with a BMI ≥ 40 kg/m² or BMI ≥ 35 kg/m² with a comorbidity, who have not been able to successfully lose weight with behavioral therapy (with or without pharmacotherapy) may be candidates for bariatric surgery.

Goals of Drug Therapy

Goals of therapy are to reduce body weight and maintain a lower body weight for the long term. A weight loss program that consists of diet, physical activity, and behavior therapy interventions typically results in a 5% to 10% weight loss in the first 6 months. However, it is important to note that sustained weight loss of even 3% to 5% can lead to beneficial effects such as reductions in triglycerides, blood glucose, hemoglobin A1C, and the risk of developing type 2 diabetes. Greater weight loss results in even greater benefits such as decreases in blood pressure, improvements in plasma lipid profiles, and the decreased need for medications to treat chronic conditions such as hypertension, dyslipidemia, and diabetes.

In order to achieve weight loss, patients should be recommended to initiate a comprehensive lifestyle intervention that includes dietary, physical activity, and behavioral therapy. However, weight loss is difficult for most patients. The addition

TABLE 54.3

Overview of Agents Prescribed for Weight Loss

Generic (Trade) Name and Dosage	Selected Adverse Events	Contraindications	Special Considerations
Appetite Suppressants			
diethylpropion (Tenuate) Start: 25 mg TID (immediate release) or 75 mg daily (controlled release)	Increased heart rate, increased blood pressure, insomnia, tremor, and headache	Advanced atherosclerosis, uncontrolled hypertension, pulmonary hypertension, hyperthyroidism, and glaucoma Approved for those aged >16 years old	Schedule IV drug
phendimetrazine (Bontril) Tablet: 17.5–35 mg 2 or 3 times daily, 1 h before meals (maximum 70 mg TID) Capsule: 105 mg every morning before breakfast	Same as above	Same as above Approved for those aged >17 years old	Schedule III drug
phentermine (Adipex-P, Suprenza) Capsule/tablet: 15–37.5 mg daily in 1–2 divided doses ODT: 15–37.5 mg every morning	Same as above	Same as above Approved for those aged >16 years old	Schedule IV drug
Lipase Inhibitor			
orlistat (Xenical, Alli) Rx: 120 mg tid with meals OTC: 60 mg tid with meals	Oily spotting, flatus with discharge, fecal urgency, and fatty/oily stool	Chronic malabsorption syndrome or cholestasis Safety in people <12 y not established	May decrease absorption of fat-soluble vitamins (A, D, E, K)
Serotonin 5-HT$_{2c}$ Receptor Agonist			
lorcaserin (Belviq) 10 mg BID	Headache, nausea, dry mouth, dizziness, fatigue, constipation, and mood changes	SSRIs, SNRIs, MAOIs, triptans, and bupropion	Schedule IV drug
Glucagon-Like Peptide-1 Receptor Agonist			
liraglutide (Saxenda) Start: 0.6 mg subcutaneously once daily; titrate up weekly to target dose of 3 mg subcutaneously daily	Nausea, vomiting, diarrhea, constipation, and pancreatitis	Medullary thyroid cancer and multiple endocrine neoplasia type 2	
Combination			
Phentermine ER/topiramate Start: phentermine ER 3.75 mg/topiramate 23 mg once daily (maximum phentermine ER 15 mg/topiramate 92 mg once daily)	Increased heart rate, insomnia, dry mouth, constipation, paresthesia, dizziness, and dysgeusia	MAOIs, hyperthyroidism, and glaucoma	Schedule IV drug
Naltrexone/bupropion Start: naltrexone 8 mg/bupropion 90 mg once daily (maximum naltrexone 32 mg/bupropion 360 mg once daily)	Increased heart rate, increased blood pressure, nausea, constipation, headache, vomiting, and dizziness	MAOIs, uncontrolled hypertension, seizure disorders, bulimia or anorexia nervosa, and drug or alcohol withdrawal	Boxed warning: suicidal ideation and serious neuropsychiatric events

of weight loss medications may actually help with adherence to behavior change by helping to create the negative energy balance needed for weight loss. In turn, this increased weight loss may potentially have positive cardiometabolic benefits as mentioned previously. However, weight loss medications should be used in combination to lifestyle changes; they do not "work on their own." It should also be noted that they also do not change the underlying physiology of weight regulation. Therefore, gradual weight gain typically occurs when the medications are stopped. Keeping this in mind, it is important to note that, previously, most weight loss medications were only approved for short-term use. Over the past several years, there have been several medications approved for chronic weight management.

Stimulants

These agents are not widely used in the treatment of obesity primarily because of their high risk of abuse and high risk of cardiovascular side effects. As Schedule II (C-II) agents, there are often restrictions on the amount and duration of therapy, and some states even prohibit these drugs from being prescribed for weight loss. These medications are not recommended. The only medication in this class is methamphetamine (Desoxyn).

Appetite Suppressants

The nonamphetamine derivatives are considered appetite suppressants. Other terms for these nonamphetamine agents include *anorexiants*. These agents (see **Table 54.3**) include diethylpropion (Tenuate) extended release (ER) or immediate release, phendimetrazine (Bontril PDM), and phentermine (Adipex-P, Suprenza oral-disintegrating tablet [ODT]). They are considered adjuncts to a comprehensive weight management program. The effects of these agents are often short lived because tolerance may develop to the anorexigenic effect after a few weeks. They are only approved for short-term use.

Mechanism of Action

The mechanism of action of appetite suppressants works to decrease appetite by stimulating the hypothalamus to release catecholamines, specifically norepinephrine. The drugs are considered short-acting agents and are often dosed three times daily but are also formulated in extended-release products for once-daily dosing. The dosing varies by individual response, but it is recommended to start at the lowest dose and increase based on weight loss and tolerance of adverse events.

Contraindications

All of these agents have a potential for abuse, and as such are classified as Schedule III (C-III) or IV (C-IV) drugs. Caution should be used when prescribing these agents in patients with a history of substance abuse.

Because they lead to increased levels of norepinephrine, these agents can result in elevations of blood pressure and heart rate. Therefore, they are contraindicated in patients with advanced atherosclerosis, uncontrolled hypertension, pulmonary hypertension, hyperthyroidism, and glaucoma. In addition, patients taking monoamine oxidase (MAO) inhibitors should not take these medications due to the potential increase in blood pressure that could lead to hypertensive crisis.

Adverse Events

Adverse events include central nervous system (CNS) stimulation such as insomnia, tremor, and headache. Overstimulation may result in an impairment of ability to perform activities requiring mental alertness (e.g., driving or operating heavy machinery). Occasionally, urinary frequency, blurred vision, and changes in libido may occur.

Other adverse effects include dry mouth and nausea as well as cardiovascular effects such as increases in blood pressure and tachycardia. For this reason, blood pressure and heart rate should be monitored on a biweekly or monthly basis and even more frequently in patients with preexisting hypertension.

Lipase Inhibitor: Orlistat

Orlistat (Xenical, Alli) differs from previously available weight loss medications in that it works nonsystemically, acting locally in the GI tract. Orlistat is a GI lipase inhibitor that facilitates weight loss by lowering the absorption of dietary fat, on average by 30%. In research, orlistat users saw small but significant drops in their total cholesterol, LDL, blood pressure, and blood sugar and insulin levels.

Dosage

Orlistat is available as a prescription or OTC medication. Prescription orlistat (Xenical) should be administered at a dose of 120 mg three times a day, while OTC orlistat (Alli) should be administered at a dose of 60 mg three times a day. The doses should be taken during or up to 1 hour after a meal containing fat. The meal should contain less than 30% fat, and orlistat should not be taken with a meal containing no fat. The maximum daily dose is 360 mg/d. A primary concern with the use of orlistat is the potential for decreased absorption of the fat-soluble vitamins A, D, E, and K. Multivitamins should be taken by all patients taking orlistat, and these should be separated from the orlistat by 2 or more hours to ensure vitamin absorption.

Contraindications/Precautions

Orlistat is contraindicated in patients with chronic malabsorption syndrome or cholestasis. In addition, orlistat is not indicated in patients younger than age 12.

Adverse Events

Because orlistat is not absorbed, the primary side effects of orlistat include diarrhea, fatty stools, and flatulence. Patients should be advised of this because the fatty stools may appear as an oily leakage, particularly after flatus, and may cause embarrassment. Nausea and abdominal pain may also occur. GI effects associated with orlistat worsen with the more fat the dieter eats. However, data suggest that concomitant administration of natural fiber (psyllium mucilloid) may significantly reduce the self-reported frequency and severity of GI side effects associated with orlistat. Caution should be used in patients taking oral warfarin (Coumadin) because orlistat may inhibit the absorption of vitamin K, resulting in an increased international normalized ratio (INR). In addition, orlistat may decrease the serum concentration of the following medications: amiodarone, cyclosporine, levothyroxine, and anticonvulsants. For amiodarone and anticonvulsants, these should be administered 2 hours before or 2 hours after the orlistat dose; cyclosporine should be dosed 3 hours after orlistat; and levothyroxine and orlistat should be dosed at least 4 hours apart.

Rarely, orlistat can result in hepatotoxicity. Patients should be advised to stop using orlistat and contact their health care provider if they experience any signs or symptoms of liver injury, such as fatigue, fever, jaundice, brown urine, nausea, vomiting, and abdominal pain.

Serotonin 5-HT$_{2c}$ Receptor Agonist: Lorcaserin

Lorcaserin (Belviq) is a serotonin 5-HT$_{2c}$ receptor agonist approved for weight loss in conjunction with comprehensive lifestyle changes.

Mechanism of Action

Lorcaserin works by acting on the serotonin 5-HT$_{2c}$ receptors. This stimulation activates pro-opiomelanocortin (POMC) neurons in the arcuate nucleus. This results in the feeling of satiety and decreased food intake.

Dosage

Although low, lorcaserin does have a potential for abuse, and as such is classified as a Schedule IV (C-IV) drug. Lorcaserin should be administered 10 mg by mouth twice daily.

Contraindications/Precautions

Lorcaserin should be used in caution with patients taking the following medications: selective serotonin reuptake inhibitors (SSRIs), serotonin norepinephrine reuptake inhibitors (SNRIs), MAOI, serotonin 5-HT$_{1B,1D}$ receptor agonists (triptans), and bupropion due to the risk of serotonin syndrome. If patient has signs and symptoms of serotonin syndrome, such as tremor, myoclonus, and agitation, discontinue treatment immediately.

Adverse Events

The most common side effects of lorcaserin include headache, nausea, dry mouth, dizziness, fatigue, and constipation. In addition, due to some of the CNS side effects, patients should use caution when performing things that may require alertness such as driving and patients should monitor signs of mood changes that may indicate depression.

While hematological side effects such as leukopenia or anemia are rare, it is recommended to monitor complete blood cell counts (CBC) during use. Hyperprolactinemia has been reported and prolactin levels should be monitored if patient experiences any signs or symptoms such as galactorrhea or gynecomastia. Finally, men have experienced priapism. If a patient experiences an erection for greater than 4 hours, he should discontinue use of lorcaserin and seek medical attention.

Glucagon-Like Peptide-1 Receptor Agonist: Liraglutide

Liraglutide (Saxenda) is a GLP-1 receptor agonist, which is a medication also used for type 2 diabetes (Victoza) and was approved by the U.S. FDA in 2014 for weight loss in conjunction with comprehensive lifestyle changes. As with other pharmacologic agents approved for weight loss, a risk evaluation and mitigation strategy (REMS) was issued due to the serious potential side effects of thyroid medullary cancer and acute pancreatitis.

Mechanism of Action

Liraglutide is a GLP-1 receptor agonist, which influences diabetes by stimulating glucose-dependent insulin secretion, decreases glucagon secretion, and slows gastric emptying. As it relates to weight loss, liraglutide also activates the POMC neurons, which results in the feeling of satiety and decreased food intake.

Dosage

Liraglutide should be titrated up over the course of 5 weeks to help minimize GI side effects. Liraglutide is dosed as 0.6 mg subcutaneously once daily for a week; then, the dose is increased by 0.6 mg subcutaneously daily at weekly intervals until the target dose of 3 mg subcutaneously daily is achieved. If the 3-mg dose cannot be achieved, then the medication should be discontinued as it has not shown efficacy at lower doses.

Contraindications/Precautions

Liraglutide has boxed warning for the potential of medullary thyroid cancer (MTC) and multiple endocrine neoplasia type 2. Both of these conditions were observed in animal studies. However, patients with a history of either of these conditions should not use liraglutide.

Adverse Events

The most common side effects experienced with liraglutide are nausea, vomiting, diarrhea, and/or constipation. The dose is titrated up at weekly intervals to help minimize these side effects. In addition to these side effects, patients have reported headache and increased heart rate. Liraglutide has been associated with pancreatitis and patients should be monitored for this.

Combination Medications

Phentermine Extended Release/Topiramate

Phentermine ER/topiramate (Qsymia) is a medication that is a combination of low-dose phentermine ER, an anorexiant medication (see above), and topiramate, an anticonvulsant medication. This medication was approved by the U.S. Food and Drug Administration (FDA) (2012) for weight loss in conjunction with comprehensive lifestyle changes. In 2014, additional REMS for Qsymia was issued to inform prescribers and female patients about teratogenic effects of the drug during pregnancy. While the drug is still available, providers must go through special training to prescribe the drug.

Mechanism of Action

As mentioned previously, the mechanism of action of phentermine works to decrease appetite by stimulating the hypothalamus to release catecholamines, specifically norepinephrine. While the mechanism of action in regard to weight loss for topiramate is not fully understood, it is believed to be due to the enhancement of gamma-aminobutyric acid (GABA) and the inhibition of kainite/alpha-amino-3-hydroxy-5-methyl-4-isoxazole propionic acid (AMPA) glutamate, which results in appetite suppression.

Dosage

Although low, phentermine ER/topiramate does have a potential for abuse, and as such is classified as a Schedule IV (C-IV) drug. Phentermine ER/topiramate should be titrated up over several weeks. The starting dose is phentermine ER 3.75 mg/topiramate 23 mg once daily for 2 weeks. If the patient is tolerating this dose, then it can be increased to phentermine ER 7.5 mg/topiramate 46 mg once daily for 12 weeks and then evaluate weight loss. If after 12 weeks, 3% of baseline body weight has not been lost, then the medication can be increased to phentermine ER 11.25 mg/topiramate 69 mg once daily for 2 weeks and then to phentermine ER 15 mg/topiramate 92 mg once daily.

Contraindications/Precautions

Phentermine ER/topiramate is contraindicated in patients with hyperthyroidism and glaucoma. In addition, patients taking MAO inhibitors should not take these medications due to the potential increase in blood pressure that could lead to hypertensive crisis. Women who are taking Qsymia and become pregnant must immediately stop the drug.

Adverse Events

The most common side effects experienced with phentermine ER/topiramate are increased heart rate, insomnia, dry mouth, constipation, paresthesia, dizziness, and dysgeusia. Due to the carbonic anhydrase inhibition of this medication, electrolytes should be monitored for hypokalemia and metabolic acidosis, and patients should be cautioned to monitor closely during strenuous exercise or extreme heat for signs of hyperthermia. In addition, be aware of any changes in behavior that may indicate any cognitive dysfunction or psychiatric disturbances. Due to the topiramate component, this medication should be withdrawn gradually as there is an increased risk of seizures with abrupt discontinuation.

Naltrexone/Bupropion

Naltrexone/bupropion (Contrave) is a medication that is a combination of naltrexone, an opioid antagonist, and bupropion, a dopamine/norepinephrine reuptake inhibitor. This medication was approved by the U.S. Food and Drug Administration in 2014 for weight loss in conjunction with comprehensive lifestyle changes.

Mechanism of Action

The exact mechanism of action of the naltrexone/bupropion combination is not fully understood. However, it is believed that together, they stimulate the POMC neurons that lead to appetite suppression.

Dosage

Naltrexone/bupropion should be titrated up over several weeks. The starting dose is naltrexone 8 mg/bupropion 90 mg to take one tablet by mouth in the morning for 1 week. Starting week 2, increase dose to 1 tablet by mouth in the morning and 1 tablet by mouth with dinner. At week 3, increase dose to 2 tablets by mouth in the morning and 1 tablet by mouth with dinner. At week 4, increase dose to 2 tablets by mouth in the morning and 2 tablets by mouth with dinner. The final target dose should be naltrexone 16 mg/bupropion 180 mg by mouth twice a day. If a patient is taking a medication that is a CYP2B6 inhibitor such as ticlopidine or clopidogrel, then the maximum dose should be naltrexone 8 mg/bupropion 90 mg by mouth twice daily.

Contraindications/Precautions

Naltrexone/bupropion is contraindicated in patients with uncontrolled hypertension, seizure disorders, bulimia or anorexia nervosa, and drug or alcohol withdrawal. In opioid-dependent patients, naltrexone/bupropion may precipitate acute withdrawal; patients should be opioid free for 7 to 10 days before starting naltrexone/bupropion. In addition, patients taking MAO inhibitors should not take these medications due to the potential increase in blood pressure that could lead to hypertensive crisis; do not start naltrexone/bupropion in a patient receiving linezolid or intravenous methylene blue.

Naltrexone/bupropion has a boxed warning for the potential suicidal ideation and serious neuropsychiatric events. Patients should be monitored for severe psychiatric changes such as depression or mania, psychosis, hallucinations, hostility, anxiety, and suicidal ideation or attempt.

Adverse Events

The most common side effects experienced with naltrexone/bupropion are nausea, constipation, headache, vomiting, and dizziness. In addition, use caution in patients with cardiovascular disease due to the potential increase in heart rate and blood pressure.

Other Medications

Some antidepressant, antiseizure, and diabetes medications have been studied for use in weight loss. The use of these medications for weight loss is considered an "off-label" use.

Anticonvulsant medications: Zonisamide (Zonegran) is an anticonvulsant medication that has resulted in weight loss. However, adverse effects of the medication seem to be limiting.

TABLE 54.4

Dietary Supplements for Weight Loss

Name	Selected Adverse Events
Bitter orange	Increased heart rate and blood pressure
Chitosan	Well tolerated: gastrointestinal side effects
Chromium	Well tolerated: gastrointestinal side effects
Conjugate linoleic acid	Dyspepsia, constipation, diarrhea
Green coffee extract	Anxiety, insomnia, agitation
Green tea extract	Insomnia, agitation, nausea, vomiting, bloating, diarrhea
Guar gum	Abdominal pain, gas, bloating
Hoodia	Headache, dizziness, nausea, vomiting
Raspberry ketone	Unknown

Diabetes medications: Metformin (Glucophage) has demonstrated the ability to help people with type 2 diabetes and obesity lose weight. In addition, pramlintide (Symlin), an amylin analog, has also demonstrated weight loss.

Alternative Medications

There are many over-the-counter weight loss products on the market. The only nonprescription product, which is regulated by the Food and Drug Administration (FDA), is orlistat (Alli), which was discussed previously. All other products on the market are dietary supplements. The manufacturer of the dietary supplement is responsible for making sure their product is safe; however, they are not reviewed by the FDA. Many of the weight loss supplements on the market do not have a lot of evidence to support their claim of weight loss. See **Table 54.4** for a summary of some of the most common dietary supplements available on the market.

Drugs That Cause Weight Gain

In addition to considering whether or not an overweight or obese patient should be started on weight loss medication, it is also important to assess their current medication profile to see if they are taking any medications that may be associated with weight gain. Whenever possible, it is recommended to use an alternative medication that may not be associated with weight gain. However, if there is no acceptable therapeutic alternative, it is advised to try and use the lowest dose to achieve the desired clinical outcome. See **Table 54.5** for a list of drugs that may cause weight gain and potential alternatives.

Selecting the Most Appropriate Agent

The selection of the most appropriate agent for treating an obese patient depends on a number of factors. In particular, the provider should use a patient-centered approach to

TABLE 54.5

Drugs That May Cause Weight Gain

Medical Condition	Drug Class or Name	Alternative Medications
Type 2 diabetes	Insulin Sulfonylureas Glitinides Thiazolidinediones	Metformin (Glucophage) Pramlintide (Symlin) GLP-1 receptor agonists
Hypertension	β-Adrenergic blockers	ACE inhibitors ARBs Calcium channel blockers
Depression	Paroxetine (Paxil) Amitriptyline Mirtazapine (Remeron)	Fluoxetine (Prozac) Sertraline (Zoloft) Citalopram (Celexa) Escitalopram (Lexapro) Bupropion (Wellbutrin)
Psychiatric disorders	Clozapine Olanzapine (Zyprexa) Quetiapine (Seroquel) Risperidone (Risperdal)	Ziprasidone (Geodon) Aripiprazole (Abilify)
Chronic inflammatory diseases (e.g., rheumatoid arthritis)	Corticosteroids	Nonsteroidal anti-inflammatory drugs Disease-modifying antirheumatic drugs

determine which medication would be best for a patient. The provider should assess the patient's other health conditions and consider both potential contraindications and benefits of certain medications as it pertains to weight loss. For example, a patient with underlying cardiovascular disease or uncontrolled hypertension would not be a good candidate for any medication that increases heart rate or blood pressure such as phentermine, phentermine ER/topiramate, or naltrexone/bupropion. On the other hand, a patient with uncontrolled type 2 diabetes may benefit from the addition of liraglutide as it may help with blood glucose control in addition to weight loss.

Finally, as mentioned previously, all pharmacotherapeutic treatment should be coupled with comprehensive lifestyle intervention that involves calorie restriction, physical activity, and behavior modification.

Special Population Considerations

Pregnancy and Breast-Feeding

All of the weight loss medications are contraindicated in pregnancy and breast-feeding. Women who are pregnant or breast-feeding and concerned with their weight should discuss this with their provider and be monitored closely.

Pediatrics

Overweight and obesity are on the rise among the youth in the United States. For people aged 2 to 19 years old, 31.8% are considered to be overweight or obese and 16.9% are considered to be obese. Young children aged 2 to 5 years old have lower rates of obesity. However, for children and adolescents aged 6 to 19 years old, almost 1 in 3, 33.2%, is considered to be overweight or obese (18.2% are obese). Obesity in childhood affects both physical and psychosocial health. Like treatment for adults, childhood obesity should be addressed with a comprehensive lifestyle intervention that targets healthy eating, physical activity, and behavioral therapy. This is the cornerstone and pharmacotherapy is not routinely recommended. In regard to pharmacotherapy, however, only a few of the aforementioned medications are approved for use in children or adolescents. Phentermine and diethylpropion are approved for children aged greater than 16 years old and orlistat (Xenical) is approved for children greater than 12 years old. Childhood obesity is complex and should be facilitated by the child's primary care provider and parents/legal guardians.

Diabetes

Caution should also be used when any of these weight loss agents are prescribed for patients with diabetes. The decrease in caloric intake may decrease a patient's blood glucose level, requiring adjustment of insulin or oral hypoglycemic agents.

Smokers

Smoking in itself is a risk factor for cardiovascular disease. The additional burden of obesity places the obese smoker in a much higher risk category for long-term cardiovascular effects. Nicotine has some thermogenic and metabolic effects, which are known to decrease appetite and often associated with a lower BMI. In comparison, smoking cessation is associated with weight gain. Therefore, the obese patient, who then quits smoking, runs the risk of gaining weight or thwarting efforts at weight loss. Special attention should be paid to this category of patient. A much greater level of attention should be paid to the lifestyle changes these patients need to make, and a continued reinforcement of the need for abstinence from smoking versus weight loss should be emphasized.

MONITORING PATIENT RESPONSE

The patient should be monitored for weight loss, decreases in BMI, and changes in waist circumference. A comprehensive lifestyle intervention is key; patients that have a high-intensity intervention (≥14 sessions in 6 months) have the greatest weight loss. However, even low to moderate interventions resulted in more weight loss than usual care (defined as limited advice or educational materials on weight loss).

For patients taking weight loss medications, it is recommended that efficacy and safety are monitored monthly for the first 3 months and then at least every 3 months thereafter. If a patient loses ≥ 5% of their body weight at 3 months and the medication is deemed safe, then the medication can be continued. However, if a patient loses less than 5% of their body weight at 3 months or if there are any issues with safety or tolerability, then the medication should be discontinued.

PATIENT EDUCATION

Patients should be educated that obesity is more than just a cosmetic problem. Patients should be educated on the fact that obesity has been linked to several serious medical conditions, such as diabetes, heart disease, high blood pressure, and stroke. It is also associated with higher rates of certain types of cancer. A patient-centered approach for weight loss is essential. The provider and the patient should determine an appropriate weight loss strategy keeping in mind health goals using a comprehensive lifestyle intervention together as a team. In addition to the weight loss strategies, the provider–patient team must also acknowledge and address the fact that weight loss maintenance is a lifelong challenge and address the challenges as they arise.

For more information regarding obesity, practitioners and patients should contact the following organizations or visit their Web sites. The Web site addresses listed below will direct people to the obesity section of the organization's Web site:

The Obesity Society
8757 Georgia Avenue
Suite 1320
Silver Spring, MD 20910
301-563-6526
www.obesity.org

Centers for Disease Control and Prevention
1600 Clifton Road
Atlanta, GA 30329
800-232-4636
www.cdc.gov/obesity/

National Institutes of Health
9000 Rockville Pike
Bethesda, MD 20892
301-496-4000
http://health.nih.gov/topic/obesity

WHO Regional Office for the Americans
525 23rd Street, NW
Washington, DC 20037
202-974-3000
www.who.int/health_topics/obesity/en/

CASE STUDY*

A.P. is a 34-year-old woman who comes into your clinic looking for a medication to help her lose weight. She states that she has tried several times to lose weight but seems to gain it back within months after stopping her dieting.

Your workup reveals a normal, young, well-developed woman in no acute distress. She is 66 inches tall and weighs 200 lb. Pertinent labs include A1c 5.9%. Her blood pressure is 128/88 and heart rate is 80. She has a history of monthly migraine headaches for which she takes sumatriptan 50 mg PO PRN headache and may repeat dose in 2 hours if there is no relief; she also has hypothyroidism for which she take levothyroxine 112 mcg PO daily. She does not smoke or drink alcohol. She works as a secretary in an office. She has a BMI of 32.3 kg/m².

DIAGNOSIS: OBESITY

1. List specific goals for treatment for **A.P.**
2. What drug therapy would you prescribe? Why?
3. The patient was prescribed phentermine ER/topiramate. What are the parameters for monitoring success of the therapy?
4. Discuss specific patient education based on the prescribed therapy.
5. Describe one or two adverse reactions for the selected agent that would cause you to change therapy.
6. What would be the alternative therapy?
7. What over-the-counter and/or alternative medications would be appropriate for **A.P.**?
8. What lifestyle changes would you recommend to **A.P.**?
9. Describe one or two drug–drug or drug–food interactions for the selected agent.

* Answers can be found online.

Bibliography

Starred references are cited in the text.

Apovian, C. M., Aronne, L. J., Bessesen, D. H., et al. (2015). Pharmacological management of obesity: An Endocrine Society clinical practice guideline. *Journal of Clinical Endocrinology, 100*, 342–362.

Budd, G. M., & Peterson, J. A. (2014). The obesity epidemic. Part 1: Understanding the origins: A review of underlying physical, psychological, and social factors. *American Journal of Nursing, 114*, 40–46.

Burke, L. E., Wang, J., & Sevick, M. A. (2011). Self-monitoring in weight loss: A systematic review of the literature. *Journal of the American Dietetic Association, 111*(1), 92–102. Retrieved from http://dx.doi.org/10.1016/j.jada.2010.10.008

Cavaliere, H., Floriano, I., & Medeiros-Neto, G. (2001). Gastrointestinal side effects of orlistat may be prevented by concomitant prescription of natural fibers (psyllium mucilloid). *International Journal of Obesity and Related Metabolic Disorders, 25*, 1095–1099.

Cizza, G., & Rother, K. I. (2012). Beyond fast food and slow motion: Weighty contributors to the obesity epidemic. *Journal of Endocrinological Investigation, 35*, 236–242.

Del Parigi, A. (2000). Definitions and classification of obesity. [Updated 2010 June 1]. In L. J. De Groot, P. Beck-Peccoz, G. Chrousos, et al. (Eds.), *Endotext [Internet].* South Dartmouth, MA: MDText.com, Inc.

Dhurandhar, E. J., & Keith, S. W. (2014). The aetiology of obesity beyond eating more and exercising less. *Best Practice and Research. Clinical Gastroenterology, 28*, 533–544.

Expert Panel on the Identification, Evaluation, and Treatment of Overweight and Obesity in Adults. (1998). Executive summary of the clinical guidelines on the identification, evaluation and treatment of overweight and obesity in adults. *Archives of Internal Medicine, 158*, 1855–1867.

Finkelstein, E. A., Kruger, E., & Karnawat, S. (2015). Cost-effectiveness analysis of Qsymia for weight loss. *PharmacoEconomics, 33*(7), 699–706. Retrieved from http://dx.doi.org/10.1007/s40273-014-0182-6

Finkelstein, E. A., Trogdon, J. G., Cohen, J. W., et al. (2009). Annual medical spending attributable to obesity: Payer-and service-specific estimates. *Health Affairs, 28*, w822–w831.

Flegal, K. M., Carroll, M. D., Ogden, C. L., et al. (2012). Prevalence and trends in obesity among U.S. adults, 1999–2010. *Journal of the American Medical Association, 307*, 491–497.

James, P. T., Leach, R., Kalamara, F., et al. (2001). The worldwide obesity epidemic. *Obesity Research, 9*(Suppl. 5), S228–S233.

Jensen, M. D., Ryan, D. H., Apovian, C. M., et al. (2013) AHA/ACC/TOS Guideline for the management of overweight and obesity in adults: A report of the American College of Cardiology/American Heart Association Task Force on Practice Guidelines and The Obesity Society. *Circulation.* Published online November 12, 2013.

Lexi-Comp Online™, Lexi-Drugs Online™, Hudson, Ohio: Lexi-Comp, Inc.; 2015; June 3, 2015.

Mayo Clinic Staff. (2014). Weight loss: The temptation to use over-the-counter weight-loss pills to lose weight fast is strong. But are these products safe and effective? Retrieved from http://www.mayoclinic.org/healthy-lifestyle/weight-loss/in-depth/weight-loss/art-20046409 on June 3, 2015.

Mitchell, N. S., Catenacci, V. A., Wyatt, H. R., et al. (2011). Obesity: Overview of an epidemic. *Psychiatric Clinics of North America, 34*, 717–732.

National Institute of Diabetes and Digestive and Kidney Diseases. (2000). Overweight, obesity, and health risk. *Archives of Internal Medicine, 160*, 898–904.

National Institutes of Health. (2012). *Overweight and obesity statistics (NIH Publication No. 04-4158).* Bethesda, MD: Author. Retrieved from http://www.nhlbi.nih.gov/health-information/healthstatistics/pages/overweight-obesity-statistics.aspx on May 22, 2015.

NDA 22580. (2014). Qsymia (phentermine and topiramate extended-release) capsules: Risk, evaluation and mitigation strategy. Retrieved at www.accessdata.fda.gov/drugsatfda_docs/rems/Qsymia%20_2014-09-26_Full%20REMS.pdf

Pi-Sunyer, X. (2009). The medical risks of obesity. *Postgraduate Medicine, 121*, 21–33.

Redman, L., Johannsen, D., Ravussin, E. (2000). Regulation of body weight in humans. [Updated 2012 January 1]. In L. J. De Groot, P. Beck-Peccoz, G. Chrousos, et al. (Eds.), *Endotext [Internet].* South Dartmouth, MA: MDText.com, Inc.

*U.S. Food and Drug Administration. (2012). FDA approves weight management drug "Qsymia". Retrieved from http://www.fda.gov/NewsEvents/Newsroom/PressAnnouncements/ucm312468.htm

*U.S. Food and Drug Administration. (2014). FDA approves weight management drug "Contrave". Retrieved from http://www.fda.gov/newsevents/newsroom/pressannouncements/ucm413896.htm

Vine, M., Hargreaves M. B., Briefel, R. R., et al. (2013). Expanding the role of primary care in the prevention and treatment of childhood obesity: A review of clinic- and community-based recommendations and interventions. *Journal of Obesity*. Article ID 172035.

Wickelgren, I. (1998). Obesity: How big a problem? *Science, 280*, 1364–1367.

World Health Organization. (2015). *Obesity and overweight: Fact sheet*. Retrieved from http://www.who.int/mediacentre/factsheets/fs311/en/ on May 22, 2015.

Yanovski, S. Z., & Yanovski, J. A. (2014). Long-term drug treatment for obesity: A systematic and clinical review. *Journal of the American Medical Association, 311*, 74–86.

UNIT 14

Women's Health

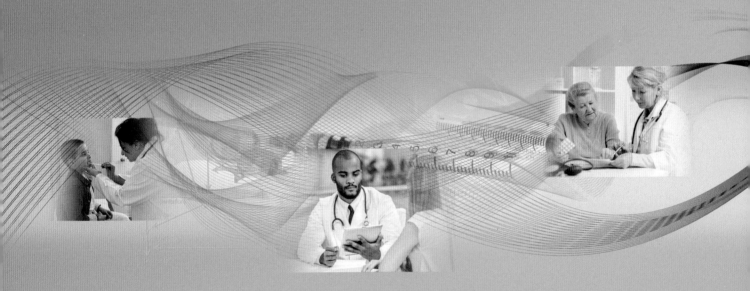

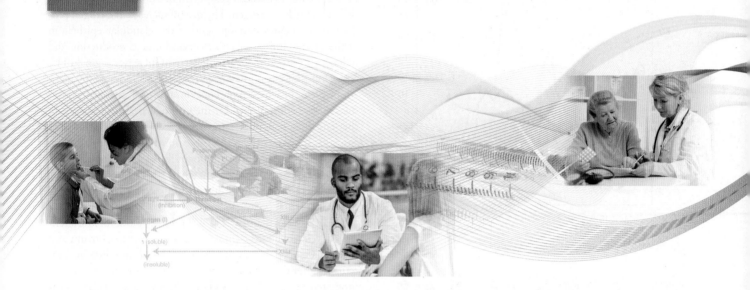

55

Contraception

Virginia P. Arcangelo

Contraception is the inhibition of pregnancy by a process, device, or method. The U.S. Food and Drug Administration (FDA) first approved oral contraception (OC), the use of hormones to prevent pregnancy, in the 1960s, and the last law prohibiting its use in the United States was overturned in 1973 (Speroff & Darney, 2000). Regardless of the type used, one of contraception's major benefits is its potential impact on the rate of unplanned pregnancies. Current estimates are that approximately half of all pregnancies in the United States are unintended. Of these, about 42% are aborted (Espey et al., 2008). Healthy People 2020 aims to reduce unintended pregnancy from 49% of pregnancies to 44% of pregnancies. Unintended pregnancies that continue, including both unwanted and mistimed pregnancies, are positively associated with late-entry prenatal care, low birth weight, child abuse or neglect, and behavioral problems in children. One way a decrease in unintended pregnancies may be achieved is through the increased awareness of contraception and the various available options. The widespread use of contraception in health care in the United States has expanded opportunities for women. Its use has allowed women to take on roles beyond (or in addition to) motherhood. Contraception has increased women's ability to decide when pregnancy and subsequent child rearing will occur.

Age and desire for future pregnancy greatly influence a woman's method of choice. Reversible forms of contraception are the regimens of choice among most women planning future pregnancies. Oral, transdermal, and vaginal hormonal contraception are a first choice because return of fertility after discontinuing use is expected. Among those 15 to 44 years old in the United States who use contraception, oral contraceptives are the most common method used (27.5%). Male condom use (16%) is the next most common at 16%. Intrauterine devices (IUDs) account for about 5% of contraception (Mosher & Jones, 2010).

At 48 months after discontinuing reversible forms of contraception, 82% of patients ages 30 to 34 have given birth. Among women ages 25 to 29, the pregnancy rate is 92% at the same time after discontinuation (Speroff & Darney, 2000).

PHYSIOLOGY

A woman's ability to reproduce begins after she has completed the developmental stage of puberty. The average age of the onset of puberty is 11.2 years, whereas the length of time for the completion of this process is 4 years. Menarche, the last step in the pubertal process, is when menses commences. The average age for menarche is 12.7 years.

The cause or trigger for the onset of puberty is not completely understood. It is thought that a decreased sensitivity of the hypothalamus and pituitary glands to already circulating sex hormones results in an increased production of luteinizing hormone (LH) and follicle-stimulating hormone (FSH). Increased LH and FSH further stimulate the gonadal response of increased secretion of estrogen, progesterone, and testosterone. LH subsequently surges, inciting the release of ova. In the absence of fertilization, menses ensues.

A woman's menstrual cycle can be described in terms of either the follicular or luteal phase. In addition, in each of these phases, endometrial, ovarian, and pituitary hormone-secreting changes occur. These two major phases and the physiologic changes occurring in each are illustrated in **Figure 55.1**.

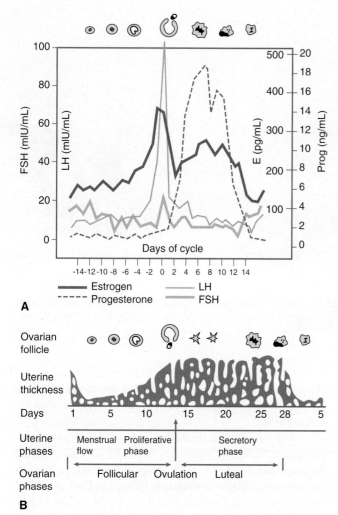

FIGURE 55.1 Comparison of the phases of the reproductive cycle. **A.** Plasma hormone concentrations in the normal female reproductive cycle. **B.** Ovarian events and uterine changes during the menstrual cycle. FSH, follicle-stimulating hormone FSH; LH, luteinizing hormone. (Reprinted from Bullock, B. A., & Henze, R. L. (2000). *Focus on pathophysiology* (p. 1100). Philadelphia, PA: Lippincott Williams & Wilkins, with permission.)

The endometrial changes can be subdivided. Menstruation, occurring on days 1 to 4 of the menstrual cycle, is the shedding of the endometrial lining. The next three phases are the proliferative phase (day 4 or 5 through ovulation), the secretory phase (immediately after ovulation), and the implantation phase (approximately days 21 to 27). During these phases, the endometrial lining is prepared for implantation of a fertilized ovum. In the event that an ovum does not implant, the next phase, endometrial breakdown, begins once again.

Relative to the ovarian changes that occur during the menstrual cycle, three major subdivisions can be identified: the follicular, ovulatory, and luteal phases. During the follicular phase, a dominant follicle is produced that will be released and await possible fertilization. The regulatory hormone largely responsible for this portion of the ovarian phase of the menstrual cycle is FSH. FSH stimulates the conversion of androgens to estrogen in the granulosa cells of the ovaries. Stimulation by FSH contributes to the development of a dominant follicle that produces further estrogen. The overall increase in estrogen production stimulates development of the glandular epithelium of the uterine lining, increases cervical mucus production and reduces the viscosity of this mucus, and increases vaginal pH.

Opposing the normal negative feedback mode of the menstrual cycle, in which high concentrations of estrogen inhibit the release of FSH and LH, the eventual peak in estrogen in this late follicular phase stimulates a surge in LH. The LH surge is subsequently responsible for the final maturation, release, and rupture of the dominant follicle. Follicular rupture and ovulation occur approximately 24 to 36 hours after the beginning of the LH surge and encompass the ovulatory phase of the menstrual cycle.

After the ovulatory phase, the luteal phase of the menstrual cycle enables the implantation of a fertilized ovum and maintenance of the uterine lining. The corpus luteum that remains after the follicle ruptures, releasing the ovum, secretes progesterone and 17-β-estradiol. The secretion of these hormones increases the secretory activity of the endometrial glands. Cervical mucus also increases in viscosity. In the event that pregnancy occurs, the life of the corpus luteum is extended to continue production of these hormones. In the absence of pregnancy, the corpus luteum dies, estrogen and progesterone levels decline, and menstruation occurs.

INITIATING DRUG THERAPY

Given the normal menstrual cycle, pregnancy can be inhibited by preventing fertilization, manipulating hormones of the menstrual cycle such that ovulation never occurs, or interfering with implantation. Contraceptive options may be nonpharmacologic or pharmacologic. **Figure 55.2** identifies these options and the failure rates of each.

Nonpharmacologic options include periodic abstinence, barrier devices, and IUDs and intrauterine systems (IUSs). Periodic abstinence, which means avoiding sexual intercourse during the period of maximum fertility, includes several assumptions. First, the viability of sperm in the female reproductive tract is 2 to 7 days. Second, the life span of the ovum is 1 to 3 days. It is assumed, therefore, that the period of maximum fertility occurs in the 5 days before ovulation and ends on the day of ovulation. Prediction of ovulation is important in recognizing the dates to avoid sexual intercourse. Several methods may be incorporated into the periodic abstinence method to identify better the time of ovulation. Examples include the use of ovulation predictor kits, monitoring of basal body temperature, and testing of cervical mucus. The increase in progesterone concentration just before the LH surge is accompanied by a 0.4°F to 0.8°F increase in basal body temperature. The woman measures her body temperature orally with a basal thermometer just before arising from bed daily.

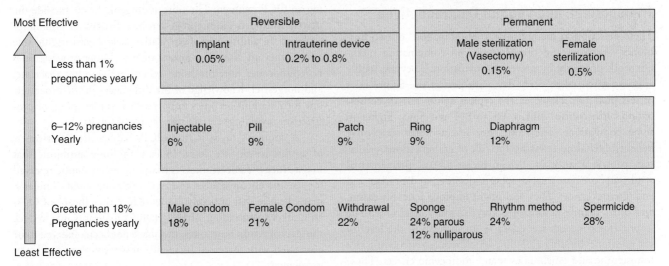

FIGURE 55.2 Effectiveness of contraceptive methods (From U.S. selected practice recommendations for contraceptive use. (2013). Adapted from the World Health Organization selected practice recommendations for contraceptive use 2nd ed. (2013). *Mortality and Morbidity Weekly Report, 62*(RR05), 1–46).

She also may observe cervical mucus as a guide to predicting ovulation. Midcycle cervical mucus, just before ovulation, is clear, thin, and stringy. Peak mucus production occurs on the day of ovulation. After this, the mucus becomes sticky and wet. Intercourse, with a low presumed risk of pregnancy, is permitted beginning on the fourth day of this sticky, wet mucus.

Other nonpharmacologic options for the prevention of pregnancy include the use of barrier devices such as condoms, diaphragms, and cervical caps. These options vary not only in their efficacy rates but in their abilities to prevent sexually transmitted infections (STIs). The male latex condom helps to prevent the spread of human papillomavirus and many other STIs. It is the only contraceptive option clinically proven to prevent the spread of the human immunodeficiency virus (HIV). The female condom has been shown to act as a barrier to most STIs. However, limitations include its cost, decrease in spontaneity, and improper placement.

The diaphragm and cervical cap are both devices that require fitting by a health care provider. The woman can insert a diaphragm up to 6 hours before intercourse and must leave it in place for at least 6 hours (but no more than 24 hours) after intercourse. The diaphragm has been shown to reduce the risk of cervical gonorrhea, pelvic inflammatory disease (PID), and tubal infertility secondary to STIs. It is not, however, effective against HIV infection, and urinary tract infections are twice as common in diaphragm users compared with nonusers. Comparably, the cervical cap may be left in place for a total of 48 hours. It must remain in place, however, for at least 8 hours after sexual intercourse. Like the diaphragm, it has not been shown to afford any protection against HIV infection.

The third major type of nonpharmacologic contraception is the IUD/IUS. Although its mechanism of action is not clearly understood, it is thought to prevent pregnancy through production of a "spermicidal intrauterine environment," interfering with sperm transport into and within the uterus. The intrauterine environment is rendered unreceptive to sperm or the implantation of a fertilized ovum should fertilization occur. In progesterone-implanted IUSs, the continued release of progesterone contributes to the contraceptive action of this device through production of viscous cervical mucus, which further impedes the sperm's ability to reach the ovum.

Both the American College of Obstetricians and Gynecologists and the North American Menopause Society recommend that women continue contraceptive use until menopause or ages 50 to 55. The median age of menopause is approximately 51 years in North America but can range from ages 40 to 60.

Goals of Drug Therapy

In addition to, or in place of, the nonpharmacologic contraceptive options available, pharmacologic options do exist. The primary mechanism by which these agents prevent pregnancy is through manipulation of the normal menstrual cycle, effects on cervical mucus, or both. Estrogen plus progesterone or progesterone alone is used to interfere with the process of ovulation, conception, or both. Optimal contraception features, as defined by the World Health Organization, include

- Safety
- Effectiveness
- Convenience
- Regular bleeding episodes
- Rapid reversibility

Combined (Estrogen and Progestin) Oral, Transdermal, and Vaginal Contraceptives

These prescription methods use a "combination" of two hormones—estrogen and progesterone. All combination methods work primarily by preventing ovulation. They are highly effective when taken every day, with perfect use failure rates of less than 1%. However, the typical failure rate of combination birth control pills is 3% to 8% and much higher in some populations. They also have several noncontraceptive benefits, including reducing the risk of endometriosis, ovulatory pain, ovarian cysts, benign breast disease, premenstrual syndrome, premenstrual dysphoric disorder, and ovarian and endometrial cancer. They also might improve acne, hirsutism, and other manifestations of polycystic ovary syndrome. The improvement occurs secondary to an increase in the level of sex-hormone–binding globulin, which reduces circulating free testosterone and ameliorates many androgenic effects. These methods are reversible and can be used by women of all ages.

The combination contraceptive agents contain estrogen, usually in the form of ethinyl estradiol. Doses of estrogen range from 20 to 35 mg; 98% of all prescribed OCs contain less than 35 mg of estrogen, and even OCs with as little as 20 mg of estrogen are considered effective. Pills with low estrogen content are considered safer than higher-dose OCs for certain patients, including perimenopausal women, those with a family history of heart disease, and smokers younger than age 35 (although women who take OCs and smoke remain at an increased risk of myocardial infarction [MI] and stroke due to OC-associated changes in coagulation factors). Progesterone is in the form of desogestrel, ethynodiol diacetate, levonorgestrel (LNG), norethindrone, norethindrone acetate, norgestimate, or norgestrel. A synthetic progesterone (drospirenone [DRSP]) is also available. It has antiandrogenic and antimineralocorticoid properties. It is associated with less water retention than other progesterones, less negative emotional affect, and less appetite increase after 6 months of use.

The mechanism of action of combination contraceptive agents is the suppression of the pituitary gonadotropins FSH and LH by the continued high concentrations of circulating estrogen and progesterone. The suppression of LH, primarily by the progesterone component, inhibits the LH surge responsible for ovulation. Progesterone also exerts its influence through its effects on increasing cervical mucus viscosity, thus impairing sperm transport. FSH suppression, largely through estrogen's influence, prevents the selection and emergence of a dominant follicle. Therefore, the combination of estrogen and progesterone inhibits selection of a dominant follicle and ovulation.

In addition to their influence on the reproductive cycle, the hormones used in OC pills (OCPs) exert other actions. All forms of progesterone exhibit some estrogenic, androgenic, or anabolic activity. For example, highly androgenic forms of progesterone affect lipid and carbohydrate metabolism and promote the appearance of acne, weight gain, and hirsutism. As such, practitioners should consider the various progesterone

formulations relative to their androgenic effects when choosing an OCP regimen. The least androgenic forms include the newer, third-generation progesterones desogestrel and norgestimate. In addition to their relative lack of androgenic side effects, they are also more potent than the other progesterones norethindrone, norethindrone acetate, ethynodiol diacetate, and norgestrel. Knowledge of the differences in the progesterone formulations becomes important when managing (or prospectively avoiding) certain side effects of OCPs.

A common myth is that OCPs reduce the effectiveness of antibiotics or vice versa. In fact, the only antibiotic that may reduce pill effectiveness is rifampin, an antibiotic reserved for specific circumstances and not commonly used. Similarly, many believe that anticonvulsants reduce the efficacy of OCs, an unlikely association. Although anticonvulsants may reduce the level of serum hormones, they have not been observed to be associated with increased incidence of ovulation or accidental pregnancy.

Many options exist when choosing an OC regimen for a patient. In general, combination OCPs are divided into monophasic, biphasic, and triphasic combinations. **Tables 55.1** and **55.2** list the available formulations. Monophasic combinations

TABLE 55.1	
Monophasic Contraception	
Brand Name	**Hormonal Components**
Alesse, Aviane, Lessina	20 μg EE, 0.1 mg levonorgestrel
Brevicon	35 μg EE, 0.5 mg norethindrone
Apri, Desogen, Ortho-Cept	30 μg EE, 0.15 mg desogestrel
Kelnor 1/35	35 μg EE, 1 mg ethynodiol diacetate
Levlen, Nordette, Portia	30 μg EE, 0.15 mg levonorgestrel
Loestrin 1/20	20 μg EE, 1.0 mg norethindrone acetate
Loestrin 1.5/30	30 μg EE, 1.5 mg norethindrone acetate
Lo/Ovral, Cryselle	30 μg EE, 0.3 mg norgestrel
Norethin 1/35E	35 μg EE, 1 mg norethindrone
Norinyl 1 + 35	35 μg EE, 0.5 mg norethindrone
Nortrel 0.5/35	30 μg EE, 3 mg drospirenone
Ocella, Yasmin	35 μg EE, 0.25 mg norgestimate
Ortho-Cyclen	35 μg EE, 1 mg norethindrone
Ortho-Novum 1/35, Nortrel	50 μg EE, 1 mg norethindrone
Ortho-Novum 1/50, Norinyl 1+50	35 μg EE, 0.4 mg norethindrone
Ovcon 35	50 μg EE, 1 mg norethindrone
Ovcon 50	50 μg EE, 0.5 mg norgestrel
Ovral	30 μg EE, 0.15 mg levonorgestrel
Seasonale	20 μg EE, 3 mg drospirenone
Yaz	35 μg EE, 1 mg norethindrone
Extended Cycle	
Jolessa, Seasonale	30 μg EE, 0.15 mg levonorgestrel
Lybrel	20 μg EE, 0.09 mg levonorgestrel

EE, ethinyl estradiol.

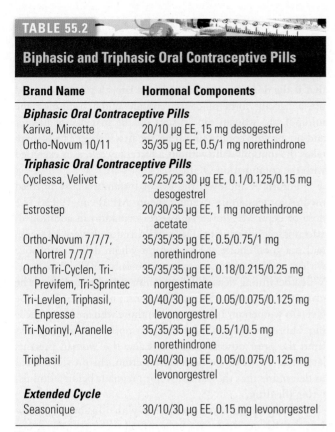

TABLE 55.2	
Biphasic and Triphasic Oral Contraceptive Pills	
Brand Name	**Hormonal Components**
Biphasic Oral Contraceptive Pills	
Kariva, Mircette	20/10 μg EE, 15 mg desogestrel
Ortho-Novum 10/11	35/35 μg EE, 0.5/1 mg norethindrone
Triphasic Oral Contraceptive Pills	
Cyclessa, Velivet	25/25/25 30 μg EE, 0.1/0.125/0.15 mg desogestrel
Estrostep	20/30/35 μg EE, 1 mg norethindrone acetate
Ortho-Novum 7/7/7, Nortrel 7/7/7	35/35/35 μg EE, 0.5/0.75/1 mg norethindrone
Ortho Tri-Cyclen, Tri-Previfem, Tri-Sprintec	35/35/35 μg EE, 0.18/0.215/0.25 mg norgestimate
Tri-Levlen, Triphasil, Enpresse	30/40/30 μg EE, 0.05/0.075/0.125 mg levonorgestrel
Tri-Norinyl, Aranelle	35/35/35 μg EE, 0.5/1/0.5 mg norethindrone
Triphasil	30/40/30 μg EE, 0.05/0.075/0.125 mg levonorgestrel
Extended Cycle	
Seasonique	30/10/30 μg EE, 0.15 mg levonorgestrel

EE, ethinyl estradiol.

provide a set amount of estrogen and progesterone daily for 21 days. Placebo or nothing is given on days 22 to 28, the days during which a woman menstruates. The monophasic combinations may be useful in managing adverse effects such as breakthrough vaginal bleeding. Also, women who are sensitive to fluctuations in hormone levels that occur with the biphasic and triphasic OCPs may respond more positively to the monophasic formulations. Side effects, including breast tenderness, nausea, headaches, and bloating, are usually limited to the first 1 to 2 months of use but may discourage continuation. A backup method of birth control, such as condoms, should be used for the first week after pills are started. Few clinical differences have been noted among the myriad different pill formulations (monophasic, biphasic, triphasic, different generation progestins, and other formulations), so it is reasonable to prescribe a generic monophasic pill containing 30 to 35 mcg of estrogen for most patients.

There is a variation to the traditional monophasic OCP. This formulation provides a constant amount of estrogen and progesterone daily on days 1 to 21. The woman takes placebo tablets on days 22 to 23. On days 24 to 28, a lower dose of estrogen alone is given. The rationale for providing estrogen on days 24 to 28 is to help manage problems in women who may have exhibited symptoms of estrogen deficiency during the traditional week-long placebo period. This includes, for example, women who experience rebound headaches in the absence of estrogen during days 22 to 28.

The biphasic and triphasic OCP combinations were developed to mimic more closely the normal fluctuations in hormones experienced during the menstrual cycle. Changes in the estrogen or progesterone components occur every 7 to 10 days in these products. The phasic OCPs have not been shown to have any proven advantages in efficacy over the monophasic products. The major difference between the biphasic and triphasic regimens and the monophasic regimens is the net amount of progesterone delivered per cycle. The biphasic and triphasic regimens contain, in general, less progesterone. (See **Tables 55.1** and **55.2**.) Therefore, for women experiencing progesterone-related side effects, changing to a regimen containing lower doses of a product with less androgenic effects may be most beneficial.

Extended-cycle OCPs are now available. During the standard 7-day hormone-free interval that occurs with the use of low-dose estrogen formulations, the function of the hypothalamic–pituitary–ovarian axis recovers rapidly, and this increases the risk of ovarian follicle development, ovulation with unintended pregnancy, and increased spotting due to endogenous estradiol production. Fluctuating hormone levels allow endometrial buildup and can exacerbate premenstrual symptoms and menstrual headaches by creating hormone excess and withdrawal states. Extended-cycle OCPs with a shorter or eliminated hormone-free interval reduce the risk of these unwanted effects by preventing endogenous estradiol production while still providing highly effective and safe contraception.

When initiating therapy for patients, a contraceptive regimen is started relative to the woman's menstrual cycle. One can initiate either a day 1 start or a Sunday start regimen. Women who follow a day 1 start regimen begin the contraceptive agent on the first day of their period, regardless of the day of the week. Likewise, women who follow Sunday start regimens begin the OCP pack on the Sunday directly after the onset of menses. This means that the woman will not menstruate on a weekend, which is desirable to many patients. OCP packs are produced with the Sunday start regimen in mind. In the event that a patient is a day 1 start, the pharmacist places a special label on the pack noting the beginning day of the pack and the end. The situation in which the day 1 versus Sunday start becomes an issue is relative to missed doses, which is discussed later in the chapter.

In reality, combined hormonal contraceptives can be initiated at any time if it is reasonably certain that the woman is not pregnant. If combined hormonal contraceptives are started within the first 5 days since menstrual bleeding started, no additional contraceptive protection is needed. If they are started more than 5 days since menstrual bleeding started, the woman needs to abstain from sexual intercourse or use additional contraceptive protection for the next 7 days.

Another form of contraception is the transdermal patch containing 75 mcg of ethinyl estradiol and 6 mg of norelgestromin. The hormones are absorbed through the skin. The patch can be applied to the abdomen, buttocks, upper outer arm, or upper torso on clean, dry, healthy skin free of lotions. The patient can bathe, shower, or swim while wearing the patch. A new patch is applied each week, worn for 7 days, and removed and replaced with a new patch. During the fourth week, no patch is worn. The first patch should be applied on the first day of menses and a new one on the same day the next week. Detachment has been shown in only 5% of cases, but if it becomes loose or falls off, it must be replaced with a new patch. If the patch is off for more than 24 hours, a new cycle is started and backup methods of birth control used for the next 7 days.

The most frequent complaint from users of the patch is reactions at the application site. Women who weigh more than 198 lb may experience a higher failure rate and should use a different form of contraception.

Combination contraceptive vaginal rings are also available. The NuvaRing is a flexible transparent device inserted into the vagina by the patient. It releases 15 mcg of ethinyl estradiol and 120 mcg of etonogestrel daily. It is removed after 3 weeks for 1 week and a new ring is inserted. Lower hormonal doses are required with the vaginal ring because there is no hepatic or gastrointestinal (GI) interference. It can remain in place during bathing, swimming, and intercourse.

It has been shown that there is a mean of 5.88 cycles for conception following discontinuation of combined OC (Stenchever et al., 2001).

Progestin-Only Hormonal Contraceptives

Progesterone alone to prevent pregnancy may be used in the dosage formulations of oral tablets, intramuscular injections, or subdermal implants. Regardless of the formulation, they are the hormonal contraceptive options of choice in women who cannot take or cannot tolerate estrogen-containing formulations. They are a better choice for women with problems, such as high blood pressure or smoking over age 35, which may be negatively impacted by estrogen-containing pills. The progestin-only pill is often recommended for breast-feeding women. In ease of administration, compliance, and efficacy, however, the formulations vary greatly.

The progesterone-only contraceptive pill, commonly referred to as the *minipill*, contains a very low dose of progesterone. **Table 55.3** lists the available formulations and active components of each. The minipills do not consistently suppress the pituitary gonadotropins LH and FSH. Their primary effect is exerted through changing the endometrial and cervical mucus environments. The time from dosing to changes

in the cervical mucus is 2 to 4 hours. The impermeability of the mucus declines 22 hours after the dose. Therefore, to help ensure maximum efficacy, it is imperative that the woman take the pill at exactly the same time daily. Recommendations are that if the dose is more than 3 hours late, the woman should use a backup form of contraception. When beginning the minipill, the woman should start on the first day of menses and use backup contraception for the first 7 days. The woman takes the minipill daily without a placebo week, as is exercised with the combination OCPs.

The FDA approved the use of intramuscularly injected medroxyprogesterone acetate (depo MPA) in 1992. The dose of depo MPA used suppresses ovulation in addition to affecting cervical mucus. Depo MPA is dosed every 13 weeks and is a good choice for women for whom daily compliance with a combination or progesterone-only OCP is an issue. When beginning depo MPA, recommendations are that it be given within the first 5 days of the onset of menses. It can be given to women postpartum and to those who are breast-feeding. Subsequent doses must be given no later than 13 weeks from the prior dose to ensure efficacy. If a woman presents later than 13 weeks for her next injection, the provider needs to determine that the patient is not pregnant before administering the drug.

Depo-Provera is safe for women with a history of cardiovascular disease, stroke, thromboembolism, or peripheral vascular disease. It is ideal for women with hemoglobinopathies, such as sickle cell disease, because these women will likely notice a decrease in painful hemolytic crises.

In addition to the positive compliance effects of this dosage formulation, women wishing future pregnancy also frequently prefer depo MPA. On discontinuation of depo MPA, 70% of women conceive within the first year and 90% within 24 months. Limitations to the use of depo MPA include the occurrence of menstrual changes in most women and episodes of unpredictable bleeding lasting more than 7 days. The latter problem occurs more commonly in the first few months of therapy. Depo-Provera reduces serum estradiol levels, and this can adversely affect bone health. Bone loss was reversible with discontinuation of Depo-Provera. The practitioner should recommend that Depo-Provera users exercise regularly and increase their intake of calcium and vitamin D.

The Intrauterine System

Another form of contraception is IUSs. These are flexible plastic devices inserted into the uterus and cause a sterile inflammatory reaction within the uterus that interferes with sperm transport into and within the uterine cavity. This is one of the most effective methods of reversible contraception. There are two types available in the United States currently. One is the Copper T380 IUD ParaGard. It is effective for at least 10 years. It can be inserted anytime it is certain the woman is not pregnant. It can be inserted within 5 days of the first act of unprotected sexual intercourse as an emergency contraceptive.

TABLE 55.3	
Progesterone-Only Oral Contraceptive Pills	
Brand Name	**Hormonal Component**
Micronor, Camila, Errin, Nor-QD	0.35 mg norethindrone
Ovrette	0.075 mg norgestrel

Another IUS is a LNG-releasing device. There are two available in the United States. One releases 20 µg/d of LNG (Mirena) and is approved for 5 years of use. The other releases 14 µg/d of LNG and is approved for 3 years of use.

Because the IUS contains no estrogen component, it is appropriate for women in whom estrogen is contraindicated. The IUS may also be an effective treatment for women with dysmenorrhea, menorrhagia, and anemia and may serve as an effective transition from contraception to hormone replacement therapy. Little maintenance is required. The patient must check the string after each menstrual period to ensure that it is still in place. For women who choose to become pregnant, the device can be removed by the clinician at any time; no waiting period is required before conception, and IUS use is not associated with a decline in fertility. This system has been shown to lessen dysmenorrhea and bleeding.

The only contraindications to the use of this method are suspected pregnancy, uterine abnormalities that cause significant distortion of the uterus, PID, or unexplained vaginal bleeding prior to insertion. Immediate postpregnancy insertion is appropriate.

Progestin-Only Implants

Nexplanon is a contraceptive device that is implanted subdermally in the upper arm and remains active for 3 years. It consists of a single rod that contains etonogestrel, which is the same progestin used in the NuvaRing. Implanon has been available for more than 10 years but has been widely marketed in the United States only since 2007.

Like other progestin-only contraceptives, Implanon works by blocking the LH surge, thereby preventing ovulation. It also thickens the cervical mucus and thins the endometrial lining. Unlike other progestin-only methods, Implanon causes estradiol to gradually increase to normal endogenous levels after an initial decrease. Progestin-only implants are extremely effective in preventing pregnancy and have an efficacy rate similar to that associated with sterilization or use of an IUD. Women experience a quick return to normal cycles after implant removal, and there have been no reports of infertility after removal. Implantation and removal of Implanon require training, but they can be performed as simple office procedures.

Progestin-only implants may cause irregular bleeding. It is contraindicated in women being treated with CYP3A-inducing or CYP3A-inhibiting medications. Inducers of CYP3A might decrease the efficacy of progestin-only implants and lead to unintended pregnancy, and inhibitors of CYP3A might increase serum etonogestrel levels and cause toxicity. It is also contraindicated in women with active liver disease or active venous thromboembolism. Progestin-only methods of contraception have long been considered safe to use in women with an increased risk of venous thromboembolism (e.g., women who smoke or have hypertension, diabetes mellitus, migraine headaches, or a history of venous thromboembolism).

Emergency Contraception

Two forms of emergency contraception (or "morning-after contraception") are available: LNG (Plan B) and ulipristal acetate (UPA) (Ella). LNG has a total of 1.5 mg LNG taken in two doses (0.75 mg taken 12 hours apart or one dose [1.5 mg LNG]). Pregnancy can be prevented if taken up to 120 hours after intercourse, but it is most effective if taken immediately. The effectiveness decreases as more time passes. It has a 94% efficacy, with efficacy decreasing between 72 and 120 hours. Effectiveness is decreased in the obese. This is available without a prescription.

UPA is a progesterone receptor antagonist. It is to be taken within 5 days (120 hours) of unprotected intercourse. It inhibits follicle rupture and is effective even near ovulation. It has a greater efficacy than LNG. It is only available by prescription.

IUDs are another form of emergency contraception. The copper IUD is the most effective and can remain in place for continued contraception. See the section on IUS for more information.

Regardless of the regimen chosen, a woman should menstruate within 21 days. If she does not, the clinician should instruct her to follow up with her provider to determine whether pregnancy has occurred. In addition, the practitioner should take this opportunity to discuss other forms of contraception so that emergency contraception does not become the woman's routine method of pregnancy prevention.

According to the American College of Obstetricians and Gynecologists and the World Health Organization, there are no absolute medical contraindications to the use of emergency contraception with the exception of pregnancy.

Drug Interactions

Any agent that increases GI motility or causes diarrhea may reduce the plasma concentration of ethinyl estradiol by decreasing its absorption. Agents, such as ascorbic acid, that inhibit sulfation of ethinyl estradiol in the GI tract may increase the bioavailability of ethinyl estradiol and lead to an increase in estrogenic adverse effects.

Ethinyl estradiol is metabolized by the cytochrome P-450 (CYP) 3A4 enzyme pathway. Drugs known to induce CYP3A4 (phenytoin, primidone, barbiturates, carbamazepine, ethosuximide, topiramate, methsuximide, rifampin, and griseofulvin) can lead to decreased plasma ethinyl estradiol levels and may cause failure of emergency contraception. Reports suggest that the enterohepatic circulation of ethinyl estradiol is decreased in women taking antibiotics, which may lead to a decrease in systemic concentrations of ethinyl estradiol. Ethinyl estradiol may interfere with the metabolism of other compounds. It can inhibit microsomal enzymes, which may slow the metabolism of other drugs (i.e., analgesic anti-inflammatory drugs such as antipyrine, antidepressant agents, theophylline, and ethanol), increasing their plasma and tissue concentrations and increasing the risk of adverse effects. There is a potential interaction between warfarin and LNG given as an emergency contraceptive. The proposed mechanism is the displacement of warfarin by LNG from the FIS binding site of human alpha$_1$-acid glycoprotein,

TABLE 55.4

Treatment Order for Available Hormonal Contraceptive Agents

Clinical Scenario	Therapeutic Options
Women wish to use hormonal contraception—adolescents; perimenopausal women; and postpartum, nonlactating women with no other medical risks	Any OCP < 50 mcg EE either continuous or cyclic
History of: • Smoking and over age 35 • Uncontrolled hypertension • Undiagnosed abnormal vaginal bleeding • Diabetes with vascular complications or more than 20 years' duration • Deep vein thrombosis or pulmonary embolism or history of ischemic heart disease • Headaches with focal neurological symptoms • History of breast cancer • Active viral hepatitis or cirrhosis History of cholestasis with OCP use or pregnancy	Consider progestin-only OCPs, Depo-Provera, Implanon, or IUD
Endometriosis	Monophasic continuous therapy
Postpartum, lactating	Progesterone-only minipill
Noncompliance	Depot medroxyprogesterone acetate *or* levonorgestrel subdermal implants
Breakthrough bleeding—first half of cycle	Change to combination pill with higher estrogen content in first half of cycle.
Breakthrough bleeding—second half of cycle	Change to combination pill with higher progestin content in second half of cycle

Data from Zieman, M., Hatcher, R., Cwiak, C., et al. (2010). *A pocket guide to managing contraception.* Tiger, GA: Bridging the Gap Foundation.

the main transport protein for drugs in the plasma. This potential interaction should be considered so that the patient's international normalized ratio levels can be monitored because the Yuzpe regimen for emergency contraception generally would not be recommended in women with a history of deep vein thrombosis who are receiving anticoagulant therapy.

Selecting the Most Appropriate Agent

When deciding which pill to select, the patient's body mass should be considered. Obese women require higher doses of estrogen and progesterone. A physical exam including blood pressure, lipid panel, and liver and renal function is important. A pregnancy test should be performed.

Most women can tolerate up to 735 µg of ethinyl estradiol for a 28-day cycle. But a 3-month trial should be done to determine tolerability. Most side effects subside after three months.

With the wide variety of forms of hormonal contraception, many questions exist about which agent should be used first and for whom. **Table 55.4** addresses some of these issues and is provided as a guide to the prescription of hormonal contraception.

MONITORING PATIENT RESPONSE

Therapeutic drug monitoring of hormonal contraception includes, primarily, monitoring for adverse effects and preventing complications from their use. Before using any of the hormonal regimens, all sexually active patients should receive a gynecologic examination with Papanicolaou smear to observe cervical cytology. They also should have a thorough physical examination before beginning use, including information such as blood pressure and weight. A lipid panel, including baseline total cholesterol, high-density lipoprotein cholesterol, and triglyceride levels, may be especially important in women with other risk factors for heart disease. Identification of blood glucose control before and after initiating hormonal contraception is important in women with diabetes mellitus.

In addition to the initial workup and physical examination, it is also important to maintain a high index of suspicion for adverse effects associated with the use of either the estrogen or progesterone components, or both, in women receiving hormonal contraception. It is estimated that 25% to 50% of women discontinue hormonal contraception within the first 12 months of use because of physical side effects. Therefore, it is important to look for these side effects and know how to manage them. **Box 55.1** identifies side effects related to excess estrogen and progesterone.

Side effects due to insufficient estrogen and progesterone, such as breakthrough bleeding, also may occur. In the first half of the menstrual cycle, breakthrough bleeding is likely due to insufficient estrogen; in the second half of the cycle, it is likely due to insufficient progesterone. Therefore, practitioners can simplify management by adding supplemental estrogen or progesterone when appropriate or changing to a new regimen with higher estrogen or progesterone as necessary.

BOX 55.1 — Causes of Side Effects of Hormone Contraception

Too Much Estrogen
Heavy bleeding
Cystic breasts
Breast enlargement
Breast tenderness
Dysmenorrhea
Bloating
Premenstrual edema
Gastrointestinal symptoms
Premenstrual headache
Premenstrual irritability
Cervical exstrophy

Too Little Estrogen
Bleeding (spotting) early in cycle
Too light bleeding
Bleeding throughout the cycle
Amenorrhea

Too Much Progestin
Increased appetite
Candidiasis
Depression
Fatigue
Cervicitis

Too Little Progestin
Bleeding fewer days
Bleeding (spotting) late in cycle
Heavy bleeding
Delayed withdrawal bleeding
Bloating
Dysmenorrhea
Premenstrual edema
Gastrointestinal symptoms
Premenstrual headache
Premenstrual irritability

TABLE 55.5 — Guidelines for Missed Pills

Number of Missed Pills	Recommended Action
One pill	Take missed pill as soon as possible and resume schedule; backup method of contraception is not necessary
Two 30- to 35-mg pills	Take missed pill as soon as possible and resume schedule; backup method of contraception is not necessary
Two 20-mg pills	Follow directions for more than two pills
More than two pills	Take pill and continue taking a pill daily. Use condom or abstinence for 7 days. If missed in week 3, finish active pills in current pack and start a new pack the next day (skip current inactive pills). If missed pills in first week and had sex, use emergency contraception (EC), then resume taking pills the next day after EC

If there is breakthrough bleeding early in the cycle, a change to a pill with more estrogen but the same level of progestin is appropriate. Breakthrough bleeding late in the cycle requires a pill with more progestin. Heavy bleeding with periods and bloating indicates the need for a pill with lower estrogen to progestin level since estrogen builds up the endometrium causing heavier bleeding. Breakthrough bleeding throughout the cycle indicated the need for more estrogen but the same amount of progestin. Elevated blood pressure and depression indicates the need for a lower progestin dose.

PATIENT EDUCATION

Poor outcomes secondary to the use of hormonal contraception may include treatment failures, potentially life-threatening side effects, or side effects beyond those commonly expected. Treatment failures frequently are related to compliance with the regimen. In the case of combination OCs, guidelines exist that explain what to do in the event of a missed pill (or pills) to help ensure continued contraceptive efficacy. **Table 55.5** illustrates these guidelines. Another cause of treatment failure includes drug interactions that may affect the efficacy of the hormonal contraceptive. Agents proven to reduce circulating estrogen concentrations, therefore affecting efficacy, include rifampin (Rifadin), phenytoin (Dilantin), and carbamazepine (Tegretol). Recommendations to reduce the risk of treatment failure relative to these agents include the use of higher daily doses of estrogen (50 mg ethinyl estradiol) or use of progesterone-only options.

Patients can best avoid life-threatening side effects of the hormonal contraceptives, especially combination OCs, if they follow the contraindications to their use. **Box 55.2** identifies absolute contraindications to the use of combination OCs. In addition, the acronym *ACHES* is useful in teaching patients

BOX 55.2 — Absolute Contraindications to the Use of Combination Oral Contraceptive Pills

- Thrombophlebitis, thromboembolic disorders, cerebral vascular disease, coronary occlusion*
- Markedly impaired liver function
- Breast cancer (known or suspected)
- Abnormal vaginal bleeding in the absence of a diagnosed cause
- Pregnancy
- Smokers older than age 35

*Includes a past history or other situations that may put the patient at risk for developing these conditions.

about the potential severe side effects that may occur with the use of OCPs. Clinicians should instruct patients to call their primary care provider if any of the following occur:

- Severe **A**bdominal pain (indicative of gallbladder disease)
- **C**hest pain (potentially related to pulmonary embolism or MI)
- **H**eadache (relative to stroke, hypertension, or migraine)
- **E**ye problems (relative to stroke or hypertension)
- **S**evere leg pain (indicative of deep vein thrombosis)

It is crucial to relay this information to the patient. Early recognition and treatment of these adverse events save lives.

Many women are unaware of the health risks and side effects of the various forms of hormonal contraception. Likewise, 25% of women are unaware that the use of combination contraceptive agents imparts benefits in addition to the prevention of pregnancy. Some of these benefits include a 50% to 60% reduction in ovarian cancer risk with 5 years of use. This benefit persists for up to 10 or more years after discontinuation. In addition, 50% to 60% reductions in PID risk and 30% to 50% reductions in the occurrence of menstrual disorders have been observed with combination agents.

Another benefit of OCPs is their use in other indications. For example, 60% to 94% of women with endometriosis who

BOX 55.3 Noncontraceptive Benefits of Combined Oral Contraceptives

- Decreased iron deficiency anemia
- Decreased dysmenorrhea
- Decreased dysfunctional uterine bleeding
- Decreased incidence of ovarian cysts
- Improvement in acne
- Decreased incidence of pelvic inflammatory disease
- Decreased risk of osteoporosis
- Decreased incidence of endometrial cancer
- Decreased risk of benign breast disease

Several Web sites contain patient information on contraception: www.contraception.net, http://www.nlm.nih.gov/medlineplus/birthcontrol.html, and www.plannedparenthood.org.

are treated with daily monophasic contraceptive agents for 6 to 9 months experience symptomatic improvement. After treatment, a 5% to 10% annual recurrence rate of the disease is noted. Benefits of contraceptive agents are listed in **Box 55.3**.

CASE STUDY*

J.L., a 27-year-old account executive, presents to the family medicine office for her annual checkup with her primary care provider. She has no significant past medical history except heavy menses. Her medications include calcium carbonate 500 mg orally twice a day and a multivitamin daily. She exercises regularly. Her family history is significant for cardiovascular disease (her father had an MI at age 54 and died of a further MI at age 63). She notes that she has been dating her current partner for approximately 5 months. She is interested in a reliable form of contraception. After discussing the various contraceptive options, she is here for contraceptive counseling.

1. Before prescribing an OCP regimen, what tests or examinations would you like to perform?
2. Identify three different contraceptive regimens that could be chosen for **J.L.** Note their differences and why you chose them.
3. Identify the potential side effects that need to be relayed to **J.L.** Note especially those side effects for which **J.L.** should seek immediate medical care.

* Answers can be found online.

Bibliography

*Starred references are cited in the text.

Ahern, R., Frattarelli, L., Delto, J., et al. (2010). Knowledge and awareness of emergency contraception in adolescents. *Journal of Pediatric and Adolescent Gynecology, 23*(5), 273–278.

Allsworth, J. E., Secura, G. M., Zhao, Q., et al. (2013). The impact of emotional, physical, and sexual abuse on contraceptive method selection and discontinuation. *American Journal of Public Health, 103*(10), 1857–1864.

Bonnema, R., Mcnamara, M., & Spencer, A. (2010). Contraceptive choices in women with underlying medical conditions. *American Family Physician, 82*(6), 621–628.

*Espey, E., Ogburn, T., & Fotieo, D. (2008). Contraception: What every internist should know. *Medical Clinics of North America, 92*(5), 1037–1058.

Hardeman, J., & Weiss, B. D. (2014). Intrauterine devices: An update. *American Family Physician, 89*(6), 445–450.

Klein, D. A., Arnold, J. J., & Reese, E. S. (2015). Provision of contraception: Key recommendations from the CDC. *American Family Physician, 91*(9), 625–637.

Lara-Torre, E. (2009). Update in adolescent contraception. *Obstetrics and Gynecology Clinics, 36*(1), 119–128.

Mosher W. D., & Jones, J. (2010). Use of contraception in the United States: 1982–2008. *Vital and Health Statistics, 29*, 1–44.

Plastino, K., & Sulak, P. (2008). New forms of contraception. *Obstetrics and Gynecology Clinics, 35*(2), 185–197.

Prine, L. (2007). Emergency contraception, myths and facts. *Obstetrics and Gynecology Clinics, 35*(2), 127–136.

Secretary's advisory committee on National Health Promotion and Disease Prevention Objectives for 2020. (2010). *Evidence-based clinical and public health: Generating and applying the evidence.* Washington, DC: CDC.

Spencer, A., Bonnema, R., & McNamara, M. (2009). Helping women choose appropriate hormonal contraception: Update on risks, benefits and indications. *American Journal of Medicine, 122*(6), 497–506.

*Speroff, L., & Darney, P. (2000). *A clinical guide for contraception* (3rd ed.). Philadelphia, PA: Lippincott Williams & Wilkins.

Steinauer, J., & Autry, A. (2007). Extended cycle combined hormonal contraception. *Obstetrics and Gynecology Clinics, 34*(1), 43–55.

*Stenchever, M. A., Droegemueller, W., Herbst, A. L., et al. (2001). *Comprehensive Gynecology* (4th ed.). St. Louis, MO: Mosby.

*U.S. selected practice recommendations for contraceptive use. (2013). Adapted from the World Health Organization selected practice recommendations for contraceptive use 2nd ed. (2013). *Mortality and Morbidity Weekly Report, 62*(RR05), 1–46.

Yen, S., Saah, T., & Adams Hillard, P. (2010). Intrauterine devices and adolescents: An underutilized opportunity for pregnancy prevention. *Journal of Pediatric and Adolescent Gynecology, 23*(3), 123–128.

Zieman, M., Hatcher, R., Cwiak, C., et al. (2010). *A pocket guide to managing contraception.* Tiger, GA: Bridging the Gap Foundation.

56 Menopause

Elena M. Umland ■ Virginia P. Arcangelo

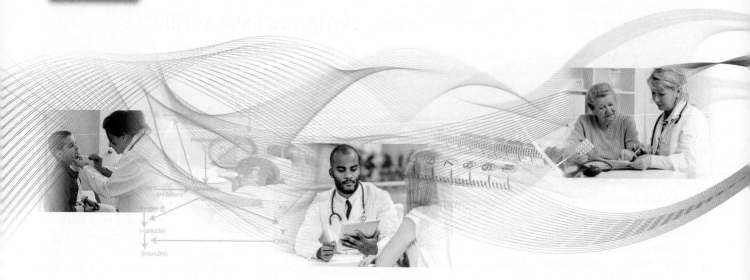

INTRODUCTION

Menopause is the permanent cessation of menstruation resulting from loss of ovarian function. It is an endocrinopathy resulting from failure of the ovary to produce estrogen. Menopause is not an acute condition but rather a gradual transition from perimenopause to menopause and finally postmenopause. The menopausal transition is defined as that period of time from the first changes in the menstrual cycle to the final menstrual period (FMP). The menopausal transition typically begins about 2 years prior to the FMP; however, this time frame varies from woman to woman (Harlow et al., 2012).

Healthy women typically spend one third of their lives in a menopausal state. According to the North American Menopause Society (NAMS), the postwar baby boom of the 1940s and 1950s has led to an absolute increase in the over-50 population (NAMS, 2010). Every day, over 6,000 women enter menopause. American women today can expect to live beyond age 80. The mean age of menopause in the United States is 51 years, with a range of 40 to 58 years. Approximately 4% of women experience their FMP before age 40. Overall, women can expect to spend approximately 30 postmenopause. By the year 2020, it is estimated that there will be greater than 50 million women in the United States who are postmenopause. Factors that contribute to menopause occurring at an earlier than average age include a history of irregular menses before the perimenopause, African American heritage, cigarette smoking, and weight reduction diets.

The increased incidence of chronic disease in postmenopausal women appears to be influenced by decreased levels of estrogen or progesterone. Following menopause, women can expect to experience an increased probability of developing coronary heart disease (CHD), stroke, hip fracture, breast cancer, colorectal cancer, and endometrial cancer. Further, postmenopausal women have a greater increased risk of Alzheimer disease over men. While efforts in preventing these disease states as well as diagnosing them in a timely manner and effectively managing them are often the focus of health care providers, it is the management of the symptoms associated with menopause directly, namely, vasomotor symptoms (VMS) and urogenital symptoms, that is the focus of this chapter.

PHYSIOLOGY

Menopause involves an age-related loss of ovarian function and a resulting decrease in estrogen secretion by the ovarian follicular unit. The ovary produces 17-β-estradiol, the major circulating estrogen. At birth, approximately 1 to 2 million ovarian follicles are present. By age 45, the number drops to approximately 10,000.

During the menopausal transition, the woman herself notices changes in her menstrual pattern. This may include a change in the time span from the first day of one menstrual period to the first day of the next (variable by greater than 7 days from what was previously considered normal for the patient); the amount of menstrual flow and the number of days of bleeding may vary from month to month, increasing or decreasing. It is expected that later in the menopausal transition, cycles become skipped with phases of amenorrhea lasting ≥60 days (Harlow et al., 2012).

Amenorrhea in menopause results from the remaining follicles becoming resistant to the effect of follicle-stimulating hormone (FSH). The ovaries begin with a large number of follicles that atrophy during the reproductive years at a steady rate until there are too few to produce significant amounts of estradiol. During the perimenopause (the time frame inclusive of the menopause transition and 1 year following the FMP), estradiol and progesterone production declines. The reduction in hormone levels reduces the negative feedback loop of the hypothalamic–pituitary system, which leads to a rise in FSH levels.

Estrogen has an impact on many body tissues and systems: bone, teeth, brain, eyes, vasomotor, heart, colon, and urogenital. Ovarian failure causes changes in many organ systems, but the changes are subtle and usually not distressing to women. The most noticeable change is amenorrhea. This is the change in reproductive function that all women experience. Women are considered postmenopause following their FMP.

Morbidity in postmenopausal women is largely the result of alterations in hormone production, notably the decline in estradiol production. During the menopause transition and early postmenopause, women seek treatment for the related occurrences of VMS insomnia, mood changes, and urogenital symptoms. The most commonly noted symptoms are the VMS. Risk factors associated with the occurrence and severity of VMS include obesity, cigarette smoking, depression, anxiety, lack of exercise, low socioeconomic status, and race, specifically African American women (Thurston & Joffe, 2011). The occurrence of VMS is felt to be due to a disruption of the thermoregulatory circuitry that functions under the influence of consistent concentrations of the neurotransmitters serotonin and norepinephrine. Changes in estradiol levels have been associated with fluctuations in serotonin and norepinephrine, thus the link between declining estradiol concentrations and the presence of VMS (Deecher & Dorries, 2007; Rossaminth & Ruebberdt, 2009). According to the American College of Obstetricians and Gynecologists (ACOG), approximately 87% of women experience these on a daily basis, occurring in the form of hot flashes or flushes, perspiration, chills, and clamminess (ACOG, 2014). These are transient sensations typically lasting from 1 to 5 minutes. Of women experiencing VMS, approximately 33% experience more than 10 hot flashes per day. They are the most annoying consequences of menopause for many women, often affecting mood and disrupting sleep.

There are also changes in the genitourinary system as a result of menopause. And it is estimated that the symptoms resulting from these changes affect up to 40% of midlife women (ACOG, 2014). The vagina, vulva, urethra, and bladder have a large number of estrogen receptors. As estrogen concentrations decline, the potential for urogenital symptoms increases. The vulva loses collagen, adipose tissue, and the ability to retain water. There is a shortening and narrowing of the vagina; the walls become thin and pale and elasticity decreases. Vaginal secretions decrease, thereby decreasing vaginal lubrication. The urethra may become irritated as well. New terminology for vulvovaginal atrophy was implemented in 2014 with this now being referred to as the genitourinary syndrome of menopause (GUSM) Portman & Gass, 2014). Unlike VMS, which do tend to improve and subside over time, menopause-related genitourinary symptoms such as vaginal dryness, itching and burning, and subsequent dyspareunia tend to be chronic and progressive and unlikely to resolve over time.

INITIATING DRUG THERAPY

Goals of Drug Therapy

In managing symptoms related to menopause, notably VMS and menopause-related genitourinary symptoms, the goal is reduction in symptom severity and frequency and a subsequent improvement in quality of life (QoL). There are many treatment options available including regimens containing estrogen with or without the addition of a progestin as well as a variety of nonhormonal options such as the selective serotonin reuptake inhibitors (SSRIs) and gabapentin, to name just two. Newer products such as estrogen agonist/antagonist agents and tissue selective estrogen complexes (TSECs) have also been recently added to the list of options. Regardless of the treatment regimen, the goals remain the same, minimizing menopause symptoms of estrogen deficiency. Contrary to the suggested findings of early observational studies, and subsequent to prospective, randomized trials, it is no longer acceptable to use estrogen with or without the addition of a progestin to prevent long-term chronic conditions, particularly CHD (Moyer, 2013).

Hormone Therapy

Estrogen decreases the frequency of night sweats and periods of wakefulness during the night, reduces sleep latency (time between going to bed and falling asleep), and improves sleep in postmenopausal women with sleeping difficulty. Estrogen regimens reduce frequency and intensity of hot flashes by 75% and 87%, respectively (ACOG, 2014). No other method provides such consistent and significant relief of menopausal symptoms as estrogen. Hormone therapy (HT) generally refers to treatment with estrogen and progestin used in women with an intact uterus and estrogen alone in women who have no uterus. See **Table 56.1** for a summary overview of select HT and related products to treat menopausal symptoms.

QOL data have been reported for the estrogen plus progestin arm of the Women's Health Initiative (WHI). Approximately 16,600 women completed surveys at baseline and year 1. About 1,500 women completed surveys at year 3. At year 1, there was statistically significant improvement in sleep disturbance, physical functioning, and bodily pain as compared with the placebo group. However, the differences were so small that there is a question about clinical significance. There was no significant difference at year 3. In women reporting moderate to severe VMS, those taking estrogen plus progestin had significant improvement in the severity of hot flashes and night sweats (WHI, 2002). Further, the Society for Women's Health Research unanimously recommends that significant improvement in health-related QOL and global QOL are provided via HT; the greatest benefits are observed when started in a timely fashion related to the onset of menopausal symptoms (Davies et al., 2013).

TABLE 56.1

Overview of Available HT and Related Agents to Treat Menopausal Symptoms

Generic (Trade) Name and Dosage	Side Effects	Contraindications	Special Considerations
Oral Menopause Hormone Therapy			
conjugated equine estrogen (CEE) (Premarin) Usual daily dose 0.3–0.65 mg Doses available: 0.3, 0.45, and 0.625 mg	Nausea, vomiting, breakthrough bleeding, edema, weight changes, swollen/tender breasts, hypertension, depression, hair loss, changes in libido, venous thromboembolic events	Estrogen-dependent neoplasia Thrombophlebitis or thromboembolic disorder Pregnancy Undiagnosed vaginal bleeding Uncontrolled hypertension Acute liver disease	May cause GI upset, may take with food Treatment should occur at the lowest effective dose for the shortest duration as needed
estradiol (Estrace) 1 mg/d	Same as above	Same as above	Same as above
Combination Products			
CEE and medroxyprogesterone acetate (MPA) (Prempro) Doses: 0.5/1.5, 0.4/1.5, 0.625/2.5, 0.625/5 mg ethinyl estradiol and norethindrone acetate (NETA)	Same as above	Same as above	Same as above
CEE and bazedoxifene (Duavee) Doses: 0.45 mg/20 mg, 0.625 mg/20 mg	Same as observed with estrogen	Same as observed with estrogen PLUS the addition of known protein C, protein S, or antithrombin deficiency	Addition of bazedoxifene further minimizes the bone loss observed with estrogen and reduces the risk for developing endometrial hyperplasia
FemHRT 1/5 5 mcg/1 ng	Same as above	Same as above	Same as above
estradiol (NETA) 1 mg/0.5 ng	Same as above	Same as above	Same as above
(Estratest) esterified estrogen 1.25 mg and methyltestosterone 2.5 mg (Estratest H.S.) esterified estrogen 0.625 mg and methyltestosterone 1.25 mg Taken daily for 3 wk and then 1 wk off	Liver function changes, nausea, breakthrough bleeding, edema, weight gain, hypertension, depression, intolerance to contact lenses, changes in libido, virilization, jaundice, gallbladder disease	Breast or endometrial cancer, undiagnosed genital bleeding, thromboembolic disease, pregnancy, lactation	Report any adverse events immediately May take at bedtime to prevent nausea
Progestins			
MPA (Amen, Curretab, Cycrin, Provera) 2.5–10 mg either daily or cyclic	Vision changes, migraine, porphyria, depression, insomnia, jaundice, nausea, thrombophlebitis, pulmonary embolism, increased blood pressure, breakthrough bleeding, breast tenderness, rash, hirsutism, increased weight, decreased glucose tolerance	Thrombophlebitis, hepatic disease, breast cancer, undiagnosed vaginal bleeding, pregnancy, lactation Caution in epilepsy, migraine, asthma, cardiac dysfunction	Report any adverse events immediately May take at bedtime to prevent nausea
norethindrone acetate (NETA) Aygestin dose: 2.5–10 mg/d	Same as above	Same as above	Same as above
Transdermal Menopause Hormone Therapy			
estradiol (Alora, Estraderm, Vivelle) Change transdermal patch twice a week Alora—0.05, 0.075, 0.1 mg/d Vivelle—0.0375, 0.05, 0.075, 0.1 mg/d	Irritation at application site, headache, breakthrough bleeding, nausea, abdominal cramps	Undiagnosed abnormal vaginal bleeding, thromboembolic disorder, pregnancy, breast or estrogen-dependent tumor	Apply to clean, dry area on lower abdomen, hips, or buttocks (not breast or waistline) Rotate application sites Use 3 wk on and 1 wk off in patient with intact uterus; continuous in patient without uterus

(Continued)

TABLE 56.1

Overview of Available HT and Related Agents to Treat Menopausal Symptoms (*Continued*)

Generic (Trade) Name and Dosage	Side Effects	Contraindications	Special Considerations
estradiol (Climara)—0.025, 0.0375, 0.05, 0.075, 0.1 mg Change transdermal patch once a week 0.05, 0.075, 0.1 mg/d	Same as above	Same as above	Same as above
estradiol and NETA (CombiPatch) Change transdermal patch twice a wk (0.05 mg estradiol and 0.14 mg norethindrone, 0.05 mg estradiol and 0.25 mg norethindrone)	Same as above	Same as above	Apply to clean, dry area on lower abdomen, hips, or buttocks (not breast or waistline) Combination therapy
Other Related Options			
ospemifene (Osphena) 60 mg daily	Vaginal discharge, hot flashes, muscle spasms	Undiagnosed, abnormal genital bleeding, known or suspected estrogen-dependent neoplasia, a history of or active thromboembolic disease	As it is an antagonist in breast cancer, it does not have the same risk as estrogen The only product in its class approved in the United States for dyspareunia associated with vulvovaginal atrophy
Vaginal Hormones			
estradiol 0.01% (Estrace Vaginal Cream) Initially 2–4 g/d for 1–2 wk, then 1–2 g/d for 1–2 wk; maintenance dose: 1 g 1–3 times/wk (3 wk on and 1 wk off)	Uterine bleeding, vaginal candidiasis	Breast or estrogen-dependent cancer, thrombophlebitis, undiagnosed genital bleeding, pregnancy, lactation, impaired liver function	Need to take progestin if uterus present
Estring (vaginal ring) 0.0015/d ring into the vagina; replaced every 90 d Femring 0.05, 0.1/d	Headache, leukorrhea, back pain, urinary tract infection, vaginitis, vaginal pain, abdominal pain, bacterial growth	Same as above	Remove while treating vaginitis Re-evaluate every 3–6 mo
Premarin vaginal cream 0.625 mg/g 0.5–2 g/d	Nausea, vomiting, breakthrough bleeding, edema, weight changes, swollen/ tender breasts, hypertension, depression, hair loss, changes in libido	Same as above	Therapeutic regimen consists of 3 wk on therapy and 1 wk off

In the women's health, osteoporosis, progestin, estrogen (HOPE) trial, healthy postmenopausal women ages 40 to 65 were randomly assigned to treatment with conjugated equine estrogen (CEE) alone (0.625, 0.45, or 0.3 mg daily), CEE plus MPA (0.625/2.5, 0.45/2.5, 0.45/1.5, or 0.3/1.5 mg daily), or a placebo. Over 13 cycles, women in all active treatment groups had a significant reduction in VMS. In women taking CEE alone, benefit increased with increased dosage. In women taking CEE plus MPA, the benefit was comparable with all doses (Utian et al., 2001).

If HT is prescribed solely for vaginal symptoms, health care providers are advised to consider the use of topical vaginal products (gel or cream applied locally) secondary to reduced systemic effects as compared to oral or transdermal formulations.

The slight decrease in testosterone production that accompanies menopause can cause a significant decrease or complete loss of libido in some women. For these women, testosterone can be added to HT in doses of 1.25 to 2.5 mg methyltestosterone. The adverse events of testosterone in these doses are hirsutism, voice change, and a decrease in the high-density lipoprotein cholesterol level. Long-term use is associated with the risk of hepatocellular neoplasm, increased edema, and possible elevation of cholesterol level. The only indication for treatment is severe vasomotor disturbances and decreased libido. The most frequent treatment choice is either Estratest, which is 1.25 mg esterified estrogen and 2.5 mg methyltestosterone, or Estratest H.S., which is 0.625 mg esterified estrogen and 1.25 mg methyltestosterone. Estratest H.S.may be used safely as long as baseline lipid levels are normal. Estratest, with its 1.25 mg esterified estrogen, is a high dose of estrogen and should be used only for short periods.

HT started after age 65 does not improve memory and, in fact, has been observed to increase the risk for developing dementia (Coker et al., 2010). While preliminary data suggest that there may be cognitive benefits when HT is used in younger women, it has not been well studied. The WHI memory study of younger women is currently underway to determine whether women ages 50 to 59 who start HT a short time after onset of menopause and who are treated for an average of 5.4 years would experience cognitive benefits (Vaughan et al., 2013).

Mechanism of Action

HT with estrogen minimizes VMS and genitourinary symptoms related to estrogen deficiency. Estrogen assists in temperature control that occurs in the anterior hypothalamus. Further, estrogen receptors are located throughout the entire female genitourinary tract. Increasing the estrogen levels that declined via menopause through estrogen replacement helps to improve the symptoms of deficiency. Progestins are added to systemic estrogen formulations (oral and transdermal) in women who have a uterus. The unopposed use of estrogen in these women can lead to endometrial hyperplasia, increasing the risk for developing endometrial cancer. However, progestins may increase the risk of breast cancer above that observed with estrogen alone (further discussed under adverse events of HT).

Dosage

Several systemic estrogen and progestin formulations (oral and transdermal) are available, and there is no strong evidence that one formulation is superior to another relative to the impact on VMS or genitourinary symptoms. Hormones delivered via a transdermal patch are associated with a lower risk of venous thromboembolism (VTE) compared to oral formulations. A reasonable starting dose of estrogen for women who are having hot flashes is 0.025 mg of transdermal estradiol, 0.5 mg of oral estradiol, or 0.3 mg of CEE. The transdermal and vaginal routes of administration of estrogen avoid first-pass hepatic metabolism and may be the reason for which reduced thromboembolic risk (VTE and stroke) is observed. In relation, there

is not an increase in C-reactive protein (perhaps contributing to this lower risk of VTE) seen with the nonoral products as is observed with oral therapy. However, no randomized controlled trials to support this concept have been published to date.

When considering the use of vaginal estrogen products, especially for the management of genitourinary symptoms, it is important to note that 10% to 15% of systemic estrogen users may not achieve adequate relief of their symptoms such that additional low-dose vaginal products can be added (NAMS, 2013). For genitourinary symptoms including vulvovaginal atrophy, recurrent urinary tract infections, and overactive bladder, low-dose vaginal estrogen is very effective; 80% to 90% efficacy is noted with vaginal products as compared to 75% efficacy with systemic estrogen formulations. Vaginal formulations are available as vaginal rings (7.5 mcg estradiol released daily over 90 days), vaginal tablets, and vaginal creams. The vaginal tablets contain 10 mcg estradiol and should be dosed one tablet daily for 2 weeks and then one tablet twice weekly thereafter. The vaginal creams contain 0.1 mg active estradiol per 1-g dose. The vaginal creams are dosed 2 to 4 g of cream vaginally per day for 1 to 2 weeks followed by 1 g of cream vaginally one to three times per week. Unlike the systemic estrogen products, the vaginal formulations appear safe alone (in the absence of a progestin) relative to endometrial hyperplasia and endometrial cancer risk; however, long-term data are lacking. Overall, the benefits of these products are dose dependent and patient specific.

In addition, and during the menopause transition in particular, low-dose oral contraceptives can be used to prevent and control symptoms until the patient reaches menopause and to ensure prevention of conception because these women are still fertile. To determine when, in fact, the patient taking oral contraceptives is postmenopausal, such that alternative treatment regimens can be considered, FSH levels can be determined on the last hormone-free day of the oral contraceptive package.

The postmenopausal estrogen progestin intervention (PEPI) trial showed that CEE with cyclic micronized progesterone had the best lipid profile of any of the combined regimens. Micronized progesterone and norethindrone acetate (NETA) have better side effect profiles than MPA and should be considered when choosing a progestin (PEPI Writing Group, 1995).

Time Frame for Response and Treatment Duration

Overall, it is recommended that HT should be used at the lowest effective dose and for the shortest duration possible. Improvement in symptoms may be realized over a short period of time, days to weeks. Symptom improvement is dose related. Owing to the long-term effects such as increased risk of breast cancer, CHD, and VTE, duration of HT should be limited to 3 to 5 years for estrogen plus progestin or an average of 7 years for estrogen alone (i.e., status post hysterectomy). Women with premature menopause who are candidates for HT can use this treatment until the median age of menopause, 51 years, with longer treatment considered if needed for symptom management (NAMS, 2012).

Contraindications

The WHI was a large, 8- to 10-year study of healthy, post-menopausal women with a randomized controlled component of 27,347 postmenopausal women, ages 50 to 79 years (WHI Writing Group, 2002). They were randomized to HT (estrogen alone, estrogen plus progestin) or placebo. The estrogen used was continuous-combined CEE 0.625 mg daily and 2.5 mg MPA daily. The estrogen plus progestin arm was stopped early (after about 5.2 years). This group also had increased risk of coronary events, stroke, pulmonary embolism, and invasive breast cancer. The thought is that because there was an increased incidence of invasive breast cancer, HT promotes the growth of existing breast cancer rather than causing cancer. There was a reduced risk of colorectal cancer and hip fractures. Many of the risks appeared in year 1 (coronary and venous thromboembolic events) and year 2 (stroke). It was determined based on the data that the risk–benefit profile of estrogen plus progestin was such that its use for primary prevention of chronic conditions was not validated and it should not be prescribed to prevent chronic conditions. The study was stopped in 2002. Poststopping, and representing 13 years of cumulative follow-up for the WHI, there continues to be (1) lack of support for the use of HT for chronic disease prevention and (2) acknowledgment that the lowest risks of long-term negative effects occur in younger women with hysterectomy receiving CEE alone. Additional subanalyses focusing on the younger cohort of the WHI (estrogen alone or HT) have failed to find adverse cardiac outcomes among this subset. In fact, women in their 50s who took estrogen appear to have less coronary artery calcification than controls (Manson et al., 2013).

Box 56.1 identifies specific contraindications to the use of HT in postmenopausal women; in addition, oral contraceptives are contraindicated in smokers older than 35 years of age.

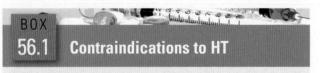

BOX 56.1 Contraindications to HT

ABSOLUTE CONTRAINDICATIONS

- Known or suspected breast cancer
- Known or suspected endometrial cancer
- Untreated endometrial hyperplasia
- Uncontrolled hypertension
- Acute liver disease
- Active thromboembolic disease or history of thromboembolic disease
- Known or suspected pregnancy

RELATIVE CONTRAINDICATIONS

- Chronic, mild liver dysfunction
- Smoking (cigarettes, marijuana)
- Acute intermittent porphyria

Adverse Events

The routine physical examination for a postmenopausal woman should include the patient's measured height, a gynecologic examination, and clinical breast examination. Investigative studies should include a pregnancy test, mammogram, and Papanicolaou (Pap) smear. Conditions that predispose women to increased risk of endometrial cancer include a lifelong history of irregular menses, polycystic ovary disease, or a recent history of irregular menses occurring closer than 21 days apart or menses lasting longer than 10 days. These women should have an endometrial biopsy before beginning HT. Adverse events include intolerance to contact lenses from steepening of corneal curvature, headache, and gallbladder disease, an increase in serum triglycerides, nausea, vomiting, abdominal cramps, increased blood pressure, thromboembolic disease, edema, breast cancer, breast tenderness, and breakthrough bleeding. **Table 56.1** identifies side effects associated with various elements of HT.

All continuous HT regimens can cause breakthrough bleeding. About 30% of all women who are recently menopausal have some breakthrough bleeding; this decreases with women who are more than 3 years postmenopausal. Amenorrhea usually occurs within 1 year of initiating therapy.

Relative to the longer term, more serious adverse events, data from the WHI show that short-term use of combined estrogen and progestin increases the incidence of breast cancer and abnormal mammograms. Those women in the study taking HT were diagnosed at a more advanced stage of breast cancer. In the WHI, this risk was an additional eight cases of breast cancer per 10,000 women using estrogen plus progestin for 5 or more years.

The results of the WHI showed that for every 10,000 women taking MHT for 1 year, there was an increase of eight strokes, seven cases of CHD, eight more invasive breast cancers, and eight additional pulmonary embolisms (Manson et al., 2013).

Interactions

Drug interactions with CEE include increased effects of corticosteroids and decreased levels of estrogen with barbiturates, phenytoin, and rifampin. Patients taking phenytoin metabolize estrogen more quickly. An increased dose of estrogen may be needed in smokers because only half the serum level achieved in nonsmokers is reached. However, any changes in CEE dose should be based upon symptom response, not anticipated responses. Alternatively, alcohol increases the circulating levels of estrogen due to the liver's preoccupation with metabolizing the alcohol at the expense of the estrogen.

Additional/Summary Recommendations

The Endocrine Society issued conclusions on the use of HT (Santen, 2010). Select conclusions with "A level" of evidence include the following:

- "Standard-dose" estrogen used with or without a progestogen is associated with marked reduction in frequency and severity of hot flashes. For many women, lower doses of estrogen are also effective.

- For symptoms of vaginal atrophy, very low doses of vaginal estradiol are effective.
- Symptoms of overactive bladder may be reduced by estrogen given vaginally or systemically.
- Vaginal estrogen is associated with lower rates of recurrent urinary tract infections.
- For women in late postmenopause, estrogen given with or without a progestogen is as effective as bisphosphonate therapy for preventing early postmenopausal bone loss and increasing bone mass.
- Use of estrogen alone and estrogen plus a progestogen is associated with a lower incidence of hip and vertebral fractures.
- Use of HT containing estrogen plus a progestogen is linked to a lower risk of colon cancer.
- Mammographic density is increased in women taking estrogen alone or with a progestogen.
- Risk for venothrombotic episodes is approximately doubled in women using HT, and this risk is multiplicative with baseline risk factors such as age, increased body mass index, thrombophilias, surgery, and immobilization.
- Although continuous estrogen plus a progestogen does not cause endometrial cancer, estrogen alone without a progestogen is associated with an increased incidence of endometrial cancer.
- The risk of gallbladder disease is increased in women using estrogen alone or with a progestogen.

Estrogen Agonist/Antagonist

Ospemifene (Osphena), the only agent in this class of drugs approved for postmenopausal symptom management, notably for the treatment of the genitourinary symptom of dyspareunia, is an alternative to HT for this indication. Further, it is recommended by the NAMS for moderate to severe dyspareunia.

Mechanism of Action

Ospemifene binds to both estrogen receptor alpha (ERα) and estrogen receptor beta (ERβ). It acts as an agonist in some tissues and as an antagonist in other tissues. Specifically, it acts similarly to estrogen in vaginal tissues (i.e., minimizing dyspareunia) and has very weak estrogen activity in the uterus (i.e., minimal role in contributing to endometrial hyperplasia). It is a triethylene derivative, similar to tamoxifen, and as such may also have antiestrogenic activity in breast tissue therefore lacking the increased risk of breast cancer observed with traditional HT. Similar to HT, it has been shown to reduce bone turnover as measured by biochemical markers of bone turnover.

Dosage

Ospemifene is administered orally at a dose of 60 mg daily. It is recommended that it be taken with food to maximize its absorption from the gut.

Time Frame for Response

Clinical trials evaluating ospemifene have included those of 12 weeks duration and out to 52 weeks. While a meaningful response was not noted to occur before two weeks of treatment, clinical efficacy was realized by 12 weeks and observed to continue through to 52 weeks.

Contraindications

Ospemifene use should be avoided in women with undiagnosed, abnormal vaginal bleeding, women with known or suspected estrogen-dependent neoplasia, and women with a history of or active thromboembolic disease.

Adverse Events

Overall, in studies with ospemifene, 61% of women experienced an adverse event. Among these, the most common were vaginal discharge, muscle spasms, hot flashes, and hyperhidrosis. In particular, the rate of hot flashes observed with ospemifene was more than double than that observed in the placebo groups (8% vs. 3%). To date, there are no studies exceeding 1 year in duration such that any long-term side effects are yet to be identified.

The labeling for ospemifene includes a boxed warning for increased risk of VTE events, cardiovascular disease, and endometrial cancer with its use. And while the U.S. Food and Drug Administration currently recommends the concomitant use of a progestin in women receiving ospemifene who have an intact uterus, there is currently no study to evaluate this combination.

Interactions

Ospemifene is metabolized by the cytochrome (CYP) P-450 isoenzyme system and is a highly protein-bound agent. Its concurrent use with other drugs that are inhibited or induced by CYP 3A4, 2C9, or 2C19 or that are greater than 89% protein bound may significantly alter ospemifene's effects. The manufacturer specifically recommends avoiding the concomitant use of fluconazole and rifampin.

Tissue Selective Estrogen Complex

TSEC describes the combination of CEE and bazedoxifene, an estrogen agonist/antagonist. This product is currently marketed under the brand name Duavee and is approved for the treatment of moderate to severe VMS.

Mechanism of Action

Like ospemifene, bazedoxifene acts as an estrogen agonist in some tissues and an antagonist in others. In particular, it acts as an antagonist in uterine tissue, reducing the risk for developing endometrial hyperplasia. Its effect as an estrogen agonist is responsible for its role in minimizing bone loss. When bazedoxifene is combined with CEE, the effects include a further reduction in bone mineral density loss, a reduction in VMS, and no greater increased risk of VTE (compared to the combination of CEE and progestin).

Dosage

The recommended dose following dose-ranging studies and based upon safety and efficacy data is 20 mg bazedoxifene plus 0.45 mg OR 0.625 mg CEE by mouth daily.

Time Frame for Response

A significant 74% to 80% reduction in the severity and frequency of hot flashes (compared to placebo) was observed following 12 weeks of treatment. A secondary outcome of improvement in sleep symptoms was also observed.

Contraindications

Use of the combination of bazedoxifene plus CEE should be avoided in patients with active or past history of VTE disorder, active or past history of an arterial thromboembolic disorder, a history of or current breast cancer, hepatic impairment or disease, and protein C and S or antithrombin deficiency that would predispose a woman to clot formation.

Adverse Events

In clinical trials, the adverse events observed with the combination of bazedoxifene plus CEE were comparable to those observed in the placebo treatment groups.

Interactions

The concomitant use of bazedoxifene and ospemifene is to be avoided. Other interactions with this combination product include those noted with estrogen in the HT treatment section of this chapter.

Selective Serotonin Reuptake Inhibitors and Selective Serotonin–Norepinephrine Reuptake Inhibitors

Agents including paroxetine, sertraline, venlafaxine, desvenlafaxine, citalopram, and escitalopram have been evaluated for their efficacy in reducing VMS associated with menopause. Only paroxetine, marketed as Brisdelle, has received FDA approval for the treatment of moderate to severe VMS.

Mechanism of Action

The preoptic area of the anterior hypothalamus, responsible for temperature regulation, is under the influence of serotonin and norepinephrine. The action of these two neurotransmitters at the hypothalamus is negatively affected by fluctuating estrogen levels. Therefore, the use of the SSRIs and selective

serotonin–norepinephrine reuptake inhibitors (SNRIs) reestablish the neurotransmitters in the thermoregulatory center of the hypothalamus, improving VMS.

Dosage

Recommended starting doses of the abovementioned agents for the management of VMS associated with menopause are citalopram 10 mg by mouth daily, escitalopram 10 mg by mouth daily, venlafaxine 37.5 mg by mouth daily, desvenlafaxine 100 mg by mouth daily, sertraline 50 mg by mouth daily, and paroxetine 7.5 mg by mouth daily. The doses of citalopram, escitalopram, and venlafaxine can be increased to 30, 20, and 75 mg, respectively.

Time Frame for Response

While maximal dose–response effect to HT occurs in approximately 4 weeks, improvement in symptoms may be observed within the first week of treatment. To the contrary, the effects of the SSRIs and SNRIs are typically not realized until several weeks of therapy have been completed. After 4 to 8 weeks of treatment, an overall 30% to 75% reduction in hot flashes compared to placebo has been observed.

Contraindications

The SSRIs and SNRIs are not to be used within 14 days of the use of any of the monoamine oxidase inhibitors as such use may result in the development of serotonin syndrome.

Adverse Events

The most common adverse events observed with the use of the SSRIs and SNRIs include nausea, dizziness, dry mouth, nervousness, constipation, and sexual dysfunction.

Interactions

As noted under contraindications, the concomitant use of this class of drugs and a monoamine oxidase inhibitor may result in the development of the serotonin syndrome. Carbamazepine may increase the metabolism of the SSRIs/SNRIs and, conversely, the SSRIs/SNRIs may reduce carbamazepine metabolism. Cimetidine reduces the metabolism of the SSRIs/SNRIs. The SSRIs/SNRIs enhance the antiplatelet effects of nonsteroidal anti-inflammatory agents.

Gabapentin
Mechanism of Action

Gabapentin is an anticonvulsant that has been used to treat VMS associated with tamoxifen treatment in breast cancer patients as well as those associated with menopause. The mechanism of action of gabapentin for these purposes is unknown.

Dosage

Trials of gabapentin in postmenopausal women have utilized starting doses of 600 to 900 mg gabapentin in divided doses daily. Doses have been titrated to effect to a maximum total daily dose of 2.7 g.

Time Frame for Response

While efficacy may be appreciated at approximately 4 to 6 weeks of treatment, full effects may not be observed until as late as 12 weeks. In clinical trials, hot flash frequency was reduced by 45% and the composite hot flash score (including frequency and severity) was reduced by as much as 54% when compared to placebo.

Contraindications

Gabapentin should not be used in women with a history of hypersensitivity to gabapentin or any of its components.

Adverse Events

Somnolence, fatigue, dizziness, rash, and peripheral edema have been observed in women taking gabapentin for the treatment of VMS.

Interactions

Antacids may significantly reduce the absorption of gabapentin such that gabapentin should be dosed 2 hours after any antacids.

Clonidine

Clonidine is a centrally acting α-2 agonist used in the management of hypertension that has also been observed to treat VMS associated with menopause.

Mechanism of Action

The exact mechanism of clonidine in treating VMS is unclear but thought to be related to its central activity and potential impact on the thermoregulatory center in the hypothalamus.

Dosage

The recommended dose of clonidine for postmenopausal VMS is 0.1 mg by mouth daily.

Time Frame for Response

Improvement in VMS may be experienced following 4 to 6 weeks of clonidine treatment. Overall, clinical trial data for clonidine used to minimize VMS are lacking. What is available illustrates that clonidine is more effective than placebo but less effective than HT.

Contraindications

As clonidine is an antihypertensive agent, women with baseline low blood pressure would not be candidates for its use in managing VMS.

Adverse Events

The most common side effects noted with clonidine use include dry mouth, insomnia, drowsiness, and increased risk for hypotension.

Interactions

Clonidine may potentiate the effects of other central nervous system depressants.

SELECTING THE MOST APPROPRIATE THERAPY

The options for managing VMS and the GUSM are varied, and there is not one regimen that fits all patients. The regimens vary in dosage formulation as well as active drug. In addition, nondrug recommendations should also be considered. Regardless, a patient-centered approach identifying the potential benefits and risks of each regimen as well as patient preference(s) and potential for regimen adherence for each patient must be considered. The choice of regimen should be arrived at by the "team" of patient and provider.

The Patient-Centered Approach

The decision of how to manage VMS or symptoms of the GUSM is one that must be reached by both patient and provider. While HT remains the most effective treatment modality, its duration of use must be limited and many women do not view its benefits to outweigh its risks, such that alternative modalities are desired. Any treatment agreed to should be in addition to the lifestyle changes identified later in this chapter. **Figure 56.1** illustrates a decision tree that can be used in determining initial treatment modalities for women presenting with menopause-related symptoms. As noted, and included within the previous text of this chapter, whether or not a woman has had any history of estrogen-dependent cancer is a factor that contributes to the final management decision. Debate still exists over the short-term use of HT in women following treatment of estrogen-dependent cancers including breast, ovarian, and endometrial. One retrospective study found that in spite of being treated for an estrogen-dependent cancer, 19.5% of women chose to take estrogen for menopause-related symptoms (primarily VMS) in spite of the contraindications to its use (Sekar et al., 2013). In addition, while there appears little question or controversy surrounding the use of HT in younger women at the time of menopause as having a very positive benefit to risk profile and being the most effective treatment for VMS, the increasing evidence of the risks and benefits of HT beyond the age of 65 years makes HT as an initial treatment choice in this older population a much less clear decision. Alternative treatments to HT should be carefully considered in this population (Davies et al., 2013; Moyer, 2013).

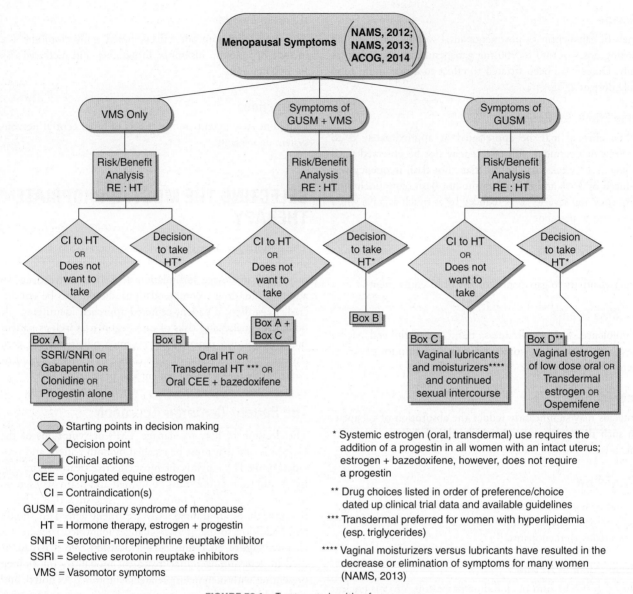

FIGURE 56.1 Treatment algorithm for menopause.

MONITORING PATIENT RESPONSE

The decision to continue HT should be revisited yearly, and therapy should be discontinued when symptoms resolve—usually in 1 to 3 years after menopause. And owing to an increase in breast cancer risk, its use beyond 3 to 5 years is not recommended (NAMS, 2012). The patient should be seen 4 to 8 weeks after starting therapy to evaluate response and make any necessary dosage adjustments and then in 3 to 6 months to monitor continued response to therapy, the need for any further dosage adjustments, and the occurrence of any side effects. After that, annual visits are required.

The health status of a woman on HT must be evaluated annually. Their medical history for the past year should be reviewed, including questions about vaginal bleeding. The woman should have an annual clinical breast examination and

mammogram if she is older than age 40. Any woman on continuous-combined HT who has vaginal bleeding beyond the first year of treatment should be evaluated with an endometrial biopsy. The physical examination should include:

- Height and weight measurements to screen for osteoporosis and obesity
- Fasting lipid panel according to recommendations
- Blood pressure evaluation to screen for cardiovascular disease
- Clinical breast examination and review of procedures for breast self-examination
- Full pelvic examination, including a Pap smear

Prescriptions for HT should not be renewed without a full annual history and physical. Discontinuing HT should be done gradually as abrupt discontinuation may lead to a rebound of symptoms. This may be done in several ways. The patient may begin to skip more days between doses or the daily dose may be decreased at 4- to 6-week intervals.

PATIENT EDUCATION

Following publication of many prospective, randomized trials in the late 1990s and early 2000s, and the subsequent unbalanced media coverage that ensued, many women abruptly discontinued their HT (resulting in a plethora of women with rebounding symptoms of menopause). This only further illustrated the need for practitioners to remain current with the HT research and be able to put the clinical trial data in a balanced light for their patients. It also illustrated the need for practitioners to be more aware than ever of the alternatives that exist to HT and to effectively communicate this to their patients without overwhelming them. Menopause is a natural part of the aging process and women need to know that their providers realize the gravity of the impact its consequences may have on QoL and trust that their providers will assist them in managing this part of their life.

Drug Information

Several options are available for the postmenopausal woman with VMS. If she decides to begin HT, the decision must be an informed decision. To make an informed decision, the patient must be provided with detailed information on the risks and benefits of therapy and other options available. It is also important to understand the side effects and that there may be monthly bleeding. General key teaching points include the following:

- The patient must be aware that it may take up to 4 weeks or more (depending on treatment option chosen) before symptoms to respond to treatment. Efficacy of the treatment chosen is typically dose dependent.
- Encourage patients to be aware of and communicate with their provider the occurrence of potential adverse events as, in some instances, there may be ways to minimize them. For example, HT can be taken with food or at bedtime to prevent nausea. For other, more severe adverse events such as VTE, patients should be educated regarding the signs and

symptoms and be encouraged to contact their provider in a very timely manner or seek emergency treatment as needed.
- Patients should be instructed to never, in the event of missed doses, double the next dose.
- Patients should be aware that the management of menopause-related symptoms is at the lowest necessary dose for the shortest duration as is needed; and they should be empowered to follow up with their provider regarding potential discontinuation of treatment in a timely manner.

Patient information sources for menopause include:

- The American Congress of Obstetricians and Gynecologists: http://www.acog.org/Patients
- Harvard Health Publications: http://www.health.harvard.edu/topics/womens-health
- The North American Menopause Society: http://www.menopause.org/for-women

Nutrition/Lifestyle Changes

The reduction in intake of refined carbohydrates, caffeine, and alcohol has been reported by women to result in minimizing hot flashes. Wearing only cotton clothing and maintaining low environmental temperatures may also allow women to feel more comfortable during hot flashes. Further recommendations to reduce VMS include dressing in layers, smoking cessation, and weight loss. The latter two suggestions are also beneficial to overall good health.

For genitourinary symptoms associated with menopause, specifically the symptoms of atrophy, regular sexual activity should be encouraged.

Complementary and Alternative Medications

In women not wishing to take pharmacologically active agents to minimize the symptoms of vaginal atrophy, the use of long-acting vaginal moisturizers and lubricants is an option. Such agents may increase the vaginal pH to premenopausal levels, and their use during intercourse may reduce friction-related effects worsened by atrophy.

Women are also turning to other herbs, such as soy or black cohosh, or the phytoestrogens for managing menopausal symptoms, specifically VMS (**Table 56.2**). Phytoestrogens,

TABLE 56.2

Herbal Treatment of Menopausal Symptoms

Menopausal Symptom	Herbal Treatment	Usual Dose	Adverse Events and Contraindications
Hot flashes	Black cohosh (*Cimicifuga*)	40–200 mg/d; not to be taken for >6 mo	Not to be used during pregnancy Potential side effects: GI disturbances, hypotension
Mood swings	Isoflavones (soy) St. John wort (*Hypericum*)	20–40 mg/d 300 mg tid	Flatulence Do not take with any antidepressant May cause sun sensitivity

CASE STUDY*

E.P., a 51-year-old Asian woman who is 68 inches tall and weighs 130 pounds, presents complaining of amenorrhea for the past 8 months. She wakes up at least 5 times a night with hot flashes and experiences them at least 10 times a day. She is very uncomfortable and sleep deprived. At the visit, a Pap smear is done and a mammogram is negative. Her FSH level is 32 international units/mL. She has no family history of breast cancer, but her mother has osteoporosis.

1. List specific goals for treatment for **E.P.**
2. What drug therapy would you prescribe? Why?

3. What are the parameters for monitoring success of the therapy?
4. Discuss specific patient education based on the prescribed therapy.
5. List one or two adverse reactions for the selected agent that would cause you to change therapy.
6. What would be the choice for second-line therapy?
7. What over-the-counter and/or alternative medications would be appropriate for **E.P.**?
8. What lifestyle changes would you recommend to **E.P.**?
9. Describe one or two drug–drug or drug–food interactions for the selected agent.

* Answers can be found online.

estrogens obtained from plant sources, are marketed in oral formulations for the management of VMS. An example of this is the brand-named product Promensil. Phytoestrogens are also found in a number of common foods including soybeans and soy products, cashews, peanuts, oats, corn, wheat, flaxseeds, and sunflower seeds. While phytoestrogens appear to lack the negative effects of estrogen relative to stimulation of the breast and uterus, they must be used for 4 to 6 weeks, before any improvement may be noticed. Soy, chickpeas, and other legumes contain isoflavones, which exhibit estrogenic properties. They can provide some VMS relief, although their effectiveness in menopause is still being investigated.

Another option is vitamin E. While vitamin E has been evaluated, the results have illustrated that the treatment group had minimal to no positive impact on daily hot flashes compared to placebo (Loprinzi et al., 2008). Some clinical trials have shown improvement of hot flashes with soy and black cohosh and some have shown no improvement (Faure et al., 2002).

And while black cohosh is also used to treat menopause, specifically purportedly inducing vaginal maturation and improving VMS, no long-term scientific data are available and concern regarding the development of hepatitis and myopathy with long-term use exists.

Bibliography

Starred references are cited in the text.

*American College of Obstetricians and Gynecologists. (2014). Practice Bulletin No. 141: Management of menopausal symptoms. *Obstetrics and Gynecology, 123*(1), 202–216.

Barnes, K. N., Pearce, E. F., Yancey, A. M., et al. (2014). Ospemifene in the treatment of vulvovaginal atrophy. *Annals of Pharmacotherapy, 48*(6), 752–757.

Carris, N., Kutner, S., Reilly-Rogers, S. (2014). New pharmacological therapies for vasomotor symptoms management: Focus on bazedoxifene/conjugated equine estrogens and paroxetine mesylate. *Annals of Pharmacotherapy, 48*(10), 1343–1349.

Carroll, D. G., Lisenby, K. M., & Carter, T. L. (2015). Critical appraisal of paroxetine for the treatment of vasomotor symptoms. *International Journal of Women's Health, 7*, 615–624.

*Coker, L. H., Espeland, M. A., Rapp, S. R., et al. (2010). Postmenopausal hormone therapy and cognitive outcomes: The Women's Health Initiative Memory Study (WHIMS). *The Journal of Steroid Biochemistry and Molecular Biology, 118*(4–5), 304–310.

*Davies, E., Mangongi, N. P., & Carter, C. L. (2013). Is timing everything? A meeting report of the Society for Women's Health Research roundtable on menopausal hormone therapy. *Journal of Women's Health, 22*(4), 303–312.

*Deecher, D. C., & Dorries, K. (2007). Understanding the pathophysiology of vasomotor symptoms (hot flushes and night sweats) that occur in perimenopause, menopause, and postmenopause. *Archives of Women's Mental Health, 10*, 247–257.

Eder, S. E. (2014). Ospemifene: A novel selective estrogen receptor modulator for treatment of dyspareunia. *Women's Health, 10*(5), 499–503.

*Faure, E., Chantre, P., & Mares, P. (2002). Effects of a standardized soy extract on hot flushes: A multicenter, double-blind randomized, placebo-controlled study. *Menopause, 9*, 329–334.

*Harlow, S. D., Gass, M., Hall, J. E., et al. (2012). Executive summary of the Stages of Reproductive Aging Workshop +10: Addressing the unfinished agenda of staging reproductive aging. *Menopause, 19*(4), 1–9.

Krause, M. S., & Nakajima, S. T. (2015). Hormonal and nonhormonal treatments of vasomotor symptoms. *Obstetric and Gynecologic Clinics of North America, 42*, 163–179.

*Loprinzi, C. L., Barton, D. L., Sloan, J. A., et al. (2008). Mayo Clinic and North Central Cancer treatment group hot flash studies: A 20-year experience. *Menopause, 15*, 655–660.

*Manson J. E., Chlebowski, R. T., Stefanick, M. L., et al. (2013). Menopausal hormone therapy and health outcomes during the intervention and extended poststopping phases of the Women's Health Initiative randomized trials. *Journal of the American Medical Association, 310*(13), 1353–1368.

McLendon, A. N., Clinard, V. B., & Woodis, C. B. (2014). Ospemifene for the treatment of vulvovaginal atrophy and dyspareunia in postmenopausal women. *Pharmacotherapy, 34*(10), 1050–1060.

Mirkin, S., Komm, B., & Pickar, J. H. (2014). Conjugated estrogen/bazedoxifene tablets for the treatment of moderate-to-severe vasomotor symptoms associated with menopause. *Women's Health, 10*(2), 135–146.

*Moyer, V. A., on behalf of the U.S. Preventive Services Task Force (2013). Menopausal hormone therapy for the primary prevention of chronic conditions: U.S. Preventive Services Task Force Recommendation Statement. *Annals of Internal Medicine, 158*(1), 47–54.

*North American Menopause Society. (2010). Overview of menopause. In *Menopause practice: A clinician's guide* (4th ed., Chapter 1). Retrieved from http://menopause.org/publications/other-resources/terms-statistics# on June 19, 2015.

North American Menopause Society. (2011). The role of soy isoflavones in menopausal health: Report of the North American Menopause Society/Wulf H. Utian Translational Science Symposium in Chicago, IL (October 2010). *Menopause, 18*(7), 732–753.

*North American Menopause Society. (2012). The 2012 hormone therapy position statement of the North American Menopause Society. *Menopause, 19*(3), 257–271.

*North American Menopause Society. (2013). Management of symptomatic vulvovaginal atrophy: 2013 position statement of the North American Menopause Society. *Menopause, 20*(9), 888–902.

*Portman, D. J., & Gass, M. L. (2014). Genitourinary syndrome of menopause: New terminology for vulvovaginal atrophy from the International Society for the Study of Women's Sexual Health and the North American Menopause Society. *Menopause, 21*(10), 1–6.

Rao, S., Singh, S., Parker, M., et al. (2008). Health maintenance for postmenopausal women. *American Family Physician, 78*(5), 583–591.

Reed, S., Newton, K., LaCroix, A., et al. (2007). Night sweats, sleep disturbances and depression associated with diminished libido in late menopausal transition and early postmenopause: Baseline data from the Herbal Alternatives for Menopause Trail (HALT). *American Journal of Obstetrics and Gynecology, 196*(6), 1–7.

*Rossaminth, W. G., & Ruebberdt, W. (2009). What causes hot flashes? The neuroendocrine origin of vasomotor symptoms in the menopause. *Gynecological Endocrinology, 25*(5), 303–314.

*Santen, R. J. (2010). Postmenopausal hormone therapy: An Endocrine Society scientific statement. *Journal of Clinical Endocrinology and Metabolism, 7*(Suppl. 1), S1–S66.

*Sekar, H., Singhal, T., Holloway, D., et al. (2013). The use of hormone therapy and its alternatives in women with a history of hormone dependent cancer. *Menopause International*, 1–6. doi: 10.1177/1754045312473874.

*Thurston, R. C., & Joffe, H. (2011). Vasomotor symptoms and menopause: Findings from the Study of Women's Health Across the Nation. *Obstetrics and Gynecology, 38*, 489–501.

Umland, E. M., & Falconieri, L. (2012). Treatment options for vasomotor symptoms in menopause: Focus on desvenlafaxine. *International Journal of Women's Health, 4*, 305–319.

*Utian, W. H., Shoupe, D., Bochman, G., et al. (2001). Relief of vasomotor symptoms and vaginal atrophy with lower doses of conjugated equine estrogen and medroxyprogesterone acetate. *Fertility Sterility, 75*, 1065–1079.

*Vaughan, L., Espeland, M. A., Snively, B., et al. (2013). The rationale, design, and baseline characteristics of the Women's Health Initiative Memory Study of Younger Women (WHIMS-Y). *Brain Research, 1514*, 3–11.

*Writing Group for the PEPI Trial. (1995). Effects of estrogen or estrogen/progestin on heart disease risk factors in post menopausal women. *Journal of the American Medical Association, 273*, 199–208.

*Writing Group for the Women's Health Initiative. (2002). Risks and benefits of estrogen plus progestin in healthy postmenopausal women. *Journal of the American Medical Association, 288*, 321–333.

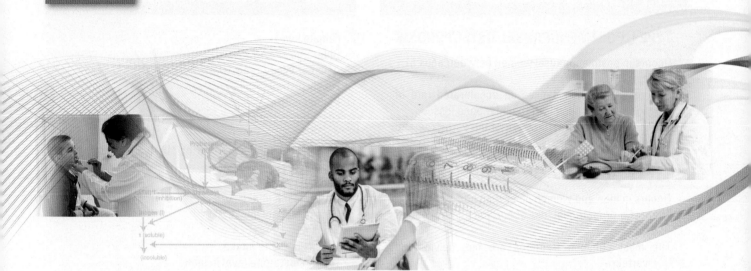

57 Osteoporosis

Virginia P. Arcangelo

Osteoporosis is a progressive systemic disease characterized by a decrease in bone mass and microarchitectural deterioration of bone tissue, resulting in bone fragility and increased susceptibility to fractures. Bone loss occurs at about 10% each 10 years after the age of 30. Each decade after 40 years is associated with a fivefold increase in the incidence of osteoporosis. Osteoporosis, or low bone mass (osteopenia), is estimated to occur in approximately 54 million Americans aged 50 years and older, 80% of whom are women (National Osteoporosis Foundation, 2014). Women are more likely than men to develop osteoporosis because of thinner, lighter bones, changes associated with menopause, and greater longevity than men.

One in four men will have an osteoporotic-associated fracture. Men develop osteoporosis because of the inability to convert testosterone into estrogen through enzyme deficiency leading to decreased bone mass. They also may develop it because of medication side effects.

Osteoporosis affects 10.2 million adults, and another 43.4 million have low bone mass; more than one half of the total U.S. adult population is currently affected (http://nof.org/news/2948, accessed 3/28/2015). Based on these statistics, it is predicted that by 2020, the number of adults over age 50 with osteoporosis is 64.4 million, and by 2030, the number will increase to 71.2 million (http://nof.org/news/2948, accessed 3/28/2015).

Bone fracture is the major cause of mortality and morbidity in patients with osteoporosis. The most common fractures are vertebral compression fractures and fractures of the distal radius and proximal femur.

CAUSES

The three types of osteoporosis are postmenopausal, senile, and secondary (**Box 57.1**). Many risk factors are associated with osteoporosis (**Box 57.2**).

Skeletal growth and the majority of bone mass are achieved during the first two decades of life, with bone density peaking around age 30. Between age 30 and menopause, bone mass remains relatively stable. At menopause, women have a period of 5 or more years during which there is an accelerated rate of bone loss. Some women lose up to 5% of their bone mass per year during this time.

PATHOPHYSIOLOGY

Two types of bone are discerned at the macroscopic level: cortical bone and trabecular bone. Cortical bone has a dense structure, whereas trabecular bone has a spongy appearance. Long bones have a thick outer layer of cortical bone and a thin inner layer of trabecular bone, whereas short bones consist of mostly trabecular bone with a thin layer of cortical bone.

The skeleton undergoes continuous remodeling throughout life. Bone remodeling involves the removal of mineralized bone by osteoclasts followed by the formation of bone matrix through the osteoblasts that become mineralized. There are three phases of remodeling: resorption, during which osteoclasts digest old bone; reversal, when mononuclear cells appear on the bone surface; and formation, when osteoblasts lay down new bone until the resorbed bone is completely replaced. Bone remodeling serves to maintain skeletal integrity and repairs microdamages in bone matrix preventing the accumulation of old bone. Additionally, it serves to maintain plasma calcium homeostasis. Bone remodeling takes place at the systemic and local level. The major systemic regulators include parathyroid hormone (PTH), calcitriol, and other hormones such as growth hormone, glucocorticoids, thyroid hormones, and sex hormones. Factors such as insulin-like growth factors (IGFs),

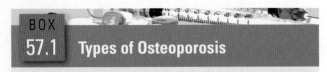

BOX 57.1 Types of Osteoporosis

TYPE I: POSTMENOPAUSAL OSTEOPOROSIS

Occurs in postmenopausal women between ages 51 and 75.
Decreased estrogen causes an accelerated rate of bone loss, especially trabecular bone loss.
The most common fractures are of the vertebrae and distal femur. There is also tooth loss.

TYPE II: SENILE OSTEOPOROSIS

Occurs in men and women older than age 70.
There is a proportional loss of cortical and trabecular bone.
The most common fractures are hip, pelvic, and vertebral.

TYPE III: SECONDARY OSTEOPOROSIS

Occurs in men and women at any age.
Secondary to other conditions such as drug therapy and other diseases.

BOX 57.2 Risk Factors for Osteoporosis

Female sex
Older age
Asian or White race
Family history
Petite stature
Low body weight
Amenorrhea
Menopause (either natural or surgical) without hormone replacement
Sedentary lifestyle
Low calcium intake
Excess alcohol intake
Smoking
Excess caffeine intake
Low testosterone level in men
Drugs
    Thyroid replacement drugs
    Lithium
    Glucocorticoids
    Anticonvulsants
    Chemotherapy
    Heparin
    Cyclosporin
    Depot medroxyprogesterone (Depo-Provera)
    Tamoxifen, before menopause
    Pioglitazone (Actos) and rosiglitazone (Avandia)
Disease states
    Anorexia/bulimia
    Cushing syndrome
    Thyrotoxicosis
    Rheumatoid arthritis
    Type 1 diabetes mellitus
    Thalassemia

prostaglandins, tumor growth factor-beta (TGF-beta), bone morphogenetic proteins (BMPs), and cytokines are involved as well. At the local level, there are cytokines and growth factors that affect bone cell functions. Through the RANK/receptor activator of NF-kappa B ligand (RANKL)/osteoprotegerin (OPG) system, the processes of bone resorption and formation are closely interwoven allowing bone formation to follow each cycle of bone resorption to maintain skeletal integrity.

An imbalance in bone remodeling causes osteoporosis. This can be due to numerous factors targeting both osteoblasts and osteoclasts that result in greater resorption than formation. One cause is the decreased estrogen levels during menopause causing an up-regulation of RANKL. OPG secretion is suppressed. Because of this, there is greater osteoclastogenesis and accelerated bone resorption. Because bone formation is coupled to resorption, the entire remodeling unit is activated. Bone resorption is a rapid process, taking about 2 weeks for the osteoclasts to attach and resorb matrix. Formation is much more deliberate, meaning that with the release of soluble cytokines, an imbalance in remodeling immediately occurs, and this favors bone resorption. The loss is faster than remodeling causing bone loss. Estrogen administration can prevent bone loss by enhancing OPG production as well as by suppressing RANKL expression.

Bone is in a constant state of remodeling (reforming). Osteoblasts are responsible for bone formation and osteoclasts for bone resorption. A balance is normally achieved between osteoblast and osteoclast activity. When bone resorption occurs at a faster rate than bone remodeling, osteoporosis is the result because the bones then become brittle and prone to fracture. Bone loss is greater in trabecular bone than in cortical bone.

Maximal mineral content of cortical bone occurs between the second and fourth decades of life, followed by a slow decline. In general, women have less bone mass than men, so even a small loss is more significant in women. Cortical bone loss in women is approximately 3% per decade until menopause, when the rate of bone loss accelerates to 9% per decade. Women lose approximately 15% of trabecular bone during the first 5 to 7 years after menopause. The rate returns to normal approximately 20 years after menopause. Generalized bone loss in men occurs at a rate of approximately 4% per decade throughout life.

Diagnostic Criteria

Medical history and a drug history are essential in the diagnosis. Bone mineral density (BMD) is related to bone mass at maturity and subsequent bone loss. Dual-energy x-ray absorptiometry (DEXA) scan measures BMD and is used to diagnose osteoporosis. A BMD of –1 to –2.5 standard deviations (SD) signifies osteopenia. A BMD of –2.5 SD, or lower than the mean for a normal 30- to 35-year-old woman, is diagnostic of osteoporosis. Initial screening is recommended for:

- All women older than age 65
- Younger perimenopausal or postmenopausal women and men who have any medical condition or are taking medication associated with bone loss
- Any adult older than age 50 with a fracture
- Anyone being treated for osteoporosis
- Men age 50 and older at risk

For every 1 SD decrease in bone mass, the relative risk of fracture increases by 1.5 to 3 SD.

The guidelines use fracture risk calculations derived from a new computerized model developed by the World Health Organization (WHO). FRAX, or "WHO Fracture Risk Assessment Tool," is a free online tool. It assesses the likelihood a patient will experience an osteoporotic fracture within 10 years. FRAX considers 10 risk factors in addition to the BMD T-score so it will aid in the decision-making process of who to treat. The risk factors are age, gender, fracture history, parental hip fracture history, oral steroid therapy, low body mass index, femoral neck BMD, secondary osteoporosis, current smoking, and alcohol intake. FRAX is available for download at http://www.shef.ac.uk/FRAX/.

INITIATING DRUG THERAPY

Prevention of osteoporosis should begin early in life with adequate intake of calcium and vitamin D. Children ages 9 to 18 should consume 1,300 mg of calcium daily. Adults ages 19 to 50 need 1,000 mg of calcium per day, and those age 51 and older require 1,200 mg each day. Because it is difficult to ingest that amount, supplements are usually needed. Weight-bearing exercise enhances bone mass and thereby helps prevent osteoporosis. Alcohol intake should be minimal, and those who smoke should stop.

Drugs used for the prevention and treatment of osteoporosis decrease bone resorption. They are called resorption-inhibiting drugs and include estrogens, bisphosphonates, calcitonin, and selective estrogen receptor modulators (SERMs). When these drugs are given, the rate of bone resorption decreases within weeks and the rate of bone formation increases within months. Remodeling spaces fill in, and an increase of BMD of 5% to 10% occurs with treatment. This process takes 2 to 3 years.

The National Osteoporosis Foundation (NOF) recommends that health care providers should consider U.S. Food and Drug Administration (FDA)–approved medical therapies in patients with:

1. Low bone mass (T-score from –1.0 to –2.5 at the femoral neck, total hip, or spine) and 10-year probability of hip fracture of 3% or more or a 10-year probability of any major osteoporosis-related fracture of 20% or more
2. T-score of 2.5 or less at the femoral neck, total hip, or spine after appropriate evaluation to exclude secondary causes
3. Low bone mass (T-score from –1.0 to –2.5 at the femoral neck, total hip, or spine) and secondary causes associated with high fracture risk (such as glucocorticoid use or immobilization)
4. A hip or vertebral (clinical or morphometric) fracture
5. Other prior fractures and low bone mass (BMD T-score from –1.0 to –2.5 at the femoral neck, total hip, or spine).

Goals of Drug Therapy

The goals of drug therapy are minimizing bone loss, delaying the progression of osteoporosis, and preventing fractures and fracture-related morbidity and mortality. Once osteoporosis is diagnosed and drug therapy is started, it is continued for life. **Table 57.1** provides an overview of the drugs used in treatment.

Calcium Supplements

There has been recent discussion about calcium supplements increasing cardiovascular risk.

Data have been analyzed and it has been determined that there is no strong evidence that calcium supplement intake increases CVD risk in women (Paik et al., 2014).

Sufficient calcium intake is necessary for the prevention of osteoporosis. Postmenopausal women should take 1,200 to 1,500 mg of calcium a day. This can be achieved through dietary intake or supplements. Calcium is absorbed most effectively when taken in small amounts throughout the day. Patients should not take calcium with meals that are high in fiber or with bulk-forming laxatives because such materials decrease absorption. The over-the-counter (OTC) antacid Tums is an excellent and inexpensive source of calcium.

Most brand-name calcium products are absorbed easily in the body. If the product information does not state that it is absorbable, how well a tablet dissolves can be determined by placing it in a small amount of warm water for 30 minutes, stirring occasionally. If it hasn't dissolved within this time, it probably will not dissolve in the stomach. Chewable and liquid calcium supplements dissolve well because they are broken down before they enter the stomach. Calcium carbonate is absorbed best when taken with food. Calcium citrate can be taken any time. Calcium, whether from the diet or supplements, is absorbed best by the body when it is taken several times a day in amounts of 500 mg or less, but taking it all at once is better than not taking it at all.

TABLE 57.1

Overview of Selected Agents Used to Prevent or Treat Osteoporosis

Generic (Trade) Name and Dosage	Selected Adverse Events	Contraindications	Special Considerations
Bisphosphonates			
alendronate (Fosamax) Prevention: 5 mg/d or 35 mg once a week Treatment: 10 mg/d or 70 mg once a week	GI upset, abdominal pain, gastroesophageal reflux disease, esophagitis, headache	Esophageal abnormalities, inability to be upright for 30 min, hypocalcemia, creatinine clearance <30	Swallow whole Take with 8 oz of water 30 min before eating or drinking Sit or stand for 30 min after taking (do not lie down until after eating) Calcium supplements and aluminum- or magnesium-containing antacids may interfere with absorption, so it should be given at a different time
risedronate (Actonel) 5 mg/d or 35 mg once a week	Arthralgia, GI disturbances, headache, abdominal pain, rash, edema, chest pain, bone pain, dizziness, leg cramps, infection	Same as above	Same as above This drug is more tolerable for patients with GI problems than alendronate
ibandronate (Boniva) 2.5 mg PO daily or 150 mg PO once a month or 3 mg/3 mL IV every 3 mo	Same as above	Same as above	If taken monthly, take the same day each month IV medication is given in a bolus over 15–30 s
zoledronic acid (Reclast) 5 mg/100 mL once a day	Same as above	Same as above	Infusion must be given over at least 15 min
Selective Estrogen Receptor Modulators			
raloxifene (Evista) 60 mg qd	Hot flashes, leg cramps	Pregnancy, history of thromboembolic events	Medication is to be stopped 72 h before surgery or prolonged immobilization
RANK Ligand Inhibitor			
denosumab (Prolia) 60 mg subq q 6 months	Musculoskeletal pain, infection, arthralgia, myalgia, and abdominal pain	Pregnancy, low calcium	Caution in creatinine clearance <30, immunosuppression, small bowel excision
Other			
calcitonin (Miacalcin) 200 U (1 spray) daily 100 U IM or SC daily	Rhinitis, GI upset, back pain, facial flushing (with injection)	Allergy to salmon or fish products, lactation Caution in renal deficiencies	Perform periodic nasal examinations to check for ulceration Stop if nasal ulceration results Switch nostrils each day Injection recommended at bedtime because of possible facial flushing and nausea
Hormone Modifiers			
teriparatide (Forteo) 20 mcg daily SC	Hypercalcemia, dizziness, hyperuricemia, leg cramps, nausea, arthralgia	Paget disease, previous bone radiation, skeletal malignancy, hypercalcemia, hyperparathyroidism; caution with kidney stones	Used in women with a high risk of fracture or who have failed other therapies

While calcium supplements are a satisfactory option for many people, certain preparations may cause side effects, such as gas or constipation, in some individuals. If simple measures such as increased fluids and fiber intake do not solve the problem, another form of calcium should be tried. Also, it is important to increase supplement intake gradually; take 500 mg/d for a week, then add more calcium slowly.

Even if calcium supplements are not taken, vitamin D intake is important. Vitamin D is responsible for the maintenance of an adequate concentration of calcium and phosphorus in the extracellular fluid. It also works with PTH to regulate calcium movement across the gastrointestinal (GI) tract. The recommendation is 800 to 1,000 international units of vitamin D_3.

LEAVE ALL OF THIS IN Estrogen administration can prevent bone loss by enhancing OPG production as well as by suppressing RANKL expression.

Bisphosphonates

Alendronate (Fosamax), risedronate (Actonel), ibandronate (Boniva), and zoledronic acid (Reclast) are bisphosphonates used for preventing and treating osteoporosis.

Mechanism of Action

These drugs inhibit bone resorption and increase bone density. They are deposited in the bone at sites of mineralization and in resorption lacunae. The bone resorption and fracture rates decline, whereas bone density increases. In studies of alendronate, an increase in bone mass was shown in the spine and hip, with a 48% decrease in the rate of vertebral compression fractures. Bone turnover increases to previous levels after 6 to 9 months when the patient takes alendronate for 6 months and then stops. If the patient takes alendronate for 6 years, no decrease in bone mass is noted for 2 years after therapy stops. These drugs have been used successfully for prevention and treatment of decreased bone mass as a result of long-term use of glucocorticoids.

In large, randomized, controlled trials, alendronate showed consistent increases in BMD irrespective of the severity of the underlying bone density levels, and it reduced the incidence of both vertebral and nonvertebral fractures (Cummings et al., 1998; Liberman et al., 1995). Among women with osteoporosis, the incidence of symptomatic vertebral fractures was decreased by 44% over 4 years and clinical fractures were reduced by 36% (Cummings et al., 1998). Risedronate similarly reduced the incidence of vertebral fractures by 41% over 3 years (Harris et al., 1999) and reduced hip fractures by 40% in elderly women who had low BMD but not in women who had risk factors alone (McClung et al., 2001).

Dosage

The dosage for alendronate is 5 mg/d for prevention and 10 mg/d for treatment. It has also been approved for use once a week at 35 mg for prevention and 70 mg for treatment. Intestinal absorption of the drug is poor, so patients should take it on awakening with 8 ounces of water and 30 minutes before consuming any food or other drink. The dosage for risedronate is 5 mg/d or 35 mg once a week for prevention and treatment. The dosage for ibandronate is 2.5 mg daily or 150 mg once a month. There is also a 3 mg/3 mL solution for intravenous (IV) use every 3 months. Zoledronic acid is an IV medication given once a year. The dose is 5 mg/100 mL.

Contraindications

Bisphosphonates are not prescribed to patients with a history of esophageal problems, gastritis, or peptic ulcer disease. Adverse events include GI disturbance, esophagitis, diarrhea, and abdominal pain. Absorption increases with intravenous administration of ranitidine. Bisphosphonates should be prescribed with caution when the patient also is using nonsteroidal anti-inflammatory drugs. Absorption decreases when these drugs are taken with food, calcium, or iron, so patients should take the medication at different times from these substances (i.e., at least 30 minutes before or after taking food or liquid nourishment).

Adverse Events

Alendronate can cause esophagitis, usually within the first month of therapy. Ways to diminish esophagitis as well as to increase drug absorption include taking alendronate and risedronate with 8 ounces of water and remaining upright for 30 minutes after administration. Risedronate has fewer harsh effects on the GI system.

Calcitonin

Salmon calcitonin (Miacalcin) is another drug used in treating osteoporosis.

Mechanism of Action

Calcitonin works by inhibiting the action of osteoclasts. It is available in injectable form and as a nasal spray. It is not effective in preventing bone loss early in the postmenopausal period, but studies have shown that it increases bone mass in the spine and decreases the risk of vertebral compression fractures. Calcitonin also has an analgesic effect on pain associated with vertebral compression fractures.

In one study of postmenopausal women who used calcitonin daily, new vertebral fractures were decreased by 33% compared with placebo, though only a small increase was noted in BMD (Chesnut et al., 2000).

Dosage

The intranasal dosage of calcitonin is 200 U/d. The patient should alternate nostrils each day. The injectable dosage is 100 U subcutaneously or intramuscularly each day.

Adverse Events

An adverse event with the use of nasal calcitonin is rhinitis. The nasal mucosa should be inspected every 6 months for ulceration. Injection can cause local irritation. With both inhalation and injection, GI upset, flushing, rash, and back pain may occur. Recommendations are for patients to perform injections at bedtime because facial flushing and nausea may occur.

Selective Estrogen Receptor Modulators

SERMs are indicated for treating and preventing osteoporosis. They reduce the risk of vertebral fractures but do not appear to have an effect on hip fractures.

Mechanism of Action

SERMs mimic the effects of estrogen on bones without replicating the stimulating effects of estrogen on the breasts and uterus. They decrease bone resorption and bone turnover. These agents also decrease total cholesterol and low-density lipoprotein cholesterol levels.

Dosage

Raloxifene (Evista) is the only available SERM. The dose is 60 mg/d. Supplemental calcium and vitamin D are recommended.

Contraindications

Raloxifene is contraindicated in women who are lactating or who may become pregnant. It is also contraindicated in women who have a history of thromboembolic events. The patient must discontinue the drug 72 hours before prolonged immobilization, such as surgery requiring bed rest.

Adverse Events

Adverse events include hot flashes, GI distress, flu-like symptoms, leg cramps, deep vein thrombosis, and arthralgias. When taken with cholestyramine, absorption is disrupted.

Hormone Modifiers

Hormone modifiers contain recombinant human PTH. Teriparatide (Forteo) is the only PTH recombinant currently available.

Mechanism of Action

PTH is the primary regulator of calcium and phosphate metabolism and regulates bone metabolism, renal tubular reabsorption of calcium and phosphates, and intestinal calcium absorption. It stimulates new bone formation in trabecular and cortical bone surface by preferential stimulation of osteoblastic activity over osteoclastic activity. This causes an increase in skeletal mass and an increase in markers of bone formation and resorption and bone strength.

A study showed women using teriparatide had an increased density of the spine of 10% to 14% and of the hip of 5%. In 18 months, vertebral fractures were reduced 60% to 70% and nonvertebral fractures 55% (Dempster et al., 2001). It has been shown that teriparatide can prevent back pain in women with osteoporosis for up to 18 months beyond the end of treatment.

Dosage

Teriparatide is the only agent in this class currently. It is administered subcutaneously at a dosage of 20 mcg daily. This is used in women at high risk for fracture or those who have failed to respond to or who are intolerant of other therapies.

Contraindications

Teriparatide is contraindicated in the following circumstances: Paget disease, children, previous bone radiation therapy, history of skeletal malignancy, metabolic bone disease, hypercalcemia (which is usually transient), and hyperparathyroidism. It should be used cautiously in patients with a history of kidney stones.

Adverse Events

Teriparatide may increase calcium levels and increase the risk of digoxin toxicity if used together. Common adverse events include dizziness, nausea, leg cramps, arthralgia, and hyperuricemia.

RANK Ligand Inhibitor

Denosumab (Prolia) is a RANK ligand inhibitor.

Mechanism of Action

RANK ligand is an essential mediator of osteoclast activity. In postmenopausal osteoporosis, decreased estrogen leads to increased RANK ligand, an essential mediator of osteoclast activity. Increased osteoclast activity leads to increased bone loss and fracture risk. A RANK ligand inhibitor targets and binds to RANK ligand, inhibiting osteoclast formation, function, and survival, keeping osteoclasts from resorbing bone.

Dosage

The dosage is 60 mg subcutaneously every 6 months.

Contraindications

Denosumab is contraindicated in pregnancy and hypocalcemia, Caution should be used if the creatinine clearance is greater than 30, immunocompromised patients, and those who have had small bowel excision.

Adverse Events

Denosumab can cause musculoskeletal pain, infection, arthralgia, myalgia, and abdominal pain.

Selecting the Most Appropriate Agent

The patient needs an intake of calcium and vitamin D in addition to any other drug selected. Results of the DEXA scan guide the provider's decision in selecting therapy for osteoporosis. If the T-score is less than –1 SD from the norm, the patient is said to have no osteoporosis or osteopenia, but calcium intake and weight-bearing exercise are encouraged. A T-score below –1 SD or less than –2.5 SD from the mean indicates osteopenia, and treatment with calcium and vitamin D should begin. Also, the practitioner should consider preventive resorption-inhibiting therapy. The risk of fracture almost doubles for each BMD decrease of 1 SD. The DEXA scan should be repeated in 2 years or sooner if the patient experiences menopause. The NOF recommends pharmacologic treatment if the T-score is below –2 SD from the mean, if the T-score is –1.5 with other risk factors for osteoporosis or fracture, and if the woman is older than age 70 with multiple risk factors, especially previous fractures (**Figure 57.1**).

First-Line Therapy

Raloxifene or bisphosphonate therapy is used for prevention; bisphosphonates are used for treatment (**Table 57.2**). Patients should have calcium and vitamin D supplementation. Treatment decisions are based on patient history. For instance, if the patient has a history of esophagitis, alendronate is not the best choice; if the patient has a history of thromboembolic disease, raloxifene is not the appropriate therapy.

Second-Line Therapy

Calcitonin, a hormone modifier or RANK ligand inhibitor, is recommended for second-line therapy in women who have failed to respond to first-line therapy or who cannot tolerate hormone replacement therapy, bisphosphonates, or SERMs.

MONITORING PATIENT RESPONSE

The DEXA scan should be repeated every 2 years. Measurement of the density of the proximal femur is most helpful in predicting fractures, and measurement of the density of the lumbar

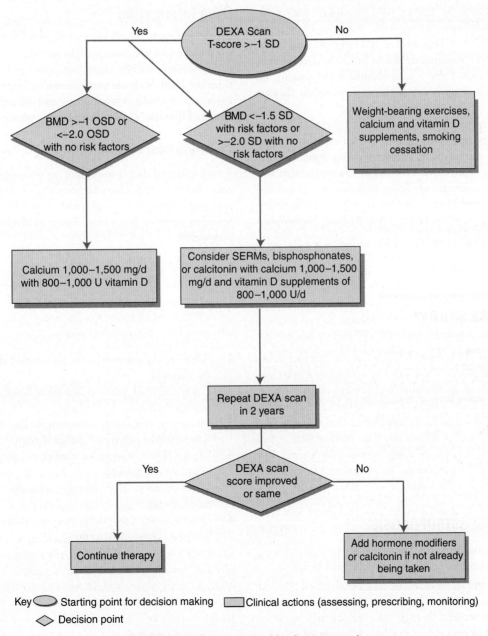

FIGURE 57.1 Treatment algorithm for osteoporosis.

TABLE 57.2		
Recommended Order of Prevention and Treatment for Osteoporosis		
Order	**Agents**	**Comments**
First line	Prevention: raloxifene, alendronate, ibandronate, zoledronic acid, or risedronate plus calcium and vitamin D	Treatment may be lifelong.
	Treatment: raloxifene, alendronate, risedronate, ibandronate, zoledronic acid, or calcitonin	
Second line	Addition of hormone modifiers or calcitonin if not being taken	

spine is most effective in measuring the response to therapy. Within 2 years, resorption-inhibiting drugs increase the BMD of the lumbar spine by 5% to 10% in women with post-menopausal osteoporosis, causing the incidence of fractures to decrease by 50% (Cummings et al., 1998; Melton et al., 1993). Follow-up is recommended 1 to 2 months after the start of therapy and then every 3 to 6 months if the patient has osteoporosis. Follow-up is necessary every year if the therapy is prophylactic

Even if the medication is stopped, its positive effects can persist. That's because after taking a bisphosphonate for a period of time, the medicine remains in your bone. Because of this lingering effect, there is a belief by the experts that it is reasonable for people who are doing well during treatment—those who have not broken any bones and are maintaining bone density—to consider taking a holiday from bisphospho-nate after taking it for 5 years.

PATIENT EDUCATION

Drug Information

Bisphosphonates should be taken with 8 ounces of water, and the patient should remain upright for 30 minutes after administration. Information about osteoporosis can be obtained from the NOF Web site (http://www.nof.org) or the National Institutes of Health Osteoporosis and Related Bone Disease National Resource Center (http://www.osteo.org).

Lifestyle/Nutritional Changes

A well-balanced diet is important, as are weight-bearing exercises. Safety strategies are necessary, such as removing unstable rugs and keeping items that could cause a fall out of the way. Smoking cessation is essential. Excessive alcohol intake should be avoided.

CASE STUDY*

J.S., a 72-year-old woman of Asian descent, has just transferred to your practice. She had a hysterectomy 8 years ago and has not been on hormone replacement therapy. She is 5 ft 2 inches tall and weighs 102 lb. She has had a sedentary lifestyle (she was a secretary and retired 2 years ago). She drinks four glasses of wine a day. Her mother died at age 62 from complications of a hip fracture. **J.S.'s** sister was just diagnosed with metastatic breast cancer. You prescribe a DEXA scan, and the T-score is –2.6 SD.

DIAGNOSIS: OSTEOPOROSIS

1. List specific goals of therapy for **J.S.**
2. What drug therapy would you prescribe? Why?

3. What are the parameters for monitoring the success of the therapy?
4. Discuss specific patient education based on the prescribed therapy.
5. List one or two adverse reactions for the selected agent that would cause you to change therapy.
6. What OTC or alternative medicines might be appropriate for this patient?
7. What dietary and lifestyle changes might you recommend?
8. Describe one or two drug–drug or drug–food interactions for the selected agent.

* Answers can be found online.

Complementary and Alternative Therapy

Supplemental calcium and vitamin D are important adjuncts to therapy. Patients without osteopenia or osteoporosis should ingest 1,200 mg of calcium a day, and those with osteopenia or osteoporosis should ingest more—1,500 mg calcium daily and 800 to 1,000 U of vitamin D to facilitate the absorption of calcium.

Bibliography

Starred references are cited in the text.

Bolland, M. J., Grey, A., Reid, I. R. (2013). Calcium supplements and cardiovascular risk: 5 years on. *Therapeutic Advances in Drug Safety, 4*(5), 199–210.

*Chesnut, C. H., III, Silverman, S., Andriano, K., et al. (2000). A randomized trial of nasal spray salmon calcitonin in postmenopausal women with established osteoporosis: The Prevent Recurrence of Osteoporotic Fractures Study. PROOF Study Group. *American Journal of Medicine, 109,* 267–276.

*Cummings, S. R., Black, D. M., Thompson, D. E., et al. (1998). Effect of alendronate on risk of fracture in women with low bone density but without vertebral fractures: Results from the Fracture Intervention Trial. *Journal of American Medical Association, 280,* 2077–2082.

*Dempster, D. W., Cosman, F., & Kurland, E. S. (2001). Effects of daily treatment with parathyroid hormone on bone microarchitecture and turnover in patients with osteoporosis: A paired biopsy study. *Journal of Bone and Mineral Research, 16,* 1846–1853.

*Harris, S. T., Watts, N. B., Genant, H. K., et al. (1999). Effects of risedronate treatment on vertebral and nonvertebral fractures in women with postmenopausal osteoporosis: A randomized controlled trial. Vertebral Efficacy with Risedronate Therapy (VERT) Study Group. *Journal of American Medical Association, 282,* 1344–1352.

*Liberman, U. A., Weiss, S. R., Broll, J., et al. (1995). Effect of oral alendronate on bone mineral density and the incidence of fractures in postmenopausal osteoporosis. The Alendronate Phase III Osteoporosis Treatment Study Group. *New England Journal of Medicine, 333,* 1437–1443.

*McClung, M. R., Geusens, P., Miller, P. D., et al. (2001). Effect of risedronate on the risk of hip fracture in elderly women. *New England Journal of Medicine, 344,* 333–340.

*Melton, L. J., Atkinson, E. J., O'Fallon, W. M., et al. (1993). Long-term fracture prediction by bone mineral assesses at different skeletal sites. *Journal of Bone and Mineral Research, 8,* 1227–1233.

*National Osteoporosis Foundation. (2014, June 2). 54 million Americans affected by osteoporosis and low bone mass. Retrieved from http://nof.org/news/2948

Nelson, H. D. (2014). Osteoporosis. In H. Sloane, et al., (Ed.), *Ham's Primary Care Geriatrics* (pp. 445–455). Philadelphia, PA: W.B. Saunders.

*Paik, J. M., Curhan, G. C., et al. (2014). Calcium supplement intake and risk of cardiovascular disease in women. *Osteoporosis International, 25*(8), 2047–2056.

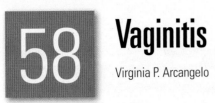

58 Vaginitis

Virginia P. Arcangelo

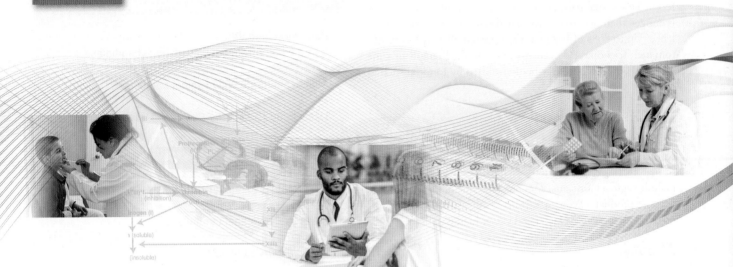

Vaginitis is one of the most common gynecologic complaints. The most common causes of vaginitis are vulvovaginal candidiasis (VVC), bacterial vaginosis (BV), and *Trichomonas vaginalis*. The presentation is often vaginal or perineal itching, burning, vulvar or vaginal irritation, and abnormal vaginal discharge. Many women may be asymptomatic. Other causes of vaginal irritation or inflammation include allergic reactions and atrophic changes in the vaginal mucosa.

CAUSES

Candidiasis

Most vaginal yeast infections are caused by *Candida albicans*, although other organisms, such as *Candida tropicalis* and *Candida glabrata*, are seen, especially in recurrent candidiasis. Colonization of Candida at other sites, such as the oral mucosa and the gastrointestinal (GI) tract, may be associated with recurrent vaginitis. Candidal vaginitis is often accompanied by vulvitis, so the term *vulvovaginal candidiasis* may better describe this disorder.

Behavioral factors may cause VVC. Sexual factors, in particular orogenital sex, may contribute to the introduction of microorganisms or cause microtrauma to the vulva and vestibule. Contraceptive practices may contribute to VVC; oral contraceptives, use of a diaphragm and spermicide, and the use of an intrauterine device are associated with an increased risk of infection.

Bacterial Vaginosis

BV is a polymicrobial vaginal infection that occurs when the hydrogen peroxide–producing *Lactobacillus* normally present in the vagina diminishes, allowing other bacteria to proliferate.

Bacteria, such as *Gardnerella vaginalis*, *Prevotella* species, *Mobiluncus* species, and *Mycoplasma hominis*, are responsible for BV. Although the cause of BV is not well understood, some studies suggest that causes may include complications of pregnancy and infections associated with gynecologic procedures, pelvic inflammatory disease, and cervical intraepithelial neoplasia. It is unclear whether BV is only sexually transmitted.

Although BV in the past frequently has been ignored, it is considered the most common form of vaginitis and affects approximately 30% of women. The prevalence of BV among U.S. women aged 14 to 49 is about 29% (Koumans et al., 2007).

Because most women who have BV exhibit no or minor symptoms, there is a tendency to overlook this condition. Sociodemographic factors associated with BV include younger age, being non-Hispanic Black or Mexican American, having less than a high school education, living at or near the federal poverty level, and douching. Sexual risk factors, such as being sexually active, age of first sexual intercourse, and having multiple male lifetime sexual partners, particularly multiple over the past year, all are risk factors for BV. In lesbian women, female partners of women who have BV have a higher incidence of BV. Despite the sexual risk factors associated with BV, however, BV is considered sexually associated but not sexually transmitted. While infection is rare in women who have never been sexually active, treatment of male sex partners has not proven to be beneficial in preventing recurrence.

Trichomoniasis

Trichomonas vaginalis, an anaerobic protozoan, is one of the most commonly sexually transmitted organisms. Practitioners have long recognized that some asymptomatic women may harbor the organism. The organism, which can apparently survive in the environment for several hours, may be transmitted by contact, particularly with moist objects (e.g., underclothing and towels). Increased numbers of sexual partners, a recent new sexual partner, or early initiation of sexual activity (younger than age 16) is associated with an increased prevalence. Up to 86% of trichomoniasis infections may be asymptomatic. Trichomonads can live for a limited length of time on moist surfaces and may be transmitted by fomites, such as towels or sexual toys.

Allergies and Irritants

Conditions or products that irritate the vulva or the vaginal epithelium or local allergic reactions may produce symptoms similar to those of infectious vaginitis. Examples of irritants include vaginal lubricants, condoms, spermicides, and feminine hygiene products. Women who have other atopic skin conditions may experience vaginal and vulvar manifestations as well.

Atrophy

Low levels of estrogen in a postmenopausal woman may lead to atrophy of the vaginal epithelium and subsequent irritation and inflammation, which also may predispose the woman to vaginitis.

PATHOPHYSIOLOGY

A review of the normal physiology of the vaginal environment forms the basis for understanding the possible causes and pathophysiology of vaginitis. In postpubertal women, both anaerobic and aerobic bacteria make up the normal vaginal flora. These include potential pathogens, such as *Staphylococcus*, *Streptococcus*, and *Bacteroides* species, and nonpathogens, such as lactobacilli and diphtheroids. *Candida albicans* is a saprophytic fungus that is a normal vaginal inhabitant in 15% to 25% of women.

One of the most important factors in the defense against infection is an acidic vaginal pH, which may be influenced by the acidic by-products produced by the normal vaginal flora. Hydrogen peroxide–producing strains of lactobacilli in vaginal secretions have been associated with protection against some vaginal infections as well. Therefore, variables that alter the vaginal pH or destroy lactobacilli may predispose a woman to vaginal infection. Among these variables are pregnancy, diabetes, sexual activity, hormonal changes, antibiotic therapy, and the use of feminine hygiene products. The thickness of the vaginal epithelium may also influence antimicrobial defenses.

DIAGNOSTIC CRITERIA

Candidiasis (VVC)

Symptoms of VVC include intense pruritus and erythema, dysuria, and a thick, white, curdlike vaginal discharge that tends to adhere to the vaginal walls. Diagnosis is made on the basis of presenting complaints, physical findings, and observation of pseudohyphae on potassium hydroxide (KOH) wet

---

> ### BOX 58.1 CDC Classification of Vulvovaginal Candidiasis (VVC)
>
> **Uncomplicated VVC**
> Sporadic or infrequent vulvovaginal candidiasis
> *or*
> Mild to moderate vulvovaginal candidiasis
> *or*
> Likely to be *C. albicans*
> *or*
> Nonimmunocompromised women
>
> **Complicated VVC**
> Recurrent vulvovaginal candidiasis
> *or*
> Severe vulvovaginal candidiasis
> *or*
> Non-*albicans* candidiasis
> *or*
> Women with uncontrolled diabetes, debilitation, or immunosuppression, or those who are pregnant

mount slide. Gram stain and culture of the vaginal discharge are other methods that may be employed in the diagnosis of VVC. Vaginal cultures can confirm the diagnosis and identify the species of *Candida* causing infection. Since 10% to 20% of women harbor *Candida* in the vagina, it is not recommended that asymptomatic women be treated. If the vaginal pH is tested, the value in candidiasis is usually less than 4.5. *Candida* may also be identified on Papanicolaou (Pap) smears of symptomatic or asymptomatic women. VVC may be classified as complicated or uncomplicated (**Box 58.1**).

Bacterial Vaginosis

Routine cultures are not helpful in diagnosing BV because up to 50% of women who harbor *G. vaginalis* vaginally are asymptomatic. When symptomatic, a woman may complain of a fishy odor, yellow or grayish discharge, and vaginal irritation. A yellow discharge increases the likelihood of BV fourfold but also can indicate a *Trichomonas* infection. A white discharge makes BV less likely. A clinical diagnosis of BV requires three out of four Amsel criteria, which are 92% sensitive but only 77% specific. Amsel criteria are abnormal grayish homogenous discharge, vaginal pH greater than 4.5, positive amine or "whiff test" ("fishy" odor with KOH applied to discharge), and more than 20% positive clue cells (epithelial cells surrounded by adherent coccobacilli) on microscopy (**Box 58.2**). Treatment reduces symptoms, yet recurrences are common, with 23% at 1 month and 58% at 12 months.

Trichomoniasis

Patients with vaginitis caused by *Trichomonas* organisms report a profuse, frothy, yellowish vaginal discharge, vaginal and vulvar

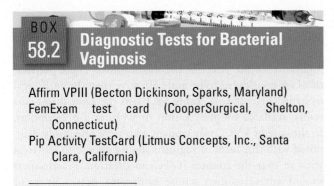

Affirm VPIII (Becton Dickinson, Sparks, Maryland)
FemExam test card (CooperSurgical, Shelton, Connecticut)
Pip Activity TestCard (Litmus Concepts, Inc., Santa Clara, California)

CDC, 2010

irritation, dysuria, and dyspareunia. Microscopic identification of the motile organism on a wet mount slide usually confirms the diagnosis. *Trichomonas* organisms may also be identified on a Pap smear. Because the organism may be recovered from male partners of infected women, this form of vaginitis is considered to be sexually transmitted.

Occasionally, asymptomatic women are diagnosed with trichomoniasis by routine Pap smear, which is reported to be 57% sensitive and 97% specific. If symptomatic, trichomoniasis presents as vaginal itching, burning, vaginal discharge (frequently profuse, yellowish-green, and malodorous), or postcoital bleeding. Trichomonads often appear in motion on a vaginal secretion saline wet mount, "swimming" with the flagella in a jerking or tumbling action. The sensitivity of detecting trichomonads on saline wet mount is estimated at 62% with a specificity of 97% and a positive predictive value of 75%. Culture is very sensitive (95%) and specific (greater than 95%) but delays diagnosis and is not routinely performed.

Allergic Vaginitis

Vaginitis resulting from allergy or irritants may be characterized by pruritus, discharge, and dyspareunia. The diagnosis often relies on exclusion. Although vaginal discharge may be increased, the secretions, when examined microscopically, do not harbor candidal organisms, trichomonads, or clue cells.

Atrophic Vaginitis

Vaginitis associated with atrophy of the vaginal walls produces pruritus, discharge, dryness, and dyspareunia. Physical examination reveals thinning of the vaginal walls with a characteristic shiny-smooth appearance. Introduction of the speculum into the vaginal introitus may cause bleeding. Microscopic examination reveals no candidal organisms, trichomonads, or clue cells.

INITIATING DRUG THERAPY

When considering pharmacotherapy for vaginitis, the practitioner explores lifestyle choices that may predispose the patient to infection or inflammation. Questions to ask regard the use of douches or other feminine hygiene products, sexual practices and partners, the possible relationship between sexual activity and appearance of symptoms, and recent antibiotic or oral contraceptive use. The practitioner should perform a thorough assessment to identify other possible irritants or complaints.

Before choosing a plan of therapy, the practitioner and patient also need to consider the issue of recurrent infection. In the case of recurrent VVC (four or more symptomatic episodes annually), the practitioner should be alert to the possibility of diabetes, and the need for screening should be discussed. In the case of recurrent trichomonal infection, sex partners should be examined and treated if they are found to be transmitting the organisms. It also is not uncommon for BV to recur.

Goals of Therapy

The primary goal of therapy in treating infectious vaginitis is eradication of the offending organism. The primary goals of therapy for allergic vaginitis include reducing inflammation and avoiding irritants. Addressing the hypoestrogenic state of postmenopausal women with hormone replacement therapy alleviates the symptoms of atrophic vaginitis. (Refer to Chapter 56 for a discussion of these treatment options.)

Another important goal of therapy is relief of symptoms. Vaginitis can cause considerable discomfort, both physically and emotionally. Women with vaginitis often experience embarrassment and even fear, particularly of the implications of a sexually transmitted disease. The frustration associated with recurrent infection may lead women to repeated attempts to self-treat, which delays proper evaluation by their primary care provider. For more information on self-treatment, see **Box 58.3**.

In the treatment of BV, additional goals of therapy include reduction of the risk of complications following gynecological procedures (e.g., abortion and hysterectomy) and reduction in the risk of acquiring other sexually transmitted infections. Adverse pregnancy outcomes have been associated with BV and trichomoniasis. The treatment of asymptomatic women with BV is not recommended, but some specialists recommend that women at high risk for preterm delivery be screened and treated for BV during the first prenatal visit.

Topical Azole Antifungals

Topical vaginal preparations for treating VVC include the following azoles: clotrimazole, butoconazole, tioconazole, miconazole, and terconazole. Treatment duration with these agents varies from 1 to 3 to 7 days. Response to treatment varies according to the duration of therapy. Types of topical preparations include creams, ointments, tablets, and suppositories. Oral fluconazole is also available for treatment in a one-time dose.

Time Frame for Response

The cure rates for topically applied azoles have long been established at between 80% and 90%. It can take up to 3 days to see the effect of the medications. These preparations are considered to be more effective than the antifungal nystatin (Mycostatin). **Table 58.1** lists the azole drugs currently available by prescription or without a prescription. In the case of VVC, only women who were previously diagnosed with this form of vaginitis should choose to self-treat with an over-the-counter (OTC) medication. Practitioners should advise women whose symptoms persist or recur within 2 months of self-treatment to seek medical care. In general, the only contraindication to the topical antifungals is hypersensitivity to the azole or components of the cream or gel.

TABLE 58.1

Overview of Antifungal Agents

Generic (Trade) Name and Dosage	Selected Adverse Events	Contraindications	Special Considerations
OTC Preparations			
butoconazole 2% cream (Femstat) 1 applicatorful intravag. qhs for 3 d	Vaginal irritation, skin rash, hives	Allergy	Oil based; might weaken latex condoms and diaphragms
butoconazole 2% cream (sustained release) 1 applicatorful qhs for 3 d	Refer to product labeling for more information		
clotrimazole 1% cream (Gyne-Lotrimin, Mycelex-G) 1 applicatorful intravag. qhs for 7–14 d	Same as above	Same as above	Same as above
clotrimazole 100-mg vaginal tablets (Gyne-Lotrimin, Mycelex-G) 1 tab intravag. qhs for 7 d or 2 tabs intravag. qhs for 3 d	Same as above	Same as above	Same as above
miconazole 2% cream (Monistat 7) 1 applicatorful intravag. qhs for 7 d	Same as above	Same as above	Same as above
miconazole 200-mg suppository (Monistat 3) 1 suppository intravag. qhs for 3 d	Same as above	Same as above	Same as above
miconazole 100-mg suppository (Monistat 7) 1 suppository intravag. qhs for 7 d	Same as above	Same as above	Same as above
tioconazole 6.5% ointment (Vagistat) 1 applicatorful intravag. qhs, single dose	Same as above	Same as above	Same as above
Prescription Preparations			
terconazole 0.4% cream (Terazol 7) 1 applicatorful intravag. qhs for 7 d	Same as above	Same as above	Same as above
terconazole 0.8% cream (Terazol 3) 1 applicatorful intravag. qhs for 3 d	Same as above	Same as above	Same as above
terconazole 80-mg suppositories (Terazol 3) 1 suppository intravag. qhs for 3 d	Same as above	Same as above	Same as above
fluconazole 150-mg tablet (Diflucan) 1 tablet orally, single dose	Headache, abdominal pain, nausea Rare: hepatic injury	Same as above	May interact with oral hypoglycemics, anticoagulants, cyclosporine, rifampin, theophylline, calcium channel antagonists, cisapride, astemizole, phenytoin, protease inhibitors, tacrolimus, terfenadine, trimetrexate

CDC recommendations, 2010.

Adverse Events

Topical azoles seldom cause systemic adverse events, although they may cause local irritation. Unfortunately, these effects may be difficult to distinguish from the conditions for which they are being used. Less common events may include penile irritation of the sex partner, abdominal cramps, or headache.

Interactions

Since these preparations are oil based, they may weaken latex condoms and diaphragms.

Oral Azole Antifungal Agents

Fluconazole, the only oral azole to be recommended by the Centers for Disease Control and Prevention (CDC) for treating uncomplicated VVC, is available by prescription in a single 150-mg dose. It is as effective as topical azoles. The findings of a study evaluating the acceptance of single-dose oral fluconazole by patients and physicians showed that most participants believed the drug to be effective in relieving or alleviating the symptoms of VVC. Oral fluconazole maintenance therapy for recurrent VVC should be extended for 6 months, but caution should be used with long-term ketoconazole therapy since hepatotoxicity may occur.

Contraindications

Contraindications to oral azole antifungals include known hypersensitivity to these azoles and the concomitant use of drugs with which they interact.

Time Frame for Response

Because patients treated with oral antifungals may not obtain relief of symptoms for 2 or 3 days, they may need to use an OTC antifungal cream for a few days. Failure to respond necessitates re-evaluation.

Adverse Events

The most commonly reported adverse events noted in patients treated with oral fluconazole are headache, nausea, and abdominal pain. Ketoconazole and itraconazole can cause GI disorders, headache, and pruritus. Hepatotoxicity may also occur, especially with ketoconazole. Liver enzyme levels may need to be monitored, especially with long-term use. Adverse effects tend to be dose related. Interactions may occur because oral azoles are cytochrome P-450 inhibitors.

Antibacterials/Antibiotics

Metronidazole (Flagyl) may be used orally or intravaginally for treating BV. Oral metronidazole 500 mg twice daily for 7 days is the standard treatment for BV, and only the oral form is effective in treating trichomonal infection. Tinidazole 2 g in a single dose is also used (see **Table 58.2** for specific dosages). Topical clindamycin cream 2% (Cleocin) should be used in patients who are allergic to metronidazole. Clindamycin 300 mg twice daily may also be used orally for a 7-day course. It is contraindicated in patients with hypersensitivity to it or to other preparations containing lincomycin. Cleocin ovules intravaginally are also effective if inserted at bedtime for three nights.

Contraindications

Metronidazole is no longer thought to be teratogenic, and therefore, it is not contraindicated in the first trimester of pregnancy. It is contraindicated, however, in patients with a known hypersensitivity to it or other nitroimidazoles.

TABLE 58.2			
CDC* Recommendations for Treating Bacterial Vaginosis			
Generic (Trade) Name and Dosage	**Selected Adverse Events**	**Contraindications**	**Special Considerations**
Recommended Regimens			
metronidazole 500-mg tablets (Flagyl) 1 tab PO bid for 7 d	Metallic taste, headache, GI distress	Allergy (no longer contraindicated in pregnancy)	Avoid alcohol during therapy and for 24 h after stopping (will cause nausea and vomiting) May potentiate the anticoagulant effects of warfarin and other anticoagulants
clindamycin 2% cream (Cleocin) 1 applicatorful intravag. qhs for 7 d Clindamycin ovules 100 g intravaginally once qhs for 3 d	Vaginal irritation, skin rash, hives	Allergy	Oil based; may weaken latex condoms and diaphragms Refer to product labeling for more information
metronidazole gel 0.75%. (MetroGel) 1 applicatorful intravag. bid for 5 d	Vaginal irritation, skin rash, metallic taste, GI distress	Same as above	Although blood levels are lower than with the use of oral metronidazole, alcohol still should be avoided
clindamycin 300-mg tablets (Cleocin) 1 tablet orally bid for 7 d	GI distress	Same as above	None

*CDC recommendations as of 2010.

Adverse Events

Metallic taste, headache, and GI distress are common side effects of metronidazole. To avoid the disulfiram-like effect of nausea and vomiting, patients must not consume alcohol during treatment and for 24 hours after treatment stops.

Interactions

Metronidazole may potentiate the anticoagulant effect of warfarin (Coumadin) and other oral anticoagulants. Although some animal studies have linked metronidazole to cancer, no current evidence indicates that the drug has a similar effect on humans.

Estrogens

Treatment of atrophic vaginitis consists of systemic estrogen replacement or topical estrogen creams administered externally or intravaginally. Refer to Chapter 56 for a complete discussion of these therapies.

Anti-Inflammatories

Mild topical steroid preparations can be used on a short-term or episodic basis. Careful monitoring of the patient's response is advised.

Selecting the Most Appropriate Agent

First-Line Therapy: Candidiasis

In an attempt to guide therapeutic options, the CDC classifies VVC as either uncomplicated or complicated (see **Box 58.2**).

OTC topical antifungals are typical first-line therapy of uncomplicated VVC and can be used before the patient seeks professional treatment. Women experiencing typical symptoms such as pruritus and vaginal discharge can obtain relief of symptoms promptly without the expense of a visit to the practitioner. Appropriate therapy consists of 1 to 7 days of treatment with the topical antifungals. It is recommended that self-treatment with OTC antifungals be reserved for women who have been previously diagnosed with VVC and who have not experienced a recurrence within 2 months.

Single-dose oral antifungals are an alternative first-line therapy in uncomplicated VVC, especially because the ease of administration may ensure therapeutic adherence. Fluconazole is the oral azole of choice. The patient's sex partners need not be treated because candidiasis is not sexually transmitted. However, consideration may be given to treating male sex partners of women with recurrent infection. Male sex partners who have symptoms of balanitis may benefit from the use of topical antifungals. See **Figure 58.1** and **Table 58.3** for an overview of VVC treatment.

Second-Line Therapy: Candidiasis

If symptoms persist beyond the recommended course of therapy with first-line agents, second-line therapy involves assessing for possible recurrent VVC or infection with non-*albicans Candida*, such as *C. glabrata*. Vaginal cultures should be obtained to confirm the diagnosis and identify the species of *Candida* involved.

If an oral antifungal was not the first-line therapy, the practitioner may opt to treat with oral fluconazole as second-line therapy or extend the course of topical or oral therapy. It has been suggested that 7- to 14-day treatment with topical agents or a 150-mg dose of oral fluconazole repeated 3 days later may achieve remission in patients with recurrent VVC. Maintenance regimens are recommended for patients with recurrent VVC and include clotrimazole (500-mg suppositories once weekly), ketoconazole (100-mg dose once daily), fluconazole (100- to 150-mg dose once weekly), or itraconazole (100-mg dose once monthly). These maintenance therapies should be continued for 6 months. Hepatotoxicity may occur in long-term treatment with ketoconazole, and these patients should be monitored accordingly.

Second-line therapy for patients with non-*albicans* VVC consists of 7- to 14-day treatment with a non-fluconazole azole drug followed by boric acid suppositories (600 mg in a gelatin capsule intravaginally once daily for 14 days), if the infection recurs. Topical flucytosine 4% and nystatin 100,000-unit vaginal suppositories are additional options in the treatment of non-*albicans* VVC. However, consultation with a specialist is recommended. Women who are immunocompromised also benefit from the prolonged therapy (7 to 14 days) with either topical or oral agents.

In complicated cases, a second dose of oral fluconazole 150 mg given at day 3 yields an 80% cure rate versus 67% with a single dose. In women who have more than four infections a year, a 7- to 14-day course of oral fluconazole may be needed to suppress the *Candida*. Suppression therapy with fluconazole 150 mg weekly for 6 months controls symptomatic episodes in 90% of women, and one half have prolonged symptom relief. A treatment failure may indicate infection with *C. glabrata*, which does not respond well to azoles. Boric acid 600-mg capsules given intravaginally for 14 days may be effective.

First-Line Therapy: Bacterial Vaginosis

Oral metronidazole (500 mg twice daily) 7-day therapy has long been considered standard first-line treatment for BV. However, the CDC (2010) also recommends topical clindamycin cream 2% (intravaginally for 7 days) or metronidazole gel 0.75% (intravaginally for 5 days) as acceptable first-line therapy. Alternative regimens for first-line therapy include clindamycin 300 mg twice daily orally for a 7-day course or clindamycin ovules 100 g intravaginally at bedtime for 3 days. Once-daily dosing with metronidazole 750-mg extended-release tablets has been approved by the U.S. Food and Drug Administration for the treatment of BV, but data are not available regarding the efficacy of this regimen (CDC, 2006). Treatment of sex partners is not recommended because clinical trials have not shown a relationship between treatment of partners and recurrence of BV. See **Figure 58.2** and **Table 58.4** for an overview of treatment.

Second-Line Therapy: Bacterial Vaginosis

Treatment reduces symptoms, yet recurrences are common, with 23% at 1 month and 58% at 12 months. Recurrent BV should be treated. One randomized trial for persistent BV indicated that metronidazole gel 0.75% twice per week for 6 months after completion of a recommended regimen was effective in maintaining a clinical cure for 6 months (Sobel et al., 2006).

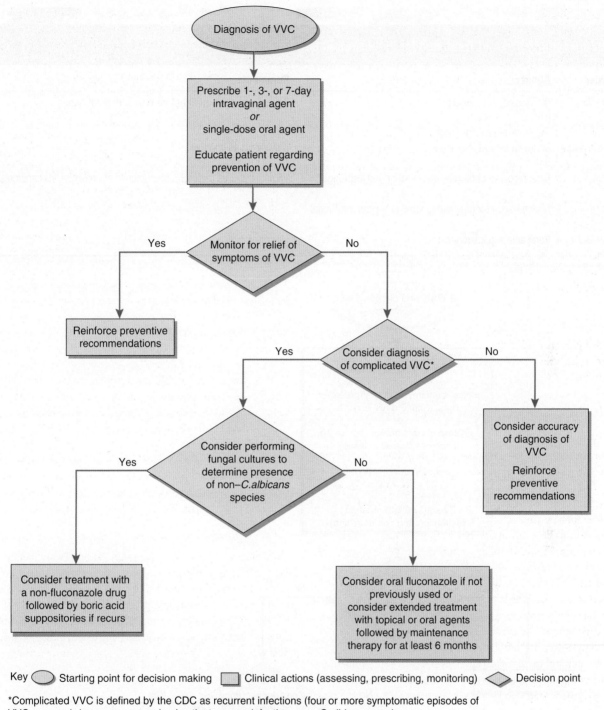

Key ⬭ Starting point for decision making   ▭ Clinical actions (assessing, prescribing, monitoring)   ◇ Decision point

*Complicated VVC is defined by the CDC as recurrent infections (four or more symptomatic episodes of VVC per year), immunocompromised patient, severe infection, non–*C.albicans* species.

FIGURE 58.1   Treatment algorithm for vaginitis known as vulvovaginal candidiasis (VVC).

Clinical trials indicate that a woman's response to therapy and the likelihood of relapse or recurrence are not affected by treatment of her sex partner(s). Therefore, routine treatment of sex partners is not recommended.

First-Line Therapy: Trichomoniasis

Only one treatment regimen is considered to be clinically efficacious for trichomoniasis: metronidazole or tinidazole given as a single 2-g dose. An alternative regimen is metronidazole 500 mg twice daily for 7 days. Treatment of male sex partners (who are usually asymptomatic) is recommended, and patients and their partners should avoid intercourse until they have completed therapy and are symptom free. Patients should be cautioned to avoid alcohol, as previously described. See **Figure 58.3** and **Table 58.5** for an overview of treatment.

TABLE 58.3

Recommended Order of Treatment for Vulvovaginal Candidiasis

Order	Agents	Comments
First line	OTC topical antifungals *or* Single-dose oral antifungal	Patients may self-treat before visit with practitioner
Second line	Single-dose oral antifungal *or* Extend course of therapy of topical or oral antifungal *or* Maintenance therapy with an oral or topical antifungal *or* Boric acid suppositories	If not used as first line Vaginal cultures to determine presence of non-*albicans* candidiasis

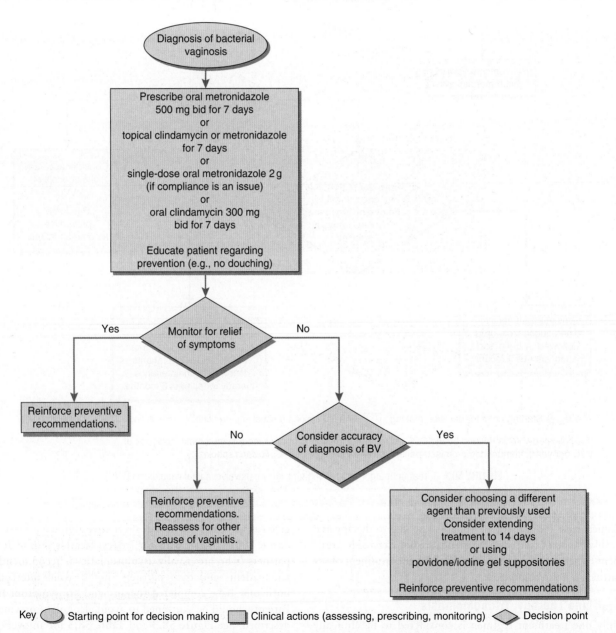

FIGURE 58.2   Treatment algorithm for bacterial vaginosis (BV).

TABLE 58.4

Recommended Order of Treatment for Bacterial Vaginosis

Order	Agents	Comments
First line	Oral metronidazole *or* clindamycin cream 2% *or* metronidazole gel 0.75% *or* clindamycin orally *or* clindamycin ovules	Traditionally used as first line
Second line	Extend duration of above agents *or* povidone–iodine gel suppositories *or* choose different agent	*May* be effective

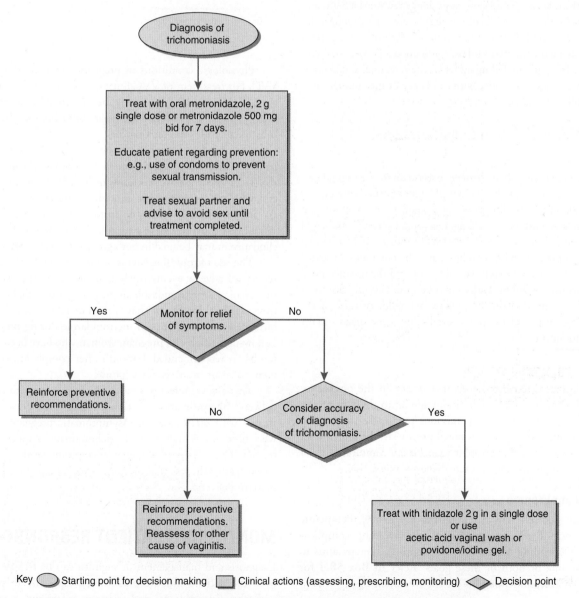

FIGURE 58.3   Treatment algorithm for vaginitis resulting from *Trichomonas* organisms.

TABLE 58.5
Recommended Order of Treatment for Trichomonal Infection

Order	Agents	Comments
First line	Metronidazole Single dose of 2 g	
Second line	Extend the course of metronidazole *or* Acetic acid vaginal wash or povidone–iodine solutions	*May* be effective

Second-Line Therapy: Trichomoniasis

Some strains of *T. vaginalis* can have diminished susceptibility to metronidazole but respond to tinidazole or higher doses of metronidazole. Tinidazole has a longer serum half-life and reaches higher levels in genitourinary tissues than metronidazole. If treatment fails and reinfection is excluded, the patient can be treated with metronidazole 500 mg orally twice daily for 7 days. For patients failing either of these regimens, clinicians should consider treatment with tinidazole or metronidazole at 2 g orally for 5 days.

Special Population Considerations
Pediatric

Before menarche, when estrogen levels are low, the vaginal epithelium is thin and the vaginal pH tends to be between 6.0 and 7.0. These conditions create a vaginal environment that is more susceptible to invading anaerobic bacteria if the child is exposed. Infections may be sexually transmitted or caused by contamination with fecal flora, and the possibility of sexual abuse must be considered. Poor hygiene and the use of vaginal irritants such as bubble baths and other products may also contribute to infections in the prepubertal child. Because of the high vaginal pH of the prepubertal child, candidiasis usually does not occur.

Postmenopausal Women

The decline in estrogen levels that occurs in the postmenopausal woman produces conditions similar to those in prepubertal children, and these conditions predispose the woman to infection and atrophy. As noted previously, the practitioner needs to be aware that atrophic vaginitis is a common cause of vaginal symptoms, and accurate diagnosis is essential.

Pregnant Women

Because vaginitis may occur during pregnancy, therapeutic goals include relieving symptoms and avoiding complications. Depending on the cause of vaginitis, therapy aims to achieve one or both of these goals. Refer to **Box 58.4** for the CDC recommendations for the treatment of vaginitis in pregnancy.

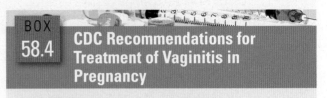

BOX 58.4   CDC Recommendations for Treatment of Vaginitis in Pregnancy

VULVOVAGINAL CANDIDIASIS

Topical azole therapies, *only*, for 7 days (most effective: butoconazole, clotrimazole, miconazole, terconazole)

BACTERIAL VAGINOSIS

Recommended: metronidazole 250 mg PO tid for 7 days *or* clindamycin 300 mg PO bid for 7 days

TRICHOMONIASIS

Metronidazole 2 g orally single dose

Data are current for 2010.

Physiologic conditions of pregnancy increase the risk of VVC. For treatment of VVC during pregnancy, the CDC recommends that only topical azoles be used for a 7-day course of therapy. The most effective agents are butoconazole, clotrimazole, miconazole, and terconazole.

Because adverse pregnancy outcomes have been reported in patients with BV, it is recommended that women who are at high risk (i.e., those who have previously delivered a premature infant) and who are asymptomatic should be treated. Symptomatic BV in women at low risk (no history of premature delivery) should be treated to relieve symptoms. Oral metronidazole and clindamycin may be used in both groups (see **Table 58.3**).

The use of topical agents is not recommended because of reports of adverse events, such as premature birth. Although the use of oral metronidazole in pregnancy had long been controversial, multiple studies have found no relationship between birth defects and the use of metronidazole during pregnancy. Follow-up of high-risk pregnant women who have been treated for BV is recommended 1 month after completion of treatment to ensure a successful response.

Trichomonas infections have been associated with preterm delivery. Symptomatic infections during pregnancy can be treated with metronidazole. Asymptomatic pregnant women who have incidentally noted trichomonads should not be treated. The severity of a woman's symptoms needs to be balanced against the risk that metronidazole therapy may increase preterm delivery.

MONITORING PATIENT RESPONSE

Diagnosis and management of vaginitis can be frustrating for both the patient and the practitioner, especially in patients with chronic symptoms and recurrent infections. Symptoms may recur or persist despite adherence to prescribed therapy. The practitioner should consult an expert if the patient fails to respond to current treatment recommendations.

The use of fungal cultures to assess response to therapy and to identify the offending candidal species is beneficial in assessing and treating patients with recurrent VVC. Fungal cultures play a role in detecting non-*albicans* candidal infections that may require second-line therapy.

Practitioners need to individualize the plan of care with each patient. They also need to maintain current knowledge of research regarding alternative therapies and to inform patients of findings. In many situations, yogurt and similar products may cause no harm and may provide patients with a perception of control over a frustrating condition.

Because of the increased risk of postoperative infectious complications associated with BV, some specialists suggest that before performing surgical abortion or hysterectomy, providers should screen for and treat women with BV in addition to providing routine prophylaxis. However, more information is needed before recommending treatment of asymptomatic BV before other invasive procedures. Routine treatment of sex partners is not recommended because studies have shown that treatment of partners does not reduce the incidence of recurrence or relapse.

PATIENT EDUCATION

Drug Information

Metronidazole and tinidazole can cause nausea and vomiting if alcohol is ingested during therapy and up to 24 to 72 hours after therapy stops. Patients should be instructed to adhere to the directions included with the product. In patients taking oral azole and oral antibiotic medications, the practitioner should reinforce the importance of following directions carefully and completing the full course of antibiotic therapy even if symptoms subside earlier.

Lifestyle Changes

The patient should avoid tight-fitting clothing, should wear undergarments that allow adequate vaginal ventilation, and should avoid douches and other feminine hygiene products that may alter the normal vaginal pH. The possibility that sexual activity may be associated with the onset of symptoms should be discussed, and the patient should be instructed to monitor these patterns. The patient should use condoms to protect against sexually transmitted disease. Because the use of antibiotics and oral contraceptives may be factors that predispose patients to vaginitis, other treatment options should be explored.

Receiving orogenital sex and using any form of contraceptive, having a high body mass index, having impaired glucose tolerance, consuming excessive sweets, and having high stress levels are some of the risk factors for recurrent vulvovaginal candidiasis.

Complementary and Alternative Medicine

Probiotics are supplements that contain live bacteria. They promote healthy normal flora. Ingesting yogurt or inserting in intravaginally (to promote vaginal recolonization) may be effective in preventing VVC. The true benefit of colonization with lactobacilli as protection against VVC or BV, however, has not been established.

CASE STUDY*

R.S. is a 32-year-old woman who seeks treatment for a vaginal discharge that she has had for the past month. She is sexually active and has had the same partner for the past 6 months. She reports noticing an odor, especially after sexual intercourse. Her history reveals that she has been using a commercial douche on a biweekly basis during the past year for hygienic purposes in an attempt to prevent vaginal infections. She denies any other associated symptoms. The physical examination reveals a white vaginal discharge. Microscopic examination of the vaginal discharge shows clue cells, and the pH is 5.5.

DIAGNOSIS: BACTERIAL VAGINOSIS

1. List specific goals of treatment for this patient.
2. What drug therapy would you prescribe? Why?

3. What are the parameters for monitoring the success of the therapy?
4. Discuss specific patient education based on the prescribed therapy.
5. List one or two adverse reactions for the selected agent that would cause you to change therapy.
6. What would be the choice for second-line therapy?
7. What OTC or alternative medications would be appropriate for this patient?
8. What dietary or lifestyle changes should be recommended?
9. Describe one or two drug–drug or drug–food interaction for the selected agent.

* Answers can be found online.

Bibliography

Starred references are cited in the text.

Biggs, W., & Williams, R. (2009). Common gynecological infections. *Primary Care; Clinics in Office Practice, 36*(1), 33–51.

*Centers for Disease Control and Prevention. (2010). Sexually transmitted treatment guidelines, 2010. *Morbidity and Mortality Weekly Reports, 59*(RR-12), 1–110.

*Ferris, D. G., Dekle, C., & Litaker, M. (1996). Women's use of over the counter antifungal medications for gynecological symptoms. *Journal of Family Practice, 42*, 595–600.

Hainer, B. L., & Gibson, M. V. (2011). Vaginitis. *American Family Physician, 83*(7), 807–815.

*Koumans, E., Steinberg, M., Bruce, C., et al. (2007). Prevention of bacterial vaginosis in the United States 2001–2004 associated with symptoms, sexual behavior and reproductive health. *Sexually Transmitted Diseases, 34*(1), 844–869.

Nyirjesy, P. (2008). Vaginovulvar candidiasis and bacterial vaginosis. *Infectious Disease Clinics of North America, 22*(9), 637–652.

Nyirjesy, P. (2014). Management of persistent vaginitis. *Obstetrics and Gynecology, 124*(6), 1135–1146.

*Nyirjesy, P., Weitz, M. V., Grody, M. H. T., et al. (1997). Over the counter and alternative medicines in the treatment of chronic vaginal symptoms. *Obstetrics and Gynecology, 90*, 50–53.

Sheth, S., & Keller, J.M. (2015). Infections of the genital tract. In C. T. Johnson, J. L. Hallock, J. L. Bienstocek, et al., (Eds.), *The Johns Hopkins manual of gynecology and obstetrics* (5th ed., pp. 356–378). Philadelphia, PA: Walter Kluwer.

*Sobel, J. D., Ferris, D., Schwebke, J., et al. (2006). Suppressive antibacterial therapy with 0.75% metronidazole vaginal gel to prevent recurrent bacterial vaginosis. *American Journal of Obstetrics and Gynecology, 194*, 1283–1289.

UNIT 15

Integrative Approach to Patient Care

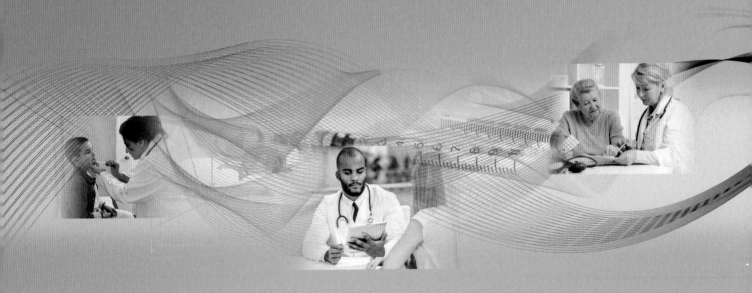

59 The Economics of Pharmacotherapeutics

Samir K. Mistry ■ Briana L. Santaniello ■ Joshua J. Spooner

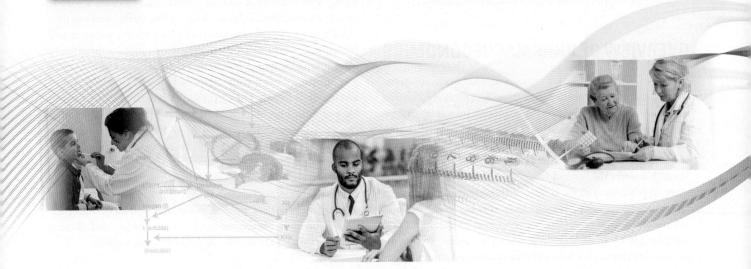

As little as 100 years ago, health insurance in the United States was scarce. Although President George Washington signed a law establishing prepaid health care in 1798, health insurance plans were slow to develop. Traditionally, patients in the United States paid health care providers and hospitals directly for their services on a fee-for-service basis. This system worked well for patients in times of good health; however, a serious injury or illness could place the patient in severe financial risk.

The goal of this chapter is to provide a fundamental understanding of the principles used by managed care organizations (MCOs) and pharmacy benefit managers (PBMs) to manage pharmacy costs while providing access to appropriate patient care. This chapter provides a brief review of pharmacoeconomic principles, educates the reader about the strategies used by MCOs and PBMs to manage health care expenditures, explains how these strategies are developed and implemented, and reviews how MCOs evaluate the performance of contracted providers. Through a better understanding of the practices, benefits, and challenges of MCOs and PBMs, practitioners can better prescribe appropriate and cost-effective medications for their patients.

ORIGINS OF MANAGED CARE

Modern health insurance's origins can be traced to 1929, when the Baylor University Hospital in Dallas, Texas, began to offer 1,500 school teachers up to 21 days of hospital care a year for $6 per person (Starr, 1982). Other groups also entered into agreement to prepay for Baylor's services. Shortly thereafter, several other Dallas-area hospitals followed suit and offered similar plans. Other early health insurance plans included the Kaiser Health Plans (early to mid-1930s) and the Group

Health Association in Washington, DC (1937). As the country slid into the depression and hospital revenues plummeted by 75% per patient, hospitals began to rely on insurance payments for a greater proportion of their operating budget (Starr, 1982).

Most health plans offered indemnity insurance (also known as *fee-for-service insurance*), in which patients paid for health care expenses out of their own pockets and then requested reimbursement from the insurer (often receiving reimbursement for 80% of incurred expenses). However, indemnity insurance did little to control health care expenditures because physicians and hospitals received payments proportional to the volume of services they provided. Concerned with the rising cost of providing health care, insurance providers sought ways to slow the increases in health care expenditures. After extensive lobbying and negotiations in Congress, President Richard Nixon signed the federal Health Maintenance Organization (HMO) Act into law in 1973. This act encouraged the growth of managed care by providing grants and loans to develop HMOs, overturned restrictive state laws regulating health providers, defined a basic package of services that HMOs were required to offer, and established procedures by which HMOs could become federally qualified.

Because HMOs could deliver cost-effective health care benefits while maintaining a reasonable quality of care, they were viewed as an attractive health insurance alternative for employers. The rate of enrollment in HMOs grew rapidly during the 1980s and 1990s, growing to rival preferred provider organizations (PPOs) as the leading source of employer-sponsored health insurance in the United States in the late 1990s. The federal government also encouraged the use of HMOs to manage the health care costs of Medicare-eligible beneficiaries; HMOs were reimbursed on a prospective basis by the government. The states soon followed suit, offering HMO-based options to Medicaid recipients. Of late, there has been a significant decline in employer-sponsored HMO enrollment, with a shift in favor of other health insurance plan types (Kaiser Family Foundation, 2014).

OVERVIEW OF PHARMACOECONOMICS

When MCOs make decisions related to what medications are covered and placed on formularies, those decisions could impact thousands of members. Applying economic principles to analyze the impact of a medication on the MCO's overall health care cost and disease management of the patient population is essential to appropriate decision making. *Pharmacoeconomic* research assesses the "overall value" of medications in the treatment or prevention of the disease(s) they are intended to treat (Navarro et al., 2009). Because they evaluate both cost and human data, studies on pharmacoeconomics are important tools for MCOs in making drug therapy decisions. To provide an overview, some different pharmacoeconomic study designs are described in the following sections.

Cost–Benefit Analysis

A cost–benefit analysis is used to determine the overall cost of a particular intervention or protocol by evaluating all pertinent data and converting the data to a monetary end point (e.g., U.S. dollars or EU Euros). Most often, this type of analysis is used to compare two different programs that also have different units for end points because the data can then be converted to one common unit (usually the dollar). The limitation to this analysis involves the evaluation of "intangible" end points or data that cannot be equated to a monetary value.

Cost Minimization Analysis

A cost minimization analysis evaluates the cost of two or more interventions with equivalent components or end points and determines which intervention is least costly. The most appropriate use for such analyses involves situations in which every aspect of compared interventions is identical except the cost of the intervention. Because efficacy and safety are identical, the cost of each intervention becomes the differential outcome. The outcomes of these analyses are also expressed in a monetary end point.

Cost-Effectiveness Analysis

A cost-effectiveness analysis may help determine the best program or intervention, where the desired outcome is a combination of both a monetary end point and a nonmonetary end point relative to an improvement in health (e.g., life expectancy, blood glucose measurements). An example of this would be dollars per life-year saved.

Cost–Utility Analysis

A cost–utility analysis, which is closely related to a cost-effectiveness analysis, measures data in terms of quality of life.

Quality of life is an assessment of a patient's well-being and social functioning, which can assist practitioners in determining a patient's response to drug therapy (Hunter et al., 2015). Along with traditional clinical results (e.g., laboratory values, blood pressure, serum glucose level), a cost–utility analysis provides a more complete evaluation of a patient's progress and compares the cost of an intervention or program in terms of more intangible end points, rather than dollars. These analyses predominantly use quality-adjusted life-years (QALYs) gained as a major outcome. The QALY is symbolic of healthy years of life and is the unit of measurement that encompasses outcomes (e.g., morbidity and mortality) in preferential sequence. This method has been very successful in evaluating various procedures compared with drug therapy in which a patient's quality of life is the chosen outcome (Hunter et al., 2015).

Pharmacoeconomic research compares cost and consequence with respect to pharmaceutical products and their impact on individuals, the health care system, and society. Such parameters are seldom analyzed in most studies.

FORMULARIES AND PHARMACY AND THERAPEUTICS COMMITTEES

An evaluation of American health expenditures identified $2.9 trillion in total health care spending in 2013 (Centers for Medicare and Medicaid Services [CMS], 2014a), which accounted for 17% of the national gross domestic product (GDP). Of this $2.9 trillion in health expenditures, $271.1 billion (9.3%) was spent on prescription drugs. Although this represents a minor portion of overall health care expenditures, it is a target for intervention by MCOs due to large annual increases in prescription drug spending. Prescription drug spending in the United States increased 13.1% in 2014, driven by demand for newer treatments for cancer, multiple sclerosis, and hepatitis C (IMS Health, 2015).

Formularies

One of the most effective methods by which an MCO can improve the quality of care provided to patients and mitigate the increasing costs of providing a prescription benefit is by implementing a formulary. Also known as a *preferred drug list*, a medication formulary is simply a list of preferred medications approved for use within an HMO, third-party payer, or PBM (Navarro et al., 2009). Formularies are usually organized by therapeutic area and medication class, with the formulary status and reimbursement category listed for each medication.

Formularies encourage the use of medications considered to be safer, more clinically effective, or more cost-effective than other medications within the same therapeutic category. When an MCO wants to limit the use of a drug for a specific reason (safety, efficacy, or cost), the formulary allows the flexibility to implement restrictions or limitations on utilization. Examples of such restrictions include prior authorizations, step therapies, quantity limitations, and tiered copayments.

Evolution of Formularies

The use of formularies can be traced back to 1925, when the physicians and pharmacists of Syracuse University Hospital collaborated to establish a formulary system to monitor drug use and reduce therapeutic duplication (the unnecessary use of two or more medications to treat the same condition) in its drug therapy program (Sonnedecker, 1976). By the 1960s, formularies were being implemented in hospitals throughout the country with the guidance of the *American Hospital Formulary Service*, a prominent set of formulary development materials published by the American Society of Hospital Pharmacists. Following the HMO Act of 1973, many HMOs adopted the hospital formulary to monitor medication use. Formularies were initially used by managed care as an inventory control mechanism for staff model HMOs (Navarro et al., 2009), but they have evolved into effective tools for monitoring and regulating medication utilization for all types of MCOs.

Structure of Formularies

Although formats may differ among plans, a formulary usually contains the same fundamental information. Formularies usually begin with a basic plan summary and detailed key points of reference and then proceed to the list of drugs. The drugs are most often categorized within their respective therapeutic classes with the therapeutic classes listed in alphabetic order. The order of the drugs within each therapeutic class can vary but are often listed alphabetically, either in complete alphabetical order (generic and brand drugs intermixed) or generic drugs listed before brand-name drugs. Additional information usually detailed for each drug includes the brand/generic status; the drug's relative cost, which is most often symbolized by relative $ signs; copay tier; and any potential utilization management programs. An example of a formulary is shown in **Table 59.1**. A "formulary medication" is a drug that is covered (reimbursed) by the health plan; formulary medications can be subdivided into different groups such as preferred and nonpreferred agents. "Preferred" agents are drugs that the health plan would prefer the practitioner to prescribe, due to safety, efficacy, and/or relative cost. "Nonpreferred" drugs are not the preferred drugs of the health plan but will nonetheless be covered by the plan at a higher out-of-pocket cost to the patient. Most formularies have different tiered copays for preferred and nonpreferred drugs, in which preferred drugs have a lower-cost tiered copay than the nonpreferred drugs. "Nonformulary medications" are drugs that are excluded from the formulary; health plans generally do not publish nonformulary medications on their formularies. Prescribers must usually provide exception justification for a patient to receive reimbursement for nonformulary medications.

Formularies can be grouped into three different categories: closed, open, and tiered formularies. Closed formularies limit clinicians to prescribing from a limited list of preferred agents (Edlin, 2015). Open formularies usually do not involve a preferred group of agents; instead, they allow the prescriber to select any covered medication. Tiered formularies are essentially the compromise between closed and open formularies. Tiered formularies are open formularies that set different copay tiers for generic, preferred, and nonpreferred medications (Edlin, 2015).

Impact of Formularies on Patients

The price that consumers pay for prescription medications varies from plan to plan. Patients are commonly required to pay a portion of the cost of the prescription, also known as the *copayment*, or *copay*. Copay amounts can differ from plan to plan and by geographic region. Closed and open formularies usually only have two copays: one for generic drugs and brand drugs, respectively. Tiered formularies have more than two copays, and each tier is related to a copay amount. Tiered formularies usually have three tiers: generic drugs, preferred brand drugs, and nonpreferred brand drugs.

Most copays are set to cover up to a 1-month supply of medication (28 to 34 days of therapy, depending on the health plan). Thus, a patient who received a prescription for a 7-day course of therapy of prednisone for an acute allergic reaction would likely have the same copayment as a patient who received a prescription for a 30-day course of therapy of prednisone for chronic use.

Some plans may allow patients to get more than a 1-month supply of medication at a time for a maintenance medication (medications used for chronic conditions). For maintenance medications, most health plans allow patients to receive a 90-day supply of medication. Health plans usually charge patients three copays for a 90-day supply (three 1-month supply copays). For example, if a patient paid a $10 copay for a 1-month supply, then the 90-day supply would cost $30. Health plans often offer reduced copayments as an enticement for patients to order their maintenance medications from a mail-order pharmacy service; a 90-day supply of medication might only cost the patient one or two copayments instead of three.

In the rigid formulary systems utilized in the 1990s, a two-tiered prescription copayment system was used by most health plans and pharmacy benefits manager (PBM); the lower

TABLE 59.1				
Example of a Formulary				
Drug Name	**Brand/Generic**	**Relative Cost**	**Tier**	**Edits**
Drug A	Generic	$	Tier 1	
Drug B	Generic	$	Tier 1	QL
Drug C	Brand	$$	Tier 2	QL, ST
Drug D	Brand	$$	Tier 2	
Drug E	Brand	$$$	Tier 3	ST
Drug F	Brand	$$$$	Tier 3	PA
Drug G (specialty injectable)	Brand	$$$$$$	Tier 4	QL, ST

Key: PA, prior authorization; QL, quantity limits; ST, step therapy; Tier 1, generic; Tier 2, preferred brand drug; Tier 3, nonpreferred brand drug; Tier 4, specialty injectable.

copayment tier was used for generic medications, whereas the higher copayment tier was used for formulary brand-name medications. Nonformulary medications were rarely covered by health plans or PBMs without prior approval; if granted, the prescription would fall into the higher copayment tier. Nonformulary medications that were not approved by the health plan were not covered; either the patient paid the full retail price for the prescription or the prescription was switched to a formulary agent by the prescriber.

Fueled by unsustainable prescription cost increases, MCOs abandoned the two-tiered formulary system in favor of higher tiered formulary designs, ranging from three-tiered systems up to the more recently used four- to six-tiered systems. Within the generally utilized three-tiered formulary system, the first two tiers are set up the same as the previous two-tiered system, with the first (lowest) tier copayment reserved for generic products and the second-tier copayment reserved for preferred brand-name products. Agents in the third tier are the nonpreferred brand-name products; the copayment is substantially higher than the second-tier copayment. Some plans include a fourth tier to their formulary for high-cost specialty medications with the highest prescription copayments. Three- and four-tiered formularies have introduced value considerations to patients: Do they value a specific third-tier or fourth-tier product enough to pay the higher copayment or will a second-tier product (with a lower copayment) be suitable for their needs? The multiple-tiered copayment has been proven to successfully move patients to products in the first and second tiers of the formulary without restricting access to prescription products (Edlin, 2015).

Functions of Formularies

Formularies have been used to promote the prescribing of safe, efficacious, and cost-effective medications. Formularies' main functions are to promote the use of less costly and equally efficacious medications (which are most often generic medications). For brand-name medications, formularies financially incentivize the use of preferred brand drugs over nonpreferred brand drugs or place barriers that prevent nonpreferred branded medications from being covered by the MCO. MCOs also implement policies or programs with their formularies to promote appropriate drug utilization and the use of generic drugs and preferred brand drugs prior to nonpreferred and nonformulary drugs. Examples of such policies or programs include generic substitution, therapeutic interchange, prior authorization, step therapy, medical necessity, and dispensing limitations around quantity, duration of therapy, age and gender.

Generic Substitution

A highly effective method of reducing the cost of the pharmacy benefit is generic substitution. Generic substitution is the process of dispensing an appropriate generic equivalent of a prescribed brand-name drug. Prescribing generic products can reduce the cost of providing prescription medications for patients; generic medication use reduced prescription drug

expenses by an estimated $239 billion in 2013 (IMS Health, 2014). Generic substitution has been supported by cost minimization analyses; as the brand and generic agents are considered identical in composition and activity, cost becomes the contributing factor for an agent's selection.

A generic medication is considered equal, or bioequivalent to its parent brand-name medication, and must undergo stringent safety and equivalency testing and comply with specific criteria established by the U.S. Food and Drug Administration (FDA). The FDA has set certain therapeutic equivalence evaluation codes to show the relative bioequivalence of generic agents to the brand-name drugs (FDA, 2014). There are two basic rating codes: A and B. The "A" rating indicates that the drug is considered therapeutically equivalent to other pharmaceutically equivalent products. The "B" rating indicates that the agent is not therapeutically equivalent to other pharmaceutically equivalent agents. Both A- and B-rated drugs are further differentiated based on dosage form. An "AB" rating states that the product's bioequivalence problems have been resolved, and evidence exists supporting the bioequivalence to pharmaceutically equivalent agents.

An example of generic substitution is dispensing the diuretic furosemide when the prescriber writes the prescription for Lasix, and the prescriber has not indicated that the brand-name product is medically necessary. In such a situation, the pharmacist is filling the prescription with an FDA-approved, bioequivalent form of the brand-name drug. Some insurance plans may allow the patient or prescriber to request the brand-name agent, but this often results in a higher copayment for the patient (Navarro et al., 2009). The increase in copayment may be as large as the difference in cost to the health plan between the brand and generic agents.

To maximize generic substitution, plans may use restrictive strategies such as "dispense as written" (DAW) blocks. A DAW code describes the rationale for the drug's selection and is entered into the prescription claim by the pharmacist before it is transmitted to the health plan for adjudication. There are DAW codes for "substitution permissible" (DAW 0), "dispense as written" (DAW 1), "patient requests brand" (DAW 2), as well as other choices to provide a rationale for the chosen agent. A health plan can require that the patient receive an acceptable generic substitution for a brand-name product unless a suitable DAW code has been entered. A DAW code of 7 is used for products with a narrow therapeutic index. Due to the risk of disrupting the level of drug in the patient's blood, drugs with a narrow therapeutic index may not have to be automatically substituted for an equivalent generic agent. A DAW of 7 informs the health plan that the physician, pharmacist, or patient has elected to continue use of the brand-name product. Drugs in this category include warfarin (Coumadin) and levothyroxine (Synthroid).

Therapeutic Interchange

Therapeutic interchange is defined as the procedure of dispensing prescribed medications that are chemically different but deemed therapeutically similar to the medication prescribed

(Holmes et al., 2011). In general, therapeutic interchange involves the substitution of drugs that are different chemical compounds but are considered to exert the same therapeutic effect and have similar toxicity and side effect profiles (e.g., HMG-CoA reductase inhibitors: substitution of generic atorvastatin [Lipitor] for Crestor). The use of therapeutic interchange has increased significantly because of a large influx of new medications that do not offer any therapeutic advantages over existing therapies but are priced much higher than the established products. These medications are commonly known as *me too drugs*. Some popular examples of therapeutic categories that contain me too drugs include proton pump inhibitors (PPIs), HMG-CoA reductase inhibitors (statins), angiotensin receptor blockers, and bisphosphonates.

Pharmaceutical manufacturers offer rebates to health plans to compete for preferred status on formularies, which lowers the prescription benefit cost. Controversies tend to arise when discounts are used to exchange one drug over another when the drugs are in different classes. If a therapeutic interchange involves two drugs of the same therapeutic class, it can be considered an example of therapeutic minimization because the only difference between the two agents is cost (assuming that the relative safety/efficacy data for the two agents are similar).

Therapeutic interchange is used for reasons other than controlling costs, including promoting the use of agents associated with fewer drug–drug interactions (e.g., substitution of fluconazole for ketoconazole) or of agents with a more convenient dosing schedule (e.g., once-daily enalapril instead of two- to three-times daily captopril). These interventions may prevent unnecessary drug–drug interactions or enhance medication compliance, which could, in turn, improve care and decrease overall health care costs.

In the outpatient pharmacy setting, therapeutic interchange must be verified and accepted by the prescribing practitioner. In the institutional setting, therapeutic interchange does not necessarily require a prescriber's approval if the institution's pharmacy and therapeutics (P&T) committee approves the specific interchange protocol. The American Medical Association (AMA) endorses the practice of therapeutic interchange in settings that have an organized medical staff and a functioning P&T committee (AMA, 1994).

Drug-Dispensing Limitations

Limitations regarding dispensing drugs are developed and implemented to promote appropriate prescribing of medications and are often structured around FDA-approved labeling and evidence-based medical data. Examples of drug limitations include drug quantity limits, duration of therapy limits, age limits, and gender limits. Drug quantity limitations are used to promote the appropriate quantity of medication that should be prescribed. There are two main types of quantity limits: quantity per filled prescription and quantity per days. Quantity per filled prescription limits are implemented for drugs that are prescribed for short-term use, such as analgesics and antibiotics. An example of such a quantity limit would be limiting the prescribing of addictive, high-potency narcotic analgesics

indicated for acute pain to 10 tablets per prescription. Quantity per days limits are utilized for chronically used (maintenance) medications. An example of this type of quantity limit would be limiting the prescribing of simvastatin to one tablet per day. Duration of therapy limits are implemented to manage how long a drug should be used, especially for medications that are not considered maintenance medications. An example of a duration of therapy limit would include a 3-month duration of therapy limit for the prescribing of PPI agents. Age limitations prevent the use of medications either above or below what is recommended by the FDA. An example of an age limit would be to prevent the use of barbiturates in members greater than 65 years of age. Gender limits prevent the use of medications for a gender when prescribing would not be safe and/or appropriate; an example of which would prevent prescriptions of oral contraceptives for males.

Prior Authorization and Step Therapy Programs

Prior authorization refers to the approval process that health plans may require for certain medications before they will be covered. The primary purpose of a prior authorization process is to control the use of and prevent the overuse of nonformulary, hazardous, or inappropriately prescribed medications. Prior to the recent move by health plans toward increasingly open formularies with three and four tiers of copayments, health plans would require prior authorizations for most nonformulary drugs, expensive drugs, newly approved drugs, and drugs with less expensive alternatives (Navarro et al., 2009). Over 80% of commercial health plans used prior authorization programs in 2014 (Takeda Pharmaceuticals, 2014), and prior authorizations are used by a majority of the states in their Medicaid programs (National Conference of State Legislatures, 2010).

The criteria for approval of each drug undergoing the prior approval process will depend on the drug, the patient, the disease state involved, and the prescribing practitioner. Some prior authorizations may require a diagnosis along with pertinent laboratory values, whereas others may require a patient to fail therapy with certain drugs that are indicated to treat the same disease as the restricted agent. Other criteria may include patient demographics, such as age or gender limits, or prescriber limits, where only specific specialty types are allowed to prescribe for certain medications (e.g., only allowing dermatologists to prescribe isotretinoin).

The usual chain of events involving prior authorization starts with a patient presenting a pharmacist with a prescription for a newly prescribed medication. The pharmacist, after submitting a claim and having it rejected, learns that the medication requires prior authorization (often from a message sent with the rejected claim). The pharmacist or patient then contacts the prescriber, tells the prescriber that the medication requires prior authorization, and requests that the prescriber contact the MCO to explain why the patient requires that medication. Either prescribers can decide to contact the MCO and pursue prior authorization or they may choose not to pursue prior authorization and select an alternative agent.

MCOs often accept prior authorization requests from practitioners by mail, fax, telephone, or Internet. Completing the prior authorization process may result in the drug's approval for use in that patient, or the MCO may again reject the claim and offer a list of alternative medications that are covered by the plan.

If the prescriber knows that the drug requires prior authorization, the necessary paperwork can be completed to have the drug approved for the patient before the patient enters the pharmacy. Problems arise when the patient and prescriber are unaware of which agents on the MCO's formulary require prior authorization. This confuses many patients, possibly leading them to think that the prescriber ordered the wrong medication or the pharmacist made an error in filling the prescription (Bendix, 2013).

Step therapy programs are utilization management programs that are a version of prior authorization, in which they promote the use of one drug before another (Navarro et al., 2009). There are two main types of step therapy programs: those driven by cost-effectiveness and those that promote more clinically effective medications before less effective medications. The cost-effectiveness step therapy programs promote the use of cost-effective generic medication before the use of an expensive branded medication. They can be implemented using drugs within the same therapeutic class or different categories. An example of a step therapy within a therapeutic class would be to require the use of a generic HMG-CoA reductase inhibitor, such as atorvastatin, before the approval of a branded HMG-CoA reductase inhibitor like Crestor. An example of a step therapy using different categories would be to require the use of metformin before the approval of DPP4 inhibitors like sitagliptin and saxagliptin. Step therapy programs implemented for the purpose of promoting clinical effectiveness are usually based on practice guidelines or evidence-based medical data. An example of this type of program would be to require the use of nasal corticosteroids or nonsedating antihistamines before the approval of leukotriene inhibitors for the treatment of allergic rhinitis.

MCOs have increased their efforts to prospectively review prescriptions requiring prior authorization during the claim adjudication process. When a pharmacy sends a claim for a prior authorization drug to the PBM for adjudication, the PBM can review the patient's prescription claim history and the claim itself to determine if the prior authorization criteria have been met. This step can decrease the number of rejected prescription claims and minimize the time and efforts of prescribers, pharmacists, and patients in obtaining prior authorizations. When initiated effectively by informing practitioners of the drug's status and the preapproval process, prior authorization can become a very efficient mechanism for controlling costs and drug use.

Medical Necessity

Some MCOs use the term *medical necessity* interchangeably with *prior authorization*. In most settings, a medication considered a medical necessity is a nonformulary drug that is usually extremely expensive and usually has less expensive generic

and branded alternatives or is considered a relatively unsafe medication compared to available alternatives (Navarro et al., 2009). Some MCOs make medical necessity drugs available only after failure of drug therapy with a drug requiring prior authorization. MCOs carefully evaluate drugs before classifying them as medical necessity drugs, knowing that the drugs will be restricted if they are covered. Like the criteria for medications requiring prior authorization, the criteria for coverage vary from drug to drug.

PHARMACY AND THERAPEUTICS COMMITTEE

Structure and Function

A P&T committee is a group that meets periodically to review and revise the organization's formulary. The committee is composed primarily of physicians and pharmacists and may also include nurses, nurse practitioners, physicians' assistants, and members of the organization's administration. The physicians on the committee often comprise a diverse group from various fields of practice, with general practitioners and multiple specialists represented. The committee should be a well-balanced mix of practitioners who can view health care policies from different perspectives and provide sound recommendations.

Formulary Management

The main responsibilities of a P&T committee are to develop and revise the formulary, create and implement medication use policies, and provide education for practitioners. Formulary reviews include evaluating new medications for formulary consideration, periodic drug class reviews, and utilization analyses. A major goal of the P&T committee is to provide cost-effective, clinically safe, and effective therapy. Frequent formulary revisions are needed for several reasons: the introduction of new products into the marketplace, modifications to a product's labeling to include new treatment indications, emerging research indicating a previously unknown benefit or risk of therapy, changes in consensus disease treatment guidelines, and changes in the brand/generic status of a product or other pricing concerns.

The inclusion and exclusion of agents are time-intensive processes for P&T committees. As such, many P&T committees elect to delay their consideration of a new product until it has a sufficient body of evidence to perform a review and/or it has been on the market for a sufficient length of time (e.g., 1 year) to provide an opportunity for any adverse events undetected in clinical trials to be noticed. P&T committees may consider a wide variety of information when evaluating a new product, including peer-reviewed clinical trials, adverse event/safety data, patient-oriented health outcomes (e.g., the ability of an antihypertensive to reduce the risk of myocardial infarctions, not merely to lower blood pressure), the FDA-approved product labeling for the new agent, quality-of-life research,

BOX 59.1 Information Considered by a Pharmacy and Therapeutics Committee When Reviewing a Product for the Formulary

1. FDA-approved indications
2. Pharmacology/mechanism of action
3. Pharmacokinetic/pharmacodynamic data
4. Dosing and administration, including special monitoring or drug administration requirements
5. Adverse effect profile, warnings, precautions, contraindications, and black box warnings
6. Drug interactions (with other drugs, foods, or medical conditions)
7. Clinical evidence: clinical trials, health outcomes research, retrospective database analyses, quality-of-life research
8. Risks versus benefits regarding clinical efficacy and safety of a particular drug relative to other drugs with the same indication
9. Pharmacoeconomic data and modeling
10. Off-label uses
11. Cost comparisons against other drugs available to treat the same medical condition(s)
12. Source of supply and reliability of manufacturer and distributor

and pharmacoeconomic data (**Box 59.1**). The committee must consider the issue of bias when evaluating results provided by any research sponsored by the pharmaceutical manufacturer. Literature that includes data comparing the new agent with an agent currently used to treat the same disorder is prized by P&T committees for its utility in comparing one drug with another. If the new agent offers a clinical, safety, or economic advantage to existing formulary agents, the P&T committee may place the agent on the formulary and can do so by adding the new product with or without removing an existing product or products. Further, committees can add the drug to the formulary unconditionally or may recommend implementation of certain restrictions on the coverage (prior authorization, quantity limitations, step therapy) of the new agent to allow its inclusion in the formulary.

Because of the increase in prescription drug spending by health plans, cost now plays a more significant role in formulary status, although many organizations claim that cost is considered only after safety and efficacy data have been evaluated. Pharmacoeconomic modeling allows an organization to estimate the impact of a formulary change on both the health outcomes experienced by their members and total prescription drug and health care spending. To improve the likelihood of a drug's addition to a formulary, pharmaceutical manufacturers may offer prescription volume-dependent rebates to MCOs as incentives.

Development of Disease Management Programs or Treatment Protocols

Another responsibility of a P&T committee is to develop or approve disease management programs or treatment protocols for the organization. These programs and protocols provide useful recommendations for practitioners treating various diseases. They may be based on current consensus practice guidelines, or they may be developed by the P&T committee using current clinical data. A main purpose of guidelines or algorithms is to minimize treatment variations and improve patient outcomes while reducing costs (Navarro et al., 2009).

ENSURING FORMULARY AND PRACTICE GUIDELINE COMPLIANCE

One of the primary reasons that MCOs develop formularies and practice guidelines is to help lower the cost of the prescription drug benefit. Unfortunately, merely printing and distributing formularies and algorithms often are not enough to alter prescribing practices. Patients and pharmacists may also be wary of the formulary system, failing to understand both its necessity and utility. While educational programs (including seminars, newsletters, provider peer-to-peer communications, and one-on-one meetings) are useful, these tools alone do not ensure improved formulary compliance. MCOs have developed a variety of payment and reimbursement strategies to improve compliance. The following sections describe the ways that MCOs evaluate formulary and treatment guideline compliance and how MCOs use different levels of payments to improve compliance.

Prescriber Incentives for Compliance

MCOs can monitor compliance to the formulary and treatment protocols with a variety of tools. Many MCOs use the level of peer compliance to determine the amount of a prescriber's or practice's year-end incentives. Prescribers can be eligible for financial incentives if their compliance to the formulary or treatment protocols meets the threshold established by the MCO (Navarro et al., 2009).

Some MCOs may tie a portion of a provider's compensation to the level of compliance. If a practitioner fails to follow treatment protocols closely and inexplicably high prescription costs result, an MCO may withhold a portion of the provider's compensation. In a capitated plan, the provider receives a fixed, predetermined, per-member payment by the MCO to provide services for members, regardless of how much or how frequently a member uses service. Providers can reap financial reward if they can provide services at a cost lower than their level of payment but are responsible for all costs if expenses should rise above their level of payment. While capitation remains a frequently utilized tool by MCOs to manage medical costs (Kaiser Family Foundation, 2010), few (if any) health plans utilize a capitated pharmacy benefit.

Evaluating Compliance: Percentage Formulary Compliance

The simplest way for an MCO to evaluate formulary compliance is to determine the prescriber's percentage of prescriptions for generic and branded formulary products. Although this method is useful for determining formulary compliance (e.g., the use of generic and branded formulary angiotensin receptor blockers (ARBs) compared with nonformulary-branded ARBs), it does not evaluate the quality of prescribing; just because a formulary agent is prescribed does not make the prescription appropriate. It may be more important to determine if the prescriber is following consensus disease treatment guidelines. A prescriber who prescribes a formulary agent but is not following treatment guidelines may have the same percentage formulary compliance as a prescriber who uses a different and potentially less expensive or more appropriate formulary medication by following treatment guidelines. Also, prescribers who use medically necessary or appropriate nonformulary drugs are penalized in this system. Many MCOs have initiated programs to evaluate the quality of prescriber by implementing practitioner profiling programs, where MCO clinicians evaluate questionable prescribing with the provider.

Because of the aforementioned limitations with percentage formulary compliance, MCOs also use another tool to evaluate compliance: per-member–per-month (PMPM) reports.

Health Care Trend Reporting

When analyzing health care trends for an MCO, many variables are reviewed and factored in to evaluate and justify the trends during any particular year. The PMPM reports are a unit of measure related to each enrollee for each month. When used to evaluate prescribing practices, average PMPM prescription costs are determined for each provider. Theoretically, prescribers who adhere to formulary and practice guidelines will achieve lower PMPM prescription costs than their peers who do not. This is not a foolproof method to evaluate compliance because a small number of patients requiring expensive therapy (e.g., chemotherapy, antipsychotics) can substantially increase a prescriber's PMPM amount. More frequently, MCOs use PMPM reports to evaluate prescription costs for a specific disease. An example of a disease-specific PMPM report appears in **Table 59.2**. Although prescriber A is responsible for the highest dollar expenditure on antihyperlipidemics, his or her PMPM prescription cost is close to the average of the prescriber's peers. On the other hand, despite prescriber C's low overall dollar expenditure on lipid agents, his or her PMPM prescription cost is the highest.

Another factor that is considered in evaluating health care trends is drug cost. Monitoring the rate of increase in drug cost has become a significant factor in overall health care spending. As the prices of prescription medications increase, MCOs are adjusting their overall plan designs to compensate for that increase. These adjustments may include changes in product status on drug formularies, implementation of prior authorization

TABLE 59.2

Per-Member–Per-Month (PMPM) Prescription Costs for Patients Receiving Antihyperlipidemic Therapy

Prescriber	Number of Member Months	Lipid Prescription Costs ($)	PMPM Prescription Costs ($)
A	561	45,183	80.54
B	240	18,818	78.41
C	285	25,639	89.96
D	496	36,248	73.08
E	357	30,780	86.22
F	489	40,223	82.31

and step therapy programs for expensive products, increases in member copayments, or increases in member premiums.

Improving Formulary Compliance

In addition to prescribers, MCOs have an opportunity to improve formulary and practice guideline compliance by providing financial incentives or disincentives to other players: the prescription dispenser (pharmacist) and the prescription recipient (patient). These financial incentives include bonuses, differential reimbursement rates, and different levels of prescription copayment.

Pharmacist Reimbursement

An MCO can influence pharmacists as a secondary step in limiting the use of nonformulary medications. As a part of the contracting process, MCOs may impose requirements on pharmacies if the pharmacy wishes to serve members of the plan. MCOs can require that pharmacies dispense generic products when available, unless the prescriber requires the prescription to be DAW or the medication has a narrow therapeutic index (e.g., phenytoin [Dilantin], warfarin). Many states already require automatic generic substitution when applicable. To reduce wasted or unused medication, MCOs often impose a limit on the amount of medication that a community pharmacist can dispense—usually no more than 1 month's worth at a time. Once a patient is stabilized on a maintenance dose for medications used to treat chronic illnesses (e.g., hypertension, diabetes), MCOs may require that patients receive a 3-month supply of medication from a mail-order pharmacy; this can be done at a lower expense to the MCO.

Pharmacies that are successful in increasing formulary compliance or reducing member pharmacy costs may be eligible for bonuses or they may receive a higher reimbursement rate. Alternatively, pharmacies that fail to meet the requirements of the contract may receive a lower reimbursement rate or have their contract terminated altogether. MCOs frequently audit the claims of pharmacies with a higher-than-average number of DAW orders to ensure that the prescriber does in fact require the brand-name drug be dispensed to the patient.

Patient Prescription Copayment

The impact of prescription copayment on patients was reviewed earlier in this chapter. In summary, as formularies have progressively become more open, health plans have responded by using differential copayments with significant price differentials between tiers in an effort to encourage patients to use lower-cost generic or preferred brand medications. Patients who are hesitant to pay a high prescription copayment when lower priced alternatives are available frequently ask their provider to prescribe the product with the lower copayment; the provider will often comply with the patient's request if they believe the change can be made without adversely affecting the outcome of care.

ELECTRONIC PRESCRIBING AND ELECTRONIC HEALTH RECORDS

Before the introduction of electronic prescribing, practitioners were faced with a variety of options by which they could prescribe medications: written orders on prescription pads, typed orders sent via fax, or verbal orders communicated through telephone calls. These prescribing options leave room for error, as there is the potential for illegible handwriting, poorly scanned images, and inaudible messages. Furthermore, these options are not exempt from tampering or fraud, as individuals can alter handwritten prescriptions, send falsified prescriptions via fax, or call in fake prescriptions over the phone. With the advent of electronic prescribing, practitioners were presented with an additional option that has the potential to save time and money, as well as reduce medication errors and fraud.

Electronic prescribing, or e-prescribing, is the process whereby a prescriber orders and submits a prescription through an application that electronically transmits the prescription to a pharmacy in real time (CMS, 2014b). A variety of e-prescribing software programs exist, and thus, there may be differences in functionality among the e-prescribing software programs available to clinicians. Ideally, the software programs should allow the prescribers to view a patient's current medication list, medication history, available pharmacy, and prescription insurance plan (Health Resources and Services Administration [HRSA], 2015).

E-prescribing software requires a user (the prescriber or an authorized representative) to log in to a secure system and verify his/her identity using a username and password combination. After authentication, the prescriber can search for and select a patient record within the e-prescribing system using patient-specific information (i.e., first name, last name, date of birth, etc.). The prescriber can then choose to review the patient's records and begin to enter and edit a prescription (HRSA, 2015).

After entering the intended prescription information, the prescriber can send the order to the transaction hub, which links the prescriber to both the pharmacy and the PBM. This interoperability allows for the verification of patient eligibility

for prescription coverage by submitting the prescription information to the PBM before the e-prescription arrives at the pharmacy. Once the information has been submitted, the PBM determines if the drug is a covered benefit for the member. The prescriber then receives a message regarding the drug's coverage status. If the drug is covered, the prescriber may choose to send the prescription to the pharmacy for it to be filled. On the other hand, if the drug is not covered, the prescriber has the option of ordering a different medication or contacting the PBM for prior authorization of the drug (HRSA, 2015).

The ability of prescribers to directly transmit prescriptions from the office to the pharmacy eliminates the need for the patient to take it to the pharmacy to be filled. Since patients are not required to take electronically transmitted prescriptions to the pharmacy, there are increased chances that the prescriptions actually arrive at the pharmacy. Surescripts, an e-prescribing software vendor, released a report that showed that e-prescribing increases the number of first fills of prescriptions that actually reach the pharmacy by 11.7% and the number of prescriptions picked up at the pharmacy by 10% (Surescripts, 2012).

E-prescribing has also been shown to reduce prescribing errors. Researchers at Weill Cornell Medical College found 37 errors for every 100 prescriptions written by hand, but only 7 errors for every 100 prescriptions ordered via e-prescribing software (Kaushal et al., 2010). These benefits, along with the potential for time and cost savings, explain the rationale behind the "meaningful use" incentive payments program offered by the Centers for Medicare and Medicaid Services (CMS), which began in 2009 and ended in 2013 (CMS, 2014c).

E-prescribing represents only one part of a greater change to the health care system: electronic health records. Electronic health records, or EHR, are digital versions of patient-centered medical records, which can be updated in real time (HealthIT, 2013). In 2009, the American Recovery and Reinvestment Act (ARRA) authorized CMS to offer financial incentives to providers and hospitals that exhibit "meaningful use" of EHR technology (AMA, 2014). With the recent advances in technology, many providers have already adopted the software necessary to maintain electronic health records. However, these systems can impart challenges to smaller practices because of the significant cost to upgrade technology and the operational changes needed to use the system. Aside from the large costs associated with the purchase of EHR software, the universal implementation of EHR represents an opportunity for enhanced interoperability, improved continuity of care, and medical error reduction.

CURRENT ISSUES IN MANAGED CARE

One cause of discontent among health care purchasers is the cost of insurance premiums, which began to rise at a rate greater than that of inflation starting in the mid-1990s. The average family's annual premium costs were nearly $17,000 in 2014, with covered workers paying 29% of the premium (Kaiser Family Foundation, 2014). A portion of the price increase is attributed to increased costs of medications, which increased an average of 9.9% a year during the 10-year period ending in 2007 and increased 13.1% in 2014 (Aitken et al., 2009; Kaiser Family Foundation, 2014). The increase in expenditures for prescription drugs is the effect of three factors: price inflation, increased utilization, and the increased availability of high-cost specialty medications. If prescription drug spending continues to increase at the 5.7% annual rate forecast for the next decade as projected (Sisko et al., 2014), MCOs will be forced to modify the extent to which they cover prescription drugs through coverage limits, establish more rigid formulary systems, and increased cost shifting to consumers.

In March 2010, the U.S. Congress passed the Affordable Care Act, commonly known as either the Healthcare Reform Bill or "ObamaCare." The premise for the act was to ensure accountability of MCOs, lower health care costs, improve quality of care, and provide improved consumer choice for health care services (U.S. Department of Health & Human Services, 2010). Components of the Affordable Care Act include provisions requiring insurers to provide coverage for individuals with preexisting conditions, allowing individuals under the age of 26 years to remain on a parent's insurance plan, an elimination of lifetime and annual dollar limits for essential health benefits, and requirements for specific preventive services (e.g., colorectal cancer screening for adults over 50, breast cancer mammography screening for women over 40, vision screening for children) without having to pay a copayment or coinsurance when delivered by a network provider (U.S. Department of Health & Human Services, 2015). A mandate written into the act requires individuals not covered by an employer-sponsored health plan or a public insurance plan to obtain an approved private insurance policy or pay a penalty. This individual mandate provision of the act was upheld by the U.S. Supreme Court in June 2012 as a constitutional action under Congress's taxation powers (National Federation of Independent Businesses vs. Sebelius, June 28, 2012). The act established health insurance exchanges to facilitate the purchase of health insurance by citizens; the rollout of the federally operated exchange in October 2013 to serve the citizens of the 36 states that opted not to establish their own state-specific exchanges was marred by technological issues that took several months to resolve. The act continues to face legal and legislative challenges in its funding and implementation, and the regulations and provisions noted here may be modified or eliminated in the future.

Despite its critics and shortcomings, managed care is likely to remain the leading manner of financing and delivering health care in the United States. Through more effective communication and cooperation, practitioners and MCOs may someday resolve their conflicting issues. It is imperative for practitioners and MCOs to understand each other's role in health care. Although practitioners and MCOs have quite different responsibilities in health care, both groups share a common goal: the delivery of high-quality care to patients.

Bibliography

Starred references are cited in the text.

Academy of Managed Care Pharmacy. (2013). *AMCP format for formulary submissions, version 3.1.* Alexandria, VA: Author.

*Aitken, M., Berndt, E. R., & Cutler, D. M. (2009). Prescription drug spending trends in the United States: Looking beyond the turning point. *Health Affairs, 28,* w151–w160.

*American Medical Association. (1994). AMA policy on drug formularies and therapeutic interchange in inpatient and ambulatory patient care settings. *American Journal of Hospital Pharmacy, 51,* 1808–1810.

*American Medical Association. (2014). Medicare/Medicaid HER Incentive and Penalty Programs. Retrieved from http://www.ama-assn.org/ama/pub/advocacy/topics/digital-health/medicare-medicaid-incentive-programs.page on April 27, 2015.

*Bendix, J. (2013) Curing the Prior Authorization Headache. *Medical Economics.* Retrieved from http://medicaleconomics.modernmedicine.com/medical-economics/content/tags/americas-health-insurance-plans/curing-prior-authorization-headache?page=full on May 10, 2015.

Campbell, G., & Sprague, K. L. (2001). The state of drug decision-making: Report on a survey of P&T committee structure and practices. *Formulary, 36,* 644–655.

*Centers for Medicare and Medicaid Services. (2014a). *Office of the Actuary, National Health Statistics Group. National health expenditures fact sheet.* Washington, DC: Author.

*Centers for Medicare and Medicaid Services. (2014b). *Electronic prescribing (eRx) incentive program.* Baltimore, MD: Author. Retrieved from https://www.cms.gov/Medicare/Quality-Initiatives-Patient-Assessment-Instruments/ERxIncentive/index.html on April 27, 2015.

*Centers for Medicare and Medicaid Services. (2014c). *E-prescribing.* Baltimore, MD: Author. Retrieved from https://www.cms.gov/Medicare/E-Health/Eprescribing/index.html?redirect=/eprescribing on April 27, 2015.

*Edlin, M. (2015). Closed formularies hold the line on costs: One of a number of strategies in use. *Managed Healthcare Executive, 25*(3), 48.

Fairman, K. A., Motheral, B. R., & Henderson, R. R. (2003). Retrospective, long-term follow-up study of the effect of a three-tier prescription drug co-payment system on pharmaceutical and other medical utilization and costs. *Clinical Therapeutics, 25,* 3147–3161.

Fins, J. J. (1998). Drug benefits in managed care: Seeking ethical guidance from the formulary? *Journal of the American Geriatrics Society, 46,* 346–350.

*Food and Drug Administration. (2014). Electronic Orange Book preface 34th edition. http://www.fda.gov/Drugs/DevelopmentApprovalProcess/ucm079068.htm. Accessed May 9, 2015.

Fullerton D. S., & Atherly D. S. (2004). Formularies, therapeutics, and outcomes: New opportunities. *Medical Care, 42*(4 Suppl.), 39–44.

*Health Resources and Services Administration. (2015). How does e-prescribing work? http://www.hrsa.gov/healthit/toolbox/HealthITAdoptiontoolbox/ElectronicPrescribing/epreswork.html. Accessed May 30, 2015.

*HealthIT.gov. (2013). What is an electronic health record (EHR)? http://www.healthit.gov/providers-professionals/faqs/what-electronic-health-record-ehr. Accessed April 27, 2015.

*Holmes, D. R., Becker, J. A., Granger, C. B., et al. (2011). ACCF/AHA 2011 health policy statement on therapeutic interchange and substitution. *Circulation, 124,* 1290–1310.

*Hunter, R. M., Baio, G., Butt, S., et al. (2015). An educational review of the statistical issues in analysing utility data for cost utility analysis. *Pharmacoeconomics, 33,* 355–366.

*IMS Health. (2015). *Press release: IMS Health Study: 2014 a record-setting year for U.S. medicines.* Parsippany, NJ: Author.

*IMS Institute for Healthcare Informatics. (2014). *Medicine use and shifting costs of healthcare: A review of the use of medicines in the United States in 2013.* Parsippany, NJ: Author.

*Kaiser Family Foundation. (2010). *Medicaid and managed care: Key data, trends, and issues. (Publication No. 8046).* Washington, DC: Author.

*Kaiser Family Foundation and Health Research Educational Trust. (2014). *Employer health benefits 2014 annual survey. (Publication No. 8625).* Menlo Park, CA: Author.

*Kaushal, R., Kern, L. M., Barron, Y., et al. (2010). Electronic prescribing improves medication safety in community-based office practices. *Journal of General Internal Medicine, 6,* 530–536.

Keech, M. (2001). Using health outcomes data to inform decision-making. *Pharmacoeconomics, 19,* 27–31.

Lisi, D. (1997). Ethical issues for pharmacists in managed care. *American Journal of Health-System Pharmacy, 54,* 1041–1045.

Luce, B. R., Lyles, A. C., & Rentz, A. M. (1996). The view from managed care pharmacy. *Health Affairs, 15,* 168–176.

Lyles, A., & Palumbo, F. B. (1999). The effect of managed care on prescription drug costs and benefits. *Pharmacoeconomics, 15*(2), 129–140.

Monane, M., Nagle, B., & Kelly, M. (1998). Pharmacotherapy: Strategies to control drug costs in managed care. *Geriatrics, 53*(9), 53–63.

*National Conference of State Legislatures. (2010). State Pharmaceutical Assistance Programs 2010. Retrieved from http://www.ncsl.org/default.aspx?tabid=14334. Denver, CO: Author.

*National Federation of Independent Businesses vs. Sebelius, 567.U.S. 2012, 132 S. Ct 2566. June 28, 2012.

*Navarro, R. P., Dillon, M. J., & Grzegorczyk, J. E. (2009). Role of drug formularies in managed care organizations. In R. P. Navarro (Ed.). *Managed care pharmacy practice* (2nd ed., pp. 233–252). Sudbury, MA: Jones and Bartlett Publishers.

Penna, P. M. (2002). AMCP format for formulary submissions: Who is using them, who will be evaluating them, and what regulatory concerns do they raise?. International Society for Pharmacoeconomics and Outcomes Research Seventh International Meeting, Arlington, VA

*Sisko, A. M., Keehan, S. P., Cuckler, G. A., et al. (2014). National health expenditure projections, 2013–23: Faster growth expected with expanded coverage and improving economy. *Health Affairs, 33,* 1841–1850.

*Sonnedecker, G. (1976). *Kremer's and Urdang's history of pharmacy.* Madison, WI: American Institute of the History of Pharmacy.

*Surescripts (2012). Study: E-Prescribing shown to improve outcomes and save healthcare system billions of dollars. Retrieved from http://surescripts.com/news-center/press-releases/!content/212_eprescribing on April 27, 2015.

*Starr, P. (1982). *The social transformation of American medicine.* New York: Basic Books.

Sweet, B. T., Wilson, M. W., Waugh, W. J., et al. (2002). Building the outcomes-based formulary. *Disease Management and Health Outcomes, 10,* 525–530.

*Takeda Pharmaceuticals. (2014). *2014–2015 Prescription drug benefit cost and plan design report.* Plano, TX: Pharmacy Benefit Management Institute.

*U.S. Department of Health & Human Services. (2010). Understanding the affordable care act: About the law. Retrieved from http://www.hhs.gov/healthcare/rights/index.html on April 27, 2015.

*U.S. Department of Health & Human Services. (2015). Understanding the Affordable Care Act: Read the Law. Retrieved from http://www.hhs.gov/healthcare/rights/law/ on April 27, 2015.

60 Integrative Approaches to Pharmacotherapy— A Look at Complex Cases

Virginia P. Arcangelo ■ Andrew M. Peterson ■ Jennifer A. Reinhold ■ Veronica F. Wilbur

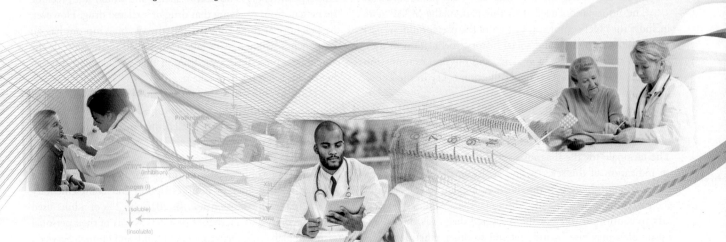

The cases presented in each of the disorders-focused chapters were designed to help the learner think through the process of evaluating patient-specific drug therapy needs. The cases were simple ones, typically involving a single problem related to the disorders discussed in the chapter. This chapter, however, uses cases involving patients with multiple problems, which encourages the learner to assess the problems and prioritize them. When managing multiple problems in a single patient, the practitioner must evaluate possible medication therapies and select the best patient-specific option. This level of complexity is reflective of real-life situations and requires a systematic approach to the patient to manage the complexities.

THE COMPLEXITY OF PATIENTS

The reality of life is that patients are complex individuals with multiple competing issues and priorities. Patients have economic, social, emotional, and cultural issues that affect their medical conditions.

Chronic medication therapy can be costly, even in instances when patients are prescribed generic medications exclusively. Nearly two thirds of elderly patients use medications on a daily basis with an average of eight prescription medications per person. The average yearly cost for a single generic drug in 2013 was more than $280, which can be cost prohibitive for some patients, particularly those on multiple medications. In the same year, the average annual cost associated with brand name medications was more than 10 times higher than that of generic medications (Schondelmeyer & Purvis, 2014). The selection of treatment options must include consideration of the cost, because if patients cannot afford the treatment, they will not follow the plan.

In addition, the social and emotional impact of a diagnosis must be considered. Patients requiring insulin injections to maintain adequate blood glucose levels need assistance in making the lifestyle change necessary to incorporate the injections as well as the monitoring into their daily routine. The emotional reminder of "illness associated with chronic medication-taking behavior" must be addressed at the initial and subsequent visits. Last, culturally accepted treatment options are important considerations; injectable medications containing human blood products (e.g., albumin) may not be acceptable to patients who are of the Jehovah's Witness faith. Asian cultures view illness as an inevitable consequence of life and, as a result, may not seek care or may refuse treatment.

GENERAL OVERVIEW OF METHODS FOR ASSESSING PATIENTS AND DRUG THERAPY

One of the more common methods for organizing medical information is the problem-oriented medical record (POMR). Each of the patient's medical problems is identified and prioritized in order of importance. The order of the problems depends on the acuity and severity of the situation. Typically, the most severe and acute problems are listed first, followed by the chronic conditions, and then problems requiring preventive measures (e.g., smoking cessation).

In addition to the prioritized problem list, the POMR system uses the "SOAP" note technique for organizing information associated with each problem. The acronym *SOAP* stands for (S)ubjective, (O)bjective, (A)ssessment, and (P)lan. The subjective and objective components are the data that support the identification of the prioritized problem. The subjective data refer to information provided by the patient (or other individual) that cannot be independently verified. The objective data often are laboratory data or health assessments (e.g., blood pressures) performed or observed by the practitioner.

The information needed in this part of the SOAP note includes the chief complaint, history of the present illness, past medical history, family and social history, medication history, the results of the review of systems, and physical examination and laboratory results. This data collection is key in the assessment of the patient.

The assessment section of the SOAP note integrates the subjective and objective information and is where the practitioner delineates the potential diagnosis related to the problem. The rationale for the diagnosis should be included as well as an indication of the severity and acuity of the problem. The last portion of the note is the therapeutic plan. In this section, the practitioner may include additional diagnostic tests necessary to confirm or rule out the suspected diagnosis. This diagnostic plan may also include referral to other practitioners as necessary. The other portion of the plan section should include information about changes in therapeutic plans such as adding or discontinuing drug therapy, identifying therapeutic goals, and establishing monitoring parameters.

Anticipating Problems

One of the key elements of a good practitioner is the ability to plan for unintended consequences. A patient may become noncompliant with a medication due to an adverse event and not report the event or the noncompliance before your next scheduled visit. The result is the patient forgoes treatment for an identified problem for an unknown period of time. When addressed, the patient will admit to the noncompliance but may indicate unawareness of the severity of self-discontinuing drug therapy. Proactive discussions regarding potential consequences (adverse reactions, noncompliance) will help reduce the frequency of these types of encounters. As a practitioner, one should always consider what to do if the patient has an adverse drug reaction, takes an interacting drug, or even stops taking the drug.

Other Information Needed Before Prescribing

When taking a medication history, the practitioner needs to assess specific information related to drug therapy. An inventory of patient-reported allergies is vital to a good medication history. These allergies include an assessment of drug allergies. A

patient may report a symptom as an allergy, but the clinician must assess the validity of the report. For example, a patient may report abdominal discomfort as an allergy to erythromycin, but in reality, the reported symptom is an adverse effect of the drug. This type of report is not a true allergy and would not preclude the patient from receiving that drug or a related drug. However, the practitioner must consider the impact the symptom has on the patient's willingness to take a prescribed medication. If the patient was prescribed a medication that would cause distress, the patient is less likely to take it.

Food allergies are also important to assess. Reports of allergies to shellfish or other iodine-containing foods are important to know when prescribing medications such as intravenous contrast dyes.

Further, within this section of the patient history, the practitioner must not only assess prescription medication use but also obtain a good history of nonprescription and complementary and alternative medication use. In 2012, 33.2% of adults used complementary and alternative products as part of their personal treatment plan (U.S. Department of Health and Human Services, 2015), representing a decrease as compared to 2002 through 2007 and 2007 through 2012. The most commonly used products were fish oil; glucosamine/chondroitin products are consistently among the most popular. As compared to previous years' trends, there was a meaningful increase in the use of melatonin and a meaningful decrease in the use of echinacea. The potential for drug–drug and drug–disease interactions with these and other agents exists and must be considered as part of the treatment plan.

Questions

As noted earlier, each disorder chapter had a simple case with a series of questions designed to help you work through the pharmacotherapeutic approach to the patient. These nine questions are indicative of a thought process that should be followed when developing the pharmacotherapeutic aspect of the care plan. The following real-life cases are more complex than those in the disorder chapters and are designed to help the learner integrate the treatment plan for patients with multiple disorders and multiple medication needs. We use the same nine questions, in varying forms, to illustrate the thought process. The answers provided may not be the only "correct" answers. Other choices of drug therapy may clearly be available, or as time progresses, we may learn that there are better choices due to new drug development and new research on existing drugs. We encourage you to use this process to help you think through the problem, not solely finding the answer.

CASE STUDY 1*

DEPRESSION/ANXIETY/RHEUMATOID ARTHRITIS

J.R. is a 48-year-old Caucasian male who is employed as a college professor and has been diagnosed with depression and anxiety in the last year. At the time of diagnosis, the Hamilton

Depression Rating Scale score was 18 (moderate depression), and the Hamilton Anxiety Rating Scale score was 20 (moderate anxiety). Though he had vague complaints of mood disturbances and sad mood, he resisted medication therapy. His past medical history is also significant for rheumatoid arthritis, which has been managed with weekly methotrexate (7.5 mg every week). Recent personal issues (divorce, a new boss) have prompted **J.R.** to seek some assistance with his depressed and anxious symptoms. Currently, **J.R.** complains of staying awake at night worrying, lack of pleasure or joy in daily activities, decreased desire to socialize and lack of interest in his hobbies, and increase in napping during the weekends. In addition, **J.R.** complains about an increase in his normal daily pain rating (normal for **J.R.** = 2/10, but in the last few weeks, it has consistently been 4/10).

Weight: 250 lb (an increase of 20 lb since his last visit 6 months ago)

Height: 64 inches

BP: 140/80 mm Hg

Pulse: 72 bpm

Current medications:

    Methotrexate: 7.5 mg every Friday

    Naproxen: 500 mg bid, as needed

Lab values:

    Glucose: 107 mg/dL (fasting)

HbA_{1c}: 6.5%

Total cholesterol: 250 mg/dL

LDL: 169 mg/dL

HDL: 30 mg/dL

Triglycerides: 290 mg/dL

Creatinine: 1.0 mg/dL

BUN: 14 mg/dL

AST: 15

ALT: 20

Urine microalbumin (–)

Issues: **J.R.** has an established diagnosis of rheumatoid arthritis that had been previously controlled with drug therapy. In addition to complaints of less optimal pain control, **J.R.** also has had an exacerbation of his mood and anxiety symptoms, which has prompted him to seek help. Some new metabolic issues have also emerged as he has gained a significant amount of weight in a short time and his blood glucose and HbA_{1c} are no longer at goal. The challenge will be to determine which complaints and lab abnormalities are independent problems and which are potentially consequences of another issue.

* Answers can be found online.

List specific goals for treatment for J.R.

There are two distinct types of outcomes that should be expected for **J.R.**; clinical and quality of life related. The current complaints are primarily related to depressed mood and anxiety, which consequently impact his social and occupational quality of life. The rating scales that would be used to measure response to treatment will yield quasiobjective information, which can be considered a clinical outcome. Additional clinical outcomes related to the anxiety and depression would be prevention of serious outcomes (suicidality, worsening depression, or anxiety). **J.R.**'s pain complaint is a subjective parameter. The abnormal lab values are suggestive of an emerging metabolic problem, and the related goals would be clinical. An important consideration in this case is determining whether to treat all problems as independent or to approach treatment systematically, assuming that the weight gain and associated metabolic changes as well as the increase in pain rating may be a result of the worsened depression and anxiety. It is also a reasonable possibility that the increase in pain is also elevating his blood pressure.

Specific goals of therapy would reasonably include:

- HAM-D response (a ≥50% reduction in HAM-D score = 9)
- HAM-A response (a ≥50% reduction in HAM-A score = 10)
- Return to baseline function (subjective)
- Improvement in quality of life (subjective)
- Reduction in pain level (subjective)
- BMI: 18.5 to 24.9
- Blood glucose (fasting): less than 100 mg/dL
- Reduction in 10-year cardiovascular risk (no longer driven by LDL goals)

What drug therapy would you prescribe? Why?

One approach to drug therapy would be to treat the depression and anxiety first and then evaluate the impacts on the other problems (weight gain, metabolic disturbances, pain). An alternate and possibly less conservative approach would be to initiate medication therapy for the blood glucose, lipids, and pain. Though, starting multiple drug therapies simultaneously for problems that are likely dependent on one another is probably not optimal. Targeting the mood and anxiety first is recommended. In the absence of contraindications, a medication from the SSRI or SNRI class is recommended as first-line drug therapy for depression as well as anxiety. This patient has no contraindications; therefore, he is a candidate for these drug classes. One possible choice would be duloxetine (Cymbalta) 30 mg. The rationale would be that it is indicated for both depression and anxiety and also for neuropathic pain. **J.R.**'s pain results from rheumatoid arthritis and would not be classified as neuropathic; however, some patients report improvement in pain rating regardless of the etiology. There is a risk of weight gain with almost all of the medications in the SSRI and SNRI class, with a few exceptions. This risk does exist with duloxetine, but it is potentially less so as compared to other medications. There is less of a risk of increases in blood pressure as compared to venlafaxine (Effexor); the other SNRI indicated for anxiety. Sertraline (Zoloft) is a weight neutral SSRI, but the risk of sexual dysfunction is higher than that of the SNRIs, and though the patient is divorced, adding an additional potential life stressor may not be in his best interest. Bupropion (Wellbutrin) would have been a great choice secondary to its alerting properties and potential weight loss, but the patient has comorbid anxiety and bupropion may worsen it.

What are the parameters for monitoring success of the therapy?

Assuming that the anxiety and depression are treated first, and then any additional potentially remaining problems are treated after resolution of the psychiatric complaints, the HAM-A and HAM-D would be the most likely instruments. After 4 to 8 weeks of drug therapy with duloxetine (or alternate SSRI or SNRI), the patient should be reevaluated using both of these rating scales. A response to drug therapy is defined (based on these rating scales) as a 50% or greater reduction in baseline score. This equates to a nine or less on the HAM-D (baseline was 18) and a 10 or less on the HAM-A (baseline was 20).

Discuss specific patient education based on the prescribed therapy.

Adherence is especially important in the context of depression and anxiety medication therapy. Discussion regarding the importance of taking the medication daily and not skipping doses should occur. In addition, there needs to be explanation about the expected delay to therapeutic effect. These medications generally take four or more weeks to exert a therapeutic effect and it's important (particularly with regard to adherence) to let patients know that they should not expect to feel "better" within the first few weeks of therapy. Once patients do feel a therapeutic effect, it is important that they do not self-discontinue the drug and assume that they are "cured." Drug therapy typically extends for 6 to 12 months beyond symptom resolution. Duloxetine can cause weight gain. All SSRIs and SNRIs carry warnings for worsening depression and risk of suicidality; therefore, the patient needs to be told to report any worsened or emerging symptoms to the provider.

List one or two adverse reactions for the selected agent that would cause you to change therapy.

Any significant worsening of depressive or anxious symptoms or any change in personality or thoughts of suicide would warrant a change in therapy.

What would be the choice for second-line therapy?

In the event that duloxetine failed to produce a therapeutic effect after an appropriate trial (8 to 12 weeks), then another medication from the SSRI or SNRI class would be appropriate.

What over-the-counter and/or alternative medications would be appropriate for J.R.?

There are no nonprescription products that have been shown to be safe and effective in the treatment of depression or anxiety.

What lifestyle changes would you recommend to J.R.?

Seeking counseling or therapy would be an appropriate treatment option in addition to drug therapy. J.R. should also increase his physical activity to 30 or more minutes most days of the week while also limiting high-fat and processed foods.

Describe one or two drug–drug or drug–food interaction for the selected agent.

Other medications that are serotonergic (other SSRIs or SNRIs, TCAs) should not be used in combination with duloxetine. Some over-the-counter products, like St. John's wort, are known to interact with duloxetine as both are serotonergic.

CASE STUDY 2*

SEIZURE DISORDER/HEADACHE/INSOMNIA

R.M. is a 32-year-old female who presents with a 6-week history of brief periods of "blanking out" and having a bilateral, rhythmic, mild "jerking" of her arms. These episodes, which have occurred approximately six times, last from 30 seconds to about 1 minute, and consciousness is not lost. She worries that she might be hypoglycemic and is seeking help. Her past medical history is significant for migraine headaches and insomnia. R.M. has been self-managing her infrequent migraines with ibuprofen (doses as high as 800 mg once and then repeating in 4 hours up to three times) but reports that they are now increasing in frequency with approximately 4 to 5 per month. She is currently not treated for her insomnia, which she categorizes as difficulty staying asleep. Though in the office R.M.'s EEG is normal (as would be expected since it would only be abnormal during an actual seizure), her provider diagnoses her with complex partial seizures, as her complaints are consistent with this diagnosis. There are no metabolic abnormalities that could explain the seizure activity.

Weight: 140 lb
Height: 68 inches
BP: 112/76 mm Hg
Pulse: 68 bpm
Current medications:
    Ibuprofen as needed for migraine (usual doses during headache are 800 mg two to three times)

Issues: R.M. is newly diagnosed with complex partial seizures and requires initiation of drug therapy. She has two additional diagnoses; migraine headaches (which are increasing in frequency) and insomnia, which are not formally treated with prescription drug therapy. She currently manages her migraines with over-the-counter ibuprofen at higher than recommended doses for self-treatment. There are no additional medications or lab abnormalities that complicate this clinical picture. There is an opportunity to minimize the pill burden for R.M. as there is some overlap in terms of the drug therapy that can be used for at least two of her complaints.

List specific goals of treatment for R.M.

- Reduce seizure frequency, ideally to zero seizures.
- Reduce the number of migraine headaches per month to zero.
- Minimize adverse effects and drug interactions.
- Improve sleep quality and maintain sleep through the night.

What drug therapy would you prescribe? Why?

There are a number of medications that are indicated for the treatment of complex partial seizures. Monotherapy is recommended, and therefore, a medication indicated as monotherapy should be considered. Since the efficacy of most antiepileptic medications is comparable, adverse effects, drug interaction potential, and practical considerations (the need to monitor blood levels, frequency of administration, etc.) are at the forefront of selecting drug therapy for seizures. Considering that based on the frequency of her migraine headaches, **R.M.** is also a candidate for prophylactic therapy for her migraines. Both topiramate and valproic acid are indicated for the monotherapy treatment of complex partial seizures as well as the prophylactic treatment of migraine headaches; these two drugs should be considered possible options. A rationale to initiate topiramate instead of valproic acid is that valproic acid needs to be monitored and topiramate does not. Also, though most seizure medications are contraindicated or strongly not recommended in pregnancy, valproic acid is the medication that is associated with the most risk of fetal harm. The patient is not pregnant currently but she is of childbearing age. An appropriate starting dose of topiramate would be 50 mg daily for 1 week with a weekly increase by 50 mg daily up to 200 mg once daily (maximum of 400 mg daily). This plan is driven by the dosing for seizures and not migraine prophylaxis. If **R.M.** had been on interacting medications or if she has existing metabolic issues, the drug initiated could be different (e.g., if she had risk factors for kidney stones or a history of kidney stones, topiramate would not be the best choice).

Topiramate may cause unwanted sedation initially, which could ultimately be beneficial given the presence of insomnia. But since topiramate can be sedating, initiating a medication for insomnia at this time would not be recommended. Once **R.M.** was stable on her chronic topiramate dose and was no longer experiencing daytime sedation (assuming that this occurs), and if her insomnia complaint persists, then drug therapy could be initiated. Since her insomnia complaint involves waking in the middle of the night, a medication with a longer duration of action is warranted. Zolpidem ER 5 mg would be an appropriate choice since it is a first-line medication and it would be expected to exert an effect through the night.

What are the parameters for monitoring success of the therapy?

After approximately 1 week, topiramate dosing can be adjusted so 1-week postinitiation of medication therapy would be an appropriate time for a follow-up. At 1 week, an assessment of seizure frequency is made. Ideally, there have been no additional episodes of complex partial seizures by this time. Assuming that there has been no seizure activity and the medication has been well tolerated, the dose should be titrated upward as detailed above. Absence of seizure activity will remain the parameter by which success of therapy is measured. If a drug that needs to be monitored had been chosen, then therapeutic level would also be part of the monitoring plan for efficacy.

Discuss specific patient education based on the prescribed therapy.

Adherence to drug therapy for seizure disorder is critical, as noncompliance is the most common reason for treatment failure and subsequent seizure activity. Topiramate is a pregnancy category D (according the current rating structure) and is not recommended during pregnancy. If **R.M.** decides to start a family, she needs to inform her provider. Additionally, if she is in a sexual relationship with a male partner, she must be counseled on what constitutes effective contraception.

List one or two adverse reactions for the selected agent that would cause you to change therapy.

Topiramate is associated with a risk of nephrolithiasis and metabolic acidosis. Baseline and periodic monitoring of serum bicarbonate, electrolytes, and ammonia are recommended. Emergence of nephrolithiasis or metabolic acidosis may warrant a change in drug therapy.

What would be the choice for second-line therapy?

Assuming that the plan remained to treat the seizure disorder and provide migraine prophylaxis with a single drug, then valproic acid would be the next best choice. Periodic monitoring of the level is required (50 to 100 mg/L), and the risk of fetal malformation is higher with valproic acid. The dosing is weight based and should be initiated at 15 mg/kg/d and adjusted by 5 to 10 mg/kg/d at weekly intervals until therapeutic levels are achieved (maximum of 60 mg/kg/d). The initial dose for this patient would be 954 mg/d, which would be accomplished by administering a 500-mg tablet twice daily. If the migraine prophylaxis and seizure treatment were separated, then multiple other antiepileptics would be considered appropriate for this patient (e.g., lamotrigine). A new prophylactic and/or abortive therapy for the migraines would need to be initiated with this plan.

What over-the-counter and/or alternative medications would be appropriate for R.M.?

Aside from the current periodic use of ibuprofen during episodes of migraine headache, there are no additional nonprescription products that would be recommended for any of **R.M.**'s diagnoses.

What lifestyle changes would you recommend to R.M.?

With regard to insomnia, **R.M.** needs to establish a regular routine and initiate sleep hygiene measures in addition to any subsequent medication therapy that may be initiated. This should occur regardless of whether or not a drug is started. In terms of the migraines and seizure disorder, **R.M.** should keep a headache and seizure diary in an attempt to capture a pattern and, especially, any triggers that may contribute to headache or seizure episodes.

Describe one or two drug–drug or drug–food interaction for the selected agent.

Topiramate may interact with other medications that depress the central nervous system and/or cause sedation. If zolpidem (or a similar medication for insomnia) is eventually initiated, this will become a very important counseling point and the zolpidem would need to be started at a lower dose (half of a 5-mg tablet). Splitting the tablet would preclude the use of the extended-release product, also. Alcohol may increase the serum concentration of topiramate and may result in increased sedation as well as toxic effects associated with higher serum concentrations of topiramate. If the patient decided to initiate the ketogenic diet for seizures (which is not recommended), her risk of kidney stones with topiramate would be increased.

CASE STUDY 3*

ATTENTION DEFICIT HYPERACTIVITY DISORDER (ADHD)/ANXIETY/ASTHMA

C.P. is a 16-year-old high school student presenting with complaints of not being able to concentrate in class. The patient is seen with her mother who confirms the patient's concerns and narrative. The issues related to attention have been present since **C.P.** was about 8 years old, though they have never been problematic as her grades have always been good. This year, however, her grades have worsened considerably, and there is a possibility that **C.P.** may not progress to her senior year. Her main complaints include an inability to focus in class, challenges with maintaining focus while studying at home, avoidance of homework, failure to follow through on school assignments and personal obligations, forgetfulness, losing her belongings, organizational deficits, and "zoning out" while she is engaged in conversation. These symptoms also have emerged at her part-time job as well, and her supervisor has needed to speak to her about it several times. **C.P.** has gotten a tutor, studies in silence, and uses a calendar to help organize her responsibilities but without success. During the last 9 months, she has also begun to feel "nervous" and reports some trouble sleeping, excess worrying, restlessness, and frequent stomach upset that she can't control. **C.P.**'s past medical history is significant for asthma, which is currently treated with an albuterol inhaler. She also indicates that she has had to use her inhaler more frequently than in the past (once per day for an asthma exacerbation), and she is running out of her medication in 3 weeks instead of 4. The worsening of asthma symptoms began 3 months ago and has persisted ever since.
Weight: 186 lb
Height: 63 inches
BP: 118/80 mm Hg

Pulse: 72 bpm
EKG: normal
HAM-A: 12
Current medications:
  Albuterol inhaler 90 mcg/actuation: two inhalations every 4 to 6 hours as needed

Issues: C.P. meets the DSM-5 criteria for the diagnosis of ADHD since she has six or more symptoms of inattention, the symptoms occur in more than one domain (home, school, work), symptoms were present before the patient was 12, and the symptoms are causing clinically significant impairment. Since she has already instituted nondrug approaches (keeping a calendar, studying in an appropriate environment, getting a tutor) without success, a medication is warranted. She also *may* meet the DSM-5 criteria for generalized anxiety disorder (6-month duration of symptoms, excessive worry, trouble concentrating, and presence of somatic symptoms). This is arguable because she has an identifiable stressor (possibility of not passing the school year, poor grades) and the symptoms emerged after the symptoms of ADHD. The HAM-A score suggests the presence of an anxiety disorder as well. This needs to be evaluated again at another time when the ADHD is controlled. The anxious symptoms may be the result of the ADHD and the associated academic and social consequences of the ADHD. C.P. has an established diagnosis of asthma, but her symptoms have worsened, and she is using her rescue inhaler (her only prescribed drug for asthma) more frequently than prescribed. C.P. is also obese, though this was not one of her complaints. At this time, this issue should not be addressed with drug therapy, but with lifestyle changes (not covered in detail in this case).

List specific goals for treatment for C.P.

- Resolution of ADHD symptoms (no longer meeting diagnostic criteria)
- Improvement in academic, social, and occupational performance and quality of life
- Resolution of anxious symptoms (worrying, restlessness, stomach ache, trouble sleeping)
- Reduced utilization of her asthma rescue medication

What drug therapy would you prescribe? Why?

C.P. meets the diagnostic criteria for ADHD, as referenced above. As discussed, it is common for ADHD to cooccur with depression, anxiety, substance use disorders, and other psychiatric comorbidities. There is also significant symptom overlap, which may complicate the accurate diagnosis and appropriate treatment of some patients. The anxious symptoms emerged after the onset of the ADHD symptoms, and it is reasonable to assume that the anxious symptoms are actually a product of ADHD (and the subsequent stressors of possibly not passing her classes, etc.). It is possible that a separate anxiety disorder is present, but it is more likely that it is a result of the ADHD and not independent. A diagnosis of generalized anxiety disorder is precluded when the symptoms are better explained by a different disorder. In this particular case, it is best to treat the ADHD and then reevaluate any residual anxious symptoms if they persist.

First-line drug therapy for ADHD, in the absence of contraindications, is a stimulant. This patient has no contraindications. Since the attention-related symptoms occur throughout the day, choosing a long-acting medication is optimal. This reduces the number of times per day the medication needs to be administered and improves convenience and compliance. In addition, it also minimizes the severity of the perceived onset and offset of the drug (feeling a rush when blood levels climb and feeling a "crash" when they decline). Lastly, the longer-acting drugs are less likely to be abused or diverted than the shorter-acting medications, though this risk is never truly absent.

Many of the long-acting products, which last at least 8 hours (because of the average school and workday or evening study time), would be appropriate. An example of a once-daily, long-acting medication with minimal abuse potential is lisdexamfetamine (Vyvanse). A starting dose of 20 or 30 mg is appropriate and can be titrated up to a maximum daily dose of 70 mg as needed and as tolerated.

Since **C.P.** is having daily symptoms of asthma, she is classified as moderate persistent and requires daily scheduled medication therapy. At this severity of asthma, she is a candidate for a low-dose inhaled corticosteroid with a long-acting beta agonist. An example of a possible product would be salmeterol 21 mcg and fluticasone 45 mcg MDI (Advair HFA): two inhalations twice daily.

What are the parameters for monitoring success of the therapy?

A 1-month follow-up period would be appropriate and that is more than adequate time for the drug to have a meaningful effect. Theoretically, there should be improvement within the first day or so of therapy, but meaningful, measurable markers of efficacy (like improved grades, reduced work tension, etc.) may take more time to emerge. By the end of the first month, however, the patient should report improvements in ability to focus, concentrate, and engage in tasks that require attention, reduced forgetfulness, and complete projects.

In terms of the asthma control, patient reports of decreased frequency of use of her recue inhaler would indicate effectiveness. In addition, in-office assessments of FEV1, FVC, and PEF would indicate whether the drug has improved her respiratory function.

Discuss specific patient education based on the prescribed therapy.

The patient needs to be educated about adverse effects and also what substances cannot be consumed concurrently with lisdexamfetamine. If the patient experiences any changes in mood or personality, the provider needs to be notified. Secondary to the ability of stimulants to cause weight loss, the patient should be encouraged to maintain a healthy diet and not skip meals (as appetite may be decreased). This patient is obese, and therefore, weight loss will not necessarily be detrimental; however, she should not use this drug for weight loss. Lifestyle changes should be encouraged, and the patient should be counseled on stimulant abuse for purposes of weight loss. **C.P.** can also be educated about keeping her treatment confidential, as sometimes peers may pressure patients being treated for ADHD to share or sell their medications.

C.P. should rinse her mouth after using her new daily inhaler as the steroid component may result in oral candidiasis.

List one or two adverse reactions for the selected agent that would cause you to change therapy.

Adverse effects that would warrant a change in therapy include clinically significant increases in blood pressure, panic attacks, frequent tachycardia, significant weight loss, or serious changes in sleep patterns. The baseline EKG was normal, and so the risk of the stimulant causing a conduction disturbance is minimal but not nonexistent. If tachycardia emerges or the patient feels an abnormal rhythm ("racing heart," "strange thumping pattern"), then the drug should be discontinued and a different stimulant would not be started. Significant weight loss is of concern even in an obese patient if there is no evidence to suggest that a lifestyle change resulted in the weight loss and it is purely the result of a stimulant.

What would be the choice for second-line therapy?

If lisdexamfetamine failed to produce an acceptable therapeutic effect, then another longer-acting stimulant can be chosen. Examples might include the extended-release mixed amphetamine salts or an extended-release methylphenidate product. If the lisdexamfetamine produced intolerable adverse effects or a serious adverse effect emerged, then another stimulant would be avoided, and potentially, atomoxetine (Strattera) would be next line. Atomoxetine has the added benefit of potentially alleviating anxious symptoms as well as ADHD symptoms. If there is concern about the presence of an anxiety disorder, then bupropion would not be appropriate as it can exacerbate anxiety.

What over-the-counter and/or alternative medications would be appropriate for C.P.?

There would not be any nonprescription products that are proven to be safe or efficacious for the treatment of ADHD, anxiety, or asthma.

What lifestyle changes would you recommend to C.P.?

Aside from continuing her structured studying and time management strategies, there are no additional life-style recommendations with regard to the ADHD. She should avoid taking pseudoephedrine due to its stimulant effects.

Describe one or two drug–drug or drug–food interactions for the selected agent.

C.P. should not take any additional stimulant products (like pseudoephedrine as mentioned above) and should obviously not ingest any illicit drug substances.

CASE STUDY 4*

ASTHMA/ADHD/ALLERGIES WITH EXACERBATION OF ALLERGY

N.J. is an 11-year-old boy with a 5-year history of ADHD and a 7-year history of asthma. He also experiences peren-nial allergic rhinitis. **N.J.**'s mother is bringing him into your office due to an exacerbation of this allergy. The symptoms he presents with include increased cough and runny nose and sneezing. He has no other medical history. The follow-ing is his current list of medications:

Concerta: 36 mg every morning
Albuterol inhaler, two puffs as needed (uses one to two times a day)
Singulair: 5 mg PO daily
Zyrtec: 5 mg PO daily

* Answers can be found online.

List specific goals of treatment for N.J.

The obvious goal is to decrease the coughing and other allergic symptoms. However, it is not clear if the cough is a secondary manifestation of the uncontrolled asthma or as a result of the rhinorrhea associated with the allergies. Therefore, an addi-tional goal would be to improve the asthma control. Specific goals related to asthma would be a decrease in the frequency of use of the albuterol inhaler.

What drug therapy would be appropriate for N.J.? Why?

The National Asthma Education and Prevention Program update of 2007 recommends that all persons with persistent asthma be prescribed a low-dose inhaled corticosteroid con-troller balancing the availability on the patient's formulary and the convenience of administration (bid vs. qid). He should also remain on the Singulair daily and the albuterol as needed.

What are the parameters for monitoring success of the therapy?

For the allergies, a reduction in the rhinorrhea and, if appropri-ate, a decrease in the cough would be good clinical markers of success. For the asthma, the primary indicator of stable asthma would be a decreased use of the short-acting beta agonist to less than twice weekly as well as improved lung function such as improved peak flow readings or improved exercise tolerance.

Discuss specific patient education based on the prescribed therapy.

An investigation of the potential changes in the household or other environmental changes should be part of the workup. Discussion with the mother and child regarding triggers is a key to preventing these exacerbations.

Finally, the patient needs to be educated about the use of this agent as a long-term controller and not a symptom reliever. The inhaled corticosteroid is not intended to relieve acute symptoms of asthma. The clinician should also observe **N.J.**'s use of the inhaler to assure proper technique.

List one or two adverse reactions for the selected agent that would cause you to change therapy.

When considering alternative therapy, a thorough review of the use of short-acting β_2 agonists must also be considered because these will also produce palpitations, chest pain, and tachycardia. Further, an increasing need for short-acting β_2 agonists or a perceived lack of benefit of short-acting β_2 ago-nists may be a sign of seriously worsening asthma, and the patient should notify the clinician immediately.

What would be the choice for the second-line therapy for treating N.J.?

If **N.J.**'s symptoms are not resolved, a second-line therapy would be to move up to moderate-dose corticosteroid with or without the Singulair. Alternatively, a long-acting beta agonist such as salmeterol can be added to the regimen.

What over-the-counter or alternative medications would be appropriate for N.J.?

For treating the rhinorrhea, over-the-counter antihistamines may be used additively, but the sedating effects need to be taken into consideration.

What dietary and lifestyle changes should be recommended for N.J.?

Avoidance of allergen triggers should be considered one of the primary lifestyle changes. Removal of carpets from the bedroom, keeping pets out of rooms in which **N.J.** spends time, and washing sheets/linens in hot water weekly are some of the strategies for reducing environmental allergens. Exposure to second-hand smoke should also be minimized.

CASE STUDY 5*

DEPRESSION/GASTROESOPHAGEAL REFLUX DISEASE (GERD)

M.M. is a 60-year-old African American man who presents with a 3-month history of lack of sleep because he awakens every 2 hours and cannot get back to sleep. He lacks desire to do anything that he previously enjoyed, has an increased appetite, and does not want to leave his house. It is an effort for him to go to work every morning. Additionally, he says that when he eats anything, he gets burning in his stomach and esophagus and is awakened at night with indigestion.

Social history: Married for 35 years to the same woman. Two grown children. His 15-year-old dog died 3 months ago. He took the dog everywhere with him. He smokes 1/2 pack of cigarettes a day.

BP: 126/80
Pulse: 76
Weight: 204 lb
Height: 67 inches
Rest of physical exam: WNL
Labs:
  TSH: 3.4
  PSA: 0.6
  Cholesterol: 212 mg/dL
  LDL: 128 mg/dL
  HDL: 40 mg/dL

Issues: **M.M.** has symptoms of depression. Insomnia is an issue. He also has the symptoms of new-onset GERD.

* Answers can be found online.

List specific goals for treatment for M.M.

The goals of therapy for **M.M.** relate to quality of life as well as clinical goals. Relieving the depressive symptoms should help **M.M.** enjoy life and feel better, but the time frame for response is 4 to 6 weeks, provided the initial therapy works. This should be discussed with **M.M.** as therapy is initiated. A depression scale, such as the Hamilton Depression Scale (HAM-D), might be given to determine a baseline level of depression and as a means of monitoring progress as treatment continues. A specific goal might be a 50% decrease or better from the baseline HAM-D score.

However, relief of indigestion and providing adequate sleep are more immediate goals that should be achievable within the first week of therapy. Progress on these short-term goals is likely to help **M.M.** continue with the therapy for relieving the long-term problem of depression. Therefore, specific goals are:

- Relief of symptoms of depression
- Provision of adequate sleep
- Relief of reflux symptoms
- Smoking cessation.

What drug therapy would you prescribe for M.M.? Why?

Paroxetine is a good choice because it promotes better sleep. It is best to give this agent in the evening due to slight sedative effects. If another agent is on formulary at a substantially lower cost, such as sertraline, it can be prescribed and taken in the morning. Typically, a sleeping aid is prescribed in patients such as **M.M.**, but the sedative effects of paroxetine might be sufficient. If the insomnia persists after 4 to 6 weeks, an additional hypnotic may be considered. A proton pump inhibitor (PPI) would be a reasonable choice for relief of his GERD now, and if it persists after 3 months, endoscopy would be indicated.

What are the parameters for monitoring success of the therapy?

Follow-up history is the best way to monitor therapy for depression. Readministration of a depression scale with an improved score would indicate successful therapy. Also, indication of 8 hours of sleep a night demonstrates successful therapy. Patient-reported frequency and severity of GERD episodes is a good tool to determine success of therapy for GERD.

Discuss specific patient education based on the prescribed therapy.

The overall premise is the promotion of "good sleep habits," which include setting a routine bedtime, instituting regular exercise habits, using the bed for sleeping only, and getting in bed only when ready for sleep. Occasional completion of a sleep log is an important tool for the clinician to evaluate the effectiveness of therapy.

Lifestyle changes are as important as drug therapy in managing GERD. Discussion with the patient and family should cover the following important dietary changes: avoidance of excess alcohol and food intake; decreased amounts of chocolate and spicy, fried, or fatty foods; and avoidance of the recumbent position for at least 3 hours after meals. Because these recommended changes involve many activities or foods that are pleasurable for the patient, they should be eliminated gradually—one at a time. A nutritionist can be consulted to help the patient learn to choose and prepare less problematic foods.

Additional measures include teaching the patient to elevate the head of the bed approximately 4 to 6 inches (using blocks); to avoid tight, restrictive clothing; and to lose weight if necessary.

The patient needs to be counseled on the risks of continued smoking. The patient's readiness for change must be ascertained, and he needs to be educated on the poor health consequences associated with continued smoking.

List an adverse reaction for the selected agents that would cause you to change therapy.

If **M.M.** complains of decreased libido from the paroxetine, then consideration should be given to lowering the dose or changing to a nonselective serotonin receptor inhibitor. This is particularly important if it becomes upsetting to him because he and his wife have a very satisfying sexual relationship.

What would be the choice for second-line therapy?

Lowering the dose of paroxetine might help with the side effects. However, if this is not possible, bupropion is an appropriate choice for second-line therapy for the depression, particularly as it relates to sexual side effects.

What over-the-counter or alternative medications would be appropriate for M.M.?

Some patients, especially those with delayed sleep phase insomnia, may benefit from the administration of exogenous melatonin; however, further study is necessary.

Aloe vera juice may help in the healing of gastrointestinal tract irritation. Other herbs, such as catnip, fennel, ginger, and marshmallow root, as well as papaya juice, may help stop heartburn. Licorice is used to treat both heartburn and stomach and esophageal ulcers.

What lifestyle changes would you recommend to M.M.?

Lifestyle modifications are essential for the patient with GERD. Although drug therapy will help reduce the level of acid in the stomach and promote healing, lifestyle changes will aid in preventing the symptoms from returning. These lifestyle changes include dietary changes, such as avoiding irritating foods like caffeine, alcohol, and spicy foods. Further, refraining from eating at least 3 hours before bedtime and elevating the head of the bed by at least 6 inches will help reduce nighttime symptoms. Weight loss will also reduce the frequency of GERD symptoms. Lastly, smoking cessation will reduce the frequency of GERD symptoms.

The overall premise is the promotion of "good sleep habits," which include setting a routine bedtime, instituting regular exercise habits, using the bed for sleeping only, and getting in bed only when ready for sleep. Occasional completion of a sleep log is an important tool for the clinician to evaluate the effectiveness of therapy.

Describe one or two drug–drug or drug–food interactions for the selected agents.

Paroxetine is an inhibitor of the cytochrome P-450 (CYP) 2D6 system and might increase the serum concentrations of cough suppressants such as dextromethorphan and codeine, so care must be taken when using these agents during cough/cold season. The PPIs omeprazole, lansoprazole, and pantoprazole are inhibitors of the CYP2C19 system and would increase levels of drugs such as diazepam, phenytoin, or amitriptyline.

CASE STUDY 6*

ACUTE CARE VISIT SCHEDULED FOR A COLD; DISCOVERED TO HAVE HYPERTENSION

J.F. is a 41-year-old white male who presents with a cold that he has had for about 4 days. He has a runny nose, cough that is annoying, and periodic headache. He has not tried any over-the-counter medicines. He wants an antibiotic for the cold because he is going skiing this weekend.

While in the office, he says he needs a note saying he is well enough to use the gym. He has no known health problems but has not seen a health professional in over 4 years. *Social history:* Single. Elementary school teacher. Multiple sexual partners. Strong family history of heart disease. His father and uncle died before age 50 of an acute myocardial infarction. Does not smoke. Drinks socially but may have 10 beers on the weekend.

Physical exam:
BP: 150/100
Pulse: 70 RRR
Weight: 250 lb
Height: 70 inches
Nasal mucosa: red and swollen

Ears: normal
No lymphadenopathy
Lungs: clear to auscultation

Issues: **J.F.** presents with symptoms of a viral upper respiratory infection. He wants antibiotics for a quick fix. He also wants clearance for the gym. Physical exam shows that he is overweight and has hypertension. He also has a strong family history of heart disease at an early age.

* Answers can be found online.

List specific goals for treatment for J.F.

The cold appears to be viral in nature. Symptoms of a cold consist primarily of clear nasal discharge, sneezing, nasal congestion, cough, low-grade fever (below 102°F), scratchy or sore throat, mild aches, chills, headache, watery eyes, tenderness around the eyes, full feeling in the ears, and fatigue. Symptoms usually resolve in approximately 1 week, but they may linger for 2 weeks.

Specific goals are:

- Relief of symptoms
- Reduction of the risk of complications
- Prevention of spread to others

The fact that **J.F.** has an elevated blood pressure is concerning, especially in light of his family history. At this time, clearance for the gym cannot be given until there is further cardiac testing completed.

There are other issues that need to be addressed, such as his alcohol intake and multiple sexual partners.

What drug therapy would you prescribe for J.F.? Why?

Nonpharmacologic alternatives to treating the common cold are the first line. For example, rest allows the body to gain strength and be more effective in defending itself against the pathogen. The body can then dictate the increase in activities. An alternative to decongestants and expectorants is increasing water or juice intake. This assists in liquefying tenacious secretions; making expectoration easier; soothing scratchy, sore throats; and relieving dry skin and lips. Saline gargles also are effective for soothing sore throats.

Coughing caused by chest congestion can cause a muscular chest pain. Menthol rubs can soothe this ache and open airways for some congestion relief. Menthol lozenges also have been effective in soothing scratchy throats and clearing nasal passages. Saline nasal flushes are also effective for clearing nasal passages without the rebound side effect. Petrolatum-based ointments for raw and macerated skin around the nose and upper lip ease the drying effects of dehydration and the use of multiple tissues.

Other measures, such as drinking chicken soup, taking a hot shower, or using a room humidifier, may prove helpful. Inhaling warm, moist heat helps raise the temperature of the nasal mucosa to at least 37 °C, a temperature at which the virus does not replicate so readily.

Expectorants, including water, increase the output of respiratory tract fluid by decreasing the adhesiveness and surface tension of the respiratory tract and by facilitating removal of viscous mucus. The effect is noted within 1 to 2 hours.

J.F.'s symptoms appear viral in nature so an antibiotic is not indicated at this time. Decongestants are not recommended for **J.F.** because of his elevated blood pressure.

What are the parameters for monitoring success of the therapy?

Follow-up is the best way to monitor therapy. Acute sinusitis often results from progression of the common cold (5% to 10% of cases). **J.F.** should be seen back in 1 week to evaluate symptoms. At that time, his other issues, such as blood pressure, multiple sexual partners, and alcohol intake, need to be addressed.

If the infection has failed to resolve or improve after 7 to 10 days, he may have sinusitis. Major symptoms include facial pain, pressure, congestion, fullness, obstruction, blockage, or discharge with a temperature greater than 38°C. Purulent drainage in the middle meatus may be a strong indicator of acute sinus disease; however, nasal purulence does not differentiate viral from bacterial infection. Symptoms may include headache, fatigue, dental pain, halitosis, otalgia, or cough. Other symptoms include toothache and a poor response to decongestants. There is usually edema of the mucous membranes upon examination and tenderness over the sinus areas upon percussion.

Characteristic signs are purulent, green or yellow nasal discharge and abnormal sinus illumination. Acute bacterial sinusitis is a consideration in patients who report cold symptoms lasting more than 8 days or with prolonged nasal obstruction or a cold that seems to have gotten better but returns with more severe symptoms.

Discuss specific patient education based on the prescribed therapy.

J.F. needs to be educated not to take decongestants that might increase his blood pressure. He should increase fluids and humidity for symptom relief. If symptoms do not get better within 1 to 2 weeks, he needs to follow up. Education should be included as to how to prevent spread of germs.

However, **J.F.** needs to schedule a visit within 1 to 2 weeks to address his other issues. He needs a cardiac workup and probably an antihypertensive. Since his hypertension is presumed to be stage 1, the recommended antihypertensive is a thiazide diuretic.

List one or two adverse reactions for the selected agent that would cause you to change therapy.

Adverse reactions from expectorants include drowsiness, headache, and GI symptoms. Decongestants are not used because they can increase blood pressure.

What would be the choice for second-line therapy?

An antibiotic would be considered if symptoms do not resolve in 1 to 2 weeks since it has probably become sinusitis.

The recommended length of antibiotic therapy for acute bacterial sinusitis is at least 14 or 7 days beyond the resolution of symptoms, whichever is longer. Amoxicillin is appropriate for the initial treatment of acute, uncomplicated, mild sinusitis in patients with no recent antibiotic use. Antimicrobial agents with more broad-spectrum activity may be indicated as initial therapy for patients who have more severe infection, comorbidity, or risk factors for bacterial resistance or who have not responded to amoxicillin therapy. These agents include

amoxicillin and clavulanic acid, the newer quinolones (e.g., levofloxacin, gatifloxacin, moxifloxacin), and some second- and third-generation cephalosporins (cefdinir, cefuroxime axetil, and cefpodoxime proxetil). Patients who are allergic to penicillin may be treated with a macrolide, trimethoprim–sulfamethoxazole, tetracyclines, or clindamycin.

If **J.F.**'s blood pressure is not controlled on the diuretic, it is recommended to start a second antihypertensive agent in addition to the diuretic.

What over-the-counter or alternative medications would be appropriate?

Increased humidification is recommended. Also, **J.F.** should increase fluid intake to loosen secretions. A hot shower helps to relieve sinus congestion.

What dietary and lifestyle changes should be recommended?

J.F. needs to decrease sodium intake because of his elevated blood pressure. He needs to lose weight and increase physical activity after a cardiac evaluation.

J.F. needs counseling in safe sexual practices, such as the use of condoms. These issues can be handled at another visit when he follows up.

CASE STUDY 7*

ADOLESCENT WITH DYSMENORRHEA/ACNE AND SEXUALLY ACTIVE

S.S. is a 16-year-old presenting with severe dysmenorrhea. She began menstruating at age 13. Her periods have been irregular. Each month she misses a day of school because of severe cramps and heavy bleeding with her menses. She also has a moderate case of acne, which is very disturbing to her. She has tried topical preparations and antibiotic therapy for the acne without results. She has no history of gallbladder disease, migraine headaches, or chest pain.

Social history: **S.S.** is a sophomore in high school. She is sexually active but does not use condoms. She has

had two sexual partners, although now she is in a monogamous relationship with a senior at her high school. She lives with her mother and younger brother. She does not smoke or drink.

Issues: **S.S.** has dysmenorrhea that affects her quality of life. In addition, she has acne, which is disturbing to her self-image. **S.S.** is sexually active and does not use condoms. This puts her at risk for pregnancy and sexually transmitted infections (STIs).

* Answers can be found online.

List specific goals for treatment.

Goals of treatment for **S.S.** relate to quality of life as well as clinical goals. Relief of dysmenorrhea is paramount. It will decrease absences from school and improve overall well-being. Additionally, treatment of acne is important because that affects her self-image.

Another goal is prevention of pregnancy and STIs. Therefore, specific goals are:

- Relief of dysmenorrhea
- Treatment of acne
- Prevention of pregnancy
- Prevention of STIs.

What drug therapy would you prescribe? Why?

NSAIDs can be used for treatment of dysmenorrhea. However, oral contraceptives (OCs) are the drug of choice for **S.S.** since she is sexually active and has acne unresponsive to other treatment. OCs prevent pregnancy and reduce the risk of endometriosis, ovulatory pain, dysmenorrhea, ovarian cysts, benign breast disease, premenstrual syndrome, premenstrual dysphoric disorder, and ovarian and endometrial cancer. They also might improve acne. The improvement occurs secondary to an increase in the level of sex-hormone–binding globulin, which reduces circulating free testosterone and ameliorates many androgenic effects. It is reasonable to prescribe a generic monophasic OC pill containing 30 to 35 mcg of estrogen.

In addition, **S.S.** should receive quadrivalent human papillomavirus (HPV) vaccine. This provides protection against the four types of HPV most commonly associated with clinical diseases. It is recommended for females ages 13 to 26. It is a series of three doses.

Ideally, vaccine should be administered before potential exposure to HPV through sexual contact. The second dose is administered 1 to 2 months after the first dose, and the third dose is administered 6 months after the first dose.

What are the parameters for monitoring success of therapy?

Follow-up history is the best way to monitor success of the OCs for dysmenorrhea. Resolution of acne can be determined by examination of the skin.

Discuss specific patient education based on the prescribed therapy.

OCs can have either a day 1 start or a Sunday start regimen. Women who follow a day 1 start regimen begin the contraceptive agent on the first day of their period, regardless of the day of the week. Likewise, women who follow Sunday start regimens begin the OC pill pack on the Sunday directly after the onset of menses. This means that the woman will not menstruate on a weekend, which is desirable to many patients. **S.S.** may experience some breakthrough bleeding for the first 3 months of therapy.

OCs should be taken at the same time every day. It can be recommended to place them with **S.S.**'s toothbrush so she takes them when she brushes her teeth. If a pill is missed, **S.S.** should follow this regimen:

One pill	Take missed pill as soon as possible and resume schedule; backup method of contraception is not necessary.
Two 30- to 35-mg pills	Take missed pill as soon as possible and resume schedule; backup method of contraception is not necessary
Two 20-mg pills	Follow directions for more than two pills
More than two pills	Take pill and continue taking a pill daily
	Use condom or abstinence for 7 d
	If missed in week 3, finish active pills in current pack and start a new pack the next day (skip current inactive pills)
	If missed pills in first week and had sex, use emergency contraception (EC) and then resume taking pills the next day after EC

It is imperative to discuss the use of condoms to prevent STIs. OCs prevent pregnancy, but not STIs.

List adverse reactions for the selected agent that would cause you to change therapy.

If **S.S.** had prolonged breakthrough bleeding, a change in hormone content would be considered. In the first half of the menstrual cycle, breakthrough bleeding is likely due to insufficient estrogen; in the second half of the cycle, it is likely due to insufficient progesterone. Therefore, changing to a new regimen with higher estrogen or progesterone is recommended.

CASE STUDY 8*

DIZZINESS, INSOMNIA, STRESS

A.E. is a 56-year-old white female who presents ongoing symptoms of dizziness, inability to sleep, and recent increase in stress. She reports that these symptoms have been present off/on for at least 6 months, but worsening the last 3 weeks. The dizziness is really an off-balance sensation, and she feels weak at times going down steps. Currently sleeps only 6 hours nightly, but with many awakenings. Also, reports some ringing in her ears at times. Last full physical was 2 years ago.

Past medical history: None

Social history: Married for 30 years but recently separated from her husband. Relationship has been verbal abuse for many years, but worse recently. Current smoker of 30 pack years. Denies alcohol. Not currently working and has just moved up to live with her sister. Has three grown children, one who is disabled.

Physical exam:
BP: 140/82
Pulse: 70 RRR
Weight: 150 lb
Height: 66 inches

Alert, oriented × 3 in NAD. Eyes, PERRLA 3 mm without nystagmus, remainder. Ears, clear but some fluid present and bulging slightly. Remainder of HEENT unremarkable. CV, regular, rate, rhythm, no murmurs, rubs, gallops. Lungs, clear. Neuro, no focal deficits, negative Romberg, pronator drift, able to tandem walk, no cerebellar signs. Psych, appears anxious and fatigued. Poor self-esteem evident in conversation.

Issues: A.E. presents with symptoms of vertigo that could be caused by a variety of problems including stress reaction, acoustic neuroma, and eustachian dysfunction. She also has sleep disturbance issues that could be related to the stress.

---

* Answers can be found online.

What drug therapy would you prescribe for A.E.? Why?

The vertigo-type symptoms **A.E.** is experiencing could be something as simple as eustachian dysfunction. A trial of oral high-dose guaifenesin (Mucinex) could be helpful to improve mucous drainage from the eustachian tubes. Decongestants are not recommended for **A.E.** because her blood pressure is slightly elevated.

Concomitantly, there is a need to address the stress level of **A.E.** for pharmacologic therapy. She has been treated in the past for anxiety. Selecting an agent that addresses anxiety and depression may be helpful. A good selection for this patient is escitalopram (Lexapro), which has a minimal side effect profile. It does not causes further neurologic impairment such as drowsiness, and reports are minimal to none for worsening of suicidal ideation.

What are the parameters for monitoring success of the therapy?

Close follow-up is the best method of monitoring for success. The guaifenesin will likely help with the eustachian dysfunction in 10 to 12 days. However, the escitalopram can take up to 6 weeks for any noticeable response; however, some patients report a slight change within 2 weeks. The anticipated change is that she will feel less "off balance" and have more energy.

Discuss specific patient education based on the prescribed therapy.

A.E. needs to be educated to take the guaifenesin consistently for at least 10 to 12 days. Also, she should be advised to not to take decongestants that might increase her blood pressure until it can be ascertained that she is not truly hypertensive.

Education about healthy diet, smoking cessation, and exercise will help with her overall mood.

However, **A.E.** needs to schedule a visit within 2 to 3 weeks to evaluate the tolerance to treatment. Appropriate bloodwork should be ordered prior to screen for other disease processes such as diabetes and hyperlipidemia.

List one or two adverse reactions for the selected agent that would cause you to change therapy.

Adverse reactions from expectorants include drowsiness, headache, and GI symptoms. Common side effects from the escitalopram can include nausea (usually only initially), dry mouth, increased sweating, and dizziness (more related to missed doses).

What would be the choice for second-line therapy?

Change to another within this class of antidepressant, such as paroxetine, which also treats for anxiety.

What over-the-counter or alternative medications would be appropriate?

Guaifenesin (Mucinex) is an over-the-counter drug. While **A.E.** is on escitalopram, she should not take any alternative medications advertised for depression/insomnia such as St. John's wort or valerian root due to interactions.

What dietary and lifestyle changes should be recommended?

A.E. needs to evaluate her sleep habits including temperature of the room, darkness, and activities before bedtime. Also, counseling is highly desirable to help her find coping strategies for her abusive relationship and self-esteem.

CASE STUDY 9*

FATIGUE, HYPERTENSION, OBESITY, AND SEASONAL ALLERGIES

D.E. is a 64-year-old white female who presents ongoing symptoms of heart racing, heat intolerance, and weight loss. She has some sleep problems, but these have occurred in most of her life. She reports that these symptoms have been present off/on for at least 6 months, but worsening the last 3 weeks. Her allergy symptoms generally affect her in the fall.
Past medical history: Hypertension, obesity, seasonal allergies
Social history: Married for 35 years. Current smoker of 20 pack-years. Denies alcohol. Has three grown children.
Medications: Lisinopril 10 mg, HCTZ 25 mg, loratadine 10 mg
Physical exam:
BP: 152/82

Pulse: 110
Weight: 192 lb down from 210 lb without trying
Height: 66 inches

Alert, oriented × 3 in NAD. HEENT unremarkable. Neck, supple, no thyromegaly or nodules. CV, regular, tachycardic, rate, rhythm, no murmurs, rubs, gallops. Lungs, clear. Neuro, no focal deficits. Skin, no rashes, lesions, slightly dry but warm.
Issues: **D.E.** presents with symptoms of tachycardia that could be caused by a variety of problems including hyperthyroidism, hypothyroidism, infection with fever, and/or cardiac arrhythmias. Her hypertension could also be a component of the fast heart rate.

---

* Answers can be found online.

What drug therapy would you prescribe for D.E.? Why?

The rapid heart rate and other symptoms **D.E.** is experiencing must be evaluated further; however, adding a beta-blocker would help assist with slowing the heart rate and subsequent work of the heart. Atenolol is a good choice since it controls heart rate for 24 hours along with hypertension. It is well tolerated with a potential side effect profile of bradycardia, dizziness, and hypotension in those who do not have underlying coronary disease. A baseline 12-lead EKG is necessary before implementing treatment. If the EKG shows atrial fibrillation, **D.E.** needs more immediate follow-up in the emergency room. If the presentation is due to a transient thyroiditis, institution of antithyroid medications is not indicated at this time; the need is control the symptoms until bloodwork (TSH, T$_4$) is obtained.

What are the parameters for monitoring success of the therapy?

Close follow-up is the best method of monitoring for success. Rechecking **D.E.** in 3 to 4 days is necessary to evaluate for success of decreasing the heart rate and blood pressure.

Discuss specific patient education based on the prescribed therapy.

D.E. needs to be educated to take the medication routinely and not miss any doses, especially the atenolol; beta blockers should not be abruptly discontinued. If she experiences any worsening of the tachycardia as therapy is initiated, she should go to the emergency room. Education about healthy diet, smoking cessation, and exercise will help with her overall mood.

List one or two adverse reactions for the selected agent that would cause you to change therapy.

Post marketing, some patients have experienced elevated liver enzymes and/or bilirubin; hallucinations; headache; impotence; Peyronie disease; postural hypotension, which may be associated with syncope; psoriasiform rash or exacerbation of psoriasis; psychoses; purpura; reversible alopecia; thrombocytopenia; visual disturbance; sick sinus syndrome; and dry mouth. Atenolol, like other beta blockers, has been associated with the development of antinuclear antibodies (ANA), lupus syndrome, and Raynaud phenomenon.

What would be the choice for second-line therapy?

Since the tachycardia may be related to hyperthyroidism, verapamil would be a good second choice. It treats both the fast heart rate and also the hypertension. Lisinopril should still be maintained due its effect on the renin–angiotensin-activating system.

What over-the-counter or alternative medications would be appropriate?

No medications are appropriate, but the patient should avoid foods with high caffeine and OTC cold and cough products.

What dietary and lifestyle changes should be recommended?

Even though **D.E.** has lost weight, she is still very overweight. Ongoing counseling about dietary intake and exercise will help to enhance appropriate weight loss. Additional counseling on tobacco cessation is also important.

CASE STUDY 10*

TYPE 2 DIABETES MELLITUS, HYPERTENSION, HYPERLIPIDEMIA

M.A. is a 45-year-old African American male who presents for follow-up on his diabetes. Reports to have lost a few pounds but is finding it difficult to control his diet. Performs home glucose monitoring periodically, but only at the same time of day in the morning. The results are consistently 180 to 200 mg/dL. Otherwise, he feels generally healthy. Reports taking all his medications routinely and has no problem with obtaining the drugs.
Past medical history: Type 2 diabetes mellitus × 10 years, hypertension, obesity, hyperlipidemia
Social history: Married for 20 years. Current smoker of 20 pack years. Socially drinks beer on the weekends. Has three children: one adolescent and two younger children. He does not routinely exercise. Works at the USPS in maintenance of vehicles.
Medications: Metformin 1,000 mg bid, lisinopril 10 mg, HCTZ 25 mg, simvastatin 40 mg
Physical exam:
Pertinent recent lab work: HgA$_{1c}$ 8.0%, FBS 192, Chol 178 mg/dL, HDL 45 mg/dL, LDL 70 mg/dL, eGFR 98 mL/min/1.73 m^2

BP: 132/82
Pulse: 70
Weight: 220 lb
BMI: 30.9%
Height: 71 inches

Alert, oriented × 3 in NAD. HEENT unremarkable. Neck, supple, no thyromegaly or nodules. CV, regular, tachycardic, rate, rhythm, no murmurs, rubs, gallops. Lungs, clear. Neuro, no focal deficits. Skin, no rashes, lesions, slightly dry but warm.
Issues: M.A. presents for routine maintenance of his diabetes, hypertension, and hyperlipidemia. His lab works show uncontrolled diabetes but without current complications of CKD. Blood pressure is within normal expected range with appropriate medications. Cholesterol is well controlled with the simvastatin. Addressing his blood sugar control is the most urgent priority today.

---

* Answers can be found online.

What drug therapy would you prescribe for M.A.? Why?

At this point, it may be appropriate to prescribe INVOKANA (canagliflozin) tablets. Sodium–glucose cotransporter 2 (SGLT2), expressed in the proximal renal tubules, is responsible for the majority of the reabsorption of filtered glucose from the tubular lumen. Canagliflozin is an inhibitor of SGLT2. By inhibiting SGLT2, canagliflozin reduces reabsorption of filtered glucose and lowers the renal threshold for glucose (RTG) and thereby increases urinary glucose excretion (UGE). **M.A.**'s kidney function meets the criteria for administration.

What are the parameters for monitoring success of the therapy?

Decrease in HgA_{1c} to $\leq 7.0\%$, 45% of those taking 100 mg daily within 26 weeks. This means that daily blood sugar monitoring would have a decrease on average to 130 mg/dL.

Discuss specific patient education based on the prescribed therapy.

M.A. needs to be educated to take the medication routinely with the first meal of the day. Canagliflozin will cause sugar to be excreted in the urine. In some cases, the medication can cause hypoglycemia, so routine blood sugar monitoring, especially with hypoglycemic symptoms, is important. **M.A.** needs to continue all other medications for his hypertension and hyperlipidemia. Caution should be exercised with administration of diuretics, phenytoin or phenobarbital, digoxin, rifampin, or ritonavir.

List one or two adverse reactions for the selected agent that would cause you to change therapy.

This class of drug can cause hyperkalemia, mycotic infections, urinary tract infections, and renal insufficiency. The mycotic infections are more common in women than men. Monitoring of renal function is a necessity as the drug must be stopped for decreasing glomerular filtration rate. Elevation in potassium would also be another indication to change therapy.

What would be the choice for second-line therapy?

Starting basal insulin would be a second-line therapy given the persistent elevation in blood sugar and HgA_{1c}. Using any of the insulin glargine preparations (Levemir, Lantus, etc.) with a bedtime dose.

What over-the-counter or alternative medications would be appropriate?

There are no OTC medications for diabetes. Although there are some small studies with cinnamon, they have proven small increases in blood sugar control. Therefore, taking cinnamon daily would not be harmful.

What dietary and lifestyle changes should be recommended?

M.A. needs to continue to watch his carbohydrate intake. Instructions of carb counting and calorie control, with continual reinforcement at each visit. Daily exercise is beneficial for helping blood sugar control and overall well-being.

CONCLUSION

These are just a few examples of the decision-making process involved in prescribing medications. Most patients do not present with just one diagnosis and are taking several medications, and these factors must be considered in deciding on the best pharmacologic approaches. The intent of these examples is to help the reader understand *possible* solutions to some common problems. With advances in pharmacotherapy and in evidence-based medicine, the potential approaches to these cases are expected to change. The complexity of patients requires the practitioner to prioritize problems, develop a systematic approach to resolving the problems pharmacotherapeutically, and anticipate how to manage the plan prospectively.

Bibliography

Starred references are cited in the text.
*Schondelmeyer, S. W. & Purvis, L. (2014). Rx Price Watch Report: Trends in Retail Prices of Brand Name Prescription Drugs Widely Used by Older Americans: 2006 to 2013. *AARP Public Policy Institute,* November.
*U.S. Department of Health and Human Services. (2015) Centers for Disease Control and Prevention. Trends in the Use of Complementary Health Approaches Among Adults: United States, 2002–2012. No. 79; February 10.

Note: Page numbers followed by "f" denote figures; those followed by "t" denote tables; and those followed by "b" denote boxes.

drug interactions with, 138
for erectile dysfunction, 541–542
for GERD, 459
for gout, 609
for headache, 652
herbs used in, 138, 139t–140t, 141, 142
for herpes simplex virus infections, 178
for herpes zoster, 178
for hyperthyroidism, 820
increasing awareness of, 143
for inflammatory bowel disease, 514, 514t
information sources for, 138b, 143
for insomnia, 732
label requirements for, 136–137, 137t
for menopausal symptoms, 981–982, 981t
for migraine headache, 652
national center for, 135
for nausea and vomiting, 445
for obesity, 952
for osteoarthritis, 601
for osteoporosis, 993
otitis externa, 252
for pain management, 98b, 99
for Parkinson disease, 779
patient education on, 138, 138b
for peptic ulcer disease, 463
for psoriasis, 205
reasons for using, 135, 136b
regulation of, 136–137, 136b
for rheumatoid arthritis, 625
risks of, 137–138, 137b
for skin infections, 194
for upper respiratory infections, 362t–363t, 373
for vaginitis, 1005
warfarin interactions with, 886
Complementary medicine. See also
  Complementary and alternative
  medicine
  definition of, 135
Complex cases, 1021–1036
  allergies, 1028
  anxiety asthma with ADHD, 1026
  arthritis, 1022–1024
  assessment of, 1021–1022
  depression with GERD, 1029–1030
  diabetes mellitus with associated conditions, 1035
  dizziness, insomnia and stress, 1033–1034
  urinary tract infection, 1036
Complex partial (psychomotor) seizures, 657
Compliance
  with practice guidelines and formularies, 1015–1017, 1016t
  with treatment (See Adherence issues)
Complicated lesions, in atherosclerosis, 291–292
Computed tomography
  in pulmonary embolism, 868
  in seizures, 657
  in stroke, 869
Concentration, drug, 37
Concerta (methylphenidate)
  for ADHD, 748t, 749, 749t
Condoms, 961
Conduction system, dysrhythmias arising in, 325, 326, 326b
Condyloma acuminata. See Human papilloma
  virus infections

Condylox (podofilox), for human papilloma virus
  infections, 584, 585t
Congenital disorders, hypothyroidism, 814
Congestive heart failure. See Heart failure
Conjugated equine estrogen, for menopausal
  symptoms, 973t, 974–978
Conjunctivitis, 224–231
  algorithm for, 230f
  allergic, 226, 226t–227t, 228, 840–842
  causes of, 224
  diagnosis of, 225
  in dry eye syndrome, 231–234, 233t
  giant papillary, 224, 229, 231
  pathophysiology of, 232
  patient education on, 231
  pediatric patients, 226
  therapeutic monitoring of, 231
  treatment of, 222t–224t, 225, 226t–228t, 229–231, 230f
Constipation, 465–475
  algorithm for, 473f
  causes of, 465, 466b
  complementary and alternative medicine for, 475
  definition of, 465, 466
  diagnosis of, 466, 466b
  disorders associated with, 465, 466b
  drug-induced, 465, 466b
  in elderly persons, 83, 474
  information sources for, 475
  in irritable bowel syndrome, 485–489, 488t, 493t
  lifestyle changes for, 475
  nutrition for, 466, 475
  pathophysiology of, 466
  patient education on, 475
  in pediatric patients treatment of, 474
  in pregnancy, 474
  prevalence of, 465
  therapeutic monitoring of, 475
  treatment of, 473f, 473t, 478–483
  in women, 474
Contact dermatitis, 155–160
  allergic, 155
  causes of, 155
  complementary and alternative medicine for, 160
  diagnosis of, 156
  in elderly persons, 160
  irritant, 155
  pathophysiology of, 155, 828
  patient education on, 160
  pediatric patients, 159
  therapeutic monitoring of, 160
  treatment of, 155–160, 157t–159t, 159f
Contact lenses, conjunctivitis with, 224–225, 229, 229t
Contraception
  oral (See Oral contraceptives)
Contraception combined products for, 961–964, 963t
  definition of, 959
  emergency, 965–966
  failure rates of, 961f
  intrauterine systems for, 964–965
  methods for, 959, 961f
  nonpharmacologic, 960, 961f

optimal features of, 961
oral (See Oral contraceptives)
physiology of, 959–960, 960f
progestin-only, 964–965, 964t
reversible forms of, 959
usage of, 959
vaginal devices for, 964
Contrast-enhanced venography, in venous thromboembolism, 868
Contrave (naltrexone/bupropion)
  in obesity, 951
Controlled Substances Act of 1970, 4, 4b
COPD. See Chronic obstructive pulmonary
  disease
Cordarone (amiodarone)
  for dysrhythmias, 328, 335–337
  for heart failure, 318–319
Coreg (carvedilol)
  for heart failure, 315, 316
  for hypertension, 263t, 266
Corlanor (ivabradine)
  for heart failure, 319
Coronary artery(ies), vasospasm of, 293
Coronary heart disease
  after menopause, 971
  hyperlipidemia and, 277, 277b
  pathogenesis of, 276–277
  premature, 289
  prevention of, 278
  risk assessment for, 277–278
  risk factors for, 290–291, 290b
Corticosteroids
  for allergic conjunctivitis, 841
  for allergic rhinitis, 837–838, 838t
  for anaphylaxis and anaphylactoid
    reactions, 829
  for asthma, 378t–379t, 380, 382, 382t–383t,
    385–386, 388–389
  for conjunctivitis, 227t–228t, 228–229
  for contact dermatitis, 156–158, 157t, 158t
  for COPD, 400–401
  for dry eye syndrome, 231, 233t
  for gout, 605, 606
  immunization and, 913
  for inflammatory bowel disease, 501t,
    504, 508, 511
  for migraine headache, 643t, 647
  for nausea and vomiting, 435t, 438–439, 441t
  for osteoarthritis, 596, 599
  for otitis externa, 250
  potency of, 156, 157t
  for psoriasis, 200
  for rheumatoid arthritis, 623–624
Cortisporin (hydrocortisone and combinations)
  for otitis externa, 250, 250t
Corvert (ibutilide), for dysrhythmias, 330t, 338
Coryza. See Common cold
Cost analyses, for managed care, 1009–1010
Cost factors, in adherence, 78–80
Cough
  from angiotensin-converting enzyme
    inhibitors, 313
  in bronchitis, 407–409
  in common cold, 362t, 364, 367
  for COPD, 395–396
Coumadin. See Warfarin
Covera (verapamil), for hypertension, 264t, 267

Phillips Milk of Magnesia (magnesium hydroxide), for constipation, 468t, 470
Phosphate(s), for constipation, 468t, 470
Phosphodiesterase 5 inhibitors, for erectile dysfunction, 539–540, 540t, 541t
Phospholipid bilayer
absorption through, 21
receptors on, 27
Phospholipid(s), in lipoprotein transport, 275–276
Physical therapy
for osteoarthritis, 593
for rheumatoid arthritis, 612
Physicochemical properties, absorption and, 56
Phytoestrogens, 981, 981t, 982
Pigmentation, loss of, in tinea versicolor, 169, 169t
Pilocar (pilocarpine), for glaucoma, 237t, 239
Pilocarpine
for dry eye syndrome, 231, 234t
for glaucoma, 237t, 239
Piloptic (pilocarpine), for glaucoma, 237t, 239
Pilostat (pilocarpine), for glaucoma, 237t, 239
Pimecrolimus
for contact dermatitis, 158, 158t
Pindolol, for hypertension, 263t, 266
Pioglitazone, for diabetes mellitus, 790t, 793
Piperacillin, 113t, 116t
Piperacillin–tazobactam, 117t
sensitivity of, 113t
Pityriasis versicolor, 169, 169t
Placebo effect, 8
Placenta, drug transfer across, 65–66, 66t
Plantar warts, 178, 179f, 179t
Plaque, atherosclerotic, 276–277, 291–292
Plaque psoriasis, 197
Plaquenil (hydroxychloroquine)
for rheumatoid arthritis, 614t, 618
Platelet(s), in clotting cascade, 866, 866f
Plavix (clopidogrel)
for chronic stable angina, 294t, 299–300
coagulation disorders, 882–883
Plegine (phendimetrazine), for obesity, 948t, 949
Plendil (felodipine)
for hypertension, 264t, 267
Plummer disease, 815
Pneumococcal vaccine, 251, 915, 915b, 916
Pneumococcus infections, conjunctivitis, 225
Pneumonia
algorithm for, 420f
causes of, 433b
diagnosis of, 419–420, 420f, 421b, 421t–423t
in elderly persons, 83
pathophysiology of, 419
patient education on, 424
therapeutic monitoring of, 424
treatment of, 419–420, 421b, 421t–423t
Podofilox, for human papilloma virus infections, 566t, 584, 585t
Podophyllin resin, for human papilloma virus infections, 566t, 584, 585t
Poison ivy, 155
Polio vaccine, 924b
Pollen allergy. *See* Allergic rhinitis
Polycarbophil
for constipation, 467t, 469, 487t
for diarrhea, 480t, 481
Polyethylene glycol 3350, for constipation, 489

Polyethylene glycol/electrolyte solution, for constipation, 469–470
Polygenic disorders, 146
Polymorphisms, 145, 146b
Polymyxin B
for otitis externa, 250, 250t
Polypharmacy, in elderly persons, 76–78
Polysomnography, in sleep disorders, 724
Pomade acne, 207
Positron emission tomography, in seizures, 657
Postantibiotic effect, 116b
Posthemorrhagic anemia, 894
Postherpetic neuralgia, 174, 178
Postinfarction chronic stable angina, 289, 290b
Postmenopausal osteoporosis, 985, 986b
Postoperative nausea and vomiting, 429
Postpartum depression, 683, 697
Postpartum thyroiditis, 822
Potassium channel blockers, for dysrhythmias, 333b, 335, 337–339
Potassium hydroxide test
in candidiasis, 996
in tinea, 163
Potassium-sparing diuretics
for heart failure, 310t, 314
for hypertension, 261, 262t
Potty training, constipation in, 474
Povidone–iodine suppositories, for bacterial vaginosis, 1000–1001
Practice guidelines, 1015–1017
Pramipexole (Mirapex)
for restless legs syndrome, 734
Prasugrel (effient), for coagulation disorders, 876t, 882
Pravachol (pravastatin), for hyperlipidemia, 278t, 286
Pravastatin
for hyperlipidemia, 278t, 286
Prazosin
for benign prostatic hyperplasia, 534
for hypertension, 265t, 267
Precose (acarbose), for diabetes mellitus, 790t, 794
Prednisone
asthma in, 385, 386
for gout, 606
for inflammatory bowel disease, 501, 504
for nausea and vomiting, 438
for rheumatoid arthritis, 614
for tinea capitis, 167
Preferred drugs, in formularies, 1010–1011
Preferred provider organizations, 1009
Pregestational diabetes mellitus, 802
Pregnancy, 65–68
acne in, 210
allergic rhinitis in, 840
anemia in, 904
asthma in, 400
Chlamydia trachomatis infections in, 565, 569
constipation in, 474
diabetes mellitus in, 787, 802
diarrhea in, 492
drug use in, 65
metabolism of, 67
physiologic changes and, 65–66, 66t
placental transfer of, 66–67, 67t

risk categories of, 68t
teratogenic, 67, 68t
GERD in, 456
gonorrhea in, 572
headache in, 651–652
heart failure in, 321
herpes simplex virus infections in, 580
HIV infection in, 855–856
human papilloma virus infections in, 587
hyperlipidemia in, 279, 281
hypertension in, 270
hyperthyroidism in, 809
hypothyroidism in, 814
immunization during, 922
inflammatory bowel disease in, 512
insomnia in, 732
menopause, 973t–974t, 976, 976b, 981t
migraine headache in, 651–652
nausea and vomiting in, treatment of, 444
in obesity, 952
for osteoarthritis, 600
postpartum depression after, 683, 697
prescription considerations for, 11
rheumatoid arthritis, 625
skin infections in, 193
smoking cessation in, 940
syphilis in, 576
unintended, 959
urinary tract infections in, 525
vaginitis in, 1004, 1004b
venous thromboembolism in, 877
Prehypertension, 258
Prelu-2 (phendimetrazine), for obesity, 948t, 949
Premarin (conjugated equine estrogen), for menopausal symptoms, 973t–974t, 974
Premature infants
definition of, 54
gastric emptying time in, 55
gastrointestinal enzymes of, 55
immunization of, 913
pharmacokinetics in, 54
Premature ventricular contractions, treatment of, 347t, 350
Prescribing of drugs
adherence issues in, 13, 13b
authority for, 8
for elderly persons, 89
errors in, 9
ethical considerations in, 7–8
from formularies (*See* Formularies)
patient education in, 8
practical issues in, 7
refills, 12
selection in, 7, 7b, 9, 10b
steps of, 9–10, 10b, 10f
writing prescription in, 11–13, 12f
Prescription Drug Marketing Act of
Prescription drugs, *vs.* nonprescription drugs, 5
Prevalite (cholestyramine), for hyperlipidemia, 281t, 282
Prevotella infections, bacterial vaginosis, 995
Primary open-angle glaucoma. *See* Glaucoma
Primaxin (imipenem), 114t, 119–120, 120t
Primidone, for seizures, 661t, 666, 668
Primsol (trimethoprim), 126, 126t